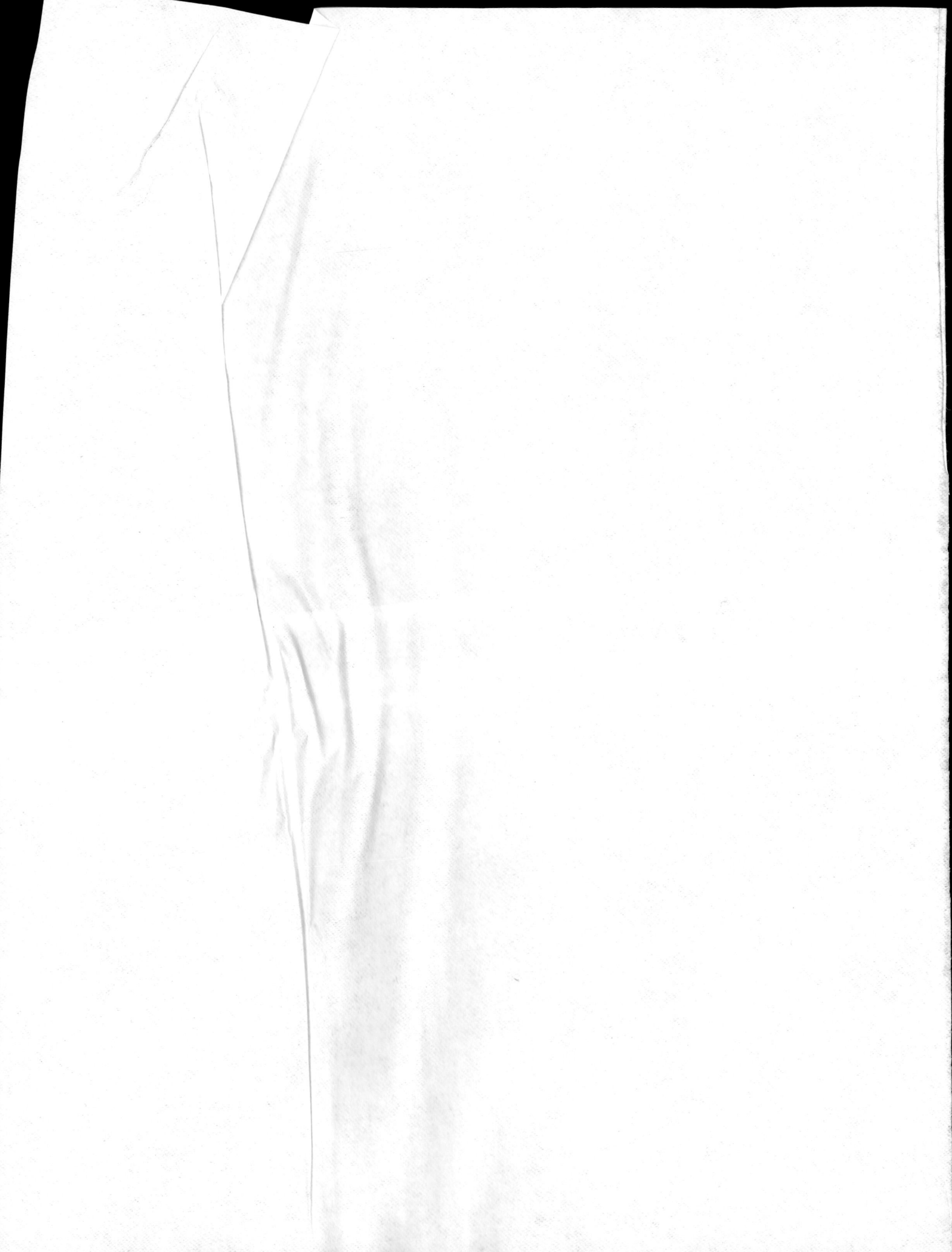

THE
HEART
Arteries and Veins

THE HEART

Arteries and Veins

Fifth Edition

Editor-in-Chief

J. Willis Hurst, M.D.
Candler Professor of Medicine (Cardiology)
Chairman of the Department of Medicine
Emory University School of Medicine
Chief of the Medical Service, Emory University
Hospital and Grady Memorial Hospital
Chief, Medical Section, Emory University Clinic
Atlanta, Georgia

Editors

R. Bruce Logue, M.D.
Professor of Medicine (Cardiology) Emeritus
Emory University School of Medicine
Director, Carlyle Fraser Heart Center
Crawford W. Long Memorial Hospital
Atlanta, Georgia

Charles E. Rackley, M.D.
Professor of Medicine
Division of Cardiology
Department of Medicine
University of Alabama Medical Center
Birmingham, Alabama

Robert C. Schlant, M.D.
Professor of Medicine (Cardiology)
Director, Division of Cardiology
Emory University School of Medicine
Atlanta, Georgia

Edmund H. Sonnenblick, M.D.
Professor of Medicine
Chief, Division of Cardiology
Department of Medicine
Albert Einstein College of Medicine
Bronx, New York

Andrew G. Wallace, M.D.
Professor of Medicine
Associate Vice President for Health Affairs
Chief Executive Officer
Duke University Medical Center
Durham, North Carolina

Nanette Kass Wenger, M.D.
Professor of Medicine (Cardiology)
Department of Medicine
Emory University School of Medicine
Director, Cardiac Clinics, Grady Memorial Hospital
Atlanta, Georgia

MCGRAW-HILL BOOK COMPANY
New York St. Louis San Francisco Auckland
Bogotá Guatemala Hamburg Johannesburg
Lisbon London Madrid Mexico Montreal New Delhi
Panama Paris San Juan São Paulo Singapore
Sydney Tokyo Toronto

NOTICE

Medicine is an ever-changing science. As new research and clinical experience broaden our knowledge, changes in treatment and drug therapy are required. The editors and the publisher of this work have made every effort to ensure that the drug dosage schedules herein are accurate and in accord with the standards accepted at the time of publication. Readers are advised, however, to check the product information sheet included in the package of each drug they plan to administer to be certain that changes have not been made in the recommended dose or in the contraindications for administration. This recommendation is of particular importance in regard to new or infrequently used drugs.

THE HEART
Arteries and Veins

Copyright © 1982, 1978, 1974, 1970, 1966 by McGraw-Hill, Inc. All rights reserved. Printed in the United States of America. Except as permitted under the Copyright Act of 1976, no part of this publication may be reproduced or distributed in any form or by any means, or stored in a data base or retrieval system, without the prior written permission of the publisher.

1 2 3 4 5 6 7 8 9 0   DODO   8 9 8 7 6 5 4 3 2 1

ISBN 0-07-031481-0
ISBN 0-07-031483-7
ISBN 0-07-031484-5
ISBN 0-07-079033-7

This book was set in Baskerville by Waldman Graphics, Inc. The editors were Richard S. Laufer, Ellen Warren, and Moira Lerner; the production supervisors were Jenet C. McIver and Jeanne Skahan; the design was done by Caliber Design Planning, Inc.; the index was prepared by Philip James.

R. R. Donnelley & Sons Company was printer and binder.

Library of Congress Cataloging in Publication Data
Main entry under title:

The Heart, arteries and veins.

Issued also in 2 v.
Includes bibliographical references and index.
1. Cardiovascular system—Diseases. I. Hurst, J. Willis (John Willis),   date
RC667.H42 1982   616.1   81-13641
ISBN 0-07-031481-0   AACR2

LC CIP DATA (2 vol. ed.)
RC667.H42 1982b   616.1   81-13642
ISBN 0-07-031483-7 (vol 1)   AACR2
ISBN 0-07-031484-5 (vol 2)
ISBN 0-07-079033-7 (set)

To those who are in the profession* of serving the sick.

*"The essential characteristic of a profession is the dedication of its members to the service they perform." M. J. Adler, *Great Ideas from the Great Books,* Washington Square Press, Inc., New York, 1961, p. 282.

Also see the quotation from Judge Elbert Tuttle at the beginning of Chapter 6.

Contents

Francois M. Abboud, M.D.
Professor and Chairman, Department of Medicine; Professor of Physiology, Department of Internal Medicine, University of Iowa Hospitals and Clinics, Iowa City, Iowa

Walter H. Abelmann, M.D.
Professor of Medicine, Harvard Medical School; Physician, Beth Israel Hospital, Boston, Massachusetts

James K. Alexander, M.D.
Professor of Medicine, Baylor College of Medicine; Chief of Cardiology, Ben Taub General Hospital, Houston, Texas

Joseph S. Alpert, M.D.
Professor of Medicine; Director, Division of Cardiovascular Medicine, University of Massachusetts Hospital, Worchester, Massachusetts

W. Banks Anderson, Jr., M.D.
Professor of Ophthalmology, Duke University Eye Center, Durham, North Carolina

Daniel Arensberg, M.D.
Assistant Professor of Medicine (Cardiology), Department of Medicine, Emory University School of Medicine, Atlanta, Georgia

Donald S. Baim, M.D.
Fellow in Cardiology, Stanford University Medical Center, Stanford, California

Giorgio Baroldi, M.D., F.A.C.C.
Director, Department of Pathology, Institute of Clinical Physiology Medical School, University of Pisa, Pisa, Italy; Director, Special Program on Atherosclerosis, National Research Council, Rome, Rome, Italy; Professor of Pathologic Anatomy, Institute of Pathologic Anatomy Medical School, University of Milan, Milan, Italy

Arthur C. Beall, Jr., M.D.
Professor of Surgery, Baylor College of Medicine, Houston, Texas

Harvey J. Berger, M.D.
Assistant Professor of Diagnostic Radiology and Medicine; Director of Cardiovascular Imaging, Yale University School of Medicine, New Haven, Connecticut

S. Gilbert Blount, Jr., M.D.
Professor of Medicine, Division of Cardiology, Department of Medicine, University of Colorado Health Sciences Center, Denver, Colorado

David K. Bone, M.D.
Assistant Professor of Surgery (Cardio-Thoracic), Department of Surgery, Emory University School of Medicine, Atlanta, Georgia

Harisios Boudoulas, M.D.
Chief, Cardiovascular Diagnostic and Training Center; Professor of Medicine, Wayne State University School of Medicine, Detroit, Michigan

W. Scott Brooks, Jr., M.D.
Assistant Professor of Medicine (Digestive Diseases), Department of Medicine, Emory University School of Medicine, Atlanta, Georgia

James C. Buell, M.D.
Chief, Cardiology, Omaha Veterans Administration Medical Center; Assistant Professor of Medicine, Cardiovascular Center, University of Nebraska Medical Center, Omaha, Nebraska

Bernadine H. Bulkley, M.D.
Associate Professor, Medicine; Assistant Professor, Pathology; Assistant Dean, Postdoctoral Programs and Faculty Development, The Johns Hopkins Hospital, Baltimore, Maryland

Howard B. Burchell, M.D.
Emeritus Professor of Medicine, University of Minnesota, Minneapolis, Minnesota

Agustin Castellanos, M.D.
Professor of Medicine; Director, Clinical Electrophysiology, University of Miami/Jackson Memorial Medical Center, Miami, Florida

Nisha Chandra, M.D.
Assistant in Medicine, Johns Hopkins Medical Institutions, Baltimore, Maryland

James T. T. Chen, M.D.
Professor of Radiology; Director of Cardiopulmonary Radiology, Duke University Medical Center, Durham, North Carolina

James H. Christy, M.D.
Professor of Medicine (Endocrinology), Department of Medicine, Emory University School of Medicine, Atlanta, Georgia

Stephen D. Clements, Jr., M.D.
Associate Professor of Medicine (Cardiology), Department of Medicine, Emory University School of Medicine, Atlanta, Georgia

Leonard A. Cobb, M.D.
Director, Division of Cardiology, Harborview Medical Center; Professor of Medicine, University of Washington, Seattle, Washington

Jay N. Cohn, M.D.
Professor of Medicine; Head, Cardiovascular Division, University of Minnesota Hospital, Minneapolis, Minnesota

Denton A. Cooley, M.D.
Chief, Division of Surgery, Texas Heart Institute; Consultant, Cardiovascular Surgery, St. Luke's Episcopal-Texas Children's Hospitals; Clinical Professor, Department of Surgery, The University of Texas Medical School, Houston, Texas

Ernest Craige, M.D.
Professor of Medicine; Henry A. Foscue Distinguished Professor of Cardiology; Attending Physician–Director, Cardiac Graphics Laboratory, North Carolina Memorial Hospital, Chapel Hill, North Carolina

Joseph M. Craver, M.D.
Associate Professor of Surgery (Cardio-Thoracic), Department of Surgery, Emory University School of Medicine, Atlanta, Georgia

I. Sylvia Crawley, M.D.
Associate Professor of Medicine (Cardiology), Department of Medicine, Emory University School of Medicine; Chief, Cardiology Section, Atlanta Veterans Administration Hospital, Atlanta, Georgia

James E. Dalen, M.D.
Professor of Medicine; Physician-in-Chief, University of Massachusetts Hospital, Worcester, Massachusetts

Michael E. DeBakey, M.D.
President, Chancellor, and Chairman, Department of Surgery, Baylor College of Medicine, Houston, Texas

Antonio C. deLeon, Jr., M.D.
Professor of Medicine; Associate Director, Division of Cardiology, Georgetown University Medical Center, Washington, D.C.

Regis A. DeSilva, M.D.
Research Associate in Cardiology, Harvard University School of Public Health, Boston, Massachusetts

Victor G. deWolfe, M.D.
Senior Physician, Department of Peripheral Vascular Disease, Cleveland Clinic Foundation, Cleveland, Ohio

Lewis Dexter, M.D.
Emeritus Professor of Medicine, Harvard Medical School, Boston, Massachusetts

Edward R. Dorney, M.D.
Professor of Medicine (Cardiology), Department of Medicine, Emory University School of Medicine, Atlanta, Georgia

John S. Douglas, Jr., M.D.
Associate Professor of Medicine (Cardiology) and Radiology (Cardiac Radiology), Emory Univesity School of Medicine, Atlanta, Georgia

David T. Durack, M.B., D. Phil.
Associate Professor of Medicine; Associate Professor of Microbiology and Immunology; Chief, Division of Infectious Diseases, Duke University Medical Center, Durham, North Carolina

Harriet P. Dustan, M.D.
Professor of Medicine, Department of Medicine; Director, Cardiovascular Research and Training Center, University of Alabama Hospitals and Clinics, Birmingham, Alabama

Jesse E. Edwards, M.D.
Professor of Pathology, University of Minnesota, Minneapolis, Minnesota; Senior Consultant, Anatomic Pathology, Miller Hospitals, St. Paul, Minnesota

Robert S. Eliot, M.D., F.A.C.C.
Professor of Medicine; Director of Cardiovascular Center and Division of Cardiovascular Medicine and Monsour Medical Foundation Professor of Cardiovascular Medicine, The University of Nebraska Medical Center, Omaha, Nebraska

Susan K. Fellner, M.D.
Associate Professor of Medicine (Nephrology), Department of Medicine, Emory University School of Medicine, Atlanta, Georgia

Joel M. Felner, M.D.
Associate Professor of Medicine (Cardiology), Emory University School of Medicine; Teaching Scholar, American Heart Association; Director, Graphics Laboratory and Coronary Care Unit, Grady Memorial Hospital, Atlanta, Georgia

Charles Fisch, M.D.
Distinguished Professor of Medicine; Director, Krannert Institute of Cardiology and Division of Cardiology, Indiana University School of Medicine, Indianapolis, Indiana

Noble O. Fowler, M.D.
Professor of Medicine; Director, Division of Cardiology, University of Cincinnati College of Medicine, Cincinnati, Ohio

Robert H. Franch, M.D.
Professor of Medicine (Cardiology) and Radiology (Cardiac Radiology), Emory University School of Medicine, Atlanta, Georgia

Gottlieb C. Friesinger, M.D.
Professor of Medicine; Director, Division of Cardiology, Vanderbilt University School of Medicine, Nashville, Tennessee

Victor F. Froelicher, M.D.
Associate Professor of Medicine; Director, Cardiac Rehabilitation and Exercise Testing, University Hospital and Veterans Administration Hospital, San Diego, California

John J. Gallagher, M.D., F.A.C.C.
Director, Clinical Electrophysiology Laboratory; Edward S. Orgain, Professor of Medicine, Duke University Medical Center, Durham, North Carolina

Peter C. Gazes, M.D.
Professor of Medicine; Director, Cardiovascular Division, Medical University of South Carolina, Charleston, South Carolina

John A. Glomset, M.D.
Professor of Medicine, Department of Medicine, University of Washington School of Medicine, Seattle, Washington

J. F. Goodwin, M.D.
Professor of Clinical Cardiology; Consultant Physician, Royal Postgraduate Medical School, London, England

Richard Gorlin, M.D.
Murray M. Rosenberg Professor of Medicine; Chairman, Department of Medicine, The Mount Sinai Medical Center, New York, New York

Robert F. Grover, M.D., Ph.D.
Professor of Medicine; Director, Cardiovascular Pulmonary Research Laboratory, University of Colorado Health Sciences Center, Denver, Colorado

Andreas R. Grüntzig, M.D.
Professor of Medicine (Cardiology) and Radiology, Emory University School of Medicine; Director of Interventional Cardiovascular Medicine, Emory University Hospital, Atlanta, Georgia

J. Caulie Gunnells, Jr., M.D.
Professor of Medicine, Duke University Medical Center, Durham, North Carolina

Robert J. Hall, M.D.
Clinical Professor of Medicine, Baylor College of Medicine and the University of Texas Medical School at Houston; Medical Director, Texas Heart Institute; Director, Division of Cardiology, St. Luke's Episcopal Hospital, Houston, Texas

W. Dallas Hall, Jr., M.D.
Professor of Medicine (Hypertension); Director, Division of Hypertension, Director, Division of General Medicine, Department of Medicine, Emory University School of Medicine, Atlanta, Georgia

Donald C. Harrison, M.D.
Professor and Chief, Division of Cardiology, Stanford University School of Medicine, Stanford, California

W. Proctor Harvey, M.D.
Professor of Medicine; Director, Division of Cardiology, Georgetown University Medical Center, Washington, D.C.

Charles R. Hatcher, Jr., M.D.
Professor of Surgery (Cardio-Thoracic); Chief of Cardio-vascular Surgery, Division of Cardio-Thoracic Surgery, Emory University School of Medicine, Director, Emory University Clinic, Atlanta, Georgia

Carl C. Hug, Jr., M.D., Ph.D.
Professor of Anesthesiology and Pharmacology, Emory University School of Medicine; Associate Director, Division of Cardiothoracic Anesthesia, Emory University Hospital, Atlanta, Georgia

J. O'Neal Humphries, M.D.
Professor of Medicine; Chairman of the Department of Medicine, University of South Carolina School of Medicine, Columbia, South Carolina

J. Willis Hurst, M.D.
Candler Professor of Medicine (Cardiology); Chairman of the Department of Medicine, Emory University School of Medicine; Chief of the Medical Service, Emory University Hospital and Grady Memorial Hospital; Head of the Medical Section, Emory University Clinic, Atlanta, Georgia

Thomas N. James, M.D.
The Mary Gertrude Waters Professor of Cardiology and Chairman of the Department of Medicine, University of Alabama Medical Center, Birmingham, Alabama

Robert B. Jennings, M.D.
Professor and Chairman, Department of Pathology, Duke University Medical Center, Durham, North Carolina

Ellis L. Jones, M.D.
Associate Professor of Surgery (Cardio-Thoracic), Department of Surgery, Emory University School of Medicine, Atlanta, Georgia

William B. Kannel, M.D., M.P.H.
Professor of Medicine; Chief of Section, Preventive Medicine and Epidemiology, Boston University School of Medicine, Boston, Massachusetts

Joel A. Kaplan, M.D.
Associate Professor of Anesthesiology, Emory University School of Medicine; Director, Division of Cardiothoracic Anesthesia, Emory University Hospital, Atlanta, Georgia

Robert B. Karp, M.D.
Professor of Surgery, Department of Surgery, University of Alabama School of Medicine, Birmingham, Alabama

Spencer B. King III, M.D.
Professor of Medicine (Cardiology); Associate Professor of Radiology, Emory University School of Medicine; Director of Cardiac Laboratory, Emory University Hospital, Atlanta, Georgia

Edward S. Kirk, Ph.D.
Associate Professor of Medicine and Professor of Physiology, Albert Einstein College of Medicine, Bronx, New York

John W. Kirklin, M.D.
Fay Fletcher Kerner Professor; Chairman, Department of Surgery, University of Alabama School of Medicine, Birmingham, Alabama

Hiroshi Kuida, M.D.
Professor of Medicine and Physiology, University of Utah College of Medicine, Salt Lake City, Utah

Lynn M. Kutsche, M.D.
Research Fellow, Cardiology, Department of Pediatrics, University of Florida College of Medicine, Gainesville, Florida

Aubrey Leatham, F.R.C.P.
Physician to St. George's Hospital and the National Heart Hospital, London, England

Graham J. Leech, M.A.
Physicist, St. George's Hospital, London, England

Richard P. Lewis, M.D.
Professor of Medicine, Ohio State University College of Medicine, Columbus, Ohio

Joseph Lindsay, Jr., M.D.
Professor of Medicine, The George Washington University; Director, Noninvasive Laboratory, Washington Hospital Center, Washington, D.C.

R. Bruce Logue, M.D.
Professor of Medicine (Cardiology) Emeritus, Emory University School of Medicine; Director, Carlyle Fraser Heart Center; Crawford W. Long Memorial Hospital, Atlanta, Georgia

Bernard Lown, M.D.
Professor of Cardiology, Harvard University School of Public Health; Physician, The Peter Bent Brigham Hospital, Boston, Massachusetts

John H. McAnulty, M.D.
Associate Professor of Medicine, University of Oregon Health Sciences Center, Portland, Oregon

Terence B. McGhee, M.D.
Mountain Neurological Center, Asheville, North Carolina

Kamal A. Mansour, M.D.
Associate Professor of Surgery (Cardio-Thoracic), Department of Surgery, Emory University School of Medicine, Atlanta, Georgia

Henry J. L. Marriott, M.D.
Clinical Professor of Medicine (Cardiology), Department of Medicine, Emory University School of Medicine, Atlanta, Georgia

James Metcalfe, M.D.
Professor of Medicine, Oregon Heart Association Chair of Cardiovascular Research, University of Oregon Health Sciences Center, Portland, Oregon

Joseph I. Miller, M.D.
Assistant Professor of Medicine (Cardio-Thoracic), Department of Surgery, Emory University School of Medicine, Atlanta, Georgia

Howard E. Morgan, M.D.
Evan Pugh Professor of Physiology, The Pennsylvania State University College of Medicine, Hershey, Pennsylvania

Douglas C. Morris, M.D.
Associate Professor of Medicine (Cardiology), Department of Medicine, Emory University School of Medicine, Atlanta, Georgia

Robert J. Myerburg, M.D.
Professor of Medicine and Physiology; Director, Division of Cardiology, University of Miami Medical Center, Miami, Florida

James R. Neely, Ph.D.
Professor of Physiology, The Pennsylvania State University College of Medicine, Hershey, Pennsylvania

R. Joe Noble, M.D.
Clinical Professor of Medicine, Indiana University School of Medicine, Indianapolis, Indiana

Elizabeth W. Nugent, M.D.
Associate Professor of Pediatrics, Division of Pediatric

Cardiology, Emory University School of Medicine, Atlanta, Georgia

Donald O. Nutter, M.D.
Professor of Medicine (Cardiology); Associate Professor of Physiology; Executive Associate Dean, Emory University School of Medicine, Atlanta, Georgia

Edward S. Orgain, M.D.
Professor (Emeritus) of Medicine, Duke University Medical Center, Durham, North Carolina

Robert A. O'Rourke, M.D.
Professor of Medicine; Chief of Cardiology, University of Texas Teaching Hospitals, San Antonio, Texas

Philip E. Oyer, M.D., Ph.D.
Assistant Professor of Cardiovascular Surgery, Stanford University Medical Center, Stanford, California

Garland D. Perdue, M.D., F.A.C.S., F.A.C.C.
Professor of Surgery; Chief, Vascular Surgery, Emory University School of Medicine, Atlanta, Georgia

Joseph K. Perloff, M.D.
Professor of Medicine and Pediatrics, Center for the Health Sciences, School of Medicine, University of California, Los Angeles, Los Angeles, California

William H. Plauth, Jr., M.D.
Professor of Pediatrics; Director, Division of Pediatric Cardiology, Emory University School of Medicine, Atlanta, Georgia

Edward L. C. Pritchett, M.D.
Assistant Professor of Medicine, Division of Cardiology, Duke University Medical Center, Durham, North Carolina

Raymond D. Pruitt, M.D.
Professor of Medicine, Mayo Medical School, Rochester, Minnesota

Charles E. Rackley, M.D.
Professor of Medicine, Division of Cardiology, Department of Medicine, University of Alabama School of Medicine, Birmingham, Alabama

Aidan A. Raney, M.D.
Resident in Cardiovascular Surgery, Stanford University Medical Center, Stanford, California

John T. Reeves, M.D.
Professor of Medicine, University of Colorado Health Sciences Center, Denver, Colorado

Timothy J. Regan, M.D.
Professor of Medicine; Director, Division of Cardiovascular Diseases, College of Medicine and Dentistry of New Jersey; New Jersey Medical School, Newark, New Jersey

Michael J. Reiter, M.D.
Fellow in Cardiology, Department of Medicine, Duke University Medical Center, Durham, North Carolina

Bruce A. Reitz, M.D.
Assistant Professor of Cardiovascular Surgery, Stanford University Medical Center, Stanford, California

William C. Roberts, M.D.
Chief, Pathology Branch, National Heart, Lung, and Blood Institute, National Institutes of Health, Bethesda Maryland; Clinical Professor of Pathology and Medicine (Pathology), Georgetown University, Washington, D.C.

Paul H. Robinson, M.D.
Associate Professor of Medicine (Cardiology), Emory University School of Medicine, Atlanta, Georgia

John Ross, Jr., M.D.
Professor of Medicine; Head, Division of Cardiology, University of California Medical Center, San Diego, California

Joseph C. Ross, M.D.
Chief, Pulmonary Section, VA Medical Center; Professor of Medicine, Vanderbilt University School of Medicine, Nashville, Tennessee

Russell Ross, Ph.D.
Professor of Pathology; Adjunct Professor of Biochemistry, University of Washington School of Medicine, Seattle, Washington

Loring B. Rowell, Ph.D.
Professor of Physiology and Biophysics; Adjunct Professor of Medicine (Cardiology), University of Washington School of Medicine, Seattle, Washington

Elliot L. Sagall, M.D.
Assistant Clinical Professor of Medicine, Harvard Medical School; Associate Physician, Beth Israel Hospital, Boston, Massachusetts

Herbert A. Saltzman, M.D.
Professor of Medicine, Duke University Medical Center, Durham, North Carolina

Royal S. Schaaf, M.D.
Vice President, Medical Services, Prudential Insurance Company of America (Retired)

James Scheuer, M.D.
Professor of Medicine and Physiology, Albert Einstein College of Medicine; Chief of Cardiology, Montefiore Hospital and Medical Center, Bronx, New York

Robert C. Schlant, M.D.
Professor of Medicine (Cardiology); Director, Division of Cardiology, Department of Medicine, Emory University School of Medicine, Atlanta, Georgia

Ralph Shabetai, M.D.
Professor of Medicine, University of California, San Diego; Chief, Cardiology Section of the Veterans Administration Medical School, San Diego, California

Louis C. Sheppard, Ph.D.
Professor and Chairman, Department of Biomedical Engineering; Associate Professor of Surgery, University of Alabama in Birmingham, Birmingham, Alabama

Libi Sherf, M.D.
Associate Professor of Medicine, Department of Medicine, University of Alabama School of Medicine, Birmingham, Alabama

Norman E. Shumway, M.D., Ph.D.
Professor of Cardiovascular Surgery, Stanford University Medical Center, Stanford, California

Mark E. Silverman, M.D.
Professor of Medicine (Cardiology), Department of Medicine, Emory University School of Medicine and Piedmont Hospital, Atlanta, Georgia

Robert B. Smith III, M.D., F.A.C.S.
Professor of Surgery, Emory University School of Medicine; Chief of Surgery, Atlanta Veterans Administration Medical Center, Atlanta, Georgia

Warren M. Smith, M.B., Ch.B., F.R.A.C.P.
Research Associate in Medicine; Associate Director, Clinical Electrophysiology Laboratory, Duke University Medical Center, Durham, North Carolina

Edmund H. Sonnenblick, M.D.
Professor of Medicine; Chief, Division of Cardiology, Albert Einstein College of Medicine, Bronx, New York

James F. Spann, M.D.
Professor of Medicine; Chief, Cardiology Section, Temple

University Health Sciences Center, Philadelphia, Pennsylvania

Eugene A. Stead, Jr., M.D.
Professor of Medicine; Distinguished Physician, Duke University Medical Center and Veterans Administration, Durham, North Carolina

Richard M. Steingart, M.D.
Instructor in Medicine, Albert Einstein College of Medicine, Bronx, New York

Edward B. Stinson, M.D.
Professor of Cardiovascular Surgery, Stanford University Medical Center, Stanford, California

Gene H. Stollerman, M.D.
Professor of Medicine, Boston University School of Medicine, Boston, Massachusetts

D. E. Strandness, Jr., M.D.
Professor of Surgery, University of Washington School of Medicine, Seattle, Washington

Harold C. Strauss, M.D., C.M.
Associate Professor of Medicine and Pharmacology, Duke University Medical Center, Durham, North Carolina

Harold J. C. Swan, M.D., Ph.D.
Professor of Medicine, University of California, Los Angeles, School of Medicine; Director of Cardiology, Cedars-Sinai Medical Center, Los Angeles, California

Panagiotis N. Symbas, M.D.
Professor of Surgery, Thoracic and Cardiovascular Surgery Division, Emory University School of Medicine; Director, Thoracic and Cardiovascular Surgery, Grady Memorial Hospital, Atlanta, Georgia

W. Jape Taylor, M.D.
Distinguished Service Professor of Medicine, University of Florida College of Medicine, Gainesville, Florida

James F. Toole, M.D.
Professor and Chairman, Department of Neurology, North Carolina Baptist Hospital/Bowman Gray School of Medicine of Wake Forest University, Winston-Salem, North Carolina

Elbert P. Tuttle, Jr., M.D.
Professor of Medicine (Nephrology); Director, Division of Nephrology, Department of Medicine, Emory University School of Medicine, Atlanta, Georgia

Kent Ueland, M.D.
Professor of Gynecology and Obstetrics; Chief, Section of Maternal-Fetal Medicine, Stanford University Medical Center, Stanford, California

L. H. S. Van Mierop, M.D.
Professor of Pediatrics (Cardiology) and Pathology; Graduate Research Professor, University of Florida College of Medicine, Gainesville, Florida

Andrew G. Wallace, M.D.
Professor of Medicine; Associate Vice-President for Health Affairs; Chief Executive Officer, Duke University Medical Center, Durham, North Carolina

Paul F. Walters, M.D.
Professor of Medicine (Cardiology), Department of Medicine, Emory University School of Medicine, Atlanta, Georgia

James V. Warren, M.D.
Professor of Medicine, Ohio State University Hospital, Columbus, Ohio

Myron L. Weisfeldt, M.D.
Professor of Medicine; Director, Cardiology Division, Johns Hopkins Hospital, Baltimore, Maryland

Arnold M. Weissler, M.D.
Professor and Chairman, Department of Medicine, Wayne State University School of Medicine, Detroit, Michigan

Nanette Kass Wenger, M.D.
Professor of Medicine (Cardiology), Department of Medicine, Emory University School of Medicine; Director, Cardiac Clinics, Grady Memorial Hospital, Atlanta, Georgia

Jeffrey A. Werner, M.D.
Director, Coronary Care Unit and Cardiac Ultrasound Laboratory, Harborview Medical Center; Assistant Professor of Medicine, University of Washington, Seattle, Washington

Willis H. Williams, M.D.
Associate Professor of Surgery, Division of Cardio-Thoracic Surgery, Emory University School of Medicine; Chief of Surgery, Henrietta Elgeston Hospital for Children, Atlanta, Georgia

A. Calhoun Witham, M.D.
Professor of Medicine, Medical College of Georgia, Augusta, Georgia

Gary L. Wollam, M.D.
Assistant Professor of Medicine (Hypertension), Department of Medicine, Emory University School of Medicine, Atlanta, Georgia

Jess R. Young, M.D.
Head, Department of Peripheral Vascular Disease, Cleveland Clinic, Cleveland, Ohio

Barry L. Zaret, M.D.
Associate Professor of Medicine and Diagnostic Radiology; Chief, Cardiology Branch, Yale University School of Medicine, New Haven, Connecticut

Robert F. Zelis, M.D.
Professor of Medicine and Physiology; Chief, Division of Cardiology, The Pennsylvania State University College of Medicine, Hershey, Pennsylvania

Douglas P. Zipes, M.D.
Professor of Medicine, Indiana University School of Medicine; Director of Cardiovascular Research, Division of Cardiology; Senior Research Associate, Krannert Institute of Cardiology; Indiana University Hospital, Indianapolis, Indiana

Preface

Research is endlessly seductive; writing is hard work. One has to sit down on that chair and think and transform thought into readable, consecutive, interesting sentences that both make sense and make the reader turn the page. It is laborious, slow, often painful, sometimes agony. It means rearrangement, revision, adding, cutting, rewriting. But it brings a sense of excitement, almost of rapture; a moment on Olympus. In short, it is an act of creation.

Barbara W. Tuchman[1]

The first edition of *The Heart* was conceived in 1962 and born in 1966. The objective of *The Heart* has always been to *assist physicians and other health personnel in their effort to provide excellent medical care for their patients.* From the beginning we linked basic science principles to the identification and solution of clinical problems. We included discussions of the arteries and veins, as well as all-encompassing discussions of the heart itself. *As we wrote, we had clinicians and their patients in mind.*

The four previous editions of *The Heart* were well received by physicians, students, house officers, fellows, and other personnel. Our fondest dream was exceeded when *The Heart* was chosen on several occasions by the American College of Physicians as the cardiology book that should be in every internist's library. *The Heart* achieved considerable success in this country and was translated into Italian, Spanish, Portuguese, Japanese, and Greek. Its worldwide success was then ensured.

While it is easy to be content with success, I have always held that changes in institutions, programs, and books should be made at a time when success is apparent. *I believe very strongly that the greatest peril of excellence is contentment.*[2] Accordingly, I felt *The Heart* should be revised at a time when it was enjoying its greatest success. The time had come to reorganize and to rewrite the entire book in an effort to set the tone for the teaching and practice of cardiology for the eighties.

To help in the planning and editing of this major undertaking, three eminent cardiologists—distinguished for their scientific, clinical, and educational contributions to the field—have joined the editorial board. Drs. Charles E. Rackley, Edmund H. Sonnenblick, and Andrew G. Wallace have already

1. Tuchman, B. W.: In Search of History, *Radcliffe Quarterly*, 65(1):34, 1979.
2. Hurst, J. W. (ed.): The Perils of Excellence, in "Four Hats", Year Book Medical Publishers, New York, 1970, pp. 42–44.

made substantial contributions to *The Heart*, and they are most gratefully and enthusiastically welcomed.

The fifth edition began with a two-day "think tank" in a Washington hotel, July 11 to 13, 1979, when the new editors joined the old editors for the first time. New ideas were abundant, and each new idea was examined carefully. We were determined to write a book that would assist the practicing physician in the care of his or her patients. We would continue to link basic science information to the clinical problems. *We reasoned that we should highlight the cardiovascular questions that we believed physicians should ask about their patients and discuss the new techniques used in cardiology as methods devised to answer these questions. We would deemphasize the routine use of techniques before the proper questions have been formulated in the minds of physicians.* This led to the development of the new format for the fifth edition, which included the creation of the short prefaces that introduce each of the six parts of the book. We hope the miniprefaces will be carefully read, for they will guide the reader through the book.

While we strove to eliminate unnecessary duplication in the book, there is some purposeful duplication. Unnecessary duplication in a book is like placing one shingle directly on top of another shingle on a roof. This does not guarantee that the roof will not be filled with holes. Purposeful duplication is similar to placing the end of a shingle over the end of another shingle. When this is done carefully, it produces continuity and eliminates holes. Thus, we have retained the duplication that provides continuity, eliminates holes, and reinforces the points we have tried to make.

The fourth edition of *The Heart* had "daughters." They were *Self-Assessment and Review of the Heart* and five Updates. The self-assessment book was developed so that Continuing Medical Education (CME) credit was given by the Department of Continuing Medical Education of Emory University School of Medicine. The Update series has been very popular. (An index was placed in the last Update of the series). The purpose of the Updates has been to present new ideas that updated the information presented in the previous editions of *The Heart;* old subjects that needed updating and new emphasis; and more detailed discussions of interesting subjects. The discussions in the Updates have been exciting and may not be found in other textbooks or journals.

The daughters were well received by the readership and will continue. Accordingly, a self-assessment book (permitting CME credit) and five Updates will follow this edition also. *The Heart* plus the self-assessment book plus the five Updates offer the most extensive discussions of the heart and its diseases that have ever been developed.

I want to express my appreciation to all who made this edition of *The Heart* possible. I wish to thank our predecessors in medicine. In doing so I agree with the philosopher who said, "He who drinks the water should not forget who dug the well."

I wish to thank my secretary, Carol Miller, who can type with lightning speed, edit beautifully, keep order, and smile. I also thank Paula Noriega and Mary Garner in my office for their special contribution to typing and editing the manuscripts. They are invaluable.

The secretaries of the authors deserve our gratitude. Accordingly, we have devoted a special page of the book to the acknowledgement of their help.

I thank my colleagues in the Departments of Medicine, Pediatrics, and Surgery for their help. I thank Dean James Glenn, Vice-President Garland Herndon, and President James Laney of Emory University for their encouragement and support.

I thank Rich Laufer, Dereck Jeffers, M. Lorraine Andrews, Anthony Castagna, Moira Lerner, Jenet McIver, Jeanne Skahan, and Ellen Warren of McGraw-Hill Book Company for their remarkable ability and creativity.

I thank my wife Nelie. No Nelie, no book. She has been the center of my private world since we were sixteen. I thank her for all she has done to make our life together so meaningful.

I encourage the readers to write me. Remember, the book is written for *physicians and others who take care of patients.* We hope you have as much fun reading—and studying—the book as we did writing it.

J. Willis Hurst, M.D.

ACKNOWLEDGMENTS

The people whose names are listed below contributed a great deal to the creation of this book. The authors and editors express their special thanks and gratitude to them.

Libby Adams, Emory University School of Medicine, Atlanta, Georgia

Patricia Allen, Cedars-Sinai Medical Center, Los Angeles, California

Joyce Anderson, The University of Nebraska Medical Center, Omaha, Nebraska

Marilyn K. Anderson, University of Alabama Medical Center, Birmingham, Alabama

Grace S. Antle, Emory University School of Medicine, Atlanta, Georgia

Janet L. Arntfield, Wayne State University School of Medicine, Detroit, Michigan

Patricia Bailey, Emory University School of Medicine, Atlanta, Georgia

Daniela Banti, Istituto di Fisiologia Clinica del CRN, Pisa, Italy

Yolanda M. Barcena, University of Miami School of Medicine, Miami, Florida

Lynn H. Barnes, Emory University School of Medicine, Atlanta, Georgia

Thelma Barrett, Vanderbilt University School of Medicine, Nashville, Tennessee

Betty Barron, Emory University School of Medicine, Atlanta, Georgia

Linda J. Barth, Harborview Medical Center, Seattle, Washington

Elizabeth Bashford, Royal Postgraduate Medical School, London, England

Elaine Beckham, Emory University School of Medicine, Atlanta, Georgia

Dr. Victor S. Behar, Duke University Medical Center, Durham, North Carolina

Sherri Bell, University of California School of Medicine, Los Angeles, California

Sylvia L. Bell, University of Alabama Medical Center, Birmingham, Alabama

Jane Betts, Duke University Medical Center, Durham, North Carolina

Anne Binetti, New Jersey Medical School, Newark, New Jersey

Maxine Blob, Temple University Health Sciences Center, Philadelphia, Pennsylvania

James Bradford, Ph.D., Emory University School of Medicine, Atlanta, Georgia

Alison Brown, Emory University School of Medicine, Atlanta, Georgia

Audrey Brown, New Jersey Medical School, Newark, New Jersey

Gerry Brown, Emory University School of Medicine, Atlanta, Georgia

Penny Brown, The Ohio State University College of Medicine, Columbus, Ohio

Debby Butler, Texas Heart Institute, Houston, Texas

Helen Callahan, Baylor College of Medicine, Houston, Texas

Sandra Camp, Emory University School of Medicine, Atlanta, Georgia

Emanuela Campani, Istituto di Fisiologia Clinica del CRN, Pisa, Italy

JoAnn Campbell, Washington Hospital Center, Washington, D.C.

Jennifer Carson, Emory University School of Medicine, Atlanta, Georgia

Tony Carter, Grady Memorial Hospital, Atlanta, Georgia

Marie T. Ceballos, Harborview Medical Center, Seattle, Washington

Sue Chiaramonti, Duke University Medical Center, Durham, North Carolina

Ann Clayton, Duke University Medical Center, Durham, North Carolina

Gwen Cleary, Duke University Medical Center, Durham, North Carolina

Frances C. Cohn, Emory University School of Medicine, Atlanta, Georgia

Laura Cook, R.N., Duke University Medical Center, Durham, North Carolina

Marilyn Cornwell, University of California School of Medicine, San Diego, California

Charlotte Cox, Emory University School of Medicine, Atlanta, Georgia

Brenda Coy, Northside Cardiology, Indianapolis, Indiana

Michelle Cuonzo, The Cleveland Clinic Foundation, Cleveland, Ohio

Ruth Dawson, The University of Iowa, Iowa City, Iowa

Selma DeBakey, Baylor College of Medicine, Houston, Texas

Karen Deering, Northside Cardiology, Indianapolis, Indiana

Catherine M. DeVries, Emory University School of Medicine, Atlanta, Georgia

Rebecca K. Duffy, Emory University School of Medicine, Atlanta, Georgia

Nina Eaker, Emory University School of Medicine, Atlanta, Georgia

Patricia Edwards, Cedars-Sinai Medical Center, Los Angeles, California

Dorothy M. Efland, Duke University Medical Center, Durham, North Carolina

Helen Emerick, University of Washington School of Medicine, Seattle, Washington

Michelle J. Enriquez, University of Miami School of Medicine, Miami, Florida

Donna Erickson, University of Colorado Health Sciences Center, Denver, Colorado

Judy Evans, Emory University School of Medicine, Atlanta, Georgia

Charlotte Fairchild, Georgetown University Medical Center, Washington, D.C.

Rita Feran, The Cleveland Clinic Foundation, Cleveland, Ohio

Santa L. Ferraro, University of Minnesota, Minneapolis, Minnesota

Princella Fields, Grady Memorial Hospital, Atlanta, Georgia

Helen B. Fischer, University of Oregon Health Sciences Center, Portland, Oregon

ACKNOWLEDGMENTS

Barbara Fluitt, University of Colorado Health Sciences Center, Denver, Colorado

Martha Ford, Medical University of South Carolina, Charleston, South Carolina

Mary L. Garner, Emory University School of Medicine, Atlanta, Georgia

Vittorio Gattai, Istituto di Fisiologia Clinica del CRN, Pisa, Italy

Donna Glenn, Vanderbilt University School of Medicine, Nashville, Tennessee

Thelma L. Gottlieb, University of Miami School of Medicine, Miami, Florida

Barbara Green, Emory University School of Medicine, Atlanta, Georgia

Dr. Steve Grossman, Duke University Medical Center, Durham, North Carolina

Carol Gundlach, Montefiore Hospital and Medical Center, Bronx, New York

Janan Henry, Piedmont Hospital, Atlanta, Georgia

Pamela Hill, The Johns Hopkins Medical Institutions, Baltimore, Maryland

Maureen Hiss, University of California School of Medicine, Los Angeles, California

Gail Hitchcock, Emory University School of Medicine, Atlanta, Georgia

Patricia Hodgson, Duke University Medical Center, Durham, North Carolina

Janet Holwell, Montefiore Hospital and Medical Center, Bronx, New York

Judy Holzer, The Milton S. Hershey Medical Center, Hershey, Pennsylvania

Suzanne Howatt, University of Massachusetts Medical Center, Worcester, Massachusetts

Brenda Howell, Duke University Medical Center, Durham, North Carolina

Dave Huggett, Duke University Medical Center, Durham, North Carolina

Mary C. Humphries, University of South Carolina School of Medicine, Columbia, South Carolina

Rose E. James, The Johns Hopkins Medical Institutions, Baltimore, Maryland

Susan Johanson, University of Minnesota, Minneapolis, Minnesota

Jane Jungbauer, United Hospitals of Saint Paul, St. Paul, Minnesota

Sue Kaplan, University of Tennessee College of Medicine, Memphis, Tennessee

Oonagh Kater, University of Florida College of Medicine, Gainesville, Florida

Claudia Kenney, Harvard University School of Public Health, Boston, Massachusetts

Patricia Kirby, Piedmont Hospital, Atlantic, Georgia

Denis Kohernak, USCI, Billerica, Massachusetts

Lance Laforteza, Cedars-Sinai Medical Center, Los Angeles, California

Brady Lambert, Duke University Medical Center, Durham, North Carolina

Cindy Lewis, Emory University School of Medicine, Atlanta, Georgia

Elizabeth Lindley, Emory University School of Medicine, Atlanta, Georgia

Lois Lippert, The University of Nebraska Medical Center, Omaha, Nebraska

Marlis D. McDowell, Emory University School of Medicine, Atlanta, Georgia

Friedel Madörin, Med. Pol. Clinic, Zurich, Switzerland

Beti Mallett, The Ohio State University College of Medicine, Columbus, Ohio

Jean A. Matsumoto, University of Oregon Health Sciences Center, Portland, Oregon

Carol May, Duke University Medical Center, Durham, North Carolina

Carol Miller, Emory University School of Medicine, Atlanta, Georgia

Vera Mills, Duke University Medical Center, Durham, North Carolina

Nancy Minar, The Cleveland Clinic Foundation, Cleveland, Ohio

Sandi Morris, Emory University School of Medicine, Atlanta, Georgia

Dr. Mark J. Morton, University of Oregon Health Sciences Center, Portland, Oregon

Jacqueline T. Muther, Emory University School of Medicine, Atlanta, Georgia

Carol Nicholson, Emory University School of Medicine, Atlanta, Georgia

Werner Niederhauser, Schneider Medintag, Zurich, Switzerland

Paula J. Noriega, Emory University School of Medicine, Atlanta, Georgia

Joye Nunn, Cedars-Sinai Medical Center, Los Angeles, California

Marcelino Obaya, Univesity of Miami School of Medicine, Miami, Florida

Kristina Orvis, Cedars-Sinai Medical Center, Los Angeles, California

Sarah Overaker, Duke University Medical Center, Durham, North Carolina

Dr. George A. Pantely, University of Oregon Health Sciences Center, Portland, Oregon

Marilyn Parks, University of Massachusetts Medical School, Worcester, Massachusetts

Dolores Patterson, Egleston Hospital, Atlanta, Georgia

Ann Payne, Medical University of South Carolina, Charleston, South Carolina

Judy W. Peed, Duke University Medical Center, Durham, North Carolina

Tracey Peterson, Boston University Medical Center, Boston, Massachusetts

Don Powell, Duke University School of Medicine, Durham, North Carolina

Luciana Pozzolini, Istituto di Fisiologia Clinica del CRN, Pisa, Italy

Shirley Proffitt, Indiana University School of Medicine, Indianapolis, Indiana

Carol W. Purdy, Bowman Gray School of Medicine, Winston-Salem, North Carolina

Elaine Raines, University of Washington School of Medicine, Seattle, Washington

Jean A. Reifel, University of Florida College of Medicine, Gainesville, Florida

Lola Righton, Emory University School of Medicine, Atlanta, Georgia

Martin T. Rothman, M.R.C.P., Stanford University Medical Center, Stanford, California

Emily Salhany, The University of Nebraska Medical Center, Omaha, Nebraska

Sue Konkol Sauter, University of Colorado Health Sciences Center, Denver, Colorado

Coletta Sawyer, Yale University School of Medicine, New Haven, Connecticut

Dr. Henrich Schelbert, University of California School of Medicine, Los Angeles, California

Kathleen D. Schmitt, University of Washington, Seattle, Washington

Alice Scott, Emory University School of Medicine, Atlanta, Georgia

Estelle R. Shabetai, University of California, San Diego, California

Cindy South, University of South Carolina, Columbia, South Carolina

Nancy Stamp, The University of Iowa, Iowa City, Iowa

Betty Stancik, Duke University Medical Center, Durham, North Carolina

Ellen Starrett, Emory University School of Medicine, Atlanta, Georgia

Joyce Staton, Texas Heart Institute, Houston, Texas

Barbara Sternlight, University of California School of Medicine, Los Angeles, California

Pamela Stevens, University of Washington School of Medicine, Seattle, Washington

Kay V. Stroud, Emory University School of Medicine, Atlanta, Georgia

Linda Struggs, University of Alabama Medical Center, Birmingham, Alabama

Grace M. Stuart, Temple University Health Sciences Center, Philadelphia, Pennsylvania

Lynn Fraser Surasky, Emory University School of Medicine, Atlanta, Georgia

April Swader, Crawford W. Long Memorial Hospital, Atlanta, Georgia

Cathy Sylvia, Stanford University Medical Center, Stanford, California

Stephanie Thessamboon, University of California School of Medicine, Los Angeles, California

Andrea Tillotson, Duke University Medical Center, Durham, North Carolina

Cynthia Timm, Piedmont Hospital, Atlanta, Georgia

Harriet H. Tucker, Emory University School of Medicine, Atlanta, Georgia

Laurelle Useted, Duke University Medical Center, Durham, North Carolina

Lisbeth A. Van Wyk, University of Florida College of Medicine, Gainesville, Florida

Mary Vernon, Emory University School of Medicine, Atlanta, Georgia

Dr. Jonne Walter, Georgia Baptist Hospital, Atlanta, Georgia

Roberta Waltz, University of Cincinnati College of Medicine, Cincinnati, Ohio

Deborah S. Ward, University of Washington School of Medicine, Seattle, Washington

James A. Weiss, Temple University Health Sciences Center, Philadelphia, Pennsylvania

Martha R. Welch, University of Washington School of Medicine, Seattle, Washington

Pamela Wentworth, Emory University School of Medicine, Atlanta, Georgia

Joanne Werner, Harborview Medical Center, Seattle, Washington

Connee Wethee, Piedmont Hospital, Atlanta, Georgia

Peggy N. Wilder, Medical University of South Carolina, Charleston, South Carolina

Beryl Wilson, Medical College of Georgia, Augusta, Georgia

Mary Wirt, The University of Alabama Medical Center, Birmingham, Alabama

Marguerite Wismont, The University of Nebraska Medical Center, Omaha, Nebraska

Carla Wolfe, North Carolina Memorial Hospital, Chapel Hill, North Carolina

Julia Wright, Grady Memorial Hospital, Atlanta, Georgia

Jeanette Zahler, Emory University School of Medicine, Atlanta, Georgia

THE
HEART Arteries and Veins

Prologue

PART I The Normal Heart and Blood Vessels

The purpose of Part I is to describe the normal heart. An entire book could be written on the normal heart, but the discussion has been refined herein to emphasize the body of knowledge that will interest the practicing physician. This emphasis is justified since this entire book is designed to assist the physician who cares for patients.

The science that is basic to the understanding of heart and blood vessel diseases may be approached in two different ways. Some physicians may recognize their need to know more about the science that is basic to the field of cardiology. Other physicians may begin by investigating a specific patient's problem and recognize that they cannot properly understand the disease process or its management without understanding the scientific basis for it. Part I has been designed so that it can be studied as a separate unit by those who wish to learn more about the science that is basic to the understanding of the disease that affects the heart and blood vessels. Part I has also been designed so that physicians who ask fundamental questions about the problems they encounter in their patients can find the answers to such questions with relative ease.

Prologue

The Growth of Knowledge

Howard B. Burchell, M.D.

But there is no possible knowledge, which arrives not from pre-existent knowledge, that very demonstrable.

William Harvey, M.D. (1578–1657)[1]

Advances in the understanding of cardiovascular disease and the emergence of cardiovascular specialists have paralleled one another, but these developments have not reflected identical processes, nor necessarily involved the same persons. As physicians interested in the heart, our debt to basic science investigators is a tremendous one. Not infrequently, it has been a basic scientist or a clinical investigator, not specifically categorized as "heart-oriented," who has had a new insight into, or has made observations which have clarified, a puzzling cardiovascular phenomenon. Generally, progress has occurred in the basic science field without there having been much prior thought of the practical applications. Logically, it follows that one could not predict when a scientific discovery would have therapeutic implications. However, when a real "breakthrough" in treatment became evident, basic scientists predictably have accelerated their effort to explain and assess that treatment, this activity being nurtured both from an interest of basic scientists in helping their fellow human beings and possibly an expectance of liberal financial support. The development of open heart surgery exemplifies how a therapeutic triumph required many years of work in the basic science laboratory with technological breakthroughs being mandatory before success was attained.[2]

The evolution of our knowledge of the heart and its diseases has been presented in several ways. Common approaches have been to present a condensed list of dates of the discoveries, or of the classical descriptions of disease, with the names of the investigators who were seemingly responsible. There are many alternative approaches, such as (1) biographical sketches of major contributors to knowledge of the circulation, (2) discussions concerning the emergence of new techniques and equipment (these may have been the escutcheons of a specific era), (3) studies of the histories of cardiac institutions and hospitals, or (4) singling out for detailed study the growth of knowledge of a category of cardiac disease, beginning with its earliest recognition and following, over the decades, the errors and successes in investigations of its causes and mechanisms, with the progressive fumbling to create precise therapeutic programs. Yet other approaches would be to tell the story of the cardiovascular textbooks or of the development of specialism. In a parallel approach, one can be enthralled with the tale of the appearance of the heart specialist, with surveys of those medical centers to which the heart disease–oriented students had journeyed for their graduate education over the decades. In this saga, the story of the methods of accreditation for the cardiovascular subspecialist would be unfolded.

William Harvey is properly claimed as the father of cardiology, but he belongs to no specialist sect. The quadricentennial of his birth was celebrated in 1978. It is of less importance to debate whether conceptually or experimentally Harvey was the first to *discover* the circulation than to accept the all-persuasive evidence which indicates that the quality and quantity of his theoretical calculations, logic, and experimental work *proved* the existence of the circulation. The story of his work has been told and retold. Of the voluminous literature, two appraisals I have particularly enjoyed reading are Osler's Harverian Lecture, "The Growth of Truth as Illustrated in the Discovery of the Circulation,"[3] and Bylebyl's "The Growth of Harvey's 'De Motu Cordis.' "[4] A newly edited translation of Harvey's book by Whitteridge[5] is now available and is of great help to any scholar, particularly because of the extensive footnotes.

The mechanisms of the growth of knowledge has fascinated both the scientist and philosopher. Progress in understanding has always seemed to plateau after great contributions to the sum of knowledge and momentous theories, and it takes years or centuries for a system to have so many exceptions or faults that new paradigms are made. These shifts are revolutionary, sometimes recognized as such by the perpetrator, e.g., Harvey, but usually not. Kuhn,[6] in particular, has explored such mechanisms and discussed the complex background from which discoveries evolve and are accepted as the new truths.

For the beginnings of a personal library containing accounts of the history of cardiology, there should be space, in my opinion, for *Cardiac Classics*, edited by Willius and Keys;[7] *Circulation of the Blood: Men and Ideas*, by Fishman and Richards;[8] *A Short History of Cardiology*, by Herrick;[9] *A History of Electrocardiography*, by Burch and Pasquale;[10] and *The History of Coronary Heart Disease*, by Leibowitz.[11]

To appreciate the history of cardiovascular surgery, two books I recommend are Steven Johnson's

The History of Cardiac Surgery[12] and Richardson's *The Surgeon's Heart*.[13] To learn about the beginnings of cardiac catheterization and of angiography, I have usually turned to the reports of Cournand[14] and of Doby,[15] respectively.

Physicians have been interested in the symptoms of heart disease since ancient times, and very early their attention was directed to major or minor changes in the palpable pulse. Scientific specialism began about 100 years ago. The early specialist was usually a consultant for difficult or complicated problems of virtually all varieties; later there was often gradual limitation of interests to a categorical disease. The emergence of the specialty wherein physicians concentrated upon, or limited themselves to, problems of the heart has taken place only in the last 50 years. It is in the last 25 years that cardiologists have increased greatly in numbers, and many have become further specialized, e.g., in areas of hemodynamics, electrocardiology, nuclear cardiology, and radiology. In this time, also, there evolved the pediatric cardiology subspecialty.

For me, the first comprehensive cardiologic text was that of the young James Hope,[16] first published in 1842. This stemmed directly from the work of Laennec and the introduction of the stethoscope. Since 1931, the number of textbooks on heart disease seems to have increased exponentially. After inspecting the titles along the 40 feet of shelves occupied by the cardiologic texts in the University of Minnesota Biomedical Library and scanning the pages of the texts, I cannot give good reasons why some have been more popular than others.

It was almost exactly a century after the publication of Hope's textbook that the first edition of Paul White's *Heart Disease* appeared (1931).[17] The latter was a noteworthy event, and further editions kept the book up to date for over two decades. I still recommend that this text be consulted in any special study of a problem, particularly as historic notes are appended. It is a challenge to peruse Dr. White's list of unanswered questions about heart disease in the appendix of the first edition, and to ponder the growth of knowledge, from this catechism, during the following half century.

For a young, eager American graduate, the opportunities for advanced study were minimal in the United States before the present century. Scientific treks occurred in the eighteenth century, particularly to Edinburgh, London, and sometimes Leyden. The role of Benjamin Franklin in sponsoring such trips is noteworthy.[18] Later, in the first half of the nineteenth century, there were frequent travelers to Paris, where, in particular, the clinics of Louis and of Laennec were the attractions. Among these young American medical graduate visitors to Paris was Oliver Wendell Holmes. He is well known to cardiologists, on his lighter side, for his "Stethoscope Verses," which facetiously outlined in rhyme the perils of overinterpretation of sounds heard over the heart.[19] In the mid-nineteenth century,

Dublin was attracting students of heart disease, and in the latter part of the century, the German clinics (so well-described in Osler's letters to his students in 1872 to 1874) gained a dominant position. It was from Carl Ludwig's laboratory that Bowditch returned to America to start at Harvard the first American physiologic laboratory.[20] The revolutionary clinical insights of James Mackenzie,[21] initially a general practitioner, and his crude experimental apparatus to record the pulse were outstanding contributions. Thomas Lewis[22] was one of the first true clinical investigators, and because of his laboratory base and his leadership in cardiology during the renaissance of experimental physiology, he established London as an outstanding cardiologic center after the beginnings of the twentieth century. The English specialty journal *Heart* was launched in 1909. It was in London that a large number of the American cardiologic leaders made their entrance on the cardiac stage, a fact in part determined by World War I (1914 to 1918). In the two decades following this war, the Vienna cardiologic clinic attracted many graduate students. In addition, the American cardiologic community was benefited by émigrés, both students and established physicians, from many countries. These illustrious persons have made a lasting imprint on American cardiology.

Among the institutes of cardiology that have been established over the world, the one in Mexico City has been identified as having shown a special interest in the history of cardiology, and the frescoes by Diego Rivera portraying the cardiologic "greats" are lasting memorials to the leaders in the cardiologic world and to the scientific advances in cardiology.

For the first three editions of this textbook edited by J. Willis Hurst and colleagues, Paul White wrote the first chapter, entitled "The Evolution of Our Knowledge of the Heart and Its Diseases." His view of the events will always be worthy of study. With all due respect for the physician who is dedicated to improved diagnosis and better treatment of those afflicted with heart disease, I support Paul White's emphasis on preventive cardiology. This was epitomized by his clarion challenge to the profession and the public: "Heart disease before 80 is our fault, not God's or Nature's will."

References

1. Harvey, W.: De Circulatione Sanguinis: Another Exercitation to John Riolan, tercentenary ed., in G. Keynes, "De Motu Cordis," The Nonesuch Press, London, 1928, p. 179.
2. Comroe, J. H., and Dripps, R. D.: Ben Franklin and Open Heart Surgery, *Circ. Res.*, 35:661, 1974.
3. Osler, W.: "The Growth of Truth as Illustrated by the Discovery of the Circulation of the Blood, Being the Harverian Oration Delivered at the Royal College of Physicians, London, October 18, 1906," H. Frowde, London, 1906.

4. Bylebyl, J. J.: The Growth of Harvey's "De Motu Cordis," *Bull. Hist. Med.*, 47:427, 1973.

5. Harvey, W.: "An Anatomical Disputation Concerning the Movement of the Heart and Blood in Living Creatures," G. Whitteridge (trans.), Blackwell Scientific Publications, Ltd., Oxford, 1976 (Lippincott distributors, United States).

6. Kuhn, T. S.: "The Essential Tension: Second Thoughts on Paradigms," The University of Chicago Press, Chicago, 1977.

7. Willius, F. A., and Keys, T. E. (eds.): "Cardiac Classics," The C. V. Mosby Company, St. Louis, 1941.

8. Fishman, A. P., and Richards, D. W. (eds.): "Circulation of the Blood: Men and Ideas," Oxford University Press, Fair Lawn, N.J., 1964.

9. Herrick, J.: "A Short History of Cardiology," Charles C Thomas, Publisher, Springfield, Ill., 1942.

10. Burch, G. E., and Pasquale, N. P.: "A History of Electrocardiography," The Year Book Publishers, Inc., Chicago, 1964.

11. Leibowitz, J. O.: "The History of Coronary Heart Disease," Wellcome Institute of the History of Medicine, University of California Press, Berkeley, Calif., 1970.

12. Johnson, S. L.: "The History of Cardiac Surgery, 1896–1955," The Johns Hopkins Press, Baltimore, 1970.

13. Richardson, R. G.: "The Surgeon's Heart: A History of Cardiac Surgery," Heinemann Medical Books, Ltd., London, 1969.

14. Cournand, A.: Cardiac Catheterization, *Acta Med. Scand.* (suppl.) 579:7, 1975.

15. Doby, T.: "Development of Angiography and Cardiovascular Catheterization," Publishing Sciences Group, Littleton, Mass., 1976.

16. Hope, J.: "A Treatise on the Diseases of the Heart and on the Affections That May Be Mistaken for Them," Lea and Blanchard, Philadelphia, 1842. (First available American edition based on third London edition published by C. W. Pennock.)

17. White, P. D.: "Heart Disease," The Macmillan Company, New York, 1931.

18. Larabee, L. W. (ed.): "The Papers of Benjamin Franklin," Yale University Press, New Haven, Conn., 1966, vol. 9, pp. 219, 377.

19. Holmes, O. W.: Stethoscope Verses, in F. A. Willius and T. E. Keys (eds.), "Cardiac Classics," The C. V. Mosby Company, St. Louis, 1941, pp. 831–833.

20. "Dictionary of American Biography," Charles Scribner's Sons, New York, 1927–1957, vol. I, pp. 494–496 [H. P. Bowditch (1840–1911)].

21. Mair, A.: "Sir James Mackenzie, M.D.: General Practitioner 1853–1925," Churchill and Livingstone, Edinburgh, 1973.

22. Hugh Clegg: "Dictionary of National Biography, 1941–1950," Oxford University Press, New York, 1959, pp. 501–502, [Sir T. Lewis (1881–1945)].

1

Embryology of the Heart

L. H. S. Van Mierop, M.D.
Lynn M. Kutsche, M.D.

The phylogenetic change in some groups of vertebrates from an aquatic to a terrestrial way of life was accompanied by profound structural, functional, and ontogenetic modifications of the cardiovascular system. Air-breathing lungs, apparently already present (in addition to gills) in primitive Devonian fishlike Placodermi[1] and in a few modern fishes as rather primitive accessory respiratory organs, became the sole means of gas exchange in all terrestrial amniotes. At the same time, partitioning of the originally unpaired series of cardiac chambers, progressing from the venous to the arterial end of the heart, led to increasing separation of pulmonary and systemic circulations, which reached completion in birds and mammals. Ontogenetic development of the mammalian heart is reminiscent of that which has taken place in phylogeny: the simple, essentially tubular heart of the early embryo develops into a complex, four-chambered, four-valved, double pump.

Since the metabolic and gaseous requirements of the vertebrate embryo cannot be met adequately once the volume of the embryo exceeds a few cubic millimeters, it is necessary that a functioning circulatory system is established early. In humans, the vascular system makes its appearance about 3 weeks after conception and is essentially completed 4 weeks later, before the end of the second month. Because of the precocious and rapid development of the heart and because of the complexity of the processes involved, the study of mammalian cardiovascular development is not at all easy; and certain details of cardiovascular development to this day are still inadequately known and remain controversial.

Renewed interest in the subject, not only among embryologists and anatomists, but also among clinicians, was stimulated by the rapid and spectacular advances made in the surgical treatment of congenital heart disease. With the recognition that cardiac anomalies are many and often complex came the realization that embryology of the heart, rather than being a difficult subject that had little or no relevance to clinical medicine, was of enormous value in the understanding of the nature and pathogenesis of these anomalies.

Development of the Heart

The Heart Prior to Septation

Early Vasculogenesis

The vascular system makes its appearance in embryos of about 3 weeks' ovulation age as scattered masses of cells.[2] These angiogenic cell clusters, or "blood islands," rapidly increase in size and number, acquire a lumen, and become confluent to form a vascular plexus. Part of the plexus differentiates into main channels, resulting in a bilaterally symmetrical vascular system. At the cephalic end of the embryo a section of main channel on each side of the midsagittal plane of the embryo specializes further. Each acquires contractile elements within its wall, thus producing a pair of heart tubes which come to lie parallel and close to each other within the cephalic part of the developing body cavity (intraembryonic coelom), ventral to the foregut.

Fusion of the pair of heart tubes results in the formation of a single tube (Fig. 1-1). The wall of the tube consists of an external myocardial mantle one to two cell layers thick and a single layer of endothelial cells internally, separated from each other by a relatively thick, acellular, and almost structureless third layer called *cardiac jelly*.[3,4] From this tube will develop initially the embryonic ventricle and bulbus cordis (hence it is referred to as the *bulboventricular tube*) and later the ventricles and their outflow tracts. A more detailed account of the foregoing events, only briefly described here, has been given elsewhere.[5,5a]

Formation of the Heart Loop

At the beginning of the next phase of development, the embryo is about 2 mm long and approximately 23 days old. The cephalic, extrapericardial portion of the bulboventricular tube is dilated and is called the *aortic sac*. From it originates the first pair of aortic arches and later also the second, third, fourth, and sixth pair of arches (the fifth pair of aortic arches does not normally develop in mammals or is very rudimentary). The caudal half of the bulboventricular tube expands and represents the early embryonic ventricle. The atria are still paired and lie extrapericardially, caudal to the embryonic ventricle, embedded in mesenchyme.

The growing bulboventricular tube bends to the right and anteriorly, initially in the shape of the letter C, later into a compound sigmoid structure: the *bulboventricular loop*. The deepening concavity on the left side of the bulboventricular loop is referred to as the *bulboventricular* or *conoventricular groove* or *sulcus*. Since the bending of the heart tube involves the entire cardiac wall, the bulboventricular sulcus corresponds internally to a fold, the bulboventricular (conoventricular) fold. At this stage the descending limb of the loop is called the *embryonic ventricle;* the ascending limb is the *bulbus cordis*.

Cardiac looping appears to be due to a fundamental property of the heart tube that resides in the

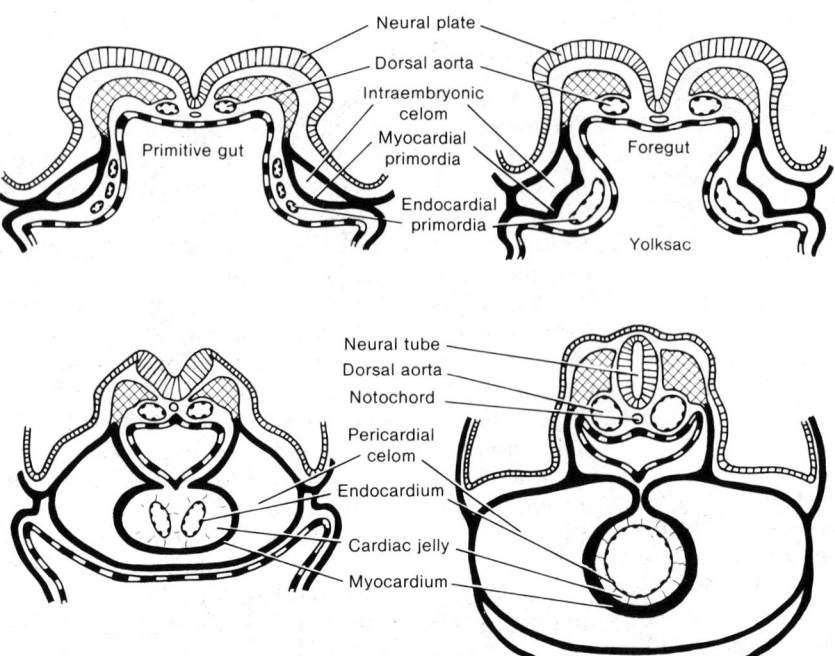

FIGURE 1-1 Schematic transverse sections through embryos of different ages, showing formation of the single heart tube. (*Adapted from several sources.*)

myocardium[6–9] and is not a passive phenomenon brought about by the necessity for the rapidly lengthening bulboventricular loop to accommodate itself to the available space in a much slower growing coelomic (pericardial) cavity, a view that has been held until recently.[10,11] Various explanations as to why looping occurs to the right have been discussed by Lepori,[12] DeHaan,[13] and Stalsberg.[8]

Since the arterial and venous poles of the heart tube are fixed, bending of the tube imparts upon it a certain amount of torsion. This torsion is at least in part responsible for the spiral disposition of the truncoconal septum, which develops later. The atrioventricular junction, which at first lies in the midline, is crowded laterally and to the left. At the same time the embryonic ventricle moves to the left side of the pericardial cavity, and the right side of this cavity is now occupied by the rapidly enlarging bulbus cordis.

Initial changes within the endocardial tube are concerned mainly with the development of local expansions throughout its length (Figs. 1-2 and 1-3). The atrial portion of the heart dilates considerably to form a large common atrium. This expansive growth of the atrial portion of the heart takes place in a dorsocephalad direction, so that the atrium appears to migrate along the dorsal wall of the pericardial cavity. The atrioventricular junction remains relatively narrow, shifts cephalad and mesiad, and is now called the *atrioventricular canal*. The ventricle and the proximal one-third of the bulbus cordis also expand, while the junction between them remains narrow and comes to lie approximately in the midsagittal plane. For reasons which will soon become apparent, it may be called the *primary interventricular foramen*[11] (Figs. 1-2 and 1-3).

Anomalies *Ventricular Inversion with Transposition of the Great Arteries*. If the cardiac loop is formed to the left and anterior, rather than to the right and anterior, then all structures derived from the bulboventricular loop, i.e., the atrioventricular valves, the ventricles, and the arterial roots, will develop in an inverted position. Since the truncoaortic sac, the atria, and the sinus venosus all lie extrapericardially, these parts of the heart will be normally located. The aorticopulmonary septum also develops in a normal fashion, but since partitioning of the inverted truncus arteriosus takes place in mirror image, the end result is a transposition of the great arteries with the aorta arising anteriorly from a left-sided, morphologically right ventricle and the pulmonary trunk posteriorly from a right-sided left ventricle; hence the term *corrected transposition* is commonly used for this anomaly.

The Primitive Ventricles, the Conus Cordis, and the Truncus Arteriosus

At the close of this phase of development, diverticula appear in two sharply defined areas along the right and left ventrolateral borders of the endocardial tube just proximal to, and distal from, the primary interventricular foramen[14] (i.e., in the early embryonic ventricle and in the proximal one-third of the bulbus cordis) (Fig. 1-3). These diverticula develop initially at the expense of the cardiac jelly, and later also penetrate the myocardium as the latter increases in thickness, producing a spongy mass of trabeculae. Thus, the capacity of the heart is increased.

Although externally the appearance of the heart has changed considerably, functionally it still consists essentially of a single tube. The trabeculated,

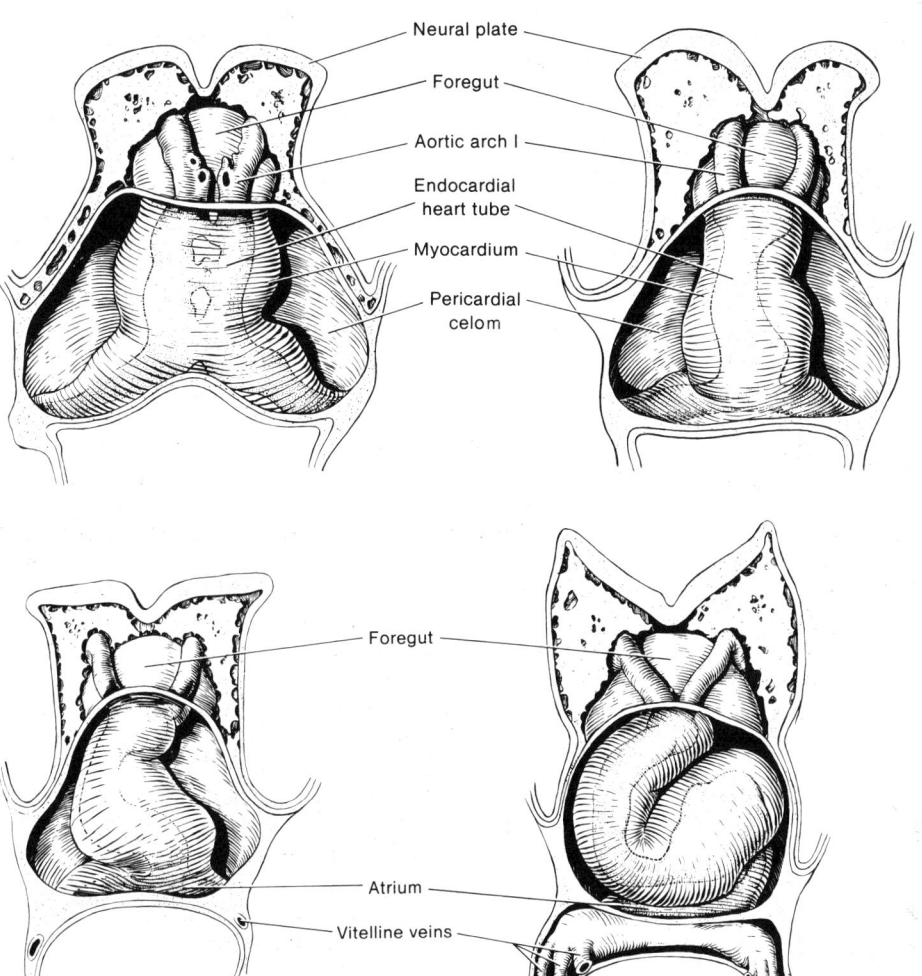

Neural plate
Foregut
Aortic arch I
Endocardial
heart tube
Myocardium
Pericardial
celom

Foregut

Atrium
Vitelline veins

FIGURE 1-2 Schematic ventral dissections of human embryos of different ages, showing formation of the heart loop. (*Adapted from Davis.[2] Reproduced with permission.*)

embryonic ventricle may now be called the *primitive left ventricle*, since it will contribute the major portion of the definitive left ventricle (Fig. 1-3). Similarly, the proximal one-third of the bulbus cordis, also trabeculated, may be called the *primitive right ventricle*.[15]

At this stage of development the embryo is approximately 3 mm long, and has an ovulation age of about 25 days.[3] The heart completely occupies the pericardial cavity, with the primitive left ventricle located on the left side and the bulbus cordis on the right. Because of future developments, it now becomes helpful to distinguish three sections in the bulbus cordis, of which the proximal trabeculated one-third is the primitive right ventricle. From the adjacent middle one-third of the bulbus, the conus cordis, the outflow portions of both ventricles will be derived. The terminal one-third of the bulbus, after partitioning, develops into the aortic and pulmonary roots and may, therefore, be appropriately called the *truncus arteriosus*. The most distal portion of the truncus arteriosus, together with the adjoining aortic sac from which the aortic arches arise, may be indicated by the term *truncoaortic sac*.

The rapid growth and expansion of the primitive atria causes the truncoconal section of the bulbus cordis to shift from its initial far lateral position to a more medial location. The result is that the truncus arteriosus comes to lie in a midsagittal position, in a depression of the atrial roof between the primitive right and left atria; the conus cordis assumes an oblique position and lies between the roof of the primitive left ventricle and the anteromedial wall of the right atrium. In an embryo of approximately 4 to 5 mm crown-rump (CR) length (ovulation age of approximately 25 days), the external shape of the heart already suggests its future four-chambered condition. The stage is now set for septation of the heart, and no major changes in the external appearance of the heart, other than size, will take place while that process goes on over the next 10 days.

Because of rapid growth and continually changing curvature of the embryo during the following period of growth and development, it becomes difficult to continue to appreciate spatial relationships. In the following discussion on cardiac septation, therefore, the diaphragm (septum transversum) is assumed to maintain an approximately horizontal

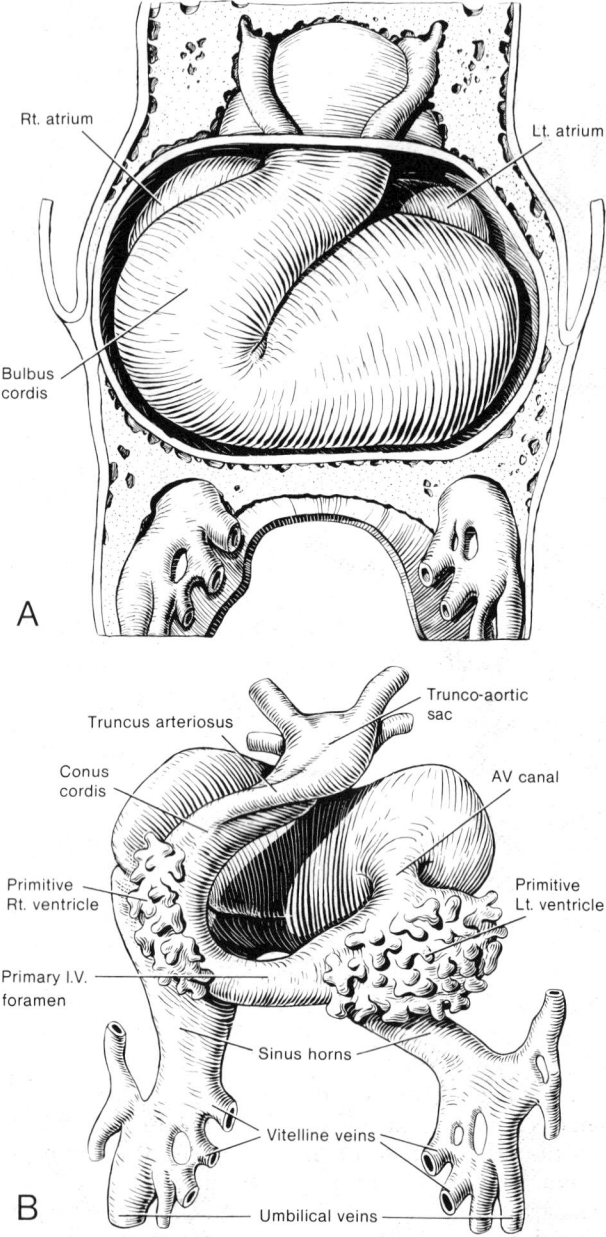

A

B

FIGURE 1-3 Twenty human somite embryos, ovulation age about 25 days. *A.* Ventral dissection. *B.* Reconstruction of cardiac lumen. (*Adapted from Davis.*[2])

position, as in the standing adult. The terms *anterior, posterior, superior,* and *inferior* are employed accordingly.

The formation of the various cardiac septa takes place more or less simultaneously; for descriptive purposes, however, it is necessary to consider their development separately.

Septation of the Heart

Mechanisms of Cardiac Septation

There are three ways in which a septum can be formed in a hollow organ such as the heart:[5]

1. A relatively narrow segment increases in diameter only slowly or not at all, while on either side of the segment, rapid and expansive growth takes place (Fig. 1-4*A* and *B*). The portion of the walls of the expanded regions on either side of the narrow intervening segment come to face each other, become apposed, and fuse. If growth takes place more or less equally everywhere, the particular portion of the heart, after fusion of the apposing walls, is transformed into a structure containing a diaphragm with a central opening. Usually, however, expansive growth takes place mainly in one direction, resulting in the formation of a septum with an eccentrically placed communication between the two adjoining chambers. It is apparent that a septum formed in this fashion is simply a reduplication of the wall of the organ and can never be complete: there is always an opening in it somewhere. If fusion of the apposing walls occurs very early and keeps pace with the expansive growth of the cardiac section involved, the fact that the septum is a reduplication may never be very obvious, and it may look more like a ridge or a membrane.

2. An entirely different mechanism of septum formation may be observed in portions of the heart that possess a well-developed layer of cardiac mesenchyme (endocardial "cushion" tissue) between the myocardium and the endocardium (e.g., the atrioventricular canal, the conus cordis, and the truncus arteriosus). This cardiac mesenchymal tissue is derived from, or at any rate

FIGURE 1-4 Mechanisms of cardiac septation. *A.* and *B.* Passively formed septum. *C.* Actively formed septum. *D.* Combination of *B* and *C.* (*From Van Mierop.*[5a] *Reproduced with permission of author and publisher.*)

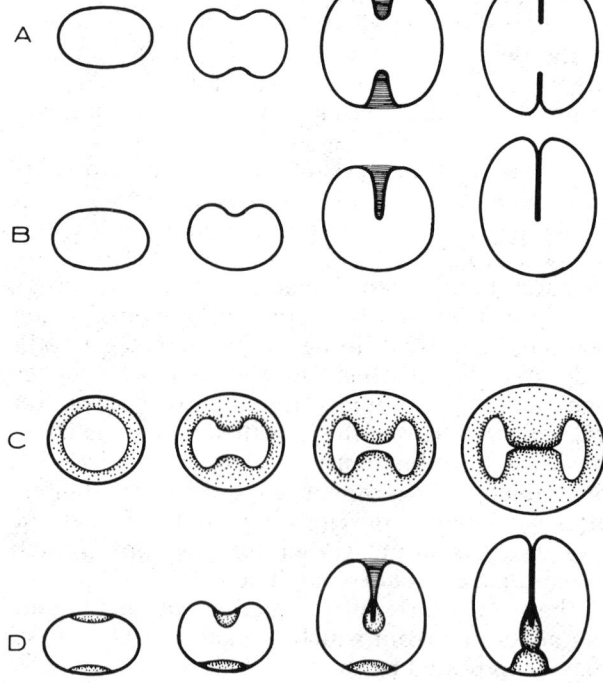

replaces, the earlier cardiac jelly. Local elaborations of such cardiac mesenchyme, forming two opposing masses of tissue, grow toward each other and fuse. These masses of actively growing mesenchymal tissue have a very characteristic appearance in microscopic sections. They stain lightly and contain relatively fewer nuclei than the surrounding tissue. They are large and bulky and are called *cushions*. When fully formed, septa developed in this manner are complete, and their thickness characteristically equals or exceeds their height in the early phases of their development (Fig. 1-4C).

3. Occasionally a septum in its initial phases of development is formed passively, but it is completed by actively growing tissue present along its free edge. Such actively growing tissue has the typical histological appearance of cushion tissue and again tends to be rather bulky (Fig. 1-4D).

Partitioning of the embryonic heart is accomplished by the formation of seven septa. Of these, three are formed passively (septum secundum of the atrium, the muscular portion of the ventricular septum, and the aorticopulmonary septum), three are formed actively (the septum of the atrioventricular canal, the conal septum, and the truncal septum), and one, the atrial septum primum, appears to start out as a passively formed septum, but it is completed by actively growing tissue along its border, probably derived from the atrioventricular endocardial cushions.

It has been held that with further growth of the heart, any septum (or atrioventricular valve cusp) formed by cardiac mesenchyme (endocardial cushion tissue) is temporarily invaded by cardiac muscle,[16–18] and that therefore the adult structure is a direct derivative of the embryonic mesenchymal septum or cusp. This, however, is not the case. Once fusion of opposing endocardial cushions has occurred, there is little, if any, further growth of the embryonic septum thus formed. This limited growth capacity of cushion tissue was already commented upon by Grant.[19] Endocardial cushion tissue eventually either disappears completely or is replaced by connective tissue. One important function of cardiac mesenchyme, therefore, appears to be to effect initial fusion and partitioning; i.e., it acts as a "glue," keeping things together while the heart continues its growth and development. The crista supraventricularis, for example, does not represent a conal septum that has been invaded by muscle secondarily, but is derived from the cardiac wall which has been drawn in, as it were, after the conus cushions have fused to form the embryonic conus septum. Nothing is normally left of the original mesenchymal conal septum. A second, important function of endocardial cushion tissue and the cardiac jelly preceding it is to act as a provisional valve apparatus.[20]

A number of factors, including cardiac looping and the development of local dilatations in the tubular heart, cause the flow of blood to break up into two spiral streams. By some authors these spiral streams are believed to have an important influence on cardiac septation.[21–24]

The Ventricles

In the 3-mm embryo, the primitive right and left ventricles are little more than local widenings of the original cardiac tube.[3] They are connected to each other by the smooth-walled, relatively narrow primary interventricular foramen, and trabeculae have just begun to make their appearance in each (Fig. 1-3).

In an embryo of about 5-mm CR length, the atrioventricular (AV) canal leads exclusively into the primitive left ventricle, and blood can reach the primitive right ventricle only by way of the primary interventricular foramen, the borders of which are formed by the developing muscular interventricular septum inferiorly and anteriorly, and by the bulboventricular fold superiorly and posteriorly (Fig. 1-5A). The interventricular septum and the bulboventricular fold are continuous with each other anterosuperiorly.

The ventricles enlarge by centrifugal growth of the myocardium, closely followed by increasing diverticulation and formation of trabeculae internally to prevent the compact outer layer of the myocardium from becoming too thick.

The medial walls of the growing and expanding ventricles appose and fuse, forming the major portion of the (passively formed) muscular ventricular septum.[11,25–27] On the right side, a large trabecula, the trabecula septomarginalis,[28] appears early (in embryos of about 9-mm CR length) and runs from the anteroinferior border of the primary interventricular foramen toward the apex, where it disappears among apical trabeculae (Fig. 1-5B).

The primary interventricular foramen never closes but actually enlarges, and in the fully developed heart gives access to the aortic infundibulum or vestibule.[11,19,26]

Anomalies *Single Ventricle, Left Ventricular Type with Rudimentary Outflow Chamber.* If the early embryonic atrioventricular canal fails to shift medially, retains its far leftward position, and goes on to divide into right and left atrioventricular ostia, then both of these ostia continue to empty into the primitive left ventricle. The proximal one-third of the bulbus (primitive right ventricle) therefore does not receive the right atrioventricular ostium, its inflow portion will not develop, and as a result it remains small. The communication between the large ventricular chamber and the rudimentary outflow chamber represents the persistent primary interventricular foramen of the young embryo heart. Because the main chamber has the morphological features of a left ventricle, this anomaly has also been referred to as *double-inlet left ventricle.*

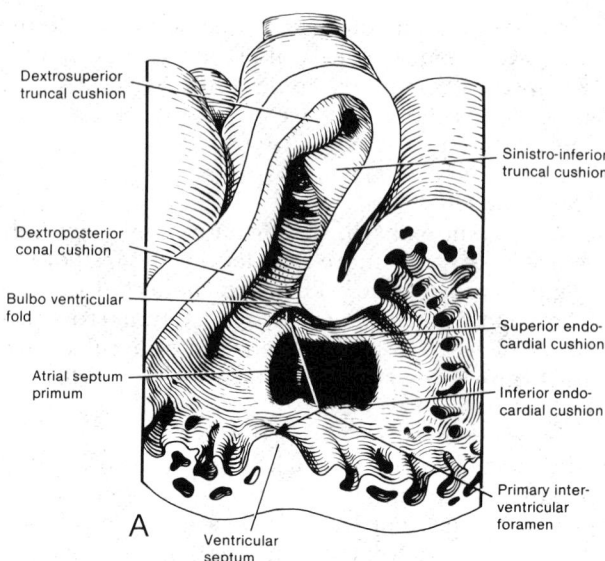

Dextrosuperior truncal cushion

Dextroposterior conal cushion

Bulbo ventricular fold

Atrial septum primum

Sinistro-inferior truncal cushion

Superior endo-cardial cushion

Inferior endo-cardial cushion

Primary inter-ventricular foramen

A

Ventricular septum

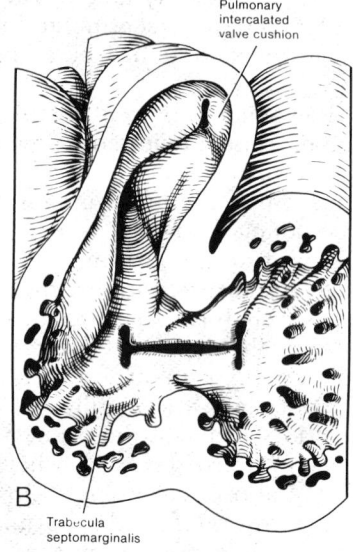

Pulmonary intercalated valve cushion

B

Trabecula septomarginalis

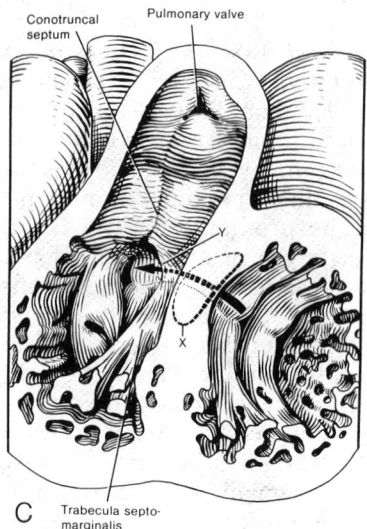

Conotruncal septum

Pulmonary valve

Y

X

C

Trabecula septo-marginalis

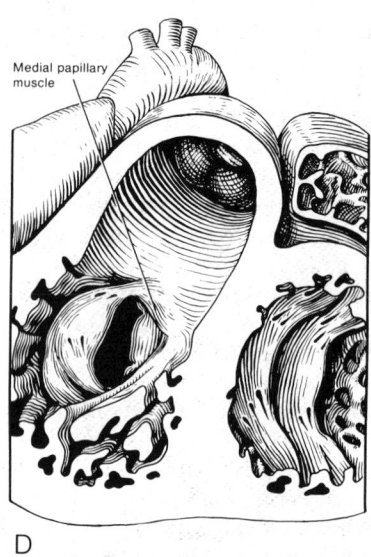

Medial papillary muscle

D

FIGURE 1-5   Schematic frontal section through the heart of embryos of various CR lengths: *A.* 6.5 mm. *B.* 9 mm. *C.* 16 mm. *D.* 40 mm. X = primary interventricular foramen; Y = secondary interventricular foramen. (*Redrawn after Van Mierop et al.*[15])

Double-Inlet Right Ventricle. In this anomaly both atrioventricular valves enter a morphologically right ventricle, and the left ventricle is a very small chamber communicating with the right ventricle by means of a basilar ventricular septal defect. This anomaly can be thought of as being due to excessive rightward shift of the atrioventricular canal. Generally, both great arteries arise from the right ventricle as well; i.e., double-outlet right ventricle is associated.

Double-Outlet Right Ventricle. This anomaly appears to be due to a lack of medial shift of the conus cordis, which retains its original embryological relationships with the right ventricle only. The bulboventricular fold is retained and separates the two arterial ostia from the atrioventricular ostia (aortic–mitral valve discontinuity).

The Atrioventricular Canal

Division of the atrioventricular canal into a right and left atrioventricular orifice is executed by a pair of opposing masses of mesenchymal tissue, the superior and inferior atrioventricular endocardial cushions, which make their appearance at the superior and inferior borders of the canal in embryos of about 6-mm CR length (Fig. 1-5). At this time, the atrioventricular canal and the truncoconal region of the heart have begun to realign themselves, and both have shifted medially from the far lateral position seen in younger specimens. At 6 mm, this shift has not been completed as yet: the atrioventricular canal still gives access to the primitive left ventricle only and is separated from the conus cordis by the bulboventricular fold. With further development, the central portion of this fold recedes, and blood can now enter the primitive right ventricle directly from the atrium (Fig. 1-5). In embryos of about 9-mm CR length, the left-sided portion of the fold is seen to terminate almost midway along the base of the superior endocardial cushion and is much less prominent (Fig. 1-5*B*); the right-sided portion becomes part of the parietal band. In older embryos, both the shift to the left and the effacement of the central part continue until this portion eventually becomes unrecognizable as such. As a result, the plane of the primary interventricular foramen (the posterosuperior border of which is formed, as we have seen, by the bulboventricular fold) inclines more and more to the left from an originally vertical position. As a further result, direct access is gained from the primitive left ventricle to the posteromedial portion of the conus cordis (by way of the primary interventricular foramen) and therefore to the aorta.

Meanwhile, the atrioventricular canal has enlarged to the right while the growing endocardial cushions project progressively into the lumen and approach each other (Fig. 1-5*B*). Similar but much smaller masses of tissue, the lateral atrioventricular cushions, appear on the right and left borders of the atrioventricular canal.

In embryos of about 10-mm CR length, the major cushions reach each other and begin to fuse, resulting in a complete division of the canal into right and left atrioventricular orifices. At the same time the cushions also bend, and after fusion they eventually form an arch which has its concavity directed anteriorly and toward the left ventricle[11,29] and its convexity directed posteriorly toward the atria (Figs. 1-5*C* and 1-8). The free margin of the atrial septum primum meets the convex atrial side of the fused endocardial cushions about midway between their extremities and fuses with them (Fig. 1-7*C*). That portion of the endocardial cushions to the left of the septum primum, i.e., the left limb of the arch, eventually becomes incorporated into the anterior or aortic cusp of the mitral valve, and therefore does not participate in the formation of the cardiac septum.

With deepening of the endocardial cushion arch or bay, the right half of the fused endocardial cushions comes to lie more and more in a sagittal plane, i.e., in about the same plane but somewhat to the right of the muscular interventricular septum. The communication still remaining between right and left ventricles, the secondary interventricular foramen, is bordered at this point by the muscular ventricular septum inferiorly and anteriorly, the right extremity of the fused endocardial cushions posteriorly, and the conal septum superiorly (Fig. 1-5*C*). The plane of the secondary interventricular foramen, therefore, inclines somewhat to the right, while that of the primary interventricular foramen, as we have seen, has come to deviate to the left. They share, however, the top of the muscular septum as part of their inferior borders. Before the closure of the secondary interventricular foramen can be discussed, it is necessary first to direct our attention to the truncus arteriosus and the developments which have taken place there.

Anomalies *Persistent Atrioventricular Canal.* There are several forms of persistent atrioventricular canal, and all are due to various degrees of failure of fusion of the superior and inferior endocardial cushions of the embryonic atrioventricular canal. Total lack of fusion results in a single atrioventricular ostium—the complete form of the anomaly. Since, in addition, the arch or bay normally formed after the fusion of the endocardial cushions fails to develop, the lower border of the atrial septum cannot fuse with the endocardial cushions. The result is a low-lying, large interatrial communication, and the atrioventricular part of the cardiac septum is absent. The upper part of the ventricular septum remains deficient to a greater or lesser degree, and there is a large interventricular communication.

In the partial forms the endocardial cushions fuse centrally only, and the arch is generally not formed. The result is an interatrial communication or so-called ostium-primum-type atrial septal defect. The upper part of the muscular ventricular septum remains deficient, but this area of the ventricular septum is closed by fibrous tissue. Because the left side of the endocardial cushions does not fuse, the anterior or aortic cusp of the mitral valve is cleft. Occasionally the arch is formed well enough so that the atrial septum does fuse with the partially fused endocardial cushions, producing a form of partial persistent atrioventricular canal with an intact atrial septum but with an interventricular communication and a cleft anterior mitral valve cusp. The aortic valve in all forms of persistent atrioventricular canal cannot descend to assume its proper position and therefore is located somewhat higher and further to the right than in a normal heart. This, in addition to the deficiency of the basilar part of the muscular ventricular septum, accounts for the elongated left ventricular outflow tract ("gooseneck" deformity) characteristic for this group of anomalies.

Ventricular Septal Defect. Some forms of perimembranous ventricular septal defect may be due to failure of fusion of the right extremity of the fused endocardial cushions and the upper border of the muscular ventricular septum and also the conal septum. Since the endocardial cushions fuse normally, there is no cleft in the anterior mitral valve cusp, nor is there an interatrial communication.

The Truncus Arteriosus

Septation of the truncoconal area of the bulbus cordis also begins in embryos of about 6-mm CR length with the appearance of two opposing truncal cushions. One of these is located on the dextrosuperior wall of the truncus (dextrosuperior truncal cushion), the other on the sinistroinferior wall (sinistroinferior truncal cushion).

The cushions rapidly enlarge and fuse to form the truncal septum, thus dividing the truncus into aortic and pulmonary channels. The truncus is the first part of the heart to become partitioned (embryos of about 7-mm CR length, Fig. 1-6A). The truncal cushions (and therefore the truncal septum) are large and bulky, and to accommodate them the initially slender truncal area of the heart expands.

Meanwhile, the truncal cushions proximally meet the distal extremities of a similar pair of mesenchymal masses developing in the conus cordis: the conal

FIGURE 1-6 Septation of the truncoconal area of the heart. View from above. Embryo CR lengths: *A.* 6.5 mm. *B.* 8 mm. *C.* 9 mm. *D.* 16 mm. (*Redrawn after Van Mierop et al.*[11])

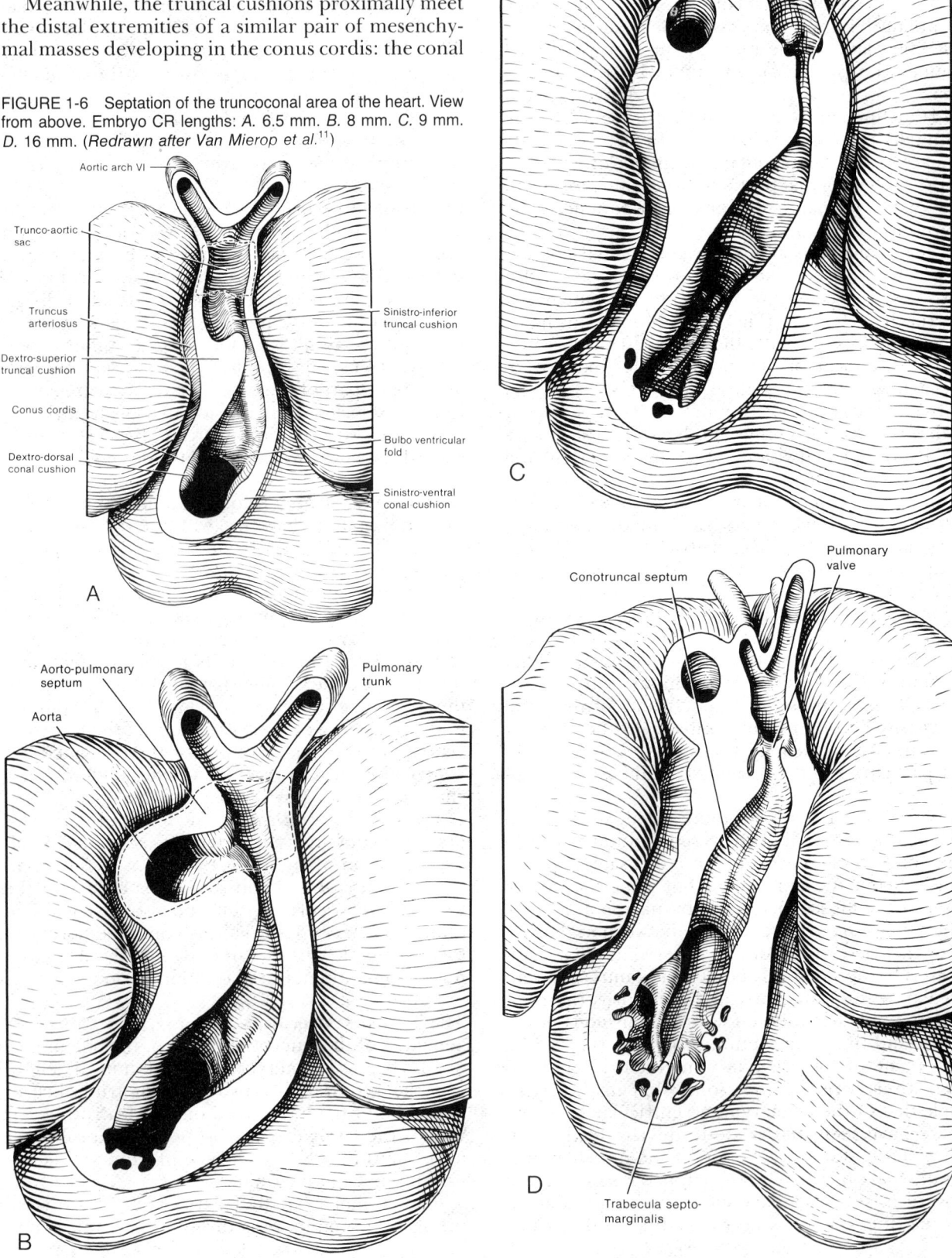

cushions. With further growth, the distal surface of the fused truncal cushions presents a front which faces the origin of the sixth aortic arches (Fig. 1-5). The distal, still undivided portion of the truncus, together with the adjacent aortic sac, dilates to form the truncoaortic sac. At the same time, the sixth arches move closer together and to the left, their most proximal portions probably fusing for a short distance. The origins of the fourth aortic arches (from the roof of the truncoaortic sac) shift somewhat to the right. As a result, the sixth arches become aligned with the pulmonary channel, and the fourth arches with the aortic channel. At the same time, the dorsal wall of the truncoaortic sac between the origins of the fourth and sixth arches invaginates to form a vertical septum, the aorticopulmonary septum, the leading edge of which approaches the distal face of the truncal septum with which it fuses (Fig. 1-6).[11,15,30,31]

Partitioning of the truncoaortic area is complete in embryos of about 9-mm CR length.

Anomalies *Persistent Truncus Arteriosus.* If the truncal cushions remain hypoplastic and fail to fuse, partitioning of the truncus arteriosus does not take place. If, in addition to the hypoplastic truncal cushions, both intercalated valve cushions are present, these structures may each form a valve cusp, and the result is a quadricuspid truncal valve. Fusion between adjacent valve anlagen may produce a tricuspid truncal valve in which one of the cusps is larger than the other two and contains a raphe, indicating its dual origin. This is the most commonly seen condition. In the great majority of cases, the aorticopulmonary septum does develop and a short common pulmonary trunk arises from the persistent trunk. In the few cases where it does not, the two pulmonary arteries arise independently from the major trunk. Usually the conal cushions also fail to fuse, and the infundibular septum therefore is absent as well. The ductus arteriosus is almost always absent, except when interruption of the aortic arch is associated.

Aorticopulmonary Septal Defect. This anomaly appears to be due to failure of fusion between the distal extremity of the truncal septum and the aorticopulmonary septum. Both arterial valves are present, but there is a communication of varying size between the ascending aorta and the pulmonary trunk.

The Conus Cordis
The conal cushions make their appearance at about the same time as do the truncal cushions (Figs. 1-5 and 1-6). One is located on the dextrodorsal wall, the other on the sinistroventral wall of the conus cordis. The dextrodorsal conal cushion becomes continuous with the dextrosuperior truncal cushion, and the sinistroventral conal cushion with the sinistroinferior truncal cushion. Fusion of the conus cushions begins proximally, progressing rapidly in a distal direction to complete the partition of the

truncoconal part of the heart in embryos of about 14- to 15-mm CR length.

With completion of the conal septum, the originally large interventricular communication becomes much reduced in size, and in a 15- to 16-mm embryo the remaining small secondary interventricular foramen is bordered by the conal septum, by the top of the muscular ventricular septum, and by the right extremities of the fused endocardial cushions, all of which contribute to its closure. This region is initially quite thick, and only much later (fetus of about 3 months), and with the formation of the anterior portion of the septal (medial) cusp of the tricuspid valve, does an area of variable extent become thin and fibrous: the interventricular part of the membranous septum. That part of the endocardial cushion arch or bay between the junction with septum primum and the ventricular septum also becomes the atrioventricular portion of the membranous septum (Fig. 1-7).

Anomalies *Ventricular Septal Defect, Eisenmenger Type.* Hypoplasia or absence of the conal cushions results in a large basilar septal defect, dextroposition of the aortic valve, and a hypoplastic or absent infundibular septum.

Ventricular Septal Defect, Supracristal Type. This type of interventricular communication is either due to simple failure of fusion of truncal and conal septa or to malalignment between these septa, which makes fusion impossible.

Tetralogy of Fallot. The basic anomaly in tetralogy of Fallot appears to be an anterior displacement of varying degree of the conal septum. This leads to unequal partitioning of the conus at the expense of the right ventricular infundibulum, hence the infundibular stenosis. The displaced conal septum cannot participate in the closure of the interventricular foramen. There is therefore a very large basilar ventricular septal defect and dextroposition of the aortic valve. Pulmonary valve anomalies, while commonly associated, are not an essential feature of tetralogy of Fallot.

The Sinus Venosus
In a 4-mm embryo, the sinus venosus consists of a central unpaired part, the transverse portion of the sinus venosus, and the right and left sinus horns (Figs. 1-3 and 1-8). It receives three pairs of veins: the omphalomesenteric veins (vitelline veins), the umbilical (allantoic) veins, and the common cardinal veins. At first, the sinus venosus is not well demarcated from the atrium; i.e., there is a wide sinoatrial ostium. Later the left horn and the transverse portion of the sinus venosus become more and more separated from the left side of the atrium by the development of a deep fold which, in the fully developed heart, represents the wall between the coronary sinus and the left atrium (Fig. 1-8*B* to *D*). The proximal portions of the umbilical veins soon disappear. Owing to the development of anastomotic channels between right and left systemic veins and

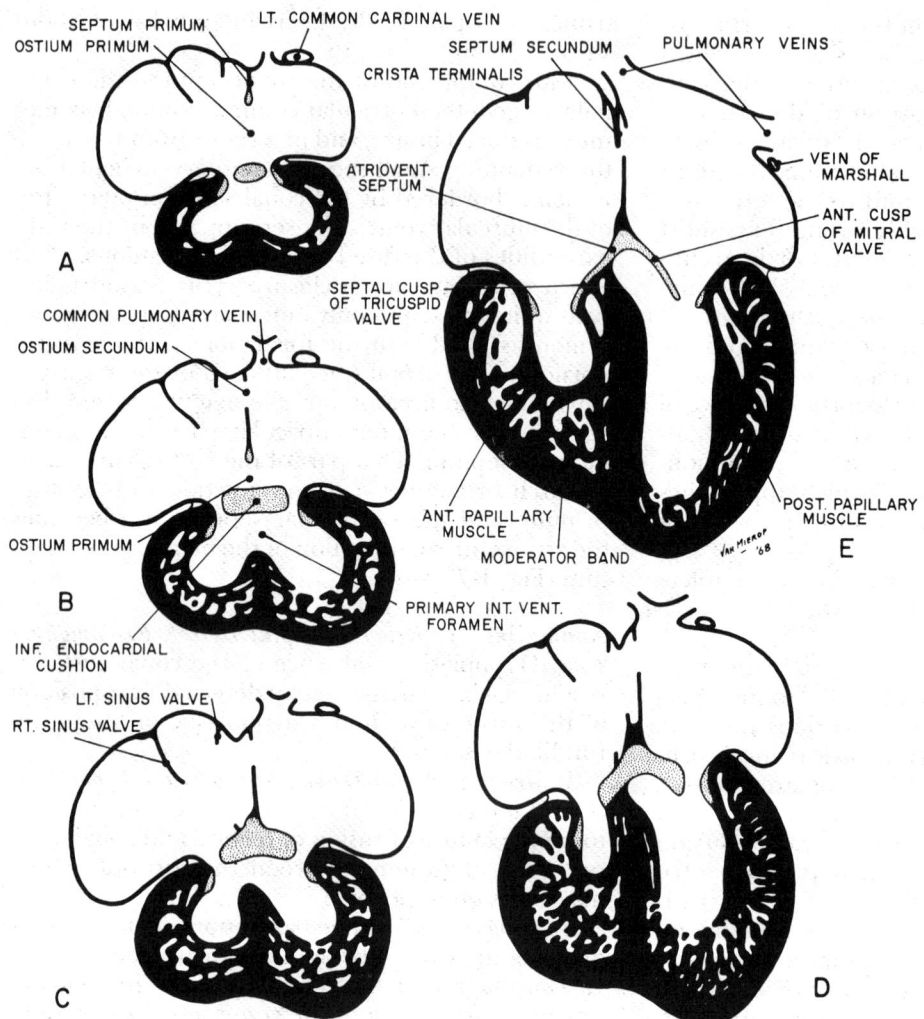

FIGURE 1-7   Sections through heart of embryos of different ages. Diagrammatic. *A.* 6 mm. *B.* 9 mm. *C.* 12 mm. *D.* 17 mm. *E.* 40 mm. *(From L. H. S. Van Mierop, Embryology of the atrioventricular canal region, in R. H. Feldt (ed.), "Atrioventricular Canal Defects," W. B. Saunders Company, Philadelphia, 1976, p. 6. Reproduced with permission of author and publisher.)*

preferential flow of blood to the right side, the right sinus horn and proximal cardinal and vitelline veins gain in size and importance, while their left counterparts become greatly attenuated. The right sinus horn attains a vertical position and becomes incorporated into the right atrium to form the smooth-walled, intercaval part of the atrium, and the communication between the sinus venosus and the atrium is now limited to this horn. The transverse portion and the proximal left sinus horn become the coronary sinus; the distal left sinus horn and left common cardinal vein normally obliterate (*ligament of Marshall*).

On the right side, the cardiac wall at the sinoatrial junction also folds in, as on the left side, and forms the right sinus valve (Figs. 1-3 and 1-7). Another, smaller fold, the left sinus valve, appears somewhat later on the left side of the sinoatrial junction, so that in a 4- to 6-mm embryo the vertical sinoatrial orifice is flanked on either side by a valvelike structure (Fig. 1-7). Superiorly, the sinus valves join to

form a single fold, the septum spurium. The sinus valves, particularly the right sinus valve, are relatively very large in a 16-mm embryo, but later they usually disappear almost completely. The left sinus valve fuses with the atrial septum. The inferior part of the right sinus valve is divided into a larger inferior vena caval (*eustachian*) valve and a smaller coronary sinus (*thebesian*) valve; the remainder usually disappears.

Anomalies   *Cor Triatriatum Dexter.* Total persistence of the very large right sinus valve of the embryonic heart produces a septum in the right atrium separating the intercaval part of the right atrium from the atrial body. The remaining opening may be quite small and restrictive, producing central venous hypertension.

Persistent Left Superior Vena Cava. Persistence of the left sinus horn and left common cardinal vein results in a left superior vena cava entering the coronary sinus.

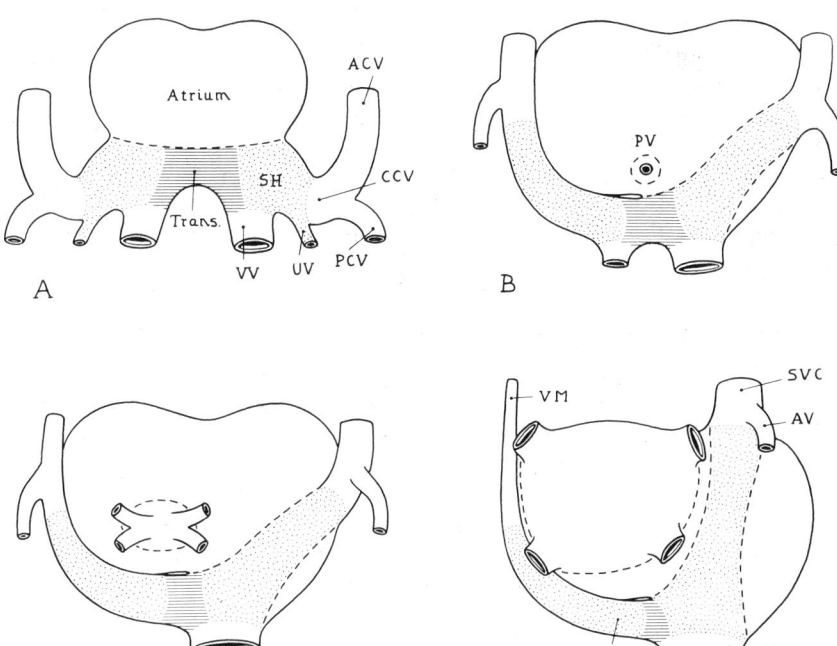

FIGURE 1-8
Posterior view of the atria and sinus venosus in embryos of the following CR lengths: *A.* 3 mm. *B.* 5 mm. *C.* 12 mm. *D.* Postnatal. Diagrammatic. A(C)CV = anterior (common) cardinal vein; AV = azygos vein; CS = coronary sinus; IVC = inferior vena cava; PCV = posterior cardinal vein; PV = pulmonary vein; SH = sinus horn; UV = umbilical vein; VM = vein of Marshall; VV = vitelline vein. (*From L. H. S. Van Mierop and F. W. Wiglesworth, Lab. Invest., 11:1303, 1962. Reproduced with permission of author and publisher.*)

The Atria, Atrial Septum, and Pulmonary Veins

In a 3-mm embryo, expansion of the atrial portion of the heart is well on its way (Fig. 1-3). Due to the presence of the truncus arteriosus, however, a depression is formed in the roof of the common atrium. As expansion proceeds, the depression deepens, corresponding internally to a more or less sickle-shaped crest. This is the first indication of the septum primum. Its free edge is directed toward the atrioventricular canal, and the foramen between the left and right primitive atria which it borders is the *ostium primum* (Fig. 1-7). Extensions from the superior and inferior endocardial cushions grow along the edge of the septum primum. Proliferation of this tissue with the concomitant fusion of the endocardial cushions brings about closure of the ostium primum, a process which is completed in embryos of about 10- to 11-mm CR length. Meanwhile, perforations have appeared in the septum primum posterosuperiorly. These rapidly coalesce to form the *ostium secundum*, thus ensuring continued free communication between the right and left primitive atria. Expansive growth of the atria and infolding of the atrial wall between the left sinus valve and septum primum produces the posterosuperior part of the *septum secundum*. The anteroinferior part of the septum secundum is believed to have a different origin.[32–34] The opening bordered by the free edge of the septum secundum is the *foramen ovale*. Postnatally, after fusion of the septum primum and the septum secundum, the foramen ovale becomes the *fossa ovalis*, and the free edge of the septum secundum is then called the *limbus fossae ovalis*.

The single embryonic pulmonary vein, already well developed in a 5- to 6-mm embryo (Figs. 1-7 and 1-8), develops as an outgrowth of the posterior left atrial wall near the atrial floor just to the left of the septum primum, and gains connections with the splanchnic plexus of veins in the region of the developing lung buds.[35–37] Later in development, the vein itself and parts of its first four branches expand tremendously and become incorporated into the embryonic left atrium to form the larger smooth part of the adult left atrium. In the fully developed heart, the original embryonic left atrium is represented by little more than the trabeculated atrial appendage. The intrapulmonary part of the splanchnic venous plexus ultimately loses its connections with the systemic veins and drains exclusively by way of the pulmonary veins.

Anomalies Atrial Septal Defect at the Fossa Ovalis. This anomaly, also often referred to as *secundum-type atrial septal defect* is due to overresorption of septum primum, producing a very large ostium secundum, which cannot be guarded adequately by septum secundum. Not infrequently, septum secundum is also hypoplastic, further enlarging the atrial septal defect. In some cases ostium secundum is normal but septum secundum is absent. Total absence of both septum primum and septum secundum (common atrium) is rare and almost always associated with a form of persistent atrioventricular canal.

Anomalous Pulmonary Venous Connection. The total form of anomalous pulmonary venous connection presumably is due either to lack of development of the embryonic common pulmonary vein or early involution and disappearance of this vein. One or more of the early embryonic channels connecting the pulmonary venous bed to the systemic venous circulation is retained. Depending upon which of these channels drains the pulmonary vascular bed, a number of types of total anomalous pulmonary venous connections are recognized. Partial anomalous pulmonary venous return is due to retention of a connection between part of the pulmonary venous system with the systemic venous circulation.

Cor Triatriatum Sinister. If incorporation of the common pulmonary vein into the left atrium does not take place and the common pulmonary venous ostium remains narrow, the result is a septum-like structure that divides the left atrium into two components, one of which receives the pulmonary veins and the other gives access to the mitral valve and left atrial appendage.

Development of the Heart Valves

The Atrioventricular Valves

In an embryo of about 10- to 12-mm CR length, both atrioventricular orifices are surrounded by mesenchymal endocardial cushion-type tissue which, as in younger embryos, has a provisional valve function.

The definitive atrioventricular valves, however, are derived only in very small part from this tissue. Nearly all the material contributing to the atrioventricular valve cusps is elaborated from the (muscular) ventricular wall, the internal layer of which is liberated by the process of diverticulation and undermining described earlier (Fig. 1-7). A "skirt" of ventricular muscle is formed at each atrioventricular orifice, originating from the atrioventricular junction and attached lower down to the ventricular walls or septum by trabeculae retained for this purpose.[5] All atrioventricular valve cusps are therefore thick and fleshy at first, and only later in development are they transformed into thin and fibrous cusps.[15]

As in the case of the cusps themselves, the chordae tendineae are initially thick, muscular, and few in number; only later are they transformed into delicate fibrous strands. The papillary muscles remain muscular.

The atrioventricular valve cusps are not all formed at the same time. The anterior cusp of the mitral valve is the first to develop (12- to 14-mm embryo), followed shortly by the anterior cusp of the tricuspid valve and by the posterior cusp of the mitral valve (14- to 16-mm embryo). The posterior and septal cusps of the tricuspid valve are "liberated" much more slowly, and even in a 10- to 12-week-old fetus (50-mm CR length) the most anterior part of the septal cusp has not been formed.[11]

Anomalies *Tricuspid Valve Atresia, Mitral Valve Atresia.* These anomalies are probably due to fusion of endocardial cushion tissue which borders the atrioventricular canal in very young embryos, usually during or shortly after partitioning of the atrioventricular canal.

Ebstein's Anomaly of the Tricuspid Valve. This anomaly is very likely due to an abnormality of the process of undermining of the myocardium.

The Arterial Valves

The primordia of the semilunar valves are already visible as small tubercles in a 9-mm embryo, just after partitioning of the truncus has been completed (Fig. 1-6). Each truncal cushion carries a tubercle on the extremity of its distal face. One of each pair is assigned to pulmonary and aortic channels, respectively. On the walls of both aortic and pulmonary channels, opposite the fused truncus cushions, a third small cushion appears. These two intercalated valve cushions[30] form the third member of each arterial valve primordium (Figs. 1-6 and 1-9). Beginning at the tubercles, the semilunar valve cusps and sinuses of Valsalva are probably formed by a process of excavation of the truncal and intercalated valve cushions in a proximal direction. This process appears well advanced in a 16-mm embryo, and is virtually completed in a 40-mm embryo. It could explain the "migration" of the arterial valves, which at first lie far distal[19,38] to the much more proximal position they occupy in the fully developed heart. Therefore, both the aortic and pulmonary roots, consisting of the sinuses of Valsalva and the semi-

FIGURE 1-9 Development of the arterial valves. Diagrammatic.

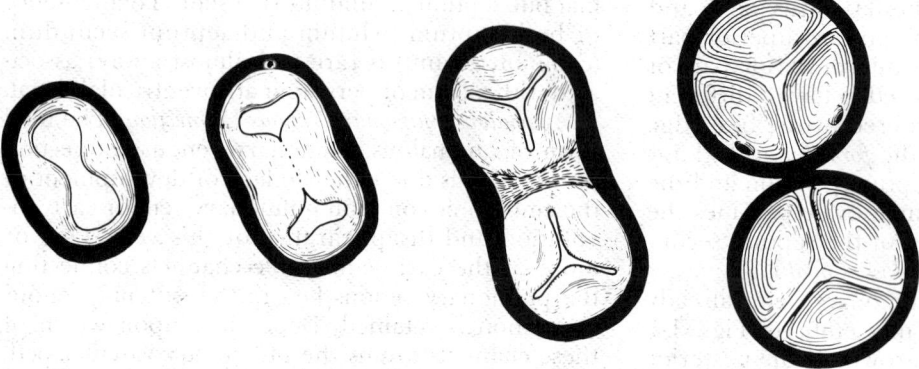

lunar valves, are derived from the truncus arteriosus and the truncal and the intercalated valve cushions.

Anomalies *Bicuspid Arterial Valves.* A bicuspid aortic or pulmonary valve is due either to failure of development of an intercalated valve cushion, resulting in a valve with two cusps of approximately equal size, neither one of which contains a raphe, or, more commonly, to fusion of adjacent valve anlagen, in which case the cusps are generally unequal in size, with the larger containing a raphe of varying height.

Arterial Valve Stenosis or Atresia. Fusion of two or all three of the arterial valve anlagen produces stenosis or atresia of the valve. Not uncommonly, the valves are dysplastic as well.

Absent Arterial Valves. Absence of the pulmonary or aortic valve is a rare anomaly, particularly the latter, and presumably is due to failure of development of arterial valve anlagen.

Development of the Aortic Arch System

In primitive chordates ciliary action induces a stream of water to enter the pharynx, from which it exits through a series of openings present bilaterally in the pharyngeal wall. Thus, food particles are strained out of the water and are then propelled backward into the gut. The bars between the pharyngeal clefts are referred to as *pharyngeal arches.* Primitively, six pairs of such pharyngeal arches are present, each containing a skeletal component for support and each possessing its own arterial and nervous supply. With the appearance of jaws in phylogeny, the first two pairs of pharyngeal arches become highly modified to form the jaws (first pair) and the jaw-suspension mechanism (second pair). In fishes the third to sixth (occasionally more or less) pharyngeal arches bear gills or branchiae and possess a respiratory as well as food-gathering function. With increasing sophistication of the jaw apparatus the latter function becomes much less important or is lost. The gill-bearing arches are then referred to as *branchial arches.* In air-breathing animals, their respiratory function is partly or completely taken over by lungs, and branchial arches as such are present only in early embryonic life; eventually they retrogress, become greatly modified, and acquire other functions. During mammalian embryonic development, the first two branchial arch arteries are present only very transiently: they retrogress almost completely, and in the adult are represented by a few small arteries in the jaws and the middle ear. The third to sixth branchial arch arteries are retained to form the large arteries of the neck and thorax. Traditionally, the branchial arch arteries are referred to as *aortic arches.*

In an embryo of about 3 mm the first pair of aortic arches is large and the second pair is just forming (Figs. 1-3 and 1-10*A*). The junction of the truncus arteriosus and the first pair of aortic arches, the aortic sac, is somewhat dilated. It is from this aortic sac that subsequent aortic arches originate, new arches being added caudally. A true ventral aorta is not present in mammalian embryos. Caudally the dorsal aortas fuse to form a single vessel; this fusion progresses craniad.

In a 4-mm embryo the first arch has largely disappeared, with only a part of it persisting as a portion of the maxillary artery (Fig. 1-10*B*). The second aortic arch has also retrogressed, and eventually all that remains is the tiny stapedial artery. The third aortic arch is well developed, and the fourth and sixth arches are being formed as ventral and dorsal sprouts of the aortic sac and dorsal aorta, respectively. The ventral portion of the sixth arch already has as its major branch the primitive pulmonary artery, even though the arch itself has not yet been completed. The fifth aortic arch in mammals is rudimentary and present only for a very brief time.

In a 10-mm embryo the first two aortic arches are no longer present as such, and the third, fourth, and sixth are large (Fig. 1-10*C*). The truncoaortic sac has been divided by the formation of aorticopulmonary septum so that the sixth arches are now continuous with the pulmonary trunk. Of the cervical intersegmental arteries the seventh pair will play an important role in the formation of the subclavian arteries. They are located at about the level where the dorsal aortas join each other.

In a 14-mm embryo the aortic arch system has largely lost its original symmetrical pattern (Fig. 1-10*D*). The segments of the dorsal aortas between the third and fourth arches, the carotid ducts, have disappeared, and the third arches begin to elongate as the heart descends further into the thorax. This descent has also caused a relative shortening of the paired portion of the dorsal aorta. The dorsal portion of the right sixth arch has disappeared, and its counterpart on the left persists until birth as the *ductus arteriosus.* The seventh intersegmental arteries have migrated craniad. The aortic sac has been "pulled out" on both sides: on the right it forms the brachiocephalic (innominate) trunk, on the left it becomes part of the definitive arch of the aorta up to the origin of the left third arch (common carotid artery).

In a 17-mm embryo the right dorsal aorta between its junction with the left dorsal aorta and the origin of the right seventh intersegmental artery has become attenuated and eventually disappears (Fig. 1-10*E*). The remainder of the right dorsal aorta persists and, with the right fourth aortic arch, persists as part of the proximal subclavian artery.

After birth the distal part of the left sixth aortic arch, the ductus arteriosus, normally also obliterates and is converted to the ligamentum arteriosum. Thus the adult aortic arch system is established. See Table 1-1 for the ultimate fate of the various components of the embryonic aortic arch system.

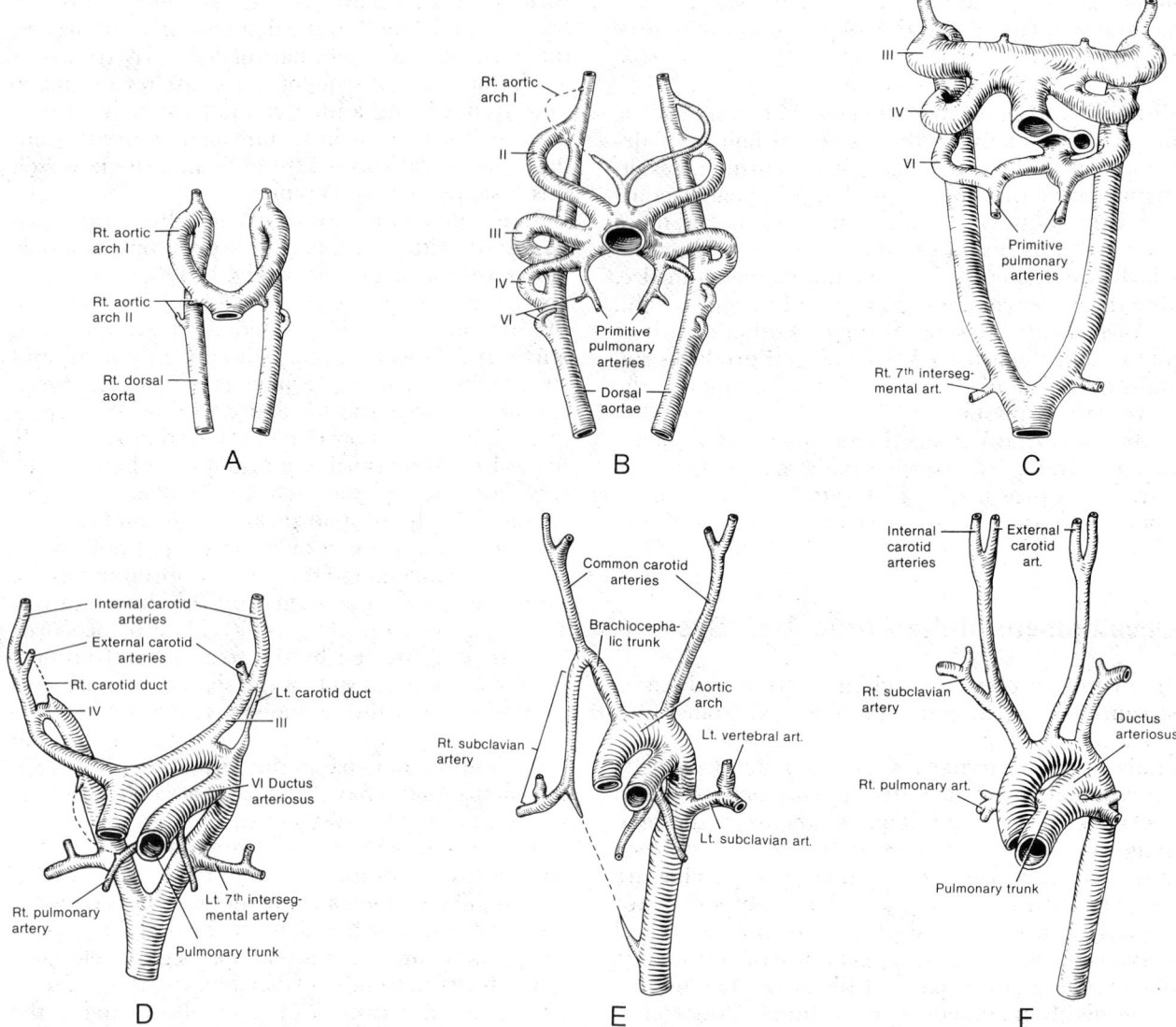

FIGURE 1-10 Development of the aortic arch system. Embryos of the following CR lengths: *A*. 3 mm. *B*. 4 mm. *C*. 10 mm. *D*. 14 mm. *E*. 17 mm. *F*. Neonate. (*After E. D. Congdon, Contrib. Embryol., 14:47, 1922.*)

Anomalies

Patent Ductus Arteriosus
A ductus arteriosus is anomalous only if it remains patent after birth.

Double Aortic Arch
This is the result of persistent and continued patency of the segment of right dorsal aorta between the origin of the right seventh intersegmental artery and its junction with the left dorsal aorta.

Right Aortic Arch
In this anomaly the right rather than left dorsal aorta is maintained in its entirety. The branching pattern of the aortic arch, therefore, will be the mirror image of normal with the brachiocephalic (innominate) artery arising as the first vessel on the left rather than the right side.

Anomalous Subclavian Artery
If the right fourth arch disappears, then the right dorsal aorta between the origin of the right seventh intersegmental artery and the junction with the left dorsal aorta is maintained to form the proximal portion of the right subclavian artery. Because of its genesis, such a subclavian artery will arise from the aortic arch distal to the left subclavian artery and will course behind the esophagus to enter the right arm.

Interrupted Aortic Arch
In this anomaly the left fourth arch disappears. The ascending aorta has no connection with the descending aorta, which receives its blood from the pulmonary trunk by way of a patent ductus arteriosus. If both fourth arches disappear, then the right subclavian artery will arise from the descending aorta, as is described above, and the ascending aorta terminates into the two carotid arteries.

TABLE 1-1 Components of the Heart and Their Embryonic Origins

Embryonic Origin	Component of the Heart
1. Truncus arteriosus	Aortic and pulmonary roots
2. Aortic sac	Ascending aorta, brachiocephalic (innominate) artery, and aortic arch up to origin of left common carotid artery
3. First arches	Parts persist as components of the maxillary arteries
4. Second arches	Parts persist as the stapedial arteries
5. Third arches	Common carotid arteries and proximal segment of internal carotid arteries
6. Fourth arches	
a. Right	Most proximal segment of right subclavian artery
b. Left	Aortic arch segment between left common carotid and left subclavian arteries
7. Fifth arches	No known derivations; transient and never well developed
8. Sixth arches	
a. Right	Proximal part becomes proximal segment of right pulmonary artery; distal part disappears early
b. Left	Proximal part becomes proximal segment of left pulmonary artery; distal part persists, until birth, as ductus arteriosus
9. Right dorsal aorta	Cranial portion becomes part of right subclavian artery; remainder disappears
10. Left dorsal aorta	Distal aortic arch
11. Right seventh intersegmental artery	Part of right subclavian artery
12. Left seventh intersegmental artery	Left subclavian artery

Absent Left Pulmonary Artery

The left pulmonary artery almost always is absent only in the sense that it arises from a left-sided ductus arteriosus (or ligamentum arteriosum). The anomaly is the result of disappearance of the proximal left sixth arch. If, in this anomaly, the aortic arch is on the left side, then the ductus arteriosus which feeds the intrapulmonary part of the left pulmonary artery arises from the usual position on the underside of the arch. If the aortic arch is on the right, then the ductus arteriosus will arise from the brachiocephalic trunk, with the left common carotid and left subclavian arteries as a trifurcation.

A discussion of the pathogenesis of many other aortic arch anomalies is beyond the scope of this chapter. It is almost always possible to deduce their genesis as being due to abnormal retention or disappearance of various segments of the aortic arch system.

References

1. Romer, A. S.: "The Vertebrate Body." Shorter version, 4th ed., W. B. Saunders Company, Philadelphia, 1971, p. 245.
2. Davis, C. L.: Development of the Human Heart from Its First Appearance to the State Found in Embryos of 20 Paired Somites, *Contrib. Embryol.*, 19:245, 1927.
3. Davis, C. L.: Description of a Human Embryo Having 20 Paired Somites, *Contrib. Embryol.*, 15:1, 1923.
4. Davis, C. L.: The Cardiac Jelly of the Chick Embryo, *Anat. Rec.*, 27:201, 1924.
5. Van Mierop, L. H. S.: Embryology of the Heart, in F. H. Netter (ed.), "The CIBA Collection of Medical Illustrations," CIBA Pharmaceutical Co., Summit, N. J., 1969, vol. 5, part I, p. 112.
*5a. Van Mierop, L. H. S.: Morphological Development of the Heart, in R. M. Berne (ed.), "Handbook of Physiology," sec. 2: "The Cardiovascular System," vol. 1: "The Heart," American Physiological Society, Bethesda, Md., 1979, p. 1. (64 references)
6. Castro-Quezada, A., Nadal-Ginard, B., and de la Cruz, M. V.: Experimental Study of the Formation of the Bulboventricular Loop in the Chick, *J. Embryol. Exp. Morphol.*, 27:623, 1972.
7. Manasek, F. J., Burnside, M. B., and Waterman, R. E.: Myocardial Cell Shape Change as a Mechanism of Embryionic Heart Looping, *Dev. Biol.*, 29:9, 1972.
8. Stalsberg, H.: Origin of Heart Asymmetry: Right and Left Contributions to the Early Chick Embryo Heart, *Dev. Biol.*, 19:109, 1969.
9. Stalsberg, H.: Mechanism of Dextral Looping of the Embryonic Heart, *Am. J. Cardiol.*, 25:265, 1970.
10. Patten, B. M.: The Formation of the Cardiac Loop in the Chick, *Am. J. Anat.*, 30:273, 1922.
11. Van Mierop, L. H. S., Alley, R. D., Kausel, H. W., and Stranahan, A.: Pathogenesis of Transposition Complexes. I. Embryology of the Ventricles and Great Arteries, *Am. J. Cardiol.*, 12:216, 1963.
12. Lepori, N. G.: Research on Heart Development in Chick Embryo under Normal and Experimental Conditions, *Monit. Zool. Ital.*, 1:159, 1967.
13. DeHaan, R. L.: Development of Form in the Embryonic Heart. An Experimental Approach, *Circulation*, 35:821, 1967.
14. Streeter, G. L.: Developmental Horizons in Human Embryos. Description of Age Groups XI, 13–20 Somites, and Age Group XII, 21–29 Somites, *Contrib. Embryol.*, 30:211, 1942.
15. Van Mierop, L. H. S., Alley, R. D., Kausel, H. W., and Stranahan, A.: The Anatomy and Embryology of Endocardial Cushion Defects, *J. Thorac. Cardiovasc. Surg.*, 43:71, 1962.
16. Goor, D. A., Dische, R., and Lillehei, C. W.: The Conotruncus. I. Its Normal Reverse Torsion and Conus Absorption, *Circulation*, 46:375, 1972.
17. Odgers, P. N. B.: The Development of the Atrioventricular Valves in Man, *J. Anat.*, 73:643, 1939.
18. Tandler, J.: The Development of the Heart, in F. Keibel and F. P. Mall (eds.), "Manual of Human Embryology," J. B. Lippincott Company, Philadelphia, 1912, p. 534.

*This article is a review of the literature and contains additional references to the literature.

19. Grant, R. P.: Embryology of Ventricular Flow Pathways in Man, *Circulation*, 25:756, 1962.
20. Patten, B. M., Kramer, T. C., and Barry, A.: Valvular Action in the Embryonic Chick Heart by Localized Apposition of Endocardial Masses, *Anat. Rec.*, 102:299, 1948.
21. Bremer, J. L.: The Presence and Influence of Two Spiral Streams in the Heart of the Chick Embryo, *Am. J. Anat.*, 49:409, 1932.
22. DeVries, P. A., and Saunders, J. B.: Development of the Ventricles and of the Spiral Outflow Tract in the Human Heart. A Contribution to the Development of the Human Heart from Age Group IX to XV, *Contrib. Embryol.*, 37:87, 1962.
23. Goerttler, L.: Durchstromungsversuche an Glasmodellen embryonaler Herzanlagen, *Verh. Dtsch. Ges. Path ol.*, 38:220, 1955.
24. Goerttler, L.: Hämodynamische Untersuchungen über die Entstehung der Missbildungen des arteriellen Herzendes, *Virchows Arch. Pathol. Anat. Physiol.*, 328:391, 1956.
25. Streeter, G. L.: Developmental Horizons in Human Embryos. Description of Age Group XV, XVI, XVII, XVIII, Being the Third Issue of a Survey of the Carnegie Collection, *Contrib. Embryol.*, 32:113, 1948.
26. Mall, F. P.: On the Development of the Human Heart, *Am. J. Anat.*, 13:249, 1912.
27. Keith, A.: The Hunterian Lectures on Malformation of the Heart, *Lancet*, 2:359, 433, and 519, 1909.
28. Tandler, J.: Anatomie des Herzens, in "Bardeleben's Handbuch der Anatomie des Menschen," Gustav Fischer Verlag, Jena, 1913, p. 1.
29. Los, J. A.: Embryology, in H. Watson (ed.), "Paediatric Cardiology," The C. V. Mosby Company, St. Louis, 1968, p. 1.
30. Kramer, T. C.: The Partitioning of the Truncus and Conus and the Formation of the Membranous Portion of the Interventricular Septum in the Human Heart, *Am. J. Anat.*, 71:343, 1942.
31. Shaner, R. F.: Anomalies of the Heart Bulbus, *J. Pediatr.*, 61:233, 1962.
32. Asami, I.: Beitrag zur Entwicklungsgeschichte des Vorhofseptums im menschlichen Herzen, eine lupenpräparatorisch-photographische Darstellung, *Z. Anat. Entwicklungsgesch.*, 139:55, 1972.
33. Christie, G. A.: Development of the Limbus Fossae Ovalis in the Human Heart—A New Septum, *J. Anat.*, 97:45, 1963.
34. Odgers, R. N. B.: The Formation of the Venous Valves, the Foramen Secundum and the Septum Secundum in the Human Heart, *J. Anat.*, 69:412, 1935.
35. Aüer, J.: The Development of the Human Pulmonary Veins and Its Major Variations, *Anat. Rec.*, 101:581, 1948.
36. Los, J. A.: The Development of the Human Pulmonary Veins and the Coronary Sinus in the Human Embryo. Thesis, Univ. of Leiden, 1958.
37. Neill, C. A.: Development of the Pulmonary Veins, *Pediatrics*, 18:880, 1956.
38. Waterston, D.: The Development of the Heart in Man, *Trans. R. Soc., Edinburgh*, 52:257, 1918.

2

Anatomy of the Heart

Thomas N. James, M.D.
Libi Sherf, M.D.
Robert C. Schlant, M.D.
Mark E. Silverman, M.D.

Structure is a sure guide to function. No physiological theory can be true unless it gives a complete and final explanation of all points of structure.

Sir Arthur Keith[1]

Gross Anatomy of the Heart and Blood Vessels

A comprehensive knowledge of gross cardiac anatomy is an indispensable foundation for the clinician who wishes to examine the patient, to understand the chest roentgenogram and the electrocardiogram, or to perform cardiac catheterization or echocardiography. This knowledge can be gained only by studying the heart at autopsy, by correlating the anatomy with the cardiac silhouette of the chest roentgenogram, and by mentally visualizing the cardiac anatomy while palpating the chest and listening to the heart.[2-8]

The heart is situated in the middle mediastinum, where it is partially overlapped by the neighboring lungs (Fig. 2-1). The sternum and costal cartilages of the third, fourth, and fifth ribs overlie the heart anteriorly. About two-thirds of the heart is left of the midline. The heart rests upon the diaphragm and is tilted forward and to the left so that the apex is anterior to the rest of the heart. The normal apex impulse can be palpated in the fourth or fifth intercostal space near the midclavicular line. The weight and size of the heart varies considerably depending on age, sex, body length, epicardial fat, and general nutrition.

The borders of the normal cardiac silhouette in a frontal view are formed by the following structures (Fig. 2-1):[8] The top of the cardiac silhouette is formed by the transverse and ascending aorta. The upper right margin is contributed by the superior vena cava. The right atrium provides the remaining right lateral cardiac border. Most of the inferior border is composed of right ventricle. The

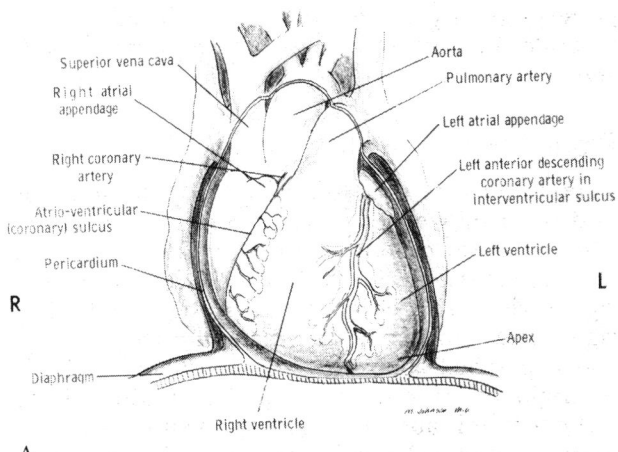

A

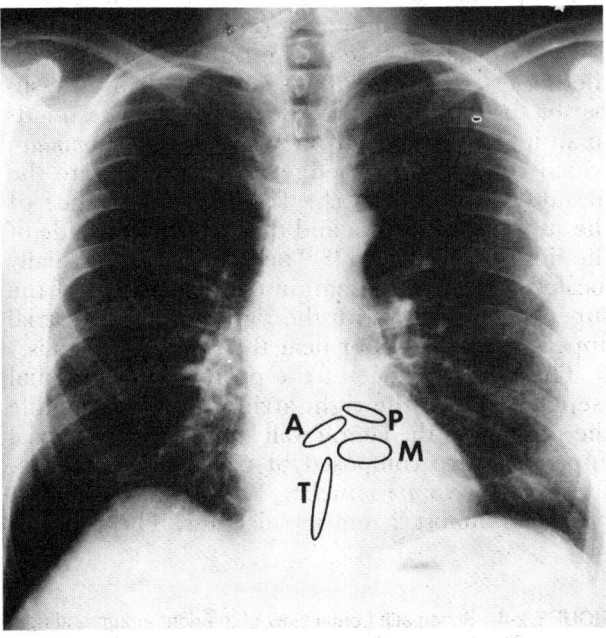

B

FIGURE 2-1 *A.* Schematic drawing showing the normal relations of the pericardium, great vessels, ventricles, and atria as viewed in the frontal position. R = right; L = left. *B.* Frontal (AP) roentgenogram of the heart. The components which form the cardiac silhouette can be readily identified from *A.* A = aortic valve ring; P = pulmonary valve ring; M = mitral valve ring; T = tricuspid valve ring.

apex and the lower left lateral cardiac border consist of left ventricle. The left atrial appendage perches atop the left ventricle and to the side of the pulmonary artery, interjecting on the cardiac border between the left ventricle and pulmonary outflow tract. The pulmonary outflow area produces the rest of the upper left border.

External Features

The atria are separated from the ventricles externally by the *coronary sulcus (atrioventricular sulcus),* which circles the heart between the atria and ventricles (Fig. 2-1). The right coronary artery, after

leaving the aorta, travels in this sulcus between the right atrium and right ventricle until it descends on the posterior surface of the heart. Similarly, the left circumflex artery is found in the coronary sulcus between the left atrium and left ventricle until the artery ramifies posteriorly.

Externally the two ventricles are delineated by *interventricular sulci,* which descend from the coronary sulcus toward the apex. Epicardial fat often obscures these landmarks. The anterior interventricular sulcus contains the *left anterior descending* coronary artery and courses over the muscular interventricular septum between the right and left ventricles to the apex. It then passes around the apex and continues as the posterior interventricular sulcus on the diaphragmatic surface of the heart (Fig. 2-1).

The posterior interventricular sulcus is the pathway for the posterior descending coronary artery, which is usually the terminal branch of the right coronary artery or, less frequently, of the left circumflex artery. The two atria may be delineated externally by a groove on the posterior surface between the right pulmonary veins and the venae cavae.

The *crux* of the heart is the area on the posterior surface where the coronary sulcus meets the posterior interventricular sulcus. Internally at this junction the interatrial septum joins the interventricular septum. The coronary artery which crosses this area makes a U turn, providing a small artery to the nearby atrioventricular node. The surface of the heart below the crux is referred to as the *diaphragmatic,* or *inferior, area* of the heart. A transverse section through the heart is extremely helpful in demonstrating the relations of the cardiac chambers (Fig. 2-2). The ventricular and atrial septa are aligned obliquely 45° to the left of the midline so that the planes of the septa are directed approximately from right scapula to left nipple.[9] The entire right side of the heart is to the right of this plane, placing most of the right atrium anterior to the left atrium and most of the right ventricle anterior to the left ventricle.

Fibrous Skeleton

A fibrous tissue framework affords a firm anchorage for the attachments of the atrial and ventricular musculature as well as the valvular tissue (Fig. 2-3). At the center of the heart the central fibrous body (right fibrous trigone) fuses together the medial aspect of the mitral, tricuspid, and aortic roots. Compact bundles of connective tissue continue posteroinferiorly from the right fibrous trigone and anteriorly and to the left as the left fibrous trigone. Continuations of fibroelastic tissue from these two bundles partially encircle the mitral and tricuspid valves. These rings of tissue are the *annuli fibrosi cordis,* which serve as attachments for the mitral and tricuspid valves as well as for the atrial and ventric-

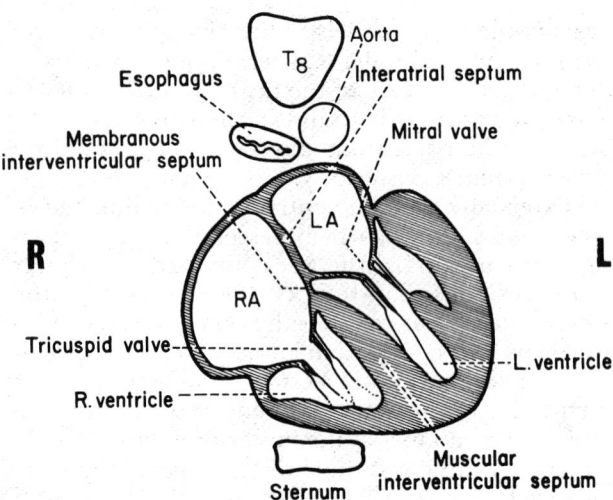

FIGURE 2-2 Schematic drawing of a transverse section through the heart at approximately the level of the eighth thoracic vertebra. The plane of the interatrial and interventricular septa slants approximately 45° to the left of the midline. RA = right atrium; LA = left atrium; R = right; L = left.

ular muscle. A triple scalloped line of heavy collagenous tissue extends anteriorly from the left and right fibrous trigones to provide a three-pointed crownlike skeletal support for the aortic root and cusps. A substantial ligament of tissue, the conus ligament, passes from the right side of the aortic root to a similar arrangement of scalloped tissue that surrounds the pulmonic root.

An important extension of the fibrous skeleton, the *membranous ventricular septum* extends inferiorly and anteriorly from the right fibrous trigone. This membranous septum is located at the summit of the muscular ventricular septum, where it provides support for the right coronary and noncoronary aortic cusps (Fig. 2-3). The membranous ventricular septum extends slightly above the tricuspid valve, forming a small portion of the medial wall of the right atrium.[10] The bundle of His penetrates the right fibrous trigone and travels along the inferior margin of the membranous portion of the interventricular septum.[11] At the crest of the muscular septum, about the level of junction of the right coronary and

posterior (noncoronary) aortic cusps, the His bundle separates into a *left bundle branch* and a *right bundle branch*.

Right Atrium

Venous blood returns to the heart via the superior and inferior venae cavae into the right atrium, where it is stored during right ventricular systole. During ventricular diastole, blood flows from the right atrium into the right ventricle (Fig. 2-4). The right atrium forms the right lateral cardiac border and is perched above, behind, and to the right of the right ventricle (Figs. 2-2 and 2-4). Most of the right atrium is anterior to the left atrium as well as to the right of it (Fig. 2-5). Anteromedially the right atrial appendage protrudes from the right atrium and overlaps the aortic root (Fig. 2-1). On the posterior external surface of the right atrium a ridge, the *sulcus terminalis*, extends vertically from the superior to the inferior vena cava. This corresponds to an internal muscular bundle, the *crista terminalis*, which runs along the edge of the opening to the atrial appendage to the front of the orifice of the superior vena cava and then to the right side of the inferior vena cava.[12] The sinus node is usually located at the lateral margin of the junction of the superior vena cava with the right atrium and atrial appendage, beneath or near the sulcus terminalis.

The inner surface of the posterior and medial (septal) walls of the right atrium is smooth, while the surfaces of the lateral wall and of the right atrial appendage are composed of parallel muscle bundles, the *pectinate muscles*. The right atrial wall measures almost 2 mm in thickness. The superior

FIGURE 2-3 Schematic anterosuperior view of the heart with the atria removed. The components of the fibrous skeleton and the orientation of the leaflets of each valve are demonstrated.

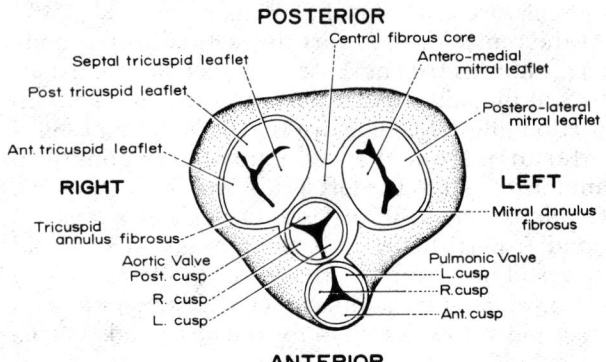

FIGURE 2-4 Schematic frontal view of the right atrium and right ventricle. The arrows indicate the general orientation of blood as it enters the right atrium and right ventricle and is ejected into the pulmonary artery. SVC = superior vena cava; ra = right atrium; rv = right ventricle; pa = pulmonary artery; R = right; L = left.

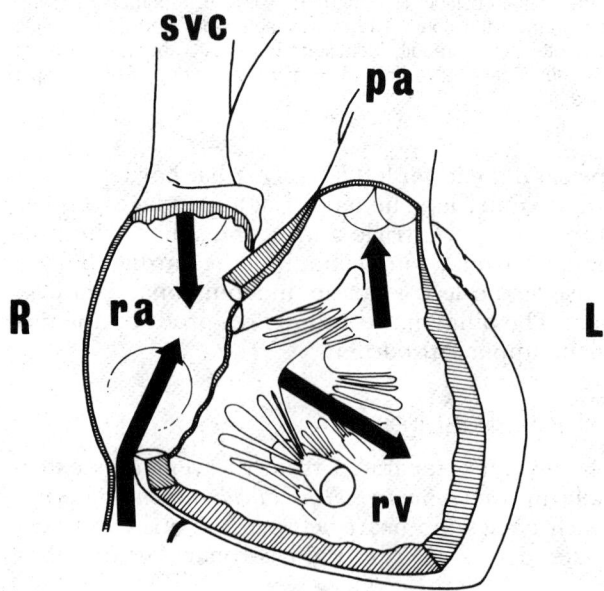

POSTERIOR

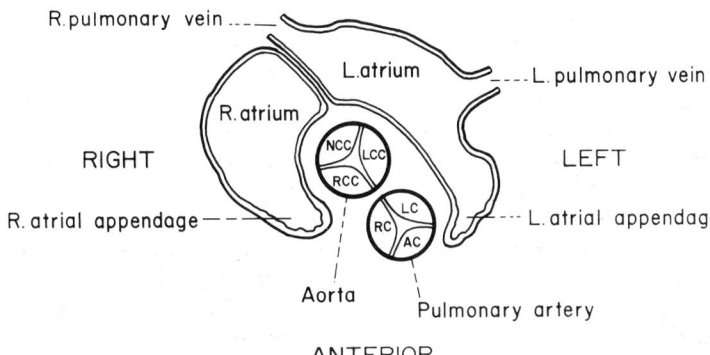

ANTERIOR

FIGURE 2-5 Schematic transverse section through the heart at approximately the level of the second intercostal space. The relation between the left and right atria and the interatrial septum is illustrated. The relative positions of the aortic and pulmonary valves and their cusps are shown. AC = anterior cusp; RC = right cusp; LC = left cusp of the pulmonary valve; LCC = left coronary cusp; RCC = right coronary cusp; NCC = noncoronary cusp of the aortic valve.

and inferior venae cavae enter the right atrium posteriorly and medially at its superior and inferior aspects. The orifice of the superior vena cava has no valve; the orifice of the inferior vena cava is flanked anteriorly by an inconstant, rudimentary valve, the *eustachian valve,* formed by a crescentic fold. The caval orifices may vary in shape and diameter depending upon the phase of respiration, the cardiac cycle, and the contraction or relaxation of surrounding muscular bands. The variation in the orifice may play some role in promoting venous return or preventing atrial reflux.

The medial wall of the right atrium is important because of its proximity to several structures.[13] Anteriorly, the posterior (noncoronary) cusp and the right coronary cusp of the aortic root lean against the medial right atrium, forming a normal slight bulge known as the *torus aorticus,* which is a useful landmark during transseptal catheterization of the left side of the heart. The proximal right coronary artery as it enters the coronary sulcus is in the immediate vicinity. The proximity of the aortic root to the right atrium permits an aneurysm of the sinus of Valsalva to rupture into the right atrium.

The *atrial septum* is found in the posteroinferior portion of the medial wall of the right atrium and extends obliquely forward from right to left (Fig. 2-5).[14] Near the center of the interatrial septum there is a shallow depression, the *fossa ovalis,* which has a prominent fold, or limbus, anteriorly. The ostium of the *coronary sinus* is located between the inferior vena cava and the tricuspid valve. The orifice of the coronary sinus is guarded by a rudimentary flap of tissue, the *Thebesian valve.*[20] The *atrioventricular (AV) node* is anterior and medial to the coronary sinus, just above the septal leaflet of the tricuspid valve. The sinus and atrioventricular nodes as well as the entire conducting pathways are not grossly visible.

Right Ventricle

The right ventricle receives venous blood from the right atrium during ventricular diastole and propels blood into the pulmonary circulation during ventricular systole (Fig. 2-4).

The right ventricle is normally the most anterior cardiac chamber, lying directly beneath the sternum (Fig. 2-2). Enlargement or hyperactivity of the right ventricle may often be detected by palpation of the sternum or the lower left sternal border. The right ventricle is partially below, in front of, and medial to the right atrium, and anterior and to the right of the left ventricle. Most of the entire inferior border of the frontal roentgenogram view of the heart consists of the right ventricle (Fig. 2-1).

The striking difference in configuration between the two ventricles is illustrated by a transverse section (Fig. 2-6). The left ventricular chamber is an ellipsoidal sphere surrounded by relatively thick (8 to 15 mm at autopsy) musculature, well suited to ejecting against the high resistance of the systemic vessels. The right ventricle, which normally contracts against very low resistance, has a crescent-shaped chamber and a thin outer wall, measuring 4 to 5 mm in thickness.[15] The anterior right ventricular wall curves over the *ventricular septum,* which bulges into the right ventricular cavity. Although the ventricular septum forms the medial wall of both ventricles, functionally it seems to belong predominantly to the left ventricle in normal subjects.

FIGURE 2-6 Schematic drawings of the heart to illustrate the differences in shape of the right and left ventricles. *A.* Ventricles in approximate anatomic position. *B.* Cross section, illustrating the more nearly circular dimensions of the left ventricle.

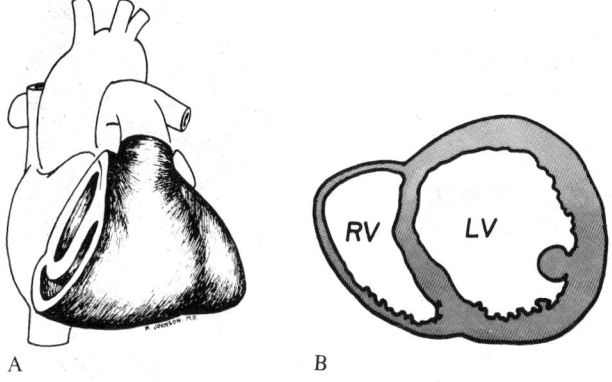

A   B

The anterior and inferior walls of the right ventricular cavity are lined by muscle bundles, the *trabeculae carneae*, which often form ridges along the inner surface of the wall or cross from one wall to the other. A rather constant muscle, the *moderator band*, crosses from the lower ventricular septum to the anterior wall, where it joins the anterior papillary muscle (Fig. 2-7). The right bundle branch, after traveling through the muscular ventricular septum, courses through the moderator muscle.

Functionally, the right ventricle can be partitioned into an inflow and an outflow tract. The inflow tract, consisting of the tricuspid valve and the trabecular muscles of the anterior and inferior walls, directs entering blood anteriorly, inferiorly, and to the left at an angle of 60° to the outflow tract (Fig. 2-4).[16] The smooth-walled outflow tract, also referred to as the *infundibulum*, forms the superior portion of the right ventricle. It is separated from the inflow tract by a thick muscle, the *crista supraventricularis*, which arches from the anterolateral wall over the anterior leaflet of the tricuspid valve to the septal (medial) wall, where it joins other constrictor bands of muscle which encircle the outflow tract (Fig. 2-7).[12] Blood entering the infundibulum is ejected superiorly and posteriorly into the pulmonary artery.

Left Atrium

The left atrium receives blood from the pulmonary veins and serves as the reservoir during left ventricular systole and as a conduit during left ventricular filling. In addition, left atrial contraction provides a significant increment of blood to the left ventricle, stretching the ventricle and priming it for ventricular ejection.

The left atrium is located superiorly, in the midline, and posterior to the other cardiac chambers (Figs. 2-2 and 2-8). As a consequence of this posterior position, the left atrium is not normally seen in the frontal roentgenogram. The esophagus abuts directly upon its posterior surface, while the aortic root impinges upon its anterior wall. The right atrium is to the right and anterior (Fig. 2-5). The left ventricle is to the left, anterior, and inferior. The posterior position of the left atrium makes it impossible to palpate externally unless it is massively dilated. With severe mitral regurgitation, however, expansion of the left atrium from the regurgitation and the ejection recoil of the anteriorly located ventricles may force the heart anteriorly, producing a late systolic sternal lift. The left atrium usually enlarges posteriorly and laterally in mitral stenosis or regurgitation, occasionally reaching the right or left lateral chest wall.

The wall of the left atrium is 3 mm, slightly thicker than that of the right atrium. Two pulmonary veins enter posterolaterally on each side, conveying oxygenated blood from the lungs. Though there are no true valves at the junction of the pulmonary veins and the left atrium, sleeves of atrial muscle extend from the left atrial wall around the pulmonary veins for 1 or 2 cm and may exert a partial sphincter-like influence, tending to lessen reflux during atrial systole or mitral regurgitation.

The endocardium of the left atrium is smooth and slightly opaque. Pectinate muscles are present

FIGURE 2-7 Schematic representation of a frontal view of the heart. The anterior right ventricular wall has been removed to demonstrate the orientation of the tricuspid leaflets and the papillary muscles. The anterior papillary muscle is sectioned. The trabeculated inflow portion of the right ventricle is contrasted with the smooth infundibular (outflow) area.

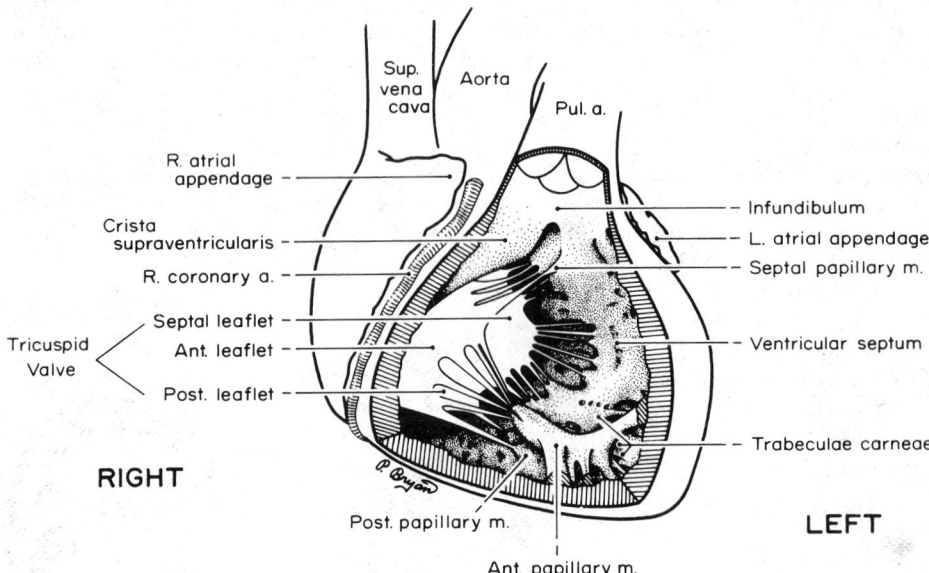

INFERIOR

only in the *left atrial appendage,* which projects from the anterolateral left atrium, alongside the pulmonary artery (Fig. 2-1). The atrial septum is smooth but may contain a central shallow area, corresponding to the *fossa ovalis.*

Left Ventricle

The left ventricle receives blood from the left atrium during ventricular diastole and ejects blood into the systemic arterial circulation during ventricular systole (Figs. 2-8 and 2-9). The left ventricle is roughly bullet-shaped with the blunt tip directed anteriorly, inferiorly, and to the left, where it contributes, with the lower ventricular septum, to the apex of the heart (Fig. 2-2).[17,18] Although the left ventricle forms the lower left lateral cardiac border in the frontal roentgenogram, the major portion of its external surface is posterolateral (Fig. 2-2). The left ventricle is posterior and to the left of the right ventricle and inferior, anterior, and to the left of the left atrium. The left ventricular chamber is approximately an ellipsoidal sphere, surrounded by thick muscular walls measuring 8 to 15 mm, or ap-

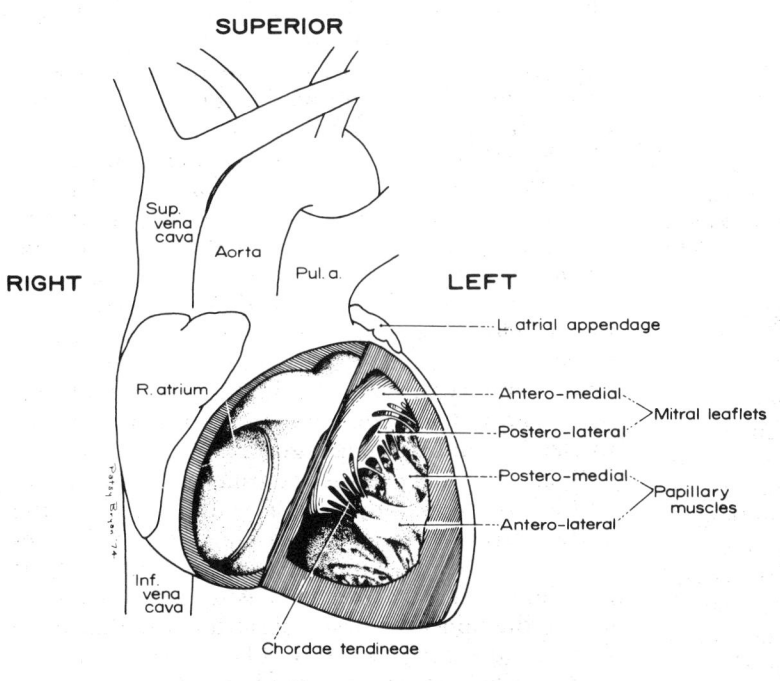

A

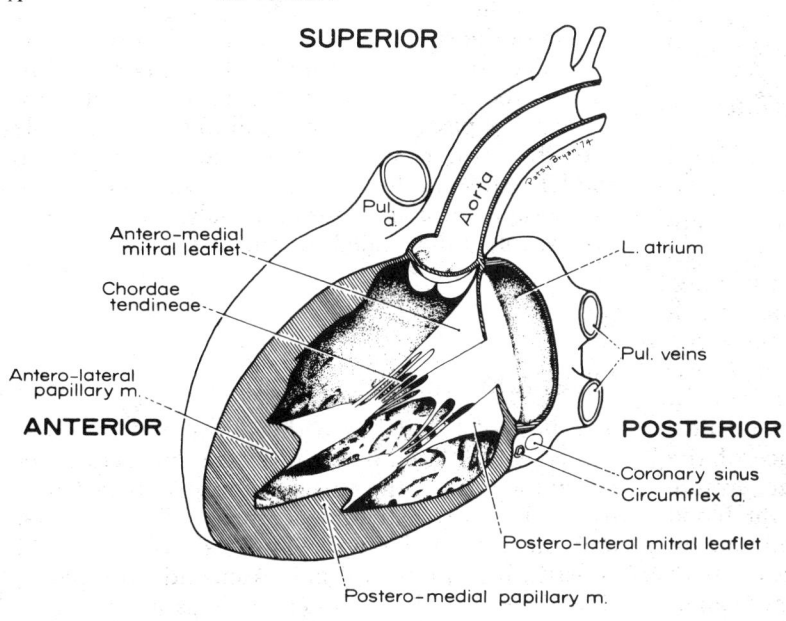

B

FIGURE 2-8 Schematic drawings illustrating the components of the mitral complex (mitral annulus, mitral leaflets, chordae tendineae, and papillary muscles). *A.* Frontal view, right ventricle and interventricular septum removed. *B.* Left lateral view, lateral wall of left atrium and left ventricle partially removed.

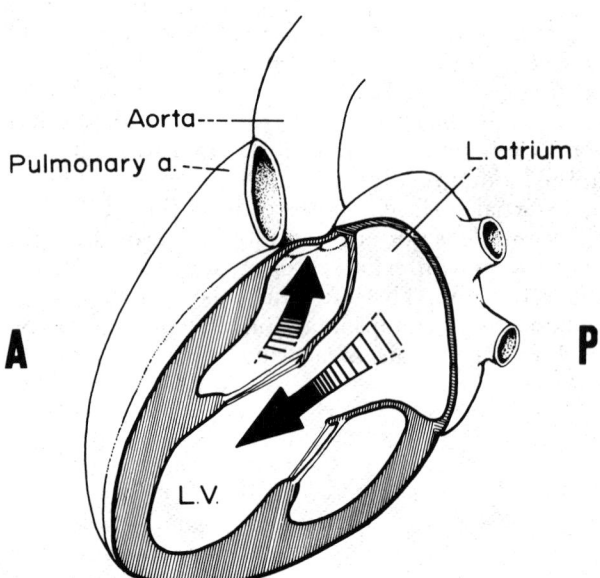

FIGURE 2-9 Schematic left lateral view of the left side of the heart. The arrows indicate the general orientation of blood flow from left atrium to left ventricle to aorta. A = anterior; P = posterior.

proximately two to three times the thickness of the right ventricular wall. The tip of the left ventricular apex is very thin, measuring 2 mm or less.[11] The medial wall of the left ventricle is the *ventricular septum*, which is shared with the right ventricle (Fig. 2-6). The septum, which is roughly triangular in shape with the base of the triangle at the level of the aortic cusps, is entirely muscular except for the small membranous septum, located superiorly just below the right coronary and the posterior cusps (Fig. 2-2).[10,11] The upper third of the septum is smooth endocardium. The remaining two-thirds of the septum and the remaining ventricular walls are ridged by interlacing muscles, the *trabeculae carneae*. The ventricular wall exclusive of the septum is often referred to as the *free wall of the left ventricle*.

The *anteromedial leaflet* of the mitral valve, which is the larger and more mobile of the two mitral leaflets, extends from the top of the posteromedial septum across the ventricular cavity to the anterolateral ventricular wall, separating the left ventricular cavity into an inflow and an outflow tract. The funnel-shaped inflow tract, which is formed by the *mitral annulus* and by both mitral leaflets and their *chordae tendineae*, directs the entering atrial blood inferiorly, anteriorly, and to the left (Fig. 2-9). The outflow tract, surrounded by the inferior surface of the anteromedial mitral leaflet, the ventricular septum, and the left ventricular free wall, orients the blood flow from left ventricular apex to the right and superiorly at an angle of 90° to the inflow tract.[19] With the onset of ventricular systole, both mitral leaflets are propelled upward, converting the entire left ventricle into an expulsion chamber.

Semilunar Valves[20,21]

The semilunar aortic and pulmonary valves are similar in configuration, except the aortic cusps are slightly thicker. They are situated at the summit of the outflow tract of their corresponding ventricle, the pulmonary valve being anterior, superior, and slightly to the left of the aortic valve (Figs. 2-3 and 2-5). Each valve is composed of three fibrous cusps. The U-shaped convex lower edges of each cusp are attached to and suspended from the root of the aorta or pulmonary artery, with the upper free valve edges projecting into the lumen. The cusps, which are often slightly unequal in width, circle the inside of the vessel root.[22] Behind each cusp the vessel wall bulges outward, forming a pouchlike dilatation known as the *sinus of Valsalva*. The free edge of each cusp is concave, with a nodular interruption at the center of the leaflet, the *noduli Arantii*. The portion of the cusp adjacent to the rim is not as thick and may normally contain small perforations. During ventricular systole the cusps are passively thrust upward, away from the center of the aortic lumen. During ventricular diastole the cusps fall passively into the lumen of the vessel as they support the column of blood above. The noduli Arantii meet in the center and contribute to the support of the leaflets. The geometry of the cusps and the strong fibrous tissue support provide excellent approximations of the leaflets and prevent regurgitation of blood.

The pulmonary cusps are called anterior, right, and left (Figs. 2-3 and 2-5). The designation of the aortic cusps is best related to the coronary arteries (Fig. 2-5). The two anterior cusps are referred to as the right and left coronary cusps. The remaining cusp is the noncoronary or posterior cusp. Since the plane of the aortic valve is oblique, with the right posterior side lower than the left anterior side, the origin of the left coronary artery is slightly superior to that of the right coronary artery. The ostia of the coronary arteries are located in the upper third of their respective sinus of Valsalva. The right coronary artery passes anteriorly and to the right, while the left coronary artery courses anteriorly and to the left. In some hearts there is a separate ostium in the right coronary sinus of Valsalva for the conus artery, sometimes called the third coronary artery.

Mitral and Tricuspid Complex[23–26]

The flow of blood across the mitral and tricuspid orifice is regulated by an intricate interaction between the atrium, the annulus fibrosus, the valvular tissue, the chordae tendineae, the papillary muscles, and the ventricular wall. These six components, constituting the mitral and tricuspid "complex," should be considered functionally as a unit, since derangement of any one part may allow serious hemodynamic consequences.

Mitral Valve

The orifice of the mitral valve faces anterolaterally and directs the left atrial blood inferiorly, anteriorly, and to the left. The fibroelastic valvular tissue, which is attached to the annulus fibrosus, completely encircles the orifice, providing a cone-shaped funnel extending into the recesses of the left ventricular cavity (Fig. 2-8). There are two major leaflets connected by bridging commissural tissue. The triangular *anteromedial leaflet* stretches diagonally from the posteromedial aspect of the muscular ventricular septum across the ventricular cavity to attach to the anterolateral wall of the left ventricle. This leaflet is continuous with supporting tissues of the noncoronary and left coronary aortic cusps which lie above. The ventricular surface of the anteromedial leaflet forms the posterosuperior portion of the left ventricular outflow tract. There are pathologic conditions in which the outflow tract may be obstructed by abnormal attachment of the anteromedial leaflet or by an eccentric pull by its papillary muscles.

The longer, less mobile quadrangular *posterolateral leaflet* encircles about two-thirds of the circumference of the mitral valve orifice. It is attached superiorly to the annulus fibrosus and circles from anterolateral to posteromedial ventricle (Fig. 2-3). This leaflet is more restricted in its movements than the anteromedial leaflet.

Though the two leaflets differ greatly in height and mobility, both contribute importantly to effective valve closure.

Tricuspid Valve[27]

The right atrioventricular (tricuspid) orifice, which is larger than the mitral orifice, is oriented with its plane in a semivertical axis, and directs the right atrial blood anteriorly, inferiorly, and to the left (Fig. 2-4). Its relatively superficial position below the lower left sternal border allows tricuspid murmurs to be heard best in this area. The tricuspid leaflets differ from the mitral leaflets in being thinner, more translucent, and less easily separated into well-defined leaflets. There are usually three major leaflets of unequal size (Fig. 2-6). The largest leaflet is the *anterior leaflet,* which stretches from the infundibular area downward to the inferolateral wall of the ventricle. The *septal (medial) leaflet* attaches to both the membranous and muscular portions of the interventricular septum. At times this leaflet may partially or completely occlude small ventricular septal defects of the outflow tract. The *posterior leaflet,* which is usually the smallest, is attached to the tricuspid ring along its posteroinferior border.

The rapid opening and closing of the mitral and tricuspid leaflets is possible because of their remarkable mobility, facilitated by attachments at only the basilar and apical aspects, a specific gravity approximating that of blood, a smooth surface minimizing friction, and a large area of coaptation between the leaflets.

Papillary Muscles[28]

The papillary muscles of both ventricles are located below the commissures of the atrioventricular valves. These muscles project from the trabeculae carneae and may be single or bifid; occasionally they are made up of a row of muscles arising from the ventricular wall. In the left ventricle the two groups of papillary muscles, located below the anterolateral and posteromedial commissures, arise from the junction of the apical and middle third of the ventricular wall (Fig. 2-10). In the right ventricle there are usually three papillary muscles (Fig. 2-7). The largest is the *anterior papillary muscle,* which is found below the commissure between the anterior and posterior leaflets, originating from the moderator band as well as from the anterolateral ventricular wall. The *posterior papillary muscle* lies beneath the junction of the posterior and septal leaflets. A small *septal papillary muscle,* originating from the wall of the infundibulum, tethers the anterior and septal leaflets high against the infundibular wall. At times this muscle is virtually absent, and the chordae tendineae arise from a small tendinous connection to the infundibulum.

The papillary muscles, because of their relatively parallel alignment to the ventricular wall and their chordal attachments to two adjacent valve leaflets, pull the leaflets of the mitral and tricuspid valves together and downward at the onset of isovolumic ventricular systole (Fig. 2-11).

Chordae Tendineae[29]

Strong cords of fibrous tissue, the chordae tendineae, spring from the tip of each papillary muscle (Figs. 2-6, 2-10, and 2-11). They often subdivide and

FIGURE 2-10 Papillary muscle of the left ventricle, demonstrating its origin from the trabeculae carneae. The chordae tendineae are shown reaching from the papillary muscle to both mitral valve leaflets. A = anteromedial mitral leaflet; P = posterolateral mitral leaflet; PM = papillary muscle.

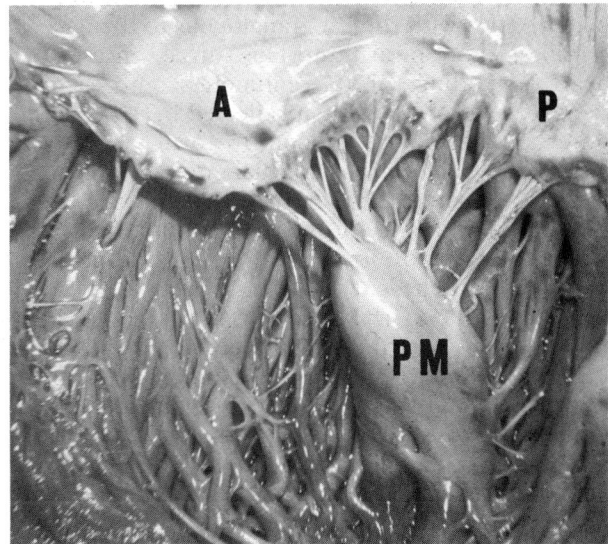

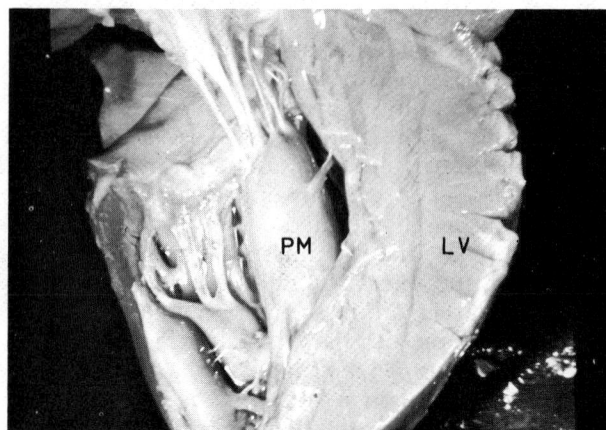

FIGURE 2-11 The left ventricular wall and papillary muscle are shown to have a parallel orientation. PM = papillary muscle; LV = left ventricle.

interconnect before they attach to the two leaflets directly above. The chordae may attach directly into a fibrous band running along the free edge of the valves, or they may become incorporated into the ventricular surface of the leaflet a few millimeters back from the edge. Additional chordae run directly from the ventricular wall into the undersurface of the posterolateral leaflet of the left ventricle and the septal and posterior leaflets of the right ventricle.

The chordae tendineae, by their attachments to most of the free valvular border and by their numerous cross connections, allow the valve leaflets to balloon upward and against each other and evenly distribute the forces of ventricular systole. Dysfunction or rupture of a papillary muscle or rupture of a chorda tendinea may undermine the support of one or more valve leaflets, producing regurgitation.

Pericardium[30]

The heart is enclosed by the pericardium, the two surfaces of which can be visualized by considering the heart as a fist which is plunged into a large balloon (Fig. 2-1). The surface of the balloon in intimate contact with the fist is analogous to the *visceral pericardium*, or epicardium. This surface encases the heart, extending several centimeters onto each of the great vessels. It is then reflected back, as is the outer surface of the balloon, to form the *parietal pericardium*. The two pericardial surfaces are lined by smooth, glistening serous tissue and are separated by a thin layer of lubricating fluid, which allows the heart to move freely within the parietal pericardium. The parietal pericardium is attached by ligaments to the manubrium, the xiphoid process, the vertebral column, and the diaphragm. There is normally about 10 to 20 ml of thin, clear pericardial fluid which moistens the contracting surfaces of the visceral and parietal pericardium.

Innervation of the Heart[31-33]

Although the SA (sinoatrial) node, AV node, and specialized conduction system of the heart possess the inherent ability for spontaneous, rhythmic initiation of the cardiac excitation impulse, the autonomic nervous system has an important role in the regulation of the rate of impulse formation. The autonomic nervous system also influences the rate of spread of the excitation impulse, depolarization and repolarization of the myocardium, and the contractility of both the atria and the ventricles. It is probable that sympathetic nerve fibers supply all areas of the atria and the ventricles, whereas vagal nerve fibers are primarily found in the SA node, atrial muscle fibers, and the AV node. Vagal fibers and vagal impulses also extend to both ventricles.

The efferent sympathetic innervation of the heart originates in the upper thoracic spinal cord and reaches the cardiac plexus via the *superior, middle,* and *inferior cervical ganglia,* and the *superior, middle,* and *inferior cardiac nerves.* The efferent parasympathetic innervation originates in the medulla oblongata and passes by way of the vagus nerves to join the sympathetic fibers in the cardiac plexus. The sympathetic and parasympathetic efferent nerves mingle together, forming the cardiac plexus, which surrounds the root and arch of the aorta near the tracheal bifurcation. From the cardiac plexus the sympathetic and parasympathetic nerves extend to the heart, richly supplying in the SA node, AV node, and the main trunks of the coronary arteries.

Sympathetic stimulation to the heart is mediated by the release of the neurohormone norepinephrine. Cardiac parasympathetic impulses are transmitted by acetylcholine. Normally the parasympathetic influence is the dominant autonomic influence on the heart rate, whereas sympathetic influence is the normal dominant influence on ventricular function.

Afferent impulses from several types of receptors in the pericardium, connective tissue, adventitia, and walls of the heart pass by peripheral sensory axons through sympathetic plexuses and through the lower two cervical and upper four thoracic sympathetic ganglia to thoracic dorsal ganglia, where the cell bodies of the neurons are located. The impulses are carried by the central axon of this neuron through the dorsal roots to the posterior gray column of the spinal cord, where the fibers synapse with the second-order neuron. From this neuron, fibers cross the median plane, ascend in the ventral spinothalamic tract, and terminate in the posteroventral nucleus of the thalamus. Some afferent vagal ganglia have been found in the left coronary artery system. Impulses passing through these neurons and ganglia are thought to be important in the Bezold-Jarisch reflex.

Aorta and Great Vessels

The origins of the aorta and pulmonary artery are similar in that they are both derived from the division of the embryonic truncus arteriosus. Although at birth the walls of these vessels are of approximately equal thickness, in the adult the wall of the aorta is considerably thicker than that of the pulmonary artery. This is presumably a result of the decreased pulmonary artery pressure in the adult state. The aorta has many elastic fibers which allow it to function as a compression chamber or reservoir for blood during the rapid ejection from the left ventricle. The term *Windkessel* (from the German word for the air-compression chamber in water pumps which converts pulsatile flow to nearly continuous flow) is customary in the literature for this function. Aging changes in the aorta may reduce the windkessel effect, resulting in a higher pulse pressure.

Arteries

The systemic arteries originate from the aorta and its branches, and they branch successively to become individually smaller. As the total cross-sectional area of the arteries, arterioles, and capillaries increases, the average velocity of blood flow decreases. The arteries eventually branch into small arterioles, which are the major areas of resistance in the systemic circulation. At the junction of the arterioles and the capillaries, there are often vascular sphincters. These precapillary sphincters have a basal myogenic tone which is continuously modified by local and systemic physical, chemical, and neural influences that profoundly affect the perfusion of the capillaries in the region. In addition, there may be small vascular shunts between small arterioles and venules which are capable of shunting blood past the capillary bed.

Capillaries

The capillaries are small vessels, usually consisting of single endothelial cells. At times the capillaries seem capable of holding several red blood cells transversely; at other times the red blood cells appear to pass singly through the capillaries. In a given capillary bed, there is frequently a stasis of flow in some capillaries while there is an active flow in other capillaries. This periodic flow through different capillary beds is thought to have a normal physiologic function of increasing nutrition in these areas. Under conditions of maximal flow, the entire capillary bed may be maximally dilated. Under normal flow conditions, there may be some gravitational layering of red blood cells, white blood cells, and plasma in the capillaries. Under certain conditions, such as acute stress, shock, toxemia, or uncontrolled diabetes, there may be a sludging or congregation of red blood cells in the capillaries. The normal capillary pressure in the systemic circulation is estimated to be approximately 25 to 35 millimeters of mercury (mmHg). In contrast, the normal pulmonary capillary pressure is 7 to 10 mmHg. It is estimated that the systemic capillary bed, under basal resting conditions, has a volume of approximately 5 percent of the total blood volume.

Veins

The veins of the body collect the blood from the capillaries and successively join one another to form progressively larger vessels that return the blood to the heart by way of the superior and inferior venae cavae. There is normally a slight pressure gradient between the systemic veins and the right atrium. In addition, the flow of blood returning to the heart is aided by the presence of valves in many of the larger veins, particularly those of the legs. This allows the muscular contraction of the arms and legs (the *muscular pump*) and the normal pressure changes in the thoracic (the *respiratory pump*) and abdominal cavities to contribute to the return of blood to the heart. Since they are normally subjected to less pressure than arteries, veins are considerably thinner-walled. Their pressure-volume characteristics are also significantly different from those of arteries. As a result, veins are capable of accommodating much larger volumes of blood with very slight changes in pressure. For this reason the veins are often referred to as *capacitance vessels*. The veins, as well as the arteries, are capable of changing their pressure-volume characteristics in response to hormonal or neural stimulation. At times this change in venomotor "tone" enables the veins to increase the return of blood to the heart and to make available blood needed in other areas. In a sense, such shifts in the distribution of blood volume are a type of internal blood transfusion. At rest, about 50 to 65 percent of the blood volume is located in the venous portions of the circulation.

Lymphatic Vessels[34–36]

Although the cardiovascular system is sometimes considered to be a closed fluid system, there is a large volume of fluid with small amounts of protein that is filtered in the renal glomeruli and a considerable quantity of similar filtration through the systemic capillaries into the interstitial spaces.

Fluid and protein filtered from blood capillaries into the interstitial fluid must return to the heart by way of either the veins or the lymphatic circulation. Generally, the smallest lymphatic vessels in the tissues are closed, permeable vessels similar to blood capillaries. Like the veins, the lymphatic vessels contain valves which allow the flow of lymph to be directed centrally. The major terminal vessel of the lymphatic system is the *thoracic duct*. The thoracic duct usually terminates by joining the left brachiocephalic vein at the junction of the internal jugular and left subclavian veins. Occasionally, it may end in branches of the left brachiocephalic vein or may even subdivide into branches ending separately in various great veins. On the right side there are three major lymphatic vessels: the right jugular, right subclavian, and right mediastinal lymphatic ducts. Although they usually enter the right internal jugular, subclavian, and brachiocephalic veins, respectively, occasionally the right jugular and subclavian ducts unite to form a *right lymphatic duct,* which usually enters the right brachiocephalic vein. The right mediastinal lymphatic vessel almost always enters the right brachiocephalic vein separately. The significance of other lymphaticovenous connections, such as those present in the abdomen, is uncertain at present.

Some of the importance of the lymphatic system becomes apparent when one realizes that in 24 h the thoracic duct alone returns to the circulation a volume of fluid about equal to the total plasma volume and containing 50 to 100 percent of the total circulating plasma protein.

The importance of the myocardial lymphatic vessels in the maintenance of normal myocardial nutrition and in the response to injury of the heart, particularly the endocardium and heart valves, has been emphasized. Undoubtedly, a more significant role will be shown for the lymphatic system in many other conditions, particularly pulmonary edema and rheumatic and infective valvulitis.

Pulmonary Circulation[37]

The basic function of the pulmonary circulation is the uptake of oxygen and the liberation of carbon dioxide by the blood. This function is efficiently accomplished by the pulmonary circuit, which normally carries all the cardiac output through the lungs at a pressure in the adult approximately one-sixth that of the systemic circulation. It is obvious, therefore, that its resistance to blood flow (the ratio of pressure difference across the pulmonary circuit to flow through the pulmonary circulation) is one-sixth that of the systemic circulation.

The pulmonary circulation differs from the systemic circulation in several important ways. The pulmonary arterial vessels have thinner walls and less medial muscle than their counterparts in the systemic circulation with the same luminal cross-sectional area. The main pulmonary artery, which in the fetus is histologically similar to the aorta, becomes much thinner-walled than the aorta after birth. There is normally a conspicuous fragmentation of the elastic fibers in the pulmonary artery following birth, unless there is a congenital heart defect that allows pulmonary hypertension to persist. In general, the pulmonary circulation may be said to be relatively passive. In comparison with systemic vessels, its blood vessels in most instances react relatively less to neural, humoral, or pharmacologic agents. In some cases the reactions are the opposite of those produced in systemic vessels; e.g., arterial hypoxia and hypercapnia may both produce vasoconstriction in the pulmonary circulation, whereas in the systemic circulation their effect is generally vasodilatation. Although pulmonary vasoconstriction has been demonstrated experimentally to occur under autonomic nervous system stimulation and as a result of carotid sinus and carotid body reflexes, the importance of these mechanisms in the normal control of the pulmonary circulation is uncertain. Two mechanisms that help to maintain the normal relation between pulmonary ventilation and blood flow in different areas of the lung (normal ventilation/perfusion ratio) are local regional vasoconstriction produced by alveolar hypoxia and local bronchoconstriction in underperfused areas, possibly produced by a lack of normal carbon dioxide concentration.

In the normal person at rest in the upright position, there is relatively little perfusion of the upper segments of the lung, and consequently there is little exchange of oxygen and carbon dioxide in these areas. This pattern of blood flow is the result of the relatively low pulmonary artery pressure, which is barely adequate to perfuse the upper areas of the lungs. When an individual lies on one side, there is correspondingly a greater flow of blood to the dependent parts of the lung.

In contrast to systemic capillaries, which have a pressure of 25 to 35 mmHg, the pulmonary capillaries at rest have a pressure of only 7 to 10 mmHg. This is of distinct advantage, since pulmonary capillary pressure must be elevated to 25 to 30 mmHg before pulmonary edema occurs if the serum proteins, capillary walls, and lymphatic drainage are normal (*pulmonary capillary reserve*). Actually, the net effect of the low pressure in the pulmonary capillaries combined with a normal oncotic pressure of blood causes the pulmonary circulation to keep the interstitial tissues of the lung in a relatively "dehydrated" state.

The total pulmonary blood volume in normal adults is probably about 500 ml. As in the systemic circulation, about 50 to 65 percent of this volume is on the venous side. Normal pulmonary capillary blood volume at rest is about 100 ml. The total surface area of the pulmonary capillaries is estimated to be 50 to 100 m².

The flow through the lungs of a normal person can increase about threefold before there is a significant increase in the required driving pressure, or pressure gradient, between the main pulmonary artery and the left atrium. This is usually attributed to the utilization of vascular channels not used at rest and to dilatation of other vessels. In the presence of pulmonary vascular disease or lung disease, this reserve may be markedly diminished.

The Coronary Arteries and Veins

Although the anatomy of the coronary arteries aroused the curiosity of Vieussens 350 years ago, it was only after a relation between disease of the coronary arteries and chest pain was established in this century that knowing about these vessels assumed more than academic importance. In recent years the rapid advances in cardiac surgery and in coronary angiography have stimulated further interest in the coronary arteries. This section will deal first with the typical course and important variations of each major artery, the anatomy of the veins and of arterial anastomoses, and the blood supply of special regions of the heart.

Left Coronary Artery

In nearly all human hearts the left coronary artery arises from a single ostium located in the middle of the upper half of the left coronary sinus of the aorta, which protrudes between the main pulmonary artery and the body of the left atrium (Fig. 2-12). There are virtually never any large branches of the main left coronary artery proximal to its division into anterior descending and circumflex rami. This stout vessel, which varies from a few millimeters to a few centimeters in length, lies free in epicardial fat. During systolic filling of the coronary arteries, it buckles easily because it is not held down to myocardium by branches like those of the anterior descending artery.

Although the division of the main left coronary artery is usually referred to as a bifurcation, three or more equally large divisions at this point are much more common (Fig. 2-13). The large branch which courses down the anterior interventricular sulcus becomes the left anterior descending artery; the one which courses into the left atrioventricular

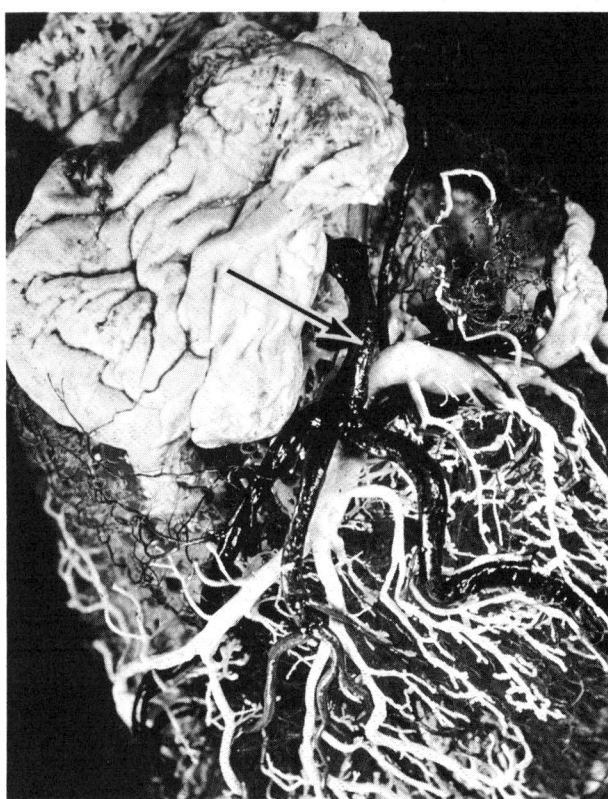

FIGURE 2-13 A Vinylite cast of the left coronary artery (arrow) appears dark in this photograph, which demonstrates the frequently complex division conventionally designated a "bifurcation." Here the left coronary artery divides into four almost equal trunks, the left anterior descending, two diagonal branches, and the left circumflex, indicated in order from the left. The left circumflex artery immediately twists beneath the great cardiac vein, which, together with all other veins and the right cardiac chambers, is cast white; the left atrium and ventricle are uncast. All the Vinylite casts illustrated in this chapter are from human hearts. (*From James.*[38] *Reproduced with permission of the publisher.*)

FIGURE 2-12 Photograph of dissected normal human heart viewed from above, demonstrating the origins of the left coronary artery (arrow with L) and right coronary artery (arrow with R) from the sinuses of Valsalva in the root of the aorta (Ao). The noncoronary sinus of the aorta bulges posteriorly into the anterior margin of the interatrial septum, dividing the left atrium and mitral valve (M) from the right atrium and tricuspid valve (T). The left coronary sinus bulges slightly between the body of the left atrium and the main pulmonary artery, which is cut flush with the right ventricle just anterior to the aorta. The right coronary sinus is not seen in this view, but with the two other sinuses occupying two-thirds of the circumference of the aortic root, its position is easy to infer. The upper half of the coronary sinus (CS) has been removed to demonstrate its course behind the left atrium; its entrance into the right atrium is marked by the inefficient semilunar Thebesian valve, which protrudes in an anterior direction. (*From James.*[38] *Reproduced with permission of the publisher.*)

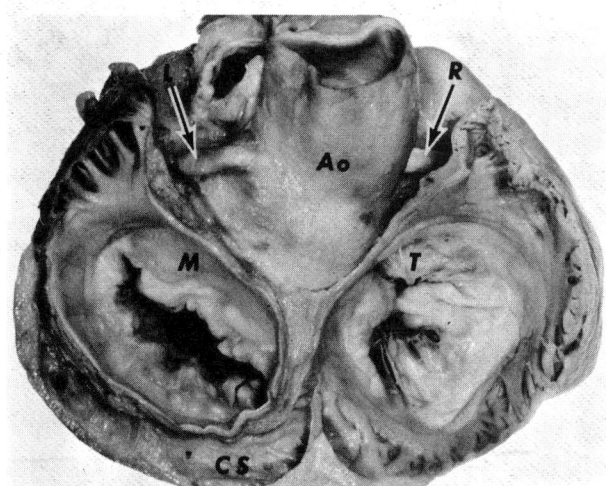

sulcus becomes the left circumflex artery. The intervening branches of the main left coronary artery distribute diagonally over the free wall of the left ventricle and are usually proportionately spaced between the anterior descending and circumflex arteries; these are commonly referred to as *diagonal* left ventricular branches, are one to three in number, and course between the anterior interventricular sulcus and the margo obtusus toward the apex of the heart.

Left Anterior Descending Artery

Viewed frontally, the left anterior descending artery appears to be a direct continuation of the main left coronary artery, the two together forming a reverse S curve,[38] the initial turn being around the base of the pulmonary artery into the anterior interventricular sulcus, and the second turn being around the apex cordis up into the posterior interventricular sulcus (Fig. 2-14). The anterior descending artery gives off major branches in two directions: those which course over the free wall of the left ventricle and those which penetrate and curve posteriorly

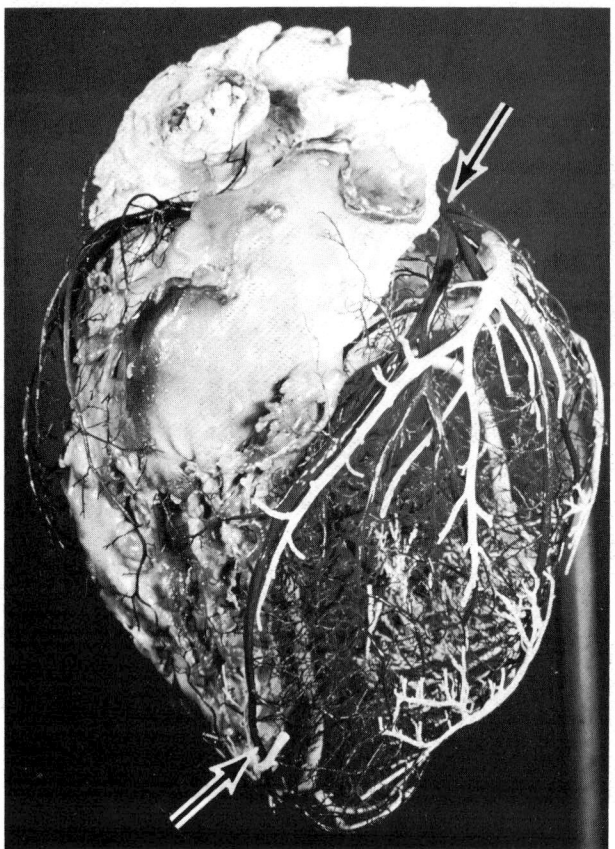

FIGURE 2-14 A Vinylite cast demonstrating the reverse S curve of the left anterior descending coronary artery, indicated by the two arrows: the upper arrow indicates the origin of the artery, and the lower indicates its course near the apex cordis. Again the right cardiac chambers and veins are cast white, while the left chambers are uncast. (*From James.[38] Reproduced with permission of the publisher.*)

into the ventricular septum. Lesser branches are distributed to the adjacent wall of the right ventricle, although in rare instances a single major vessel arises from the anterior descending artery to cross diagonally over the anterior wall of the right ventricle. At the level of the pulmonary valves a constant small artery curves about the pulmonary conus to meet a similar branch from the right side. Together these two form an important anatomic landmark first described by Vieussens.[39]

Branches of the left anterior descending artery arise at an acute angle from the parent trunk, whether distributing to the free wall of the left ventricle or to the ventricular septum. The septal branches of the anterior descending artery (numbering three to five in different hearts) fix it to the epicardium and limit its range of excursion during systolic filling. The branches to the free wall of the left ventricle (also usually three to five in number) course parallel to diagonal branches of the main left coronary artery. It is not generally appreciated that the anterior descending artery rarely terminates on the anterior surface of the apex, but nearly always curves around to the posterior interventricular sulcus and ascends for 2 to 5 cm, distributing branches

to the posterior surfaces of the apex of the left and right ventricles.[38] It is met at its termination by the distal branches of the posterior descending artery.

Left Circumflex Artery

In contrast to the left anterior descending branch, which characteristically arises as a direct continuation of the main left coronary artery, the left circumflex branch typically arises at a sharp angle of 90° or more and occasionally courses in an almost opposite direction from the main left coronary artery. The proximal portion of the left circumflex artery, as well as most of the area of the "bifurcation" of the main left coronary artery, is normally covered by the overlying left atrial appendage (Fig. 2-15). Because of the proximity of the atrial appendage, and because the left circumflex artery some-

FIGURE 2-15 A Vinylite cast demonstrating the close relation between the left atrial appendage, seen protruding down the center of the upper half of the picture, and the division of the main left coronary artery (left upper arrow) into left circumflex (right upper arrow) and left anterior descending (lower arrow) rami. Branches into the interventricular septum may be seen curving from the anterior descending artery to the viewer's left and then posteriorly. The arrow on the left circumflex artery indicates the termination of its course in the atrioventricular sulcus, just as it begins to turn down the margo obtusus. Note that most of the proximal course of the circumflex artery is covered by the atrial appendage. In this heart the left cardiac chambers were cast white and the right chambers and veins were uncast. (*From James.[38] Reproduced with permission of the publisher.*)

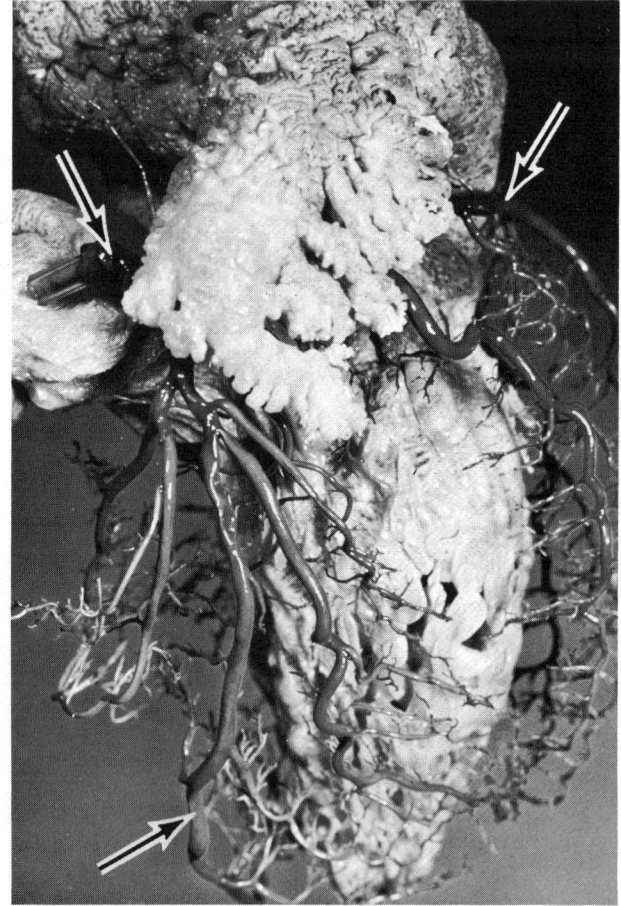

times courses within the myocardium at the base of the appendage, this artery is frequently injured during surgical procedures which ligate or amputate the left atrial appendage.

From its origin near the aorta and pulmonary artery, the left circumflex artery ascends into the left coronary sulcus and courses to the obtuse margin of the left ventricle. Just proximal to the margo obtusus it emerges from beneath the lateral margin of the atrial appendage and is then covered only by epicardial fat. At the margo obtusus it usually turns down the left ventricle toward the apex of the heart. It always provides stout branches to the posterior (diaphragmatic) surface of the left ventricle from its course along the margo obtusus, including one or more fairly large branches which continue in the atrioventricular sulcus toward the posterior interventricular sulcus, where they are met by terminal branches of the right coronary artery. In about 10 percent of human hearts the left circumflex artery itself continues in the posterior half of the left atrioventricular sulcus and crosses the crux of the heart, then turns down into the posterior interventricular sulcus to form one or more posterior descending arteries; in such hearts branches of the left coronary artery supply the entire left ventricle and interventricular system.

Branches of the left circumflex artery supply most of the left atrium and the lateral wall and part of the posterior wall of the left ventricle (Fig. 2-16). The two significant atrial branches are the one supplying the sinus node in about 45 percent of human hearts (discussed later) and the left atrial circumflex artery.[38] This latter vessel courses parallel to the main left circumflex artery, but above it, lying in the lower portion of the left atrium; it is often 1 or 2 mm in diameter and in some hearts is larger than the ventricular counterpart. Occasionally the left atrial circumflex artery, which usually terminates on the posterior wall of the left atrium, crosses back over the atrioventricular sulcus to supply the upper portion of the posterior left ventricle. The ventricular branches of the left circumflex artery arise at acute angles from the parent vessel in the same way as the branches of the anterior descending artery. These ventricular branches course toward the margo obtusus from the atrioventricular sulcus and are roughly parallel to the diagonal branches of the main left coronary artery and similar branches arising from the left anterior descending artery.

Right Coronary Artery

Whereas the left coronary artery nearly always arises from a single ostium in the aorta, in approximately half of human hearts there are two ostia in the right coronary sinus, which normally bulges from the aorta in a direction between the base of the pulmonary artery and the body of the right atrium. The smaller of these two ostia is rarely more than 1 or 2 mm from the larger, and is usually 1 mm or less in diameter. It gives rise to the conus

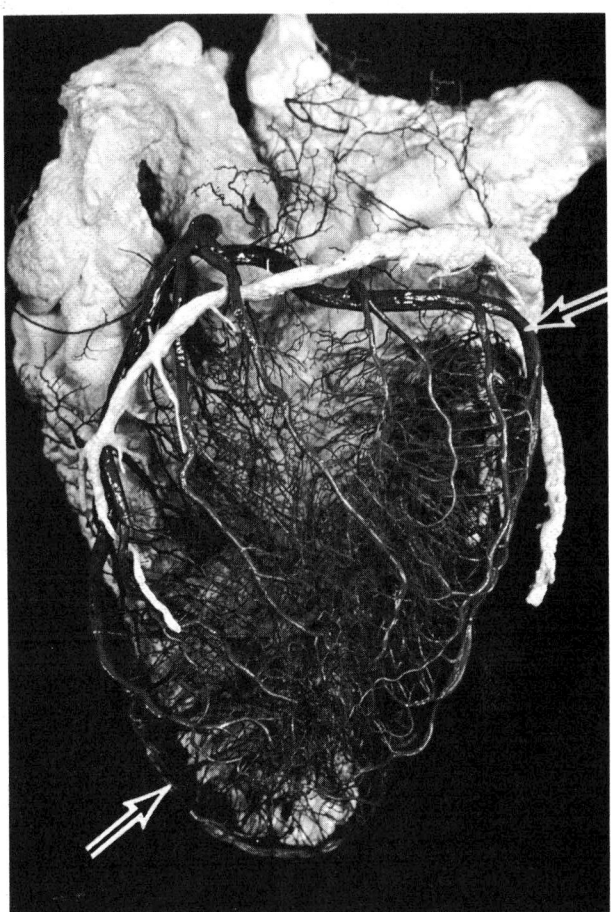

FIGURE 2-16   A Vinylite cast demonstrating the distribution of left ventricular branches from the left circumflex (right upper arrow) and left anterior descending (left lower arrow) arteries. The right cardiac chambers are cast white, but the left chambers and many of the veins are uncast. The root of the aorta, from which the main left coronary artery emerges, is also cast white and is joined with an artificial plastic bridge to the root of the pulmonary artery in the left upper corner of the photograph. (*From James.[38] Reproduced with permission of the publisher.*)

artery,[40] which forms the right half of Vieussens' ring at the level of the pulmonary valves. When the conus artery does not arise from the aorta directly, it is the first branch of the main right coronary artery. The potential importance of the conus artery as an alternate route of collateral arterial circulation is apparent from its strategic location.

The right coronary artery courses from the aorta into the right atrioventricular sulcus, lying more deeply in the fat of the sulcus than the left circumflex artery (Fig. 2-17). In 90 percent of human hearts it continues past the acute margin of the right ventricle into the posterior right atrioventricular sulcus to cross the crux of the heart and divide terminally in two directions; two or more branches descend in or near the posterior interventricular sulcus toward the apex of the heart, while another stout branch continues in the left atrioventricular sulcus about halfway to the margo obtusus, with its descending branches supplying nearly half of the diaphragmatic surface of the left ventricle (the other

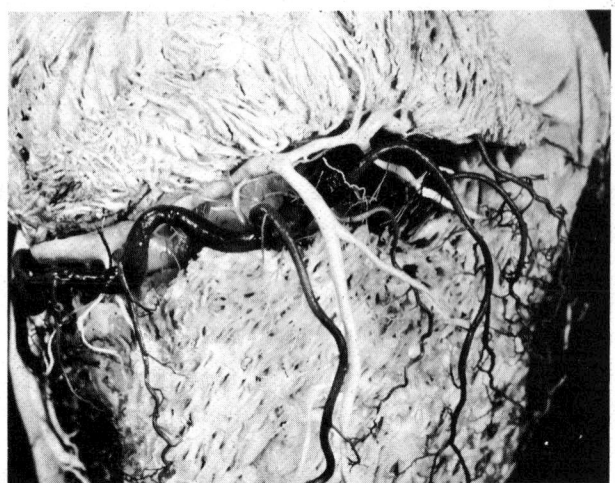

FIGURE 2-17   A Vinylite cast demonstrating the course of the right coronary artery (dark plastic) in the right atrioventricular sulcus, with the right atrium above and the right ventricle below. The pulmonary valves may be seen in the right upper corner of the picture. Anterior cardiac veins and a subintimal collecting vein are cast white and course near the artery. Note that the right coronary artery lies deep in fat of the atrioventricular sulcus, with the ventricular branches looping out to the epicardial surface. (*From James.[38] Reproduced with permission of the publisher.*)

half usually supplied by terminal branches of the left circumflex artery). Nearly all right ventricular branches of the right coronary artery arise perpendicular to the parent vessel, and those from the right atrioventricular sulcus to the anterior wall of the right ventricle have a looping exit as they emerge from their deep position in fat. The anterior right ventricular branches are three or four in number, the one coursing along the margo acutus being the dominant of these; all these branches are roughly parallel to the acute margin of the heart, coursing toward the apex and anterior interventricular sulcus. In about 55 percent of human hearts the right coronary artery provides the sinus node's arterial supply (see below), but other atrial branches are smaller and less constant.

It is the reciprocal lengths of the right coronary and left circumflex arteries in the posterior atrioventricular sulci—one being longer as the other is shorter—which led Bianchi[41] and Spalteholz[42] to classify coronary distribution in this region as right- or left-predominant. Thus, if the right coronary artery (Fig. 2-18) crossed the crux of the heart (as it does in 90 percent of human beings), it predominated. If the left circumflex artery crossed the crux

FIGURE 2-18   Drawing (*A*) and Vinylite cast (*B*) demonstrating the arterial supply to the posterior (diaphragmatic) surface of the human heart as it occurs in about 90 percent of instances. The left circumflex artery terminates at or near the margo obtusus, while branches of the right coronary artery cross the crux and supply the atrioventricular (AV) node (arrow). The crux is the arbitrary point at which the atrioventricular sulci cross the posterior margin of the interatrial and coronary sulci. Note the penetrating U turn of the artery crossing the crux of the heart, which here is the right coronary artery. Value of this U turn as an angiographic landmark is discussed in the text and further illustrated in Figs. 2-27 and 2-28. (*B, from James.[38] Reproduced with permission of the publisher.*)

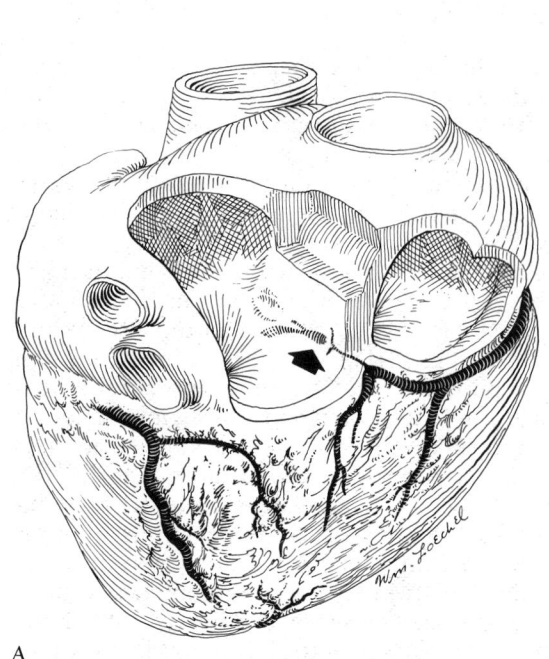

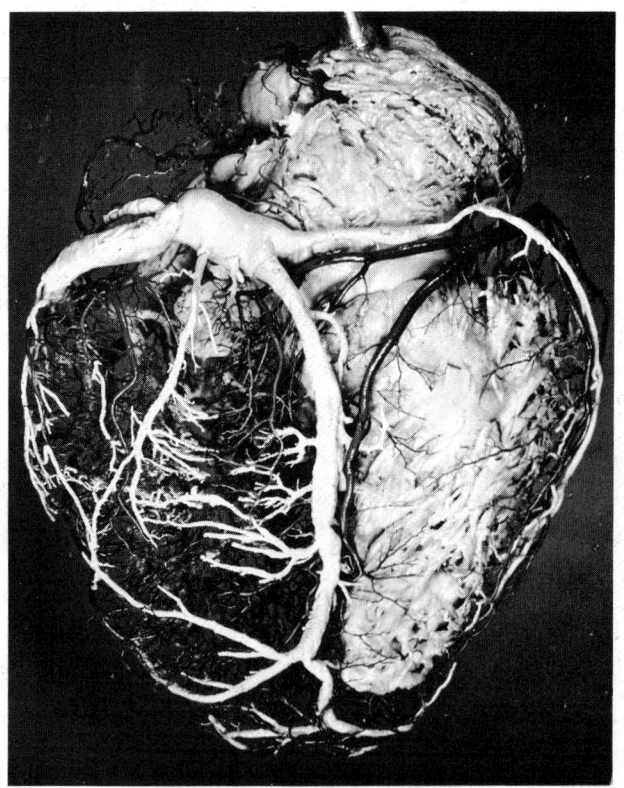

A   B

of the heart (Fig. 2-19), (as it does in 10 percent of instances), it predominated. They did not intend this classification to refer to arterial supply of the entire heart, which is the unfortunate way the classification is now commonly used. It is frequently

FIGURE 2-19 Drawing (*A*) and Vinylite cast (*B*) of the arterial supply to the posterior surface as seen in about 10 percent of human hearts. Again the artery crossing the crux makes a deep U turn and supplies the AV node (arrow). (*B, from James.*[38] *Reproduced with permission of the publisher.*)

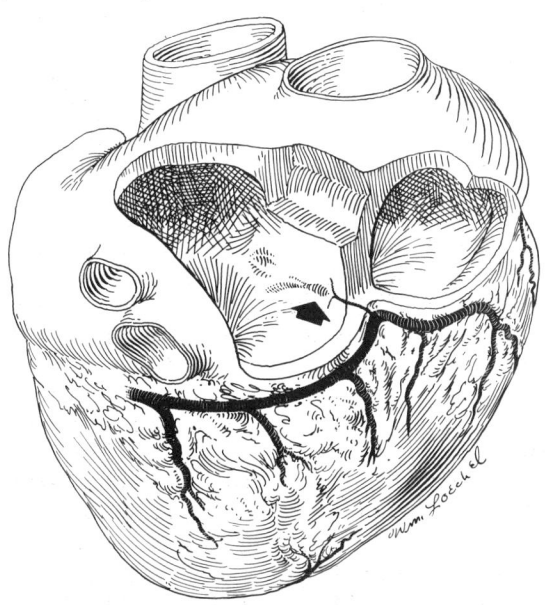

A

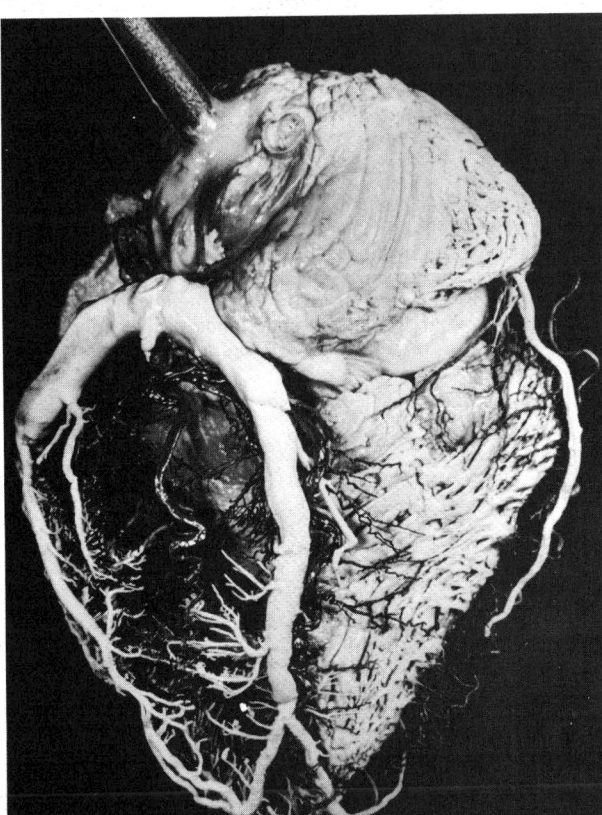

B

stated in describing angiograms, for example, that the heart may be classified as a right coronary–predominant heart, implying that the right coronary artery supplies most of the heart. Actually this is so rarely the case, considering the mass of ventricular and atrial myocardium normally supplied by the left coronary artery, that the misused terminology becomes grossly misleading. It would seem simpler and more accurate to say that the right or left coronary artery crosses the crux, as the case may be, or that the right coronary is the longer (as is usual in 90 percent of human beings), and to abandon the misleading terms *preponderant* or *predominant.*

Coronary Veins

There are three systems of veins in the human heart. The smallest of these consists of the *Thebesian veins,* which are not large and do not account for much volume of the venous drainage. They occur primarily in the right atrium and right ventricle but are occasionally demonstrable in the left side of the heart. In both sides of the heart they are more numerous near the septa than in the free walls. The intermediate system of veins is larger and more important, providing most of the venous drainage of the right ventricle. These are the *anterior cardiac veins* (Fig. 2-20), which form over the anterior wall of the right ventricle into two or three large trunks draining in the direction of the anterior right atrioventricular sulcus, which they cross either deep or superficial to the main right coronary artery to empty directly into the right atrium. In some hearts there is a collecting subintimal vein in the base of the right atrium, into which the anterior cardiac veins drain.

Venous drainage of the left ventricle is, under normal circumstances, primarily through the *coronary sinus and its tributaries,* which together form the

FIGURE 2-20 A white Vinylite cast of anterior cardiac veins. The corresponding course of the right coronary artery (dark plastic) closely follows the veins. Some veins pass beneath the artery and others over it to merge in a subintimal collecting vein, which then drains anteriorly to enter the right atrium directly beneath the atrial appendage, seen in the right upper corner of the photograph. (*From James.*[38] *Reproduced with permission of the publisher.*)

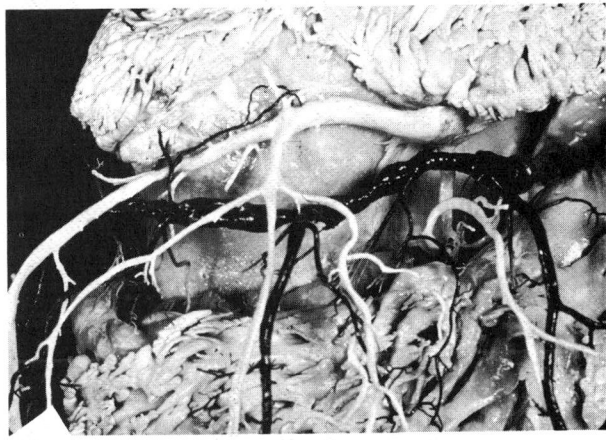

third and largest system of coronary veins (Fig. 2-21). Although there are equally large tributaries farther along its course, it is convenient to think of this system as originating with the anterior interventricular vein, which courses parallel to the left anterior descending artery in most of the anterior interventricular groove (blood flow in the two vessels being in opposite directions, however). Near the origin of the anterior descending artery, the anterior interventricular vein diverges toward the atrioventricular sulcus. At this point it becomes known as the *great cardiac vein,* receiving smaller tributary veins from the left ventricle. About midway in the course of this vein within the left atrioventricular sulcus it receives the curving entrance of a small but very important left atrial vein known as the *oblique vein of Marshall.*[43] Opposite the entrance of this vein a loose fold of endothelium commonly forms an incompe-

tent valve. This valve and the point of entrance of the oblique vein of Marshall together mark the anatomic division between the great cardiac vein and the coronary sinus (Fig. 2-22), which then extends to its point of entrance into the right atrium. Embryologically the oblique vein of Marshall represents the residual of the left superior cardinal vein and left superior vena cava, and the coronary sinus itself is the remains of the terminal portion of the left superior vena cava.

Near the junction of the great cardiac vein and coronary sinus, a large tributary vein, or more than one, enters from the lateral and posterior surfaces of the left ventricle. A large vein along the margo obtusus is the left marginal vein; a similar vein between this margin and the posterior interventricular sulcus is the left posterior ventricular vein. Frequently one or the other of these veins is absent or replaced by a number of smaller tributaries. The last major tributary of the coronary sinus is the posterior interventricular vein, which joins it just proximal to the right atrial ostium of the coronary sinus, and sometimes drains separately into the right atrium directly adjacent to the ostium of the coronary sinus. The entrance of the coronary sinus into the right atrium is guarded by an incompetent semilunar fold of endothelium known as the Thebesian valve. A number of venous lacunae or Thebesian veins drain this region of the interatrial septum directly into the right atrium, their ostia being near the coronary sinus ostium.

Anastomoses between the anterior cardiac veins and the tributaries of the coronary sinus are numerous and large, frequently measuring 1 or 2 mm in diameter in normal hearts (Fig. 2-23). There are similar anastomoses between each of the various large veins over the free walls of the right and left

FIGURE 2-21 A Vinylite cast of the veins of the left ventricle, which unite to form the great cardiac vein and coronary sinus. All the veins and the right cardiac chambers are cast white, with the left chambers uncast. The anterior interventricular vein courses parallel to the anterior descending artery along the left margin of the photograph. Near the middle of the cast the left marginal vein is seen ascending along the margo obtusus. At the right margin of the photograph the posterior vein of the left ventricle ascends to the coronary sinus. Only the apical portion of the posterior interventricular vein is well seen. Although much of the course of the venous branches is in relation to arteries, at some points there is considerable divergence, as in the region of margo obtusus. (*From James.*[38] *Reproduced with permission of the publisher.*)

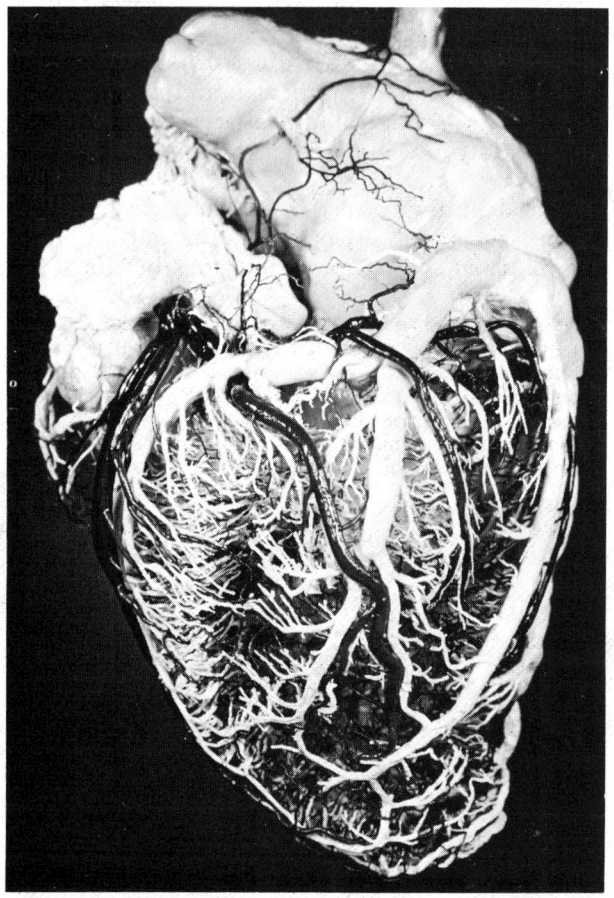

FIGURE 2-22 A Vinylite cast of the great cardiac vein (GCV) and coronary sinus (CS). The indentation at the juncture of these two structures is caused by the valve of Vieussens, and directly adjacent to this is the entrance of the oblique vein of Marshall (arrow), which descends along the posterior wall of the uncast left atrium. The embryologic and anatomic importance of this area is discussed in the text. (*From James.*[38] *Reproduced with permission of the publisher.*)

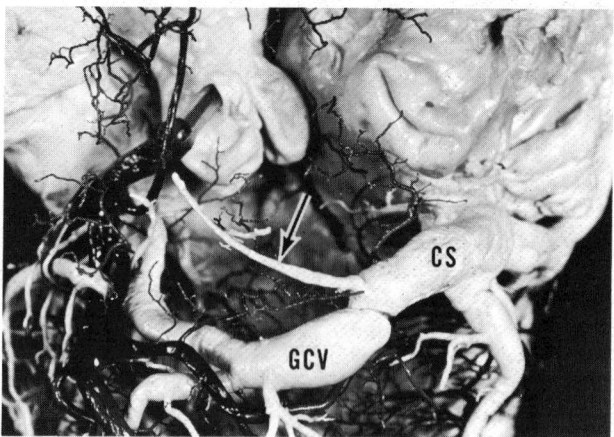

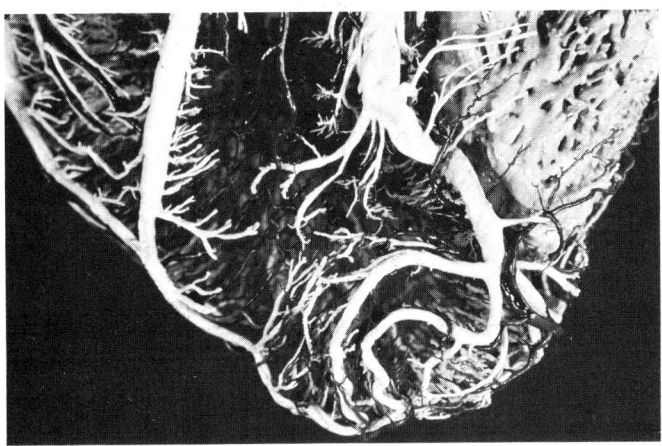

FIGURE 2-23 Venous anastomoses of the human heart are numerous and large, often being 1 or 2 mm in internal diameter, as in this photograph. The view is toward the posterior surface of the apex cordis, with white plastic filling the veins and right ventricle; the left ventricle is uncast. These normal venous anastomoses join the apical ends of the posterior interventricular and posterior left ventricular veins. (*From James.*[38] *Reproduced with permission of the publisher.*)

ventricles. Although venous flow from right ventricular myocardium is generally through the anterior cardiac veins, and that of the left ventricular myocardium generally through the coronary sinus, there is no anatomic reason why, with almost any increased resistance occurring in either of these two venous systems, the flow could not go in the opposite direction via the large anastomoses. For example, if flow in the coronary sinus were impeded by an intracardiac catheter, a variable but possible large volume of the left ventricular venous flow could shift into the anterior cardiac veins. Of further anatomic significance in physiologic studies is the fact that the tip of a catheter cannot be placed sufficiently deep into the coronary sinus in vivo to avoid right atrial mixing without being well past the entrance of the posterior interventricular vein as well as one or more of the major veins draining the posterior left ventricle.

Coronary Arterial Anastomoses

Much has been made of the size of anastomoses between the coronary arteries of the normal human heart, and too little attention has been paid to the fact that almost no one questions the existence of such anastomoses. The weight of present evidence indicates that arterial anastomoses in the normal human heart are commonly over 100 μm in diameter, and that some are several hundred microns. This has been demonstrated by injection of radiographic dyes,[44–48] perfusion of small calibrated spheres,[49] and the classic injection and corrosion technique.[38,50] In view of this demonstration by a number of different investigators employing a variety of techniques, it seems likely that the often-quoted criterion of 40 μm being the upper limit of size of normal coronary arterial anastomoses[51] is too conservative.

Arterial anastomoses occur throughout the human heart, but they are particularly numerous within the ventricular and atrial septa, at the apex of the heart, at the crux of the heart, over the anterior surface of the right ventricle, and between the

sinus node artery and other atrial arteries. The anastomoses in right ventricular epicardium become particularly important and large following an occlusion of either the left anterior descending or right coronary artery (Fig. 2-24). Although there are anastomoses in the region of the endocardium of both ventricles, they are not as numerous or large as those in the epicardium. Epicardial anastomoses on the left ventricle connect all three major coronary trunks. These epicardial anastomoses over the surfaces of both ventricles appear from an anatomic standpoint to be among the most important routes for collateral circulation, and it is therefore incongruous that a number of surgical procedures devised for "revascularizing" the heart make a particular point of producing extensive epicardial fibrosis by abrasion, talc powder, or phenol, which must of necessity obliterate a large number of the major normal routes of anastomosis.

Demonstration of the presence of anastomoses does not of course establish their functional importance. However, the excellent functional recovery of most patients who suffer coronary occlusion indicates that the collateral arterial circulation is capable of functioning efficiently in most patients. Since all human hearts possess an abundant number of coronary arterial anastomoses (of various sizes), the critical question is why some patients who develop coronary occlusion fail to utilize the anastomoses efficiently for collateral circulation.[52] A number of quickly apparent factors contribute to such failure, including the speed of development of the occlusion, its location more distally or more proximally in the artery, and the presence or absence of occlusions in neighboring arteries; but there are probably still other factors which are presently less clearly defined. Among these may be the maintenance of adequate arterial pressure to ensure a sufficient gradient across the anastomosis to permit flow from an unoccluded artery into the distal segment of the occluded artery.

There is one anatomic characteristic of coronary arterial anastomoses which may be a crude indication of whether the anastomosis functioned during

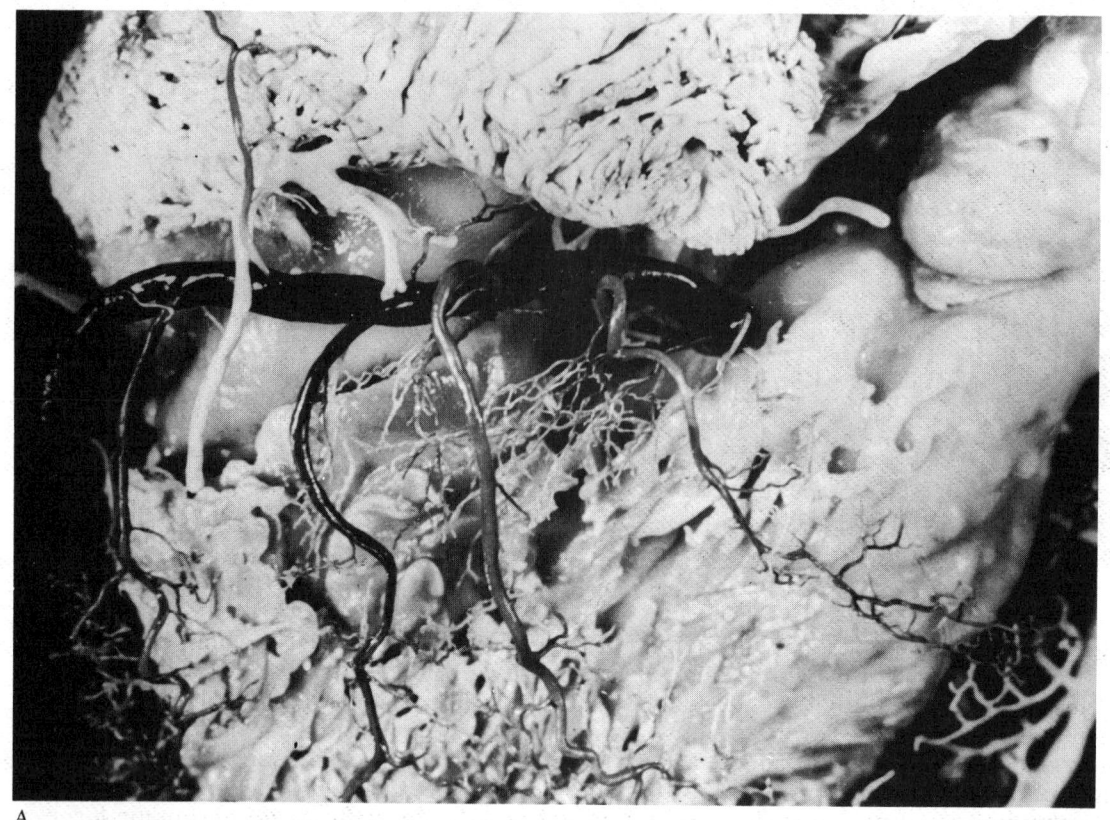

A

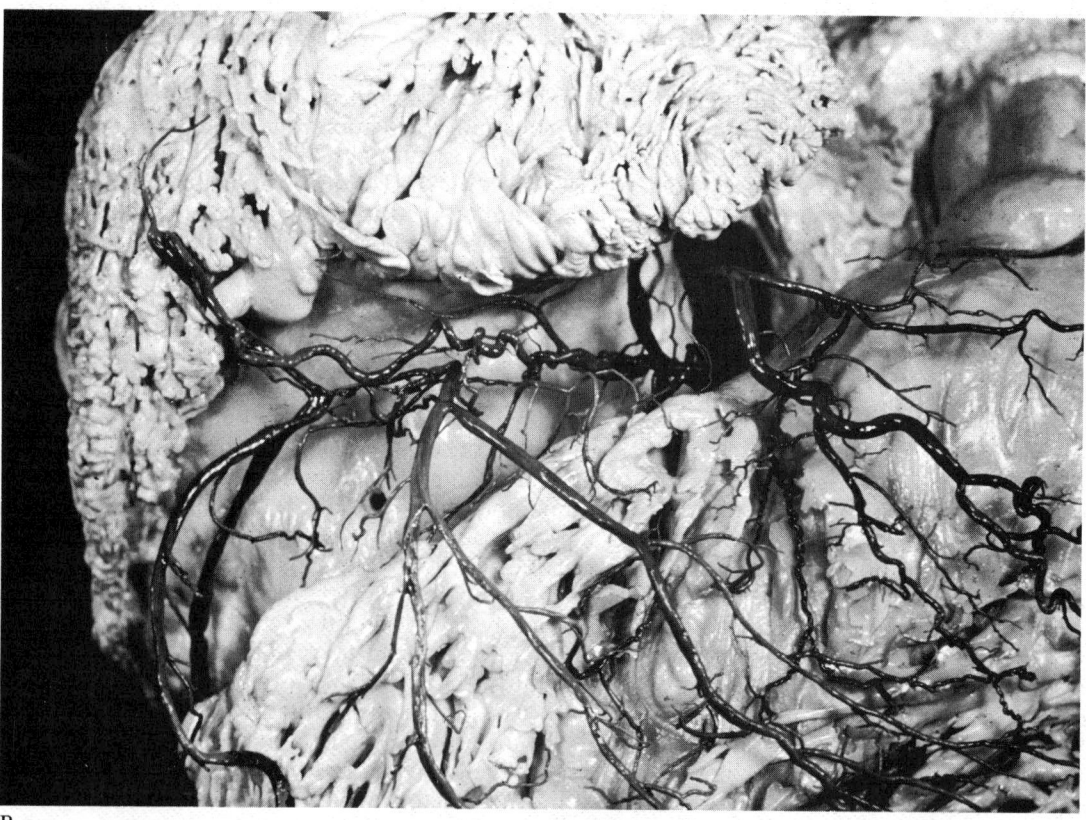

B

FIGURE 2-24 Vinylite casts comparing the same region of right coronary artery in a normal heart (*A*) and an atherosclerotic one (*B*). Note the smooth configuration of the dark plastic in the normal right coronary artery and the gradual termination of its branches in relatively straight or gently curving descent over the surface of the right ventricle. By contrast, the branches of the occluded right coronary artery are thicker distally and become extremely twisted into corkscrew shapes. A complete occlusion of the main trunk of the right coronary artery is bridged by intracoronary anastomoses, while the branches over the right ventricle course toward the anterior interventricular sulcus, where they anastomose with the left anterior descending artery (not shown). (*From James.*[38] *Reproduced with permission of the publisher.*)

life to carry collateral circulation, and this is the structure of the anastomotic artery. Coronary anastomoses in normal human hearts are generally straight or gently curving, regardless of their diameter; those in hearts with coronary occlusion (Fig. 2-24B) are extensively twisted and corkscrew in shape.[38,50] It seems likely that the normal anastomoses (not regularly participating in coronary flow) are not under much stress, while those connecting a low-pressure occluded artery with a high-pressure unoccluded artery do participate in flow, the stress of higher pressure and pulsation causing them to become elongated, enlarged, and tortuous. If this consideration is correct, then the gross morphologic characteristics of coronary anastomoses may be a reasonable indication of whether they were functioning for collateral flow in vivo.

Blood Supply of Special Areas of the Heart

Most special areas of the heart have either a dual arterial supply or a single primary supply with important secondary sources. Presenting the anatomy of the usual course of each branch of the coronary arteries in sequence still leaves the reader with a task of synthesizing in his or her mind how these branches distribute in a specific single area. To simplify such a synthesis, this section will deal with special areas of the heart and describe their usual blood supply. As a corollary, the effect of coronary occlusion at various locations will be discussed relative to the effect on each special area.

Ventricular Septum[53]

Contrary to frequent descriptions of the blood supply of the ventricular septum as being almost equally supplied by the anterior and posterior descending arteries, in human beings this supply is predominantly by branches from the anterior descending artery (Fig. 2-25). These large septal arteries in most of their course lie very close to the right ventricular myocardium, their terminal ramifications penetrating the septum itself. Only a small portion of the posterior margin of the muscular septum is supplied by the posterior descending artery. In the event of occlusion of the anterior descending

FIGURE 2-25 Drawing (A) and Vinylite cast (B) demonstrating the normal blood supply of the human interventricular septum. The lighter branches of the left anterior descending artery in the cast correspond to those labeled as such in the drawing, as do the dark but much shorter branches of the posterior descending branch of the right coronary artery. The U turn of the right coronary artery is obscured in the cast by the posterior interventricular vein, identified by its wrinkled surface. Right ventricular branches of the right coronary artery have been cut away in the cast to reveal the septal arteries, which are seen to be predominantly branches of the left anterior descending ramus. White plastic fills the left atrium and left ventricle; the right chambers are uncast. (A, from James and Burch.[53] B, from James.[38] Both reproduced with permission of the publishers.)

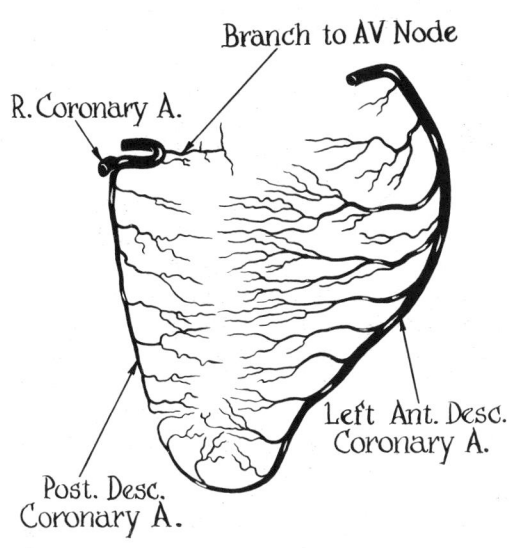

A

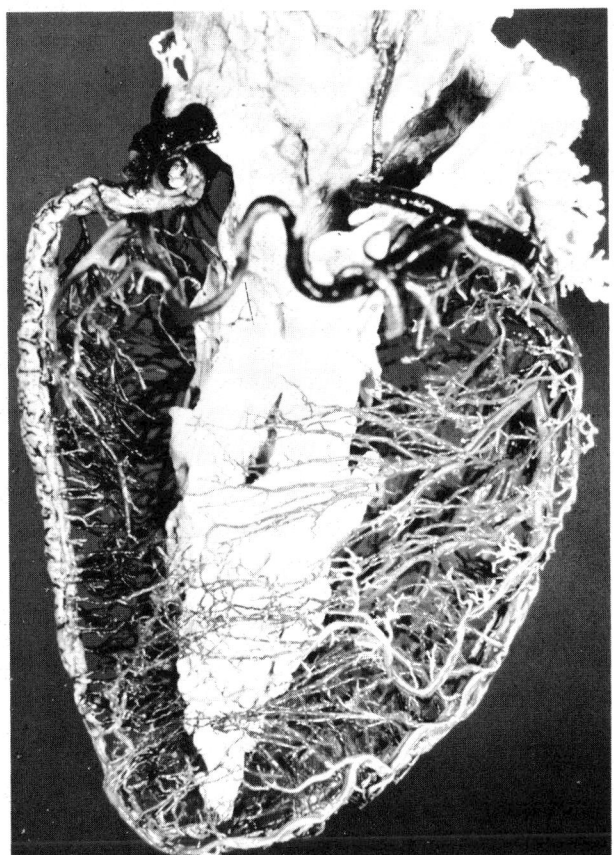

B

artery, however, the posterior artery becomes the principal route of collateral circulation. It follows logically, therefore, that most instances of perforation of the ventricular septum due to myocardial infarction occur in patients in whom both these arteries are occluded, although one occlusion may be an old one and may or may not have been associated with a previous clinically recognizable episode. When the posterior descending artery is a terminal branch of the left circumflex artery, as it is in 10 percent of human hearts, the entire septum is supplied by branches of the left coronary tree.

Crista Supraventricularis

The crista supraventricularis abuts into the ventricular septum directly under the proximal portion of the right coronary artery, and is nourished by penetrating branches from it. These are usually small branches and naturally not visible on the surface of the heart nor in ordinary dissection, as at a necropsy table. Occasionally a large branch of the right coronary artery descends directly into the crista supraventricularis and courses through it into the ventricular septum, where it may terminate by supplying a small local area of septal myocardium. In three hearts studied by the authors, this branch was sufficiently large to continue through the ventricular septum anteriorly and emerge to the cardiac surface in the anterior interventricular sulcus, where it descended and distributed branches to neighboring right and left ventricular myocardium. In one of these three hearts there was no conventional left anterior descending artery, so that the branch through the crista supraventricularis supplied a major portion of the left ventricle as well as the interventricular septum. In addition to this being an interesting anomalous distribution, there is a point of functional significance in that the patient died with progressively increasing myocardial insufficiency and ischemia. Anomalous coronary branches distributing to the left ventricle from the right coronary artery commonly follow one of three routes: in epicardium curving behind the aorta, in epicardium coursing across the pulmonary conus, or deep in myocardium via the crista supraventricularis. Since the course of most large coronary arteries is normally epicardial, this intramyocardial course by the third route may be singularly inefficient because of the compression of a large coronary trunk during ventricular systole, preventing its normal filling at a time when most coronary trunks are filled. Thus, although some variant courses for major coronary arteries may be of primarily academic interest, a course deep through the crista supraventricularis may be a slowly lethal anomaly.

Papillary Muscles of the Left Ventricle

The anterior papillary muscle is virtually always supplied by branches of the left coronary artery, while the posterior papillary muscle is usually supplied by branches of both the right and left coronary arteries. One of the diagonal branches of the main left coronary artery commonly descends over the anterior papillary muscle, but there are always major additional branches to this area from both the anterior descending artery and the marginal termination of the left circumflex artery. When the right coronary artery supplies half or more of the diaphragmatic surface of the left ventricle, as it usually does, its terminal branches end directly over the posterior papillary muscle; but again there are additional branches coursing to that area from the marginal termination of the left circumflex artery and occasionally from the posterior apical termination of the left anterior descending artery. Because both papillary muscles receive regularly multiple sources of blood supply, occlusion of a single major coronary artery rarely deprives them of all their circulation. Ruptured papillary muscles are usually due to occlusion of more than one major artery.

Interruption of the blood supply of the papillary muscles of the left ventricle may lead to papillary muscle dysfunction or rupture.

Sinus Node

In human beings the artery supplying the sinus node originates from the proximal few centimeters of the right coronary artery in about 55 percent of instances and from the proximal few millimeters of the left circumflex artery in about 45 percent (Fig. 2-26). Collateral circulation to the sinus node is provided by neighboring atrial arteries, but the primary supply is virtually always a single unilaterally derived artery.[38,54] Despite its proximity to the main left coronary artery and anterior descending ramus, the left sinus node artery virtually never arises from any but the left circumflex ramus. From either right or left origin the sinus node artery courses in the adjacent atrial epicardium to the base of the superior vena cava, which it encircles as it penetrates the center of the sinus node. In addition to being the primary supply of the sinus node, this artery is also the largest atrial artery and distributes to a major portion of the atrial myocardium and interatrial septum. It regularly provides almost the entire supply of the thickest portion of atrial myocardium, the crista terminalis. All but the smallest atrial infarctions are associated with occlusion of flow into the sinus node artery. Such occlusions also cause infarction of the sinus node and lead to atrial arrhythmias.[55] An occlusion of this type is rarely in the sinus node itself, however; it is usually in the main coronary artery proximal to the origin of the sinus node branch. Since most posterior myocardial infarctions are due to right coronary occlusion, the concurrent onset of an atrial arrhythmia indicates that the occlusion must be in the proximal few centimeters of the right coronary artery in order to block flow into the sinus node branch. Similarly, lateral myocardial infarctions due to left circumflex artery occlusion and associated with the onset of atrial arrhythmias carry a grave prognosis,[56] for the occlusion must be

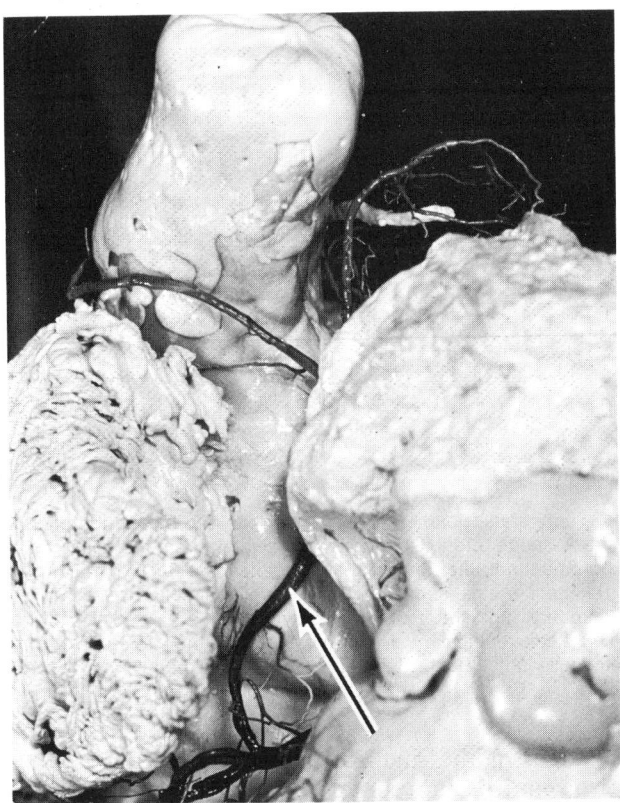 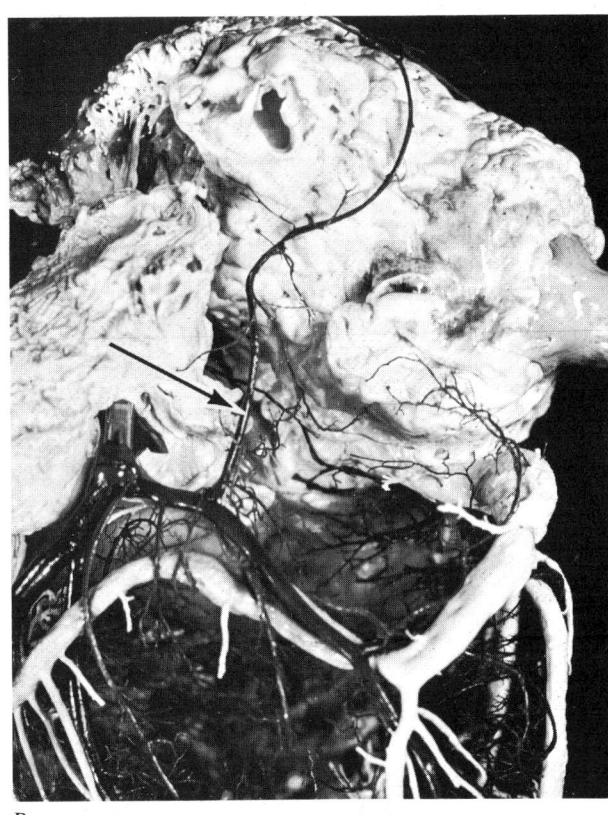

A   B

FIGURE 2-26 Two Vinylite casts showing the usual course of the sinus node artery when it originates from the right (*A*) and left (*B*). *A*. The sinus node artery (arrow) arising from the proximal portion of the right coronary artery, as it does in 55 percent of human hearts, and coursing between the right atrial appendage and root of the aorta along the medial surface of the body of the right atrium to the base of the superior vena cava, which protrudes upward in the left upper corner of the picture. As the right sinus node artery curves about the vena cava, it enters the sulcus terminalis and penetrates the sinus node. An additional large branch is seen coursing into the dorsal wall of the uncast left atrium. *B*. The sinus node artery (arrow) arising from the proximal left circumflex artery and crossing beneath the uncast left atrial appendage to the base of the superior vena cava, which protrudes toward the viewer. Here it circles counterclockwise to enter the sulcus terminalis and penetrate the sinus node. (*From James.*[38] *Reproduced with permission of the publisher.*)

in the first few millimeters of the left circumflex artery, and any proximal propagation of the occlusion would block the main left coronary artery.

The AV Node

The artery supplying the atrioventricular (AV) node arises from the apex of the penetrating U turn made by the artery (either right or left coronary) crossing the crux of the heart (Fig. 2-27). This deep turn is a useful angiographic landmark,[57] being easily visualized on good-quality coronary angiograms (Fig. 2-28), and marks the posterior junction of the interatrial and interventricular septa. The U turn additionally lies just below the ostium of the coronary sinus, and its apex is only a few millimeters from the AV node. A line drawn from the apex of this turn to the noncoronary sinus of the aorta separates the right from the left atrioventricular orifices and the interatrial septum above from the interventricular septum below. The U turn and AV node artery are provided by the right coronary artery in 90 percent of human beings and by the left circumflex artery in 10 percent. The coronary anatomy of the dog, which space does not permit us to discuss, is

quite different in this region.[38] Some collateral circulation to the AV node is provided by Kugel's artery (arteria anastomotica auricularis magna),[58] which arises from the proximal right or left coronary artery and courses posteriorly through the base of the interatrial septum. Coronary occlusions which produce posterior myocardial infarction necessarily deprive the AV node of its primary blood supply. Fainting and syncope during angina or during an acute infarct are characteristic clinical features of acute posterior infarcts,[59,60] because of transient ischemia of the AV node.

The AV Bundle and Bundle Branches

Terminal branches of the AV node artery (in 90 percent of human beings a branch of the right coronary artery) supply the AV bundle and the proximal few millimeters to the right and left bundle branches, as well as neighboring septal myocardium.[53] These arterial branches coursing inward from the posterior surface of the heart are met by the terminal branches of Kugel's artery, which enters from the anterior portion of the heart. Distal to the inferior margin of the membranous portion of

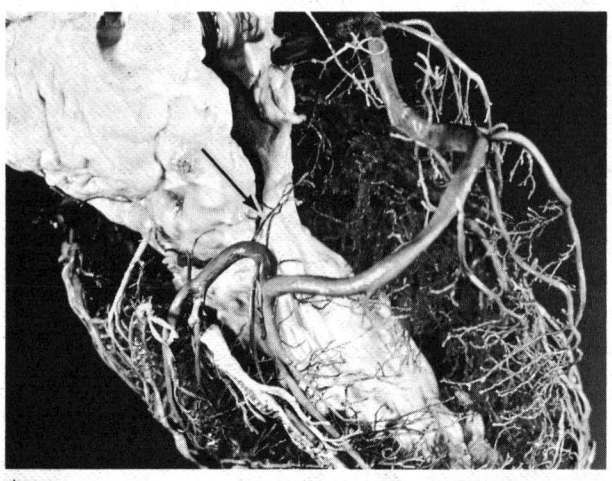
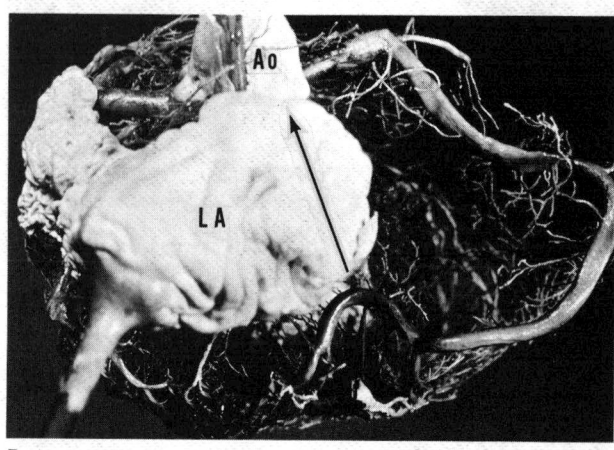

A   B

FIGURE 2-27 Two views of the U turn of the right coronary artery at the crux of the heart. *A.* View from above and behind the uncast right atrium, showing the sweep of the right coronary artery as well as the AV node artery itself (arrow), originating from the apex of the U turn. *B.* The same cast viewed from directly above, with the uncast right atrium to the right and the left atrial cast (LA) to the left. Ao = root of the aorta. The long arrow lies directly over the normal position of the interatrial septum. The left atrial cast bulges over this line because the right atrium is uncast. The usefulness to the interpreter of coronary angiograms of a line drawn from the apex of the U turn to the noncoronary sinus of the aorta is apparent. Such a line divides the right atrioventricular valve from the left, and the interatrial septum above from the interventricular septum below, thus forming almost a central axis for the heart. See Fig. 2-28. (*From James.*[38] *Reproduced with permission of the publisher.*)

the ventricular septum, the bundle branches on both sides are supplied by the septal arteries arising from the left anterior descending artery. Since the right bundle branch is a single small bundle of fibers, while the left branches occur in a large sheet of fibers, vascular and other lesions producing focal damage can more readily lead to right bundle branch block than to left bundle branch block. Conversely, the presence of left bundle branch block indicates damage to a large associated area of myocardium.

The Small Coronary Arteries

Although not generally supplying a single special area (the sinus node and AV node are exceptions), the small coronary arteries (0.1 to 1.0 mm in diameter) (Fig. 2-29) have been so frequently neglected in studies of the heart that they deserve special mention. Occlusion of one or a few of the small ventricular arteries, particularly if gradual, is usually of little clinical significance. However, there are circumstances in which occlusion of small coronary arteries is very important.[61-63] An obvious example is that in which the supply to critical centers in the conduction system is interrupted. When the process is widespread and many small arteries in the ventricular myocardium are occluded, the effect is extended to mechanical as well as electrical function of the heart.

Many different diseases affect the small coronary arteries, but they may conveniently be considered in three general categories: *embolic, inflammatory,* and *noninflammatory* (see Table 2-1). The first two groups are etiologically self-explanatory (Fig. 2-30). Among the possible causes for noninflammatory pathologic

changes of the small coronary arteries (Fig. 2-31), two require some comment:

1. In the hearts of patients with abnormal large coronary arteries conventionally classified as "atherosclerotic," the small coronary arteries are often additionally diseased.[64-66] Whether the original disturbance was the same for both large and small vessels is unknown. On the other hand, though the contrary is frequently assumed today, the exact cause and pathogenesis of atherosclerosis are also unknown, and the end result (narrowed large coronary arteries) may have begun as any of a large number of widely different abnormal changes.

2. Hereditary medial necrosis (Figs. 2-32 and 2-33) is a process most often associated with heritable neuromuscular and musculoskeletal diseases in which cardiac pathologic change is frequently present. Some of these diseases are listed in Table 2-2. Clinical features of such cardiac disease include progressive cardiac enlargement with eventual insufficiency and failure, a high percentage of arrhythmias and conduction disturbances, syncopal attacks, and often sudden death. All these features may be explained by widespread gradually progressive occlusion of many small coronary arteries, and such histopathologic change is demonstrable. The basic lesion appears to be a noninflammatory necrosis of the tunica media, and the wide variety of reparative processes secondary to this lesion includes endothelial proliferation and/or fibromuscular hyperplasia of the remaining tunica media; the end result is narrowing of the arterial lumen and fi-

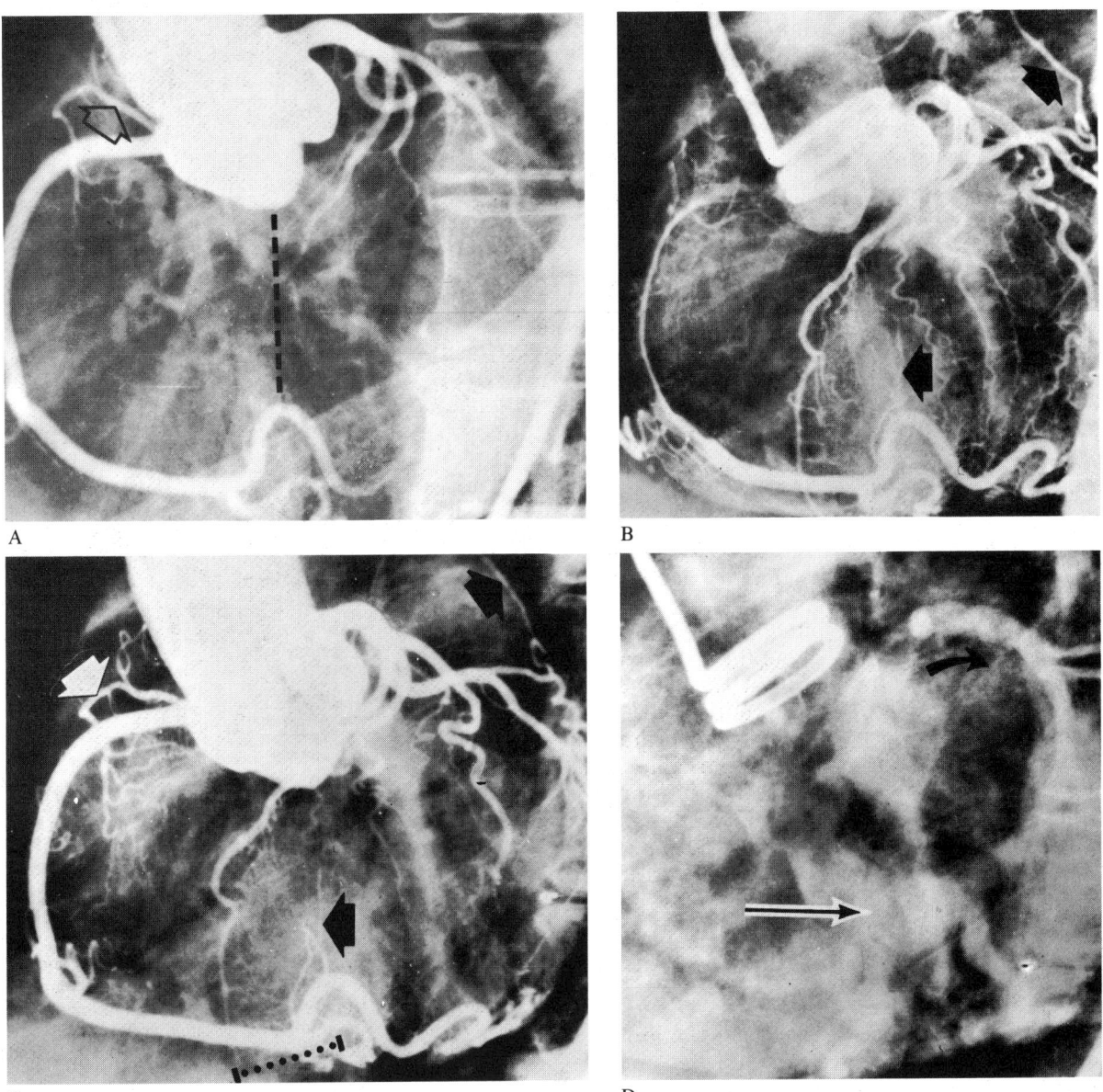

A

B

C

D

FIGURE 2-28 Coronary angiograms made with injection into the aortic root and rapid serial exposures in the LAO projection. *A.* Immediate filling of the entire right coronary artery (on the left in this photograph), with excellent demonstration of the U turn (see also Fig. 2-27); the arrow indicates the conus artery. The anatomic usefulness of the U turn is demonstrated with the dashed line drawn from the apex of the turn to the noncoronary sinus of the aorta; the tricuspid valve orifice is on one side of the line and the mitral on the other; the atrial septum is above it and the ventricular septum below; the AV node is just above the U turn, and the coronary sinus ostium is directly over it in this view. *B.* A second usefulness of the U turn, illustrated with the dotted line, which extends from the U turn to the apex of the heart, identified by the terminal portion of the left anterior descending artery. This line, corresponding to the posterior interventricular sulcus, effectively divides the right and left ventricular diaphragmatic surfaces. In *B* the AV node artery (lower dark arrow), originating from the U turn, is well visualized; the upper black arrow indicates beginning filling of the sinus node artery, here originating exceptionally far out in the left circumflex branch; the white arrow again indicates the conus branch. *C.* The AV node artery is still visible, and the sinus node artery is filled nearly all the way to the sinus node. *D.* A phase of venous filling, with the anterior interventricular vein seen end-on as a white circle, and the great cardiac vein continuing (curved arrow) from it into the atrioventricular sulcus and then on to the region of the ostium of the coronary sinus (straight arrow); on comparison with *A* to *C* one can visualize the relation of the U turn to the ostium of the coronary sinus. The usefulness of the line drawn in *B* was suggested by Dr. Sven Paulin, of the Harvard Medical School. (*Courtesy of Dr. Paulin.*)

nally occlusion. Of the noncardiac clinical features associated with hereditary medial necrosis of small coronary arteries, one of the more consistent is deformity of the chest and thoracic spine, such as kyphoscoliosis and pectus excavatum or pectus carinatum. Although the reason for this association is not presently known, the evidence suggests that the relatively obscure cardiac disease seen in many patients with such skeletal deformities is more likely due to an intrinsic disorder within the heart than to cardiac overwork because of intrathoracic distortion.

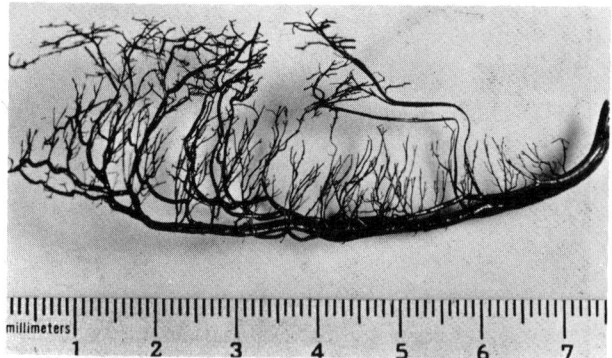

FIGURE 2-29 Vinylite cast of human coronary arteries; a segment cut from the free wall of the left ventricle and illustrating "small" branches discussed in the text. (*From James.*[38] *Reproduced with permission of the publisher.*)

The Conduction System of the Heart

Throughout recorded history, humans have been fascinated by the spontaneous beating of the heart, and many ancient rites of worship included its sacrificial excision during life. Despite this long history of curiosity, factual knowledge about the structures actually responsible for the heartbeat is relatively recent. The classic studies of His the younger,[67] Tawara,[68] and Keith and Flack[69] were only performed near the start of this century. It is remarkable in studying their papers to see how clearly the sinus node, the atrioventricular (AV) node, and the AV bundle and its branches were described. Their descriptions make all the more puzzling the current aura of mystery which seems to pervade most discussions of the conduction system of the heart.

The Sinus Node

Since the pacemaker of the heart is near the junction of both the superior vena cava and the sinus

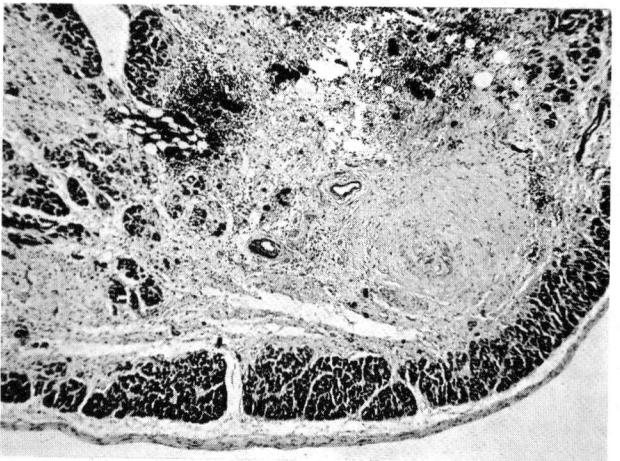

A

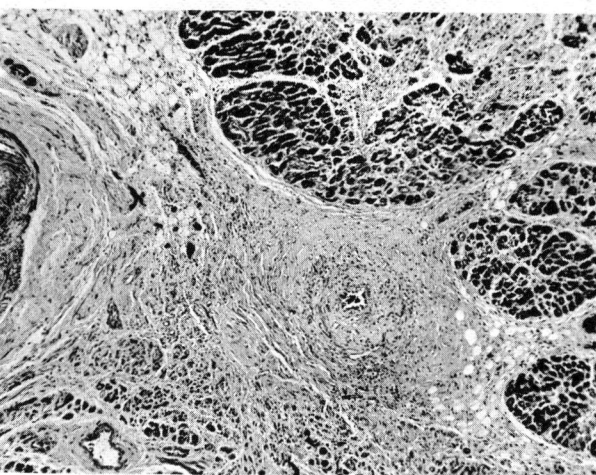

B

FIGURE 2-30 Photomicrographs illustrating typical pathologic change of the human myocardium and small coronary branches in polyarteritis nodosa. *A.* Old and recent focal myocardial damage and a sclerosed small artery, shown from the crista terminalis. *B.* More active arteritis at the margin of the sinus node. Unless otherwise indicated, all photomicrographs are from sections prepared with Goldner's trichrome stain.

TABLE 2-1 Pathology of Small Coronary Arteries*

Embolic:
  Bacterial
  Atheromatous
  Intracardiac surgical debris
  Platelets
Inflammatory:
  Polyarteritis nodosa
  Lupus erythematosus
  Rheumatoid arthritis
  Rheumatic fever
Noninflammatory:
  Thrombotic thrombocytopenia
  Amyloidosis
  Atherosclerosis (sic)
  Diabetes mellitus
  Hereditary medial necrosis
  Focal fibromuscular dysplasia

*This is not intended as an exhaustive list; it provides characteristic examples of each category.

intercavarum with both the atrium and the auricle, neither *sinoatrial* nor *sinoauricular* is a completely accurate term. It seems more suitable, as initially proposed by Walmsley,[70] to refer to this structure by the less restrictive term *sinus node,* a name which has the additional attractive advantage of brevity.

It has been suggested by Patten[71] that embryologically the sinus node and the AV node are analogous structures, arising at the junctions of the right and left superior cardinal veins, respectively, with the sinus venosus. Then as the sinus venosus ultimately becomes the medial half of the right atrium and part of the interatrial septum, the AV node migrates to the internal position it occupies in the heart of the human adult. The sinus node on the other hand remains, even in the adult heart, more nearly in its primitive position. Whether Patten's explanation is ultimately accepted as correct or not, it is a useful concept. In lower animals the entire region of the sinus venosus has been demonstrated to

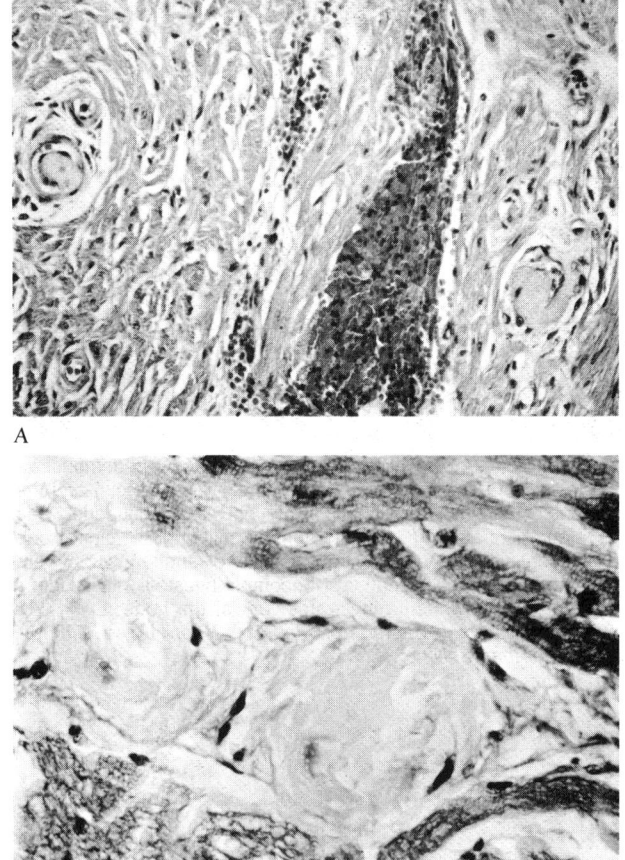

A

B

FIGURE 2-31 Noninflammatory pathologic change of small coronary arteries in photomicrographs from the AV node in thrombotic thrombocytopenic purpura in *A*, and from the right ventricular myocardium in amyloidosis in *B*. Although the occluding amorphous mass in the small arteries appears identical in both diseases here, the considerable difference is simple to demonstrate with appropriate stains.

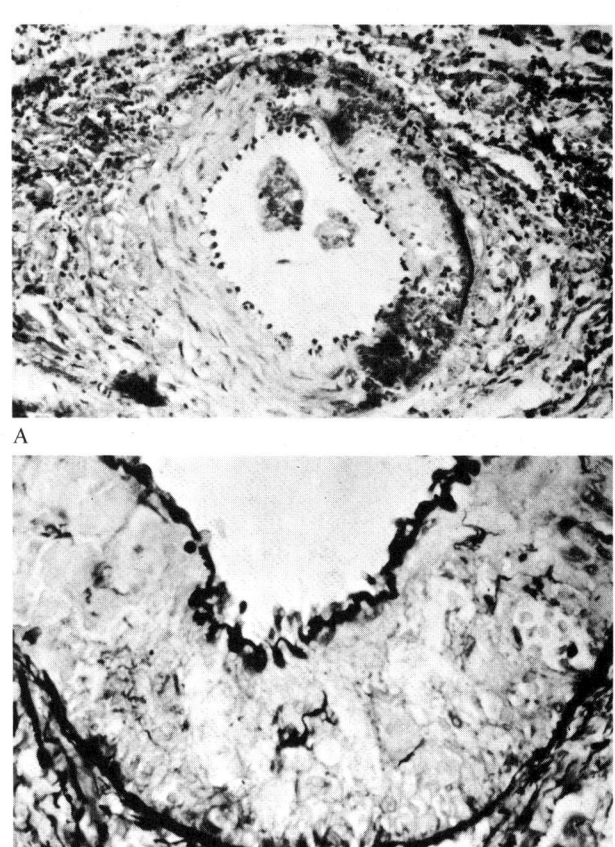

A

B

FIGURE 2-32 *A* and *B*. Typical histopathologic change of the tunica media in hereditary medial necrosis of small coronary arteries in photomicrographs from a patient dying with "primary" pulmonary hypertension. These sections are of the sinus node artery. Elastic stain. Note that the granular amorphous degeneration is confined to the media.

have special electrophysiologic properties,[72] and one may think of the two nodes as representing the opposite poles of this special region of the heart.

Grossly the sinus node lies near the junction of the superior vena cava and the right atrium (Fig. 2-34), with its anterior margin very near the crest formed by the junction of the anterior margin of the atrial appendage with the superior vena cava.[73,74] The sinus node is about 10 to 20 mm long, lying just beneath the sulcus terminalis. Its posterior portion is at the junction of the atrium with the sinus intercavarum instead of the superior vena cava. The shape of the node is roughly a flattened ellipse, and it does not have a head or tail, as is commonly alleged. Being located a millimeter or less beneath the epicardium (Fig. 2-35), it is heir to all the diseases which afflict the surface, most notably pericarditis.[75] The opposite surface of the node is slightly further from the endocardium, but the inferior margin of the node joins the free wall of the right atrium directly over the recess between the crista terminalis and the lateral wall of the atrium, an area known as

the *atrium atrii dextri*.[76] On cross section the sinus node has an approximately triangular shape with the apex pointing toward the superior vena cava and sinus intercavarum, while the base is astride the atrium atrii dextri, with angular extensions into both the free wall of the right atrium and the crista terminalis. Disease of the sinus node is commonly associated with extensive thrombus formation in the atrium atrii dextri.[76]

Internally the most intriguing feature of the sinus node is its constant relation to a disproportionately large, centrally located artery (Fig. 2-36). While some small lateral branches of this artery function to nourish the node, the large artery itself passes directly through the center of the node as if en route elsewhere. This close anatomic relation prompted Soderstrom to describe the sinus node as resembling an enormous adventitia of its artery.[76] Since the sinus node artery is regularly one of the first branches of the main coronary arteries, which are in turn the first branches of the aorta, the sinus node is in an admirable position to monitor central aortic pressure and pulsation. The possibility of a functional relation between pulsation and caliber of the

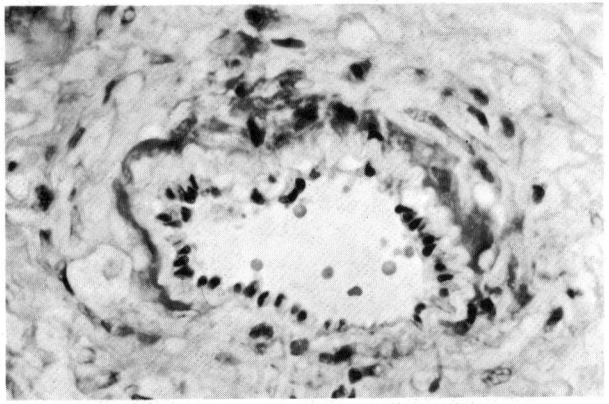

A

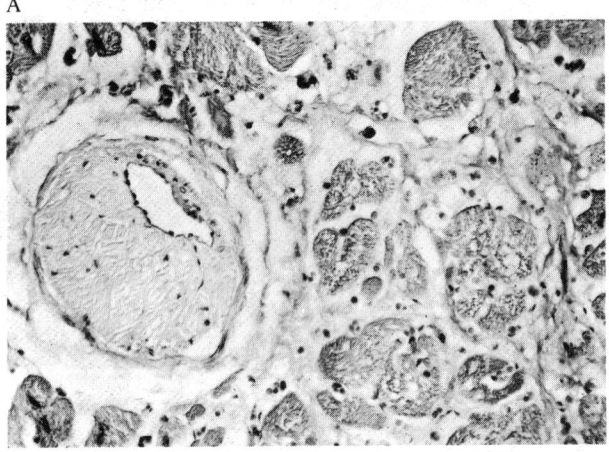

B

FIGURE 2-33 Hereditary medial necrosis of small coronary arteries from patients dying with heart failure: *A*, in progressive muscular dystrophy, and *B*, in Friedreich's ataxia. Both patients had progressively increasing cardiac enlargement and paroxysmal arrhythmias. *A.* From the sinus node; paranuclear cysts are associated with degeneration of individual smooth-muscle cells of the tunica media of the artery. *B.* From the posterior papillary muscle of the left ventricle; a large amorphous mass is deposited beneath the arterial endothelium, and the tunica media is atrophic.

intranodal artery and pacemaking by the sinus node has led to a number of physiologic and pharmacologic studies.[77–82] Observations to the present time indicate that those drugs and procedures which accelerate the sinus node may decrease the caliber of the artery, while those which slow the node may be associated with increased caliber of the artery. There is also experimental evidence of a pulse and impulse relation operating from one sinus beat to the next and serving as a servomechanism or simple feedback which tends to stabilize sinus rhythm.[82] For the concept of cardiac pacemakers behaving as

TABLE 2-2 Hereditary Medial Necrosis

Friedreich's ataxia
Marfan's syndrome
Primary pulmonary hypertension
Familial cardiomegaly
Congenital deafness
Progressive muscular dystrophy

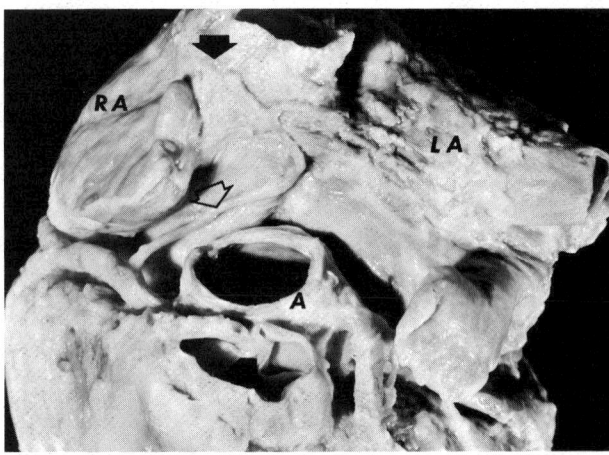

FIGURE 2-34 A dissection of a normal human heart demonstrating the course of a right sinus node artery (open arrow) and the location of the sinus node (black arrow) between the superior vena cava and right atrium (RA). Although the caliber of the sinus node artery continues the same size, the artery disappears when it enters the sinus node, because it becomes invested with a dense collagen matrix which is the framework of the node. LA = left atrium; A = aorta. (*Adapted from James.[38] Reproduced with permission of the publisher.*)

FIGURE 2-35 *A.* Low-power photomicrograph; the normal sinus node, which is the pale-staining area, about a centrally located artery. Note its proximity to the epicardium above. The free wall of the right atrium extends to the right, and the sinus intercavarum extends to the left from the node. The large mass of atrial myocardium extending to the right and below the node is a cross section of the crista terminalis. The interspaces between the crista terminalis and the free wall of the right atrium are the antrum antrii dextri. *B.* Relation of pericarditis to the sinus node. Because of its proximity to the epicardium, the node is virtually always involved during pericarditis. Orientation of structures in *B* is the same as in *A*. *A* is stained with Goldner's modification of Masson's trichrome; and *B* with the Verhoeff-Van Gieson stain.

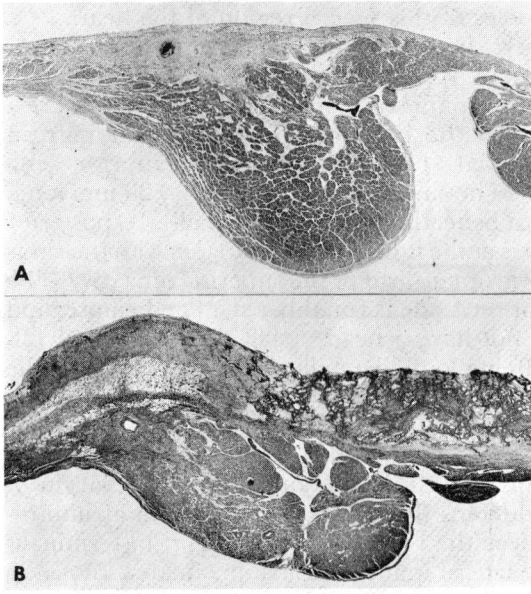

A

B

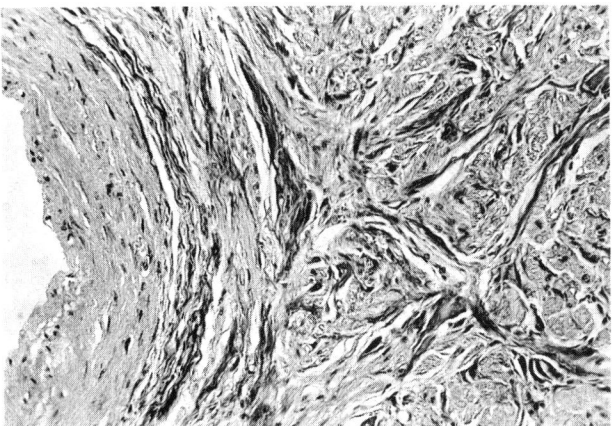

FIGURE 2-36 Photomicrograph of internal structure of the normal human sinus node and the relation between the centrally located, disproportionately large artery and the node. Darker-staining tissue is collagen; lighter-staining tissue consists of sinus node fibers, except for smooth muscle in the wall of the artery (left margin of the picture). The sinus node fibers occur in interlacing bundles, except for those nearest the artery, which encircle it (Goldner's trichrome stain).

relaxation oscillators,[83] the pulse in the sinus node artery may be the essential link closing the loop for two coupled oscillators (sinus node and AV node).

The framework of the sinus node is dense collagen which is closely attached to the entire circumference of the central artery. Within this collagen lattice, interlacing bundles of fibers also attach to this framework. These fibers are of smaller diameter and stain paler than ordinary myocardium with almost all dyes (Fig. 2-37). Nearest the central artery, the bundles of sinus node fibers tend to encircle the vessel; further out into the substance of the node the bundles interweave more at random. At the margins of the node, in nearly all directions, the sinus node fibers converge into exiting Purkinje tracts. Some sinus node fibers unite to form large Purkinje fibers, but occasionally a single small fiber

may be seen progressively to enlarge as it leaves the node.

There are numerous nerve endings but no ganglia within the sinus node.[84] At the anterior and posterior margins of the sinus node, however, there are many ganglia. Within the midportion of the sinus node is a variable number of stellate cells which have a large round nucleus (Fig. 2-38) and are now known as P cells. Sinus node fibers distribute from these cells, which are often near nerve endings. It has been suggested that these primitive-appearing cells may be the site of actual pacemaking within the sinus node.[74] More recent identification of these cells with electron microscopy strengthens the likelihood that these P cells produce the sinus impulse. Their close resemblance to the "leading cells" shown by Harary to be dominant pacemakers in myocardial fiber tissue cultures[85] further supports this likelihood.

Pathology of the sinus node is closely related to two of its anatomic features: its proximity to the epicardium and its proximity to the centrally located artery. Pericarditis almost invariably involves at least the epicardial surface of the node and often even deeper portions.[75] Vascular lesions are generally of two types: those caused by occlusion of the main coronary artery proximal to the sinus node branch, and those involving small arteries directly. The former vascular lesions are usually associated with acute ventricular myocardial infarction and commonly with atrial arrhythmias; in these lesions there is characteristically hemorrhage at the function of the sinus node and right atrium.[86] The lesions of the small arteries include all the diseases affecting such arteries, e.g., lupus erythematosus and polyarteritis nodosa. Additionally, a number of heritable disorders commonly associated with cardiomyopathy and arrhythmias or conduction disturbances

FIGURE 2-37 Photomicrograph showing details of individual human sinus node fibers. Fiber indicated by the arrow demonstrating the perinuclear bulge and clear zone, which resembles the larger conventional Purkinje fibers elsewhere in the heart (Goldner's trichrome stain with phase illumination).

FIGURE 2-38 Photomicrograph showing a stellate-shaped cell (long arrow) of the type found in the central portion of the normal human sinus node. Compare the round, relatively large nucleus with that of a conventional sinus node fiber (short arrow). Another sinus node fiber is faintly shown connected to the right upper margin of the cell and coursing toward the right upper corner of the picture, almost parallel to the indicated (short arrow) sinus node fiber (Goldner's trichrome stain).

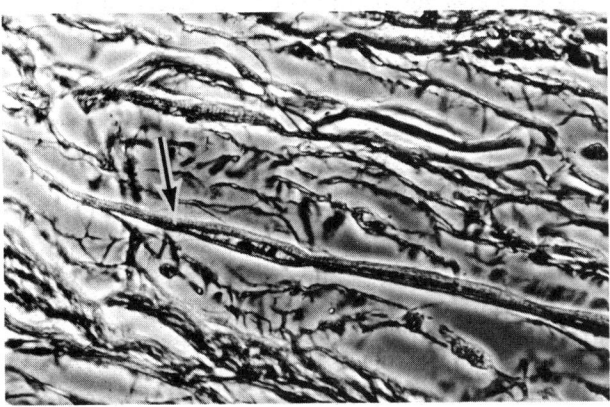

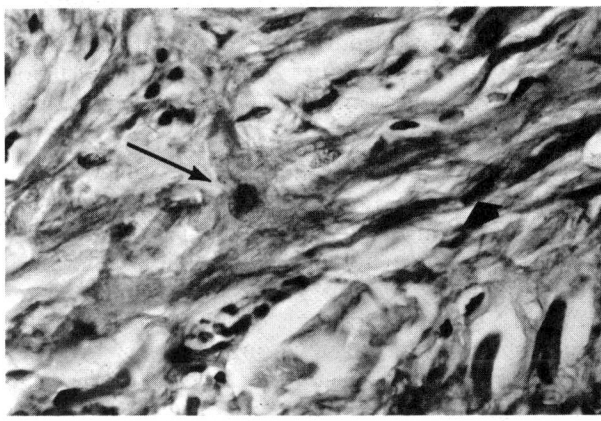

have surprisingly exhibited widespread lesions of the small arteries of the heart, including those of the sinus node and AV node.[61–63]

The AV Node

Located at a critical vantage point guarding the only normal conduction path between the atria and ventricles, the AV node is in a peculiarly strategic position. One AV nodal function is *triage* of atrial signals for transmission to the ventricles. Another function is a delay of approximately 0.04 s in AV transmission which occurs at or near the atrionodal junction.[87] There are two advantages to this normal delay: (1) postponement of ventricular excitation until the atria have had time to eject their contents into the ventricles, and (2) a coincident limitation in the maximum number of signals which can be accommodated for transmission by the AV node. An appreciation of the anatomic location and internal structure of the AV node is essential to an accurate concept of its electrophysiologic function.

The human AV node is situated just beneath the right atrial endocardium directly above the insertion of the septal leaflet of the tricuspid valve and just anterior to the ostium of the coronary sinus.[88] The surface it presents toward the right atrium is convex, and the opposite surface (concave) rests on the collagenous base of the mitral annulus (Fig. 2-39). At its posterior and superior margins the AV node receives fibers from the interatrial septum and eustachian ridge, which are the terminal portion of the internodal pathways (discussed later). In addition to these fibers which enter the margins of the AV node, a number of similar fibers course past the margins to enter the node at various points along its convex surface, including some which enter near the ventricular end of the node (Fig. 2-40). If the anatomic location of the point of normal electrophysiologic delay in AV transmission is at the proximal atrionodal junction, then these fibers entering the lateral surface of the node may function to bypass the point of normal delay.[88] The anatomy of this region therefore provides anatomic support for the concept of dual AV transmission proposed on the basis of physiologic studies by Moe et al.[89]

Although electrocardiographic phenomena such as the Wolff-Parkinson-White complexes are often attributed to rapid conduction through lateral atrioventricular connections, there are reasons to doubt this explanation:

1. Cases with accelerated conduction have been found which had no lateral atrioventricular bundles, and conversely cases with such bundles demonstrable do not always exhibit accelerated conduction.
2. Even the demonstrations of lateral atrioventricular bundles have shown only ordinary myocardium, which may or may not be capable of rapid conduction.

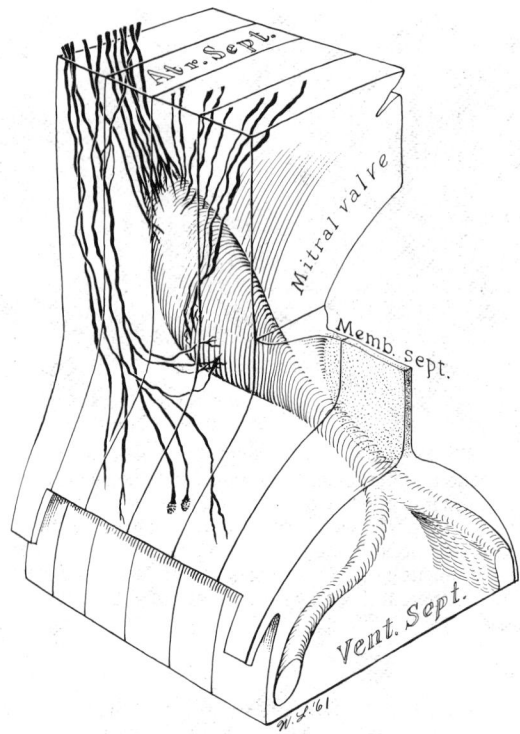

FIGURE 2-39 Schematic drawing of the human AV node and His bundle, showing their relation to the two atrioventricular valves and the interatrial and interventricular septa, including the membranous portion of the latter. As the bundle courses medially and inferiorly along the lower margin of the membranous interventricular septum, it gives rise early to a single right branch but continues providing multiple left branches, which form virtually a sheet of fibers down the left septal endocardium. Only a few fibers from the internodal pathways are shown, to avoid obscuring details of the AV node, but these may be seen entering the superior and posterior margins of the node (its crest) as well as the lower portion of the convex right atrial surface of the node. A few internodal fibers terminate in the base of the tricuspid valve, and rarely (almost exclusively in infants) a few may penetrate directly to the interventricular septum. The potential electrophysiologic significance of these multiple entrances into the AV node is discussed in the text.

3. If dual AV conduction does occur in the region of the AV node, there are more tenable explanations for intermittent occurrence of accelerated conduction, e.g., the normal and abnormal influence of the rich autonomic innervation of the node and its immediate environs.[84] On the basis of present anatomic and electrophysiologic evidence, it seems unlikely that lateral atrioventricular bundles are of any functional significance and more likely that phenomena such as ventricular preexcitation can be explained by altered conduction in or very near the AV node.[90]

Internally the AV node exhibits both similarities to and differences from the sinus node. Like those of the sinus node, slender fibers of the AV node interweave to form a meshwork, but there is much less collagen between fibers (Fig. 2-41). Although there is some variation in the size and length of AV node fibers from one heart to another, in general they are slightly thicker and shorter than those of the sinus node but not as thick as those of ordinary

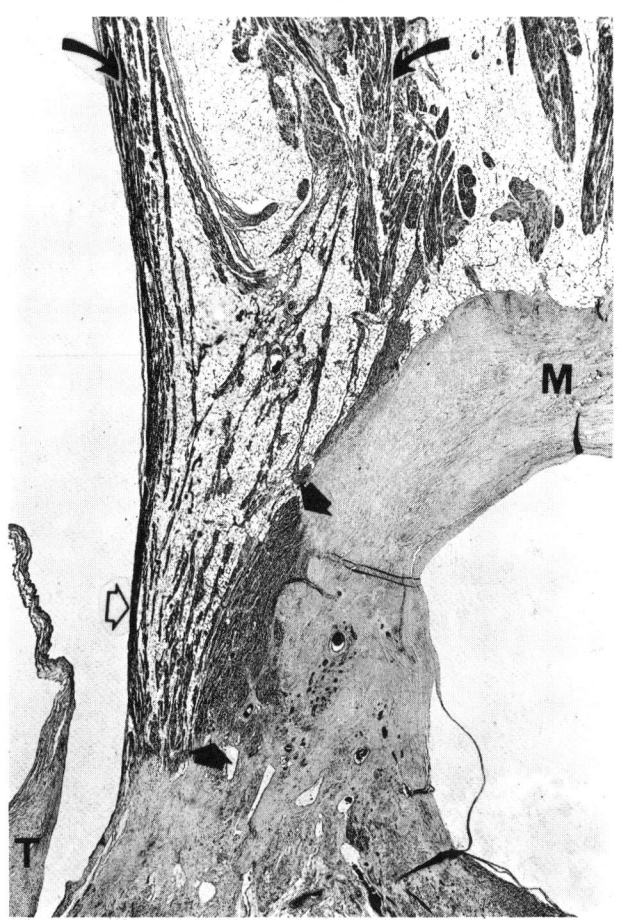

FIGURE 2-40 Low-power photomicrograph of the normal human AV node near its midportion. Decussation of internodal fibers as they approach the node from above is shown, with the fibers in the central interatrial septum (curved arrow on the left) entering predominantly the superior margin of the node, while those in the bypass region (curved arrow on the right and open arrow adjacent to the node) circumvent the crest to enter the convex surface of the node. The body of the AV node is between the two short black arrows, lying on the annulus of the mitral valve (M). A deflected leaflet of the tricuspid valve is labeled T (Goldner's trichrome stain). (*From James.*[98] *Reproduced with permission.*)

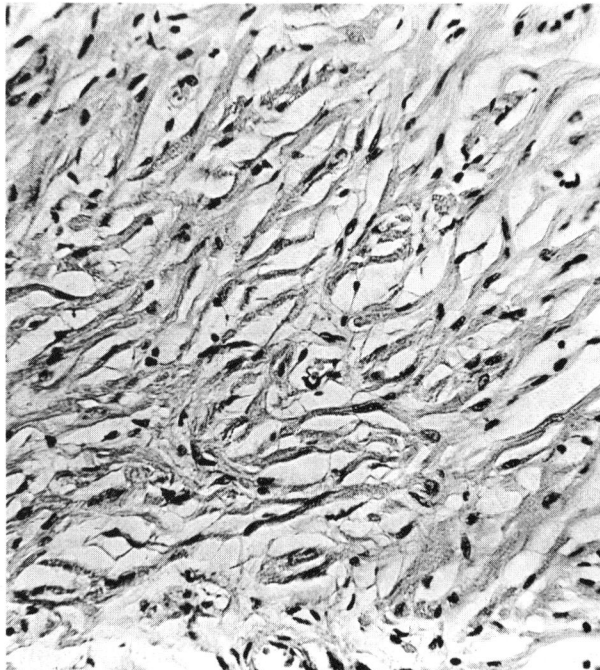

FIGURE 2-41 Photomicrograph showing details of the internal structure of a human AV node. The fibers are slightly shorter than those of the sinus node, and there is much less supporting collagen. A central artery is sometimes seen in the AV node but is not a constant feature, as it is in the sinus node. Fibers of the AV node interweave and interconnect abundantly (Goldner's trichrome stain).

myocardium. Throughout the upper and middle portions of the AV node the fibers frequently connect with one another and interweave at random, but in the anterior and inferior portions of the node they begin to orient into a longitudinal axis as they form the AV bundle. No anatomic feature of the AV node suggests a morphologic basis for the commonly used electrocardiographic terms of upper, lower, and middle AV nodal rhythm, but the history of the origin of these terms casts even greater doubt on their validity.[91] Similarly, the electrocardiographic term *coronary sinus rhythm* may serve some useful didactic purpose, but anatomically it seems unlikely that a signal originating in the coronary sinus (if indeed it does) could inscribe a significantly different peripherally recorded electrocardiographic complex on comparison with one from a signal originating in the AV node, since the coronary sinus and the AV node are virtually contiguous.

Behind the AV node, in the very small area between it and the coronary sinus, there are a number of autonomic ganglia.[84] These are presumably vagal ganglia. They and adjacent neural structures may have a receptor function[60] as well as being the probable route by which vagal stimuli of extracardiac origin arrive at the AV node. The most common pathologic change of the AV node is ischemic infarction or fibrosis due to occlusion of the main coronary artery supplying the AV node branch (Fig. 2-42). In 90 percent of human beings the AV node is supplied by the right coronary artery, the occlusion of which is associated with posterior myocardial infarction as well as with AV nodal ischemia or infarction. In addition to syncope or more prolonged loss of consciousness during angina pectoris preceding a posterior infarction, or during the actual infarction, other clinical features of this type of infarction include an uncommonly high incidence of nausea and vomiting, unusual diaphoresis, sialorrhea, tenesmus, and intense sinus bradycardia. All these symptoms can be caused by excess vagal discharge, and in the patient with acute posterior myocardial infarction they can often be promptly abolished with atropine.[60] There has been some question as to the origin of this vagotonia, but the demonstration by Juhasz-Nagy and Szentivanyi of vagal receptor sites in or near the wall of the coronary

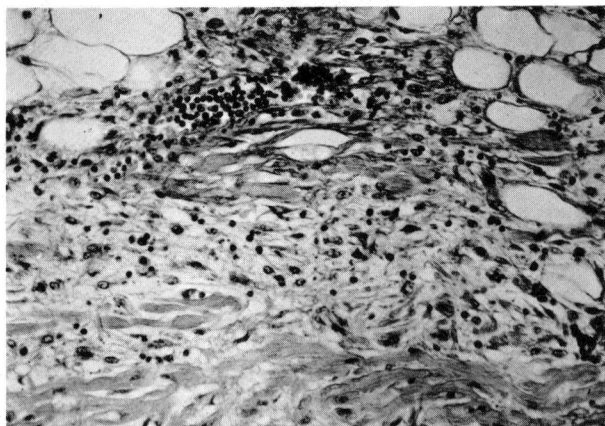

FIGURE 2-42 Photomicrograph showing an extensively infarcted AV node from a patient with acute posterior myocardial infarction and heart block. Hemorrhage and necrosis are evidence of very recent damage; the fat spaces and young connective tissue suggest older injury (Goldner's trichrome stain).

sinus[92] suggest that the neural strictures near the posterior margin of the human AV node may constitute this site.[60,84] If this is so, the vagal reflex phenomena of acute posterior myocardial infarction are the human counterpart of the Bezold-Jarisch reflex, which has heretofore been recognized and extensively studied only in experimental animals.[93,94]

The AV Bundle and Its Proximal and Distal Branches

Formed by convergence of fibers at the anterior and inferior margin of the AV node, the parallel fibers of the AV (His) bundle veer from the right atrial endocardial location of the AV node into the middle of the central fibrous body. The fibers of the AV bundle are separated by fine collagen septa.[95] From the AV node the AV bundle descends along the posterior margin of the membranous interventricular septum to the crest of the muscular septum. The AV bundle is often triangular in cross section, and the two lower corners of the triangle give rise to the right and left bundle branches (Fig. 2-43). The right bundle branch is a single slender group of fibers which leave the common bundle shortly after it reaches the muscular crest of the interventricular septum. The left bundle branch is a virtual sheet of fibers cascading down from the left margin of the common bundle through most of its course. The difference in size of the two bundle branches is a striking anatomic feature which probably accounts for the clinical observation that right bundle branch block is clinically more often an innocuous finding in the electrocardiogram, since it can be produced by such a small focal lesion, whereas block of the left bundle branches requires a much more extensive lesion.

From their origin near the membranous septum the two bundle branches both course generally in an anterior and apical direction along the endocar-

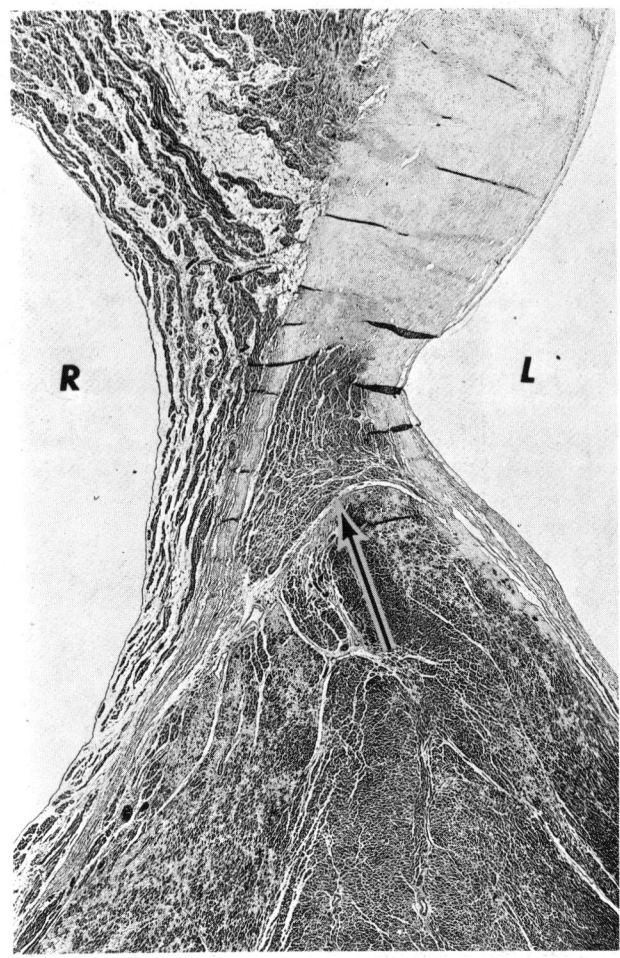

FIGURE 2-43 Photomicrograph of human AV bundle (arrow). Note the triangular shape of this cross section, with right and left bundle branches originating from its two lower corners. R = right side of the heart; L = the left. The mitral annulus and valve course from the center of the picture to the right upper corner. The tricuspid valve base is in the left lower corner; the interatrial septum above, and the interventricular septum below (Goldner's trichrome stain).

dium, rapidly fanning out in all directions to cover the ventricular endocardium.[96] After an initial undivided course of 20 to 30 mm, the left bundle branches form two relatively direct pathways to the anterior and posterior papillary muscles, in addition to spreading more diffusely. Presumably this permits delivery of a slightly earlier signal of these two structures, since their effective contraction should slightly precede contraction of the ventricular free walls in order to prevent mitral regurgitation. Peripheral divisions of the right bundle branch are fairly evenly distributed, but because the slender right bundle branch originates at a level considerably below the crista supraventricularis and courses without much branching to the moderator band near the right ventricular apex, the crista is some distance removed from the earliest contact of right bundle branch with ventricle and therefore is activated relatively late.

The noncoronary sinus of the aorta protrudes

into the interatrial septum just above the membranous interventricular septum, so that its posterior margin is in close proximity to the common AV bundle (Fig. 2-44). It is hardly surprising, therefore, that lesions causing aortic valvulitis are sometimes associated with disruption of AV conduction, as a result of associated inflammation or other pathologic change in the AV bundle. During aortic valvular bacterial endocarditis the AV bundle may even be destroyed; the AV bundle may also be destroyed in extensive calcification of the aortic valve. Occasionally inflammation of the mitral annulus may extend to involve either the AV bundle or the AV node (which are directly adjacent to the annulus), and this is particularly likely to be a consequence of calcification or abscesses of the mitral

ring. Whether inflammation of the mitral annulus may contribute to heart block sometimes seen in acute rheumatic fever may also be considered, although histopathologic studies in this stage of the disease are understandably uncommon.

Fibers in the AV bundle are larger than those in the AV node, and their parallel arrangement is entirely different from the thick interweaving of the fibers of the node. Shortly after bifurcation of the bundle into its right and left branches, the fibers become even more enlarged and are of greater diameter than ordinary myocardial fibers. Most of the fibers in the bundle branches have sparse myofibrils, rectangular or oblong nuclei, and a perinuclear clear zone and bulge; thus they resemble the classic Purkinje fibers (Fig. 2-45), which are much better seen in ungulates, where they were originally described, than in human beings. It is important to realize that, in the human heart, not even the bundle branches are composed exclusively of Purkinje fibers, and that there are many other fibers which are directly continuous with the Purkinje fibers but which are morphologically (at least by present methods) indistinguishable from ordinary myocardium. This occurs not only at the points of transition from the bundle branch area to definite ordinary myocardium, but also within the main course of the bundle branch area itself.

More peripherally, there are common areas of right and left ventricular subendocardium where many Purkinje fibers occur in a layer or small groups, but there are also areas of subendocardium where such fibers cannot be identified. Much confusion has resulted from the suggestion by some investigators that rapid conduction is an exclusive property of Purkinje fibers. The presence of fibers of ordinary appearance within the bundle branches themselves strongly suggests that some fibers also conduct rapidly. As discussed by Truex,[97] it is quite probable that rapidly conducting fibers in the human heart often exhibit classic Purkinje character-

FIGURE 2-44 Photomicrograph showing proximity of the human noncoronary sinus of the aorta (Ao) to the AV bundle (arrow). The septal leaflet of the tricuspid valve is attached to the left upper margin of the noncoronary sinus. The interatrial septum extends upward, and the interventricular septum downward. L = left side of the heart; R = the right (Goldner's trichrome stain).

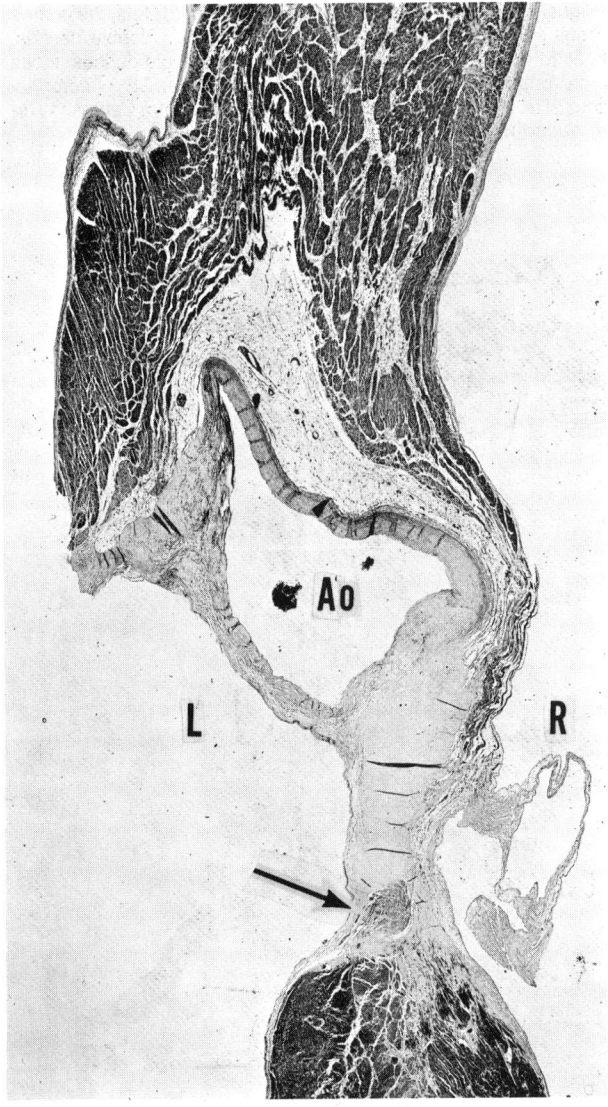

FIGURE 2-45 Photomicrograph of several human Purkinje fibers. In addition to the wispy myofibrils, note the rectangular nucleus with a perinuclear bulge and clear zone (arrow) (Goldner's trichrome stain).

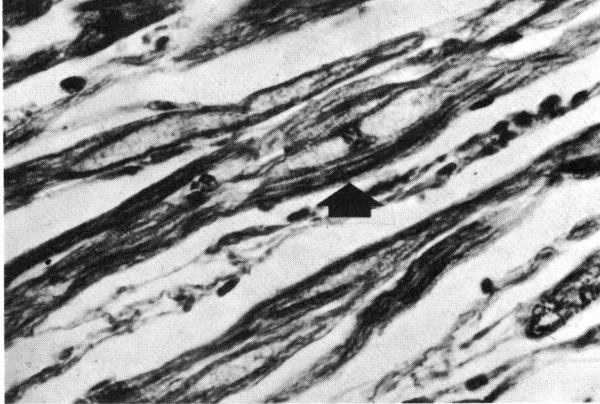

istics similar to those in ungulates, but that some fibers which we now consider morphologically as ordinary myocardium must also possess the ability to conduct rapidly.

Internodal and Interatrial Connecting Pathways

Largely because of the erroneous assumption that rapid conduction is exclusively a property of fibers with Purkinje characteristics, it has often been stated that there is no pathway of specialized tissue between the sinus node and the AV node. Since electrophysiologic studies have established beyond doubt that the impulse from the sinus node arrives at the AV node more rapidly than could occur in ordinary myocardium,[87] the question is really not whether such pathways exist but where they are. On gross dissection there are three potential pathways between the sinus node and the AV node (Fig. 2-46), the continuity of fibers being histologically demonstrable with serial sectioning. These pathways are similar in humans[98] and dogs,[99] and correspond in part to areas previously described by Wenckebach,[100] Thorel,[101,102] and Bachmann.[103] The pathway originally described by Bachmann, on the basis of both physiologic and anatomic studies, was concerned primarily with interatrial conduction, and he made no mention of its function in internodal conduction.

The *anterior internodal pathway* extends from the

anterior margin of the sinus node, curves around the superior vena cava, and enters the anterior interatrial myocardial band (*Bachmann's bundle*). Fibers in Bachmann's bundle divide near the anterior margin of the interatrial septum (Figs. 2-46 and 2-47), some continuing into the left atrium and others descending obliquely and posteriorly within the interatrial septum behind the noncoronary sinus of the aorta to enter the upper margin of the AV node. This is a well-developed pathway in almost all human hearts and can easily be demonstrated throughout its course by careful dissection. It is

FIGURE 2-46 Drawing of location and course of the three internodal pathways of the human heart. The heart is viewed from above and behind the left atrium. The open arrow indicates the sinus node, at the junction of the superior vena cava and right atrium; the black arrow indicates the AV node, lying near the junction of the interatrial and interventricular septa and between the ostium of the coronary sinus behind and the membranous interventricular septum ahead. A = the anterior internodal pathway as well as the predominant interatrial pathway, with the division occurring as they course in Bachmann's bundle; these interatrial fibers were first described by Bachmann. M = the middle internodal pathway, first described by Wenckebach; P = the posterior internodal pathway, first described by Thorel. (See text for further discussion.)

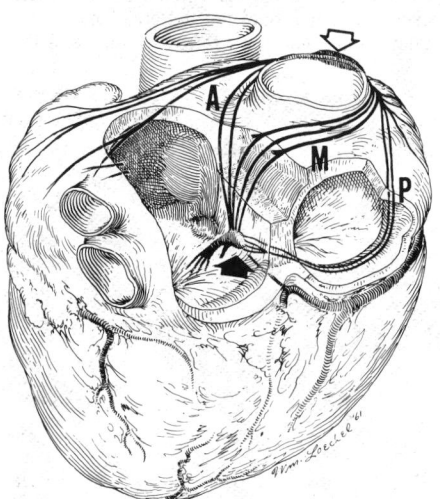

FIGURE 2-47 Gross photograph (slightly enlarged) of horizontal section through the atria and interatrial septum of a human heart, demonstrating the general location of the three internodal pathways. X, location of the sinus node, which is above the plane of this section; open arrow, approximate location of the AV node, which is below the plane of this section. Short black arrow, fibers in the posterior internodal pathway as they approach the AV node from the eustachian ridge (ER). Bachmann's bundle is indicated by the narrow black arrow and the letters BB. Note its division into fibers which continue into the left atrium and others which descend obliquely in the interatrial septum to the AV node. Dots, the course of fibers in the anterior internodal pathway; thin double dashes, those in the middle internodal pathway; bold single dashes, those in the posterior internodal pathway. Ao = aorta; CS = coronary sinus; RA = right atrium; LA = left atrium. (*From James.*[98] *Reproduced with permission.*)

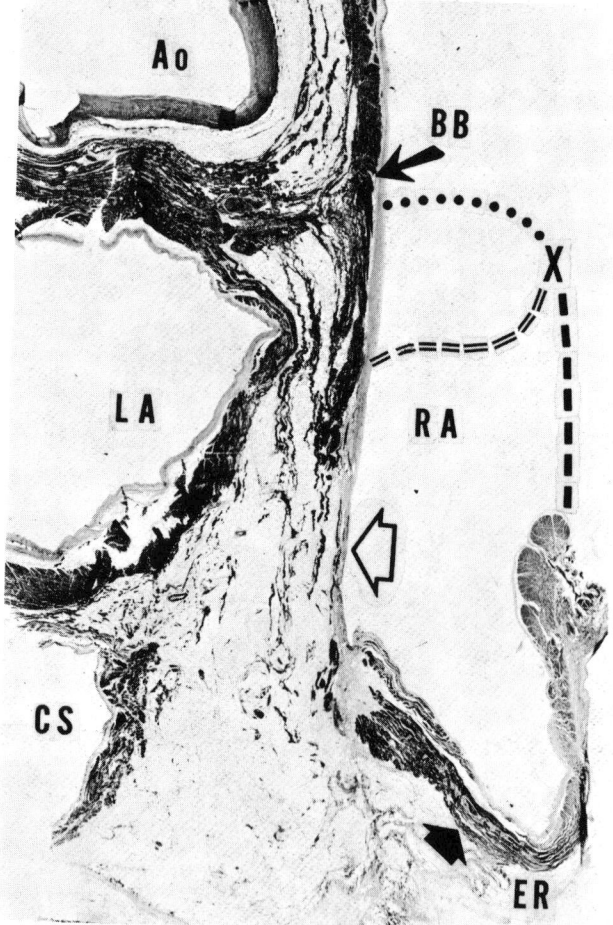

composed of both ordinary and Purkinje fibers; there are a large number of the latter but frequent intercellular continuity of both types. The initial portion of this pathway and its continuation into the left atrium are the bundle described by Bachmann, who did not indicate awareness of the division descending to the AV node.

The *middle internodal pathway* was first described by Wenckebach, who suggested that it was the route of conduction not only from node to node but also between the two atria. These fibers leave the superior and posterior margins of the sinus node to curve behind the superior vena cava and cross the sinus intercavarum to the crest of the interatrial septum. There they divide into a few sparse fibers continuing into the left atrium and a much larger number which descend within the interatrial septum to enter the top of the AV node (Figs. 2-46 and 2-48). The connections with the left atrium by this route are inconstant and seldom very extensive, suggesting that Wenckebach's concept of interatrial conduction by this route is important only in exceptional hearts.

The *posterior internodal pathway* was first described by Thorel and was more recently emphasized by Soderstrom[76] as a major route for internodal conduction. These fibers leave the posterior margin of the sinus node and continue along the crista terminalis to the eustachian ridge, in which they sweep into the interatrial septum directly above the posterior margin of the AV node (Figs. 2-46 to 2-48). There they curve down to enter the node. Like the anterior internodal pathway, this pathway is fairly constant and easily demonstrable by gross dissection, especially in hearts with a prominent eustachian ridge. When the eustachian ridge is diminutive, appearing as a thin fold, it is composed almost exclusively of fibers with Purkinje characteristics. The route of conduction in this posterior internodal pathway is similar in the human and the dog, but there is an important difference in the rabbit.[104] Instead of the fibers entering the interatrial septum above the coronary sinus and thence connecting with the AV node, those in the rabbit descend further in the crista terminalis to the level of the tricuspid ring and then course medially to enter the interatrial septum *beneath* the ostium of the coronary sinus. This important difference should be noted because of its potential significance in experimental electrophysiologic studies which commonly employ the rabbit. An additional important anatomic difference exhibited by the rabbit heart is its constant left superior vena cava, a feature first reported by Marshall.[105] In view of Patten's theory about the embryologic origin of the sinus node and AV node, the lack of attrition of the left superior vena cava in the rabbit may suggest a more primitive state of associated structures, including the AV node. Finally, the large size of the ostium of the coronary sinus in the rabbit (because it drains the left superior vena cava as well as the cardiac veins) leads to a more

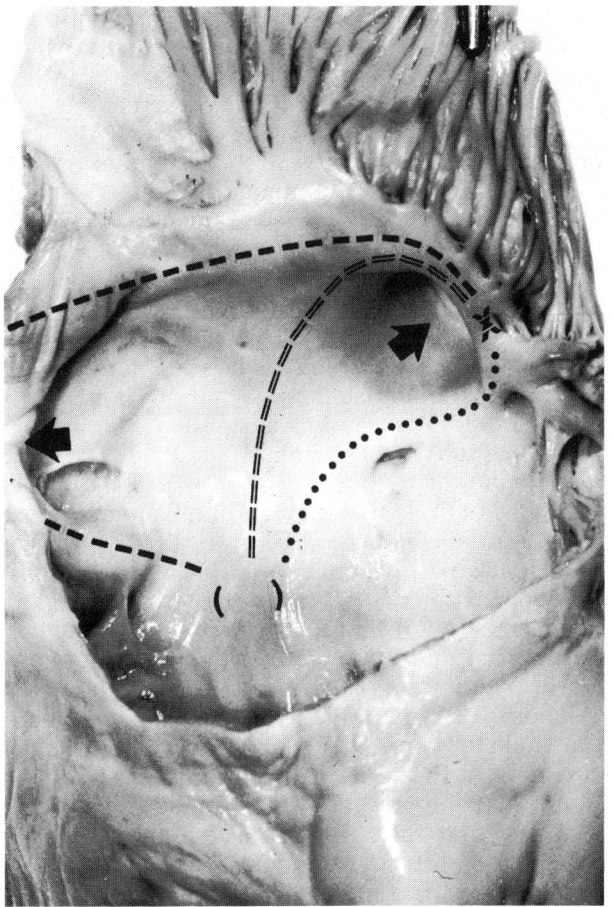

FIGURE 2-48   Interior of the right atrium: showing the relation of the three internodal pathways to internal structures. Dots and dashes are the same indicators as in Fig. 2-47. The arrow on the right is in the ostium of the superior vena cava; that on the left indicates the inferior vena cava, which has been cut open as the free wall of the right atrium was reflected upward from the coronary sulcus. The parentheses indicate the approximate location of the AV node just anterior to the ostium of the coronary sinus. The broken X indicates the location of the sinus node, which is epicardial. The anterior internodal pathway curves anteriorly about the superior vena cava through Bachmann's bundle into the interatrial septum, where it descends to the AV node. The middle pathway curves behind the superior vena cava across the sinus intercavarum to the top of the interatrial septum and then descends to the AV node. The posterior internodal pathway follows the crista terminalis to the posterior margin of the interatrial septum and AV node, crossing the top of the ostium of the coronary sinus. (*From James.[98] Reproduced with permission.*)

anterior intracardiac displacement of the AV node in the rabbit than in the human being or the dog.

As fibers of all three internodal pathways approach the AV node, some merge with one another while others enter the node directly. The septal portions of the anterior and middle internodal pathways particularly mingle to form the torus Loweri, which is at the anterior margin of the fossa ovalis. Some fibers of all three pathways bypass the superior margin of the AV node (its crest) and enter the node at various points along its convex surface. The general outline of the area encompassed by the internodal pathways indicates most of the residuum

56

of the primitive sinus venosus, another reason to anticipate that fibers within this region may have specialized conduction properties, whether these are morphologically identifiable by current methods or not. Furthermore, when one considers the merging of the three pathways in the vicinity of the AV node as well as their common origin in the sinus node, a reasonable route is presented for the circus movement so often employed in electrocardiographic theory but rarely defined anatomically.

Interatrial conduction may occur along any one of the three internodal pathways, but under normal circumstances in most hearts it is probably preferentially through Bachmann's bundle (Figs. 2-46, 2-47, and 2-49), beginning along the anterior internodal pathway. Fibers from the middle internodal pathway to the left atrium are so sparse and inconstant it is unlikely that they are of much importance in interatrial conduction. Fibers from the posterior internodal pathway have such a long interatrial route, extending from sinus node to AV node and then spreading from the AV node up the left atrial side of the interatrial septum, that they probably participate little if at all in normal interatrial conduction. During ectopic rhythm originating in the AV node, however, its septal connections to the left atrium and the posterior internodal pathway become more important routes of spread to both atria. Conduction to the right atrium from the sinus node is normally virtually direct, radiating mainly from the inferior margin of the node into the adjacent trabeculae of the free wall of the right atrium, and extending into the crista terminalis, from which more distal radiation may occur. Many fibers in both atria exhibit Purkinje characteristics, particularly in the regions of the internodal and interatrial pathways.

FIGURE 2-49 External surface of the human heart, showing the general course of the three internodal pathways. Dots and dashes are the same indicators as in Fig. 2-47. X = location of the sinus node; RA = right atrium; LA = left atrium. Compare with Figs. 2-47 and 2-48. (*From James.[98] Reproduced with permission.*)

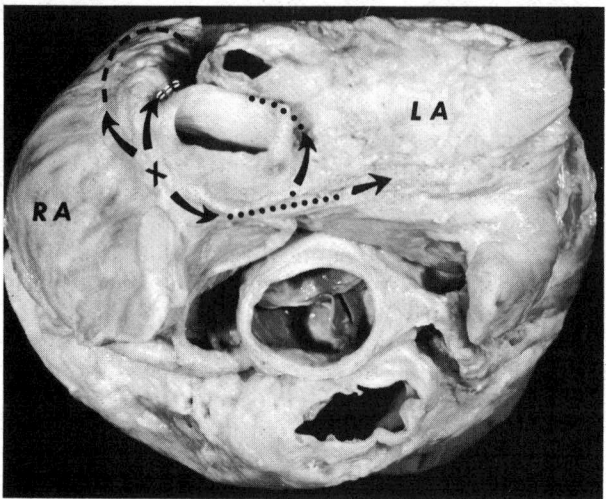

Although it may reasonably be presumed that normal spread of excitation is roughly radial from the sinus node into the right atrium and through Bachmann's bundle to the left atrium, the normal (usual) pathway for internodal conduction is not so apparent. For example, one internodal pathway may function selectively under normal conditions, with the others providing alternate routes in the case of disease. On the other hand, two or more pathways may function normally, with some means of cancellation of late-arriving impulses at the AV node or synchronization of conduction between the various pathways just prior to arrival of an impulse at the AV node. On the basis of anatomic length alone, the anterior internodal pathway is the shortest internodal pathway and under normal circumstances of sinus rhythm is probably the preferential one. Future studies on the electrophysiology of these regions will doubtless explain more clearly the functioning of what we see, but a number of these anatomic observations are already useful in clinical electrocardiography.[106,107]

Ultrastructure of the Myocardium

The functions of the heart are in general of two different types, electrical and mechanical. Certain myocardial cells are specialized for the best performances of these functions, and this specialization includes their anatomic features. The internal anatomy of myocardial cells has been explored almost since the invention of the microscope, but detailed intracellular structure has only recently begun to be defined. With electron microscopy it has become apparent that all the myocardial cells concerned primarily with mechanical function are similar, although there are slight differences between atrial and ventricular myocardium.[108,109] It has also become apparent that there are several different types of cells having electrical activity as their principal function, and they are quite different from "working myocardial cells."[74,88,110–114] An understanding of internal cellular structure is essential to an understanding of function, and in this section we shall consider the fine structure of the cells of the myocardium. First we will deal with those cells concerned with pacemaking and conduction, and then with myocardial cells doing mechanical work by contracting.

Cells Concerned with the Electrical Activity of the Heart

Although every contractile myocardial cell is activated by an electrical stimulus, certain special portions of the heart are particularly developed for the generation of an impulse and for very rapid conduction of this impulse to the working cells. Impulse formation normally occurs in the sinus node and from there is delivered to both atria and to the atrioventricular (AV) node via specialized atrial pathways.[115] In or near the AV node there is a delay in conduction of about 0.04 s, followed then by more rapid spread through the His (AV) bundle and its branches to the working cells of the ventricular myocardium. In this system of impulse formation and rapid conduction there are four types of cells, all of which are significantly different from ordinary working myocardial cells. They are *P cells, transitional cells, ameboid cells, and Purkinje cells.* P cells are found in the sinus node, AV node, and internodal pathways,[116] but they are much more numerous in the sinus node. Transitional cells are found predominantly within the two nodes and internodal pathways but also extend for considerable distances into all adjacent atrial margins of both nodes. Ameboid cells were found only in the eustachian ridge area. Purkinje cells are found at all margins of the sinus node, throughout the internodal pathways (which also contain intermingled transitional cells and ordinary working myocardial cells), at the crest and at the convex surface of the AV node, and through the His bundle and its branches. The main body of the His bundle is composed primarily of Purkinje cells, but in the bundle branches there are some intermingled cells with the anatomic appearance of ordinary working myocardium.

P Cells

These cells were so named[112,113] because they have a pale appearance both on light and electron microscopy, because in many respects they resemble primitive myocardial cells, and because correlative studies with intracellular microelectrode recording[111] suggest that they are the site of pacemaker impulse formation. The initial suggestion that these cells were the site of impulse formation[116] was based on the following anatomic features: their central location within the sinus node and appropriate connection with fibers distributing from the node, their simple (primitive) internal structure, and their proximity to numerous nerve endings. Their structural similarity to cells that became the pacing cells in myocardial tissue cultures[117,118] supported the hypothesis. Their particular abundance in the sinus node and smaller number in the AV node, which are normally the principal and alternate (subsidiary) pacemakers of the heart, further supports the assumption that P cells are the site of normal impulse formation. P cells are also found in internodal pathways.

The two most striking features of the *internal organization* of P cells are their simplicity and a cytoplasm which appears empty (Figs. 2-50 and 2-51). The simplicity is due to the relatively small number and scattered distribution of organelles, and the cytoplasmic emptiness is largely due to sparse glycogen content. This latter finding is somewhat of a paradox, since conduction tissue has classically been considered as containing large amounts of glycogen. Glycogen sparsity does not appear to be an artifact,

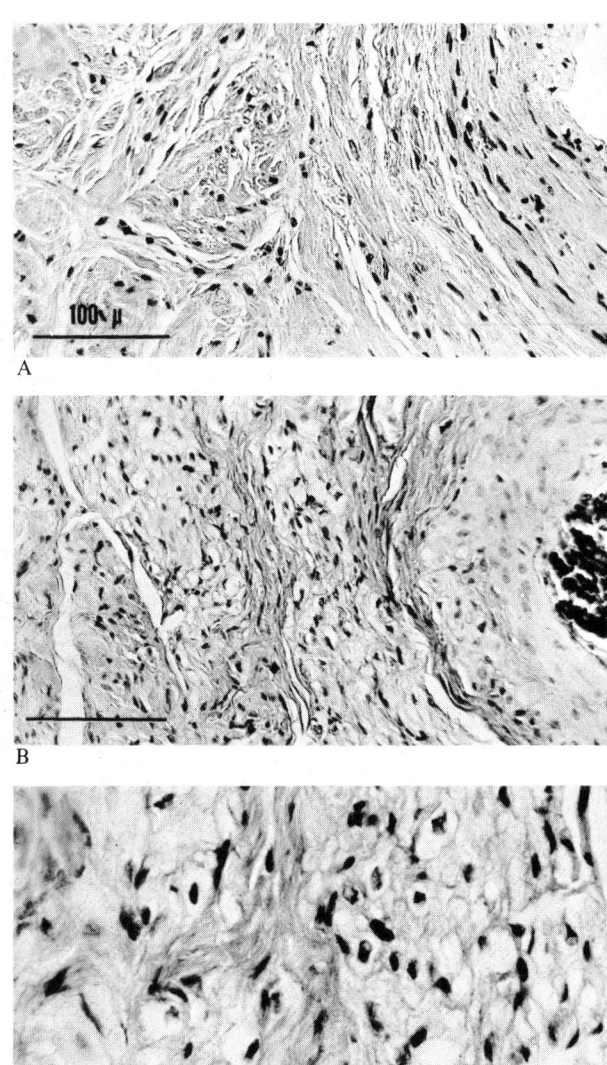

FIGURE 2-50 Light photomicrographs of sinus node, serving to orient the reader for the subsequent electron micrographs. *A.* Human sinus node. *B* and *C.* Canine sinus node. The central artery of the sinus node is to the right in *A* and *B.* Individual cells and fibers of the node interweave within collagen about the artery. High-power magnification of P cells is shown in *C*, which represents an area seen in *B* at lower magnification. Actual magnification in each is indicated by a bar representing 100 μm.

since the P cells were fixed in vivo with direct perfusion of glutaraldehyde, and the immediately neighboring working myocardial cells fixed at the same time in the same way in the same heart had abundant glycogen.[112] P cells are polyhedral and occur in clusters or rows (Figs. 2-53 and 2-54), being most abundant in the central portion of the sinus node, with decreasing numbers toward the periphery. In the AV node they are most numerous near the central fibrous body, which is the deepest portion of the AV node, but as in the sinus node, they are also scattered elsewhere; in no portion of the

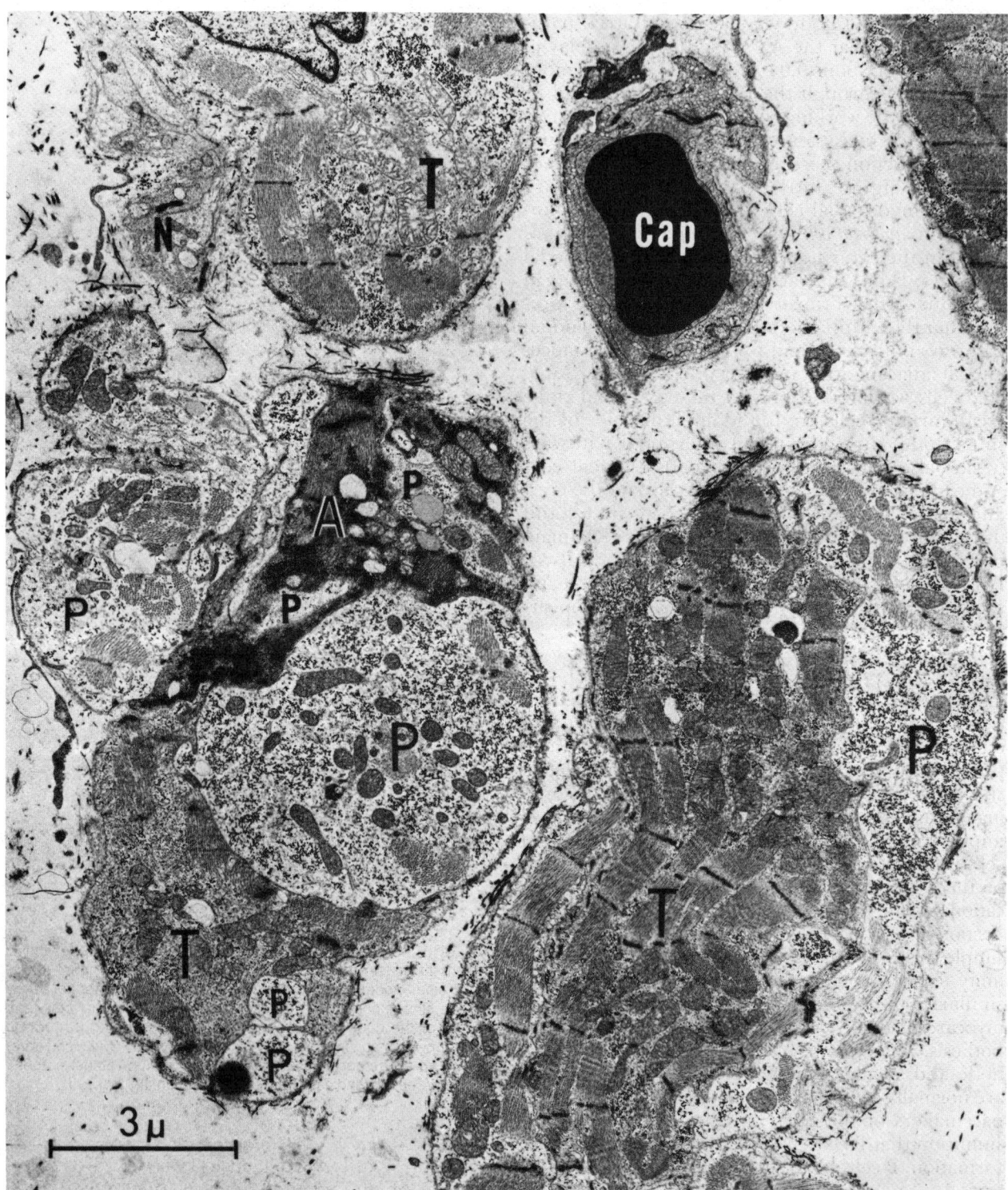

FIGURE 2-51 This single electron micrograph illustrates the characteristically complex organization around an ameboid cell of the eustachian ridge. There are numerous P cells in its vicinity, with portions of seven cells labeled P, as well as slender transitional cells (T) and nerves (N). Note the dense accumulation of very dark granules in the ameboid (A) cell, the cystic lacunae or spaces within it, and its remarkable intertwining or interdigitation among multiple P cells. This ameboid cell is shown at higher magnification in Figure 2-55.[129] Cap = capillary.

AV node are they as numerous as in the sinus node. On cross section P cells are ovoid or rounded, in contrast to the elongated shape of all other myocardial cells, and their surface is smooth. They measure 5 to 10 µm in greatest diameter, making them the smallest myocardial cells. There is no apparent difference in the internal structure of P cells in humans,[74,112] dogs,[110,112] rabbits,[104,111] and steer.[119]

P cells are bound by a double-layered *membrane* (the sarcolemma) at their surface (Figs. 2-50 to 2-56). The sarcolemma is a complex structure[120-122] containing an internal plasma membrane and an external basement membrane. The plasma membrane consists of at least two layers, but except at very high electron microscopic resolution these layers appear as a single, sharply defined electron-dense layer. The components of the plasma membrane are a biomolecular layer of lipid molecules with associated protein layers on the surface, and the total thickness is about 60 Å. External to the plasma membrane is the basement membrane, which is more fuzzy and less electron-dense, measuring about 100 Å thick. The basement membrane is in close relation to extracellular elements such as collagen and nerve endings. No nerve endings have been found to terminate directly on the surface of any myocardial cells, including P cells, and this is an important difference from the situation in skeletal muscle, where nerve endings terminate directly on the cell surface, with specialized contacts. The basement membrane of P cells is directly attached to collagen fibrils, however, and this feature is more prevalent in the sinus node than in the AV node (as already stated, there is much more collagen in the sinus node).

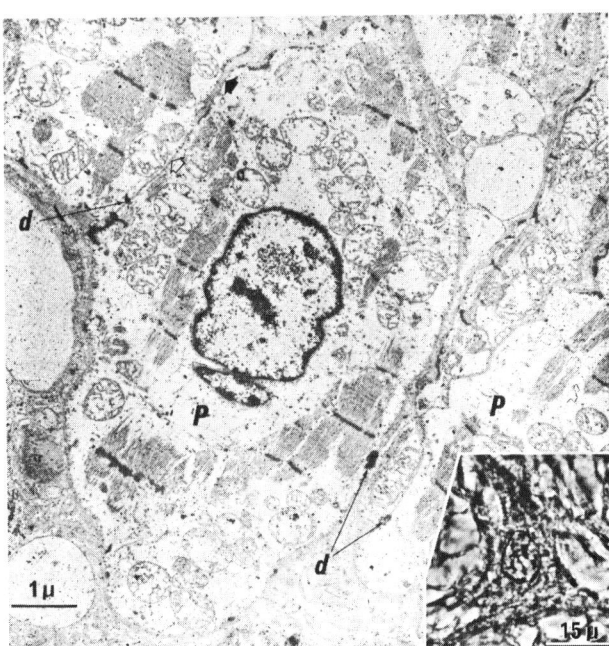

FIGURE 2-52 Electron micrograph of P cells from human sinus node. Again note the simple internal structure. Inset at the right lower corner: a similar cell, examined by light microscopy and phase illumination, from human sinus node. Intercellular junctions of P cells are by plasma membrane–to–plasma membrane apposition (small open arrow at the upper left) with a few scattered desmosomes, indicated by d. The small short black arrow in the upper left indicates an intercellular cleft just above the intercellular junction, and the double-layered sarcolemma can be seen. (*From James et al.*[112] *Reproduced with permission.*)

FIGURE 2-53 Cluster of P cells (A, B, and C) from human AV node. The arrow indicates two desmosomes on the intercellular junction line between cells B and C. The whorl of dark material near the bottom of cell A probably represents a desmosome cluster from junction with an intruding cell tip. (*From James and Sherf.*[113] *Reproduced with permission.*)

FIGURE 2-54 Electron micrograph of a variety of cells from canine sinus node fixed with direct glutaraldehyde perfusion in vivo. Two P cells are obviously paler and simpler than the other cells. At the top, a transitional cell (Tr); near the bottom, three working myocardial cells (W); C = collagen, to which the basement membrane of the P cells is directly attached. In each cell the small arrows point to mitochondria; the simpler structure of those in P cells is apparent (see also Fig. 2-58). A centriole (ce) is indicated with a narrow arrow in one P cell. The micron bar is in a cross section of one capillary. A small tip of an unlabeled P cell joins the lower margin of the Tr cell, and a long desmosome can be seen on the junction line. (*From James et al.*[112] *Reproduced with permission.*)

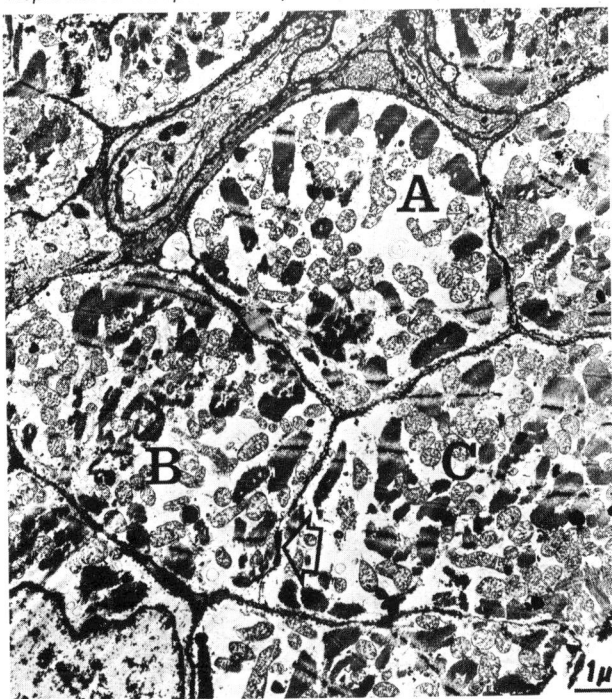

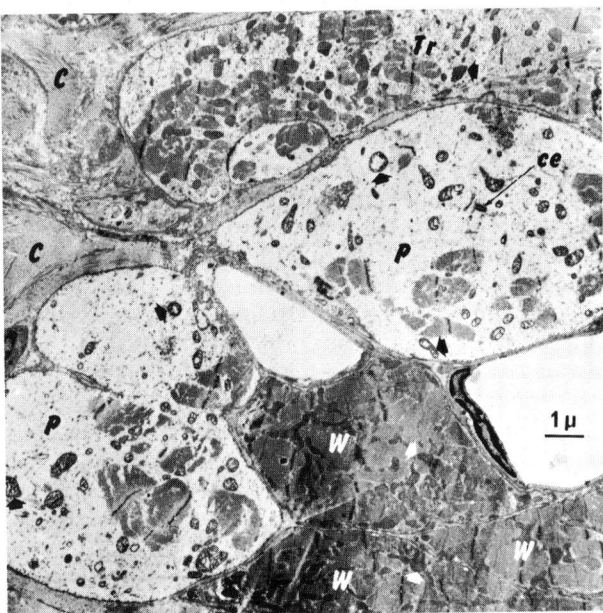

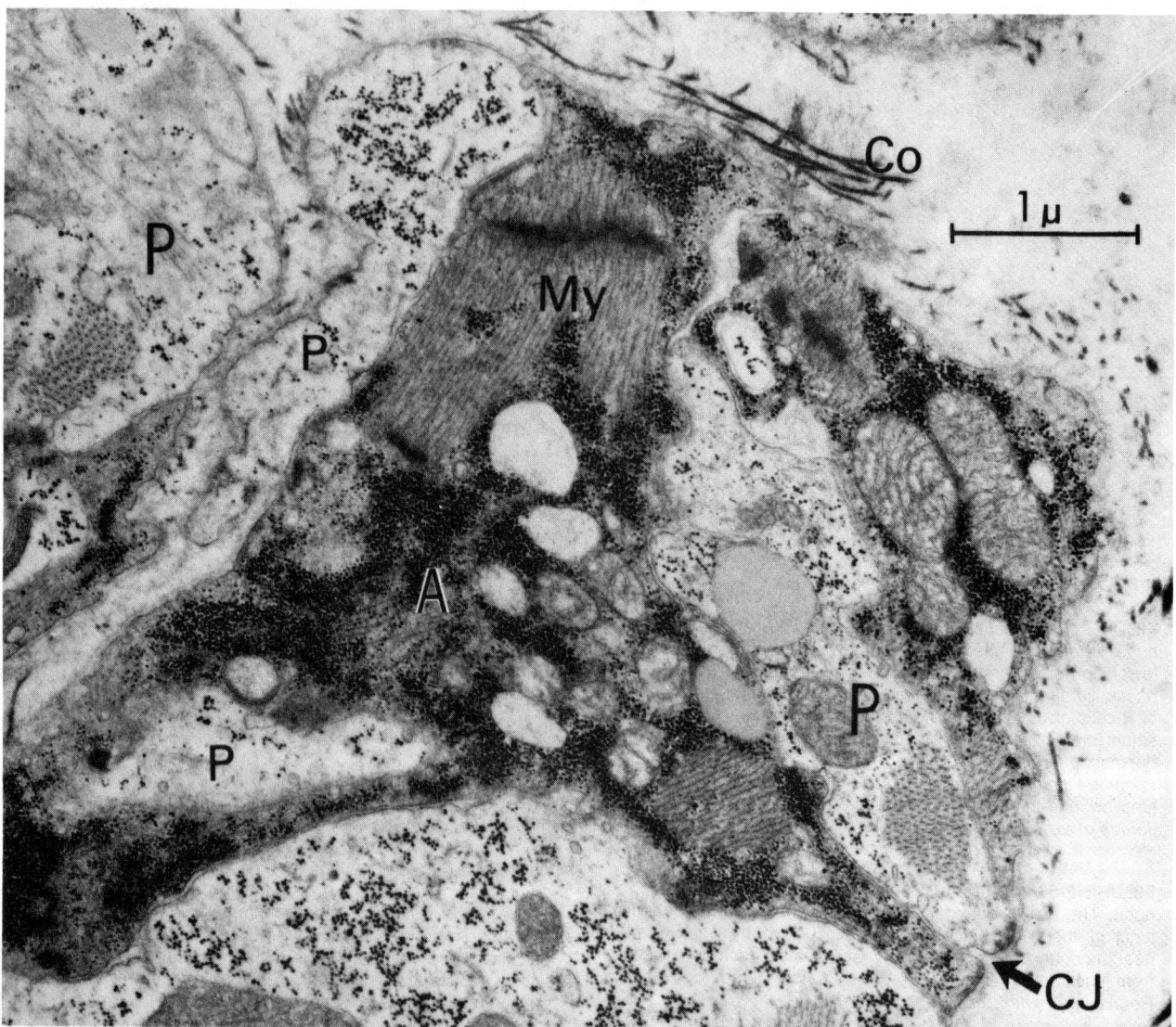

FIGURE 2-55 More details of the internal structure and the intercellular junctions of the ameboid (A) cell shown in Fig. 2-51. Although the dark granules resemble glycogen and the lacunae may be some form of expanded sarcoplastic reticulum, the identity of either of these elements is not certain. The external surface of one intercellular junction is marked CJ; on the other side of the P cell (P) joined at that point is either another ameboid cell or a twisting extension of the same one. Myofibrils within one of several profiles included in this ameboid cell are marked My. Co = collagen.[129]

The molecular structure of the sarcolemma is of great functional importance, since selective changes in its permeability are involved in the electrical and biochemical processes of depolarization and repolarization.[123] It is these changes in permeability which permit an influx of sodium into the cell, inducing the action potential. Changes in permeability of the sarcolemma also induce the efflux of potassium at the end of the action potential. An ATP-dependent "sodium pump" located in or near the sarcolemma then restores the electrolyte equilibrium during the repolarization phase.[123] The way in which these changes in membrane permeability are produced is not clear, but there are some suggestions that they may result from binding locally released acetylcholine to lipoprotein moieties, transiently disorganizing the structure of the membrane.

To understand cell function, it is essential to think of the cell membrane as an "impermanent" anatomic structure.

Along the internal surface of the sarcolemma many pinocytotic vesicles can be seen (Fig. 2-57), appearing as small pinched-off invaginations of the plasma membrane; these are generally thought to represent a means of transport for various solutes into the cell.[120] In addition to these small, shallow vesicles of relatively uniform size, much deeper invaginations into the cell (the sarcotubular system) have been described in recent years. The *sarcotubular system* (sarcoplasmic reticulum) is a complicated network of intracellular tubules, vesicles, and cisternae.[124–126] Although well developed in working myocardial cells, it is poorly developed in P cells. There is no apparent pattern for the sarcotubular system

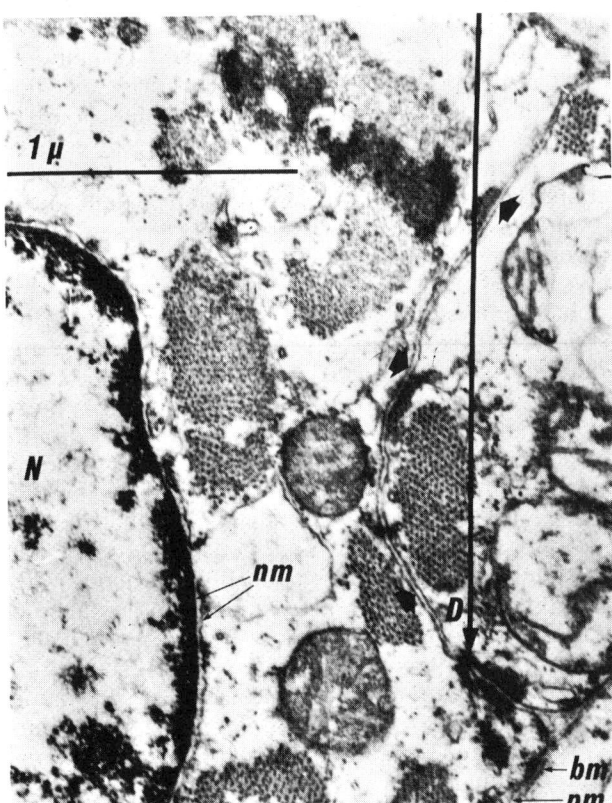

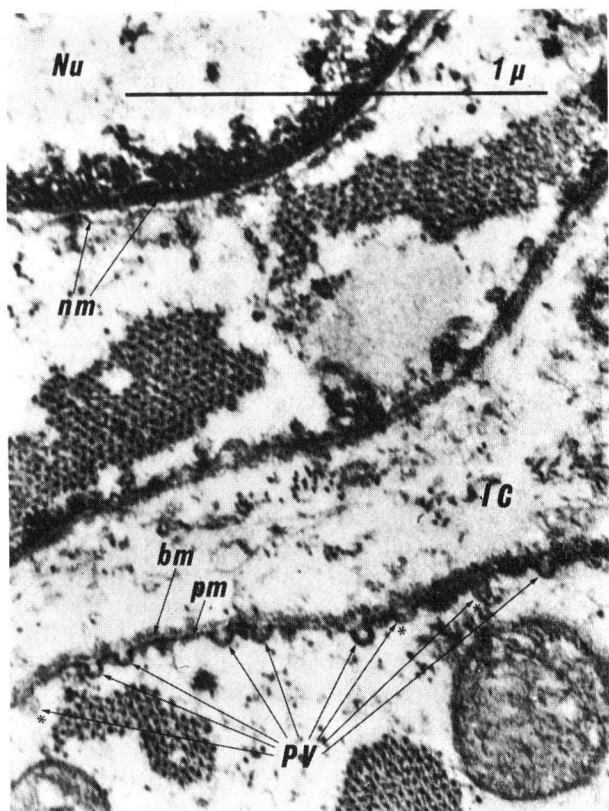

FIGURE 2-56 Illustration of the constant intermembrane distance of two apposing plasma membranes (small short black arrows). The two layers (nm) of the limiting membrane of the nucleus (N) are also shown. Right lower corner, basement membrane (bm) bridging the two cells, while their respective plasma membranes (pm) veer in from the surface. Right upper corner, a similar surface topography, unlabeled. The myofibrils are cut in cross section; the regular hexagonal geometry of the filaments can be seen. A desmosome (D) is opposite the tip of the long arrow. Clumping of the nuclear chromatin is a postmortem artifact. (*From James et al.*[112] *Reproduced with permission.*)

FIGURE 2-57 Pinocytotic vesicles (PV) invaginating into the cell from the plasma membrane (pm). The fuzzier basement membrane (bm) is adjacent to the intercellular cleft (IC). Two layers of the nuclear membrane (nm) are again indicated. Varying sharpness in outline indicates that some pinocytotic vesicles are dissolving or discharging their contents into the cytoplasm; the faintest ones in this process are indicated with asterisks. (*From James et al.*[112] *Reproduced with permission.*)

in P cells, but widely scattered profiles of varying diameters are seen, lined with both smooth and rough membranes. There appears to be more pinocytosis in P cells than in other myocardial cells, and this may be functionally related to their sparse sarcotubular system. As a corollary of the small number of intracellular tubules and myofibrils within P cells, their sarcolemma has almost no indentations or scalloping of the type characteristic of working cells.

P cells have different *intercellular connections* from those of other myocardial cells. Groups or clusters of P cells are bound by a single basement membrane, intercellular contact being direct plasma membrane–to–plasma membrane apposition (Figs. 2-52 and 2-56). In such clusters the enveloping basement membrane is pitted by numerous invaginations into the cluster, giving a spongelike organization to the multicellular unit. The distance between apposite plasma membrane is regularly constant for given cells, and it is in the range of 70 to 150 Å. There are only rare small, tight junctions or nexus formations between P cells. In contrast to the highly

specialized intercellular contact between working myocardial cells through intercalated disks, the contact between P cells is simple and appears unspecialized, containing only a few scattered desmosomes and often being only the closely apposed plasma membranes. Pinocytotic vesicles occur at such appositions as well as at the external surface of P cells, suggesting the possibility of direct intercellular exchange of contents through this mechanism. Both the simple sparse sarcotubular system and the lack of much specialized intercellular contact suggest a different type of intracellular and intercellular spread of excitation in P cells from that of working myocardium, and one which is compatible with the known difference demonstrable electrophysiologically. Slow conduction known to occur in the sinus node and AV node[127] may in part be due to the unspecialized intercellular contacts of P cells.

The *mitochondria* of P cells are fewer than in working myocardial cells; and instead of being sandwiched cells or sandwiched between myofibrils, they are randomly distributed within the cell (Figs. 2-51 to 2-54). The size and shape of P-cell mitochondria are widely varied, but their average maximal dimensions (about 0.5 μm) may be slightly smaller than those of working myocardial cells. Many factors profoundly and rapidly influence the size, shape, and internal configuration of mitochondria,[128] and functional interpretations from a structural basis must be made with more caution than is sometimes observed. In addition to such known factors as rapid swelling and distortion postmortem, and the influence of various fixatives, the presence of hypoxia or any preexisting disease or myocardial strain and the effect of many different cardiac drugs are additional factors which may profoundly influence the ultrastructural appearance of mitochondria. In particular, one must accept with reservations any functional interpretations of mitochondrial structure in human myocardium studied postmortem.

If one keeps these reservations in mind, the mitochondria of P cells in the sinus node studied from healthy dogs with in vivo fixation by direct perfusion of glutaraldehyde appear to have an unusual structure.[112] In contrast to those of working myocardial cells, the mitochondria of P cells in the sinus node appear very simply organized, with relatively few cristae and with little intercristal matrix (or else one which is not electron-dense) (Fig. 2-58). The cristae assume a number of simple patterns, including the formation of peripheral rosettes within the mitochondrion, but some of this apparent variation may be the result of the plane of sectioning. The much more complex structure of mitochondria of working myocardial cells as described by other investigators utilizing the same fixative technique is identical to that of mitochondria of working cells in our specimens, suggesting that the marked difference in internal structure of the mitochondria in directly ad-

jacent P cells is not an artifact of processing. Since it is known that pacemaking cells are unusually resistant to hypoxia and since current evidence suggests that the internal complexity of mitochondria is directly related to the level of metabolic requirement of the myocardial cell, the simplicity of mitochondria in P cells may be a reflection of their lower level of metabolic activity, or it may represent a different type of metabolism from that of working myocardial cells.

Each mitochondrion in P cells is surrounded by a double-layered membrane, each layer being sharply defined and of approximately the same thickness (30 Å), with a similar thickness of intermembrane distance. The individual cristae of mitochondria in P cells appear thicker than those of working myocardium, but this apparent difference may be exaggerated by the smaller number of cristae per mitochondrion in P cells. The cristae of P-cell mitochondria are coarsely homogeneous, with a suggestion of granularity, and each cristal fold measures from 200 to 400 Å in thickness. Interpretation of the internal structure of human P-cell mitochondria is limited by the necessity that such tissue be obtained postmortem, but allowing for this limitation, the general configuration of some mitochondria in human P cells is quite similar to that seen in the dog with in vivo fixation. Furthermore, the only cells in human myocardium in which such simple mitochondrial structure is found are P cells and, much more rarely, Purkinje cells.

The *myofibrils* of P cells are few in number, are randomly distributed and oriented within the cell, and contain relatively few filaments per fibril. Myofibrils in P cells rarely attach to the sarcolemma, although this appearance is of course in part due to planes of sectioning. The random distribution and orientation of myofibrils in P cells means that they cannot generate significant linearly oriented contractile forces. But they may be capable of generating a multidirectional wringing action within the cell, and in view of the paucity of sarcotubular system this may be an important action promoting exchange of fluid within the cell and between the cell and its environment.

Nuclei of P cells appear disproportionately large, but their actual size is comparable with that of nuclei in working myocardial cells, the apparent disproportion being due to the smaller overall size of P cells. Within the P cell the nuclei are centrally located and are usually ovoid or rounded in cross section. The nuclear chromatin quickly clumps postmortem, but in rapidly fixed P cells it is finely granular and evenly distributed. Nucleoli are found in P-cell nuclei, but their demonstration is fortuitously dependent on the plane of sectioning. Neither the nuclei nor nucleoli have any apparent special characteristics, although it must be admitted that surprisingly little is known of either nuclear structure or function. P-cell nuclei are bound by a double-layered external membrane. Double or mul-

FIGURE 2-58 Electron micrographs of typical mitochondria (M) from P cells, on the left, contrasted with those from working myocardial cells on the right. The basement membrane and pinocytotic vesicles from the plasma membrane are incidentally seen well in the P cell. Note that the cristae mitochondriales are much more numerous in mitochondria of working cells, and the intercristal matrix is more electron-dense; the cristae of P cell mitochondria are simple in configuration and few in number, although their single folds may be coarser. The two layers of the mitochondrial membrane are well shown.

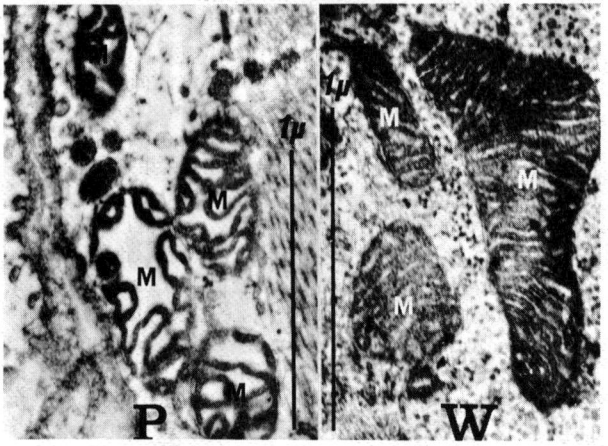

tiple nuclei within a single P cell have not been observed.

A number of *other organelles* are found in P cells, but little is known of their function. *Centrioles* are sometimes seen near the nucleus; since these structures are thought to be associated with cell division, they may have functional significance. Centrioles are so small (Fig. 2-54) that in sectioning they must be missed with far greater frequency than they are demonstrated. *Lysosomes* are found in P cells and contain a large variety of inclusions, have many different shapes and sizes, and have no apparent regularity of intracellular distribution. Numerous *membrane-bound inclusions* containing both granular and other particulate matter are present in various frequency and distribution within P cells; some have single and others two or more layers of their membranes, and some appear to be opening and discharging their contents into the cytoplasm. So little is known about these miscellaneous organelles that their true functional importance simply cannot be assessed yet. It is even likely that organelles with critically important functions have not yet been described.

Transitional Cells

The second type of cell concerned primarily with electrical activity of the heart is a heterogeneous group known as *transitional cells* (Figs. 2-59 and 2-60). This group arbitrarily contains all cells with internal fine structural details intermediate between the simple P cells and the more complex working myocardial cells. In general they are slender elongated cells which are both shorter and narrower than working myocardial cells. Transitional cells are the principal components of the slender fibers seen with light microscopy in both the sinus node and AV node, and in their environs. Since transitional cells are narrow and narrower cells are slower electrical conductors,[127] their presence may be another explanation for slow conduction velocity in the sinus node and AV node. They are more numerous than P cells in the sinus node, but they are by far the principal cell type in the AV node.

More important from a functional standpoint, the transitional cells are the *only* link between P cells and the rest of the heart. P cells make contact only with one another and with transitional cells. Transitional cells in turn contact one another and all other myocardial cells. This contact sometimes takes the form of two or more transitional cells merging to form a larger fiber, and at other times a slender transitional cell simply seems to enlarge into another fiber.

The general organization within transitional cells is one of increasing complexity. Myofibrils become larger in transitional cells than in P cells and orient in longitudinal array parallel to one another, with mitochondria sandwiched in between. The mitochondria are intermediate in internal complexity between the simple ones of P cells and those of

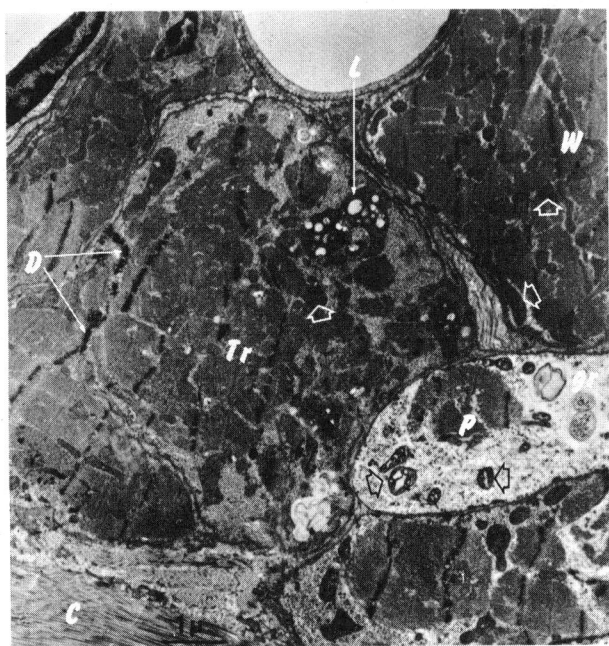

FIGURE 2-59 Electron micrograph showing several important differences among transitional cell (Tr), P cell (P), and working myocardial cell (W), from canine sinus node fixed in vivo with glutaraldehyde. Note the well-preserved abundant glycogen appearing as very fine background granules in both the Tr and W cells, but virtually absent in the P cell. The simple and randomly distributed mitochondria of the P cell can be compared with the more complex ones in the other two types of cell, fixed at the same time in the same manner in this single specimen; the mitochondria are all indicated by small open arrows. The increasing number and orderly array of myofibrils in going from the P cell to the Tr cell to the W cell are apparent, as well as the increasingly dependent association of mitochondria with adjacent myofibrils. Lumens of two transected capillaries are seen at the top of the picture. A lysosome (L) is indicated in the Tr cell, and several desmosomes (D) are seen at its junction with another cell (unidentified by probably a P cell). A number of membrane-bound granule-containing organelles of uncertain identity are labeled gr in the P cell. Collagen fibrils are labeled C.

working myocardial cells. The sarcotubular system becomes progressively more organized and extensive, and the intercellular contacts vary from the simplest in conjunction with P cells to the most complex (fully developed intercalated disks) for working myocardium. Some transitional cells are of heterogeneous internal organization, one portion of the cell having the simple appearance of a P cell and another portion of the same cell having intricately organized contents similar to working myocardium. In such heterogeneous transitional cells the external contacts are of a complexity consonant with the internal cell content adjacent to that portion of the sarcolemma; e.g., there are simple plasma membrane–to–plasma membrane contacts along the surface adjacent to the simpler internal contents.

It is the wide spectrum of degrees of internal organization which arbitrarily classifies transitional cells, and special features of this variation are indicated above. Since all the internal components of transitional cells are similar to either P cells or work-

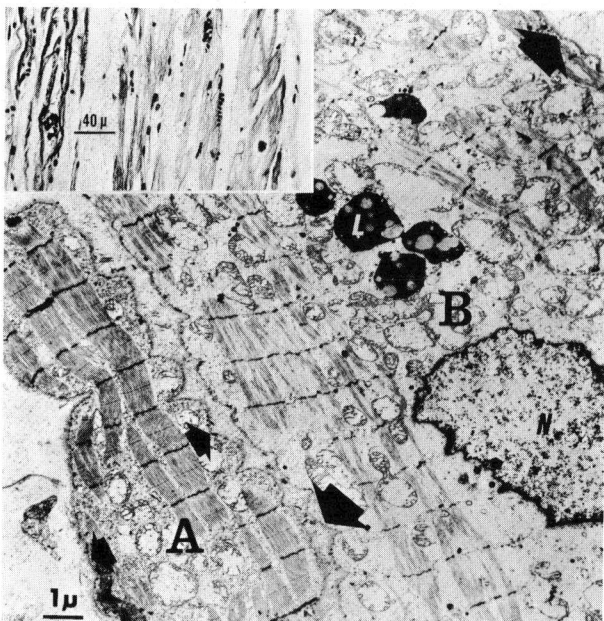

FIGURE 2-60 Electron micrograph of a typical slender transitional cell (*A*) compared with a typical Purkinje cell (*B*) in tissue from the margin of a human AV node. The Purkinje cell is from the bypass region adjacent to the AV node. Insert in the upper left: the same area (different heart) photographed with the light microscope; the transitional cells from the slender fibers are in the left half, while the paler and much broader Purkinje cells in the bypass region make up the right half of the insert. Note the direct connections of transitional cells and Purkinje cells. In the electron micrograph the smaller black arrows mark the margins of the transitional cell, and the larger ones of the margins of the Purkinje cell. L = one of a group of lysosomes; N = the nucleus of the Purkinje cell. The myofibrils of the Purkinje cell are wispy, containing far fewer myofilaments per fibril than those in the transitional cell. Note the scalloping of the sarcolemma of both cells, with the indentations in registry with the Z bands of the myofibrils. (*From James and Sherf.*[113] *Reproduced with permission.*)

ing myocardial cells, a separate description of these contents is unnecessary.

Ameboid Cells

Ameboid cells were recently described[129,130] in electron micrographs of the eustachian ridge (Fig. 2-51 and 2-55). They have a number of characteristic and unusual features: The shape may be elongated, triangular, oval, or nongeometric. All ameboid cells have pseudopodic prolongations that fill the spaces between neighboring cells (Fig. 2-57). They are filled with a heavy concentration of electron-opaque granules (possibly glycogen), which give these cells a dark appearance. Their numerous myofibrils assure the propriety of their classification as myocardial cells. They also have many mitochondria; these appear in clusters, most often without relation to myofibrils. The mitochondria have a small number of cristae arranged in a simple way, and their overall size is smaller than that of the mitochondria of neighboring cells. Ameboid cells contain multilobular nuclei, sometimes of strange form, and variable

numbers of vacuoles, vesicles, and channels. They join only with P cells or slender transitional cells by simple membrane-to-membrane apposition.

Ameboid cells are considered as active cells performing some possibly important but as yet unknown function. An attractive hypothesis would attribute an integral role in some multicellular ectopic pacemaker. For example, ameboid cells could serve as a special frame or matrix for the few adjacent P cells. Other possible functions could account for their rich accumulations of dark granules resembling glycogen and their small, simple mitochondria; that is, they might serve as a kind of storehouse for energy-rich substrates ready to be delivered to the neighbor cells. Concerning this latter possibility, we noted that in the sinus node the mitochondria of the P cells had a very simple and empty appearance, whereas in the eustachian ridge the mitochondria of local P cells had an ordinary appearance; it is the adjacent ameboid cells that had small, simple mitochondria. Still another functional possibility is that, by their proximity to nerve elements, the ameboid cells serve as some sort of special connection between nerves and P cells, an especially important advantage for ectopic automatic centers. If this were to prove to be their true role, then the dark granules may be some form of neurotransmitter substance rather than glycogen granules. Numerous nerves were near all the ameboid–P cell complexes found in the eustachian ridge (Fig. 2-51), although the only direct neuromuscular junction that we found was to a myofibril-rich cell.

Purkinje Cells

The fourth type of cell concerned primarily with electrical activity of the heart is the *Purkinje cell*. The cell to be described here is classified primarily on the basis of its ultrastructural anatomy, and less on the basis of its distribution within the heart. This is the principal cell type in the His bundle and the bundle branches, although cells with ordinary working myocardial appearance may also be found interposed in the bundle branches. Purkinje cells are numerous in the internodal pathways, but within these pathways there are many interposed cells with the internal structure of working myocardium. Finally, Purkinje cells are numerous at all margins of the sinus node and AV node, and they form the usual link between transitional cells of either node and the rest of the heart. In sequential order of impulse origin and delivery from the sinus node, the route is from P cell to transitional cell and then to Purkinje cell. Conduction in the internodal pathways probably utilizes both Purkinje cells and interposed working myocardial cells, as well as intermingled transitional cells. At the AV node the sequence is from Purkinje cell to transitional cell, then numerous interposed P cells, and then from other transitional cells to the Purkinje cells of the His bundle. The remaining route for electrical activity is through Purkinje cells (and a few interposed working cells) of the bundle branches to the typical working myocardial cells of the ventricles.

Most Purkinje cells are both broader and shorter than working myocardial cells, measuring from 10 to 30 μm in cross section and 20 to 50 μm in length (Figs. 2-60 and 2-61). Purkinje cells have fewer myofibrils than working cells, but the number of myofilaments per fibril is comparatively even less, accounting for the wispy appearance of myofibrils in Purkinje cells seen with the light microscope. In contrast to those in P cells, however, the sparse myofibrils of Purkinje cells are usually linearly arrayed and in this feature more closely resemble working myocardium. The smaller number of myofibrils and of myofilaments per fibril helps account for the paler staining characteristic of Purkinje cells in light microscopic examination. Nuclei are centrally lo-

cated in Purkinje cells and are typically surrounded by a large "clear" zone which may contain many mitochondria but may also be relatively vacant of organelles. The myofibrils appear to skirt the region of the nucleus in Purkinje cells. When myofibrils are near the sarcolemma in either transitional cells or Purkinje cells, a periodic indentation is seen in register with the Z bands. Since Purkinje myofibrils are sparse, much of the cell surface is smooth, without indentation.

Because of the few myofibrils and small number of myofilaments per fibril, contractile power of Purkinje cells does not appear anatomically to be their important action; this is in keeping with physiologic knowledge indicating that conduction is their main function. Relative to rapid conduction, three anatomic features of Purkinje cells are pertinent: (1) they are short and broad: (2) there is less scalloped

FIGURE 2-61 An electron micrograph of three canine cells: on the left a Purkinje cell (PuC) with few myofibrils (My) and randomly arranged mitochondria (M), on the right two working myocardial cells (W) separated by an intercalated disc (ID) showing the parallel orderly array of myofibrils with their dark Z bands and the interfibrillar sandwiching of mitochondria (M). Note the increased number of myofibrils in the working myocardial cells as compared with the Purkinje cell, and note the steplike progression of the wavy, intercalated disk as it crosses the cell and how it remains equally spaced between the neighboring Z bands of each sarcomere. N = nuclei; C = capillary; Co = collagen; Nv = nerve.

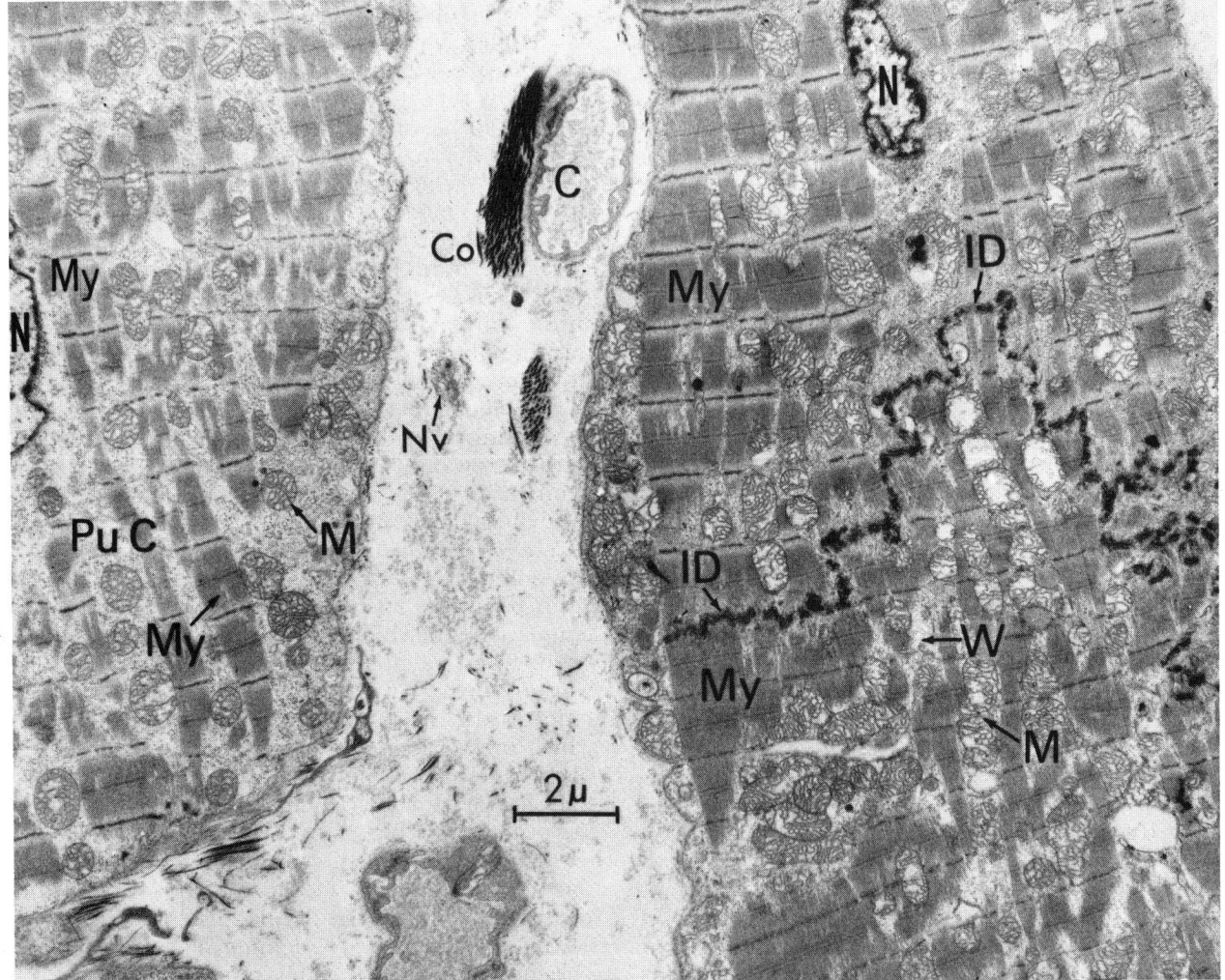

indentation of their sarcolemmae and presumably less perforation into the interior of the cells; and (3) they are joined end to end (less often end to side) through fully developed intercalated disks. The intercalated disk is also a characteristic terminal junction in working myocardial cells, which are narrower and much longer cells whose surface is more perforated for entrance of a more highly developed sarcotubular system. The functional significance of these differences can only be speculated upon at present, but it is possible that the numerous surface perforations represent sites of current leak or dilution from the surface to the interior of the cell in working myocardium. Because of its surface geometry, a broad myocardial cell probably offers less electrical resistance than a narrow cell and consequently conducts more rapidly.[127] If the intercalated disks act as points of low electrical resistance, as current physiologic evidence indicates,[131] then the larger number of these connections per fiber length for Purkinje cells may facilitate rapid conduction; for this interpretation it should be visualized that a Purkinje fiber contains many component Purkinje cells in series.

Except for their frequent dense accumulation about the nucleus, the mitochondria of Purkinje cells tend to be loosely arrayed between the sparse, thin myofibrils. Occasional simple mitochondria of the P-cell type are seen in Purkinje cells, and this may have functional significance relative to latent pacemaking activity. The sarcotubular system is more developed in regions containing more myofibrils than in other regions of Purkinje cells, but this development is seldom as extensive as in working myocardium. Anatomic features of other organelles in Purkinje cells either have been considered in the discussion of P cells or will be considered with working myocardial cells.

In both the His bundle and its proximal branches the Purkinje cells occur in longitudinally oriented strands separated by collagen. Intercellular junctions within the strands contain both desmosomes and numerous nexuses of exceptional size. These junctions are at the ends and along the sides of cells within each strand. The combination of longitudinal collagen partitions plus special junctions between cells in each strand strongly suggests normal longitudinal separation of conduction in this region.

Cells Concerned with the Mechanical Activity of the Heart

In contrast to the variety of cells concerned primarily with the heart's electrical activity, those cells concerned primarily with its mechanical activity are all of similar appearance, and this applies for both atrial and ventricular myocardium. As might be anticipated because the principal function is contraction, the large number and special arrangement of myofibrils are the most immediately apparent characteristics of working myocardial cells. However, as the fine structure is examined and studied more extensively, it is also becoming obvious that additional intricate internal organization and structure are present. For the long-continued efficient work of each myocardial cell in contraction, one might teleologically reason that a special intracellular system of structures for excitation, for excitation-contraction coupling, and for energy synthesis must be present.

The *general organization* of working myocardial cells is as follows: They are arranged longitudinally in series, with multiple cells forming a "fiber" as seen with the light microscope, and with most fibers arrayed parallel to one another. In contrast to skeletal muscle, cardiac muscle fibers have many lateral and end-to-side connections. But contrary to the prevailing interpretation prior to appropriate electron microscopic studies, the cells of the working myocardium are not an anatomic syncytium. In addition to the lateral margins (sarcolemma) of working myocardial cells, which have always been recognized, the intercalated disks which form their terminal margins and junctions are now known to be the site of a transversely oriented cell boundary which is of specialized structure.[132,133] In working myocardial cells the myofibrils insert in the region of the intercalated disk, which means that the disk must possess unusual strength to support the forces generated by constantly repeated contraction of the myofibrils. In contrast to the sparse linear myofibrils of Purkinje cells, and the sparse randomly distributed myofibrils of P cells, the myofibrils of working myocardial cells are packed into a remarkably organized linear array, with the mitochondria sandwiched in lines between the fibrils. The nucleus of working myocardial cells is centrally located and slightly elongated in the long axis of the cell. The internal features and membranes are similar to those of nuclei in other myocardial cells and, similarly, not much is known about their function. The elongated shape of working myocardial cells, which are 10 to 20 μm in diameter and 50 to 100 μm in length, is an ideal geometric shape for their main function, which is mechanical contraction.

The *membranes* of working myocardial cells are composed of the same layers as the other cells described, but along the lateral margins the sarcolemma is regularly indented in register with the Z bands to give a scalloped appearance to the typical working myocardial cell. The depth of this indentation is due in part to the state of contraction in which the working cell was fixed. From the depth of this indentation there is a special penetration into the cell, which will be discussed further on with the sarcotubular system.

At the end of each working myocardial cell the *intercalated disk* forms a characteristic "zigzag" border between cells (Fig. 2-63). At the lateral surface of this junction the sarcolemma separates into the basement membrane, which continues from one cell to the next, and the plasma membrane, which is directed at near-right angles inward to appose the plasma membrane of the other cell. Within the disk the plasma membranes of apposing cells are brought in close proximity, the intercellular space being about 100 Å. Considered in three dimensions, the intercalated disk is not a single plane but may be thought of as two interdigitated mountain ranges, with peaks of one cell thrusting into valleys of the next. The plasma membranes of the intercalated disk appear to be more electron-dense than those on the lateral surface of the cell. Areas of much closer approximation of the plasma membranes occur almost exclusively along the lateral margins of the protrusions from one cell into another, and have been called *nexus*[134] or *zonula occludens*.

Recent technical advances have led to revision of the concept that there is true fusion between the plasma membranes at the nexuses.[135] An electron-opaque tracer (lanthanum hydroxide) and the freeze-cleave technique permit demonstration of the nexus formed by close apposition of two unit membranes (plasma membranes), but with a distinct gap still interposed. On this basis the term *gap junction* is a better synonym for the nexus than is *tight junction*. Furthermore, there is suggestive evidence of central hydrophilic communication (e.g., for K^+ ions); this supports the interpretation of the nexus as a focus of low resistance to spread of the electric impulse.[136]

The position of the intercalated disk relative to the length of the working myocardial cell is always at the regular periodic location of the Z band of the myofibrils, but the disk shifts from the region of one Z band to another in a characteristic steplike manner within the cell, to continue higher or lower in an adjacent myofibril (Figs. 2-61). At the transverse portion of the cell interface, the paired plasma membranes remain separated at a fixed space, but a number of points of cytoplasmic deposits of moderate density accumulate, giving the dark appearance to the intercalated disk. When these deposits are short (along the line of the plasma membrane), they are termed *desmosomes* (macula adherens[137]). Longer membrane appositions without "fusion," and without adjacent electron-dense accumulations, have been named *fasciae occludens* by Fawcett.[138] All fine-structure features of the intercalated disk are relatively new knowledge, and much more needs to be learned about this important region.

The *sarcotubular system* of working myocardial cells (Figs. 2-62 and 2-63) is an extensive complicated network of intracellular tubules, vesicles, and cisternae.[122-126] It is composed of two principal components. The first is formed by the periodic invagination of the sarcolemma, as mentioned above, and appears as a double-layered, transversely oriented tubular system known as the T system. In the neighborhood of the Z band, focal dilatation of the T-system tubules is seen, forming a cistern-like structure known as the *intermediary vesicle*.[139] The second component of the sarcotubular system consists of a series of thin-layered interconnecting tubules longitudinally oriented parallel to and surrounding the myofibril. This component also has local dilatations, known as *lateral sacs* or *terminal cisternae*. At the level of the Z band the vesicular dilatations of the two components form a characteristic structure called a *triad*. It consists of the medially placed intermediary vesicle from the T system, flanked by the two lateral sacs of the longitudinal system. The three components of the triad are in very close apposition, but no direct communication is known to exist between the longitudinal and transverse systems;[139] and this noncommunication is important in understanding function within the working myocardial cell.

This general image of the sarcotubular system has been recently modified—it is apparently more characteristic of skeletal muscle than of mammalian myocardium. In myocardium the term *transverse tubules* accurately describes their prevailing distribution, but it is now clear that the transverse tubules also branch in a longitudinal direction and directly connect successive transverse tubules.[108,140] The longitudinal system (or sarcoplasmic reticulum), on the other hand, is a plexiform labyrinth of tubules and is *not* locally modified in relation to particular bands of the repeating cross section. In fact, this system also possesses many transversely oriented profiles.[141] Most authors agree today that no true triads exist in mammalian myocardium. Instead, one finds sites of close proximity between the sarcoplasmic reticulum (longitudinal system), and both the transverse tubules are in fact invaginations of the sarcolemma; a general term *subsarcolemma cisternae* has been suggested for both sites of proximity. This term is equally descriptive of central (T system) and peripheral (sarcolemma) sites of proximity.[108]

In recent years it has become clear that the sarcotubular system plays an important part in electric impulse conduction[142] and electromechanical coupling.[139] It was once thought that impulses flowing down the sarcolemma of the cells produced contraction of myofibrils by diffusion of calcium into the core of the fibril.[143] In 1949, however, Hill[144] demonstrated that an entire section of each cell became active in a time too short to be accounted for by diffusion of an ion over the relatively long pathway from the surface to the center of the fiber. When the transverse system was first described, the attention of many investigators was drawn to the possibility that it was involved in the more rapid channeling of the electrical excitation wave into the interior of the cell.[142,145] And indeed the continuity of these tubules with the outside of the cell was soon elegantly proved when ferritin introduced into the extracellular fluid was detected at the triad inside the cell only in the intermediary vesicles of the T system,[146] an observation subsequently confirmed using horseradish peroxidase as a tracer.[140] The inward conduction of electric impulses through the

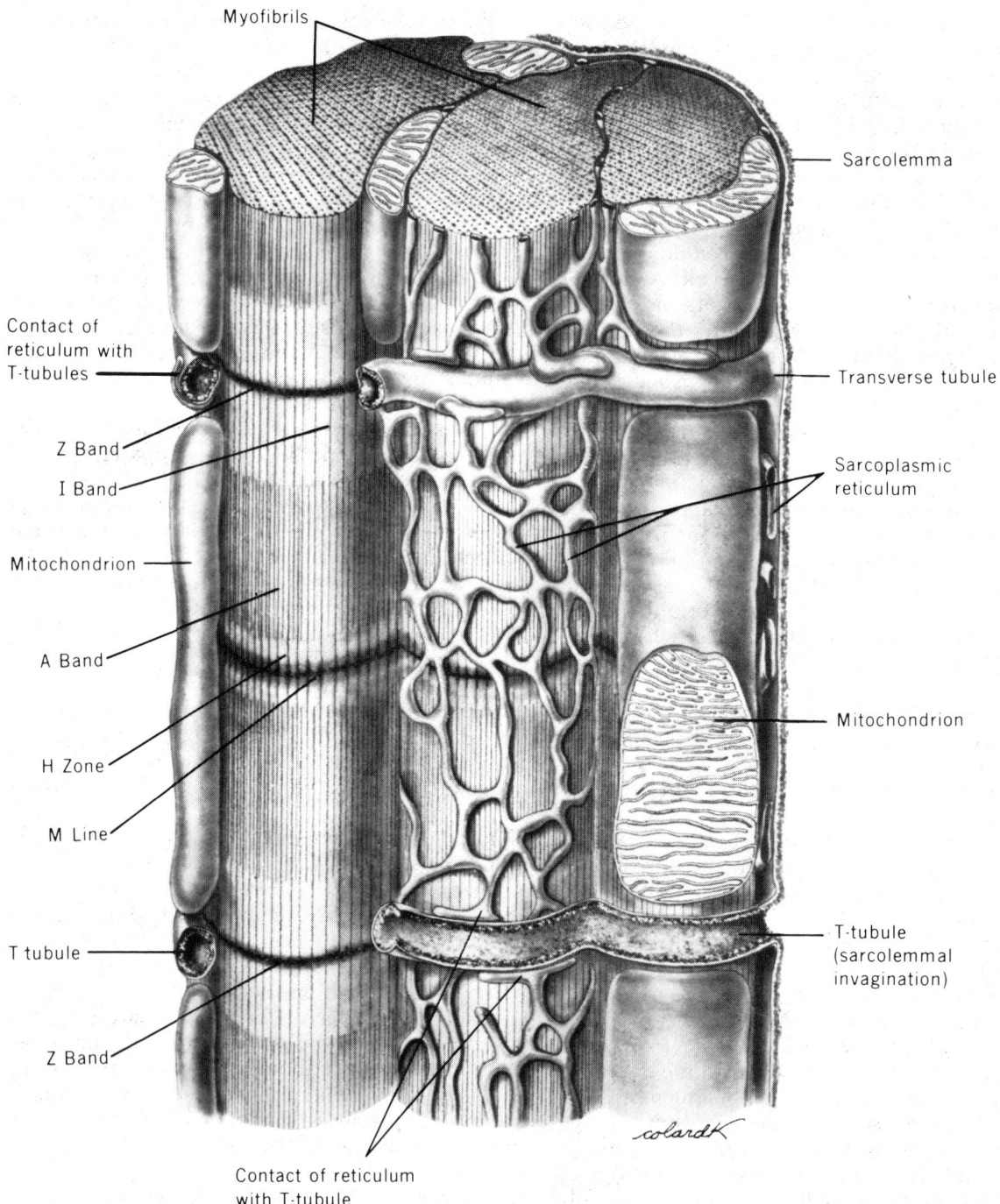

Myofibrils

Sarcolemma

Contact of reticulum with T-tubules

Transverse tubule

Z Band

I Band

Sarcoplasmic reticulum

Mitochondrion

A Band

H Zone

M Line

Mitochondrion

T tubule

T-tubule (sarcolemmal invagination)

Z Band

Contact of reticulum with T-tubule

FIGURE 2-62 Schematic representation of myocardium. Sarcomere extends from one Z band to the other. Mitochondria, sarcoplasmic reticulum, and T tubules are also shown. (*Modified from Fawcett and McNutt*[108] *and the drawing by Sylvia Colard Keene.*)

channel of the T system was convincingly demonstrated by Huxley and Taylor,[142] who were able to produce precise microcontraction in parts of a myofibril when the impulse was placed on the surface membrane at points exactly opposite to the triads (i.e., the surface entrance to the system).

While the inward spread of the electric impulse into the cell is now largely accepted as a function of the T system, increasing evidence links the longitudinal component with the process of electrome-

chanical coupling. It was recently shown that calcium, an essential factor in muscular contraction, actively accumulates in the longitudinal component at the same point where ATPase activity occurs.[147] This demonstration led investigators to suggest that an ATP-dependent "calcium pump" is active in the lateral sacs of the triad.[148] The phasic movement of calcium ions into and out of the lateral sacs may cause the cyclic variations in the concentration of calcium ions around the contractile elements nec-

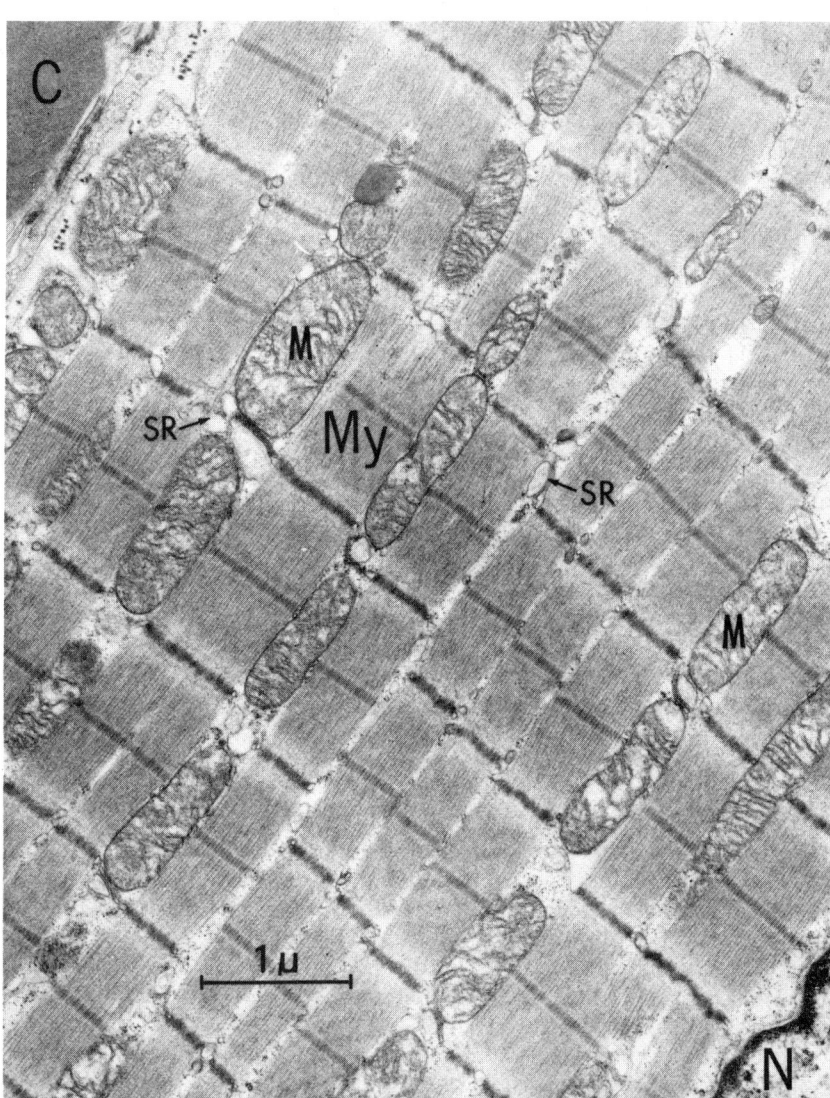

FIGURE 2-63 Electron micrograph of canine working myocardium illustrating the sandwiched array of mitochondria between myofibrils and the packed content of a working cell. My = myofibrils; M = mitochondria; SR = sarcoplastic reticulum; C = capillary; N = nucleus.

essary for muscular contraction or relaxation.[139] How the action potential transmitted through the tubules of the T system into the intermediary vesicles activates the release of calcium from the lateral sacs is not known. (See Chap. 3.)

The myofibrils are the contractile element of working myocardial cells (Figs. 2-61 to 2-63). They are long, parallel strands, longitudinally arranged inside the cell. The myofibrils exhibit a periodic pattern of dark and light areas, which are formed by a repeating morphologic and functional unit, the sarcomere.

The sarcomere is 1.5 to 2.2 μm long, depending on the degree of relaxation or contraction of the myofibril,[149] and is composed of interdigitating thick and thin protein filaments. The sarcomere is bounded at either end by a very dark line known as the Z band. Anchored on these Z bands, and extending toward the center of the sarcomere, are thin filaments measuring 1 μm in length and composed mostly of actin molecules and some tropomyosin B (another contractile protein).[150] The central part of

the sarcomere is occupied by the thick filaments, showing knoblike excrescences in their center, where cross bridges between them are seen.[148] The thick filaments measure 1.5 μm in length and are composed of still another protein, myosin.

The dark and light zones in the sarcomere are the optical counterpart of the relation between the thin and the thick filaments (Figs. 2-61 to 2-63). During a moderate stretch of the myofibrils, the following pattern is observed: Extending in either direction from the Z band (into adjacent sarcomeres) is a light area where only thin actin filaments are seen. This is the I band, so called because it is isotropic under polarized light. The broad central darker area between the two peripherally located I bands of the sarcomere is called the A band (anisotropic). A lighter one crossing the center of the A band is called the H zone, and this region contains only the thick myosin filaments; where these myosin filaments interdigitate with knoblike excrescences in the center of the H zone, there is a thin line known as the M line. Five thin lines can often be resolved within the M line. The structural basis for these periodic linear markings is probably the optical superimposition of intermyosin cross bridges occurring in lateral register at five specific sites along the M band.[108] The remainder of the A band, extending in either direction from the H zone to each adjacent I band, is darker than the H zone and contains both thin actin and thick myosin filaments, which are telescoped parallel to each other. If we inspect a sarcomere from one end to the other, we see consecutively the Z band, the I band, the A band with its lighter H zone and central M line, the next I band, and finally the second Z band. This periodicity in sarcomeres is the same in cardiac and skeletal muscle.

When the myofibril is cut transversely (Figs. 2-62 and 2-64), the two types of filaments can be seen together or alone, depending on the region of the sarcomere where the cut was made. In the H-zone and M-line area, only thick myosin filaments will be observed, arranged in a hexagonal pattern; in the I band, only thin actin filaments, which are evenly spaced, can be seen. Finally, in the A band (*except* in the H zone), interdigitation of the two types of filaments is found in the form of a regular hexagonal pattern, six thin actin filaments surrounding one thick myosin filament, with each hexagonal group in turn surrounded at its points by six other thick myosin filaments.[139] Connecting bridges between thick and thin filaments can be seen.[151]

The working myocardial cell is thus uniformly organized not only longitudinally but also transversely. A single cell contains hundreds of parallel myofibrils. Sandwiched between them are rows of mitochondria (Figs. 2-62 and 2-63). As part of the orderly arrangement, the Z bands of different myofibrils are in precise register, as are consequently the I and A bands, thus forming the characteristic cross striations noted on light microscopy. This anatomic precision in the muscle cell affords a maximal degree of synchronization during contraction.

Theories of muscle contraction have been much simplified following the introduction of Huxley and Hanson's *sliding filament hypothesis*[152] for skeletal muscle. Recent studies support the application of this theory to the myocardium as well. It was observed that while the myocardial sarcomere length shortened during contraction, by the approaching of the two opposite Z bands, neither of the two component filaments decreased in length. The length of the A band, containing all the thick filaments, remained the same; while the width of the I band decreased, that of the H zone within the A band concomitantly decreased approximately the same amount, so that the length of the thin filament also did not change.[149] What changed was only the relation between the two sets of filaments. On the basis of these observations, Huxley and Hanson[152] suggested that the muscle shortens because the two sets of filaments slide past each other. The actin filaments are pulled or propelled toward the center of

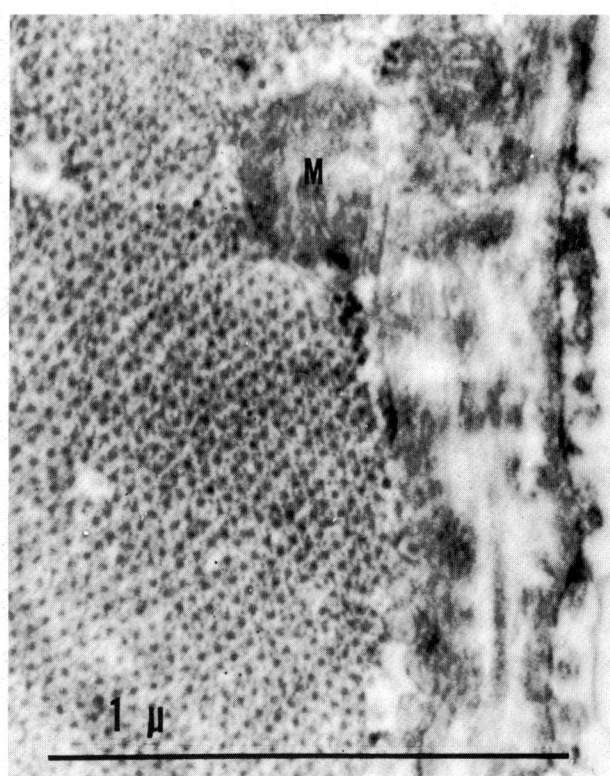

FIGURE 2-64 Electron micrograph of hexagonal array of actin and myosin filaments in cross section of canine working myocardial cell. One mitochondrion is labeled M. An intercellular cleft descends vertically in the right half of the picture. Note the geometric relation of the thin actin and thick myosin filaments.

the sarcomere by linkages between the myosin and actin filaments (actomyosin), links which are made and detached cyclically. The myosin component for the linkage is thought to be composed of a subcomponent of the myosin molecule, the heavy (H) meromyosin.[153] This H meromyosin fraction contains both the properties for combining with actin and the ATPase needed to split the ATP. Davies[154] suggested that calcium ions form chelate links between bound ATP in the H meromyosin and the bound ADP of the actin filament. When the ATP is split by ATPase, and the calcium is reaccumulated in the sarcotubular system by the calcium pump, then the link between the two filaments is broken and the cycle starts over. The ATP needed for energy is produced in the neighboring mitochondria.

The *mitochondria* of working myocardial cells (Figs. 2-62 and 2-63) are cylindrically shaped bodies, 2 by 0.5 μm, delimited by a double membrane. Numerous platelike infoldings, known as the *cristae*, project inward from the delimiting membrane. They are closely packed inside the mitochondrion and arranged in a specific order. Dense granules measuring several hundred angstroms are sometimes observed between the cristae. The mitochondria are very numerous in the myocardium, composing between 25 and 50 percent of the entire myocardial mass.[149] They are arranged in rows between the myofibrils of the working cells.

The mitochondria are the principal site of oxidative phosphorylation, the process by which ATP molecules are produced with the energy contained in carbohydrates, lipids, and proteins. The enzymes involved in oxidative phosphorylation are presumed to exist in sterically ordered arrays on the cristae, for the order needed in the step-by-step biochemical reactions. The exact way by which the ATP is then transferred from the mitochondrion to the myofibril is not known. The great number of mitochondria in the myocardium, as well as the great number of cristae inside each mitochondrion, is commensurate with the tremendous need of energy by the continuously contracting heart muscle. Fawcett and McNutt[108] have demonstrated slender prolongations of mitochondria and suggested two possible functional interpretations: the slender fronds are a form of mitochondrial reproduction by budding, or such mitochondrial branches provide a means to redistribute mitochondrial mass into narrow interfibrillar interstices for optimal diffusion.

References

1. Keith, A.: The Functional Anatomy of the Heart, Lecture before the Harveian Society of London, March 21, 1918, *Br. Med. J.,* 1:361, 1918.
*2. Walmsley, R.: The Orientation of the Heart and the Appearance of Its Chamber in the Adult Cadaver, *Br. Heart J.,* 20:441, 1958. (4 references)
3. Davies, M. J., Pomerance, A., and Lamb, D.: Techniques in Examination and Anatomy of the Heart, in A. Pomerance and M. J. Davies (eds.), "The Pathology of the Heart," Blackwell Scientific Publications, Ltd., Oxford, 1975, pp. 1–48.
4. Van Mierop, L. H. S.: Anatomy of the Heart, *Clin. Symp.,* 17:67, 1965.
5. McAlpine, W. A.: "Heart and Coronary Arteries," Springer-Verlag New York, Inc., New York, 1975.
6. Grant, R. P.: Architectonics of the Heart, *Am. Heart J.,* 46:405, 1953.
7. Burton, A. C.: The Importance of the Shape and Size of the Heart, *Am. Heart J.,* 54:801, 1957.
8. Zimmerman, J.: The Functional and Surgical Anatomy of the Heart, *Ann. R. Coll. Surg. Engl.,* 39:348, 1966.
*9. Walmsley, R., and Watson, H.: The Outflow Tract of the Left Ventricle, *Br. Heart J.,* 28:435, 1966. (13 references)
10. Rosenquist, G. C., and Sweeney, L. J.: The Membranous Ventricular Septum in the Normal Heart, *Johns Hopkins Med. J.,* 135:9, 1974.
11. Lev, M.: The Normal Anatomy of the Conduction System in Man and Its Pathology in Atrioventricular Block, *Ann. N.Y. Acad. Sci.,* 111:817, 1964.
12. Bradfield, J. W. B., Beck, G., and Vecht, R. J.: Left Ventricular Apical Thin Point, *Br. Heart J.,* 39:806, 1977.
13. Walmsley, R., and Watson, H.: The Medial Wall of the Right Atrium, *Circulation,* 34:400, 1966.

*14. Sweeney, L. J., and Rosenquist, G. C.: The Normal Anatomy of the Atrial Septum in the Human Heart, *Am. Heart J.,* 98:194, 1979. (28 references)
15. Prakash, R.: Determination of Right Ventricular Wall Thickness in Systole and Diastole: Echocardiographic and Necropsy Correlation in 32 Patients, *Br. Heart J.,* 40:1257, 1978.
16. Grant, R. P., Downey, F. M., and MacMahon, H.: The Architecture of the Right Ventricular Outflow Tract in the Normal Heart and in the Presence of Ventricular Septal Defects, *Circulation,* 24:223, 1961.
17. Grant, R. P.: Notes on the Muscular Architecture of the Left Ventricle, *Circulation,* 32:301, 1965.
18. Kennedy, J. W., Baxley, W. A., Figley, M. M., Dodge, H. T., and Blackmon, J. R.: Quantitative Angiocardiography: I. The Normal Left Ventricle in Man, *Circulation,* 34:272, 1966.
*19. Walmsley, R.: Anatomy of Left Ventricular Outflow Tract, *Br. Heart J.,* 41:263, 1979. (2 references)
20. Zimmerman, J.: The Functional and Surgical Anatomy of the Aortic Valve, *Isr. Med. J.,* 5:862, 1969.
21. Merklin, R. J.: Position and Orientation of the Heart Valves, *Am. J. Anat.,* 125:375, 1969.
22. Vollebergh, F. E. M. G., and Becker, A. E.: Minor Congenital Variations of Cusp Size in Tricuspid Aortic Valves: Possible Link with Isolated Aortic Stenosis, *Br. Heart J.,* 39:1006, 1977.
23. Silverman, M. E., and Hurst, J. W.: The Mitral Complex, *Am. Heart J.,* 76:399, 1968.
24. Ranganathan, N., Lam, J. H. C., Wigle, E. D., and Silver, M. D.: Morphology of the Human Mitral Valve. II. The Valve Leaflets, *Circulation,* 41:459, 1970.
*25. Perloff, J. K., and Roberts, W. C.: The Mitral Apparatus: Functional Anatomy of Mitral Regurgitation, *Circulation,* 46:227, 1972. (54 references)
*26. Walmsley, R.: Anatomy of Human Mitral Valve in Adult Cadaver and Comparative Anatomy of the Valve, *Br. Heart J.,* 40:351, 1978. (22 references)
*27. Silver, M. D., Lam, J. H. C., Ranganathan, N., and Wigle, E. D.: Morphology of the Human Tricuspid Valve, *Circulation,* 43:333, 1971. (15 references)
28. Estes, E. H., Jr., Dalton, F. M., Entman, M. L., Dixon, H. D., II, and Hackel, D. B.: The Anatomy and Blood Supply of the Papillary Muscles of the Left Ventricle, *Am. Heart J.,* 71:356, 1966.
29. Lam, J. H. C., Ranganathan, N., Wigle, E. D., and Silver, M. D.: Morphology of the Human Mitral Valve. I. Chordae Tendineae, *Circulation,* 41:449, 1970.
*30. Holt, J. P.: The Normal Pericardium, *Am. J. Cardiol.,* 26:455, 1970. (85 references)
31. Mitchell, G. A. G.: "Cardiovascular Innervation," The Williams & Wilkins Company, Baltimore, 1956.
32. White, J. C.: Cardiac Pain: Anatomic Pathways and Physiologic Mechanisms, *Circulation,* 16:644, 1957.
33. Hirsch, E. F.: The Innervation of the Human Heart, *Arch. Pathol.,* 75:378, 1963.
*34. Johnson, R. A., and Blake, T. M.: Lymphatics of the Heart, *Circulation,* 33:137, 1966. (25 references)
35. Rusznyak, I.: "Lymphatics and Lymph Circulation: Physiology and Pathology," L. Youlten (ed.),

*This article is a review of the literature and contains additional references to the literature.

2d English ed., Oxford, England, Pergamon Press, New York, 1967, p. 971.

36. Yoffey, J. M., and Courtice, F. C.: "Lymphatics, Lymph and Lymphomyeloid Complex," Academic Press, Inc., New York, 1970.

37. Fishman, A. P., and Hecht, H. H. (eds.): "The Pulmonary Circulation and Intestinal Space," The University of Chicago Press, Chicago, 1969, p. 432.

*38. James, T. N.: "Anatomy of the Coronary Arteries," Hoeber Medical Division, Harper & Row, Publishers, Inc., New York, 1961. (Extensively referenced)

39. Vieussens, R.: Nouvelles découvertes sur le coeur, Paris, 1706.

40. Schlesinger, M. J., Zoll, P. M., and Wessler, S.: The Conus Artery: A Third Coronary Artery, *Am. Heart J.,* 38:823, 1949.

41. Bianchi, A.: Morfologia delle arteriae coronariae cordis, *Arch. Ital. Anat. Embriol.,* 3:87, 1904.

42. Spalteholz, W.: "Die Arterien der Herzwand," S. Hirzel Verlag KG, Stuttgart, 1924.

43. Marshall, J.: On the Development of the Great Anterior Veins in Man and Mammalia; Including an Account of Certain Remnants of Foetal Structure Found in the Adult: A Comparative View of These Great Veins in the Different Mammalia, and an Analysis of Their Occasional Peculiarities in the Human Subject, *Philos. Trans. R. Soc. Lond. (Biol. Sci.),* 140:133, 1850.

44. Vastesaeger, M. M., Van Der Straeten, P. O., Friart, J., Candaele, G., Ghys, A., and Bernard, R. M.: Les Anastomoses intercoronariennes telles qu'elles apparaissent a la coronarographie post mortem, *Acta Cardiol. (Brux.),* 12:365, 1957.

45. Laubry, C. H., Soulie, P., and Thys, H.: Les Anastomoses septales, *Arch. Mal. Coeur,* 141:1, 1948.

46. Laurie, W., and Woods, J. D.: Anastomoses of the Coronary Circulation, *Lancet,* 2:812, 1958.

47. Pepler, W. J., and Meyer, B. J.: Interarterial Coronary Anastomoses and Coronary Arterial Pattern, *Circulation,* 22:14, 1960.

48. Bellman, S., and Frank, H. A.: Intercoronary Collaterals in Normal Hearts, *J. Thorac. Surg.,* 36:584, 1958.

49. Prinzmetal, M., Simkin, B., Bergman, H. C., and Kruger, H. E.: Studies on the Coronary Circulation. II. The Collateral Circulation of the Normal Human Heart by Coronary Perfusion with Radioactive Erythrocytes and Glass Spheres, *Am. Heart J.,* 33:420, 1947.

50. Baroldi, G., Mantero, O., and Scomozoni, G.: The Collaterals of the Coronary Arteries in Normal and Pathologic Heart, *Circ. Res.,* 4:223, 1956.

51. Blumgart, H. L., Schlesinger, M. J., and Davis, D.: Studies on the Relation of the Clinical Manifestations of Angina Pectoris, Coronary Thrombosis, and Myocardial Infarction to the Pathologic Findings, *Am. Heart J.,* 19:1, 1940.

52. James, T. N.: The Delivery and Distribution of Coronary Collateral Circulation, *Chest,* 58:183, 1970.

53. James, T. N., and Burch, G. E.: Blood Supply of the Human Interventricular Septum, *Circulation,* 17:391, 1958.

54. Anderson, K. R., Ho, S. Y., and Anderson, R. H.: Location and Vascular Supply of Sinus Node in Human Heart. *Br. Heart J.,* 41:28, 1979.

55. James, T. N.: Myocardial Infarction and Atrial Arrhythmias, *Circulation,* 24:761, 1961.

56. Wood, F. C., Wolferth, C. C., and Bellet, S.: Infarction of the Lateral Wall of the Left Ventricle: Electrocardiographic Characteristics, *Am. Heart J.,* 16:387, 1938.

57. James, T. N.: A Useful Landmark for Interpreting Angiocardiograms, *Radiology,* 75:804, 1963.

58. Kugel, M. A.: Anatomical Studies on the Coronary Arteries and Their Branches. I. Arteria Anastomotica Auricularis Magna, *Am. Heart J.,* 3:260, 1927.

59. James, T. N.: Posterior Myocardial Infarction, *J. Mich. Med. Soc.,* 60:1409, 1961.

*60. James, T. N.: The Coronary Circulation and Conduction System in Acute Myocardial Infarction, *Prog. Cardiovasc. Dis.,* 10:410, 1968. (95 references)

61. James, T. N.: An Etiologic Concept Concerning the Obscure Myocardiopathies, *Prog. Cardiovasc. Dis.,* 7:43, 1964.

62. James, T. N.: Pathology of the Small Coronary Arteries, *Am. J. Cardiol.,* 20:679, 1967.

63. Varnauskas, E., Ivemark, B., Paulin, S., and Ryden, B.: Obscure Cardiomyopathies with Coronary Artery Changes, *Am. J. Cardiol.,* 19:531, 1967.

64. Saphir, O., Ohringer, L., and Wong, R.: Changes of the Intramural Coronary Branches in Coronary Arteriosclerosis, *A.M.A. Arch. Pathol.,* 62:159, 1956.

65. More, B. M., and Sommers, S. C.: The Status of the Myocardial Arterioles in Angina Pectoris, *Am. Heart J.,* 64:323, 1962.

66. Donomae, I., Matsumoto, Y., Kokubu, T., et al.: Pathological Studies of Coronary Atherosclerosis: Especially of Sclerosis of Intramuscular Coronary Arteries, *Jpn. Heart J.,* 3:423, 1962.

67. His, W., Jr.: Die Thätigkeit des embryonalen Herzens und deren Bedeutung fur die Lehre von der Hersbewegung beim Erwachsenen, *Arb. Med. Klin.,* vol. 14, 1893.

68. Tawara, S.: "Das Reizleitungssystem des Saugetierherzens," G. Fischer, Jena, 1906.

69. Keith, A., and Flack, M.: The Form and Nature of the Muscular Connections between the Primary Divisions of the Vertebrate Heart, *J. Anat. Physiol.,* 41:172, 1907.

70. Walmsley, T.: Comparative Anatomy of the Heart, in "Quain's Elements of Anatomy," Longmans, Green, & Co., Ltd., London, 1929, part III, vol. 4, p. 3.

71. Patten, B. M.: "Human Embryology," 2d ed., McGraw-Hill Book Company, New York, 1953.

72. Weidmann, S.: Resting and Action Potentials of Cardiac Muscle, *Ann, N.Y. Acad. Sci.,* 65:663, 1957.

73. Hudson, R. E. B.: The Human Pacemaker and Its Pathology, *Br. Heart J.,* 2:153, 1960.

*74. James, T. N.: Anatomy of the Human Sinus Node, *Anat. Rec.,* 141:109, 1961. (26 references)

75. James, T. N.: Pericarditis and the Sinus Node, *Arch. Intern. Med.,* 110:305, 1962.

76. Soderstrom, N.: Myocardial Infarction and Mural Thrombosis in the Atria of the Heart, *Acta Med. Scand.,* 132(suppl. 217):114, 1948.

77. James, T. N., and Nadeau, R. A.: Sinus Bradycardia during Injections Directly into the Sinus Node Artery, *Am. J. Physiol.,* 204:9, 1963.

78. James, T. N., and Nadeau, R. A.: Effects of Sym-

pathomimetic Amines Studied by Direct Perfusion of the Sinus Node, *Am. J. Physiol.,* 204:591, 1963.

79. James, T. N., and Nadeau, R. A.: Selective Cholinergic Stimulation and Blockade of the Sinus Node by Direct Perfusion through Its Artery, *J. Lab. Clin. Med.,* 62:40, 1963.

80. James, T. N., and Nadeau, R. A.: Relation of Retrograde Pressure in the Sinus Node Artery to Sinus Tachycardia from Stellate Stimulation, *J. Lab. Clin. Med.,* 62:777, 1963.

81. James, T. N., and Nadeau, R. A.: The Effects of Vagal Stimulation, Eserine, and Atropine on Retrograde Pressure in the Sinus Node Artery, *Henry Ford Hosp. Med. Bull.,* 12:23, 1964.

82. James, T. N.: Pulse and Impulse of the Sinus Node, *Henry Ford Hosp. Med. J.,* 15:275, 1967.

83. Grant, R. P.: The Mechanism of A-V Arrhythmias: With an Electronic Analogue of the Human A-V Node, *Am. J. Med.,* 20:334, 1956.

*84. James, T. N.: Cardiac Innervation: Anatomic and Pharmacologic Relations, *Bull. N. Y. Acad. Med.,* 43:1041, 1967. (96 references)

85. Harary, I.: Heart Cells in Vitro, *Sci. Am.,* 206:141, 1962.

86. James, T. N.: Myocardial Infarction and Atrial Arrhythmias, *Circulation,* 24:761, 1961.

87. Hoffman, B. F., and Cranefield, P. F.: "Electrophysiology of the Heart," McGraw-Hill Book Company, New York, 1960.

*88. James, T. N.: Morphology of the Human Atrioventricular Node, with Remarks Pertinent to Its Electrophysiology, *Am. Heart J.,* 62:756, 1961. (54 references)

89. Moe, G. K., Preston, J. B., and Burlington, H.: Physiologic Evidence for a Dual A-V Transmission System, *Circ. Res.,* 4:357, 1956.

90. James, T. N.: The Wolff-Parkinson-White Syndrome: Evolving Concepts of Its Pathogenesis, *Prog. Cardiovasc. Dis.,* 13:159, 1970.

91. Brumlik, J. V.: The Sinoatrial Node, the Atrioventricular Node and Atrial Dysrhythmias, in Charles E. Kossman (ed.), "Advances in Electrocardiography," Grune & Stratton, Inc., New York, 1958, p. 252.

92. Juhasz-Nagy, A., and Szentivanyi, H.: Localization of the Receptors of the Coronary Chemoreflex in the Dog, *Arch. Int. Pharmacodyn.,* 131:39, 1961.

93. Dawes, G. S.: Studies on Veratrum Alkaloids. VII. Receptor Areas in the Coronary Arteries and Elsewhere as Revealed by the Use of Veratridine, *J. Pharmacol. Exp. Ther.,* 89:325, 1947.

94. Dawes, G. S.: Cardiovascular Reflexes and Myocardial Infarction, in T. N. James and J. W. Keyes (eds.), "The Etiology of Myocardial Infarction," Little, Brown and Company, Boston, 1961.

95. James, T. N., and Sherf, L.: Fine Structure of the His Bundle, *Circulation,* 44:9, 1971.

*96. Massing, G. K., and James, T. N.: Anatomic Configuration of the His Bundle and Bundle Branches in the Human Heart, *Circulation,* 53:609, 1976. (30 references)

97. Truex, R. C.: Comparative Anatomy and Functional Considerations of the Cardiac Conduction System, in A. P. DeCarvalho (ed.), "Specialized Tissues of the Heart," American Elsevier Publishing Company, Inc., New York, 1962, p. 22.

*98. James, T. N.: The Connecting Pathways between the Sinus Node and the A-V Node and between the Right and the Left Atrium in the Human Heart, *Am. Heart J.,* 66:498, 1963. (24 references)

99. James. T. N.: Anatomy of the Sinus Node of the Dog, *Anat. Rec.,* 143:251, 1962.

100. Wenckebach, K. F.: Beitrage zur Kenntnis der menschlichen Herztatigkeit, *Arch. Anat. Physiol.,* 3:53, 1908.

101. Thorel, C.: Vorlaufige Mittelung uber eine besondere Muskel verbindung zwischen der Cava superior und dem Hisschen Bundel, *Munch. Med. Wochenschr.,* 56:2159, 1909.

102. Thorel, C.: Uber den Aufbaum des Sinusknotens und seine Verbindung mit der Cava superior und den Wenckebachschen Bundeln, *Munch. Med. Wochenschr.,* 57:183, 1910.

103. Bachmann, G.: The Inter-auricular Time Interval, *Am. J. Physiol.,* 41:309, 1916.

104. James. T. N.: Anatomy of the Cardiac Conduction System in the Rabbit, *Circ. Res.,* 20:638, 1967.

105. Marshall, J.: On the Development of the Great Anterior Veins in Man and Mammalia; Including an Account of Certain Remnants of Foetal Structure Found in the Adult, a Comparative View of These Great Veins in the Different Mammalia, and an Analysis of Their Occasional Peculiarities in the Human Subject, *Philos. Trans. R. Soc. Lond. (Biol. Sci.),* 140:133, 1850.

*106. James, T. N., and Sherf, L.: Specialized Tissues and Preferential Conduction in the Atria of the Heart, *Am. J. Cardiol.,* 28:414, 1971. (86 references)

107. Sherf, L., and James, T. N.: QRS Abnormalities in AV Block: Variations and Their Significance, in J. W. Hurst and R. C. Schlant (eds.), "Chapters in Advanced Electrocardiography," Grune & Stratton, Inc., New York, 1972, p. 81.

*108. Fawcett, D. W., and McNutt, N. S.: The Ultrastructure of the Cat Myocardium. I. Ventricular Papillary Muscle, *J. Cell Biol.,* 42:1, 1969. (115 references)

*109. McNutt, N. S., and Fawcett, D. W.: The Ultrastructure of the Cat Myocardium. II. Atrial Muscle, *J. Cell Biol.,* 42:46, 1969. (39 references)

110. Kawamura, K.: Electron Microscope Studies on the Cardiac Conduction System of the Dog. I. The Purkinje Fiber. II. The Sinoatria and Atrioventricular Nodes, *Jpn. Circ. J.,* 25:594, 1961.

111. Trautwein, W., and Uchizono, K.: Electron Microscopic and Electrophysiolgic Study of the Pacemaker and the Sino-atrial Node of the Rabbit Heart, *Z. Zellforsch. Mikrosk. Anat.,* 61:96, 1963.

*112. James, T. N., Sherf, L., Fine, G., and Morales, A. R.: Comparative Ultrastructure of the Sinus Node in Man and Dog, *Circulation,* 34:139, 1966. (45 references)

*113. James, T. N., and Sherf, L.: Ultrastructure of the Human Atrioventricular Node, *Circulation,* 37:1049, 1968. (30 references)

*114. James, T. N., Sherf, L., and Urthaler, F.: Fine Structure of the Bundle Branches, *Br. Heart J.,* 36:1, 1974. (16 references)

*115. James, T. N.: The Connecting Pathways between the Sinus Node and the A-V Node and between the Right and the Left Atrium in the Human Heart, *Am. Heart J.,* 66:498, 1963. (24 references)

116. James, T. N., and Sherf, L.: Specialized Tissues

and Preferential Conduction in the Atria of the Heart, *Am. J. Cardiol.*, 28:414, 1971.

117. Harary, I.: Heart Cells In Vitro, *Sci. Am.*, 206:141, 1962.

118. DeHaan, R. L.: Development of Pacemaker Tissue in the Embryonic Heart, *Ann. N.Y. Acad. Sci.*, 127:7, 1965.

119. James, T. N.: Anatomy of the Sinus Node, AV Node and Os Cordis of the Beef Heart, *Anat. Rec.*, 153:361, 1965.

120. Bennett, H. S.: The Concepts of Membrane Flow and Membrane Vesiculation as Mechanisms for Active Transport and Ion Pumping, *J. Biophys. Biochem. Cytol.*, 2:99, 1956.

121. Fawcett, D. W.: Physiologically Significant Specializations of the Cell Surface, *Circulation*, 26:1105, 1962.

122. Fernandez-Moran, H.: Cell-Membrane Ultrastructure. Low-Temperature Microscopy and X-Ray Diffraction Studies of Lipoprotein Components in Lamellar Systems, *Circulation*, 26:1039, 1962.

123. Page, E.: The Electrical Potential Difference across the Cell Membrane of Heart Muscle; Biophysical Considerations, *Circulation*, 26:582, 1962.

*124. Porter, K. R., and Palade, G. E.: Studies on the Endoplastic Reticulum. III. Its Form and Distribution in Striated Muscle Cells, *J. Biophys. Biochem. Cytol.*, 3:269, 1957. (44 references)

125. Nelson, D. A., and Benson, E. C.: On the Structural Continuities of the Transverse Tubular System of Rabbit and Human Myocardial Cells, *J. Cell Biol.*, 16:297, 1963.

126. Fawcett, D. W.: Sarcolemmal Invaginations and Cell-to-Cell Contacts of Cardiac Muscle, *Anat. Rec.*, 151:487, 1965.

*127. Hoffman, B. F.: Physiology of Atrioventricular Transmission, *Circulation*, 24:506, 1961. (22 references)

128. Lehninger, A. L.: Dynamics and Mechanisms of Active Ion Transport across the Mitochondrial Membrane, *Ann. N.Y. Acad. Med.*, 137:700, 1966.

*129. Sherf, L., and James, T. N.: Fine Structure of Cells and Their Histological Organization within Internodal Pathways of the Heart. Clinical and Electrocardiographic Implications, *Am. J. Cardiol.*, 44:345, 1979. (70 references)

130. Sherf, L., and James, T. N.: Functional Anatomy and Ultrastructure of the Internodal Pathways, in R. C. Little (ed.), "Physiology of Atrial Pacemakers and Conductive Tissues," Futura Publishing Co., Inc., Mount Kisco, N.Y., 1980, p. 67.

*131. Weidmann, S.: The Diffusion of Radiopotassium across Intercalated Disks of Mammalian Cardiac Muscle, *J. Physiol.*, 187:323, 1966. (34 references)

132. Sjostrand, F. S., Andersson-Cedergren, E., and Dewey, M. M.: The Ultrastructure of the Intercalated Discs of Frog, Mouse and Guinea Pig Cardiac Muscle, *J. Ultrastruct. Res.*, 1:271, 1958.

*133. Sjostrand, F. S., and Andersson-Cedergren, E.: Intercalated Discs of Heart Muscle, in G. H. Bourne (ed.), "The Structure and Function of Muscle," Academic Press, Inc., New York, 1960, chap. 12, p. 421. (94 references)

134. Barr, L., Dewey, M. M., and Berger, W.: Propagation of Action Potentials and the Structure of the Nexus in Cardiac Muscle, *J. Gen. Physiol.*, 48:797, 1965.

135. Kawamura, K., and James, T. N.: Comparative Ultrastructure of Cellular Junctions in Working Myocardium and the Conduction System under Normal and Pathologic Conditions, *J. Mol. Cell. Cardiol.*, 3:31, 1971.

136. McNutt, N. S., and Weinstein, R. S.: The Ultrastructure of the Nexus. A Correlated Thin-Section and Freeze-Clave Study, *J. Cell Biol.*, 47:666, 1970.

137. Farquhar, M. G., and Palade, G. E.: Functional Complexes in Various Epithelia, *J. Cell Biol.*, 27:375, 1963.

138. Fawcett, D. W.: "The Cell," W. B. Saunders Company, Philadelphia, 1966.

139. Essner, E., Novikoff, A. B., and Quintana, N.: Nucleoside Phosphatase Activities in Rat Cardiac Muscle, *J. Cell Biol.*, 25:201, 1965.

140. Forssmann, W. G., and Giardier, L.: A Study of the T System in Rat Heart, *J. Cell Biol.*, 44:1, 1970.

141. Sommer, J. R., and Johnson, E. A.: A Comparative Study of Purkinje Fibers and Ventricular Fibers, *J. Cell Biol.*, 36:497, 1968.

142. Huxley, A. F., and Taylor, R. E.: Local Activation of Striated Muscle Fibres, *J. Physiol.*, 144:426, 1958.

143. Johnson, E. A., and Sommer, J. R.: A Strand of Cardiac Muscle: Its Ultrastructure and the Electrophysiological Implications of Its Geometry, *J. Cell Biol.*, 33:103, 1967.

144. Hill, A. V.: Abrupt Transition from Rest to Activity in Muscle, *Proc. R. Soc. Lond. (Biol.)*, 136:399, 1949.

145. Huxley, A. F.: The Links between Excitation and Contraction, *Proc. R. Soc. Lond. (Biol.)*, 160:486, 1964.

146. Huxley, H. E.: Evidence for Continuity between the Central Elements of the Triads and Extracellular Space in Frog Sartorius Muscle, *Nature*, 202:1067, 1964.

147. Ebashi, S., and Lipmann, F.: Adenosine Triphosphate Linked Concentration of Ca Ions in a Particulate Fraction of Rabbit Muscle, *J. Cell Biol.*, 14:389, 1962.

148. Hasselbach, W.: ATP Driven Active Transport of Ca in the Membranes of the Sarcoplasmic Reticulum, *Proc. R. Soc. London, (Biol.)*, 160:501, 1964.

149. Braunwald, E., Ross, J., Jr., and Sonnenblick, E. H.: Mechanisms of Contraction of the Normal and Failing Heart, *N. Engl. J. Med.*, 277:794, 1967.

150. Corsi, A., and Perry, S. V.: Some Observations of Localization of Myosin, Actin and Tropomyosin in Rabbit Myofibril, *Biochem. J.*, 68:12, 1958.

151. Huxley, H. E.: Structural Evidence Concerning Mechanism of Contraction in Striated Muscle, in W. M. Paul, C. M. Kay, and G. Monckton (eds.), "Muscle," Pergamon Press, Toronto, 1965, p. 3.

152. Huxley, H. E., and Hanson, J.: Changes in the Cross-Striations of Muscle during Contraction and Stretch and Their Structural Interpretation, *Nature*, 173:973, 1954.

153. Huxley, H. E.: Structural Arrangement and the Contraction Mechanism in Striated Muscle, *Proc. R. Soc. London (Biol.)*, 160:442, 1964.

154. Davies, R. E.: A Molecular Theory of Muscle Contraction: Ca-dependent Contraction with H Bond Formation plus ATP-Dependent Extensions of Part of the Myosin-Actin Bridges, *Nature*, 199:1068, 1963.

3

Normal Physiology of the Cardiovascular System

Robert C. Schlant, M.D.
Edmund H. Sonnenblick, M.D.
Richard Gorlin, M.D.

The cardiovascular system has these three basic functions: to transport oxygen and other nutrients to the cells of the body, to remove metabolic waste products from the cells, and to carry substances such as hormones from one part of the body to another. With every beat, the performance of the heart may be considered the net result of the following three major determinants: preload, afterload, and contractility (the inotropic state). The heart rate then determines the performance of the heart relative to time. Cardiac performance is further influenced by atrial function, neural control, hormones and metabolic products, the synchrony of ventricular contraction, anesthesia, and drugs. This chapter will review myocardial excitation-contraction coupling, fundamentals of muscle mechanics, the major factors influencing cardiac performance, the cardiac cycle, the major mechanisms of cardiac reserve, the response to exercise, and the coronary circulation. Detailed discussions are found in the general reference sources.[1-14] The evaluation of cardiac and myocardial function is further discussed in Chap. 18.

Myocardial Excitation-Contraction Coupling[11,15-33]

In recent years there has been a great increase in our understanding of the mechanisms by which the action potential stimulus initiates the contractile process in heart muscle. All these studies have emphasized the central role in excitation-contraction coupling of the calcium ion (Ca^{2+}), which was known to be essential for myocardial contraction since the classic studies of S. Ringer. The Ca^{2+} ion is now known to have two major roles in excitation-contraction, i.e., the initiation of contraction (trigger substance) and the regulation of myocardial contraction (regulating factor).

With the initiation of the action potential in ventricular myocardium (Fig. 3-1), there is a very rapid influx of Na^+ (or change in Na^+ *conductance*) which produces the rapid electrical spike and overshoot during phase 0 (see Chap. 4). During the plateau of the action potential (phase 2), there is a slow inward flux of Ca^{2+} across the myocardial cell membrane, or sarcolemma, into the intracellular fluid (sarco-

plasm or cytosol). One view maintains that the extracellular Ca^{2+} ions are temporarily bound on special sites on the membrane for one or more beats prior to being transported into the sarcoplasm by subsequent action potentials.[23,31] As indicated schematically in Fig. 3-2, the action potential also spreads from the myocardial cell membrane down the extensive *transverse (T) tubular system*, which consists of sarcolemma invaginations especially near the Z bands that are in direct continuity with the extracellular or interstitial space (see Chap. 2 for anatomic details). Although not definitely established, it would appear probable that during the passage of the action potential the T system contributes qualitatively to intracellular Ca^{2+} in the same manner as the regular sarcolemma. The action potential descends the T system near the Z bands into *triadic junctions* in which a single T-system tubule is in extremely close proximity to, but not in open communication with, two terminal cisternae or extensions (*lateral sacs*) of the *sarcoplasmic reticulum* (SR). The SR is an extensive system of intracellular tubules more or less floating in the sarcoplasm, with many branches near the transverse tubules and surface membranes (sarcolemma), and investing every myofibril in the cell. While the SR is present in all mammalian cardiac cells, the T system is present where the cells are relatively large and serves to take the surface membrane deep into the fiber. In small atrial fibers and the conduction system, the T system is generally absent. The exact mechanism by which the action potential "signal" is transferred from the sarcolemma and the T system to the intracellular sarcoplasmic reticulum is unknown, though it has been suggested with substantial evidence that the relatively small transsarcolemmal calcium flux mediates this role.[33] Once the sarcoplasmic reticulum is depolarized, however, the excitation spreads rapidly throughout the SR, resulting in the release into the sarcoplasma of relatively large amounts of free Ca^{2+}, which then activates the fibril to contract. It appears probable that the Ca^{2+} is released particularly from the terminal *cisternae* (or *vesicles* or *lateral sacs*) of the SR. Mitochondria can also release Ca^{2+} into the intracellular fluid, but it is doubtful that this mechanism contributes significantly to intracellular Ca^{2+} in human myocardium.[34,35] It is likely that the initiating stimulus for this calcium-triggered or "regenerative" release of Ca^{2+} from SR and mitochondria is the relatively small amount of inward Ca^{2+} movement actually produced by the action potential.[33]

The increased sarcoplasmic "free" or "activating" Ca^{2+} diffuses to the myofibrils, where it binds to subunits of troponin, troponin C, which are located periodically along the thin actin filaments. In the absence of Ca^{2+}, troponin works through tropomyosin, which courses along the actin filament, to prevent actin from acting with myosin. Once Ca^{2+} attaches to troponin C, however, the inhibitory effect of troponin and tropomyosin upon the interaction of actin and myosin is released.[36-39] This loss of in-

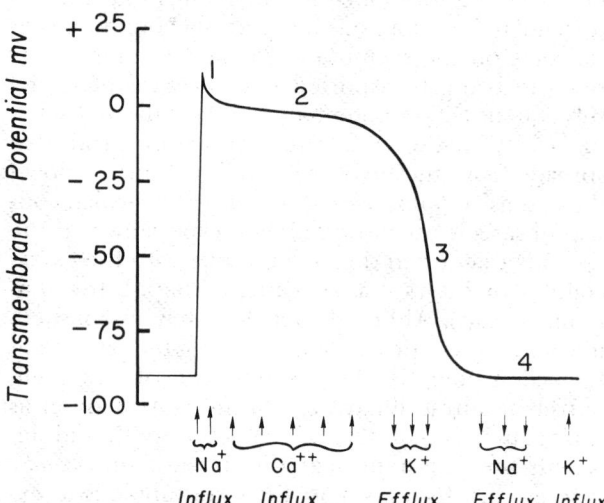

FIGURE 3-1 Ion fluxes associated with myocardial action potential. Schematic action potential of human ventricular myocardium together with probable electrolyte movements. The initial phase 0 spike and overshoot is related to a sudden influx of Na^+. This is followed by a slower, maintained influx of Ca^{2+} during the plateau phase 2. The phase of Ca^{2+} efflux is not well defined for human ventricular myocardium, but presumably it occurs during phase 4.

hibition, or "derepression," allows enzyme sites on myosin bridges to interact with actin so that the resultant actomyosin ATPase, in the presence of bound ATP and magnesium, can produce bridge motion and thus myocardial contraction by the sliding-filament mechanism. An increase in the free Ca^{2+} concentration from 5×10^{-7} to 6×10^{-6} M results in the production of approximately 90 percent of the maximum force. The exact fraction of myofibrillar Ca^{2+} bound by troponin C and necessary for activation is unknown, though about 22 μmol is needed by the myofibril for 50 percent activation and 90 μmol for maximal activation. The increased sarcoplasmic Ca^{2+} also influences myocardial metabolism by activating glycogen phosphorylase, which results in increased glycogenolysis. The energy for myocardial contraction is obtained from molecules of magnesium adenosine triphosphate (ATP) that are split by an ATPase site on the myosin filament heads during each interaction with actin (see Chap. 5).

Relaxation is initiated by an unknown stimulus (or loss of inhibition) that produces an increased binding, uptake, or sequestration of sarcoplasmic Ca^{2+}. It is not certain exactly where or how this decrease in intracellular Ca^{2+} occurs in human myocardium. It has been suggested that Ca^{2+} uptake occurs on the sarcolemma, on the sarcoplasmic surface of the longitudinal tubules of the SR, and directly back into the terminal cisternae of the SR. The route that would be taken by Ca^{2+} after being reabsorbed into longitudinal tubules at the SR is also uncertain. It may be transported or diffused back to the terminal cisternae or diffused to the T system and to the interstitial space. Relaxation of the actin-myosin myofibrils occurs as the result of an inhibi-

tion produced by the troponin-tropomyosin complex in the presence of low intracellular Ca^{2+}.

The amount of Ca^{2+} available to inhibit troponin and induce contraction of the actin-myosin myofilaments is directly related to the rate of tension developed and to the amount of tension developed. It is likely that many drugs (such as digitalis,[23,31,40–42] sympathomimetic amines,[43–45] xanthines[46]) or conditions (acidosis, an increase in heart rate,[47–48] postextrasystolic potentiation[49]) have their influence upon myocardial contractility through their effect upon available intracellular Ca^{2+}.[50,51]

It has also been suggested that there is competition between intracellular sodium (Na^+) and calcium (Ca^{2+}) ions for myocardial sarcolemma binding sites. Such competition has been used to explain the influence of extracellular and intracellular Na^+ concentration upon intracellular Ca^{2+} concentration and myocardial contractility.[10,17,19,21,23] When the heart rate is abruptly increased, there is an associated progressive increase in contractile force, known as the *Bowditch staircase* or *treppe phenomenon*. Langer has suggested that the increased heart rate results in a temporary increase in intracellular Ca^{2+} secondary to the internal shift of Na^+.[23,31] Drugs such as digitalis, which inhibit membrane sodium-potassium-activated ATPase, also might produce some of their effects by influencing intracellular Na^+, which in turn influences intracellular Ca^{2+} and contractile force.[17,23,31,40–42,52] Recent studies have also suggested that defects in the kinetics of intracellular calcium may be present in the myocardium of patients with heart failure[6,16,18,21,23,26,53] (see Chap. 22).

Muscle Mechanics

The basic mechanics of contraction of the heart is regulated by four distinct, although interrelated, factors: (1) the *preload* (Starling's law of the heart), which is the passive load that establishes the initial muscle length of the cardiac fibers prior to contraction; (2) the *afterload*, which is the sum of all the loads against which the myocardial fibers must shorten during systole, created by the end-diastolic volume of the ventricle, the aortic impedance, the arterial resistance, the peripheral vascular resistance, the mass of blood in the aorta, and the viscosity of the blood; (3) the *contractility*, or *inotropic state* of the heart, which reflects the speed and shortening capacity of the myocardium for a given set of loading conditions; and (4) the *heart rate*, or frequency of contraction. As will be described, the fiber length appears to influence quantitatively the number of active force-generating sites in the myocardium, whereas a change in the contractile state (or contractility) is related to a qualitative change in the force generated by the sites, i.e., their activations, with or without a change in their number. Before discussing these mechanisms, a very brief review of

A. Myocardial Excitation-Contraction Coupling

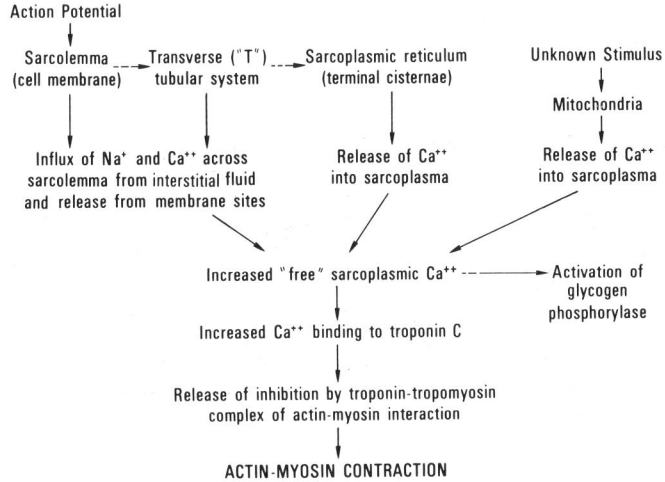

B. Myocardial Relaxation

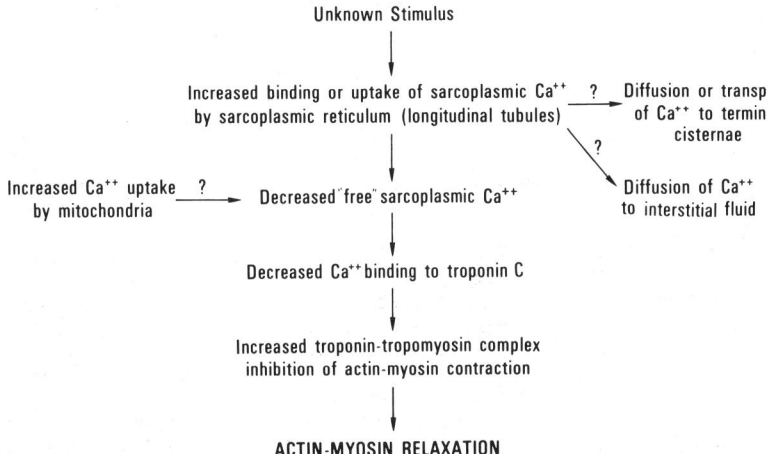

FIGURE 3-2 Schematic diagram of the events producing (A) excitation-contraction coupling and (B) relaxation in myocardium. The relative contribution of the sarcolemma, the T system, and the mitochondria to the increase in free sarcoplasmic Ca^{2+}, which is responsible for the initiation of contraction, is uncertain in human myocardium. The mechanisms and the pathways by which sarcoplasmic Ca^{2+} is taken up or sequestered during relaxation are not well defined for human myocardium.

fundamental myocardial mechanics as described by force-velocity-length relations is appropriate. More detailed discussions are presented in specialized reviews.[6,54–59]

Fundamentals of Muscle Mechanics[6,54–78]

A model for muscular contraction which has been exceedingly useful for understanding myocardial mechanics and predicting their changes under a number of different circumstances has been suggested by A. V. Hill.[79,80] In this model (Fig. 3-3) muscle contraction behaves as if there were a *contractile element* (CE), which is capable of developing force and of shortening; a *series elastic component* (SE), which is passively stretched by shortening of the CE; and a *parallel elastic component* (PE), which supports resting tension but plays little role during contraction. The anatomic sites of the components or, indeed, their exact arrangement is uncertain.

These factors may be in the contractile filaments, in the cell membranes, or in both. Several other models have been proposed using the same basic components. Although the "working" model is useful for conceptual purposes, one must recognize that anatomic reality is not implied. In isolated muscle preparations, this SE is created by damaged elastic ends of the muscle; in the intact heart, the SE includes valves and elastic structures.

After activation of a strip of heart muscle that is not allowed to shorten (*isometric contraction*, Fig. 3-4), the CE rapidly begins to shorten at its maximal velocity (V_{max}). As the CE shortens, it stretches the SE, which transmits the force to the external attachments. As the force in the SE develops, however, the velocity of shortening declines in accord with a basic inverse relation between force and velocity of muscle contraction. Because of the time required to stretch the SE, the external developed force lags behind the theoretical maximal force of the CE that

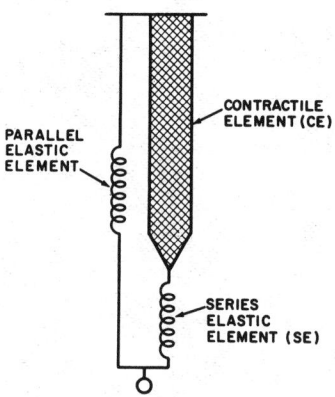

A.V. Hill 1938

FIGURE 3-3   A. V. Hill's three-component model for muscle. See text. (*From Sonnenblick.*[67] *Reproduced with permission of the publisher.*)

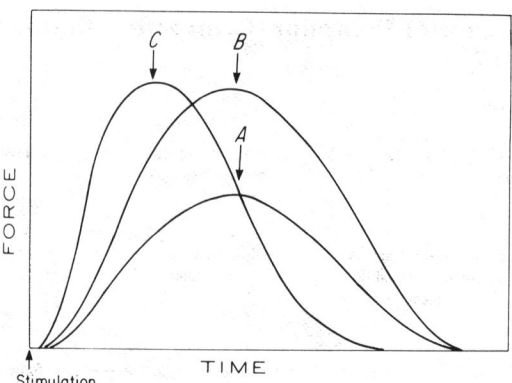

FIGURE 3-5   Hypothetical isometric force developed by three hypothetical contractions. A = control; B = increased initial muscle length; C = the muscle in curve B contracting more frequently. See text. (*From Sonnenblick.*[67] *Reproduced with permission of the publisher.*)

it could develop (P_0) if no SE were present. Three hypothetical isometric contractions under different conditions are shown in Fig. 3-5. Curve A represents the control contraction; curve B represents the changes produced by an increase in initial muscle length and is characterized by a greater peak force P_0, which occurs after about the same time interval following stimulation; and curve C represents an increased frequency of contraction from curve B, illustrating the increased contractility manifested by an increased rate of force development (increased velocity of CE shortening) and shortened duration of the active state, rather than by an increase in peak force.

The *preload* is the load that stretches the muscle to its initial length *prior* to contraction as related to the resting length-tension (load) curve of the muscle. The *afterload* is the load the muscle must move after it starts to contract.

When myocardium contracts against a constant

afterload and is allowed to shorten (an *isotonic contraction*, Fig. 3-6), the CE initially shortens and stretches the SE while developing enough external force to overcome the afterload. The initial slope of the shortening curve relative to time, shown on the right in Fig. 3-6, is used to calculate the initial velocity of shortening for the particular load P. With progressively increasing afterloads, the time interval from stimulus to the onset of shortening is prolonged, but the time to maximal shortening is unchanged (Fig. 3-7). In addition, the initial velocity

FIGURE 3-6   An afterloaded isotonic contraction of myocardium. On the left is the muscle model attached to a load P which is supported when the muscle is at rest (A). This type of load P that is encountered by the CE only when the CE attempts to shorten is termed the *afterload*, whereas the small load used to stretch the system to its initial length is termed the *preload*. With stimulation of the system, the CE begins to shorten at maximum speed, V_{max}. During the isometric portion of the contraction, between A and B, the CE shortens and the SE matches the load P, and the load starts to move. Once the load begins to move to point B, the SE remains constant in length, and shortening of the system reflects shortening of the CE alone. The curves on the right reflect force and shortening as functions of time after stimulation. The tangent to the slope of the curve of initial shortening is used to obtain the *initial velocity* of isotonic shortening for a given load. After plotting the initial velocity of shortening for different loads, one may extrapolate the curve to zero load to obtain the theoretic intrinsic or maximal velocity V_{max}. See Fig. 3-8. (*From Sonnenblick.*[67] *Reproduced with permission of the publisher.*)

FIGURE 3-4   Schematic model of an isometric contraction of a strip of heart muscle. *Left:* The muscle model with a contractile element (CE) and a series elastic component (SE). The initial length of the SE (l_0) increases by $\Delta 1$ between A and B. *Right:* The time course of development of external force together with the hypothetical instantaneous force of CE which it might develop if no SE attachments were present. Point A, the initial resting state; point B, some time during active activation. See text. (*From Sonnenblick.*[67] *Reproduced with permission of the publisher.*)

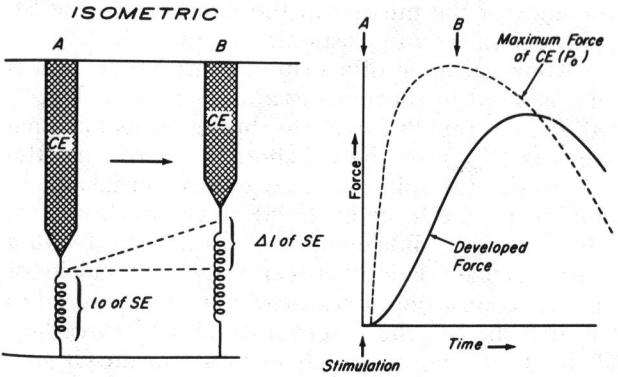

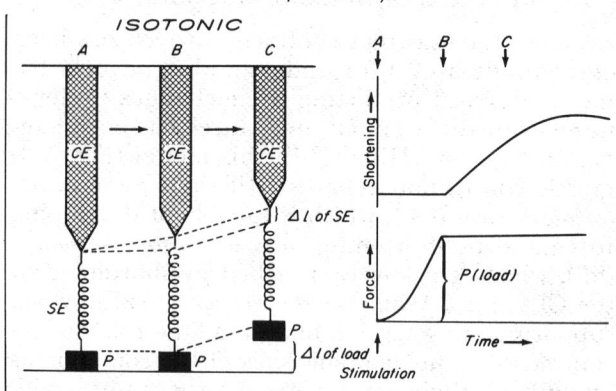

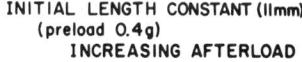

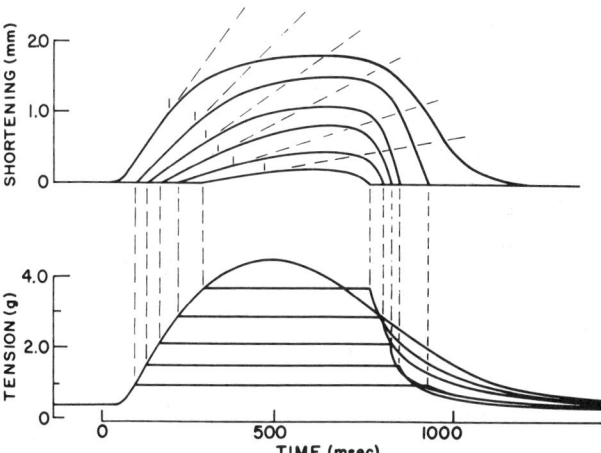

FIGURE 3-7 A series of superimposed tracings made from iso-lated papillary muscle which was arranged in such a manner that both initial isometric contraction and subsequent isotonic short-ening are possible. *Below:* Serial isometric contraction at increas-ing afterloads (horizontal lines). *Above:* Successive isotonic short-ening corresponding to the increasing afterloads in the lower tracing (dashed lines). The dashed lines on the upper tracing rep-resent the initial velocity of shortening. As the afterload increases, the initial velocity of shortening decreases, the extent of shortening decreases, but the isometric relaxation phase increases. (*From Sonnenblick.*[67] *Reproduced with permission of the publisher.*)

of isotonic shortening for each load, which is ob-tained by drawing a tangent to the initial shortening slope, decreases markedly with increasing loads. This basic relation is further illustrated in Figs. 3-8 and 3-9, in which the force-velocity relations of iso-lated papillary muscles are plotted to illustrate the basic principle of a decrease in the initial velocity of shortening with increasing loads. As shown in Fig. 3-8, extrapolation of the curve to zero load yields the theoretic maximal velocity (V_{max}) of shortening of the contractile elements in the unloaded muscle. V_{max} in turn is altered by factors that modify the activation of the muscle but not by a change in initial muscle length within physiological resting lengths. Thus, it has been a useful index of the contractility of the myocardial fibers being examined.

Preload: The Frank-Straub-Wiggers-Starling Principle

In 1871 H. P. Bowditch[81] showed that if the con-dition of the heart muscle remains unaltered, con-tractions remain equal in strength, regardless of the strength of stimuli applied. This principle, which has become known as the *all-or-nothing law of the heart,* implied that cardiac muscle either does not contract at all or responds to the fullest extent, but that the magnitude of the all-or-none response is determined by the inherent "condition" of the mus-cle. In 1884 Howell and Donaldson[82] presented unequivocal evidence that the heart itself has intrin-

sic mechanisms by which its output is adjusted to the venous input. Using a heart-lung preparation, they found that increasing the venous return in-creased cardiac output and stroke as well as right atrial pressure. In 1895 O. Frank[83] published his classical studies on the dynamics of heart muscle. His object was to correlate the reactions of cardiac muscle with the responses of skeletal muscle, the force of contraction of which had been previously shown by A. Fick,[84] J. von Kries,[85] and Blix[86] to be related to the initial length and resting tension. Frank studied the frog atria and ventricles and showed that, within limits, stepwise increases in dia-stolic volume and pressure just before contraction— the *presystolic* or *end-diastolic* volume and pressure— determine the magnitude of the all-or-none re-sponse. His studies emphasized the dependence of the cardiac response on hemodynamic events preceding excitation. In 1914 Wiggers[87] reported experiments that were the first to demonstrate that the reactions established by Frank for the frog's ven-tricle are also applicable to the naturally beating right ventricle of dogs. He concluded that the rate of isometric pressure rise and the peak systolic pres-sure are determined by changes in the initial ten-sion, as long as marked changes in inherent con-tractility are not simultaneously produced by experimental procedures. Also in 1914, Straub[88] and Starling and associates[89,90] independently re-ported their studies of the effect of changes in initial tension and length on the response of isolated hearts. The studies of Starling and associates have received the greatest amount of attention in the English-speaking areas of the world, and, in defer-ence to Otto Frank, the general principle is often referred to as the *Frank-Starling law of the heart.*[91] Starling and associates, on the basis of highly suggestive, but not quite conclusive, studies on the heart-lung preparation, concluded that, "The me-chanical energy set free on passage from the resting to the constricted state depends on the area of chemically active surfaces, i.e., on the length of the muscle fibers." Wiggers[92] has pointed out that al-though there is a general impression that the often-reproduced representation of the law by Starling and associates was based on data from their own experiments, the careful reader will discover that the published curves were acknowledged to be re-productions of graphs previously published by Blix and by O. Frank. From the earlier studies of Frank, Straub, and Wiggers, it was not certain whether the responsiveness of the heart was fundamentally re-lated to changes in presystolic pressure (initial ten-sion) or to changes in volume (initial length). The conclusion by Starling that cardiac responsiveness was primarily related to presystolic *fiber length* has been validated by nearly all investigators, but it is clear that fiber length and resting tension are inter-related. Wiggers[92] has emphasized the importance of other factors affecting the responsiveness of the myocardium and has stressed that the statement of

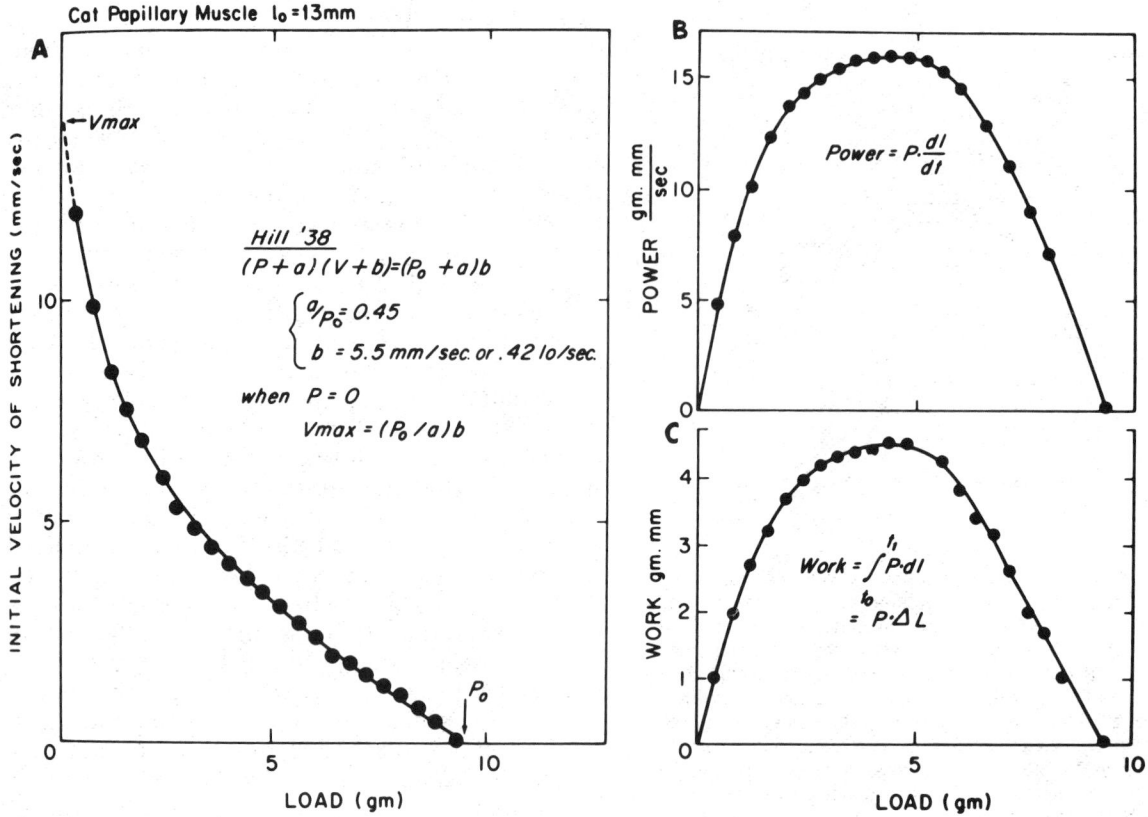

FIGURE 3-8 *A.* Force-velocity relations of a papillary muscle, illustrating the decreasing initial velocity of shortening with increasing loads. The insert gives Hill's equation for muscular contraction with the derived constants. When the curve is extrapolated to zero load, one obtains the V_{max}, or the intrinsic velocity of shortening. When the load is increased to the point at which no shortening can occur (an isometric contraction), the maximum force is manifest (P_0 or intrinsic force). *B.* The load versus the power (force versus velocity of shortening). *C.* The load versus work (force or load versus displacement). Note that peak power and work are obtained at loads approximately 50 percent of the maximal force of contraction P_0 obtained during isometric conditions. Instantaneous force-velocity curves similar to those in *A* are also obtained when the velocity of shortening is measured at a constant time after stimulation by quick-release techniques. (*From Sonnenblick.*[67] *Reproduced with permission of the publisher.*)

FIGURE 3-9   Relation between the initial velocity of isotonic shortening and afterload of a human papillary muscle stimulated at a rate of 12 stimuli per minute. Preload was 1.4 g with a muscle length of 15 mm. Note the significant decrease in initial velocity as the load increases. The insert shows four recordings with different afterloads; the decrease in rate of shortening with increasing afterload is apparent from the altered slopes of the length-time curves. (*From Sonnenblick.*[63] *Reproduced with permission of the publisher.*)

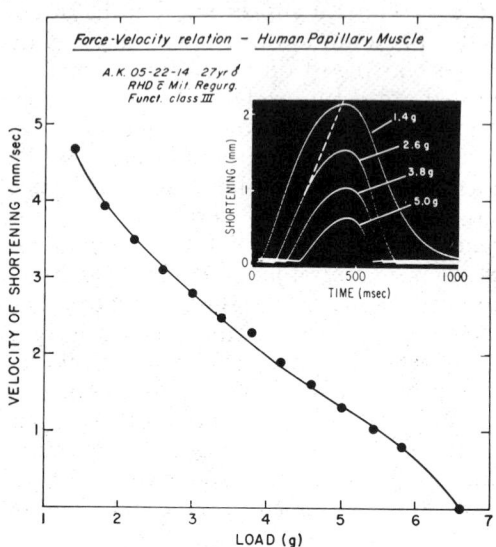

the law of the heart, in which the energy of contraction is a function of the length of the muscle fiber, should be modified by the phrase, "under equivalent states of responsiveness." Sarnoff and Berglund[93,94] demonstrated this principle by showing that a "family of curves" relating stroke work to left atrial pressure exists for each ventricle and that many other factors, such as humoral agents, neural influences, and metabolic condition of the myocardium, determine which particular "curve" the ventricle is operating on at a given moment. The studies of Braunwald and associates[6,95,96] have shown the applicability of the law of the heart in both the normal and the diseased human heart.

The fact that initial fiber length rather than intraventricular pressure is important in influencing the strength of contraction is of great significance. Although these two factors are usually related to each other, the relation may vary considerably because of changes in ventricular *distensibility* or *compliance,* i.e., the ratio of change in ventricular volume to change in ventricular diastolic pressure ($\Delta V/\Delta P$). Ventricular *stiffness* is the reciprocal or the change in pressure for a given change in volume ($\Delta P/\Delta V$).[97–106] Most of the recognized changes in ventricular compliance occur chronically as a result of ventricular distension or hypertrophy. Significant acute changes in the pressure-volume relation or distensibility of ventricles probably do not occur except in response to ischemia, nor are there changes due to inotropic agents.[97,107] On the other hand, ventricular distensibility is often significantly influenced by filling of the opposite ventricle, especially when filling pressures are elevated and within the constraints of the pericardium.[107] Thus, the pressure-volume relationships of one ventricle can be immediately influenced by acute changes in the filling of the contralateral ventricle. At cardiac catheterization it is possible to obtain reasonable estimations of ventricular end-diastolic and end-systolic volumes and very accurate measurements of end-diastolic pressure. As discussed in Chap. 22, the ventricular end-diastolic pressure may be elevated both by an altered compliance due to myocardial failure and by ventricular hypertrophy itself.[6,97–109]

The Frank-Starling law of the heart is the major mechanism by which the normal right and left ventricles maintain equal minute outputs even though their stroke outputs may vary considerably during normal respiration. Thus, if the right ventricle temporarily pumps more blood into the pulmonary circulation than the left ventricle pumps into the systemic circulation, the proper balance between the two pumps is soon achieved, since the venous return to the left atrium and ventricle causes the left ventricular end-diastolic fiber length to be greater, increasing left ventricular stroke output. In addition, a decreased left ventricular stroke output would eventually lead to decreased return of blood to the right atrium and ventricle, producing a decrease in right ventricular stroke output. By this mechanism, the two ventricles, which function as two pumps in series, are able to balance their outputs and prevent pulmonary edema, despite marked variations in stroke volumes.

A left ventricular *function curve* is shown in Fig. 3-10, in which left ventricular stroke volume is plotted as a function of left ventricular end-diastolic pressure. Although similar curves may be obtained by plotting ventricular stroke volume against left atrial mean pressure or left ventricular volume (which is more difficult to measure), the basic determinant is probably fiber length. Because end-diastolic fiber length and intraventricular pressure are normally related to each other, it is common in clinical situations to measure left ventricular end-diastolic pressure, since fiber length is difficult to determine in patients. In Fig. 3-10, curve A represents a hypothetical normal left ventricular function curve. Curve B represents a *shift to the left* of the function curve of the same ventricle under the influence of sympathetic stimulation or the infusion of epinephrine, norepinephrine, or other catecholamines. Curve C represents a *shift to the right* of curve A, such as might occur with myocardial depression from hypoxia or cardiodepressant drugs or in myocardial "failure." Note that under normal conditions (curve A) very slight changes in fiber length,

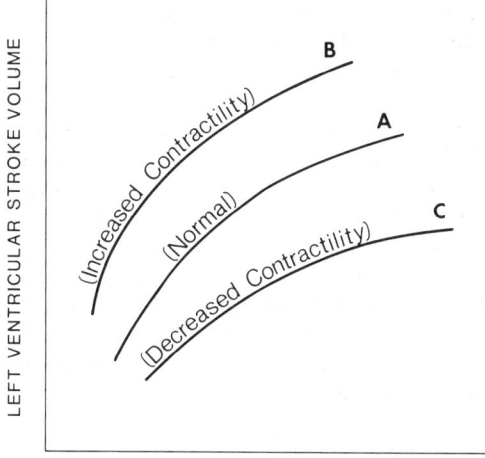

FIGURE 3-10   Relation between left ventricular end-diastolic pressure and left ventricular stroke volume. Curve A, the normal function; curve B, the shift to the left of the original curve associated with increased contractility, such as might result from sympathetic stimulation of the ventricle or the infusion of epinephrine or norepinephrine; curve C, a shift to the right of the original curve associated with decreased contractility, such as might result from ventricular failure from ischemia or myocardial-depressant drugs. A ventricle functioning on a curve C might be restored to a curve A by the action of digitalis or inotropic drugs, such as norepinephrine epinephrine. Similar but not identical curves are obtained when left ventricular stroke volume or cardiac output is plotted against left ventricular end-diastolic pressure or left atrial mean pressure. Function curves such as these may be obtained from both ventricles and both atria.

which can be produced by small changes in filling pressure, are associated with significant increases in stroke volume. As mentioned above, this is one of the major mechanisms by which the two ventricles have balanced outputs over any period of time, even though their stroke outputs may vary considerably from beat to beat, particularly during the respiratory cycle. It should be emphasized that sympathetic stimulation may increase cardiac output, not only by producing an increase in heart rate, but also by increasing the contractile force of both the atria and the ventricles, with a resultant increase in stroke volume. The increase in ventricular contractile force produced by sympathetic stimulation may be depicted graphically as a shift to the left of the ventricular function curve. Thus, sympathetic impulses can produce an increase in ventricular stroke volume without the necessity of a change in end-diastolic fiber length or pressure. While there is good evidence that the normal heart utilizes alterations in preload or the Starling law of the heart during normal resting circumstances or during exercise, the failing, dilated heart may have little such reserve remaining. Thus, the hearts of patients with heart failure and cardiac dilatation have most of their fibers chronically extended to the top (L_{max}) of their force-length curve, where sarcomere lengths are about 2.2 μm after fixation. Accordingly, many such hearts appear to be operating chronically at their ideal maximal length and therefore unable to respond significantly to increased filling or stretch with a greater force of contraction.

Figure 3-11 illustrates the interrelationships between ventricular end-diastolic volume, end-diastolic pressure, and stroke work. As indicated in Fig. 3-11A, the relationship between stroke volume and end-diastolic volume is nearly linear. On the other hand, the relationship between end-diastolic pressure and volume (Fig. 3-11B) is curvilinear, with a definite volume at zero pressure and with a rather sharp increase in pressure above a certain volume. Figure 3-11C illustrates the familiar curvilinear relationship between ventricular end-diastolic pressure and stroke volume.

FIGURE 3-11 The interrelationships between stroke work, ventricular end-diastolic volume, and end-diastolic pressure are illustrated. As indicated in the top graph, the relationship between stroke volume and end-diastolic volume is actually nearly linear. On the other hand, the relationship between end-diastolic pressure and end-diastolic volume (center), is curvilinear, with a definite volume at zero pressure and with a rather sharp increase in pressure above a certain volume. At bottom is illustrated the familiar curvilinear relationship between stroke volume and ventricular end-diastolic pressure, similar to Fig. 3-10.

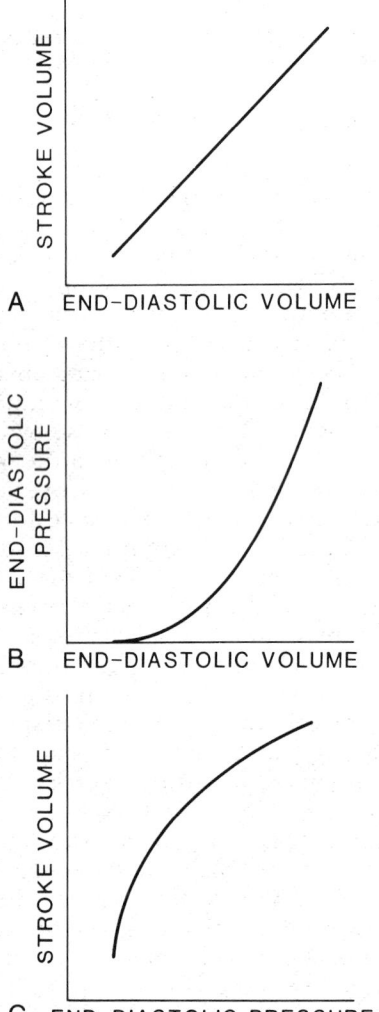

Ultrastructural Basis of Starling's Law[6,66,108–121]

The length-tension relation of a papillary muscle is shown in Fig. 3-12. The length of a myocardial sarcomere at which maximal force develops is approximately 2.2 μm after fixation, at which length the thin actin and thick myosin myofilaments are optimally overlapped to provide the greatest number of force-generating sites. When the sarcomere is stretched beyond about 2.2 μm, the developed force decreases as the myofilaments become partially disengaged and fewer contractile sites are brought into play. At a length of 3.65 μm, the actin and myosin myofilaments are completely disengaged, and developed tension drops to zero. These long sarcomeres are only seen in skeletal fibers since cardiac sarcomeres are too stiff to be that overstretched. While consistent with a sliding-filament mechanism, these longer sarcomere lengths, where force decreases, are not seen physiologically. At sarcomere lengths less than 2.2 μm, the actin myofilaments first

FIGURE 3-12 The relation between papillary sarcomere length, resting tension, and developed or active tension. Note that active tension increases up to a sarcomere length of 2.2 μm L_{max} and then decreases. The resting tension increases markedly above a sarcomere length of 2.0 to 2.2 μm, which corresponds to an end-diastolic pressure of about 10 to 12 mmHg. The course of a normal contraction is shown in ABCD. Contraction starts at point A and develops a force equal to an imposed load P, reaching point B. The fiber then shortens until the active tension curve is reached at C, when relaxation occurs and returns the course to D at the end of systole. Normally, the ventricle functions on the ascending limb of the active tension curve at length below L_{max}, where greatest active tension develops, with sarcomere lengths between 1.8 and 2.2 μm. The descending limb of the length–active tension curve occurs at sarcomere lengths greater than L_{max}. There is normally a moderate heterogeneity of sarcomere lengths in the heart, sarcomeres in the subendocardial layers tending to be longer and to shorten more than sarcomeres from the midwall or epicardium. In patients with marked ventricular dilatation, most of the dilatation is due to rearrangement and plastic "slippage" of the muscle fibers and myofibrils together with an increase in length of fibers which is due to synthesis of sarcomeres in series rather than to stretching of individual sarcomeres. (From Sonnenblick, Spotnitz, and Spiro.[121] Reproduced with permission of the authors, publisher, and the American Heart Association, Inc.)

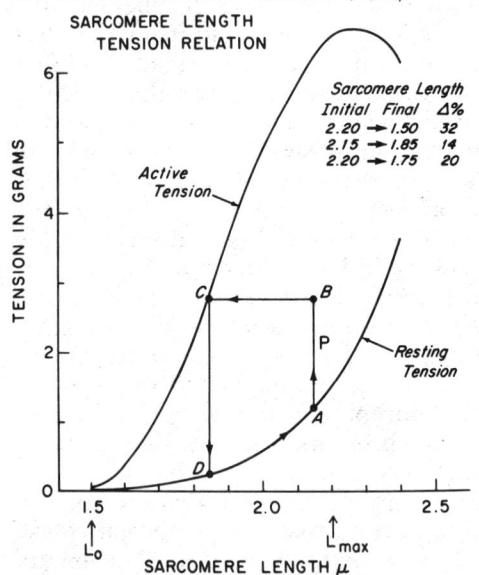

pass into the center of the sarcomere; at 2.0 μm, they bypass one another and developed tension decreases. The reason for the fall in force with shortening sarcomere length in this physiological portion of the curve is not clear. Explanations for this include the following: interference of the thin filaments, restoring forces, and a decrease in Ca^{2+} sensitivity of the sarcomere at short lengths. The last explanation has received recent support.[122] As the papillary muscle in Fig. 3-12 is increasingly stretched, the resting tension increases, at first slowly and then more markedly. The *stiffness* of myocardial muscle can be defined as the slope of the curve relating the change in resting tension (ΔT) to the change in length (ΔL).

It is also significant that a sarcomere length of 2.2 μm, which produces peak active tension (L_{max}), occurs in normal dogs at about the upper limit of normal ventricular filling pressure, 10 to 12 mmHg. Theoretically, the normal ventricle may have an ejection fraction of 55 percent, with a shortening of individual sarcomere length of only 13 percent.[6,112,113] One study has suggested that perhaps 50 percent of the normal stroke volume can theoretically be accounted for by a piston-like effect produced by ventricular thickening;[123] however, the physiological significance of this phenomenon is uncertain.

Influences of Fiber Length and Heart Rate upon Force-Velocity Relations

The influence of increased initial fiber length on the force-velocity relation of a papillary muscle is shown in Fig. 3-13. With increasing fiber length there is an increase in the maximal actively developed force which the fiber can develop (P_0) at zero velocity of shortening or isometric contraction for each fiber length. In contrast, there is little or no change in the maximal velocity of shortening (V_{max}).[124] The increase in intrinsic force P_0 with unchanged V_{max} produced by increased initial muscle length is probably related to an increased number of active contractile sites rather than to an increase in their contractility per se. The contrasting effects of an increase in muscle length and an increase in heart rate on force-velocity relations are illustrated in Fig. 3-14. As in Fig. 3-12, an increase in muscle length increases the maximum load at which no shortening occurs (i.e., increases P_0, the peak isometric tension) with no change in V_{max}; on the other hand, an increase in heart rate increases V_{max} but may occur with or without a significant change in the load at which no shortening occurs.[64] The increase in contractility associated with an increase in heart rate occurs in both atrial and ventricular muscle and is termed the *Bowditch effect*, or *treppe*.[47,48,64,66,69,125–129]

Contractility and the Inotropic State[6,10,54–78,130–163]

The second major mechanism by which myocardial function is altered is by a change in the inotropic state (contractility) of the muscle independent of a

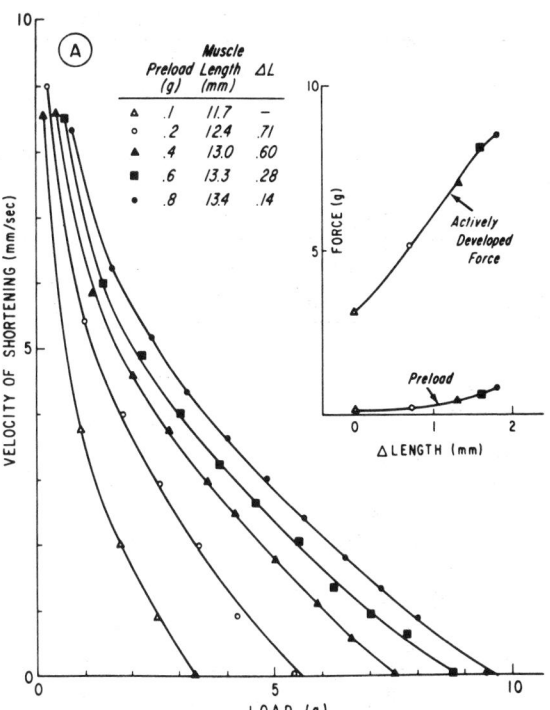

FIGURE 3-13 The effects of increasing initial muscle length on the force-velocity relation. The initial velocity of shortening is plotted against preload, increases in which increase the initial length. In the insert, the maximal force developed is plotted against the change in muscle length. It is apparent that an increased muscle length produces little or no increase in V_{max}, the velocity of shortening at zero load obtained by extrapolation, but increases the actively developed maximal force P_0, which is produced under isometric conditions when the load is increased so much that no shortening can occur. (*From Sonnenblick.*[124] *Reproduced with permission of the publisher.*)

change in fiber length. The actual biochemical events at or near the ultrastructural contractile sites that are responsible for increases in contractility, or inotropism, are the subject of very active investigation and appear related to an enhanced degree of activation of cardiac muscle for a given contraction.[27–33] Abbott and Mommaerts[161] and Sonnenblick and his associates,[6,54,60,63–71,124,130,160,162] have noted that an increase in the contractile state of a muscle is characterized by an increase in V_{max}, with or without a change in P_0, the maximal force under isometric conditions at zero velocity.

The effects of changes in heart rate and of norepinephrine on the force-velocity relation of papillary muscle are shown in Figs. 3-14 and 3-15, in which the initial velocity of shortening is plotted against the load. Both an increase in heart rate and in norepinephrine concentration increase the contractile state, as shown by an increase in the velocity of shortening at any level of tension and by changes in location of V_{max}, obtained by extrapolating to zero load, whether or not there is a change in P_0. As noted in Fig. 3-15, both strophanthidin and norepinephrine produce a significant shift to the right in the force-velocity curves, and an increase in both V_{max} and P_0 in association with a decrease in the time from stimulation to peak shortening.[65] In-

THE NORMAL HEART AND BLOOD VESSELS

FORCE-VELOCITY IN HUMAN PAPILLARY MUSCLE

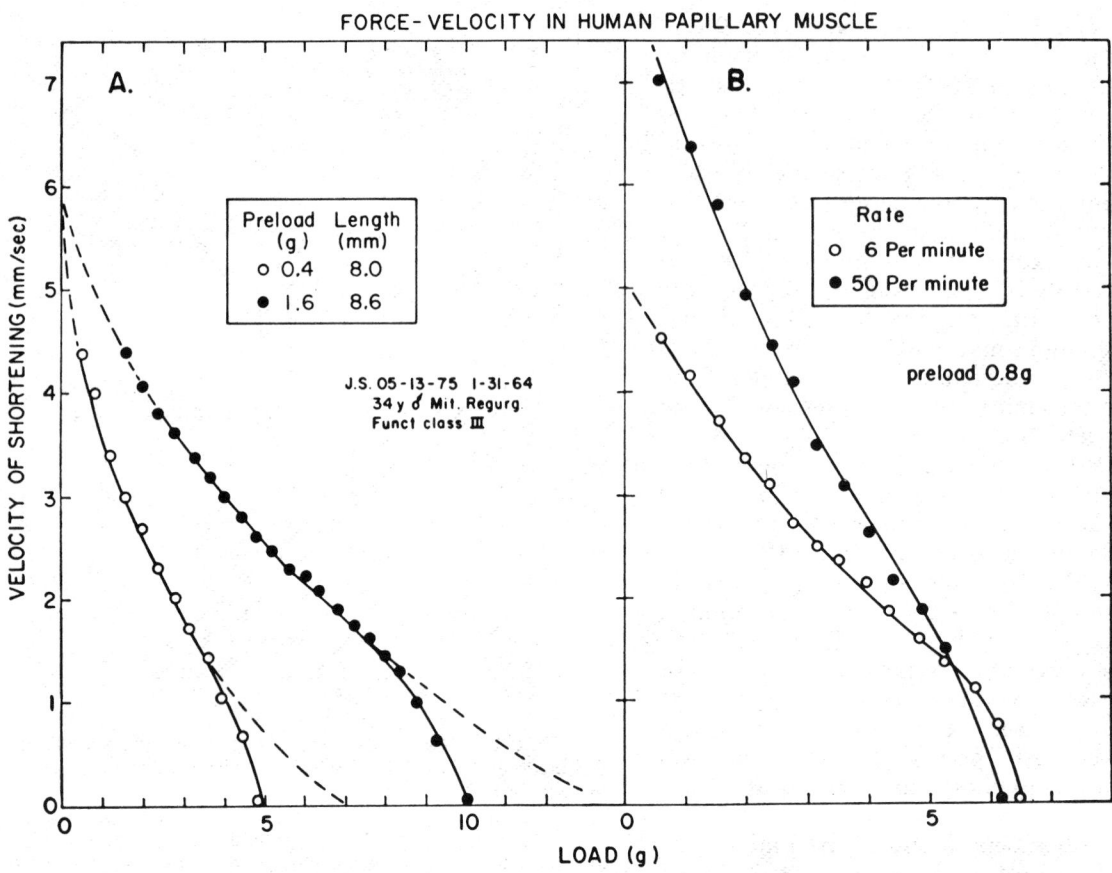

FIGURE 3-14   Force-velocity curves of human papillary muscle to illustrate the effects of (A) increasing muscle length and (B) increasing rate of contraction. Lengthening the muscle increased maximal isometric force P_0 without a change in maximal velocity of shortening (V_{max}, the velocity at zero load, obtained by extrapolation). Conversely, in the same muscle, increasing the rate of stimulation increased V_{max} without a change in P_0. (*From Sonnenblick et al.[64] Reproduced with permission of the publisher.*)

FIGURE 3-15   The increased contractility of papillary muscle produced by strophanthidin and by norepinephrine. The increased contractility produced by both drugs is reflected in a shift to the right of their force-velocity curve, with an increase in both V_{max} and in P_0. The time interval between stimulation and peak shortening was also decreased. (*From Sonnenblick et al.[64] Reproduced with permission of the publisher.*)

FORCE-VELOCITY IN HUMAN PAPILLARY MUSCLE

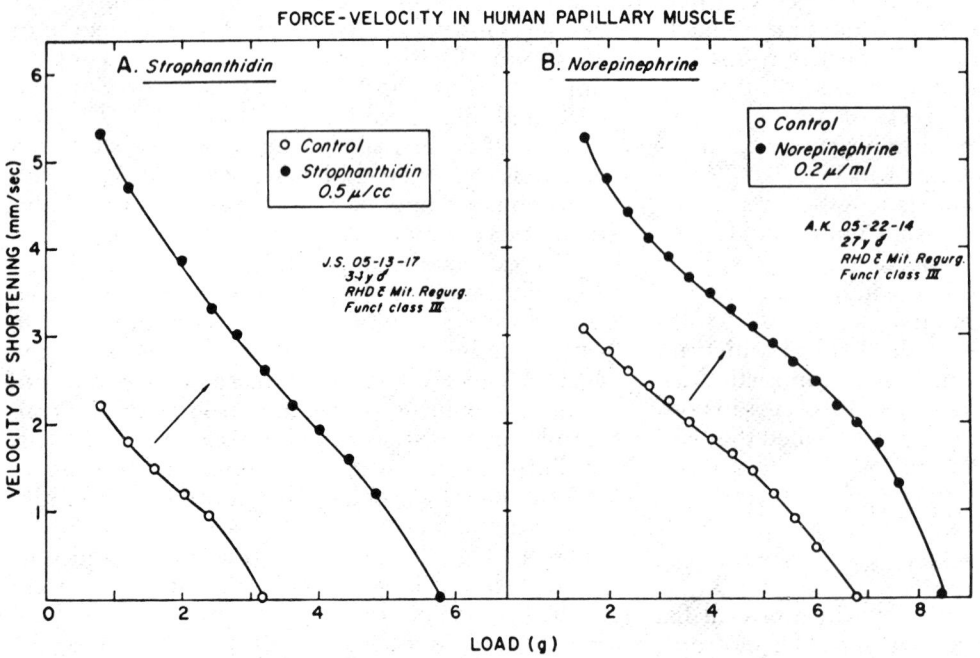

creased contractility can also be illustrated by ventricular function curves (Fig. 3-10); however, a function curve tends to be a less sensitive indicator of changes in the contractile state of the myocardium than a force-velocity curve. Thus, function curves, which relate end-diastolic pressure to stroke volume and stroke work, may show only small changes, while significant changes are apparent in the force-velocity curves.[69] Similarly, the increased contractility produced by an increase in heart rate (the *force-frequency relation* or the *Bowditch phenomenon*[47,48,68,125–129]) in effecting primarily speed of contraction may more readily be shown by force-velocity curves than by ventricular function curves. Larger amounts of norepinephrine or larger increases in heart rate may, however, influence both types of curves in the direction of increased contractility.

The complex interrelations between *force, velocity, and length* of both isolated myocardium and intact ventricles can best be represented by a three-dimensional graph.[6,67] Figure 3-16 is a diagram of such a graph for a ventricle with the superimposed course of a single contraction; Fig. 3-17 illustrates the effect of increasing preload or initial muscle length; Fig. 3-18 illustrates the effects of an increased contractile state. This indicates that when contractility is augmented, the myocardium shortens faster at any given muscle length, for any given load, and also shortens further or generates more force. It should

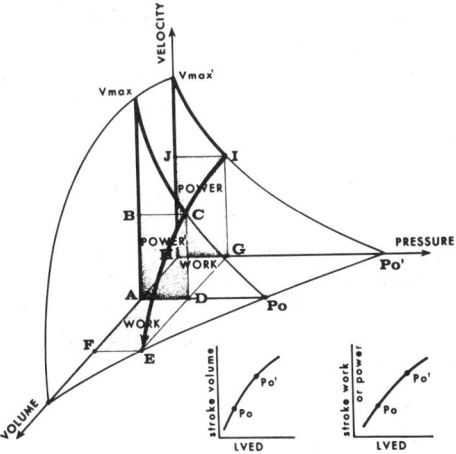

FIGURE 3-17 The effect of increasing preload (left ventricular end-diastolic pressure) on the force-velocity-volume relation (Frank-Starling law). Blood pressure remains the same. Maximum isometric force increases from P_0 to P_0': work increases from ADEF to HGEF, while power increases from ABCD to HGIJ. This increase in the end-diastolic volume of the ventricle does not represent a change in the contractile state of the myocardium, since V_{max} is not changed. The insert in the lower right shows the predicted relations of stroke volume, stroke work, and stroke power to left ventricular end-diastolic pressure (LVED), reflecting changes in work and power areas from the three-dimensional diagram. (*From Sonnenblick.*[67] *Reproduced with permission of the publisher.*)

be noted that myocardial contractility at any one moment is best defined by the three-dimensional curved surface relating force, velocity, and length.

When sympathetic stimulation causes the heart to beat with increased contractility and at a faster rate, not only is the contraction more forceful and faster, but the relaxation and elastic recoil of the ventricular musculature are also more rapid. Both these effects tend to increase stroke volume of the next beat, since the diastolic filling period is longer than

FIGURE 3-16 Force-velocity-length (force-velocity-volume) diagram of the intact ventricle. The force is the equivalent of load, which is the sum of preload (end-diastolic pressure) and afterload (aortic pressure). The length axis is derived from intraventricular volume. The superimposed dark line portrays the course of a single contraction. Starting at A, with activation, the CE velocity rises toward V_{max}. With CE shortening, force is built up and velocity of shortening decreases to C. This represents the isometric (isovolumic) phase of contraction. At C, the force equals the load, and shortening begins from C to E. During muscle shortening between C and E, velocity of shortening changes as a function of the decrease in muscle length which ensues. Shaded area on the force-velocity (vertical) plane represents calculated power (ABCD); shaded area on the base represents work for a load P (ADEF). (*From Sonnenblick.*[67] *Reproduced with permission of the publisher.*)

FIGURE 3-18 The effect of increasing the contractile state on the force-velocity-volume relation of the ventricle. Both V_{max} and P_0 are augmented, while the load (pressure) has been kept constant. Work and power are augmented. (*From Sonnenblick.*[67] *Reproduced with permission of the publisher.*)

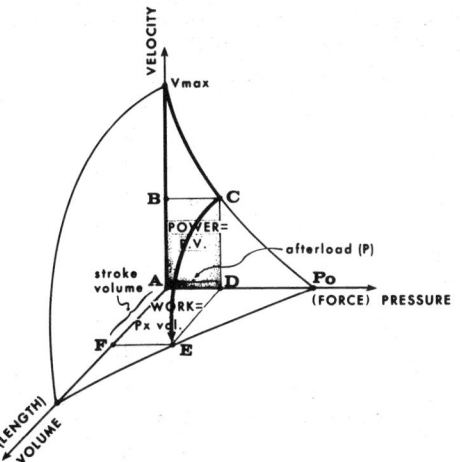

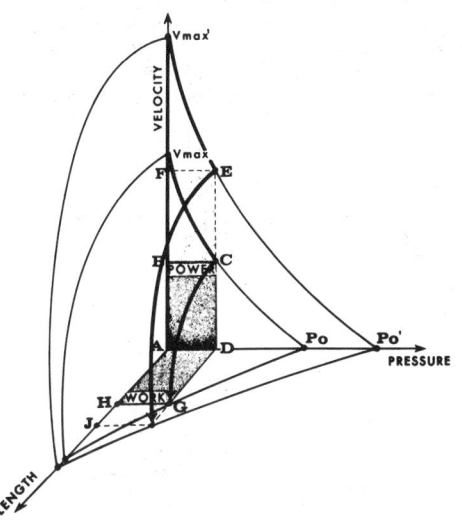

it would otherwise be and since, with the more rapid elastic recoil, the ventricular pressure will be lower earlier, and possibly lower absolutely, than it would otherwise be. The increased emptying produced by increased contractility also means that the fiber length will be less at the beginning of the next diastole. This tends to increase distensibility of the ventricle and to allow greater filling at a lower filling pressure. Figure 3-19 illustrates this important characteristic, by which very slight increases in venous pressure can markedly increase fiber length when operating at this point on the ventricular pressure–fiber length curve.

Afterload: Aortic Impedance

It has been known since O. Frank's experiments[83] that ventricular ejection and performance are importantly influenced by the resistance against which the ventricles contract.[6,54,57–65,76,87,89,92,143,144,164–170] For the left ventricle the major peripheral factors are the aortic impedance, the peripheral vascular resistance, the arterial wall (or stiffness) resistance, the mass of the column of blood in the aorta, and the viscosity of blood; the corresponding factors for the right ventricle are the main pulmonary artery impedance, the pulmonary vascular resistance, the mass of blood in the pulmonary circulation, and the viscosity of blood. In addition to these peripheral factors, the preload or end-diastolic volume of the ventricle is a major determinant of ventricular afterload. Thus, the amount of blood in the ventricle at end-diastole directly determines the radius of the ventricle at the onset of systole and thereby (by the Laplace relationship) the amount of myocardial wall tension necessary during ventricular ejection. In conditions in which the volume of blood in the left

ventricle decreases rapidly after the onset of systole (such as mitral regurgitation or ventricular septal defect), the total impedance to left ventricular emptying rapidly decreases during systole, thereby decreasing significantly the load upon the ventricle.[168] In general, the effects of afterload continuously influence the force-velocity-length-time relations throughout the course of myocardial shortening. Since afterload influences the rate and extent of systolic emptying of the ventricles, it directly influences the ventricular end-systolic volume; thus, afterload indirectly influences the diastolic characteristics (filling pressure and volume or preload) of the next beat of the ventricle. An additional influence of changes in afterload is manifest by an increase in ventricular performance several beats after aortic pressure is raised (the *Anrep effect*).[171] Some studies have indicated that it may be due to recovery from transient subendocardial ischemia caused by the sudden change in arterial pressure.[6,172]

Heart Rate

The fourth major determinant of cardiac function is the heart rate, or the frequency of cardiac contraction. This is probably the major mechanism by which most individuals increase their cardiac output during periods of modest increased demand or exercise. An increase in pulse rate may also increase myocardial contractility (Fig. 3-14); this force-interval relationship is known as *treppe, staircase phenomenon,* or *Bowditch effect*.[6,47,48,68,69,81,125–129,173] This effect is much more apparent in the anesthetized animal, or in the depressed heart, than in the intact, conscious subject.[6,127,174] Even in the intact individual, however, the duration of each systole decreases as the heart rate increases, within limits. Neverthe-

FIGURE 3-19 *Left.* The relation between left ventricular end-diastolic pressure and stroke work. *Center.* The relation between left ventricular segment length and left ventricular end-diastolic pressure. *Right.* The relation between changes in left ventricular segment length and stroke work. In the left-hand panel it is apparent that large changes in ventricular stroke work are obtained without extensive changes in the pressure necessary to fill the ventricle or the pressure in the atrium and veins behind it when the ventricle is functioning on the initial steep portion of the curve, as it probably is normally during the various phases of the respiratory cycle. In the center panel it is apparent that at low segment lengths, such as might occur after greater emptying of the ventricle, relatively large changes in fiber length are brought about by small pressure changes in the ventricle and hence in the atrium and veins behind it. In the right-hand panel it is apparent that there is a more nearly 1:1 relation than in the other panels. This supports the opinion that end-diastolic fiber length is the most appropriate factor in the analysis of ventricular function, even though other values (e.g., end-diastolic pressure) are more readily determined experimentally. (*From Sarnoff and Mitchell.*[163] *Reproduced with permission of the authors and publisher.*)

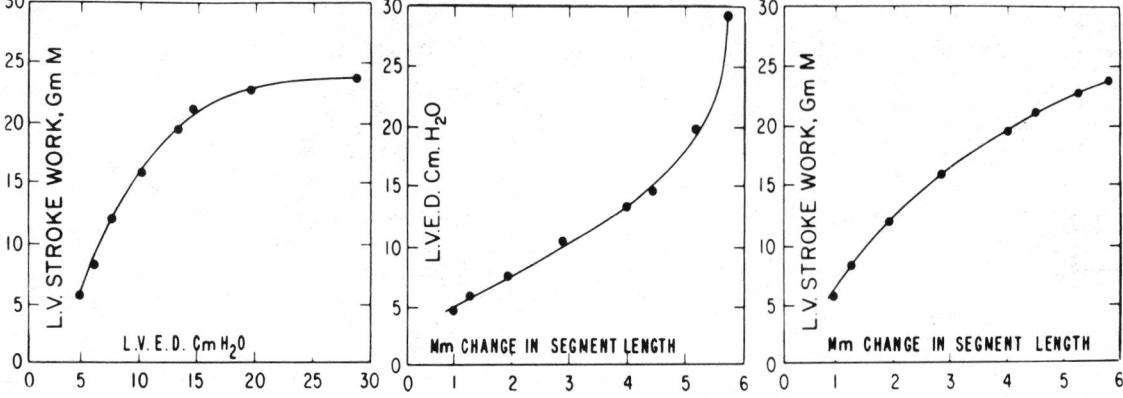

less, since there are more systoles per minute, the time per minute spent in systole increases.[175] Presumably, the increase in heart rate results in more Ca^{2+} being released from the stores within the myocardial cell, thus enhancing myofibrillar contraction. The "recuperative effect of a long pause" upon the strength of contraction is known as the *Woodworth phenomenon*, or as *negative*, or *reverse, staircase phenomenon*.[176,177]

Other Factors Influencing Ventricular Function and Contractility

Sequence of Ventricular Contraction

An additional concept of importance in the application of the law of the heart to the ventricle as a whole concerns the sequence of ventricular activation and contraction. Since the ventricular myocardial fibers contract sequentially, the strength of contraction of the later-contracting myocardial fibers is influenced by the strength, the rate, and the sequence of contraction of the fibers that contract earlier and that stretch the later-contracting fibers.[178–181] Since one aspect of increased contractility is a faster rate of contraction, an increased contractility of the initially contracting fibers may increase the end-diastolic fiber length of the myocardial fibers that have not yet begun to contract, and thereby directly increase the force of contraction of those fibers that contract later. This phenomenon has been referred to as *idioventricular kick*,[181] in analogy with the increased ventricular filling and performance, or the *atrial kick*, produced by atrial systole. An abnormal sequence of ventricular contraction or dyssynergy is also mechanically less efficient and relatively wasteful of energy, particularly if there are areas of akinesis or dyskinesis (see Chap. 44).

Ventricular Suction

Ventricular filling is enhanced by any increases in the pressure difference between the atrium and ventricle, whether produced by increased atrial pressure or by lower ventricular diastolic pressure. The latter phenomenon, which can be produced by increased elastic recoil, is referred to as *diastolic suction*. One form is present normally during early diastole, immediately following opening of the atrioventricular (AV) valve, and its extent is inversely related to ventricular volume. During this earliest phase of rapid ventricular filling, the pressure in the ventricle *decreases* despite a rapid *increase* in ventricular volume. Other forms of diastolic suction have been reviewed by Brecher,[182] although the physiological significance of the phenomena is still uncertain. This phenomenon enhances filling of the ventricle in early diastole, especially when the end-systolic volume is small.[183] Such a mechanism would be of especial value during exercise, where tachycardia may limit the time for filling. Interestingly, increases in contractility not only increase the rate of pressure

change during systole (dP/dt) but also increase the rate of relaxation, reflected as negative dP/dt.[184] In the failing ventricle, where ventricular volume is large, diastolic suction is much less, and higher mean atrial pressures are needed to fill the ventricle.

Atrial Function[2,6,185–192]

There are two main functions of the atria: a transport, or pump, function and a reservoir function to contain blood available for rapid ventricular filling. Like the ventricles, the atria respond to an increase in fiber length by an increased force of contraction. Increased atrial contractility characterized by a shift to the left of atrial function curves (or a shift to the right of their force-velocity curves) may be produced by increased sympathetic stimulation and by inotropic agents such as digitalis or catecholamines or decreased vagal stimulation. Both these mechanisms cause the atrium to pump a greater amount of blood forward into the ventricle, with a resultant increase in ventricular end-diastolic fiber length and pressure (the *atrial kick*), thereby causing the ventricle to increase its force of contraction. When the atrial transport function is lost (i.e., by atrial fibrillation) in a person with an otherwise normal heart, the normal circulatory reserve mechanisms are able to maintain the cardiac output at rest within normal limits, although the response of the cardiac output to strenuous exercise may be somewhat diminished. In a patient with ventricular disease, however, even the resting cardiac output may be diminished significantly by this form of *atrial failure* (see Chap. 22).

Nervous Control[1–10,193–201]

The nerve endings of sympathetic fibers, which lie between the myocardial fibers, synthesize norepinephrine and store it in granules. Upon stimulation, these sympathetic fibers cause the local release of norepinephrine, which acts locally upon beta receptors which are present on the fiber surface to enhance the activity of adenyl cyclase, which in turn catalyzes the conversion of adenosine triphosphate (ATP) to cyclic AMP (adenosine 3′,5′-monophosphate or "second messenger").[202–204] Once nerve stimulation stops, the same nerve endings take up and store norepinephrine for reutilization. A small amount of the norepinephrine is also metabolized locally. Sympathetic nerve fibers reach the entire atria and ventricles, as well as the sinoatrial (SA) and atrioventricular (AV) nodes, while vagal fibers, which cause the local release of acetylcholine, influence predominantly the atrial musculature and SA and AV nodes. Vagal innervation, however, has been shown to reach the ventricles, and vagal stimulation can decrease ventricular contractility to a small extent.[205] In general, sympathetic stimulation increases atrial and ventricular contractility, increases heart rate, and speeds the spread of excitation through the AV node and, very slightly, through the ventricles.[206]

Vagal stimulation generally has opposite effects to sympathetic stimulation. At any given instant, the effect of the nervous system on the heart is the net balance of these two opposing controls, which usually vary reciprocally. It is probable that the vagal parasympathetic stimulation, which is generally inhibitory, normally predominates in the conscious state and maintains the usual resting heart rate of about 65 to 75 beats per minute.[6,207] The resting bradycardia of exercise training is due predominantly to a slowing of the intrinsic rate of the pacemaker as a result of enhanced vagal activity accompanied by a decrease in the adrenergic influence.[208] Neural reflexes, particularly from stretch receptors in the carotid sinus and aorta, form a major extrinsic control mechanism that influences myocardial performance directly and indirectly.[200] When carotid sinus stretch decreases, as with arterial hypotension, a reflex venoconstriction is produced by the sympathetic nervous system that increases venous return and thereby increases ventricular end-diastolic fiber length. Simultaneously, carotid sinus hypotension produces reflex arterial vasoconstriction, increasing peripheral vascular resistance and aortic impedance. In addition, carotid sinus hypotension elicits reflexes that increase atrial and ventricular contractility. Stimulation of the carotid sinus nerve, such as might occur with carotid sinus hypertension, produces opposite effects.

Drugs and Hormones

Myocardial contractility is increased by increased activation of the myocardium, which is mediated in one form or another by an enhanced availability of Ca^{2+} ions inside the cell.[32,33] Increased Ca^{2+} bathing the heart produces this action. Catecholamines, including norepinephrine, epinephrine, and isoproterenol, act through beta receptors on the myocardial cell that activate the adenyl cyclase system, which ultimately affects membrane systems within the cells that deliver Ca^{2+} to the contractile proteins. Phosphorylation of these membranes also enhances relaxation.[10] Digitalis glycosides also enhance contractility but act by inhibiting the Na^+-K^+–stimulated ATPase in the cell surface membrane, which appears to leave larger amounts of Ca^{2+} within the fiber.[23,31,40–42] Contractility is also increased to some degree by corticosteroids, aldactone, angiotensin, serotonin,[209] and glucagon.[210–212] The physiological role of other substances, such as prostaglandins,[213–215] and polypeptide systems, such as kinekard[216] and cardioglobulin, in the regulation of myocardial contractility is unclear. The actions of thyroxine on myocardial contractile functions are complex,[218–221] but in general its effects are to increase contraction and relaxation rate. Myocardial contractility is decreased by hypoxia and by many drugs, including barbiturates, quinidine, propranolol, procainamide, and lidocaine. Acidosis also depresses myocardial

contractility, particularly if the sympathoadrenal system function is impaired.[222] Morphine produces a negative inotropic effect upon isolated myocardial strips, but in the conscious dog it produces a beta-adrenergic–mediated increase in myocardial contractility and alpha-adrenergic–mediated coronary vasoconstriction.[223]

Anesthesia

General anesthesia from halothane or pentobarbital may depress myocardial contractility significantly.[174] In addition, the reflex control mechanisms influencing heart rate may be significantly altered by anesthesia. For example, under anesthesia, the reflex bradycardia of acute hypertension is caused mainly by withdrawal of sympathetic stimulation, while in the conscious state, it is caused almost entirely by increased parasympathetic restraint.[174,193,194] In the intact conscious animal, the force-frequency relation, or the *Bowditch phenomenon,* appears to influence myocardial contractility relatively little, whereas an increase in heart rate causes a much larger increase in contractility if the base line of contractility is first depressed by generalized anesthesia.[174] Similarly, in anesthetized animals, the increase in heart rate produced by acute volume loading and presumed stimulation of low-pressure receptors in the atria (the *Bainbridge reflex*) is erratic; on the other hand, the reflex is consistently found in conscious animals and can be blocked by the combination of atropine and propranolol.[224] In contrast, the *Anrep effect,* or the positive inotropic effect of an acute increase in afterload, has been demonstrated in the anesthetized animal but is difficult to demonstrate in the conscious subject with low spontaneous heart rates.[174]

Anesthesia also influences the response to many drugs. The relative increase in myocardial contractility produced by digitalis is much less apparent in the conscious state than if the myocardium is depressed by general anesthesia or propranolol. In addition, intravenous ouabain given to the conscious subject produces substantial coronary vasoconstriction and mesenteric vasodilatation, in contrast to effects that are produced when ouabain is given during anesthesia.[174] The coronary vasoconstriction produced by norepinephrine or morphine sulfate, which is due to alpha-adrenergic stimulation, is much more apparent with the subject in the conscious state than under general anesthesia, as in the coronary vasoconstriction produced by dopamine.[174,225]

When an extraventricular depolarization is imposed or occurs spontaneously between normal beats, the subsequent normal beat is potentiated. The extent of *postextrasystolic potentiation* is generally related to the closeness of the extra beat to the prior normal beat. Advantage has even been taken clinically of this phenomenon by placing an electrically induced extra beat close to the spontaneous beat and continuing this.[226–228] This paired electrical stimulation markedly increases myocardial contractility and stroke output, although the cardiac output per minute is not increased unless it was previously decreased. The mechanism of this type of post-extrasystolic potentiation is probably related to increased availability of calcium ions near the contractile sites of the actin and myosin myofilaments. Unfortunately, the use of this mechanism for the treatment of the failing heart has the danger of inducing ventricular fibrillation.

Mechanisms of Cardiac Reserve

The normal homeostatic mechanisms regulate cardiac output to meet the demands of the body, and they can enable the heart to increase its output five- to sixfold during exercise. It is not possible to separate sharply those mechanisms by which the cardiovascular system is normally controlled and those mechanisms of *cardiac reserve* (Table 3-1) that the heart may utilize to meet increased demands on the normal heart and/or to maintain cardiac function in the presence of disease of the heart or circulatory system. Many of these homeostatic and regulatory mechanisms act synergistically in the intact organism; others, such as the sympathetic and parasympathetic nervous control of the heart, are in a state of constantly varying balance. Although it is often possible to separate and even quantify the relative contributions of each mechanism in the experimental animal, it is at present difficult, if not impossible, to separate the possible mechanisms functioning at any one instant in human beings. Indeed, the demonstration of mechanisms during physiological experiments indicates only *potential* mechanisms of reserve or control, not what actually happens in the intact organism. Furthermore, most of the mechanisms are interrelated and affect one another, so that the contribution of one mechanism depends on, and changes with, the contribution of the other mechanisms. In the following discussion, we shall consider some of these mechanisms from the standpoint of their use as forms of *cardiac reserve*, although many of these same mechanisms are utilized in the *normal circulatory regulation.*[6,144,149,229–232] (See also Chap. 22.)

The two basic mechanisms of cardiac reserve by which the heart or any other pulsatile pump can increase its minute output in the face of increased demands (or attempt to maintain output in the presence of myocardial disease) are (1) change in rate and (2) change in stroke volume.

Heart Rate

A change in pulse rate is one of the simplest and most effective ways of increasing cardiac output. It is probably the most important and most commonly employed mechanism for effecting rapid changes in cardiac output, particularly in untrained individuals under conditions of moderately increased demands. An increase in heart rate by itself may increase cardiac output about three- to fourfold in highly trained athletes. Above certain limits, however, cardiac output may actually begin to fall as heart rate rises. This rate is about 170 to 180 beats per minute for most normal young individuals, but may be 200 to 220 in trained athletes or only 120 to 140 in older, untrained persons or in patients with heart disease. The decrease in cardiac output above a certain rate is due largely to the shortening of the time of diastole, limiting the time for both adequate filling of the ventricles and for coronary blood flow, which occurs predominantly during diastole in the left ventricle. Although an increase in heart rate does produce a rather slight increase in myocardial contractility and a shortening in the absolute duration of systole,[6,47,66–68,125–129,173] negative inotropic effects of tachycardia can become apparent above a certain rate.[173] Most changes in pulse rate are effected by decrease in vagal inhibition and/or by sympathetic stimulation of the sinoatrial pacemaker of the heart.[193–201]

Stroke Volume

In a normal individual in the recumbent position, the ratio of left ventricular stroke volume (SV) to end-diastolic volume (EDV), termed the *ejection fraction,* is about 60 to 75 percent as estimated angiographically. Increased contractility may increase the ejection fraction and the stroke volume with a decreased end-systolic volume (ESV), with the end-diastolic volume (EDV) either decreasing or remaining the same. An increased stroke volume can also be produced either by a primary increase in venous return, which increases the end-diastolic fiber length of the atria and ventricles, or by a decrease in afterload, which permits enhanced emptying of the ventricle. In the early stages of heart failure, there is often an increase in end-diastolic volume and fiber length which tends to maintain the stroke volume, although the ejection fraction is decreased. A decrease in ejection fraction is a hallmark of ventricular failure (see Chaps. 18 and 22).

Increased Oxygen Extraction

When the tissue requirements for oxygen increase, or the supply of blood decreases, the tissues may, up to a point, extract more oxygen from each volume of blood passing through the tissue. The entry

TABLE 3-1   Mechanisms of Cardiac Reserve

Increased heart rate
Increased stroke volume
Increased oxygen extraction
Redistribution of blood flow
Anaerobic metabolism
Cardiac dilatation
Cardiac hypertrophy

of oxygen into myocardial cells is facilitated by myoglobin, which has oxygen-dissociation characteristics favorable to the diffusion of oxygen into the cells.[233] Increased oxygen extraction is a major reserve mechanism utilized by the tissues of the body acutely during extreme exertion or chronically when the cardiac output is diminished. This reserve mechanism is of less value to the myocardium, which even normally extracts about 75 percent of its arterial oxygen content (see Chap. 20).

Redistribution of Blood Flow[1–14,196,234–242]

The redistribution of cardiac output is a major mechanism of reserve for the body under conditions of increased demand, as during exercise or under conditions of diminished cardiac output. The general result is to maintain blood flow to the brain and the heart and to the tissues acutely requiring blood flow, while sacrificing blood flow to tissues and organs not being utilized or less essential to the immediate survival of the person. The mechanisms by which this redistribution occurs are complex. Although the following explanation is oversimplified, the redistribution may be considered to be the integrated response of two mechanisms: (1) a local autoregulation of the metabolically active tissue or organ, by which local changes in P_{O_2}, P_{CO_2}, pH, potassium ion (K^+) concentration, and other metabolic products affect the local blood vessels to reduce small-vessel resistance and increase blood flow (see below), and (2) an integrated response of the central nervous system, mediated by the sympathetic and parasympathetic nervous systems, to produce vasodilatation of the active or exercising organ and vasoconstriction of many other tissues and organs. In addition, there often appears to be a venoconstriction mediated by the sympathetic nervous system, which increases venous return to the heart and performs a type of internal transfusion or shifting of blood from the large venous reservoirs to the heart, arterial system, and active organs.

Anaerobic Metabolism

Many tissues, particularly skeletal muscle, may also utilize anaerobic metabolism as a reserve mechanism, although the value of this mechanism for the myocardium is also quite limited (see Chap. 20). In a normal individual during moderate exercise, anaerobic metabolism may account for about 5 percent of the energy utilized; patients with heart failure may obtain 30 percent of their immediate total energy requirements by anaerobic metabolism during exercise.

Dilatation and Hypertrophy

Dilatation and hypertrophy are forms of compensatory reserve, although they are also swords of Damocles for the heart. Their effects in heart fail-

ure are discussed in Chap. 22, and their significance in athletes is discussed in Chap. 68.

Sequential Phases of the Cardiac Cycle[11,243–247]

The successive mechanical events of the cardiac cycle may be described by a modification (Plate 1) of Wiggers' classic diagram, which divided the cardiac cycle into two *periods*, systole and diastole, and subdivided these periods into *phases* of cardiac activity.[243–247] In the following discussion, the cardiac cycle is divided according to events on the left side of the heart. Corresponding periods and phases may also be described for events on the right side of the heart, with some differences (see below).

The first phase of ventricular systole is *isovolumic* (*isovolumetric* or *isochoric*) *contraction*. This phase begins with the first detectable rise in left ventricular pressure after the z point; it is associated with the initial, mitral component (MC) of the first heart sound and the beginning of the isovolumic contraction (IC) wave of the apex cardiogram. The end of the isovolumic contraction phase and the beginning of the succeeding *rapid ventricular ejection* phase are indicated by the opening of the aortic valve (AO), a rise in aortic pressure, a decrease in ventricular volume, and the peak of the ejection E wave of the apex cardiogram. The onset and termination of the next phase of *reduced ventricular ejection* are less well defined; however, this phase may be said to begin when the shape of the ventricular volume curve indicates a significant decrease in the rate of ejection. This normally occurs prior to the peak systolic pressure in the left ventricle and aorta. The phase of reduced ejection lasts until the end of actual ventricular ejection with the beginning of diastole, which occurs just prior to the recording of the incisura on the aortic pressure tracing. The very brief initial phase of diastole preceding the incisura is referred to as *protodiastole* and represents the time required for the reversal of flow in the aorta and for closure of the aortic valve, which is responsible for the incisura of the aortic pressure tracing.

The beginning of the next phase of isovolumic relaxation of the left ventricle is signified by the closure of the aortic valve as indicated by the aortic component (AC) of the second heart sound and by an inward isovolumic relaxation (IR) wave of the apex cardiogram. Isovolumic relaxation lasts until the left ventricular pressure falls below the left atrial pressure and blood begins to flow from the atrium into the ventricle. Usually the left ventricular pressure falls below the left atrial pressure tracing slightly *after* the peak of the left atrial v wave, since there is a slight fall in left atrial pressure caused by a decrease in the upward bulging of the atrioventricular (AV) valve structures during ventricular isovolumic relaxation. In a sense, this is the opposite of the mechanism thought to produce the c wave in the atria during early ventricular systole.

The end of the isovolumic relaxation phase and the beginning of the *rapid ventricular filling phase* are indicated by an increase in the ventricular volume curve, and by the zero point of the apex cardiogram, which coincides with the opening of the mitral valve (MO). If the mitral valve is diseased, the opening of the valve may be audible as an "opening snap" (OS). This rapid ventricular filling phase is associated with a continuation of the decrease in atrial pressure (the *y* descent) begun during isovolumic relaxation, a rapid increase in ventricular volume, and an outward rapid-filling wave in the apex cardiogram.

The end of the rapid ventricular-filling phase and the beginning of the *slow ventricular-filling phase* are evidenced by a change in the slope of the ventricular volume curve, which indicates a change in the rate of ventricular filling. At times the end of rapid ventricular filling is associated with low-frequency vibrations or a sound, termed the S_3 or ventricular gallop, which occurs very shortly before the nadir of the *y* descent of the atrial pressure tracing. On the apex cardiogram the end of the rapid ventricular-filling phase (and the identification of S_3) is indicated at the moment when an abrupt change in slope occurs at the transition from the rapid-filling wave (RFW) to the slow-filling wave (SFW). This may be associated with a brief outward pulsation, which is referred to as an *F wave*, or *peak*, on the apex cardiogram; frequently it is both visible and palpable.

During the phase of slow ventricular filling, or diastasis, the pressures in the left atrium and left ventricle slowly increase until the next atrial systole produces the *a* wave in the left atrial pressure tracing. At times, an *h wave* is present in late diastasis prior to the *a wave*. Atrial contraction and the increased ventricular filling produced by atrial contraction are reflected in an increase in ventricular pressure, an increase in ventricular volume, and an outward *a* wave of the apex cardiogram. Toward the peak or the second half of the atrial *a* wave there may be a sound (S_4), particularly if there is a vigorous atrial contraction and relaxation. After the *a* wave of atrial contraction and relaxation, there is a very brief period or point (*z point*) when atrial and ventricular pressures are essentially equal in normal individuals. The next cardiac cycle begins when the next ventricular contraction causes a definite sharp rise in pressure from the *z* point.

As one would expect from the location of the sinus node, contraction of the right atrium and opening of the tricuspid valve occur slightly before the corresponding events on the left side of the heart (Plates 1 and 2). On the other hand, excitation and contraction of the left ventricle begin prior to contraction of the right ventricle, although the beginning of ejection of blood into the pulmonary artery slightly precedes ejection into the aorta, since the pressure in the right ventricle does not have to increase to such a high level before ejection begins (Plate 2). Interestingly, right ventricular ejection lasts beyond left ventricular ejection, producing the normal interval between the aortic component of the second heart sound (A_2) and the pulmonic component of the second heart sound (P_2). The shorter duration of left ventricular ejection is related to the greater contractile force of the left ventricle and to differences in the aorta and the pulmonary artery impedance and compression-chamber (windkessel) characteristics.

During the brief phase of left ventricular isovolumic systole, the central aortic pressure pulse may show a slight positive wave that is produced by slight bulging of the aortic valve that is due to the rapidly increasing left ventricular pressure. There is evidence that during left ventricular ejection, the left ventricular pressure exceeds aortic pressure only during the early part of ejection, and actually is slightly less than aortic pressure during most of systole.[248] It should also be noted that though several components of the first and second heart sounds are referred to by the name of the valve commonly associated with the production of that sound, the sounds are not produced by the actual closure or striking together of the valve leaflets. *The sounds are more properly considered to be produced by the sudden acceleration and deceleration of blood with tensing of the entire valve structures, and by vibrations of all cardiac structures.* Actually, there is evidence that the atrioventricular valves and the aortic valve may be closed physiologically at a different time than when these sounds occur.[249–255] In most clinical situations, the two components of the first heart sound, the mitral (M) and the tricuspid (T) component, are produced by sudden acceleration-deceleration of blood, the valves, and cardiac structures in association with closure of the mitral and tricuspid valves, respectively.

The shape of the apex cardiogram tracing varies significantly depending on the particular instrumentation used to record it. The tracing shown in Plate 1 was obtained with a piezo crystal, which is widely used for timing despite some inherent distortion (see Chaps. 11 and 85).

The Arterial Pulse

The arterial pressure pulse is produced by the ejection of blood from the left ventricle into the aorta and great vessels at a rate faster than its runoff into the peripheral circulation. In humans, an average left ventricular stroke volume of 60 to 100 ml is ejected in about 0.25 s, and of this volume, approximately two-thirds is ejected during the rapid-ejection phase. Although the peak rate of ejection of blood occurs prior to the peak pressure in the left ventricle or aorta, the pressure continues to rise in the aorta as long as blood is ejected into the aorta faster than it runs off into the peripheral arteries. Sometimes there is a slight notch in the central arterial pulse wave during or toward the end of the rapid-ejection phase. This is referred to as the *anacrotic notch,* or *shoulder;* it is accentuated in valvular aortic stenosis. At the end of ventricular ejection (and after the very brief phase of protodiastole), the aortic valve closes. In central aortic pressure tracings, this event is reflected by a sharp downward deflection, or *incisura*, on the descending limb of the pressure tracing and a gradual fall during diastole. At times left ventricular isovolumic contraction causes a slight positive deflection in central arterial tracings just prior to the onset of the main arterial pulse wave.

As the arterial pressure pulse wave passes to the periphery, there are marked changes in its form (Fig. 3-20).[256] As the pulse moves away from the heart, the initial upstroke of the pulse becomes steeper, there is normally no anacrotic pause on the ascending limb, and the systolic maximum becomes peaked and increased in magnitude. The *dicrotic notch*, or *halt*, which corresponds to the incisura recorded more centrally, tends to occur later and lower and to be smoother in contour than the incisura. The positive wave which follows the dicrotic notch is referred to as the *dicrotic wave;* in many peripheral arteries it is normally more prominent than the slight upward deflection recorded centrally following the incisura. Although the systolic pressure may increase as the wave moves to the periphery, the diastolic and mean arterial pressures decrease slightly. The major factors responsible for these changes in the arterial pulse contour are (1) distortion of the components of the pulse waves as

they travel peripherally, (2) different rates of transmission of various components of the pulse wave, (3) amplification or distortion of different components of the pulse by *standing* or *reflected waves,* (4) differences in elastic behavior and in caliber of the arteries, and (5) conversion of some kinetic energy to hydrostatic energy. Further details of the arterial pulse are discussed in Chap. 10.

The Venous Pulse[185,257]

The form of the venous pressure pulse is determined by the rate of return of the blood from the peripheral tissues into the venous segment, the pressure-volume characteristics of the segment of the vein, the nature of the resistance to flow or distensibility offered by the right atrium and ventricle during the different phases of the cardiac cycle, and, to a slight degree, the tissues overlying the veins at the point of observation. Although the venous pressure pulse wave travels peripherally away from the heart, there is at the same time a venous flow of blood in the opposite direction toward the heart.

The *a* wave of the venous pressure pulse is related to contraction of the right atrium and is followed by the *z* point immediately preceding ventricular systole. In the jugular venous pulse, the *c* wave as usually recorded is predominantly produced by

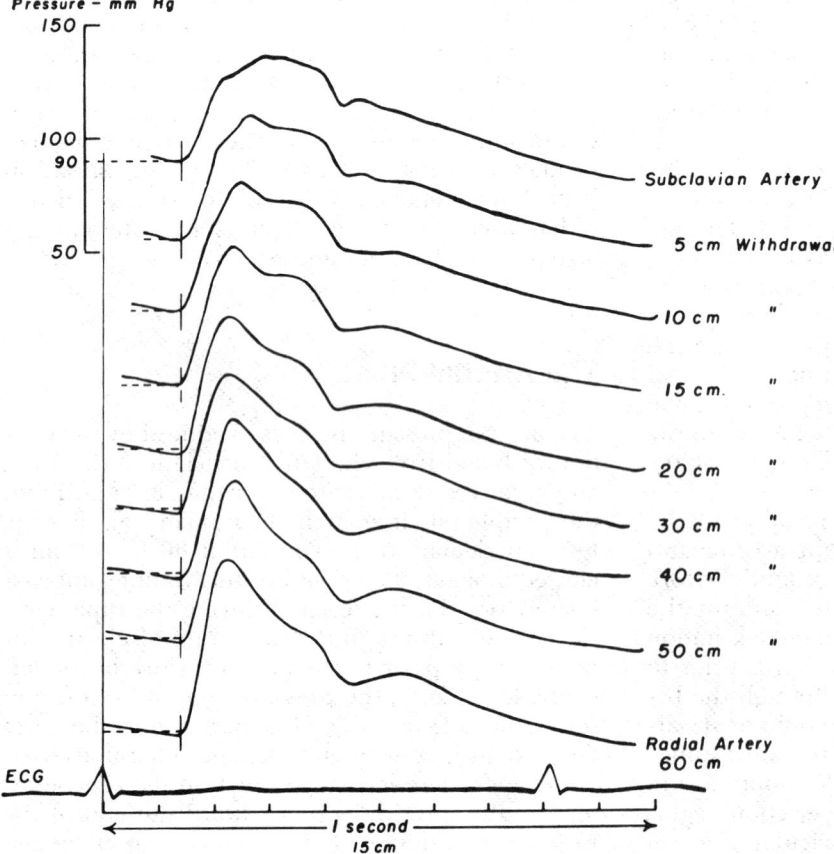

FIGURE 3-20 Pulse contours in a healthy 30-year-old man, showing transformation of pressure pulse in subclavian-radial system. Pressure pulses were recorded consecutively during withdrawal of tip of arterial catheter from subclavian artery near aorta to radial in left arm. Onsets of pressure pulses are aligned for purposes of comparison. As the pulse wave moves peripherally, initial wave steepens and increases in magnitude, dome-shaped systolic maximum becomes peaked, and dicrotic halt moves down and to the right and becomes slurred. Low-amplitude, central postdicrotic wave is not seen after catheter has been withdrawn 10 cm or more. Prominence of radial dicrotic wave is due, in part, to change in position of dicrotic halt. Horizontal broken line intersecting onset of each pulse contour is calibration reference point (90 mmHg). Interval of time from peak of R wave of electrocardiogram to onset of systolic upswing of each pulse wave is indicated by duration of each tracing to left side of short vertical lines, which mark onset of systole from each pulse. (*From Marshall, Helmholz, and Wood.*[256] *Reproduced with permission of the authors and the publisher.*)

the systolic impulse in the adjacent carotid artery with some contribution produced by right ventricular contraction and upward bulging of the tricuspid valve. In the early part of ventricular systole and following the brief c wave, there is a rapid inflow of blood to the right atrium, produced in part by descent of the tricuspid valve ring, which produces the normal negative venous wave during ventricular systole, the negative x wave, or x descent (or systolic collapse). It is also probable during this phase of systole that the ejection of blood from both ventricles decreases the intrapericardial pressure and therefore the pressure in both atria. As the venous inflow continues into the atria after the x descent, the pressure in the atria and in the veins builds up, producing the v wave during approximately the second half of ventricular systole. The v wave continues to build up until the right ventricle passes through the phase of isovolumic relaxation and begins its phase of rapid ventricular filling. The peak of the right atrial v wave occurs shortly before or simultaneously with the opening of the tricuspid valve and the beginning of the phase of rapid right ventricular filling. During early ventricular diastole, the rapid flow of blood from the great veins and right atrium into the right ventricle produces the negative y descent (or diastolic collapse) of the peripheral venous pulse wave. The venous pulse wave is somewhat damped when recorded externally, and even when recorded directly, the waves are usually less steep in rise and descent than the corresponding waves of the atria. In part this is due to the damping effect of the large veins, which can accommodate markedly different volumes of blood without a marked change in pressure. Clinically, venous pulse waves are particularly difficult to evaluate in the presence of tachycardia, obesity, or shock, or during the administration of drugs that produce venoconstriction. Further details of the venous pulse are discussed in Chap. 10.

Normal Pressures and Flow Rates in the Cardiovascular System[258-261]

In general, the pressure in the systemic arteries is about five or six times greater than the pressure in the pulmonary arteries, though the amount of blood flowing in each unit is essentially the same. The left ventricular output may be very slightly greater than the right ventricular output, because of the small amount of bronchial artery flow that returns in the pulmonary veins and the drainage of a few Thebesian veins into the left atrium and ventricle. In order to compare measurements between individuals of different sizes, measurements of flow and resistance are often expressed in terms of square meters of body surface area; i.e., instead of comparing cardiac output in absolute number of liters per minute, the output of the heart is expressed as the *cardiac index,* or liters per minute per square meter of body sur-

face area. There is still a need for additional data to establish the limits of "normal" for vascular pressures, flow, and resistance for all ages of normal individuals under conditions of rest, exercise, or emotional stress. Furthermore, some of the slight differences in normal values reported from different laboratories are related to the use of different methods of measurement or different base lines for measurement of pressure. Table 3-2 lists the mean and range of hemodynamic measurements for normal resting adults, and Table 3-3 gives the distribution of systemic blood flow and oxygen consumption in a hypothetical 70-kg normal resting male.

TABLE 3-2 Hemodynamic Values of Normal Recumbent Adults

	Mean	Range
Cardiac index, liter/min/m^2	3.4	2.8–4.2
Stroke index, ml per beat	47	30–65
Arteriovenous O$_2$ difference, ml per liter of blood	38	30–48
Arterial saturation, %	98	94–100
Pressures,* mmHg:		
Brachial artery		
Systolic	130	90–140
Diastolic	70	60–90
Mean	85	70–105
Left ventricle		
Systolic	130	90–140
End-diastolic	7	4–12
Left atrium		
Maximum	13	6–20
Minimum	3	−2–+9
Mean	7	4–12
Pulmonary artery wedge (PC)		
Maximum	16	9–23
Minimum	6	1–12
Mean	9	6–15
Pulmonary artery		
Systolic	24	15–28
Diastolic	10	5–16
Mean	16	10–22
Right ventricle		
Systolic	24	15–28
End-diastolic	4	0–8
Right atrium		
Maximum	7	2–14
Minimum	2	−2–+6
Mean	4	−1–+8
Venae cavae		
Maximum	7	2–14
Minimum	5	0–8
Mean	6	1–10
End-diastolic volume		
Left ventricular, ml/m^2	70	50–90
Resistances, dyn·s/cm^5		
Total systemic	1150	900–1400
Systemic arteriolar	850	600–900
Total pulmonary	200	150–250
Pulmonary arteriolar	70	45–120

*Base line for pressure measurements one-half of anteroposterior chest diameter. 1 mmHg = 133.332 pascal (Pa) = 0.133 kPa.

TABLE 3-3 Distribution of Systemic Blood Flow and Oxygen Consumption in a Normal Subject* at Rest in a Comfortable Environment

Circulation	Blood Flow, ml/min	Percent of Total Flow	Arteriovenous O_2 Difference, ml/dl	O_2 Consumption, ml/min	Percent of Total Consumption
Splanchnic	1400	24	4.1	58	25
Renal	1100	19	1.3	16	7
Cerebral	750	13	6.3	46	20
Coronary	250	4	11.4	27	11
Skeletal muscle	1200	21	8.0	70	30
Skin	500	9	1.0	5	2
Other organs	600	10	3.0	12	5
Total	5800	100	4.0 (mean)	234	100

*Male; weight, 70 kg; surface area, 1.7 m^2.
Source: From Wade and Bishop.[260] Reprinted with permission.

Response to Exercise[6,14,66,262–285]

The mechanisms utilized to increase the cardiac output during exercise vary, depending on the age, condition, posture, and athletic training of the person. In particular the relative contribution of heart rate and stroke volume has been the subject of considerable interest. It would appear that most normal but untrained individuals in the supine position increase their cardiac output during mild to moderate exercise predominantly by an increase in pulse rate rather than by an increase in stroke volume. With more extreme exercise, even this type of individual will increase stroke volume about 10 to 15 percent in the supine position and 30 to 100 percent in the upright position, despite a considerably shortened systolic ejection period. In normal persons who are more accustomed to physical exertion, there is an earlier and more marked increase in stroke volume in both positions, and stroke volume often doubles during extreme upright exercise. In general, pulse rate may increase threefold (or even fourfold in trained athletes), whereas stroke volume increases considerably less. With extreme increases in rate, stroke volume may even decline slightly.

Exercise results in increased sympathetic adrenergic nervous activity to the resistance vessels of the kidney and splanchnic area and to the uninvolved muscles, while it increases blood flow to the exercising muscles by sympathetic vasodilatation and, probably, by local autoregulation. The arterial systolic blood pressure often increases 40 to 60 mmHg during moderate or severe exercise, although the mean arterial blood pressure increases much less. The diastolic pressure may increase slightly, decrease slightly, or stay the same. Calculated total arterial resistance normally decreases considerably during exercise. An increase in cardiac output is further aided by an increase in venous return produced by the combination of vasodilatation of the exercising muscles and the increased

mechanical activity of the skeletal muscles, which rhythmically compress the peripheral veins, and by the rhythmic increase and decrease of the pressure in the peritoneal and thoracic cavities. The latter is sometimes referred to as the *abdominothoracic pump*. Exercise also produces a decrease in the volume of blood in venous reservoirs, especially in the splanchnic blood volume. The result of these shifts is to make more blood available to the heart, arterial vessels, and exercising muscles. On the other hand, during prolonged exercise, plasma volume may decrease significantly, with a resultant increase in hematocrit.[286,287] Isometric exercises of relatively mild degree may produce significant increases in blood pressure and pulse rate,[288–297] factors of considerable importance in patients with coronary artery disease (see Chaps. 20, 44, and 45).

During exercise, there is a significant redistribution of the elevated cardiac output. During mild to moderate exercise, coronary blood flow and blood flow to the active skeletal muscles increase, and cerebral flow is maintained, whereas renal and splanchnic flow diminish. During more severe exercise, these changes are exaggerated, and flow to the inactive muscles may decrease. During maximal exercise, cerebral flow may also decrease, because of hyperventilation and respiratory alkalosis. Skin flow may decrease initially during exercise but rises with continued exercise and contributes to the elimination of body heat.

In general, there is evidence of a generalized sympathetic discharge during exercise that is overridden in certain organs by local vasodilator metabolites and changes in P_{O_2}, P_{CO_2}, pH, and K^+. In exercising skeletal muscles, there may be increased activity of sympathetic vasodilator fibers in addition to decreased vasoconstrictor activity. Venoconstriction during exercise tends to shift blood toward the central circulation and to the active skeletal muscles. Similar venoconstriction may occur in response to cold, emotion, hyperventilation, or norepinephrine.

Myocardial Oxygen Consumption (M$\dot{V}_{O_2}$)

The hemodynamic determinant of myocardial oxygen consumption (M$\dot{V}_{O_2}$) was related in 1907 by Barcroft and Dixon to external work, or the product of aortic pressure and flow.[298] In 1912, Rohde concluded that ventricular pressure and heart rate together determined myocardial oxygen consumption,[299] and in 1915 Evans and Matsuoka[300] reported "a relation between the tension set up on contraction and the metabolism of the contractile tissue." They noted that volume work was performed more economically (i.e., with less oxygen consumed) than was an equal amount of calculated pressure work, and they also called attention to the fact that the tension change in the wall of the heart "varies roughly as the endocardiac pressure and as the square of the radius of the heart cavities," the now-familiar Laplace relation. Since their paper, many studies have confirmed the importance of active intramyocardial tension, or wall stress, developed by the ventricle, or several related variables, as a major determinant of myocardial oxygen consumption.[301–304] Some of the related variables which have been correlated with M$\dot{V}_{O_2}$ include the product of pressure and heart rate, the product of integrated ventricular pressure and heart rate (the tension-time index),[305] developed wall tension, and contractile element work. The inotropic state, or contractility, or the velocity of contraction, is the second major determinant of myocardial oxygen consumption, and it can account for the variations in M$\dot{V}_{O_2}$ when various calculations of developed tension or work, under various positive or negative inotropic interventions, either do not change or change in the opposite direction.[301–307] The results of several earlier studies relating M$\dot{V}_{O_2}$ to ventricular end-diastolic fiber length or diastolic volume were probably related to changes in developed tension or velocity of contraction. Similarly, the net effect on myocardial oxygen consumption of various positive inotropic interventions, such as sympathetic nerve stimulation or excitement, paired electrical stimulation, or the infusion of digitalis glycosides, catecholamines, or calcium, depends to a large degree on the relative effects on the tension developed and on the contractile state, as reflected in V_{max}, the maximum velocity of shortening of the unloaded muscle.[301–304] Most of the increase in myocardial oxygen uptake produced by catecholamines is related to the hemodynamic alterations which they induce, although large doses can increase uptake by a small amount in the nonbeating heart. The effect of digitalis on M$\dot{V}_{O_2}$ depends on the balance between its direct effect of increasing the contractile state of the myocardium, which increases M$\dot{V}_{O_2}$, and its indirect effect of decreasing ventricular wall tension by decreasing ventricular size and radius.[304,307,308]

As shown in Table 3-4, the seven determinants of myocardial oxygen consumption can be classified

TABLE 3-4 Determinants of Myocardial Oxygen Consumption

Major determinants:
  Myocardial mass
  Intramyocardial tension or wall stress (pressure × volume)
  Inotropic state (contractility)
  Heart rate
Minor determinants:
  External work (load × shortening)
  Basal oxygen requirements
  Activation energy

as four major determinants and three minor determinants. The oxygen cost of electrical activation is probably less than 1 percent of the total M$\dot{V}_{O_2}$, and the costs for contractile-state activation and deactivation and for the maintenance of the active state are also small.[302–305]

Coronary flow and pressure affect oxygen consumption in the nonworking heart but have variable effects in the beating heart.[309] Alcohol stimulates the myocardial uptake of oxygen, whereas hypothermia markedly decreases oxygen consumption.

Regulation of Regional Blood Flow[1–10,12,13,194,196,234,238,310–312]

The amount of blood flowing to an individual organ of the body is determined by the difference between the arterial and venous pressures in the vessels supplying the organ and by the vascular resistance of the organ. Although the arterial and venous pressures change in certain situations, such as during exercise, eating, or emotional stress, most of the alterations in the distribution of blood flow are the consequence of changes in vascular resistance of the organ.

The major mechanisms by which decreases in organ vascular resistance are effected are an increase in caliber of the vessels and an opening of new vascular channels. Since most of the vascular resistance appears to be located at the level of the small arteries and arterioles, it is probable that most of the regulation occurs by changes in caliber of these vessels, although changes in the capillaries and veins may at times play an important role.

In a consideration of the local control of blood flow, several fundamental relations and definitions should first be introduced.

The *resistance* to blood flow through a given portion of the circulation is expressed by the ratio of mean pressure difference between two points in the vascular system to the mean amount of blood passing from one point to the other. It is usually calculated using mean pressures and flows, although most vascular flow is pulsatile. If it were possible to measure accurately instantaneous pressure differences and flows, it would be theoretically more proper to calculate vascular *impedance,* which is the ratio of pulsatile pressure to pulsatile flow and which varies with the frequency of the pulse. Vascular resistance may be expressed in various units. It may be expressed in *peripheral resistance units* (PRU), i.e., pressure gradient (mmHg) per unit blood flow (ml/s); by Aperia's formula to give results in absolute units (cgs, or cm·g·s.) by multiplying PRU units by a conversion factor of 1332 to express resistance in terms of dyn·s/cm^5; or by the ratio of pressure gradient (mmHg) to blood flow expressed in liters per minute to give *R units.* R units may be converted approximately to dyn·s/cm^5 by multiplying by 80. Minor changes in calculated resistance are usually of no significance, not only because of possible errors in pressure or flow measurements, but also because changes in apparent resistance may result from the distending effect of inflow or exit pressure. Conversely, alteration in the distending force may mask changes in the vascular bed. Because of such considerations and the nonlinear relation between pressure and flow of most vascular beds, changes in calculated resistance cannot be equated simply with vasoconstriction or vasodilatation. This is particularly true if there are changes in both pressure and flow.

The relation of the various factors affecting the resistance to fluid flow in rigid tubing is expressed by Poiseuille's equation:

$$\text{Fluid flow} = \frac{(\text{pressure difference})(\text{radius})^4\,\pi}{(\text{vessel length})(\text{fluid viscosity})8}$$

Since the experiments from which the equation was derived were performed in straight rigid tubes with steady, streamlined flow of an ideal, viscous fluid, it is not possible to apply this relation directly to the vascular system, in which vessels are neither straight nor rigid, the blood is not a simple viscous fluid, and the flow is not always streamlined. Nevertheless, it is apparent that the predominant influence on flow is the radius of the vessel, which is raised to the *fourth* power in the above equation. Of the other factors, changes in vessel length are thought to be ordinarily relatively unimportant; however, changes in viscosity related to changes in hematocrit, temperature, and serum proteins are often of marked significance, particularly in small blood vessels. It should also be noted that in most vascular beds, most of the blood vessels are connected in parallel rather than in series. The total resistance of vessels connected in parallel is calculated by adding the *conductance* of each individual vessel (1/R, the reciprocal of the individual resistance) to obtain the total conductance of all the vessels (Fig. 3-21). Because of these relations for vessels in parallel and in accordance with Poiseuille's laws, the resistance of four small tubes in parallel is four times as great as that of a single large tube of equal total cross-sectional area. Actually, it requires 16 small tubes with four times the total cross-sectional area to have a resistance as low as a single wide tube or vessel.

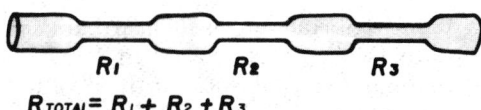

SERIES

$R_{TOTAL} = R_1 + R_2 + R_3$

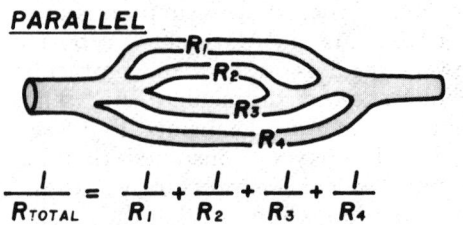

PARALLEL

$$\frac{1}{R_{TOTAL}} = \frac{1}{R_1} + \frac{1}{R_2} + \frac{1}{R_3} + \frac{1}{R_4}$$

FIGURE 3-21 Comparison of the calculation of vascular resistance of vessels in series and in parallel. In most vascular beds most of the blood vessels of the same size are connected in parallel.

Since all normal blood vessels are distensible at least to some extent, it follows that increasing the *intraluminal pressure* will increase the *transmural pressure* on the vessel wall and increase the diameter and radius of the vessel. This effect is seen in Fig. 3-22, which illustrates the pressure-flow and pressure-resistance curves of an isolated peripheral vascular bed. Note that as pressure is increased from 20 to 40 mmHg (distending the vessels), there is a marked decrease in calculated resistance associated with an increase in flow. The pressure at about 20 mmHg, at which flow ceases entirely, has been sometimes referred to as the *critical closure pressure;* however, it is perhaps better referred to as the *critical flow pres-*

FIGURE 3-22 Relations among pressure, flow, and resistance of a peripheral vascular bed. Curve A shows no apparent flow below about 20 mmHg, the critical flow pressure (critical closure pressure). At pressure above this value, the flow increases progressively more for each unit of pressure rise as the resistance of the vascular bed is decreased by the pressure within the vessels. Curve B shows marked decrease in calculated resistance. (*Adapted from Guyton.*[312] *Reproduced with permission.*)

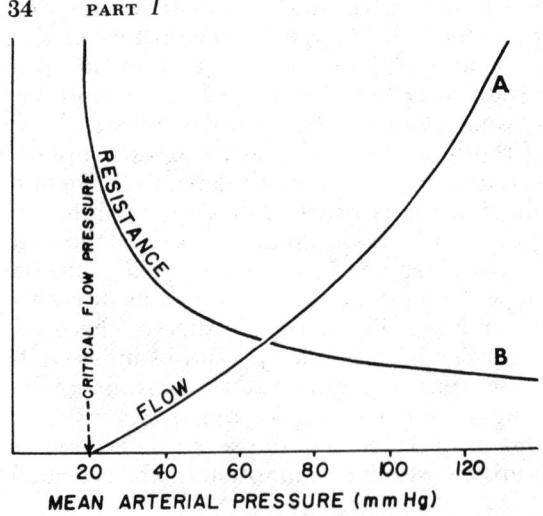

MEAN ARTERIAL PRESSURE (mm Hg)

sure, since it is unlikely that there is often complete anatomic closure of the vessels.

The amount of distension present in an individual blood vessel is dependent on the stiffness, or *tone,* of the vessel and on the *distending* or *transmural pressure,* i.e., the difference between the intraluminal pressure, which tends to expand the vessel, and the external pressure, which tends to compress the vessel. The tone, or stiffness, of a blood vessel is determined by the geometry of the vessel and the mechanical properties of the vessel wall. Important relations between the distending pressure and the tension in the wall of a blood vessel are expressed in the following form of the *law of Laplace:*

$$\text{Wall tension} = \text{distending pressure} \times \frac{\text{vessel radius}}{\text{wall thickness}}$$

From this equation it is apparent that the tension in the wall of a blood vessel tending to expand it is greater if the radius of the vessel is greater or if the blood vessel wall is thinner. Thus, veins with greater radii and thinner walls than their arterial counterparts have a greater wall tension than their arterial counterparts *at the same pressure.* The degree of stretching of the vessel wall produced by wall tension depends on the elastic stiffness of the vessel wall. The term *distensibility* is usually defined by the pressure-volume characteristics of a given vessel and is dependent on the above and other factors.

The regulation of vascular stiffness achieved by alterations in the physicochemical-mechanical properties of vascular smooth muscle is referred to as *vasomotion.* The major factors by which changes in vasomotion and changes in vessel caliber are accomplished are (1) metabolic, chemical, and hormonal substances carried in the blood and/or locally produced, and (2) the activity of fibers from the autonomic nervous system innervating the blood vessels and locally releasing norepinephrine or acetylcholine. The relative importance of these two mechanisms varies markedly from one vascular bed to another. Although it was formerly thought that the release of epinephrine and norepinephrine from the adrenal medulla played an important role in the normal physiological control of vascular tone, this mechanism is not currently thought to be important except under conditions of extreme stress, when the adrenal medulla releases significant quantities of these substances.

Most systemic arteries, and probably veins, respond to hypoxia and/or an increase in P_{CO_2} with vasodilatation.[234-236,238,241,242] The vasodilatation produced by hypoxia in many vascular beds is significantly augmented by an increase in K^+ concentration. Other substances that may be important in the local control of vasomotion include prostaglandins,[216,239,240,313] lactic acid, histamine, and unknown "metabolic products." The cerebral vessels are particularly sensitive to P_{CO_2},[237,238] whereas the coronary vessels respond strikingly to changes in P_{O_2}[314-316] although qualitatively similar changes are found in most other systemic vessels. It is probable that the myocardial vasodilatation produced by hypoxia is ordinarily mediated by the metabolite adenosine, rather than by a direct effect of lowered P_{O_2}, unless the hypoxia is extreme.[314-316] Local prostaglandins may also be important.[214,215,239,313] In most organs, the effects of P_{O_2}, P_{CO_2}, K^+, prostaglandins, and metabolic products work synergistically with the autonomic nervous system to regulate regional blood flow. In contrast to systemic vessels, the pulmonary vessels seem to respond in the opposite manner to changes in P_{CO_2}, pH, and P_{O_2}. In addition to their regional effects, P_{O_2} and P_{CO_2} in the mixed venous blood returned to the heart appear to be involved in the control of the total output of the heart through poorly understood mechanisms.

Neural Control of Blood Vessels[2,6,12,194,196,197,242,310,311]

Three main types of nerve fibers are important in the control of blood vessels: (1) sympathetic vasoconstrictor fibers, (2) sympathetic vasodilator fibers, and (3) parasympathetic vasodilator fibers.

Sympathetic vasoconstrictor fibers are found in both arteries and veins throughout the body, but not in capillaries. These fibers appear to effect vasoconstriction by the release of norepinephrine at the nerve fiber endings. Vasodilatation may be produced by inhibition of the discharge rate of these nerve fibers. These fibers are important in responding to local or regional stimuli of many types. In addition, they are the major pathways for reflex changes in peripheral resistance secondary to changes in carotid sinus and aortic stretch receptors, as well as reflex changes from the carotid body chemoreceptors and from stretch receptors in the low-pressure areas of the intrathoracic vascular bed. They are thought to be the principal mechanism by which impulses from the cortical and subcortical areas of the brain influence total and regional peripheral resistance. The effect of these nerve fibers on the coronary and cerebral blood vessels is ordinarily very slight, being overshadowed by the influence of P_{O_2} and P_{CO_2}.[237-242] The influence of sympathetic stimulation and coronary reflexes is considered in Chap. 44.

Sympathetic vasodilator fibers appear to be of importance in skeletal muscles, although it is possible that some cutaneous blood vessels and coronary vessels also receive this type of fiber. It is probable that these fibers are not normally active tonically and that they are not significantly influenced by the carotid sinus or aortic arch stretch receptors. They are thought to be important in increasing blood flow to muscles during exercise. The effector agent at the nerve fiber ending is thought to be acetylcholine.

Parasympathetic vasodilator fibers are restricted to the tongue and salivary glands and to the sacral area, particularly the erectile vessels of the genital organs. In the sacral area these nerves take part in the local regulation of blood flow according to the needs of local activity, but they are not thought to play an important role in the reflex control of major cardiovascular functions. The transmitted substance at their nerve root endings is acetylcholine.

Parasympathetic stimulation of the salivary glands causes the release of a *kallikrein*, which acts on kininogen, a plasma α_2 globulin synthesized in the liver, to form lysyl-bradykinin, which is converted by a plasma aminopeptidase to *bradykinin*, a substance with powerful vasodilator properties. There is also evidence that the sweat glands of the skin, innervated by sympathetic cholinergic fibers, may also liberate a kallikrein, as well as evidence that a kallikrein precursor in plasma may be activated by certain physical and chemical factors. In addition, the release of kallikrein and the formation of kinins have been suggested as contributing factors in the hypotension associated with endotoxin and anaphylactic shock, the dumping syndrome, and the carcinoid syndrome.[318,319]

In general, vasoconstriction occurs as the result of increased activity of the sympathetic nervous system, which causes the local release of norepinephrine at the nerve fiber endings in blood vessels, whereas vasodilatation is produced by the inhibition of sympathetic vasoconstrictor impulses and/or by metabolic products and local environmental conditions (P_{O_2}, P_{CO_2}, pH, K^+, etc.). Localized vasodilatation may also be produced in exercising muscle by sympathetic vasodilator fibers, and in the sacral area and salivary glands by parasympathetic fibers. In some areas vasodilatation may be produced by the formation of polypeptides under autonomic nervous system influence.[320] Prostaglandins are also very important in local circulatory control.[39,213–215,239]

It is not possible to present a succinct but accurate description of the anatomic pathways by which the central nervous system helps to control cardiovascular function. Even less possible is a description of the mechanisms by which the nervous system is able to integrate impulses from all levels—the cortex and limbic system, reticular system, diencephalon, mesencephalon, medulla oblongata, spinal cord, etc.—and to synthesize these impulses in order to provide the organism with responses varying from the massive sympathetic discharge associated with shock to very discrete vasomotor changes. There appear to be three major pools of spontaneously active neurons important to the control of both the heart and the peripheral blood vessels: the cardiovascular excitatory center (pressor area), which is located in the rostrolateral portion of the medulla; the cardiovascular inhibitory center (depressor area), which is located in the mediocaudal portion of the medulla; and the dorsal motor nucleus of the vagus nerve, which exerts a cardiac-inhibitory influence.[2] It is also apparent that impulses from high levels at times bypass lower integrative areas. Unfortunately there is little information regarding the nature of the processes by which conditioning involving the autonomic nervous system occurs.

Coronary Circulation

Normal Values

Coronary flow is subject to change from moment to moment to an extraordinary degree, as is cardiac output. Some estimate may be made, however, of average values. Coronary blood flow in humans has been determined almost solely by diffusible indicators, and only for the left ventricle (because coronary sinus blood is the only venous effluent readily accessible for analysis). Most workers report a flow of between 0.7 and 0.9 ml per gram of left ventricular muscle per minute.[314–317,321–324] The weight of the left ventricle in grams is approximate to the body weight of the human subject in pounds.[321,322] Thus, normal resting left ventricular coronary flow in a subject of 150 lb (68 kg) lies between 105 and 135 ml/min. Under experimental conditions, values up to two and one-half times the resting coronary flow have been recorded in human beings[324–326] and up to five times the resting flow in the dog.[327]

The arteriovenous oxygen difference averages 0.12 ml per milliliter of coronary flow,[321,322] giving an average cardiac oxygen consumption per gram of 0.08 and 0.1 ml/min. The normal heart is metabolically aerobic and normally does not exhibit anaerobic energy metabolism at rest or with usual stresses.[328]

Vascular resistance, usually calculated as mean pressure gradient divided by mean flow, is not readily estimated for the coronary system, because in the left ventricle the small vessels are closed in systole but in the right ventricle they are open (see below). One may employ an empirical calculation that considers only the resistance in small vessels of the left ventricle.[321] This is expressed as:

$$CVR = \frac{P \times T \times 1322}{CF}$$

where CVR = coronary diastolic vascular resistance
   P = arterial diastolic mean coronary venous pressure*
   T = coronary diastolic filling time
   CF = coronary flow

Thus, the pressure and cycle time directly affecting left ventricular coronary flow can be entered into the assessment of small-vessel resistance.

In order to find any pattern in the response of the coronary circulation, one must distinguish between *hydraulic* factors mechanically responsible for

---

*This value may be influenced by either the diastolic intramyocardial pressure (left ventricular diastolic pressure) and/or right atrial pressure, whichever is higher.

any given flow and *metabolic* or other factors initiating a need for a certain quantity of flow.[314–317]

Anatomic Factors

A knowledge of the anatomy of the coronary circulation is very important in the understanding of the various normal and pathologic factors that influence myocardial blood flow. After arising from the aortic root, the right and left coronary arteries subdivide into branches that follow an epicardial course over the cardiac surface. The intramural blood supply, particularly of the thick-walled left ventricle, occurs through two separate types of vessel,[329] known as A vessels and B vessels. The A vessels arise from the epicardial arteries at a shallow angle and branch within and supply the outer one-third of the myocardium. The inner portion of the myocardial wall is supplied by the B vessels, which arise at a right angle and plunge directly through the myocardial substance to ramify into the subendocardial plexus to supply the inner or deep portions of the myocardium. Thus, it can be seen that the B vessel by its very anatomic course can be compromised by changes in the balance between intramyocardial compressive forces and coronary perfusion pressure.

Hydraulic Factors

Coronary blood flow (Fig. 3-23) is phasic in nature, first because it is dependent on phasic aortic pressure, and second because the myocardium offers a variable degree of resistance to flow during systole. For those branches of the coronary arteries which supply the right ventricle, this latter factor is usually insignificant because of the low intramyocardial pressure in relation to the aortic pressure. For those branches which plunge through the left ventricular myocardium the situation is quite different, however. The heart is a thick-walled shell, and intramyocardial tension must always be greater than intracavitary pressure[330] with a steady increase from the epicardium to the endocardium. Thus, left ventricular coronary flow is virtually all diastolic (Fig. 3-24).[331] This fact places a certain premium on the time available for left ventricular coronary flow. This time can be encroached upon by either prolongation of systole or increase in cardiac rate. The effect of perfusion pressure alone is also influenced by right atrial or coronary venous exit pressure. The diastolic pressure in the left ventricle is a very important determinant of coronary blood flow to the left ventricle, particularly the subendocardium. From these simple facts, one can readily appreciate the effect which various diseases and conditions have on mechanical coronary perfusion (Fig. 3-25). Hypertension is self-compensating, whereas aortic stenosis is not. Aortic regurgitation through low aortic diastolic pressure, and tachycardia, through lessened diastolic coronary filling time, place mechanical disadvantages on the coronary perfusion system at a time when the work load may be greatly augmented by these very conditions. Similarly, right ventricular hypertension, if severe, can interfere with the normal pancyclic right coronary flow and predispose to right-sided coronary insufficiency.[321]

FIGURE 3-24 Comparison of phasic coronary blood flow in the left and right coronary arteries. Note the marked decrease in flow in the left coronary artery during systole. (*From Berne and Levy.*[332] *Reproduced with permission.*)

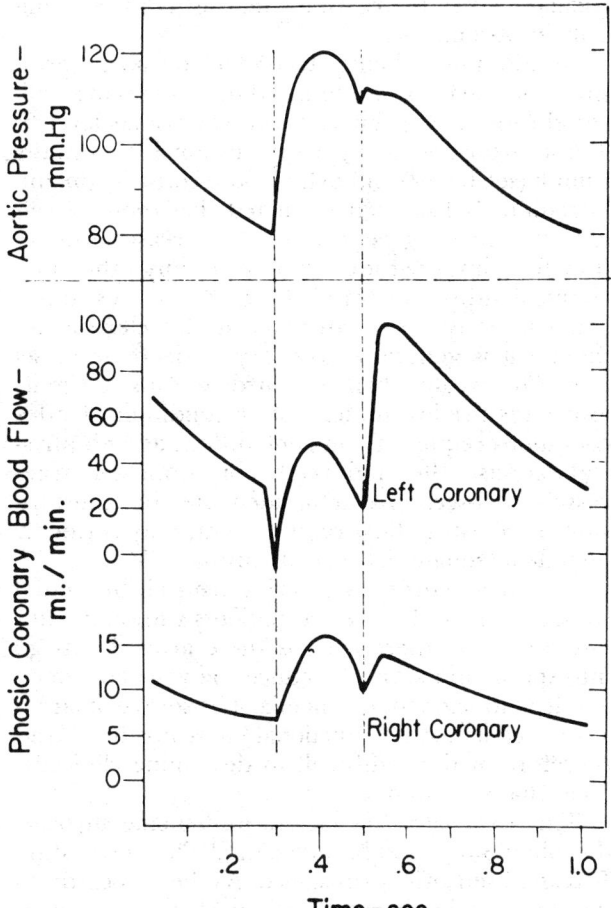

FIGURE 3-23 The mechanical factors which can affect the volume of coronary flow (C.F.). Diastolic blood pressure (BPd) is critical to left ventricular flow, as is mean blood pressure to right ventricular flow. The duration of diastole, so important to left ventricular flow, is shortened by increase in heart rate or duration of systole (as in aortic stenosis). Resistance to flow can occur in the large arteries, in the myocardium during its contraction, and in the collateral and other small vessels of the coronary tree. Change in arteriolar resistance is probably the most important regulator of coronary flow.

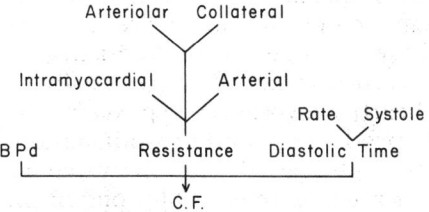

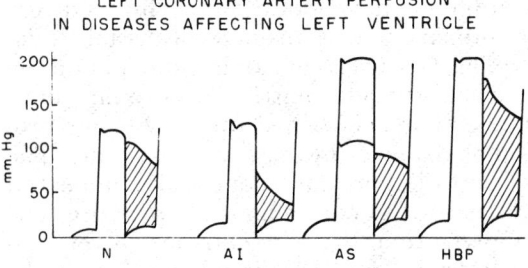

LEFT CORONARY ARTERY PERFUSION
IN DISEASES AFFECTING LEFT VENTRICLE

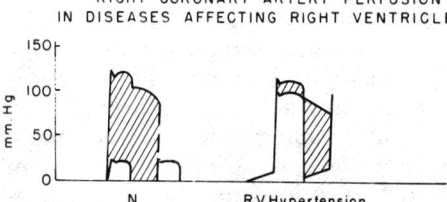

RIGHT CORONARY ARTERY PERFUSION
IN DISEASES AFFECTING RIGHT VENTRICLE

FIGURE 3-25 *Above.* Pressure-time relationships in normal individuals (N) and in those with aortic insufficiency (AI), aortic stenosis (AS), or hypertension (HBP). *Below.* Pressure-time relationships in the normal subject (N) and in the subject with right ventricular (RV) hypertension. *Hatched area* = effective perfusion pressure-time relationship.

Impedance to coronary venous exit by significant right atrial pressure elevation,[333] as with right ventricular failure or tricuspid stenosis, is rarely clinically important.

In addition to being dependent on aortic pressure, coronary flow is regulated by changes in small-vessel resistance, primarily at the arteriolar level.[322] These arterioles are greatly responsive to many stimuli (see below) and exhibit both constriction and dilatation. It has been estimated that these vessels can dilate to a degree sufficient to increase coronary flow five times without changes in any other mechanical supply factor.[327] Large-artery resistance can also occur, as in coronary atherosclerosis, although it is generally necessary to decrease vessel lumen by greater than two-thirds to cause a significant pressure loss under resting conditions. Under conditions requiring augmented flow, as with physical exercise, the moderately compromised large-vessel cross-sectional area, adequate for transmission of a resting flow requirement, may seriously impede adequate delivery of coronary flow.

The large coronary arteries are rich in medial smooth muscle. In selected patients with and without coronary atherosclerosis these arteries can go into spasm and severely reduce the vascular lumen and lead to segmental ischemia. The source of large-vessel resistance is "functional" and not fixed and therefore at times difficult to determine clinically. (See Chaps. 20 and 44.)

The *depth-dependent* factors influencing myocardial blood flow must be stressed:[334] The perforating B vessel itself offers resistance. As the myocardium develops tension in systole, the perforating vessel is compressed.[335] Since this tension progressively increases toward the endocardial surface, it is here that the resistance to flow during systole will be greatest. Since diastolic intramyocardial pressure can be no lower than intracavitary diastolic pressure, the degree to which left ventricular diastolic pressure is altered will increase tissue resistance during diastole when perfusion is maximum. The development of cardiac failure with a markedly elevated diastolic left ventricular diastolic pressure can have deleterious effects on perfusion and result in subendocardial ischemia, particularly if concomitant arterial hypotension is present. The process of ventricular hypertrophy can elongate the perforating vessel as well as cause an increase in the muscle mass to be perfused. Thus, these depth-distribution factors can affect myocardial function so that there can be "shells" of dysfunction, particularly at the inner surface of the left ventricle.[336]

No discussion of coronary vessel resistance would be complete without mention of collateral vascular pathways.[337–340] These structures are anatomically present from early life but become large and significant only if the need for coronary flow exists in some region of the heart. They serve as alternative, and sometimes as solitary, routes of blood flow around stenotic or occluded arteries.

These collateral vessels may occur either in series, so that the bypass around an occlusion occurs from the proximal to the distal portion of the same coronary artery, or in parallel, so that collaterals come across from another coronary artery to the postocclusion segment of the artery. The collaterals may be large structures (100 to 500 μm in diameter) coursing over the epicardium, commonly anteriorly over the right ventricle from right to left, posteriorly from left to right, or transseptally in either direction. There are also pathways which utilize the subendocardial network, so that perforating vessels communicate from the epicardium to subendocardium on both sides of the obstruction. The volume flow in collateral vessels, though considerable, rarely is enough to prevent myocardial glycolysis from occurring with stress (see below).

Oxygen Requirement

The heart extracts approximately 70 percent of the oxygen in every milliliter of blood, leaving venous blood about 30 percent saturated at a P_{O_2} of 18 to 20 mmHg.[338] This is the lowest value for venous oxygen in the body and is matched only by exercising skeletal muscle (Fig. 3-26). The heart functions almost solely on aerobic metabolic pathways (contrary to skeletal muscle), and the deprivation of oxygen for more than 2 min results in total cessation of mechanical activity. As a result, the most urgent stimulus to increased coronary flow (regionally or throughout the heart) is myocardial hypoxia.[333] Hypoxia invariably produces prompt vasodilatation. This is evident from the fact that coronary venous oxygen saturation remains remarkably constant in

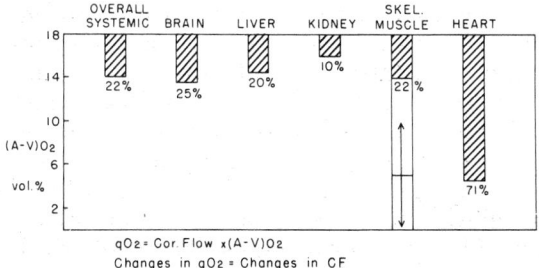

FIGURE 3-26 Arteriovenous oxygen difference and percentage extraction (of original arterial oxygen concentration) for each of the various organs at rest. Note that the high myocardial and exercising skeletal muscle bar represents the somewhat greater variability seen in venous oxygen content here as compared with the heart.

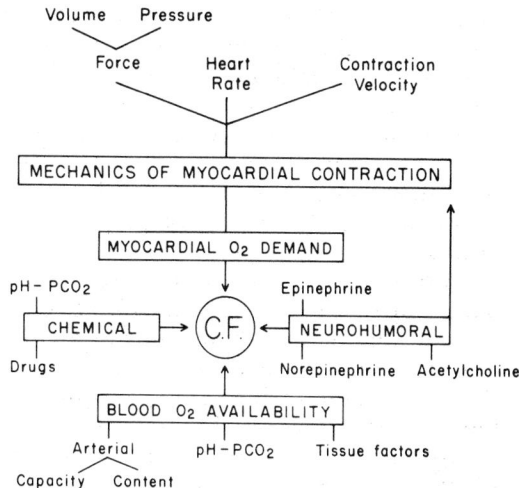

FIGURE 3-27 Factors affecting coronary flow (C.F.) through neurometabolic pathways. The factors are arranged in four groups: chemical, blood oxygen availability, neurohumoral, and myocardial oxygen demand. These are further broken down into subcategories. Note in particular the factors which affect myocardial mechanics. Note also that neurohumoral agents (the catecholamines in particular) exert effects on the coronary circulation both directly in the arteriole and indirectly through induced changes in mechanical modalities of contraction.

a given patient over a wide range of spontaneous or induced hemodynamic variables.[341] The "hypoxic feedback" may be initiated in the following situations:

1. *Regional.* Decreased oxygen tension distal to an obstruction or stenosis can cause local vasodilatation and variable restoration of segmental flow.[333]
2. *General.* Reduced oxygen tension can result from:
   a. Reduced arteriovenous extraction, as with arterial hypoxia or anemia. Change in pH and P_{CO_2} can have minor but definite effects on oxygen extraction through change in the oxygen dissociation curve. Shifts can also occur with altered concentration of red blood cell 2,3-diphosphoglyceric acid or carboxyhemoglobin.
   b. Increase in mechanical activity of the heart. Energy consumption of any pump is usually related directly to the work done, with a fixed efficiency. This does not appear to be true for the heart, primarily for two reasons: heart size, and therefore the pump itself, is constantly changing; and external work (i.e., that volume of blood moved out of the heart at any pressure) is not necessarily the same as internal work (i.e., that performed by the contractile element itself).[342] Muscle shortening is not directly equatable with contractile-element shortening, because there is an elastic component acting in series with the contractile element.[342] Despite these theoretical problems, certain empirical variables of cardiac action seem to relate well to changes in cardiac oxygen requirement, and hence to affect coronary flow (Fig. 3-27). These are:
   (1) Time integral of ventricular systolic pressure. Acute changes in blood pressure can affect oxygen consumption and, hence, coronary flow. This is also seen with aortic stenosis and systemic hypertension. In the latter condition, however, some self-compensation occurs solely through increased

diastolic coronary perfusion pressure (Fig. 3-23).
   (2) Heart rate.[343] Tachycardia, by increasing time spent in contraction, increases oxygen consumption and the need for coronary flow. The product of items 1 and 2, variously called *tension-time index*[344] and *pressure time per minute,*[345] correlates well with oxygen consumption in most situations.
   (3) Cardiac size.[346] Increased cardiac size results in increased ventricular wall tension per unit systolic pressure developed. With increased cardiac volume, oxygen consumption increases; usually the increase is out of proportion to the increase in mechanical work induced by increased fiber length.
   (4) Cardiac fiber-shortening velocity or contractility.[347,348] There is an energy cost associated with this factor. Increased contraction velocity occurs particularly with sympathetic or catecholamine stimulation and is the mechanism for increasing or maintaining stroke volume at unchanged end-diastolic cardiac size. This kinetic change has an energy cost of its own (to be differentiated from the increased stroke volume which occurs with increased cardiac end-diastolic volume). This has been shown to be a relatively "cheap" action and has given rise to a distinction between costly "high-pressure" and efficient "high-flow" work. This probably occurs

because when heart size is increased by increased stretch, more blood will be ejected per unit fiber shortening.*,[349] Thus, stroke volume can increase with relatively minor changes in mean systolic cardiac volume and tension and no change in kinetics of fiber shortening—therefore, with little increase in oxygen consumption or coronary flow.

In this regard, it is perhaps relevant to point out that catecholamines affect oxygen consumption predominantly by an induced change in mechanical activity.[347] With norepinephrine, for example, if blood pressure rises, then oxygen consumption follows this change; if fiber shortening increases also, then energy cost will be proportionately greater, and so on.

c. Chemical uncoupling of oxidative phosphorylation, as with dinitrophenol, or cytochrome enzymatic block, as with cyanide, can greatly increase coronary flow. Neither the naturally occurring catechols[350] nor thyroid hormone[351] acts upon the heart through these mechanisms.

Local or Circulating Metabolites

Coronary flow is increased and oxygen extraction decreased in beriberi[352] and to some extent in thyrotoxicosis.[353] Rather than a metabolic block to oxygen uptake,[354] this may be the participation of the coronary system in a generalized circulatory vasodilatation, possibly induced by some metabolic substance.

Neurohumoral Factors

The coronary system contains epicardial muscular arteries. These arteries as well as the arterioles possess both alpha- and beta-adrenergic receptors and parasympathetic receptors.

Under most circumstances, coronary flow is metabolically autoregulated, and this *local* effect supersedes central neurogenic influences. Thus, flow will be redistributed selectively to zones of myocardium which are rendered ischemic for any reason.

There are certain situations, however, in which primary vasoconstriction of the muscular arteries and/or arterioles can occur. As discussed in Chaps. 20 and 44, this constriction can be so profound as to cause spastic closure of the vessels and severe segmental ischemia (Prinzmetal's variant angina). A suggested mechanism has been excessive or extremely sensitive alpha-adrenergic stimulation of coronary smooth muscle or an equivalent *reduction* in beta-adrenoreceptor function.

---

*$dv = 4\pi r^2$, where v = stroke volume and r = ventricular radius. Thus, small changes in radius have exponential effects on stroke volume.

Norepinephrine is a primary coronary vasoconstrictor[355–357] and almost invariably causes an increase in oxygen extraction and a drop in coronary venous oxygen saturation.[356,357] The increased mechanical activity of the heart induced by norepinephrine acts as a secondary and competing dilator stimulus through the hypoxic mechanism.[355,357] Norepinephrine activates alpha, or vasoconstrictor, receptors. On the other hand, isoproterenol, which affects only beta, or dilator, receptors, causes a rise in coronary venous oxygen saturation.[326] Epinephrine has only a secondary dilator action. Pitressin is a naturally occurring hormone which has a profound constrictor influence on the coronary circulation.[358] The prostaglandins also possess powerful vasomotor properties. The myocardium and the arteries themselves synthesize selectively a variety of these compounds.[213–216,239,313,359] Thus, smooth muscle of the arteries may be dilated by locally produced prostacyclin (PGI_2) and constricted by thromboxane A_2, a prostaglandin found in platelets and released if a platelet binds to endothelium and intima. There also are weak effects of the renin-angiotensin constrictor system on the coronary vascular bed. How these substances function under physiological conditions or in the presence of disease is currently unknown.

One can see, then, that analysis of any given coronary blood flow response becomes extremely complex. A catecholamine, for example, can change from one to four mechanical variables of cardiac action with a subsequent change in oxygen requirements. Satisfaction of these increased coronary flow requirements will be mechanically aided if catechol action induces diastolic hypertension but will be hindered if a primary vasoconstrictor action is exerted upon the coronary arterioles themselves. By contrast, during physical exercise, apparently only the hypoxic feedback from the working myocardium is initiated. Coronary venous oxygen saturation and oxygen extraction remain constant, and coronary flow rises *pari passu* with cardiac oxygen requirements.[341,361] The flow increment occurs primarily through dilatation of arterioles, because the diastolic perfusion pressure-time factor usually remains constant.[360]

Coupling of Supply-Demand Mechanisms

In certain situations, increased demand is met directly by the involved variable. Specifically, in hypertension, the increase in coronary flow and oxygen consumption needed to keep up the increased systolic pressure load is brought about directly by the simultaneous increase in diastolic perfusion pressure.

In most circumstances, however, there is believed to be a direct chemical mediator that acts either through the neural receptors, as with norepinephrine, epinephrine, and acetylcholine, or directly on the arteriolar wall, as has been suggested for bradykinin,[361] lactic acid,[362] or the adenine nucleotides.[363,364] With the exception of Berne's work,[314,316,355,364] relatively little information has been forthcoming to indicate the link between demand and supply on the heart. Berne has suggested that with hypoxia there is an immediate local breakdown of adenine nucleotides (Fig. 3-28). Some of these are known potent vasodilators. A new steady state with increased flow and no hypoxia is established and maintained by local biochemical feedback. It may even be that the myocardium is peculiarly responsive because P_{O_2} is about 18 to 20 mmHg, or only 10 mmHg above the level[365] at which anaerobic metabolism sets in (presumably because of shift in cell redox potential).

Coronary Insufficiency

Coronary insufficiency results whenever the demand for energy exceeds the supply. As described earlier, this can be generalized or localized within the heart. Whether generalized, as in the patient with aortic valvular disease,[366] or localized, as in coronary atherosclerosis, coronary insufficiency manifests itself physiologically in the following ways: (1) reduction in coronary venous oxygen saturation and increase in oxygen extraction over previous values;[341] and (2) appearance of myocardial anaerobic metabolism.[367,368] There are other abnormalities peculiar to the patient with coronary heart disease, because of the patchy distribution of ischemia and

scarring. Often the mixed coronary venous oxygen saturation is higher than normal at rest, possibly from shunts through scar tissue or inappropriate vasodilatation.[341] Also, coronary blood flow determinations may vary, depending on the region of the heart studied. This, in all probability, may represent not only varying rates of perfusion but also delayed onset of perfusion of different parts of the myocardium because of the devious collateral pathways. A particular characteristic of the coronary heart disease condition is that stress evokes a greater than normal increase in coronary flow, presumably as a result of inefficient contractile mechanisms in the ischemically damaged myocardium.[369] Those portions of the myocardium that are normally perfused must have adequate contractile state to compensate for those regions of myocardium that have previously been damaged and do not participate as effectively in contraction. While flow to the latter region may rise inadequately during stress, flow to normal muscle must increase excessively in relation to its augmented regional activity. This, of course, uses up the available coronary reserve for lesser degrees of stress than in the normal subject, thus potentiating coronary insufficiency.

As mentioned before, the depth-dependent aspects of the coronary circulation render the deep layers most susceptible to ischemia whenever the supply-demand balance is altered. This depth dependence is manifest by the detection of subendocardial ischemia by ST-segment depression on the

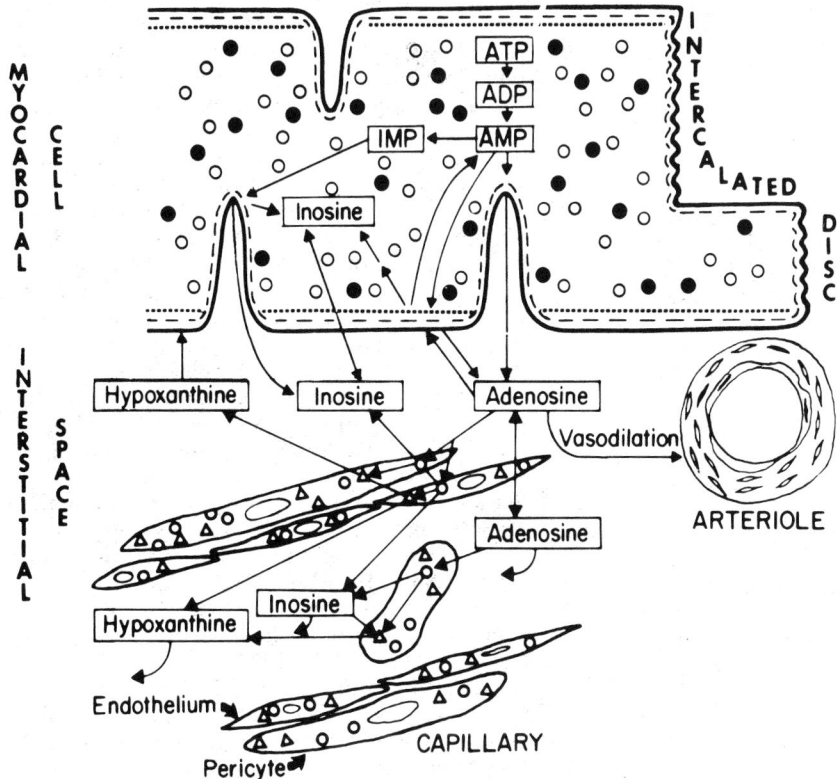

FIGURE 3-28 Schematic drawing depicting a myocardial cell, interstitial space, an arteriole, and a capillary with the localization of enzymes involved in formation and fate of adenosine. Adenosine formed by 5′-nucleotidase from AMP (which in turn arises from ATP) can enter the interstitial space. There it can induce arteriolar dilatation and reenter the myocardial cell, where it is either phosphorylated to AMP by adenosine kinase or deaminated to inosine by adenosine deaminase, or it can enter the capillaries and leave the tissue. A large fraction of adenosine that crosses the capillary wall is deaminated to inosine, which in turn is split to hypoxanthine and ribose-1-phosphate by nucleoside phosphorylase located in the endothelial cells, pericytes, and erythrocytes. Most of the adenosine is taken up by the myocardial cells, and that escaping in the circulation is largely in the form of inosine and hypoxanthine. Since adenylic acid deaminase (which deaminates AMP to IMP) is in low concentration in heart muscle, the major degradative pathway from AMP is via dephosphorylation to adenosine. $\bigcirc$ = adenosine deaminase; $\bullet$ = adenylic acid deaminase; Δ = nucleoside phosphorylase; dashes = 5′-nucleotidase; dots = adenosine kinase. (*From Berne and Rubio.[316] Reproduced with permission of the authors and publishers.*)

electrocardiogram. Griggs et al. demonstrated a difference in the metabolic activity of the deep compared with the superficial layers of the myocardium.[370] In the presence of coronary obstruction, the deep layers showed augmented glycolysis. Similarly, Forman et al. have shown that there are shells of contractility within the myocardium, the subendocardial layer being the most sensitive to decreased blood flow.[371] In this study, any changes which interfered with perfusion, such as a slight reduction in arterial pressure or increase in heart rate, decreased both deep flow and contractile force of the inner layer, even when coronary stenosis was only moderate.

A major consequence of the local inadequacy in energy supply is local disturbance in contractile state. Regions of the myocardium contract less effectively or not in unison with the remaining ventricle. The result, loss of coordinated effort, has been termed *asynergy* and may give rise to either topographic or temporal abnormalities in contraction.[372] Asynergic contraction may occur even in the presence of viable-looking muscle and is not the same as fibrous aneurysm. This asynergy probably underlies the development of congestive failure in many patients with coronary heart disease and may explain why there may be a morphologic reason for failure in one patient but not in another.

In summary, the human coronary circulation is unique in that (1) flow through a part of the system occurs predominantly during one phase of the cardiac cycle; (2) oxygen extraction is high and flow relatively low; (3) flow is exquisitely sensitive to change in oxidative energy need and therefore to any change in cardiac mechanical activity; and (4) flow requirements and supply mechanisms can be simultaneously affected, and often in opposite directions, by a single variable.[314–317]

References

1. Hamilton, W. F., and Dow, P. (eds.): "Handbook of Physiology," sec. 2: "Circulation," vols. 1–3, American Physiological Society, Washington, D.C., 1962–1965.
2. Guyton, A. C., Jones, C. E., and Coleman, T. G.: "Circulatory Physiology: Cardiac Output and Its Regulation," 2d ed., W. B. Saunders Company, Philadelphia, 1973.
3. Guyton, A. C., and Jones, C. E. (eds.): "Cardiovascular Physiology," vol. I, University Park Press, Baltimore, 1974.
4. Guyton, A. C., Taylor, A. E., and Granger, H. J.: "Circulatory Physiology," vol. II: "Dynamics and Control of the Body Fluids," W. B. Saunders Company, Philadelphia, 1975.
5. Guyton, A. C., and Young, D. B.: "Cardiovascular Physiology," vol. III: "Arterial Pressure and Hypertension," University Park Press, Baltimore, 1979.
*6. Braunwald, E., Ross, J., Jr., and Sonnenblick, E. H.: "Mechanisms of Contraction of the Normal and Failing Heart," 2d ed., Little, Brown and Company, Boston, 1976, p. 417. (Extensively referenced)
7. Rushmer, R. F.: "Cardiovascular Dynamics," 4th ed., W. B. Saunders Company, Philadelphia, 1976.
8. Levine, H. J. (ed.): "Clinical Cardiovascular Physiology," Grune & Stratton, Inc., New York, 1976.
9. Vasalle, M. (ed.): "Cardiac Physiology for the Clinician," Academic Press, Inc., New York, 1976.
10. Katz, A. M.: "Physiology of the Heart." Raven Press, New York, 1977.
11. Noble, M. I. M.: "The Cardiac Cycle," Blackwell, Oxford, 1979.
*12. Berne, R. M. (ed.): "Handbook of Physiology," sec. 2: "The Cardiovascular System," vol. 1: "The Heart," American Physiological Society, Bethesda, Md., 1979. (Extensively referenced)
13. Shepherd, J. T., and Vanhoutte, P. M.: "The Human Cardiovascular System. Facts and Concepts," Raven Press, New York, 1979.
*14. Braunwald, E., and Ross, J., Jr.: Control of Cardiac Performance, in R. M. Berne (ed.), "Handbook of Physiology," sec. 2: "The Cardiovascular System," vol. 1: "The Heart," American Physiological Society, Bethesda, Md., 1979, p. 533. (299 references)
15. Ebashi, S., and Endo, M.: Calcium Ion and Muscle Contraction, *Prog. Biophys. Mol. Biol.*, 18:123, 1968.
16. Harris, P., and Opie, L.: "Calcium and the Heart," Academic Press, Inc., New York, 1971.
17. Kones, R. J.: The Molecular and Ionic Basis of Altered Myocardial Contractility, *Res. Commun. Chem. Pathol. Pharmacol.*, vol. 5 (suppl. I), 1973.
18. Inesi, G.: Active Transport of Calcium Ion in Sarcoplasmic Membranes, *Ann. Rev. Biophys. Bioenerget.*, 1:191, 1973.
19. Morad, M., and Goldman, Y.: Excitation-Contraction Coupling in Heart Muscle: Membrane Control of Development of Tension, *Prog. Biophys. Mol. Biol.*, 27:257, 1973.
20. Trautwein, W.: Membrane Currents in Cardiac Muscle Fibers, *Physiol. Rev.*, 53:793, 1973.
21. Reuter, H.: Exchange of Calcium Ions in the Mammalian Myocardium: Mechanisms and Physiological Significance, *Circ. Res.*, 34:599, 1974.
22. Levy, M. N., and Martin, P. J.: Cardiac Excitation and Contraction, in A. C. Guyton and C. E. Jones (eds.), "Cardiovascular Physiology," University Park Press, Baltimore, 1974, vol. I, p. 49.
23. Langer, G. A.: Ionic Movements and the Control of Contraction, in G. A. Langer and A. J. Brady (eds.), "The Mammalian Myocardium," John Wiley & Sons, Inc., New York, 1974.
24. Schwartz, A.: Active Transport in Mammalian Myocardium, in G. A. Langer and A. J. Brady (eds.), "The Mammalian Myocardium," John Wiley & Sons, Inc., New York, 1974.
25. Nayler, W. G., and Seabra-Gomes, R.: Excitation-Contraction Coupling in Cardiac Muscle, *Prog. Cardiovasc. Dis.*, 18:75, 1975.
26. Katz, A. M., Tada, M., and Kirchberger, M. A.: Control of Calcium Transport in the Myocardium by the Cyclic AMP Protein Kinase System, *Adv. Cyclic Nucleotide Res.*, 5:453, 1975.

*This article is a review of the literature and contains additional references to the literature.

27. Ebashi, S.: Excitation-Contraction Coupling, *Ann. Rev. Physiol.*, 38:293, 1976.

*28. Fozzard, H. A.: Heart: Excitation-Contraction Coupling, *Ann. Rev. Physiol.*, 39:201, 1977. (100 references)

*29. Endo, M.: Calcium Release from the Sarcoplasmic Reticulum, *Physiol. Rev.*, 57:71, 1977. (198 references)

*30. Fabiato, A., and Fabiato, F.: Calcium Release from the Sarcoplasmic Reticulum, *Circ. Res.*, 40:119, 1977. (72 references)

*31. Langer, G. A.: Ionic Basis of Myocardial Contractility, *Ann. Rev. Med.*, 28:13, 1977. (44 references)

*32. Winegrad, S.: Electromechanical Coupling in Heart Muscle, in R. M. Berne, (ed.), "Handbook of Physiology," sec. 2: "The Cardiovascular System," vol. 1: "The Heart," American Physiological Society, Bethesda, Md., 1979, p. 393. (288 references)

*33. Fabiato, A. and Fabiato, F.: Calcium and Cardiac Excitation-Contraction Coupling, *Ann. Rev. Physiol.*, 41:473, 1979. (63 references)

34. Lehninger, A. L.: Ca^{2+} Transport by Mitochondria and Its Possible Role in the Cardiac Contraction-Relaxation Cycle, *Circ. Res.*, 35:83, 1974.

35. Carafoli, E., Tiozzo, R., Lugli, G., Crovetti, F., and Kratzing, C.: The Release of Calcium from Heart Mitochondria by Sodium, *J. Mol. Cell. Cardiol.*, 6:361, 1974.

36. Young, M.: The Molecular Basis of Muscle Contraction, *Ann. Rev. Biochem.*, 38:913, 1969.

37. Katz, A. M.: Biochemical Basis for Cardiac Contraction, in I. Mirsky, D. N. Ghista, and H. Sandler (eds.), "Cardiac Mechanics: Physiological, Clinical, and Mathematical Considerations," John Wiley & Sons, Inc., New York, 1974.

38. Katz, A. M.: Contractile Proteins, in G. A. Langer and A. J. Brady (eds.), "The Mammalian Myocardium," John Wiley & Sons, Inc., New York, 1974, p. 51.

*39. Noble, M. I., and Pollack, G. H.: Molecular Mechanisms of Contraction, *Circ. Res.*, 40:333, 1977. (74 references)

40. Akera, T.: Membrane Adenosine Triphosphatase: A Digitalis Receptor, *Science*, 198:569, 1977.

41. Akera, T., and Brody, T. M.: The Role of Na^+, K^+-ATPase in the Inotropic Action of Digitalis, *Pharmacol. Rev.*, 29:187, 1977.

42. Langer, G. A.: Relationship between Myocardial Contractility and the Effects of Digitalis on Ionic Exchange, *Fed. Proc.*, 36:223, 1977.

43. Katz, A. M., Bailin, G., Kirchberger, M. A., and Today, M.: Regulation of Myocardial Cell Function by Agents That Increase Cyclic AMP Production in the Heart, in A. P. Fishman (ed.), "Heart Failure," Hemisphere Publishing Corp., Washington, D.C., 1978, pp. 11–28.

44. Keely, S. L., and Corbin, J. D.: Involvement of cAMP-Dependent Protein Kinase in the Regulation of Heart Contractile Force, *Am. J. Physiol.*, 233:H269, 1977.

45. Hicks, M. J., Shigekawa, M., and Katz, A. M.: Mechanism by Which Cyclic Adenosine 3′,5′-Monophosphate-Dependent Protein Kinase Stimulates Calcium Transport in Cardiac Sarcoplasmic Reticulum, *Circ. Res.*, 44:384, 1979.

46. Luttgau, H. C.: Caffeine, Calcium, and the Activation of Contraction, in A. W. Cuthbert (ed.), "Calcium and Cellular Function," St. Martins Press, Inc., New York, 1970.

47. Arentzen, C. E., Rankin, J. S., Anderson, P. A. W., Feezor, M. D., and Anderson, R. W.: Force-Frequency Characteristics of the Left Ventricle in the Conscious Dog, *Circ. Res.*, 42:64, 1978.

*48. Johnson, E. A.: Force-Interval Relationship of Cardiac Muscle, in R. M. Berne (ed.), "Handbook of Physiology," sec. 2: "The Cardiovascular System," vol. I: "The Heart," American Physiological Society, Bethesda, Md. 1979, p. 475. (134 references)

49. Hoffman, B. F., Bindler, E., and Suckling, E. E.: Postextrasystolic Potentiation of Contraction in Cardiac Muscle, *Am. J. Physiol.*, 185:95, 1956.

50. Langer, G. A.: Heart: Excitation-Contraction Coupling, *Ann. Rev. Physiol.*, 35:55, 1973.

51. Sperelakis, N., and Schneider, J. A.: A Metabolic Control Mechanism for Calcium Ion Influx That May Protect the Ventricular Myocardial Cell, *Am. J. Cardiol.*, 37:1079, 1976.

52. Schwartz, A.: Is the Cell Membrane Na^+,K^+-ATPase Enzyme System the Pharmacologic Receptor for Digitalis?, *Circ. Res.*, 39:2, 1976.

*53. Schwartz, A., Sordahl, L. A., Entman, M. L., et al.: Abnormal Biochemistry in Myocardial Failure, in D. T. Mason (ed.), "Congestive Heart Failure: Mechanisms, Evaluation and Treatment," Yorke Medical Books, New York, 1976, p. 25. (91 references)

54. Brutsaert, D. L., and Sonnenblick, E. H.: Cardiac Muscle Mechanics in the Evaluation of Myocardial Contractility and Pump Function: Problems, Concepts, and Directions, *Prog. Cardiovasc. Dis.*, 16:337, 1973.

55. Langer, G. E., and Brady, A. J.: "The Mammalian Myocardium," John Wiley & Sons, Inc., New York, 1974, p. 310.

56. Mirksy, I., Ghista, D. N., and Sandler, H.: "Cardiac Mechanics: Physiological, Clinical, and Mathematical Considerations," John Wiley & Sons, Inc., New York, 1974.

57. Skelton, C. L., and Sonnenblick, E. H.: Physiology of Cardiac Muscle, in H. J. Levine (ed.), "Clinical Cardiovascular Physiology," Grune & Stratton, Inc., New York, 1976, p. 57.

*58. Brady, A. J.: Mechanical Properties of Cardiac Fibers, in R. M. Berne (ed.), "Handbook of Physiology," sec. 2: "The Cardiovascular System," vol. 1: "The Heart," American Physiological Society, Washington, D.C., 1979, p. 461. (74 references)

*59. Alpert, N. R., Hamrell, B. B., and Mulieri, L. A.: Heart Muscle Mechanics, *Ann. Rev. Physiol.*, 41:521, 1979. (74 references)

60. Sonnenblick, E. H.: Implications of Muscle Mechanics in the Heart, *Fed. Proc.*, 21:975, 1962.

61. Fry, D. L., Griggs, D. M., Jr., and Greenfield, J. C., Jr.: Myocardial Mechanics: Tension-Velocity-Length Relationships of Heart Muscle, *Circ. Res.*, 14:73, 1964.

62. Evans, J. R., (guest ed.): Symposium: Structure and Function of Heart Muscle, *Circ. Res.*, 15(suppl. 2):1, 1964.

63. Sonnenblick, E. H.: Instantaneous Force-Velocity-Length Determinants in the Contraction of Heart Muscle, *Circ. Res.*, 16:441, 1965.

64. Sonnenblick, E. H., Braunwald, E., and Morrow, A. G.: The Contractile Properties of Human Heart Muscle: Studies on Myocardial Mechanics of Surgically Excised Papillary Muscles, *J. Clin. Invest.,* 44:966, 1965.

65. Glick, G., Sonnenblick, E. H., and Braunwald, E.: Myocardial Force-Velocity Relations Studied in Intact Unanesthetized Man, *J. Clin. Invest.,* 44:978, 1965.

66. Sonnenblick, E. H., Braunwald, E., Williams, J. F., Jr., and Glick, G.: Effects of Exercise on Myocardial Force-Velocity Relations in Intact Unanesthetized Man: Relative Roles of Changes in Heart Rate, Sympathetic Activity, and Ventricular Dimensions, *J. Clin. Invest.,* 44:2051, 1965.

*67. Sonnenblick, E. H.: The Mechanics of Myocardial Contraction, in S. A. Briller and H. L. Conn, Jr. (eds.), "The Myocardial Cell: Structure, Function, and Modification by Cardiac Drugs," University of Pennsylvania Press, Philadelphia, 1966, p. 173. (93 references)

68. Sonnenblick, E. H., Morrow, A. G., and Williams, J. F., Jr.: Effects of Heart Rate on the Dynamics of Force Development in the Intact Human Ventricle, *Circulation,* 33:945, 1966.

69. Covell, J. W., Ross, J., Jr., Sonnenblick, E. H., and Braunwald, E.: Comparison of the Force-Velocity Relation and the Ventricular Function Curve as Measures of the Contractile State of the Intact Heart, *Circ. Res.,* 19:364, 1966.

70. Braunwald, E., Sonnenblick, E. H., Ross, J., Jr., and Gault, J. H.: Insights into Cardiovascular Physiology Derived from Muscle Mechanics, *Am. J. Cardiol.,* 20:705, 1967.

71. Pool, P. E., and Sonnenblick, E. H.: Mechanochemistry of Heart Muscle. I. The Isometric Contraction, *J. Gen. Physiol.,* 50:951, 1967.

72. Gault, J. H., Ross, J., Jr., and Braunwald, E.: Contractile State of the Left Ventricle in Man: Instantaneous Tension-Velocity-Length Relations in Patients with and without Disease of the Left Ventricular Myocardium, *Circ. Res.,* 22:451, 1968.

73. Pool, P. E., Chandler, B. M., Seagren, S. C., and Sonnenblick, E. H.: Mechanochemistry of Cardiac Muscle. II. The Isotonic Contraction, *Circ. Res.,* 22:465, 1968.

74. Barnes, J. W., Covell, J. W., and Ross, J., Jr.: The Mechanics of Isotonic Left Ventricular Contractions, *Am. J. Physiol.,* 224:725, 1973.

75. Huxley, A. F.: Muscular Contractions, *J. Physiol. (Lond.),* 243:1, 1974.

76. Mahler, F., Ross, J., Jr., O'Rourke, R. A., and Covell, J. S.: Effects of Changes in Preload, Afterload and Inotropic State on Ejection and Isovolumic Phase Measures of Contractility in the Conscious Dog, *Am. J. Cardiol.,* 36:626, 1975.

77. Abbott, B. C., and Gordon, D. G.: A Commentary on Muscle Mechanics, *Circ. Res.,* 36:1, 1975.

78. Jewell, B. R.: A Re-examination of the Influence of Muscle Length on Myocardial Performance, *Circ. Res.,* 40:221, 1977.

79. Hill, A. V.: The Heat of Shortening and the Dynamic Constants of Muscle, *Proc. R. Soc. Lond. (Biol.),* 126:136, 1938.

80. Hill, A. V.: "First and Last Experiments in Muscle Mechanics," University Press, Cambridge, 1970, p. 141.

81. Bowditch, H. P.: Ueber die Eigenthumlichkeiten der Reizbarkeit, welche die Muskelfasern des Herzens zeigen, *Verh. K. Sachs Ges. Wochenshr. Leipzig Math. Phys. Cl.,* 23:652, 1871.

82. Howell, W. H., and Donaldson, F., Jr.: Experiments upon the Heart of the Dog with Reference to Maximum Volume of Blood Sent Out by Left Ventricle in a Single Beat, *Philos. Trans. R. Soc. Lond. (Biol. Sci.),* 175:139, 1884.

83. Frank, O.: Zur Dynamik des Herzmuskels, *Z. Biol.,* 32:370, 1895, translated by C. B. Chapman and E. Wasserman, *Am. Heart J.,* 58:282, 467, 1959.

84. Fick, A.: "Mechanische Arbeit und Warmeentwickelung bei der Muskeltatigheit," F. A. Brockhaus, Leipzig, Germany, 1882.

85. von Kries, J.: Untersuchungen zur Mechanik der quergestreiften Muskels, *Arch. Physiol. (Leipzig),* 1880, p. 348; 1885, p. 67.

86. Blix, M.: Die Lange und die Spannung des Muskels, *Skand. Arch. Physiol.,* 5:173, 1895.

87. Wiggers, C. J.: Some Factors Controlling the Shape of the Pressure Curve in the Right Ventricle, *Am. J. Physiol.,* 33:382, 1914.

88. Straub, H.: I. Dynamik des Saugetierherzens, *Dtsch. Arch. Klin. Med.,* 115:531, 1914; II. Mitteilung Dynamik des Rechten Herzens, *Dtsch. Arch. Klin. Med.,* 116:409, 1914.

89. Patterson, S. W., and Starling, E. H.: On the Mechanical Factors Which Determine the Output of the Ventricles, *J. Physiol.,* 48:357, 1914.

90. Patterson, S. W., Piper, H., and Starling, E. H.: The Regulation of the Heart Beat, *J. Physiol.,* 48:465, 1914.

91. Starling, E. H.: "The Linacre Lecture on the Law of the Heart," Longmans, Green & Co., Ltd., London, 1918.

92. Wiggers, C. J.: Determinants of Cardiac Performance, *Circulation,* 4:485, 1951.

93. Sarnoff, S. J., and Berglund, E.: Ventricular Function. I. Starling's Law of the Heart Studied by Means of Simultaneous Right and Left Ventricular Function Curves in the Dog, *Circulation,* 9:706, 1954.

94. Sarnoff, S. J.: Myocardial Contractility as Described by Ventricular Function Curves: Observations on Starling's Law of the Heart, *Physiol. Rev.,* 35:107, 1955.

95. Braunwald, E., and Ross, J., Jr.: Applicability of Starling's Law of the Heart to Man, in J. R. Evans (guest ed.), Symposium: Structure and Function of Heart Muscle, *Circ. Res.,* 15 (suppl. 2): 169, 1964.

96. Braunwald, E.: The Control of Ventricular Function in Man, *Br. Heart J.,* 27:1, 1965.

97. Levine, H. J.: Compliance of the Left Ventricle, *Circulation,* 46:423, 1972.

98. Templeton, G. H., Ecker, R. R., and Mitchell, J. H.: Left Ventricular Stiffness during Diastole and Systole: The Influence of Changes in Volume and Inotropic State, *Cardiovasc. Res.,* 6:95, 1972.

99. Covell, J. S., and Ross, J., Jr.: Nature and Significance of Alterations in Myocardial Compliance, *Am. J. Cardiol.,* 32:449, 1973.

100. Grossman, W., McLaurin, L. P., Moos, S. P., Stefandouros, M. A., and Young, D. T.: Wall Thickness and Diastolic Properties of the Left Ventricle, *Circulation,* 49:129, 1974.

101. Gaasch, W. H., Cole, J. S., Quinones, M. A., and Alexander, J. K.: Dynamic Determinants of Left Ventricular Diastolic Pressure-Volume Relations in Man, *Circulation,* 51:317, 1975.

102. Mirsky, I.: Assessment of Passive Elastic Stiffness of Cardiac Muscle: Mathematical Concepts, Physiologic and Clinical Considerations, Directions for Future Research, *Prog. Cardiovasc. Dis.,* 18:277, 1976.

*103. Grossman, W., and McLaurin, L. P.: Diastolic Properties of the Left Ventricle, *Ann. Intern. Med.,* 84:316, 1976. (101 references)

104. Gaasch, W. H., Levine, H. J., Quinones, M. A., and Alexander, J. K.: Left Ventricular Compliance: Mechanisms and Clinical Implications, *Am. J. Cardiol.,* 38:645, 1976. (35 references)

105. Wisnecki, J. A., and Bristow, J. D.: Left Ventricular Stiffness, *Ann. Rev. Med.,* 29:475, 1978.

*106. Lewis, B. S., and Gotsman, M. S.: Current Concepts of Left Ventricular Relaxation and Compliance, *Am. Heart J.,* 99:101, 1980. (74 references)

107. Bemis, C. E., Serur, J. R., Borkenhagen, D., Sonnenblick, E. H., and Urshel, C. W.: Influence of Right Ventricular Filling Pressure on Left Ventricular Pressure and Dimension, *Circ. Res.,* 34:498, 1974.

108. Braunwald, E., and Ross, J., Jr.: The Ventricular End-Diastolic Pressure: Appraisal of Its Value in the Recognition of Ventricular Failure in Man, *Am. J. Med.,* 34:147, 1963.

109. DiDonna, G., LeWinter, M., Johnson, A., and Peterson, K.: Effects of Left Ventricular Hypertrophy on Diastolic Wall Stiffness, *Circulation,* 50(suppl. 3):45, 1974.

110. Spiro, D., and Sonnenblick, E. H.: The Structural Basis of the Contractile Process in Heart Muscle under Physiological and Pathological Conditions, *Prog. Cardiovasc. Dis.,* 7:295, 1965.

*111. Spiro, D.: The Fine Structure and Contractile Mechanism of Heart Muscle, in S. A. Briller and H. L. Conn, Jr. (eds.), "The Myocardial Cell: Structure, Function, and Modification by Cardiac Drugs," University of Pennsylvania Press, Philadelphia, 1966, p. 13. (93 references)

112. Ross, J., Jr., Sonnenblick, E. H., Covell, J. W., Kaiser, G. A., and Spiro, D.: Architecture of the Heart in Systole and Diastole: Technique for Rapid Fixation and Analysis of Left Ventricular Geometry, *Circ. Res.,* 21:409, 1967.

113. Sonnenblick, E. H., Ross, J., Jr., Covell, J. W., Spotnitz, H. M., and Spiro, D.: The Ultrastructure of the Heart in Systole and Diastole: Changes in Sarcomere Length, *Circ. Res.,* 21:423, 1967.

114. Sonnenblick, E. H., and Ross, J., Jr.: Some Ultrastructural Considerations in Myocardial Failure: Sarcomere Overextension and Length Dispersion, in R. D. Tanz, F. Kavaler, and J. Roberts (eds.), "Factors Influencing Myocardial Contractility," Academic Press, Inc., New York, 1967, p. 43.

115. Leyton, R. A., and Sonnenblick, E. H.: The Sarcomere as the Basis of Starling's Law of the Heart in the Left and Right Ventricles, in E. Bajusz and G. Jasmin (eds.), "Methods and Achievements in Experimental Pathology," S. Karger A. G., Basel, 1971, vol. 5, p. 22.

116. Spotnitz, H. M., Leyton, R. A., Kelly, D. T., et al.: "Outstretched" Sarcomere in Subacute Volume Pressure Loading of Dog Right Ventricle, *Circulation,* 46(suppl. 2):44, 1972.

117. Sonnenblick, E. H., Skelton, C. L., Spotnitz, W. D., and Feldman, D.: Redefinition of the Ultrastructural Basis of Cardiac Length-Tension Relations, *Circulation,* 48(suppl. 4):65, 1973.

118. Yoran, C., Covell, J. W., and Ross, J., Jr.: Structural Basis for the Ascending Limb of Left Ventricular Function, *Circ. Res.,* 32:197, 1973.

*119. Sonnenblick, E. H., and Skelton, C. L.: Reconsideration of the Ultrastructural Basis of Cardiac Length-Tension Relations, *Circ. Res.,* 35:517, 1974. (53 references)

120. Skelton, C. L., Sponitz, W. W., Feldman, D., Serur, J. R., Mirsky, I., and Sonnenblick, E. H.: Ultrastructural and Functional Correlates of Acute Cardiac Distention, *Clin. Res.,* 22:304a, 1974.

121. Sonnenblick, E. H., Spotnitz, H. M., and Spiro, D.: Role of the Sarcomere in Ventricular Function and the Mechanism of Heart Failure, *Circ. Res.,* 15 (suppl. 2):70, 1964.

122. Allen, D. G., and Kurihara, S.: Calcium Transients at Different Muscle Length in Rat Ventricular Muscle, *J. Physiol. (London),* 292:68P, 1979.

123. Dodge, H. T., Frimer, M., and Stewart, D. K.: Functional Evaluation of the Hyperthrophied Heart in Man, *Circ. Res.,* 35(suppl. 2):122, 1974.

124. Sonnenblick, E. H.: Series Elastic and Contractile Elements in Heart Muscle: Changes in Muscle Length, *Am. J. Physiol.,* 207:1330, 1964.

125. Vatner, W. F. and Braunwald, E.: Cardiac Frequency: Control and Adjustments to Alterations, *Prog. Cardiovasc. Dis.,* 14:431, 1972.

126. Anderson, P. A. W., Manring, A., and Johnson, E. A.: Force-Frequency Relationship: A Basis for a New Index of Cardiac Contractility?, *Circ. Res.,* 33:665, 1973.

127. Higgins, C. B., Vatner, S. F., Franklin, D., and Braunwald, E.: Extent of Regulation of the Heart's Contractile State in the Conscious Dog by Alteration in the Frequency of Contraction, *J. Clin. Invest.,* 52:1187, 1973.

128. Mahler, F., Yoran, C., and Ross, J., Jr.: Inotropic Effect of Tachycardia and Poststimulation Potentiation in the Conscious Dog, *Am.J. Physiol.,* 227:569, 1974.

129. Stone, H. L.: Effect of Heart Rate on Left Atrial Systolic Shortening in the Dog, *J. Appl. Physiol.,* 38:1110, 1975.

130. Tanz, R. D., Kavaler, F., and Roberts, J. (eds.): "Factors Influencing Myocardial Contractility," Academic Press, Inc., New York, 1967.

131. Mason, D. T., Spann, J. F., and Zelis, R.: Quantification of the Contractile State of the Intact Human Heart: Maximal Velocity of Contractile Element Shortening Determined by the Instantaneous Relation between the Rate of Pressure Rise and Pressure in the Left Ventricle during Isovolumic Systole, *Am. J. Cardiol.,* 26:248, 1970.

132. Sonnenblick, E. H., Parmley, W. W., Urschel, C. W., and Brutsaert, D. L.: Ventricular Function: Evaluation of Myocardial Contractility in Health and Disease, *Prog. Cardiovasc. Dis.,* 12:449, 1970.

133. Mason, D. T., Spann, J. F., Jr., Zelis, R., and Amsterdam, E. A.: Alterations of Hemodynamics and Myocardial Mechanics in Patients with Congestive Heart Failure: Pathophysiologic Mechanisms and

Assessment of Cardiac Function and Ventricular Contractility, *Prog. Cardiovasc. Dis.*, 12:507, 1970.

134. Mirsky, I., Ellison, R. C., and Hugenholtz, P. G.: Assessment of Myocardial Contractility in Children and Young Adults from Ventricular Pressure Recordings, *Am. J. Cardiol.*, 27:359, 1971.

135. Braunwald, E.: On the Difference between the Heart's Output and Its Contractile State, *Circulation*, 43:171, 1971.

136. Mason, D. T., Braunwald, E., Covell, J. W., Sonnenblick, E. H., and Ross, J., Jr.: Assessment of Cardiac Contractility: The Relation between the Rate of Pressure Rise and Ventricular Pressure during Isovolumic Systole, *Circulation*, 44:47, 1971.

137. Karliner, J. S., Gault, J. H., Eckberg, D., Mullins, C. B., and Ross, J., Jr.: Mean Velocity of Fiber Shortening: A Simplified Measure of Left Ventricular Myocardial Contractility, *Circulation*, 44:323, 1971.

138. Graham, T. P., Jr., Jarmakani, J. M., Canent, R. V., Jr., and Anderson, P. A. W.: Evaluation of Left Ventricular Contractile State in Childhood: Normal Values and Observations with a Pressure Overload, *Circulation*, 44:1043, 1971.

139. Grossman, W., Brooks, H., Meister, S., Sherman, H., and Dexter, L.: New Technique for Determining Instantaneous Myocardial Force-Velocity Relations in the Intact Heart, *Circ. Res.*, 28:290, 1971.

140. Wolk, M. J., Keefe, J. F., Bing, O. H. L., Finkelstein, L. J., and Levine, H. J.: Estimation of V_{max} in Auxotonic Systoles from the Rate of Relative Increase of Isovolumic Pressure: (dp/dt)kP, *J. Clin. Invest.*, 50:1276, 1971.

141. Mirsky, I., Pasternac, A., and Ellison, R. C.: General Index for the Assessment of Cardiac Function, *Am. J. Cardiol.*, 30:483, 1972.

142. Noble, M. I. M.: Problems Concerning the Application of Concepts of Muscle Mechanics to the Determination of the Contractile State of the Heart, *Circulation*, 45:252, 1972.

143. Mitchell, J. H., Hefner, L. L., and Monroe, R. G.: Performance of the Left Ventricle, *Am. J. Med.*, 53:481, 1972.

144. Ross, J., Jr., and Sobel, B. E.: Regulation of Cardiac Contraction, *Ann. Rev. Physiol.*, 34:47, 1972.

145. Mason, D. T., Zelis, R., Amsterdam, E. A., and Massumi, R. A.: Clinical Determination of Left Ventricular Contractility by Hemodynamics and Myocardial Mechanics, in P. N. Yu and J. F. Goodwin (eds.), "Progress in Cardiology," Lea & Febiger, Philadelphia, 1972, vol. I, p. 121.

146. Blinks, J. R., and Jewell, B. R.: The Meaning and Measurement of Myocardial Contractility, in D. H. Bergel (ed.), "Cardiovascular Fluid Dynamics," Academic Press, Inc., New York, 1972, p. 225.

147. Ross, J., Jr., and Peterson, K. L.: On the Assessment of Cardiac Inotropic State, *Circulation*, 47:435, 1973.

148. Dodge, H. T., Kennedy, J. W., and Peterson J. L.: Quantitative Angiocardiographic Methods in the Evaluation of Valvular Heart Disease, *Prog. Cardiovasc. Dis.*, 16:1, 1973.

149. Mason, D. T.: Regulation of Cardiac Performance in Clinical Heart Disease: Interactions between Contractile State Mechanical Abnormalities and Ventricular Compensatory Mechanisms, *Am. J. Cardiol.*, 32:437, 1973.

150. Benzing, G., III, Stockert, J., Nave, E., and Kaplan, S.: Evaluation of Left Ventricular Performance: Circumferential Fiber Shortening and Tension, *Circulation*, 49:925, 1974.

151. Peterson, K. L., Skloven, D., Ludbrook, P., Uther, J. B., and Ross, J., Jr.: Comparison of Isovolumic and Ejection Phase Indices of Myocardial Performance in Man, *Circulation*, 49:1088, 1974.

152. Morkin, E., and LaRaia, P. J.: Biochemical Studies on the Regulation of Myocardial Contractility, *N. Engl. J. Med.*, 290:445, 1974.

153. Davidson, D. M., Covell, J. W., Malloch, C. I., and Ross, J., Jr.: Factors Influencing Indices of Left Ventricle Contractility in the Conscious Dog, *Cardiovasc. Res.*, 8:299, 1974.

154. Mirsky, I., and Parmley, W. W.: Force-Velocity Studies in Isolated and Intact Heart Muscle, in I. Mirsky, D. N. Ghista, and H. Sandler (eds.), "Cardiac Mechanics: Physiological, Clinical, and Mathematical Considerations," John Wiley & Sons, Inc., New York, 1974, p. 87.

155. Mirsky, I., Pasternac, A., Ellison, R. C., and Hugenholtz, P. G.: Clinical Applications of Force-Velocity Parameters and the Concept of a "Normalized Velocity," in I. Mirsky, D. N. Ghista, and H. Sandler (eds.), "Cardiac Mechanics: Physiological, Clinical, and Mathematical Considerations," John Wiley & Sons, Inc., New York, 1974, p. 293.

156. Mirsky, I.: Review of Various Theories for the Evaluation of Left Ventricular Wall Stresses, in I. Mirsky, D. N. Ghista, and H. Sandler (eds.), "Cardiac Mechanics: Physiological, Clinical, and Mathematical Considerations," John Wiley & Sons, Inc., New York, 1974, p. 381.

157. Brady, A. J.: Mechanics of the Myocardium, in G. A. Langer and A. J. Brady (eds.), "The Mammalian Myocardium," John Wiley & Sons, Inc., New York, 1974, p. 163.

158. Abel, F. L.: Comparative Evaluation of Pressure and Time Factors in Estimating Left Ventricular Performance, *J. Appl. Physiol.*, 40:196, 1975.

159. Naqvi, S. Z., Chisholm, S. Z., Standen, J. R., and Shane, S. J.: Relative Insensitivity of Isovolumic Phase Indices in Assessment of Left Ventricular Function, *Am. Heart J.*, 91:577, 1976.

160. Sonnenblick, E. H., and Strobeck, J. E.: Derived Indices of Ventricular and Myocardial Function, *N. Engl. J. Med.*, 296:978, 1977.

161. Abbott, B. C., and Mommaerts, W. F. H. M.: A Study of Inotropic Mechanisms in the Papillary Muscle Preparation, *J. Gen. Physiol.*, 42:533, 1959.

162. Parmley, W. W., Chuck, L., and Sonnenblick, E. H.: Relation of V_{max} to Different Models of Cardiac Muscle, *Circ. Res.*, 30:34, 1972.

163. Sarnoff, S. J., and Mitchell, J. H.: The Control of the Function of the Heart, in W. F. Hamilton and P. Dow (eds.), "Handbook of Physiology," sec. 2; "Circulation," vol. 1, American Physiological Society, Washington, D.C., 1962, p. 489.

164. Imperial, E. S., Levy, M. N., and Zieske, H. J., Jr.: Outflow Resistance as an Independent Determinant of Cardiac Performance, *Circ. Res.*, 9:1145, 1961.

165. Sonnenblick, E. H., and Downing, S. E.: Afterload as a Primary Determinant of Ventricular Performance, *Am. J. Physiol.*, 204:604, 1963.

166. Levine, H. J., Forwand, S. A., McIntyre, K. M.,

and Schecter, E.: Effect of Afterload on Force-Velocity Relations and Contractile Element Work in the Intact Dog Heart, *Circ. Res.*, 18:729, 1966.

167. Evans, G. L., Smulyan, H., and Eich, R. H.: Role of Peripheral Resistance in the Control of Cardiac Output, *Am. J. Cardiol.*, 20:216, 1967.

168. Urschel, C. W., Covell, J. W., Sonnenblick, E. H., Ross, J., Jr., and Braunwald, E.: Myocardial Mechanics in Aortic and Mitral Valvular Regurgitation: The Concept of Instantaneous Impedance as a Determinant of the Performance of the Heart, *J. Clin. Invest.*, 47:867, 1968.

169. MacGregor, D. C., Covell, J. W., Mahler, F., Dilley, R. B., and Ross, J., Jr.: Relations between Afterload, Stroke Volume, and the Descending Limb of Starling's Curve, *Am. J. Physiol.*, 227:884, 1974

170. Milnor, W. R.: Arterial Impedance as Ventricular Afterload, *Circ. Res.*, 36:565, 1975.

171. Von Anrep, G.: On the Part Played by Suprarenals in the Normal Vascular Reactions of the Body. *J. Physiol.*, 45:307, 1912.

172. Vatner, S. F., Monroe, R. G., and McRitchie, R. J.: Effects of Anesthesia Tachycardia and Autonomic Blockade on Anrep Effect in Intact Dogs, *Am. J. Physiol.*, 226:1450, 1974.

173. Koch-Weser, J., and Blinks, J. R.: The Influence of the Interval between Beats on Myocardial Contractility, *Pharmacol. Rev.*, 15:601, 1963.

174. Vatner, S. F., and Braunwald, E.: Cardiovascular Control Mechanisms in the Conscious State, *N. Engl. J. Med.*, 293:970, 1975.

175. Boudoulas, H., Rittgers, S. E., Lewis, R. P., Leier, C. V., and Weissler, A. M.: Changes in Diastolic Time with Various Pharmacologic Agents: Implications for Myocardial Perfusion, *Circulation*, 60:164, 1979.

176. Woodworth, R. S.: Maximal Contraction, "Staircase" Contraction, Refractory Period, and Compensatory Pause of the Heart, *Am. J. Physiol.*, 8:213, 1902.

177. Hajdu, S.: Mechanism of the Woodworth Staircase Phenomenon in Heart and Skeletal Muscle, *Am. J. Physiol.*, 216:206, 1969.

178. Hawthorne, E. W.: Instantaneous Dimensional Changes of the Left Ventricle in Dogs, *Circ. Res.*, 9:110, 1961.

179. Schlant, R. C., Dixon, F., Elson, S. H., Rawls, W. J., and Williamson, F. R., Jr.: Modification of the Law of the Heart: Influence of Early Contracting Areas, *Circulation*, 30(suppl. 3):153, 1964.

180. Schlant, R. C., Rawls, W. J., Dixon, F., and Elson, S.: Intraventricular Kick: An Additional Determinant of Ventricular Performance, *Clin. Res.*, 13:62, 1965.

181. Schlant, R. C.: Idioventricular Kick, *Circulation*, 34(suppl. 3):209, 1966.

182. Brecher, G. A.: Experimental Evidence of Ventricular Diastolic Suction, *Circ. Res.*, 4:513, 1956.

183. Sonnenblick, E. H.: The Structural Basis and Importance of Restoring Forces and Elastic Recoil for the Filling of the Heart, *Eur. Heart J.*, 1(supp. A):107, 1980.

*184. Weisfeldt, M. L., Scully, H. E., Frederiksen, J., et al.: Hemodynamic Determinants of Maximum Negative DP/DT and the Periods of Diastole, *Am. J. Physiol.*, 227:613, 1974. (30 references)

185. Brecher, G. A., and Galletti, P. M.: Functional Anatomy of Cardiac Pumping, in W. F. Hamilton and P. Dow (eds.), "Handbook of Physiology," sec. 2, "Circulation," vol. 2, American Physiological Society, Washington, D.C., 1963, p. 759.

186. Mitchell, J. H., Gilmore, J. P., and Sarnoff, S. J.: The Transport Function of the Atrium: Factors Influencing the Relation between Mean Left Atrial Pressure and Left Ventricular End Diastolic Pressure, *Am. J. Cardiol.*, 9:237, 1962.

187. Braunwald, E.: Hemodynamic Significance of Atrial Systole, *Am. J. Med.*, 37:665, 1964.

188. Burchell, H. B.: A Clinical Appraisal of Atrial Transport Function, *Lancet*, 1:775, 1964.

189. Williams, J. F., Jr., Sonnenblick, E. H., and Braunwald, E.: Determinants of Atrial Contractile Force in the Intact Heart, *Am. J. Physiol.*, 209:1061, 1965.

190. Mitchell, J. H., Gupta, D. N., and Payne, R. M.: Influence of Atrial Systole on Effective Ventricular Stroke Volume, *Circ. Res.*, 17:11, 1965.

191. Payne, R. M., Stone, H. L., and Engelken, E. L.: Atrial Function during Volume Loading, *J. Appl. Physiol.*, 31:326, 1971.

192. Suga, H.: Importance of Atrial Compliance in Cardiac Performance, *Circ. Res.*, 35:39, 1974.

193. Higgins, C. B., Vatner, S. F., and Braunwald, E.: Parasympathetic Control of the Heart, *Pharmacol. Rev.*, 25:119, 1973.

194. Sagawa, K., Kumada, M., and Schramm, L. P.: Nervous Control of the Circulation, in A. C. Guyton and C. E. Jones (eds.), "Cardiovascular Physiology," Physiology Series I, vol. 1, University Park Press, Baltimore, 1974, p. 197.

*195. Linden, R. J.: Reflexes from the Heart, *Prog. Cardiovasc. Dis.*, 18:201, 1975. (110 references)

*196. Abboud, F. M., Heistad, D. D., Mark, A. L., and Schmid, P. G.: Reflex Control of the Peripheral Circulation, *Prog. Cardiovasc. Dis.*, 18:371, 1976. (182 references)

197. Kirchheim, H. R.: Systemic Arterial Baroreceptor Reflexes, *Physiol. Rev.*, 56:100, 1976.

198. Randall, W. C. (ed.): "Neural Regulation of the Heart," Oxford University Press, New York, 1977, p. 440.

*199. Levy, M. N., and Martin, P. J.: Neural Control of the Heart, in R. M. Berne (ed.), "Handbook of Physiology," sec. 2: "The Cardiovascular System," vol. 1: "The Heart," American Physiological Society, Bethesda, Md., 1979, p. 581.(294 references)

*200. Brown, A. M.: Cardiac Reflexes, in R. M. Berne (ed.), "Handbook of Physiology," sec. 2: "The Cardiovascular System," vol. 1: "The Heart," American Physiological Society, Bethesda, Md. 1979, p. 677. (104 references)

*201. Korner, P. I.: Central Nervous Control of Autonomic Cardiovascular Function, in R. M. Berne (ed.), "Handbook of Physiology," sec. 2: "The Cardiovascular System," vol. 1, "The Heart," American Physiological Society, Bethesda, Md. 1979, p. 691. (452 references)

202. Sutherland, E. W.: On the Biological Role of Cyclic AMP, *J. Am. Med. Assoc.*, 214:1281, 1970.

203. Hardman, J. G., Robison, G. A., and Sutherland, E. W.: Cyclic Nucleotides, *Ann. Rev. Physiol.*, 3:311, 1971.

204. Sobel, B. E., and Mayer, S. E.: Cyclic Adenosine Monophosphate and Cardiac Contractility, *Circ. Res.*, 32:407, 1973.

205. DeGeest, H., Levy, M. N., Zieske, H., and Lipman, R. I.: Depression of Ventricular Contractility by Stimulation of the Vagus Nerves, *Circ. Res.*, 17:222, 1965.

206. Wallace, A. G., and Sarnoff, S. J.: Effects of Cardiac Sympathetic Nerve Stimulation on Conduction in the Heart, *Circ. Res.*, 14:86, 1964.

207. Glick, G., and Braunwald, E.: Relative Roles of the Sympathetic and Parasympathetic Nervous Systems in the Reflex Control of Heart Rate, *Circ. Res.*, 16:363, 1965.

208. Badeer, H. S.: Resting Bradycardia of Exercise Training: A Concept Based on Currently Available Data, in P. E. Roy and G. Rona (eds.), "The Metabolism of Contraction," vol. 10: "Recent Advances in Studies on Cardiac Structure and Metabolism," University Park Press, Baltimore, 1975, p. 553.

209. Buccino, R. A., Covell, J. W., Sonnenblick, E. H., and Braunwald, E.: Effects of Serotonin on the Contractile State of the Myocardium, *Am. J. Physiol.*, 213:483, 1967.

210. Parmley, W. W., Glick, G., and Sonnenblick, E. H.: Cardiovascular Effects of Glucagon in Man, *N. Engl. J. Med.*, 279:12, 1968.

211. Glick, G., Parmley, W. W., Wechsler, A. S., and Sonnenblick, E. H.: Glucagon: Its Enhancement of Cardiac Performance in the Cat and Dog in Persistence of Its Inotropic Action Despite Beta-Receptor Blockade and Propranolol, *Circ. Res.*, 22:789, 1968.

212. Glick, G.: Glucagon: A Perspective, *Circulation*, 45:513, 1972.

213. Higgins, C. B., and Braunwald, E.: The Prostaglandins: Biochemical, Physiologic and Clinical Considerations, *Am. J. Med.*, 53:92, 1972.

*214. Dusting. G. J., Moncada, S., and Vane, J. R.: Prostaglandins, Their Intermediates and Precursors: Cardiovascular Actions and Regulatory Roles in Normal and Abnormal Circulatory System, *Prog. Cardiovasc. Dis.*, 21:405, 1979. (256 references)

215. Bloor, C. M., White, F. C., and Sobel, B. E.: Coronary and Systemic Haemodynamic Effects of Prostaglandins in the Unanaesthetized Dog, *Cardiovasc. Res.*, 7:156, 1973.

216. Lowe, T. E.: The Clinical Significance of Kinekard, *Am. J. Cardiol.*, 20:304, 1967.

217. Leonard, E., and Hajdu, S.: Cardioglobulin: Clinical Correlations, *Circ. Res.*, 9:891, 1961.

218. Gold, H. K., Spann, J. F. J., and Braunwald, E.: Effect of Alterations in the Thyroid State on the Intrinsic Contractile Properties of Isolated Rat Skeletal Muscle, *J. Clin. Invest.*, 49:849, 1970.

219. Gunning, J. F., Harrison, C. E., Jr., and Coleman, H. J., III: Myocardial Contractility and Energetics Following Treatment with D-Thyroxine, *Am. J. Physiol.*, 226:1166, 1974.

220. Strauer, B. E., and Scherpe, A.: Experimental Hyperthyroidism. I. Hemodynamics and Contractility In Situ, *Basic Res. Cardiol.*, 70:115, 1975.

221. Skelton, C. L., Su, J. Y., and Pool, P. E.: Influence of Hyperthyroidism on Glycerol-Extracted Cardiac Muscle from Rabbits, *Cardiovasc. Res.*, 10:380, 1976.

222. Rocamora, J. M., and Downing, S. E.: Preservation of Ventricular Function by Adrenergic Influences during Metabolic Acidosis in the Cat, *Circ. Res.*, 24:373, 1969.

223. Vatner, S. F., Marsh, J. D., and Swain, J. D.: Effects of Morphine on Coronary and Left Ventricular Dynamics in Conscious Dogs, *J. Clin. Invest.*, 55:207, 1975.

224. Horwitz, L. D., and Bishop, V. S.: Effect of Acute Volume Loading on Heart Rate in the Conscious Dog, *Circ. Res.*, 30:316, 1972.

225. Vatner, S. F., Higgins, C. B., and Braunwald, E.: Effects of Norepinephrine on Coronary Circulation and Left Ventricular Dynamics in the Conscious Dog, *Circ. Res.*, 34:812, 1974.

226. Frommer, P. L., Robinson, B. F., and Braunwald, E.: Paired Electrical Stimulation: A Comparison of the Effects on Performance of the Failing and Nonfailing Heart, *Am. J. Cardiol.*, 18:738, 1966.

227. Cranefield, P. F., and Hoffman, B. F.: The Physiologic Basis and Clinical Implications of Paired Pulse Stimulation of the Heart, *Dis. Chest*, 49:561, 1966.

228. Braunwald, E., Sonnenblick, E. H., Frommer, P. L., and Ross, J., Jr.: Paired Electrical Stimulation of the Heart: Physiologic Observations and Clinical Implications, *Adv. Intern. Med.*, 13:61, 1967.

229. Braunwald, E.: Regulation of the Circulation, *N. Engl. J. Med.*, 290:1124, 1974.

*230. Neill, W. A.: Regulation of Cardiac Output, in H. J. Levine (ed.), "Clinical Cardiovascular Physiology," Grune & Stratton, Inc., New York, 1976, p. 121. (63 references)

231. Oberg, B.: Overall Cardiovascular Regulation, *Ann. Rev. Physiol.*, 38:537, 1976.

*232. Parmley, W. W., and Talbot, L.: Heart as a Pump, in R. M. Berne, (ed.), "Handbook of Physiology," sec. 2: "The Cardiovascular System," vol. 1: "The Heart," American Physiological Society, Bethesda, Md. 1979, p. 429. (132 references)

233. Wittenberg, J. B.: Myoglobulin-Facilitated Oxygen Diffusion: Role of Myoglobin in Oxygen Entry into Muscle, *Physiol. Rev.*, 50:559, 1970.

234. Rodbard, S. (guest ed.): Local Regulation of Blood Flow, *Circ. Res.*, 18–19(suppl. I):1,1971 (AHA Monograph No. 33).

235. Shepherd, A. P., Granger, H. J., Smither, E. E., and Guyton, A. C.: Local Control of Tissue Oxygen Delivery and Its Contribution to the Regulation of Cardiac Output, *Am. J. Physiol.*, 225:747, 1973.

236. Hutchins, P. M., Bond, R. F., and Green, H. D.: Participation of Oxygen in the Local Control of Skeletal Muscle Microvasculature, *Circ. Res.*, 34:85, 1974.

237. Lassen, N. A.: Control of Cerebral Circulation in Health and Disease, *Circ. Res.*, 34:749, 1974.

*238. Korner, P. I.: Control of Blood Flow to Special Vascular Areas: Brain, Kidney, Muscle, Skin, Liver, and Intestine, in A. C. Guyton and C. E. Jones (eds.), "Cardiovascular Physiology," Physiology Series I, University Park Press, Baltimore, 1974, vol. 1, p. 123. (252 references)

239. Berger, H. J., Zaret, B. L., Speroff, L., Cohen, L. S., and Wolfson, S.: Regional Cardiac Prostaglandin Release during Myocardial Ischemia in Anesthetized Dogs, *Cir. Res.*, 38:566, 1976.

240. Messina, E. J., Weiner, R., and Kaley, G.: Prostaglandins and Local Circulatory Control, *Fed. Proc.*, 35:2367, 1976.

*241. Abboud, F. M., Schmid, P. G., Heistad, D. D., and Mark, A. L.: Regulation of Peripheral and Coronary Circulation, in H. J. Levine (ed.), "Clinical Cardiovascular Physiology," Grune & Stratton, Inc., New York, 1976, p. 143. (219 references)

*242. Zelis, R. (ed.): "The Peripheral Circulations," Grune & Stratton, Inc., New York, 1975, p. 417. (Extensively referenced)

243. Wiggers, C. J.: Studies on the Consecutive Phases of the Cardiac Cycle. I. The Duration of the Consecutive Phases of the Cardiac Cycle and the Criteria for Their Precise Determination, *Am. J. Physiol.*, 56:415, 1921.

244. Wiggers, C. J.: Studies on the Consecutive Phases of the Cardiac Cycle. II. The Laws Governing the Relative Durations of Ventricular Systole and Diastole, *Am. J. Physiol.*, 56:439, 1921.

245. Braunwald, E., Fishman, A. P., and Cournand, A.: Time Relationship of Dynamic Events in the Cardiac Chambers, Pulmonary Artery and Aorta in Man, *Circ. Res.*, 4:100, 1956.

246. Wooley, C. F., Levin, H. S., Leighton, R. F., Goodwin, R. S., Ryan, J. M., and Rieser, G. F.: Intracardiac Sound and Pressure Events in Man, *Am. J. Med.*, 42:248, 1967.

247. Schlant, R. C.: Events during Cardiac Cycle, in P. L. Altman and D. S. Dittmer (eds.), "Respiration and Circulation," 2d ed., *Fed. Proc.*, Bethesda, Md., 1973, p. 304.

248. Spencer, M. P., and Greiss, F. C.: Dynamics of Ventricular Ejection, *Circ. Res.*, 10:274, 1962.

249. Grant, C., Greene, D. G., and Bunnell, I. L.: The Valve-Closing Function of the Right Atrium: A Study of Pressures and Atrial Sounds in Patients with Heart Block, *Am. J. Med.*, 34:325, 1963.

250. MacCanon, D. M., Arevalo, F., and Meyer, E. C.: Direct Detection and Timing of Aortic Valve Closure, *Circ. Res.*, 14:387, 1964.

251. Piemme, T. E., Barnett, G. O., and Dexter, L.: Relationship of Heart Sounds to Acceleration of Blood Flow, *Circ. Res.*, 18:303, 1966.

252. Delman, A. J.: Hemodynamic Correlations of Cardiovascular Sounds, *Ann. Rev. Med.*, 18:139, 1967.

253. Craige, E., and Fortuin, N. J.: Genesis of Heart Sounds and Murmurs as Demonstrated by Echocardiography, in C. R. Joyner (ed.), "Ultrasound in the Diagnosis of Cardiovascular-Pulmonary Disease," Year Book Medical Publishers, Inc., Chicago, 1974, p. 119.

254. Burgraf, G. W., and Craige, E.: First Heart Sound and Ejection Sounds: Echocardiographic and Phonocardiographic Correlation with Valvular Events, *Am. J. Cardiol.*, 35:346, 1975.

255. Chandraratna, P. A. N., Lopez, J. M., and Cohen, L. S.: Echocardiographic Observations on the Mechanism of Production of the Second Heart Sound, *Circulation*, 51:292, 1975.

256. Marshall, H. W., Helmholz, H. F., and Wood, E. H.: Physiologic Consequences of Congenital Heart Disease, in W. F. Hamilton and P. Dow (eds.), "Handbook of Physiology," sec. 2: "Circulation," vol. 1, American Physiological Society, Washington, D.C., 1962, p. 417.

257. Mackay, I. F. S.: The True Venous Pulse Wave, Central and Peripheral, *Am. Heart J.*, 74:48, 1967.

258. Barratt-Boyes, B. G., and Wood, E. H.: Cardiac Output and Related Measurements and Pressure Values in the Right Heart and Associated Vessels, Together with an Analysis of the Hemodynamic Response to the Inhalation of High Oxygen Mix-

tures in Healthy Subjects, *J. Lab. Clin. Med.*, 51:72, 1958.

259. Braunwald, E., Brockenbrough, E. C., Frahm, C. J., and Ross, J.: Left Atrial and Left Ventricular Pressures in Subjects without Cardiovascular Disease, *Circulation*, 24:267, 1961.

260. Wade, O. L., and Bishop, J. M.: "Cardiac Output and Regional Blood Flow," Blackwell Scientific Publications, Ltd., Oxford, 1962.

261. Grossman, W.: "Cardiac Catheterization and Angiography," 2d ed., Lea & Febiger, Philadelphia, 1980.

262. Dexter, L., Whittenberger, J. L., Haynes, F. W., Goodale, W. T., Gorlin, R., and Sawyer, C. G.: Effect of Exercise on Circulatory Dynamics of Normal Individuals, *J. Appl. Physiol.*, 3:439, 1951.

263. Barratt-Boyes, B. G., and Wood, E. H.: Hemodynamic Response of Healthy Subjects to Exercise in the Supine Position while Breathing Oxygen, *J. Appl. Physiol.*, 11:129, 1957.

264. Wang, Y., Marshall, R. J., and Shepherd, J. T.: The Effect of Changes in Posture and of Graded Exercise on Stroke Volume in Man, *J. Clin. Invest.*, 39:1051, 1960.

265. Braunwald, E., Goldblatt, A., Harrison, D. C., and Mason, D. T.: Studies on Cardiac Dimensions in Intact, Unanesthetized Man. III. Effects of Muscular Exercise, *Circ. Res.*, 13:460, 1963.

266. Ross, J., Jr., Gault, J. H., Mason, D. T., Linhart, J. W., and Braunwald, E.: Left Ventricular Performance during Muscular Exercise in Patients with and without Cardiac Dysfunction, *Circulation*, 34:597, 1966.

267. Epstein, S. E., Beiser, G. D., Stampfer, M., Robinson, B. F., and Braunwald, E.: Characterization of the Circulatory Response to Maximal Upright Exercise in Normal Subjects and Patients with Heart Disease, *Circulation*, 35:1049, 1967.

268. Braunwald, E., Sonnenblick, E. H., Ross, J., Jr., Glick, G., and Epstein, S. E.: An Analysis of the Cardiac Response to Exercise, *Circ. Res.*, 20(suppl. 1):1, 1967.

269. Chapman, C. B. (ed.): Physiology of Muscular Exercise, *Circ. Res.*, 20(suppl. 1):1, 1967.

270. Bevegard, B. S., and Shepherd, J. T.: Regulation of the Circulation during Exercise in Man, *Physiol. Rev.*, 47:178, 1967.

271. Ekelund, L. G.: Circulatory and Respiratory Adaptation during Prolonged Exercise, *Acta Physiol. Scand.*, vol. 70 (suppl. 292), 1967.

272. Astrand, P. O., and Rodahl, K.: "Textbook of Work Physiology: Physiological Bases of Exercise," 2d ed., McGraw-Hill Book Company, New York, 1977.

273. Luepker, R. V., Holmberg, S., and Varnauskas, E.: Left Atrial Pressure during Exercise in Hemodynamic Normals, *Am. Heart J.*, 81:494, 1971.

274. Shappell, S. D., Murray, J. A., Bellingham, A. J., Woodson, R. C., Detter, J. C., and Lenfant, C.: Adaptation to Exercise: Role of Hemoglobin Affinity for Oxygen and 2,3-diphosphoglycerate, *J. Appl. Physiol.*, 30:827, 197.

275. Simonson, E.: Evaluation of Cardiac Performance in Exercise, *Am. J. Cardiol.*, 30:722, 1972.

276. Vatner, S. F., Franklin, D., Higgins, C. B., Patrick, T., and Braunwald, E.: Left Ventricular Response to Severe Exertion in Untethered Dogs, *J. Clin. Invest.*, 51:3052, 1972.

277. Horwitz, L. D., Atkins, J. M., and Leshin, S. J.: Role of the Frank-Starling Mechanism in Exercise, *Circ. Res.*, 31:868, 1972.

278. Guyton, A. C., Jones, C. E., and Coleman, T. G.: Cardiac Output in Muscular Exercise, in A. C. Guyton, C. E. Jones, and T. G. Coleman (eds.), "Circulatory Physiology: Cardiac Output and Its Regulation," 2d ed., W. B. Saunders Company, Philadelphia, 1973, p. 436.

279. Randall, D. C., and Smith, O. A.: Ventricular Contractility during Controlled Exercise and Emotion in the Primate, *Am. J. Physiol.*, 226:1051, 1974.

280. Scheuer, J., Penpargkul, P., and Bhan, A. K.: Experimental Observations on the Effects of Physical Training upon Intrinsic Cardiac Physiology and Biochemistry, *Am. J. Cardiol.*, 33:744, 1974.

*281. Scheuer, J., and Tipton, C. M.: Cardiovascular Adaptations of Physical Training, *Ann. Rev. Physiol.*, 39:221, 1977. (211 references)

282. Adams, W. C., McHenry, M. M., and Bernauer, E. C.: Long-Term Physiologic Adaptations to Exercise with Special Reference to Performance and Cardiorespiratory Function in Health and Disease, *Am. J. Cardiol.*, 33:765, 1974.

283. Vatner, S. F.: Effects of Exercise on Distribution of Regional Blood Flows and Resistances, in R. Zelis (ed.), "The Peripheral Circulations," Grune & Stratton, Inc., New York, 1975, p. 211.

284. McRitchie, R. J., Vatner, S. F., Boettcher, D., Heyndricks, G. R., Patrick, T. A., and Braunwald, E.: Role of Arterial Baroreceptors in Mediating Cardiovascular Response to Exercise, *Am. J. Physiol.*, 230:85, 1976.

*285. Smith, E. E., Guyton, A. C., Manning, R. D., and White, R. J.: Integrated Mechanisms of Cardiovascular Response and Control during Exercise in the Normal Human, *Prog. Cardiovasc. Dis.*, 18:421, 1976. (102 references)

286. Astrand, P. O., and Saltin, B.: Plasma and Red Cell Volume after Prolonged Severe Exercise, *J. Appl. Physiol.*, 19:819, 1964.

287. Lundvall, J., Mellander, S., Westling, H., and White, T.: Fluid Transfer between Blood and Tissues during Exercise, *Acta Physiol. Scand.*, 85:258, 1972.

288. Lind, A. R., Taylor, S. H., Humphreys, P. W., Kennelly, B. M., and Donald, K. W.: The Circulatory Effects of Sustained Voluntary Muscle Contraction, *Clin. Sci.*, 27:299, 1964.

289. Lind, A. R., and McNicol, G. W.: Local and Central Circulatory Responses to Sustained Contractions and the Effect of Free or Restricted Arterial Inflow on Postexercise Hyperaemia, *J. Physiol.*, 192:575, 1967.

290. Lind, A. R., and McNicol, G. W.: Circulatory Responses to Sustained Hand-Grip Contractions Performed during Other Exercise, Both Rhythmic and Static, *J. Physiol.*, 192:595, 1967.

291. Lind, A. R., and McNicol, G. W.: Cardiovascular Responses to Holding and Carrying Weights by Hand and by Shoulder Harness, *J. Appl. Physiol.*, 25:261, 1968.

292. Nutter, D. O., Schlant, R. C., and Hurst, J. W.: Isometric Exercise and the Cardiovascular System, *Mod. Concepts Cardiovasc. Dis.*, 41:11, 1972.

293. Fisher, M. L., Nutter, D. O., Jacobs, W., and Schlant, R. C.: Haemodynamic Responses to Isometric Exercise (Handgrip) in Patients with Heart Disease, *Br. Heart J.*, 35:422, 1973.

294. Haissly, J. C., Messin, R., Degre, S., Vandermoten, P., Demaret, B., and Denolin, H.: Comparative Response to Isometric (Static) and Dynamic Exercise Tests in Coronary Disease, *Am. J. Cardiol.*, 33:791, 1974.

295. Martin, C. E., Shaver, J. A., Leon, D. F., Thompson, M. E., Reddy, P. S., and Leonard, J. J.: Autonomic Mechanism in Hemodynamic Responses to Isometric Exercise, *J. Clin. Invest.*, 54:104, 1974.

296. Stefadouros, M. A., Grossman, W., Shahawy, M. E., and Whitham, A. C.: The Effect of Isometric Exercise on the Left Ventricular Volume in Normal Man, *Circulation*, 49: 1185, 1974.

297. McCloskey, D. I., and Streatfield, K. A.: Muscular Reflex Stimuli to the Cardiovascular System during Isometric Contractions of Muscle Groups of Different Mass, *J. Physiol.*, 250:431, 1975.

298. Barcroft, J., and Dixon, W. E.: The Gaseous Metabolism of the Mammalian Heart, *J. Physiol.*, 35:182, 1907.

299. Rohde, E.: Über den Einfluss der mechanischen Bedingungen auf die Tatigkeit und den Sauerstoffverbrauch des Warmblüterherzens, *Arch. Exp. Pathol. Pharmakol.*, 68:401, 1912.

300. Evans, C. L., and Matsuoka, Y.: The Effect of Various Mechanical Conditions on the Gaseous Metabolism and Efficiency of the Mammalian Heart, *J. Physiol.*, 49:378, 1915.

301. Graham, T. P., Jr., Covell, J. W., Sonnenblick, E. H., Ross, J., Jr., and Braunwald, E.: Control of Myocardial Oxygen Consumption: Relative Influence of Contractile State and Tension Development, *J. Clin. Invest.*, 47:375, 1968.

302. Sonnenblick, E. H., Ross, J., Jr., and Braunwald, E.: Oxygen Consumption of the Heart: Newer Concepts of Its Multifactoral Determination, *Am. J. Cardiol.*, 22:328, 1968.

303. Braunwald, E.: Control of Myocardial Oxygen Consumption: Physiologic and Clinical Consideration, *Am. J. Cardiol.*, 27:416, 1971.

304. Sonnenblick, E. H., and Skelton, C. L.: Oxygen Consumption of the Heart: Physiological Principles and Clinical Implications, *Mod. Concepts Cardiovasc. Dis.*, 40:9, 1971.

305. Sarnoff, S. J., Braunwald, E., Welch, G. H., Case, R. B., Stainsby, W. N., and Macruz, R.: Hemodynamic Determinants of Oxygen Consumption of the Heart with Special Reference to the Tension-Time Index, *Am. J. Physiol.*, 192:148, 1958.

306. Sonnenblick, E. H., Ross, J., Jr., Covell, J. W., Kaiser, G. A., and Braunwald, E.: Velocity of Contraction as a Determinant of Myocardial Oxygen Consumption, *Am. J. Physiol.*, 209:919, 1965.

307. Covell, J. W., Braunwald, E., Ross, J., Jr., and Sonnenblick, E. H.: Studies on Digitalis. XVI. Effects on Myocardial Oxygen Consumption, *J. Clin. Invest.*, 45:1535, 1966.

308. Coleman, H. N., III: Role of Acetylstrophanthidin in Augmenting Myocardial Oxygen Consumption: Relation of Increased O_2 Consumption to Changes in Velocity of Contraction, *Circ. Res.*, 21:487, 1967.

309. Gregg, D. E.: Effect of Coronary Perfusion Pressure or Coronary Flow on Oxygen Usage of the Myocardium, *Circ. Res.*, 13:497, 1963.

*310. Shepherd, J. T., and Vanhoutte, P. M.: "Veins and

Their Control," W. B. Saunders Company, Philadelphia, 1975, p. 269. (Extensively referenced)

*311. Abboud, F. M., Schmid, P. G., Heistad, D. D.,
Mark, A. L., and Barnes, R.: The Venous System,
in H. J. Levine (ed.): "Clinical Cardiovascular
Physiology," Grune & Stratton, Inc., New York,
1976, p. 207. (125 references)

312. Guyton, A. C.: "Textbook of Medical Physiology,"
2d ed., W. B. Saunders Company, Philadelphia,
1961, p. 347.

313. Needleman, P.: The Synthesis and Function of
Prostaglandins in the Heart, *Fed. Proc.*, 35:2376,
1976.

*314. Rubio, R., and Berne, R. M.: Regulation of Coro-
nary Blood Flow, *Prog. Cardiovasc. Dis.*, 18:105,
1975. (69 references)

*315. Klocke, F.: Coronary Blood Flow in Man, *Prog.
Cardiovas. Dis.*, 19:117, 1976.

*316. Berne, R. M. and Rubio, R.: Coronary Circulation,
in R. M. Berne (ed.), "Handbook of Physiology,"
sec. 2: The Cardiovascular System, vol. 1: "The
Heart," American Physiological Society, Bethesda,
Md., 1979, p. 873. (600 references)

*317. Klocke, F. J., and Ellis, A. K.: Control of Coronary
Blood Flow, *Ann. Rev. Med.*, 31:489, 1980. (74 references)

318. Kellermeyer, R. W., and Graham, R. C., Jr.: Kinins—Possible Physiologic and Pathologic Roles in
Man, *N. Engl. J. Med.*, 279:754, 1968.

319. Schachter, M.: Kallikreins and Kinins, *Physiol. Rev.*,
49:509, 1969.

320. Sander, G. E., and Huggins, C. G.: Vasoactive Peptides, *Ann. Rev. Pharmacol.*, 12:227, 1972.

321. Gregg, D. E., and Fisher, L. C.: Blood Supply to
the Heart, in W. F. Hamilton and P. Dow (eds.),
"Handbook of Physiology," sec. 2: "Circulation,"
vol. 2, American Physiological Society, Washington, D.C., 1963, p. 1517.

322. Gorlin, R.: Measurement of Coronary Blood Flow
in Health and Disease, in A. Morgan Jones (ed.),
"Modern Trends in Cardiology," 34:251, 1974.

323. Rowe, G. G.: Nitrous Oxide Method for Determining Coronary Blood Flow in Man, *Am. Heart
J.*, 58:268, 1959.

324. Berne, R. M.: Regulation of Coronary Blood Flow,
Physiol. Rev. 44:1, 1964.

325. Krasnow, N., Rolett, E. L., Yurchak, P. M., Hood,
W. B., Jr., and Gorlin, R.: Isoproterenol and Cardiovascular Performance, *Am. J. Med.*, 37:514,
1964.

326. Braunwald, E.: Control of Myocardial Oxygen
Consumption: Physiologic and Clinical Consideration, *Am. J. Cardiol.*, 27:416, 1971.

327. Case, R. B., Berglund, E., and Sarnoff, S. J.: Ventricular Function. VII. Changes in Coronary Resistance and Ventricular Function Resulting from
Acutely Induced Anemia and the Effect Thereon
of Coronary Stenosis, *Am. J. Med.*, 18:397, 1955.

328. Krasnow, N., Neill, W. A., Messer, J. V., and Gorlin, R.: Myocardial Lactate and Pyruvate Metabolism, *J. Clin. Invest.*, 41:2075, 1962.

329. Estes, E. H., Jr., Entman, M. L., Dixon, H. B., II,
and Hackel, D. B.: The Vascular Supply of the
Left Ventricular Wall: Anatomic Observations,
plus a Hypothesis Regarding Acute Events in
Coronary Artery Disease, *Am. Heart J.*, 71:58,
1966.

330. Pflugge, W.: "Stresses in Shells," Springer-Verlag
DHG, Berlin, 1960, p. 18.

331. Laszt, L., and Muller, A.: Pressure and Velocity
Conditions in the Coronary Circulation of the Dog,
Helv. Physiol. Acta, 15:38, 1957.

332. Berne, R. M., and Levy, M. N.: "Cardiovascular
Physiology," 2d ed., The C. V. Mosby Company,
St. Louis, 1972.

333. Gregg, D. E.: "Coronary Circulation in Health and
Disease," Lea & Febiger, Philadelphia, 1950.

*334. Hoffman, J. I. E.: Determinants and Prediction of
Transmural Myocardial Perfusion, *Circulation*,
58:381, 1978. (56 references)

335. Downey, J. M., and Kirk, E. S.: Distribution of the
Coronary Blood Flow across the Canine Heart
Wall during Systole, *Circ. Res.*, 34:251, 1974.

336. Kirk, E. S., Turbow, M. E., Urschel, C. S., and
Sonnenblick, E. H.: Non-uniform Contractility
across the Heart Wall Caused by Redistribution of
Coronary Flow, *J. Clin. Invest.*, 49:51A, 1970.

*337. Wechsler, A. S.: Development of Coronary Collat-
eral Circulation, *Ann. Rev. Med.*, 28:341, 1977. (29
references)

338. Brachfeld, N., Bozer, J., and Gorlin, R.: Action of
Nitroglycerin on the Coronary Circulation in Normal and in Mild Cardiac Subjects, *Circulation*,
19:697, 1959.

*339. Schaper, W.: Collateral Circulation, in W. Schaper
(ed.), "The Pathophysiology of Myocardial Perfusion," Elsevier/North Holland Biomedical Press,
Amsterdam, 1979. (59 references)

340. Gregg, D. E., and Patterson, R. D.: Functional Importance of the Coronary Collaterals, *N. Engl. J.
Med.*, 303:1404, 1980.

341. Messer, J. V., Wagman, R. J., Levine, H. J., Neill,
W. A., Krasnow, N., and Gorlin, R.: Patterns of
Myocardial Oxygen Extraction during Rest and
Exercise, *J. Clin. Invest.*, 41:725, 1962.

342. Britman, N. A., and Levine, H. J.: Contractile Element Work: A Major Determinant of Myocardial
Oxygen Consumption, *J. Clin. Invest.*, 43:1397,
1964.

343. Hill, A. V.: The Abrupt Transition from Rest to
Activity in Muscle, *Proc. R. Soc. London (Biol.)*,
136:399, 1949.

344. Gorlin, R.: Studies on the Regulation of the Coronary Circulation in Man. I. Atropine Induced
Changes in Cardiac Rate, *Am. J. Med.*, 25:37, 1958.

342. Sarnoff, S. J., Braunwald, E., Welch, G. H., Jr.,
Case, R. B., Stainsby, W. N., and Macruz, R.:
Hemodynamic Determinants of Oxygen Consumption of the Heart with Special Reference to
the Tension Time Index, *Am. J. Physiol.*, 192:148,
1958.

345. Neill, W. A., Levine, H. J., Wagman, R. J., and
Gorlin, R.: Left Ventricular Oxygen Utilization in
Intact Dogs: Effect of Systemic Hemodynamic Fac-
tors, *Circ. Res.*, 12:163, 1963.

346. Rolett, E. L., Hood, W. B., and Gorlin, R.: Pressure
Volume Correlates of Left Ventricular Oxygen
Consumption in the Hypervolumic Dog, *Circ. Res.*,
17:499, 1965.

347. Gorlin, R., Yurchak, P. M., Rolett, E. L., Elliott, W.
C., and Cohen, L. S.: Inferential Evidence for the
Fenn Effect in the Human Heart, *J. Clin. Invest.*,
42:939, 1963.

348. Sonnenblick, E. H., Ross, J., Jr., Covell, J. W., Kai-

ser, G. A., and Braunwald, E.: Velocity of Contraction as a Determinant of Myocardial Oxygen Consumption, *Am. J. Physiol.*, 209:919, 1965.

349. Gorlin, R., Rolett, E. L., Yurchak, P. M., and Eliott, W. C.: Left Ventricular Volume in Man Measured by Thermodilution, *J. Clin. Invest.*, 43:1244, 1964.

350. Lianides, S. P., and Beyer, R. E.: Oxidative Phosphorylation in Liver Mitochondria Prepared from Adrenal-Demedullated and Epinephrine-Treated Rats, *Biochim. Biophys. Acta*, 44:356, 1960.

351. Lee, C. W.: Effect of Hyperthyroidism on Oxidative Phosphorylation in the Rat Heart, master's thesis, University of Pittsburgh Graduate School of Public Health, 1958.

352. Hackel, D. B., and Kleinerman, J.: Effects of Thiamin Deficiency on Myocardial Metabolism in Intact Dogs, *Am. Heart J.*, 46:1, 1953.

353. Leight, L., Defazio, V., Talmers, F. N., Regan, T. J., and Hellems, H. K.: Coronary Blood Flow, Myocardial Oxygen Consumption and Myocardial Metabolism in Normal and Hyperthyroid Human Subjects, *Circulation*, 14:90, 1956.

354. Olson, R. E.: Myocardial Metabolism in Congestive Heart Failure, *J. Chronic Dis.*, 9:442, 1959.

355. Berne, R. M.: Effect of Epinephrine and Norepinephrine on the Coronary Circulation, *Circ. Res.*, 6:664, 1958.

356. Yurchak, P. M., Rolett, E. L., Cohen, L. S., and Gorlin, R.: Effects of Norepinephrine on the Coronary Circulation in Man, *Circulation*, 30:180, 1964.

357. Sullivan, J. M., and Gorlin, R.: Effect of L-Epinephrine on the Coronary Circulation in Human Subjects with and without Coronary Artery Disease, *Circ. Res.*, 21:919, 1967.

358. Corliss, R. J., McKenna, D. H., Sigler, S., O'Brien, G. S., and Rowe, G. G.: Systemic and Coronary Hemodynamic Effects of Vasopressin, *Am. J. Med. Sci.*, 5:293, 1968.

*359. Needleman, P., and Kaley, S.: Cardiac and Coronary Prostaglandin Synthesis and Function, *N. Engl. J. Med.*, 298:1122, 1978. (85 references)

360. Gorlin, R., Krasnow, N., Levine, H. J., and Messer, J. V.: Effect of Exercise on Cardiac Performance in Human Subjects with Minimal Heart Disease, *Am. J. Cardiol.*, 13:293, 1964.

361. Hilton, S. M., and Lewis, G. P.: Relationship between Glandular Activity, Bradykinin Formation and Functional Vasodilatation in the Submandibular Salivary Gland, *J. Physiol.*, 134:471, 1956.

362. Lundholm, L.: Mechanism of the Vasodilator Effect of Adrenaline. I. Effect on Skeletal Muscle Vessels, *Acta Physiol. Scand.*, 39(suppl. 133):1, 1956.

363. Berne, R. M.: Nucleotide Degradation in the Hypoxic Heart and Its Possible Relation to Regulation of Coronary Blood Flow, *Fed. Proc.*, 20:101, 1961.

*364. Berne, R. M.: The Role of Adenosine in the Regulation of Coronary Blood Flow. *Circ. Res.*, 47:807, 1980. (61 references)

365. Shea, T. M., Watson, R. M., Piotrowski, S. F., Dermksian, G., and Case, R. B.: Anaerobic Myocardial Metabolism, *Am. J. Physiol.*, 203:463, 1962.

366. Fallen, E. L., Elliott, W. C., and Gorlin, R.: Mechanisms of Angina in Aortic Stenosis, *Circulation*, 36:480, 1967.

367. Cohen, L. S., Eliott, W. C., Klein, M. D., and Gorlin, R.: Coronary Heart Disease: Clinical, Cinearteriographic and Metabolic Correlations, *Am. J. Cardiol.*, 17:152, 1966.

368. Herman, M. V., Elliott, W. C., and Gorlin, R.: Electrocardiographic, Anatomic and Metabolic Study of Zonal Myocardial Ischemia in Coronary Heart Disease, *Circulation*, 35:834, 1967.

369. Messer, J. V., Levine, H. J., Wagman, R. J., and Gorlin, R.: Effect of Exercise on Cardiac Performance in Human Subjects with Coronary Artery Disease, *Circulation*, 28:404, 1963.

370. Griggs, D. M., Jr., Tchokev, V. V., and DeClue, J. W.: Effect of Beta-Adrenergic Receptor Stimulation on Regional Myocardial Metabolism: Importance of Coronary Vessel Patency, *Am. Heart J.*, 82:492, 1971.

371. Forman, R., Kirk, E. S., Downey, J. M., and Sonnenblick, E. H.: Nitroglycerine and Heterogeneity of Myocardial Blood Flow: Reduced Subendocardial Blood Flow and Ventricular Contractile Force, *J. Clin. Invest.*, 52:905, 1973.

372. Herman, M. V., Heinle, R. A., Klein, M. D., and Gorlin, R.: Localized Disorders in Myocardial Contraction, *N. Engl. J. Med.*, 277:222, 1967.

4

Electrical Activity of the Heart

Andrew G. Wallace, M.D.

Each contraction of the heart is initiated by an electrical event that occurs because cardiac muscle is an excitable tissue. There is a difference in electrical potential between the inside and the outside of nearly all cells of the body. This difference is called the *transmembrane potential*. In the heart, the transmembrane potential is substantial in size and the cells are also excitable: that is, an appropriate stimulus leads to a change in membrane properties as a consequence of which ions flow across the membrane and elicit an *action potential.*

Certain cells in the heart do not require an external stimulus to initiate the membrane changes that lead to an action potential. Such cells undergo slow, spontaneous diastolic depolarization; and when membrane potential has fallen to threshold, an action potential ensues. The property by which excitation is initiated in the absence of an external stimulus is referred to as *automaticity*. Numerous regions throughout the specialized conduction system are capable of automatic behavior under normal physiological conditions. The frequency of automatic impulse formation is greatest in the sinoatrial node, and for this reason the sinus node normally functions as the pacemaker of the heart.

When current is injected into any single cardiac cell through a microelectrode, membrane potential is displaced not only in that cell, but also in neighboring cells over some distance from the electrode. This phenomenon demonstrates that heart cells are connected through couplings that offer a low resistance to the flow of electric current, and as a consequence an action potential elicited in one cell is capable of being transmitted to another and to another, that is, conducted.

The atrial chambers are thin-walled and contain orifices for the entrance of systemic and pulmonary veins. Specialized fibers are found in the atria, but they are not organized into specialized tracts or bundles as they are within the ventricles. Rather, in certain locations working atrial musculature becomes more densely packed and longitudinally oriented, creating routes of preferential impulse propagation at a velocity greater than observed in thinner, less organized parts of the atrial chambers. (See also Chap. 2.) Activation of the atrial musculature is responsible for the P wave on the surface electrocardiogram. The morphology of the P wave is determined primarily by the site of impulse formation within the sinoatrial (SA) node. A second factor in determining the morphology of the P wave is the relative mass of the two atria. Finally, the preferential routes of atrial propagation play an important role in intraatrial conduction, influencing the conduction time from sinus node to atrioventricular (AV) node and from sinus node to left atrium.

The atrioventricular node is an important structure because it is the only normal avenue over which an impulse can be transmitted from atrium to ventricle. It has a number of unique structural and functional properties, the most important of which is its exceedingly low conduction velocity. The long time required for conduction through the atrioventricular node is responsible for the delay between atrial and ventricular activation, the PR interval of the electrocardiogram.

In the ventricles, specialized cells called *Purkinje fibers* are organized into a system that programs the sequence of activation of working muscle. Purkinje cells and their organization confer upon the system the property of high conduction velocity. The Purkinje system rapidly distributes the electrical impulse to the endocardial shells of both ventricles; subsequent activation of the large mass of working ventricular muscle is responsible for generating the QRS complex on the surface electrocardiogram. In general, the form of the QRS complex is determined by the sequence of ventricular activation and by the respective mass of the two ventricles.

The specialized conduction system plays a key role in initiating and coordinating the activity of a complex and very nonhomogeneous organ (Fig. 4-1). It is remarkable, indeed, that we know as much as we do about disturbances of cardiac rhythm and activation since the activity of the specialized conduction system is silent on the ordinary surface electrocardiogram. Studies in animals, and more recently in human beings, have been able to record the activity of these specialized tissues. These recordings have contributed importantly to clarifying the role of the specialized conduction system in the normal heart and elucidating the mechanisms responsible for many electrocardiographic abnormalities.

Transmembrane Potential

In the heart, as in all other living cells, ions are distributed unequally between the inside and outside of the cell. The disequilibrium of ions has two principal features. First, there are large differences in the concentration of any given ion across the membrane; and second, there is a transmembrane difference in electrical potential.[1] Ions in solution tend to migrate from regions of higher concentration to regions of lower concentration. Hence, differences in ionic concentration represent a passive diffusion force that will tend to promote ionic movement. The magnitude of this force is proportional to the concentration gradient. For charged particles, movement in a solution is also affected by electric forces. In a resting cardiac cell, the intracellular space has a negative potential of approximately 90 mV rela-

THE NORMAL HEART AND BLOOD VESSELS

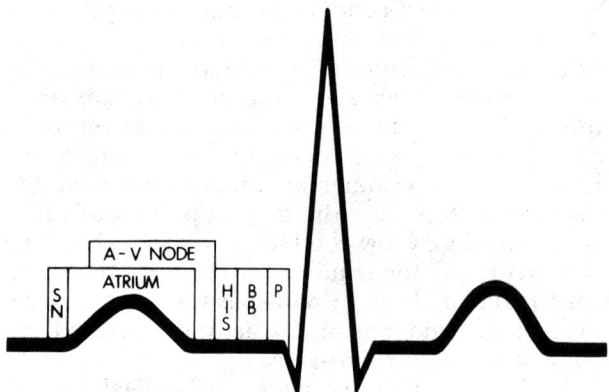

FIGURE 4-1 Normal electrocardiographic complex. Also shown is the sequence of activity in the specialized conducting system. SN = sinus node; HIS = His bundle; BB = bundle branches; P = peripheral Purkinje tissue.

tive to the extracellular space (Fig. 4-2). This difference in electrical potential acts as a second passive force so that positively charged ions tend to migrate to the inside of the cell and negatively charged ions tend to migrate to the outside. The potential energy of any ion on either the inside or outside of the cell membrane is the net result of diffusion and electric forces. When the potential energy of an ion is the same on the inside and outside of the cell, no net

movement will occur and the inside and outside of the cell are said to be in a *steady state* with respect to the ion in question. The transmembrane electrical potential that exactly counteracts the force attributable to a difference in concentration is referred to as the *equilibrium potential* for that ion.

Potassium exists at a concentration approximately 35 times greater on the inside of the cell than on the outside, while the sodium concentration is approximately 4.5 times greater on the outside of the cell than on the inside. The diffusion force tending to move potassium out of the cell (P_c) is proportional to the concentration gradient, and the potential energy attributable to this force can be expressed quantitatively by the equation:

$$P_c = RT \log_e \frac{[K]_i}{[K]_o} \tag{1}$$

where R = the gas constant
T = the absolute temperature
K_i = intracellular K^+ concentration
K_o = extracellular K^+ concentration
e = 2.718 (the base of natural logarithms)

The inside of the cell, however, is 90 mV negative with respect to the outside. This electric force will

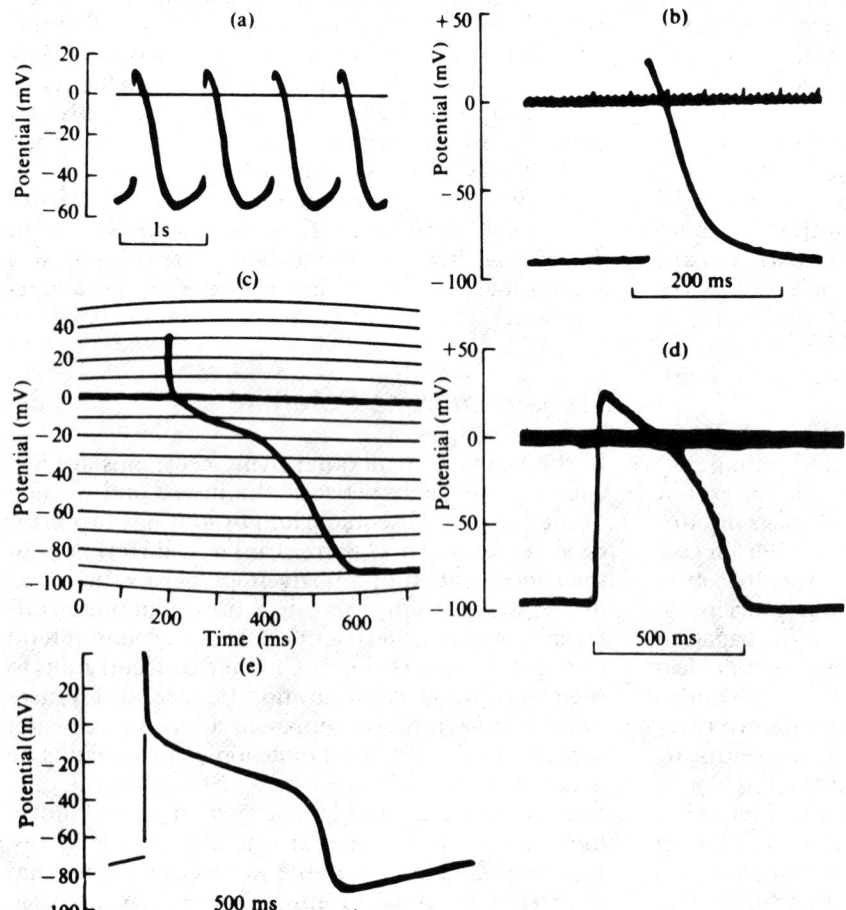

FIGURE 4-2 Action potentials recorded from different parts of the heart. *a.* Sinus node. *b.* Atrium. *c.* Quiescent Purkinje fiber. *d.* Ventricle. *e.* Automatic Purkinje fiber. Transmembrane potential at rest varies from −50 mV in SA node to −95 mV in atrium, Purkinje, and ventricle. (*From Noble.*[1] *Reproduced with permission.*)

tend to move potassium to the inside of the cell in proportion to the voltage gradient. The potential energy (PE) attributable to this force can be expressed quantitatively by the equation

$$PE = ZFE_m \qquad (2)$$

where Z = the valence of the ion in question
F = 96,500 (the Faraday number)
E_m = the transmembrane potential difference

In a steady state the potential energy attributable to diffusion and electric forces is equal and no net ionic movement occurs. Thus

$$ZFE_m = RT \ln \frac{[K]_i}{[K]_o} \qquad (3)$$

or at 37°C,

$$E_k = 61.5 \log \frac{[K]_i}{[K]_o} \qquad (4)$$

This is the Nernst equation, which describes the membrane potential that must exist for potassium to be in equilibrium across the membrane of a resting cardiac cell. When Eq. 4 is solved using known values for intracellular and extracellular potassium concentration, $E_k = -90$ mV, which is nearly identical to the observed membrane potential across the resting cell. This finding suggests that the potassium equilibrium potential is the major factor responsible for resting transmembrane potential.

Whenever membrane potential is stable, as it is in most cardiac cells during diastole, the sum of all ionic currents moving across the cell membrane must equal zero. Furthermore, the passive movement of any ion across the membrane is influenced not only by the concentration gradient, but also by the permeability of the membrane to the ion in question. These considerations lead to a more general description of membrane voltage, the Hodgkin and Katz modification of Goldman's constant field equation, where

$$V_m = \frac{RT}{F} \log \left[\frac{P_K[K]_i + P_{Na}[Na]_i + P_{Cl}[Cl]_o \cdots}{P_K[K]_o + P_{Na}[Na]_o + P_{Cl}[Cl]_i \cdots} \right] \quad (5)$$

If Eq. 4 is solved for the sodium equilibrium potential, a value of +50 mV is obtained. Since this is oppositely directed and far from the observed resting membrane potential, it is very unlikely that the sodium potential contributes to resting potential. The explanation lies in Eq. 5 if we assume that the resting membrane is permeable to potassium but impermeable to sodium. Solution of Eq. 5 gives a V_m of 90 mV, i.e., the equilibrium potential for K^+.

The sodium and potassium concentration gradients across the cell membrane are created by the activity of a Na^+-K^+ exchange pump that accumulates K inside the cell and pumps Na to the outside. The pump includes an enzyme that requires ATP for its activity and is subject to inhibition by uncoupling oxidative phosphorylation or by perfusion with a solution deficient in oxygen.[2] The activity of the enzyme is stimulated by Na and K through two separate loci (an internal site with high affinity for Na and an external site with high affinity for K). The activity of the enzyme is further dependent on pH and is inhibited by high concentrations of ouabain. For many years, the Na and K exchange was felt to be tightly coupled and thus electroneutral. Recent data, however, indicate that more Na is pumped out than K is pumped in and hence there is a net outward current that contributes to the negative intracellular potential. This interpretation implies that the Na^+-K^+ pump is electrogenic, that it contributes to the transmembrane potential, and that transmembrane potential can be changed by agents that affect the activity of the pump.

Excitability and the Action Potential

The term *excitability* is used to describe the fact that when a resting cardiac cell is depolarized to a critical level (called *threshold*), the membrane becomes permeable and a regenerative inward current causes an action potential. It is well known that cells found in different parts of the heart have different transmembrane potentials, different thresholds, and action potentials of different shapes (Fig. 4-3). Recently these action potentials have been grouped into two general types: fast and slow responses (Fig. 4-4). Fast responses are characteristic of ordinary working atrial and ventricular muscle cells and of Purkinje fibers. In these fibers resting membrane potential is −80 to −90 mV, the upstroke velocity of the action potential is 100 to 500 V/s, and conduction velocity is rapid.[3] Slow responses are characteristic of the normal sinus and AV nodal cells. In these fibers, resting potential is −40 to −70 mV, upstroke velocity of the action potential is 1 to 10 V/s, and conduction velocity is very slow.[4] The membrane properties and ionic currents responsible for each type of action potential are different.

Much of what is known about excitable cells was initially derived from studies of squid axon and cardiac Purkinje fibers, both of which have fast responses. Consequently, we know more about the ionic basis for the action in fast cells. It is of great interest and importance, however, that when fast-responding cardiac cells become depressed and depolarized, they assume many of the characteristics of slow cells. Thus, mechanisms responsible for the slow response are relevant to both the normal and abnormal function of the heart.

In Purkinje fibers, threshold potential is approximately −70 mV, and when the cell is depolarized to that level either by a stimulus or by a propagated action potential, membrane sodium conductance

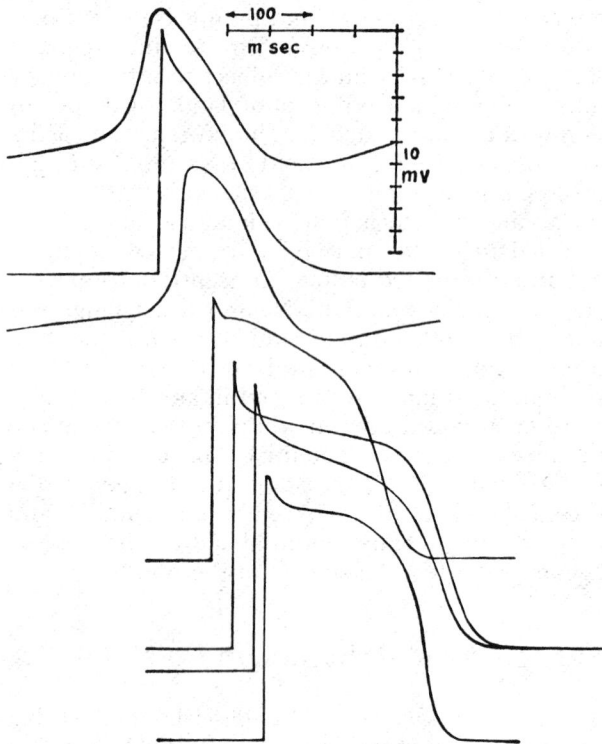

FIGURE 4-3 Transmembrane action potentials recorded from (top to bottom) SA node, atrium, AV node, His bundle, false tendon, peripheral Purkinje, ventricle. Note differences in shape, amplitude, and duration of action potentials. (*From B. F. Hoffman, and P. F. Cranefield, "Electrophysiology of the Heart," McGraw-Hill Book Company, New York, 1960, p. 261. Reproduced with permission.*)

(permeability) increases abruptly. As a consequence, positively charged sodium ions enter the cell rapidly, causing further depolarization (phase 0 of the action potential). Membrane potential reaches approximately +20 mV, but never quite equals the +50-mV value predicted by the sodium equilibrium potential (Fig. 4-5). This is because activation of the fast channel for sodium conductance lasts only a millisecond or two and then becomes at least partially inactivated.[5]

The fast sodium channel is currently viewed as being guarded by a mechanism that functions as a gate that probably represents a charged electric field

between components of the phospholipid matrix of the membrane.[1] The gate is closed in a resting fiber because of the orientation of charged phospholipids that block the entry of positively charged ions. With depolarization, the lipids reorient and the gates open, allowing sodium to move inside the fiber (Fig. 4-5). The sodium current is described by the equation

$$I_{Na} = g_{Na} (V_m - V_{Na})$$

where g_{Na} = the sodium conductance of the channel
V_m = the membrane potential
V_{Na} = the sodium equilibrium potential

g_{Na} is a variable parameter expressed by the equation

$$g_{Na} = \overline{g}_{Na} \, m^3 h$$

where $\overline{g}_{Na}$ = the maximal sodium conductance
m = a voltage-dependent variable describing activation (opening) of the gates
h = a voltage- and time-dependent variable describing inactivation or closing of the gates

In this two-component model of the sodium channel, m changes much more rapidly than h in response to a change of membrane potential (V_m). Assume for illustrative purposes that at a resting potential of −90 mV, $h = 1$ (open) and $m = 0$ (closed). With depolarization, m changes very rapidly to 1 and the channel is maximally open. Once the cell is depolarized, h changes more slowly from 1 to 0, reducing the value m^3h and hence g_{Na}. The rapid sodium channel in heart cell appears to have great similarity to that in nerve cell.

In addition to this early inward sodium current, there is a second and much more slowly inactivated inward current that appears to contribute to the plateau of the action potential in cardiac fibers. Current evidence suggests that this inward current develops about 10 ms after phase 0 and is most likely attrib-

A.

B.

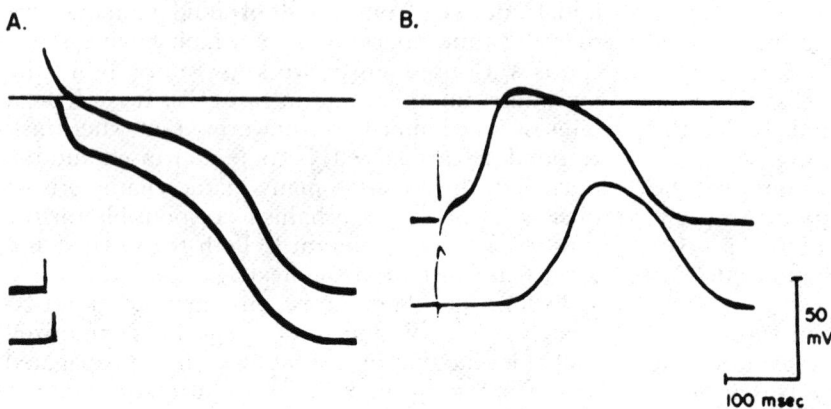

50 mV

100 msec

FIGURE 4-4 Action potentials typical of fast (*A*) and slow (*B*) responses.

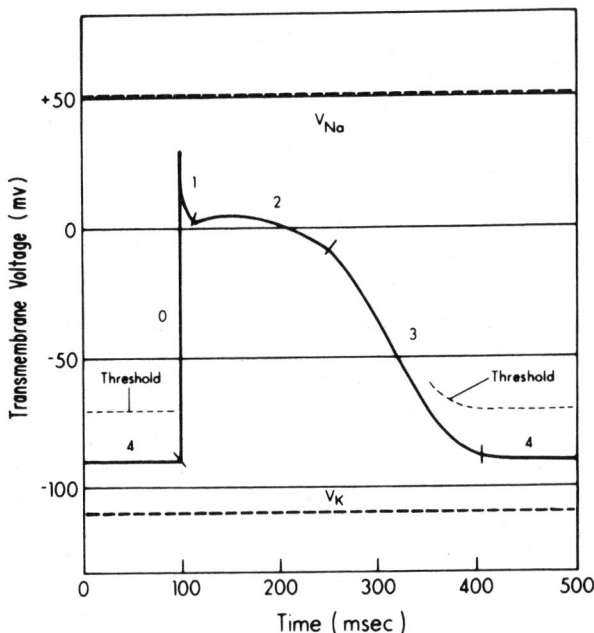

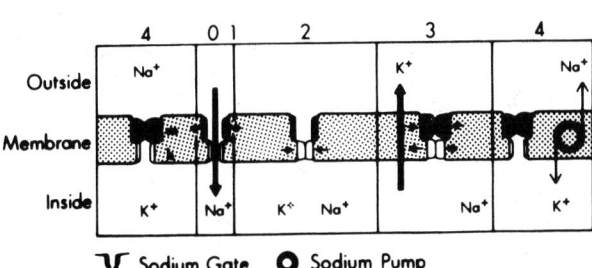

]C Sodium Gate **O** Sodium Pump

FIGURE 4-5 A schematic of the cardiac action potential and the sequence of events that determine the time change in voltage. V_{Na} = sodium equilibrium potential; V_K = potassium equilibrium potential. The four phases of the action potential are noted above. Below are shown the cardiac membrane, the gates which open and close to allow Na and K ions to move across the membrane, causing depolarization and then repolarization. Finally, the activity of the pump which restores Na and K during phase 4 is illustrated. *(Redrawn from T. Bigger, Antiarrhythmic Drugs in Ischemic Heart Disease, in "The Myocardium: Failure and Infarction," H. P. Publishing Company, Inc., New York, 1974, p. 296. Reproduced with permission.)*

utable to calcium ions[6] or to a separate slow sodium channel.

Most investigators agree that following the plateau of the action potential, potassium conductance, which had been reduced by depolarization and had remained low during the plateau, returns to its higher level. This rising potassium conductance allows potassium to move out of the cell:

$$I_K = g_K (V_m - V_K)$$

where I_K = the potassium conductance
of the channel
V_m = the membrane potential
V_K = the potassium equilibrium
potential

As a consequence of the egress of positively charged potassium, the cell repolarizes (Fig. 4-6). In cardiac fibers the onset and rate of repolarization are influenced primarily by agents that increase or decrease potassium conductance.[1]

In summary, in muscle and Purkinje fibers the action potential is brought about by an initial fast inward movement of sodium (phase 0) that ends abruptly (phase 1). During the plateau of an action potential (phase 2), membrane voltage is influenced by slow inward currents carried by calcium and/or sodium and an outward potassium current (ix_1). This latter current (ix_1) is slow to start but turns on in a time-dependent manner and, when maximal, causes the cell to rapidly repolarize (phase 3).

Recall that the variables m and h which determine rapid sodium conductance were reversed from their normal values as a consequence of depolarization, and that the membrane is unresponsive during the plateau. As the membrane repolarizes, the values of m and h, which are dependent on membrane potential, return to the levels that existed before depolarization. Current evidence suggests that the values for m and h follow membrane potential closely, but that recovery of h is dependent on both potential and time. Under normal circumstances, recovery of the sodium-carrying system is closely coupled to repolarization. However, under the influence of a number of agents, including reduced temperature and drugs that alter the kinetics of h, repolarization and recovery of responsiveness can be dissociated in

FIGURE 4-6 A model of the cardiac action potential based on modifications of the Hodgkin-Huxley theory. The action potential is shown above. Change in sodium conductance (g_{Na+}), solid curve, and potassium conductance (g_{K+}), dashed curve, are shown below. See text for description. *(From Noble.[1] Reproduced with permission.)*

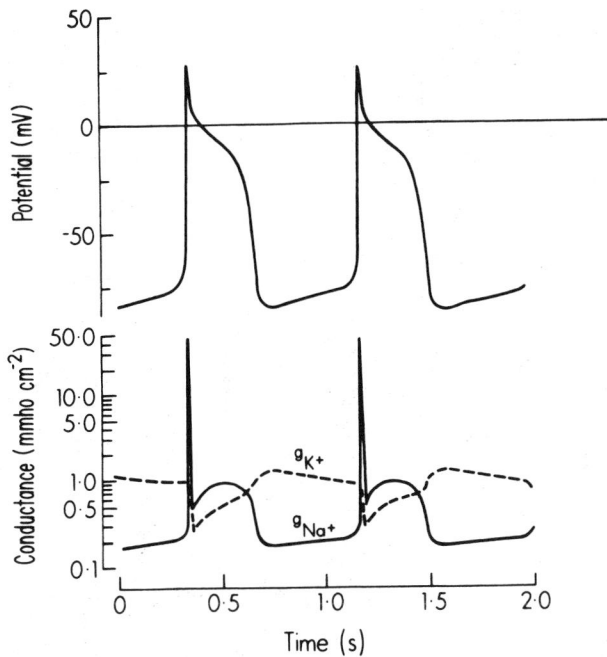

time such that recovery from inactivation occurs only long after repolarization.

We have already noted that in normal Purkinje fibers there is evidence of a second inward current that is delayed in onset and is carried by calcium and/or sodium through a slow channel (Fig. 4-7). When a Purkinje fiber becomes depolarized, either by an applied voltage or by a high external potassium concentration, the rapid sodium channel, which is normally responsible for phase 0, is inactivated (i.e., the gates or channels are closed). Under these circumstances an action potential can still be elicited, and it is attributable solely to the slow channel (Fig. 4-8). A slow-response action potential has the following characteristics: (1) threshold is in the range of −50 to −35 mV, (2) upstroke velocity is 1 to 10 V/s, (3) action potential amplitude is reduced, (4) action potential duration is short, and (5) recovery of excitability is delayed long after repolarization. The slow-response action potential is not altered by tetrodotoxin (which blocks the fast channel), but is abolished by manganese or by verapamil (which block the slow channel). In the sinus node and in the N region (middle) of the AV node normal cells typically have resting potentials of −50 to −60

FIGURE 4-7 A model of the cardiac action potential, similar to that shown in Fig. 4-6, except that changes in calcium conductance (g_{Ca2+}) have been added to indicate the slow-channel current. S and X_1 are variables which control potassium conductances (g_{K+}) and are analogous to m and h, which control sodium conductance (g_{Na+}). (*From Noble.*[1] *Reproduced with permission.*)

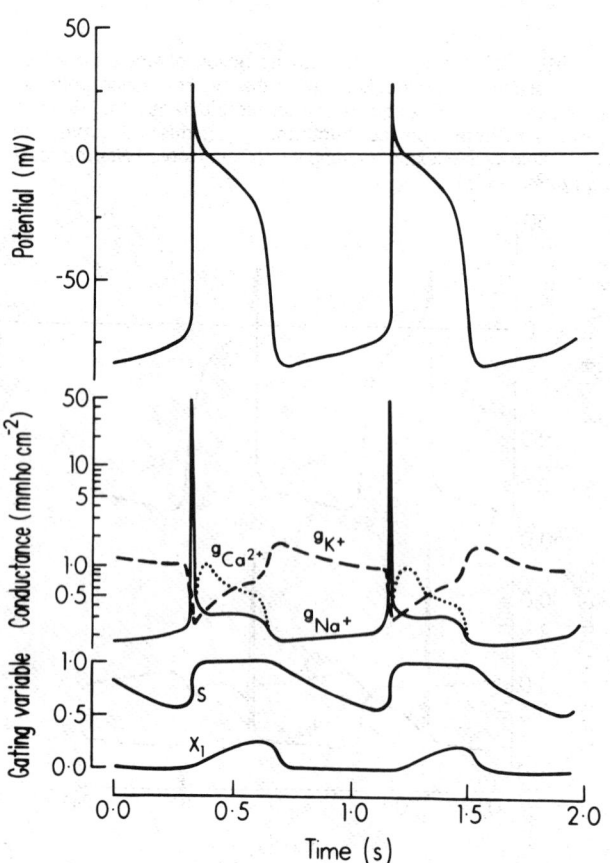

mV, a slow upstroke, and short duration and are sensitive to verapamil and insensitive to tetrodotoxin. These and other features suggest that the action potential of sinus and AV node cells is due solely to a slow inward current,[7] while Purkinje and muscle fibers have both fast and slow channels.

Automaticity

The term *automaticity* has been used to describe a property of certain cardiac cells to initiate an action potential spontaneously. Many cells within the specialized conducting system have the capacity of becoming automatic, but only the cell or group of cells that initiate a propagated impulse are referred to as the *pacemaker* of the heart.

There is an important difference in the characteristics of the transmembrane action potential recorded from automatic cells and from ordinary working myocardium which is nonautomatic. In automatic cells the membrane potential is not steady, but rather undergoes slow, spontaneous diastolic depolarization. When this slow decrease in membrane potential reaches threshold, an action potential is initiated (Fig. 4-9).

Automatic behavior is clearly evident under normal conditions in the sinus node and in Purkinje fibers. On the other hand, the maximal diastolic potential, the rate of spontaneous depolarization, and other features of the action potential are distinctly different in sinus node and in Purkinje fibers. It follows that the mechanisms responsible for automaticity in the sinus node and in Purkinje fibers are not necessarily the same.

The mechanisms responsible for automaticity and its control have been reviewed recently.[8] It should be recalled that in all cardiac cells there is an inward (leakage) current, which is presumably carried by positively charged sodium ions. If this leakage current is not offset in diastole by an electrically equal outward ion flux, then diastolic depolarization will ensue.

In the sinus node the action potential is short. Potassium conductance is activated by depolarization and increases further with time to cause repolarization. The subsequent diastolic decrease of the outward potassium current (ix_1), especially at a low membrane potential, allows the inward sodium leakage current to dominate membrane potential and cause diastolic depolarization.

In Purkinje fibers the action potential is long. Furthermore, the cells repolarize to a membrane potential of −85 to −95 mV. Voltage clamp studies have shown that when a Purkinje fiber is clamped at −60 mV an outward potassium current $i_{K,2}$ is maximally activated. At −90 mV, however, $i_{K,2}$ is completely inactivated, although this deactivation is slow and time-dependent. Thus, during repolarization when membrane potential reaches −60 mV, $i_{K,2}$ is maximal. Further repolarization to −90 mV

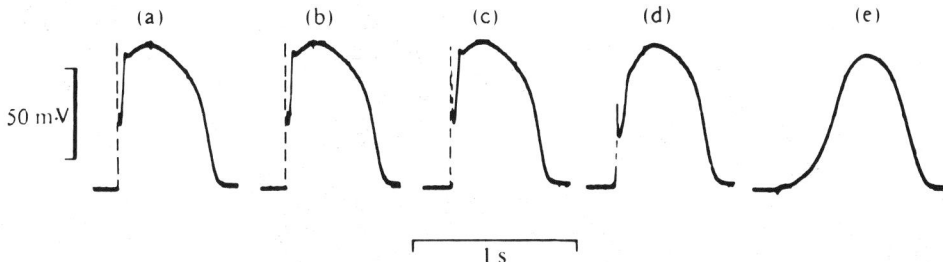

FIGURE 4-8 Action potential recorded from a calf Purkinje fiber in the presence of adrenalin. Panel *a* is control. Panels *b* to *e* show action potentials recorded in the presence of increasing concentrations of tetrodotoxin. Tetrodotoxin blocks the fast sodium channel, and the residual action potential (*e*) is due entirely to the slow channel. (*From Noble.*[1] *Reproduced with permission.*)

deactivates $i_{K,2}$ but only with a time delay (Fig. 4-10). Hence in Purkinje fibers there is a slow fall of potassium conductance in diastole, as in sinus node, which allows the inward sodium current to cause spontaneous diastolic depolarization. In the sinus node it is delayed inactivation of ix_1, while in Purkinje fibers it is delayed inactivation of $i_{K,2}$, that causes the pacemaker current.

Vagal nerve stimulation slows impulse initiation by the sinus node, while sympathetic nerve stimulation speeds impulse formation. The major consequence of vagal nerve stimulation is hyperpolarization of sinus node cells. This hyperpolarization is induced by acetylcholine, which increases potassium conductance. Both hyperpolarization and a reduced rate of spontaneous diastolic depolarization contribute to a reduced frequency of sinus node firing (Fig. 4-11). The ionic basis for the ability of adrenergic

stimuli to enhance firing in the sinus node is not known.

Conduction

Once an action potential has been initiated at any given site in the heart, excitation is propagated away from that site and is referred to as *conduction*. Because the resistivity of the cytoplasm is low by comparison with the membrane, current flows with ease through the cytoplasm from excited to unexcited regions of the cell. This flow of current is sufficient to discharge the capacitance of distal membrane and hence to bring the membrane to threshold, where its resistance drops, allowing more inward current as a source to discharge still more distant units of membrane. As noted previously, propagation from

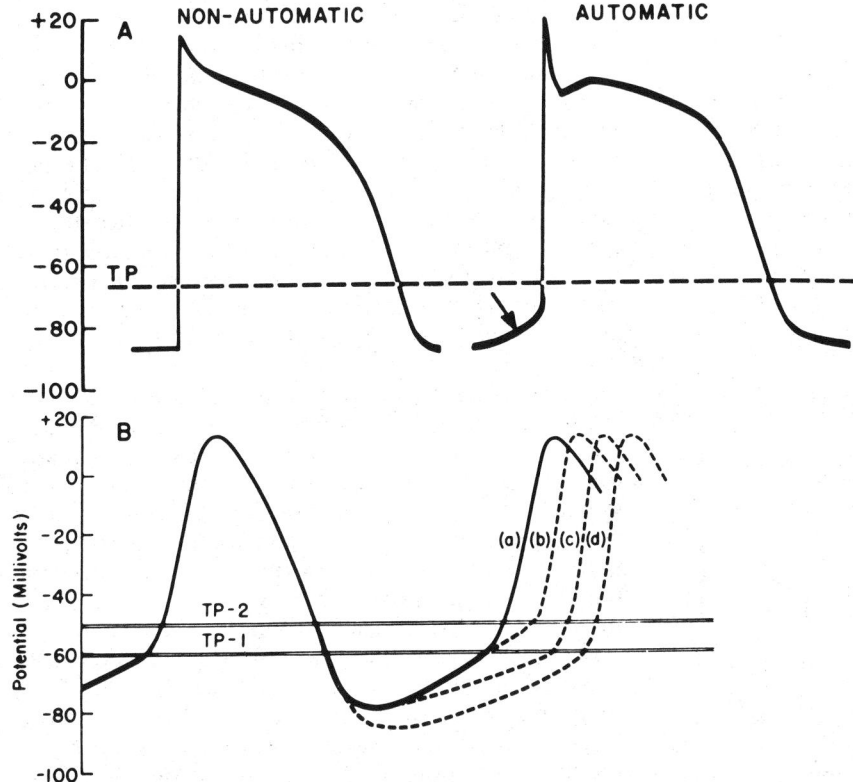

FIGURE 4-9 Schematic showing the difference in action potential characteristics of a nonautomatic and automatic cell (upper panel). The lower panel shows that changes in the rhythmicity of an automatic cell can result from a change in threshold (*b*), a reduced rate of diastolic depolarization (*c*), or hyperpolarization (*d*).

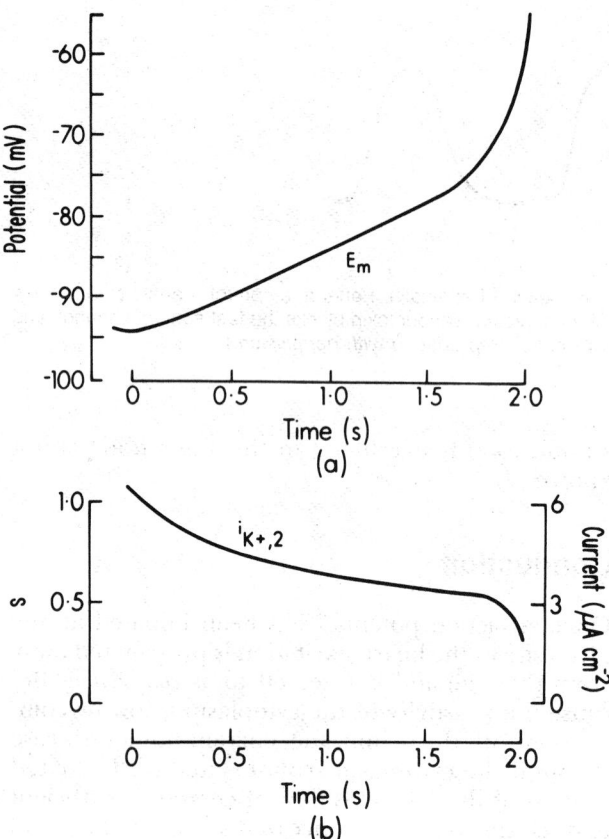

FIGURE 4-10 Mechanism of pacemaker activity in Purkinje fibers. The upper panel shows diastolic depolarization of the transmembrane potential (E_m) characteristic of a pacemaker potential. The lower curve depicts the slow diastolic decrease in outward potassium current ($i_{K+,2}$). The decrease in this outward potassium current allows the inward sodium leakage current to depolarize the cell. See text. (*Redrawn from Noble.[1] Reproduced with permission.*)

one fiber to another occurs at sites of low-resistance coupling between cells, allowing current derived from one cell to discharge an adjacent cell. In a system of cells, the conduction velocity between two points in the system will be influenced by the dimensions and geometry of the cells, by the nature and frequency of connections, by the passive or cable properties of the fiber, by the threshold potential, and by the amplitude and velocity of phase 0 of

FIGURE 4-11 Membrane potential recorded from pacemaker cell of the frog sinus venosus during vagal nerve stimulation. Note that hyperpolarization and a reduced slope of diastolic depolarization both contribute to the slowing of the pacemaker. (*From Hutter and Trautwein, J. Gen. Physiol., 39:715, 1956. Reproduced with permission.*)

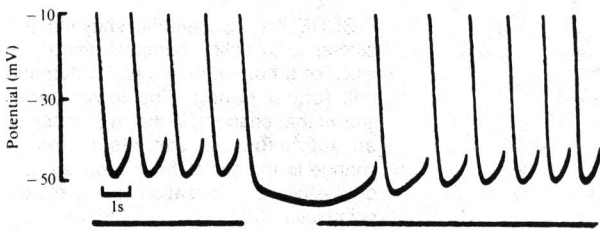

the action potential.[9] These relationships are expressed by the formula

$$\theta = \sqrt{\frac{a \; d^2V/dt^2}{2R_i \; (C_m \; dV/dt + I_m)}}$$

where θ = conduction velocity
a = fiber radius
V = membrane potential
R_i = the specific resistance of the cytoplasm
C_m = the specific capacitance of the membrane
I_m = the active membrane current density

If we assume that individual cells constituting a system are normal, a strong case has been made for the fact that differences in apparent conduction velocity in different regions of the heart are attributable primarily to geometry and to the nature and frequency of intercellular connections.

In its simplest and theoretical form the cardiac cell in a steady state has been viewed as behaving as though it were a segment of a cable. This cable is made up of a membrane (the sarcolemma) surrounding the myoplasm. The membrane has a resistance (i.e., the inverse of conductance), and conductance reflects permeability to the ion in question. Membrane conductance is small (i.e., resistance is high) in the resting fiber and attributable primarily to potassium. The cell membrane also behaves like a capacitor, evident from the fact that when a step function of current is applied across the membrane, transmembrane potential changes more slowly. Membrane capacitance is presumed to reflect primarily the structure and composition of the sarcolemma. The resistivity of the cytoplasm and of the extracellular fluid are considered constant and small relative to membrane resistance. Although the geometry of cardiac tissue and the nature of intercellular connections may seem to make it difficult to treat the preparation as though it were a cable (and in fact such treatments are fraught with interpretive difficulty), one important conclusion seems inescapable: cardiac cells are joined to each other by low-resistance couplings that allow current to flow from one cell to the next with minimal impediment.

During normal rhythm, impulse formation takes place in the sinoatrial node. The sinus node usually dominates other potentially automatic regions of the specialized conduction system, and therefore it acts as the pacemaker. One reason for this dominance is that impulses formed in the sinus node are initiated at a greater frequency than other latent pacemakers and the spread of the impulse from the node discharges these other latent pacemaker cells before their own inherent rhythmicity would result in spontaneous discharge. A second reason is the interaction between pacemaker regions of different inherent rhythmicity. When a frequency of excitation greater than that which is inherent to one group of cells is superimposed on that group, their own rate of firing is suppressed. This phenomenon is referred to as *overdrive suppression.*

Recordings from the region of the atrioventricular node in mammalian hearts have revealed that slow propagation of the impulse is the basis for the normal delay between excitation of the atria and of the ventricles. A functional description of the atrioventricular node has been formulated on the basis of the timing of excitation at various regions and the characteristics of locally recorded cellular transmembrane action potentials. The node can be divided into three regions: AN (atrionodal junction), N (nodal), and NH (nodal-His junction). These regions progress from superficial to deep as the atrioventricular junctional zone is viewed from the right atrium; they represent the sequence of excitation as a normal impulse propagates through the atrioventricular junction. Conduction velocity is slowest in the N region. Transmembrane recordings from cells in the N zone reveal no rapid upstroke or overshoot, but rather a very slowly rising action potential in which the upstroke velocity is insensitive to tetrodotoxin. Furthermore, anatomic studies show a paucity of intercellular connections and a more or less random arrangement of very slender cells. These structural and electrophysiologic facts appear sufficient to account for exceedingly slow conduction velocity through the N region.

Genesis of the Electrocardiogram

The activity of the heart creates an electric field that is distributed throughout the body. These currents produce potentials on the body surface, and when two electrodes are placed on the body and connected through an appropriate amplifier, an electrocardiogram or graphic recording of the potential difference between sites is obtained. Ordinarily, voltage is plotted on the vertical axis and time on the horizontal axis over an interval of time that is equal to at least one complete cardiac cycle. Voltage displacements with respect to time occur during excitation and recovery of the atrium and ventricle.

The form of the electrocardiogram is determined by the sequence of excitation and recovery, by the resulting potential differences on the surface of the heart (i.e., the generator), and by factors that determine current flow within a three-dimensional, bounded, nonhomogeneous conductor such as the torso. These latter factors help to explain the relation between epicardial potentials and their projection onto the body surface.

During normal rhythm, excitation of the atrium begins in the region of the sinus node high in the right atrium (Fig. 4-12). The excitation wave spreads outward over the right atrium, from the head of the sinus node into the left atrium, and down the interatrial septum.[10] Because all three of

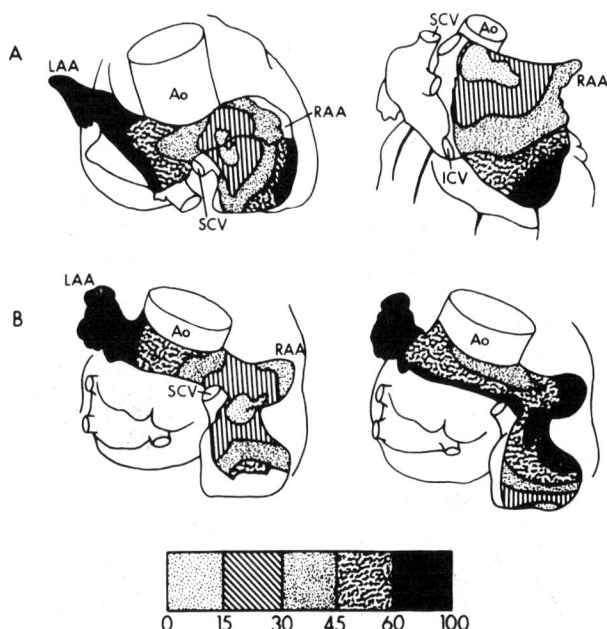

FIGURE 4-12   Sequence of atrial activation in two human hearts. *A.* The left side shows a superior view and the right side a posterior view of atrial activation. The little stippling over the SA node is the earliest area, and the black solid tone shows the latest area. *B.* This is from a second heart. The left side is again portrayed during sinus rhythm. The right side shows retrograde activation during ventricular pacing. (*Redrawn from Durrer.*[11] *Reproduced with permission.*)

these structures have a thin wall, the wave front is best viewed as a surface phenomenon. Endocardial to epicardial spread is an insignificant factor in determining P-wave morphology. Since there are areas of preferential impulse propagation in the atrial walls and septum (see Chap. 2), the advancing wave front on any one of the atrial surfaces is irregular, with projecting pseudopods of early activity and valleys of delayed excitation. The overall direction of the wave front, however, is downward and from right to left. During the earliest portions of the P wave the dominant wave front is advancing from the sinus node, down the right atrial wall along the sulcus terminalis. Shortly thereafter, two widely separated activation fronts develop, one moving laterally in the right atrial free wall and a second in the upper portion of the left atrium near the entrance of the pulmonary veins. While these two excitation waves persist, activity begins in the central portion of the interatrial septum, spreading the terminal portion of the P wave. There are colliding wave fronts in the posterior regions of the left atrium.

Ventricular activation proceeds in an orderly sequence, and, as might be expected from the anatomic distribution of the Purkinje system, the general order is from apex to base.[11] Initial excitation begins on the left side of the interventricular septum near the apex (Fig. 4-13). This is followed within a few milliseconds by activation of the endocardial surface of the right ventricle near the apex. Within

THE NORMAL HEART AND BLOOD VESSELS

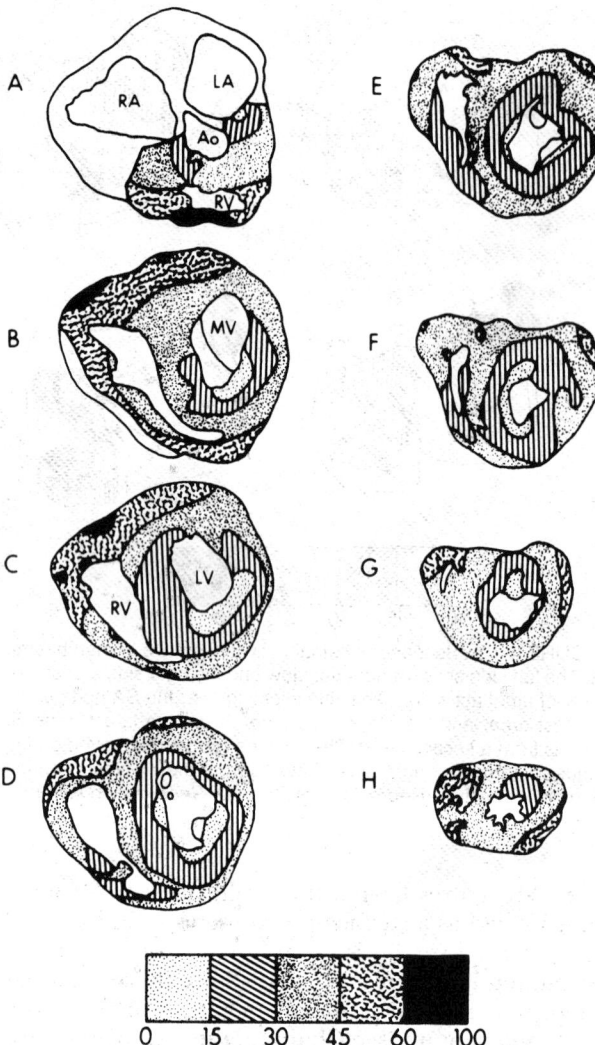

FIGURE 4-13 The normal sequence of activation of the human ventricle. *A* to *H*. Transverse sections from base to apex. In each section regions of similar activation times are enclosed by isochronous lines, and the temporal sequence is depicted in the legend. RA = right atrium; LA = left atrium; Ao = aorta; MV = mitral valve; RV = right ventricle. See text. (*From Durrer.*[11] *Reproduced with permission.*)

ner right ventricle. The terminal portions of the QRS complex arise almost solely from persisting activity in the basal regions of the left ventricle and upper interventricular septum.

The traditional approach for relating the activation sequence of the heart to the electrocardiogram is to assume (1) that the boundary between excited and still unexcited cells is a smooth, continuous surface, and (2) that any component of this surface is a potential dipole, one side of which is a source and the other a sink for current flow. The dipole theory also assumes that current flow is oriented perpendicular to the direction of propagation and that the strength of the dipole is related to its surface area. The potential at any site remote from the dipole is then proportional to the solid angle subtended by that dipole surface.

Recent work has indicated that this theory is inadequate to explain the electrocardiogram.[12,13] The critical problem is that the theory was developed for isotropic tissues in which electrical properties such as conductivity are the same in all directions. Heart muscle, however, is anisotropic. In the heart the relation between the spatial intracellular potential gradient and extracellular potential is the opposite of that predicted from studies of isotropic tissue. As a consequence, extracellular potential is directly related to conduction velocity and the orientation of a dipole is perpendicular to a slowly moving wave front but parallel to a high-velocity wave front. Because of these considerations, most current analyses that view the heart as a generator of electrocardiographic potentials use the measured epicardial potential rather than isochrones demarcating the activation fronts to simulate potentials on the body surface.[14]

Maps of epicardial potential distribution are obtained by placing electrodes at multiple epicardial sites and recording the instantaneous voltage with respect to some remote site such as the left leg. At any given instant, regions of similar potentials are enclosed by *isopotential lines;* a region of maximal positive potential is called a *maximum,* and a region of peak negative potential is called a *minimum.*

During sinus rhythm a negative potential (minimum) develops over the sinus node with surrounding positive potentials over the right atrial free wall. During subsequent parts of the P wave, the epicardial potentials are exceedingly complex, with irregular minima extending along the sulcus of the right atrium, into the left atrium over Bachman's bundle, and into the right atrial appendage, each surrounded by areas of positive potential. At the end of the P wave, there is a maximum in the inferolateral portion of the left atrium, surrounded by negative potentials that gradually converge upon and extinguish the left atrial maximum.

During early ventricular activation, there are positive potentials recorded from most of the epicardial surface except for the lateral left ventricle

5 to 10 ms of the onset of the QRS complex the impulse spreads rapidly over the Purkinje network and there are shells of depolarized endocardial muscle that encircle the cavities of both right and left ventricles. These shells are closed near the apex, but they are open posteriorly and at the base near the AV valves. Fusion of these shells progresses within the septum from the apex to the base while activity spreads in an endocardial to epicardial direction in the free wall of each ventricle. Excitation first reaches the epicardial surface of the anterior right ventricle at its margin with the interventricular septum. At the same time, wave fronts in the left ventricle are still confined to the intramural portions of the free wall. Midway through the QRS, epicardial breakthrough has been completed around the thin-

(Fig. 4-14). The maximum is over the anterior right ventricle. With the onset of epicardial excitation, negative potentials are recorded from the surface of the right ventricle, positive potentials are recorded from the left ventricle, and the maximum is on the diaphragmatic surface. The area of negative potential gradually expands over both ventricles, generally from apex to base, leaving a positive potential over only the lateral left ventricle. Finally, a positive potential over the posterobasal portion of the left ventricle becomes extinguished by the converging negative potentials as a result of epicardial breakthrough.

Throughout the cardiac cycle, whenever areas of

FIGURE 4-14 Epicardial potential distributions throughout the QRS complex. *a.* Very early ventricular activation. *b.* Approximately 20 ms into QRS. *c.* Approximately 50 ms into QRS. *d.* During terminal ventricular activation. Adapted from data regarding detailed isopotential maps of chimpanzee. See text. (*From Spach et al.*[14] *Reproduced with permission.*)

ANTERIOR   **POSTERIOR**

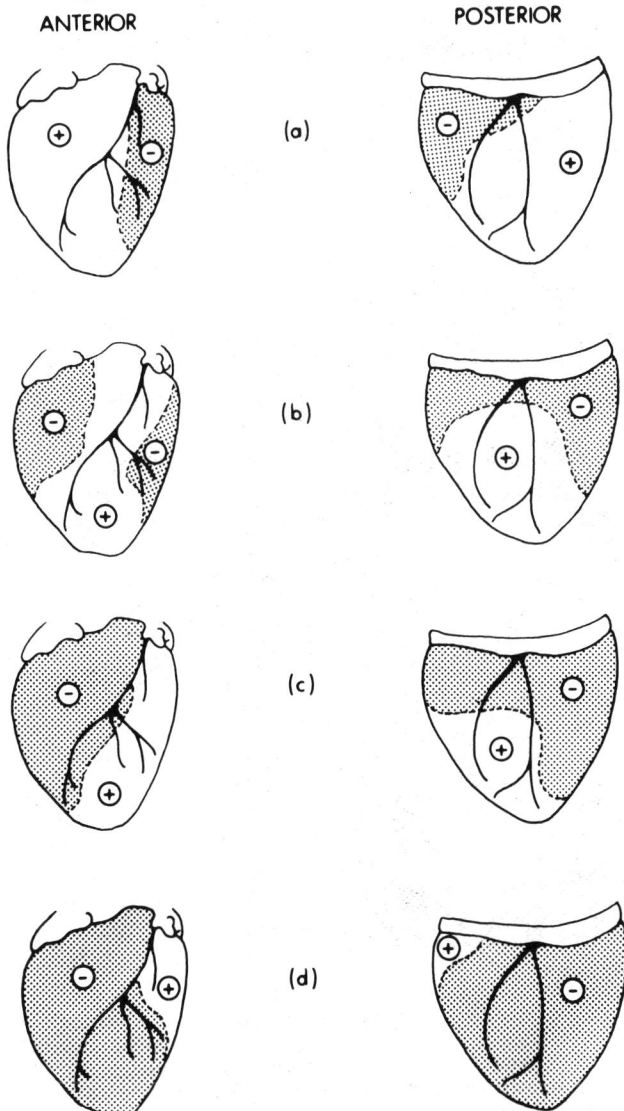

voltage difference exist on the epicardial surface, an electric field is generated in the body. The heart, therefore, can be considered as a current source (generator) within the body (a volume conductor). At any point in time during activation, regions of maximal epicardial potential (maxima) act as a source for current flow and areas of peak negative potential (minima) act as a sink for current.

On the body surface regions close to a source are in the positive portion of the field while areas close to the sink are in the negative portion of the field. All points of equal potential on the body describe an equipotential surface. The region of maximal positive potential at any instant is opposite the source, and the region of maximal negative potential is opposite the sink. Surrounding these maxima and minima are concentric regions of equal potential, but as the distance from source and sink increases, the current density, and hence the magnitude of the potential, decreases toward zero. There are many additional factors that influence the relation between potentials generated by the heart and those recorded on the body surface. Diminishing the conductivity of lung tissue (as in emphysema) decreases surface potentials. Obesity per se has a very slight effect, but the location of the heart within the torso has a major effect on surface potentials and their distribution.[15]

The location of maxima and minima on the epicardium changes during the process of excitation, and these regions also change in size (Fig. 4-15). Thus, at any point on the body surface, the potential with respect to any other point varies in sign and amplitude throughout excitation. The sign of the potential will be positive if the recording point faces the source, and negative if it faces the sink. The amplitude of the potential will be determined by the distance of the recording point from the source or sink and the conductivity of the tissues between the electrode and the source of potential.

In general, because atrial activation starts in the sinus node and progresses over the atria and septum toward the atrioventricular valves, the sinoatrial node regions are a sink and the atrial margins of the atrioventricular rings act as a source. Hence, the right shoulder tends to be in the negative portion of the field throughout most of atrial activation, and the left lower chest is in the positive portion of the field. Thus, the normal P wave is negative in lead aV_R and upright in electrocardiographic leads II, III, aV_F, and V_4 to V_6.

With ventricular activation the initial situation is one of left-to-right activation across the septum, producing positive potentials over the right anterior chest and negative potentials over the left shoulder and back. Subsequently, the maximal positive potentials move to the left side of the chest and negative potentials develop over the anterior chest. Finally as epicardial breakthrough develops over the apex of the left ventricle, the lower chest develops

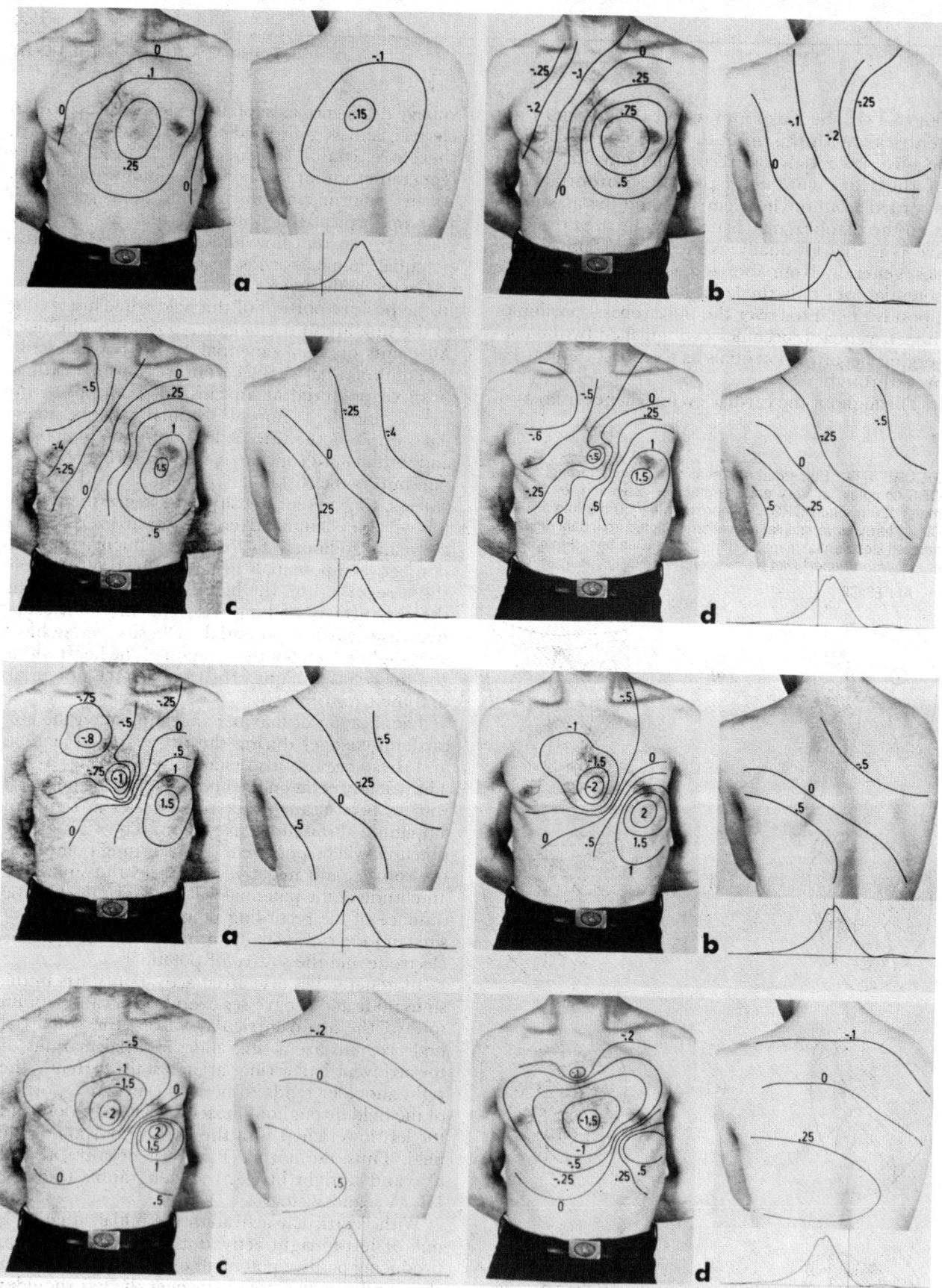

FIGURE 4-15   Isopotential maps of the thoracic surface in normal subject. Top: *a*. Onset of ventricular activation. There is one anterior maximum and one dorsal minimum. *b*. Early activation, dorsal minimum moves to right shoulder. *c*. The anterior maximum moves to the left nipple and negative potentials appear over the right anterior chest. *d*. A new minimum appears on right anterior chest. *Bottom* (continued from same subject): *a*. There are two anterior minima. *b*. The two anterior minima merge. *c*. Late QRS. *d*. Terminal QRS with maximum at lower left anterior axillary line and lower left back. See text. (*From B. Taccardi, Distribution of Heart Potentials on the Thoracic Surface of Normal Human Subjects, Circ. Res., 12:341, 1963. Reproduced with permission.*)

negative potentials and positive potentials shift to the left shoulder and back. This sequence produces a QRS complex which is predominantly positive in leads II, III, aV_F, and V_4 to V_6, and predominantly negative in leads aV_R and V_1.

In ventricular muscle, the action potential has a duration of 250 to 300 ms and a plateau phase during which membrane potential is relatively stable. Yet, the entire process of ventricular activation and inscription of the QRS complex is completed in 80 to 90 ms. As a consequence, there is an interval after the QRS when nearly all cells are in the same state of depolarization (phase 2 of the action potential), the potential difference between cells is negligible, and no appreciable electric field is created or recordable on the body surface. This interval corresponds to the isoelectric period (the ST segment) on the ECG separating the end of the QRS and the onset of the T wave.

When individual cells enter the phase of rapid repolarization (phase 3 of the action potential), a situation again exists in which regions of the heart in different stages of repolarization create an epicardial potential distribution and a consequent electric field in the volume conductor, resulting in potential difference on the body surface. Generally, the amplitude of the T wave is less than that of the QRS because the strength of potentials is somewhat less than during excitation. The duration of the T wave is greater than that of the QRS because repolarization is of longer duration, and because the process of repolarization is not propagated; hence, cells repolarize at their own intrinsic rate. An interesting feature of ventricular repolarization is that the process seems to start later and last longer in endocardium than in epicardium. As a consequence, the sequence of recovery is opposite to the sequence of excitation. If the sequence of repolarization were the same as depolarization, one would expect the T wave to be directed opposite to the QRS in most ECG leads. The fact that the sequence of repolarization is the reverse of excitation explains a characteristic feature of the normal electrocardiogram, where the polarity of the QRS and the T wave is the same in most leads. During repolarization positive potentials develop early in the T wave over the anterior right ventricle, with negativity recorded over the atria. Positive potentials persist over the anterior surface of right and left ventricles throughout the T wave, with the maxima moving superiorly and then simply collapsing at the end of the T wave as surrounding areas drop toward zero potential and engulf the maxima.

References

*1. Noble, D.: "The Initiation of the Heart Beat," Clarendon Press, Oxford, 1975. (Extensively referenced)
2. Carmeliet, E.: Cardiac Transmembrane Potentials and Metabolism, *Circ. Res.*, 42:577, 1978.
3. Cranefield, P. F.: "The Conduction of the Cardiac Impulse," Futura, Mt. Kisco, N.Y., 1975.
4. Zipes, D. P.: Recent Observations Supporting the Role of Slow Currents in Cardiac Electrophysiology, in J. J. J. Wellens, K. I. Lee, and M. J. Janse (eds.), "The Conduction of the Cardiac Impulse," Stanfertdroese, B.V., Leiden, 1976.
5. McAllister, R. E., Nobel, D., and Tsien, R. W.: Reconstruction of the Action Potential of Cardiac Purkinje Fibers, *J. Physiol.*, 251:1, 1975.
6. Beeler, G. W., and Reuter, H.: Reconstruction of the Action Potential of Ventricular Myocardial Fibers, *J. Physiol.*, 268:177, 1977.
7. Wit, A. L., and Cranefield, P. F.: Effect of Verapamil on the Sinoatrial and Atrioventricular Nodes of the Rabbit and the Mechanism by Which It Arrests Reentrant Atrioventricular Nodal Tachycardia, *Circ. Res.*, 35:413, 1974.
8. Vassalle, M.: Cardiac Automaticity and Its Control, *Am. J. Physiol.*, 233:H625, 1977.
9. Lieberman, M., Kootsey, J. M., Johnson, E. A., and Sawanobori, T.: Slow Conduction in Cardiac Muscle, *Biophys. J.*, 13:37, 1973.
10. Boineau, J. P., Moone, C. R., Hudson, R. D., Hughs, D. G., Erdin, R. A., Jr., and Wylds, A. C.: Observation in Reentrant Excitation Pathways and Refractory Period Distributions in Spontaneous and Experimental Atrial Flutter, in H. Kulbertus (ed.), "Reentrant Arrhythmias: Mechanisms and Treatment," University Park Press, Baltimore, Md., 1976, chap. 6.
11. Durrer, D., Van Dam, R. T., Freud, G. E., Janse, M. H., Meijler, F. L., and Arzbaecher, R. C.: Total Excitation of the Human Heart, *Circulation*, 41:899, 1970.
12. Corbin, L. A., and Scher, A. M.: The Canine Heart as an Electrocardiographic Generator: Dependence on Cell Orientation, *Circ. Res.*, 41:58, 1977.
13. Spach, M. S., Miller, W. T., Jones, E. M., Warren, R. B., and Barr, R. C.: Extracellular Potentials Related to Intracellular Action Potentials during Impulse Conduction in Anisotropic Cardiac Muscle, *Circ. Res.*, 45:188, 1979.
14. Spach, M. S., Barr, R. C., Lanning, C. F., and Tucek, P. C.: Origin of Body Surface QRS and T Wave Potentials from Epicardial Potential Distributions in the Intact Chimpanzee, *Circulation*, 55:268, 1977.
15. Rudy, Y., Plonsey, R., and Liebman, J.: The Effects of Variations in Conductivity and Geometric Parameters on the Electrocardiogram Using an Electric Sphere Model, *Circ. Res.*, 44:104, 1979.

*This article is a review of the literature and contains additional references to the literature.

5

Metabolic Regulation and Myocardial Function

Howard E. Morgan, M.D.
James R. Neely, Ph.D.

Cardiac metabolism is a dynamic process that regulates production of high-energy phosphates on a beat-to-beat basis and turnover of heart proteins within periods of a few hours to several days. Energy reserves within the heart are severely limited; for example as much as 5 percent of the total of ATP and creatine phosphate are consumed per beat, and the glycogen and triglyceride contents are able to support high levels of ventricular pressure development for no more than 6 and 12 min, respectively. As a result, the heart is dependent upon a continuous supply of substrate from the plasma to maintain energy production. Furthermore, both oxygen and substrates must be available because production of ATP by anaerobic glycolysis is limited to no more than 5 to 7 percent of normal energy production. The dynamics of energy production and utilization are best illustrated by measuring changes in high- and low-energy phosphate compounds during the cardiac cycle. Measurements of this type have not been technically feasible in mammalian hearts in the past because of the lack of methods to stop cardiac contraction during various phases of the cycle and the relatively small changes in total high-energy phosphate content that occur with each beat. The ability to make measurements during defined portions of the cycle has been obtained by use of phosphorus nuclear magnetic resonance (^{31}P-NMR) spectroscopy.[1] With this technique, the nuclei of phosphate compounds within the heart are induced to resonate by placement of the heart in a high magnetic field where it is bombarded with bursts of radio waves. Time resolution using this technique is approximately 2 ms, and potentially allows for 100 estimates to be made during each cardiac cycle. In well-oxygenated hearts that are perfused in vitro and supplied only glucose as substrate, ATP and creatine phosphate levels are maximal during diastole and lowest during systole (Fig. 5-1). Conversely, inorganic orthophosphate (P_i) and the sum of low-energy compounds, P_i, sugar phosphates, and NAD, are highest during systole and lowest during diastole. These data emphasize the dynamic nature of cardiac energy production and demonstrate directly the utilization and production of ATP and creatine phosphate during each beat of the heart.

Although turnover of protein and other macromolecular components of the heart occurs on a much longer time base than the high-energy phosphate reserves, the half-time for turnover of heart proteins and RNA varies from 1 h to several days.[2] The significance of the rapid turnover rate is that myofibrillar or enzymatic components of the heart can change in quantity or in type of isozyme over short time periods. For example, if synthesis of a specific cardiac protein with a half-life of 2 h were inhibited in ischemic hearts while normal rates of protein degradation were maintained, more than 95 percent of that protein would disappear after 12 h. If this protein were an essential component in energy production or contractile activity, functional capacity would be severely compromised. Fortunately, both synthesis and degradation of proteins are energy-requiring processes. Consequently, degradation of existing protein is reduced at the same time that synthesis of new protein is inhibited, and turnover rate is slowed greatly.

This chapter will focus on the biochemical mechanisms that sustain energy production and macromolecular synthesis and degradation by the heart. Fine control of the regulatory mechanisms is necessary to sustain the function of this vital organ.

General Features of Metabolic and Functional Alterations

Cardiac metabolism is regulated in a manner that sustains production of high-energy phosphate and contractile and synthetic activity despite large fluctuations in availability of carbohydrates, lipids, amino acids, and hormones. The metabolic versatility of the heart allows a wide range of substrates to be oxidized for energy production. Increased cardiac work stimulates substrate uptake and oxidation as well as biosynthetic processes in proportion to the need of the tissue.[3,4] As a result, metabolic and functional alterations that threaten cell survival occur only when coronary flow is reduced to the point that oxygen delivery and removal of metabolic products is severely compromised. However, lesser degrees of impairment can result from marked hormonal deficiency or during hypertrophy that is associated with overload of the left ventricle.

Modification of Function by Availability of Oxidative Substrates and Hormones

Fatty acids are the major fuel of the heart in normal animals, but glucose and lactate can make a large contribution following a meal that elevates insulin levels. When insulin is lacking, as in the diabetic, fatty acids and ketone bodies account for practically all of the oxidative fuel of cardiac muscle. Glucose utilization in the diabetic heart is impaired both by insulin lack and by indirect inhibitory effects of oxidation of fatty acids and ketone bodies on entry of glucose into the cell, on the glycolytic pathway, and on mitochondrial oxidation of pyruvate, the product of glycolysis. As a result, the small amount of

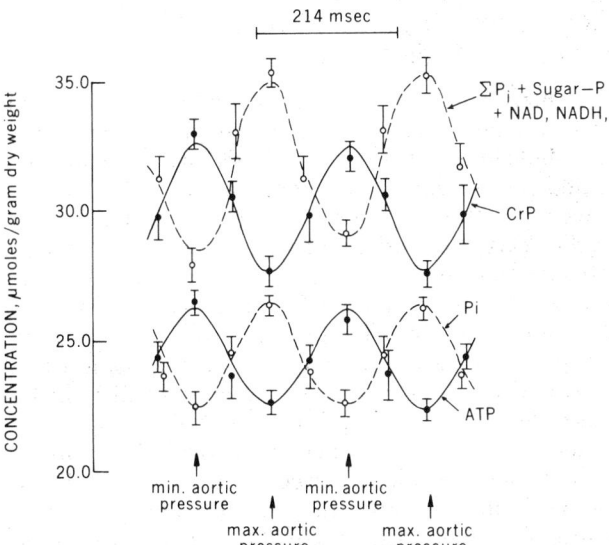

FIGURE 5-1   Concentration of ATP, creatine phosphate, P_i, and the sum of P_i plus sugar phosphates, NAD, and NADH in isolated working rat hearts that were perfused at an aortic pressure of 115/70 mmHg and provided 11 mM glucose in Krebs-Henseleit bicarbonate buffer. Maximal and minimal aortic pressures occurred at the times indicated. *(Adapted from Fossel, Morgan, and Ingwall.[1] Reproduced with permission.)*

glucose that is taken up is diverted to glycogen, and glycogen levels increase. The increased plasma levels of fatty acid lead to higher triglyceride content of the heart and may contribute to more rapid onset of irreversible damage if severe ischemia ensues. Functional consequences of insulin lack may be observed when energy generation is dependent on glucose uptake and oxidation. An impairment of function has been observed in vitro when hearts from diabetic animals are supplied only glucose as exogenous substrate,[5] and an improvement of function has been observed in human diabetics who had impaired ventricular function following cardiac surgery and were treated with glucose and insulin.[6]

Modification of Function Mediated by Altered Protein Turnover and Gene Expression

Heart proteins have half-lives averaging approximately 5 days.[2] As a result, a complete complement of new protein is synthesized about every 3 weeks; from this point of view, a person has essentially a "new heart" each month. Maintenance of constant cardiac mass depends on equal rates of synthesis and degradation of protein. Similarly constant levels of a specific enzyme or myofibrillar protein indicates that rates of synthesis and degradation of that particular protein are the same. Insulin, fatty acids, oxygen availability, and cardiac work affect rates of both synthesis and degradation. Synthetic rates can be modified by availability of ribosomes, messenger RNA, and enzymatic components (capacity for synthesis) or by the rate at which the components that

are present are used to form protein (efficiency of synthesis). Efficiency of synthesis generally is well-maintained, and changes in cardiac mass are accounted for by modifications in the capacity of the pathway. It should be noted that cellular components with short half-lives are particularly susceptible to derangements in protein synthesis or degradation. In hypoxic muscle, for example, degradation of mitochondria is accelerated; restoration of normal oxidative capacity is dependent upon rapid resynthesis of these organelles when normoxia is restored.

Gene expression also is under hormonal and metabolic control in heart muscle. Perhaps the best example of these changes occurs in relation to the isozymes of myosin.[7] The Ca^{2+}- and actin-activated splitting of ATP by one isozyme is faster than with the other. Speed of contraction in muscle correlates closely with myosin ATPase activity. Expression of the gene for the isozyme with high as compared with low ATPase activity is dependent upon the presence of physiological levels of thyroid and adrenocortical hormones and upon development of normal levels of ventricular pressure. For example, Ca^{2+}-activated myosin ATPase and speed of contraction are reduced in hypertrophied or hypothyroid hearts. However, the mechanisms that control expression of myosin genes are not understood.

General Mechanisms of Metabolic Control

Regulation of flux through a metabolic pathway occurs by four major mechanisms: (1) changes in levels of enzymes in the pathway, (2) changes in substrate availability, (3) allosteric control of key enzymes, and (4) covalent modification of enzymes.

Regulation Dependent upon Enzyme Levels

This type of regulation involves changes in the rate of synthesis and/or degradation of the enzyme and generally occurs after exposure for a few hours to several days to altered substrate or hormone availability or work load.[2] As noted above, however, levels of enzymes with short half-lives can change rapidly. For example, the synthesis of ornithine decarboxylase, an enzyme associated with rapid formation of polyamines in hypertrophying hearts, increases within a few hours following imposition of increased afterload or induction of hyperthyroidism. In addition, availability of substrates or other substances that bind to the substrate site of an enzyme can decrease degradation and lead to increased tissue levels. An example of this type of regulation is provided by another enzyme in the synthetic pathway for polyamines, *S*-adenosylmethionine decarboxylase. In this case, a substrate analogue, methylglyoxal-bis(guanylhydrazone) (MGBG) binds to the substrate site, inhibits degradation, and leads to a 10-fold increase in tissue levels of the protein after 24 h.

Regulation Dependent upon Substrate Availability

If a substrate is present at concentrations below that required for saturation of the pathway, substrate concentration can influence the rate of its utilization. For example, relative rates of glucose and fatty acid utilization depend to a large extent on the plasma concentrations of fatty acids. Fatty acid oxidation is increased when the plasma concentration is elevated above the usual physiological level and inhibition of glucose utilization occurs. On the other hand, rates of glucose utilization depend more upon availability of insulin and fatty acids and the levels of ventricular pressure development than upon the plasma levels of carbohydrate.

Regulation Dependent upon Allosteric Modification of the Enzyme

Various metabolites may bind to a site on an enzyme other than the substrate site and either increase or decrease the catalytic activity.[3,4] The rate of several glycolytic enzymes, including phosphofructokinase and phosphorylase *b* (Fig. 5-2), is controlled, at least in part, by this mechanism. Tissue levels of metabolites that increase in hypoxic muscle, including inorganic phosphate, 5'-AMP, ADP, and fructose-1,6-diphosphate, enhance catalytic activities of these enzymes, while metabolites that are present in high amount in well-oxygenated muscle inhibit catalytic activity. The rate that is expressed in vivo depends on the relative amounts of activators and inhibitors. This type of regulation is rapid and accounts for much of the fine control of metabolism.

Regulation Dependent upon Covalent Modification

The activities of several glycolytic enzymes, as well as other enzymes that are involved in amino acid metabolism and protein synthesis, are regulated by a phosphorylation-dephosphorylation mechanism.[3,4,8] Several of the enzymes are phosphorylated by the cyclic AMP–dependent protein kinase, but protein kinases that are regulated by Ca^{2+} and metabolic intermediates are involved in many cases (Fig. 5-3). Activation of glycogen phosphorylase is mediated by phosphorylase kinase, but this kinase is, in turn, activated by the cyclic AMP–dependent protein kinase. On the other hand, cyclic AMP has not been demonstrated to influence the activity of pyruvate dehydrogenase, either directly or indirectly. Phosphorylation may either increase the catalytic activity (phosphorylase, phosphorylase kinase, or phosphofructokinase) or inhibit the enzyme (glycogen synthase and pyruvate dehydrogenase). Although covalent modification is involved, the phosphorylation-dephosphorylation reactions are rapid and account for changes in catalytic activity over periods of seconds to minutes.

Regulation of the Glycolytic Pathway

Utilization of glucose and glycogen by heart muscle is regulated at a number of steps in the conversion of these substrates to acetyl CoA or lactate,[3,4] the final products of the pathway (Fig. 5-4). The activities of glucose transport, phosphofructokinase, glyceraldehyde-3-phosphate dehydrogenase, pyruvate dehydrogenase, glycogen synthase, and glycogen phosphorylase have been identified as regulatory sites that are affected by factors such as insulin, epinephrine, cardiac work, ischemia, availability of fatty acids, and diabetes.

Effector	Change in concentration in hypoxic heart	Effect on catalytic activity	
		Phosphofructokinase	Phosphorylase b
Inorganic phosphate	↑	↑	↑
5' - AMP	↑	↑	↑
ADP	↑	↑	↔
ATP	↓	↓	↓
Glucose - 6 - P	↓	↔	↓
Fructose - I, 6 - P	↑	↑	↔
Citrate	↓	↓	↔

FIGURE 5-2 Factors accounting for allosteric activation of phosphofructokinase and phosphorylase *b* in hypoxic heart.

Enzyme	Protein kinase	Effect of phosphorylation on catalytic activity
Glycogen phosphorylase	Phosphorylase kinase	↑
Phosphorylase kinase	Cyclic AMP - dependent protein kinase	↑
Glycogen synthase	Cyclic AMP - dependent protein kinase	↓
Phosphofructokinase	Cyclic AMP - dependent protein kinase	↑
Pyruvate dehydrogenase	Pyruvate dehydrogenase kinase	↓

FIGURE 5-3 Effect of covalent modification on the activities of glycolytic enzymes.

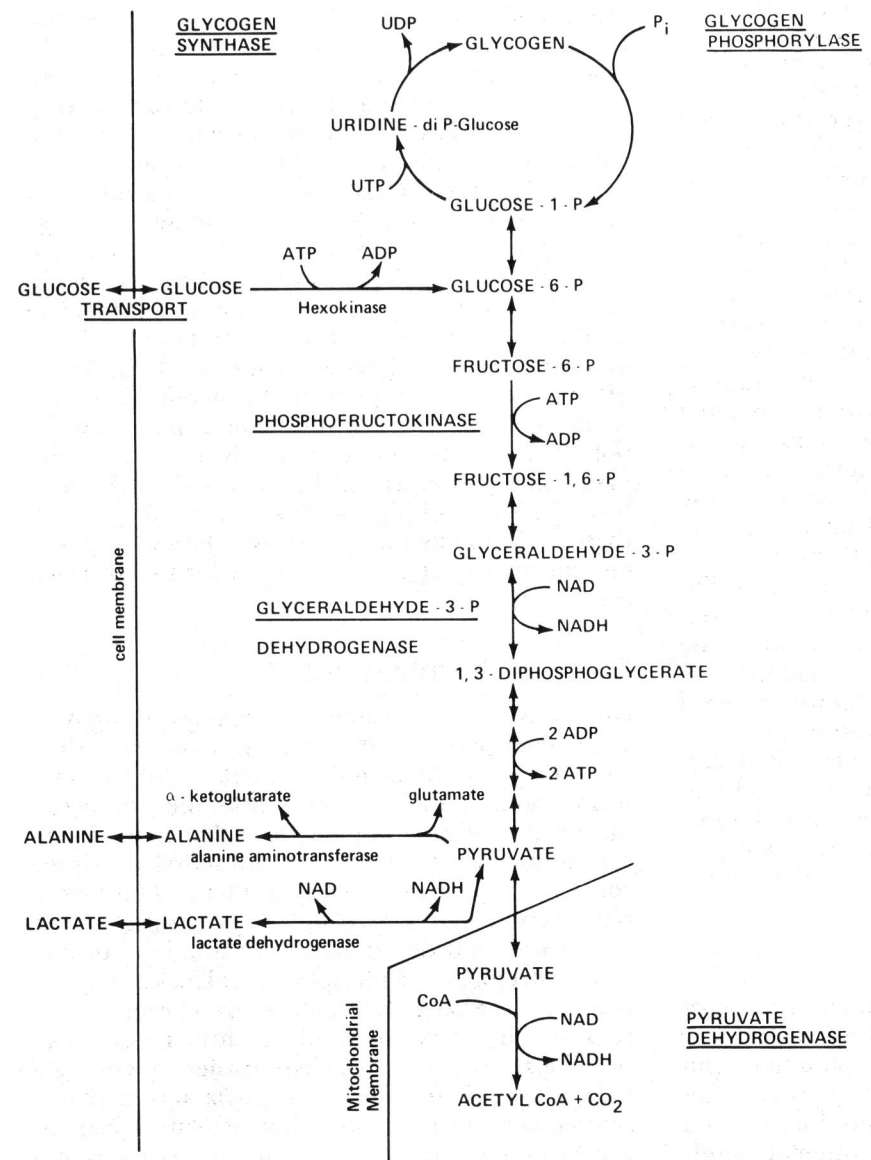

FIGURE 5-4 Simplified pathway of glucose and glycogen metabolism in heart and sites of metabolic regulation.

Glucose Transport

Glucose movement across the cell membrane of heart muscle involves carrier-mediated transport of sugar down a concentration gradient and, as such, may only equilibrate intracellular and extracellular glucose concentrations (Fig. 5-4). The transport system shows saturation kinetics, stereospecificity, and competition between different sugars, suggesting that binding of sugar to a membrane component involves a limited number of binding sites which behave in a manner similar to substrate binding to an enzyme.[3,4] Binding of insulin or an increase in ventricular pressure development somehow alters the rate of movement of glucose across the membrane. In the absence of insulin, the rate of transport is slow, intracellular glucose concentrations are low, and transport represents the major restriction to glucose utilization. When insulin is present, transport is accelerated and intracellular glucose concentrations approach the extracellular value. In these circumstances, intracellular phosphorylation of sugar restricts the overall rate of utilization. In the diabetic heart, transport is less sensitive to stimulation by insulin; for example, a given concentration of insulin within the physiological range results in less acceleration of transport in diabetic as compared with normal hearts. Transport is inhibited in normal hearts by oxidation of fatty acids, and the decreased sensitivity to insulin in diabetic hearts has been associated with increased plasma and tissue levels of fatty acid. Hypophysectomy of diabetic animals restores insulin sensitivity perhaps because there is less mobilization of fatty acid from adipose tissue. Inhibition of fatty acid oxidation in isolated hearts restores insulin sensitivity toward normal. Increased cardiac work accelerates transport both in the presence and absence of insulin, but not in the presence of high concentrations of fatty acid. The mechanism of this work effect is not known.

In addition to increased cardiac work and insulin, hypoxia accelerates glucose transport in hearts from normal animals. In addition, hypoxia renders the transport system more sensitive to stimulation by insulin. In hearts of diabetic animals, however, there is less acceleration of transport as a result of hypoxia or increased cardiac work. These observations suggest that hypoxia, increased cardiac work, and oxidation of fatty acids exert control on glucose transport principally by altering insulin sensitivity rather than through direct effects on the carrier system.

Glycogen Metabolism

Glycogen synthesis and degradation occur by separate pathways (Fig. 5-4). Synthesis involves transfer of the glucose moiety from uridine diphosphate glucose to glycogen and is catalyzed by glycogen synthase. Glycogen synthase occurs in two forms, a and b. Conversion of one form to the other depends upon a phosphorylation-dephosphorylation mech-

anism.[3,4,8] The a, or active, form is dephosphorylated (Fig. 5-3). Synthase a is converted to the b form by phosphorylation that is catalyzed by a cyclic AMP–dependent protein kinase. The activities of both forms are increased by glucose-6-phosphate, but the activity of the b form is completely dependent upon this allosteric effector.

Phosphorylase catalyzes the transfer of a glucose residue from glycogen to glucose-1-phosphate. Phorphorylase also occurs in two forms, a and b. The a form is the phosphorylated form of the enzyme and is active in the absence of AMP (Fig. 5-3). Activity of the b form is dependent upon AMP for activity, and the activity is inhibited by ATP and glucose-6-phosphate (Fig. 5-2). Conversion of phosphorylase b to phosphorylase a is catalyzed by phosphorylase kinase, an enzyme whose activity also is controlled by phosphorylation-dephosphorylation (Fig. 5-3).

Turnover of glycogen is regulated both by hormonal and nonhormonal factors. Epinephrine and glucagon activate adenylate cyclase, increase cyclic AMP levels, and result in conversion of phosphorylase to the a form and synthase to the b form.[8] Glycogen breakdown ensues. Insulin increases the fraction of synthase in the a form and raises glycogen levels. Hypoxia also results in b-to-a conversion and, in addition, activates the b form by a decrease in ATP and in increase in 5′-AMP and P_i concentrations. Glycogenolysis is rapid under these conditions. Myocardial glycogen metabolism differs from that of skeletal muscle in that starvation and diabetes increase the glycogen concentration. These effects appear to depend upon increased plasma levels of free fatty acids and ketone bodies. Oxidation of these substrates increase tissue levels of glucose-6-phosphate, as will be discussed in the next section. Glucose-6-phosphate activates glycogen synthase and inhibits phosphorylase; these changes in enzyme activity appear to account for the glycogen accumulation.

Glucose Phosphorylation

Glucose is phosphorylated by hexokinase using ATP as the energy donor.[3,4] The enzyme occurs both in soluble (30 percent) and particulate (70 percent) forms; both forms are inhibited by the product of the reaction, glucose-6-phosphate. The major factor regulating the rate of glucose phosphorylation is the concentration of glucose-6-phosphate. The principal reaction that controls glycolysis and glycogen metabolism and determines the tissue level of glucose-6-phosphate is phosphofructokinase. The activity of this enzyme is regulated by allosteric effectors and by covalent modification. In general, situations that lead to decreased tissue levels of high-energy phosphates, such as hypoxia and increased cardiac work, increase phosphofructokinase activity, while conditions that increase energy levels and provide alternative oxidative substrates, such as diabetes and elevated plasma levels of fatty acid, decrease activity. These inhibitory effects appear to be mediated both by higher energy levels and accumulation of citrate, a product of fatty acid oxidation. Intracellular pH also appears to have a large effect on phosphofructokinase activity. As pH decreases from 7.3 to 6.9, enzyme activity falls, and control by allosteric effectors is much more marked. In contrast to regulation of phosphofructokinase activity by allosteric effectors, the physiological role of covalent modification is not understood at present.

Activation of phosphofructokinase leads to accumulation of fructose-1,6-diphosphate, and a shift in the rate-limiting step of glycolysis to glyceraldehyde-3-phosphate dehydrogenase in hearts that are perfused under anoxic or ischemic conditions and in aerobic hearts at very high levels of cardiac work. Factors that restrict activity of the dehydrogenase include accumulation of NADH, H^+, and lactate. Because high levels of these intermediates accumulate during ischemia, glycolysis may be blocked at the dehydrogenase step. In these cases, increased cytosolic NADH appears to be most important in restricting the rate.

Pyruvate Metabolism

Pyruvate that is formed by glycolysis can be released from the heart as lactate or alanine or can be oxidized within the mitochondria to acetyl CoA and CO_2 (Fig. 5-4). Both lactate dehydrogenase and alanine aminotransferase catalyze near-equilibrium reactions that are dependent upon the levels of NAD, NADH, α-ketoglutarate, and glutamate in the cytosol. When NADH and pyruvate levels are increased, such as in hypoxic muscle, production of lactate and alanine are raised. Oxidation of pyruvate to acetyl CoA is an intramitochondrial reaction that is catalyzed by the pyruvate dehydrogenase complex.[3,4] Because of its localization, the complex is in direct competition with β oxidation of fatty acids for CoA and NAD.

Pyruvate dehydrogenase is a complex of five enzymes, three of which are involved with pyruvate metabolism (pyruvate dehydrogenase, dihydroxylipoyltransacetylase and dihydroxylipoyl dehydrogenase). The other two enzymes modify the activity of the pyruvate dehydrogenase component by phosphorylation and dephosphorylation of the enzyme (pyruvate dehydrogenase kinase and pyruvate dehydrogenase phosphatase). Phosphorylation decreases the activity, while dephosphorylation by the phosphatase activates. High NADH/NAD and acetyl CoA/CoA ratios decrease the activity of the complex. This effect is due, in part, to product inhibition (NADH and acetyl CoA are both inhibitors) and to inactivation by phosphorylation. Pyruvate dehydrogenase kinase is activated by acetyl CoA and NADH and is inhibited by CoA and NAD; the active kinase inhibits pyruvate dehydrogenase by phosphorylation.

In hearts from normal animals, approximately 20 percent of pyruvate dehydrogenase is in the active form. Activity is decreased in hearts from diabetic animals, in association with higher tissue levels of acetyl CoA and NADH. This effect of diabetes probably is another example of a secondary alteration in glucose metabolism of the heart that results from increased fatty acid mobilization in the periphery and oxidation of the fatty acid by the heart. Inhibition and inactivation of pyruvate dehydrogenase can be produced in hearts from normal animals by perfusion with fatty acids or ketone bodies; these conditions result in high mitochondrial levels of acetyl CoA and NADH.

Integrated Control of Carbohydrate Metabolism in Heart

Both in vivo and in isolated hearts, fatty substrates are used in preference to glucose and glycogen. In well-oxygenated hearts that are developing normal levels of ventricular pressure, glucose transport is the major restriction to utilization of exogenous glucose, and glycogen breakdown is restrained at the phosphorylase reaction. The rate of transport depends upon the levels of insulin bound to the tissue and the availability of fatty substrates. Glycogen breakdown is restrained because phosphorylase is almost entirely in the *b* form and the activity of this form is inhibited by high levels of ATP and glucose-6-phosphate and low levels of 5'-AMP and P_i. The activity of phosphofructokinase is very low because of high levels of ATP and citrate. Under these circumstances glucose utilization is markedly reduced and most of the substrate that is taken up is diverted to glycogen. The final site at which fatty acid restrains glycolysis is at the pyruvate dehydrogenase reaction. Increased levels of acetyl CoA and NADH, products of the oxidation of fatty acids, inhibit the enzyme and lead to conversion of a larger fraction of the pyruvate that is formed to lactate.

An increase in ATP and O_2 consumption in heart muscle accompanies increased ventricular pressure development, or heart rate, or the presence of inotropic agents, such as epinephrine or glucagon. When plasma fatty acid levels are low, an increase in ventricular pressure development accelerates glucose uptake and oxidation. This effect is accounted for by more rapid rates of glucose transport, glucose phosphorylation, and phosphofructokinase. Activation of phosphofructokinase is accounted for by lower tissue levels of creatine phosphate, ATP, and citrate and higher levels of P_i. In these circumstances, pyruvate dehydrogenase is activated as a result of low NADH/NAD and acetyl CoA/CoA ratios in the mitochondria, and glucose oxidation is rapid. When plasma fatty acid levels are high, the heart preferentially utilizes this substrate because of the inhibition of pyruvate dehydrogenase, phosphofructokinase, phosphorylase, and glucose transport. Pyruvate dehydrogenase is inhibited by higher levels of NADH and acetyl CoA, while phospho-fructokinase is inhibited by elevated levels of citrate and lower concentrations of P_i. Glucose phosphorylation and glycogen breakdown are restrained by higher tissue levels of glucose-6-phosphate that are secondary to inhibition of phosphofructokinase.

The most common causes of decreased ATP production in heart muscle are restriction of oxygen supply by hypoxia (decreased oxygen tension) or ischemia (decreased coronary flow of well-oxygenated blood).[3] Hypoxia results in a 10-fold increase in glucose uptake and a rapid rate of glycogen breakdown. These effects are accounted for by acceleration of glucose transport, hexokinase, phosphorylase, and phosphofructokinase as a result of increased intracellular levels of ADP, AMP, and P_i, and decreased levels of ATP and glucose-6-phosphate. Because of lack of oxygen, conversion of pyruvate to lactate and alanine is rapid. It should be emphasized that the accelerated rate of glycolytic flux in the hypoxic tissue generates only 5 to 7 percent of the ATP that is formed in well-oxygenated hearts. As a result, tissue levels of high-energy phosphates fall. Ventricular failure is rapid in severe hypoxia.

In contrast to the sustained increase in glycolytic flux in hypoxic muscle, ischemia results in only a transient elevation that is followed by inhibition.[3,9] Inhibition occurs despite higher tissue levels of ADP, AMP, and P_i. Inhibition of the glycolytic rate is not overcome by insulin. In this circumstance, the rate-controlling step appears to be glyceraldehyde-3-phosphate dehydrogenase, whose activity is restricted by high levels of NADH, lactate, and H^+. In ischemic muscle, accumulation of lactate and hydrogen ions is more marked than in hypoxic hearts. Intervention to improve glycolytic rate in ischemic hearts should be directed toward accelerating release of lactate, increasing intracellular pH, and providing other hydrogen acceptors for reoxidation of NADH.

Regulation of Fatty Acid Metabolism

The rate of fatty acid uptake and utilization by the heart depends to a large extent on the concentration of fatty acid in the blood, but even more upon the metabolic activity of the myocardium.[10] The fatty acid that is taken up may be used for synthetic purposes, but in the heart it is used primarily for oxidation to produce energy. Cardiac muscle oxidizes fatty acids as the principal fuel for ATP production.

Because the overall rate of fatty acid utilization is determined primarily by the energy demands of the heart, an increased supply in the plasma has a limited ability to accelerate fatty acid uptake. The upper limit is reached when the supply exceeds the capacity of the cells to bind the fatty acids and to convert them to CO_2 and, to a much less extent, to form complex lipids and metabolic intermediates. The control of uptake by the heart will be discussed

for three conditions: (1) increased availability of extracellular fatty acids as a determinant of fatty acid uptake at low levels of cardiac work, (2) increased fatty acid oxidation that results from increased cardiac work, and (3) decreased oxidation that results from restriction of oxygen availability in ischemic muscle.

Fatty Acid Uptake and Activation

Fatty acids are supplied to the heart from the blood, where they are carried either as the free acid, bound to albumin, or as triglycerides in chylomicrons and lipoproteins (Fig. 5-5). The free fatty acid (FFA) is the principal form that is utilized by heart. The triglycerides are hydrolyzed to FFA by lipoprotein lipase prior to their utilization. The majority of plasma FFA is bound to albumin. The amount that is free in solution is small and is determined by the FFA/albumin molar ratio; the portion that is free is less than 1 percent of the total. The unbound pool of FFA is in equilibrium with albumin-bound plasma FFA and a tissue pool of FFA (Fig. 5-5). The exact nature of the tissue pool is not known, but probably is composed of FFA in the cytoplasm and FFA bound to intracellular membranes and soluble proteins. The uptake of FFA by cells does not require energy and functions only to maintain an equilibrium between plasma and cellular pools of FFA. When plasma FFA is raised to about 0.5 mM, uptake increases in proportion. With further elevations in plasma concentration, uptake is not proportional to concentration and finally reaches a plateau. Because the net rate of FFA uptake depends on the concentration gradient across the cell membrane, the rate of uptake is increased when removal of intracellular FFA is increased by raising the rate of oxidation, as with increased ventricular pressure development. Thus, the predominant control of fatty acid uptake in the heart appears to be related to the plasma content of unbound fatty acid, which is determined by diet and hormonal control of fatty acid mobilization from liver and adipose tissue, and the level of intracellular fatty acid, which is determined by the rates of FFA removal by cellular metabolism.

The first step in the cellular metabolism of fatty acids is their conversion to long-chain fatty acyl CoA (FACoA) esters. This process, referred to as *activa-*

FIGURE 5-5 Fatty acid uptake and activation.

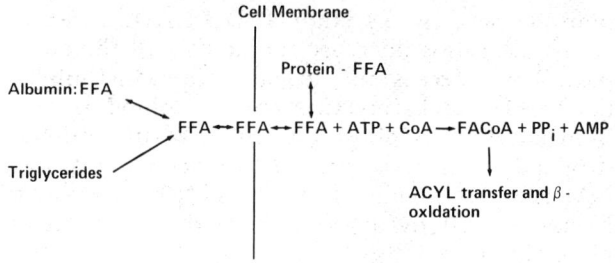

tion, is catalyzed by long-chain acyl CoA synthases (Fig. 5-5). In heart muscle, these enzymes are located on the outer mitochondrial membrane. Fatty acyl CoA is relatively insoluble in water and is bound to cellular proteins and lipid membranes. The activities of the synthases are inhibited by all three of their products and are restrained by the low concentration of CoA in the cytosol. As a result, fatty acid activation is controlled by the FACoA/CoA and ATP/AMP ratios.

Mitochondrial Transport of Fatty Acyl Residues and β Oxidation

After FACoA is formed, it can be used either for synthesis of complex lipids in the cytosol or for oxidation in the mitochondria. Prior to mitochondrial oxidation, the fatty acyl moiety undergoes reactions that function to move the acyl group from the site of activation on the outer mitochondrial membrane to the mitochondrial matrix, where it is oxidized (Fig. 5-6). First, the acyl group is transferred from CoA to carnitine, and second, it is transported across the inner mitochondrial membrane. Transport of acylcarnitine involves an exchange reaction in which acylcarnitine moves across the mitochondrial membrane in exchange for free carnitine and is independent of metabolic energy. The third reaction in this segment is the transfer of the acyl group from carnitine to matrix CoA and forms FACoA in the matrix that is used for β oxidation. In hearts that are developing low levels of ventricular pressure and are perfused with a range of palmitate concentrations in the buffer, the ratios of FACoA/CoA and fatty acylcarnitine/carnitine vary over a wide range, but a linear relationship exists between the fractions of CoA and carnitine in the fatty acyl forms, suggesting that the transfer and transport systems are in equilibrium in the intact cell. With higher levels of pressure development and more rapid oxidation, however, the tissue level of fatty acylcarnitine (FACarn) increases while that of FACoA decreases. This observation suggests that, with rapid rates of oxidation, β oxidation removes

mitochondrial FACoA faster than either acylcarnitine transport or the transferase in the inner mitochondrial membrane can replenish the supply. If β oxidation is inhibited, as occurs in ischemic hearts, most of the total CoA and carnitine are converted to their long-chain acyl derivatives within 5 min. Under ischemic conditions, the increase in FACoA/CoA is linearly related to the rises in FACarnitine/carnitine, again indicating that the system of transferases, as a whole, remained in equilibrium. Therefore, changes in the rates of these reactions on a short-term basis are most likely brought about by increased levels of substrates and/or faster rates of product removal. On a longer time scale, the activities of the enzymes that are involved in these reactions may be increased by synthesis of more enzyme, as has been demonstrated in exercising skeletal muscle.[11]

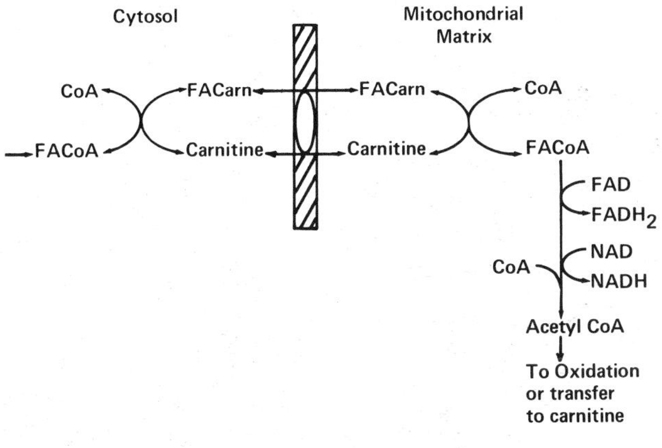

After production of FACoA in the matrix, the next major sequence of reactions involved in the oxidation of fatty acids is the β-oxidation system that leads to production of acetyl CoA (Fig. 5-6). The most likely means of controlling these reactions is through the availability of one or more of the substrates: FACoA, CoA, NAD, or FAD. For example, acceleration of β oxidation that results from increased work in cardiac muscle is associated with a decrease in the acetyl CoA/FACoA and NADH/NAD ratios. In ischemic hearts, levels of acetyl CoA decrease and levels of FACoA increase, indicating that β oxidation is inhibited in association with a large increase in the NADH/NAD ratios. These observations indicate that the rate of β oxidation depends on rates of oxidation of NADH and $FADH_2$ by electron transport and of acetyl CoA by the citric acid cycle.

In heart muscle, acetyl CoA that is produced by β oxidation is used at appreciable rates only for oxidation by the citric acid cycle. The only alternative route for disposal of mitochondrial acetyl CoA is to transfer the acetyl unit across the mitochondrial membrane to cytosolic carnitine, where it is stored as acetylcarnitine. The acetyl transferase system has a very high activity in cardiac muscle, but the purpose of storing acetylcarnitine is not clear. Because there is about 10 times as much carnitine as CoA in the heart, storage of excess acetyl units as cytosolic acetylcarnitine may provide a buffer against large changes in mitochondrial acetyl CoA and may act as a reservoir of readily available substrate for oxidation.

FIGURE 5-6 Acyl transfer, transport, and oxidation.

Integrated Control of Fatty Acid Metabolism in Heart

The entire pathway of fatty acid oxidation is geared to replenish acetyl CoA, as this intermediate is oxidized in the citric acid cycle. Flux through the citric acid cycle is coupled to the rate of myocardial oxygen consumption through feedback control of the

THE NORMAL HEART AND BLOOD VESSELS

cycle by changes in levels of high-energy phosphates and NADH. When hearts are perfused with high levels of fatty acids at low levels of cardiac work (Fig. 5-7), flux through the citric acid cycle occurs at a constant rate. Under these conditions, the rate of FFA oxidation is limited by the rate of acetyl CoA oxidation, and, as a result, acetyl CoA accumulates. Excess acetyl units that are produced from β oxidation are transferred to the cytosol and stored there as acetyl derivatives of CoA and carnitine. Long-chain acyl derivatives of both CoA and carnitine also accumulate, but to a lesser extent than the acetyl derivatives. As a result of increased levels of acetyl and long-chain derivatives of CoA and carnitine, the levels of free CoA and carnitine decrease and limit activation and transfer of acyl units. Higher tissue levels of FFA result.

When cardiac work is accelerated and the rate of substrate oxidation increases, flux through the citric acid cycle is faster and levels of acetyl CoA and acetylcarnitine are diminished rapidly (Fig. 5-8); β oxidation is stimulated and levels of long-chain acyl CoA decrease. Simultaneously, levels of free CoA and free carnitine increase, the rate of FFA activation accelerates, and FFA uptake increases in association with decreased cellular levels of fatty acids. Under these conditions, the slowest step for fatty acid utilization appears to be the capacity of the cells to transport acyl units across the inner mitochondrial membrane. The rise in FACarn most likely occurs in the cytosol, and this increase probably accounts for faster rates of transport into the mitochondria because of a higher cytosolic-to-matrix gradient.

Under oxygen-deficient conditions, i.e., ischemia and hypoxia, the amount of oxygen that is available to support oxidation by the citric acid cycle is reduced. Levels of $FADH_2$ and NADH increase, and β oxidation is inhibited. Long-chain acyl derivatives of CoA and carnitine increase to very high levels (Fig. 5-9), and activation and uptake of FFA is reduced. High levels of fatty acyl CoA inhibit enzymes in both a specific and nonspecific manner.[12] Free fatty acids and long-chain acylcarnitine have a detergent effect at high concentrations and inhibit Na-K-ATPase.[13,14] Therefore, in addition to reducing capacity for ATP synthesis, myocardial ischemia also results in accumulation of compounds that potentially are detrimental to myocardial function and metabolism.

As mentioned above, the heart of a diabetic animal oxidizes almost entirely fatty acids and ketone bodies for energy production. Alterations of fatty acid metabolism in the diabetic heart include increased tissue levels of long-chain acyl CoA and acylcarnitine esters, increased rates of esterification to complex lipids, and higher tissue levels of triglycerides. The increased acyl CoA and acylcarnitine esters result, at least in part, from a greater supply of plasma fatty acids. But, in addition to increased fatty acid supply, the tissue content of total CoA increases by 40 to 50 percent. Insulin is a strong inhibitor of CoA synthesis; and in the diabetic animal, increased synthesis of CoA probably results from insulin deficiency. This increase in total CoA may also contribute to the higher levels of long-chain acyl CoA and, because of the equilibrium position of the transferase enzymes, to higher acylcarnitine. The high levels of acyl CoA could account for increased triglycerides as a result of a mass action effect on triglyceride synthesis and an inhibition of triglyceride lipase.

FIGURE 5-7 Pathway for fatty acid oxidation in heart muscle. Metabolic intermediates that are elevated when hearts are perfused with 1.2 mM fatty acid at 60 mmHg ventricular pressure development are shown in boldface. This figure illustrates the two transferase systems for acyl units, each located on the inner and outer surfaces of the inner mitochondrial membrane. It includes compartmentation of CoA in two nonexchangeable pools (cytosolic and mitochondrial matrix); carnitine translocase is shown on the inner mitochondrial membrane between the two transferase systems. At low rates of energy utilization and excess fatty acid supply, most of the CoA and carnitine are converted to their acetyl derivatives. (See text for additional discussion.) (*From Idell-Wenger and Neely.*[10] *Reproduced with permission.*)

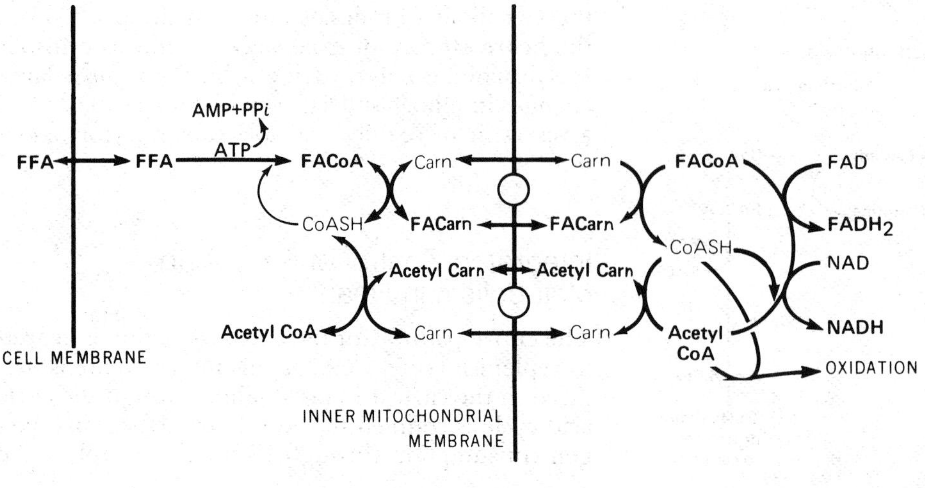

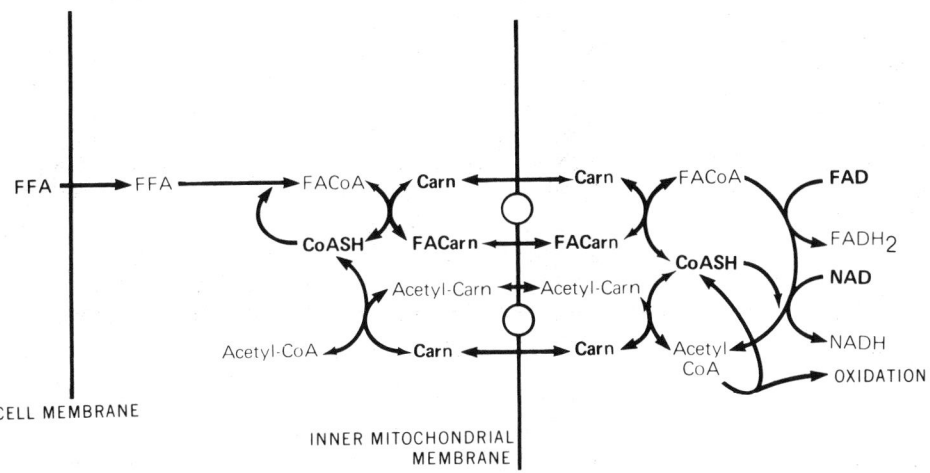

FIGURE 5-8 Pathway for fatty acid oxidation in which metabolic intermediates that are elevated when hearts are perfused with 1.2 mM fatty acid at 120 mmHg ventricular pressure are shown in heavier print. Levels of FACarn increased, but it is uncertain if the increase occurs in both cellular compartments. Most, if not all, of the increase was restricted to the cytosolic compartment. (See text for additional discussion.) (*From Idell-Wenger and Neely.*[10] *Reproduced with permission.*)

Regulation of Protein Turnover

Disorders of ventricular function, high-energy phosphate formation, and substrate oxidation may result from inhibition of synthesis or accelerated degradation of specific heart proteins. Hypertrophy and reduction in cardiac mass depend upon changes in the relative rates of synthesis and degradation of all heart proteins. As mentioned earlier in this chapter, turnover of heart proteins is a dynamic process that results in rapid replacement of proteins. The $t_{\frac{1}{2}}$ for turnover of cardiac myosin is 5 to 6 days. Protein turnover in the heart is affected by availability of hormones, oxidative substrates, and oxygen. Decreased availability of these factors may perturb protein balance of the heart.

Regulation of Protein Synthesis

The pathway of protein synthesis is shown in Fig. 5-10.[2] Transport of amino acids into the intracel-

lular pool is considered to be the first step in protein synthesis. On the other hand, extracellular availability of amino acids does not appear to restrain protein synthesis in the heart when normal plasma levels of amino acids are present. At least six transport systems for various classes of amino acids are present in most cell types:

1. The A system transports alanine, glycine, and other neutral amino acids with short side chains. It is Na^+-dependent and transports amino acids against a concentration gradient.
2. The L system is leucine-preferring, is not Na^+-dependent, and has highest affinity for neutral amino acids with branched-chain or aromatic rings.
3. The ASCP system transports alanine, serine, cysteine, and proline and is Na^+-dependent.
4. Basic amino acids, such as lysine, arginine, and ornithine, are transported by the lysine system.
5. Acidic amino acids, such as glutamic and aspartic

FIGURE 5-9 Pathway for fatty acid oxidation illustrating metabolic intermediates that are elevated during ischemia in hearts perfused with 1.2 mM fatty acid. (See text for additional discussion.) (*From Idell-Wenger and Neely.*[10] *Reproduced with permission.*)

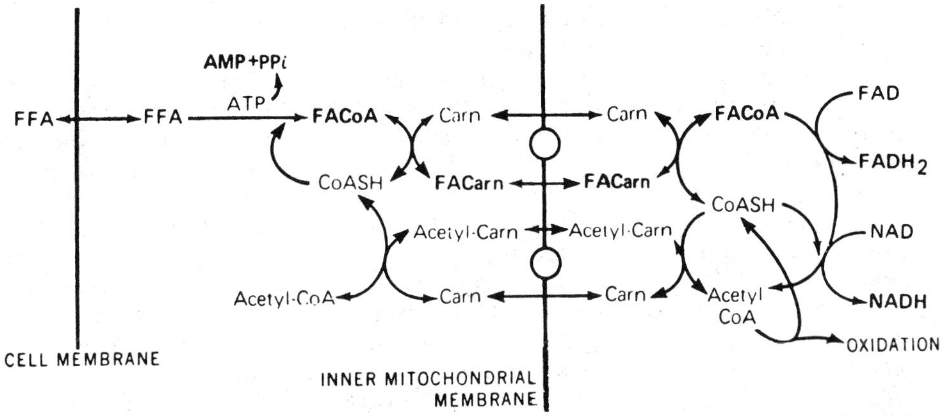

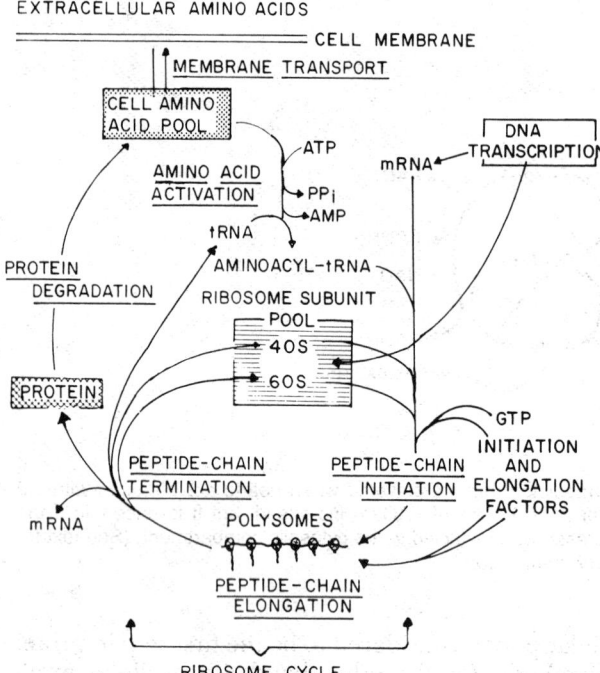

FIGURE 5-10 Pathway of protein turnover. Amino acids are supplied to the intracellular pool by either membrane transport or protein degradation. Intracellular amino acids are activated to form aminoacyl derivatives by combination with transfer RNA (tRNA). Polymerization of activated amino acids into protein is catalyzed by a series of ribosome-catalyzed reactions that make up the ribosome cycle. These reactions include initiation of peptide chains on the ribosomes and elongation and termination of chains. Peptide-chain initiation refers to binding of messenger RNA (mRNA) and initiator tRNA (methionyl tRNA$_f$) to the small ribosomal subunit (40 S), followed by the binding of the large subunit (60 S). Both steps require GTP and initiation factors. Peptide-chain elongation refers to successive addition of activated amino acids as determined by the code contained within mRNA. This process is dependent on elongation factors. When the protein is complete, the peptide chain and ribosomal subunits are released into the cytoplasm. Protein degradation refers to reactions catalyzed by proteases and results in the release of free amino acids into the intracellular pool. (See text for additional discussion.) (*From Morgan, Rannels, and McKee.*[2] *Reproduced with permission.*)

acids, are transported by the dicarboxylate carrier.

6. The β system is a low-affinity system that transports β-alanine and taurine.

The contents of amino acids within the intracellular pool are determined by (1) the rate of entry from the extracellular space, (2) the rate of exit from the cell, (3) rates of formation or destruction of the compound by transamination, oxidation, or other metabolic processes; and (4) rates of protein synthesis and degradation. As a result, intracellular levels of amino acids may fall even though protein synthesis is accelerated. These findings, in addition to the observation that 90 percent of the tRNA is in the aminoacyl form, indicates that steps that occur later in the protein synthetic pathway, such as peptide-chain initiation and elongation, are rate-limiting for protein synthesis in vivo.

The heart contains a pool of ribosomes that is present either as subunits or polysomes. These particles cycle from the subunit pool into polysomes through the peptide-chain initiation reactions. Initiation consists of the binding of mRNA, an initiator tRNA, and 40- and 60-S subunits, and is followed by translation of the mRNA to form a protein. Initiation of peptide chains in the heart is controlled by insulin, epinephrine, glucagon, and the availability of amino acids, fatty substrates, and oxygen. As a result of the breadth of factors that regulate initiation, these reactions remain sufficiently rapid to keep most of the ribosomal subunits in polysomes and to shift the rate-limiting step to elongation and termination of peptide chains. These reactions are limited by the supply of ribosomes, elongation factors, aminoacyl tRNA, and guanosine triphosphate (GTP). In anoxic or ischemic hearts, high-energy phosphate reserves are depleted, including the GTP levels, and rates of protein synthesis are inhibited at the level of these ribosome-catalyzed reactions.

Regulation of Protein Degradation

The exact pathway by which proteins are degraded to free amino acids is not known, but lysosomes appear to be involved.[2] These organelles contain a number of hydrolytic enzymes, including acid proteases that are capable of degrading protein to free amino acids. Wildenthal et al. demonstrated that chloroquine, a drug that is sequestered by lysosomes and inhibits their function, lowers the rate of proteolysis in fetal mouse hearts.[15] Lysosomal proteases have pH optima that are in the range of 2 to 4, a value much lower than the overall intracellular pH. One mechanism of the energy requirement of protein degradation appears to involve maintenance of low intralysosomal pH. Lysosomes often appear in the perinuclear region of myocardial cells and in the rows of mitochondria.

Changes in the total activity of lysosomal enzymes and the morphology of cardiac lysosomes are found to accompany a number of physiological and pathological changes in the heart.[16] The total activity of cathepsin D, a lysosomal protease, changes during thyrotoxic cardiac hypertrophy and its regression.[17] These findings suggest that changes in the lysosomal system are linked to physiological events that modify protein turnover.

In addition to acid proteases, proteolytic enzymes that have pH optima in the neutral and alkaline range are present in the heart. These enzymes include a soluble Ca^{2+}-activated protease that removes Z lines from myofibrils and particulate proteases that degrade protein to free amino acids. The physiological role of these particulate proteases is in doubt, however, because much of the activity appears to be localized in a nonmuscle cell, the mast cell. This finding illustrates one of the difficulties in defining the proteolytic pathway, namely, the presence within the heart of a variety of cell types, including fibroblasts, endothelial cells, mast cells, and phagocytic cells. Some of these cells are rich in proteolytic enzymes, but these proteases may play little or no role in normal protein turnover.

The energy requirement for proteolysis may involve not only maintenance of intralysosomal pH, but other steps in the proteolytic pathway. These steps include internalization of cytoplasmic components in lysosomes and an ATP-dependent proteolytic system in the cytosol.[18] The latter system has been investigated, particularly in reticulocytes, where it is active in the hydrolysis of abnormal proteins, for example, those that contain amino acid analogues. The energy requirement appears to involve initial steps in the proteolytic pathway because factors that reduce levels of high-energy phosphates, such as anoxia and ischemia, prevent the loss of activity of a specific enzyme, S-adenosylmethionine decarboxylase, and do not lead to the accumulation of the products of proteolysis, peptides and free amino acids, within the heart. In regard to effects of reduced oxygen delivery on protein degradation in the heart, it is important that the initial step in the pathway be blocked. Otherwise, proteolysis would proceed and result in inactivation of enzymes and contractile proteins and would contribute to irreversible damage in ischemic myocardium.

Factors other than activity or availability of proteases affect rates of protein degradation. Susceptibility of individual proteins to proteolytic attack is correlated with molecular weight, isoelectric point, and conformational state. In general, large proteins are degraded more rapidly than smaller ones; more acidic proteins have shorter half-lives; and alteration of conformation by cofactor or substrate binding decreases the degradative rate.

Integrated Control of Protein Metabolism in Heart

A wide range of factors affect either protein synthesis or degradation in heart muscle. These include (1) availability of amino acids, and particularly leucine, (2) supply of oxidative substrates, (3) availability of hormones, (4) adequacy of oxygen delivery, and (5) the level of ventricular pressure development. Many of these factors have opposite effects on the synthetic as compared with the degradative pathway; for example, insulin accelerates synthesis and inhibits degradation. These combined changes result in a marked reduction in net amino acid release.

Over long periods of time, protein synthesis depends on the availability of free amino acids in the plasma. Over short time intervals, however, the content of amino acids in the heart is usually well beyond what is required to saturate the synthetic pathway. Leucine appears to play a unique role in accelerating synthesis and inhibiting degradation. Plasma concentrations of leucine are increased during fasting and in diabetic animals and contribute

to maintenance of cardiac mass in these insulinopenic states. The leucine effect may involve a direct effect of the amino acid on enzymes in the pathway or may result indirectly through its oxidation.

Both protein synthesis and degradation are energy-requiring processes, and, as a result, oxidizable substrate must be supplied to maintain energy levels for both processes. Glucose can serve as a satisfactory substrate for ATP synthesis but is unable to support control rates of protein synthesis or degradation. On the other hand, fatty acids and other similar substrates are able to both support energy generation and maintain equal rates of protein synthesis and degradation and nitrogen balance. Effects of these substrates appear to be important in insulin-deficient states, such as diabetes, in which plasma levels of fatty acids and ketone bodies are elevated.

For nearly 50 years, insulin has been recognized as an important factor that affects nitrogen balance in heart and many other tissues. Early studies attributed the effects of insulin on protein synthesis to an accelerated rate of amino acid transport and increased formation of aminoacyl tRNA. Further investigation revealed, however, that the major effect of the hormone is to sustain optimal rates of peptide-chain initiation and, as a result, to keep the pool of ribosomes in the form of polysomes that are active in synthesizing protein. In addition, insulin inhibits protein degradation and prevents formation of autophagic vacuoles from primary lysosomes. In the presence of physiological levels of the hormone, rates of synthesis and degradation are equal and the heart is in nitrogen balance.

Hypertrophy that results from increased ventricular pressure development results from greater efficiency and capacity of the synthetic pathway. As shown in Table 5-1, Langendorff preparations that develop peak systolic pressures of about 70 mmHg have a rate of protein degradation that is about 40 percent faster than the rate of synthesis. In working hearts that are developing peak systolic pressures of about 145 mmHg, synthesis is increased 40 percent while rates of degradation are unchanged. The more rapid rates of synthesis indicate improved efficiency. A more important factor accounting for growth of the heart is increased concentration of RNA within the heart. RNA levels are elevated within 1 to 3 days after imposition of a high work load, and increased capacity for synthesis is a major factor leading to increased cardiac mass. Whether the increase in RNA concentration is due to faster synthesis and processing of precursor forms of RNA or to reduced RNA degradation is unresolved. After the phase of rapid growth is over, RNA concentrations return to their original value.

As described above, both protein synthesis and degradation are energy-requiring processes and are inhibited in tissues that are depleted of ATP and other high-energy compounds. After 1 h of ischemia (Table 5-1), rates of both synthesis and deg-

TABLE 5-1 Effects of Increased Ventricular Pressure Development, Myocardial Ischemia, and Diabetes on Protein Turnover*

Conditions of Perfusion and Animal	Langendorff Preparation		Working Heart	
	Protein Synthesis	Protein Degradation	Protein Synthesis	Protein Degradation
Aerobic perfusion, control	683 ± 40	1012 ± 37	954 ± 25	1022 ± 58
Ischemic perfusion			220 ± 5	214 ± 63
Aerobic perfusion, diabetic	483 ± 21	1093 ± 37	636 ± 22	1304 ± 64

*Rat hearts were perfused in vitro as Langendorff ischemic or working preparations with buffer that simulated the substrate and hormone levels of normal plasma.[19,20] Synthesis was measured by following incorporation of ^{14}C-phenylalanine into protein, and degradation was assessed by measuring release of phenylalanine. Rates are expressed as nanomoles of phenylalanine per gram of dry heart per hour.

radation are inhibited about 80 percent; but these rates are equal, indicating that loss of rapidly turning over proteins will be no greater in ischemic than in well-oxygenated tissue.

In hearts of diabetic animals, rates of protein synthesis are lower than in control aerobic hearts (Table 5-1). This reduction is present in both Langendorff preparations and working hearts and is due to reduced capacity (decreased RNA) for synthesis. The negative nitrogen balance of the diabetic heart is intensified by an increase in the rate of proteolysis in the working preparation. Furthermore, high levels of insulin are unable to normalize rates of protein synthesis in diabetic hearts. These findings indicate the precarious nature of the balance that maintains heart size in severely diabetic animals.

Relationship of Metabolic Disorders to Myocardial Function

The ability of the heart to utilize a variety of carbon substrates helps to ensure a constant supply of ATP to support mechanical function even under adverse conditions of substrate supply. In addition, a disorder in one pathway is less likely to limit ATP production because the heart simply uses another substrate. The switch in metabolism of hearts in diabetic animals, as discussed above, is an example of the benefits derived from diverse metabolic capacities. The central role of oxygen and the complete dependence of the heart on oxidative production of ATP, however, makes this tissue particularly susceptible to decreased oxygen supply. Thus, hypoxia or ischemia greatly affect mechanical function. Other examples of metabolic disorders that affect mechanical activity are the alterations of protein metabolism that develop in different thyroid states. These two conditions, i.e., decreased oxygen supply and altered protein metabolism, will be discussed below.

Myocardial Ischemia

Cardiac muscle has the highest rate of oxygen consumption and the largest fractional extraction of arterial oxygen of any tissue in the body.[3,4] The ex-

traction of oxygen is about 70 percent compared with less than 10 percent for carbon substrates. Therefore, oxygen is the first substrate whose supply becomes limited when coronary flow is reduced. The small fractional extraction of carbon substrates coupled with decreased utilization of these substrates during ischemia (see above) suggests that their supply would never limit ATP production. Although the primary metabolic disorder of ischemic tissue is a subnormal oxygen supply, the metabolism and function of the heart is disrupted at all levels. The reduced oxygen supply results in a cascade of events that eventually affect every metabolic and functional process of the heart. In addition to reduced ATP production, slow flux through electron transport causes an accumulation of NADH in both the mitochondrial and cytosolic compartments. In the mitochondria, increased NADH inhibits the citric acid cycle, pyruvate oxidation, and β oxidation of fatty acids. The slowed rate of β oxidation results in accumulation of FACoA and FACarn (Fig. 5-9), and potential detrimental effects of these naturally occurring detergents are discussed above. In the cytosol, elevated NADH causes increased lactate production and inhibits anaerobic production of ATP by glycolysis. The lower oxidative neutralization of H^+ also results in decreased cellular pH, which affects a number of enzymes and cellular functions.

Perhaps the most significant secondary consequence of reduced oxidative metabolism is the net loss of adenine nucleotides from the total pool of ATP, ADP, and AMP. ATP is hydrolyzed to ADP, which cannot be rephosphorylated by either oxidative phosphorylation or glycolysis. Tissue levels of AMP increase because adenylate kinase converts 2ADP to ATP and AMP. Associated with this increase in AMP, production of its degradation products (adenosine, inosine, and hypoxanthine) is accelerated. In contrast to the phosphorylated nucleotides, these dephosphorylated degradation products can penetrate cell membranes and are lost from the cells. The removal of nucleotide products results in a net loss of the adenine nucleotides. Mechanical function of the heart depends on an adequate supply of ATP, and the loss of nucleotides is associated with onset of irreversible damage to the tissue. Unfortunately, cardiac muscle cannot rapidly restore the nucleotide pool, and tissue levels of ATP remain low with reperfusion of ischemic tissue. Several hours to days are required for restoration of normal ATP levels. Thus, one of the major advances in open heart surgery in recent years has been the use of cardioplegic solutions to preserve ATP levels during exposure of the heart to ischemia.

Cardioplegic solutions vary considerably, depending on the institution, but the most important common ingredient is high $[K^+]$ to achieve cardiac arrest. Maintenance of contractility in the first few seconds of ischemia consumes large amounts of ATP at a time when production is suppressed. Cardiac arrest prior to inducing ischemia prevents this energy wasting, and maintenance of arrest preserves adenine nucleotide levels. Hypothermic conditions also reduce ATP utilization by cellular processes other than mechanical contraction and help to preserve cellular ATP. Many combinations of substrates have been employed in attempts to improve anaerobic production of ATP, but these can be expected to have little beneficial effects on energy levels. Not only are the substrate-utilizing pathways inhibited by ischemia as discussed above, but hypothermic conditions have the same slowing effect on energy-producing as on energy-utilizing pathways. Attempts to preserve the viability of ischemic tissue should, however, include measures to prevent metabolic products from accumulating.

Myosin ATPase Activity and Cardiac Function

Velocity of contraction in skeletal muscle correlates with myosin ATPase activity. In cardiac muscle, myosin ATPase activity is highest in those species that have the fastest heart rate. Increased cardiac contractility is associated with elevated myosin ATPase activity in hyperthyroid animals.[7] In addition, decreased contractility is associated with depressed myosin ATPase in a number of pathological conditions.[21] These alterations in myosin ATPase activity and mechanical function of the heart are due to control of gene expression that results in a change in the content of the various myosin isoenzymes.

The myosin molecule consists of two heavy chains (subunits) that contain a tail region and a globular head region which possesses the actin-binding sites and the ATPase activity. The molecule also contains two light chains which are noncovalently bound to the head region of the heavy chains and may be important in controlling the ATPase activity. Ventricular muscle contains three isoenzymes of myosin that are referred to as V_1, V_2, and V_3. These isoenzymes are structurally distinct because they consist of different combinations of the two heavy-chain subunits. The ATPase activity is greatest for V_1 and

least for V_3. The activity that is expressed in the intact muscle depends on the ratio of the different isoenzymes that are present.

Hyperthyroidism is associated with increased contractility of the heart in those species with low ATPase activity and slow heart rate, and hypothyroid states result in depressed myosin ATPase activity and contractility.[7] The ratio of V_1 to V_3 isoenzymes is highest in hyperthyroid animals and lowest in hypothyroid states. Thyroxine increases the synthesis of V_1 and suppresses synthesis of V_3.[22] Thus, effects of thyroxine on cardiac contractility are mediated through control of gene expression, which, in turn, determines the type of myosin isoenzyme that is present and, therefore, the activity of actin-activated myosin ATPase.

Concluding Remarks

The obvious question that arises from a more comprehensive understanding of myocardial metabolism is how this information can be used to describe the pathophysiology of heart disease and to plan therapy. In this section, three examples will be considered that represent either practical or potential applications of metabolic principles.

Perhaps the best example of a practical use of an understanding of metabolism is in the intraoperative protection of ischemic myocardium. As outlined above, therapy must be planned to reduce energy utilization rather than to increase high-energy phosphate production via greater substrate availability. This conclusion is based on the facts that substrate availability does not limit ATP synthesis in ischemic hearts and that factors such as hypothermia reduce both ATP utilization and production at the same time. Only increased oxygen delivery or agents that stop mechanical activity of the heart can be expected to prevent irreversible damage.

A second area in which an understanding of metabolic principles is of value is cardiomyopathies that are dependent on endocrine disorders. In the diabetic heart, optimal contractility is dependent upon substantial levels of free fatty acids or ketone bodies in plasma or upon adequate treatment with insulin. This situation results from the inability of the heart of severely diabetic animals to utilize glucose at a sufficient rate to support ATP production. In hypothyroid animals, contractility can be restored as a result of an effect of thyroid hormone on expression of the genes for myosin isoenzymes.

Finally, the potential exists for facilitating hypertrophy of muscle cells in response to an increased afterload or to loss of myocardial mass as a result of infarction. An improved understanding of factors that regulate RNA synthesis and protein turnover should aid in providing optimal conditions for growth of muscle cells and for recovery of ventricular function.

References

1. Fossell, E. T., Morgan, H. E., and Ingwall, J. S.: Measurement of Changes in High-Energy Phosphates in the Cardiac Cycle Using Gated P-31 Nuclear Magnetic Resonance, *Proc. Nat. Acad. Sci. U.S.A.,* 77:3654, 1980.
*2. Morgan, H. E., Rannels, D. E., and McKee, E. E.: Protein Metabolism of the Heart, in R. M. Berne (ed.), "Handbook of Physiology—The Cardiovascular System," American Physiological Society, Bethesda, Md., 1979, p. 845. (281 references)
*3. Neely, J. R., and Morgan, H. E.: Relationship between Carbohydrate and Lipid Metabolism and Energy Balance of Heart Muscle, *Ann. Rev. Physiol.,* 36:413, 1974. (241 references)
*4. Randle, P. J., and Tubbs, P. K.: Carbohydrate and Fatty Acid Metabolism, in R. M. Berne (ed.), "Handbook of Physiology—The Cardiovascular System," American Physiological Society, Bethesda, Md., 1979, p. 805. (224 references)
5. Miller, T. B. Jr.: Cardiac Performance of Isolated Perfused Hearts from Alloxan Diabetic Rats, *Am. J. Physiol.,* 236:4808, 1979.
6. Muller, J. E., Mochizuki, S., Koster, J. K., Collins, J. J., Cohn, L. H., and Neely, J. R.: Insulin Therapy for the Syndrome of Low Cardiac Output Following Cardiopulmonary Bypass, *Am J. Cardiol.,* 41:1215, 1978.
*7. Morkin, E.: Stimulation of Cardiac Myosin Adenosine Triphosphatase in Thyrotoxicosis, *Circ. Res.,* 44:1, 1979. (51 references)
*8. Stull, J. T., and Mayer, S. E.: Biochemical Mechanisms of Adrenergic and Cholinergic Regulation of Myocardial Contractility, in R. M. Berne (ed.), "Handbook of Physiology—The Cardiovascular System," American Physiological Society, Bethesda, Md., 1979, p. 741. (306 references)
9. Rovetto, M. J., Whitmer, J. T., and Neely, J. R.: Comparison of the Effects of Anoxia and Whole Heart Ischemia on Carbohydrate Utilization in Isolated Working Rat Hearts, *Circ. Res.,* 32:699, 1973.
*10. Idell-Wenger, J. A., and Neely, J. R.: Regulation of Uptake and Metabolism of Fatty Acids by Muscle, in J. M. Dietschy, A. M. Gotto, Jr., and J. A. Ontko (eds.), "Disturbances in Lipid and Lipoprotein Metabolism," American Physiological Society, Bethesda, Md., 1978, p. 269. (41 references)
11. Mole, P. A., Oscai, L. B., and Holloszy, J. O.: Adaptations of Muscle to Exercise: Increase in Levels of Palmitoyl-CoA Synthetase, Carnitine Palmityl-Transferase and Palmityl-CoA Dehydrogenase and in the Capacity to Oxidize Fatty Acids, *J. Clin. Invest.,* 50:2323, 1971.
12. Morel, F., Lanquin, G., Lumardi, J., Duszynski, J., and Vignais, P. V.: An Appraisal of the Functional Significance of the Inhibitory Effect of Long Chain Acyl-CoA's on Mitochondrial Transports, *FEBS Lett.,* 39:133, 1974.
13. Lamers, J. M. J., and Hulsmann, W. C.: Inhibition of $(Na^+ + K^+)$-Stimulated ATPase of Heart by Fatty Acids, *J. Mol. Cell. Cardiol.,* 9:343, 1977.
14. Wood, J. M., Busch, B., Pitts, B. J. R., and Schwartz, A.: Inhibition of Bovine Hearts Na^+,K^+-ATPase by Palmityl Carnitine and Palmityl-CoA, *Biochem. Biophys. Res. Commun.,* 74:677, 1977.
*15. Wildenthal, K., and Crie, J. S.: Lysosomes and Cardiac Protein Catabolism, in K. Wildenthal (ed.), "Degradative Processes in Heart and Skeletal Muscle," North-Holland Biomedical Press, Amsterdam, 1980, p. 113. (55 references)
*16. Morgan, H. E., Chua, B., and Beinlich, C. J.: Regulation of Protein Degradation in Heart, in K. Wildenthal (ed.), "Degradative Processes in Heart and Skeletal Muscle," North-Holland Biomedical Press, Amsterdam, 1980, p. 87. (133 references)
*17. Wildenthal, K.: Lysosomes and Lysosomal Enzymes in the Heart, in J. T. Dingle and R. T. Dean (eds.), "Lysosomes in Biology and Pathology," North-Holland Publishing Company, Amsterdam, 1975, p. 167. (114 references)
18. Hershko, A., Ciechanover, A., Heller, H., Haas, A. L., and Rose, I. A.: Proposed Role of ATP in Protein Breakdown: Conjugation of Proteins with Multiple Chains of the Polypeptide of ATP-Dependent Proteolysis, *Proc. Nat. Acad. Sci. U.S.A.,* 77:1783, 1980.
19. Williams, I. H., Chua, B. H. L., Sahms, R. H., Siehl, D., and Morgan, H. E.: Effects of Diabetes on Protein Turnover in Cardiac Muscle, *Am. J. Physiol.,* 239:E178, 1980.
20. Chua, B., Kao, R. L., Rannels, D. E., and Morgan, H. E.: Inhibition of Protein Degradation by Anoxia and Ischemia in Perfused Rat Hearts, *J. Biol. Chem.,* 254: 6617, 1979.
*21. Scheuer, J., and Bhan, A. K.: Cardiac Contractile Proteins, Adenosine Triphosphatase Activity and Physiological Function, *Circ. Res.,* 45:1, 1979. (110 references)
22. Hoh, J. F. Y., and Egerton, L. J.: Action of Triiodothyronine on the Synthesis of Rat Ventricular Myosin Isoenzyme, *FEBS Lett.* 101:143, 1979.

*This article is a review of the literature and contains additional references to the literature.

PART II Examination of the Heart and Blood Vessels

The physician examines the heart and blood vessels in order to answer several questions. First of all, the physician asks, "Is heart disease present?" If heart disease is present, it is then necessary to ask, "What is the cause? What structural abnormalities are present and how severe are they? Is there an abnormality of myocardial contractility and how severe is it? Is there an abnormality of heart rhythm or conduction? Is there a metabolic abnormality such as myocardial ischemia, and how severe is it?" And finally, the physician asks, "What is the prognosis, and how do the disease process and its consequences affect the life of the patient?" The physician who asks and answers this question can then proceed with appropriate treatment of the patient.

Certain data are acquired from all patients (or potential patients) by utilizing the history, physical examination, electrocardiogram, and chest roentgenogram. The questions listed above can usually be answered by using these methods of examination. The data and the skills required to collect the data by using the history, physical examination, electrocardiogram, and chest roentgenogram are discussed in Sec. A of Part II.

In some patients the questions listed above cannot be answered by utilizing the history, physical examination, electrocardiogram, and chest roentgenogram. When such is the case, the physician must ask whether it is absolutely necessary to answer the questions. This is proper since there are times when answering the questions does not enable the physician to manage the patient's conditions in a new and different manner.

When the physician makes the clinical judgment that he or she must know the answers to the questions listed above in order to care for the patient, *then* additional, carefully selected tests should be ordered. Accordingly, the purposes of Sec. B of Part II are to categorize the questions in a problem-oriented way and to describe the tests that may be used to answer the questions; to give the indications for the selected tests; to give the sensitivity, specificity, and predictive value of the results of the tests; and to suggest the appropriate strategy for getting definitive answers from the tests, and to do so with the lowest possible risk and cost to the patient. The discussion of equipment and techniques is presented in Part VI.

The organization of Parts II and VI of *The Heart* was created in an effort to *inhibit* a trend of modern cardiology to become technique-oriented and -dominated. *This unique organization is utilized in order to emphasize that specialized tests and procedures must be used to answer the specific questions of a perceptive physician and should not be used before the questions have been brought into proper focus.*

6

The Physician's Approach to the Patient with Heart Disease

J. Willis Hurst, M.D.

The professional man is in essence one who provides service. But the service he renders is something more than that of the laborer, even the skilled laborer. It is a service that wells up from the entire complex of his personality. True, some specialized and highly developed techniques may be included, but their mode of expression is given its deepest meaning by the personality of the practitioner. In a very real sense his professional service cannot be separate from his personal being. He has no goods to sell, no land to till; his only asset is himself. It turns out that there is no right price for service, for what is a share of a man worth? If he does not contain the quality of integrity, he is worthless. If he does, he is priceless. The value is either nothing or it is infinite.

So do not try to set a price on yourselves. Do not measure out your professional services on an apothecary's scale and say, "Only this for so much." Do not debase yourselves by equating your souls to what they will bring in the market. Do not be a miser, hoarding your talents and abilities and knowledge, either among yourselves or in your dealings with your clients, patients, or flock. Rather be reckless and spendthrift, pouring out your talent to all to whom it can be of service. Throw it away, waste it; and in the spending it can be of service. Do not keep a watchful eye lest you slip and give away a little bit of what you might have sold. Do not censor your thoughts to gain a wider audience. Like love, talent is useful only in its expenditure, and it is never exhausted. Certain it is that man must eat, so set what price you must on your service. But never confuse the performance, which is great, with the compensation, be it money, power, or fame, which is trivial.

Judge Elbert P. Tuttle, Sr., 1957[1]

From its beginning in 1966, *The Heart* has been written for physicians who take care of patients who have heart disease. Accordingly, it seems appropriate to set down some of the attributes of good physicians that I believe are timeless and to highlight some of the concerns of patients that are also timeless. The diseases of the heart and their treatment should then be viewed in the context of the performance of good physicians.

Attributes of Good Physicians[1]

I have always viewed the practice of medicine—the care of patients—as a linkage between competence in medicine and compassion. Compassionate physicians care about their patients and strive to be competent in what they do. In other words, compassion stimulates good physicians to be competent.

- Good physicians are trustworthy. Patients often assume that all physicians upon graduating from medical school are equally competent. This indicates that our predecessors produced a record of excellence that is transferred to all of us. Whether or not we are competent can only be answered by each individual and by colleagues, but the trust patients have in physicians must not be violated by any of us.
- Good physicians are intelligent, but they must be more than memory experts. The modern definition of intelligence is the ability to learn how to learn. Good physicians appreciate the essence of self-education. They are constantly asking themselves questions and pursuing the answers.
- Good physicians have an interest in scientific matters and are greatly interested in how the body works. The latter includes an intense interest in human behavior.

Physicians of today must know more about experimental design, statistics, Bayes' theorem, and the sensitivity, specificity, predictive value, and efficiency of test results, etc., than the physicians of yesterday. *Sensitivity* indicates the frequency of a positive test result in a population of patients with a certain disease. *Specificity* indicates the frequency of a negative test result in a population of patients without a certain disease. The *predictive value* of a positive test result indicates the frequency of diseased patients in a population of patients in which all of the test results are positive. The predictive value of a negative test result indicates the frequency of nondiseased patients in a population of patients in which all of the test results are negative. The *efficiency* of a test indicates the percentage of patients correctly classified by the test. *Bayes' theorem* states that the predictive value of a test result is predetermined by the prevalence of the disease in the population being studied.

Physicians have learned to apply these descriptive terms to laboratory tests. The same descriptive terms should be applied to the results of the history and physical examination. For example, every story of chest discomfort does not have the same predictive value as a diagnostic marker of coronary atherosclerosis, and rales in the lungs are not perfect markers of heart failure. The reader may say that I have gone too far, that I am describing the attributes of a scientist. Not so. The attributes I have just listed are necessary for modern physicians to read and understand the medical literature, to use test results properly, and to discuss medical matters with their colleagues. Tutors are not always available. Accordingly, physicians must be able to think and learn on their own. The medical literature becomes increasingly important to physicians who are sufficiently compassionate to wish to remain competent. Obviously then, physicians must be able to interpret what they read or hear. Furthermore, they must be able to apply what they read or hear to their daily work with patients.

- Good physicians are highly motivated people. They stand in awe at the wonders of the human body and how it works. They want to understand it. They care about the welfare of their patients and want to do all they can to help them. Their motivation is stimulated by their innate curiosity about body functions and the compassion they feel for their patients.
- Good physicians aspire to have good common sense. Anyone who uses the term *common sense* is obligated to define it. Common sense in medicine implies that physicians have sound pathophysiological or biochemical bases for their ideas and actions. This is very important, for all physicians must deal with variations of illnesses that are not exactly similar to those reported in the latest medical journal. Common sense in medicine can also be defined as a logical and defensible extension of the medical concepts that have been passed on to us by our predecessors. This implies that physicians who have a scholarly view of their profession trace the origin of the great ideas in medicine. They learn about the men and women who had the ideas and how their ideas were challenged by some and accepted by others. They learn that what we say and do now has come to us over the centuries and after much debate. Therefore, if one knows the origin of an idea, it is possible to extend it a bit, feeling that another step along a path that has stood the test of time is a reasonably safe step compared with a lateral step into the unknown.
- Good physicians have a sense of pertinence. They can separate trivia from meaningful material. Winston Churchill once said, "I did not do very well in my early schooling. My teachers learned, however, that I did awfully well in those things that really mattered."
- Good physicians have a highly developed sense of priority. They can receive all the scientific and emotional stimuli that bombard them during a busy day and determine what they should do first, next, or last. This ability is extremely important since many, many lab tests can be ordered and many things can be done. The list of possible diagnoses may be long, and the physicians must determine the order in which each possibility should be explored.
- Good physicians recognize that it is necessary to establish realistic goals for patients. Is the goal to cure, to relieve, to stand by until the end comes, to enable patients to return to work, or to enable patients to simply feed themselves?
- Good physicians have good clinical judgment. Like common sense, this term is difficult to define. Physicians who display good clinical judgment seem to have considerable common sense (as defined above), a refined sense of pertinence, and a keen sense of priority. In addition, they have a demonstrated track record of making sound decisions in complex situations.
- Good physicians keep good records. Their records need not be long, but they should indicate what they found in the patient, the data they used to make decisions, what they did for the patient's problems, and how they followed up on what they did (see later discussion).
- Good physicians have considerable organizational ability. Physicians recognize that it is not possible to render the proper medical care unless they can lead nonphysicians to assist them in accomplishing their goals in the care of patients and in medicine generally. This attribute is more important now than it was in the past because medicine is more complex and more people are required to deliver proper care.
- Good physicians make themselves available. There is, of course, a limit to endurance, and good physicians must have appropriate rest. The patients of good physicians know that their physicians want to be available to them and, when they are not available, appropriate "coverage" has been arranged.
- Good physicians are professionals. Judge Elbert P. Tuttle, Sr., offers us the finest definition of professionalism I know.[1] This definition is recorded at the beginning of this chapter.

I have not listed qualities such as honesty, integrity, and kindness as being attributes of good physicians. They are, they are. But they are the attributes of all good people. What I have discussed here are the attributes of good physicians. I have assumed that good people have chosen medicine and that many fine qualities were learned in the home long before medical school matriculation. Older physicians in medical schools and hospitals should, however, teach by their actions how the kindness one possesses can be translated to the care of the patient.

Concerns of Patients

Some years ago, I had a serious illness. Therefore, I qualify as a patient and can express my concerns from that point of view.

- As a patient I do not like to be called a *consumer of health care*. This statement is dehumanizing. At the same time I do not want the physicians who care for me and my disease to be called *purveyors of health care* for the same reason.
- I believe that most patients want a physician they can talk to and who cares about their well-being and sees them as human beings.
- Patients want physicians to be honest, but they do not demand that every rare and unusual complication be discussed to the point that they see themselves as exceptions who are doomed to the ravages of every simple illness.
- Patients can identify good physicians by the fre-

quency the physicians state they do not know. No physician knows everything, and it is arrogant to present such a picture. Patients can identify good physicians by the sensitivity they have to the need for another medical opinion. Patients expect their physicians to assist them in their health problems, and this includes obtaining proper consultation. It is amazing how the respect for physicians by patients is increased when the physicians express by words and actions that they want the best for their patients.

- Patients want their physicians to be available. They know that every human needs rest. They do not object to that. They do object to a poorly defined system of coverage when their physician is unavailable.
- Patients trust their physicians. This places the weight on medical schools, house staff and fellow programs, licensing agencies, and hospital staffs to determine whether individual physicians can do what they claim they can do.

The Whole is Greater Than the Part

Mortimer Adler points out that truth is difficult to define but offers "the whole is greater than the part" as an example of the truth that is self-evident.[2] The human body is made up of organs, and the whole body is greater than any organ. This is my way of emphasizing that the identification and management of the diseases of an organ (such as the heart) should not be the specific goal of any physician. The proper perspective should be to view problems related to one organ in the context of the problems of all other organs. Coronary arteries are not admitted to coronary care units—people with coronary arteries are admitted to coronary care units. Many decisions regarding the management of heart disease are influenced by the diseases that are present in the other organs and by the personality of the patient. This is why physicians who have good clinical judgment manage the same disease differently in different patients.

Data Collection, Problem Formulation, Planning, and Follow-Up[3]

The medical data that physicians collect from their patients is determined by the goals they set for themselves and their patients. If physicians are to render primary comprehensive care to patients, they must collect medical data that permits them to do that. If physicians are called upon to give opinions about the heart and blood vessels, they must collect data which will give insight about these structures. They must also collect data about all other organs and about the personality of the patient that may be useful in making a decision about the heart and circulation. The data to be collected on every patient can be defined in advance. *An example of a defined data base designed to identify and manage heart disease is shown in the appendix.*

A *defined data base* includes those items that are collected on every patient. After the facts (data) have been collected, the physician must analyze them and synthesize them into a list of "problems." The problems may be highly resolved (diagnoses), and no additional diagnostic work may be needed. On the other hand, the problems may be poorly resolved and may represent a symptom, a structural abnormality, a physiological derangement, a biochemical abnormality, etc. It is very useful to list and number the problems on a single sheet of paper, which should be the first item in the office or hospital record.

The *problem list* serves as the table of contents to the health of the patient. It makes it possible for a physician to view one problem in the context of all other problems. The solution to the problems that are poorly understood may require further diagnostic workup. As poorly resolved problems are solved, the new formulation is added to the problem list.

Once the problem list has been carefully formulated, listed, and numbered, it is then essential to develop and record the *initial plans* for each problem or to state why plans should not be developed for a certain problem. The plans for each problem should be numbered and titled to correlate with the problem list. It is useful to develop a differential diagnosis for those problems that are poorly resolved and to develop and record the *diagnostic workup* that is planned for each possibility. The physician's sense of priority determines the sequence in which a workup progresses. The initial plans for each problem must indicate what *therapy* is to be used at that point in time. In many instances the physician should record the *instructions* given the patient (education of the patient). For example, the operative risks for coronary bypass surgery should be recorded as follows: "The patient and the family have been instructed that the operative risk in our hospital is about 1 percent."

Progress notes should be written for appropriate problems. They too should be numbered and titled to match the number and titles on the problem list and initial plans. Such notes should include the subjective and objective data related to the specific problem, the assessment of the new data, and new plans.

This is not the place to discuss the value of organizing data and action in the manner described above. The virtue of having a system in one's work is self-evident. The system discussed above is teachable and serves to link data gathering and data analysis to the plans that are designed to improve a patient's well-being. In this sense the system highlights the patient's problems and permits the physician to direct his or her attention toward the solution of the problems (including management of the problems).

The miniprefaces recorded on the first page of each part of this book should be read carefully. The minipreface at the beginning of Part II is germane to the discussion being presented here. The defined data base indicates the information that should be gathered on every patient. The tools used to gather the information are the history, physical examination, chest x-ray, electrocardiogram, and other laboratory tests. This data-gathering process can be implemented in almost all offices and hospitals. This technique permits the physician to identify the patient's cardiovascular problem at a high level of resolution most of the time. The types of data to be gathered are discussed in Sec. A of Part II. If the problem is identified at a low level of resolution, the physician should ask whether further refinement of the problem is necessary. If the answer is yes, then the physician should ask, What question am I trying to answer? Questions should be phrased as follows: Is there an abnormal structure or flow? Is there an abnormality of cardiac performance? Is there an electrical problem (arrhythmias)? Is there a problem of ischemia or some other metabolic abnormality? In other words, after a physician has analyzed the data which has been collected, he or she should either know what is wrong with the patient or phrase the questions in such a way that it is clear what test or procedure should be done next. Thus, the tests and procedures are chosen in order to answer specific questions. Accordingly, the tests and procedures that yield results that have predictive values that are sufficiently great to make decisions are utilized. This very important strategy is discussed in Sec. B of Part II. This approach makes technology the physician's servant rather than the reverse. This approach inhibits the approach in which the physician learns certain techniques and then tries to apply them and hopes that the results are useful. A discussion of the techniques used to answer questions can be found in Part VI.

The Cardiac Appraisal

The physician must ask the following questions: Is heart or blood vessel disease present? What other diseases or disorders does the patient have that require treatment or modify the treatment that would ordinarily be used for the patient's heart disease? Do I really know all that I need to know about the patient's heart disease? This latter question leads to the purpose of the discussion in this section.

Dr. Paul White highlighted the elements of a "complete cardiac diagnosis" in 1914. He translated his concept into action when he designed special cards that were to be filled out on every patient. The original cards had four surfaces, but later he designed the cards so that a defined data base was displayed on six surfaces. The faces of the cards showed his concept of a complete cardiac diagnosis. This idea was further developed by the Criteria

Committee of the New York Heart Association. The Committee wrote the first edition of *Criteria for the Classification and Diagnosis of Heart Disease* in 1928.[4] This magnificent book was published by Little, Brown and Company. There have been eight editions of this book. The title has changed a little over the years. The eighth edition was published by Little, Brown and Company in 1979 and is titled *Nomenclature and Criteria for Diagnosis of Diseases of the Heart and Great Vessels*.

The series of eight editions of this book has had an enormous impact on the practice of medicine generally and cardiology specifically. I recommend the book to all students, house officers, cardiac fellows, and physicians who are interested in the diseases of the heart and blood vessels. The book emphasizes correct nomenclature (which is essential for communication) and throws a spotlight on the elements of a complete cardiac diagnosis. The first six editions required the physician to establish the *etiology* of the heart disease; the altered *anatomy* of the heart disease; the altered *physiology* of the heart disease; and the *functional capacity* of the patient. The latter was determined by assessing the degree of symptoms expressed by the patient. Class 1 implied the patient had no symptoms. Class 2 implied that the patient had symptoms with more-than-usual activity. Class 3 implied that the patient had symptoms with usual activity. Class 4 implied the patient had symptoms at rest. The prognosis was then based on the functional classification. While the presence of symptoms is very important, symptoms do not always determine the seriousness of a disease process or enable one to determine whether a patient can work. Therefore the Criteria Committee of the New York Heart Association made a rather marked change in the seventh edition of *Nomenclature and Criteria for the Diagnosis of Diseases of the Heart and Great Vessels*. The following paragraphs are reproduced from the seventh edition and indicate in more detail the method of determining the *cardiac status and prognosis* of a patient.[5] (Remember these new categories have replaced the functional and therapeutic classification that was presented in earlier editions.)

The following excerpts are reprinted below with the permission of the New York Heart Association and its Criteria Committee and Little, Brown and Company.

From the preface:

The Functional and Therapeutic Classification of previous editions required that the physician classify the patient's cardiac status on the basis of symptoms alone, without regard to the etiologic, anatomic, or physiologic diagnoses. Although a consideration of symptomatology is essential for a correct physiologic diagnosis, it is now recognized that a classification of cardiac status based on symptoms alone may be misleading. Symptoms may be absent in the presence of serious anatomic and physiologic abnormalities, and the necessity for medical or surgical intervention may not be appreciated. In addition, symptoms may appear only after serious changes have taken place in the heart and lungs, which can prevent an effective attack upon the underlying defect. Further, some therapies may alter the symptoms and the course of the disease only briefly, whereas others may fundamentally change the course of the disease. Recommendations for therapy can rarely be based on a single diagnostic category; the implications of the other two categories also must be considered.

With these considerations in mind, a new classification, Cardiac Status and Prognosis, is presented. This classification should reflect an accurate assessment of each patient based on the etiologic, anatomic, and physiologic diagnoses and on an understanding of the benefits of present therapies.[5]

From the introduction:

The *etiologic, anatomic,* and *physiologic* diagnoses of cardiovascular disease depend upon a careful analysis of the patient's history, a thorough physical examination, and, when indicated, a variety of laboratory examinations. Some of the latter are not specific for evaluation of the cardiovascular system, but represent an attempt to delineate the major problem. Others, such as electrocardiography, phonocardiography, echocardiography, cardiac catheterization, and a variety of radiologic techniques, are employed to detect the cause of heart disease or to identify specific anatomic and physiologic abnormalities.

The diagnostic categories are frequently dependent upon one another and, in the final synthesis, their compatibility should be examined.

The *etiology* of heart disease should be determined by considering both structural and functional disturbances. If two or more possible causes of heart disease are present, each should be mentioned. Chapter 1 delineates the etiologies of the known major structural and functional disorders of the heart, although the detailed mechanisms by which the various diseases ultimately affect the heart are not all completely understood.

Anatomic lesions of the heart and great vessels usually can be recognized clinically. In some instances their manifestations are so specific that the anatomic abnormality is easily identified. Frequently, however, the presence of a structural lesion is inferred from a recognition of the cause of the heart disease, the identification of a physiologic disturbance known to result from it, or both. More than one anatomic abnormality may be present in any one patient; each should be included in the anatomic diagnosis.

Different *physiologic* disturbances often have similar clinical manifestations; the identification of the cause of the disturbance may therefore rest upon knowledge of the etiologic or anatomic diagnoses. Frequently, more than one physiologic abnormality is present; all should be included in the physiologic diagnosis. If no disturbance is present, the physiologic diagnosis is simply: Normal Sinus Rhythm.

Each of the diagnostic items has been assigned a code number. The grading of *Cardiac Status and Prognosis* is also coded numerically.

A complete cardiac diagnosis should include one or more titles from each of the principal diagnostic categories of this nomenclature: *etiologic, anatomic, physiologic,* and *cardiac status* and *prognosis.*

Certain patients may have symptoms, abnormal physical signs, or both which are referable to the heart, but which after detailed study cannot be ascribed with certainty to structural or functional cardiac disease. In such cases the diagnosis should be No Heart Disease, Unexplained Manifestation. Patients who have a disease such as systemic arterial hypertension, which can cause heart disease but which at the time of observation has not done so, are to be designated as having No Heart Disease, Predisposing Etiologic Factor (systemic arterial hypertension).[5]

From the discussion regarding the cardiac status and prognosis:

The purpose of this classification, "Cardiac Status and Prognosis," is to assess the present cardiac status of the patient and to make a prognosis of the future status as modified by optimal therapy. *Cardiac status* represents a total assessment of the etiologic, anatomic, and physiologic diagnoses. *Prognosis* is based on an assessment of the potential effects of optimal current medical and surgical therapies. The classification should be reviewed frequently and revised when indicated. This appraisal should communicate to others the physician's opinion of the patient's status and prognosis without consideration of details of management.

Recommendations for further diagnostic procedures, medical and surgical therapies, and limitation of physical activity should be detailed at the end of this classification.

Cardiac Status	Prognosis
1 Uncompromised	1 Good
2 Slightly compromised	2 Good with therapy
3 Moderately compromised	3 Fair with therapy
4 Severely compromised	4 Guarded despite therapy

Specific Recommendations: (Further diagnostic procedures; medical or surgical correction of the underlying defect; limitation of physical activity; use of antibiotics, digitalis glycosides, diuretics, dietary restrictions; and so forth.)[5]

The changes made in the seventh edition (1973) and carried on in the eighth edition (1979) of the book are very significant.[5,6] In years to come the change will be viewed as the time in history physicians began to accept the new information made possible by the technology of the era. It will represent the time when physicians recognized that physiological abnormalities, discovered only in the laboratory, should be used to determine the severity and natural history of certain disease processes.

The proper understanding of a cardiovascular problem requires that the physician establish the etiologic, anatomic, and physiologic diagnoses. After that is completed, the physician should review *all* the data (not just the patient's symptoms) and establish the patient's cardiac status and prognosis.

The following example serves to make the point. A 54-year-old man had mild, recent-onset, angina pectoris. The patient continued to work as a machinist and developed angina with moderate exercise.

Prior to 1973, when the seventh edition of *Nomenclature and Criteria for Diagnosis of Diseases of the Heart and Great Vessels* was published, one would view and record the complete diagnosis of a patient as follows:

Etiology: Coronary atherosclerosis.
Anatomy: Obstruction of coronary arteries (location and extent of disease unknown).
Physiology: Unstable angina pectoris (recent onset).
Function: Class 1.
Therapeutic: Good with drug therapy and avoidance of moderate activity. (This assumption was based on the fact that the angina was mild and could be prevented by avoiding moderate exercise.)

Now, one would view the same patient very differently. A coronary arteriogram would be ordered even though the angina was mild. Let us suppose the arteriogram showed 95 percent cross-sectional obstruction of the left main coronary artery (as it is likely to do in more than 10 percent of such patients). *The new perception would be:*

Etiology: Coronary atherosclerosis.
Anatomy: Ninety-five percent cross-sectional obstruction of the left main coronary artery. Good contractility.
Physiology: Unstable angina pectoris (recent onset).
Cardiac Status: Class 4. Severely compromised. (Even though the symptoms are mild and controllable, it has been clearly established that left main coronary artery obstruction is a potentially lethal lesion.)
Prognosis: Class 2. Good with surgical therapy. (Five-year survival is about 90 percent in patients who have successful bypass surgery.)
Specific Recommendations: Coronary bypass surgery plus medical management.

Summary

This chapter is merely one person's approach to patients with heart disease. There are, I am sure, many other equally good approaches to the problem. The approach described here is all-encompassing since it describes: some of the attributes of a good physician; some concerns of patients; the heart and its diseases viewed in the context of all organs and their diseases; data collection, problem formulation, planning, and follow-up of the patients' problems; and an approach to the patient based on the concepts which were emphasized in the seventh and eighth editions of *Nomenclature and Criteria for Diagnosis of Diseases of the Heart and Great Vessels.*

This approach, I hope, will serve as a goal for all of us. It links the good physician to a concerned patient and translates medical knowledge to medical care.

References

1. Hurst, J. W.: "Four Hats," Year Book Medical Publishers, Inc., Chicago, 1970.
2. Adler, M. J.: "Great Ideas from the Great Books," Washington Square Press, Inc., New York, 1963.
3. Hurst, J. W., and Walker, H. K.: "The Problem-Oriented System," MEDCOM, New York, 1972.
4. The Criteria Committee for the New York Heart Association: "Criteria for the Classification and Diagnosis of Heart Disease," 1st ed., New York Heart Association, Inc., New York, 1928.
5. The Criteria Committee of the New York Heart Association: "Nomenclature and Criteria for Diagnosis of Diseases of the Heart and Great Vessels," 7th ed., New York Heart Association, Inc., New York, 1973.
6. The Criteria Committee of the New York Heart Association: "Nomenclature and Criteria for Diagnosis of Diseases of the Heart and Great Vessels," 8th ed., New York Heart Association, Inc., New York, 1979.

7

The History: Symptoms Due to Cardiovascular Disease

J. Willis Hurst, M.D.
Douglas C. Morris, M.D.
I. Sylvia Crawley, M.D.

The due appreciation of the patient's sensations is essential to a knowledge of the condition of the heart.
Sir James Mackenzie, M.D., 1916[1]

The purpose of this chapter is to discuss history taking and the symptoms patients may have as the result of cardiovascular disease. The discussion is not intended to be more than an overview of the subject since the symptoms related to cardiovascular disease are discussed in detail in the chapters dealing with the conditions that cause them.

There are three methods of collecting medical information from the patient. They are the history, the physical examination, and the laboratory examination. While an abnormality may be revealed by only one of these methods, it is important for the physician to correlate the abnormalities found by one method of examination with the abnormalities found in one or both of the other two methods. For example, the patient's historical account of syncope may correlate with the physical findings of brady-cardia and variation of intensity of the first heart sound and the laboratory finding of complete heart block (by electrocardiography).

The History: General Comments

The Purpose of History Taking

The objective of history taking is to collect medical information from the patient and to establish a doctor-patient relationship.

Eliciting the History

The art and science of obtaining an accurate medical history, including the symptoms of a patient, is the hallmark of an excellent physician. History taking is often viewed by students as being easier than performing a physical examination and laboratory evaluation. With more experience they learn the enormous value of the medical history and also learn that it is not always easy to obtain an accurate description of the symptoms felt by the patient.

Dr. Paul White, the master clinician, made the following points regarding history taking.

First and most important of all is the story of the patient together with a careful consideration of his personality and reactions as he himself tells the story. If told by someone else, especially in the absence of the patient, the story has a certain amount of value dependent on the narrator's intelligence and the closeness of his acquaintanceship with the patient, but this procedure prevents insight into the case that may come only by listening to the patient's own discussion of his history and symptoms.

If the confidence of the patient is secured at the start and he is put at once at his ease, the results for both patient and doctor may mean the difference between success and failure in the proper handling of the case, which is more than simply the establishment of the correct diagnosis and the outline of the special cardiovascular treatment. Sometimes trivial remarks, actions, or occurrences may destroy the confidence or ease of the patient and so prevent the successful evolution of the case. It is at the very outset that the physician must use the greatest care.[2]

Dr. Paul Wood, the brilliant cardiologist, expressed his view of history taking as follows.

> To take an accurate and relevant history is one of the most difficult and important arts in medicine. Sometimes, a complete diagnosis can be made from the history alone, and not infrequently the possibilities can be whittled down to two or three. A good history should at least indicate the system involved, or it should point unerringly to some group or groups of diseases. A common mistake is the failure to analyze any given symptoms sufficiently; in cardiovascular work this applies especially to pain, breathlessness, palpitations, and syncope. The student is usually taught to encourage the patient to tell his story in his own words, and to record them more or less verbatim. Yet such an account may be verbose, irrelevant, inaccurate, and misleading. It is an axiom that the leading questions must be avoided at all cost; yet again, an experienced physician must know that the ability to put the appropriate leading question at the right moment, and the intelligent interpretation of its reply, are invaluable. It is not pretended that leading questions may not lead to false information, if the power of their suggestion is not appreciated by the questioner; and it is agreed that much may be lost by failure to allow the patient freedom and time to express his complaints in his own way; but the average patient will not mention half the available information until he is pressed, and the data freely given must be checked as at the bar. For example, in the differential diagnosis between a neural and non-neural somatic lesion, an accurate description of the quality of the pain may determine the issue immediately; yet the majority of patients will volunteer no information concerning the quality of pain, and if asked to describe it will do so inadequately. They may say it is aching or sharp, but fail to enlarge on this, even when urged to do so. In answer to the leading question, "Does it tingle?" however, they may reply at once in the affirmative. It is essential to realize that the matter does not end there: that such a positive reply to a leading question is satisfied that the pain really does tingle, and that the patient is not merely saying so because it seems the easier answer. It is scarcely too much to say that the best history taker is the one who can best interpret the answer to a leading question. Appropriate leading questions can only be asked, however, when the proffered history has provided sufficient data upon which to work, and if the physician has sufficient knowledge of the possibilities then entailed. It is this latter factor which makes it easier for the expert than for the student.[3]

Errors Made in History Taking

The Inhumane Interview
As stated above, one of the objectives of history taking is to establish a doctor-patient relationship. When the history-taking period is over, patients should realize that the physician knows a lot about them and cares a lot about their well-being. When patients perceive that physicians give of themselves, they will, in return, give their trust to the physician.

Unfortunately, history taking does not always accomplish the goal of creating a good and proper doctor-patient relationship. In fact, the interview may establish advisory roles for the physician and the patient. The interview will fail if the interviewer is too hurried; demands precise answers and displays irritation when such are not given; shows disdain when the answers to questions are not known; insists on probing deeper in certain areas when he or she should realize that the subject is too emotionally painful to be discussed; fails to look up from the desk; receives multiple telephone calls during the interview; seems to treat dreaded diseases casually; gives nonverbal signals of personal unhappiness; and seems to be automated rather than understanding. In fact, should this occur, the interview will be perceived by the patient as the most inhumane and cruel portion of the entire medical workup. Today we hear a great deal about the inhumanness of medicine. The inhumanness is usually blamed on machines and technology. One does not have to reflect very long on the subject to realize that machines just sit there until used or misused by physicians and their helpers; that machines do not talk, people do; and that considerable inhumanness can be displayed during the "old-fashioned" interview a physician has with a patient. When the medical interview fails, the physician will have no workable relationship established with the patient and the medical "facts" will often be wrong because the patient wishes to avoid the cold questioning of the unpleasant interrogation.

The "Flaw" in Dealing with the Chief Complaint
Physicians are taught to ask the patient to state their "chief complaint." Sometimes the physician forgets that the patient's chief complaint may not be of assistance in identifying the patient's most serious complaint. The physician must always deal with the patient's chief complaint. Make no mistake about that. Not to do so will lead to instant patient dissatisfaction since the patient perceives his or her chief complaint as the serious one and feels the physician is calloused when it is ignored. The physician must not fail to find and pursue other complaints that are more serious. For example, a lady complained bitterly of degenerative arthritis of the knees (her chief complaint), and she and many physicians had ignored her angina pectoris due to atherosclerotic coronary heart disease.

The "Flaw" in Dealing with the Present Illness
Physicians have been taught to elicit the details related to the chief complaint. The details indicate the sequence of events related to the chief complaint and all aspects of the complaint itself. The details related to the chief complaint are labeled the *present illness*. Should the interviewer's mind be dominated by this lockstep sequence, he or she may not pursue all of the patient's complaints. It is far better to ask the patient to enumerate *all* of the complaints and

establish present illnesses for the complaints the physician judges to be of significance.

The Use and Abuse of Medical Questionnaires
A medical questionnaire, such as the one shown in the Appendix, can be helpful or harmful depending upon the manner in which the physician uses it.

The questionnaire is helpful when it is given to (or sent to) the patient well in advance of the interview. When this occurs, the patient can record certain data more accurately because time may be needed to think about the question, ask others about the question, and look up details about the question in personal papers. The physician should review the questionnaire carefully and spend some time personalizing the interview. The abnormalities perceived by the patient should be probed, and many additional areas can be pursued by the physician.

The medical questionnaire may be harmful if the physician allows it to substitute for the patient as a person; if the physician fails to show the patient that the data submitted has been reviewed; if the physician fails to pursue the complaints in a humane way; or if the physician fails to show the patient that the completed questionnaire becomes part of a very important item—the medical record.

Failure to Properly Interpret the "Past History"
Physicians may make an error when they accept a past event as fact. We seem willing to accept a past history of rheumatic fever as fact but demand very strict criteria for the current diagnosis of the disease. We seem willing to accept the past diagnosis of myocardial infarction when the basis of the belief may be hearsay evidence. The past history is very important, but, at times, it can mislead the physician.

Failure to Talk with the Family
Every experienced physician knows that the care of the patient is frequently determined by the physician's relationship with members of the patient's family. An essential part of doctoring is to establish a physician-family relationship as well as a doctor-patient relationship. It is also important to obtain information from family members about the patient's symptoms and the patient's reaction to the illness.

Failure to Assess the Patient's Feelings
The history can be obtained, and the physician may or may not really know the patient. Good historians will know their patients. They will know their reactions to illness, their feelings about disability, their feelings about surgical intervention, and their emotional responsiveness; they will know them as human beings. The physician should remember that when the interview is over, the patient will have some perception of the physician. Obviously, physicians want to be perceived as knowledgeable and caring people. The point is that the patient's perception of the physician begins with the interview; the patient "examines" the physician while the physician is examining the patient.

"Live through a Day" with the Patient
It is important for the physician to live through a day with the patient. This is accomplished by simply asking the patient to enunciate the activities of the day, beginning with getting up in the morning and ending with getting up 24 h later. When this is done, many new insights about the patient and the patient's life will be discovered.

The Value and Limitations of Symptoms as Diagnostic Markers

The Predictive Value of Symptoms
Many years ago, the experts of the day emphasized the value of the patient's medical history (including symptoms) by stating that 70 percent of the useful medical information was contained in the medical history; 20 percent of the useful medical information was contained in the physical examination; and 10 percent of the useful medical information was found in the results of the laboratory procedures. This concept did not survive because laboratory technology, including electrocardiography, roentgenography, and cardiac catheterization were developed and the value of laboratory tests became apparent. The statement was misleading even before new laboratory procedures became available. Whereas the statement does emphasize the general value of the medical history, the concept could not be applied to individual patients. The fact is that the diagnostic value of the medical history (including symptoms) is predetermined by the type of disease that the patient happens to have. For example, faint aortic regurgitation is usually identified by hearing the heart murmur with the stethoscope. The history in such a patient might reveal no information regarding the patient's heart disease. The Wolff-Parkinson-White syndrome might be suspected in a patient with a history of paroxysmal atrial tachycardia, but the electrocardiographic evidence of a short PR interval with a wide QRS duration can only be identified by inspecting the electrocardiogram. Angina pectoris due to myocardial ischemia secondary to coronary atherosclerosis can only be recognized by eliciting the appropriate symptom.

The proper way to view the various methods of data collection (history, physical examination, and laboratory examination) is to recognize that all three methods are needed to detect the presence and severity of cardiovascular disease. Which method or methods yields the answer is largely predetermined by the nature and severity of the disease process. The challenge of the day is to determine the proper content of the history, physical examination, and laboratory studies. This is why the defined data base is so important (see Appendix). As a rule, the proper analysis of the data collected in the defined data base will identify the patient's cardiovascular problem. If the data gathered by completing the defined data base does not enable a physician to make a complete diagnosis (as described in Chap. 6), it is essential to ask whether the patient's problems should be refined to a higher level of understanding. If the answer is yes, then the physician should ask: Do I suspect an abnormality of structure or flow? Do I suspect an abnormality of contractility? Do I suspect an electrical abnormality? Do I suspect myocardial ischemia or some other disorder of myocardial metabolism? The challenge then is to select the procedure or procedures that will most likely answer the question. In other words, it is proper to choose the procedure or procedures that will give a result that has a very high predictive value in giving an accurate answer to the question (see preface to Part II).

Physicians have an enormous respect for the diagnostic value of the patient's symptoms. In fact, the respect borders on reverence. To challenge the value of using symptoms as perfect diagnostic markers will often produce a reaction in which the one challenged accuses the challenger of being a "laboratory person" who is unable to elicit and interpret symptoms. Such a response is, of course, not justified since there is ample evidence to prove that symptoms do not always reveal the presence or seriousness of disease.

Modern medicine requires that physicians understand the sensitivity, specificity, and predictive value of test results. (See Chap. 6.) Physicians, as a rule, apply these standards to laboratory test results, but have not applied them to symptoms and physical signs. It is just as important to know the sensitivity, specificity, and predictive value of the result obtained by asking a question or by seeking the presence or absence of a physical phenomenon as it is to know the sensitivity, specificity, and predictive value of laboratory test results.

For example, all medical histories do not have the same predictive value as diagnostic markers. Suppose one is trying to determine whether a patient's chest discomfort is angina pectoris due to atherosclerotic coronary heart disease. There is a type of chest discomfort that has a predictive value of about 90 percent, whereas other types of chest discomfort have a predictive value of about 50 percent. (See Chap. 45.) In other words, all histories of chest discomfort do not have the same predictive value. How does the physician use such information? The physician must learn the predictive value of symptoms and determine whether the history obtained is sufficiently adequate to be used in the decision-making process about the patient. The physician then adds this information to the results (with their predictive value) obtained from the physical examination, electrocardiogram, and chest x-ray and determines whether a definite decision can be made. If definitive decisions cannot be made, the physician asks whether more information is really needed. If the answer is yes, the physician determines what should be done next (see preface to Part II and Chap. 20).

Do the Presence and Magnitude of Symptoms Always Parallel the Seriousness of Heart Disease?

If the absence of symptoms always signified the absence of heart disease and the presence of certain symptoms always signified the presence and severity of heart disease, all a physician would have to do would be to ask, "How do you feel?" If the patient answers "Fine," the physician could pronounce the patient well. The ridiculous nature of this approach is highlighted when we remember that many patients who have sudden death due to atherosclerotic coronary heart disease have *no* warning symptom before the tragic event occurs. Patients with treacherous ventricular rhythm disturbances may not know that the abnormal rhythm is occurring. Patients with evidence of pulmonary congestion on the chest x-ray may not have dyspnea. Patients with high-grade obstruction of the left main coronary artery due to coronary atherosclerosis (a very dangerous lesion) may have *mild* symptoms of angina pectoris.

Patients may, however, have many symptoms as the result of minor disorders. For example, a patient with occasional premature ventricular contractions may feel each abnormal beat and be petrified with the fear of death. The patient with severe and terrifying angina pectoris due to coronary atherosclerosis may have only a high-grade obstruction of the right coronary artery. Such a lesion is accompanied by a fairly good long-term prognosis compared to the very poor long-term prognosis of a patient with high-grade obstruction of the left main coronary artery.

Some patients deny the presence of symptoms. The patients may deny the presence of symptoms at a deep psychological level since they cannot face the reality of the problems, while others may willfully withhold information from the physician because they might lose their job if the truth were known.

Some patients whose symptoms are dependent on effort will have no symptoms because they do not do enough to produce them. Elderly patients, sedentary patients, and patients whose physical activity is limited by another illness fall into this category. Some patients with angina pectoris due to coronary atherosclerosis or shortness of breath due to mitral stenosis may consciously or unconsciously walk more slowly in order to avoid symptoms. In fact, physicians frequently advise such patients to do less walking in order to avoid symptoms. The patient follows the physician's advice and then returns for follow-up examination, and sometimes the physician erroneously concludes that the patient is "better" because he or she is having fewer symptoms.

Elderly patients with cerebral atrophy may not be able to recall symptoms and may become frustrated when the details of symptoms are pursued. Patients who are psychiatrically disturbed may be unable to perceive symptoms or give a meaningful account of their symptoms.

One must conclude that symptoms are extremely important in the recognition of heart disease and its complications. One must also conclude that the absence of symptoms does not guarantee the absence of heart disease and that the presence and magnitude of symptoms do not always parallel the seriousness of the heart disease.

The Interpretation of Symptoms

The interpretation of symptoms is not always easy. Symptoms considered to be due to heart disease may in reality be arising from another system in the body. For example, dyspnea may be due to pulmonary disease, not heart disease. Symptoms attributed to noncardiovascular disease may in reality be due to heart disease. For example, pain in the jaw may be considered to be due to a toothache when it is actually due to angina pectoris secondary to coronary atherosclerosis.

The Determinants and Value of Symptoms

The determinants and value of symptoms depend upon the presence of cardiovascular disease that has reached a level of severity that can produce symptoms; the ability of the patients to perceive, observe, and relate their symptoms; the ability of physicians to elicit the symptoms from their patients without misleading the patients; the physicians' ability to interpret the meaning of patients' symptoms; the ability of physicians to determine the predictive value of various types of symptoms; and the ability of physicians to integrate the symptoms with the results of the physical examination and laboratory data.

Pain

The ability to evaluate pain and discomfort is a direct index of the expertise of the physician. This is especially true of the pain and discomfort related to cardiovascular disease. In order for the physician to evaluate pain it is necessary to determine its location, its radiation, its quality, how long it has been present, how long each episode lasts, the factors that produce it, and the factors that relieve it.

Chest Pain

Pain Due to Myocardial Ischemia

The most common cause of myocardial ischemia is atherosclerotic coronary heart disease (see Chap. 45). Other causes include aortic stenosis and regur-

gitation (Chap. 38), cardiomyopathy (Chap. 56), mitral valve prolapse (Chap. 39), and rare forms of coronary artery disease including coronary artery spasm (Chap. 47).

Chest pain or discomfort occurs when coronary atherosclerosis reaches a critical degree of severity and the lumen of the coronary arteries becomes sufficiently narrow to cause ischemia of the cardiac muscle. Angina pectoris may develop when the coronary flow is adequate at rest but is not adequate when the demands of the heart are increased. The altered physiology responsible for myocardial ischemia due to coronary atherosclerosis is discussed in Chap. 44. Myocardial ischemia due to valve disease or cardiomyopathy is also an indication of the severity of the conditions. (See Chaps. 38, 39, and 56.)

Angina Pectoris The diagnosis of angina pectoris may be missed if the physician inquires only about pain. Many patients with angina pectoris deny pain but complain of an aching, heavy, or squeezing sensation in the chest; chest pressure; chest tightness and dyspnea; or indigestion located in the chest. Angina pectoris occurs during effort; is precipitated by emotions, especially anger, and exposure to cold; and may follow meals. The unpleasant sensation is usually located in the substernal region of the chest or across the anterior portion of the upper part of the chest. The discomfort usually affects an area about the size of a clenched fist. As a matter of fact, the patient frequently clenches his or her fist and places it on the region of the chest where the discomfort is located. It is always useful to have the patient circumscribe the extent of the pain by indicating its location, using a single finger. The pain may radiate to the neck, jaw, hard palate, tongue, left arm, right arm, shoulder, elbow, wrist, back, or upper part of the abdomen. On rare occasions the discomfort may be more pronounced in these areas or may be felt only in one or more of the areas mentioned. The pain usually lasts from 1 to 3 min if the provoking effort is discontinued. Patients soon learn to stop walking or to slow their pace when they feel this discomfort. The duration of the angina pectoris provoked by anger is perhaps longer; it may be as long as 10 min. Angina pectoris is usually relieved promptly after nitroglycerin is placed under the tongue. There are many subsets of the brief pain of myocardial ischemia known as angina pectoris. Angina pectoris may be aggravated by many other medical conditions, including all types of emotional stress, obesity, anemia, and thyrotoxicosis.

Angina pectoris may be *stable* or *unstable*. *Prinzmetal's angina (variant angina)* does not follow the pattern described above in one major respect. This type of angina usually occurs at rest and is accompanied by ST-segment elevation in the electrocardiogram. The syndrome is thought to be due to coronary artery spasm with or without fixed obstructive coronary disease. (See Chaps. 45 and 47.)

Prolonged Pain Due to Myocardial Ischemia
Prolonged pain due to myocardial ischemia is said to be present when the chest discomfort lasts longer than 10 to 20 min. The discomfort may develop when the patient is doing very little. In fact, it may awaken the patient from sleep. He or she may become restless and occasionally walk the floor in search of comfort. It is commonly—but not always—more severe than the discomfort of angina. The pain of prolonged myocardial ischemia is rarely aggravated by deep breathing or turning. Many patients with prolonged pain due to myocardial ischemia may have *no* abnormalities demonstrated in the electrocardiogram, and the blood level of cardiac enzymes may not become elevated. Some patients may, however, exhibit only ST-T wave changes in the electrocardiogram, ST-T wave changes with elevation of blood cardiac enzymes, or QRS changes with elevation of cardiac enzymes. *Infarction* of the myocardium is said to occur when two of the following three conditions exist: a history of prolonged chest discomfort characteristic of myocardial ischemia, abnormal ST-T or Q waves in the electrocardiogram, and elevation of blood cardiac enzymes.

Patients with chest discomfort due to myocardial ischemia may fall into one of several subsets (see Chap. 45). *It is mandatory to identify the subset of chest pain due to myocardial ischemia to which the patient belongs because treatment is usually linked to a particular subset (see Chap. 45).*

Pain Due to Dissecting Aneurysm of the Aorta
Acute dissection of the aorta is usually associated with excruciating pain. The pain is usually located in the anterior portion of the chest, lasts for hours, and is frequently of maximal intensity at the onset. More than the usual amount of opiates may be needed for relief. This pain tends to radiate into the thoracic portion of the back more often than the pain of myocardial infarction, and it may be felt predominately in the back. It is not aggravated by deep breathing or turning. It may be located in the abdomen if the arteries of the abdominal viscera are involved. Occasionally, the pain seems to shift from one area in the chest to a lower portion as the dissection progresses.

The other diagnostic markers of aortic dissection are discussed in Chap. 62.

Pain Due to Aortic Aneurysm
A thoracic aortic aneurysm may erode a vertebral body and produce constant severe pain (Chap. 62).

Pain Due to Acute Pericarditis
The pain of acute pericarditis is not related to effort but is usually aggravated by deep breathing at the very beginning of the illness. It is often described as feeling "sharp." It is usually located in the precordial area and may radiate to the upper portion of the shoulders or sides of the neck. The patient tends to avoid deep breaths or even normal respiration because of the intense aggravation of the discomfort associated with this activity. Turning the body from side to side may aggravate the pain, as may swallowing. Leaning forward may occasionally relieve the discomfort. The absence of a pericardial friction rub does not exclude pericarditis.

The other diagnostic markers of pericarditis are discussed in Chap. 58.

Pain Due to Pulmonary Emboli
The majority of small pulmonary emboli produce no chest pain. In fact, the patient may not identify any symptoms that are directly due to pulmonary emboli. This is why the majority of emboli are not diagnosed. The pain of pulmonary embolism may, at times, be similar to that of myocardial ischemia. Acute distressing dyspnea may be the only clue to pulmonary embolism. The diagnosis is frequently based on circumstantial evidence. When pulmonary infarction develops, pleuritis may be identified. The pain in such cases is located in the lateral portion of the chest and is aggravated by breathing.

The other diagnostic markers of pulmonary emboli are discussed in Chap. 52.

Chest Pain Related to Pulmonary Hypertension
The chest pain associated with pulmonary hypertension may simulate angina pectoris and occurs, most often, in patients with mitral stenosis or Eisenmenger's syndrome. The pain has been thought to be due to dilatation of the pulmonary artery, but we believe it is due to right ventricular myocardial ischemia.

Chest Discomfort Due to Noncardiovascular Causes
The most common cause of chest pain is not related to cardiovascular disease but is associated with *anxiety*. The discomfort is usually located in the left inframammary region and rarely radiates to other locations. The pain does not occur during effort but may occur after effort. It is not aggravated by breathing but is associated with other signs of anxiety such as periodic deep-sighing respiration, hyperventilation, sinus tachycardia, fatigue, and a fear of "closed in" places. The discomfort may be characterized as a series of short sticks and stabs lasting no longer than it takes to snap one's fingers, or it may be a dull ache lasting for hours to days at a time. This type of discomfort may be disabling to patients and may consume their every thought. The discomfort may also be located in the retrosternal area and anterior chest region (Chap. 45). The discomfort may be so similar to myocardial ischemia that it is not possible to separate the two conditions without a coronary arteriogram.

Since angina pectoris and the discomfort associated with anxiety may—and frequently do—coexist, great care and skill are needed to clarify such problems. The medical history offers the major diagnostic clues in such a situation because the patient's major complaints may be due to anxiety even if obstructive coronary disease is found on coronary arteriography.

The chest discomfort of anxiety is discussed in detail in Chap. 78.

The chest pain associated with the *shoulder-hand syndrome; esophageal rupture; esophageal spasm; esophageal reflux; diseases of the spine, shoulder girdle, pleura, lung,* and *mediastinum* (including *mediastinal emphysema*); *stomach and duodenal disorders; gallbladder disease; thrombophlebitis of the chest wall; herpes zoster;* and *other chest wall syndromes* must be considered in the differential diagnosis.

These conditions and others are discussed in Chap. 45.

Pain in the Extremities

Intermittent claudication of the lower extremities due to peripheral atherosclerosis is frequently overlooked because the physician demands that the discomfort be localized in the calf of the leg. Whenever discomfort develops in the arch of the foot, calf of the leg, thighs, hips, or gluteal region during effort, then peripheral arterial vascular disease must be considered.

The symptoms associated with acute arterial occlusion of the lower extremities may at the onset be no more than the effects of hypesthesia (interpreted by the patient as "the leg going to sleep").

Intermittent claudication of the upper extremities and masseter muscle may occur. This symptom is usually due to a nonatherosclerotic cause of arterial disease such as arteritis.

These symptoms and others related to arterial and venous diseases of the extremities are discussed in Chap. 63.

Head Pain

The pain of myocardial ischemia may be felt in the jaw, hard palate, cheek, and rarely even deep in the ear canal.

The pain of temporal arteritis may be localized to the temporal region and be associated with visual difficulty and polymyalgia rheumatica.

Migraine headache is vascular in origin and may be quite severe. Nausea, scotoma, and intolerance to light are commonly present.

Hypertension does not usually produce headache, but severe headache may occur in patients with severe hypertension (diastolic pressure above 140).

Pain in the Abdomen

The pain due to an expanding or rupturing atherosclerotic abdominal aneurysm is discussed in Chap. 62.

Abdominal angina due to vascular disease of the mesenteric arteries is discussed in Chap. 65.

The pain of myocardial ischemia may be located in the upper portion of the abdomen. The same is true for pericarditis.

The liver may become painful and tender as a result of heart failure. Liver discomfort may be aggravated by effort in such patients.

Dyspnea (Difficult Breathing)

Dyspnea is a very distressing symptom. The patient complains of "shortness of breath" or that he or she "can't get enough breath."

There are many causes of dyspnea. The investigation of dyspnea must include a search for the factors that precipitate and relieve dyspnea and must identify the body position associated with the complaint.

Obviously, an infant or small child does not complain of shortness of breath. Therefore, other clues to respiratory distress are required (Chap. 36). The rate of breathing is greatly increased in this age group when there is heart failure or acute lung disease. The respiratory rate of adults with heart failure is not as greatly increased as would be expected from the degree of dyspnea noted by the patient.

Dyspnea is always abnormal when it occurs at rest or when it occurs with slight activity. Dyspnea at rest but not with effort suggests an emotional cause of the shortness of breath.

Chronic dyspnea can be caused by heart failure, pulmonary disease, obesity, poor physical fitness, pleural effusions, and effort asthma.

Acute dyspnea may occur with acute pulmonary edema, hyperventilation, pneumothorax, pulmonary embolus, pneumonia, and airway obstruction.

Dyspnea on Effort

Dyspnea on effort is a common complaint. It is usually due to congestive heart failure or chronic pulmonary disease (Chaps. 23 and 53). It is necessary to establish the degree of activity required to produce dyspnea. This may be done by inquiring about the daily activity of each patient. It is useless to ask, "Do you get short of breath climbing stairs?" when the patient never climbs stairs. The patient may, however, climb a nearby hill every day. It is also valuable to determine when the patient began to notice increasing dyspnea. For example, if the patient has only recently had difficulty climbing a hill near home, the dyspnea is more likely to be due to heart failure than to lung disease. On the other hand, the dyspnea could be related to chronic lung disease, but it would then be wise to look for recent complications such as pneumothorax, atelectasis, and asymptomatic pulmonary infection in order to explain the recent increase in symptoms.

Dyspnea related to effort may be the equivalent

of angina pectoris in some patients with coronary atherosclerosis who develop transient global ischemia of the myocardium during effort.

Wheezing

When a patient complains of wheezing associated with dyspnea, he or she may have lung disease or heart disease (Chaps. 23 and 53). If the patient is an adult, especially over the age of 40, heart failure should be foremost in the mind of the physician, and this should prompt a search for other clues indicating heart disease. When the wheezing is due to heart disease, the patient is said to have cardiac asthma. If there is a history of periodic wheezing and dyspnea since childhood, then, of course, bronchial asthma and lung disease are more likely to be the cause. One must remember, however, that patients who have had bronchial asthma for many years may also develop heart disease and heart failure. When this occurs, the heart failure may precipitate more bronchial asthma, but the physician may be misled into assuming the patient's problem remains that of uncomplicated bronchial asthma. The point is that the patient who wheezes from bronchial asthma may wheeze more when he or she develops left ventricular failure. Wheezing on effort may be due to either heart failure or chronic lung disease. Wheezing due to the latter becomes apparent because the effort evokes deeper respiratory excursions.

Orthopnea

Orthopnea is a special type of dyspnea (Chap. 23). It implies that patients have less dyspnea in the sitting position as compared with the recumbent position. The patient relates that two or three pillows under the head are required in order to have a restful night. This symptom is often associated with congestive heart failure but may also be associated with severe chronic lung disease. The fatigue associated with the exertion of breathing seems to be less when the dyspnea is due to chronic pulmonary disease than when it is due to heart failure.

Paroxysmal Nocturnal Dyspnea

Paroxysmal nocturnal dyspnea is a very important variety of shortness of breath (Chap. 23). The predictive value of this symptom as a sign of heart failure is excellent but not perfect. Characteristically, patients have little difficulty falling asleep in the recumbent position. One or two hours later they are awakened from sleep with acute shortness of breath. They seek relief by sitting upright, perhaps on the side of the bed, or even in a chair. They occasionally go to the open window searching for air. After a time, they become comfortable and return to bed. They may then sleep comfortably the remainder of the night. The only other causes for this unusual

sequence of events are pulmonary emboli and the hyperventilation syndrome due to anxiety. It would be most unusual for pulmonary emboli to occur for very many nights at the same hour. The hyperventilation syndrome due to anxiety is not so clearly relieved by sitting up and is associated with other signs suggesting this syndrome, such as tingling of the arms and hands and other evidence of anxiety.

Acute Pulmonary Edema

Acute pulmonary edema is usually due to disease of the left ventricle or to mitral valve disease (Chap. 23). The patient experiences the sudden development of dyspnea and cough and may produce frothy, blood-tinged sputum. The symptom may occur without previous warning, as in myocardial infarction, or it may be preceded by dyspnea on effort or cardiac asthma.

Cheyne-Stokes Breathing

Cheyne-Stokes breathing is characterized by periods of hyperpnea which alternate with periods of apnea. This type of breathing usually occurs in older patients with heart failure (Chap. 23). Patients with Cheyne-Stokes respiration usually have cerebral vascular disease, and the heart disease is on the left side of the heart. Patients with Cheyne-Stokes respiration rarely complain of dyspnea, perhaps because they are so sick. They are occasionally aware of acute shortness of breath during the hyperpneic phase of the cycle. The type of breathing associated with the hypoventilation syndrome of obesity, or the Pickwickian syndrome, may be periodic in nature but is not identical with Cheyne-Stokes breathing. Cheyne-Stokes respiration rarely occurs in children or in patients with cor pulmonale.

Dyspnea Due to Pulmonary Embolism

The sudden dyspnea of acute pulmonary embolism may be profound and is often the only symptom associated with this sneaky, catastrophic event. This condition should be suspected when sudden dyspnea occurs during the postsurgical or postpartum period or in a patient who has heart failure (Chap. 52).

Dyspnea Due to Anxiety

Dyspnea due to anxiety, a common cause of breathing difficulty, has no relation to heart disease but is often, by patient and physician alike, mistakenly thought to be due to heart disease (see Chap. 45). The shortness of breath associated with anxiety assumes two forms (Chap. 78), both of which may be terrifying to patients. They may simply feel as though the air "does no good," or "does not go down far enough"; or they may say that they "can't get a good satisfying breath." Normal breathing is interrupted by deep sighs. Some patients experience an element of claustrophobia. Fatigue, palpitation, and precordial "aching" or "sticks" may also be present. The patient may develop prolonged periods of hyperventilation which are frequently associated with numbness of the arms, hands, and lips; tetany; and an unreal sensation. This type of dyspnea can occur in patients who also have pulmonary or heart disease, thereby testing the diagnostic acumen of the physician.

Dyspnea Due to Hypoxia

The dyspnea associated with congenital heart disease with right-to-left shunt is related to hypoxia (Chap. 36). The dyspnea is usually related to effort, but the young child may have episodes of breathlessness and increased cyanosis. The child may become unconscious during the terrifying episodes (Chap. 36).

Severe anemia may be the sole cause of dyspnea on effort and is a frequent contributing factor (Chap. 26).

Methemoglobinemia may also be responsible for dyspnea on effort and, like anemia, may be a contributing factor.

Dyspnea Due to Thyrotoxicosis

The dyspnea of thyrotoxicosis is due to an increase in the body's need for oxygen and associated myopathy.

The "Dyspnea" of Pregnancy and Acidosis

The full-term pregnant female may "huff and puff" with effort but has a curious reaction to the audible respiratory effort. She seems quite conscious of her labored breathing but is rarely, if ever, alarmed by it (Chap. 67). Accordingly, she is not truly dyspneic.

Patients with compensatory hyperpnea associated with metabolic acidosis due to diabetes mellitus or uremia rarely complain of true dyspnea.

Cough

A dry, nonproductive cough may be related to the pulmonary congestion associated with heart failure. It may develop with effort but may also occur at rest. Although dyspnea is usually present, cough may dominate the clinical picture.

The cough which accompanies pulmonary edema is often associated with frothy, pink-tinged sputum, while the sputum of chronic bronchitis is usually white and mucoid. The sputum of pneumonia is often thick and yellow. The sputum of pulmonary infarct may be bloody, as may the sputum of cancer of the lung or bronchiectasis.

Palpitation (Throbbing)

The term *palpitation* is used by patients to describe a disagreeable awareness of the heartbeat. The patient may use some other term and report a "pounding," "stopping," "jumping," or "racing" in the chest. A parent may observe an abnormal heart rhythm when looking at or feeling a child's precordium.

The sensitivity of the nervous system determines whether the patient complains of palpitation. The complaint is not directly related to the seriousness of the heart disease or to the exact type of arrhythmia. For example, one patient may feel every premature contraction when there is no evidence of heart disease while another patient may not detect ventricular tachycardia associated with serious heart disease.

When a patient feels a premature cardiac contraction, he or she rarely feels the early beat which has occurred out of cadence and usually feels the subsequent beat which is associated with an overfilled heart and large stroke volume. On rare occasions a patient may be aware of his or her heartbeat after digitalis medication has been given because of the increased force of contraction induced by the drug. When this occurs, ectopic beats due to digitalis intoxication may also be noted by the patient. A patient may be aware of a cardiac arrhythmia by detecting an uncomfortable sensation in the neck. This is probably due to distension of the neck veins when the right atrium contracts against a closed tricuspid valve.

Patients may complain when the heartbeat is slow or fast and when the heartbeat is regular or irregular. The patient may detect whether the onset and offset of the rapid beat is abrupt or gradual. The patient may complain of forceful, regular heartbeats. Conditions associated with an increased stroke output may produce a feeling of forceful contraction of the heart. The best example of this is perhaps found in patients with aortic regurgitation. Ectopic beats, atrial fibrillation, and other arrhythmias are perhaps more troublesome to patients with aortic regurgitation because in such cases the variations of the stroke output are so radically different from normal.

Patients may complain of palpitation of the heart when the rhythm and rate are entirely normal or when the regular cadence of the rhythm is interrupted by ectopic contractions, paroxysmal rapid heartbeat, or extreme bradycardia, including complete heart block. The rhythm responsible for the palpitation may not be present when the patient is seen. Accordingly, it is valuable for the physician to have the patient mimic normal heart action with the finger and then request that the patient simulate the event responsible for the palpitation. At times, the patient will give a dramatic reproduction of an ectopic beat or paroxysmal atrial tachycardia.

It is useful to ask if anyone counted the patient's pulse during an episode of tachycardia. The heart rate of 150 beats per minute suggests atrial flutter or sinus tachycardia. A heart rate of 180 suggests atrial tachycardia. The patient may know if the Valsalva maneuver aborted an attack of regular tachycardia. The patient may give a history of an increased urine output during atrial tachycardia, atrial fibrillation, and flutter.

The recognition of cardiac arrhythmias is discussed in Chaps. 19, 28, and 88.

Syncope

Syncope is defined as the transient loss of consciousness as a result of an inadequate cerebral blood flow (Chap. 30). *Near syncope* may be applied to the clinical situation in which the patient feels dizzy, feels weak, and tends to lose postural tone but does not lose consciousness. Although epilepsy may produce similar symptoms, cerebral vascular disease is a more common problem in differential diagnosis.

Although some patients seek medical advice because of frequent episodes of syncope, many others do not give such a history spontaneously. In such cases the patient has either forgotten the episodes or has been unaware of their occurrence. Also it is not uncommon for the physician to forget to inquire about the occurrence of syncope while interviewing the patient and the family. When a patient gives a definite history of one episode of syncope, it is wise to assume that more than one episode has occurred.

Syncope may occur in many types of heart disease and circulatory states, including atherosclerotic coronary heart disease, aortic stenosis, aortic regurgitation, mitral stenosis, idiopathic hypertrophic cardiomyopathy, left atrial tumor, primary pulmonary hypertension, pulmonary arteriolar disease secondary to left-to-right shunts, pulmonary stenosis, tetralogy of Fallot, paroxysmal rapid heartbeat, sinus arrest ("sick-sinus" syndrome), ventricular standstill or fibrillation related to atrioventricular block (Adams-Stokes attacks due to coronary atherosclerosis or perhaps more commonly Lev's disease or Lenègre's disease), carotid sinus syncope, cough syncope, micturition syncope, vagovagal syncope, vasodepressor syncope, acute blood loss, pulmonary embolism, etc. (Chaps. 28, 30, 38, 45, 56, and 60).

Other Symptoms That Worry Patients

Patients may hear or feel several worrisome cardiovascular events other than palpitation. (See later discussion.) Patients with severe tricuspid regurgitation may feel the expanding venous pulse in the neck. Some feel the pulse wave hit the ear, and others note that their collar is "too tight" when the heart beats. Patients may complain of recurring single or double sounds in the head that are synchronous with the heartbeat. These sounds are usually heard at night; the cause is not known. Patients with aortic regurgitation may feel a throbbing sensation in the neck. Benign venous hums may cause a distracting noise in the ear. Patients may hear their own intracerebral arteriovenous malformation or fistula.

History of "Swelling of the Legs," Weight Gain, or Enlarging Girth

Edema may be found on physical examination, although the patient may be unaware of its existence (Chaps. 14 and 23). On the other hand, there may be a history of "swelling," and edema may not be found at the time of examination.

Ages ago generalized edema was required before a diagnosis of heart failure could be made. Although this extreme degree of edema is not required to establish the diagnosis of heart failure today, it is unfortunate that many physicians still demand the presence of at least some edema before seriously considering the diagnosis of congestive heart failure. Of course, patients are seen today with considerable peripheral edema due to heart failure, but it must be stated emphatically that edema is a late sign of congestive heart failure. Many other subtle signs of heart failure are usually present before the appearance of edema.

Considerable weight gain due to retention of extracellular fluid may occur without associated edema. This may, at times, be as much as 10 to 15 lb. On the other hand, there are numerous causes of edema other than congestive heart failure, and its presence is not diagnostic of congestive heart failure. If the diagnosis of heart failure is delayed until edema develops or if heart failure is diagnosed simply because edema is present, then the approach to the problem is clearly superficial.

Local factors play a major role in determining the distribution of fluid in the body. Pulmonary edema due to mitral stenosis provides a good illustration of the importance of local factors. When ventricular diastole is shortened to a critical point, pulmonary edema develops because the right ventricle continues to pump more blood into the lungs than can pass the stenosed mitral valve. Under these circumstances there will be no weight gain or peripheral edema. The body fluid has simply been redistributed and it accumulates in the lungs. The patient with chronic congestive heart failure who has gained weight because of retention of sodium and water secondary to altered renal function may detect edema of the ankles and lower legs during the day and note that it subsides during the night. This occurs because of local hydrostatic factors which are related to the upright position.

It is important to ascertain whether edema of the extremities preceded or followed dyspnea on effort. Although there are many exceptions, the edema due to poor function of the left ventricle, mitral stenosis, or cor pulmonale is usually preceded by dyspnea.

Edema may be due to hypoproteinemia such as occurs in nephrosis and starvation. As with heart failure, the edema may occur in the dependent portion of the body. Such edema usually occurs when the total blood protein is below 5 g/dl.

Edema of one leg is usually due to local factors such as varicose veins, thrombophlebitis, or lymphedema. When there is bilateral leg edema due to heart failure, there may be more on one side than the other if a local factor is also present. Edema may shift from the extremities to the sacral region when a patient is confined to bed.

Periorbital edema is more common in children than in adults. Although this finding on history of physical examination is more often due to renal disease, it also occurs in heart failure. It simply indicates that salt and water have been retained and that the tissue pressure around the eyes of the child is low. Rare causes include trichinosis and superior vena caval obstruction.

Ascites may be recognized by the patient as an increase in girth or swelling of the abdomen. Ascites due to congestive heart failure is not common today and invariably follows peripheral edema. A local factor, such as cirrhosis, is also suggested when ascites, associated with heart failure, seems to be out of proportion to peripheral edema. Constrictive pericarditis should also be thought of in this setting. Heart failure due to restrictive cardiomyopathy produces ascites out of proportion to lower-extremity edema. The distribution of extracellular fluid is somewhat different in the child with heart failure as compared with the adult. The child with heart failure forms ascites more readily than does the adult.

Hemoptysis (Coughing Up Blood)

When a patient gives a history of "coughing blood," it is necessary to ascertain the exact nature of the sputum. When a patient is seen during such an episode, the sputum must be examined grossly and microscopically as part of the examination of the patient.

It is useful to determine whether the material that is coughed up contains large volumes of liquid blood (hemoptysis), which indicates brisk bleeding, or whether it contains smaller quantities of dark or clotted blood, which would indicate slow bleeding from low-pressure vessels or subsiding bleeding. Brisk bleeding, for example, is commonly associated with specific focal ulceration of the bronchus, such as bronchogenic carcinoma, a foreign body, bronchiectasis, or a bleeding aortic aneurysm. Slow bleeding strongly suggests venous bleeding and is more likely to be the result of increased pulmonary vascular resistance, with secondary increase in flow

through the bronchial venous system such as may occur as a result of mitral stenosis or bronchiectasis.

It is also helpful to notice whether the expectorated blood is intimately mixed (blood-streaked sputum) with sputum or pus, because this is a valuable clue to the possible site of the origin of the bleeding. Intimate mixtures of blood and pus are eloquent signs pointing to a deep-seated site of pulmonary suppuration.

At times, posterior epistaxis associated with systemic hypertension may cause blood-streaked sputum. On rare occasions localized disease of the nose may give a similar clinical picture. As a rule, however, epistaxis is obvious and is not usually confused with bloody sputum.

Pink, frothy sputum is frequently associated with acute pulmonary edema. Blood-streaked sputum may occur with acute pulmonary congestion when the classic findings of acute pulmonary edema are not fully developed. The blood comes from pulmonary capillaries which have ruptured under high intravascular pressure.

Hemoptysis may be due to pulmonary tuberculosis, pneumonia, bronchiectasis, bronchogenic carcinoma, primary pulmonary hemosiderosis, Osler-Rendu-Weber disease with a pulmonary arteriovenous aneurysm, and necrotic pulmonary arterial lesions due to periarteritis nodosa and lupus erythematosus. Four cardiovascular conditions must never be overlooked as causes of hemoptysis. They are mitral stenosis, pulmonary infarction, Eisenmenger physiology, and aortic aneurysm.

Mitral Stenosis

Hemoptysis due to mitral stenosis is frequently induced by physical exercise, sexual intercourse, or marked excitement. It may be the first symptom of mitral stenosis and may occur during pregnancy. The blood comes from a break in the pulmonary veins which have ruptured under very high pressure. The bleeding is due to rupture of endobronchial vessels that form collateral channels between the bronchial veins and pulmonary venous system. Episodes of pulmonary hemorrhage of this type tend to subside as the veins adapt to the high pressure and as pulmonary arteriolar disease develops (Chap. 39).

Pulmonary Infarction

Many pulmonary emboli do not lead to pulmonary infarction, but when they do, frank hemoptysis occurs in the minority of instances. Despite this, when hemoptysis occurs in a patient with heart failure, pulmonary infarction is likely. The bloody sputum usually appears from a few hours to a day after the embolus and is due to necrosis and hemorrhage into the alveoli (Chap. 52).

Eisenmenger Physiology

Patients with severe pulmonary hypertension associated with an interventricular septal defect or patent ductus arteriosus may have hemoptysis presumably secondary to rupture of pulmonary capillaries (Chap. 36).

Aortic Aneurysms

An aortic aneurysm may rupture into the tracheobronchial tree and produce lethal hemoptysis. Aneurysms due to syphilis, atherosclerosis, and dissection may cause this catastrophic event (Chap. 62).

Fatigue and Weakness

There are many causes of fatigue and weakness, and therefore these symptoms are not specific for heart disease. The most common cause of these symptoms is anxiety and increased emotional tension. Anemia and other chronic disease states may be associated with fatigue and weakness. The least common cause is Addison's disease.

When a patient with heart disease is waterlogged or when there is pulmonary congestion due to heart disease, the patient is likely to complain of dyspnea. Now, with modern therapy, these complaints may be supplanted by the feeling of fatigue and weakness. The actual physiologic mechanism of the fatigue associated with heart failure is not known, but it is probably related to an inadequate cardiac output (Chaps. 22 and 23). The heart fails in its prime objective of nourishing all the tissues and organs of the body, including the skeletal muscles. Potassium depletion due to the use of diuretics without adequate potassium may be the cause of weakness.

A patient may experience exhaustion related to effort as a manifestation of transient global myocardial ischemia due to atherosclerotic coronary heart disease (Chap. 45). Dyspnea and hypotension may also occur at the time such a patient detects the exhaustion. The complaint of exhaustion may occur before, during, or following myocardial infarction (Chap. 45).

A patient may feel weak after massive diuresis. In this case the symptom relates to potassium depletion, altered blood volume, and postural hypotension (Chap. 23). Patients on antihypertensive therapy may complain of weakness because of postural hypotension.

Fatigue and weakness may be due to anxiety rather than to heart disease. As a rule, the fatigue due to heart disease is related to effort, whereas the fatigue of anxiety occurs continuously.

A History of Cyanosis

Patients or their family members may detect cyanosis of the lips and relate their observation to the physician. Four grams per deciliter of reduced hemoglobin are needed for cyanosis to occur. Arterial oxygen saturation must be about 85 percent or less for cyanosis to develop. Cyanosis cannot occur when the hemoglobin is less than 33 percent of normal since reduced hemoglobin cannot be produced in an amount sufficient to cause the bluish color. When the hemoglobin is normal, about one-third of it must be in the reduced form for the bluish color to appear. Accordingly, family members cannot detect minor degrees of cyanosis. Physicians have the same problem. This explains why errors are made when congenital heart disease is divided into cyanotic and noncyanotic groups. Such a division may be useful when cyanosis is definitely present, but lesser degrees of arterial oxygen unsaturation are not recognized with regularity.

A bluish tint to the skin may not be due to a right-to-left shunt or pulmonary disease; it may be due to argyria or methemoglobinemia.

Cyanosis in the patient with chronic congestive heart failure should suggest the possibility of associated pulmonary embolism.

The patient or a family member may detect that the cyanosis is more intense in the feet than the hands (Chap. 36). This suggests a right-to-left shunt through the patent ductus arteriosus. Cyanosis may be associated with clubbing of the fingers (Chap. 36).

Cyanosis will be discussed more fully in the chapters dealing with congenital heart disease (Chap. 36), congestive heart failure (Chap. 23), and cor pulmonale (Chap. 53).

Squatting

Young children with tetralogy of Fallot learn that their dyspnea is relieved when they squat. Squatting increases peripheral arterial resistance, which decreases the right-to-left shunt and increases pulmonary blood flow. This compensatory mechanism does not occur when such a patient is submerged in water (Chap. 36).

Recurrent Bronchitis and Pulmonary Infection

Recurrent cough due to heart failure is often thought to be due to bronchitis. Patients with chronic bronchitis may have more cough when heart failure ensues. Patients with increased blood flow to the lungs as a result of left-to-right shunts are subject to severe attacks of pulmonary infection. Patients with high pulmonary venous pressure are more prone to the development of pulmonary edema when they have viral pneumonitis than are patients with normal pulmonary venous pressure. This is especially true in patients with mitral stenosis. The high pulmonary venous pressure plus injury to the alveolar wall by the virus increases the transudation of fluid into the alveoli.

Insomnia

There are many causes of insomnia. Although heart failure may cause insomnia, the most common causes are mental conflict, emotional disturbances, and depression. The patient with Cheyne-Stokes respiration may sleep during the apneic phase and wake during the hyperpneic phase of the condition. Patients with pulmonary congestion due to heart failure as a result of disease of the left ventricle or mitral stenosis may have insomnia before they detect nocturnal dyspnea.

Cerebral Symptoms

Patients may have dizziness, near syncope, and syncope, as discussed under "Syncope," earlier in this chapter.

Patients with decreased cardiac output secondary to heart failure may become mentally confused and disoriented. This may be due to hypoxia, drugs that are invariably prescribed for such patients, or renal or hepatic failure.

Patients may have the symptoms and signs associated with a transient ischemic attack of the brain; a cerebral vascular accident due to lacunar infarcts; cerebral hemorrhage; a cerebral embolus from an atheromatous ulcer in the carotid system, infective endocarditis, recent myocardial infarction, atrial fibrillation with or without mitral stenosis, or clots on a prosthetic valve.

Convulsions rarely occur as a result of heart disease. Convulsions may be related to cardiac standstill when unilateral intracranial disease or unilateral carotid disease makes localizing signs possible.

Coma rarely occurs as a result of heart disease. The patient in shock or the patient with violent tachycardia who also has considerable intracranial or extracranial vascular disease may have such severe cerebral hypoxia that coma occurs. Hypoxic coma may follow cardiac resuscitation.

The History of Hoarseness

Hoarseness is usually unrelated to cardiovascular disease. It can occur in patients with an aortic aneurysm that involves the left recurrent laryngeal nerve. Mitral stenosis may occasionally produce hoarseness, but this is rarely seen today since mitral stenosis is usually corrected surgically before it produces such a symptom. The hoarseness in such patients is due to the pressure of a large pulmonary artery or left atrium on the recurrent laryngeal nerve.

Pericardial effusion may be related to myxedema, which may produce a coarse, low-pitched voice. A woman with myxedema may be disturbed when her voice is mistaken for a man's voice, especially on the telephone.

Hoarseness and loss of voice may occur following the use of an endotracheal tube during cardiac surgery.

The History of Epistaxis

Severe nosebleed may occur in patients with hypertension. This disturbs the patient a great deal. This can, on rare occasions, be so severe as to place the life of a patient in danger because of exsanguination. Epistaxis was once said to occur in acute rheumatic fever, but this is rarely seen in the United States today. Trauma is the most common cause of nosebleed.

Anorexia, Nausea, and Vomiting

Nausea and vomiting are often due to digitalis in patients with heart disease. Patients with myocardial infarction may complain of nausea and exhibit vomiting, but opiates may, and often do, cause the symptoms in such patients. Patients with heart failure may have anorexia and nausea without any other apparent cause.

Indigestion

Many patients with angina pectoris due to coronary atherosclerosis attribute their symptoms to "indigestion" or "heartburn," while patients with heartburn, esophageal reflux, and esophageal spasm often believe they have angina pectoris (Chap. 45).

Hiccups

Hiccups may occur in patients with myocardial infarction and are not rare during the postoperative period after cardiac surgery.

Jaundice

Jaundice may be detected by the patient or a member of the family. As a rule, hepatic congestion due to heart failure will not produce jaundice. When jaundice does occur in a patient with heart failure, it is appropriate to consider pulmonary infarction in addition to the hepatic congestion or cirrhosis of the liver. The hemolysis of red cells may occur in patients with prosthetic valves, and this may produce jaundice. On rare occasion hemolytic anemia and jaundice may be caused by severe aortic valve stenosis.

Weight Loss, Malnutrition, and Cachexia

Patients with long-standing heart failure may give a history of poor appetite and weight loss. Therefore, caloric, protein, and vitamin malnutrition may occur.

Urinary Symptoms

Patients with chronic heart failure may note oliguria during the day and polyuria at night. Men with borderline urinary tract obstruction due to enlargement of the prostate may have more difficulty voiding when heart failure ensues, and this in turn may make the heart failure worse. Polyuria may occur during atrial tachycardia, atrial fibrillation, or flutter.

Fever and Chills

Patients with rheumatic fever do not have chills unless aspirin has been used for treatment. Chills are common in patients with bacterial endocarditis. Fever may also be due to pericarditis. Myalgia, chills, and fever may, on very rare occasions, be related to myocardial infarction presumably due to some form of autoimmune response to necrotic myocardial tissue.

It is important to inquire whether there has been any recent dental work (including cleaning) in patients with heart murmurs and fever, since this may be a clue to the diagnosis of endocarditis.

Noises Heard by the Patient

A loud heart murmur may be heard by a patient or a member of the family. For example, the murmur of interventricular septal defect is often heard by the patient. A patient may hear the murmur associated with retroversion of an aortic valve cusp or rupture of the chordae tendineae of the mitral valve. Some noises from the chest can even be heard at a considerable distance. It is not uncommon for an individual to become aware of his or her heartbeat by hearing arterial bruits or heart sounds when the side of the head is placed on a pillow. The murmur of an arteriovenous fistula located near the ear or a cervical venous hum may be heard by the patient.

Abnormal Movements

Patients may complain that their neck veins are distended or move vigorously, and patients with aortic regurgitation may complain that their head "bobs."

When Patients Say They Have Had a Heart Attack

Many patients state that they have had a heart attack because, to them, any abrupt incident thought to be related to the heart is considered to be a heart attack. This includes prolonged myocardial ischemia, a cardiac arrhythmia, pulmonary edema, or hyperventilation. Accordingly, one should not automatically conclude that a patient had a myocardial infarction when a patient says he or she has had a heart attack.

References

1. Mackenzie, J.: "Principles of Diagnosis and Treatment in Heart Affections," Oxford Medical Publications, London, 1916, p. 48.
2. White, P. D.: "Heart Disease," The Macmillan Company, New York, 1931, pp. 4, 9.
3. Wood, P. D.: "Diseases of the Heart and Circulation," 2d ed., J. B. Lippincott Company, Philadelphia, 1957, p. 1.

8

Inspection of the Patient

Mark E. Silverman, M.D.
J. Willis Hurst, M.D.

There is no more difficult art to acquire than the art of observation.

Sir William Osler[1]

Today, just as in 1903 when Osler made the above statement, the physician may fail to appreciate the value of careful observation. This section details many of the findings that an astute diagnostician can harvest from a visual search for the presence and etiology of heart disease.

Body Configuration

In Marfan's syndrome the findings include an arm span greater than the body height, an upper segment/lower segment ratio less than 0.85, kyphoscoliosis, pectus excavatum, and pectus carinatum.[2–4] Patients with homocystinuria may also have long extremities, pectus carinatum, and kyphoscoliosis.[4] The cardiac involvement differs. Homocystinuria is associated with thrombosis of intermediate-sized arteries; while patients with Marfan's syndrome may suffer aortic, mitral, or tricuspid regurgitation, aortic dilatation or dissection, coronary artery involvement, pulmonary artery dilatation, redundant chordae tendineae, calcified mitral annulus, or aneurysms of the sinus of Valsalva or descending aorta.

Exogenous obesity presents no difficulty in recognition. Biventricular cardiac hypertrophy, arrhythmias, particularly during sleep, and increased cardiac output may be present.[5] With extreme obesity the Pickwickian syndrome may occur, with somnolence, respiratory acidosis, and cor pulmonale.

The Ellis–van Creveld syndrome is characterized by dwarfism due to short extremities. A large atrial septal defect or atrioventricular (AV) canal defect is frequent.[6] In osteogenesis imperfecta the legs are short with marked bowing, saber shins, and pseudoarthroses. Calcification of the arteries and aortic and mitral regurgitation may occur.[3,4,7]

Congenital heart disease has been noted in Klinefelter's syndrome.[8] This syndrome may be recognized because of gynecomastia, tall stature, long extremities, and eunuchoid configuration of the body.

Skin

The cream-colored plaques of xanthelasma may warn of hyperlipidemia as a cause of atheroma lining or occluding coronary arteries. Aortic stenosis may also occur.[9] Xanthoma may present as lumps over the Achilles tendons, over the knuckles, and along the tendons of the arms (Fig. 8-1A and B). The implication is also an abnormal lipid metabolism.[10] Xanthoma and a yellow hue to the skin are physical findings in Cori's disease (type III glycogenosis). This disease may involve the myocardium.[9] Infarctions of the skin, nodules, petechiae, livedo reticularis, cyanosis, and gangrenous changes in the extremities may be due to polyarteritis, which may produce myocardial infarction, congestive heart failure, and pericarditis (Fig. 8-2).[11]

The contracted smooth skin of scleroderma can give the face a tight, bony appearance and contract the fingers. Cor pulmonale secondary to pulmonary fibrosis or pulmonary artery involvement is the most common cardiac difficulty; however, myocardial fi-

FIGURE 8-1 Xanthomatosis. *A.* Large xanthomatous masses located in the Achilles tendon, associated with coronary atherosclerosis. *B.* Xanthoma around the knuckles.

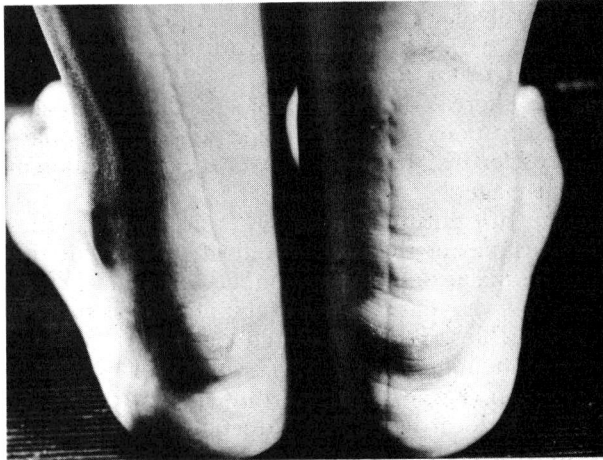

A

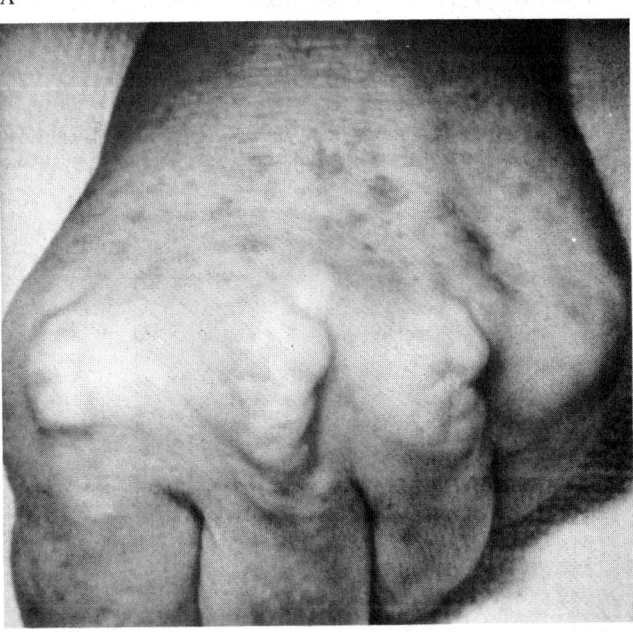

B

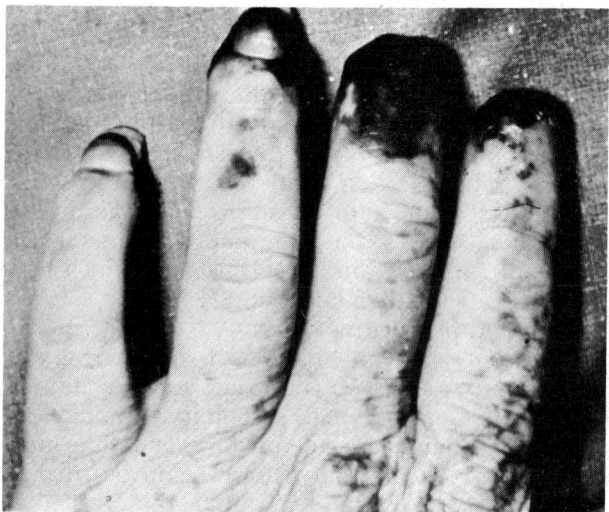

FIGURE 8-2 Polyarteritis. Distal gangrene of the fingers may be associated with coronary arteritis. *(From M. E. Silverman and J. W. Hurst.[75] Reproduced with permission of the publisher.)*

brosis, valvular thickening, and pericarditis may occur (Fig. 8-3).[12] In Werner's syndrome the skin appears atrophic and is tightly stretched over the bones. There is marked loss of subcutaneous tissue, and ulcerations occur over the legs. Severe coronary atherosclerosis often causes myocardial infarction at an early age.[13]

The presenting sign of systemic lupus erythematosus may be the typical butterfly-shaped inflammation, malar depigmentation, erythema of the fingertips, a vascular blush over the phalanges sparing the knuckles, a brownish-red palmar rash, Raynaud's phenomenon, urticaria, vitiligo, or hyperpigmentation (Fig. 8-4). Pericarditis, myocarditis, verrucous endocarditis, and conduction defects are the cardiovascular abnormalities.[14] Congenital complete heart block is now recognized as a complication in the newborn of mothers with lupus erythematosus.[15]

FIGURE 8-3 Scleroderma. Indurated, depigmented skin with flexion contractures of the fingers associated with severe systemic hypertension.

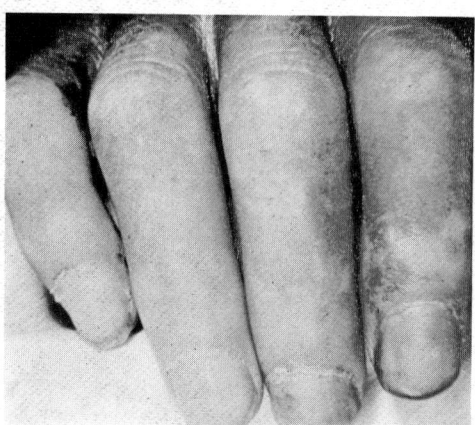

Hyperelastic, velvety skin that rebounds to its original position after being stretched, "cigarette paper" scars, and hyperextensible joints are found in the Ehler-Danlos syndrome (Fig. 8-5A and B). Mitral and tricuspid valve prolapse, dilatation of the aorta and pulmonary artery, arterial rupture, and a variety of congenital heart diseases may accompany this syndrome.[16] A progressive looseness of skin allowing pendulous folds and droopy eyelids can be due to cutis laxa, a generalized elastolysis which can cause aortic dilatation and rupture, congestive heart failure, and cor pulmonale.[17]

Tuberous sclerosis can reveal itself by subungual fibromas of the fingers, café au lait spots, subcutaneous nodules, and a scattering of yellow-brown angiofibromas on the face (Plate 3A).[18] Rhabdomyomas are found in the heart and may cause heart failure, obstruction, or arrhythmia. Café au lait spots have been seen in association with pheochromocytoma, renal artery stenosis, and pulmonic valve stenosis. Sweating is an important sign of congestive heart failure in an infant, as well as a clue to a pheochromocytoma in an adult.

In hemochromatosis the skin may develop a speckled, bronze, or slate-gray coloration. Myocardial or pericardial infiltration with iron deposits may cause arrhythmias, restrictive cardiomyopathy, congestive heart failure, or pericarditis.[9,19]

The rash of dermatomyositis is scaly and red, and is often localized over the joints of the fingers. The

FIGURE 8-4 Systemic lupus erythematosus. Butterfly rash. Associated with pericardial, myocardial, and endocardial disease. *(From M. E. Silverman and J. W. Hurst.[75] Reproduced with permission of the publisher.)*

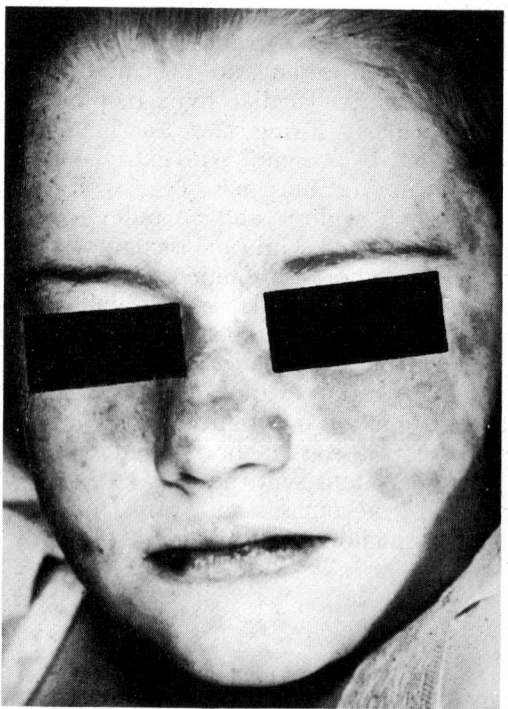

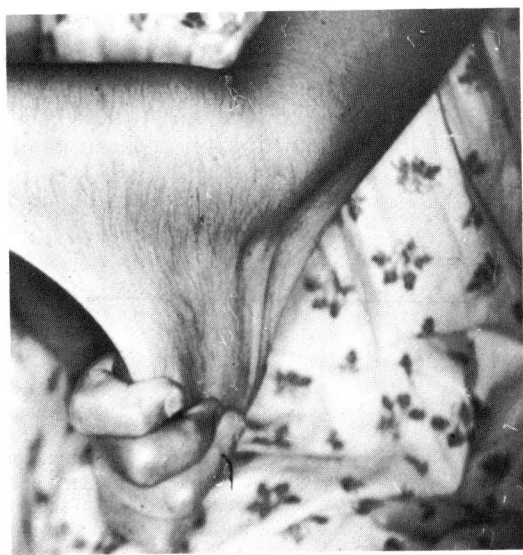

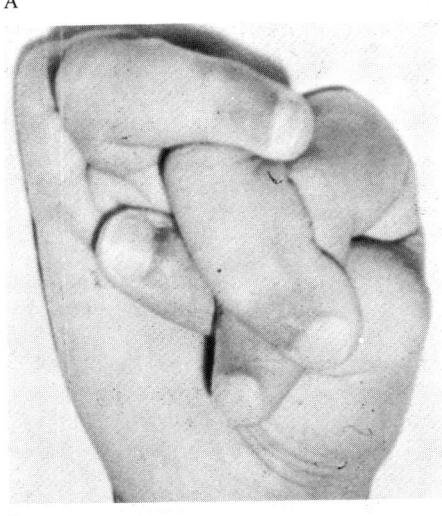

FIGURE 8-5   Ehlers-Danlos syndrome. *A.* Hyperextensible skin. *B.* Lax joints. Redundant chordae tendineae and arterial rupture may occur.

ened. Angina pectoris and claudication are frequent symptoms.[4,22]

Elevated, waxy nodules of the skin and eyelids that may become hemorrhagic when stroked may be associated with conduction abnormalities or myocardial disease due to amyloidosis.[23]

Degos' disease (malignant atrophic papulosis) is announced by a crop of asymptomatic, oval cutaneous lesions which have a white center and surrounding erythema. Occlusive fibrosis of small- and medium-sized arteries causing pleuritis and pericarditis is part of this rapidly fatal problem.[24]

Vitiligo, typically on the palms and soles, is a sign of Graves' disease.

Extensive skin lesions, particularly Kaposi's sarcoma or exfoliative dermatitis due to psoriasis, may divert enough of the vascular supply through shunts in the skin to produce high-output cardiac failure.[25] Hemangiomas of the skin may also signify multinodular hemangiomatosis of the liver, a cause of high-output congestive heart failure in infancy. An underlying arteriovenous fistula with high-output failure may be evidenced only by a barely discernible scar or by a surgical incision (Fig. 8-7). Port wine stains, hemangioma of the skin, and varicose veins may be accompanied by asymmetric lengthening and overgrowth of an extremity or digit as a result of congenital peripheral arteriovenous fistulas (Fig. 8-8A and B).[26]

Telangiectasia of the fingertips, lips, and tongue and pulmonary and hepatic arteriovenous fistulas are associated with hereditary hemorrhagic telangiectasia (HHT).[27] (See Plate 3C and D.)

The skin involvement in sarcoidosis may include lupus pernio, erythema nodosum, plaques, pigmentary changes, subcutaneous nodules, and alopecia. Cardiac involvement may be present but is usually silent. On occasion, however, arrhythmias, altered conduction, congestive heart failure, and sudden death can occur.[28]

Erythema marginatum, a migratory, annular eruption, and subcutaneous nodules may herald the

eyelids may be decorated by a lavender discoloration (Plate 3B). Pericarditis, heart block, and myocardial disease are the cardiac findings.[20]

Intense flushing episodes, a chronic reddish cyanotic hue, and telangiectasia of the face are part of the dramatic presentation of the carcinoid syndrome. The usual cardiac lesions are a combination of stenosis and regurgitation of the tricuspid and pulmonary valves; however, with a patent ductus arteriosus, lung metastases, or a patent foramen ovale, lesions can also occur on the left side of the heart.[21]

The skin in pseudoxanthoma elasticum is thickened, lax, and yellowish, particularly over the axillary folds, antecubital area, and neck (Fig. 8-6). The skin around the mouth may sag. The arteries may be calcified, and the aortic and mitral valves thick-

FIGURE 8-6   Pseudoxanthoma elasticum. Grooved, lax skin in a typical location. Arterial calcification may occur.

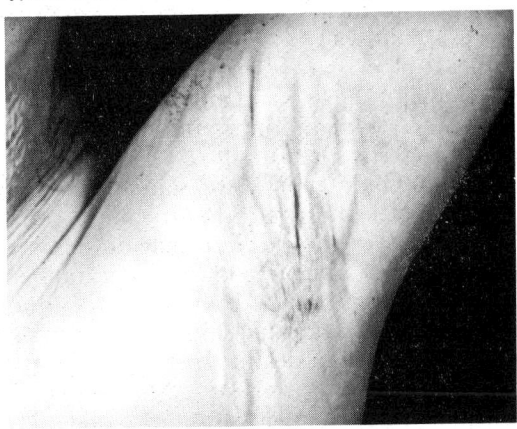

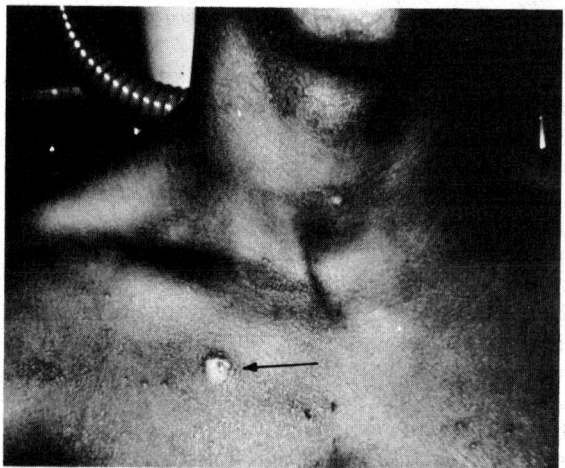

FIGURE 8-7 Bullet wound (arrow). High-output cardiac failure due to a brachiocephalic-artery–to–brachiocephalic-vein fistula.

appearance of acute rheumatic fever. Pericarditis, myocarditis, and valvular inflammation are the well-known cardiac possibilities. An expanding skin rash, erythema chronicum migrans, precedes the joint involvement and possible AV block or bundle branch block that is seen in Lyme arthritis.[29]

The multiple lentigines syndrome, consisting of small dark-brown macular lesions of varying size on the neck and trunk, has been associated with abnormal electrocardiographic conduction, T-wave changes, pulmonic stenosis, hypertrophic subaortic stenosis, and a leftward or superior mean QRS axis (Fig. 8-9).[30]

The purplish, pinpoint angiokeratomata of Fabry's disease are present on the mucous membrane surface of the lip and on the trunk. Involvement of the myocardium and blood vessels with glycolipid deposits is common and results in angina pectoris, myocardial infarction, mitral regurgitation, congestive heart failure, and arrhythmias.[9,31]

The skin lesion known as *keratosis blennorrhagica* is almost pathognomonic for Reiter's syndrome. This rash begins as erythematous macules progressing to hyperkeratotic papules which coalesce and crust over the palms and soles. Arthritis, conjunctivitis, iritis, and urethritis complete the clinical presentation. Pericarditis, myocarditis, aortic regurgitation, and heart block may be sequelae.[31a]

Pitting edema of the legs and engorgement of the neck veins are two of the most familiar changes wrought by congestive heart failure.

Urochrome pigmentation of the skin and uremic frost are cutaneous findings of far-advanced renal disease. Patients on chronic dialysis may develop severe atherosclerosis and metastatic calcification of the myocardium, resulting in heart failure, conduction disturbances, pericarditis, severe coronary artery disease, and sudden death.[32]

Cyanosis of the skin often suggests congenital heart disease with right-to-left shunt of blood.

Gait

An unusual gait can suggest a neuromuscular disorder that may also involve the heart.[33] An ataxic, wide-based gait associated with kyphoscoliosis, hammertoe, equinovarus, nystagmus, and oscillation of the head and trunk is seen in Friedreich's ataxia (Fig. 8-10). Heart disease is virtually always present and includes myocardial disease, angina pectoris, hypertrophic subaortic stenosis, sinus node artery

FIGURE 8-8 Congenital peripheral arteriovenous fistulas. Asymmetric enlargement of an extremity or digit associated with unusual varicose veins may occur in patients with congenital peripheral arteriovenous fistulas. A. Grotesque enlargement of the toes and foot on the right. B. Peculiar location of "masses" due to dilatation of the veins on the lateral aspect of the lower leg and on the posterior surface of the upper leg. In addition, this young female had multiple pulmonary emboli.

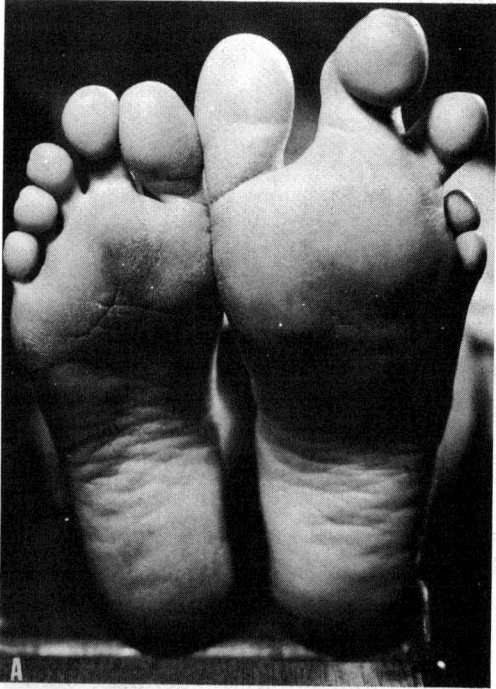

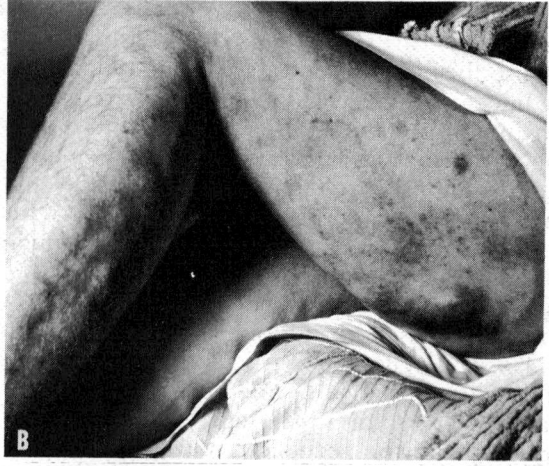

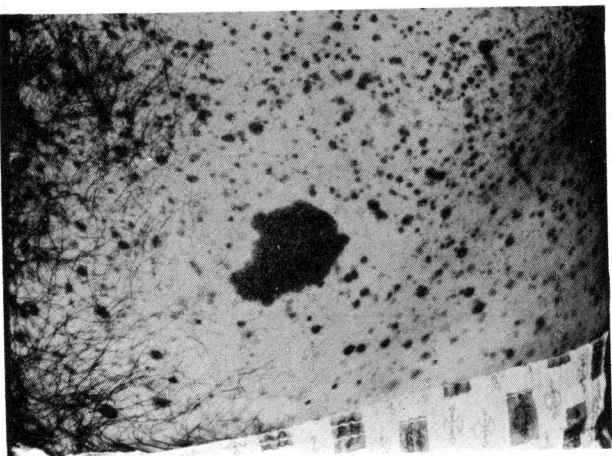

FIGURE 8-9 Multiple lentigines syndrome. Dark-brown muscular lesions on the abdomen associated with hypertrophic subaortic stenosis.

occlusion, and arrhythmias.[33,34] Refsum's disease, a lipidosis characterized by high levels of phytanic acid, associates cerebellar ataxia, night blindness, deafness, ichthyosis, cataracts, and polyneuropathy with myocardial disease and conduction abnormalities.[35] Patients with muscular dystrophy of the Duchenne type walk in a slow, waddling, awkward fashion. Myocardial disease, often diagnosable by distinctive electrocardiographic changes, tachycardia, and arrhythmias, are relatively common.[33,36] The patient with ankylosing spondylitis walks slowly and stiffly because of a rigid, painful spine. Heart block and aortic and rarely mitral regurgitation appear in the advanced stages of this illness.[37]

Squatting is a classic sign of tetralogy of Fallot.

Face[38]

In the mucopolysaccharidoses, the head is large and boat-shaped. The nose is broad and the nostrils flare. Large lips, small and widely spaced teeth, and a large protuberant tongue are oral findings.[3,9] Hurler's syndrome has a high incidence of heart disease because of mucopolysaccharide deposition in the coronary arteries, endocardial fibroelastosis, and thickening of the valves (Fig. 8-11).[39] Primary myocardial disease and aortic regurgitation are the cardiovascular abnormalities in Morquio's syndrome. Aortic regurgitation also occurs in Scheie's syndrome.

The head in Marfan's syndrome and homocystinuria is long and narrow (Fig. 8-12A). The palate is often arched. Ectopia lentis may be obvious or may be detected by finding a tremulous iris when the head is shaken from side to side (Fig. 8-12A to D).

The Cornelia de Lange syndrome is a rare disorder displaying mental retardation; bushy, con-

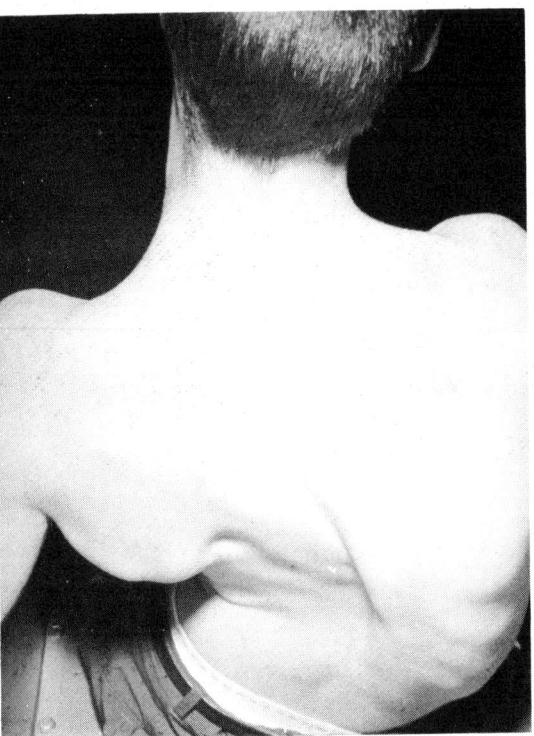

FIGURE 8-10 Friedreich's ataxia with secondary kyphoscoliosis. Severe cardiomegaly occurred before the kyphoscoliosis developed.

fluent eyebrows; long eyelashes; a small mandible; a broad, flat upturned nose; and an antimongoloid slant to the eyes in conjunction with a variety of congenital heart defects (Fig. 8-13).

In Werner's syndrome the patients have a beaked nose and premature graying and balding.

The alterations in the Rubinstein-Taybi syndrome include a prominent forehead; a thin, beaked nose or a broad nasal bridge; large low-set

FIGURE 8-11 Hurler's syndrome. Coarse features and bushy eyebrows. Mucopolysaccharides may be abnormally deposited in the valves, coronary arteries, and aorta.

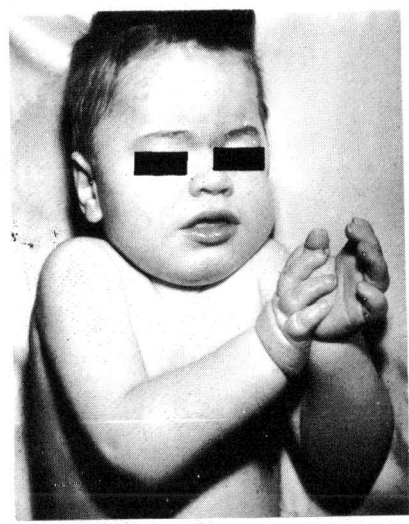

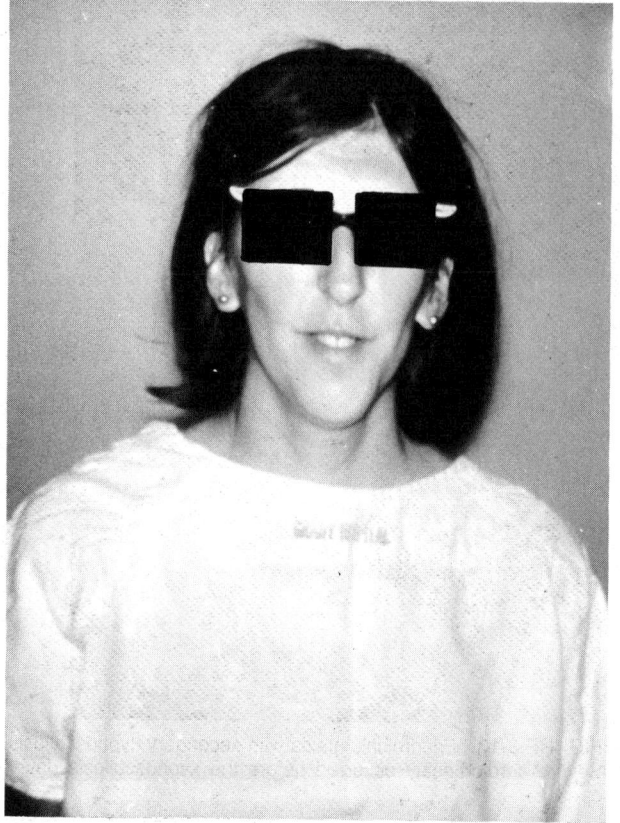

A

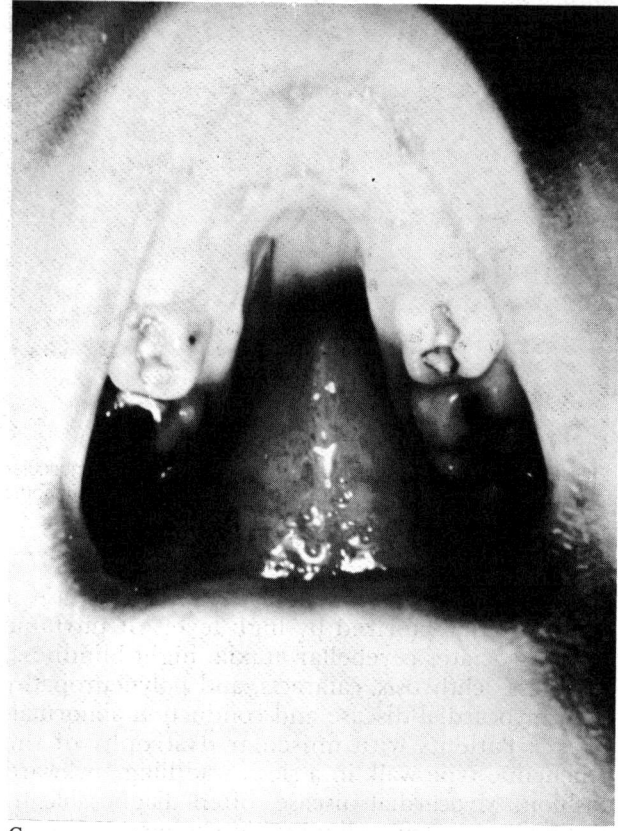

C

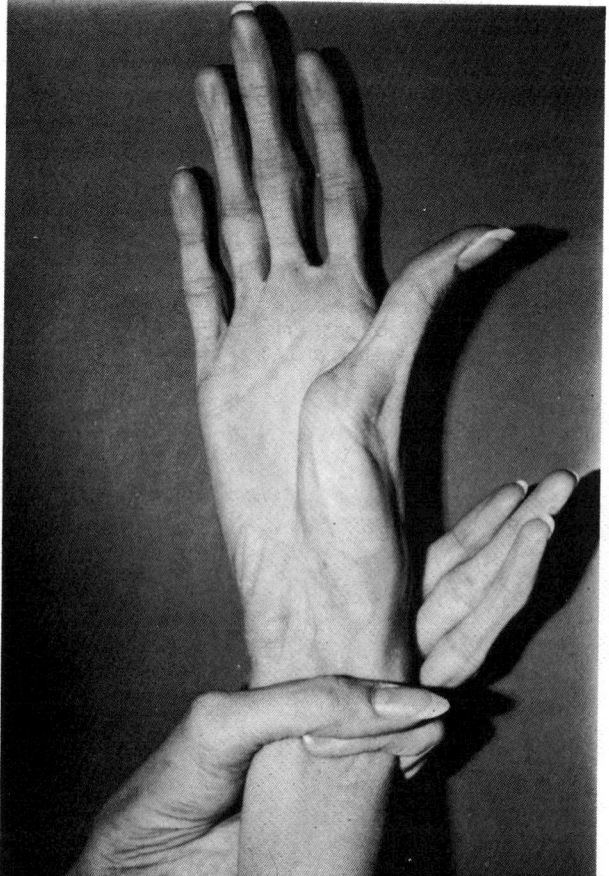

B

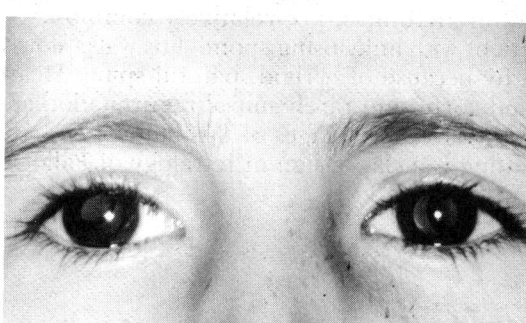

D

FIGURE 8-12 Marfan's syndrome. *A.* Long, narrow face. *B.* Arachnodactyly and positive wrist sign. *C.* High arched palate. *D.* Ectopia lentis associated with aortic aneurysm and severe aortic regurgitation in a teenage girl.

ears; and an antimongoloid slant of the eyes. A variety of congenital heart defects occur.[40]

The trisomy syndromes offer almost pathognomonic facial clues, and all have a high association with cardiovascular anomalies.[41] In trisomy 13–15 syndrome the infants have a cleft palate and lip. The ocular tissue and the nose may be missing. The features of trisomy 18 are a small triangular mouth with a receding chin, a small mandible, and a webbed neck.[42]

The familiar face of Down's syndrome (trisomy 21) is recognized because of the small head; small orbits; epicanthal folds; hypertelorism; cataracts; Brushfield's spots of the iris; large, protruding, fis-

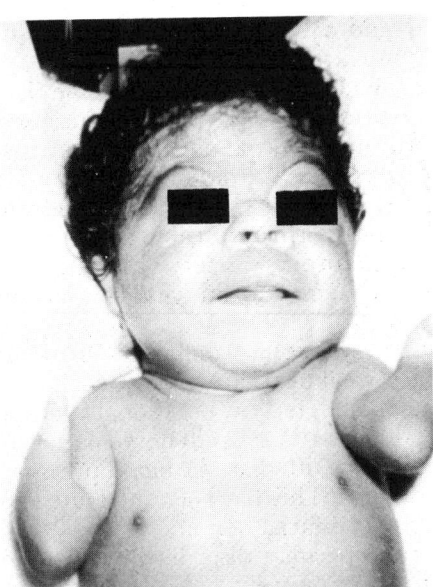

FIGURE 8-13 Cornelia de Lange syndrome. Low hairline, hirsutism, bushy eyebrows, phocomelia, and a single thumblike digit. May be associated with ventricular septal defect.

sured tongue; and small nose. The most common lesions are atrioventricular canal and ventricular septal defect.[43]

A low hairline, a small jaw, and a short, webbed neck are physical findings in both Turner's syndrome and the Klippel-Feil syndrome. Turner's syndrome also includes epicanthal folds, hypertelorism, pigmented moles, and ptosis (Fig. 8-14). Coarctation of the aorta, aortic stenosis, and hypertrophic cardiomyopathy are the usual cardiovascular considerations.[44]

Patients with Noonan's syndrome are sometimes confused with those having Turner's syndrome because they may have in common shortness of stature, webbed neck, and hypogonadism. They differ, however, in that they are often mentally retarded and have dental malocclusion, antimongoloid slanting of the eyes, and normal chromosomes. Valvular pulmonic stenosis is the defect most likely to be present. Obstructive and nonobstructive cardiomyopathy and other congenital defects have been recognized (Fig. 8-15).[44,45] The Klippel-Feil syndrome may also cause facial asymmetry, cleft palate, torticollis, deafness, strabismus, and hydrocephaly (Fig. 8-16). Ventricular septal defect is the usual cardiac problem.[46]

The term *mulibrey nanism* has been coined to describe a syndrome which involves muscle, liver, brain, and eyes. These patients have a triangular face, bulging forehead, low nasal bridge, growth retardation, pigmentary changes in the fundus, and hemangiomas. The cardiac lesion is constrictive pericarditis.[47]

In myotonia dystrophica the patient may have a masklike expression, drooping eyelids, sunken cheeks, a receding hairline, and cataracts. Conduc-

tion disturbances, arrhythmias, or myocardial disease may be present.[48] Permanent atrial paralysis has been documented in patients who have facio-scapulohumeral muscular dystrophy.

The origin of a harsh systolic murmur over the upper right chest may be resolved in favor of supravalvular aortic stenosis if the characteristic face, consisting of a wide mouth with large lips, widely spaced teeth, elfin features, a broad forehead, depressed nasal bridge, long philtrum, full cheeks, and prominent ears, is recognized (Fig. 8-17).[49]

Dysplasia of the pulmonary valve may be familial and is suggested by a triangular-shaped face, hypertelorism, ptosis, mental and growth retardation, and low-set ears. A similar dysplastic pulmonic valve is described in Noonan's, Watson's, and the multiple lentigines syndrome.[50]

A variety of congenital heart defects are associated with the Smith-Lemli-Opitz syndrome. The clinical findings are mental and growth retardation, hypertonia, anteverted nares, micrognathia, broad maxillary ridge, ptosis, epicanthal folds, cleft palate, and cataracts.[51]

Inflammatory destruction of the cartilage of the face resulting in a saddle-shaped collapse of the

FIGURE 8-14 Turner's syndrome. Epicanthal folds, pigmented moles, hypertelorism, and scars on the neck where webs have been removed may be associated with coarctation of aorta.

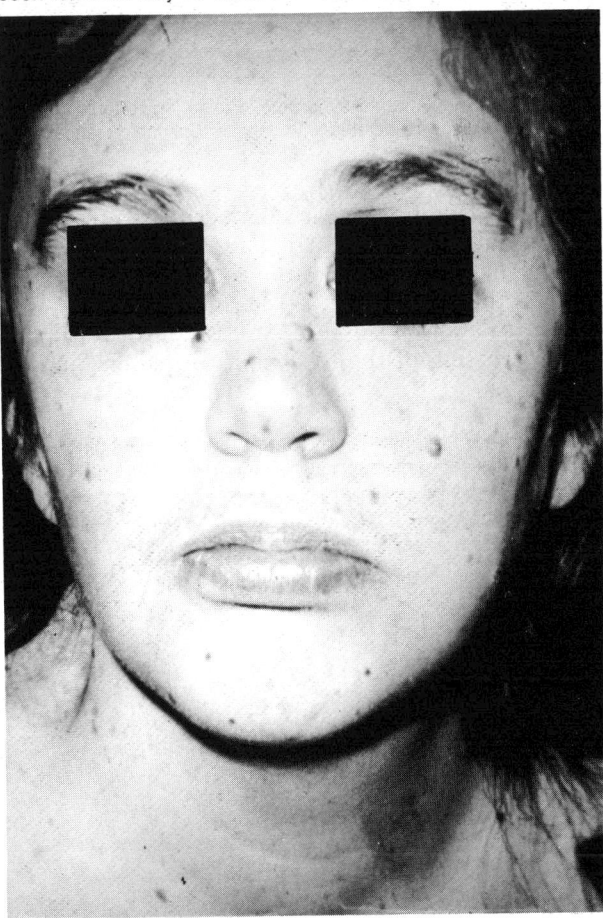

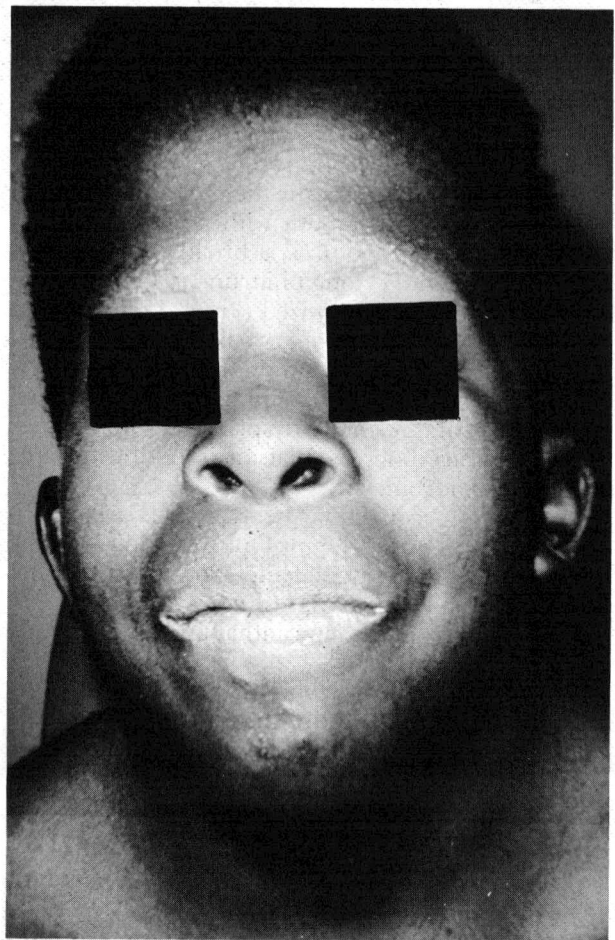

FIGURE 8-15 Noonan's syndrome. Ptosis, hypertelorism, and low-set ears were associated with valvular pulmonic stenosis.

nose or a cauliflower ear may occur together with inflammation of the aortic ring, pericarditis, and aneurysm or dissection of the aorta when polychondritis is the culprit (Fig. 8-18*A* and *B*).[52]

The calamitous onset of cyanosis of the head and neck, sweating of the forehead, prominent jugular

FIGURE 8-16 Klippel-Feil syndrome. Marked webbing of the neck and low-set ears associated with a ventricular septal defect.

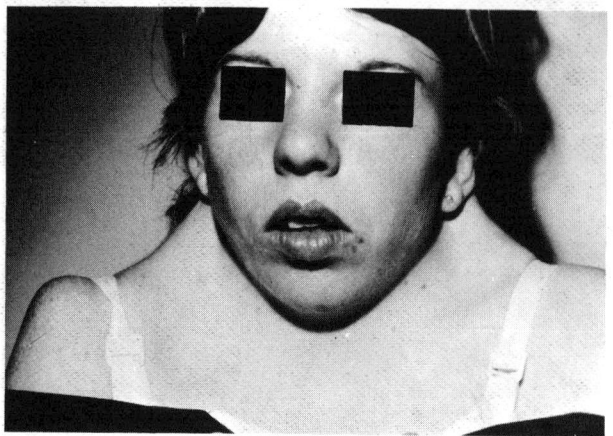

venous *a* waves, and dyspnea is almost always diagnostic of a pulmonary embolus.

The mucocutaneous lymph node syndrome (Kawasaki's disease) presents with conjunctivitis; erythema of the oral mucosa, palms, and fingertips; fissuring of the lips; cervical adenopathy; and a polymorphous rash in infants and young children. A diffuse perivasculitis is responsible for the frequent occurrence of coronary artery obstruction or aneurysm, pericarditis, myocarditis, and conduction disturbance.[53]

The cardiofacial syndrome combines unilateral partial lower-face weakness, apparent on crying, with ventricular septal defect or, occasionally, other congenital heart defects.[54] A seventh nerve palsy has been noted in children with diastolic blood pressure exceeding 120 mmHg. This has been attributed to hemorrhage within the facial nerve.[55]

Progeria is a rare, peculiar disorder in which the face is small and prematurely aged, the eyes are bulging, and the nose is beaked. Severe atherosclerosis with myocardial infarction is a common cause of death in the early years.[56]

An excessive growth of the facial bones provides the protruding mandible and broad forehead in acromegaly. Conduction defects, myocardial hyper-

FIGURE 8-17 Supravalvular aortic stenosis. Turned up nose, broad cheeks, large mouth with peg-shaped teeth, and large ears.

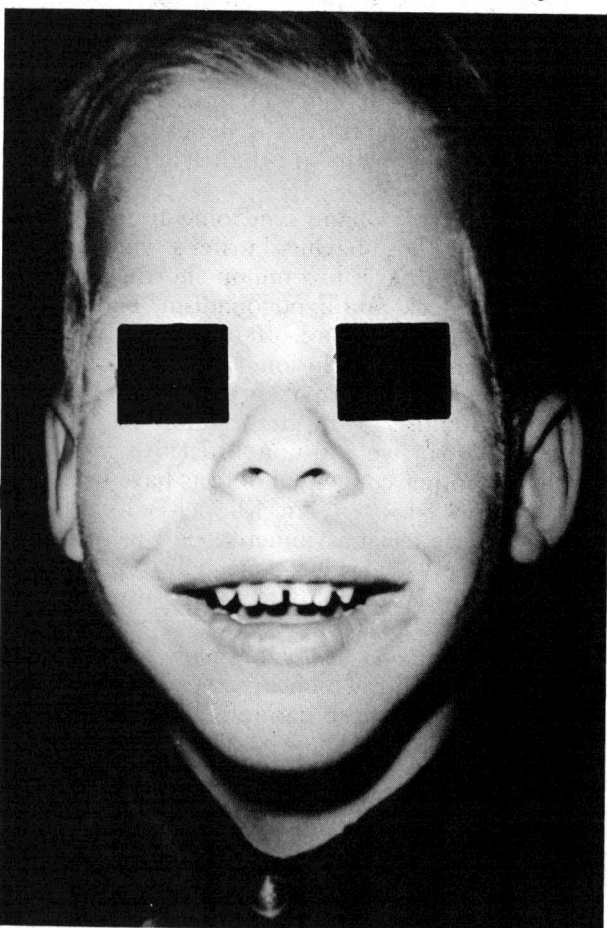

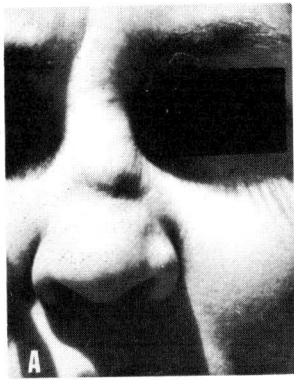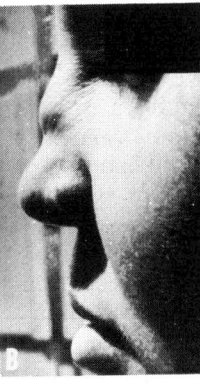

FIGURE 8-18 Polychondritis. *A.* Destruction of cartilage of nose, producing a "saddle nose" (*B*), in association with aortic regurgitation. (*Courtesy of Dr. Warren Sarrell, Anniston, Ala.*)

trophy and fibrosis, and coronary atherosclerosis may be the cardiac consequences.[57]

Hypothyroidism offers a face that is distorted by thickened skin, dry hair, puffy eyelids, and an enlarged tongue. Pericardial effusion, hypercholesterolemia, and possibly premature myocardial infarction are the cardiac possibilities.[58]

Blue sclerae may be found in osteogenesis imperfecta. The patients may have aortic regurgitation, mitral regurgitation, deafness, and a history of numerous fractures.[59]

Patients under age 40 who have arcus senilis should be evaluated for hyperlipidemia.[60]

The differential diagnosis of cataracts includes myotonia dystrophica, Marfan's syndrome, homocystinuria, Down's syndrome, Laurence-Moon-Biedl-Bardet syndrome, Friedreich's ataxia, Werner's syndrome, polychondritis, Refsum's disease, Hallerman-Streif syndrome, rubella syndrome, and diabetes. The Laurence-Moon-Biedl-Bardet syndrome and the Hallerman-Streif syndrome display a variety of congenital heart defects.[61] Diabetes is a strong risk factor for coronary atherosclerosis.[62] The association of cataracts, deafness, nystagmus, and patent ductus or pulmonary artery stenosis constitutes the rubella syndrome (Fig. 8-19). A fibrous stenosis of cerebral, renal, and aortic vessels is a late aftermath.[63]

A coloboma (fissure) of the iris and choroid is a major sign of the "cat eye" syndrome and is found with various cardiac defects.[64]

External ophthalmoplegia, ptosis, myocardial disease, and complete heart block (Kearns-Sayre syndrome) may all be due to ocular muscular dystrophy.[65]

In severe right-sided congestive heart failure or massive tricuspid regurgitation the venous pressure may be so elevated that the eyes protrude or even pulsate. Exophthalmos may also be secondary to hyperthyroidism and lead to the etiologic diagnosis of unexplained tachycardia, tricuspid regurgitation, atrial arrhythmias, or high-output congestive heart failure.[66] In the elderly patient with apathetic thyrotoxicosis the expected physical findings may not

be present. Instead these patients have a small thyroid, marked temporal muscle wasting, altered mentation, sunken eyes, and atrial fibrillation.

Patients with bacterial endocarditis may present with severe ophthalmitis as the initial sign. Persistent searching of the upper and lower eyelids for subconjunctival hemorrhage or petechiae may lead to the diagnosis of bacterial endocarditis (Fig. 8-20*A*).[67] Conjunctivitis may be associated with Reiter's syndrome and the mucocutaneous lymph node syndrome.

Ears

Low-set ears are a nonspecific congenital abnormality and are common to syndromes which have a high cranial vault, a short mandibular ramus, a short neck, or a hyperextended head. This is a finding in Down's, Noonan's, Cornelia de Lange, Turner's, and Rubinstein-Taybi syndromes, trisomy 8 mosaicism, and trisomy 13–15, trisomy 18, and the Smith-Lemli-Opitz, Klippel-Feil, and Pierre Robin syndromes.[68] The ear may be malformed in trisomy 13–15 syndrome, Klippel-Feil syndrome, Turner's syndrome, Goldenhar (oculoauriculovertebral dysplasia) syndrome,[69] chromosome 9 and 22 abnormalities, and polychondritis.

Deafness is common to Hurler's syndrome, Klippel-Feil syndrome, Turner's syndrome, osteogenesis imperfecta, rubella syndrome, familial pulmonic stenosis, the multiple lentigines syndrome, and familial mitral regurgitation with skeletal anomalies. Deafness together with a prolonged QT interval on the electrocardiogram may be familial and forewarn of arrhythmias and sudden death.[70]

An increased incidence of a diagonal earlobe crease is a curious observation in patients with coronary artery disease.[71]

Mouth

An enlarged tongue may be an important clue that amyloidosis or glycogen storage disease is the cause

FIGURE 8-19 Rubella syndrome. Cataracts associated with peripheral pulmonic stenosis.

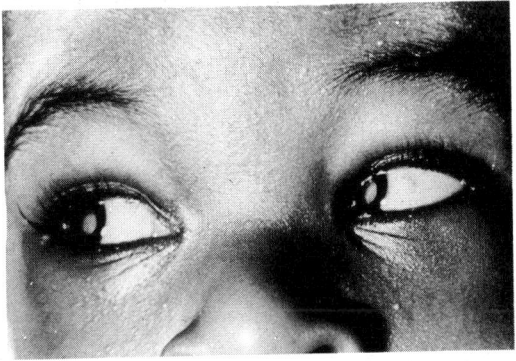

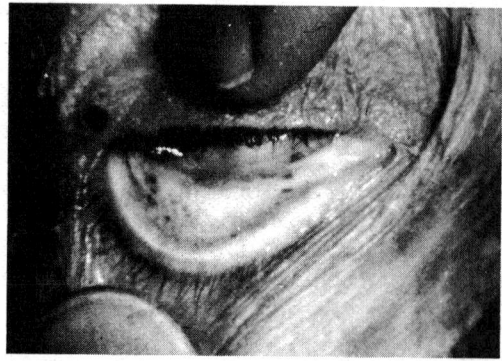

A

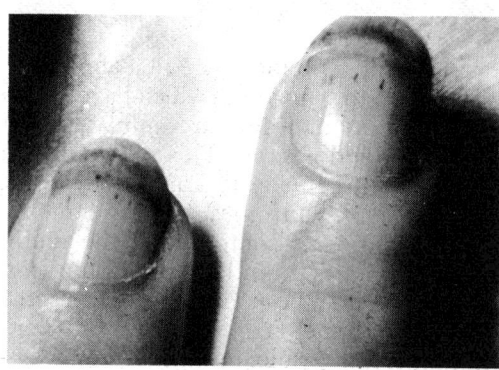

B

FIGURE 8-20 Bacterial endocarditis. *A.* Petechial hemorrhages of the lower eyelid of a patient with bacterial endocarditis. *B.* Splinter hemorrhages beneath the nails may occur in bacterial endocarditis. This example, however, is due to trichinosis.

of an unexplained cardiomyopathy.[9] The amyloid deposits may also depress the submaxillary glands, giving a misleading impression of lymphadenopathy. The tongue is also enlarged in Hurler's syndrome, Down's syndrome, and in hypothyroidism.

Orange, large lobulated tonsils are a prime feature of Tangier disease, a type of hyperlipidemia in which there is a deficiency of high-density lipoprotein and an incidence of coronary artery disease.[9]

The upper lip may be tied down to the alveolar ridge in the Ellis–van Creveld syndrome (Fig. 8-21A). The teeth may be absent, dysplastic, or peg-shaped.

Enlarged tonsils and adenoids may blockade the airways enough to result in respiratory acidosis. Infants with this problem often have flaring nostrils and an adenoidal expression. Cor pulmonale secondary to pulmonary hypertension, which is reversible following extirpation of the tonsils and adenoids, is the recently recognized cardiac manifestation.[72] Upper airway obstruction may produce increased vagal tone, sinus bradycardia, and first-degree heart block particularly in the massively obese.[73]

A high arched palate can be observed in Marfan's syndrome (Fig. 8-12B), Cornelia de Lange syndrome, trisomy 18 syndrome, Rubinstein-Taybi syn-

drome, Turner's syndrome, and the Pierre Robin syndrome.

There appears to be an increased incidence of congenital heart disease with cleft palate or lip. The exact type is variable.[74]

A cleft palate is also a common occurrence in the Pierre Robin syndrome. The invariable feature of this syndrome is a hypoplastic mandible with a "shrewlike" face (Fig. 8-22). The posteriorly displaced tongue produces severe respiratory problems. Cardiovascular disease is frequent.

Extremities[75]

The upper extremities may have a greater muscular development than the legs in coarctation of the aorta. Underdevelopment of musculature is seen in large left-to-right intracardiac shunts. Pseudohypertrophy of the calves is a manifestation of muscular dystrophy (Fig. 8-23).

Warm, moist hands with a fine tremor and occasionally with clubbing of the fingers suggest hyperthyroidism. A cold hand with coarse, puffy skin may be due to hypothyroidism.

A spadelike hand with "sausage" fingers is one of the many flagrant external changes in acromegaly.

FIGURE 8-21 Ellis–van Creveld syndrome. *A.* Typical "lip tie" due to multiple frenulum. *B.* Polydactyly. This patient had a large atrial septal defect.

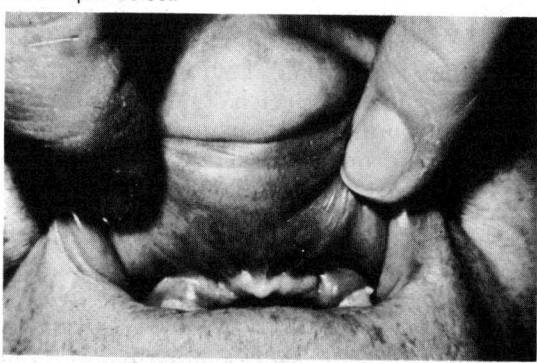

A

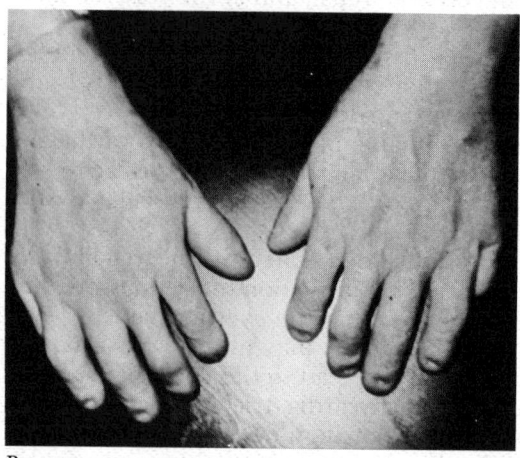

B

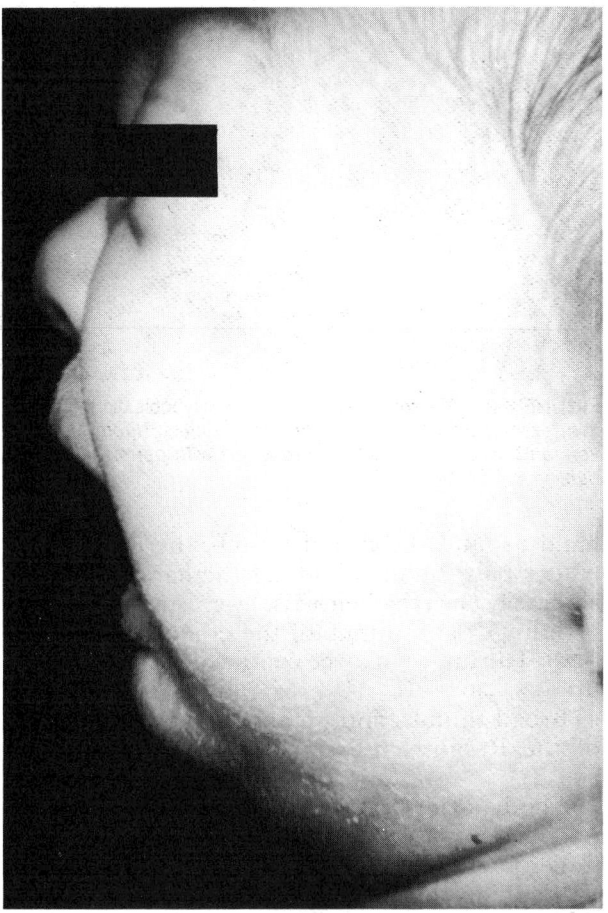

FIGURE 8-22   Pierre Robin syndrome. Hypoplastic mandible associated with a ventricular septal defect.

A myocardial infarction or arterial occlusion may be followed by the development of the shoulder-hand syndrome, which displays a hand that is swollen, shiny, discolored, and stiff. Painful swelling of the dorsal surface of the hands and feet is an early clinical sign of sickle-cell disease. High-output cardiac failure with cardiomegaly, systolic and occasionally diastolic murmurs, and pulmonary vascular thromboses are the cardiovascular complications.[76]

Hypoplastic fingernails, lymphedema, clinodactyly, and a shortened fifth finger are found in Turner's syndrome.

Clubbing of the fingers and cyanosis are typical of congenital heart disease or pulmonary arteriovenous fistulas with a right-to-left shunt (Plate 4A). Red fingertips, "tuft erythema," may signify small or intermittent right-to-left shunts with only slight reduction in arterial oxygen saturation (Plate 4B).

Cyanosis and clubbing with a high cardiac output, presumably related to small arteriovenous shunts in the lung, are infrequent physical signs of cirrhosis of the liver. Diseases of the lungs, such as emphysema, scleroderma, and sarcoidosis, may produce clubbing and may also lead to cor pulmonale. Acute painful clubbing or hypertrophic osteoarthropathy is a manifestation of bronchogenic carcinoma, which

may invade or metastasize to the heart or pericardium.

Very specific physiological implications can be made when differential cyanosis is found.[77,78] Cyanosis of the fingers greater than that of the toes suggests complete transposition of the great vessels with either a preductal coarctation or complete interruption of the aortic arch, pulmonary hypertension, and a reversed shunt through a patent ductus arteriosus delivering oxygenated blood to the lower extremities (Plate 4C). In this abnormality the presence of coarctation of the aorta can be separated from complete interruption of the aortic arch. Slightly less cyanosis of the left arm when compared with the right arm favors coarctation of the aorta, while intense, symmetric cyanosis of both arms is seen with complete aortic interruption.

Cyanosis and clubbing of the toes associated with pink fingernails of the right hand and minimal cyanosis and clubbing in the left hand are due to pulmonary hypertension with normally related great vessels and a reversed shunt through a patent ductus arteriosus bringing unoxygenated blood to the left arm and lower extremities (Plate 4D). This is also true with interruption of the aortic arch and a patent ductus arteriosus delivering unoxygenated blood to the legs. If the right subclavian artery arises proximal to the aortic obstruction, then the right hand may be pink and the left hand cyanotic. When the right subclavian artery originates anomalously from the descending aorta, then both hands are cyanotic.

Pallor of the nail bed suggests anemia and possible high-output cardiac failure or a superimposed burden on an ischemic myocardium.

FIGURE 8-23   Duchenne's muscular dystrophy. Pseudohypertrophy of the calves associated with complete heart block.

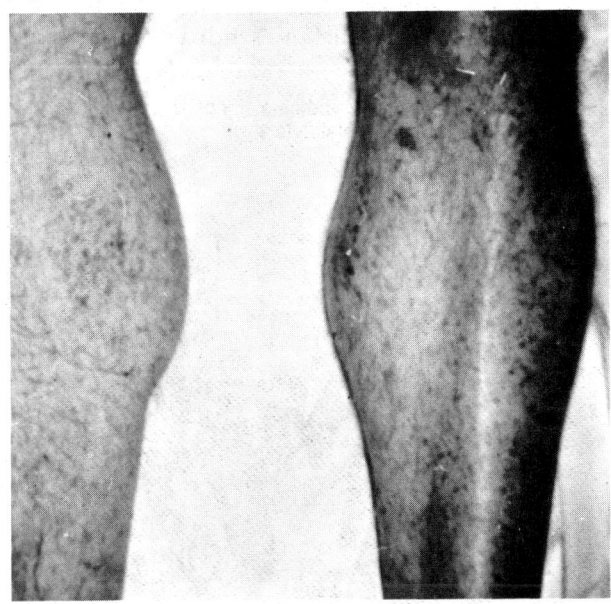

EXAMINATION OF THE HEART AND BLOOD VESSELS

Splinter hemorrhages of the nails may lead to the diagnosis of bacterial endocarditis (Fig. 8-20B).[79] Splinter hemorrhages may also occur in a wide variety of unrelated diseases, in embolism from other sources, and in healthy people. Other clues to bacterial endocarditis in the hand include Osler's nodes, Janeway's lesions, petechiae, and clubbing of the fingers (Plate 3E and F).[67] Osler's nodes are typically reddish-purple, raised, tender nodules in the distal pad of the finger or toe. There may be a white center. Janeway's lesions appear in the palms or soles. They are nontender, hemorrhagic, and slightly raised. Petechiae may be hidden in the mucous membranes of the mouth, around the clavicle, or on the legs.

A variation in the size or number of fingers is an excellent indication of congenital or inherited heart disease. In the Ellis–van Creveld syndrome polydactyly and dystrophic nails are found (Fig. 8-21B).[6] Polydactyly is part of the Laurence-Moon-Biedl-Bardet syndrome. Polydactyly in combination with retroflexible thumbs, transverse creases, hyperconvex narrow nails, and flexion of the fingers and hands is classic for trisomy 13–15 syndrome.[41]

Hypoplasia or absence of the radial aspect of the hand has a very striking connection with defects of the atrial or ventricular septum. In the Holt-Oram syndrome, which is transmitted as an autosomal dominant disorder, the thumbs may resemble a finger, being hypoplastic and in the same plane as the rest of the fingers, or they may be triphalangeal, absent, or longer than normal (Fig. 8-24). The forearms are short, and supination and pronation are limited. The usual cardiac defect is a secundum atrial septal defect.[80] An identical thumb, or absence of the thumb or radius, occurs with a ventricular septal defect in ventriculoradial dysplasia; this is not felt to be a heritable disorder (Fig. 8-25).[81]

Arachnodactyly and lax joints are salient features of both Marfan's syndrome and homocystinuria.[3] When patients with Marfan's syndrome clench their

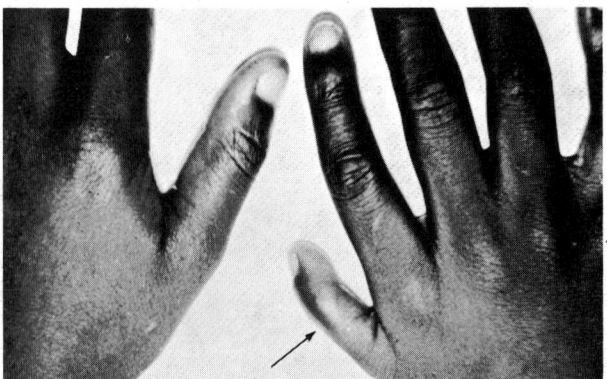

FIGURE 8-25   Ventriculoradial dysplasia. Hypoplastic thumb (arrow) associated with a ventricular septal defect. (*From M. E. Silverman and J. W. Hurst.*[75] *Reproduced with permission of the publisher.*)

hand around the flexed thumb, the thumb protrudes past the ulnar side of the hand. They can also easily encircle their wrist by grasping it with the fifth finger and thumb of the other hand (Fig. 8-12B). The fingers may be contracted in homocystinuria.

Broad thumbs and great toes are the hallmark of the Rubinstein-Taybi syndrome (Fig. 8-26A and B).[40]

The hand in trisomy 18 syndrome is characteristic, consisting of a tightly clenched fist, an index finger overlapping the third finger, a fifth finger overlapping the fourth finger, and stubby fingers (Fig. 8-27).[41,42]

Transverse creases of the palms are not diagnostic but are common in Down's syndrome (Fig. 8-28).

The Cornelia de Lange syndrome is a rare disorder featuring a "chicken wing" appendage, or a proximal thumb, or short, tapering digits (Fig. 8-13).[13]

Ulnar deviation of the fingers, thickening of the middle interphalangeal joints, boxing of the wrists, and subcutaneous nodules typify rheumatoid arthritis, which has a high incidence of cardiac disease including pericarditis, coronary arteritis, or granulomatous inflammation involving the myocardium or the base or cusps of the aortic and mitral valves.[82] Jaccoud's arthritis is almost always due to repeated attacks of rheumatic fever and may cause marked ulnar deviation at the metacarpophalangeal joints, resembling rheumatoid arthritis (Fig. 8-29).[83] The deformity, however, is due to periarticular fascial and tendon fibrosis, rather than to synovitis, and the fingers can be moved freely into a correct alignment. Acute rheumatic fever may express itself by inflammation of the joints.

The diagnosis of Whipple's disease may be neglected unless the polyarthritis is connected to the abdominal pain and diarrhea. Pericarditis and endocarditis may be present and may antedate the malabsorption.[84]

The deposition of uric acid crystals causing gouty arthritis may also occur in the heart, resulting in

FIGURE 8-24   Holt-Oram syndrome. Fingerized thumb (arrow) associated with an atrial septal defect.

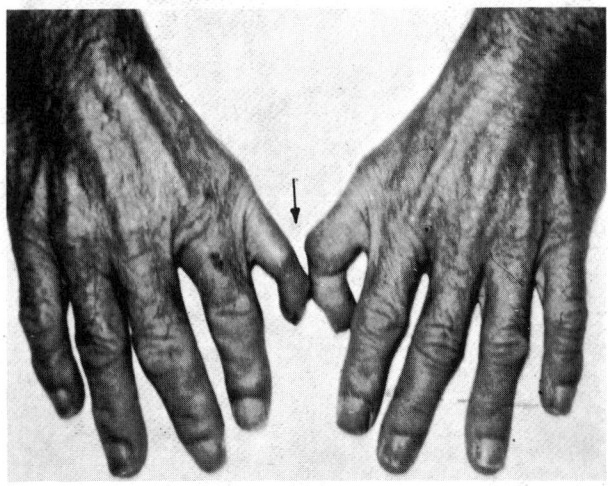

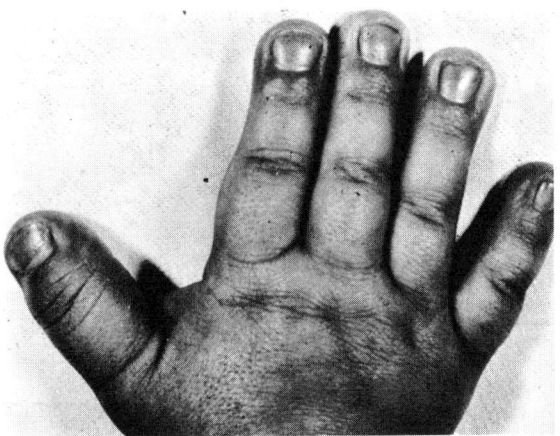

A

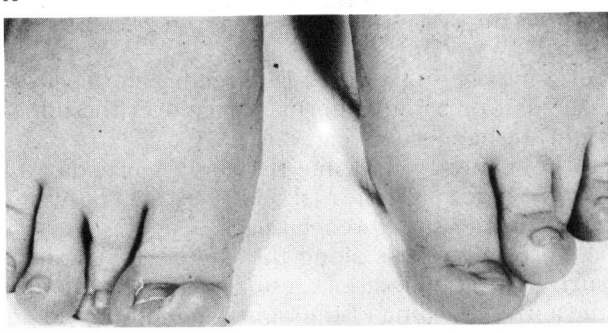

B

FIGURE 8-26 Rubinstein-Taybi syndrome. *A.* Broad thumb. *B.* Broad great toe. May be associated with variety of congenital heart defects. (*A, from M. E. Silverman and J. W. Hurst.*[75] *Reproduced with permission of the publisher.*)

gouty nodules in the myocardium, valves, or conducting system.[85]

Blue-black pigmentation of atheroma, mitral and aortic valvulitis, myocardial infarction, and arthritis can be due to an accumulation of homogentisic acid in alkaptonuria.[9]

Arthritis is also common to lupus erythematosus, polychondritis, polymyositis, sickle-cell disease, and Lyme arthritis.

FIGURE 8-27 Trisomy 18 syndrome. Tightly clenched fist with overlapping index and fifth fingers. A ventricular septal defect was present.

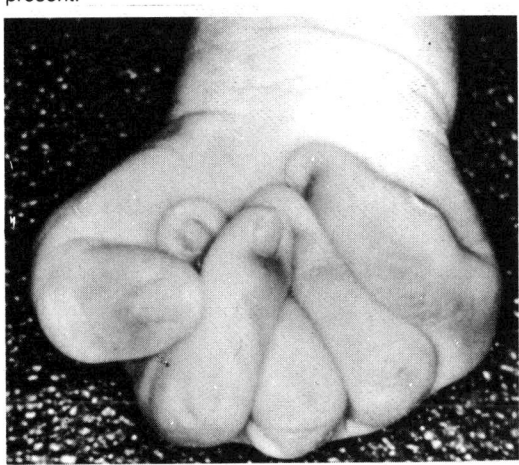

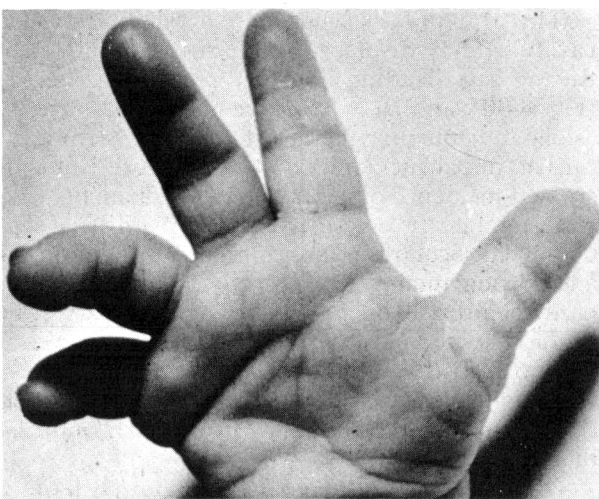

FIGURE 8-28 Down's syndrome. Simian crease associated with an atrioventricular defect. (*From M. E. Silverman and J. W. Hurst.*[75] *Reproduced with permission of the publisher.*)

Thorax and Neck

Structural deformity and neuromuscular disorders of the thorax may alter normal respiration, leading to hypoxia and vasoconstriction, distortion of the pulmonary vasculature, and impedance to pulmonary blood flow.[86] Cor pulmonale may be the consequence of this elevation in pulmonary vascular resistance. This is particularly true in kyphoscoliosis; however, cor pulmonale may also develop because of rheumatoid spondylitis, osteogenesis imperfecta, thoracoplasty, poliomyelitis, muscular dystrophy, and spinal cord disease.

In the mucopolysaccharidoses the deformities include kyphoscoliosis, pectus carinatum, and a barrel-shaped chest with a short neck.[3] The Klippel-Feil syndrome is identified by a short neck due to congenital fusion of the cervical vertebrae and scoliosis, in addition to many other bony deformities.[46]

FIGURE 8-29 Jaccoud's arthritis. Ulnar deviation of the fingers suggesting rheumatoid arthritis; however, the fingers could be freely moved back into a normal alignment. (*Courtesy of Dr. Albert Raizner, Baylor University, Houston, Texas.*)

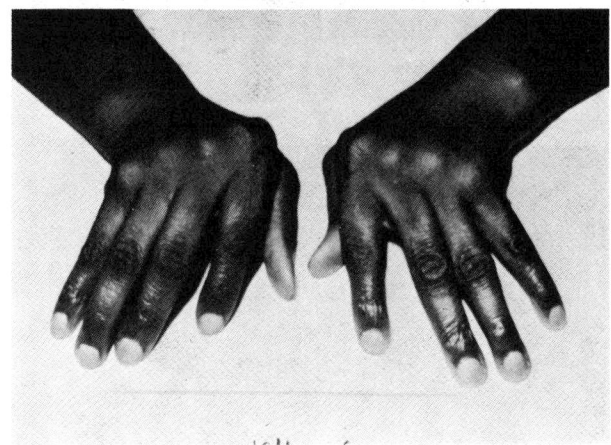

EXAMINATION OF THE HEART AND BLOOD VESSELS

The straight-back syndrome, as well as pectus excavatum, may displace the heart to the left, producing a misleading impression of cardiomegaly (Fig. 8-30*A* and *B*).[87,88] Systolic and even a rare diastolic murmur may be heard, although significant cardiac impairment rarely occurs. There is an increased incidence of a straight back in patients with congenital heart disease, particularly with atrial septal defects. Scoliosis is also commonly present in cyanotic congenital heart disease.[89] There is a significant incidence of pectus excavatum, straight thoracic spine, and scoliosis in patients with mitral valve prolapse.[90]

Ankylosing spondylitis may be associated with aortic regurgitation, complete heart block, and cardiomyopathy.[90a]

Other important clues may be gained from a closer scrutiny of the thorax. Bilateral prominence of the anterior part of the chest, with bulging of the upper two-thirds of the sternum and indrawing of the lower one-third, is an effect of ventricular septal defect in children. A unilateral bulge at the fourth and fifth intercostal spaces at the lower left sternal border is frequently found in adults with ventricular septal defects. A bulge in the area of the second and third intercostal spaces at the left sternal border may be due to an underlying atrial septal defect (Fig. 8-31).[91] An underlying aneurysm of the ascending

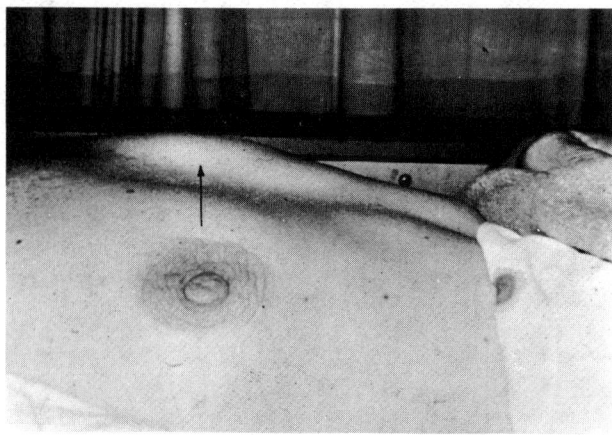

FIGURE 8-31 Atrial septal defect. A bulge over the left sternal border (arrow) is an excellent clue to congenital heart disease.

aorta may be suggested by a pulsating sternoclavicular joint or by an abnormal bulge over the upper right sternal border (Fig. 8-32).

In Turner's syndrome the chest is broad, with widely spaced nipples (shield chest), hypoplastic breast tissue, and a webbed neck.

Tortuous vessels along the lateral chest wall or surrounding the scapula result from coarctation of the aorta. Buckling of the right common carotid artery is often mistaken for an aneurysm. Distension of the left external jugular vein may develop when the aorta becomes enlarged and sclerotic or dissected, compressing the left brachiocephalic vein against the sternum (Fig. 8-33). Unilateral distension of the neck veins may lead to a diagnosis of mediastinal tumor. Bilateral distension of the neck veins, plus evidence of collateral venous circulation over the upper part of the chest, suggests superior vena cava obstruction.

Tachypnea may be an early sign of congestive heart failure, particularly in infants. Sighing respirations or tachypnea may heighten the suspicion that an atypical chest pain or dizzy spells are related to hyperventilation. The respirations in patients

FIGURE 8-30 Chest deformities that may produce murmurs. *A.* Straight-back syndrome. *B.* Pectus excavatum. (*A, from A. C. De Leon, Jr., J. K. Perloff, H. Twigg, and M. Majd, The Straight Back Syndrome. Clinical Cardiovascular Manifestations, Circulation, 32:193, 1965. Reproduced with permission.*)

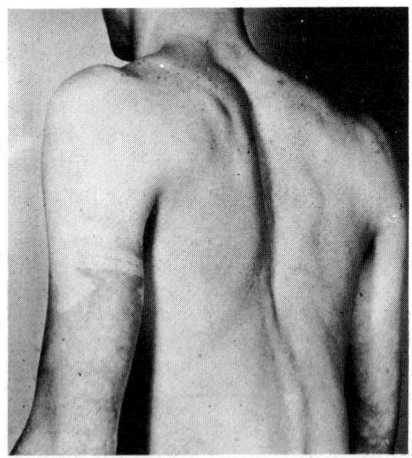

A

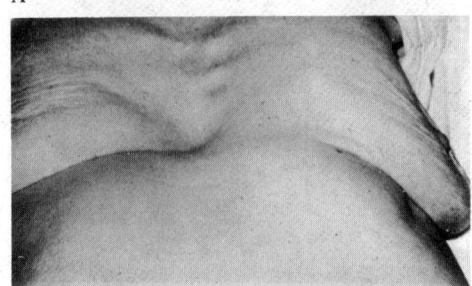

B

FIGURE 8-32 Syphilis. Syphilitic aneurysm, producing a pulsating bulge over the upper right sternal border (arrow).

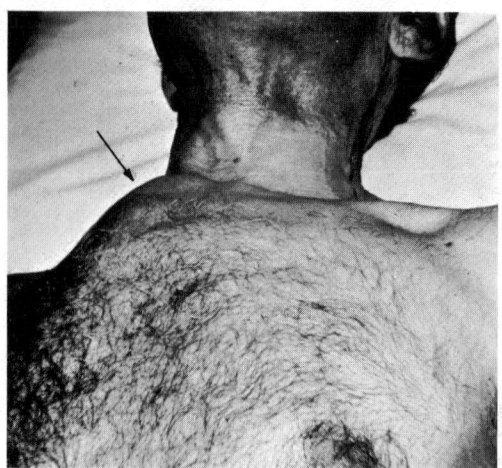

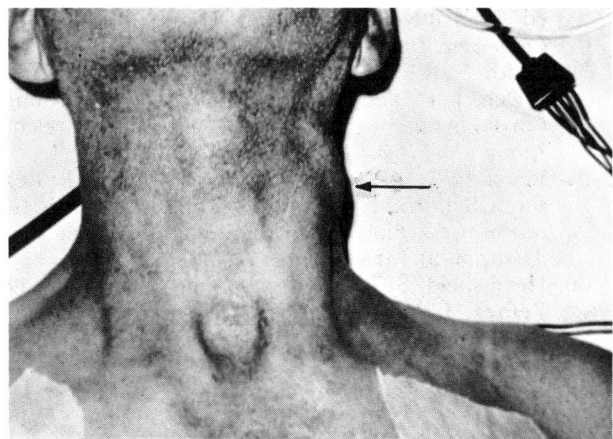

FIGURE 8-33 Dissection of the aorta. Distension of the external jugular vein on the patient's left (arrow) but not on the right, secondary to an aortic dissection compressing the left brachiocephalic vein.

with pericarditis and pulmonary infarction are shallow, because the patient is afraid of increasing the pleuritic pain. In pulmonary edema, the respirations are desperately deep and labored. Wheezing may be audible in patients suffering from a pulmonary embolus or pulmonary edema.

Miscellaneous

An imperforate anus may be associated with a cardiovascular malformation.[92] This may occur as an isolated finding or as a component of the Vater association, the asplenia syndrome, and the cat eye syndrome. The Vater association also includes vertebral defects, tracheoesophageal fistula, and radial and renal dysplasia.[93] The asplenia syndrome has a striking incidence of complex congenital heart disease.[94] Cardiovascular malformations are found in 15 to 25 percent of newborns with omphalocele.[95]

Abnormalities involving chromosomes 1, 9, 11, and 22 have been described with congenital heart disease.[96] The findings in chromosome 1 include a peaked nose, micrognathia, and long, tapering fingers. Chromosome 9 children have a prominent forehead, hypertension, anteverted nostrils, long upper lip, short neck, mental retardation, and external ear malformations. Chromosome 11 shares similar features, and, in addition, there is retraction of the lower lip. Psychomotor retardation, coloboma, hypertelorism, antimongoloid slanting of the eyes, and preauricular tags or fistulas are clues to a chromosome 22 defect.

Congenital heart disease, primarily patent ductus arteriosus, has now been linked to the 49,XXXXY syndrome. This rare syndrome is suspected when the infant has psychomotor retardation, hypoplastic genitals, prognathism, clinodactyly, and radioulnar synostoses.

Offspring of chronic alcoholic mothers have been observed to share similar characteristics. These include microcephaly, short palpebral fissures, hypoplastic face with thinned vermilion border and diminished to absent philtrum, epicanthal folds, growth deficiency, joint anomalies, and septal defects.[97]

The presence of any congenital somatic abnormality should always stimulate a search for heart disease. In a recent study extracardiac abnormalities were found in 25 percent of infants seen during the first year for significant cardiac disease. The defects were commonly found in the musculoskeletal system or associated with a specific syndrome.[98,99]

References

1. Osler, W.: Aequanimatas, with Other Addresses, "On The Educational Value of the Medical Society," 2d ed., P. Blakiston's Son & Company, Philadelphia, 1906, p. 357.
*2. Pyeritz, R. E., and McKusick, V. A.: The Marfan Syndrome, *N. Engl. J. Med.*, 300:772, 1979. (29 references)
3. McKusick, V. A.: "Heritable Disorders of Connective Tissues," 4th ed., The C. V. Mosby Company, St. Louis, 1972.
4. Beighton, P.: The Inherited Disorders of Connective Tissue. I. Pseudoxanthoma Elasticum, Ehlers-Danlos, Marfan's Syndrome, Homocystinuria, Osteogenesis Imperfecta, *Bull. Rheum. Dis.*, 23:696, 1972–1973 series.
*5. Washington University School of Medicine: Massive Obesity and Cardiac Failure, *Am. J. Med.*, 64:827, 1978. (10 references)
6. Blackburn, M. G., and Belliveau, R. E.: Ellis-van Creveld Syndrome: A Report of Previously Undescribed Anomalies in Two Siblings, *Am. J. Dis. Child.*, 122:267, 1971.
7. Stein, D., and Kloster, F. E.: Valvular Heart Disease in Osteogenesis Imperfecta, *Am. Heart J.*, 94:637, 1977.
8. Rosenthal, A.: Cardiovascular Malformations in Klinefelter's Syndrome: Report of Three Cases, *J. Pediatr.*, 80:471, 1972.
*9. Blieden, L. C., and Miller, J. H.: Cardiac Involvement in Inherited Disorders of Metabolism, *Prog. Cardiovasc. Dis.*, 16:1615, 1974. (72 references)
10. Wennevold, A., and Jacobsen, J. G.: Acquired Supravalvular Aortic Stenosis in Familial Hypercholesterolemia, *Am. J. Med.*, 50:822, 1971.
*11. Fauci, A. S., Haynes, B. F., and Katz, P.: NIH Conference: The Spectrum of Vasculitis, *Ann. Intern. Med.*, 89:660, 1978. (139 references)
12. Gottdiener, J. S., Moutsopoulos, H. M., and Decker, J. L.: Echocardiographic Identification of Cardiac Abnormality in Scleroderma and Related Disorders, *Am. J. Med.*, 66:391, 1979.
*13. Nakao, Y., Kishikara, M., Yoshimi, H., Inoue, Y., Tanaka, K., Sakamoto, N., et al.: Werner's Syndrome. In Vivo and In Vitro Characteristics As a Model of Aging, *Am. J. Med.*, 65:919, 1978. (37 references)

*This article is a review of the literature and contains additional references to the literature.

14. Borenstein, D. G., Fye, W. B., Arnett, F. C., and Stevens, M. B.: The Myocarditis of Systemic Lupus Erythematosus, *Ann. Intern. Med.*, 89:619, 1978.
15. Hess, E. V., and Spencer-Green, G.: Congenital Heart Block and Connective Tissue Diseases, *Ann. Intern. Med.*, 91:645, 1979.
16. Lier, C. V., Call, T. D., Fulkerson, P. K., and Wooley, C. F.: The Spectrum of Cardiac Defects in the Ehlers-Danlos Syndrome, Types I and III, *Ann. Intern. Med.*, 92:171, 1980.
17. Harris, R. B., Heaphy, M. R., and Perry, H. O.: Generalized Elastolysis (Cutis Laxa), *Am. J. Med.*, 65:815, 1978.
18. Fenoglio, J. J., Jr., McAllister, H. A., Jr., and Ferrans, V. J.: Cardiac Rhabdomyoma: A Clinicopathologic and Electron Microscopic Study, *Am. J. Cardiol.*, 38:241, 1976.
*19. Milder, M. S., Cook, J. D., Stray, S., and Finch, C. A.: Idiopathic Hemochromatosis, *Medicine*, 59:34, 1980. (103 references)
*20. Bohan, A., Peter, J. B., Bowman, R. L., and Pearson, C. M.: A Computer-Assisted Analysis of 153 Patients with Polymyositis and Dermatomyositis, *Medicine*, 56:255, 1977. (106 references)
21. Trell, E., Rausing, A., Ripa, J., Torp, A., and Waldenstrom, J.: Carcinoid Heart Disease: Clinicopathologic Findings and Follow-Up in 11 Cases, *Am. J. Med.*, 54:433, 1973.
22. Bete, J. M., Banas, J. S., Jr., Moran, J., Pinn, V., and Levine, H. J.: Coronary Artery Disease in an 18 Year Old Girl with Pseudoxanthoma Elasticum: Successful Surgical Therapy, *Am. J. Cardiol.*, 36:515, 1975.
23. Rubinow, A., and Cohen, A. S.: Skin Involvement in Generalized Amyloidosis, *Ann. Intern. Med.*, 88:781, 1978.
24. Pierce, R. N., and Walker Smith, G. J.: Intrathoracic Manifestations of Degos' Disease (Malignant Atrophic Papulosis), *Chest*, 73, 1979.
25. Hecht, H.: On Cardio-cutaneous Syndromes, *Trans. Assoc. Am. Physicians*, 80:91, 1967.
26. Lindemauer, S. M.: The Klippel-Trenaunay Syndrome, *Ann. Surg.*, 162:303, 1965.
27. Hodgson, C. H., Burchell, H. B., Good, C. A., and Clagett, O. T.: Hereditary Hemorrhagic Telangiectasia and Pulmonary Arteriovenous Fistula: Survey of a Large Family, *N. Engl. J. Med.*, 261:625, 1959.
*28. Roberts, W. C., McAllister, H. A., and Ferrans, V. J.: Sarcoidosis of the Heart, *Am. J. Med.*, 63:86, 1977. (94 references)
29. Hardin, J. A., Steere, A. C., and Malawista, S. E.: Immune Complexes and the Evolution of Lyme Arthritis, *N. Engl. J. Med.*, 301:1358, 1979.
*30. Voron, D. A., Hatfield, H. H., and Kalkhoff, R. K.: Multiple Lentigines Syndrome: Case Report and Review of the Literature, *Am. J. Med.*, 60:447, 1976. (49 references)
31. Becker, A. E., Schoori, R., Balk, A. B., and van der Heide, R. M.: Cardiac Manifestations of Fabry's Disease, *Am. J. Cardiol.*, 36:829, 1975.
31a. Unverferth, D. V., Beman, F. M., Ryan, J. M., and Whisler, R. L.: Reiter's Aortitis with Pericardial Fluid, Heart Block and Neurologic Manifestations, *J. Rheum.*, 6:2, 1979.
*32. Scharf, S., Wexler, J., Longnecker, R. E., and Blanfox, M. D.: Cardiovascular Disease in Patients on Chronic Hemodialytic Therapy, *Prog. Cardiovasc. Dis.*, 22:343, 1980 (104 references)
33. Perloff, J. K.: Cardiomyopathy Associated with Her-edofamilial Neuromyopathic Diseases, *Mod. Concepts Cardiovasc. Dis.*, 40:23, 1971.
34. Smith, E. R., Sangalang, V. E., Heffernan, L. P. P., Welch, J. P., and Flemington, C. S.: Hypertrophic Cardiomyopathy: The Heart Disease of Friedreich's Ataxia, *Am. Heart J.*, 94:428, 1977.
35. Lewis, H. D., Jr., White, H. H., and Dunn, M.: Refsum's Syndrome: A Neurological Disease with Interesting Cardiovascular Manifestations, *Circulation*, 34(suppl. 3):157, 1966.
36. Heymsfield, S. B., McNish, T., Perkins, J. V., and Felner, J. M.: Sequence of Cardiac Changes in Duchenne Muscular Dystrophy, *Am. Heart J.*, 95:283, 1978.
37. Roberts, W. C., Hollingsworth, J. F., Bulkley, B. H., Jaffe, R. B., Epstein, S. E., and Stinson, E. B.: Combined Mitral and Aortic Regurgitation in Ankylosing Spondylitis: Angiographic and Anatomic Features, *Am. J. Med.*, 56:237, 1974.
38. Goodman, R. M., and Gorlin, R. J.: "Atlas of the Face in Genetic Disorders," 2d ed., The C. V. Mosby Company, St. Louis, 1977.
39. Renteria, V. G., Ferrans, V. J., and Roberts, W. C.: The Heart in the Hurler Syndrome: Gross, Histologic and Ultra-structural Observations in Five Necropsy Cases, *Am. J. Cardiol.*, 38:487, 1976.
40. Gellis, S. S., and Feingold, M.: Rubinstein-Taybi Syndrome, *Am. J. Dis. Child.*, 121:327, 1971.
41. Warkany, J., Passarge, E., and Smith, L. B.: Congenital Malformation in Autosomal Trisomy Syndromes, *Am. J. Dis. Child.*, 112:502, 1966.
42. Kurien, V. A., and Duke, M.: Trisomy 17-18 Syndrome, *Am. J. Cardiol.*, 21:431, 1968.
43. Greenwood, R. D., and Nadas, A. S.: The Clinical Course of Cardiac Disease in Down's Syndrome, *Pediatrics*, 58:893, 1976.
44. Van der Hauwaert, L. G., Fryns, J. P., Dumoulin, M., and Logghe, N.: Cardiovascular Malformations in Turner's and Noonan's Syndrome, *Br. Heart J.*, 40:500, 1978.
45. Pearl, W.: Cardiovascular Anomalies in Noonan's Syndrome, *Chest*, 71:677, 1977.
46. Falk, R. H., and Mackinnon, J: Klippel-Feil Syndrome Associated with Aortic Coarctation, *Br. Heart J.*, 38:1220, 1976.
47. Turiteri, L., Perheentupa, J., and Rapola, J.: The Cardiopathy of Mulibrey Nanism: A New Inherited Syndrome, *Chest*, 65:628, 1974.
48. Motta, J., Guilleminault, C., Billingham, M., Barry, W., and Mason, J.: Cardiac Abnormalities in Myotonic Dystrophy. Electrophysiologic and Histopathologic Studies, *Am. J. Med.*, 67:467, 1979.
49. Jones, K. L., and Smith, D. W.: The Williams Elfin Facies Syndrome, *J. Pediatr.*, 86:718, 1975.
50. Yurchak, P. M.: A Nine-Year-Old Girl with Congenital Heart Disease and Dysmorphic Facies, *N. Engl. J. Med.*, 295:92, 1976.
51. Robinson, C. D., Perry, L. W., Barlee, A., and Mella, G. W.: Smith-Lemli-Opitz Syndrome with Cardiovascular Abnormality, *Pediatrics*, 47:844, 1971.
*52. McAdam, L. P., O'Hanlan, M. A., Bluestone, R., and Pearson, C. M.: Relapsing Polychondritis: Prospective Study of 23 Patients and a Review of the Literature, *Medicine*, 55:193, 1976. (116 references)
53. Fukushige, J., NiHill, M. R., and McNamara, D. G.: Spectrum of Cardiovascular Lesions in Mucocutaneous Lymph Node Syndrome, *Am. J. Cardiol.*, 45:98, 1980.

54. Cayler, G. G., Blumenfeld, C. M., and Anderson, R. L.: Further Studies of Patients with the Cardiofacial Syndrome, *Chest*, 60:161, 1971.

55. Gellis, S. S., and Feingold, M.: Peripheral Facial Paralysis and Hypertension, *Am. J. Dis. Child.*, 119:59, 1970.

56. DeBush, F. L.: The Hutchinson-Gilford Progeria Syndrome: Report of Four Cases and Review of the Literature, *J. Pediatr.*, 80:697, 1972.

57. Smallridge, R. C., Rajfer, S., Davia, J., and Schaaf, M.: Acromegaly and the Heart: An Echocardiographic Study, *Am. J. Med.*, 66:22, 1979.

58. Kerber, R. E., and Sherman, B.: Echocardiographic Evaluation of Pericardial Effusion in Myxedema: Incidence and Biochemical and Clinical Correlations, *Circulation*, 52:823, 1975.

59. Mausolf, F. A. (ed.): "The Eye and Systemic Disease," The C. V. Mosby Company, St. Louis, 1979.

60. Hickey, N., Maurer, B., and Mulcahy, R.: Arcus Senilis: Its Relation to Certain Attributes and Risk Factors in Patients with Coronary Heart Disease, *Br. Heart J.*, 32:449, 1970.

61. Nadjmi, B., Flanagan, M. J., and Christian, J. R.: Laurence-Moon-Biedl Syndrome, *Am. J. Dis. Child.*, 117:352, 1969.

62. Crall, F. A., Jr., and Roberts, W. C.: The Extramural and Intramural Coronary Arteries in Juvenile Diabetes Mellitus, *Am. J. Med.*, 64:221, 1978.

63. Fortuin, N. J., Morrow, A. G., and Roberts, W. C.: Late Vascular Manifestations of the Rubella Syndrome: A Roentgenographic-Pathologic Study, *Am. J. Med.*, 51:134, 1971.

64. Ho, C. K., Kaufman, R. L., and Podos, S. M.: Ocular Colobomata, Cardiac Defect, and Other Anomalies, *J. Med. Genet.*, 12:289, 1975.

65. Roberts, N. K., Perloff, J. K., and Kark, R. A. P.: Cardiac Conduction in the Kearns-Sayre Syndrome (A Neuromuscular Disorder Associated with Progressive External Ophthalmoplegia and Pigmentary Retinopathy): Report of 2 Cases and Review of 17 Published Cases, *Am. J. Cardiol.*, 44:1396, 1979.

*66. Davis, P. J., and Davis, F. B.: Hyperthyroidism in Patients Over the Age of 60 Years, *Medicine*, 53:161, 1974. (90 references)

67. Kaye, D.: "Infective Endocarditis," University Park Press, 1976.

68. Robinow, M., and Roche, A. F.: Low-Set Ears, *Am. J. Dis. Child.*, 125:482, 1973.

69. Friedman, S., and Saraclar, M.: The High Frequency of Congenital Heart Disease in Oculo-auriculo-vertebral Dysplasia (Goldenhar's Syndrome), *J. Pediatr.*, 85:873, 1974.

70. Crampton, R.: Preeminence of the Left Stellate Ganglion in the Long Q-T Syndrome, *Circulation*, 59:769, 1979.

71. Lichstein, E., Chadda, K. D., Nark, D., and Gupta, P. K.: Diagonal Ear-Lobe Crease: Prevalence and Implications as a Coronary Risk Factor, *N. Engl. J. Med.*, 290:615, 1974.

72. Levin, D. L., Muster, A. J., Pachman, L. M., Wessel, H. V., Paul, M. W., and Koshaba, J.: Cor Pulmonale Secondary to Upper Airway Obstruction, *Chest*, 68:167, 1975.

73. Tilkian, A. G., Guilleminault, C., Schroeder, J. S., Lehrman, K. L., Simmons, F. B., and Dement, W. C.: Sleep-Induced Apnea Syndrome. Prevalence of Cardiac Arrhythmias and Their Reversal after Tracheostomy, *Am. J. Med.*, 63:348, 1977.

74. Shah, C. V., Pruyansky, S., and Harris, W. S.: Cardiac Malformations with Facial Clefts, *Am. J. Dis. Child.*, 119:238, 1970.

75. Silverman, M. E., and Hurst, J. W.: The Hand and the Heart, *Am. J. Cardiol.*, 22:718, 1968.

76. Ries, A. H., Stefadouros, M. A., Strong, W. B., Miller, M. D., Gilman, P., Rigby, J. A., and Mc-Farlane, J.: Left Ventricular Performance in Children with Homozygous Sickle Cell Anaemia, *Br. Heart J.*, 40:690, 1978.

77. Aziz, K., Sanyal, S. K., and Goldblatt, E.: Reversed Differential Cyanosis, *Br. Heart J.*, 30:288, 1968.

78. Chesler, E., Moller, J. H., and Edwards, J. E.: Anatomic Basis for Delivery of Right Ventricular Blood into Localized Segments of the Systemic Arterial System, *Am. J. Cardiol.*, 21:72, 1968.

79. Heath, P., and Williams, D. R.: Nail Haemorrhages, *Br. Heart J.*, 40:1300, 1978.

80. Smith, A. T., Sack, G. H., Jr., and Taylor, G. J.: Holt-Oram Syndrome, *J. Pediatr.*, 95:538, 1979.

81. Harris, L. C., and Osborne, W. P.: Congenital Absence or Hypoplasia of the Radius with Ventricular Septal Defect, *J. Pediatr.*, 68:265, 1966.

82. John, J. T., Jr., Hough, A., and Sergent, J. S.: Pericardial Disease in Rheumatoid Arthritis, *Am. J. Med.*, 66:385, 1979.

83. Ignaczak, T., Espinoza, L. R., Kantor, O. S., and Osterland, C. K.: Jaccoud Arthritis, *Arch. Intern. Med.*, 135:577, 1975.

84. McAllister, H. A., Jr., Fenoglio, J. J., Jr.: Cardiac Involvement in Whipple's Disease, *Circulation*, 52:152, 1975.

85. Pund, E. P., Jr., Hawley, R. L., McGee, H. J., Blount, S. G., Jr.: Gouty Heart, *N. Engl. J. Med.*, 263:835, 1960.

86. Bergofsky, E. H.: Cor Pulmonale in the Syndrome of Alveolar Hypoventilation, *Prog. Cardiovasc. Dis.*, 9:414, 1967.

87. Matsuo, S., Yoshioka, M., Yano, K., and Hashiba, K.: Straight Back Syndrome: Clinical and Hemodynamic Study of 9 Cases, *Am. Heart J.*, 86:828, 1973.

88. Beiser, G. D., Epstein, S. E., Stampfer, M., Goldstein, R. E., Noland, S. P., and Levitsky, S.: Impairment of Cardiac Function in Patients with Pectus Excavatum, with Improvement after Operative Correction, *N. Engl. J. Med.*, 287:267, 1972.

89. Jordan, C. E., White, R. I., Jr., Fischer, K. E., Neill, C., and Dorst, J. P.: The Scoliosis of Congenital Heart Disease, *Am. Heart J.*, 84:463, 1972.

90. Udoshi, M. B., Shah, A., Fisher, V. J., and Dolgin, M.: Incidence of Mitral Valve Prolapse in Subjects with Thoracic Skeletal Abnormalities—A Prospective Study, *Am. Heart J.*, 97:303, 1979.

90a. Roberts, W. C., Hollingsworth, J. F., Buckley, B. H., Jaffe, R. B., Epstein, S. E., and Stinson, E. B.: Combined Mitral and Aortic Regurgitation in Ankylosing Spondylitis: Angiographic and Anatomic Features, *Am. J. Med.*, 56:237, 1974.

91. Arosemena, E., Elliot, L. P., and Eliot, R. S.: Chest Deformity in Adults with Congenital Heart Disease, *Am. J. Cardiol.*, 20:309, 1967.

92. Greenwood, R. D., Rosenthal, A., and Nadas, A. S.: Cardiovascular Malformations Associated with Imperforate Anus, *J. Pediatr.*, 86:576, 1975.

93. Quan, L., and Smith, D. W.: The Vater Association, *J. Pediatr.*, 82:104, 1973.

94. Freedom, R. M.: The Asplenia Syndrome: A Review

of Significant Extracardiac Structural Abnormalities in 29 Necropsied Patients, *J. Pediatr.*, 81:1130, 1972.

95. Greenwood, R. D., Rosenthal, A., and Nadas, A. S.: Cardiovascular Malformations Associated with Omphalocele, *J. Pediatr.*, 85:818, 1974.

96. Lewandowski, R. C., Jr., and Yunis, J.: New Chromosomal Syndromes, *Am. J. Dis. Child.*, 129:515, 1975.

*97. Steeg, C. N., and Woolf, P.: Cardiovascular Malformations in the Fetal Alcohol Syndrome, *Am. Heart J.*, 98:635, 1979. (45 references)

98. Greenwood, R. D., Rosenthal, A., Parisi, L., Fyler, D. C., and Nadas, A. S.: Extracardiac Abnormalities in Infants with Congenital Heart Disease, *Pediatrics*, 55:485, 1975.

99. Jaigesimi, P., and Antia, A. V.: Extra Cardiac Defects in Children with Congenital Heart Disease, *Br. Heart J.*, 42:475, 1979.

9

Measurement of the Systemic Blood Pressure

Donald O. Nutter, M.D.

In December I caused a Mare to be tied down alive on her back, she was fourteen Hands high, and about fourteen Years of Age, had a Fistula on her Withers, was neither very lean, nor yet lusty: Having laid open the left crural Artery about three Inches from her Belly, I inserted into it a brass Pipe whose bore was one sixth of an Inch in Diameter; and to that, by means of another brass Pipe which was fitly adapted to it, I fixed a glass Tube, of nearly the same Diameter, which was nine Feet in Length: Then untying the Ligature on the Artery, the Blood rose in the left Ventricle of the Heart: But it did Not attain to its full Height at once; rushed up about half way in an Instant, and afterwards gradually at each Pulse twelve, eight, six, four, two and sometimes one Inch: When it was at its full Height, it would rise and fall at and after each Pulse two, three, or four Inches; and sometimes it would fall twelve or fourteen Inches, and have there for a time the same Vibrations up and down at and after each Pulse, as it had, when it was at its full Height; to which it would rise again, after forty or fifty pulses.

Stephen Hales, 1733[1]

Blood pressure is a measure of arterial potential energy, or the lateral force per unit area of vascular wall, and is expressed in units of dynes per square centimeter in the metric system. The amplitude and configuration of the pressure pulse are dependent on the functional state of the left ventricle, the physical characteristics of the blood and arterial wall, and the peripheral resistance to blood flow. Hence, peak systolic pressure is determined by the volume and velocity of ventricular ejection, the peripheral arteriolar resistance, the distensibility of the arterial wall, the viscosity of the blood, and the end-diastolic volume in the arterial system. The magnitude of the decline in pressure during diastole is in turn determined by viscosity, arterial distensibility, peripheral resistance to flow, and the cardiac cycle length. The important physical properties which influence arterial distensibility are (1) the elastic modulus of the vessel wall, which is the ratio of stress (force acting to deform the wall) to strain (the proportional deformation produced) and (2) the geometry of the vessel wall, or more specifically, the internal radius and wall thickness which govern vascular wall tension according to the modified Laplace equation

$$T = \frac{Pr}{h}$$

where T = wall tension
P = intravascular pressure
r = internal radius
h = wall thickness

A decrease in elasticity or an increase in radius results in decreased distensibility and a greater rise in pressure per unit volume of blood.

Blood pressure measurements date back to Stephen Hales' recordings of the direct arterial pressure in animals obtained by cannulation and a blood-filled glass column (1733). The history of direct pressure measurement has been chiefly concerned with the evolution of manometers and recording devices and the development of safe, efficient methods of arterial cannulation. The mercury or saline-filled gravity manometer, still the standard for static pressure measurement, was unsuited to the quantitation of pulsatile pressures and was followed by the development of mechanical, optical, and finally electronic manometers and recorders. Indirect blood pressure measurement has also undergone a long history of technical development, highlighted by the invention of the inflatable cuff manometer (Riva-Rocci, 1896) and the discovery and application of the arterial sounds (Korotkov, 1905). The instrumentation and techniques for the measurement of blood pressure are the subject of a monograph by Geddes.[2]

Direct Methods

Present-day techniques for the direct and continuous measurement of arterial pressure utilize the electromanometer, a transducer which serves to convert mechanical pressure energy into an electric signal suitable for amplification, display, and recording. The method requires cannulation of the artery with a saline-filled catheter or needle, which mechanically couples the circulation to the arterial manometer. Pressures are conventionally recorded using atmospheric pressure as the "zero" reference level, and intravascular pressures are further referenced to the level of the heart by the addition or subtraction of a gravitation (hydrostatic) factor. The gravitational factor is expressed by the notation pgh, where p is the density of blood (1 g/ml), g is the acceleration due to gravity (980 cm/s), and h is the transducer height (cm) above or below the horizontal plane of the heart.

The most frequently used transducer is the strain gauge manometer, an instrument with acceptable linearity, sensitivity, stability, and frequency response for the precise and accurate measurement of blood pressure. However, a significant source of error may reside in the catheter or coupling system, in which the properties of inertia (fluid mass), friction (tube resistance), and elasticity (volume distortion due to air bubbles or elastic tubing) all interact to produce damping of the frequency response. Systems may be overdamped (i.e., there may be a marked decrease below desired maximum frequency response) or underdamped (i.e., there may be a tendency to oscillate as the natural frequency of the system is approached), and both conditions will result in signal distortion. The appropriate combination of catheter, fluid, and manometer characteristics results in a compromise condition of optimal or "critical" damping in which the system response is constant to some desirable frequency level. The use of a standard inelastic cardiac catheter and connecting tube filled with bubble-free fluid is usually quite adequate for the clinical recording of intravascular pressures when qualitative waveform analysis is not desired.

A different type of measurement error may occur when an end-hole catheter is positioned axial to flow in a vessel. When the catheter faces flow (and also when the catheterization procedure occludes a smaller artery), kinetic energy is converted to potential pressure energy, artifactually elevating the measured blood pressure. When the catheter points away from flow, the Bernoulli effect produces a low-pressure zone at the orifice, resulting in artifactually low pressure measurements. Although seldom of practical importance, these errors may be of significant magnitude under the conditions of high arterial flow when kinetic energy may exceed 10 percent of the total fluid energy. The use of a side-hole catheter positioned in a large, patent artery allows measurement of the true blood pressure. A second factor which can elevate the pressure reading is the motion (including acceleration) due to catheter whip. Pressure transients of significant amplitude may be regularly superimposed on the aortic or central arterial pulse under conditions of vigorous cardiac contraction or in response to sudden catheter movement.

Recently developed, miniature, self-flushing strain gauge manometers which can be attached directly to an intravascular catheter or needle may eliminate some of the problems related to transducer mounting and flushing, and overdamping by connective tubing. The most promising step in the elimination of measurement error due to damping and acceleration artifact has been the development of intravascular electromanometers suitable for mounting on cardiac catheters or for surgical implantation in the vascular wall.

Indirect Methods

The universally accepted method for the indirect measurement of arterial blood pressure is sphygmomanometry. This technique is based on the auscultatory detection of the Korotkov sounds over a peripheral artery at a point distal to cuff compression of the artery. The Korotkov sounds are low-frequency vibrations (with predominant energy content below 200 Hz) originating in the blood and vessel walls. Analysis of these sounds by McCutcheon and Rushmer[3] has demonstrated the presence of two major components: the initial transient (K_i) and the compression murmur (K_c), which correspond to the opening tap sound and the rumble sound described by Rodbard.[4] The initial transient occurs at the instant cuff pressure reaches arterial pressure and is probably caused by an acceleration transient accompanying abrupt arterial opening and vascular distension. The intensity of this initial sound is dependent on the slope of the pressure pulse and the level of the distal arterial pressure at the time of arterial opening. Increases in pressure pulse slope or decreases in distal pressure, such as might occur with vasodilatation and high-velocity flow, will increase the sound intensity. The opposite effects, such as might occur during vasoconstriction, venous congestion, or circulatory collapse, will decrease the sound intensity. The initial transient is probably caused by oscillation of the arterial wall as the occluded segment is suddenly opened by systolic pressure. The compression murmur is probably due to a turbulent jet of flow distal to the partially compressed segment, an explanation which would account for its presence only in the pressure range at which a significant volume of blood is moving through a moderate vascular constriction.

On the basis of their acoustic qualities, the Korotkov sounds have been divided into five phases occurring in sequence as the occluding pressure declines. Phase I consists of clear, tapping sounds (K_i)

which occur when the cuff pressure has fallen to the arterial peak systolic level. These sounds are initially soft, since the pulse slope is small at peak pressure, and gradually increase in intensity as cuff pressure falls into the range where the pressure pulse slope is steep. Phase II consists of K_i sounds followed by swishing sounds or murmurs (K_c). Phase III is an accentuation of the phase II sounds which occurs when cuff pressure is low enough to allow a sizable volume of blood to pass through the partially compressed artery. Phase IV is signaled by the abrupt, distinct muffling of the sounds which produces a blowing quality that gradually decreases in intensity. These characteristics are the result of diminution and loss of component K_i as cuff pressure approaches arterial diastolic levels, and diminution of component K_c as the flow period lengthens and the flow velocity decreases. Phase V, marked by complete disappearance of sound, occurs when the vessel is no longer compressed to a degree which can produce turbulent flow. The cuff pressure at which sound disappears may be extremely low, or nonexistent, when high-flow velocities already exist in the circulation, e.g., in the presence of exercise, anemia, fever, thyrotoxicosis, or arteriovenous fistulas.

Proper technique is necessary to obtain accurate measurements of blood pressure by the indirect method. The inflatable rubber bag within the compression cuff should have a width that is 20 percent greater than the limb diameter and a length adequate to encompass at least half of the limb. The cuff should be applied snugly, with the inflatable bag positioned over the artery, at the level of the heart. Before auscultation the peak systolic pressure should be estimated by determining the cuff pressure which obliterates the distal arterial pulse. The stethoscope is then applied lightly but firmly over the artery, and auscultatory pressure is determined by inflating the cuff to a level approximately 30 mmHg above the peak systolic pressure and noting the appearance and behavior of the Korotkov sounds as the cuff is deflated at a rate of 2 to 3 mmHg/s. When the sounds disappear, the bag should be rapidly decompressed and 1 or 2 min allowed to pass before repeat determinations are made. The 1967 American Heart Association subcommittee report on the determination of human blood pressure by sphygmomanometer[5] recommends that the systolic pressure be recorded as the point at which the first tapping sound occurs for two consecutive beats (phase I), and that the diastolic pressure be recorded as the point at which abrupt muffling of the sounds occurs (onset of phase IV). It is also recommended that the pressure at which the sounds are noted to disappear (phase V) be recorded. The mean blood pressure can be estimated by the addition of one-third the pulse pressure (systolic minus diastolic) to the diastolic pressure.

The method of sphygmomanometry contains several sources of error related to inadequate apparatus, inaccurate detection of the Korotkov sounds, and observer techniques. It has been reported frequently that a cuff of less than the recommended width may inadequately transmit pressure to the artery and falsely elevate the recorded blood pressure. In this respect, a cuff which bulges beyond its covering or is applied too loosely and "balloons" within the covering will act as a narrow cuff and elevate pressure. The standard blood pressure cuff may frequently be inadequate for pressure measurement in the arms of very obese subjects or in the leg. Numerous observers have noted higher blood pressures in obese subjects than in lean ones and have attributed this to the use of a cuff too narrow for the increased arm girth. However, several investigators employing both clinical observations and mechanical models of the upper arm have indicated that when the inflatable bag completely encircles the arm, there is no variation in pressure due to arm circumference and only minimal variation in pressure due to cuff width.[6-8] When the bag fails to enclose the arm, as is so often the case when the standard commercial cuff is applied to adult subjects, the pressure is falsely elevated and varies with arm circumference, cuff width, and the level of blood pressure. When the cuff is deflated too slowly or is immediately reinflated for multiple pressure determinations, the resultant venous congestion may artifactually elevate the diastolic pressure and may falsely decrease the systolic pressure by decreasing the intensity of phase I or phase II sounds to an inaudible level. This serves to emphasize the value of determining systolic pressure by palpation when the arterial sounds are faint because of circulatory collapse or marked venous congestion. With some training, the method of palpation can also be used to estimate diastolic pressure by detecting a peculiar snapping quality to the pulse as cuff pressure nears the diastolic level. This may be of particular value when the sounds are faint or when phases IV and V are widely separated, as in severe anemia or aortic valvular insufficiency. Rapid deflation of the cuff may also cause the first (systolic) sounds to be missed. An erroneously low systolic pressure may also result from the failure to detect the presence of an auscultatory gap, a silent interval occasionally present just below the systolic pressure level.

Studies correlating direct and indirect blood pressure measurements have been characterized by considerable variability between individual subjects but in general have shown a good correlation between indirect and direct measurements of blood pressure in the arm.[8] The observed trend has been for the indirect method to underestimate systolic pressure by several millimeters of mercury, to overestimate diastolic pressure by several millimeters of mercury when phase IV is used as an end point, and to slightly underestimate diastolic pressure in normal individuals when phase V is taken as the end point. A study which recorded the direct (catheter) and indirect pressures simultaneously from the same arm in young, normal women indicated that indirect measurements underestimate direct systolic pressures and overestimate direct diastolic pressure when either phase IV or phase V is used as an endpoint.[9] The correlation between direct systolic pressure and the onset of phase I sounds was good, although several pressure pulses could be detected by a catheter distal to the cuff before an audible sound occurred. Direct diastolic pressure correlated somewhat better with the disappearance of sound than with muffling.

Normal Blood Pressure

The normal range has often been chosen by performing a frequency distribution on a population sample and defining arbitrary percentages of subjects above and below the mean as normal, borderline, or abnormal. Since blood pressure varies with age, sex, and socioracial grouping, the normal range will vary with these factors. In the United States the pressure increases rapidly over the first few days of life and then increases gradually, with a slightly greater increment in systolic than in diastolic values, throughout life. The pressure tends to be higher in Western, industrialized societies than in Afro-Asian and technically underdeveloped societies.

The normal blood pressure limits for adults (less than 45 years old and of mixed sex and race) living in our society are approximately 100 to 140 mmHg systolic and 60 to 90 mmHg diastolic. In an individual subject, however, base-line pressures above or below these normal levels do not define the pathophysiological state of hypertension or hypotension or an abnormality of physiological regulation, since the physiological range of normal for an individual may extend into the statistic range of abnormality.

It has been demonstrated in mildly to moderately hypertensive persons that the blood pressure "casually" recorded in the laboratory by a physician is significantly higher than the average value of a series of intermittent indirect determinations[10] or continuous direct recordings[11] made during the course of daily activities. In an attempt to eliminate the variability present in casual pressures, and to obtain pressures which could be referenced to the statistic norms or used as a base line for subsequent studies of an individual, the concept of basal blood pressure was introduced. The basal pressure is that recorded when all stimuli or factors which might increase the arterial pressure above the level established by resting vasomotor tone are eliminated. True basal pressures are seldom recorded; indeed, they probably rarely exist except under certain conditions of sleep. Several methods have been used to estimate basal blood pressure, they include measurements obtained (1) during sleep, (2) when the subject first

awakens in the morning and is still recumbent, or (3) after several hours of reclining.

Many factors acting through the pressure regulatory system vary the individual's blood pressure during the course of daily activities; these factors include (1) body posture, (2) the state of muscular, cerebral, or gastrointestinal activity, (3) emotional or painful stimuli (endogenous or exogenous), (4) environmental physical factors such as temperature and noise level, and (5) the use of tobacco, coffee, or other drugs with direct or neurally mediated vasomotor properties. Twenty-four-hour pressures, obtained from normal and hypertensive subjects with an automatic recorder, have shown striking variability with activity and emotional stimuli (with little effect produced by eating).[11,12] The degree of variability was not significantly influenced by age, sex, or the level of pressure. The average diurnal pattern of blood pressure is characterized by an increase throughout the day and early evening and a significant, rapid, decline to a low point during the early, deep stage of sleep. The decline with sleep has been described by several investigators and has been related to a decrease in cardiac output and the presence of cutaneous vasodilatation.[13]

Dynamic exercise in both the supine and upright positions produces a modest increase in blood pressure that is dependent on total work load. The response is characterized by systolic > mean > diastolic pressure. The response is not significantly changed by training, but increasing age results in a higher slope of the pressure pulse and higher amplitude for systolic and mean pressures. Sustained or static muscular contractions produce an abrupt and significant increase in systolic, mean, and diastolic blood pressure that is dependent on the proportionate strength of contraction and independent of the muscle mass involved.[14] The observed systolic and diastolic elevations may exceed those resulting from dynamic exercise at equivalent oxygen consumptions. It should be emphasized that the pressure effects of muscular activity vary with the sampling site, as do resting blood pressures. Rowell et al. have documented significant differences between aortic and radial artery pressures during treadmill exercise, with the rise in radial pulse pressure exceeding aortic pulse pressure by a factor of 2.6 to 1.95.[15]

Clinical Application of Sphygmomanometry

Increased Pulse Pressure

An increase in pulse pressure is commonly observed during routine sphygmomanometric recordings. This is usually the result of an increase in stroke volume and ejection velocity and/or an attendant decrease in peripheral resistance. Fever, anemia, hot weather, and exercise, and occasionally hyperthyroidism or arteriovenous fistulas, may produce this change. Organic lesions of the heart, such as aortic insufficiency, often result in a widened peripheral pulse pressure. An increased pulse pressure related to an increased stroke volume may occur with complete heart block or marked sinus bradycardia.

Degenerative and/or atherosclerotic changes in the blood vessel wall contribute to decreased compliance, in which a normal or even decreased stroke volume can result in elevation of systolic pressure. The so-called systolic hypertension of the elderly does not necessarily represent a change in small-vessel resistance; therefore, attempts to lower this type of systolic pressure elevation can significantly reduce peripheral perfusion. Less common, but of critical diagnostic importance, is the increased pulse pressure associated with systemic arteriovenous fistula, where a relative tachycardia and the pulse pressure may offer the only clinical clues.

Decreased Pulse Pressure

A narrow pulse pressure is not commonly observed in normal subjects. This phenomenon may be expected to occur with (1) increased peripheral resistance, (2) decreased cardiac ejection volume, or (3) markedly decreased intravascular volume.

A striking increase in peripheral resistance may occur in response to cold, endogenous or exogenous elevations of circulating norepinephrine, or severe congestive heart failure where arterial wall stiffness and resting sympathetic vasoconstrictor tone are increased.

The conditions which result in diminished ejection volume are of more diagnostic importance. In conditions producing mechanical obstruction, the narrowing of pulse pressure generally correlates with the severity of the specific disease process. An exception is sometimes observed in young people with aortic stenosis in whom severe obstruction is present without significant narrowing of pulse pressure.

The narrowing of pulse pressure in metabolic acidosis can be related to (1) increased peripheral resistance (as in lactic acidosis or cholera), (2) decreased intravascular volume (as in diabetic ketoacidosis or cholera), or (3) decreased myocardial performance (following cardiac arrest). As the degree of acidosis increases, the myocardium becomes less responsive to the stimulus of catecholamines; i.e., the diminished inotropic response results in progressive myocardial failure, as evidenced by decreasing stroke volume and ejection velocity.

Pressure Difference between the Arms

The diagnostic importance of blood pressure differences between right and left arms has been enhanced in recent years by the recognition of two conditions: supravalvular aortic stenosis (primarily in children) and the subclavian steal syndrome (in adults). Other clues to the recognition of these states may be inadequate without the characteristic blood pressure changes. More than half the patients with supravalvular aortic stenosis have been found to have a greater than 20 mmHg difference in arm pressures (the right greater than the left except in the presence of dextrocardia.[16] The subclavian steal syndrome may be accompanied by symptoms of cerebrovascular insufficiency without overt manifestations of ischemia of the involved extremity; however, a pronounced lowering or absence of brachial artery pressure is often found in the ipsilateral extremity.[17]

Pressure Differences between Arms and Legs

Progressive systolic pressure amplification occurs as the point of measurement is moved peripherally from the supravalvular aortic area to the extremities. However, the increment in systolic pressure is equivalent in the large arteries of the upper arm and the thigh. Direct recordings of femoral and brachial arterial pressures (systolic, diastolic, and mean) in adults[18] and children[19] and indirect measurement of popliteal and brachial pressures using appropriate pressure cuffs [20] have demonstrated that pressures are equal in these sites. In addition, direct measurements of systolic and pulse pressure in the femoral and brachial arteries have failed to show a difference between the arm and leg in patients with significant, isolated aortic regurgitation.[21] A difference in arm and leg pressures may occur due to congenital aortic obstruction (coarctation) or to acquired problems such as aortic dissection, aortic arch syndrome, and the subclavian steal syndrome.

Pulsus Paradoxus (See Chap. 57)

Pulsus paradoxus can be elicited by inflating the blood pressure cuff to a level greater than systolic pressure with the patient breathing normally. (Care must be taken to prevent the patient from performing Valsalva's maneuver during the respiratory cycle.) As cuff pressure is slowly released, Korotkov sounds become audible during expiration. The pressure difference between the first discernible sound (on expiration) and the pressure level at which Korotkov sounds are audible during all phases of respiration gives a quantitative estimate of the degree of "arterial paradox." This finding may be especially useful in detecting acute cardiac tamponade; but care must be taken to rule out other causes of paradox.

During inspiration, arterial pressure decreases because increased negative intrathoracic pressures delay pulmonary venous return to the left side of the heart. Normal individuals may demonstrate an 8- to 12-mmHg drop in systolic pressure during inspiration. An exaggerated response is observed in tense pericardial effusion, constrictive pericarditis, restrictive cardiomyopathy, severe chronic obstructive lung disease, and hypovolemia (e.g., hemorrhagic shock).

Pulsus Alternans (See Chap. 10)

Beat-to-beat variations in systolic pressure can be readily appreciated by palpation of the femoral arterial pulse and, when it is prominent, can be quantitated by sphygmomanometry.

Beat-to-beat alteration of the pulse may occur (1) in tachypnea if the respiratory rate is half the heart rate, (2) in bigeminal rhythm, (3) immediately following ventricular ectopic contractions, or (4) in severe organic heart disease manifesting myocardial failure. Transient interruption of respirations will eliminate the first cause of alteration. In bigeminal rhythm the ectopic beats are generally out of phase with normal heart cadence; therefore, the Korotkov sounds will be of two intensities. A slight pause will be noted following the softer Korotkov sound. Normal persons may have true pulsus alternans for several beats following an ectopic contraction, but this rarely persists for more than 10 to 12 beats. Persistent pulsus alternans suggests organic disease and incipient myocardial failure. Pulsus alternans occasionally follows rapid atrial tachycardia.

References

1. Hales, S.: "Statistical Essays: Containing Haema-staticks; or, an Account of Some Hydraulick and Hydrostatical Experiments Made on the Blood and Blood-Vessels of Animals," W. Innys and R. Manby, London, 1733.

*2. Geddes, L. A.: "The Direct and Indirect Measurement of Blood Pressure," Year Book Medical Publishers, Inc., Chicago, 1970.

3. McCutcheon, E. P., and Rushmer, R. F.: Korotkov Sounds: An Experimental Critique, *Circ. Res.,* 20:149, 1967.

4. Rodbard, S.: The Components of the Korotkov Sounds, *Am. Heart J.,* 74:278, 1967.

5. Kirkendall, W. M., Burton, A. C., Epstein, F. H., and Freis, E. D.: Recommendations for Human Blood Pressure Determination by Sphygmomanometers, *Circulation,* 36:980, 1967.

6. King, G. E.: Errors in Clinical Measurement of Blood Pressure in Obesity, *Clin. Sci.,* 32:223, 1967.

7. Steinfeld, L., Alexander, H., and Cohen, M. L.: Updating Sphygmomanometry, *Am. J. Cardiol.,* 33:107, 1974.

8. Nielsen, P. E., and Janniche, H.: The Accuracy of Auscultatory Measurement of Arm Blood Pressure in Very Obese Subjects, *Acta. Med. Scand.,* 195:403, 1974.

9. Raftery, E. B., and Ward, A. P.: The Indirect Method of Recording Blood Pressure, *Cardiovasc. Res.,* 2:210, 1968.

10. Kain, H. K., Hinman, A. T., and Sokolow, M.: Arterial Blood Pressure Measurements with a Portable Recorder in Hypertensive Patients: I. Variability and Correlation with "Casual" Pressures, *Circulation,* 30:882, 1964.

11. Littler, W. A., Honour, A. J., Pugsley, D. J., and Sleight, P.: Continuous Recording of Direct Arterial Pressure in Unrestricted Patients, *Circulation,* 51:1101, 1975.

12. Richardson, D. W., Honour, A. T., Fenton, D. W., Stott, F. H., and Pickering, G. W.: Variation in Arterial Pressure throughout the Day and Night, *Clin. Sci.,* 26:445, 1964.

13. Khatri, I. M., and Freis, E. D.: Hemodynamic Changes during Sleep, *J. Appl. Physiol.,* 22:867, 1967.

14. Donald, K. W., Lind, A. R., McNicol, G. W., Humphreys, P. W., Taylor, S. H., and Staunton, H. P.: Cardiovascular Responses to Sustained Contractions, *Circ. Res.,* 20(suppl. 1):15, 1967.

15. Rowell, L. B., Brengelmann, G. L., Blackmon, T. R., Bruce, R. A., and Murray, T. A.: Disparities between Aortic and Peripheral Pulse Pressure Induced by Upright Exercise and Vasomotor Changes in Man, *Circulation,* 37:954, 1968.

16. Wooley, C. F., Hosier, D. M., Booth, R. W., Molnar, W., Sirak, H. D., and Ryan, J. M.: Supravalvular Aortic Stenosis, *Am. J. Med.,* 31:717, 1961.

17. Patel, A., and Toole, J. F.: Subclavian Steal Syndrome: Reversal of Cephalic Blood Flow, *Medicine (Baltimore),* 44:289, 1965.

18. Pascarelli, E. F., and Bertrand, C. A.: Comparison of Blood Pressure in the Arms and Legs, *N. Engl. J. Med.,* 270:693, 1964.

19. Park, M. K., and Guntheroth, W. G.: Direct Blood Pressure Measurements in Brachial and Femoral Arteries in Children, *Circulation,* 41:231, 1970.

20. Felix, W. R., Hochberg, H. M., George, M. E. D., Schmalzbach, E. L., and Vaserberg, R.: Ultrasound Measurement of Arm and Leg Blood Pressures, *J. Am. Med. Assoc.,* 226:1096, 1973.

21. Pascarelli, E. F., and Bertrand, C. A.: Comparison of Arm and Leg Blood Pressures in Aortic Insufficiency: An Appraisal of Hill's Sign, *Br. Med. J.,* 2:73, 1965.

*This article is a review of the literature and contains additional references to the literature.

10

Physical Examination of the Arteries and Veins

Robert A. O'Rourke, M.D.

The Arterial Pulse

The examination of the arterial pulse was one of the earliest forms of physical diagnosis, and there is still no physical sign more basic or important in clinical medicine. A description of the arterial pulse must consider recent advances in measurement of arterial hemodynamics, assessment of the arterial wave contour, and frequency analysis of the pressure pulse.[1-5]

Physical Determinants of the Arterial Pulse

Origin of the Arterial Pulse

Pressure and blood flow measurements in the ascending aorta result from the interaction between the heart and arterial system. The rise in left ventricular pressure, upon exceeding the aortic pressure, becomes the driving force for the movement of blood into the ascending aorta.[6,7] This driving force is opposed by several forces which impede the development of flow and are interrelated in a complex manner. The driving forces are dependent upon the intrinsic contractility of ventricular muscle, the size and shape of the heart, and the heart rate. Three major factors contributing to arterial impedance include (1) resistance, (2) inertia, and (3) compliance. Resistance is related to blood viscosity and the geometry of the vasculature, opposes flow, and is unaffected by changes in heart rate. Inertia is related to the mass of the blood, opposes the rate of change of arterial blood flow (i.e., acceleration), and is heart rate–dependent. Compliance is related to the distensibility of the vascular walls, opposes changes in arterial blood volume, and is also heart rate–dependent. The rate dependency of inertia and compliance introduces phase shifts between instantaneous pressure and flow in a pulsatile system.[6] Inertia and compliance are important determinants of the character of ventricular ejection, especially in early systole when flows and pressures are changing rapidly.

The arterial pulse wave begins with aortic valve opening and the onset of left ventricular ejection. Aortic pressure rises rapidly in early systole since the left ventricular stroke volume enters the aorta faster than it flows to distal sites. The rapid-rising portion of the arterial pressure curve is often termed the *anacrotic* limb (cf. Greek, "upbeat").[8] Recent studies in experimental animals and in patients indicate that peak proximal aortic flow velocity occurs slightly earlier than peak pressure.[2] After its peak, aortic pressure declines as ventricular ejection slows and peripheral blood flow continues. During isovolumic relaxation, there is a transient reversal of flow from the central arteries toward the ventricle just prior to aortic valve closure which is associated with an incisura on the descending limb of the aortic pressure pulse. The subsequent smaller, secondary positive wave has been attributed to the elastic recoil of the aorta and aortic valve but is partially due to reflected waves from more distal arteries. Beyond this, aortic pressure decreases again as further "runoff" in the peripheral circulation occurs in diastole.

The proximal aortic pulse pressure is directly proportional to the ratio of stroke volume to arterial distensibility, but multiple factors influence this complex relationship.[8] Arterial distensibility diminishes as the distending arterial pressure increases. Accordingly, the pulse pressure for a constant stroke volume will be larger if the mean blood pressure is elevated. In addition, arterial distensibility varies inversely with the rate of rise of intraluminal pressure. When the systolic ejection rate increases, the stiffer arterial wall results in a greater pulse pressure. Finally, the arterial pulse pressure may be modified by reflected pressure waves and by the rate of blood flow from arterioles to veins.

Arterial Pulse Contour

Pulsatile changes in arterial diameter are virtually identical to the pressure pulse, with minor differences explained in terms of nonlinear elasticity and viscosity of the arterial wall. In 1939, Hamilton and Dow explained the pressure wave contour in different arteries in terms of wave reflection between the aortic valve and peripheral sites.[9] They likened the arterial system to a tube with two closed ends, one representing the aortic valve and the other the resultant of all peripheral reflecting sites. In their hypothesis, the arterial pulse bounded back and forth between these sites, setting up a system of "standing waves" in the aorta. However, the standing wave hypothesis is not completely accurate since some attenuation of the wave in travel occurs and there is incomplete reflection of the wave.[10]

More precise information about the arterial pulse has been obtained from quantitative studies in which a regularly repeated pressure or flow wave is considered as a series of harmonics.[1,11] Each harmonic component has a definite modulus (amplitude) and a definite phase (delay) from a set point of reference. Given modulus and phase of the different harmonics of the pulse, the original wave can be resynthesized, and corresponding components of waves recorded simultaneously can be compared. By measuring and correlating mean values of the waves, vascular resistance can be calculated and the resistance properties of vessels downstream can be interpreted. The corresponding frequency components of pressure and flow can be compared in order to determine vascular impedance, the relationship of pressure to flow at frequencies which are multiples of heart rate.[1]

Usually, there is a linear relationship between pressure and flow at the same point in an artery and between pressure and pressure at different points in the arterial system. From impedance curves, it is possible to identify the factors responsible for the relationship between pulsatile pressure and flow.[2,3,7,12,13] Furthermore, the coefficient of reflection in peripheral vessels can be calculated from the relationship of resistance to the minimal and subsequent values of impedance modulus. The peripheral arterial pressure wave recorded is the summation of the incident (initial) and reflected waves. If the coefficient of reflection is 0.8, the wave reflected from the peripheral bed has an amplitude which is 80 percent of the incident wave.[1] The systemic circulation may be represented by a simple asymmetric T-tube model which emphasizes the importance of wave reflection at two arteriolar reflecting sites in the upper and lower parts of the body.[1,4] Such a model provides logical explanations for many of the features of arterial pressure waves recorded in humans under different conditions.

Peripheral Transmission of the Arterial Pulse

The arterial pulse wave at any site is influenced by many factors, including the left ventricular stroke volume, the rate of ejection, the compliance of the aorta and large vessels, the peripheral vascular resistance, the pulse rate, the systolic and diastolic blood pressure, the distance from the heart, the blood viscosity, and the size and pressure-volume characteristics of the vessel. As the normal aortic pulse wave is transmitted peripherally, significant changes in its contour occur due to (1) distortion and damping of pulse wave components; (2) different rates of transmission of various components; (3) distortion or exaggeration by reflected, resonant, or standing waves; (4) conversion of kinetic energy into hydrostatic or potential energy; (5) differences in distensibility and caliber of the arteries; and (6) changes in the vessel wall due to age and/or disease.[14]

The arterial pressure pulse enters the proximal aorta and travels distally at a velocity many times faster than maximum blood flow. The pressure wave is accompanied by a traveling wave distending the arterial wall, the pulse wave velocity increasing as arterial wall distensibility diminishes.[8] This normally occurs distally, as the arteries branch into smaller channels and their walls become stiffer. However, with increasing age and with systemic hypertension, arterial wall distensibility diminishes and pulse wave velocity is correspondingly greater.[1,15,16]

The pulse wave arrives at progressively later times at more peripheral sites when timed from the QRS complex on the electrocardiogram. Representative time delays are as follows: carotid, about 30 ms; brachial, 60 ms; radial, 80 ms; and femoral, 75 ms.

The arterial pulse wave undergoes a progressive change in shape during its transmission distally (Fig. 10-1). The pulse pressure and systolic amplitude increase, and the ascending limb of the pulse wave becomes steeper. The incisura of the central aortic pulse is gradually replaced by a smoother, somewhat later, dicrotic notch which occurs at lower pressure levels. The dicrotic notch and the following positive secondary or dicrotic wave probably result from the summation of the forward pulse wave and reflected waves from the peripheral vessels. The propagated pulse wave and reflected waves are affected by viscous damping, the extent of damping increasing as the velocity of the various components of the pressure waves become greater. The changes in pulse contour that are due to reflections would be even more marked if the damping were less.[8]

Examination of the Arterial Pulse

In a complete physical examination, all major arterial pulses are examined bilaterally both for patency and for waveform characteristics. The thickness and hardness of the arterial walls often can be assessed by "rolling" the vessel against underlying tissue. A pulse in the foot should not be considered absent unless examined in the dependent position. Other-

FIGURE 10-1 Systemic arterial pressure waveforms vs. location. Changes in the contour of the arterial pressure pulse in a normal subject during a pull back of a micromanometer catheter from central aorta to brachial artery. (*Courtesy of Joseph Murgo, M.D.*)

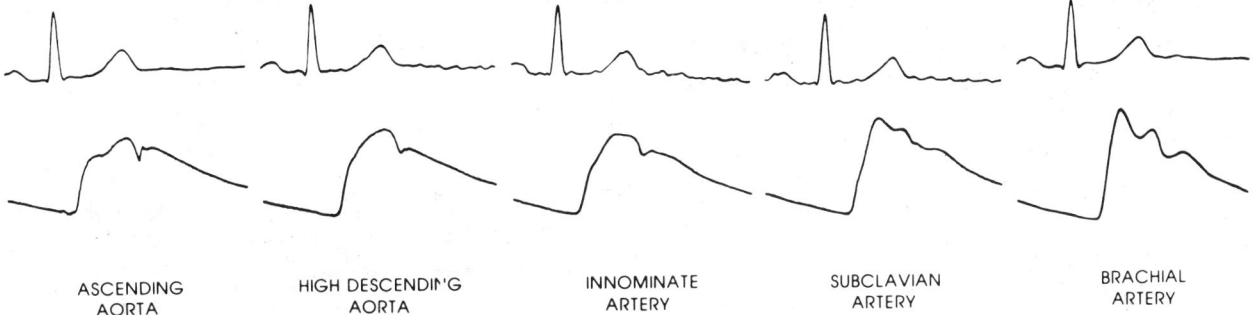

ASCENDING AORTA HIGH DESCENDING AORTA INNOMINATE ARTERY SUBCLAVIAN ARTERY BRACHIAL ARTERY

wise, the arterial pulses usually are examined with the patient supine and with the trunk of the body slightly elevated.

The examiner uses tactile receptors in the tips of the fingers to sense movement of the arterial wall associated with the pressure pulse as it passes the site of palpation. Measurements in the proximal aorta show cyclic movement in both diameter and length proportional to the pulse pressure.[17] However, in more peripheral arteries with connective tissue attachments, the detectable movement is small and variable, with radial expansion by only about 2 percent of the end-diastolic cross-sectional area.[18]

The usual technique for palpating the arterial pulse is to press with the examining fingers until the maximum pulse is sensed. The pulse is felt as changing displacement superimposed on the "base-line" displacement produced by compressing the artery. The examiner should apply varying degrees of pressure while concentrating on the separate phases of the pulse wave. This method, referred to as *trisection*, is useful for assessing the upstroke, systolic peak, and diastolic slope of the arterial pulse.[14] Controversy exists as to how many fingers should be used to palpate the pulse, and the examiner should use whichever method he or she prefers, being careful not to perceive the examining fingertip pulse as well.

Palpation of the carotid artery is preferred for assessing cardiac performance, since the carotid pulse corresponds more closely to the central aortic pressure. However, in certain cardiac diseases (e.g., aortic regurgitation), the abnormalities detected in the carotid pulse are accentuated in the peripheral pulses. For determining the cardiac rate and rhythm, the radial pulse is most often used, but if it is irregular, palpation of the left ventricular apex and cardiac auscultation often provide more reliable information. To evaluate the integrity of the peripheral arterial blood supply and to localize any lesions that exist, the arterial pulses in all four extremities should be examined and compared.

Inspection of the carotid arterial and jugular venous pulsations should be performed at the same time. The carotid pulse usually is best examined with the sternocleidomastoid muscles relaxed and with the head rotated slightly toward the examiner.

The carotid pulse may be timed from the first heart sound which is heard slightly before the pulsation. The carotid pulse should be palpated in the lower half of the patient's neck in order to avoid carotid sinus compression. Occasionally, it is useful to palpate two arteries simultaneously (e.g., femoral and radial) to detect an apparent pulse wave delay such as occurs in patients with coarctation of the aorta.

The examination of arterial pulses in the abdomen and upper and lower extremities should be performed carefully in all patients and compared using a scale such as 0 = complete absence of pulsation; $1+$ = small or reduced pulsation; $2+$ = normal or average pulsation; and $3+$ = large or bounding pulsation. Furthermore, auscultation over the major arteries should be performed since an audible bruit may be a clue to partial occlusion or may (e.g., carotid) indicate transmission from a cardiac murmur.

Normal Arterial Pulse

The normal carotid arterial pulse begins about 40 to 80 ms after the initial component of the first heart sound. The exact interval depends on the duration of isovolumic systole and the transmission time from the central aorta.

The normal carotid pulse has a smooth, rapid upstroke or ascending limb to a smooth, dome-shaped summit (Fig. 10-2). The summit of the pulse is sustained momentarily, then a downstroke occurs which is somewhat less rapid than the upstroke. The dicrotic notch and secondary diastolic wave usually are not felt, but may be palpable in some normal individuals or during fever, exercise, or excitement. The dicrotic notch usually occurs about 300 ms (range 260 to 340 ms) after the onset of the pulse wave when corrected for heart rate.

In arteries distal to the carotid, the pulse wave arrives later and has a steep initial wave that rises to a high peak pressure, whereas the diastolic pressure and the mean pressure are slightly lower. The systolic upstroke time (onset of pulse wave to its peak) tends to be shorter and the left ventricular ejection time (onset of pulse wave to incisura) longer in more peripheral arterial pulses. In the brachial artery, the heart rate–corrected systolic upstroke time averages

A. Hyperkinetic Pulse

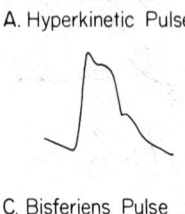

Normal

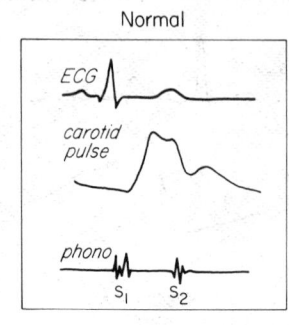

B. Hypokinetic Pulse

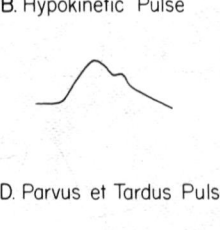

C. Bisferiens Pulse

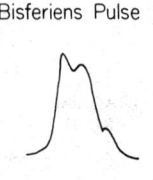

D. Parvus et Tardus Pulse

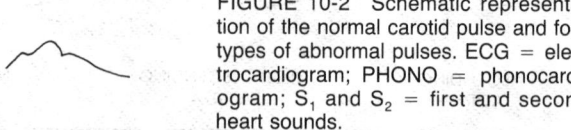

FIGURE 10-2 Schematic representation of the normal carotid pulse and four types of abnormal pulses. ECG = electrocardiogram; PHONO = phonocardiogram; S_1 and S_2 = first and second heart sounds.

120 ms (range 90 to 160 ms) and the systolic ejection phase about 320 ms (range 280 to 360 ms).

Graphic recordings of the arterial pulses frequently show two positive deflections during systole, the first shoulder being referred to as the *percussion wave* and the second as the *tidal wave*. In the normal proximal aortic pulse, the percussion wave is due to arrival of the impulse generated by left ventricular ejection, the tidal wave is its echo from the upper part of the body, and the dicrotic or diastolic wave is its reflection from the lower part of the body.[1] The contour of the distal pulses can be explained in similar terms with altered time relationships between incident and reflected waves at different distances from peripheral reflecting sites.

Characteristic changes in arterial pulsation occur with aging.[15,16,19,20] There is a relative increase in the second (tidal) systolic wave and the height of the incisura relative to the first systolic wave. The systolic upstroke time is longer, and the amplitude and duration of the diastolic wave tends to be less prominent.

Abnormal Arterial Pulses

In hypertension and arteriosclerosis, the pressure pulse amplitude is increased, the tidal wave is prominent, and the diastolic wave is absent. All features of the pulse can be explained by the increased wave velocity.[1,15] The reflected wave from the lower body returns to the proximal aorta during late systole, where it merges with the echo from the upper body sites to augment the tidal wave and increase systolic pressure.[1] With systemic hypotension, the pulse wave velocity is decreased and the tidal and diastolic waves of the pulse are further displaced from the percussion wave. The tidal wave is often less obvious but the diastolic wave more prominent than normal.[1]

Impairment of one or both carotid arteries usually is produced by atherosclerosis, but multiple other causes include thrombosis, embolus, arteritis, and diseases of the aortic arch. Kinking of the carotid or brachiocephalic artery is relatively frequent, particularly in hypertensive patients, and may simulate aneurysmal dilatation. Femoral pulses may be diminished in the child and young adult as a result of coarctation of the aorta. However, in most adults it is caused by atherosclerosis of the abdominal aorta, aortic bifurcation, or the ileofemoral vessels.

Hyperkinetic Arterial Pulse

Large, bounding arterial pulses usually indicate the rapid ejection of an increased volume of blood from the left ventricle (Fig. 10-2). Commonly, the arterial pulse pressure is increased and the peripheral arterial resistance is diminished. The hyperdynamic arterial pulse is sometimes referred to in terms which describe a particular component of the pulse wave. Thus, the *water-hammer pulse,* named after a Victorian toy, refers to an extremely rapid, forceful ascending limb of the arterial pulse wave.[21] By contrast, the term *collapsing pulse* refers to a quick, marked decrease in the arterial pulse wave following its peak. Hyperkinetic pulses often are more prominent in the brachial, radial, or femoral arteries than in the carotid artery. The term *Quincke pulse* refers to visible small pulsations in the nail beds of patients with hyperdynamic arterial pulses from any cause, including aortic regurgitation.

Hyperkinetic arterial pulses occur in normal subjects with a hyperkinetic circulation (e.g., exercise, fever), patients with cardiovascular diseases associated with increased stroke volume, and patients with marked bradycardia compensated for by an extremely large stroke volume. A hyperdynamic arterial pulse also occurs in patients with an abnormally rapid runoff of blood from the arterial system (e.g., patent ductus arteriosus, peripheral arteriovenous fistulas). Patients on chronic hemodialysis often have hyperdynamic pulses produced by the combination of a surgical arteriovenous fistula, anemia, and hypertension.

In aortic regurgitation, the rapid-rising, bounding arterial pulse results from an increase in stroke volume and the rate of left ventricular ejection. The early systolic flow often produces palpable vibrations manifested as a thrill on the steep ascending limb. Later in systole, the rate of left ventricular ejection and the arterial pulse wave decrease sharply, often resulting in systolic collapse.[8] The rapid runoff of blood from the aorta during both systole and diastole has been attributed in part to peripheral arterial vasodilatation; the regurgitation of blood into the left ventricle contributes only to the diastolic collapse. When patients with aortic regurgitation develop severe left ventricular failure, the hyperkinetic arterial pulse state often disappears.

Bisferiens Arterial Pulse

The bisferiens (cf. Latin, "twice beating") pulse has a waveform characterized by two positive waves during systole (Fig. 10-2). The pulse wave upstroke rises rapidly and forcefully, producing the first systolic peak. A brief decline in pressure is followed by a smaller and somewhat slower-rising positive pulse wave (tidal wave). Abnormalities of left ventricular ejection and reflected waves from peripheral arteries both contribute to the prominence of the second systolic wave in the bisferiens pulse. The bisferiens pulse is usually felt in the carotid artery, but frequently is palpated more easily in a brachial or radial artery. Bisferiens pulse often occurs in patients with aortic regurgitation and is common in patients with combined aortic stenosis and moderately severe aortic regurgitation.[22–25] However, it also occurs commonly in other conditions associated with the rapid ejection of an increased stroke volume from the left ventricle (e.g., exercise, fever, patent ductus arteriosus).

The bisferiens pulse often is present in patients

with idiopathic hypertrophic subaortic stenosis (also called hypertrophic obstructive cardiomyopathy).[26] In this syndrome, the midsystolic negative wave usually coincides with a marked decrease in the rate of left ventricular ejection. The second systolic wave, or tidal wave, most likely is produced by reflected waves from the periphery. In these patients, the bisferiens pulse may be elicited by maneuvers that decrease the left ventricular size or increase its contractility. However, the most characteristic aspect of the arterial pulse in hypertrophic obstructive cardiomyopathy is its rapid rate of rise. A physical finding nearly specific for hypertrophic cardiomyopathy is a much smaller arterial pressure pulse in the cardiac cycle following a premature ventricular contraction.

Hypokinetic Arterial Pulse

A small, weak arterial pulse frequently is present in patients with a diminished left ventricular stroke volume (Fig. 10-2). In most instances, the decreased stroke output is associated with both a decreased rate and duration of left ventricular ejection, and there is a narrow arterial pulse pressure despite an increased arterial resistance. Common causes include hypovolemia, left ventricular failure, and mitral or aortic valve stenosis. It is frequent in patients with valvular aortic stenosis.

Parvus et Tardus Pulse

Patients with moderate or severe valvular aortic stenosis often have an arterial pulse that is small and has a delayed systolic peak.[27,28] Occasionally, there may be a detectable shoulder on the upstroke of the carotid pulse, referred to as *anacrotic* (Fig. 10-2).[29] Palpable coarse vibrations are often present as a systolic thrill over the slowly rising carotid pulse. The parvus et tardus pulse is much easier to detect in the carotid arteries than in more distal arteries.

Most middle-aged patients with uncomplicated severe aortic stenosis have a parvus et tardus pulse; but this pulse may also occur in relatively mild stenosis. Furthermore, an apparently normal arterial pulse is not unusual in elderly patients with severe aortic stenosis. This is due to the decreased distensibility of the peripheral arteries, which alters the character of the arterial pulse. Severe left ventricular failure from any cause often results in a small, weak pulse which may be difficult to distinguish from that in aortic stenosis.

An important diagnostic clue in patients with supravalvular aortic stenosis is the finding of a larger arterial pulse in the right carotid and a systolic blood pressure that is significantly higher in the right arm.

Dicrotic Arterial Pulse

The dicrotic (cf. Greek, "double beating") pulse is a twin-peaked pulse with one peak in systole and the second in diastole, the latter due to an accentuated and palpable dicrotic wave that follows the second heart sound (Figs. 10-2 and 10-3).[30] It is usu-

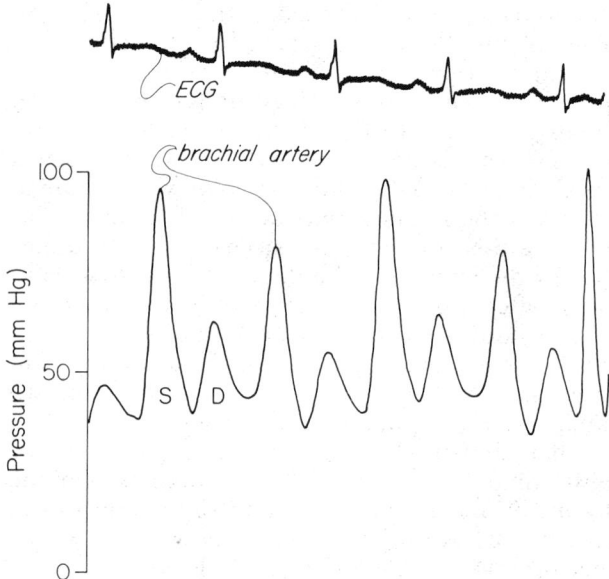

FIGURE 10-3   Intraarterial pressure curve showing both pulses alternans and a dicrotic waveform in a patient with congestive cardiomyopathy. ECG = electrocardiogram; BA = brachial artery; S = systole; D = diastole.

ally felt best in the carotids, although it may also be palpated over more peripheral arteries. Major abnormalities in the dicrotic pulse include a large diastolic wave, a low dicrotic notch, a short systolic ejection phase, a narrow pulse pressure, a diminished rate of rise of the pulse, and the lack of distinct percussion and tidal waves. The dicrotic pulse is most common in young or middle-aged patients with poor left ventricular performance. It is usually associated with a low cardiac output, markedly diminished stroke volume, elevated left ventricular end-diastolic pressure, and high systemic arterial resistance. In general, the dicrotic wave becomes less prominent with age, hypertension, generalized atherosclerosis, and diabetes. Rarely, the dicrotic wave can be palpated in young febrile patients in whom none of the other abnormal features of the dicrotic pulse are present.

Pulsus Alternans

Pulsus alternans is a characteristic pulse pattern in which the beats occur at regular intervals but in which there is a regular attenuation of the height of the pressure pulses (Fig. 10-3).[31,32] Rarely, the pulsus alternans is so marked that the weaker pulses are not felt at all. When pulsus alternans is noticed first after a premature contraction, the extent of the difference in systolic pressure in alternating beats declines for several cycles until the pulse amplitude is again constant. The initiation of post–premature ventricular contraction (post-PVC) pulsus alternans is probably related to the increased duration of left ventricular filling after the extrasystole, resulting in a greater end-diastolic volume and hence increased contractile force due to the Frank-Starling mechanism.[33] This phenomenon usually does not occur in the normal left ventricle because contractile force is much less dependent on end-diastolic volume.

Severe depression of left ventricular performance often results in sustained pulsus alternans. There is an alteration in aortic flow, systolic left ventricular pressure, aortic systolic pressure, left ventricular dP/dt, and left ventricular end-diastolic pressure. It has been postulated that sustained pulsus alternans is due to alteration of the contractile state of at least part of the myocardium, which may be caused by the failure of electromechanical coupling in some cells during the weaker contraction. A subsequent stronger contraction would then represent contraction of all cells, some of which were potentiated.[34]

Pulsus alternans may be better appreciated when palpating a distal artery that has a slightly wider pulse pressure than the carotid artery. The patient's respiration should be held since the small changes in arterial pressure caused by normal respiration may obscure the recognition of pulsus alternans. Pulsus alternans can be confirmed by using a sphygmomanometer and is usually associated with a left ventricular third heart sound.

Pulsus Paradoxus

A paradoxical pulse is defined as a marked decrease in the pulse amplitude during normal quiet inspiration or a decrease in the systolic arterial pressure by more than 10 mmHg. The normal small decline in systolic blood pressure probably is produced predominately by relative pooling of blood in the pulmonary vessels during inspiration, and may also reflect the delayed transmission through the lungs of the preceding expiratory fall in venous pressure and right ventricular cardiac output.[14]

In patients with pericardial tamponade, fluid accumulation in the pericardium increases intrapericardial pressure, and the heart's filling capacity is reduced. During inspiration, the expected augmentation of venous return to the right side of the heart occurs despite the elevated intrapericardial pressure.[35] The diminished thoracic pressure also causes a pooling of blood in the pulmonary capillary bed and diminishes pulmonary venous return to the left atrium. Since the high intrapericardial pressure limits flow to the heart and the total cardiac filling capacity is limited, the increase in right-sided heart volume with inspiration causes an obligatory decrease in left-sided heart filling. This, and the pooling of blood in the pulmonary bed, produces a decline in left ventricular stroke volume and systolic blood pressure during inspiration.[36] Pulsus paradoxus is common with cardiac tamponade but infrequent with restrictive pericardial disease.

Different hemodynamic mechanisms contribute to the production of paradoxical pulse in certain patients with superior vena cava obstruction, asthma, or obstructive airway disease, and in some patients with pulmonary embolism, shock, or post thoracotomy.[14]

Effects of Arrhythmias on the Arterial Pulse

Premature Ventricular Contractions

A premature ventricular contraction may be associated with no pulse, a small amplitude pulse, or normal arterial pulse depending upon its timing and whether the left ventricular pressure generated is able to open the aortic valve. The arterial pulse following a premature contraction is usually greatly enhanced because of decreased aortic impedance, increased left ventricular filling, and augmented left ventricular contractility. At times, premature ventricular contractions are so common as to produce an irregularly irregular pulse. Then, the presence of cannon a waves in the jugular venous pulse should alert one to the correct diagnosis.

Tachyarrhythmias

The electrocardiogram is usually needed for the definitive diagnosis of any abnormality of heart rate or rhythm. However, careful observation of the arterial and jugular venous pulses frequently leads to the correct diagnosis.

Most tachycardias associated with a regular pulse are of supraventricular origin. In sinus tachycardia, the arterial pulse will gradually slow with carotid sinus pressure and then again gradually increase. Paroxysmal atrial tachycardia has an "all-or-none" response. Carotid sinus pressure will increase the block at the AV junction in patients with atrial flutter, the pulse rate slowing and subsequently returning to its original rate in a "jerky" fashion.

In patients with ventricular tachycardia and AV dissociation, the variation in atrial-ventricular sequence of contraction and resulting pulse amplitude may often be detected by palpation.

An irregularly irregular pulse with a varying pulse pressure is usually the result of atrial fibrillation. However, multifocal atrial tachycardia is also a common cause of this finding in patients with severe chronic obstructive lung disease.

Bradyarrhythmias

An unusually slow heart rate is frequently associated with a decrease in the rate of rise and amplitude of the arterial pressure pulse. A resting rate below 60 beats per minute is expected in athletic individuals, patients receiving beta-adrenergic blocking drugs, hypothyroid patients, and many elderly patients with increased vagal tone. Complete heart block is readily diagnosed by the variability in the arterial pulse amplitude, the changing intensity of the first heart sound, and intermittent cannon a waves in the jugular venous pulse.

Venous Pulse

The evaluation of the venous pulse is an integral part of the physical examination, the venous pulse reflecting both the right atrial pressure and the hemodynamic events in the right atrium. Factors influencing the right atrial and central venous pressure include the total blood volume, the distribution of blood volume, and right atrial contraction.

Venous blood returning from the systemic capillaries has a nonpulsatile flow. Changes in volume flow created by skeletal muscles and respiratory pump are nonsynchronous with the pulsatile activity of the heart. However the changes in flow and pressure, caused by right atrial and ventricular filling, give rise to pulsations in the central veins that are transmitted toward the peripheral veins, opposite to the direction of blood flow. With the possible exception of the *c* wave, which is the combined result of carotid arterial impact and an upward movement of the tricuspid valve, the pulsations observed in the neck are produced by right atrial and ventricular activity.[37]

Examination of the Jugular Venous Pulse

The two main objectives of the bedside examination of the neck veins are the estimation of the central venous pressure (CVP) and the inspection of the waveform. In most cases, the *right internal jugular vein* is superior for both purposes. In most normal subjects, the maximum pulsation of the internal jugular vein is observed when the trunk is inclined by less than 30°. In patients with an elevated venous pressure, it may be necessary to elevate the trunk further, sometimes to as much as 90°.[38] When the neck muscles are relaxed, shining a beam of light gently across the skin overlying the internal jugular vein exposes its pulsations. Simultaneous palpation of the left carotid artery aids the examiner in deciding which pulsations are venous.

Measurements of Venous Pressure
The difference between venous distension and venous pressure elevation must be considered. Veins may be markedly dilated with minimal increase in pressure, or may not be visibly distended despite a very high venous pressure. Venous pressure may be estimated by examining the veins in the dorsum of the hand. With the patient sitting or lying at a 30° elevation or greater, the arm is slowly and passively raised from a dependent position. When the venous pressure is normal, the veins collapse when the dorsum of the hand reaches the level of the sternal angle of Lewis. Unfortunately, local venous obstruction or augmented peripheral venous constriction may affect adversely the accuracy of estimating CVP by this method.

The external or internal jugular veins may also be used to estimate venous pressure. The absence of valves and the more direct route to the right atrium make the *internal jugular vein* superior for the estimation of venous pressure and assessment of the venous waveform.[39] The patient is examined at the optimum degree of trunk elevation for visualization of venous pulsations (Fig. 10-4). In the average patient, the center of the right atrium lies approximately 5 cm below the sternal angle regardless of body position. The vertical distance from the top of the oscillating venous column to the level of the sternal angle is determined and generally found to be less than 3 cm (3 cm + 5 cm = 8 cm). Severely elevated venous pressure may be missed by failing to elevate adequately the patient's head. It may be necessary to actually have the patient sit upright. If the "pulsating meniscus" is very high, pulsations may be inapparent in the lower neck. When venous engorgement is marked, the patient's earlobe may pulsate and even the veins on the top of the head may be distended.

In patients suspected of right ventricular failure, but who have normal resting venous pressures, the hepatojugular reflux test is useful. With the patient breathing normally, firm pressure is applied with the palm of the hand to the upper quadrant of the abdomen for 30 to 60 s. Normally, the jugular venous pressure is not altered significantly. However, the abnormal right ventricle is unable to accept the increase in blood volume due to enhanced venous return without a marked increase in its filling pressure, which is transmitted to the neck veins. Thus, in a positive test, the upper level of venous pulsation increases during abdominal compression.

Analysis of Venous Waveforms
Again, the patient's trunk should be inclined to whatever elevation is necessary to reveal the top of

FIGURE 10-4 Method of measuring the mean jugular venous pressure as the vertical distance above the sternal angle of Lewis, the latter being 5 cm above the mid right atrium regardless of trunk elevation.

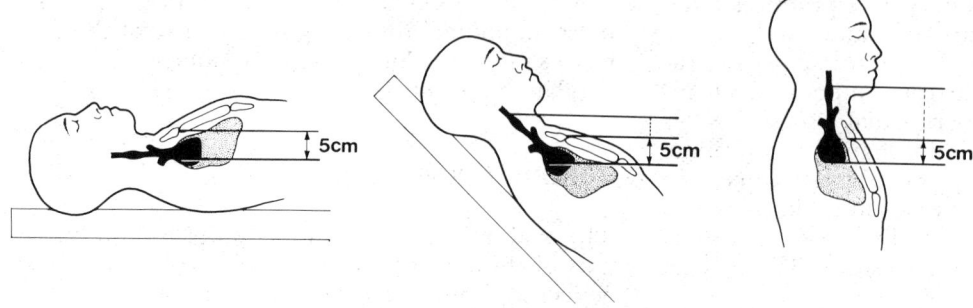

the oscillating venous column.[40] Having the patient take a slow, deep inspiration will increase the amplitude of the presystolic *a* wave while decreasing the mean right atrial pressure. This is also a useful technique for identifying the site at which the pulsations will be best visualized. Simultaneous palpation of the left carotid artery aids the examiner in relating the venous pulsations to the timing of the cardiac cycle.

Normal Venous Pulse

The normal jugular venous pulse (JVP) reflects phasic pressure changes in the right atrium and consists of three positive waves and two negative troughs (Fig. 10-5). In considering this pulse, it is useful to refer to the events of the cardiac cycle. The positive presystolic *a* wave is produced by right atrial contraction and is the dominant wave in the JVP, particularly during inspiration. If a right-sided fourth heart sound is heard, it occurs at the moment the peak of the *a* wave is recorded.

During atrial relaxation, the venous pulse descends from the summit of the *a* wave. Depending on the PR interval, this descent may continue until a plateau (*z* point) is reached just prior to right ventricular systole. More often, the descent is interrupted by a second positive venous wave, the *c* wave, which is produced by bulging of the tricuspid valve into the right atrium during right ventricular isovolumetric systole and by the impact of the carotid artery adjacent to the jugular vein.[41] Following the summit of the *c* wave, the JVP contour declines, forming the normal negative systolic wave, the *x* wave. The *x* descent is due to a combination of atrial relaxation and the downward displacement of the tricuspid valve during right ventricular systole.

The positive late systolic *v* wave in the JVP results from the increase in blood volume in the venae cavae and right atrium during ventricular systole when the tricuspid valve is closed. After the peak of the *v* wave is reached, the right atrial pressure decreases because of the diminished bulging of the tricuspid valve into the right atrium and the decline in right ventricular pressure which follow tricuspid valve opening. The latter occurs at the peak of the *v* wave in the JVP. Following the summit of the *v*

wave, there is a negative descending limb, referred to as the *y* descent or *diastolic collapse,* which is due to tricuspid valve opening and the rapid inflow of blood into the right ventricle. The initial *y* descent corresponds to the right ventricular rapid-filling phase. The trough of the *y* wave occurs in early diastole and is followed by the ascending limb of the *y* wave which is produced by continued diastolic inflow of blood into the right side of the heart. The velocity of this ascending pressure curve depends on the rate of venous return and the distensibility of the right heart chambers. When diastole is long, the ascending limb of the *y* wave is often followed by a small, brief, positive wave, the *h* wave, which occurs just prior to the next *a* wave. At times, there is a plateau phase rather than a distinct *h* wave. With increasing heart rate, the *y* trough and *y* ascent are followed immediately by the next *a* wave.

Usually, there are three visible major positive waves (*a, c, v*) and two negative waves (*x, y*) when the pulse rate is below 90 beats per minute and the PR interval is normal. With faster heart rates, there is often fusion of some of the pulse waves, and an accurate analysis of the waveform is more difficult.

Abnormal Venous Pulse

Elevated Venous Pressure
The most common cause of an elevated jugular venous pressure is an elevated right ventricular pressure such as occurs in patients with pulmonic stenosis, pulmonary hypertension (often due to left-sided heart failure), or right ventricular failure secondary to right ventricular infarction. The venous pressure also is elevated when obstruction to right ventricular inflow occurs, such as with tricuspid stenosis or right atrial myxoma, or when constrictive pericardial disease impedes right ventricular inflow. It may also result from vena cava obstruction and, at times, an increased blood volume. Patients with obstructive pulmonary disease may have an elevated venous pressure only during expiration.

Kussmaul's Sign
Normally there is an increase in the *a* wave of the JVP but a decrease in the mean jugular venous pres-

A. Tricuspid Regurgitation
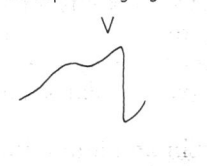

C. Constrictive Pericarditis
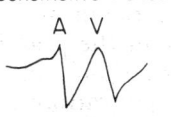

Normal
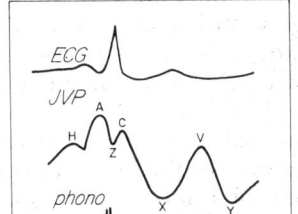

B. Tricuspid Stenosis
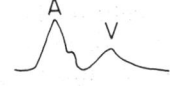

D. Atrial Septal Defect
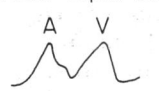

FIGURE 10-5 The normal jugular venous pulse (JVP) and four types of abnormal JVP. See text for definition of A, Z, C, X, V, Y, and H.

sure during inspiration as a result of the increased filling of the right side of the heart associated with the decline in intrathoracic pressure. However, an inspiratory increase in the venous pressure occurs in patients with severe constrictive pericarditis when the heart is unable to accept the increase in right ventricular volume without a marked increase in the filling pressure.[42] However, while Kussmaul's sign was first described in patients with constrictive pericarditis, its most common cause is severe right-sided heart failure, regardless of etiology.

Abnormalities of the *a* Wave (Fig. 10-6)

The *a* wave in the JVP is absent when there is no effective atrial contraction, such as in atrial fibrillation. In certain other conditions, the *a* wave may not be apparent. In sinus tachycardia the *a* wave may fuse with the preceding *v* wave, particularly if the PR interval is prolonged. In some patients with sinus tachycardia, the *a* wave may occur during the *v* or *y* descent and be small or absent. In the presence of first-degree AV block a discrete *a* wave with ascending and descending limbs is often completed prior to the first heart sound and the *ac* interval is prolonged (Fig. 10-6*B*).

Large *a* waves are of considerable diagnostic value (Fig. 10-5). When giant *a* waves are present with each beat, the right atrium is contracting against an increased resistance. This may result from obstruction at the tricuspid valve (tricuspid stenosis or atresia, right atrial myxoma) or increased resistance to right ventricular filling. A giant *a* wave is more likely to occur in patients with pulmonic stenosis or pulmonary hypertension in whom both the atrial and ventricular septum are intact.

Cannon *a* waves occur when the right atrium contracts while the tricuspid valve is closed during right ventricular systole. The resultant jugular venous cannon wave is the result of fusion of the giant *a* wave with some part of the usual JVP wave during ventricular systole. Cannon waves may occur either regularly or irregularly and are most common in the presence of arrhythmias (Fig. 10-6*C*).

Abnormalities of the *x* Wave

The most important alteration of the normally negative systolic collapse (*x* wave) of the JVP is its obliteration or even replacement by a positive wave. This is usually due to tricuspid regurgitation.[43,44] Although atrial relaxation may contribute to the normal *x* descent, the development of atrial fibrillation does not obliterate the *x* wave except in the presence of tricuspid regurgitation. Accordingly, the occurrence of a positive wave in the JVP during ventricular systole is strong evidence of tricuspid regurgitation (Figs. 10-5 and 10-7). Mild tricuspid regurgitation lessens and shortens the downward *x* wave as the regurgitation of blood into the right atrium produces a positive wave which diminishes the usual systolic fall in venous pressure. In some patients with moderate tricuspid regurgitation,

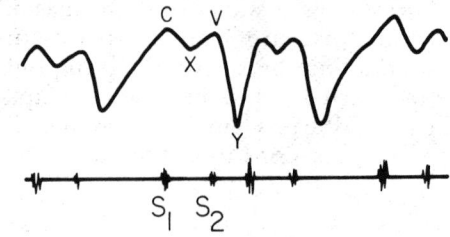

A. Atrial Fibrillation

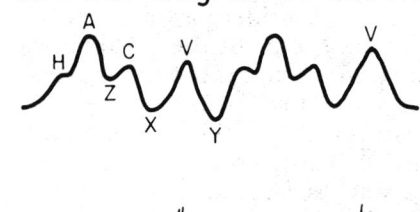

B. First Degree AV Block

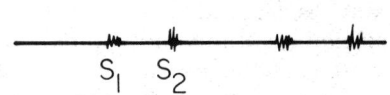

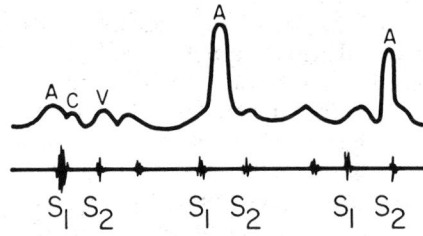

C. Complete AV Block

FIGURE 10-6 Abnormal jugular venous pulse in three common arrhythmias (see text).

there is a fairly distinct positive wave during ventricular systole between the *c* and *v* waves.

In patients with constrictive pericarditis, the *x* descent wave during systole is often more prominent than the early diastolic *y* wave (Fig. 10-5).[45]

Abnormalities of the *v* Wave

The positive, late systolic *v* wave results from the increasing right atrial blood volume during ventricular systole when the tricuspid valve normally is closed. With mild tricuspid regurgitation, the *v* wave becomes more prominent, and when tricuspid regurgitation becomes severe, the prominent *v* wave and the obliteration of the *x* descent result in a single, large, positive systolic wave (ventricularization) (Figs. 10-5 and 10-7).

Normally, the *v* wave is lower in amplitude than the *a* wave in the JVP. However, in patients with an atrial septal defect, the higher left atrial pressure is transmitted to the right atrium and the *a* and *v* waves are often equal in the right atrium and the JVP.[45] In patients with constrictive pericarditis and

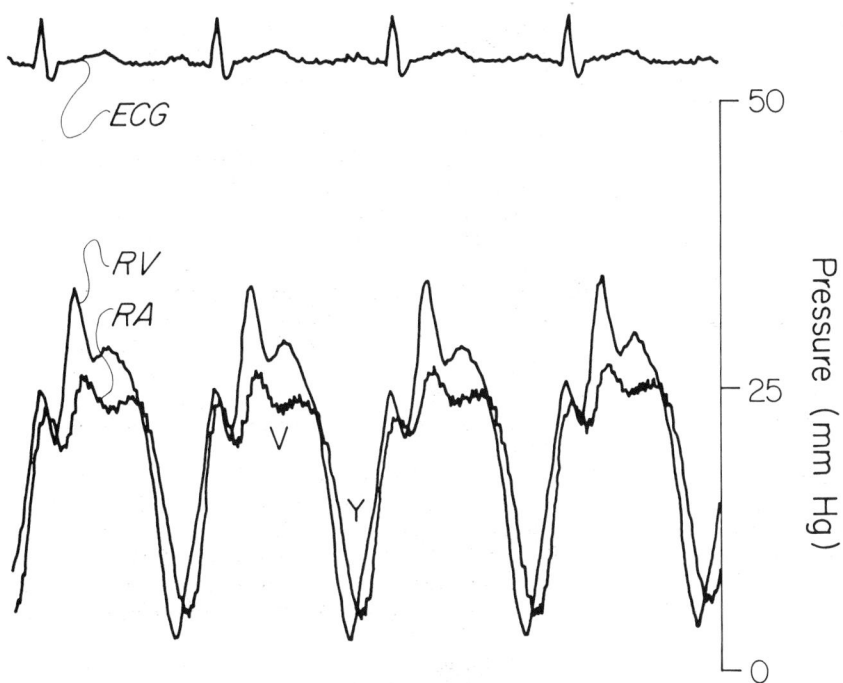

FIGURE 10-7 Right atrial (RA) and right ventricular (RV) pressure curves in a patient with severe tricuspid regurgitation. Note ventricularization of RA pressure curve. ECG = electrocardiogram.

sinus rhythm, the right atrial *a* and *v* waves may also be equal, but the venous pressure is increased, which is not the usual case with atrial septal defect. In patients with constrictive pericarditis who are in atrial fibrillation, the *cv* wave is prominent and the *y* descent rapid.

Abnormalities of the *y* Trough

The *y* descent, or diastolic collapse, is produced mainly by tricuspid valve opening and the rapid inflow of blood into the right ventricle. A rapid deep *y* descent in early diastole occurs with severe tricuspid regurgitation (Fig. 10-5). A venous pulse characterized by a sharp *y* descent, a deep *y* trough, and a rapid ascent to the base line is seen in patients with constrictive pericarditis or with severe right-sided heart failure. A slow *y* descent in the JVP suggests an obstruction to right ventricular filling and may be the only abnormal finding in patients with tricuspid stenosis or right atrial myxoma (Fig. 10-5).[46] In both constrictive pericarditis and severe right-sided heart failure, the venous pressure is elevated with a sharp *y* dip in the JVP. The presence of a large positive systolic venous wave favors the diagnosis of severe heart failure.

Effects of Arrhythmias of the Venous Pulse

Large *a* waves in the JVP during arrhythmias equate with the *P* wave (atrial contraction) occurring between the onset of the QRS complex and the termination of the T wave (Fig. 10-6). Such cannon *a* waves may occur regularly in junctional rhythm. More commonly, they occur irregularly when AV dissociation accompanies premature ventricular contractions, ventricular tachycardia, or complete heart block. The *a* wave is absent in patients with atrial fibrillation, and flutter *a* waves at a regular rate of 250 to 300 per minute frequently are observed in patients with atrial flutter and varying degrees of AV block. Patients with multifocal atrial tachycardia often have prominent and somewhat variable *a* waves in the JVP. In these patients, many of whom have pulmonary hypertension secondary to lung disease, the *a* waves are often very large.

References

*1. O'Rourke, M. F.: The Arterial Pulse in Health and Disease, *Am. Heart J.*, 82(5):687, 1971. (60 references)

2. Murgo, J. P., Westerhof, N., Giolma, J. P., and Altobelli, S. A.: Aortic Input Impedance in Normal Man: Relationship to Pressure Wave Shapes, *Circulation*, 62:105, 1980.

3. O'Rourke, M. F.: Pressure and Flow Waves in Systemic and the Anatomical Design of the Arterial System, *J. Appl. Phys.*, 23:139, 1967.

4. O'Rourke, M. F., and Auido, A. P.: Pulsatile Flow and Pressures in Human Systemic Arteries: Studies in Man and in a Multibranched Model of the Human Systemic Arterial Tree, *Circ. Res.*, 46:363, 1980.

5. Murgo, J. P., Westerhof, N., Giolma, J. O., and Altobelli, S. A.: Effects of Exercise on Aortic Impedance and Pressure Wave shapes in Normal Man, *Circ. Res.*, in press.

6. Murgo, M. P., Altobelli, S. A., Dorethy, J. F., Logsdon, J. R., and McGranahan, G. M.: Normal Ventricular Ejection Dynamics in Man during Rest and Exercise, *Circulation*, 46:92, 1975.

*7. Westerhof, N., Murgo, J. P., Sipkema, P., Giolma,

*This article is a review of the literature and contains additional references to the literature.

J. P., and Elzingor, G.: Arterial Impedance, N. H. C. Hwang, D. R. Gross, and D. J. Patel (eds.), "Quantitative Cardiovascular Studies," University Park Press, Baltimore, 1979, pp. 111–150. (77 references)

*8. Marx, H. J., and Yu, P. N.: Clinical Examination of the Arterial Pulse, *Prog. Cardiovasc. Dis.,* 10:207, 1967. (87 references)

9. Hamilton, W. F., and Dow, P.: An Experimental Study of the Standing Waves in the Pulse Propagated through the Aorta, *Am. J. Physiol.,* 125:48, 1939.

10. McDonald, D. A., and Taylor, M. G.: The Hydrodynamics of the Arterial Circulation, *Prog. Biophys.,* 9:105, 1959.

11. McDonald, D. A.: The Relation of Pulsatile Pressure to Flow in Arteries, *J. Physiol.,* 127:533, 1955.

12. Taylor, M. G.: Input Impedance of an Assembly of Randomly Branching Elastic Tubes, *Biophys. J.,* 6:29, 1966.

13. O'Rourke, M. F., and Taylor, M. G.: Input Impedance of the Systemic Circulation, *Circ. Res.,* 20:365, 1967.

14. Schlant, R. C., and Felner, J. M.: The Arterial Pulse—Clinical Manifestations, *Curr. Prob. Cardiol.,* 2(5):1, 1977.

15. O'Rourke, M. F., Blazek, J. V., Morreels, C. L., Jr., and Krovetz, L. J.: Pressure Wave Transmission along the Human Aorta. Changes with Age and Hypertension, *Circ. Res.,* 23:567, 1968.

16. Freis, E. D., Heath, W. C., Luchsinger, P. C., and Snell, R. E.: Changes in the Carotid Pulse Which Occur with Age and Hypertension, *Am. Heart J.,* 71:757, 1966.

17. Patel, D. J., Greenfield, J. C., Jr., and Fry, D. L.: In Vivo Pressure Length-Radius Relationships of Certain Blood Vessels in Man and Dog, in E. O. Attinger (ed.), "Pulsatile Blood Flow," McGraw-Hill Book Company, New York, 1964, chap. 17, p. 293.

18. Stead, E. A., and Greenfield, J. C.: Pressures and Pulses, *Physiol. Physicians,* 2:1, 1964.

19. Herron R. E., Dontas, A. S., Karvonen, M. J., and Keys, A. J.: Effects of Aging on the Carotid Pulse in Two Finnish Populations, *Acta Med. Scand.,* 182 (suppl. 472):125, 1967.

20. Freis, E. D., and Kyle, M. C.: Computer Analysis of Carotid and Brachial Pulse Waves. Effects on Age in Normal Subjects, *Am. J. Cardiol.,* 22:691, 1968.

21. Corrigan, D. J.: On Permanent Patency of the Mouth of the Aorta, or Inadequacy of the Aortic Valves, *Edinburgh Med. Surg.,* 37:225, 1832.

22. Clarke, J. M.: On the Pulsus Bisferiens of Aortic Regurgitation, *Lancet* 2:1529, 1894.

23. Broadbent, W.: Pulsus Bisferiens, *Br. Med. J.,* 1:75, 1899.

24. Fleming, P. R.: The Mechanism of the Pulsus Bisferiens, *Br. Heart J.,* 19:519, 1951.

25. Ikram, H., Nixon, P. G. F., and Fox, J. A.: The Hemodynamic Implications of the Bisferiens Pulse, *Br. Heart J.,* 26:452, 1964.

26. Wigle, E. D.: The Arterial Pressure Pulse in Muscular Subaortic Stenosis, *Br. Heart J.,* 25:97, 1963.

27. Steell, G.: The Pulse in Aortic Stenosis, *Lancet,* 2:1206, 1894.

28. Feil, H. S., and Katz, L. N.: The Transformation of the Central into the Peripheral Pulse in Patients with Aortic Stenosis, *Am. Heart J.,* 2:12, 1926.

29. Dow, P.: The Development of the Anacrotic and Tardus Pulse of Aortic Stenosis, *Am. J. Physiol.,* 131:432, 1940.

30. Ewy, G. A., Rios, J. C., and Marcus, F. I.: The Dicrotic Arterial Pulse, *Circulation,* 39:655, 1969.

31. White, P. D.: Alternation of the Pulse: A Common Clinical Condition, *Am. J. Med. Sci.,* 150:82, 1915.

32. Cohn, K. E., Sandler, H., and Hancock, E. W.: Mechanisms of Pulsus Alternans, *Circulation,* 36:372, 1967.

33. Mitchell, J. H., Sarnoff, S. J., and Sonnenblick, E. H.: Alternating End-Diastolic Fiber Length as a Causative Factor, *J. Clin. Invest.,* 42:55, 1963.

34. Pace, J. B., Priola, D. V., and Randall, W. C.: Alterations in Cardiac Synchrony and Contractility during Induced Pulsus Alternans, *Physiologist,* 9:259, 1966.

35. Shabetai, R., Fowler, N. O., Fenton, J. C., and Masangkay, M.: Pulsus Paradoxus, *J. Clin. Invest.,* 44:1882, 1965.

36. Shabetai, R., Fowler, N. O., and Guntheroth, W. G.: The Hemodynamics of Cardiac Tamponade and Constrictive Pericarditis, *Am. J. Cardiol.,* 20:480, 1970.

37. Hurst, J. W., and Schlant, R. C.: "Examination of the Veins in the Heart," 4th ed., McGraw-Hill Book Company, New York, 1977, chap. 5, pp. 81–92.

38. Fowler, N. O., and Marshall, W. J.: Cardiac Diagnosis from Examination of Arteries and Veins, *Circulation,* 30:272, 1964.

39. Ewy, G. A., and Marcus, F. I.: Bedside Estimation of the Venous Pressure, *Heart Bull.,* 17:41, 1968.

40. Fowler, N. O.: Inspection and Palpation of Venous and Arterial Pulses, in "Examination of the Heart," American Heart Association, New York, 1972, pp. 1–41.

41. Wood, P.: "Diseases of the Heart and Circulation," 2d ed., J. B. Lippincott Company, Philadelphia, 1957, p. 47.

42. Kussmaul, A.: Über Schwielige Mediastino-pericarditis und Den Paradoxen Puls, *Berl. Klin. Wochenschr.,* 10:433, 1873.

43. Messer, A. L., Hurst, J. W., Rappaport, M. B., and Sprague, H. B.: A Study of the Venous Pulse in Tricuspid Valve Disease, *Circulation,* 1:388, 1950.

44. Mueller, O., and Shillingford, J.: Tricuspid Incompetence, *Br. Heart. J.,* 16:195, 1954.

45. Dexter, L.: Atrial Septal Defect, *Br. Heart J.,* 18:209, 1956.

46. Perloff, J. K., and Harvey, W. P.: Clinical Recognition of Tricuspid Stenosis, *Circulation,* 22:346, 1960.

11

Inspection and Palpation of the Precordium

Ernest Craige, M.D.

Quod erigitur cor, et inmucronem se sursum elevat, sic ut illo tempore ferire pectus, et foris sentiri pulsatio possit.

The heart erects, and raises itself into a point, so that at this moment it strikes the chest wall, and externally a pulsation can be felt.

William Harvey, M.D., 1628[1]

In these days of increasing dependence on expensive technological methods in cardiac diagnosis, there is a tendency to give only passing attention to the physical examination. Even among the traditional features of the physical examination, inspection and palpation are often passed over as the physician limits the examination of the heart to laying on the stethoscope. This trend is unfortunate since a great deal of information of diagnostic value can be obtained by simple bedside methods which are rapid, inexpensive, and nontraumatic. Inspection, palpation, and auscultation can often lead one toward an accurate diagnosis, or, even when further technological studies are required, the questions to be asked and the protocol to be followed can be worked out with greater precision and economy.

Inspection of the Precordium

Many valuable clues in cardiac diagnosis are provided by inspection of the neck and thorax. This has been described in Chap. 8. Attention to the precordium in particular can be rewarding. Pulsations in this area can best be appreciated with the help of a light beam directed tangentially across the surface. Another simple method utilizes a wand—a cotton-tipped swab impaled in the hole of a pediatric suction electrode used in precordial electrocardiography. The suction electrode is attached to the moving chest wall and the exaggerated movements imparted to the cotton-tipped end of the swab may provide vivid clarification of an otherwise confusing undulation. Asymmetry of the thorax can often be detected by inspecting the patient from the foot of the bed. A convex bulging of the precordium suggests the presence of heart disease beginning early in life while the thorax was still capable of being molded to accommodate a dilated right ventricle, as in atrial septal defect. Generalized cardiac enlargement due to rheumatic heart disease in early childhood can result in a similar configuration.

Pulsations Due to the Heartbeat

Precordial pulsations occur principally in five areas:

1. The cardiac apex which is normally occupied by the left ventricle
2. The left sternal border at third and fourth interspaces, where a visible heave in systole may represent right ventricular enlargement
3. Higher along the left border in the second intercostal space where pulsation of the pulmonary artery may be seen when that vessel is dilated
4. Upper right sternal border, occasionally the site of pulsations due to dilatation or aneurysm of the aortic root
5. The midprecordium, third or fourth intercostal spaces at the midclavicular line, where bulging of the ischemic or aneurysmal anterior surface of the left ventricle may be perceptible

The precordium may less commonly be drawn inward during systole, as with constrictive pericarditis or isolated tricuspid regurgitation.

All of these visible signs are also palpable and will therefore be considered in greater detail below.

Palpation of the Precordium

Physiology of Tactile Perception

Physiologists have demonstrated that the human hand is endowed with certain neurons which are primarily sensitive to *positional change* and others that are sensitive to the time rate of positional change, or *velocity*.[2] Information has, however, been very limited with respect to the frequency response of the human hand, especially in the spectrum of frequencies encountered in precordial motion. This problem has recently been investigated by Smith and Craige using an in vitro palpating device in which amplitude and frequency of a sinusoidal waveform can be independently manipulated.[3] Their results show that the fingers are insensitive to movements of relatively large *amplitude* when frequency is very low (<5 Hz). Sensitivity improves with increasing frequency, where presumably neurons activated by changes in *velocity* assume a larger role in tactile perception. These observations are supported by clinical observations: for instance, the stethoscope can be *seen* to ride up and down with movements of the precordium, but, with the eyes averted, these same movements of the precordium may be imperceptible by *palpation*. On the other hand, higher-frequency phenomena such as thrills and the "shocks" associated with aortic or pulmonary components of the second sound of exaggerated intensity are easily palpable although the *amplitude* of their movement is insufficient to be visible. In palpating the impulse at the cardiac apex, ordinarily only the initial brisk outward component is perceptible. This portion of the apical motion is characterized by a major contribution of higher-fre-

199

quency vibrations. The low-frequency diastolic phenomena—filling wave and *a* wave—are usually imperceptible except when greatly exaggerated in amplitude or composed of higher-frequency elements as in some pathologic states.[4]

It is apparent therefore that the fingers represent a very imperfect transducer for transferring the information contained in precordial movement to our centers of perception in the brain. It also becomes clearer that in the design of graphic methods to represent precordial movement it is probably futile to try for a system that simulates on paper exactly what one perceives by palpation. Tactile perception by even the most experienced bedside clinician is still a very primitive form of examination. Thus, the analogy from auscultation-phonocardiography that the most useful phonocardiograms for clinical purposes are those which most nearly reproduce what one hears is not transferable to palpation and its graphic counterpart. Despite these limitations in the information which one can hope to obtain from palpation, the method provides definite advantages which continue to warrant its inclusion in the physical examination.

The Apex Beat

Source of the Apex Beat
The apex beat results from the impact of the left ventricle against the chest wall in early systole. It is affected by the pressure pulse in the left ventricle, the stroke volume, and a kaleidoscopic complex effect of ballistic recoil and torsion of the heart during systole further modified by chest wall thickness, fluid, emphysema, etc. Palpable phenomena in diastole are principally the result of ventricular filling. From the location of the apex beat one can make an estimate of heart size, and from its character one can sometimes obtain clues regarding physiologic or morphologic abnormalities.

Technique of Palpation
For the most accurate appraisal of heart size it is best to feel for the apex impulse with the patient sitting up, leaning forward in expiration. The center (not the outermost border) of the point of maximal impulse will be found to correlate within approximately 1 cm with the outer border of the heart as measured in a standard chest roentgenogram. The position of the apex impulse should be described in terms of its distance from the midsternal line and the intercostal space in which it is located. Normally the impulse of the cardiac apex lies at or medial to the midclavicular line.

The apex impulse is often palpated, for convenience, with the patient supine. In this position its pulsations are feeble because of the heart's having fallen away from contact with the chest wall and the location of the apex may be displaced upward and laterally by the higher position of the diaphragm. For optimal appreciation of the waveforms constituting the apex impulse, and particularly for its diastolic constituents, it is best to palpate with the patient in the left lateral decubitus.[5] The observer should stand at the right side of the bed. It is often very helpful to magnify the apical movements by holding the base of a wand—a Bic pencil is ideal—in the interspace where the impulse has been located, with the impulse itself acting as a fulcrum and the point thus providing a moving indicator of pulsatile systolic and diastolic phenomena. If there is any doubt about the timing of palpable movements, one should *listen* with the stethoscope while feeling the precordium. If S_1 and S_2 are clearly identified, the timing of palpable events should not be difficult.

Character of the Impulse
The normal apex beat usually consists merely of a thrust at the beginning of systole during the period of isovolumic contraction. The impulse is small in amplitude and brief in duration. It is exaggerated in thin, youthful subjects and with the patient in the left lateral decubitus. Therefore, as with other physical signs, one must make observations in a large number of individuals in order to appreciate the wide range of normalcy and the alterations that may be expected with age, body build, pregnancy, etc. Diastolic waves are usually imperceptible in normal individuals.

A hyperkinetic cardiac impulse is characterized by an increase in amplitude but retention of the brief duration that is found in the normal beat. The hyperdynamic impulse occurs in a variety of circumstances where the stroke volume is augmented, as with mitral regurgitation, thyrotoxicosis, severe anemia, and left-to-right shunts such as ventricular septal defect or patent ductus arteriosus.[6,7] The same type of exaggerated impulse may be found in young, thin normal individuals, especially with exercise and excitement. Not infrequently, where the stroke volume is increased, a filling wave may be palpable in early diastole, with the patient lying in left lateral decubitus position. This corresponds to the audible third heartbeat sound.

A hypokinetic or imperceptible apical impulse may be encountered with obesity, emphysema, pericardial effusion, or constriction. In shock also the apical impulse may be very feeble or absent.

A sustained apex beat is a heave that has greater duration than the impulses previously described. It is swift in upstroke and exaggerated in amplitude. This type of powerful thrust of the left ventricle is seen in association with aortic stenosis, systemic hypertension, and idiopathic hypertrophic subaortic stenosis—all conditions characterized by left ventricular hypertrophy.[7,8] Usually a palpable *a* wave is perceptible in presystole with the patient lying on the left side.[4,5,9] A sustained thrust can also be felt with cardiomyopathy, but its amplitude is less and the velocity of its upstroke is lower, giving the impression of a weaker impulse. Prominent waves in diastole corresponding to third and fourth sounds are a frequent accompaniment in cardiomyopathy.

Right Ventricular Impulse

In the presence of right ventricular hypertrophy (RVH) there may be a sustained thrust at the left sternal edge. This is usually best appreciated as a systolic heave in the third and fourth left intercostal spaces.[10,11] This type of impulse occurs in association with high systolic pressures in the right ventricle, as in pulmonary hypertension or pulmonary stenosis. A hyperkinetic impulse characterized by increased amplitude but brief duration may be appreciated in the same location in conditions where there is an increased stroke volume but without excess pressure as in atrial septal defect[12] or pulmonary regurgitation. It should be noted that in tetralogy of Fallot, despite the presence of systemic pressures in the right ventricle, one does not encounter a right ventricular heave. There may be brief palpable vibrations at the time of S_1 and S_2, but the precordium is motionless during systole.[13] Absence of a sustained right ventricular thrust in the tetralogy is apparently due to the escape route for blood from right ventricle to aorta in this condition in contrast to the obstructive situation in pulmonary stenosis with intact ventricular septum. Another congenital cardiac condition affecting the right ventricle, but characterized by absence of a precordial heave or thrust, is Ebstein's anomaly of the tricuspid valve.[14]

Ectopic Impulses

Precordial Bulges in Ischemic Heart Disease
Precordial bulges in the third or fourth interspaces several centimeters from the sternum may occur in ischemia of the left ventricle.[15] They may be noted occasionally during an attack of angina pectoris, presumably as a result of transitory dyskinesis of the ventricular wall. With aneurysm of the anterior surface of the left ventricle a systolic bulge may persist in this location. A prominent presystolic *a* wave is an almost invariable accompaniment.

Mitral Regurgitation
In severe mitral regurgitation, in addition to the hyperkinetic impulse at the cardiac apex described above, there may be a generalized heave in systole over the whole precordium.[16] This movement is distributed over a wider area of the chest wall than the localized thrust of RVH, and it peaks later in systole. This delayed systolic wave mimics in timing the *v* wave in the left atrium and, like the *v* wave, is thought to be due to expansion of the left atrium by the regurgitant mass of blood and consequent lifting of the whole heart forward during systole.

Pulmonary Arterial Pulsation
Where the pulmonary artery is greatly swollen due to increased flow or pressure or poststenotic dilatation, there may be a palpable systolic bulge in the second left intercostal space.[17] However, a pulsation in this area is occasionally encountered in a young normal subject with a thin chest wall and hyperactive circulation.

Pulsation at Second Right Intercostal Space
In the presence of a dilated or aneurysmal aortic root there may be a systolic pulsation at the upper right sternal edge or sternoclavicular junction.

Exaggerated Movements in Diastole

Diastolic waves may be encountered in a variety of circumstances where their audible counterparts (third and fourth heart sounds or gallops) occur. These diastolic movements may be of large amplitude, as for instance in cardiomyopathy, but owing to their low velocity, they may not be readily perceived in a casual examination. The method described above of using a wand as a lever or visible marker at the apex beat provides a vividly exaggerated manifestation of these diastolic movements that may be edifying to the observer and a readily available method of demonstrating bedside diagnostic phenomena to others.

Inward Retraction of the Precordium in Systole

An inward movement of the precordium during systole occurs principally in two situations: (1) constrictive pericarditis[18,19] and (2) pure tricuspid regurgitation, i.e., incompetence of the valve as a primary abnormality rather than secondary to pulmonary hypertension and right ventricular failure. When the precordium moves *inward* during systole, it moves *outward*, of course, in early diastole at the time of ventricular filling. A careless observer utilizing palpation by itself can easily fall into the trap of reversing systole and diastole. If, however, one *listens* while palpating, the thrust of the diastolic heartbeat should be obvious.[20]

Palpable Heart Sounds

Heart sounds are frequently palpable in normal, young, thin individuals, as when exaggerated in disease states. For example, S_1 becomes snapping and accentuated in mitral stenosis and is responsible for the "tapping" apical impulse which is characteristic of that condition. A similarly accentuated and palpable S_1 is encountered in left atrial myxoma.

S_2 is increased and palpable in conditions associated with elevated pressures in the great vessels. Thus, A_2 may be palpable at the second right intercostal space in systemic hypertension or coarctation of the aorta. P_2 may be palpable at the second left intercostal space in pulmonary hypertension. An exaggerated single second sound palpable in this location but of aortic origin occurs in the uncommonly encountered corrected transposition of the great vessels where the source of the vibration lies close to the chest wall. The high-frequency vibrations associated with closure of the semilunar valves are sometimes called *shocks* because of their percussion quality and brief duration. They must be differentiated from the more sustained movements described above that are due to ventricular contractions.

Thrills

A *thrill* by definition is a palpable sensation resulting from the intense vibration of a loud murmur. It provides no specific diagnostic information beyond that yielded by the murmur itself. Thrills are often most readily perceived by applying the sensitive area of the hand at the base of the fingers, whereas all the other palpable phenomena described above are best appreciated by the fingertips.

References

1. Harvey, W.: "Exercitatio Anatomica de Motu Cordis et Sanguinis in Animalibus," Frankfort, 1628.
2. Kneibestol, M., and Vallbo, A. B.: Single Unit Analysis of Mechanoreceptor Activity from the Human Glabrous Skin, *Acta Physiol. Scand.*, 80:178, 1970.
*3. Smith, D., and Craige, E.: Enhancement of Tactile Perception as Employed in Palpation, *Circulation*, 62:1114, 1980. (8 references)
4. Denef, B., DeGeest, H., and Kesteloot, H.: The Clinical Value of the Calibrated Apical A Wave and its Relationship to the Fourth Heart Sound, *Circulation*, 60:1412, 1979.
*5. Bethell, H. J. N., and Nixon, P. G. F.: Examination

*This article is a review of the literature and contains additional references to the literature.

6. Craige, E., and Sutton, G. C.: Quantitation of Precordial Movement. II. Mitral Regurgitation, *Circulation*, 35:483, 1967.
*7. Sutton, G. C., Prewitt, T. A., and Craige, E.: Relationship between Quantitated Precordial Movement and Left Ventricular Function, *Circulation*, 41:179, 1970. (29 references)
8. Benchimol, A., Legler, J. F., and Dimond, E. G.: The Carotid Tracing and Apex Cardiogram in Subaortic Stenosis and Idiopathic Myocardial Hypertrophy, *Am. J. Cardiol.*, 11:427, 1963.
9. Gibson, T. C., Madry, R., Grossman, W., McLaurin, L. P., and Craige, E.: The A Wave of the Apex Cardiogram and Left Ventricular Diastolic Stiffness, *Circulation*, 49:441, 1974.
10. Schmidt, R. E., and Craige, E.: Precordial Movements over the Right Ventricle in Children with Pulmonary Stenosis, *Circulation*, 32:241, 1965.
11. Kesteloot, H., and Willems, J.: Relationship between the Right Apexcardiogram and Right Ventricular Dynamics, *Acta Cardiol.*, 22:64, 1967.
12. Eddleman, E. E., Holt, J. H., and Bancroft, W. H., Jr.: Computer Analysis of the Kinetocardiogram from Patients with Atrial Septal Defects, *Am. Heart J.*, 71:435, 1966.
13. Craige, E.: Apexcardiography, in A. M. Weissler (ed.), "Noninvasive Cardiology," Grune & Stratton, Inc., New York, 1974, p. 30.
14. Genton, E., and Blount, S. G., Jr.: The Spectrum of Ebstein's Anomaly, *Am. Heart J.*, 73:395, 1967.
15. Eddleman, E. E., Jr., and Harrison, T. R.: The Kinetocardiogram in Patients with Ischemic Heart Disease, *Prog. Cardiovasc. Dis.*, 6:189, 1963.
*16. Basta, L. L., Wolfson, P., Eckberg, D. L., and Abboud, F. M.: The Value of Left Parasternal Impulse Recordings in Assessment of Mitral Regurgitation, *Circulation*, 48:1055, 1973. (42 references)
17. Sakamoto, T., Matuhisa, M., Inoue, K., Hayashi, T., and Ito, U.: Clinical and Hemodynamic Observation of Indirect Pulmonary Artery Pulse Tracing, *Cardiovasc. Sound Bull.*, 3:127, 1973.
18. Boicourt, O.W., Nagle, R. E., and Mounsey, J. P. D.: The Clinical Significance of Systolic Retraction of the Apical Impulse, *Br. Heart J.*, 27:379, 1965.
19. El-Sherif, A., and El-Said, G.: Jugular, Hepatic and Precordial Pulsations in Constrictive Pericarditis, *Br. Heart J.*, 33:305, 1971.
*20. Mounsey, J. P. D.: Inspection and Palpation of the Cardiac Impulse, *Prog. Cardiovasc. Dis.*, 10:187, 1967. (20 references)

12

Auscultation of the Heart

I was consulted in 1816 by a girl who presented the general symptoms of heart disease and in whom palpation and percussion gave little information on account of the patient's obesity. Her age and sex forbade an examination [by direct auscultation]. Then I remembered a well-known acoustic fact, that if the ear be applied to one end of a plank it is easy to hear a pin's scratching at the other end. I conceived the possibility of employing this property of matter in the present case. I took a quire of paper, rolled it very tight, and applied one end of the roll to the precordium; then inclining my ear to the other end, I was surprised and pleased to hear the beating of the heart much more clearly than if I had applied my ear directly to the chest.

Rene Theophile Hyacinthe Laennec, 1826[1]

The Principles of Auscultation

Aubrey Leatham, F.R.C.P., and
Graham J. Leech, M.A.

The Evolution of Cardiac Auscultation

Modern auscultation began with the advent of phonocardiography and the ability to produce objective evidence of the timing of heart sounds and murmurs and their relation to other hemodynamic events. Landmarks were the monograph by Orias and Menendez, and the identification of the components of the second heart sound in left bundle branch block by Wolferth and Margolies, resulting in reversal of the previously held electrocardiographic interpretation. Long before this time, the audibility of vibrations produced by contractions of the heart had been appreciated, certainly by Harvey (1628). Following the introduction of the stethoscope by Laennec in 1826 (see quotation above) remarkably accurate observations were made, including an accurate account of the variations in splitting of the second heart sound with respiration (Potain, 1866); late systolic murmurs were attributed to mitral regurgitation as early as 1892 by Griffith of Philadelphia. An account of the history of auscultation is given in the previous (fourth) edition of this textbook, and greater detail is given in McKusick's scholarly monograph *Cardiovascular Sound in Health and Disease.*[2]

In the last 30 years, the origin of the high-frequency components of heart sounds has been attributed by most practicing physicians to the final halt of closing valves; this theory was compatible with the effects of asynchronous left and right ventricular contractions as with bundle branch block, ventricular ectopics, and pacing. This view was challenged by Luisada and coworkers, but in the last decade echocardiography, with its ability to time valve movements exactly, has confirmed the valve theory.

Basic Physics of Sound Waves

The word *sound* describes a sensation produced when pressure waves having certain characteristics strike the eardrum. Pressure waves are generated by a vibrating object that disturbs the particles of the medium surrounding it. The particles pass the vibrations on to their neighbors, and the disturbance is propagated through the medium as ripples spreading out across a pond. The particles do not travel through the medium but simply vibrate to and fro. The disturbance or wave travels in a direction parallel to that of the particle vibrations and is transmitted by the elastic coupling between them.

If waves are generated continuously in a regular pattern by a vibrating piston, the resulting alternating compressions and rarefactions can be represented diagrammatically as in Fig. 12-1. The *wavelength* is the distance between two successive peaks or troughs; the *amplitude* is the difference between maximum and minimum pressures. A complete segment comprising one peak and one trough is called a *cycle*. The number of cycles passing a particular point in one second is the *frequency*. Frequency, wavelength, and propagation velocity are related as follows:

Frequency × wavelength = propagation velocity

For a given medium, propagation velocity is fixed, and so frequency and wavelength are inversely related. In air, pressure waves travel 300 m/s; in soft tissue, about 1550 m/s; and in bone, 4000 m/s. Thus, at a frequency of 256 Hz (Hz = cycles per second), which is the pitch of middle C on a piano, the wavelength of sound in air is about 1.3 m.

Waves from a small source surrounded by a uniform medium radiate outward in all directions, the intensity diminishing as the square of the distance. Intensity is further diminished by imperfect transfer of energy within the medium; water for example is a very good transmission medium, but air is some five times less efficient.

Pressure waves exhibit the same properties as other wave phenomena (e.g., light), the apparent differences being due to the relative sizes of the wavelength (100 cm for sound, compared with 0.000005 cm for light). Thus, when waves encounter an extensive boundary between two different transmission media, some of the energy is reflected and some transmitted, the path of the latter being deviated by refraction. Small obstacles scatter some of the incident energy in all directions. Diffraction allows waves to "bend" around a large obstacle; waves can also interact to produce interference ef-

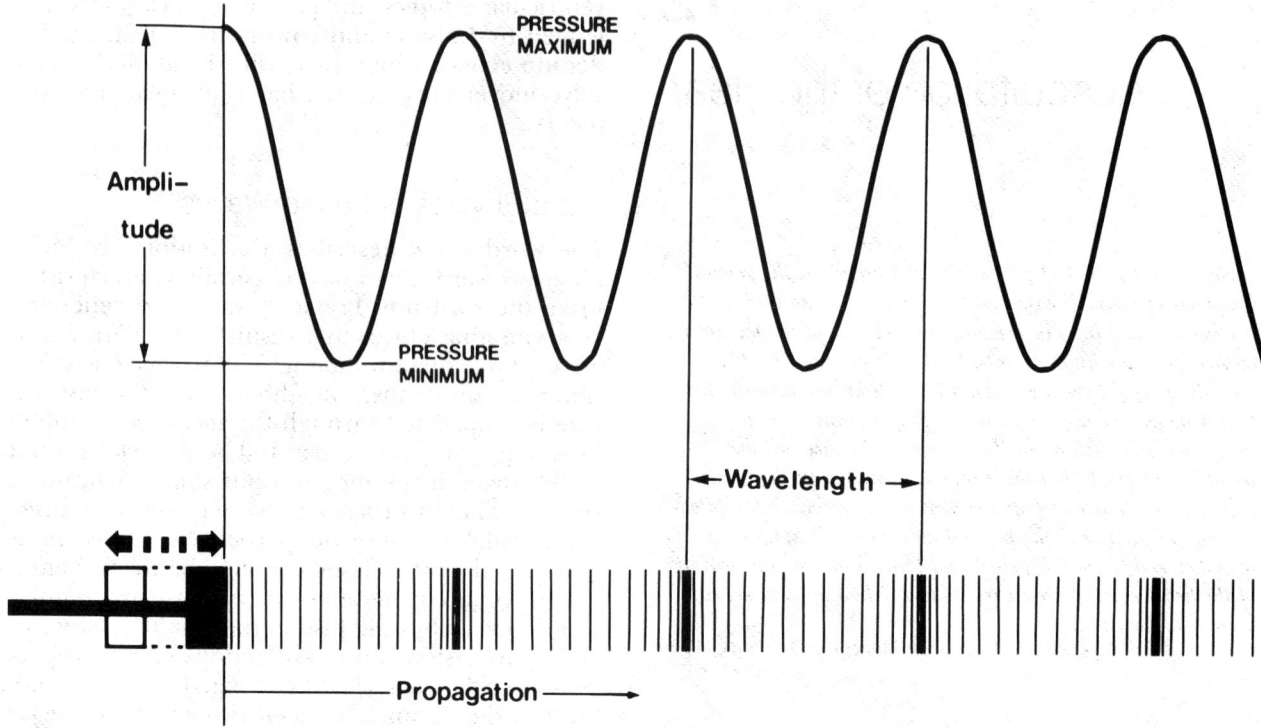

FIGURE 12-1   Diagrammatic representation of compression waves showing the nomenclature used to describe them.

fects and generate *standing waves,* i.e., zones of maximum and minimum amplitude.

If pressure waves encounter an object that is free to move in the direction of wave propagation, the object is caused to oscillate at the wave frequency. If an object that is constrained by some elastic force is disturbed, it vibrates at a frequency determined by its mass, the spring characteristics, and the degree of frictional damping present. This effect is called *resonance.* If such an object is disturbed by a wave train with a frequency that is identical to the resonant frequency, the resulting oscillations will have a very large amplitude. Thus, if for example a bank of tuning forks is placed in the path of sound waves, all the forks will vibrate a little, but the one with a resonant frequency that is closest to the wave frequency will "sing."

The Human Ear

The human hearing apparatus is very complex. It comprises the ear, which can be divided into the external, middle, and inner ears; the cochlear nerve; and those portions of the brain concerned with hearing perception.

Incoming pressure waves are collected by the pinna and led into the external auditory canal, which slopes forward and downward and is terminated by the eardrum. The waves cause the eardrum to vibrate, and the vibrations are transmitted to the oval window of the cochlea across the middle ear cavity by the three ossicles. The relatively small area of the oval window coupled with the large area

of the eardrum improves energy transfer across the impedance mismatch between the air and the fluid within the cochlea.

The cochlea is a spiral canal rather like a snail shell and is separated along its length by two membranes into three compartments, the outer two of which join at its apex. The oval window connects to one of the outer compartments, which are filled with perilymph. The channel winds up the spiral, then down the other side, terminating in the round window which connects to the middle ear again. Between the two outer sections is the cochlear duct, filled with endolymph. Within the cochlear duct is the organ of Corti containing some 25,000 fine, hairlike fibers which form the terminal elements of the cochlear nerve. Pressure waves are transmitted from the perilymph, across the separating membrane, into the endolymph. The nerve fibers act rather like the array of tuning forks described earlier. Those near the bottom of the spiral are stimulated by high-frequency vibrations; those near the apex, by lower frequencies.

The fibers of the cochlear nerve lead, via several synaptic junctions, to the primary auditory reception center in the anterior transverse temporal gyrus; the neurons of this center fire at rates corresponding to the amplitude and frequency of the pressure waves. Through complex and little-understood interaction between these cells and those of the associated cerebral cortex, the sensation of sound is generated.

Sound perception is a complex subject, but some aspects relevant to cardiac auscultation must be mentioned. The most striking feature of human hearing is its almost incredible sensitivity; at its best it can detect pressure levels of 0.0002 dyn/cm² (equivalent to 10^{-16} W/cm²). Although relatively crude by the standards of the animal kingdom, this is far superior to any manufactured microphone and amplifier. The sensitivity of the ear is, however, greatly influenced by wave frequency. It performs best between 2 and 4 kHz; outside this range, sensitivity falls progressively, and below 30 Hz or above 18 kHz is effectively zero. The manner in which sensitivity varies with frequency depends on the amplitude of the waves. As shown in Fig. 12-2, for very high amplitudes, sensitivity varies little within the overall frequency range; but for lower amplitudes, the variation is greater. Heart sounds and murmurs generally have very low intensity, close to the threshold of hearing; and furthermore, most lie in the frequency range of 1 to 500 Hz, well below the optimal range of the ear. In this region, the response characteristically approximates a straight line with a slope of 15 dB per octave. This means that if one tone has half the frequency of another, it must have 5.6 times the amplitude in order to appear to be equally loud. The substantial proportion of the heart's vibrational energy that lies below 30 Hz cannot be heard at all (though high-amplitude components may be detected by palpation).

Another psychoacoustic perception peculiarity of the ear is that it takes up to 1 s after the onset of a sound for its full intensity to be perceived, and this serves to lower the effective sensitivity for brief noises. Similarly, once the ear is accustomed to a relatively loud sound, a softer sound is not well heard. Thus, in a patient with a ventricular septal defect, it may be difficult to hear a faint P_2 component immediately after the loud systolic murmur. The smallest time interval that the ear can resolve is about 20 ms (0.02 s), so splitting of the first heart sound will only be apparent if the interval between the two components exceeds this amount. Finally, the ear has a remarkable ability to separate "wanted" from "unwanted" sounds. Thus, although a quiet environment is undoubtedly best for auscultation, the skilled practitioner can to a large extent ignore interference from extraneous sources and from respiratory noise and borborygmi which would render a phonocardiographic recording useless.

The Origin of Cardiac Sounds and Murmurs

The vibratory phenomena associated with the action of the heart can broadly be divided into *heart sounds*, brief noises which generally mark the beginning or end of phases of the cardiac cycle, and *murmurs*, which last longer and are associated with blood flow.

Although heart sounds have been studied for

FIGURE 12-2   Fletcher-Munson curves showing contours of equal perceived loudness as amplitude and frequency are varied. At high intensities (above 100 dB) there is little change in loudness (measured in phons) with frequency. At the lowest limit of hearing sensitivity (0 phons), the relationship is very nonlinear. The heavy line therefore represents the frequency response characteristic of the ear for the purposes of cardiac auscultation.

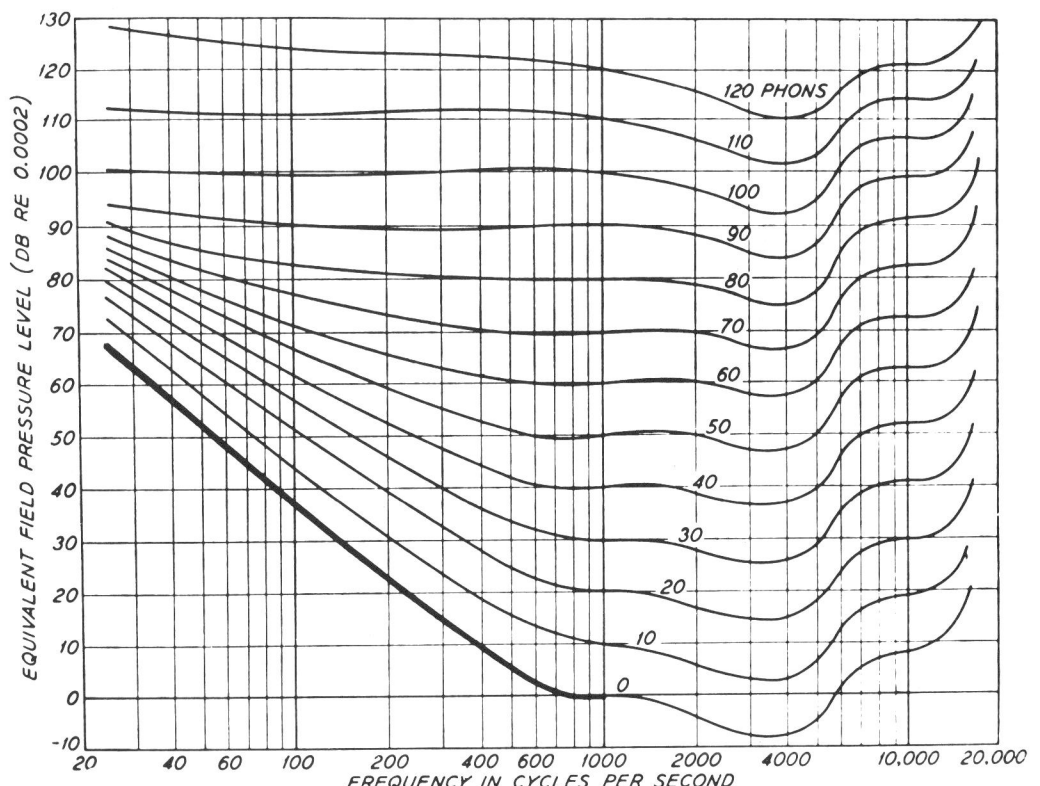

EXAMINATION OF THE HEART AND BLOOD VESSELS

over 150 years, there is no universally accepted theory for their origin. In 1830, Rouanet[3] pumped water through an animal heart while holding it to his ear to listen to the sounds generated. He observed that there were two major noises from each side of the heart, one at the beginning and one at the end of systole. He attributed these to "tensioning" of the leaflets of the atrioventricular and semilunar valves, respectively. Similar experiments by Dock[4] and others supported this view. Thus the *valvular* theory holds that the first heart sound has two major components, associated with mitral and tricuspid closure, and similarly the second sound has aortic and pulmonary components.

Although satisfactory for clinical purposes, the valvular theory came under attack in the 1960s as a result of studies of intracardiac pressures using high-fidelity micromanometers. These showed that the timing of reversal of the pressure gradient across valves did not coincide with the associated sound components, and, since the valves are passive structures, it was assumed that they opened and closed at the moment of gradient reversal. Thus, it appeared that valve closure was not synchronous with the sound events, and so alternative mechanisms involving the tensioning of the ventricles and great vessels were proposed.[5] There is fallacy in this argument, however, since blood flowing through an open valve has momentum and the reversed pressure gradient takes a finite time to halt flow before the valve can close. Gradient crossover thus precedes valve closure by a variable interval influenced by the flow rate and the impedance characteristics of the downstream vessels.

More recently, echocardiography has provided a method for timing the motions of valves directly against sound phenomena and has vindicated the valvular theory by demonstrating invariable coincidence between the sound components and the abrupt halting of the valve leaflets as they tense under the influence of moving masses of blood (Figs. 12-3 and 12-4). Thus, the components of the first and second heart sounds, opening snaps, early systolic ejection clicks, and prolapse clicks all have the same underlying mechanism.[6,7]

This concept does not, however, fully explain the early systolic "root" sounds sometimes heard in systemic or pulmonary hypertension and thought to arise from sudden distension of an enlarged artery. Their timing is identical to that of valve ejection sounds, and this makes the root theory difficult to accept, since at the moment when valve opening becomes maximal, ejection has already begun but has not yet achieved maximum velocity. It may be that some fibrous thickening of the semilunar cusps, known to occur in hypertensive states, and a high rate of increase of accelerating pressure gradient, which is due to late onset of ejection, combine to generate an audible sound in these patients.

There are also the third and fourth (ventricular filling) sounds. The former is approximately coincident with the transition from rapid to slow ventricular filling, and the latter occurs about 150 ms after the ECG P wave. Their precise origin is not certain, although they appear to arise as a result of a "shudder" of the left ventricular muscle in reaction to a sudden change in filling rate. In support of this concept is the fact that a sharp deflection of the interventricular septum coincident with a third sound can sometimes be seen on echocardiographic recordings.

When fluid flows through a pipe, if the flow velocity exceeds a certain value, flow becomes turbulent and some energy is dissipated in vortices which generate audible vibrations. Unstable flow can also arise when fluid passes through a small hole in a plate which partly occludes a pipe, when the pipe diameter changes abruptly, when a jet impinges on

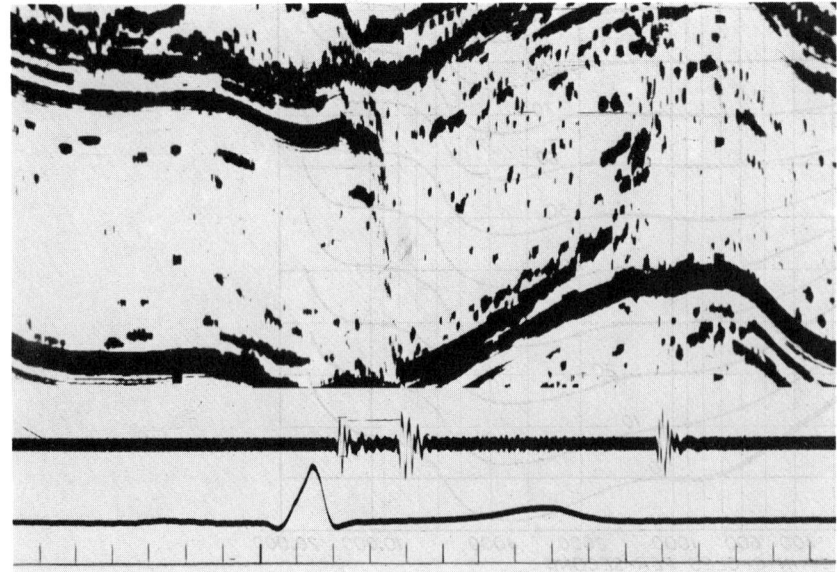

FIGURE 12-3 High-speed echophonocardiograms showing the relationship of heart sounds to valve movements. The upper tracing shows a mitral valve echo in a patient with mild mitral stenosis, and the lower nonstenotic bicuspid aortic valve. The onset of the vibrations of the opening snap and ejection sound both occur precisely at the moment when the motion of the diseased valve is suddenly halted. See also Fig. 12-4.

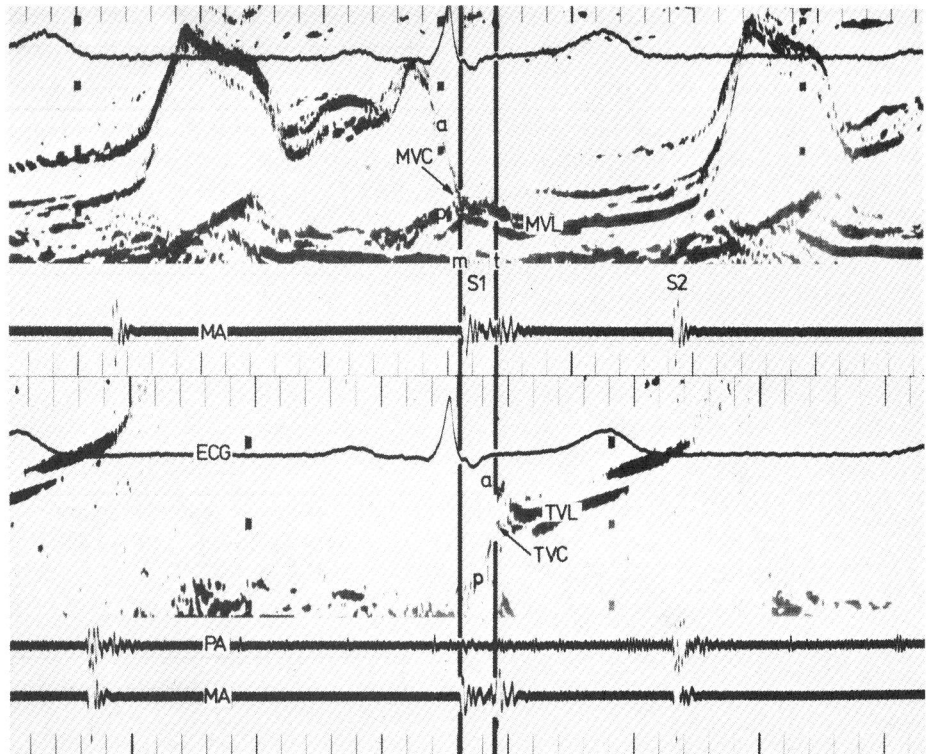

FIGURE 12-4 Echophonocardiogram from a normal subject with physiological splitting of the first heart sound. The tracings from the mitral and tricuspid valve were not recorded simultaneously, but the subject was in regular rhythm, and the tracings were aligned using the electrocardiogram. It will be seen that the first component of the first sound coincides with the terminal halt of the closing mitral valve (MVC) and the second component with that of the tricuspid valve (TVC).

a surface, or when two streams having different directions of flow interact. Similar mechanisms underlie the generation of cardiac murmurs, although the complex geometry of the cardiohemic system, together with the nonlinear mechanical properties of blood vessels and pulsatile flow, makes mathematical analysis very difficult.

The audible characteristics of a murmur are determined mainly by the size and velocity of the jet. Thus, a high-velocity jet associated with ventricular septal defect or aortic or mitral regurgitation produces a high-frequency murmur, whereas a low-velocity jet in mitral stenosis generates a low-frequency murmur. Unfortunately, murmur intensity does not necessarily indicate flow volume. Thus, although a very small jet does not usually generate a loud murmur, torrential flow through a large hole, as in a large ventricular septal defect, can produce no murmur at all. It must be remembered also that the ear perceives higher-frequency noises as being louder than those of the same amplitude but of lower frequency.

Finally, murmurs can arise from secondary phenomena such as vibrations of chordae tendineae or torn semilunar cusps. These murmurs often have a characteristic "musical" quality. Other sources of noises within the heart, such as pericardial friction rubs, generally have different audible characteristics and are best not considered as murmurs at all.

Transmission of Sounds and Murmurs

The vibrations generated within the heart are transmitted throughout the tissues of the thorax, and some of them reach the outer chest wall with sufficient amplitude to be audible. Blood transmits pressure waves very well. Thus, the murmurs of aortic or pulmonary stenosis are transmitted along the appropriate artery and are best detected at the point where they come closest to the chest surface (Fig. 12-5). In ventricular septal defect, the murmur arises within the right ventricle, close to the chest wall, and is easy to hear. In contrast, the jet in mitral regurgitation is directed backwards into the left atrium, the most distant of the four chambers, but the mass of blood within the left side of the heart still conducts the sounds fairly well to the apex, where they are best heard.

Transmission is aided by bringing the heart into contact with the chest wall without intervening lung tissue, which strongly attenuates sound waves. Thus, it helps to lean the patient forward and listen during held expiration to hear the murmur of aortic regurgitation, and to turn the patient to the left so that the apical beat can be palpated, indicating that the heart is in contact with the chest wall, when listening to the diastolic murmur of mitral stenosis.

The chest wall itself has relatively high attenuation and is far from homogeneous, with the result

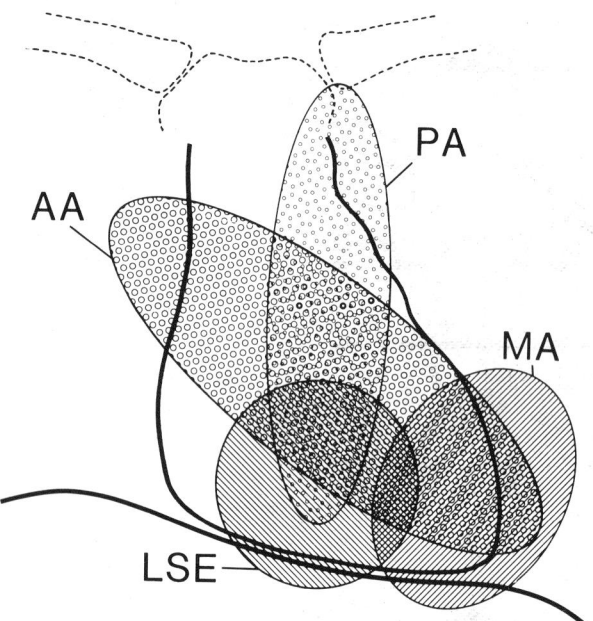

FIGURE 12-5 Sites for auscultation and nomenclature. PA = pulmonary area. Pulmonary sounds or murmurs are usually maximal in the second or third left spaces but may extend inferiorly; LSE = lower left sternal edge or tricuspid area; AA = aortic area; MA = mitral area. (*From A. Leatham, "Examination of the Cardiovascular System," 2d ed., Oxford Medical Publications, Oxford, 1979. Reproduced with permission.*)

these components do not excite resonant vibrations within the large masses of the heart and chest structures, and they die away very rapidly. Thus, if one wants to identify precisely the timing of transient events, it is best to remove all the low-frequency components. This is particularly necessary when two or more events occur in rapid succession, such as the closure of the atrioventricular or semilunar valves. The low-frequency vibrations merge together; but if they are eliminated and only the high-frequency components are detected, the vibrations from the first event end before those from the second begin, and the two can be distinguished (Fig. 12-6).

The Physical Principles of Auscultation

Most sound energy reaching our ears is transmitted under so-called free field conditions in which the intensity diminishes as the square of the distance from the source. Waves arising from very low amplitude vibrations, such as those of the precordium, would thus be audible only if the ear were placed very close to the chest. As Laennec found, however, this is not always practical, so he rolled some paper to form a tube, one end of which he held on the patient's chest and the other he applied to his ear.

that significant losses occur at interfaces between bones and muscle. The structure of the chest wall is such that most transmission is probably not via compression waves but via longitudinal shear waves, which transfer energy less effectively. Finally, the characteristics of the chest wall are somewhat frequency-dependent, with optimal transmission occurring between 100 and 200 Hz.[8]

For practical purposes, modification of heart sounds during transmission to the precordium is uncontrollable and largely unknown, so auscultatory findings are based on the characteristics of the vibrations as they appear on the chest surface. However, the build of the patient should be borne in mind when assessing their significance. Thus, a soft ejection murmur in a thin adolescent in whom the main pulmonary artery lies directly beneath the chest wall is less likely to be pathological than a murmur of the same intensity heard in an obese patient.

Vibrations reaching the chest wall, from whatever origin, combine to produce a compound wave. This can be considered on the basis of Fourier analysis to be comprised of a series of pure tones. The lowest frequency present, called the *fundamental,* is the frequency of the heart rate, typically 1 Hz (60 beats per minute). Added to it are numerous harmonics, with frequencies that are exact multiples of the fundamental and amplitudes that generally decrease with increasing frequency. The higher-frequency harmonics are most evident at the time of transient events like halting of blood masses associated with valve closures. Because of their high frequency,

FIGURE 12-6 Phonocardiograms recorded from a normal subject to illustrate the effect of electronic filtering. At the top, there is very little filtering, so low-frequency sound components dominate the tracing. The center and bottom tracings have progressively greater attenuation of low frequencies and correspond approximately to the stethoscope bell and diaphragm, respectively. Physiological splitting of the first heart sound is revealed only when the low-frequency aftervibrations are totally eliminated.

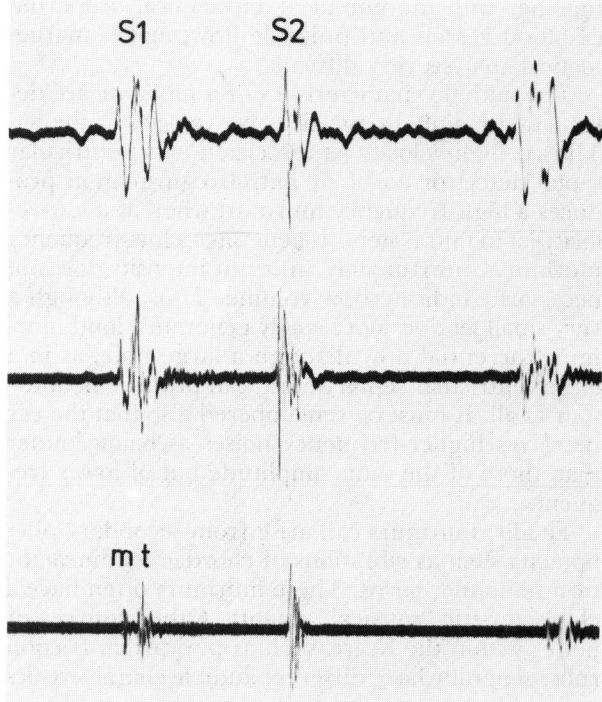

The stethoscope channels almost all the vibrational energy from the area of the precordium underneath the chest piece directly to the observer's eardrum. It is analogous to the catheter manometer system used to measure intravascular pressures, in which pressure signals are conducted along a fluid-filled tube to a remote sensing gauge. The following general principles govern the operation of the stethoscope. It should contact as large an area of the chest wall as possible, since by this means a given amplitude of precordial vibration will generate the greatest air volume displacement within the stethoscope. The internal volume of the tubing should be small, and its walls as rigid as possible, consistent with maneuverability, so that the volume displacement is converted into the maximum pressure fluctuation. It must make a perfect air seal against the chest wall, and the earpieces must fit perfectly into the external auditory canal, otherwise the pressure fluctuations will "leak out" and not be transmitted to the eardrum at maximal amplitude.

The frequency characteristics of the sounds are somewhat modified by the stethoscope tubing, which behaves rather like an organ pipe and resonates at certain frequencies determined primarily by its length.[9] However, the relatively low compliance of even thick-walled rubber tubing damps the resonant peaks considerably. Greater control of frequency response can be achieved by the use of different types of chest pieces. With an open funnel, all frequencies are transmitted into the tubing, and so the lower components, which have relatively much greater amplitudes, tend to predominate. By covering the end of the funnel with a thin rigid diaphragm of stainless steel, which has a high resonant frequency, the lower components are effectively filtered out, leaving only the high frequencies, which are important for precise timing of transients and detection of splitting of the first and second heart sounds.

The Ideal Stethoscope

The stethoscope is divisible into the earpieces, the head frame, the flexible tubing, and the chest piece.

The earpieces should fit exactly so that external noise is greatly reduced; the correct size for a particular individual should be carefully chosen; and, above all, there should be a comfortable fit. The angulation and pressure exerted by the head frame is of equal importance. The combination of a perfect fit with complete comfort is essential. The tubing should be as short and rigid as possible to reduce transmission loss, and yet should be sufficiently flexible to allow varying angulation of the chest piece without movement of the earpieces in the external meatus; this movement not only interferes with a close fit but may also cause meatitis. It is seldom practical to reduce the length of the tubing to less than 12 in, and double tubing is apparently more

efficient than single tubing for transmitting high frequencies.[10]

The greatest variations occur in the stethoscope chest piece. The essential principle is that a rigid diaphragm transmits the high frequencies preferentially by resonating with them, thus acting as a filter. On the other hand, a bell transmits all frequencies with minimal loss, provided that it is not applied so firmly to the chest wall that the skin acts as a diaphragm. The larger the bell, the greater the intensity of sound collected, but the limiting factor with a large bell is the difficulty in obtaining a good fit over the rib cage of thin individuals; thus, ideally both a large and a small bell are required, and it is possible for the two to be combined.

The small bell has an additional advantage for localization of sounds and murmurs, particularly in pediatric cardiology. The diaphragm chest piece can cover a large area, since a perfect fit on the chest wall is not needed, and should be rigid (0.003-in stainless steel is as good as anything so far known). It should now be clear that the minimum requirement for an efficient stethoscope for cardiac auscultation is the combination of a bell chest piece and a diaphragm chest piece in a single instrument with a good changeover switch. Unfortunately, most popular stethoscopes have small and inefficient bells and large floppy diaphragms passing a high volume of sound, but with no filtration. It is strongly emphasized that a diaphragm with great rigidity is required for listening to high-frequency sounds, splitting of sounds, and high-frequency murmurs, and that a bell, which should be as large as possible, should be used for listening to low-frequency sounds and murmurs. Since auscultation of the heart is normally conducted near the lower threshold of the human hearing mechanism, an efficient stethoscope carries a great advantage in the practice of clinical cardiology. It might be thought that electronic amplification would be useful for bedside auscultation, but unfortunately no portable apparatus is yet as efficient as a good stethoscope. The greatest problem is the enormous variation in amplitude of vibrations useful for diagnosis in a typical heart cycle. Thus, high gain is required for low-intensity vibrations, and loud vibrations then produce distortion.

The Technique of Auscultation

Auscultation is the most difficult part of examination of the cardiovascular system but is greatly simplified if the physician knows what to listen for. It should therefore be preceded by the history and physical examination. For example, a history of paroxysmal nocturnal dyspnea should direct attention to listening for an opening snap or mitral diastolic murmur as evidence of mitral stenosis, or for a third heart sound as evidence of left ventricular failure. The finding of a slow-rising carotid pulse helps immensely in the interpretation of an apical systolic murmur when the decision as to whether or not it is a pansystolic regurgitant murmur or a midsystolic aortic ejection murmur is impossible because of inaudibility of the second heart sound.

A quiet room is essential for accurate auscultation, and it is equally important that the patient be relaxed and comfortable. Often a background noise from contraction of chest wall muscles can be reduced by asking the patient to relax. Poor transmission of sound occurs with obesity and with hyperinflation. Particularly with the latter, aortic systolic murmurs are distant in the aortic and pulmonary areas.

At the start of auscultation, the patient is usually reclining comfortably at an elevation of 30 to 40°, as for the preceding examination of the venous and arterial pulses, and it is convenient to start auscultation in the pulmonary area, i.e., second and third left spaces. Figure 12-5 shows the usual auscultatory areas—note the considerable overlap between the aortic and mitral areas. The first and second heart sounds should be identified easily enough in most cases since systole is shorter than diastole. With tachycardia, systole and diastole may be of the same duration; accordingly, the carotid pulse should be palpated since its upstroke occurs very soon after the first heart sound. Auscultation in the pulmonary area using the diaphragm of the stethoscope usually reveals splitting of the second heart sound during the inspiratory phase of phasic respiration. The first and greater component is due to closure of the aortic valve (A_2), and the second and smaller component is due to closure of the pulmonary valve (P_2). The sounds should fuse in the expiratory phase of continuous respiration when the patient is reclining at 30 to 40°. If splitting remains obvious in expiration, the patient should be requested to breathe a little slower and deeper; fusion should then occur. Persistence of splitting suggests that there is prolongation of right ventricular systole or shortening of left. Appreciation of normal and abnormal splitting of the second sound is the single most important step in the examination of children, since physiological right ventricular outflow ejection systolic murmurs are frequently present and cause difficulty in diagnosis.

If the order of valve closure is reversed (P_2 before A_2), the splitting is maximal in expiration and disappears on inspiration as P_2 delays, and this indicates prolongation of left ventricular systole. The pulmonary component of the second sound in a normal subject may be transmitted to the lower left sternal edge, but seldom to the apex.

The diaphragm of the stethoscope should then be moved to the lower left sternal edge, where the first heart sound is usually split in normal subjects into mitral and tricuspid components. These are both high-pitched sounds, and the interval between them is very small. The first component is usually louder and is due to closure of the mitral valve; the second component is usually much softer, sometimes inaudible, and is due to closure of the tricuspid valve. The splitting is particularly obvious in patients with sternal depression, owing to the juxtaposition of the heart to the stethoscope.

The diaphragm is then moved to the apex or mitral area, where the dominant component of the first heart sound is mitral closure and tricuspid closure is difficult to hear. In fact, obvious "splitting of the first heart sound" at the apex, particularly when separation of the two components is a little more than usual, should suggest audibility of an early systolic ejection sound from the aortic valve. The second heart sound at the apex should be single and is solely due to closure of the aortic valve. In diastole in a normal subject, careful auscultation of the apex with the bell gently but accurately applied to the skin should reveal a low-pitched sound, which is the third heart sound and is due to rapid ventricular filling. This sound is obvious in thin children, progressively tends to become softer with increasing age, and disappears to auscultation (but not to a phonocardiogram) after the age of 40 to 45 years. The rapid ventricular filling sound is heard more easily if the patient leans to the left in the reclining position.

Many physicians prefer to reverse the order for auscultation, starting with the bell and then the diaphragm at the apex and continuing with the diaphragm at the lower left sternal edge and pulmonary areas.

Auscultation should now be directed toward hearing abnormal sounds. Preceding the first sound, there may be a low-pitched sound due to ventricular filling following atrial contraction. This is easily confused with splitting of the first heart sound but is maximal at the apex (when left ventricular in origin) with the patient lying on the left side, and it is best heard with the bell rather than with the diaphragm. The aortic ejection sound, best recognized at the apex, has already been mentioned. In the pulmonary area, an early systolic sound will suggest the presence of a pulmonary ejection sound. Soon after the second heart sound, there may be an opening snap of the mitral valve. This is of high frequency, best heard with the diaphragm, and resembles P_2 in quality but is heard over a wider area, including the apex; during inspiration it should be possible to hear A_2, P_2, and the snap all close together. Attention is then paid to the possibility of a systolic murmur: its site of maximum intensity is noted and its intensity is graded. Even more important is the decision as to whether or not the murmur is a midsystolic ejection murmur or a pansystolic regurgitant murmur which extends to the relevant component of the second heart sound, since the site of maximum intensity may be misleading (Fig. 12-5) and aortic murmurs are often maximal at the mitral area, particularly in elderly subjects.

In diastole, there may be a high-pitched early diastolic murmur from aortic or pulmonary regurgitation starting with the relevant component of the second heart sound. It should be remembered that the aortic valve underlies the third or fourth left intercostal space, and an aortic diastolic murmur is usually heard in this area with the diaphragm; often it is best heard with the patient upright and in held expiration since respiration mimics the quality of the murmur. An aortic diastolic murmur may also be transmitted to the apex. Maximal intensity in the aortic area to the right of the sternum suggests that the aorta is dilated. A pulmonary diastolic murmur secondary to pulmonary hypertension (the usual cause) is indistinguishable in site, timing, and quality from an aortic diastolic murmur, and should only be diagnosed if there is clinical and electrocardiographic evidence of right ventricular hypertrophy, a loud P_2 on auscultation, and a large pulmonary artery on x-ray.

Ventricular filling murmurs due to flow through the mitral or tricuspid valves occur a little later in diastole. They are low-pitched because of the much lower velocity of flow and therefore are best heard with the bell gently but accurately applied to the apex with the patient inclined to the left in the case of a mitral murmur or applied at the lower end of the sternum particularly during inspiration in the case of a tricuspid murmur. It is important to grade the intensity of the murmur, and particularly its duration, since these approximate measures of the degree of obstruction. Next, it is important to listen in other areas, particularly at the aortic area to the right of the upper sternum where aortic systolic murmurs may be maximal, and also below the left clavicle where the murmur of patent ductus arteriosus is maximal and may be confined to that area; an identical continuous murmur may, however, be due to normal return of venous blood from the head and neck (venous hum), but this disappears in the horizontal position. When congenital heart disease is suspected, it is necessary to listen to the whole chest since, for example, the continuous murmur found in pulmonary atresia may be maximal posteriorly; in coarctation of the aorta, the systolic murmur is usually as loud over the spine as it is over the front of the chest. Most murmurs are heard best when the patient is horizontal, since this causes increased venous return, or after exercise in this position. The patient should also be examined in the upright position for systolic sounds or murmurs secondary to a floppy mitral valve, since diminished stroke volume in the upright position may allow greater prolapse of floppy cusps. Left ventricular outflow obstruction and the resulting systolic murmur in obstructive cardiomyopathy also increase with diminished stroke volume when the patient assumes the upright position.

The First and Second Heart Sounds

Aubrey Leatham, F.R.C.P., and
Graham J. Leech, M.A.

Heart sounds are of two varieties: those due to halting of closing or opening valves, and those due to halt-

ing of the ventricular walls at their limit of filling. Not surprisingly, the quality and timing of each group are completely different.

Valve closing and opening sounds result from the sudden halt of valve cusps which were moving at high velocity, and for this reason they are composed of high-frequency vibrations which sound high-pitched and are relatively loud because of the ear's great sensitivity to high frequencies.

The valve origin of the high-frequency heart sounds was described by Dock[4] nearly 50 years ago and has been accepted by many clinicians for the last 30 years mainly for indirect reasons[11] and particularly because of the findings with asynchronous ventricular contraction in bundle branch block, ventricular ectopic beats, and pacing.[12] This concept was challenged by Luisada and coworkers,[13] but the development of cineangiography and later of echocardiography permitted for the first time an exact relationship to be established between valve motion and heart sounds. Echoes taken synchronously with phonocardiograms at fast paper speeds have now established that the final halting of closing and opening valves is exactly coincident with the major high-frequency heart sounds.[14–16]

The First Heart Sound

Physiological Splitting of the First Heart Sound
Contraction of the left ventricle closely precedes that of the right.[17] Thus, the first valve to halt after closure as a result of the rise of ventricular pressure in early systole is the mitral, and this is responsible for the initial major components of the first heart sound. The first heart sound is maximal at the apex or mitral area where the apex of the left ventricle strikes the chest wall as it rotates in early systole. Fractionally later, the tricuspid valve closes, and this coincides with a rather smaller high-frequency vibration that is maximal at the lower left sternal edge over the tricuspid valve. This asynchrony of mitral and tricuspid valve closure accounts for the normal splitting of the first heart sound (Fig. 12-7), which can usually be heard at the lower end of the sternum, particularly in thin patients and children. The origin of the second component of the first heart sound had been controversial for many years; it was stated that closure of the tricuspid valve was noiseless and that the second component of the first sound arose on the left side of the heart, but echophonocardiography has now firmly established the tricuspid origin of this sound (Fig. 12-4).[14,16,18] Splitting of the first heart sound in normal subjects measures 20 to 50 ms and is wider than would be expected from the slight asynchrony of onset of left and right ventricular contraction. It appears that at normal PR intervals, the preceding atrial contraction has not only reopened the mitral valve but in addition has nearly closed it so that the slightest rise of the first part of the left ventricular (LV) pressure pulse is sufficient to complete closure. The tricuspid

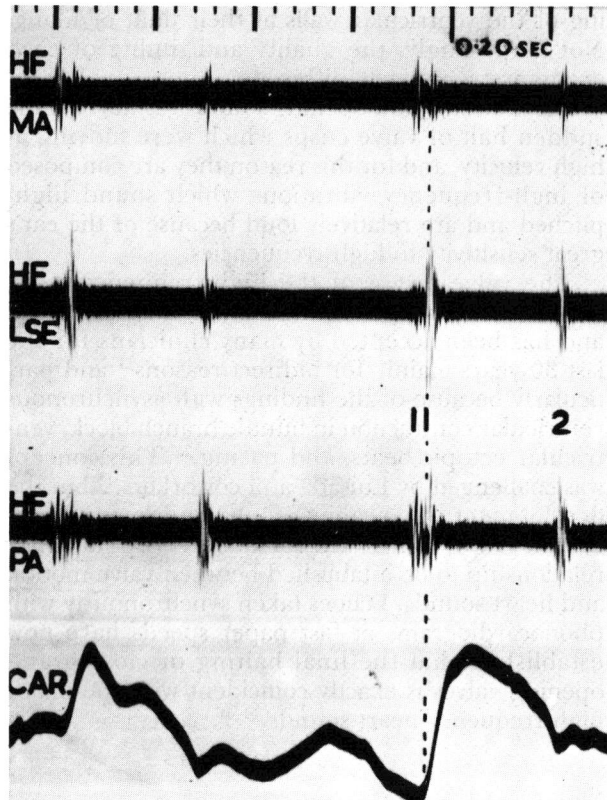

FIGURE 12-7 Physiological splitting of the first sound by 20 ms, best heard over the tricuspid valve at the lower left sternal edge where the second component (tricuspid closure) is maximal. The first component is much the louder sound in all other areas, particularly the mitral area. Echophonocardiography (Fig. 12-4) has confirmed the strong clinical suspicion that the first component is due to closure of the mitral valve, the second to the tricuspid valve.

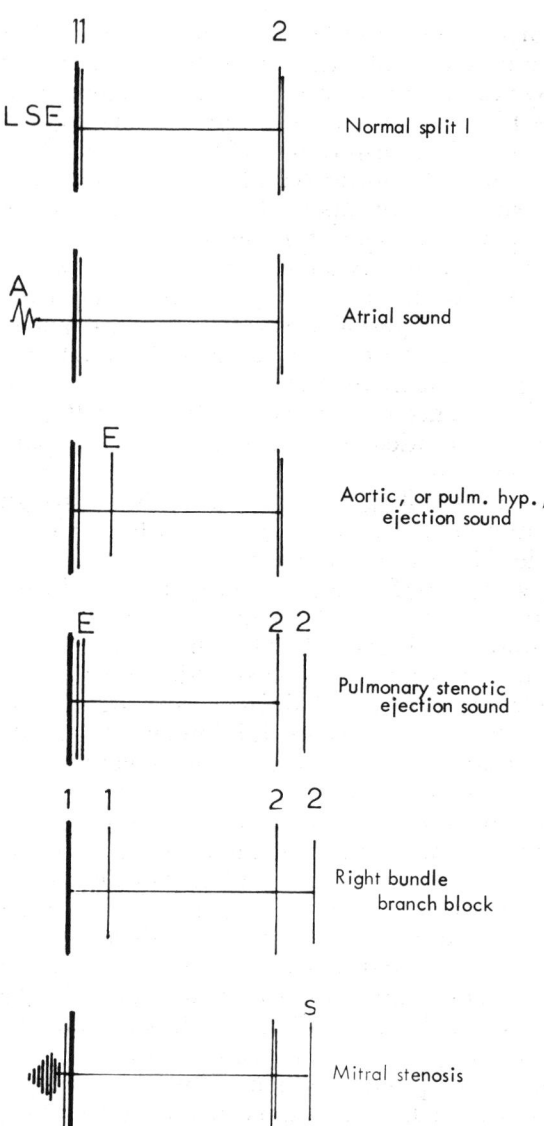

FIGURE 12-8 Differential diagnosis of physiological splitting of first sound.

valve, however, starts from a wide-open position (right atrial contraction is less efficient than left in exerting closure forces) and thus takes longer to reach its final closed position.[19]

The differential diagnosis of splitting of the first heart sound is shown in Fig. 12-8.

Abnormally Wide Splitting of the First Heart Sound

Delay in onset of right ventricular contraction, causing delay in onset of tricuspid closure, is the usual cause of abnormally wide splitting of the first heart sound. It is found in most cases of complete right bundle branch block, particularly when this is an isolated finding, and also when ventricular contraction is initiated by an ectopic or pacemaker impulse arising in the left ventricle.[12] Late tricuspid closure cannot always be heard, however, in complete right bundle branch block, and the echo shows that in these cases tricuspid closure is not delayed and produces only minor vibrations; presumably this indicates that the block is peripheral with slowing of the right ventricular upstroke rather than delay in onset.[20] Peripheral block seems more likely to be associated with advanced myocardial or conducting

tissue disease. In keeping with the division of right bundle branch block into proximal and peripheral block, depending on the timing of tricuspid closure, a loud late tricuspid closure sound is the almost invariable finding in Ebstein's anomaly[18] (Fig. 12-9), in which the right bundle is stunted and the peripheral branches fail to develop. In partial right bundle branch block, there may be slight delay of tricuspid closure; but when an electrocardiogram of similar pattern denotes hypertrophy, as in atrial septal defect, there is no delay of tricuspid closure and no abnormally wide splitting of the first heart sound.[27]

In left bundle branch block, abnormal splitting of the first heart sound is rare because there is usually no delay in onset of mitral closure and the block seems to be at arborization level in most cases.[12] High left atrial pressure, as in mitral stenosis or myxoma, may cause reversed splitting of the first sound, with tricuspid closure preceding the greatly

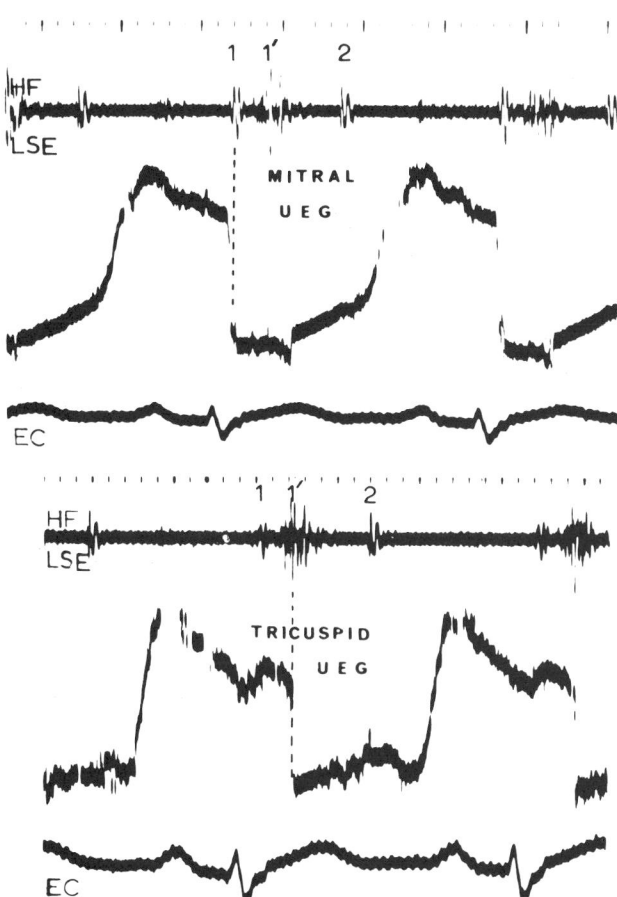

FIGURE 12-9 Ebstein's anomaly of the tricuspid valve with right bundle branch block. The first component of the first sound (1) coincides with the ultrasonic deflection from mitral valve closure [mitral ultrasound echocardiogram (UEG)]. The second component of the first sound (1) is abnormally loud and coincides with the ultrasonic deflection from tricuspid valve closure (tricuspid UEG).

delayed mitral closure, which is also extremely loud (see below).

In patients with pacemakers, we were puzzled by the frequent finding of a high-frequency sound preceding not only the first sound but also the ventricular pressure pulse. On investigation it was found to be due to contraction of chest wall skeletal muscle, which has a shorter electromechanical interval than cardiac muscle.[21]

Intensity of the First Heart Sound

The intensity of the mitral and tricuspid valve closure sound depend on several factors:

1. Adequacy of atrioventricular cusps to halt ventricular flow.
2. Mobility of cusps.
3. Position of cusps and rate of ventricular contraction.

Regurgitation has to be very severe for deficiency of cusp tissue to fail to cause an abrupt halt of closing cusps with ventricular contraction. Fibrosis or calcification of the mitral valve cusps is a much more

common cause of a faint first heart sound (and absent opening snap) and may produce difficulty in the diagnosis of mitral stenosis, which is invariably present under these conditions and would be expected to cause a loud first sound.

The position of the atrioventricular cusps, whether wide open or semiclosed, has long been known to be the most important factor responsible for the intensity of the first heart sound.[22–25] The distance of travel of flimsy cusps with little mass did not seem to be an adequate explanation; but it has recently been shown that the variable delay in closure, depending on the distance of travel, is the basic underlying factor.[26] A valve which is semiclosed at the end of diastole will come to its final halt at the very beginning of the left ventricular pressure pulse when the rate of rise is slow; the resulting sound is soft. A valve that is wide open at the end of diastole takes longer to come to its final halt, which occurs on a later and steeper part of the left ventricular pressure pulse; the resulting sound is loud.

The loudest first heart sounds are found with mitral stenosis (and mobile left atrial myxoma). Delay of mitral valve closure has been known since the beginnings of phonocardiography to be due to the longer time required for the rising of left ventricular pressure pulse to exceed the elevated left atrial pressure.[28] It is only recently, with the advent of high-speed echophonocardiography, that it has been shown that the same principle of the relation between the halt and the ventricular pressure pulse accounts for nearly all variations in intensity of the first heart sound.[26] Echocardiography has shown that when the left atrial contraction precedes ventricular contraction by a moderate or long interval (PR interval > 0.16 s), the mitral valve has not only been reopened at the end of diastole but eddies from ventricular filling have almost completely closed the valve so that its final halt occurs at the very beginning of the left ventricular pressure pulse at a low rate of pressure change and generates a soft sound. With shorter PR intervals, the valve is still wide open from the closely preceding atrial contraction; it therefore takes longer to reach its final halt position, which then occurs later at a more steeply rising part of the left ventricular pressure pulse, so the greater rate of pressure change generates a loud sound. Other causes of a wide-open valve at the end of diastole and consequently a loud first sound are high-output states, left-to-right shunts, and tachycardia, which shortens ventricular filling time.

With shunts, either the mitral or the tricuspid valve may be selectively affected; so, for example, a loud tricuspid component of the first heart sound is the rule in atrial septal defect.[27] It is also possible that the condition of the ventricular wall plays a part in the intensity of the first sound. In aortic stenosis, the first sound tends to be faint for a given PR interval; perhaps atrial contraction is unusually effective in closing the mitral valve because of its increased force of contraction in the face of inelastic ventricle.

The Second Heart Sound

The physiological asynchrony of the left and right ventricles becomes even more important with the second heart sound. Separation of its aortic (A_2) and pulmonary (P_2) components is the key to auscultation of the heart. Once A_2 and P_2 have been found, their intensities can be compared, nearby sounds and murmurs can be identified, the duration of right and left ventricular systole in the same heart cycle can be compared, and an estimate can be made of the effect of respiration on the loading of right and left ventricles.

Normal splitting of the second heart sound in the pulmonary area, well known to Potain (Fig. 12-10),[29] is confined to the height of the inspiratory phase of free respiration, when it may be very wide (e.g., 0.10 s). It is more difficult and usually impossible to detect two distinct components in the expiratory phase of continuous respiration when the subject is examined in the semiupright position (30 to 40° from the horizontal, Fig. 12-11). Simultaneous phonocardiograms from the pulmonary and mitral areas and a carotid pulse tracing were used to identify the two components of the second sound, and it was found that aortic normally precedes pulmonary closure (Fig. 12-11).

A_2 is much the louder sound, being heard in all areas; it usually exceeds the pulmonary component in intensity even in the pulmonary area, and is normally the only component of the second sound transmitted to the mitral area. P_2 is much softer and normally is confined to the pulmonary area and nearby, though often heard at the aortic area and lower left sternal edge.

Transmission of P_2 to the apex is usually abnormal in adults. Fusion or close splitting of the second sound in the expiratory phase of continued respiration *almost* excludes right-sided lesions, such as atrial septal defect and pulmonic stenosis, and thus has great practical importance in the examination of children referred because of a systolic murmur. If there is doubt about too obvious splitting of the second sound in expiration, the splitting will disappear in almost all normal subjects in the semi-

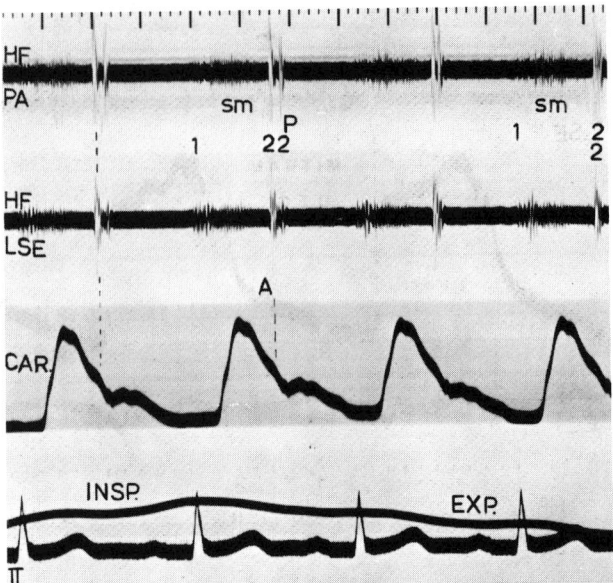

FIGURE 12-11 Physiological splitting of the second sound during inspiration, with A_2 preceding P_2, as shown by simultaneous indirect carotid tracing and high-frequency phonocardiograms from the pulmonary area and lower left sternal edge. During the expiratory phase of continuous respiration the two components are normally fused completely or nearly completely in the semiupright posture. A_2 is louder than P_2 even in the pulmonary area. P_2 is seen to be fainter than A_2 at the lower left sternal edge, and is not normally transmitted to the apex. (*From Leatham.*[11] *Reproduced with permission.*)

upright position (about 40° from the horizontal), especially when respiration becomes a little slower and deeper; splitting may persist, however, in normal subjects during expiration in the recumbent position, because of increased venous return, or during held expiration. There are a few normal subjects, however, with obvious expiratory splitting of the second sound (normal inspiratory increase) and unusually wide splitting of the first sound, suggesting delay in contraction of the right ventricle, yet with a normal electrocardiogram. When catheterization was performed in two patients to exclude atrial septal defect, a delayed onset of the right ventricular pressure pulse was found. In a few other normal subjects, unusually wide splitting of the first and second sounds appeared to be associated with a depressed sternum, but this was probably simply due to increased audibility of sounds from proximity.

The variations in splitting of the second sound are probably caused by ventricular increase in stroke volume causing delay in valve closure. During inspiration, blood is drawn by the negative pressure in the chest into the right side of the heart from the extrathoracic venous reservoir, but not immediately into the left side where the venous reservoir is intrathoracic. The splitting during inspiration has been thought to be caused mainly by the inspiratory increase in stroke volume of the right ventricle with consequent delay in pulmonary closure.[11,16,30] How-

FIGURE 12-10 Potain's diagram showing normal inspiratory splitting of the second sound during "free" respiration.

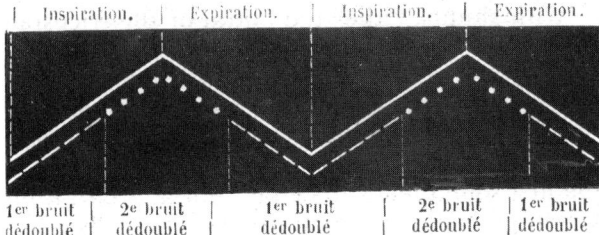

ever, aortic closure also moves with respiration,[31] though only slightly (35 percent of total movement).[32] It must be appreciated that the immediate inspiratory increase in stroke volume of the right ventricle is followed after 1 to 3 s by a similar increase in stroke volume of the left ventricle, and that it is necessary to study the effect of inspiration after a period of apnea to prevent superimposition of one respiratory cycle on another.[33] This concept was applied to the second heart sound in adult subjects by Shafter,[34] and similar results have been produced in children.[35] Following halted respiration, inspiration has no effect on A_2, but causes an immediate delay in P_2 because of increased stroke volume of the right ventricle as blood is drawn from the extrathoracic venous reservoir; 1 to 3 s later, there is a delay in A_2 as the inspiratory increase in stroke volume reaches the left ventricle (Fig. 12-12). At normal respiratory rates, diminished stroke volume of the left ventricle with earlier A_2 coincides with the inspiratory increase in stroke volume of the right ventricle and later P_2 (wide split). Increased stroke volume of the left ventricle and later A_2 coincides with the expiratory diminution in stroke volume of the right ventricle and earlier P_2 (narrow split or fusion). It should be mentioned, however, that changes in capacitance of the pulmonary vascular tree with respiration have also been suggested as the cause of variations in splitting of the second heart sound.

Thus, we are testing first the ability of the right ventricle to increase its stroke volume; provided that the right ventricle achieves this, we are then testing the function of the left ventricle in the same way. To enable the individual variations in stroke volume of the two ventricles to take place, the interatrial septum must be intact.

It follows that fixed splitting of the second heart sound may be due either to inability of the right ventricle to vary its stroke volume, causing a constant duration of systole (Fig. 12-13), or to approximately equal inspiratory delay of A_2 and P_2, indicating that the two ventricles share a common

FIGURE 12-12 Mechanism of normal splitting of the second sound.

<u>Halted respiration</u>

<u>Inspiration</u>

1) <u>Immediate</u> increase in stroke volume of R. V. - delay in P2

2) <u>Later</u> increase in stroke volume of L. V., delay in A2, diminishing stroke volume of R. V. - earlier P2.
At normal respiratory rates this coincides with expiration.

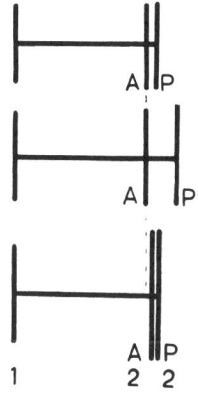

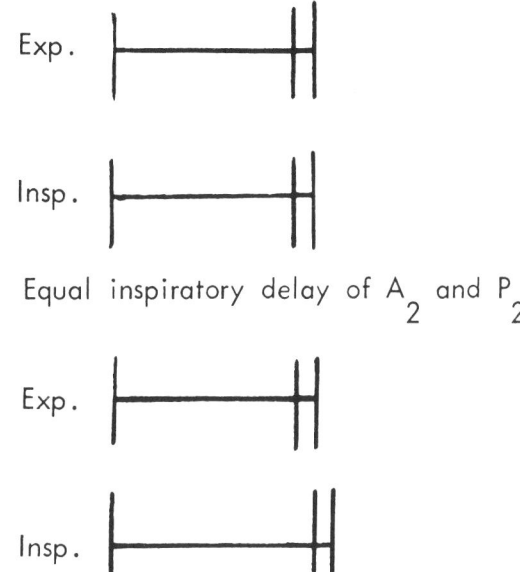

Right ventricle unable to increase stroke vol.

Exp.

Insp.

Equal inspiratory delay of A_2 and P_2

Exp.

Insp.

FIGURE 12-13 Fixed splitting of second sound.

venous reservoir (Fig. 12-13). Right ventricular failure or disease may produce true fixed splitting of the second sound. Inability of the right ventricle to vary its stroke volume means that a constant flow reaches the left ventricle, which will not therefore vary its stroke volume either, even if it has normal function. In right ventricular failure, fixed splitting of the second sound is often obvious, particularly as P_2 may be a little late. It was puzzling that in constrictive pericarditis, with its fixed ventricular capacity, inspiratory splitting of the second sound appeared to be retained, but it has now been shown[36] that although P_2 is fixed, A_2 becomes earlier on inspiration (Fig. 12-14), fitting in with the known in-

FIGURE 12-14 Constrictive pericarditis. Splitting of the second sound increases on inspiration, but the mechanism is abnormal, since it is caused by inspiratory shortening of left ventricular systole $(1 - A_2)$. Right ventricular systole $(1 - P_2)$ remains constant.

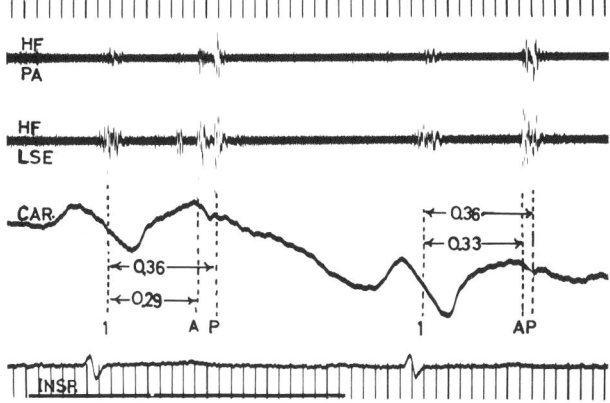

spiratory diminution in left ventricular stroke volume with pericardial constriction.

In atrial septal defect, either with normal or with high pulmonary vascular resistance (including an Eisenmenger's reaction), the fixed or nearly fixed splitting of the second sound is a highly valuable physical sign (Figs. 12-13, 12-15, and 12-16). The key point is that aortic closure usually delays *immediately* with inspiration,[34] simultaneously with the normal delay of pulmonary closure; this indicates that the stroke volume of the left ventricle is increasing at the same time as the right, either because of a transient right-to-left shunt or because of lessening of the left-to-right shunt at that moment. With anomalous venous return and an intact interatrial septum, one would not expect fixed splitting from simultaneous inspiratory delay of A_2 and P_2; in the rare patients who have been studied, no such fixed splitting has been found. Thus, with the relatively common sinus venosus type of defect, in which the interatrial communication is small, there is usually some respiratory variation in splitting of the second sound.[34] With interventricular communications it is only with very large defects or a single ventricle, always with extreme pulmonary hypertension (Eisenmenger's syndrome), that both A_2 and P_2 delay immediately on inspiration,[37] thus accounting for the single second sound (Fig. 12-17). A complicating factor is that extreme increase in stroke volume may not allow further inspiratory delay.

Wide Splitting of Second Heart Sound

Splitting of the second sound which is too wide in the expiratory phase of phasic respiration to be physiological is usually due to delay in pulmonary closure from right-sided lesions or disease (Fig. 12-18). Identification of the two components is usually

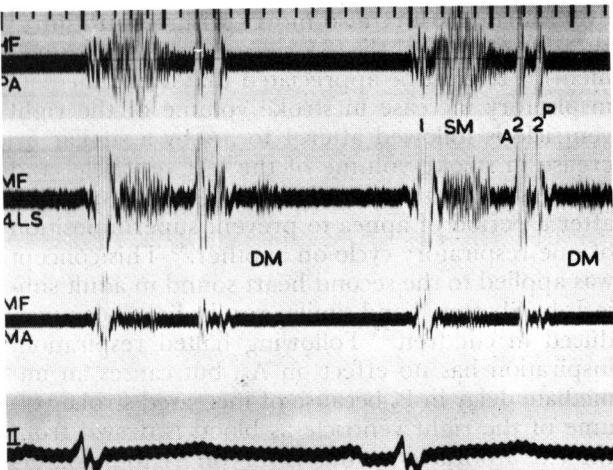

FIGURE 12-16 Atrial septal defect with left-to-right shunt (pulmonary artery pressure 22.6 mmHg). Despite the low PVR, P_2 is as loud as A_2 in the pulmonary area and is transmitted to the mitral area. (*From Leatham and Gray.*[27] *Reproduced with permission*).

easy, especially when respiratory variations are retained (i.e., when there is no right ventricular failure or atrial septal defect), for P_2 will be later on inspiration, increasing the splitting; in addition, P_2 is usually the fainter component and is usually not transmitted to the mitral area. In complete right bundle branch block, the electrical delay in activation of the right ventricle usually results in a late rise of the right ventricular pressure pulse, and the whole of

FIGURE 12-17 Pulmonary hypertension. Eisenmenger's ventricular septal defect. Complete fusion of A_2 and P_2 in expiration and inspiration (when A_2 and P_2 delay equally) is found only where there is a large ventricular septal defect or single ventricle *and* equal pulmonary and systemic vascular resistances.

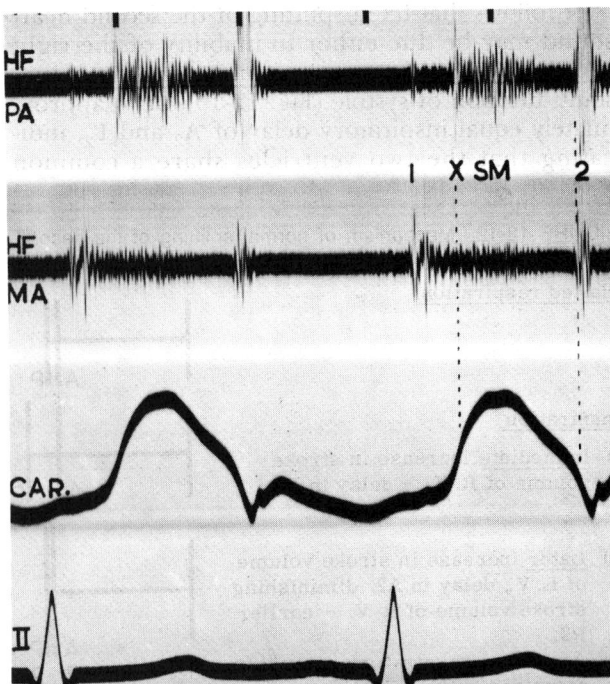

FIGURE 12-15 Atrial septal defect (normal low pulmonary vascular resistance). Wide splitting of the second sound due to delay of P_2 with little variation ("fixed split") throughout the respiratory cycle, shown by measurement from the onset of systole to be due to nearly equal delay of both A_2 and P_2 on inspiration. (*From Leatham and Gray.*[27] *Reproduced with permission.*)

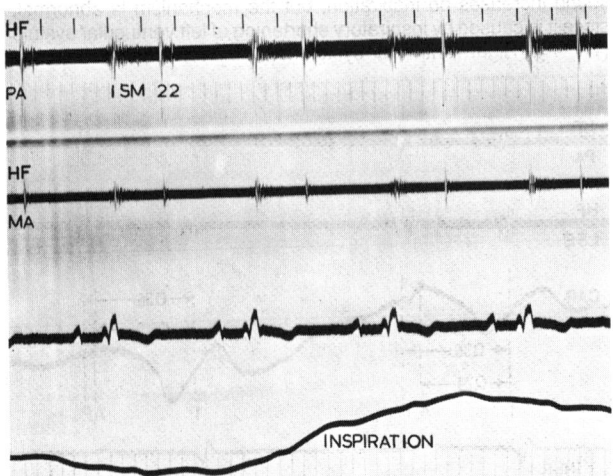

AUSCULTATION OF THE HEART

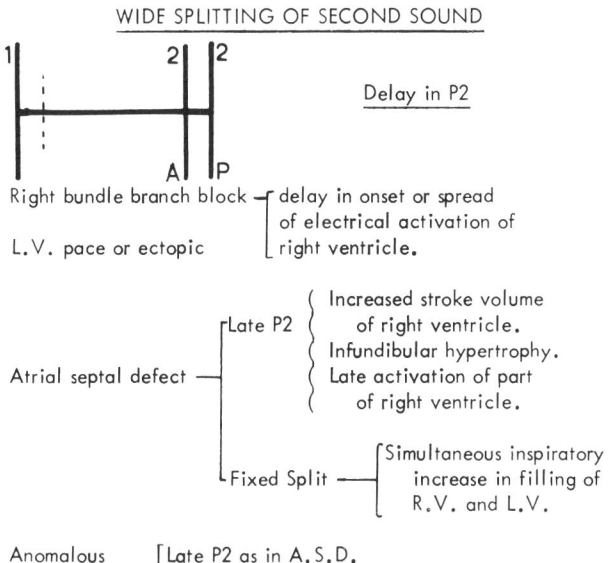

FIGURE 12-18 Right-sided heart abnormalities causing delay of P₂ and thus abnormally wide splitting of second sound.

right ventricular systole is late, resulting in late pulmonary closure. The normal respiratory variations can usually be detected, though sometimes with great difficulty, and a further clue to the diagnosis is usually given by the abnormally wide splitting of the first sound due to delayed tricuspid closure. Occasionally, in a subject who is normal or who has a small ventricular septal defect, abnormally wide splitting is a sign of right-sided electromechanical delay (prolonged Q-RV upstroke) without an electrocardiographic abnormality. In incomplete right bundle branch block accompanying right ventricular hypertrophy, there is usually no abnormality of the second (or the first) heart sound, and the Q-RV time is normal.

In atrial septal defect (Fig. 12-15), the abnormal behavior of the second sound with respiration has already been considered, but a second abnormality is delay in pulmonary closure. This is probably due in most cases to the large stroke volume of the right ventricle compared with the left, and there is a similar delay in P₂ with anomalous venous return. Following repair of an interatrial defect, respiratory variations in splitting appear at once; but in some cases delay in pulmonary closure persists for a time (without complete right bundle branch block), and there must be less easily reversible changes in the right ventricle to account for this.

In pulmonary valve stenosis with intact ventricular septum, the right ventricular pressure can rise above systemic level and achieve almost normal resting pulmonary flow and pressure. A faint and greatly delayed pulmonary closure sound can usually be heard and recorded at the pulmonary area,

except in some extremely severe cases. The earlier aortic closure sound is frequently drowned in the pulmonary systolic murmur but can be identified at the apex (Fig. 12-19). These findings are similar in pure infundibular stenosis (Fig. 12-20). In the presence of an associated right-to-left shunt through a ventricular septal defect (cyanotic tetralogy of Fallot), pulmonary flow and pressure are so greatly reduced that it is rare to hear or record pulmonary closure (Fig. 12-21)[38] (a useful point in identifying pure pulmonic stenosis with cyanosis due to a reversed interatrial shunt), though it may first appear in tetralogy of Fallot as a late sound following a Blalock operation or valvotomy (Fig. 12-22). In infants with tetralogy of Fallot, before or soon after the development of cyanosis, P₂ can often be heard and recorded,[39] especially in the reclining position. Indeed the late P₂ at the acyanotic stage in infancy may be the only way to differentiate this potentially fatal abnormality from a small and unimportant ventricular septal defect, since the electrocardiogram may be equivocal at this age. In so-called acyanotic tetralogy of Fallot (moderate pulmonic stenosis with ventricular septal defect), the pulmonary flow is not greatly reduced, and late P₂ can usually be heard and recorded, though it is notably absent in some cases. Thus, though pulmonary flow and pressures are probably the main factors in the production of an audible P₂, another factor, such as the relation of the pulmonary valve to the chest wall, may be important, for the outflow tract in tetralogy of Fallot is often directed posteriorly and the large aorta overlies it anteriorly, both to a variable degree. The valve anatomy may be a third factor. P₂ may also be audible in tetralogy of Fallot if the pressure

FIGURE 12-19 Isolated pulmonary valve stenosis (RVp., 100 mmHg—A₂ to P₂, 0.09 s). Because of prolongation of right ventricular ejection, compared with left, the pulmonary systolic murmur may drown A₂ in the pulmonary area, but stops before the greatly delayed P₂, which is usually audible or at least recordable. A₂ may be heard and recorded at the mitral area so that A₂ to P₂ interval can be measured and gives a surprisingly accurate assessment of the severity of the stenosis.

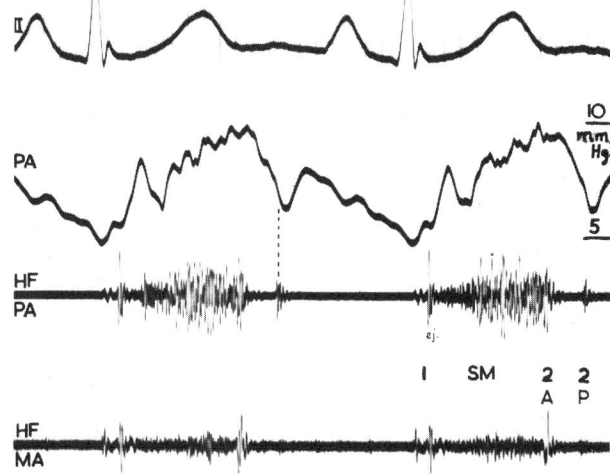

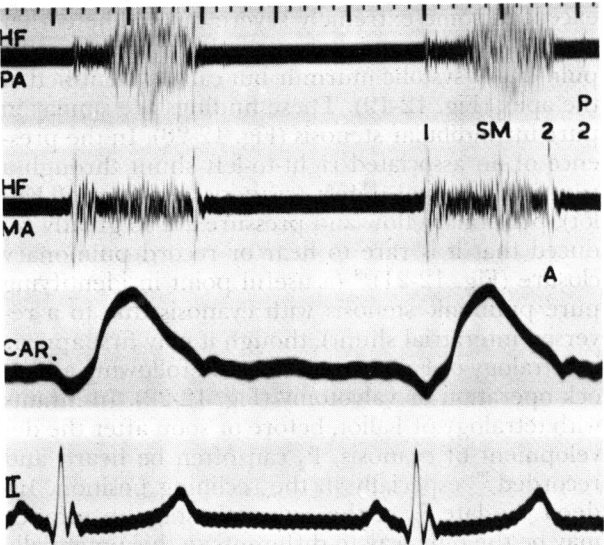

FIGURE 12-20 Isolated pulmonary infundibular stenosis. Prolongation of right ventricular systole and delay of P_2 (0.09 s after A_2), as with valve stenosis (but no ejection sound).

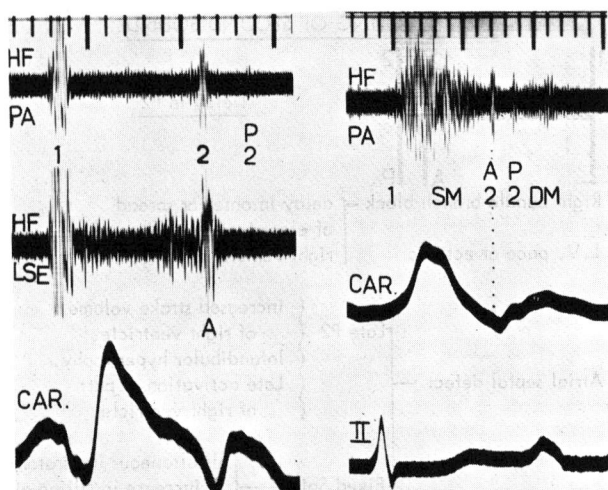

FIGURE 12-22 Tetralogy of Fallot. The delayed P_2 (0.1 s after A_2) appeared first after a successful Blalock operation, presumably because of an increase in pulmonary flow. Later a pulmonary valvotomy reduced the pressure gradient and P_2 became earlier. (*From Leatham and Weitzman.*[38] *Reproduced with permission.*)

in the main pulmonary artery is elevated by bilateral pulmonary artery branch stenosis, and it can sometimes be recorded if venous return is increased in the horizontal position. The width of splitting of the second sound (i.e., the delay of P_2 in relation to A_2 in the same heart cycle) is closely associated with the pressure difference across the valve and thus with the severity of the pulmonic stenosis (Fig. 12-23).[38] This may be particularly useful in children when

FIGURE 12-21 Severe pulmonic stenosis with ventricular septal defect and right-to-left shunt (tetralogy of Fallot), P_2 cannot be heard or recorded even with extra gain in channel 2 (+ voltage limitation distorting murmur).

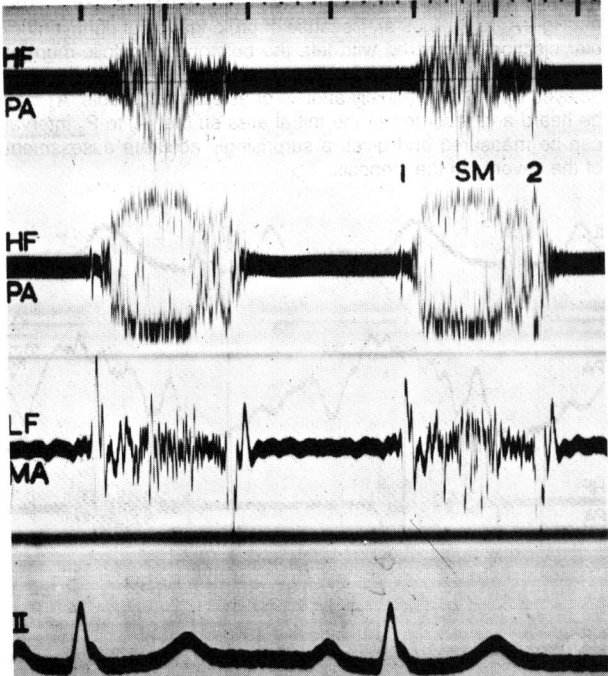

the electrocardiogram may be difficult to interpret; it also obviates the need for repeated catheterization when following the course of stenosis too mild for surgery or when judging the effect of surgery which should result in a return to a normal duration of right ventricular systole and physiological splitting. Some delay of P_2 is often found, however, with the very mild pressure differences associated with idiopathic dilatation of the pulmonary artery or minimal pulmonic stenosis, so that an elasticity factor has been invoked as another cause of delay.[40] In only one or two cases over the last 15 years has there been expiratory fusion of A_2 and P_2 with pulmonic stenosis, and the right ventricular pressure has always been less than 50 mmHg.

Though delay of P_2 compared with A_2 is frequent when there is right-sided heart failure with raised venous pressure and may be transient (e.g., with pulmonary embolism), it may occur with right ventricular disease without failure. A late P_2 may persist after successful pulmonary valvotomy (even with abolition of the gradient and no right bundle branch block, Fig. 12-24) and also after complete closure of an atrial septal defect, particularly when the shunt has been large and the patient is relatively old; presumably, persistence of a late P_2 in these cases is due to irreversible, or only slowly reversible, changes in the right ventricle or pulmonary vasculature.

Abnormally wide splitting of the second sound with the normal order of valve closure, A_2 before P_2, is sometimes due to left-sided abnormalities (Fig. 12-25). In left-to-right shunting ventricular septal defect, even when small, pulmonary closure is often abnormally late, though with normal respiratory variation; this appears to be mainly because of delayed activation of the right ventricle, even without delay on the electrocardiogram, and also because of shortening of the isovolumic time of the left ventri-

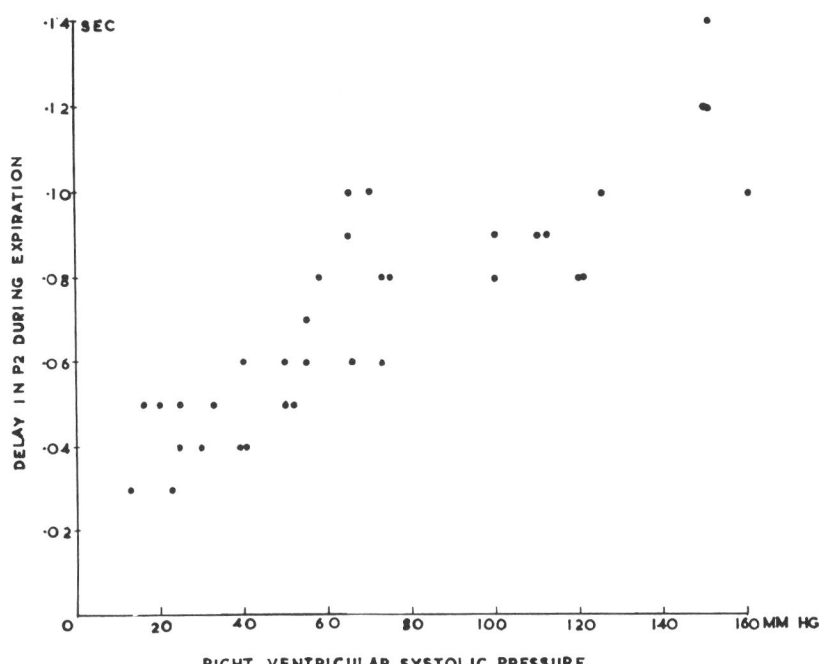

FIGURE 12-23 In pulmonic stenosis there is an approximate but useful correlation between the delay of P_2 (width of splitting) and the right ventricular systolic pressure. (*From Leatham and Weitzman.*[38] *Reproduced with permission.*)

cle from diastolic overloading. The loud pansystolic murmur may make it difficult to hear aortic closure, and an apparently single second sound (thought to be A_2) then raises the possibility of pulmonic stenosis; but a search around the pulmonary area and above it, using a rigid stethoscope diaphragm, is usually successful in picking up two components of the second sound in ventricular septal defect, even in very young infants, with insufficient splitting for the loud murmur to be due to pulmonic stenosis (Fig. 12-26). As mentioned earlier, a P_2 with only slight or moderate delay may be the only characteristic differentiating a harmless ventricular septal defect from early tetralogy of Fallot in an infant whose

only obvious physical sign is a loud systolic murmur. In mitral regurgitation, there is frequently wide splitting of the second sound (Fig. 12-27); this can be attributed to shortening of left ventricular ejection time resulting from the diminished resistance to left ventricular outflow,[41] a physical sign which may disappear when the left ventricle is more severely affected.

Reversed Splitting of Second Heart Sound

Delay in aortic closure sufficient to allow P_2 to precede A_2 results in reversed splitting of the second heart sound. The splitting will then be maximal on

FIGURE 12-24 Postpulmonary valvotomy. Two years after abolition of the pressure gradient, P_2 remains 0.08 s after A_2, presumably because of irreversible changes in the right ventricle. Preoperatively the patient had a greatly raised venous pressure.

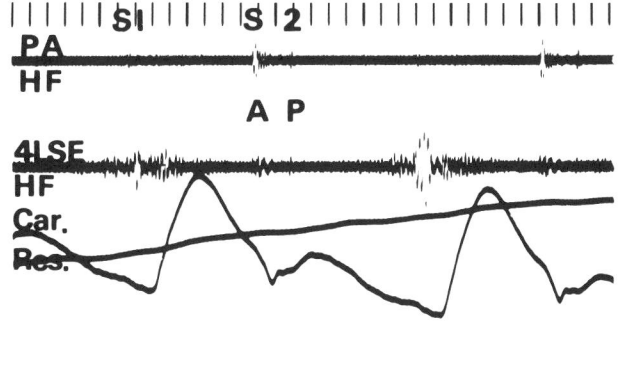

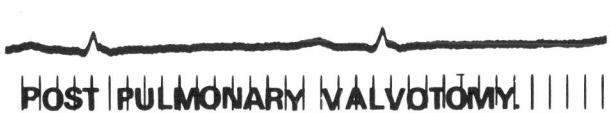

FIGURE 12-25 Left-sided heart abnormalities, causing early A_2 or late P_2 and thus abnormally wide splitting of second sound.

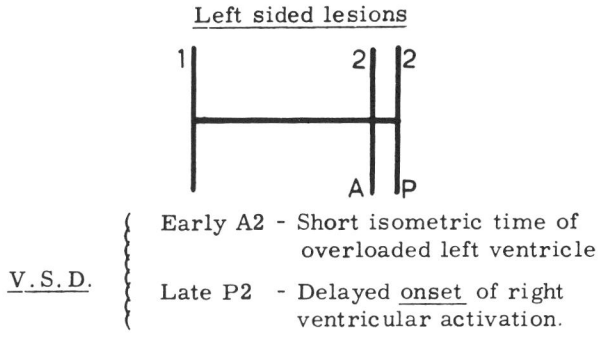

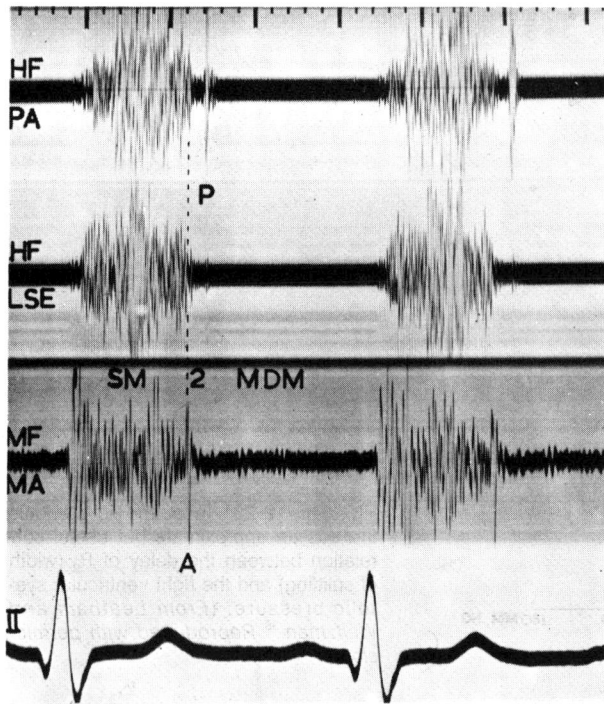

FIGURE 12-26 Ventricular septal defect with large left-to-right shunt. The loud pansystolic murmur tends to drown A_2 except at the mitral area, but the very wide splitting can usually be detected. P_2 is much louder than A_2 in the pulmonary area, and this was a useful indication of pulmonary hypertension, mainly hyperkinetic in this case (pulmonary artery systolic pressure 50, PVR 5 units). (*From Leatham.[56] Reproduced with permission.*)

REVERSED SPLITTING OF SECOND SOUND

(P_2 BEFORE A_2)

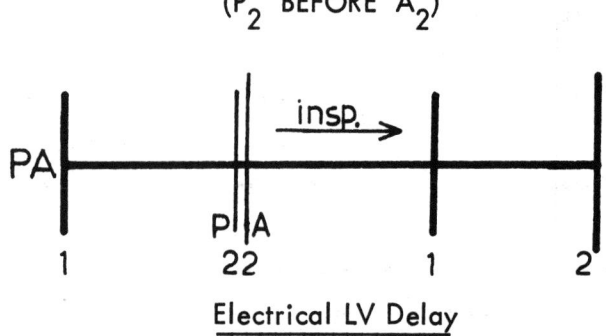

Electrical LV Delay

Lt. BBB – delayed spread of LV activation
WPW   – early RV activation
RV pace or ectopic

Mechanical LV Delay

Aortic outflow stenosis
Aorto pulmonary shunt $\binom{+}{-}$
Systolic hypertension
LV failure or disease
LV ischaemia

FIGURE 12-28 Prolongation of left ventricular systole (or delay in onset of left ventricular systole) causes reversed splitting of the second sound, P_2 before A_2 in expiration. The inspiratory delay of P_2 will cause lessening of the split or fusion of A_2 and P_2 paradoxically, on inspiration.

expiration and disappear or lessen on inspiration, with delay of pulmonary closure (Fig. 12-28).[11,42]

The most common cause of obvious reversed splitting of the second sound is left-sided electrical delay from left bundle branch block; the width of splitting is in keeping with the width of the QRS

complex and may be very great. Identification of the reversed order of valve closure may be possible by judging intensity and distribution of each component, but often P_2 is as loud as A_2 because of pulmonary hypertension from left ventricular failure. The narrowing or disappearance of the split on

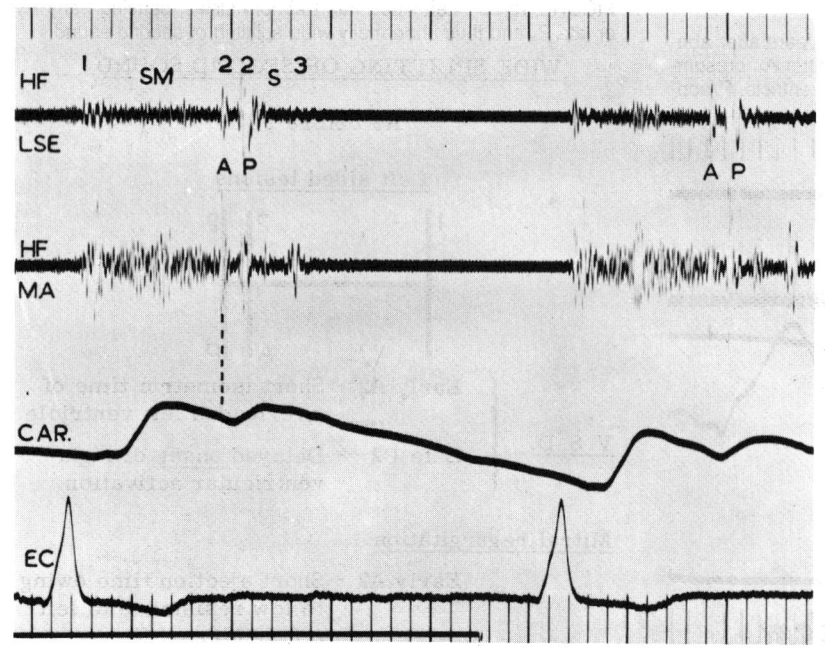

FIGURE 12-27 Mitral regurgitation. Abnormally wide splitting of second sound due to shortening of left ventricular ejection time from diminished resistance to left ventricular outflow, which is both into the aorta and into the left atrium.

inspiration is of much greater help in diagnosing reversed splitting by auscultation, but disappearance of a soft P_2 may be due to inspiratory insulation rather than to fusion with A_2. Lesser degrees of left-sided delay or preexcitation of the right ventricle (Wolff-Parkinson-White syndrome) may result in only slight precedence of P_2 in expiration (reversed split) but normal splitting (P_2 last) on inspiration (Fig. 12-29).

Delayed electrical activation of the left ventricle from a right ventricular ectopic beat or pacing usually causes reversed splitting of both first and second sounds as expected; but with right ventricular endocardial pacing, splitting is sometimes physiological, suggesting prior stimulation of left bundle fibers in the septum.

Mechanical prolongation of left ventricular systole, resulting in reversed splitting of the second sound, may be caused by obstruction to left ventricular outflow (Fig. 12-30). It may be difficult to distinguish the earlier pulmonary component because it may be drowned in the prolonged aortic ejection murmur, unless it is accentuated by pulmonary hypertension secondary to left ventricular failure. Furthermore, in calcific aortic stenosis, the aortic component may be inaudible. In the absence of bundle branch block and aortic stenosis, reversed splitting may be a sign of prolongation of left ventricular systole because of cardiac ischemia, nicely documented by Yurchak and Gorlin,[43] or because of myocardial disease. Unfortunately, reversed splitting also occurs not infrequently with unimportant systolic hypertension. Often in such cases the delay is slight and the splitting is reversed only on expiration, becoming physiological on inspiration, when P_2 is delayed.

Relative Intensity of A_2 and P_2 and Pulmonary Hypertension

Comparison of the intensity of the undivided second sound in various areas has little significance, since even in the pulmonary area, aortic closure usually contributes more than pulmonary closure, except in neonates.[44] Separation of the two components during respiration, however, allows a

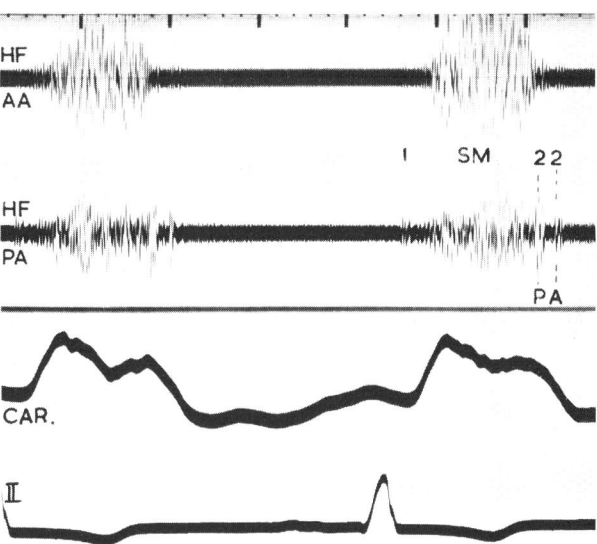

FIGURE 12-30   Aortic stenosis. Prolongation of left ventricular systole with delay in A_2, causing reversal of the normal order of valve closure. P_2, however, may be drowned in the murmur and difficult to hear unless accentuated from pulmonary hypertension secondary to left ventricular failure.

comparison to be made of their relative intensities. In the pulmonary area (second left space) of normal subjects, A_2 was never exceeded by P_2 in size on a high-frequency sound recording (resembling auscultation with a diaphragm stethoscope); and A_2 equaled P_2 in only 3 of 162 normal subjects, and these 3 subjects were all less than 20 years old.[45] P_2 is so much the lesser component that transmission to the mitral area was found in only 9 of the 162 normal subjects, and these 9 subjects were all less than 20 years old also. Thus, splitting of the second sound at the mitral area should immediately suggest that P_2 is abnormally loud.

In atrial septal defect with normal pulmonary arterial pressure, P_2 is abnormally loud; it equals or exceeds A_2 in the pulmonary area in most patients and is transmitted to the mitral area in about half of them (Fig. 12-16).[37] In normotensive atrial septal defect, the increased intensity and wide transmission of P_2—easily heard because of the wide "fixed" splitting—may be a function of the sharp pulmonary arterial pulse, because of the abnormally low pulmonary vascular resistance; an additional factor is probably the dilated right ventricle reaching to the apex.

Concerning pulmonary hypertension, lip service is still being paid to "accentuation of the second sound in the pulmonary area" by those who do not understand the large contribution of A_2 to this sound. Occasionally, however, when splitting cannot be detected, one has to fall back on this sign, which may be cautiously interpreted as suggesting pulmonary hypertension if the second sound is sufficiently intense to be palpated selectively in the pulmonary area. The widespread idea that splitting of

FIGURE 12-29   Wolff-Parkinson-White preexcitation of the right ventricle with left bundle branch block pattern in the left chest leads, causing reversed splitting of the second sound. P_2 slightly before A_2 in expiration, but physiologic splitting. A_2 before P_2 on inspiration owing to delay of P_2.

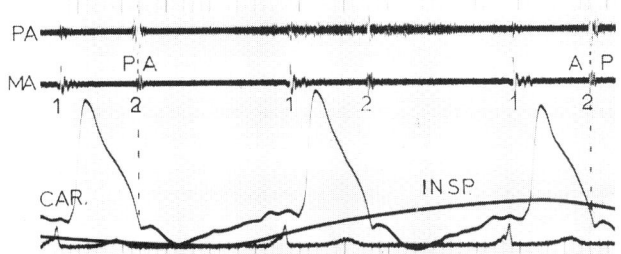

the second sound disappears in pulmonary hypertension is incorrect; this splitting disappears only in patients with a large ventricular septal defect or a single ventricle who have equal pulmonary and systemic vascular resistance and bidirectional shunt and in whom the left and right ventricles have been undertaking the same work for years and function as a single chamber. It was found that A_2 and P_2 fused together delayed equally on inspiration.[37] Otherwise, in pulmonary hypertension, the second sound splits normally on inspiration. In the pulmonary area, however, it may be difficult to detect a relatively soft A_2 preceding a very loud P_2, but in the mitral area the two components are often similar in size (Fig. 12-31) and can be heard more easily, which also indicates that P_2 is abnormally loud (as in atrial septal defect or pulmonary hypertension). However, wide splitting of the second sound, as in some normal subjects during deep inspiration, is rare with pulmonary hypertension, unless there is right ventricular failure. In contrast to the single second sound of Eisenmenger's ventricular septal defect, there is physiological splitting with Eisen-

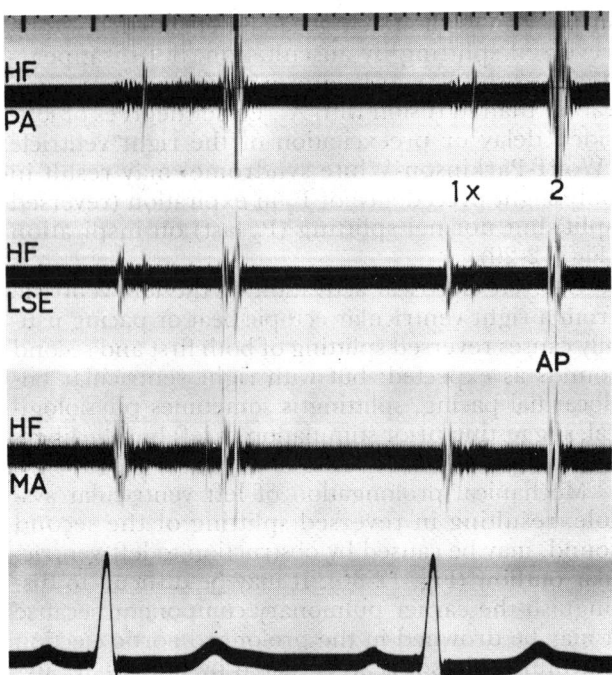

FIGURE 12-32 Pulmonary hypertension. Eisenmenger's atrial septal defect. There is wide fixed splitting of the second sound, with accentuation of P_2 as with left-to-right shunting atrial septal defect.

menger's patent ductus (Fig. 12-31), and wide fixed splitting with Eisenmenger's atrial septal defect (Fig. 12-32); these differences are often the only way of diagnosing the underlying defect in Eisenmenger's syndrome, as pointed out by Paul Wood in 1958 without the aid of phonocardiography.[46]

P_2 greater than A_2 in the pulmonary area, or transmitted to the mitral area, is a useful physical sign of pulmonary hypertension from mitral valve disease or from left-to-right shunting ventricular septal defect (Fig. 12-26), and of primary, embolic, or respiratory pulmonary hypertension. It is not a sign of pulmonary hypertension in atrial septal defect, in which pulmonary hypertension may be difficult to diagnose unless a delayed ejection sound is present. An abnormal A_2/P_2 ratio ($A_2 = P_2$ or $A_2 < P_2$) in the pulmonary area is more useful in the detection of pulmonary hypertension in mitral stenosis and ventricular septal defect than transmission of P_2 to the mitral area, which is surprisingly rare in these two situations.[37] In mitral regurgitation, P_2 may exceed A_2 in the pulmonary area without pulmonary hypertension, possibly because A_2 is reduced in intensity.

Single Second Heart Sound

A single second heart sound (Table 12-1) throughout the respiratory cycle is usually a result of the relatively faint pulmonary component being inaudible. Such inaudibility is rare in healthy children and young adults, and is uncommon even in older persons, under good auscultatory conditions, if a

FIGURE 12-31 Pulmonary hypertension. Eisenmenger's patent ductus arteriosus. Physiological splitting of second sound. P_2 is abnormally loud and dwarfs A_2 at the pulmonary area, causing difficulty in perception of the two components. The transmission of P_2 to the mitral area is also abnormal. The split can be detected more easily at the mitral area, where the two components are similar in size.

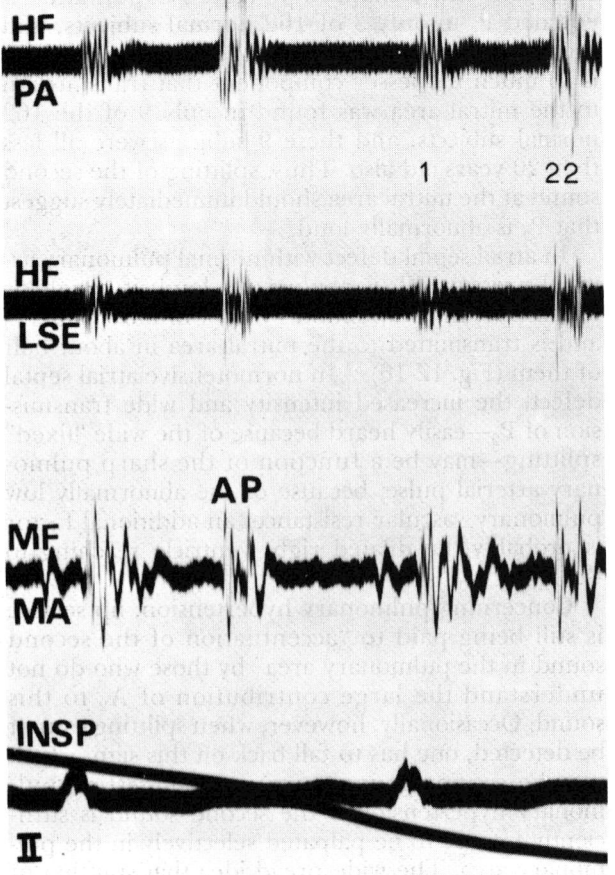

rigid stethoscope diaphragm is used. Respiration must be slow and adequate in depth, and the patient must remain relaxed while the search is made at and around the pulmonary area and lower left sternal edge. Hyperinflation, making the heart sounds distant, is perhaps the most common cause of inability to hear pulmonary closure, and a misdiagnosis of reversed splitting must be avoided when inspiratory insulation causes a soft P_2 to disappear. Separation of the components without the inspiratory loss of intensity may sometimes be achieved with increased venous return in the reclining position. Pulmonary closure is completely fused with aortic closure throughout the respiratory cycle only in Eisenmenger's syndrome, with a large ventricular septal defect or single ventricle. Otherwise, in pulmonary hypertension splitting is retained (even with a single ventricle if pulmonary vascular resistance is less than systemic), though it may be difficult to detect in the pulmonary area. With chronic right ventricular failure, the right ventricle is usually unable to increase its stroke volume with inspiration, and fusion of P_2 is abnormally late and easily detectable throughout the respiratory cycle. With constrictive pericarditis and fixed stroke volume of the right ventricle, inspiratory splitting can be detected because A_2 comes earlier. Drowning of the relatively early P_2 by a prolonged left-sided ejection murmur in patients with aortic stenosis has already been stressed (Fig. 12-30). Inaudibility of P_2 because of true diminution in intensity is relatively rare and suggests tetralogy of Fallot or pulmonary atresia. Even in neonates and infants, physiological splitting of the second sound can usually be detected by an experienced observer, and a single second sound should arouse suspicion if other signs suggest congenital heart disease.

TABLE 12-1 Single Second Heart Sound

1. P_2 *not detected* despite rigid stethoscope diaphragm, relaxation of subject, adequate respiration, search in many areas, reclining position of patient
   a. Because its intensity is diminished
      (1) Poor transmission (hyperinflation + inspiration)
      (2) Tetralogy of Fallot (severe) or pulmonary atresia, etc. (rarely pure pulmonic stenosis)
   b. Because it is synchronous with A_2
      (1) Eisenmenger's ventricular septal defect or single ventricle
   c. Because it is concealed by systolic murmur: aortic stenosis
2. A_2 *not detected*
   a. Because its intensity is diminished: calcific aortic stenosis
   b. Because it is synchronous with P_2
      (1) Eisenmenger's ventricular septal defect or single ventricle
   c. Because it is concealed by
      (1) Loud P_2 (in pulmonary area only) in pulmonary hypertension
      (2) Loud pansystolic murmur (mitral regurgitation and ventricular septal defect)
      (3) Loud prolonged ejection systolic murmur (pulmonic stenosis)

Failure to detect aortic closure in any area is much less common. In pulmonary hypertension, the fainter earlier sound (A_2) may be dwarfed and rendered inaudible by a greatly accentuated P_2 at the pulmonary area, and the splitting may then be easier to detect at the mitral area. Aortic closure may be drowned by a loud systolic murmur, but only at the site of maximum intensity of the murmur. Thus, in the pulmonary area, the loud prolonged ejection systolic murmur of pulmonary stenosis may drown an earlier A_2 which, however, is audible in the mitral area. In the mitral area, a loud regurgitant pansystolic murmur may drown A_2, but not at the base, where both A_2 and P_2 are clear and often widely separated. Finally, it is only with severe aortic stenosis (usually calcific) that A_2 may become truly inaudible.

Mistaken Diagnosis of Abnormal Splitting of Second Heart Sound

Very wide inspiratory separation of the two components can of course be found in many normal subjects at certain respiratory rates, but obvious splitting of the second sound (>0.02 s) in the expiratory phase of *continued* respiration in the semiupright position is most unusual in healthy patients, particularly when respiration is slow and deep. It is more common to make a misdiagnosis of abnormal *fixed* splitting of the second sound (Table 12-2). This is particularly likely in infants when a rapid respiratory rate causes less variation in right ventricular stroke volume. The addition of many ventricular ectopic beats may cause difficulty, particularly when irregularity from atrial fibrillation is added. Though the ear can easily detect the respiratory variations between a narrow and a wide split, a wide split increasing still further on inspiration (e.g., in isolated complete right bundle branch block) may be thought to be fixed. Finally, a late systolic click preceding A_2 and an opening snap following A_2 may be misdiagnosed as fixed splitting of the second sound, if inspiratory splitting (or at least slurring) of the second sound has been missed.

Auscultation of the heart should start with identification of aortic and pulmonary closure and their separation in relation to respiration. It is then possible to identify other sounds and relate murmurs to sounds, and make a comparison of the duration of systole of the right and left ventricles as a test of ventricular function and of an intact interatrial septum.

TABLE 12-2 Conditions Misdiagnosed as Fixed Split of Second Heart Sound

1. Rapid respiration in children, e.g., inspiration coinciding with alternate beats
2. Many ectopic beats
3. Wide split, e.g., right bundle branch block, especially if stroke volume is varying (atrial fibrillation)
4. Close opening snap or late systolic click

EXAMINATION OF THE HEART AND BLOOD VESSELS

The Normal Third Heart Sound and Gallops

W. Proctor Harvey, M.D., and
Antonio C. deLeon, Jr., M.D.

But the one which I propose to study at this moment presents itself with special characteristics that render it absolutely distinct, and upon which I will lay stress in a moment. You will comprehend, gentlemen, why I decide to reserve exclusively for it such an expressive name created by my venerable master, Professor Bouillaud. This denomination adapts itself marvelously to the sound which it designates and it should be singularly useful in distinguishing a category of facts which are very particular and quite worthy, as you shall see, of a special designation. Besides, it is this very variety which M. Bouillaud already imparted to us in applying to it this name bruit de galop [gallop rhythm].

This is the way the rhythm of which I speak to you now is constituted. One distinguishes therein three sounds, namely: two normal sounds of the heart and a super added sound. Most often the two normal sounds conserve their usual characteristics without any modification. The first, in particular, keeps its usual relationships with the apex thrust and with the arterial pulse. As to the abnormal sound, it takes place immediately before it, preceding it by a rather short interval sometimes; always notably longer, however, than that which separates the two parts of a reduplicated sound; in general, and almost always significantly shorter than the short silence. This sound is dull, much more so than the normal sound. It is a shock, a perceptible elevation; it is hardly a sound. If one applies the ear to the chest it is affected by a tactile sensation, perhaps more so than an auditory one. And, if one attempts to hear it with a flexible stethoscope little is lacking, almost always, of its disappearing entirely. The point at which it is best perceived is a little above the apex of the heart, verging somewhat towards the right. But one can sometimes distinguish it over the entire precordial region.

An elevation felt by the hand usually coincides with this sound and this, as you shall presently see, may be also clearly indicated by registering instruments. The heave is felt above all toward the middle of the precordial region and a little below; but it is vague, extensive, and does not at all resemble the clear and well delineated impulse of the apex which ordinarily accompanies the first sound.

In addition to the two normal sounds, this bruit completes the triple rhythm of the heart. It thus produces a rhythm of three sounds unequally distinct, and occasionally unequally distant, a rhythm which the ear seizes with extreme facility, provided that it had once perceived it distinctly. This is the bruit de galop.

Pierre C. Potain, 1875[47]

Ventricular Filling Sounds

The ventricular filling sounds may occur in either or both ventricles. They include the atrial (S_4) gallop sound; the ventricular (S_3) gallop sound; the summation gallop sound; and the normal physiological third heart sound. Most commonly these sounds originate in the left ventricle, but when the total evaluation of the patient is considered, right-sided filling sounds (gallops) may be properly identified. A helpful clue is the fact that the right-sided filling sounds of the right ventricle may selectively increase with inspiration.

The mechanism of production of these filling sounds is probably related to the cessation of filling of blood from the atria to the ventricles, probably resulting in distension and vibrations of the ventricular wall, papillary muscles, and chordae. The valves apparently are not implicated in production of these low-frequency sounds since the echocardiogram does not show specific valvular movement at this time. As a rule, these are low-frequency vibrations producing the sounds that we detect with our stethoscope. One should use the bell of the stethoscope (barely making an air seal with the skin) and listen over a very localized spot in order to hear these important sounds. The filling sounds of the left ventricle (atrial S_4) and ventricular (S_3) gallops (physiological third heart sounds) can best be heard by placing the bell of the stethoscope on the apical impulse.

The physician can usually palpate these filling sounds with the examining fingers. It is often said that these sounds (vibrations) can be felt (and sometimes seen) better than they can be heard. If one listens carefully and specifically for the filling sounds, however, they will generally be heard.

The ventricular filling sounds are sometimes picked up by the phonocardiogram, since the low-frequency vibrations can be accentuated to such an extent that the phonocardiogram records what the human ear cannot hear. It is important to remember, however, that the audible and palpable sounds have more clinical relevance than do inaudible sounds recorded on the phonocardiogram.

Gallop Rhythm

The term *gallop rhythm* describes an auscultatory phenomenon in which a tripling or quadrupling of heart sounds resembles the canter of a horse. Almost a century ago, Potain presented to the Medical Society of the Hospital of Paris a paper entitled "Du rhythme cardiaque appelé bruit de galop."[47] (See quotation at the beginning of this section.) In this paper he acknowledged that his professor Bouillaud was the one who gave this rhythm the name by which it is still known today.

Although gallop rhythm was described 100 years ago, the great majority of gallops go unrecognized, are misinterpreted, or are considered unimportant. This is unfortunate because a gallop sound, depending on the type, is often one of the earliest clinical clues to heart disease and affords valuable bedside information concerning diagnosis, prognosis, and treatment.[48,49] Gallops are diastolic events and appear to be related to two periods of filling of the ventricles: the rapid-filling phase (the ventricular diastolic gallop) and the presystolic filling phase related to atrial systole (atrial gallop). Since gallops are diastolic sounds, extra sounds occurring in the heart cycle must therefore be separated into being systolic or diastolic events. In the past a sound occurring in systole was often referred to as a *systolic gallop*. It is wise to abandon this label in favor of more descriptive terminology, such as systolic sound, ejection sound, or systolic click. Thus, the application of the term *gallop rhythm* is restricted to diastolic events. Whether extra sounds are systolic or diastolic is readily determined by a simple technique known as *inching* (Fig. 12-33).[48,49] The stethoscope is moved, or "inched," from the aortic area of the heart to the apex, and at the same time attention is focused on the second heart sound. If the extra sound is noted to occur in systole before the second heart sound, it is obviously a systolic sound.

FIGURE 12-33 The stethoscope is "inched" from the aortic area to the apex. The extra sound (C) is systolic and is louder at the apex.

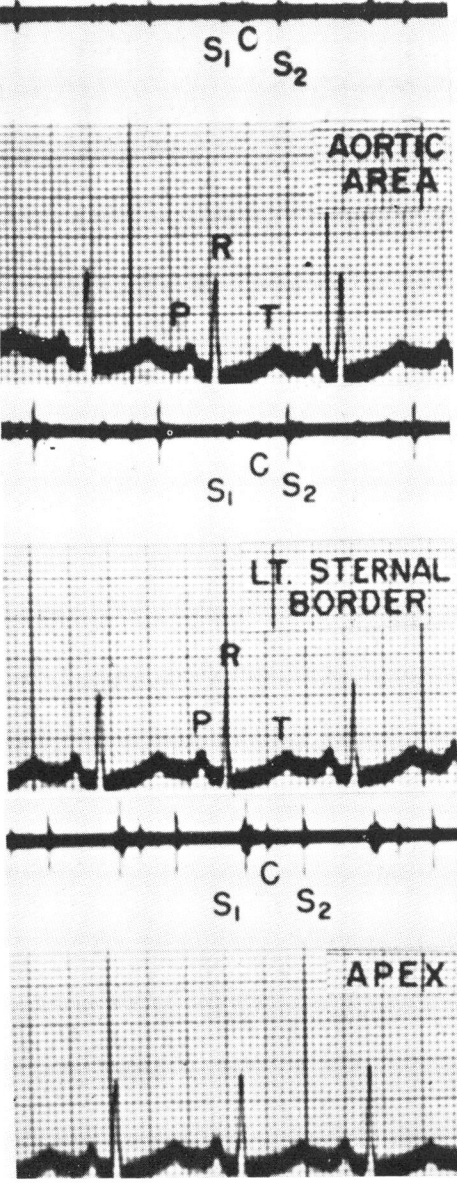

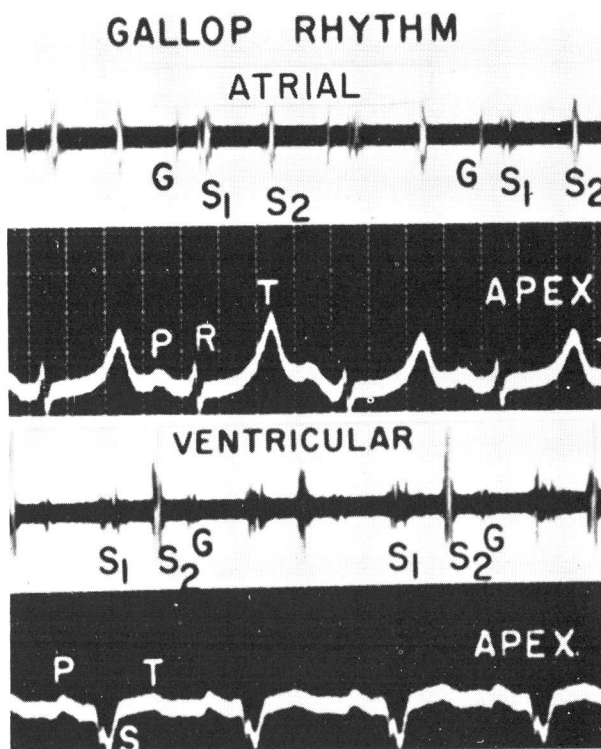

FIGURE 12-34 Gallops are diastolic sounds. The atrial gallop (G, upper tracing) is related to atrial systole. The ventricular gallop (G, lower tracing) occurs in early diastole at the end of rapid ventricular filling.

On the other hand, if the extra sound comes after the second sound or before the first heart sound, then it is in diastole and represents a diastolic event. Even with a heart rate more rapid than normal, the inching technique permits easy and accurate timing of this sound. Sounds occurring in diastole, then, are identified as to their timing and possible etiology.

Although both gallops are sounds resulting from filling of the ventricles, the atrial gallop, generally in presystole, is related to atrial contraction and can be identified on the phonocardiogram following the P wave of the electrocardiogram (Fig. 12-34). The atrial gallop is not present with atrial fibrillation since there is no atrial contraction. A ventricular diastolic gallop, on the other hand, occurs 0.14 to 0.16 s after the second heart sound (Fig. 12-34). Both atrial and ventricular diastolic gallops frequently occur in the same patient. When the two gallops occur in close proximity, low-frequency vibrations with duration may result in a diastolic rumble. Rarely both gallop sounds occur at the exact same time, producing what is known as a *summation gallop*. This summation gallop can be prominent, even at times louder than either the first or second sounds.

Atrial (S₄) Gallop[50]
An atrial (S_4) gallop sound (Fig. 12-35) is related to atrial contraction and may occur with or without any

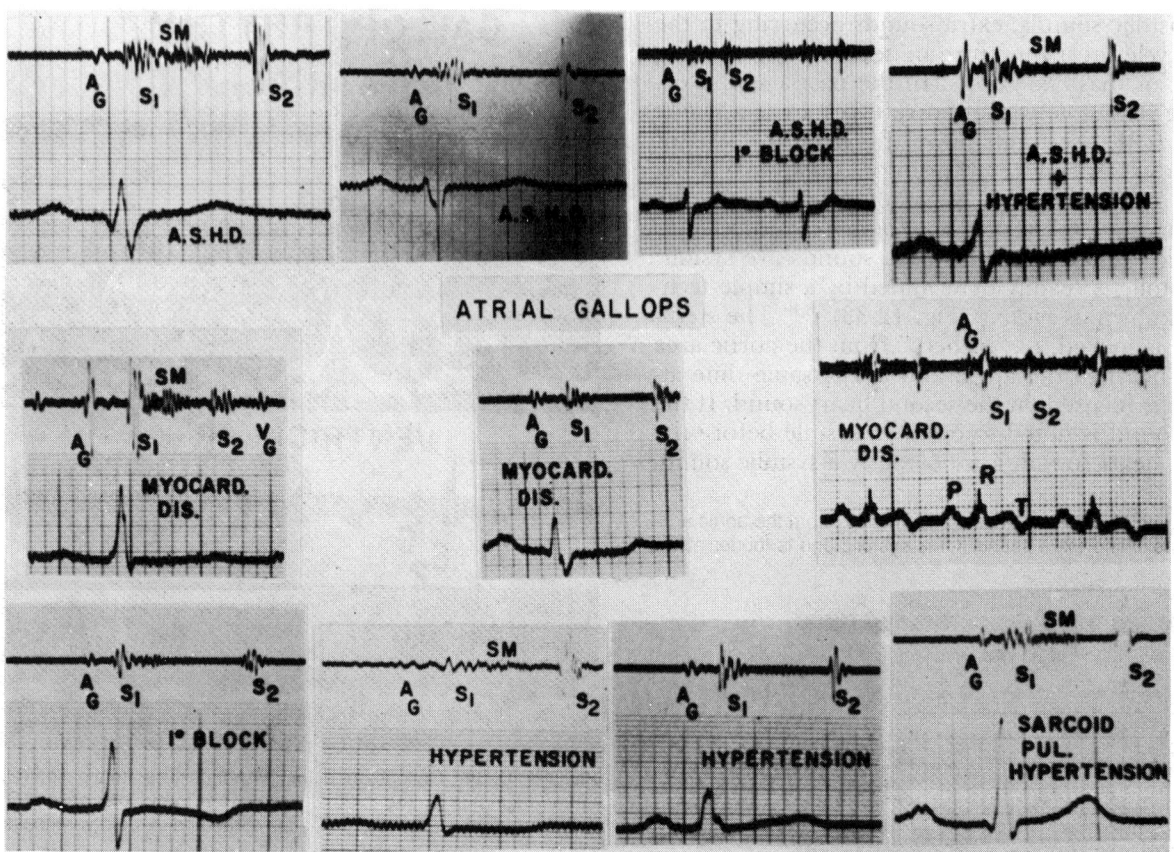

FIGURE 12-35   Composite of various atrial gallops which represent a common, although often overlooked, finding.

clinical evidence of cardiac decompensation. A left ventricular atrial gallop sound is heard at the apex and a right ventricular atrial gallop sound is heard over the right ventricle. The latter may be louder during inspiration. An atrial gallop sound (S_4) is a frequent finding in patients with cardiomyopathy (primary myocardial disease), coronary artery disease, hypertension (systemic and pulmonary), and with the more severe degrees of aortic and pulmonic stenosis. It can also occur when there is a delay in atrioventricular conduction (prolongation of the PR interval on the electrocardiogram) and, in addition, may be heard in some normal hearts. If one searches carefully for an atrial sound or gallop, it is most commonly heard in patients with coronary artery disease, and at times this may be one of the first clues from the physical examination as to the presence of underlying heart disease. It would be unusual not to hear a faint atrial gallop sound in a patient who has had a previous myocardial infarction. In a study of 107 patients with recently documented myocardial infarction, an atrial gallop was detected in 105 on clinical auscultation as well as on the phonocardiogram.[51] Of the two patients who did not have an atrial gallop, one had mitral stenosis in addition to myocardial infarction. The other patient had atrial infarction with extensive fibrosis of the left atrium documented at postmortem examination. In the same series of cases of acute myocardial infarction, an atrial gallop was present (i.e., noted clinically with the stethoscope and also documented on the phonocardiogram) in all of the 20 patients examined within an hour of admission to the hospital.

The atrial gallop sound associated with myocardial infarction may be easily heard, or it may be faint—more commonly, it is faint. The sound is often louder during an episode of acute myocardial ischemia and pain, or during the initial phases of myocardial infarction. Subsequently, usually with improvement of the patient, the gallop sound becomes fainter but, if carefully searched for, can generally be heard. It is worthy of emphasis, however, that special techniques are often necessary to "bring out" or detect a faint gallop. Listening at the point of maximum impulse of the left ventricle, with the patient turned to the left lateral position, is often necessary to adequately detect the gallop (Fig. 12-36). The gallop sound equivalent can also be palpated by the physician's examining fingers placed over the point of maximum impulse, again with the patient in the left lateral position. Careful inspection of the precordium with the naked eye, or observing the movements of a lightweight pencil, wooden stick, or broom straw held or taped over the point of maximum impulse, will also demonstrate the precordial movements which correlate with gallop sounds heard with the stethoscope.

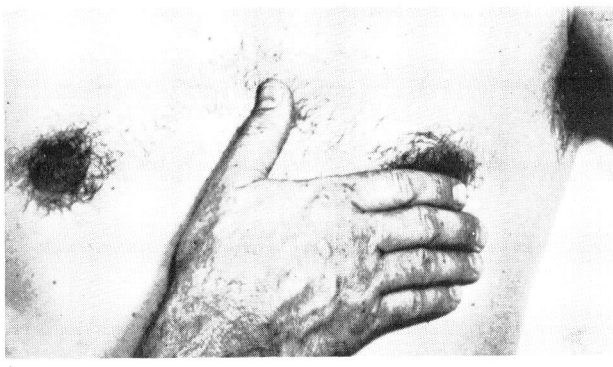

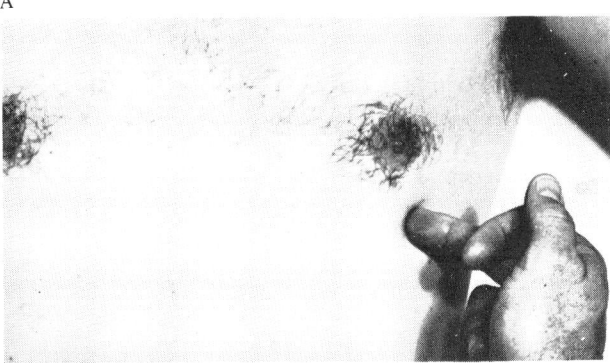

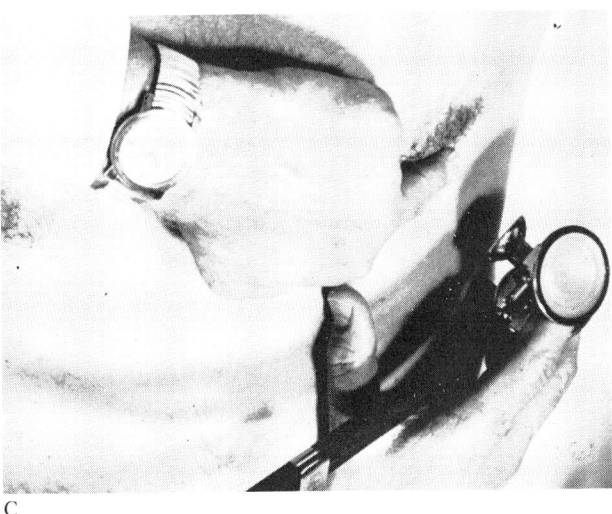

FIGURE 12-36 *A.* The patient is turned to the left lateral position, and the point of maximal impulse of the left ventricle is palpated by the physician's hand. *B.* The localized spot of the impulse is marked by a finger. *C.* The bell of the stethoscope is placed lightly over this localized area, barely making an air seal. This maneuver combines palpation and auscultation to permit better detection of faint gallops or diastolic rumbles.

An atrial gallop sound is heard in the majority of patients with cardiomyopathy who have normal sinus rhythm.[52] (Ventricular gallops are also frequent.) As a rule, the atrial gallop persists in patients with cardiomyopathy, although in some, with clinical improvement, the gallop may become faint and occasionally disappear. With the exacerbation of symptoms it generally becomes louder.

Atrial gallop sounds are common in patients with systemic arterial hypertension and are more likely to be a constant finding in a patient who has persistent blood pressure elevation. With sustained significant hypertension, an atrial gallop sound may be present for years even though there may be no evidence of heart failure.

Aortic stenosis, particularly in those patients having higher degrees of aortic valve obstruction, is associated with an atrial gallop sound. The results of the study indicated that an atrial gallop sound with aortic stenosis appeared to correlate with a systolic gradient of 70 mmHg or more and with a left ventricular end-diastolic pressure of 15 mmHg or more.[53] Personal observations, particularly in the older age group, indicate that an atrial sound may be misleading when one attempts to relate it to severity of aortic stenosis. Older patients may have an atrial gallop sound when there is a minimal or moderate aortic valve gradient, indicating that an additional myocardial disease factor, such as coronary artery disease, is obviously playing a significant role in the production of the atrial gallop. In a patient under 40 years of age, however, there seems to be a better clinical correlation of an atrial gallop sound with the severity of stenosis.[54]

A right ventricular atrial gallop sound may occur in patients with pulmonary valve obstruction.[8,9] The more severe the obstruction is, the more likely it is to be associated with an atrial gallop sound. Also, the atrial gallop sound is not unusual in patients with pulmonary hypertension from various causes, such as atrial septal defect, ventricular septal defect, patent ductus arteriosus, recurrent pulmonary emboli, and primary pulmonary hypertension. The atrial gallop sound appears, therefore, to be related to changes in the myocardium—either the left or the right ventricle, or both—in which there is a change in ventricular compliance and increased resistance to filling.

In addition, an atrial gallop sound may be heard when cardiac output and stroke volume are increased, as in some patients with thyrotoxicosis, anemia, and large arteriovenous fistulas. It is also a common finding in patients with first-, second-, or third-degree heart block.[2] Usually, an atrial gallop sound is not normally detected, since in patients with a normal PQ (PR) interval on the electrocardiogram [normal atrioventricular (AV) conduction], the atrial gallop sound occurs at an interval after atrial contraction (approximately 0.16 s after the beginning of the P wave of the electrocardiogram). Although a faint sound may normally be present, it is often not specifically identified or is merged with the first heart sound. When the PR interval is prolonged, i.e., 0.22 to 0.26 s, an atrial gallop sound is usually heard in addition to a faint first heart sound. (These two simple auscultatory findings provide the physician with an immediate bedside clue to first-degree heart block.) With second-degree block, the atrial gallop sound is easily heard. In patients with a constant 2:1 AV block, the atrial sound often occurs at the approximate timing of the normal third heart sound of ventricular diastole, resulting in a prominent sound in the early part of diastole. In complete heart block, in which there is AV dissociation, atrial gallop sounds are frequently heard. Careful auscultation in a quiet room is usually necessary to detect these sounds, which resemble faint footsteps on a carpet.

The importance of the atrial gallop sound is not sufficiently appreciated, and only in recent years has its value in assessing the various types of heart disease been realized.

Ventricular (S_3) Diastolic Gallop (Fig. 12-34)

The ventricular (S_3) diastolic gallop has clinical connotations different from those of the atrial (S_4) gallop.[48,49] It is frequently one of the first signs that one can detect indicating serious heart disease and/or cardiac decompensation. This gallop appears in the early part of diastole, later than the opening snap of mitral stenosis but at the same time as the normal physiological third heart sound heard in the young. If searched for, the ventricular diastolic gallop is a common finding and can appear in a great variety of diseased states of the heart, including those due to coronary disease; hypertensive, rheumatic, and congenital heart disease; cardiomyopathy; and others. A ventricular diastolic gallop is usually present in patients with cardiac decompensation. *In fact, it may be one of the earliest clinical findings of cardiac dysfunction.* The majority of these gallop sounds are faint, and because of this they are frequently overlooked.

Since most gallop sounds are faint, a special technique must be employed to detect them. The patient should be recumbent and examined in a quiet room. Closing the door that leads to the corridor of the hospital, closing windows, or turning off fans or the air conditioner may make the difference as to whether a gallop is heard or not. If one exerts normal pressure with the flat diaphragm of the stethoscope, the gallop, though present, may not be heard, or may be greatly diminished (Fig. 12-37). Very light pressure with the bell of the stethoscope is necessary to hear the low-frequency vibrations. Gallop sounds from the left ventricle are often best heard by having the patient turn to the left lateral position; the physician then listens at the point of maximum impulse in the apical area (this is similar to the maneuver that one uses when listening for the localized rumble of mitral stenosis) (Fig. 12-36). It is of great importance to use palpation first to detect this point of maximum impulse of the left ventricle after the patient has turned to the left lateral position. The stethoscope is then placed over this localized area, and the gallop sound is either heard for the first time or is accentuated in intensity. At times, however, a ventricular gallop sound is well heard along the lower left sternal border and apex and with the patient recumbent. This usually indicates the gallop sound originates in the right ventricle. Right ventricular (S_3) gallop sounds usually

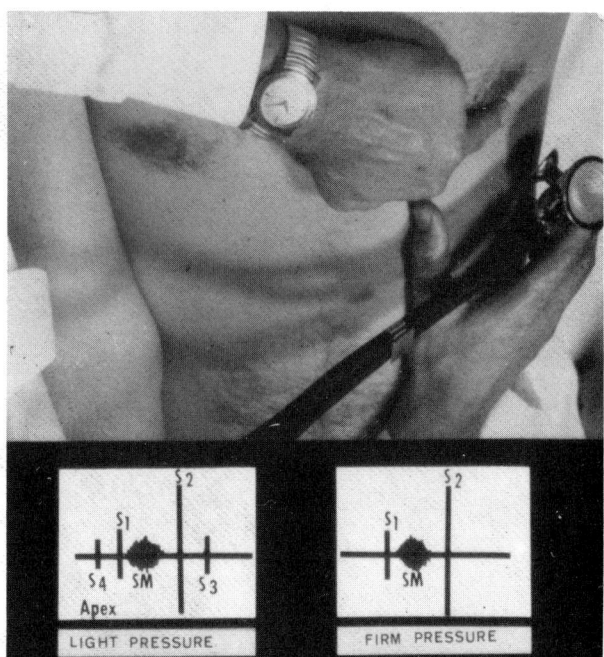

FIGURE 12-37 Note disappearance of S_3 and S_4 with firm pressure of stethoscope.

become louder with inspiration. Both atrial and ventricular gallops generally become fainter when the patient sits or stands. At times the gallop sounds are better heard after slight physical effort, and when the blood flow and heart rate are somewhat accelerated. Having the patient cough five or six times may bring out the faint gallop. Occasionally, a gallop sound is detected when one listens after the patient has had brief exertion, such as walking, climbing a flight of stairs, or performing a number of sit-ups on the examining table. The quality of sounds simulating a horse galloping is more likely to be noticed when the heart rate is increased. It should be emphasized, however, that a gallop occurring at a slow rate still has the same significance that it would have when heard at a faster rate.

Gallops frequently wax and wane with normal phases of respiration; this is particularly true of ventricular gallops. At times, instead of being detected with every heartbeat, they are heard with every third or fourth beat. If the patient has any degree of emphysema or increase in anteroposterior diameter of the chest, the gallop sound is damped. In such instances auscultation over the xiphoid process or just under the rib cage at the attachment of the diaphragm may be advantageous. The same gallop which is easily heard during sinus tachycardia (e.g., 100 to 120 beats per minute) may be poorly heard at a rate of 70 beats per minute, unless one mentally "tunes in" to this low-frequency sound and uses the above-described techniques.

When atrial and ventricular diastolic gallops occur in close proximity to each other, although not exactly simultaneously, a diastolic rumble can thereby be produced; this is not an uncommon finding in a patient with cardiomyopathy, or in others in whom myocardial dysfunction presents a problem. It is more common in patients with a sinus tachycardia, and the two gallop sounds merge closer together and may produce a diastolic rumble. This combination of low-pitched sounds may simulate the murmur of mitral stenosis. The authors have personally observed several patients referred for surgery of mitral stenosis who, instead, had cardiomyopathy with atrial and ventricular diastolic gallops producing a rumble.

Prognosis of Ventricular Diastolic Gallops To date, there has been no satisfactory study of life expectancy once a gallop sound is detected. Modern therapy has prolonged the life of cardiac patients, and in many earlier studies only the louder type of gallop was observed. As has been previously emphasized, the prognosis depends on the type of gallop present. It is obvious that the atrial diastolic gallop which occurs in the absence of cardiac decompensation does not carry as grave a prognosis as that associated with the ventricular diastolic gallop. In general, it appears that the average life expectancy after a persistent ventricular gallop has been found is approximately 4 to 5 years. There are, of course, individual variations, with some patients dying weeks or months later and still others living 10 years or longer. Some clinical points concerning gallops are worthy of discussion. The louder the gallop, the poorer the prognosis. The prognosis is worse if gallop rhythm persists despite adequate medical management. For example, it is relatively common to hear a ventricular diastolic gallop following acute myocardial infarction during the earlier stages. In the usual case, the gallop disappears in time (several days to several weeks). When it is particularly loud and persists months after the acute episode, however, it generally is associated with significant permanent heart damage and chronic cardiac decompensation, thus indicating a poorer prognosis. Another patient with an acute myocardial infarction may have a ventricular diastolic gallop during the acute phase, but subsequently no ventricular gallop or other signs of heart failure may be evident. This represents a temporary sign of heart failure with subsequent recovery, and indicates a better myocardial reserve. The prognosis in such an individual would then be related to other aspects of the underlying heart disease, rather than to congestive heart failure. It also appears that loud persistent gallops, together with slight sinus tachycardia, are additional evidence of serious heart failure, the elevation of heart rate being a further sign of compensatory mechanism for the cardiac dysfunction.

The faint ventricular gallop that has the better prognosis is the one which is detected as an early sign of congestive heart failure and which disappears after treatment for the failure. As a rule, such treatment needs to be continued. A ventricular diastolic gallop is frequently associated with a slight

pulsus alternans. On the other hand, the finding of a definite pulsus alternans is almost always associated with a ventricular diastolic gallop. Both these findings indicate a failing myocardium, and too little attention has been paid to them in the past. In addition, alternation of the intensity of heart sounds and/or murmurs is frequent when a ventricular diastolic gallop and pulsus alternans are present. Nearly all these findings are clues indicating some degree of cardiac decompensation. The patient may have a gallop rhythm and concomitant extrasystoles. For a few beats following the extrasystoles, the intensity of the gallop sound is often accentuated. This is known as *postextrasystolic accentuation* of the gallop. On the other hand, after extrasystoles, an occasional patient with a normal heart will have a few transient beats with an early diastolic third sound which is of no prognostic significance. In addition, coincident with and sometimes persistent for a period after cessation of the tachycardia, such as in atrial tachycardia, a gallop rhythm may be heard temporarily. This is likewise usually benign.

Normal Physiological Third Heart Sound

A ventricular diastolic gallop occurs with the same timing as the normal physiological third sound, approximately 0.14 to 0.16 s after the second heart sound (Fig. 12-38). The technique employed to discover the normal third sound is the same as the technique used to find a ventricular gallop sound. The third sound is a normal finding in young adults. Members of our division of cardiology examined approximately 1200 school children, ages about 8 to 12. Approximately 100 of these were personally examined by one of the authors (W.P.H.). All of the subjects had a normal third heart sound and a venous hum; an innocent systolic precordial murmur was heard in approximately 80 percent of the subjects. Short innocent bruits were heard in the neck of more than one-third of the subjects.

The normal third sound waxes and wanes in intensity with respiration. It is therefore preferable to listen while the patient continues to breathe in a normal fashion, since this aids left ventricular blood flow and production of the third sound. It is not heard as well when the patient is sitting or standing.

FIGURE 12-38 Note variation in intensity of normal third sound (S₃).

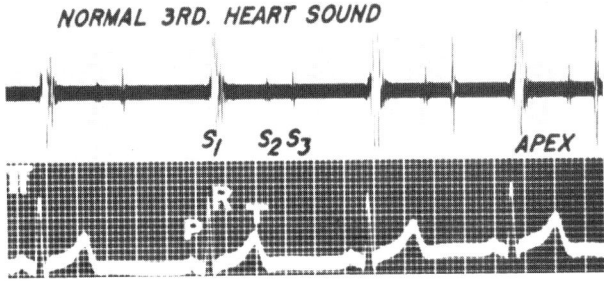

At times, the low-frequency vibrations that constitute a normal physiological third sound may be of sufficient length to produce a short rumble; this can be misinterpreted as the rumble of mitral stenosis. The third heart sound becomes less frequent in the years 20 to 30 and less frequent still after 30. Most men have lost their normal third heart sound by the age of 40; occasionally women at this age retain this normal sound. As a rule, a low-pitched sound with this timing in a person in the forties, fifties, or over represents a ventricular diastolic gallop. It is ironic that a sound which in youth represents a normal, healthy condition should in later years be an unhealthy sign denoting a failing heart. Since this diastolic sound occurs at the time of the normal physiological third sound, it is frequently asked how one can tell the difference between a normal physiological third sound and a ventricular diastolic gallop. Practically, this differentiation is not difficult: after putting together all aspects of the cardiovascular evaluation, and considering the patient's age, one can generally make a correct identification. For example, a patient at the age of 23 having a third heart sound occurring 0.15 s after the aortic component of the second sound, no history or symptoms of heart disease, a normal electrocardiogram and roentgenogram, and no other laboratory evidence indicating a heart problem, is assumed to have a normal physiological third heart sound. On the other hand, a faint heart sound occurring with the identical timing in a man aged 55 would immediately alert the physician to the presence of underlying heart disease. A total cardiovascular evaluation of such a patient will generally afford confirmatory evidence of heart disease in the history, electrocardiogram, x-ray, etc.

Timing of Atrial and Ventricular Diastolic Gallops

When the heart rate is slow or normal, the timing of gallops is not difficult. The atrial gallop sound follows the atrial contraction in presystole and therefore precedes the first heart sound. The ventricular gallop sound occurs at the time of the physiological third sound in early diastole and is easily identified when the rate is normal. With a more rapid heart rate, however, differentiation of the atrial gallop sound from the ventricular gallop sound may be difficult, if not impossible, until the heart rate becomes slower. For this differentiation, stimulation of the carotid sinus has been valuable. When slowing is produced with carotid sinus pressure, the atrial gallop will be heard in relation to the first heart sound in presystole, whereas the ventricular gallop remains in conjunction with the second heart sound, occurring shortly after it. Frequently when carotid sinus pressure causes a sudden slowing of the heart rate, there may be a temporary period of several beats when neither the atrial nor the ventricular gallop is detected; but with the gradual resumption of the faster rate, the extra sound can be identified without difficulty in its proper place. This test should not be used unless it is deemed important to obtain the information and the information cannot be obtained by other safer means.

Combination of Gallops

Not uncommonly one hears two sounds in diastole producing not a triple rhythm but a quadruple rhythm (Fig. 12-39). An atrial gallop can be heard for a number of years in a person who has hypertension but no signs or symptoms of cardiac decompensation. Once failure ensues, however, a ventricular gallop may also become evident—thus making two gallop sounds in addition to the two normal sounds. Or an individual who has coronary artery disease may have an atrial gallop in the absence of other evidence of cardiac disease, and may keep the atrial gallop for a number of years before a ventricular diastolic gallop appears. Both atrial and ventricular diastolic gallop sounds occurring in the same person can be identified by first focusing one's attention on a sound in presystole and then concentrating on a sound occurring in the early part of diastole. As previously discussed, when both atrial and ventricular diastolic gallops occur in close proximity, although not simultaneously, a rumble may be heard which simulates a rumble of mitral stenosis, or a flow rumble such as may occur with left-to-right shunts.

Summation Gallops

Uncommonly, the atrial and ventricular diastolic gallop sounds occur simultaneously. This often results in a very loud diastolic gallop sound, which may be louder than either of the two normal heart sounds. When this situation is analyzed on the phonocardiogram, it may be seen that the two gallop sounds occur at exactly the same time; for this reason, the condition is designated as a *summation gallop*. When the heart rate slows (normally or with carotid sinus pressure), it may be possible to separate the atrial from the ventricular gallop sounds, neither of which is as loud as the summation gallop made by both of them.

Classification of Gallop Rhythm

Some physicians have suggested abandoning the term *gallop rhythm* in favor of *filling sounds*. However, it is doubtful this will take place, since gallop rhythm is firmly ingrained in our medical terminology and it is "catchy" and descriptive.

Use of the terms such as *protodiastolic*, *mesodiastolic*, and *presystolic* has been purposely avoided in this discussion because it appears that this terminology has contributed to the present and past con-

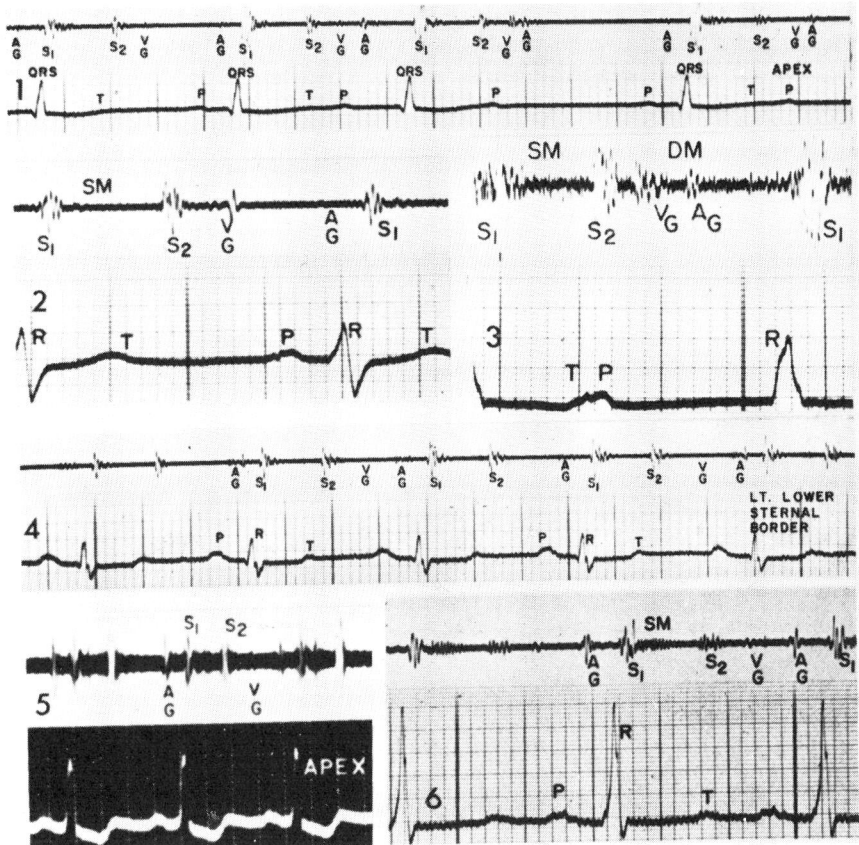

FIGURE 12-39 Composite of a group of patients having both atrial gallops (AG) and ventricular gallops (VG). (1) Wegener's necrotizing granulomatosis. (2) Chronic cardiomyopathy. (3) Cardiomyopathy—lupus erythematosus. (4) Sarcoidosis with pulmonary hypertension. (5) Malignant hypertension. (6) Hyperthyroidism.

fusion about gallop rhythm. For example, in a patient with atrial fibrillation three observers listening to the same gallop sound in diastole may each call it a different type of gallop. Depending on the length of the diastolic pause when the first observer listens, the diastolic sound may be termed protodiastolic by this observer. The next observer may concentrate on the same sound, feel that it is mid-diastolic, and thus term it mesodiastolic. If the third observer decides that the diastolic sound is closer to the first sound, he or she will designate it a presystolic gallop. Actually, the same gallop is heard by each person. If the diastolic gallops were classified as atrial or ventricular, such confusion would not exist since there is no atrial contraction. If atrial fibrillation is present, the gallop is necessarily ventricular in type. If the rhythm is regular and the rate somewhat rapid, slowing the rate makes it possible to identify the sound as either atrial or ventricular, or both.

Another terminology used today, and apparently gaining in popularity, is that of labeling the sounds as third and fourth heart sounds (S_3 and S_4 gallops). At times, however, one may hear five or six sounds in the heart. The terminology of atrial and ventricular gallop is a personal preference, as it appears to have a more physiological basis.

Ejection Sounds: Systolic Clicks, Systolic "Whoops," Opening Snaps, and Other Sounds

W. Proctor Harvey, M.D., and
Antonio C. deLeon, Jr., M.D.

Ejection Sounds[38,55]

An ejection sound is produced in early systole at the time of ejection of blood from the left ventricle into the aorta, or from the right ventricle into the pulmonary artery.[56]

Pulmonary Ejection Sound

A pulmonary ejection sound is usually heard in patients with valvular pulmonic stenosis.[57] It occurs in early systole when forward motion of the stenotic valve abruptly halts. The pulmonary ejection sound is best heard over the pulmonary area or third left intercostal space near the sternal border and is often misinterpreted as the first heart sound. To avoid this confusion one should always keep this possibility in mind and remember that the first heart sound is not well heard in this area. The pulmonary ejection sound, however, is usually poorly heard or absent at the apex. It is characteristic for the pulmonary ejection sound to diminish in intensity (Fig. 12-40) or disappear with inspiration and become louder with expiration. During inspiration, the right ventricular end-diastolic pressure exceeds the pressure in the main pulmonary artery, and no ejection sound can be heard or recorded.[11] With expiration, the right ventricular end-diastolic pressure is lower and an ejection sound can be heard. These findings support a previous suggestion[58] that during inspiration the inflow of blood to the right ventricle may move the stenotic pulmonary valve leaflets to the forward, more "open," position, thereby resulting in less movement with systole. During expiration, the valve leaflets are in a "closed" position, and with systole the stenosed valve is forced forward until it abruptly stops, producing the systolic ejection sound. An ejection sound is a common finding in pulmonary valve stenosis, particularly of the mild to moderate degrees. It may not be detected in the more severe forms of stenosis, or it may occur close to the first heart sound, thereby making specific identification difficult. An ejection sound is not heard with isolated infundibular stenosis.

The pulmonary ejection sound is useful in differentiating between atrial septal defect and mild pulmonic stenosis. At times this differential may be difficult, since both conditions may have a grade 2 to 3 systolic murmur over the pulmonary area in addition to a wide "fixed" splitting of the second heart sound. It is useful to recall that an ejection sound occurs frequently in patients with mild to moderate pulmonic stenosis but is uncommon in patients with atrial septal defect. When it is heard in a patient with an atrial septal defect, it is more likely to be associated with a variable degree of pulmonary hypertension. As a rule, a pulmonary ejection sound is not heard in the uncomplicated ostium secundum atrial defect, although exceptions have been observed. Since atrial septal defect and mild pulmonic stenosis may occur together, a pulmonary ejection sound in a patient displaying the typical clinical features of atrial septal defect should suggest the possibility of an associated pulmonic stenosis. A pulmonary ejection sound may be heard in patients with pulmonary hypertension associated with various conditions (Fig. 12-40), including ventricular septal defect, primary pulmonary hypertension, and recurrent pulmonary emboli. With pulmonary hypertension, the second sound is usually closely split and the pulmonic component of the sound is accentuated.

A pulmonary ejection sound may also be heard

FIGURE 12-40 Composite of various pulmonary ejection sounds (E). *Left.* Pulmonic stenosis (PS), mild with small ventricular septal defect (VSD). Note striking decrease in ejection sound (E) with normal inspiration. *Upper middle.* Patent ductus arteriosus with pulmonary hypertension. *Upper right.* Idiopathic dilatation of the pulmonary artery. *Right middle.* Eisenmenger's syndrome. *Right lower.* Pulmonic stenosis (PS).

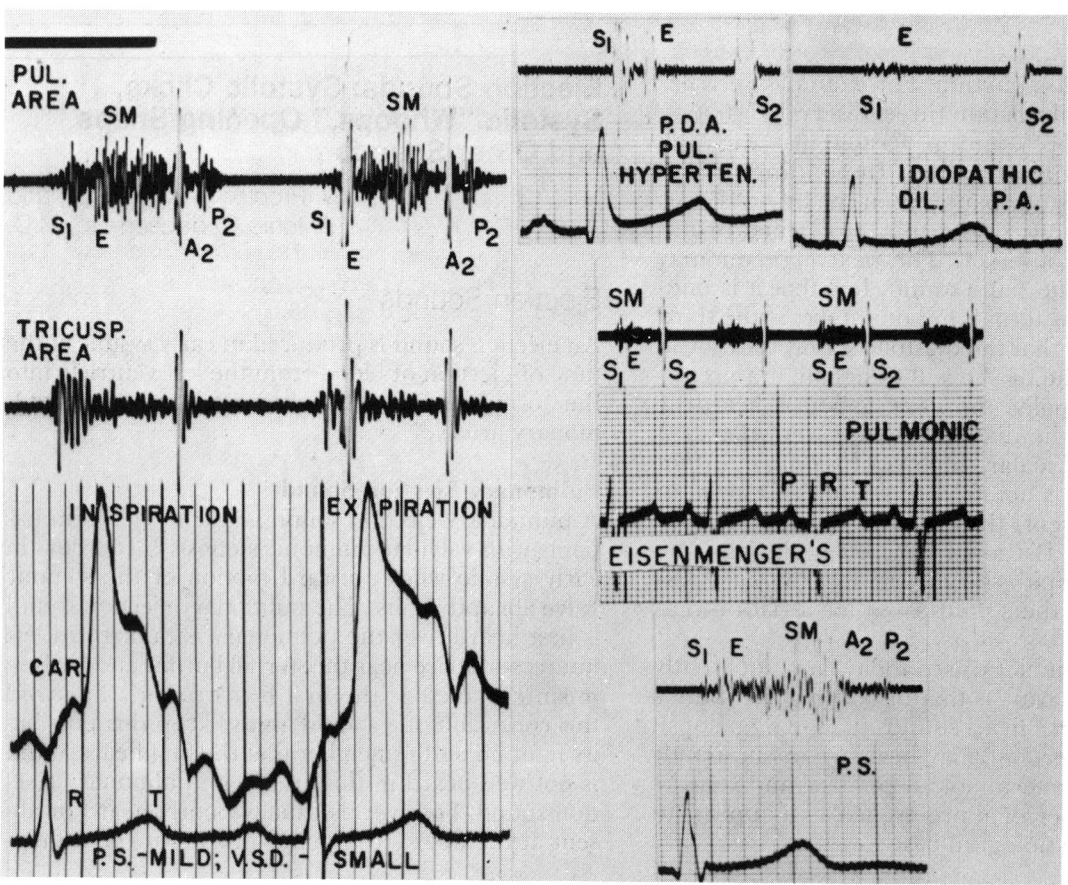

in patients who do not have pulmonary hypertension or valvular stenosis. It may occur in patients with hyperthyroidism, idiopathic dilatation of the pulmonary artery, or other conditions, including aneurysmal dilatation, that cause enlargement of the pulmonary artery.[59] In these instances, the cause of the ejection sound cannot be related to the abrupt stopping of a stenotic valve, as in congenital valvular pulmonic stenosis.

Aortic Ejection Sound

The aortic ejection sound (Fig. 12-41)[48,56,60] is heard in patients with valvular aortic stenosis. Such a sound is heard in patients with congenital bicuspid aortic valve stenosis. It may also be heard in some patients with rheumatic aortic stenosis of a milder or moderate degree in which the valve is still mobile. The ejection sound is not heard in patients with severely calcified valve leaflets.

The congenital bicuspid aortic valve is one of the most common congenital heart lesions. It presents with a spectrum of findings. An ejection sound may be heard in a patient with a bicuspid valve when no murmur is audible. The ejection sound may be heard at the apex as well as at the base. More commonly, a short midsystolic murmur of grade 2 or 3 intensity is heard, together with the ejection sound and a prominent aortic valve closure sound. An early blowing aortic diastolic murmur plus an ejection sound and easily heard aortic valve closure may be present. Bicuspid aortic valve stenosis may progress over the years. The valve may become heavily calcified in the fifth to seventh decades of life, producing symptoms of congestive failure, syncope, dizziness, and myocardial ischemia, and aortic valve replacement may then be necessary.

An ejection sound can also be heard with aortic regurgitation, coarctation of the aorta, aneurysm of the ascending aorta, and occasionally tetralogy of Fallot. If a systolic ejection sound is heard at the apex and/or over the aortic area in a patient who has coarctation of the aorta, an associated bicuspid

aortic valve is likely to be present. The ejection sound is usually produced by the bicuspid valve and not by the coarctation; however, an ejection sound can occur with coarctation and appears related to dilatation of the descending aorta. An aortic ejection sound with aortic stenosis provides clinical support of the likelihood that the stenosis is of valvular type rather than infundibular, supravalvular, or idiopathic hypertrophic subaortic stenosis. Aortic ejection sounds, in contrast to the pulmonary ejection sounds, are usually well heard at the apex and have no respiratory variation. The aortic ejection sound occurs at the time of the abrupt stopping of the forward motion of the valve in early systole. With a stenotic bicuspid valve, it coincides with the "doming" of the valve in systole as seen on cineangiograms. The aortic ejection sound is composed of higher frequencies than the ventricular filling sounds (gallops), from which it can usually be differentiated by simple techniques (to be discussed later). The aortic ejection sound is often better heard at the apex than at the base of the heart. A harsh midsystolic ejection murmur of aortic stenosis over the aortic area may compete with detection of the ejection sound, or even mask it in some patients.

Systolic Clicks

The systolic click is an extra sound occurring in systole[48] (Figs. 12-33 and 12-42, upper tracing). Usually only a single click is heard; however, at times, several or even multiple, rapidly occurring clicking sounds can be detected. Although the position of the click in the cardiac cycle is usually constant, occasionally it may vary slightly.

Change in position can alter the click-murmur auscultatory findings. For example, clicks may move toward the latter part of systole in the squatting position and return to early or midsystole on standing. Systolic clicks may be heard at early, mid-, or late systole, although most commonly they occur at midsystole. Though they are often found in otherwise

FIGURE 12-41 Examples of aortic ejection sounds (E). Note that the ejection sound is well heard at the apex, as well as over the aortic area.

FIGURE 12-42 Asymptomatic patient with a systolic click (C) and musical systolic "whoop" (W) sound. Note in the lower tracing that whoop occurred in latter part of systole.

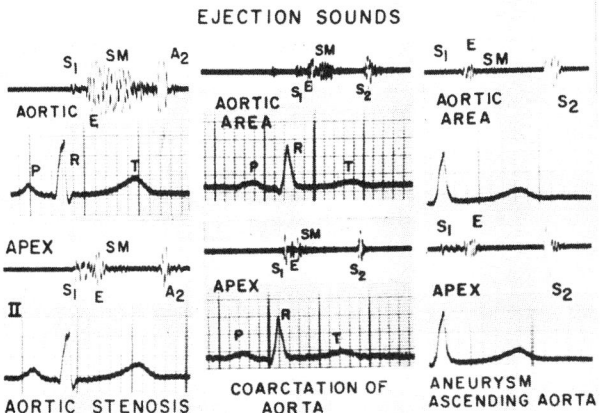

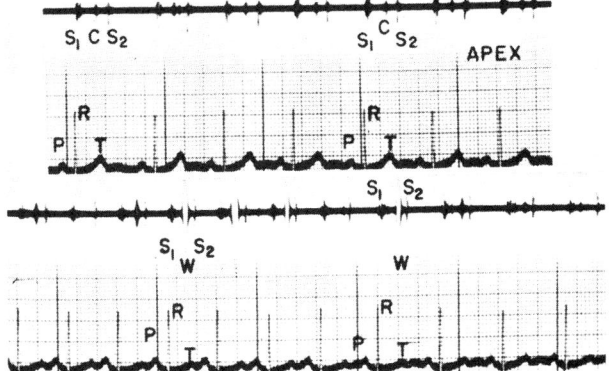

normal patients, they are frequently overlooked and sometimes misinterpreted as murmurs or friction rubs. They are very common, particularly in young females. It is now well established that these auscultatory findings are related to systolic prolapse of the mitral valve leaflets (generally posterior, although the anterior leaflet can also prolapse).[61–68] Prolapse of the tricuspid valve also occurs. A systolic click is usually decreased in intensity or is absent at the base of the heart (Fig. 12-33); it is seldom heard over the aortic area. Having the patient recumbent and in the left lateral position often helps in finding clicks; also some clicks are better heard when the patient is sitting, standing, or squatting. Systolic clicks were formerly considered to be benign or even extracardiac in origin. A possible relation to pericardial disease had also been postulated. Various descriptive terms have been used, such as systolic click–murmur syndrome, prolapsing mitral leaflet syndrome, Barlow's syndrome, "billowing" mitral valve, posterior leaflet deformity, or "floppy" valve. Of great importance and still not fully appreciated, however, is the fact that bacterial endocarditis may occur on the mitral valve in such cases.[61,67]

Sudden death has occurred, although it is rare, and too much emphasis has been placed on the possibility of this dire event; as a result many patients have been unnecessarily frightened and made unduly anxious. Rupture of chordae tendineae spontaneously or with infective endocarditis has evolved as the most serious complication, but this too is uncommon. Patients with Marfan's syndrome, or variants of this syndrome, may have varying degrees of mitral valve involvement. A systolic click, or clicks, may be the only indication of a minimal involvement, or the click sounds may be associated with the late apical systolic murmur; other patients have severe mitral insufficiency with a pansystolic murmur, a result of rupture of chordae tendineae.

For a number of years it has been known that patients having auscultatory findings of mitral valve prolapse (systolic clicks and/or a late apical systolic murmur) usually have a good prognosis and have been able to live essentially normal lives.

Systolic Whoops

Systolic whoops[48,66] are characterized by a loud, sometimes inconstant, short musical murmur heard at the apex and occurring in the latter part of systole, often without other evidence of significant heart disease (Fig. 12-42). Preceding the whoop there is often a systolic sound or click, which also, like the whoop, is sometimes transient. As with the late apical systolic murmur and systolic click, the whoop was for years considered benign, the postulation being that it was related either to a vibrating portion of the valve structure or to an extracardiac phenomenon. However, during follow-up periods of a decade or more, the whoop in some patients has been observed to develop the usual character-

istics of a systolic murmur, although it is more prominent in the latter part of systole. The whoop, therefore, is usually due to pathologic change in the mitral valve. Another term given this peculiar murmur is "precordial honk,"[69,70] since the sound is reminiscent of that made by a goose. There is evidence that the descriptive terms *whoop* and *honk* refer to similar pathological change, most frequently in the mitral valve. Evidence for this probability was a report on eight patients with precordial honks or whoops who were studied with complete catheterizations of the right and left side of the heart and left ventricular cineangiography.[70] Five patients had no other evidence of heart disease. Ballooning of the mitral valve into the left atrium during ventricular systole was seen on the cineangiogram and was associated with late systolic mitral regurgitation in four of the five patients. It is likely that what would be described as a whoop by some would be designated as a honk by others, and that the difference in terms probably has been a matter of semantics. These patients are also subject to bacterial endocarditis.

Opening Snaps

Opening Snap of the Mitral Valve

The opening of a normal mitral valve is acoustically silent. However, in the presence of disease caused by the pathologic changes of rheumatic mitral stenosis, a clear sound is definitely audible in early diastole, occurring 0.04 to 0.12 s after the aortic valve closure of the second heart sound. It is best heard at the apex but is usually widely transmitted. It can be heard in the aortic area (second right intercostal space near the sternum) and the pulmonary area (second and third left intercostal space near the sternum) where it is misinterpreted as a split second sound. This is the *opening snap of mitral stenosis;* the term is now well ingrained in the literature and is in common usage today. When students are first introduced to the term, however, it should be emphasized that this is not the first heart sound, but rather a third sound associated with mitral stenosis. The opening snap occurs in early diastole when there is a sudden halt of a downward movement of the mitral valve structure. This occurs when the left ventricular pressure is falling. The higher the atrial pressure is, the more rapid the downward descent of the mitral valve structure, and in turn, the earlier the opening snap. This sound occurs later than the usual splitting of the second heart sound but earlier than the physiological third heart sound. The opening snap often affords the first clue to the diagnosis of mitral stenosis; further supporting evidence is a loud first heart sound and an accentuated pulmonary valve closure of the second heart sound. Listening at a localized area at the point of maximum impulse of the left ventricle, with the patient turned to the left lateral position, one may hear the characteristic and diagnostic rumble of mitral stenosis (Fig. 12-36). Remember, the rumble of mitral stenosis may be localized to the apex, but the opening snap is widely transmitted.

The opening snap is present in normal sinus rhythm as well as in atrial fibrillation. It persists after mitral commissurotomy (although there may be a decrease in its intensity) and usually occurs later after the second heart sound compared to before the operation. The opening snap is present in well over 90 percent of patients with mitral stenosis; rarely, when absent, it is likely to be associated with heavily calcified, thickened immobile stenotic valves. The second heart sound associated with mitral stenosis is often loud and closely split, with the degree of splitting increasing slightly coincident with inspiration. The opening snap heard over the pulmonary area is sometimes misinterpreted as a split second sound. By focusing attention carefully on the components of the second heart sound, however, one may note that three components are heard coincident with inspiration; this "trill" effect of three sounds is the result of slightly wider splitting of the second heart sound, coincident with inspiration, plus the opening snap. This simple auscultatory point is often of important diagnostic application in the differential diagnosis of atrial septal defect versus mitral stenosis. In some cases of atrial septal defect, a diagnostic flow rumble may be heard, the second heart sound is accentuated, and the wide splitting of the second heart sound is misinterpreted as a second sound and an opening snap. In fact, a number of cases of congenital atrial septal defect have for many years been labeled as rheumatic heart disease. By paying strict attention to the splitting of the second heart sound, an important clue as to the correct diagnosis can be made. If only two components of the second heart sound persist, then the diagnosis of atrial septal defect should be entertained. On the other hand, the presence of the three components, i.e., the split second sound plus the opening snap, would be confirmatory evidence of rheumatic heart disease.

Opening Snap of the Tricuspid Valve

The characteristics of the opening snap of tricuspid stenosis are similar to those of the opening snap of mitral stenosis. The opening snap of the tricuspid valve is best heard along the lower left sternal border. Occasionally it is better heard along the lower right sternal border. Since practically all patients with rheumatic tricuspid stenosis have concomitant mitral stenosis, the possibility of confusing the two snaps always exists. In addition, the tricuspid opening snap is more likely to occur later after the second sound than the mitral opening snap; because of this, the mitral diastolic rumble may "drown out" the tricuspid opening snap, making identification difficult. An occasional rare case of tricuspid stenosis occurs unassociated with mitral stenosis, however, and the opening snap can then be easily identified as tricus-

pid. The clinical diagnosis of tricuspid stenosis is obviously better made by the combination of all the clinical findings. These include the observation of a large *a* wave in the jugular venous pulse; a slow *y* descent, suggesting obstruction at the tricuspid valve; and an increase in intensity of the diastolic rumble coincident with inspiration.

Occasionally, an opening snap of the tricuspid valve is heard in a patient with atrial septal defect.

Other Sounds

Pericardial Knock

The pericardial knock[48,71] occurs early in diastole, generally 0.10 to 0.12 s after the second heart sound, and is common in patients with constrictive pericarditis (Fig. 12-43). It has also been termed the *early diastolic sound* or the *third heart sound of constrictive pericarditis*. In a study of 26 patients with constrictive pericarditis, the pericardial knock was the

FIGURE 12-43 Pericardial knock: constrictive pericarditis.

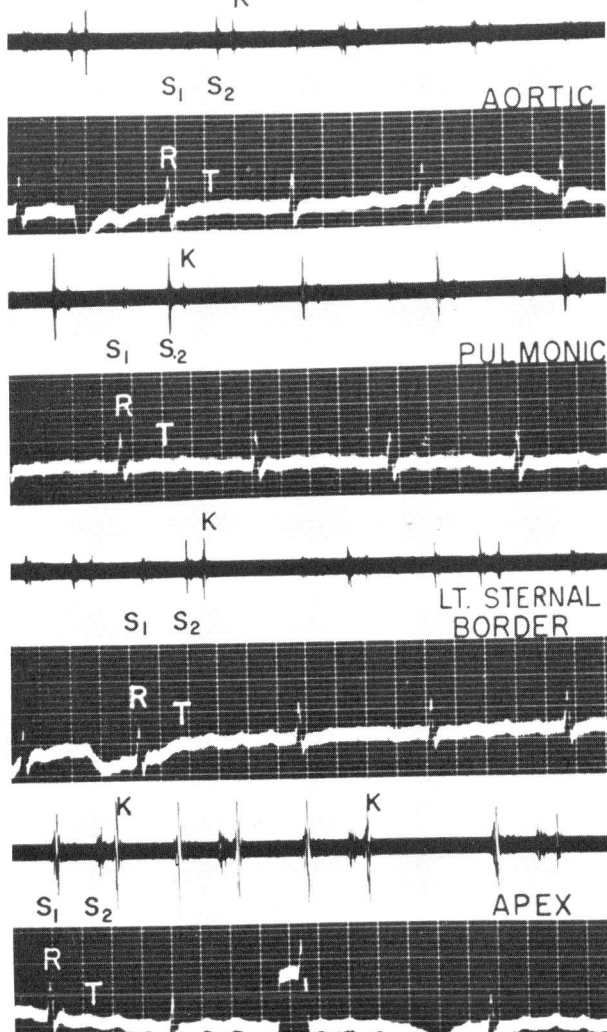

most common clinical finding, being heard in 24 of 26 patients.[72] The knock, which may be present with or without calcification of the pericardium, is produced in the rapid-filling phase of ventricular diastole. The extra sound is a filling sound, with the pericardium acting as a constricting shell, preventing the usual relaxation of the ventricles in diastole. The pericardial knock occurs in the early part of diastole, usually slightly later than the opening snap of mitral stenosis but earlier than the normal physiological third sound or the ventricular diastolic gallop sound. Occasionally, the pericardial knock comes earlier, thereby simulating the opening snap of mitral stenosis. The typical rumble of mitral stenosis, however, is generally absent. Detection of this early diastolic sound in a patient who does not have the customary signs of coronary, hypertensive, or rheumatic valvular disease should always make one suspect the presence of pericardial disease. The pericardial knock sound may be single and sharp, or occasionally it may show considerable variation in intensity as well as in the number of components. It may also vary with normal respiration. The sound or sounds may persist after surgery on the pericardium, although to a lesser degree, or they may be absent. In other patients, a diastolic sound occurs later after the second sound, simulating the timing of the ventricular diastolic gallop or a normal physiological third sound. It is likely that the pericardial knock and ventricular diastolic gallops are related to similar mechanisms concerned with the filling of the ventricles in early diastole; when the constriction is removed and the myocardium is still in a state of decompensation, the filling sound comes later, consistent with the timing of a ventricular diastolic gallop.

Artificial Valve Sounds[48,73]

Since the beginning of the use of prosthetic valves in human beings in 1951 by Hufnagel, whose artificial ball valve was placed in the first portion of the descending aorta, there has been a succession of various types of prosthetic and other valves, including artificial leaflets, caged-ball valves of the Starr-Edwards type, disk valves, homografts, heterografts, and many variants and modifications of these (Fig. 12-44). Artificial valves have usually been inserted in the aortic and mitral valve areas, but occasionally and less commonly, the tricuspid valve has also been replaced. In some cases, three artificial valves have

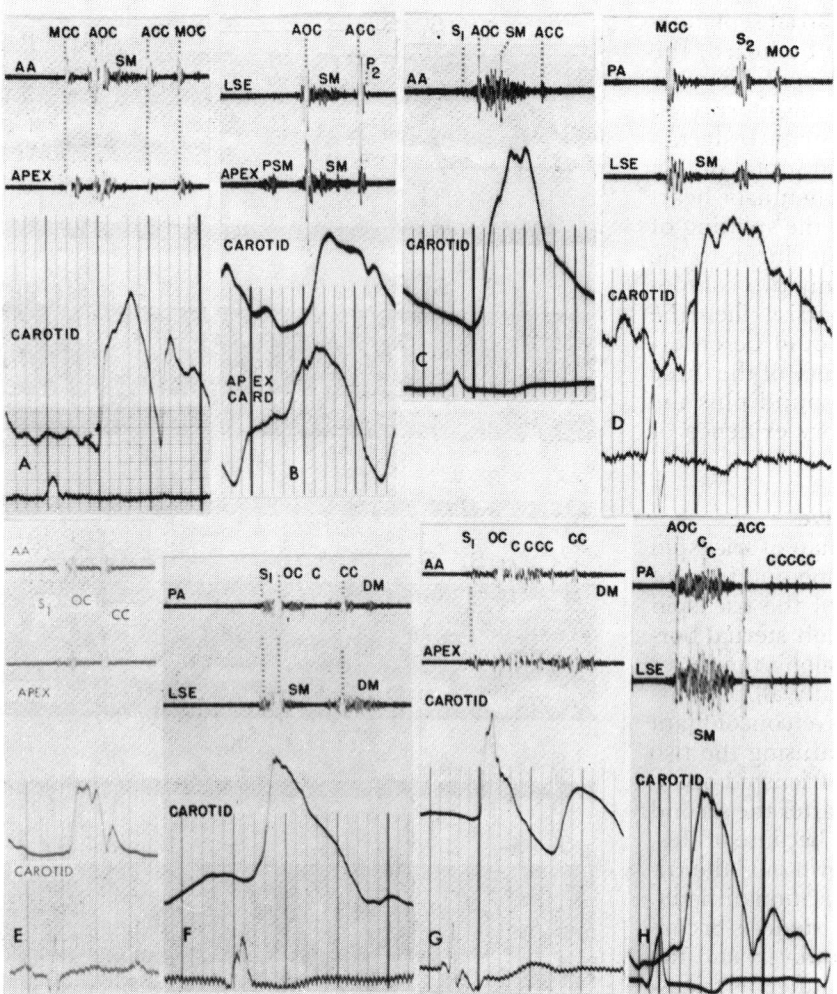

FIGURE 12-44 Composite of patients with various artificial prosthetic valves. AA, aortic area; MCC, mitral closing click; AOC, aortic opening click; ACC, aortic closing click; MOC, mitral opening click; SM, systolic murmur; DM, diastolic murmur. A. Aortic and mitral valves replaced with Starr-Edwards prostheses. B. Original Hufnagel ball valve (inserted in first portion of descending aorta). C. Aortic leaflets (three). D. Mitral discoid valve. Note interval from second sound (S_2) to mitral opening click. E. Trileaflet "unitized" aortic valve. Opening click (OC) resembles ejection sound. F. Hufnagel aortic discoid valve. Note systolic click (C) in addition to opening (OC) and closing (CC) clicks. G. Ball valve. Multiple extra sounds (CCCC) occur in systole. H. Aortic discoid valve. Extra prosthetic valve sounds (CCCCC) are heard in diastole.

been used as replacement. The caged-ball or disk valve has an opening sound and a closing sound. These sounds vary considerably with the different types of prosthetic valves. Some are louder than the normal heart sounds and have a different quality; others are more like the sounds of a normal heart. With a double valve replacement, each valve has an opening sound and a closing sound. At times, more than one sound of a normally functioning valve is made at the time of opening and/or closing.

The physician should become familiar with the characteristics of the sounds made by the various artificial valves. Complications following surgery include infection and dislodgment of the valve. Clot formation and emboli have unfortunately been frequent. *Ball variance,* a term used to describe physical changes in a caged ball, may occur. This includes changes in the ball's contour and size. Disintegration of the ball may also take place. Various unusual sounds may occur when the valve is not functioning properly. Therefore, a series of rattles or clicks, which may simulate the rolling of dice or a ball traversing a roulette wheel, may be heard. At times the sounds are multiple rather than single, occurring in systole and/or diastole. When such sounds are present, the possibility of clot formation or some other complication of the artificial valve must be suspected. Multiple sounds are more common when the ball is enclosed in a case. More than one sound coincident with opening and closing might be expected with any changes in contour of the ball, or when the ball seats itself in the cage that contains it. It should be emphasized, however, that multiple sounds can occur in a normally functioning prosthetic valve. This is particularly more likely to occur with an aortic caged-ball prosthesis during systole. Cineangiograms in such instances may show the ball "bobbing" against the top of the cage during systole. A change in the time of occurrence or intensity of the normally functioning prosthetic valve sounds may be the first sign of malfunction. This was illustrated by a patient who had an opening click sound (of her mitral prosthetic valve) that was so close to the second heart sound it gave the initial impression of being the aortic component of a widely split second sound. However, this short interval between this opening sound and the second sound indicated restricted movement of her caged-ball mitral prosthesis. This was confirmed at surgery, when ball variance was noted. A new mitral valve replaced the old one, with prompt relief of her severe congestive heart failure. On the other hand, if there is a delayed opening sound of a Starr-Edwards mitral prosthetic valve, this may also be an indication of valve malfunction. The late opening sound after the second sound can be caused by a clot or by ball variance; it also may result from obstruction to movement of the prosthetic ball (or disk) by the ventricular wall or septum, when the left ventricular cavity is too small for the size of the prosthetic valve. Disruption of sutures of a prosthetic valve can occur,

resulting in disappearance of the valve sounds. When this complication follows insertion of a mitral valve prosthesis, with resulting deterioration of the patient's condition, the opening click sound and a systolic murmur may be absent.[74] At times, a prosthetic valve, such as a discoid type of mitral valve, may get stuck in its open position; the murmur of mitral regurgitation may again be regularly heard, or heard intermittently if the valve only occasionally sticks in its open position.

Extracardiac Sounds Produced by Cardiac Pacemakers

It is now well established that the pacemaker can produce a sound in presystole that is related to skeletal muscle contraction rather than being of cardiac origin.[75] At times one can see precordial muscle contraction coincident with the sound, and the patient may be aware of it, occasionally feeling some discomfort. Also, uncommonly, the pacemaker can produce unusual auscultatory findings. This may result in peculiar musical murmurs such as a whoop or honk. These are often loud and occur in late systole. In one patient personally observed, a murmur having a musical quality resembling a "grunt" or "groan" (also described as sounding like "the croaking of a frog") was heard in systole, and at times in diastole. Apparently this was related to the position of the pacing catheter across the tricuspid valve, since repositioning it resulted in disappearance of the murmurs.

Murmurs

W. Proctor Harvey, M.D., and
Antonio C. deLeon, Jr., M.D.

Murmurs are audible successive sounds with distinct duration, as opposed to "heart" sounds such as the first or second heart sounds, which are short, transient auditory events. The currently accepted pathogenetic mechanism of cardiac murmurs is that they are the result of turbulence created by blood flow.[76] A critical level of turbulence must be achieved to produce a sound that is clinically appreciated. The characteristics of the murmur depend upon the velocity of blood flow and the surrounding structures which are caused to vibrate.

It is useful to categorize murmurs according to their location in the cardiac cycle. Accordingly, murmurs are identified as being systolic, diastolic, or continuous.

Systolic Murmurs

The classification of systolic murmurs[77] into (1) systolic ejection murmurs and (2) pansystolic, or regurgitant systolic, murmurs has proved to be of great clinical usefulness. These two broad categories are usually readily recognized and immediately en-

EXAMINATION OF THE HEART AND BLOOD VESSELS

able the clinician to limit diagnostic considerations (Fig. 12-45).

Systolic Ejection Murmurs

A systolic ejection murmur implies turbulent blood flow at the time of right and/or left ventricular ejection into its corresponding great vessel. Its origin is therefore likely to be along the ventricular outflow, at the semilunar valve level, or at the immediate great vessel. Since actual blood flow is an essential ingredient to the genesis of turbulence responsible for the murmur, the murmur starts after semilunar valve opening (i.e., after isometric period of ventricular contraction) and ends upon cessation of flow with closure of the same semilunar valve. The characteristics of the left ventricular pressure curve (Fig. 12-45) causes the murmur to be typically crescendo-decrescendo or diamond-shaped. Peak intensity of the murmur could be in early, mid-, or late systole, depending upon the factors influencing turbulent blood flow, i.e., large volume and/or rapid velocity of ventricular ejection or turbulence created by varying degrees of obstruction to ventricular outflow.

The Innocent Systolic Ejection Murmur (Fig. 12-46)

Data from intracardiac phonocardiography suggest that turbulent flow (and hence murmur) is invariably present in the great vessels at the time of ventricular ejection.[78] The intensity of the murmur, as influenced by stroke volume and/or velocity of ejection, and proximity of the great vessels to the chest wall (influenced by body build) determines whether the murmur is audible with the stethoscope. These factors are most often met in children and young adults; i.e., they tend to have a brisk

circulation and a smaller chest cage with a narrow anteroposterior (AP) diameter. Hence, systolic murmurs are most commonly encountered as normal findings. The murmur tends to be of medium frequency, peaks in early to midsystole, usually ends well before the second heart sound, and is best heard along the left sternal border or at the left or right second interspace. It may be the result of turbulent flow into the pulmonary artery,[79] the aorta,[80] or both (Fig. 12-46). On occasion, a musical or groaning murmur is noted along the left sternal border—the Still's murmur; the sound is distinctive and, once heard, is easily recognized as a variation of the innocent systolic murmur. The exact genesis of the Still's murmur has not been conclusively established. It has been proposed to originate from the right heart and result from vibrations of the right ventricular moderator band or pulmonary valve,[62] and more recently, the aortic or subaortic region has been proposed as its source.[81]

There are also several forms of extracardiac innocent systolic murmurs. One form is the systolic murmur which originates from branches of the aortic arch and presents as a cervical systolic murmur[82] from the increased vascularity which occurs in lactating breast or toxic goiter.[48]

FIGURE 12-46 Examples of innocent systolic murmurs.

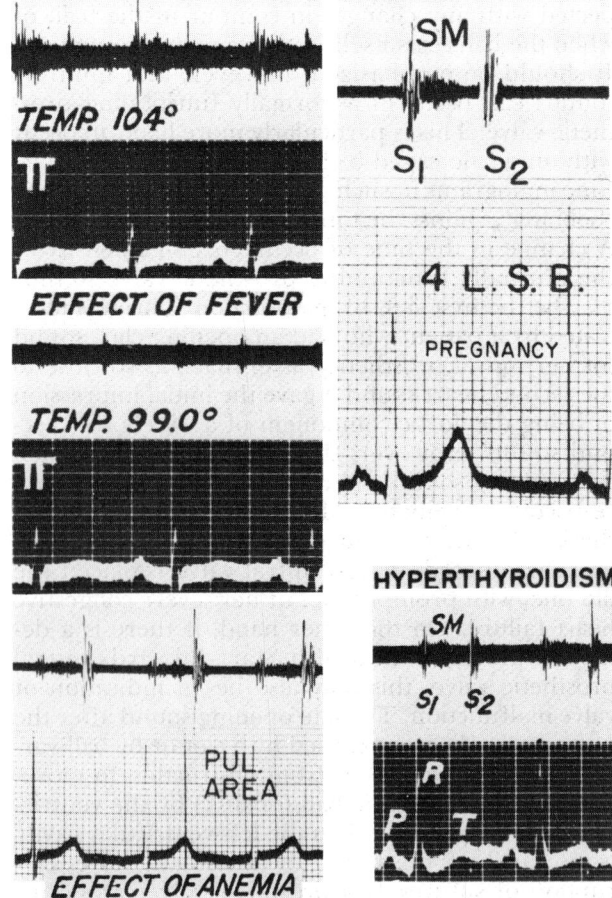

FIGURE 12-45 Characteristics of a systolic ejection murmur and a holosystolic (pansystolic) regurgitant systolic murmur.

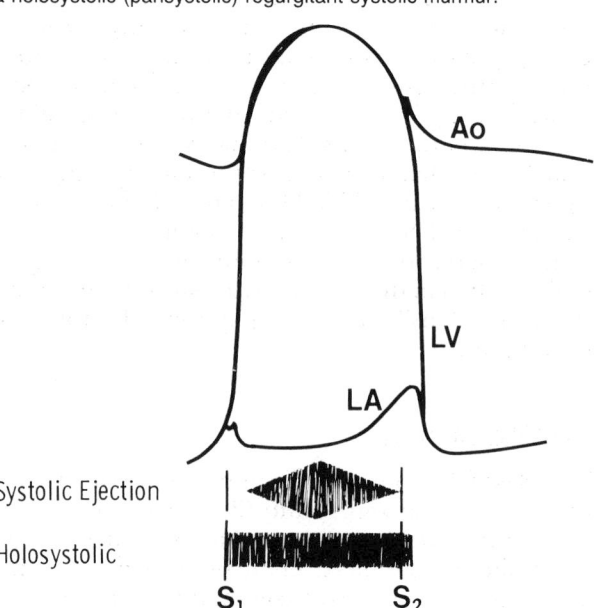

Systolic Murmurs Due to Obstruction of Right Ventricular Outflow (Pulmonic Stenosis) A useful clinical correlation has been demonstrated between the length and peak of the systolic murmur and the severity of obstruction in isolated pulmonic stenosis.[83,84] In mild stenosis, the murmur is short and peaks in early systole. With severe obstruction, the duration of right ventricular ejection is prolonged, thus resulting in delay of the pulmonic closure sound (P_2), which is also diminished in intensity. The murmur is long, and while it does end with the pulmonic closure sound (P_2), it can extend beyond the aortic closure sound (A_2). The peak of the murmur's intensity occurs in late systole (Fig. 12-47). A valvular location of the obstruction is usually indicated by the presence of a pulmonic ejection sound immediately preceding the onset of the ejection systolic murmur. A pulmonic ejection sound is not heard when the obstruction is at the infundibular portion of the right ventricle. The site of maximal murmur intensity in valvular pulmonic stenosis is the left second interspace, with radiation to the left side of the neck and clavicular area. With infundibular obstruction, the murmur may be maximal in intensity at the third left interspace.

Significant pulmonic stenosis occurring in association with a large ventricular septal defect (tetralogy of Fallot) results in a systolic ejection murmur across the obstruction which must be interpreted in a manner directly opposed to isolated pulmonic stenosis.[85] In this instance, more severe pulmonic stenosis results in more right-to-left shunting across the ventricular septal defect, and hence a smaller volume of flow across the obstruction. The converse occurs with a lesser degree of obstruction. Thus, in tetralogy of Fallot, the systolic murmur tends to get shorter with more severe degrees of cyanosis and is longest in the patient with minimal or no detectable cyanosis.

Several recognized pathological entities are associated with a systolic ejection murmur across the right ventricular outflow tract. As a rule, the murmur is short and limited to early or midsystole, heard best at the second left intercostal space. Among the conditions are: atrial septal defect,[86] idiopathic dilatation of the pulmonary artery,[87] and congenital low-pressure pulmonary valve regurgitation.[88] Their specific recognition is determined not by the systolic murmur but by other auscultatory events: "fixed splitting" of the second heart sound, a pulmonic ejection sound with physiological S_2 and radiologic evidence of a dilated pulmonary artery, or a medium- or low-frequency early to middiastolic murmur, respectively.

Pulmonary artery branch stenosis is also often associated with a systolic ejection murmur (rarely, a continuous murmur). Its length varies according to the degree of pulmonary artery constriction. The diagnostic hallmark at the bedside is the wide distribution of the murmur throughout the thoracic cage—such that it is equally well heard posteriorly, in both midaxillary regions, as well as anteriorly.[89] Occasionally, patients with a large shunt due to an atrial septal defect will have a similar, widely distributed peripheral pulmonary arterial systolic murmur as a result of increased pulmonary blood flow.[90]

Systolic Murmur Due to Obstruction of Left Ventricular Outflow (Aortic Stenosis) There is a general correlation between the length of the murmur across a fixed obstruction to left ventricular outflow and the severity of obstruction (Fig. 12-48).[91] The murmur tends to be harsh, has a crescendo-descrescendo configuration, and ends at or before aortic valve closure. With *supravalvular* obstruction, the murmur tends to be louder and best heard higher, i.e., at the suprasternal notch and carotid arteries. In fixed *subvalvular* obstruction, it may be loudest along the third left sternal border and is frequently associated with aortic regurgitation. With *dynamic obstruction* such as occurs with idiopathic hypertrophic subaortic stenosis (IHSS), the murmur is loudest at the apex and left sternal border, with poor radiation to the second interspace. Responses to bedside maneuvers, which are discussed later in this chapter, also aid in recognition. *Valvular* aortic stenosis on a congenital basis is usually preceded by an aortic ejection sound, unless the aortic valve is calcified to the extent of rendering it immobile. The murmur may be loudest at the cardiac apex, al-

FIGURE 12-47 Comparison with innocent systolic murmur. Composite of several systolic ejection murmurs. Note the ejection sound preceding the murmur (AS and PS) and the fixed split second sound (ASD).

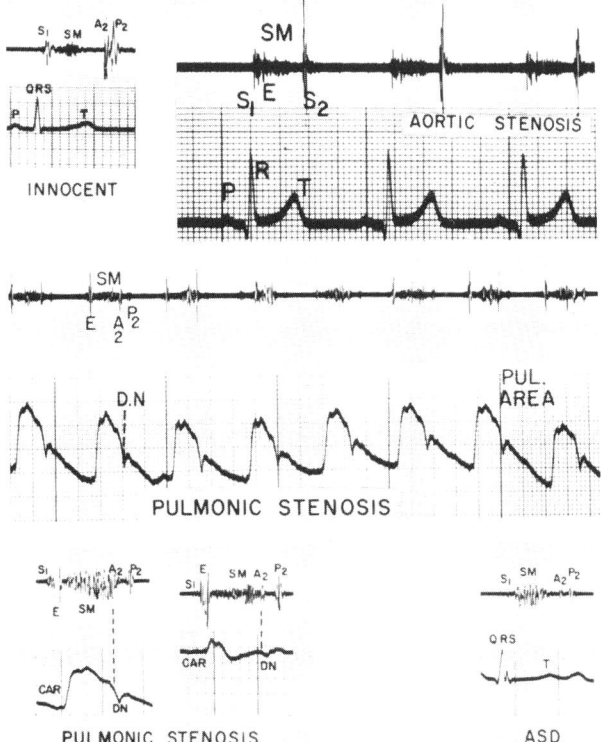

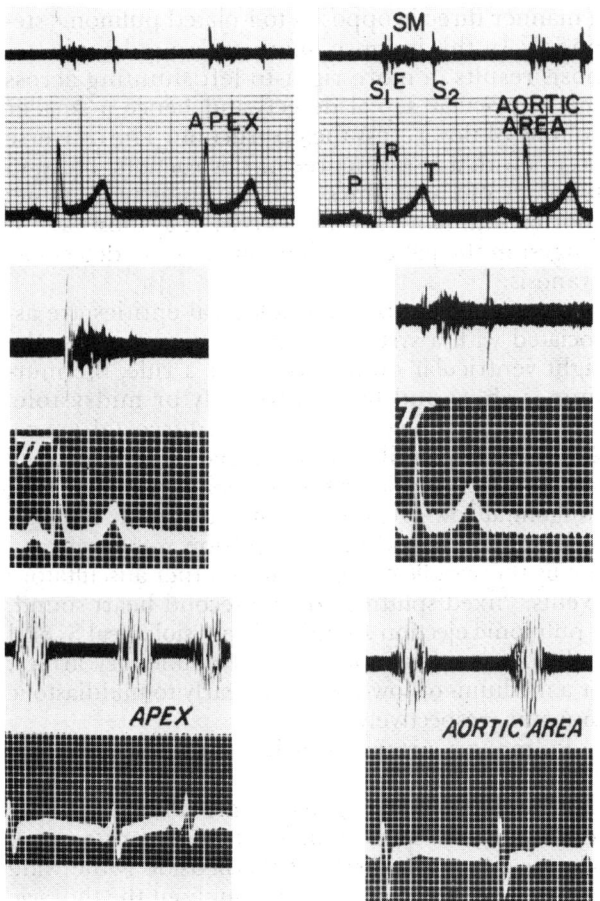

FIGURE 12-48 *Top.* Mild congenital aortic valvular stenosis—aortic ejection sound followed by a very short ejection murmur. *Middle.* Moderate aortic stenosis—longer systolic murmur occupying one-half to two-thirds of systole. *Bottom.* Severe aortic stenosis with long ejection systolic murmur occupying almost all of systole.

though it is also heard at the second right interspace, suprasternal notch, and carotid arteries. A long murmur, especially associated with a paradoxical second heart sound [no left bundle branch block (LBBB)], implies severe obstruction (Fig. 12-49). A short, early-peaking systolic murmur is expected with mild obstruction. It should be remembered, however, that in severe stenosis with left ventricular failure and diminished cardiac output, the murmur may be short and, in a few instances, even absent.

Holosystolic (Pansystolic) Murmurs

These murmurs represent *regurgitant murmurs*, i.e., mitral regurgitation, tricuspid regurgitation, and ventricular septal defect (Fig. 12-50). The murmur begins as soon as the AV valve closes and continues beyond semilunar valve closure. Because the pressure difference (gradient) between ventricle and recipient chamber [atrium or right ventricle (RV)] is considerable throughout systole, the murmur tends to have an even or plateau configuration.

Variants Mitral valve regurgitation may be present with a variety of murmur configurations. In acute, severe mitral regurgitation, the giant left atrial *v* wave results in a smaller late systolic left ventricular to left atrial (LA) gradient. Hence, the murmur tends to decrease in intensity or be absent in late systole.[92] Mitral valve prolapse frequently presents with a late systolic murmur that is crescendo-decrescendo or crescendo up to the second heart sound.[93] When holosystolic, a late systolic accentuation may be present. Papillary muscle dysfunction may present as a holosystolic, midsystolic, late systolic, or early systolic murmur (Fig. 12-51).[94]

The murmur of tricuspid regurgitation may also be altered from its typical holosystolic configuration. It may decrease in late systole, and in wide-open tricuspid regurgitation the murmur may be absent or confined to early systole. Selective inspiratory increase in intensity of the murmur is typical of this lesion.

The typical holosystolic murmur of ventricular septal defect may also be modified by the onset of pulmonary hypertension. This results in the progressive shortening of the systolic murmur as the degree of pulmonary hypertension increases.[95] In small muscular ventricular septal defects, physiological closure of the defect toward the latter part of systole accounts for the less than holosystolic murmur in some cases.[96]

Diastolic Murmurs

Murmurs in diastole can occur across two locations: (1) across the AV valves (mitral or tricuspid) or (2) across the semilunar valves (aortic and pulmonic).

Diastolic Murmurs across the AV Valves

Mitral Diastolic Murmurs Mitral diastolic murmurs begin after mitral valve opening and hence do not start immediately after the second heart sound. The onset is more in middiastole and is the result of turbulent blood flow across the valve; the murmur is usually low-frequency or rumbling in character. Certain lesions of hemodynamic severity result in increased diastolic mitral blood flow which result in a middiastolic rumble in the absence of mitral valve obstruction. Included in these lesions are *ventricular septal defect, patent ductus arteriosus,* and *mitral regurgitation* (Fig. 12-52). On the other hand, rheumatic or congenital *mitral valve stenosis* produces a diastolic rumbling murmur (Fig. 12-52).[97] In this instance, the turbulent blood flow results from the pressure gradient between left atrium and left ventricle, and hence the length of the rumble can reflect the severity of obstruction. In normal sinus rhythm, the diastolic murmur increases in intensity at the time of atrial contraction (presystolic crescendo).

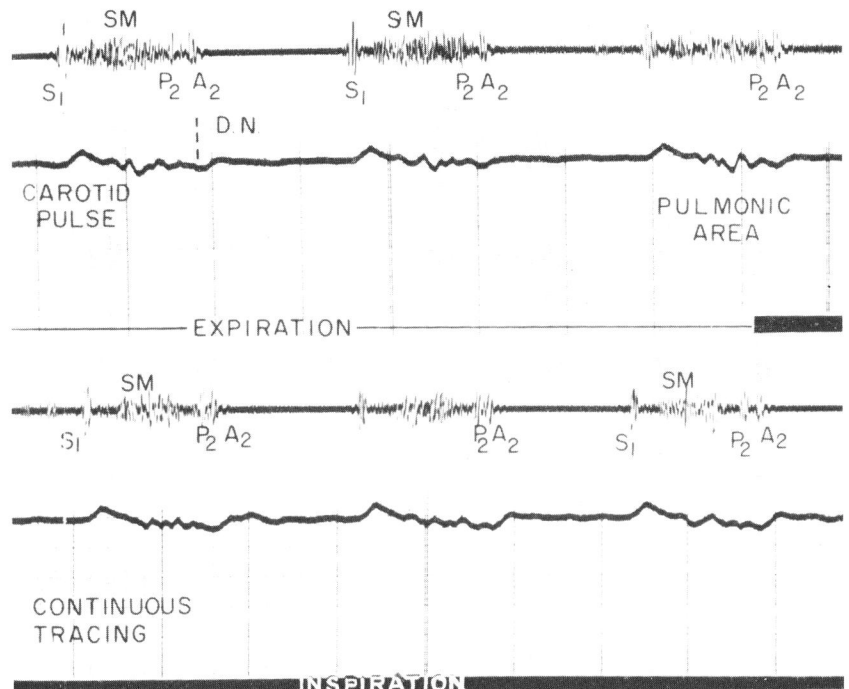

FIGURE 12-49   Severe aortic stenosis with paradoxical second sound splitting.

FIGURE 12-50   *Top.* Holosystolic murmur of chronic mitral regurgitation. *Middle.* Holosystolic murmur of ventricular septal defect. *Bottom.* Holosystolic murmur of tricuspid regurgitation with inspiratory augmentation of murmur.

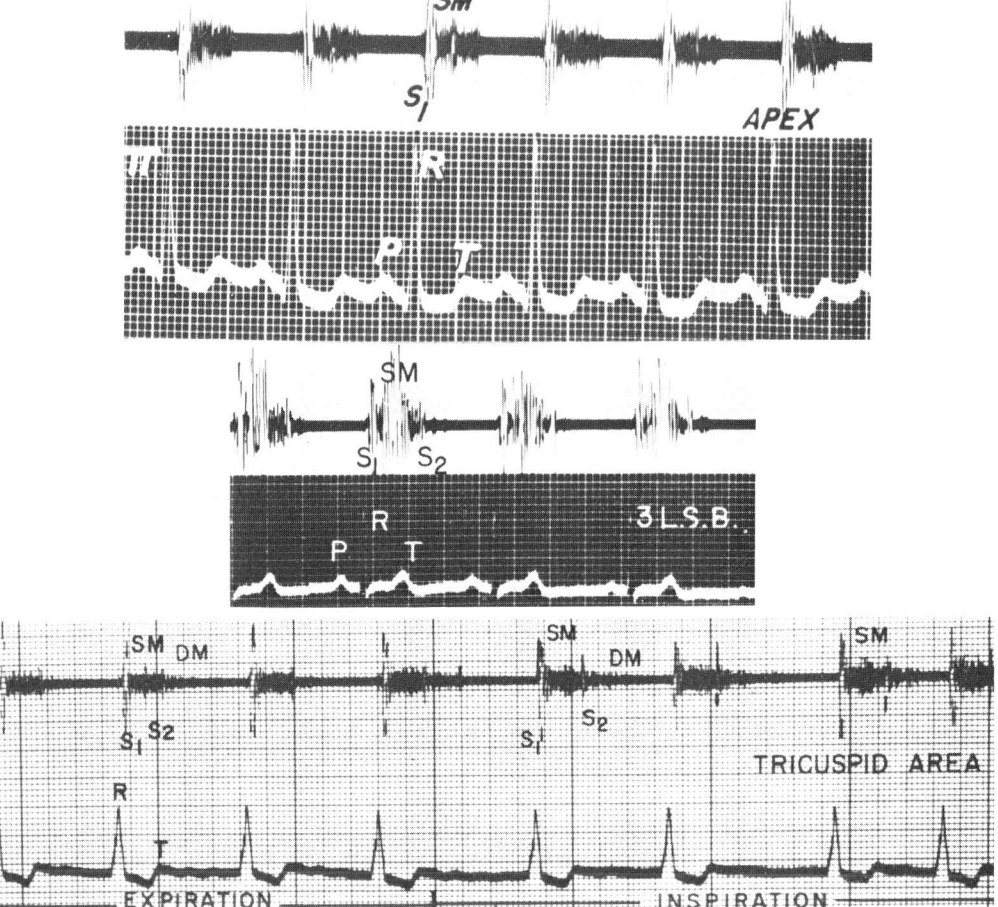

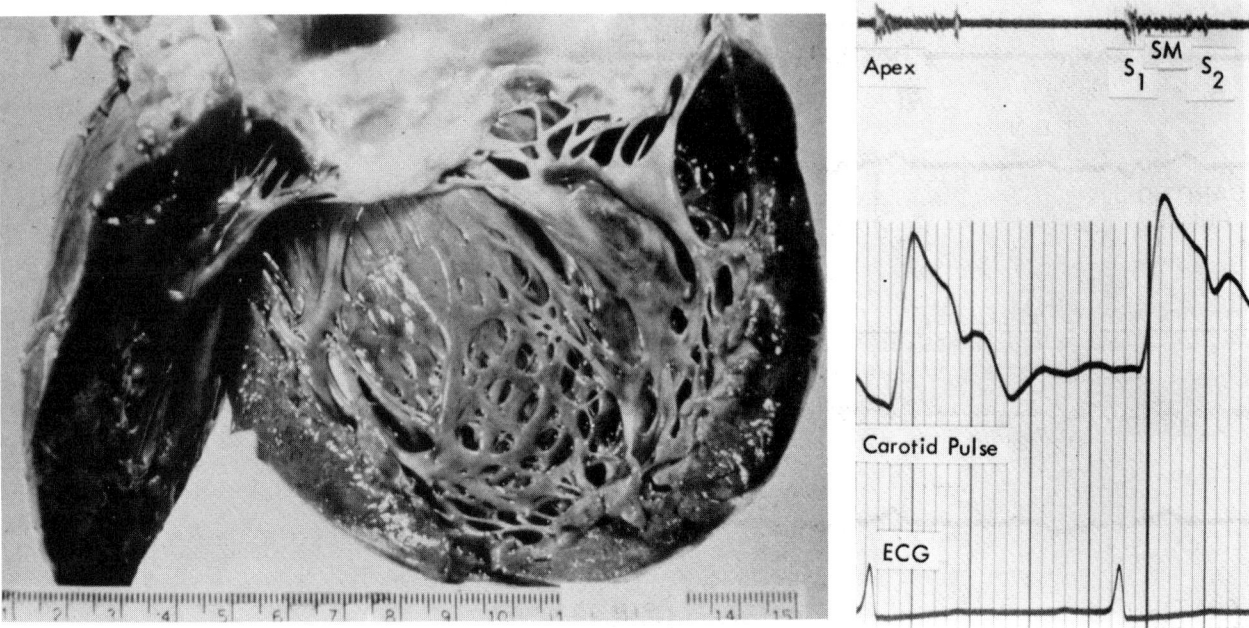

FIGURE 12-51 Posterolateral myocardial infarction with involvement of papillary muscle (left), resulting in apical systolic murmur of mitral insufficiency (right).

FIGURE 12-52 *Top.* Mitral stenosis. Loud first sound (S₁); diastolic rumble with presystolic crescendo. *Middle.* Severe mitral regurgitation with loud S₃ followed by middiastolic flow rumble. *Bottom.* Severe aortic insufficiency with apical diastolic rumble (Austin Flint) mimicking mitral stenosis.

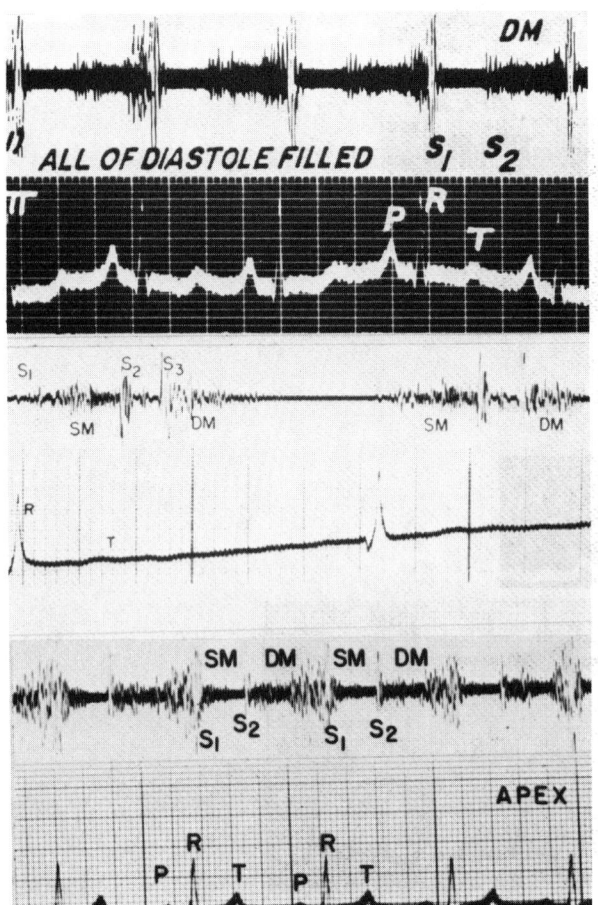

Tricuspid Diastolic Murmurs   Like its mitral valve counterpart, these murmurs are of low frequency but differ in that they are usually best heard at the lower left sternal border (vs. the apex for mitral murmurs) and may selectively increase in intensity with respiration.[98] A murmur caused by an increased volume of blood flow without valve obstruction occurs with a large left-to-right shunt in *atrial septal defect* and *tricuspid valve regurgitation*. Tricuspid stenosis also results in a diastolic rumbling murmur which can have a late diastolic (presystolic) crescendo-decrescendo component as a result of right atrial systole (Fig. 12-53).

Diastolic Murmurs across the Semilunar Valves

Aortic Valve Regurgitation   The murmur of aortic regurgitation begins immediately after the aortic valve closure sound (A₂) and typically is of high frequency with a decrescendo configuration. It is usually best heard along the left sternal border but may also be noted at the second right interspace and cardiac apex. In cases due to dilatation or aneurysm of the ascending aorta, the diastolic murmur may be louder at the right second, third, and fourth interspaces compared with the left (Fig. 12-54).[99]

With significant aortic regurgitation, a medium- to low-frequency, blubbery type of diastolic murmur with or without presystolic crescendo may be noted at the cardiac apex (Austin Flint murmur) (Fig. 12-55).

Pulmonary Valve Regurgitation   The murmur of *pulmonary valve regurgitation* in the presence of *pulmonary hypertension* results in a high-frequency, decrescendo diastolic murmur starting from the pul-

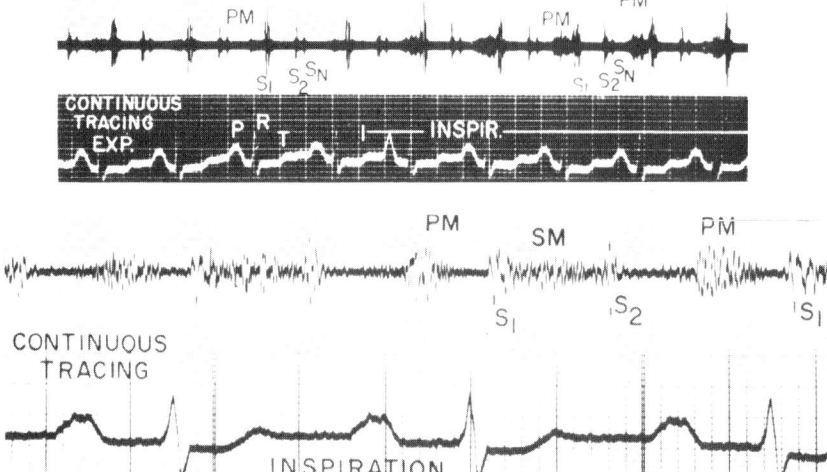

FIGURE 12-53 *Top.* Tricuspid stenosis with inspiratory increase of presystolic murmur. *Bottom.* Tricuspid stenosis and insufficiency with 1° AV block showing presystolic murmur during atrial systole well before S₁.

monic valve closure sound (P₂) and best heard along the second and third left sternal border (Graham Steell murmur) (Fig. 12-56). It may also show a selective inspiratory increase in intensity.

Low-pressure pulmonary valve regurgitation results in a low- or medium-pitched murmur. Often, the onset is at some interval after the pulmonic valve closure (P₂), resulting in the middiastolic rather than early diastolic murmur. In some cases, the murmur starts just after the pulmonic valve closure (P₂), but the low-frequency characteristic of the murmur makes it distinctive.[88]

Continuous Murmurs

Murmurs which extend from systole into diastole, thus going beyond the second heart sound, are called *continuous murmurs*. For such a murmur to occur, blood flow must be able to continue from a high pressure to a lower pressure area despite semilunar valve closure. Thus, the location or source of the murmur determines to a large extent whether the murmur itself peaks in intensity in systole, at the second heart sound, or in diastole.

Patent ductus arteriosus is the prototype of an entity causing a continuous murmur that peaks at the second heart sound (Fig. 12-57). Usually, it is loudest beneath the left clavicle, and if large, will have sharp sounds (eddy sounds) interspersed within the murmur. When small, it tends to be high-pitched.

Significant systemic arterial stenosis is the prototype of a condition which can result in a continuous murmur that peaks in systole. The greater pressure difference across the obstruction is during systole rather than diastole.

The venous hum is a prototype of a continuous murmur that tends to peak in intensity during diastole. This is so since flow through the internal jugular veins is greatest during diastole (Fig. 12-57). Some continuous murmurs will have two periods of peak intensity, one in systole and another in diastole (Figs. 12-57 and 12-58).

Among the other causes of continuous murmurs are *ruptured sinus of Valsalva aneurysm into the right heart, coronary arteriovenous fistula, pulmonary arteriovenous fistulas, systemic arteriovenous fistulas, some cases of branch stenosis of the pulmonary artery, collaterals (such as in coarctation of the aorta) and surgically induced shunts such as the Blalock-Taussig anastomosis, Waterston shunt, and the arteriovenous shunt for renal hemodialysis.*

The Grading of Murmurs

The most commonly utilized method of grading the intensity of murmurs is based upon the recommendation of Levine.[48] Murmur intensity is divided into six grades:

Grade 1 is a faint murmur heard only after a period of concentration or "tuning in."

Grade 2 is a faint murmur heard immediately on auscultation.

Grade 3 is a moderate-intensity murmur.

Grade 4 is a loud murmur associated with a thrill.

Grade 5 is a loud murmur, but it cannot be heard unless the stethoscope is touching the chest wall.

Grade 6 is a loud murmur which can be heard with the entire stethoscope chest piece held off the chest wall.

Aids to Auscultation

Cycle Length

The ejection systolic murmur caused by obstruction to the right or left ventricular outflow tract (with intact interventricular septum) increases in intensity after a long diastolic filling period. Thus, in the beat following a premature beat with a compensatory pause, the murmur increases in intensity. This can be useful in distinguishing a long ejection systolic

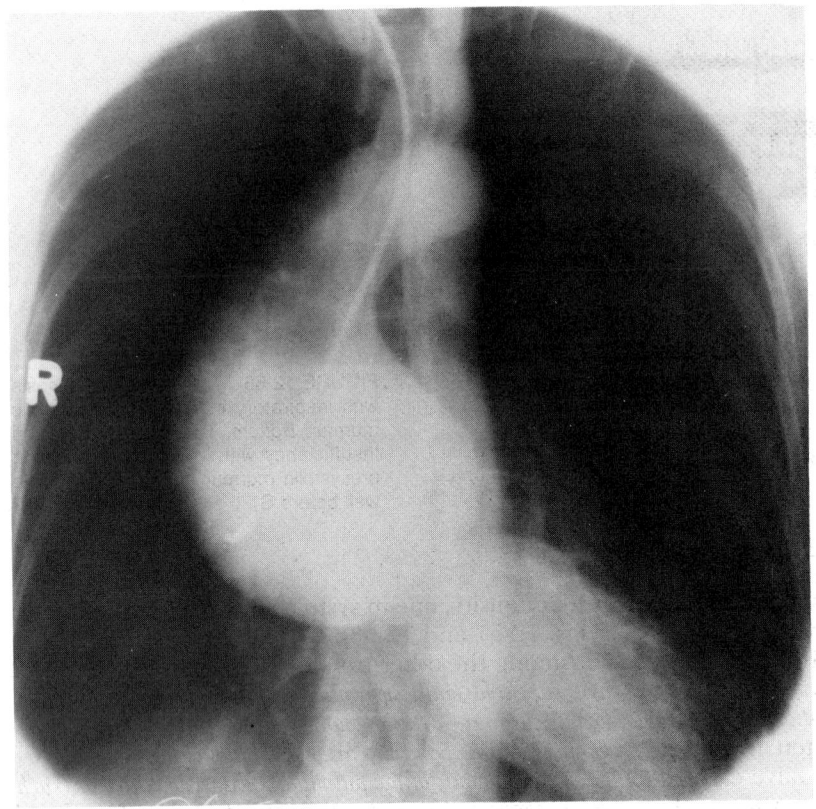

A

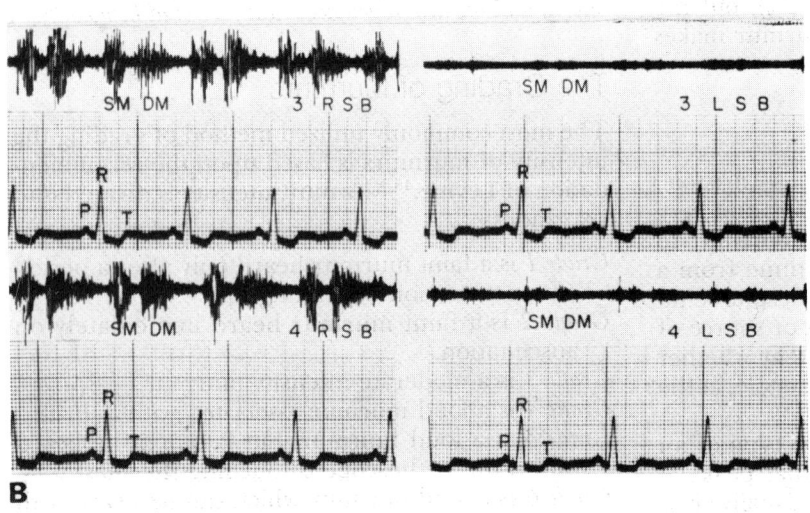

B

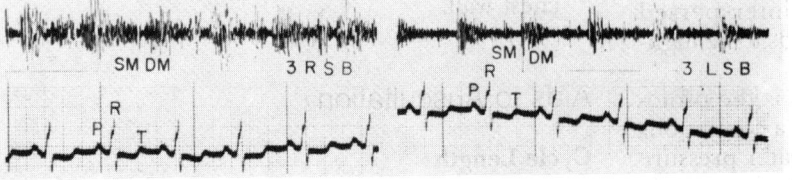

FIGURE 12-54 *A.* Aneurysm of sinus of Valsalva with severe aortic regurgitation murmurs, best heard along right sternal border. *B.* Dissectng aneurysm, first portion of ascending aorta.

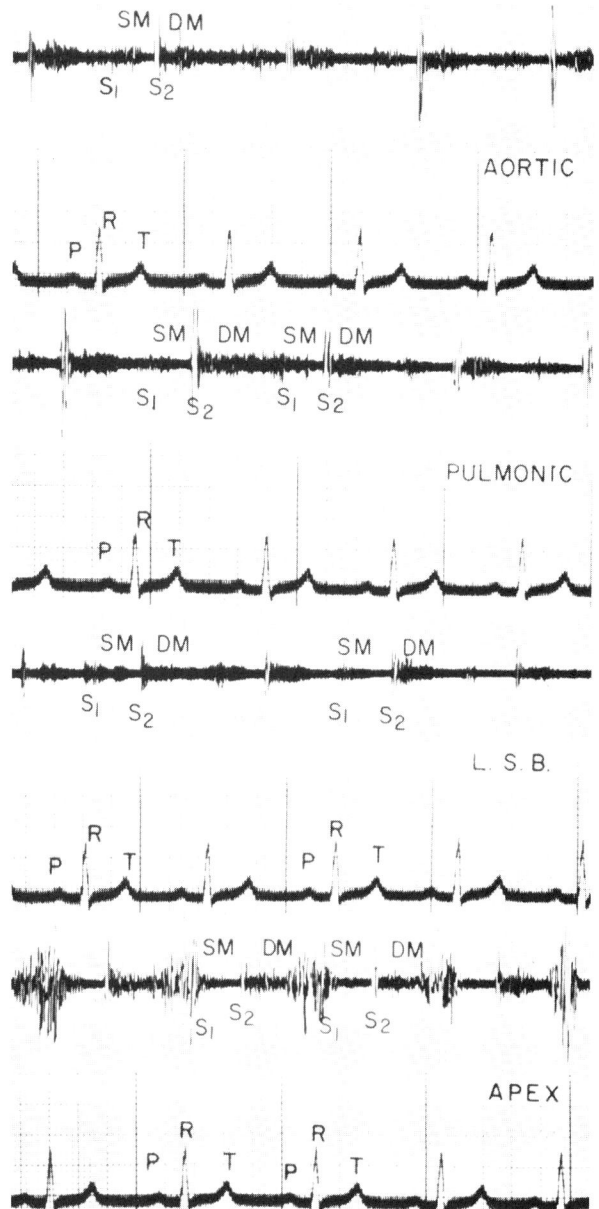

FIGURE 12-55 Phonocardiogram of a patient with severe aortic insufficiency showing a diastolic rumble (Austin Flint) at apex.

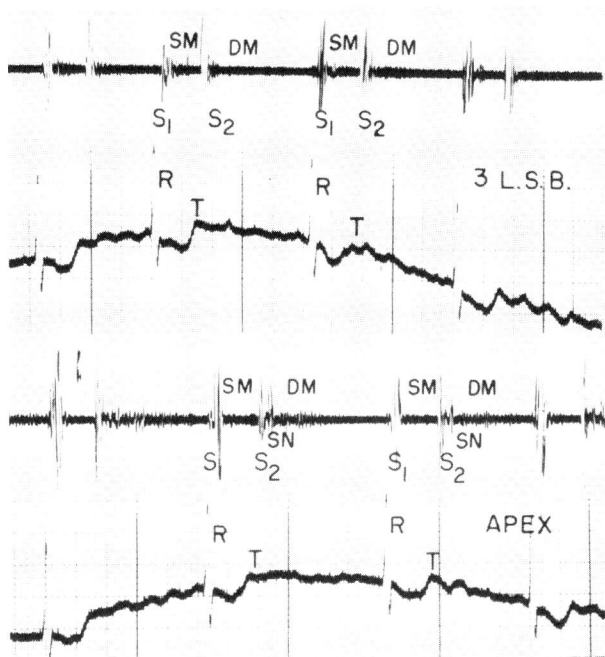

FIGURE 12-56 Graham Steell murmur, mitral stenosis.

murmur (especially when loudest at the cardiac apex) from a holosystolic or regurgitant murmur. The latter does not appreciably change in intensity following a premature beat.

Valsalva Maneuver[100]

A sustained Valsalva maneuver causes a decrease in venous return, a fall in systemic arterial pressure, and a small ventricular volume (phase 2 of the maneuver). Hence, such a maneuver results in intensification of the murmur of hypertrophic subaortic stenosis, and can also bring out a late systolic murmur or convert one into a holosystolic murmur in mitral valve prolapse.

Isometric Handgrip

This maneuver results in the elevation of systemic resistance and blood pressure. Thus, in hypertrophic subaortic stenosis, the murmur may diminish in intensity. The diastolic murmur of aortic regurgitation increases, and the click in mitral valve prolapse may occur later in systole.

Prompt Squatting

This maneuver results in an initial increase in venous return and elevation of systemic arterial pressure. Accordingly, the murmur of hypertrophic subaortic stenosis tends to decrease or may be abolished. In some cases of mitral valve prolapse, it also can result in the decrease or abolition of the late systolic murmur. In tetralogy of Fallot, the maneuver results in less right-to-left shunting and thus an increase in the length and intensity of the murmur across the stenotic right ventricular infundibular and/or pulmonary valve.

Pharmacologic Agents[100,101]

Two agents are commonly employed: one is a vasodilator, amyl nitrite; the other is a vasopressor, usually methoxamine or phenylephrine.

Amyl nitrite causes systemic vasodilatation and hence a fall in systemic blood pressure. This is promptly followed by a reflex tachycardia and increased venous return to the right heart. Thus, administration of the drug results in a decrease in intensity of the murmurs of *mitral regurgitation, ventricular septal defect, aortic regurgitation, and the Austin Flint rumble.* Conversely, it results in an *increase in intensity of the murmurs of obstruction to right (intact sep-*

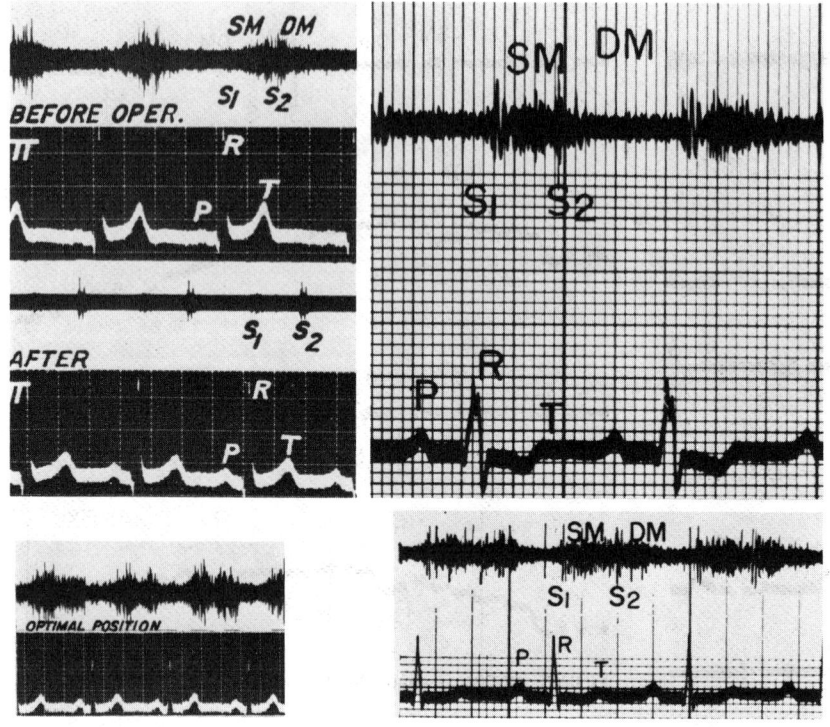

FIGURE 12-57 *Top left.* Patent ductus arteriosus. Continuous murmur peaking at the second sound (before) absent postoperatively (after). *Top right.* Pulmonary emboli producing occlusive pulmonary artery disease and resulting in a continuous murmur which peaks in systole. *Bottom left.* Venous hum. Continuous murmur peaking in systole and diastole. *Bottom right.* Coronary arteriovenous fistula; continuous murmur peaks both in systole and diastole.

FIGURE 12-58 Systolic and diastolic murmur of ventricular septal defect and aortic insufficiency (top) may be mistaken for the continuous murmur of patent ductus arteriosus (middle) and arteriovenous fistula (bottom).

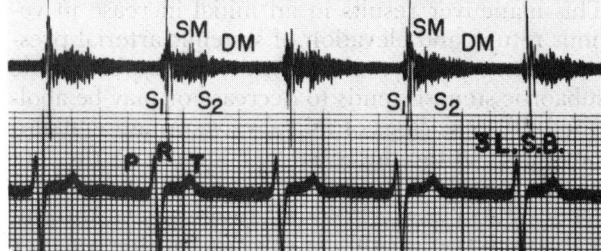

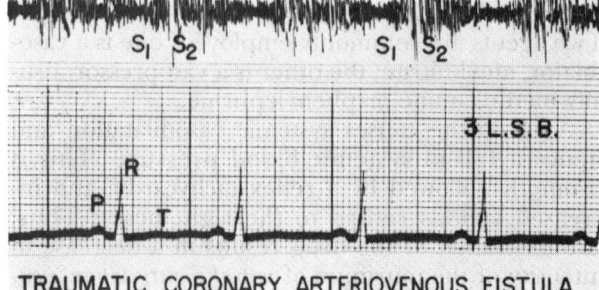

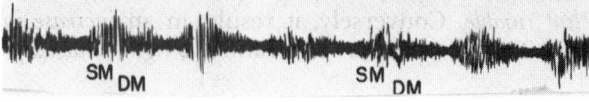

tum) and left ventricular outflow (IHSS and aortic stenosis), tricuspid stenosis and regurgitation, and mitral stenosis.

Drugs, such as methoxamine and phenylephrine, have an effect that is opposite to that caused by amyl nitrite inhalation and is similar to that obtained by a properly performed isometric handgrip or prompt squatting.

References

1. Laennec, R. T. H.: "Traité de l'auscultation médiate," 2d ed., Brosson et Chaude, Paris, 1826, vol. 1, p. 5.
2. McKusick, V. A.: "Cardiovascular Sound in Health and Disease," The Williams & Wilkins Company, Baltimore, 1958.
3. Rouanet, J.: Analyse des bruits de coeur, Thesis 252, Paris, 1832.
4. Dock, W.: Mode of Production of First Heart Sound, *Arch. Intern. Med.,* 50:737, 1933.
5. Luisada, A., MacCanon, D. M., Kumar, S., et al.: Changing Views on the Mechanism of the First and Second Heart Sounds, *Am. Heart J.,* 88:503, 1974.
6. Mills, P. G., Chamusco, R., Moos, S., et al.: Echophonocardiographic Studies of the Contribution of the Atrioventricular Valves to the First Heart Sound, *Circulation,* 54:944, 1976.
7. Leech, G., and Leatham, A.: Correlation of Heart Sounds and Valve Motion, in P. Hanrath and D. Mathey (eds.), "Evaluation of Cardiac Dynamics by Ultrasound," Springer, Berlin, 1980.
8. Zalter, R., Hardy, H. C., and Luisada, A.: Acoustic

Transmission Characteristics of the Thorax, *J. Appl. Physiol.*, 18:428, 1963.

9. Ertel, P. Y., Lawrence, M., Brown, R. K., et al.: Stethoscope Acoustics. I. The Doctor and His Stethoscope, *Circulation*, 34:889, 1966.

10. Ertel, P. Y., Lawrence, M., Brown, R. K., and Stern, A. M.: Stethoscope Acoustics. II. Transmission and Filtration Patterns, *Circulation*, 34:899, 1966.

11. Leatham, A.: Splitting of the First and Second Heart Sounds, *Lancet*, 2:607, 1954.

12. Haber, E., and Leatham, A.: Splitting of Heart Sounds from Ventricular Asynchrony in Bundle Branch Block, Ventricular Ectopic Beats, and Artificial Pacing, *Br. Heart J.*, 27:691, 1965.

13. Luisada, A. A.: Tricuspid Component of the First Heart Sound, in D. F. Leon and J. A. Shaver (eds)., "Physiologic Principles of Heart Sounds and Murmurs," American Heart Association, New York, 1975, p. 19.

14. Leatham, A., and Leech, G.: Observations on the Relationship between Heart Sounds and Valve Movements by Simultaneous Echo and Phonocardiography, *Br. Heart J.*, 37:557, 1975. (Abstract.)

15. Waider, W., and Craige, E.: First Heart Sound and Ejection Sounds: Echocardiographic and Phonocardiographic Correlation with Valvular Events, *Am. J. Cardiol.*, 35:3, 1975.

*16. Leatham, A.: "Auscultation of the Heart and Phonocardiography," 2d ed., J. & A. Churchill, Ltd., London, 1975. (Extensively referenced)

17. Braunwald, E., Fishman, A., and Cournand, A.: Time Relationship of Dynamic Events in the Cardiac Chambers, Pulmonary Artery and Aorta in Man, *Circ. Res.*, 4:100, 1956.

18. Crews, T., Pridie, R., Benham, R., and Leatham, A.: Auscultatory and Phonocardiographic Findings in Ebstein's Anomaly: Correlation of First Heart Sound with Ultrasonic Recordings of Tricuspid Valve Movement, *Br. Heart J.*, 34:681, 1972.

19. Brooks, N., Leech, G., and Leatham, A.: Factors Responsible for Normal Splitting of First Heart Sound. High Speed Echophonocardiographic Study of Valve Movement, *Br. Heart J.*, 42:695, 1979.

20. Brooks, N., Leech, G., and Leatham, A.: Complete Right Bundle Branch Block. Echophonocardiographic Study of First Heart Sound and Right Ventricular Contraction Times, *Br. Heart J.*, 41:637, 1979.

21. Harris, A.: Pacemaker "Heart Sound," *Br. Heart J.*, 29:608, 1967.

22. Wolferth, C., and Margolies, A.: Certain Effects of Auricular Systole and the Prematurity of Beat on the Intensity of the First Heart Sound, *Trans. Assoc. Am. Physicians*, 45:44, 1930.

23. Levine, S., and Harvey, W.: Clinical Auscultation of the Heart, W. B. Saunders Company, Philadelphia, 1949.

24. Shah, P., Kramer, D., and Gramiak, R.: Influence of the Timing of Atrial Systole on Mitral Valve Closure and on the First Heart Sound in Man, *Am. J. Cardiol.*, 26:231, 1970.

25. Burgraaf, G. W., and Craige, E.: The First Heart

Sound in Complete Heart Block: Phonoechocardiographic Correlations, *Circulation*, 50:17, 1974.

26. Leech, G., Brooks, N., Green-Wilkinson, A., and Leatham, A.: Mechanism of Influence of PR Interval on Loudness of First Heart Sound, *Br. Heart J.*, 43: 138, 1980.

27. Leatham, A., and Gray, I.: Auscultatory and Phonocardiographic Signs of Atrial Septal Defect, *Br. Heart J.*, 18:193, 1956.

28. Weiss, O., and Joachim, G.: Registrierung von Herztonen und Herzgeraischen mittels des Phonoskops und ihre Beziehungen zum Elektrokardiogramm, *A. klin Med.*, 73:240, 1911.

29. Potain, C.: Note sur les dédoublements normales des bruits du coeur, *Bull. Soc. Méd. Hôp. Paris.* ser. 2, 3:138, 1866.

30. Leatham, A., and Towers, M.: Splitting of the Second Heart Sound in Health, *Br. Heart J.*, 13:575, 1951.

31. Boyer, S. H., and Chisholm, A. W.: Physiologic Splitting of the Second Heart Sound, *Circulation*, 18:1010, 1958.

32. Castle, F. R., and Jones, K. L.: The Mechanism of Respiratory Variations in Splitting of the Second Heart Sound, *Circulation*, 24:180, 1961.

33. Dornhorst, A. C., Howard, P., and Leathart, G. L.: Respiratory Variations in Blood Pressure, *Circulation*, 6:553, 1952.

34. Shafter, H. A.: Splitting of the Second Heart Sound, *Am. J. Cardiol.*, 6:1013, 1960.

*35. Leatham, A., Segal, B., and Shafter, H.: Auscultatory and Phonocardiographic Findings in Healthy Children with Systolic Murmurs, *Br. Heart J.*, 4:451, 1963. (27 references)

36. Beck, W., Schrire, V., and Vogelpoel, L.: Splitting of the Second Heart Sound in Constrictive Pericarditis, with Observations on the Mechanism of Pulsus Paradoxus, *Am. Heart J.*, 64:765, 1962.

*37. Sutton, G., Harris, A., and Leatham, A.: Second Heart Sound in Pulmonary Hypertension, *Br. Heart J.*, 30:743, 1968. (21 references)

*38. Leatham, A., and Weitzman, D. W.: Auscultatory and Phonocardiographic Signs of Pulmonary Stenosis, *Br. Heart J.*, 19:303, 1957. (20 references)

39. Tofler, O. B.: The Pulmonary Component of the Second Heart Sound in Fallot's Tetralogy, *Br. Heart J.*, 25:509, 1963.

40. Schrire, V., and Vogelpoel, L.: The Role of the Dilated Pulmonary Artery in Abnormal Splitting of the Second Heart Sound, *Am. Heart J.*, 63:501, 1962.

41. Brigden, W., and Leatham, A.: Mitral Incompetence, *Br. Heart J.*, 15:55, 1953.

*42. Gray, I.: Paradoxical Splitting of the Second Heart Sound, *Br. Heart J.*, 18:21, 1956. (9 references)

43. Yurchak, P. M., and Gorlin, R.: Paradoxical Splitting of the Second Heart Sound in Coronary Heart Disease, *N. Engl. J. Med.*, 269:741, 1963.

44. Craige, E., and Harned, H. S.: Phonocardiographic and Electrocardiographic Studies in Normal Newborn Infants, *Am. Heart J.*, 65:180, 1963.

*45. Harris, A., and Sutton, G.: Second Heart Sound in Normal Subjects, *Br. Heart J.*, 30:739, 1968. (15 references)

46. Wood, P.: The Eisenmenger Syndrome or Pulmonary Hypertension with Reversed Central Shunt, *Br. Med. J.*, 2:701. 1958.

*This article is a review of the literature and contains additional references to the literature.

47. Potain, Pierre C.: Du rhythme cardiaque appelé bruit de gallop, in A. Ruskin (ed.), "Classics in Arterial Hypertension," Charles C Thomas, Publisher, Springfield, Ill., 1956. (Reference, courtesy of Dr. Robert C. Tarazi.)

*48. Levine, S. A., and Harvey, W. P.: "Clinical Auscultation of the Heart," 2d ed., W. B. Saunders Company, Philadelphia, 1959. (Extensively referenced)

49. Harvey, W. P., and Stapleton, J.: Clinical Aspects of Gallop Rhythm with Particular Reference to Diastolic Gallops, *Circulation*, 18:5, 1017, 1958.

50. Leonard, J. J., Weissler, D. M., and Warren, J. V.: Observations on the Mechanism of Atrial Gallop Rhythm, *Circulation*, 17:1007, 1958.

51. Hill, J. L., O'Rourke, R. A., Lewis, R. P., and McGranahan, G. M.: The Diagnostic Value of the Atrial Gallop in Acute Myocardial Infarction, *Am. Heart J.*, 78:194, 1969.

52. Harvey, W. P., Segal, J. P., and Gurel, T.: The Clinical Spectrum of Primary Myocardial Disease, *Prog. Cardiovasc. Dis.*, 7:17, 1964.

53. Goldblatt, A., Aygen, M. M., and Braunwald, E.: Hemodynamic-Phonocardiographic Correlations of the Fourth Heart Sound in Aortic Stenosis, *Circulation*, 26:92, 1962.

54. Caulfield, W. H., de Leon, A. C., Perloff, J. K., and Steelman, R. B.: The Clinical Significance of the Fourth Heart Sound in Aortic Stenosis, *Am. J. Cardiol.*, 28:179, 1971.

*55. Perloff, J. K.: Recognition and Differential Diagnosis of Pulmonary Stenosis, in B. L. Segal (ed.), "The Theory and Practice of Auscultation," F. A. Davis Company, Philadelphia, 1959. (Extensively referenced)

56. Leatham, A.: Auscultation of the Heart, *Lancet*, 2:793, 1958.

57. Hultgren, H. N., Reeve, R., Cohn, K., and McLeod, R.: The Ejection Click of Valvular Pulmonic Stenosis, *Circulation*, 40:631, 1969.

58. Reeve, R.: Variations of the Ejection Click in Valvular Pulmonic Stenosis, *Clin. Res.*, 14:129, 1966. (Abstract.)

59. Leatham, A., and Vogelpoel, L.: The Early Systolic Sound in Dilatation of the Pulmonary Artery, *Br. Heart J.*, 16:21, 1954.

60. Hancock, E. W.: Origin of the Ejection Sound in Aortic Stenosis, *Clin. Res.*, 13:209, 1965.

61. LeBauer, E. J., Perloff, J. K., and Keliher, T. F.: Isolated Systolic Click with Bacterial Endocarditis, *Am. Heart J.*, 73:534, 1967.

62. Humphries, J. O., and McKusick, V. A.: Differentiation of Organic and "Innocent" Systolic Murmurs, *Prog. Cardiovasc. Dis.*, 5:152, 1962.

63. Leon, D. F., Leonard, J. J., Kroetz, F. W., Page, W. L., Shaver, J. A., and Lancaster, J. F.: Late Systolic Murmurs, Clicks, and Whoops Arising from the Mitral Valve: Transseptal Intracardiac Phonocardiographic Analysis, *Am. Heart J.*, 72:325, 1966.

64. Ronan, J. A., Perloff, J. K., and Harvey, W. P.: Systolic Clicks and the Late Systolic Murmur: Intracardiac Phonocardiographic Evidence of Their Mitral Valve Origin, *Am. Heart J.*, 70:319, 1965.

65. Barlow, J. B., and Bosman, C. K.: Aneurysmal Protrusion of the Posterior Leaflet of the Mitral Valve: An Auscultatory-Electrocardiographic Syndrome, *Am. Heart J.*, 71:166, 1966.

66. Harvey, W. P.: Some Newer or Poorly Recognized Findings on Clinical Auscultation, *Mod. Concepts Cardiovasc. Dis.*, 37:85, 1968.

*67. Lachman, A. S., Bramwell-Jones, D. M., Lakier, J. B., Pocock, W. A., and Barlow, J. B.: Infective Endocarditis in the Billowing Mitral Leaflet Syndrome, *Br. Heart J.*, 37:326, 1975. (34 references)

68. Harvey, W. P., and Capone, M. A.: Bacterial Endocarditis Related to Cleaning and Filling of Teeth: With Particular Reference to the Inadequacy of Present-Day Knowledge and Practice of Antibiotic Prophylaxis for All Dental Procedures, *Am. J. Cardiol.*, 8:793, 1961.

69. Rackley, C. E., Whalen, R. E., Floyd, W. L., Orgain, E. S., and McIntosh, H. D.: Precordial Honk, *Am. J. Cardiol.*, 17:609, 1966.

70. Behar, V. S., Whalen, R. E., and McIntosh, H. D.: Ballooning Mitral Valve in Patients with the "Precordial Honk" or "Whoop," *Am. J. Cardiol.*, 20:789, 1967.

71. Mounsey, P.: The Early Diastolic Sound of Constrictive Pericarditis, *Br. Heart J.*, 17:143, 1955.

72. Dayem, M. K. A., Wasfi, R. M., Bentall, H. H., Goodwin, J. F., and Cleland, W. P.: Investigation and Treatment of Constrictive Pericarditis, *Thorax*, 22:242, 1967.

73. Dayem, M. K. A., and Raftery, E. B.: Phonocardiogram of the Ball-and-Cage Aortic Valve Prosthesis, *Br. Heart J.*, 29:446, 1967.

74. Leachman, R. D., and Cokkinos, D. V. P.: Absence of Opening Click in Dehiscence of Mitral Valve Prosthesis, *N. Engl. J. Med.*, 281:461, 1969.

75. Kramer, D. H., Moss, A. J., and Shah, P. M.: Mechanisms and Significance of Pacemaker-Induced Extracardiac Sound, *Am. J. Cardiol.*, 25:367, 1970.

*76. Sabbah, H. N., and Stein, P. D.: Turbulent Flow in Humans: Its Primary Role in the Production of Ejection Murmurs, *Circ. Res.*, 38:513, 1976. (32 references)

77. Leatham, A.: A Classification of Systolic Murmurs, *Br. Heart J.*, 17:574, 1955.

78. Lewis, D. H.: "Phonocardiography: Handbook of Physiology," sec. 2: "Circulation," vol. 1, chap. 22. American Physiologic Society, Washington, D. C., 1962.

79. de Leon, A. C., Perloff, J. K., Twigg, H., and Majd, M.: The Straight Back Syndrome, *Circulation*, 32:193, 1965.

80. Stein, P. D., and Sabbah, H. N.: Aortic Origin of Innocent Murmurs, *Am. J. Cardiol.*, 39:665, 1977.

81. Wennevold, A.: The Origin of the Innocent "Vibratory" Murmur Studied with Intracardiac Phonocardiography, *Acta Med. Scand.*, 181:1, 1967.

82. Fowler, N. O., and Marshall, W. S.: The Supraclavicular Arterial Bruit, *Am. Heart J.*, 69:410, 1965.

83. Vogelpoel, L., and Schrire, V.: Auscultatory and Phonocardiographic Assessment of Pulmonary Stenosis with Intact Ventricular Septum, *Circulation*, 22:55, 1960.

84. Gamboa, R., Hugenholtz, P. E., and Nados, A. S.: Accuracy of the Phonocardiogram in Assessing Severity of Aortic and Pulmonic Stenosis, *Circulation*, 30:35, 1964.

85. Vogelpoel, L., and Schrire, V.: Auscultatory and Phonocardiographic Assessment of Fallot's Tetralogy, *Circulation*, 22:73, 1960.

86. Barber, J. M., Magidson, O., and Wood, P.: Atrial Septal Defect with Special Reference to Electrocardiogram, Pulmonary Artery Pressure, and Second Heart Sound, *Br. Heart J.*, 12:277, 1950.

87. Deshomukh, M., Guvenc, S., Bartivoglio, L., and Goldberg, H.: Idiopathic Dilation of the Pulmonary Artery, *Circulation*, 27:710, 1960.

88. Criscitiello, M. G., and Harvey, W. P.: Clinical Recognition of Congenital Pulmonary Valve Insufficiency, *Am. J. Cardiol.*, 20:765. 1967.

89. D'Cruz, I. A., Agustsson, M. H., Bicoff, J. P., Weinberg, Jr., M., and Arcilla, R. A.: Stenotic Lesions of the Pulmonary Arteries, *Am. J. Cardiol.*, 13:441, 1964.

90. Perloff, J. K., Caulfield, W. H., and de Leon, A. C.: Peripheral Pulmonary Artery Murmur of Atrial Septal Defect, *Br. Heart J.*, 29:411, 1967.

91. Oakley, C. M., and Hallidic-Smith, K. A.: Assessment of Site and Severity in Congenital Aortic Stenosis, *Br. Heart J.*, 29:367, 1967.

92. Ronan, Jr., J. A., Steelman, R. B., de Leon, Jr., A. C., Waters, T. J., Perloff, J. K., and Harvey, W. P.: The Clinical Diagnosis of Acute Severe Mitral Insufficiency, *Am. J. Cardiol.*, 27:284, 1971.

93. Barlow, J. B., Bosman, C. K., Pocock, W. A., and Marchand, P.: Late Systolic Murmurs and Nonejection (Mid-Late) Systolic Clicks, *Br. Heart J.*, 30:203, 1968.

94. Burch, G. E., DePasquale, N. P., and Phillips, J. H.: The Syndrome of Papillary Muscle Dysfunction, *Am. Heart J.*, 75:399, 1968.

95. Perloff, J. K.: Auscultatory and Phonocardiographic Manifestations of Pulmonary Hypertension, *Prog. Cardiovasc. Dis.*, 9:303, 1967.

96. Nadas, A. S., Scott, L. P., Hauck, A. J., and Rudolph, A. M.: Spontaneous Functional Closure of Ventricular Septal Defects, *N. Engl. J. Med.*, 264:309, 1961.

*97. Wood, P.: An Appreciation of Mitral Stenosis, *Br. Med. J.*, 1:1051, 1954. (26 references)

98. Perloff, J. K., and Harvey, W. P.: Clinical Recognition of Tricuspid Stenosis, *Circulation*, 22:346, 1960.

99. Harvey, W. P., Corrado, M. A., and Perloff, J. K.: "Right-Sided" Murmurs of Aortic Insufficiency, *Am. J. Med. Sci.*, 245:533, 1963.

*100. Dohan, M. C., and Criscitiello, M. G.: Physiological and Pharmacological Manipulations of Heart Sounds and Murmurs, *Mod. Concepts Cardiovasc. Dis.*, 39:121, 1970. (15 references)

101. de Leon, Jr., A. C., and Harvey, W. P.: Pharmacologic Agents and Auscultation, *Mod. Concepts Cardiovasc. Dis.*, 44:23, 1975.

13

Examination of the Retina

W. Banks Anderson, Jr., M.D.

The study of retinal changes associated with vascular disease is of unusual importance, interest and difficulty. Of importance, because of the unique opportunities offered in the eye of observing . . . the intimate changes in the vascular tree. Of interest, because many of the most fascinating and complicated problems in medicine are bound up in the derangements of the cardiovascular system. . . . Of difficulty, because today, after more than a century of research and study, we are still far from possessing the plan of the maze into which the search for ultimate causes of these extremely common problems had led us.

Sir Stewart Duke-Elder[1]

Inspection of the smaller vessels of the body is possible in only three areas: the retina, the conjunctiva, and the nail beds. Helmholtz's gift of the ophthalmoscope has made the retina by far the easiest and most rewarding of these observation sites. Viewing this two-dimensional vascular display is generally much easier, especially in the aged, if the pupils are dilated. One drop of tropicamide 1% ophthalmic solution (Mydriacyl) will dilate the pupils in 15 or 20 min. Care should be taken to make pulse and blood pressure determinations prior to instillation of such rapidly acting mydriatics as both the pulse and the blood pressure may increase after absorption of the drops. Although complications of mydriasis are rare, patients in whom the iris seems closely apposed to the cornea or those with a history of closed-angle glaucoma are best left undilated.

Examination of the retina should proceed methodically. Best pupillary dilation is maintained if the optic disk is observed first. Look for evidence of edema and blurred margins and for cupping with sharp contours. Rule out neovascularization or the pallor of optic atrophy. Next scan along the superior temporal arcade, inspecting the arteries carefully for embolic plaques at each bifurcation. Note the arteriovenous crossings for evidence of obscuration of the vein and for pronounced nicking and banking of the vessels. The lower arcade and the nasal vessels may be inspected next. Avoid the macular area until all else has been viewed, as the pupil constricts most intensely when this area is illuminated. To find diabetic microaneurysms early, look just temporal to the fovea along the horizontal raphe. To discover cotton-wool infarcts, look circularly around the disk two disk diameters out. With such a plan in mind the retina can be efficiently searched for evidence of cardiovascular disease.

An appreciation of the pathophysiological variations in retinal architecture is essential for recognizing its disease processes. The following sections describe morphologic changes helpful in assessing the cardiac patient.

Retinal Vessel Caliber Changes

Caliber changes along the course of a single artery or vein are of much greater significance than are estimates of arteriovenous ratios or absolute vascular diameter. Estimates of the degree of tortuosity or straightening are also generally valueless, except in the situation where the veins are large, dark, and tortuous. This constellation of findings implies outflow obstruction, arterial inflow obstruction, hypoxia, or all three. Such dark and dilated veins may occur in patients with large left-to-right shunts and in the leukemias and hyperviscosity syndromes.

Autonomic innervation of the retinal vessels does not exist.[2] Nevertheless the retinal vessels may change in caliber both acutely and chronically. Autoregulation of the retinal vessels does occur, and oxygen is the most active vasomotor substance. With hyperoxia there is rapid constriction of both the arteries and veins, while in hypoxia vasodilatation occurs.[3] Elevated carbon dioxide tension is also a retinal vasodilator.[4] A striking clinical example of these combined effects is the vasodilatation, darkening of the blood column, and retinal and disk edema seen in patients with marked pulmonary insufficiency and right-sided cardiac failure.[5] At the opposite extreme the marked vasoconstrictor effect of oxygen may produce retinal vasoobliteration in immature infants with resulting retrolental fibroplasia.

Estimates of arteriovenous ratios are of little clinical utility.[6] Of much greater significance are variations in the caliber of a single vessel. These changes may take the form of focal narrowing, sometimes called *beading* or *spasm*. Beading is produced by an abnormal constriction which may be contiguous with an abnormally dilated segment. Usually seen in the venous system where there is venous outflow obstruction, such beading is particularly common in diabetic retinopathy. Beading of the arteries is *not* generally associated with systemic disease but is seen in congenital conditions such as von Hippel angiomatosis, Coats's disease, and Leber's miliary aneurysms.

Segmental narrowing or spasm of the retinal vessels has been much described in the older literature. Most descriptions of rapid waves of "spasm" were probably observations of patients with moving fibrin or platelet emboli. Narrowing of the retinal vessels has been observed in response to injections of norepinephrine and angiotensin.[7] Autoregulatory narrowing of the retinal vessels is a response to hypertension, and upon occasion may be focal. This narrowing is chronic, and *spasm* is not an apt description.

Vascular Wall Thickening

Normally only the blood column is visible when the retinal vessels are viewed. When changes in the walls do occur, they are most visible along the sides of the vessels since in this location the tangential line of sight presents a greater thickness to the viewer. Vessels at the disk often appear sheathed. This normal variant may be associated with a veil of tissue in front of the disk (Bergmeister's papilla). More peripheral retinal vessels become sheathed or cuffed in response to intraocular inflammation, vasculitis, or multiple sclerosis. Fatty exudate (hard exudate) may collect along venous walls (never arteries), particularly in diabetic exudative retinopathy. These deposits are not intrinsic to the wall itself. After venous obstructive disease of some duration, a white uniform line may develop along either side of the retinal veins in the involved area. Ballantyne terms this *halo sheathing*,[8] and Kennedy and Wise have found it to consist of increased collagen deposition in the vessel wall.[9]

Arteriosclerosis

Should the retinal arterial circulation be considered arterial or arteriolar? If one accepts the criteria of Bloom and Fawcett[10] that blood vessels less than 0.3 mm in diameter are arterioles, then all of the retinal arterial circulation may be considered arteriolar. Nevertheless Hogan and Feeney have demonstrated smooth-muscle cells several layers thick in the media of the retinal arterial vessels both posteriorly and in the periphery.[11] These authors suggest that the term *arteriole* be applied only to the smallest precapillary vessels. We will use the term *arteriosclerosis* rather than *arteriolosclerosis* and *artery* rather than *arteriole* without respect to the size of the vessel.

In arteriosclerosis the medial smooth muscle (which may hypertrophy in chronic hypertension) becomes hyalinized with the deposition of collagen. As the wall thickens, the light reflex broadens and the vessel takes on a burnished coppery luster which, with further thickening, may transmute to silver. Obscuration of the venous blood column at arterial crossings is early evidence of this process. Even when the artery walls have become so thick as

TABLE 13-1   Retinal Topography

Finding	Most Common Location
Arteriovenous crossings	Upper temporal quadrant
Cotton-wool spots	Around optic disk
Hard exudates	Between disk and fovea
Microaneurysms	Temporal to fovea
Emboli	Arterial bifurcations
Diabetic new vessels	Nerve head and arcades

to look like "silver wires," flow can ordinarily still be demonstrated by fluorescein angiography.

Arteriovenous Compression

Arteriovenous compression or "nicking" has as its histologic basis the sharing by the artery and vein of a common adventitial sheath at their crossings. Arteriosclerotic thickening impedes venous outflow at these locations with venous tortuosity, engorgement, and darkening of the blood column distal to the compression. Where the vein dives beneath the thick artery wall, sometimes "banking" to intersect at right angles, its blood column is obscured and it appears nicked.

Atherosclerosis

Atherosclerosis or fatty infiltration of the intima was once thought not to occur in the retina. Clinico-pathologic confirmation of retinal atherosclerosis has been obtained.[12] Retinal atheromata have a predilection for the bifurcations and bends within the first two branches of the central retinal artery, appearing as segments of irregular yellowish sheathing and having the crystalline knobbiness of a salted pretzel stick. On occasion the thickening may progress to the point where no blood column is visible, although total obstruction is rare.

Cotton-Wool Spots

Cotton-wool spots are generally a sign of serious systemic disease. They may be seen in patients with severe hypertension, blood dyscrasias, collagen diseases, or hemorrhagic shock. They are almost invariably found within three disk diameters of the optic disk and have a feathery, woolly character because of their anterior involvement of the nerve fiber layer. See Plates 5B and 5C. Cotton-wool spots may at times be confused with persistent myelinization of the nerve fiber layer. Cotton-wool "exudates" are *not* exudates but consist of a cluster of cell-like swollen ends of fragmented axons (cytoid bodies) in an area of edematous retina. They are evanescent and will often disappear in a few weeks, leaving behind no observable trace of their presence. Ischemia is almost certainly the cause of these spots, which may occur secondary to occlusion of peripapillary capillaries or occlusion of a small artery, or secondary to hypoxia. The presence of these cotton-wool spots is usually indicative of serious systemic disease.

Hard Exudates

Hard exudates are most probably edema residues. They occur in situations where the vessels become leaky and, as the more watery component of the extravasation is resorbed, the lipid residue forms hard, yellow, waxy deposits. They may surround the leaking vessel in a circinate ring or may accumulate in the macula, radiating from the fovea in the spokes of a macular "star." Histologically found deep in the retina, these exudates will disappear in some months if the source of the leakage is eliminated. These exudates indicate a loss of vascular wall integrity and are associated with hypertension, diabetes, venous outflow obstruction, and retinal angiomas. They are not ischemic in origin but indicate chronic fluid extravasation and retinal edema.

Microaneurysms

Microaneurysms are not unique to diabetes but occur in many disease states, including retinal venous obstructive disease, sickle-cell disease, the dysproteinemias, Behçet's disease, sarcoidosis, and other forms of uveitis. A common factor in all these conditions seems to be the presence of both retinal hypoxia and viable capillary endothelial cells. Microaneurysms are outpouchings in capillary walls that range in size from 20 to 100 μm. Commonly found adjacent to zones of capillary obliteration or "dropout," it has been suggested that they represent abortive attempts at revascularization of a compromised capillary bed. Their etiology is, however, still unknown.

Neovascularization

Neovascularization also occurs in conditions where microaneurysms are found. The new vessels generally originate from capillaries or from the venous side of the circulation and are associated with greater or lesser degrees of fibrosis. In all cases, however, the new vessels are incorporated in an associated fibrous membrane. Some of the channels appear to function as shunts, and in cases of venous outflow obstruction may serve to bypass the obstructed site. Other neovascular channels branch in a fanlike fashion toward an avascular zone or forward into the vitreous cavity proliferating along a posterior hyaloid membrane. Such a rete mirabile does not appear to have any shunting function and is more suggestive of an attempt at revascularization of an unperfused tissue. Clinically the likelihood of blinding vitreous hemorrhage is greatly increased in the presence of such neovascularization.[13]

Retinal Vessel Leakage

Normally the retinal vessels are permeable only to quite small molecules. This *blood retinal barrier* is analogous to that in the brain and is facilitated by the overlapping of the endothelial cells and the tight endothelial cell junctions in retinal vessels. Enclosed within the basement membrane of the capillary is an intramural pericyte whose investment may contribute to the relative impermeability of these vessels.

The sodium fluorescein molecule normally does not traverse this vascular barrier, and by fluorescein angiography abnormal sites of leakage can be conveniently defined. With this technique, neovascular channels are found to leak profusely, as do microaneurysms. In severe hypertension small areas of leakage may be seen along tiny arteries in the vicinity of cotton-wool spots.[14] Vessels damaged by emboli may leak, as do obstructed veins or inflamed vessels. Retinal edema and hard exudates are the consequences of this leakage.

Retinal Hemorrhage

Hemorrhage into the retina indicates further breakdown in the integrity of the vascular wall. When the hemorrhage occurs in the inner retina, as in hypertension, it assumes a feathery flame shape as it is molded and dispersed by the nerve fibers coursing toward the disk. Deeper hemorrhages, such as those in diabetics, take on a more rounded dot or blot shape. Diabetic neovascularization may result in large hemorrhages beneath the retinal internal limiting membrane or into the vitreous, which obscure the underlying retina. In obstructions of the central retinal vein, the fundus may be splattered with blood as if a tomato had ruptured on the disk. See Plate 6A. Small hemorrhages are difficult to differentiate from microaneurysms, but hemorrhages usually fade within several weeks while microaneurysms may persist for months to years.

Hemorrhage may occur *beneath* the retina and usually originates not from the retinal vessels but from proliferation of a choroidal neovascular membrane growing through Bruch's membrane. These hemorrhages commonly occur beneath the macula and may destroy central vision. They have the appearance of a gray-black mass with a red fringe and have been mistaken for malignant melanomas of the choroid.

Vascular Occlusion

When the central artery or one of its branches is occluded, the nonperfused retinal area becomes cloudy in a matter of minutes. At the fovea where the retina is one-cell-layer thick and nourished by the choroid, the normal color and transparency persist. By contrast with the surrounding pallor, the fovea then has a cherry-red appearance. Occlusion at the capillary level is identified by the surrounding microaneurysms or adjacent cotton-wool spots. With fluorescein angiography such areas can be directly identified by their lack of perfusion.

Occlusion of the central retinal vein results in ret-inal edema and the "squashed tomato" hemorrhages as noted above (Plate 6A). Occlusions of branches of the central vein produce edema and hemorrhage in the drained area. These branch vein occlusions always occur at arteriovenous crossings. Examination of the retina of the opposite eye of such patients will generally reveal significant arteriovenous compression. As collateral drainage channels develop, the edema and hemorrhagic retinopathy subside, leaving white-walled veins, neovascularization, and microaneurysms in the affected area. Hemorrhage into the vitreous may occur as a late complication from the neovascularization. There is a very high incidence of hypertension in patients with venous obstructive disease,[15] and retinal and systemic arteriosclerosis is usually present.

Optic Disk Edema

Increased intracranial pressure, retinal venous outflow obstruction, inflammation, and ischemia are the four major causes of optic disk edema. The term *papilledema* is reserved by ophthalmologists and neurologists for that form of disk edema which is the result of increased intracranial pressure. It therefore has an etiologic connotation and is not used generally to mean optic disk edema. Patients with papilledema see well, while other forms of disk edema are associated with poor vision. *Papillitis* is the term applied to inflammatory disk edema. Patients with ischemic optic neuritis commonly have a pale edematous disk with an altitudinal field defect. When associated with elevations of the sedimentation rate, such patients should be suspected of having giant-cell arteritis (temporal arteritis). If this diagnosis can be established, steroid therapy is indicated to prevent visual loss in the opposite eye.

Optic Atrophy

With the resolution of disk edema in papillitis or ischemic optic neuritis, the disk will become flat and pale. Both pallor and impaired visual function are necessary for the diagnosis of optic atrophy since both the color and vascularity of the disk are highly variable. If the disk is atrophic and cupped with a shift of the vessels to the nasal side, glaucoma should be suspected. Optic atrophy without cupping may indicate intracranial tumor and should be investigated. It is unlikely that tumor has caused the atrophy if vision was once poor and has returned to near-normal levels. This is the situation often observed in patients with demyelinating disease.

Embolism

Embolism from the heart and great vessels occurs more commonly than is generally appreciated. A sudden increase in tinnitus in one ear, a fleeting woozy sensation, a scintillating scotoma, a transient monocular visual loss, all may be symptoms of embolic ischemia. This clinical suspicion may be confirmed by ophthalmoscopy. In Table 13-2 we have listed characteristics of retinal emboli of cardiovascular significance. Of these, platelet emboli are at once the most common and the most evanescent. Within minutes after vision has returned, platelet emboli have usually broken into fragments too small to identify ophthalmoscopically. Most other emboli persist for days or years and are more lasting evidence of an embolic episode. Hollenhorst cholesterol plaques may be identified at the same bifurcations for months to years after the embolic shower.

Platelet emboli, Hollenhorst plaques (Fig. 13-1), and calcium emboli are usually seen along the course of a retinal artery. Roth spots (see Plate 6C) and fat emboli may not appear to be intravascular and may not be associated with a vessel which is ophthalmoscopically visible.

Diseases

The eye is a major target for two extremely common diseases of cardiovascular significance: diabetes and hypertension. Blindness from the former now ranks as the second leading cause of acquired adult blindness in the United States, and these diabetic changes are commonly paralleled by severe renal and cardiac vasculopathy.

Diabetes

The average diabetic develops ophthalmoscopically visible retinal changes after 16 years of the disease. Focal loss of a portion of the capillary bed is followed by microaneurysm formation and vascular

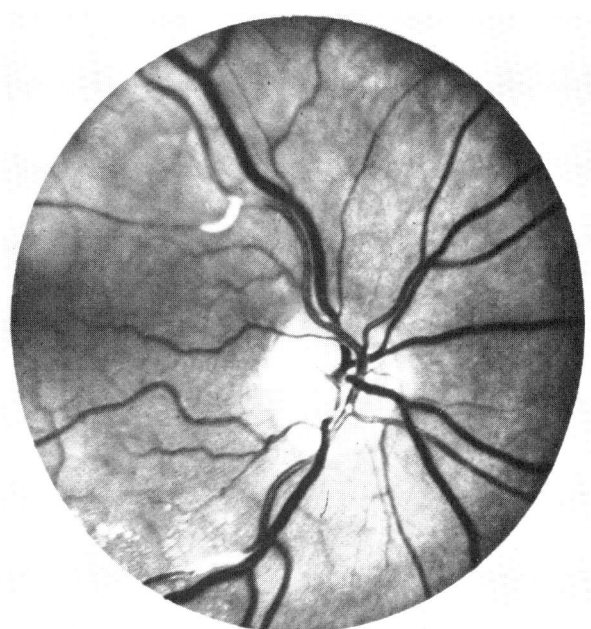

FIGURE 13-1 Retinal emboli often lodge at bifurcations, as in this patient with carotid atherosclerosis. Note that the embolic material often seems larger than the containing vessel, as in the embolus at the lower left edge of the photograph. Emboli may damage the vessel wall and cause leakage, as can be seen by the exudate deposited about the inferior embolus. Hollenhorst cholesterol plaques rarely completely obstruct arterial flow, and this patient maintained vision.

dilatation around the borders of the area of capillary drop-out. Vascular leakage occurs with dot and blot hemorrhages and deposits of hard exudate (Fig. 13-2). New blood vessels develop along the vascular arcades and at the optic nerve head (Fig. 13-

FIGURE 13-2 Exudative diabetic retinopathy, right eye, illustrating microaneurysms, dot and blot hemorrhages, and venous engorgement with extensive deposits of hard, yellow exudate.

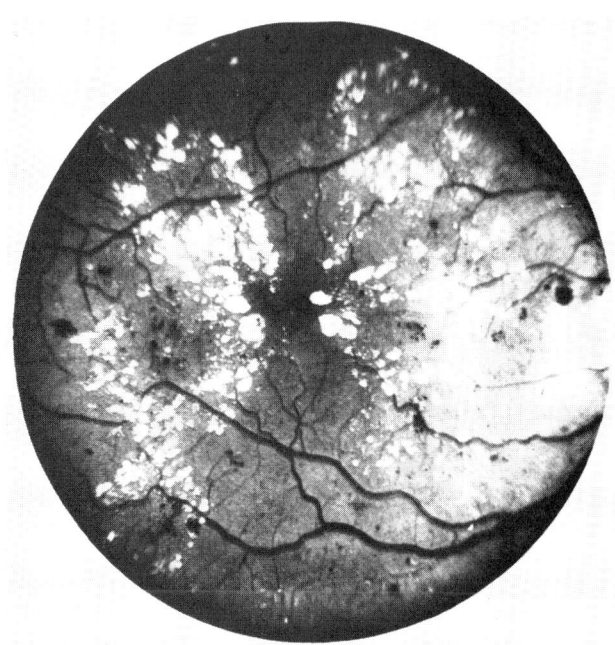

TABLE 13-2 Emboli of Cardiovascular Significance

Type	Appearance	Significance
Platelet	Dull pink to gray often with associated fibrin	Downstream vegetations, mural thrombi
Hollenhorst plaque	Glistening yellow-orange plaques at bifurcations	Downstream atheroma (containing cholesterol)
Calcium plaque	Glistening white plaques	Calcific aortic stenosis
Roth spot	Hemorrhage with gray-white center (Plate 6C)	Blood dyscrasia or septic embolus as in SBE
Fat embolus	Fuzzy-bordered gray-white spot without hemorrhage	Severe trauma with long bone fractures; prognosis grave
Myxoma	Disk edema, retinal edema in arterial supply zone	Life-threatening atrial myxoma

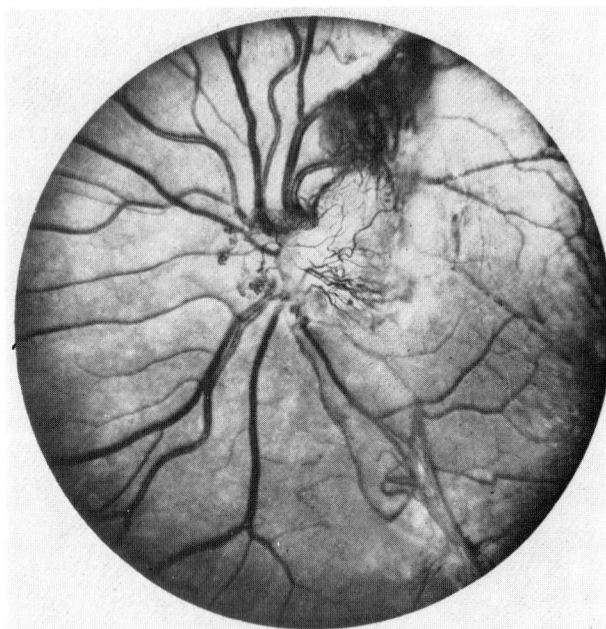

FIGURE 13-3 Proliferative diabetic retinopathy, left eye. There is extensive neovascularization of the disk with an associated small intravitreal hemorrhage which obscures the upper temporal vessels. Along the inferior temporal arcade is another area of neovascularization. These new vessels are incorporated in fibrous membranes which may tent up the vessels and cause traction detachments of the retina, as at the lower right edge of the photograph.

3). The proliferation of new blood vessels with their associated membranes often results in blinding hemorrhage into the vitreous cavity and tractional detachment of the retina.

The clinician must recognize early proliferative diabetic retinopathy, for not only are these changes associated with renal and cardiac disease but immediate laser photocoagulation of the retina may be sight-saving.[16] Control of the hypertension which is commonly associated is also of great importance, as elevations of systemic blood pressure compound the difficulty in controlling retinal vascular leakage.

Hypertension (Plates 5A to D and 6B and D)

When the systemic blood pressure rises, the retinal circulation becomes especially vulnerable since its capillary pressure floor is determined by the intraocular pressure (about 16 mmHg) and not by the jugular or cavernous sinus pressure. The intraocular pressure does not increase in hypertension, and increases in systemic blood pressure would be directly reflected in increased retinal capillary perfusion pressure were it not for the homeostatic responses of the retinal vasculature. Vasoconstriction of the arterial tree and thickening of the arterial vessel walls with consequent reduction in lumen diameter are homeostatic responses to hypertension. Arteriosclerotic narrowing of the vessels acts to insulate the capillary bed from the elevated arterial

supply pressure. These arteriosclerotic changes are visible as narrowing, increases in central light reflexes, and copper and silver wiring of the arteries. See Plate 5C. If, however, increases in the systemic blood pressure are either very marked or very rapid, these homeostatic mechanisms are overwhelmed. The resulting decompensation of the capillary bed results in accumulations of fluid in the retina and optic nerve head. The aqueous portion of the fluid is more rapidly cleared than the lipid component, which accumulates as hard exudate. Hemorrhage may occur in the inner retinal layers in a characteristic flame pattern, and focal ischemia in the nerve fiber layer may result in cotton-wool microinfarcts. In severe hypertensive decompensation the optic nerve head becomes swollen and edematous. In the Scheie[17] and Keith-Wagener[18] classifications, patients with disk edema would be assigned to the grade IV category. See Plate 5C. Patients with eclampsia or pheochromocytoma may have such marked and rapid elevations of capillary pressure that edema fluid floats the retina off the choroid, producing an exudative (nonrhegmatogenous) detachment of the retina.

Such retinal signs of capillary bed decompensation are usually paralleled by severe renal vasculopathy, and aggressive therapeutic efforts are indicated immediately. The likelihood that the patient suffers from a nonessential variety of hypertension is also markedly increased, especially if the patient is Caucasian.[19] It is clinically useful therefore to categorize hypertensive patients as to whether or not their retinal circulation is compensated, or has decompensated with observable edema, cotton-wool spots, flame hemorrhages, or swelling of the optic disk.

References

1. Duke-Elder, S.: "System of Ophthalmology," The C. V. Mosby Company, St. Louis, 1967, Vol. X, p. 277.
2. Laties, A. M.: Central Retinal Artery Innervation. Absence of Adrenergic Innervation to the Intraocular Branches, *Arch. Ophthalmol.,* 77:405, 1967.
3. Cusick, P. L., Benson, O. O., and Boothby, W. M.: Effect of Anoxia and of High Concentrations of Oxygen on the Retinal Vessels, *Proc. Mayo Clin.,* 15:500, 1940.
4. Frayser, R., and Hickam, J. B.: Retinal Vascular Response to Breathing Increased Carbon Dioxide and Oxygen Concentrations, *Invest. Ophthalmol.,* 3:427, 1964.
5. Stevens, P. M., Austen, F., and Knowles, J. H.: Prognostic Significance of Papilledema in Course of Respiratory Insufficiency, *J. Am. Med. Assoc.,* 183:161, 1963.
6. Stokoe, W. L., and Turner, R. W.: Normal Retinal Vascular Pattern. Arteriovenous Ratio as a Measure of Arterial Caliber, *Br. J. Ophthalmol.,* 50:21, 1966.
7. Dollery, C. T., Hodge, J. V., and Hill, D. W.: The Response of Normal Retinal Blood Vessels to An-

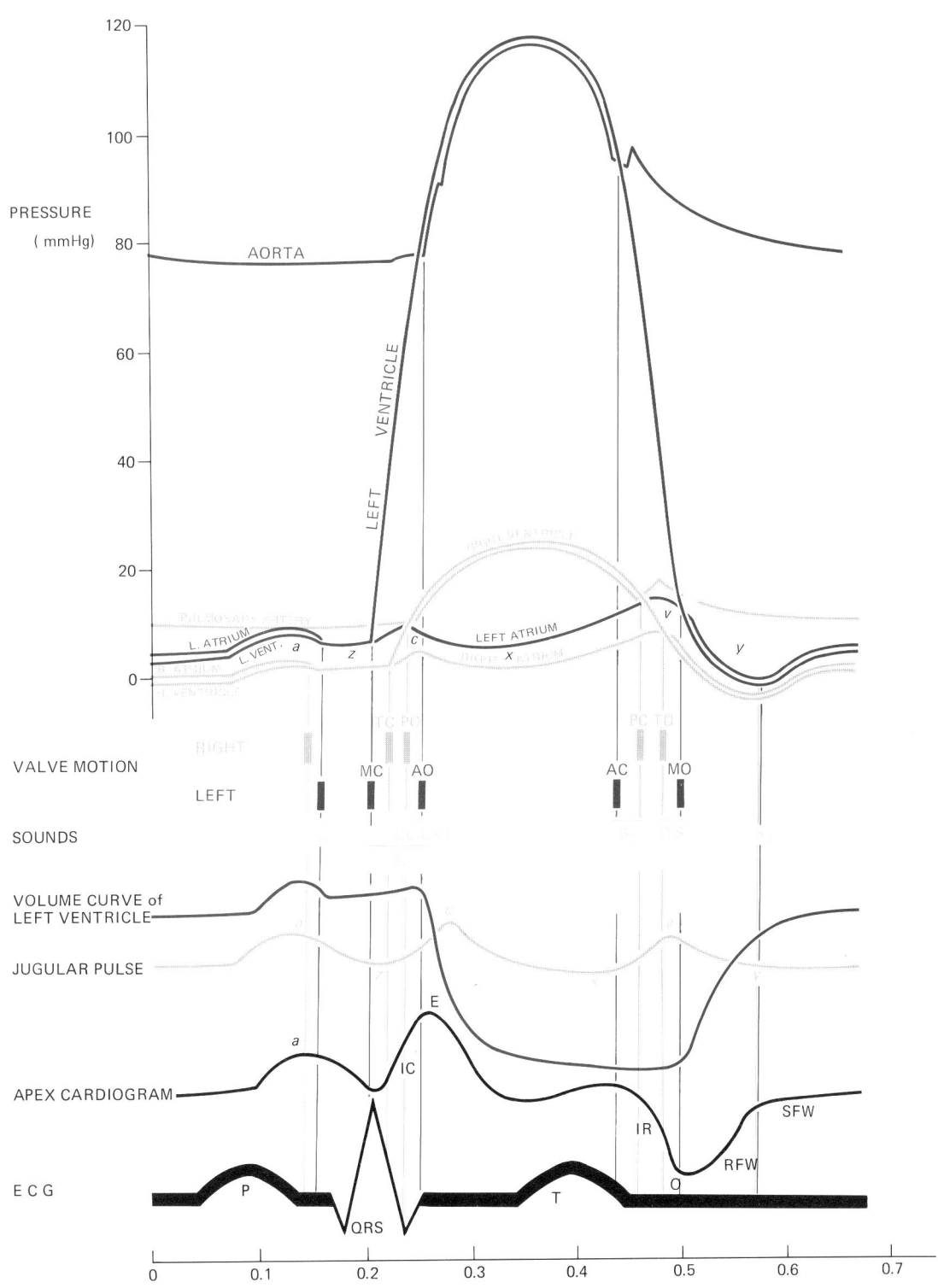

Diagram of the cardiac cycle, showing the pressure curves of the great vessels and cardiac chambers, valvular events and heart sounds, left ventricular volume curve, jugular pulse wave, apex cardiogram (Sanborn piezo crystal), and the electrocardiogram. For illustrative purposes, the time intervals between the valvular events have been modified and the z point has been prolonged. Valve motion: MC = mitral component of the first heart sound; MO = mitral valve opening; TC = tricuspid component of the first heart sound; TO = tricuspid valve opening; AC = aortic component of the second heart sound; AO = aortic valve opening; PC = pulmonic valve component of the second heart sound; PO = pulmonic valve opening; OS = opening snap of atrioventricular valves. Apex cardiogram: IC = isovolumic or isovolumetric (isochoric) contraction wave; IR = isovolumic or isovolumetric (isochoric) relaxation wave; O = opening of mitral valve; RFW = rapid-filling wave; SFW = slow-filling wave. (See text in Chap. 3.)

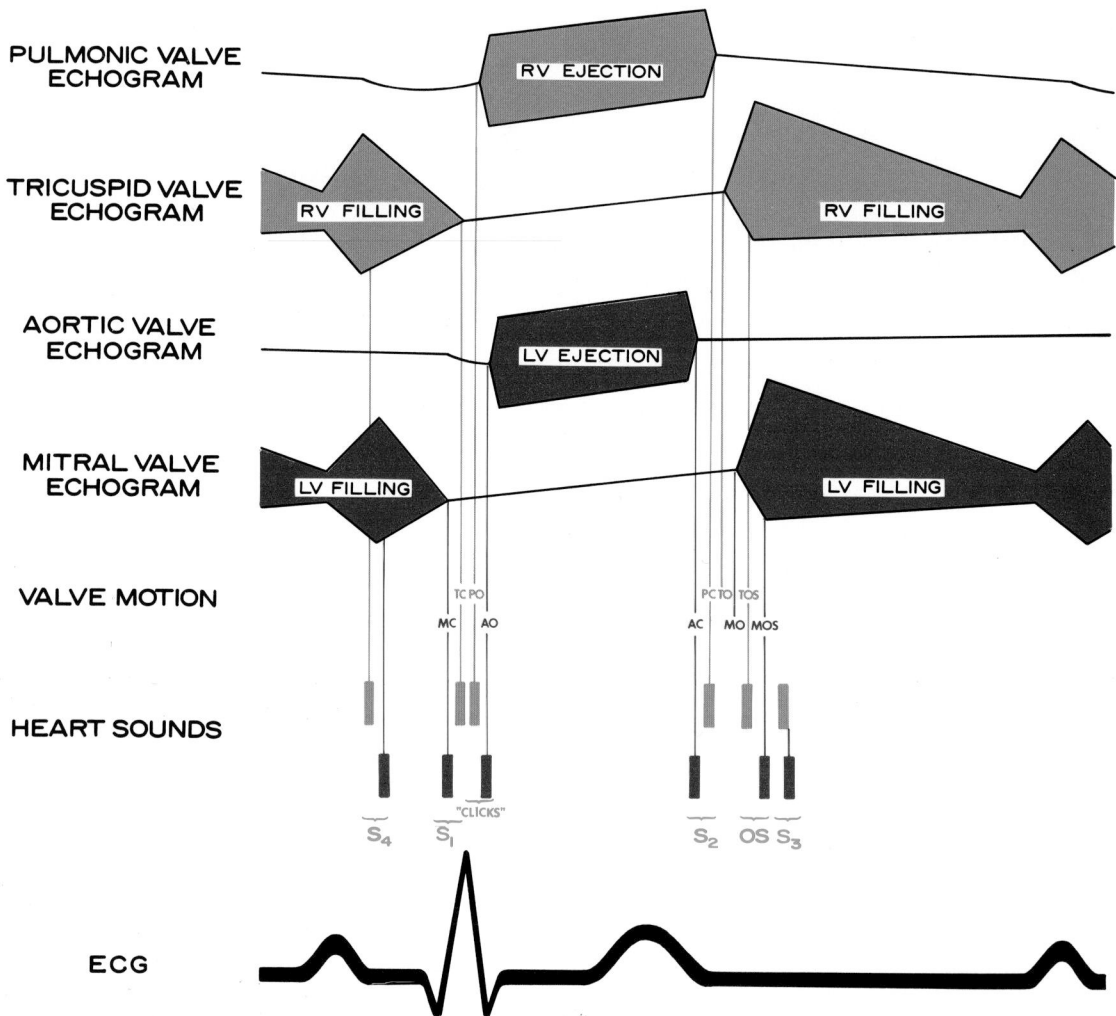

Schematic presentation of the relationships between electrical and mechanical events and heart sounds during the cardiac cycle. The sequence of ejection from, and of filling of, the right ventricle is indicated by the schematic echograms of the pulmonic valve and the tricuspid valve. The corresponding phases of the left ventricle are indicated by the schematic echograms of the aortic valve and the mitral valve. The isovolumic contraction phase for each ventricle occurs in the short phase between the end of filling and the onset of ejection, whereas isovolumic filling occurs in the brief phase between the end of ejection and the onset of filling.

The right atrium starts contracting before the left atrium; on the other hand, the left ventricle starts contracting prior to the contraction of the right ventricle. Because of the relatively higher pressure in the aorta than in the pulmonary artery, the phases of isovolumic contraction and isovolumic relaxation of the left ventricle are much longer than for the right ventricle. As a result, although left ventricular contraction begins first, right ventricular ejection begins prior to left ventricular ejection and also ends after that of left ventricular ejection. Thus, the phase of active ejection for the right ventricle is longer than that of the left ventricle. On the other hand, the total duration of systole, including isovolumic contraction and relaxation, is normally longer for the left ventricle.

The normal sequence of heart sounds and valve motion is schematically depicted: MC = the mitral component of the first heart sound (S_1); TC = the tricuspid component of the first heart sound (S_1); PO = pulmonic valve opening; AO = aortic valve opening; AC = aortic component of the second heart sound (S_2); PC = pulmonic component of the second heart sound (S_2); TO = tricuspid valve opening; TOS = tricuspid opening snap; and MOS = mitral valve opening snap. Normally, the sound produced by the opening of the cardiac valves is not audible; however, in disease states the opening of the mitral or tricuspid valve may produce an "opening snap" which usually occurs about the moment when the respective valve leaflets just reach maximal opening. Similarly, very vigorous tensing and opening of the aortic and pulmonic valves can produce ejection or opening "clicks" or sounds analogous to the opening snaps of the AV valves. An aortic and pulmonic valve opening click or sound may occur anywhere between the onset of valve opening, as illustrated, and the point of maximal opening of the respective valve, where it more commonly occurs. The sound occurring at the end of the rapid-filling phase of the ventricle is referred to as a *third heart sound (S_3)*, *ventricular filling sound*, or *ventricular gallop*. The sound that occurs during or shortly after the P wave on the electrocardiogram and that is associated with an atrial contribution to ventricular filling is referred to as the *fourth heart sound (S_4)*. Both third (S_3) and fourth (S_4) heart sounds may originate from either ventricle. The motion of the valve leaflets is depicted schematically in the valve echograms; for illustrative purposes, not all time intervals are depicted proportionately. See text for details.

PLATE 3   Tuberous sclerosis; dermatomyositis; hemorrhagic telangiectasia under fingernails; hemorrhagic telangiectasia on tongue and lips; clubbing of the fingers; Osler's node.

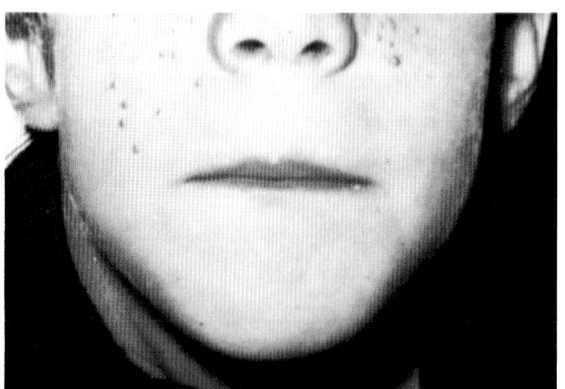

A Tuberous sclerosis. Adenoma sebaceum, may be associated with rhabdomyomas of the myocardium.

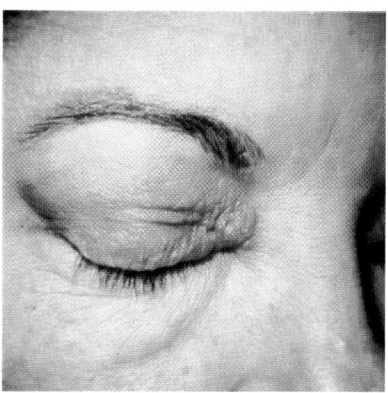

B Dermatomyositis. A violaceous hue and edema of upper eyelid, may be associated with myocardial disease.

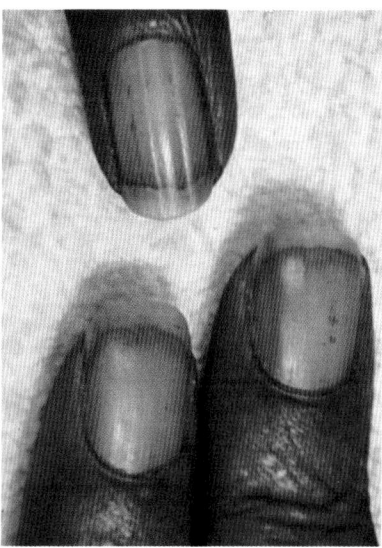

C Hereditary hemorrhagic telangiectasia. Telangiectasia under nails. *(With permission of publisher, from Silverman and Hurst, The Hand and the Heart, Am. J. Cardiol., 22:609, 1968.)*

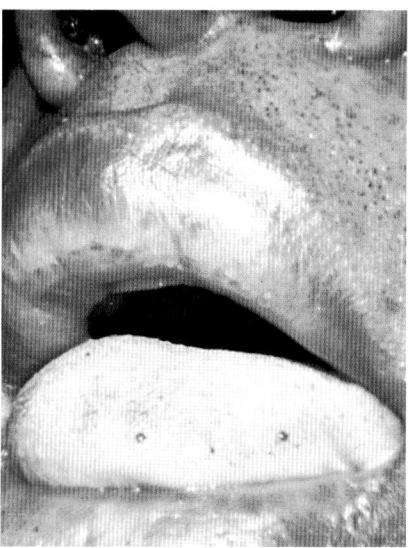

D Hereditary hemorrhagic telangiectasia. Telangiectasia on tongue and lips, may be associated with a pulmonary arteriovenous fistula.

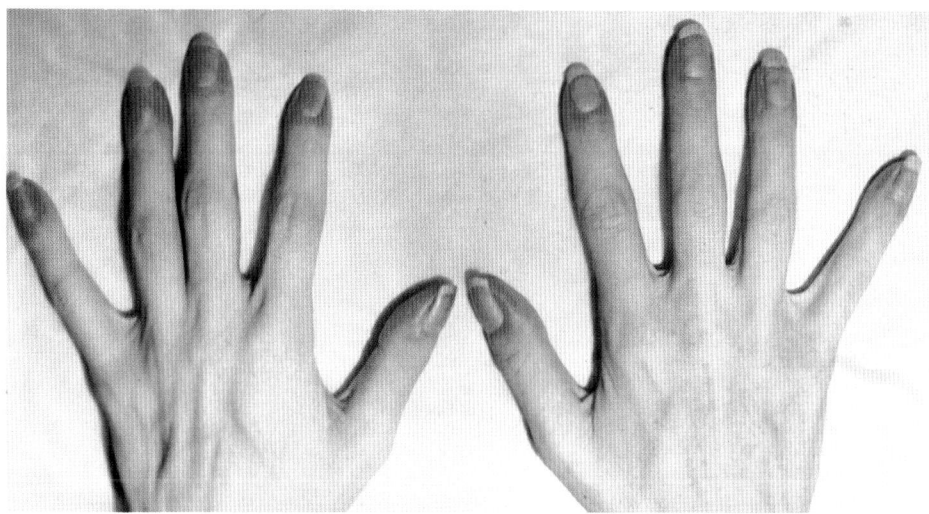

E Clubbing due to bacterial endocarditis.

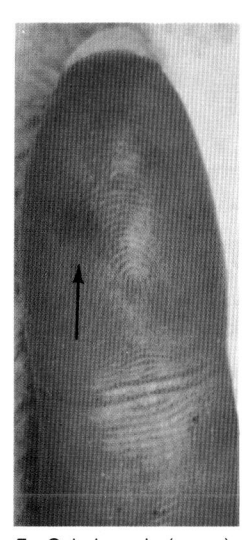

F Osler's node (arrow).

PLATE 4   Symmetric cyanosis; cyanosis of fingers greater than that of toes; cyanosis of left hand and all toes; and tuft erythema.

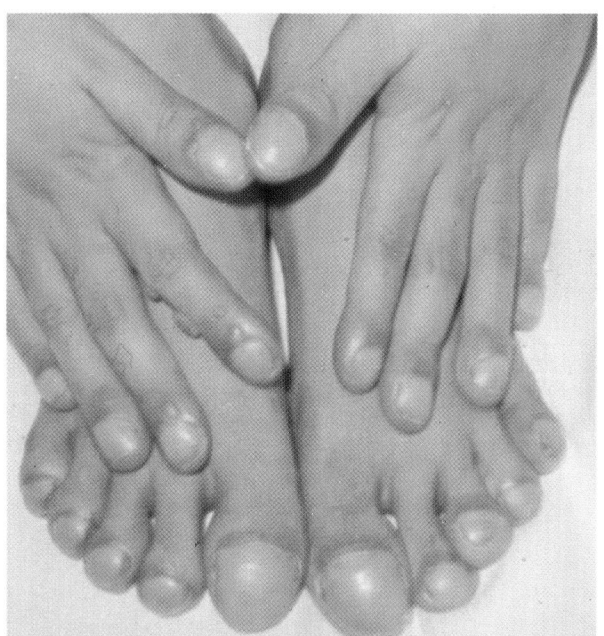

A   Symmetric cyanosis. Equal cyanosis and clubbing of hands and feet, due to transposition of great vessels and a ventricular septal defect *without* patent ductus arteriosus.

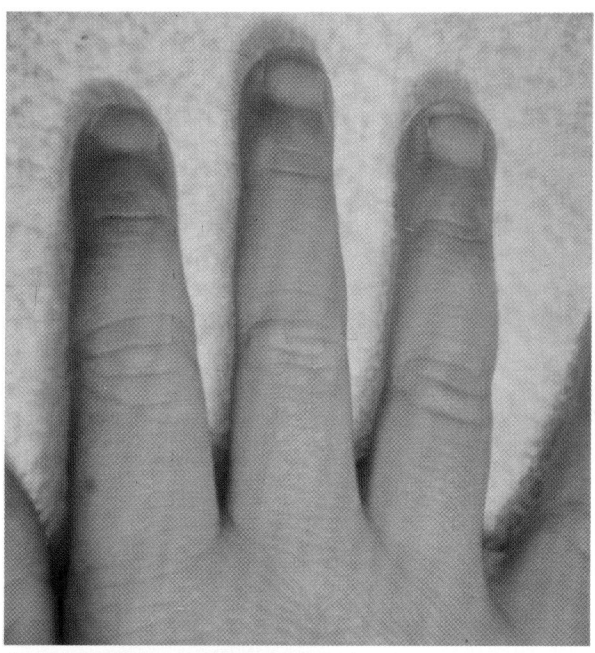

B   Tuft erythema. Erythema of fingertips, due to small right-to-left shunt from an AV canal defect.

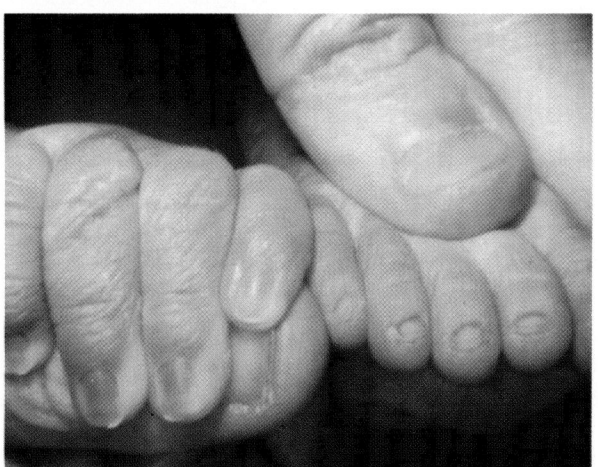

C   Differential cyanosis. Cyanosis of fingers (left) greater than that of toes, due to transposition of great vessels *with* patent ductus arteriosus.

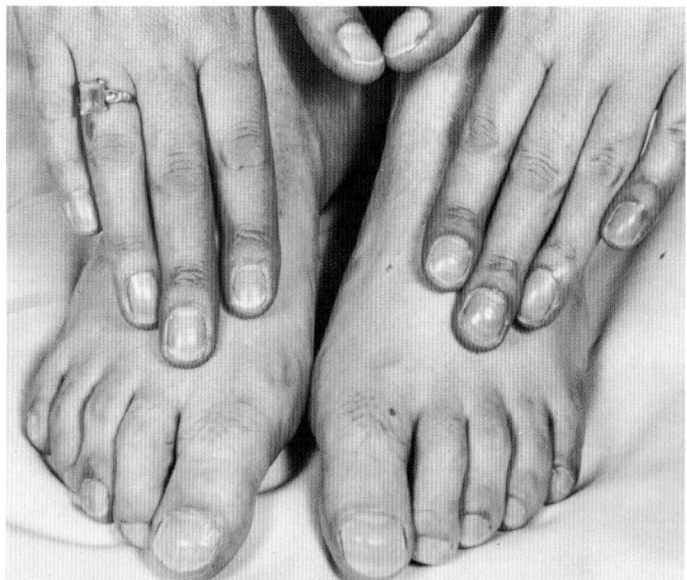

D   Differential cyanosis. Clubbing of left hand (compare thumbs) and cyanosis of left hand and all toes, due to patent ductus arteriosus with pulmonary hypertension and normally related great vessels. *(Courtesy of Dr. Joseph K. Perloff, University of California, Los Angeles.)*

PLATE 5   Retinal changes associated with systemic hypertension.

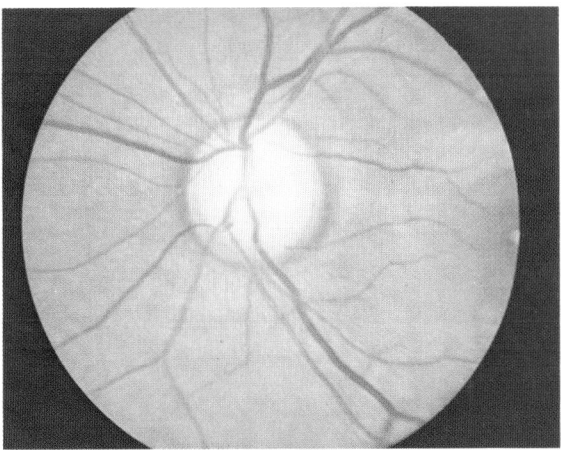

A The retina of a 49-year-old Negro woman with asympto-matic "essential hypertension" of at least 10 years' duration, showing arteriolar narrowing and straightening, increased light reflex, irregular caliber, loss of small arteriolar branches, and early AV crossing changes.

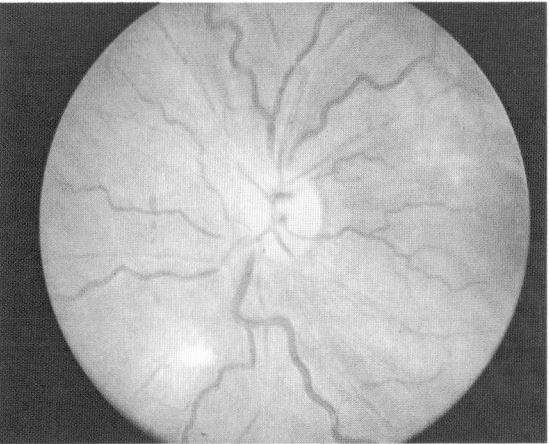

B The retina of a 42-year-old Negro woman with essential hypertension and blood pressure levels averaging 260/130. She was asymptomatic except for headaches. Note the se-vere vascular sclerosis seen as marked irregularity of arter-iolar caliber, "sheathing," and nearly complete loss of trans-parency of the arterioles. A "cotton wool" exudate is seen at 7 o'clock. The nasal disk margin is blurred, which may occur normally.

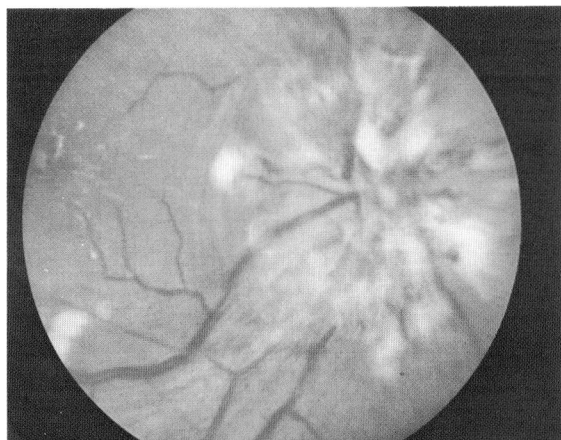

C The retina of a 38-year-old Negro man with malignant hypertension and with bilateral papilledema and azotemia. There was no visual disturbance. Note the massive edema, hemorrhages, and exudates, completely obscuring the disk and burying the blood vessels. The veins are congested and the arterioles show diffuse thickening ("copper wire"). There are hard exudates (edema residues) forming in the nerve bundle grooves in the macular region at 10 o'clock.

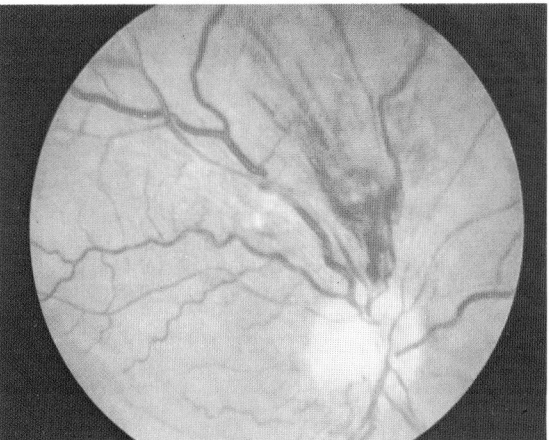

D The retina of a 50-year-old Negro woman with severe hypertension of 25 years' duration. Arteriolar sclerosis is shown by the marked narrowing, irregular caliber, increased light reflex, and AV crossing changes. Atherosclerosis is sug-gested by the large fanshaped superficial hemorrhage, due to occlusion of a branch of the superior temporal vein as it enters the disk region.

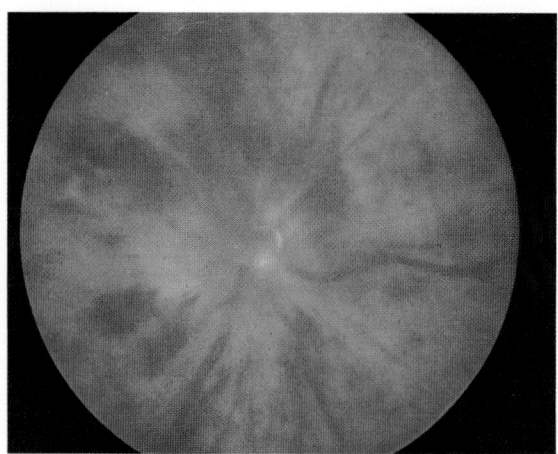

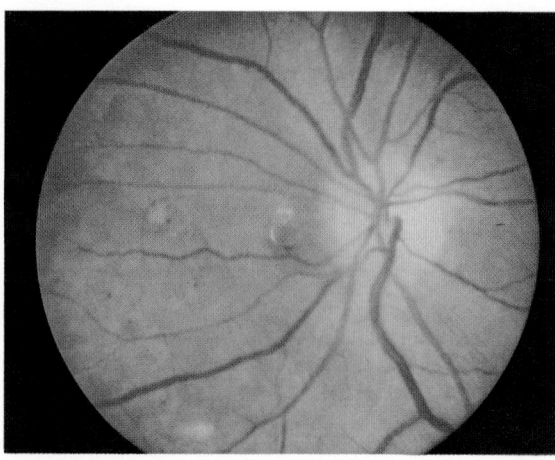

A   The retina of a 74-year-old white man with normal blood pressure who complained of sudden loss of vision in one eye. This shows the typical picture of central retinal vein occlusion, probably due to atherosclerosis of its adjacent artery behind the disk. Diffuse edema (loss of retinal detail), massive hemorrhages, and papilledema are present.

B   The retina of a 68-year-old white man with hypertension and mild diabetes mellitus. Note the very small red dots, or capillary aneurysms, scattered between the disk and the macular region. There is also a faint "cotton wool" exudate at 7 o'clock.

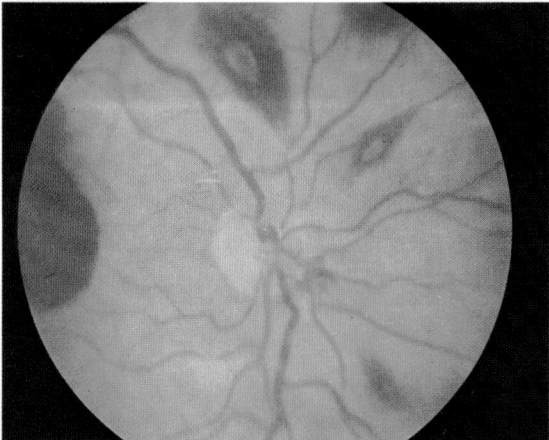

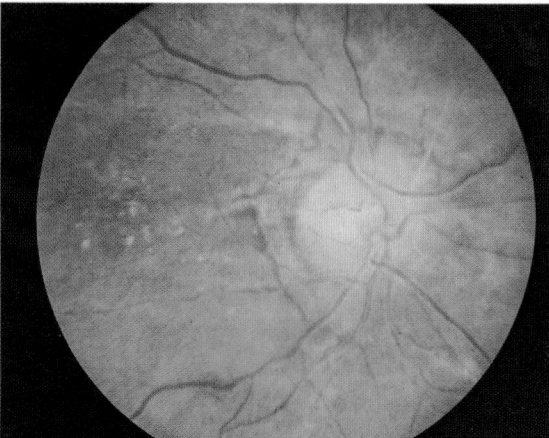

C   The retina of a 24-year-old white woman with acute myeloblastic leukemia and severe anemia; the blood pressure was normal. Note the scattered hemorrhages, some with whitish centers (Roth spots), and the portion of the large preretinal hemorrhage at 9 o'clock. The blood vessels are pale but otherwise normal.

D   The retina of a 36-year-old white woman with pseudoxanthoma elasticum. Severe hypertension, marked visual disturbance, and renal insufficiency were present. Note the characteristic brownish angioid streaks around the disk and extending toward the macula. Also seen are marked retinal arteriolar sclerotic changes, sheathing, irregular caliber, occluded vessels, and hard exudates with a "smudge" hemorrhage at 7 o'clock.

PLATE 7 Bacterial endocarditis and nonbacterial thromboendocarditis.

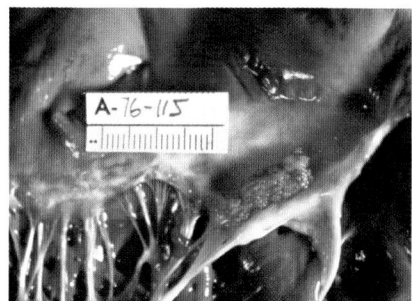

A Typical vegetation of nonbacterial thrombotic endocarditis, found at necropsy in a cachectic patient who died with disseminated lung cancer.

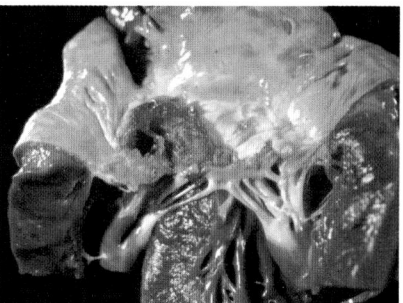

B Typical vegetation of bacteria endocarditis, complicated by perforation of the anterior mitral valve leaflet. Note that the valve shows preexisting chronic rheumatic disease, with thickening, deformity, and fusion of chordae tendineae.

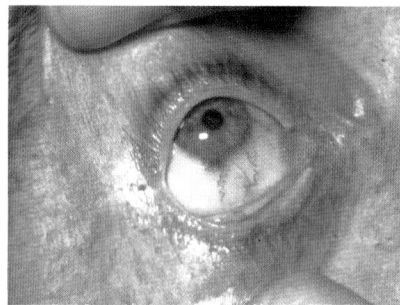

C Typical conjunctival petechia in a patient with SBE due to *Streptococcus sanguis*.

The consequences of embolization from the vegetation shown in a patient with subacute bacterial endocarditis (SBE).

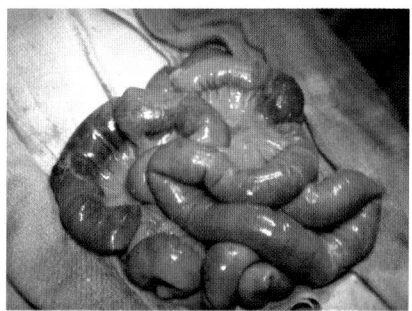

D Segmental ischemia and necrosis in the gut, presenting as acute abdomen.

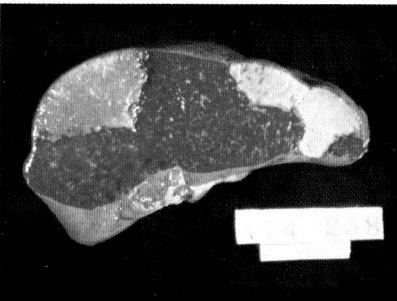

E Infarctions in the spleen.

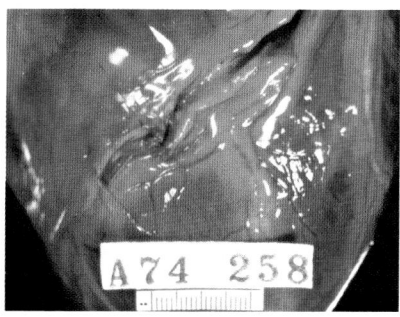

F An infected embolus in a coronary artery.

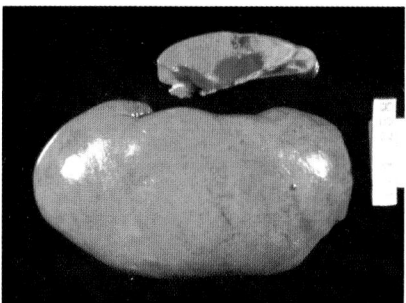

G Kidney from a case of subacute bacterial endocarditis, showing two abnormalities: (1) typical ischemic infarctions due to emboli, (2) swelling and petechiae ("flea-bitten kidney") due to immune-complex glomerulonephritis.

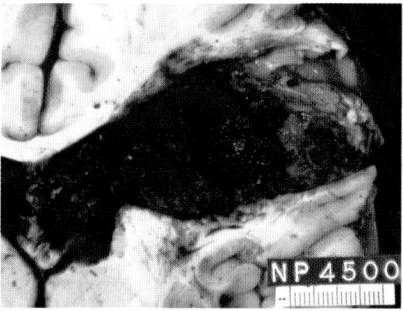

H Massive cerebral hemorrhage with intraventricular extension due to rupture of a small, peripheral mycotic aneurysm (arrowed). The patient had been *bacteriologically* cured of *Staphylococcus epidermidis* endocarditis several weeks previously. Cultures of the blood, valve, and aneurysm taken at necropsy were negative.

PLATE 8   Myocarditis of varying etiology.

A Toxoplasmosis of the heart in a 27-year-old man with acute lymphocytic leukemia. *Upper.* Area of focal myocarditis associated with *T. gondii* organisms. *Lower.* Close-up view of the encysted organisms. H&E: ×120 (upper), ×366 (lower). (*Reproduced from Chap. 55 Ref. 13 with permission of authors and publisher*).

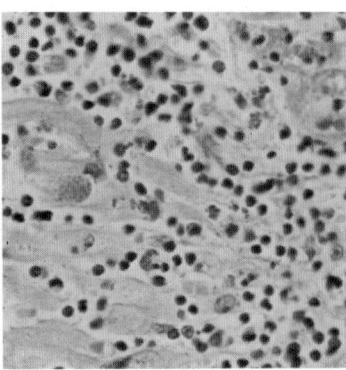

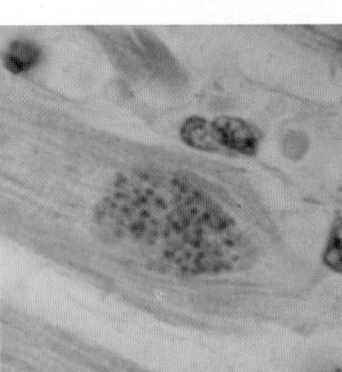

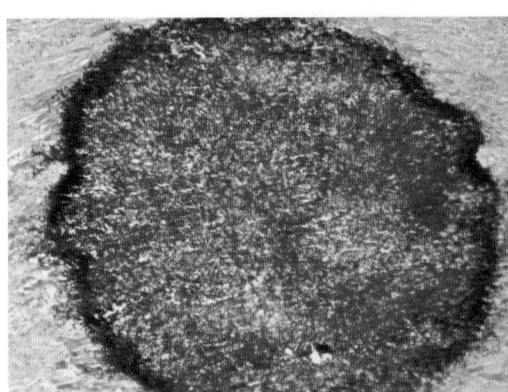

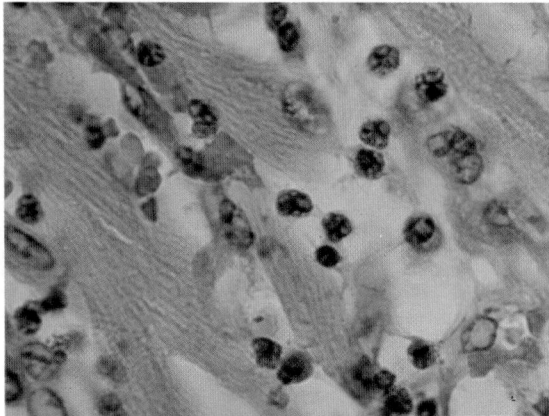

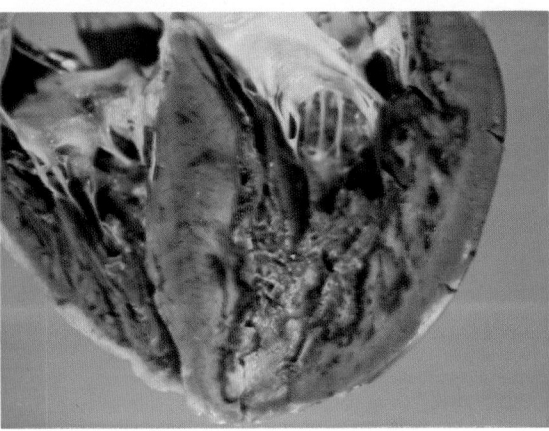

B Trichinosis involving the heart of a 46-year-old woman who lived 13 days after the onset of illness. At necropsy, the heart weighed 260 g; its myocardial walls were filled with extravasated inflammatory cells, mainly eosinophils. H&E: ×353 (upper). (*Reproduced from Chap. 55 Ref. 15 with permission of author and publisher*).

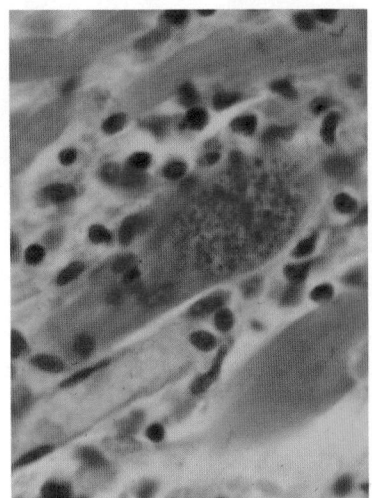

D *Trypanosoma cruzi* in its leishmanial state parasitizing the sarcoplasm of the myocardial cell. The surrounding fiber edema and acute inflammatory reaction are indicative of rupture of the myocardial cell. H&E: ×48. (*Courtesy of Dr. M. Gravanis, Professor of Pathology, Emory University School of Medicine*).

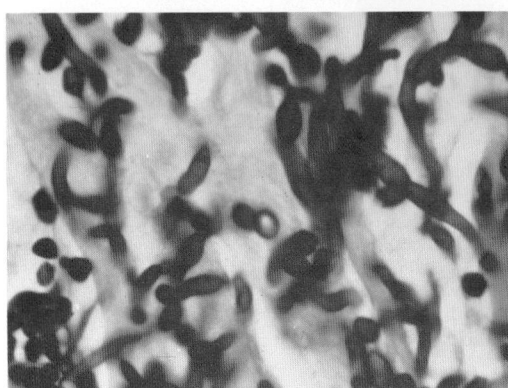

C Cardiac candidiasis in a 20-year-old man with acute myeloblastic leukemia. Large myocardial abscess containing massive numbers of *Candida* organisms (upper). Close-up of the *Candida* organisms (lower). PAS: ×5 (upper), ×133 (lower). (*Reproduced from Chap. 55 Ref. 18 with permission of author and publisher*).

giotensin and Noradrenaline, *J. Physiol.*, 165:500, 1963.

8. Ballantyne, A. J.: The State of the Retina in Diabetes Mellitus, *Trans. Ophthalmol. Soc. U.K.*, 66:503, 1966.

9. Kennedy, J. E., and Wise, G. N.: Clinicopathologic Correlation of Retinal Lesions. 2. Retinochoroidal Vascular Anastomosis in Uveitis, *Am. J. Ophthalmol.*, 71:1221, 1971.

10. Bloom, W., and Fawcett, D. W.: "A Textbook of Histology," 10th ed., W. B. Saunders Company, Philadelphia, 1975, p. 397.

11. Hogan, M. J., and Feeney, L.: The Ultrastructure of the Retinal Blood Vessels, *J. Ultrastruct. Res.*, 9:10, 1963.

12. Brownstein, S., Font, R. L., and Alper, M. G.: Atheromatous Plaques of the Retinal Blood Vessels. Histologic Confirmation of Ophthalmoscopically Visible Lesions, *Arch. Ophthalmol.*, 90:49, 1973.

*13. The Diabetic Retinopathy Study Research Group: Four Risk Factors for Severe Visual Loss in Diabetic

*This article is a review of the literature and contains additional references to the literature.

Retinopathy. The Third Report, *Arch. Ophthalmol.*, 97:654, 1979. (2 references)

14. Hodge, J. V., and Dollery, C. T.: Retinal Soft Exudates. A Clinical Study by Color and Fluorescence Photography. *Q. J. Med.*, 33:117, 1964.

15. Klien, B. A., and Olwin, J. H.: A Survey on the Pathogenesis of Retinal Venous Occlusion, *Arch. Ophthalmol.*, 56:207, 1956.

*16. The Diabetic Retinopathy Study Research Group: Photocoagulation Treatment in Proliferative Diabetic Retinopathy. The Second Report of Diabetic Retinopathy Study Findings, *Ophthalmology*, 85:82, 1978. (6 references)

17. Scheie, H. G.: Evaluation of Ophthalmoscopic Changes of Hypertension and Arteriolar Sclerosis, *Arch. Ophthalmol.*, 49:117, 1953.

18. Keith, N. M., Wagener, H. P., and Barker, N. W.: Some Different Types of Essential Hypertension. Their Course and Prognosis., *Am. J. Med. Sci.*, 197:332, 1939.

19. Davis, B. A., Crook, J. E., Vestal, R. E., Oates, J. A.: Prevalence of Renovascular Hypertension in Patients with Grade III or IV Hypertensive Retinopathy, *N. Engl. J. Med.*, 301:1273, 1979.

14

Physical Examination of the Lungs, Abdomen, and Extremities

J. Willis Hurst, M.D.
Paul H. Robinson, M.D.

This is not the proper place to discuss the details of the physical examination of the lungs, abdomen, and extremities. This important subject is discussed in other books.[1] It *is* the place to emphasize that portion of the examination that relates to the cardiovascular system and to clarify a few common misconceptions that are related to it.

The Physical Examination of the Lungs

The physical examination of the lungs is a crude method for detecting disease, but it must be learned and utilized for two reasons: (1) It is painless and noninvasive; it is easy to percuss the chest and listen to the lungs since no special equipment other than a stethoscope is needed. Since a chest x-ray cannot be made hourly or even daily, the abnormalities found on physical examination often determine *when* an x-ray of the chest should be made. (2) The chest x-ray is superior to the physical examination in detecting the presence of congestive heart failure, pleural fluid, pulmonary infiltrates, and pneumothorax. On the other hand, the chest x-ray will not detect wheezing or a pleural rub. The latter two conditions are detected only by auscultation of the lungs.

The patient with pulmonary infarction may have a pleural friction rub. Pleural fluid may be produced by pulmonary infarction or heart failure. Pleural fluid due to heart failure is usually located in the right pleural space. When pleural fluid is located on the left side or is predominant on the left, it is wise to consider a cause other than (or in addition to) heart failure. For example, pulmonary infarction may be responsible for such a clinical finding. A pneumothorax may develop as part of spontaneous mediastinal emphysema or may be secondary to a procedure. Increased resonance and decreased breath sounds may be due to pulmonary emphysema. Signs of pulmonary consolidation may be due to pneumonia or pulmonary infarction. Wheezing and rales may be due to bronchial disease. Heart failure may be associated with rales in the lung bases, wheezing, and pleural fluid. On the other hand, heart failure is frequently not associated with rales. In fact, interstitial pulmonary edema does not produce rales. Experienced and skilled clinicians rarely use the presence of rales to diagnose heart failure. They use other clues that have a higher predictive value to determine the presence or absence of heart failure.

The Physical Examination of the Abdomen

The size of the abdominal aorta must be determined in every patient. The technique of doing this is discussed in Chap. 62. An abdominal aortic aneurysm may be overlooked because the physician may ignore the area above the umbilicus and concentrate on the area below the umbilicus.

Patients with heart disease may develop certain abnormalities of the abdomen. The liver may become large and tender in patients with heart failure or constrictive pericarditis. The liver edge may move in patients with tricuspid regurgitation. Such movement is due to downward displacement of the liver by a column of regurgitant blood and to engorgement of the liver during systole.

The spleen may become palpable in patients with severe heart failure and in patients with infective endocarditis. Splenomegaly is not a good sign of heart failure or endocarditis since heart failure must be severe and endocarditis must be present a long time before the spleen enlarges. An x-ray of the abdomen may detect splenomegaly that is not detected on physical examination.

When ascites occurs, one should consider cirrhosis of the liver since this is the most common cause of the condition. Patients with heart failure alone may have ascites, but this is less common today than it was prior to the modern era of diuretic therapy. Patients with destruction of the tricuspid valve by infective endocarditis may develop grotesque systolic pulsation of the internal jugular veins in the neck; a large, moving, and pulsating liver; and ascites. When there is evidence of minimal heart failure and considerable ascites, it is wise to consider the presence of both heart failure and separate cirrhosis of the liver. Constrictive pericarditis is still common, but it is discovered earlier now than it was formerly, and therefore ascites is not commonly due to this condition. The "old-fashioned" variety of constrictive pericarditis still occurs, however, and it is wise to consider the possibility of its presence when ascites is out of proportion to the peripheral edema, the heart is of normal size or only slightly enlarged, a pericardial "knock" is heard, and there are strutted external neck veins with a rapid x or y descent in the internal jugular vein pulsation. Restrictive cardiomyopathy can mimic constrictive pericarditis in that there may be ascites, strutted neck veins, and little or no leg edema. The heart is usually quite large in patients with restrictive cardiomyopathy.

A peripheral arteriovenous fistula produces a continuous murmur. When the fistula is in the abdomen, the murmur may be heard over the abdomen. Fistulas due to trauma and surgery may occur. For example, a fistula between the renal artery and renal vein may produce a continuous murmur which is heard in the region of the kidney. The best example of a continuous murmur heard in a region which is adjacent to the abdomen is the one heard over the lumbar area following lumbar disk surgery.

A systolic bruit may be heard over the kidney areas and may signify obstructive lesions in the renal arteries. A systolic bruit may be heard over the abdominal aorta, but its presence is not sufficient to make a diagnostic decision regarding disease of the aorta.

The Physical Examination of the Extremities

The physical examination of the aorta and the arteries and veins of the upper and lower extremities is discussed in Chaps. 62, 63, and 66.

Edema of the lower extremities has been the time-honored sign of heart failure. Edema is a late sign of heart failure, and its predictive value as a diagnostic sign is poor. Edema of the lower extremities may be due to local factors such as varicose veins or thrombophlebitis. Under such circumstances, the edema may occur only in one leg. Edema may be the result of tight garters and venous stasis secondary to a long trip in an airplane. Edema may be due to primary kidney disease with its associated salt and water retention. When edema is found, the physician should think first in terms of local factors and, if local factors can be excluded, then think in terms of salt and water retention. It is then necessary to determine the cause of the salt and water retention by finding evidence of heart disease and other signs of heart failure or evidence of primary renal disease. The salt and water retention of heart failure is due to renal dysfunction related to a poor cardiac output and the alteration of certain levels of hormones. (See Chap. 22.) The salt and water retention due to primary renal disease is due to disease within the kidney itself.

References

1. Walker, H. K., Hall, W. D., and Hurst, J. W.: "Clinical Methods: The History, Physical, and Laboratory Examination," 2d ed., Butterworths, Boston, 1980.

15

The Resting Electrocardiogram

Agustin Castellanos, M.D.
Robert J. Myerburg, M.D.

Professor Einthoven has always acknowledged with utmost frankness that his own work was the direct continuation of mine, and that this string-galvanometer was invented with the direct object of providing a more adequate recording of the human electrocardiogram than was afforded by the capillary electrometer.

Augustus Waller, 1922[1]

Much has been written about the resting electrocardiogram, and the following discussion should be viewed as merely an introduction to the subject. This chapter introduces the reader to the ventricular electrocardiogram. The electrocardiographic features of cardiac arrhythmias are discussed in Chap. 28. The reader is referred to one or more of the currently available textbooks on the subject for additional information.

In the early 1930s Frank Wilson and his coworkers began the difficult task of incorporating conventional electrocardiographic theory into clinical medicine.[2,3] These workers made significant practical applications of their knowledge, so that today a large body of clinical electrocardiographic concepts can be traced directly to them.

The electrocardiogram (ECG) deals with the study of the electric forces produced by the heart muscle during the cardiac cycle as recorded from the body surface. The source of cardiac electrical activity resides at a cellular level, as discussed in Chap. 4.

Generalities

After emerging from the sinus node the cardiac impulse propagates throughout the atria in its journey toward the AV node. The *normal* P wave (resulting from activation of both atria) is a consequence of, but does not directly represent, sinus node activity. Because the impulse reaches the AV node while parts of the atria are still being activated, arrival of excitation at the AV node occurs at an undetermined point within (before the end of) the P wave.

As the impulse penetrates deeper into the AV node, it becomes weaker and weaker as it propagates into areas which are less responsive. Should this sequence continue, conduction would eventually cease. Actually, at some point within the AV node this process reverses, responses to weakly conducted impulses becoming stronger, as propagation into more responsive tissue occurs, until the His bundle is reached. Rapid propagation through the His bundle is followed by conduction through the bundle branches and their ramifications.

Activation of the ordinary ventricular muscle (onset of the QRS complex) starts as soon as the impulse emerging from the most distal ramifications of the bundle branches depolarizes a sufficiently large number of cells. Therefore, the PR interval (used to estimate AV conduction time) includes conduction through the "true" atrioventricular structures (AV node, His bundle, bundle branches, and main divisions of the left bundle branch) as well as through those parts of the atria located between sinus and AV nodes.

Conventional ECG theory holds that the onset of ventricular depolarization (given by the beginning of the normal Q wave) reflects activation of the left side of the interventricular septum. This has been attributed to the fact that the left bundle has terminal ramifications which activate the septum at a higher level than those of the right bundle branch.[4-7] But in addition, the large fanlike distribution of these terminal ramifications on the left septal surface produces activation of a greater number of ordinary muscle cells per unit of time.

The most distal ramifications of both bundle branches (Purkinje fibers) form networks within the subendocardial regions of the free ventricular walls. The latter are activated as soon as the multiple wave fronts emerge from the Purkinje fibers. Again the greater number of ordinary muscle fibers on the left ventricular free wall explain why left ventricular events predominate (therefore overpower) those from the right ventricular free wall.

The ventricular depolarization process starts in the endocardium and spreads toward the epicardium as a wave front having the positive electrical charges in front of the negative charges. That the depolarization wave front tends to produce positivity in those areas (more toward the epicardium) to which it is approaching and negativity in those regions (toward the endocardium) which it is leaving constitutes one of the most important concepts of clinical electrocardiography.

The ventricular repolarization process, on the other hand, starts in the epicardium and spreads (more slowly) toward the endocardium as a wave front having the negative charges in front (facing the endocardium). This earlier epicardial onset has been attributed to the shorter duration of repolarization that the epicardial cells have as compared with the endocardial cells.[6,8,9] Repolarization starts later and ends earlier in the epicardium than in the endocardium. The negative charges travel in front because the repolarization wave front tends to reestablish the resting polarized state of the cells which had been previously depolarized.

In the surface ECG the QRS complex reflects ventricular depolarization; the ST segment and T and U waves, ventricular repolarization; and the

EXAMINATION OF THE HEART AND BLOOD VESSELS

horizontal base line, the normal resting polarized state. The QT and/or QU interval are used as a measure of both depolarization and repolarization conduction time.

Einthoven Triangle Hypothesis

The magnitude and direction of the electrical activity on the body surface may be viewed conveniently as an average of the individual instantaneous events occurring at the cellular level. The numerous cells being depolarized or repolarized at a given instant result in the vast majority of the electrical activity being canceled out by opposing forces, but the surface recording is a reasonably reproducible and accurate approximation of net instantaneous cardiac electrical activity. For these reasons Einthoven popularized the concept that the human body represents a large volume conductor having the source of cardiac electrical activity at its center.[10] While this theory is not strictly true, it provides the clinician with a practical point from which to work. As an extension of this concept, the net electrical activity at any instant in the cardiac cycle may be viewed as originating from a point source at a theoretical "electrical center" of the heart.

The original three-lead system developed by Einthoven is based on assumptions of (1) the homogeneity of the body volume conductor; (2) the symmetry of the leads; and (3) a single equivalent dipole at the center of the volume conductor. The standard limb leads (I, II, III) are composed of three permutations of the right arm (RA), left arm (LA), and left leg (LL) electrodes. Lead I records the potential difference between the left arm and the right arm, the positive electrode on the left arm. Einthoven arbitrarily selected the relationship between positive and negative electrodes in the three leads in order to have the major deflection of the QRS complex moving in an upward direction in most normal individuals.[10]

Wilson Central Terminal

The sum of the potentials from the right arm, left arm, and left leg is equal to zero throughout the cardiac cycle with respect to any point at the body surface. If leads are attached to electrodes in these points, their potential is zero with respect to any other electrode on the body surface.[2,3] When this common point, *Wilson's central terminal,* is connected to the negative pole of the electrocardiographic machine through 5000-Ω resistors and an "exploring" electrode is attached to the positive pole, the potential variations recorded will be those of the latter only. A lead taken by this method (Fig. 15-1) is called a *unipolar lead.* Actually, the central terminal is not zero because the right arm, left arm, and left leg are not equidistant from each other and from

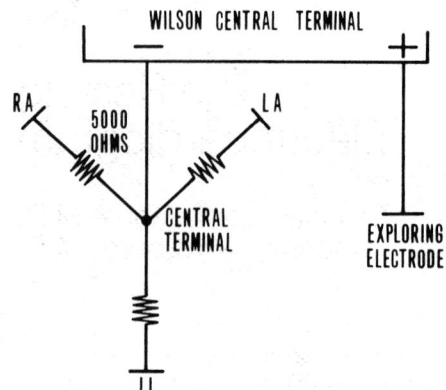

FIGURE 15-1 Diagram of the Wilson central terminal.

the heart, the body tissues vary in resistance, and the heart and the extremities do not lie in the same plane in the body. The potential of the central terminal has been said to average around 0.3 mV.[9]

Unipolar Extremity Leads

Unipolar extremity leads were initially recorded by a system in which the central terminal of Wilson constituted the indifferent electrode and the exploring electrode was placed on one of the extremities. These leads were known as V_R, V_L, and V_F. At present, unipolar extremity leads are obtained by disconnecting the input to the central terminal of Wilson from the extremity being explored. This results in a one and one-half increase in the magnitude of the wave form. These augmented (a) extremity leads are the ones usually used for clinical electrocardiography and are labeled aV_R, aV_L, and aV_F (Fig. 15-2).

Electrical Axis

The electrical axis (EA) may be defined as a vector which originates in the center of Einthoven's equilateral triangle.[2,3,6] A vector is a mathematical value expressed as a line which has direction, sense, and magnitude. The direction of the EA is also the di-

FIGURE 15-2 Connections employed in the making of augmented unipolar extremity leads.

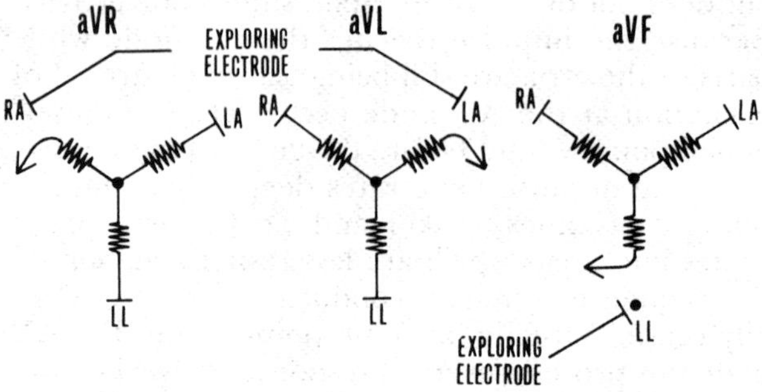

rection of activation process as projected in the plane of the limb leads. Its length represents the manifest potential of the dipole in the center of the triangle.

These general considerations apply to both the instantaneous EA (vector indicating the direction of the impulse at the instant at which it is determined) as well as the mean EA (which is the resultant of all instantaneous electrical axes). Although the mean EA can be calculated from any of the deflections of the electrocardiogram (P, T, or QRS), it generally is used in reference to the QRS.

There are many methods for determining the mean EA. The one recommended by electrocardiographers of the classical school consists of calculating the net areas enclosed by the QRS complexes in leads I, II, and III. The net area is the absolute sum of the positive and negative areas of the QRS complex in the corresponding lead. One of the drawbacks of this method is that the absolute values of the net area cannot be determined *accurately* by inspection. Since the absolute magnitude of the EA is not of fundamental clinical importance, it has been recommended that arbitrary units be used.

When this is done, the results can be counterchecked by using Einthoven's law. For example, if in a given case lead I is +4 units, lead II is +2 units, and lead III is −2 units, the calculation was accurate since the sum of leads I and III (+4 plus −2) equals lead II (+2). After having determined the net area, the results are plotted on the sides of the triangle and perpendiculars dropped from two or all three leads. The perpendiculars will meet at a point away from the center of the triangle. A line drawn from the latter to the former defines the mean EA.

A simpler, though less precise, method of calculating the quadrant (or parts of a quadrant) in which the EA is located consists of using the maximal QRS deflections in leads I and aV_F and, when necessary, lead II. This method is inexact from the mathematical viewpoint, but has the value of simplicity (Fig. 15-3).[11]

Precordial (Chest) Leads

These unipolar (V) leads are obtained by placing the exploring electrode on the various points of the chest, with the central terminal used as an indifferent electrode. According to Wilson, when a unipolar electrode is moved away from the surface of the heart (point a in Fig. 15-4) the potentials produced by the underlying myocardium decrease inversely as the cube of the distance.[2,3] In addition, the area from which potentials are recorded increases. Wilson considered that this increase was proportional to the solid angle subtended by the electrode with the heart.[2,3] A solid angle is merely an imaginary cone, with the electrode at the apex and the base being the myocardial regions from which the potentials are recorded. As the electrode is moved away

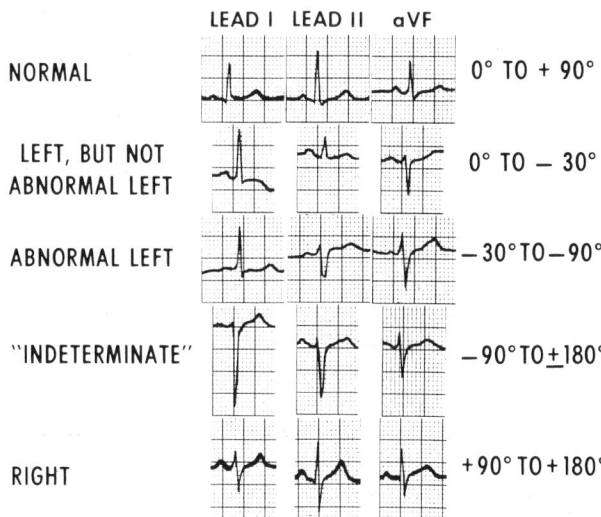

FIGURE 15-3   Determination of the quadrant, or parts of a quadrant, in which the electrical axis is located according to maximal QRS deflections.

(from a to d), the solid angles become smaller, but the corresponding bases (vertical lines b, c, and d) increase.

Considerable confusion has existed throughout the years between the concept of precordial leads as introduced by Wilson and the current (vectorial) method of precordial lead interpretation. Since the dipolar theory was, from the early days of electrocardiography, applied to the standard leads, it appeared logical to extrapolate the vectorial concept to precordial leads as well. Thus arose the vectorial approach to the precordial leads, which, when applied to the 12-lead ECG, can be properly called *vectorial electrocardiography*. This method is, no doubt, the most widely used in ECG teaching and ECG interpretation throughout the world.

Yet, it should be stated that the interpretation of Wilson's concept of precordial leads is somewhat in conflict with the vectorial concept. "Strangely enough," writes Simonson, "attempts have been made to combine the basic conflicting concepts of *unipolar* electrocardiography and *vector*cardiogra-

FIGURE 15-4   Solid angles subtended by unipolar extremity leads located at different distances from the epicardial surface of the heart (a). Vertical lines b, c, and d represent the corresponding portions of the heart from which electrical potentials are recorded by unipolar electrodes placed in the corresponding b, c, and d positions.

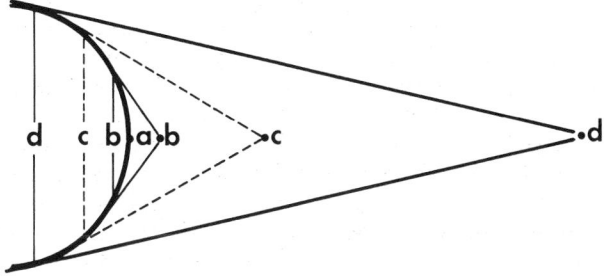

phy [as well as of *scalar* electrocardiography, we may add] in most ECG textbooks written after 1950."[12]

The vectorial concept presupposes that precordial leads record mainly electric forces moving in an anteroposterior (or posteroanterior) and in a left-to-right (or right-to-left) direction, since theoretically they are placed at (or close to) the horizontal level of the electrical center. Since in practice this does not always occur, it has to be accepted, to "understand" some of the actual morphologies, that precordial leads record forces moving toward (or away from) the electrode not only in an anteroposterior or left-to-right direction but in an inferosuperior (or superoinferior) direction as well.

For example, inadvertent or intentional recording of a "high" V_1 or of a "low" V_6 lead can result in morphologies "similar" to those recorded on aV_R and aV_F. This occurs because, regardless of the exact location (or even the existence) of the electrical center of the heart, all unipolar leads (properly or improperly placed) show upright deflections when the positive electric charges of the moving (depolarization or repolarization) wave fronts face the electrodes and show downward (below the base line) deflections when the negative charges are oriented toward the electrode.

Electrocardiographic Manifestations of Myocardial Injury, Necrosis, and Ischemia

In orthodox electrocardiograpic language injury implies *abnormal* ST-segment shifts; necrosis, *abnormal* Q waves; and ischemia, *symmetrical* T-wave inversion (or elevation).[2–4,6–9,13,14]

Electrocardiographic Signs of Injury

Following the work of Wilson several authors consider that electrocardiographic signs of injury occur because the affected cells are unable to maintain their normal polarization during diastole.[6–9,11,13,14] Various hypotheses have been postulated to explain how this diastolic hypopolarization,[7] or generalized diastolic depolarization,[15] is manifested as abnormal ST-segment shifts in the surface ECG.

One hypothesis, based on the existence of a diastolic current of injury, is depicted in Fig. 15-5. During the control (diastolic) period both membrane resting potential and surface ECG base line are at their normal level. At the onset of injury the resting intracellular potential decreases (for example from −90 mV to −70 mV) and the ECG base line shifts below its preinjury level. Because the injured cells leak negative ions, their *exterior* becomes relatively negative (or less positive) than that of the normal cells. Thus a current of injury flows between the negative (injured) zone and the positive (normal) region. This produces a negative displacement of the base line in the leads facing the injured region.

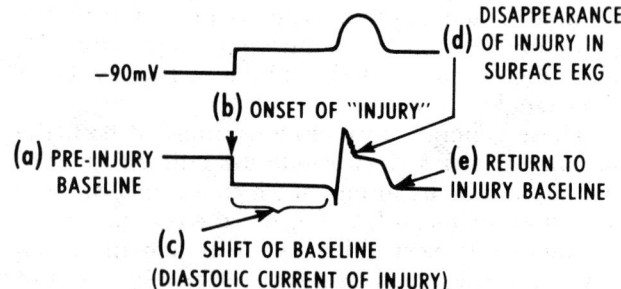

FIGURE 15-5 Genesis of the ST-segment changes due to electrical injury according to the diastolic current of injury hypothesis. The upper tracing is an intracellular recording from an injured cell. The bottom shows the precordial (body surface) changes recorded by a unipolar lead placed over the injured area.

Depolarization, beginning at the end of diastole, is characterized by an abnormal intracellular action potential (because of its takeoff at a lower than normal level) with delayed phase 0 and short duration. The surface QRS complex, representing the activity of multiple noninjured and injured cells, shows some slurring and notching due to the intrainjury conduction delay resulting from the delayed conduction occurring within the affected cells (acute, intrainjury, "focal" block). In the surface ECG, depolarization (by virtue of the electrical negativization of the nonaffected area) practically reduces the potential difference between noninjured and injured regions. Therefore, the ST segment remains at the preinjury level, which is relatively elevated in reference to the injury base line. In consequence, the ST segment appears to be abnormally displaced above the latter. Note that the apparent presence of a systolic current of injury actually reflects disappearance of the diastolic current of injury. Finally, after the end of repolarization the current of injury between injured and noninjured regions is reestablished and the ECG base line is again depressed (as it was immediately before depolarization) (Fig. 15-5). Since the precise moment at which injury starts is not recorded in the surface ECG, the base line that is almost invariably recorded is the postinjury base line which has been placed at an apparently adequate position by the recording instrument or by the ECG technician.

Very recent ingenious studies have corroborated that the elevated ST-segment displacement does not merely represent the (passive) return of the base line to its preinjury level, but that it reflects a true, active positive displacement.[16] According to this concept, when depolarization of both normal and injured regions has occurred, the surface of the normal cells will (on account of their greater initial polarization) be able to accumulate more negative ions. Hence, the normal regions become more negative than the injured regions, which are relatively more positive. In consequence, the ST segment becomes actively elevated above and beyond the preinjured base line because of the relative potential difference existing at the end of depolarization. It is likely that transmural injury reflects both disappearance of diastolic base-line shifts plus active ST elevation.[16]

Electrocardiographic Signs of Necrosis

Abnormal Q waves appearing early in the course of the infarction need not be due to anatomic necrosis. For instance, when the degree of injury is severe enough to produce a significant degree of hypopolarization (to, let us say, around -60 mV), the cells become electrically inexcitable even though they are not anatomically (irreversibly) necrotic. Hence, abnormal Q waves occur. Because the cells are only severely affected (significantly hypopolarized) but not necrotic, interventions (pharmacological or mechanical) which improve cellular metabolism and oxygenation can restore the normal polarization. If these cells can again become excitable, the abnormal Q waves disappear or "vanish."[11,13] These interventions can also be of benefit when performed before the appearance of abnormal Q waves, since they can reduce the extent and (perhaps) degree of injury (ST-segment shifts), thereby limiting the number of cells which can be electrically, or anatomically, necrotic. Of course, after anatomic necrosis has occurred, the cells cannot recuperate.

Abnormal Q waves occurring in the late (chronic) stages of myocardial infarction are due to fibrosis or scar formation. They can also disappear, but for other reasons (occurrence of some conduction disturbances or of areas of necrosis in other regions of the heart, electrode misplacement, "shrinking of the scar," etc.).

Electrocardiographic Signs of Ischemia

Symmetrical T waves (inverted or upright) characteristic of electrocardiographic ischemia have been considered to reflect a type, or degree, of cellular affection resulting only in action potentials of increased duration. Because the QT interval recorded at the body surface can be considered as the sum of all action potentials (that is, of QT intervals of individual cells), any process (such as electrocardiographic ischemia) which increases action potential duration will cause prolongation of ventricular repolarization and QT interval.

The previously mentioned (normal) shorter repolarization of epicardial cells (due to their shorter action potentials in comparison with that of the endocardial cells) and the concomitant epicardial-to-endocardial spread of repolarization with the negative charge in front (and the positive charge facing the epicardium) explain why V_5 and V_6 normally show positive T waves.

Thus, in subendocardial "ischemia" the increased duration of the action potentials occurs in a group of cells where they were already longer than in the

epicardium (Fig. 15-6). Repolarization, though more delayed than usual, still spreads from endocardium to epicardium. In consequence, the QT interval is prolonged and the T wave appears symmetrically positive. On the other hand, the increase in action potential duration that occurs in epicardial ischemia results not only in delayed repolarization (QT prolongation) but also in a change in the sequence of repolarization, which now starts at the earlier repolarized endocardium, thereafter spreading toward the epicardium with the negative charges in front. The latter produces the characteristic symmetrical T-wave inversion.

Acute Transmural Myocardial Infarction

Classically an area of transmural necrosis is surrounded by a layer of injured tissue which in turn has an ischemic zone around it (Fig. 15-7). Because of the solid angle that it subtends, the left precordial lead depicted in this figure shows the characteristic abnormal Q wave, the abnormal ST-segment elevation, and a terminally inverted T wave. Leads placed directly over different points of the epicardium may (because of their different solid angles) only reflect the necrosis, or the injury, or the ischemia. When the myocardial infarction is very large, there are distinctive changes in the leads recording the electrical activity of the affected regions. A lead displaying any of these morphologies is of course comparable to the epicardial leads shown in Fig. 15-7.

FIGURE 15-6 Genesis of QT prolongation and T-wave changes produced by (sub)endocardial and (sub)epicardial ischemia. The term *ischemia* is an electrocardiographic term which is used in reference to a type or degree of cellular affectation, not necessarily due to decreased blood supply.

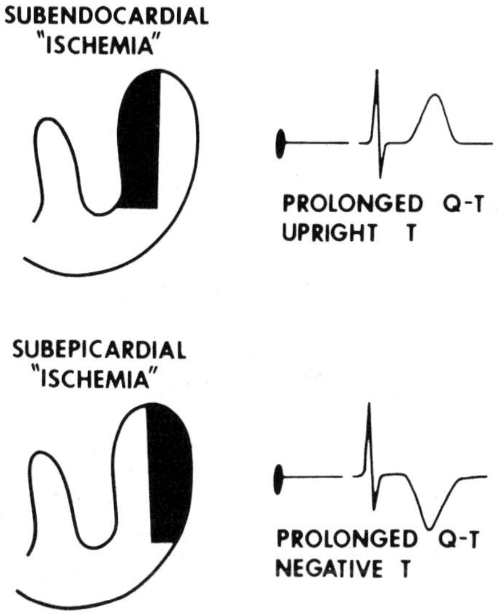

SUBENDOCARDIAL "ISCHEMIA"

PROLONGED Q-T UPRIGHT T

SUBEPICARDIAL "ISCHEMIA"

PROLONGED Q-T NEGATIVE T

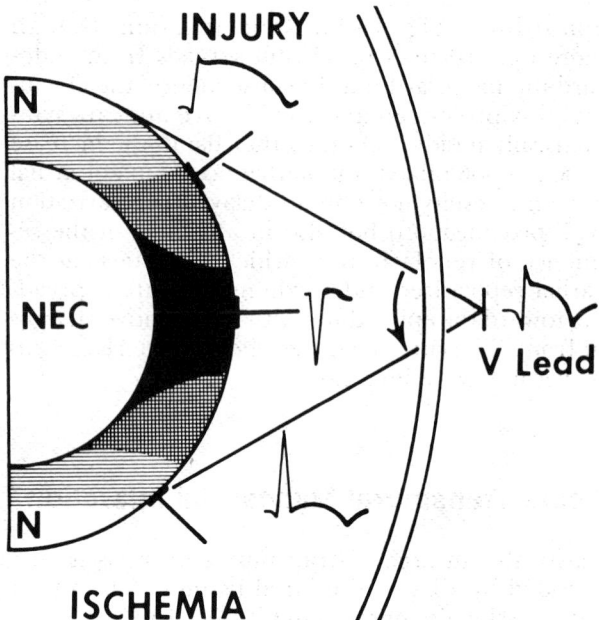

FIGURE 15-7 *Unipolar epicardial and body surface electrodes from a section of the left ventricle containing a transmural myocardial infarction. Electrodes over the necrotic (NEC) area record a QS complex; over the injured area, a significant ST-segment displacement; and over the area of ischemia, T-wave inversion. The corresponding precordial (V) lead, because of the greater solid angle which it subtends, records potentials from necrotic, injured, ischemic, and normal (N) areas.*

Location of the Site of Myocardial Infarction

According to Schamroth, changes recorded by leads overlying the affected regions are referred to as *indicative* changes, whereas those recorded by leads facing the opposite (unaffected) regions are known as *reciprocal* changes.[8] For example, in inferoposterior myocardial infarction (MI) leads II, III, and aV_F show indicative ST-segment changes (Fig. 15-8) and leads aV_L and V_2 show reciprocal changes (to the inferior and posterior walls, respectively).

True posterior MI (manifested by an increase in size of the R waves in V_1 and V_2 with large positive T waves) usually is associated with inferior or lateral MI. In adults the differential diagnosis of true posterior MI includes right ventricular hypertrophy; "atypical" Wolff-Parkinson-White syndromes (due to Kent or Mahaim bundles), and some (also "atypical") "incomplete" right bundle branch block patterns.

The term *apical* MI has been used in reference to MI affecting only leads V_2, V_3, and V_4 (localized anterior MI) or those affecting leads II, III, aV_F, V_5 and V_6 (inferolateral MI).

In anteroseptal MI, QS complexes will be found in leads V_1, V_2, and V_3.[17] False patterns of anteroseptal MI occur in patients with left anterior hemi-

FIGURE 15-8 *Inferoposterior myocardial infarction. The ECG of 11/29 shows minor nonspecific ST-T wave changes. On 12/5 an acute myocardial infarction occurred. There are pathological Q waves (1), ST-segment elevation (2), and terminal T-wave inversion (3) in leads II, III, and aV_F, indicating the location of the infarct on the inferior wall. Reciprocal changes in aV_L (small arrow). Increasing R-wave voltage with ST depression and increased voltage of the T wave in V_2 is characteristic of true posterior wall extension of the inferior infarction. (From R. J. Myerburg, Electrocardiography, in Harrison's "Principles of Internal Medicine," 9th ed., McGraw-Hill Book Company, New York, 1980, p. 999. Reproduced with permission of author and publisher.)*

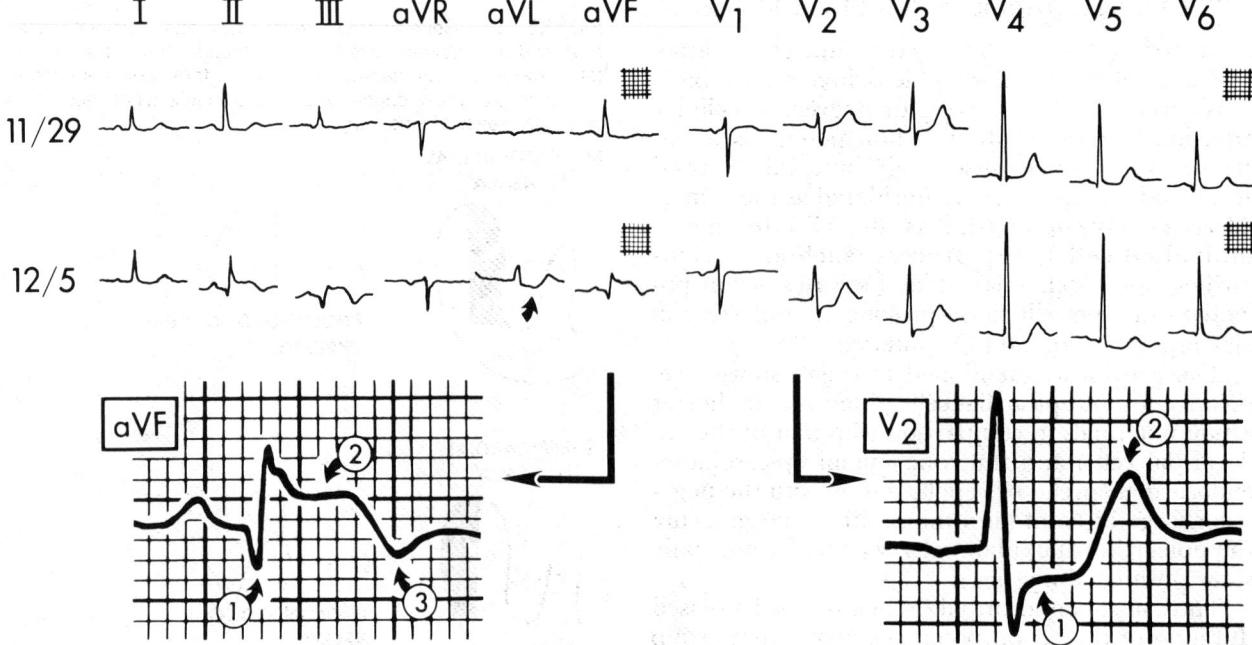

block, left bundle branch block, extensive septal fibrosis, and massive left ventricular enlargement (generally pressure overloading in type).

Anterolateral MI produces the characteristic changes in leads V_4, V_5, and V_6 as well as in leads I, II, and aV_L. However, similar patterns can occur in patients without coronary artery disease who had primary cellular necrosis and replacement fibrosis due to noncoronary artery disease–induced cellular affectation. Large Q waves in these leads (usually preceding large R waves) occur in idiopathic hypertrophic subaortic stenosis, glycogen storage disease, and certain muscular dystrophies.

Extensive anterior MI affects all chest leads, as well as leads I, II, and aV_L. Localized anterior MI is said to produce changes in V_2, and V_3, and V_4 only.[17]

The diagnosis of nontransmural (often called subendocardial) MI is based on the clinical history obtained by the physician and by the interpretation of the enzyme patterns. Since there are no characteristic electrocardiographic changes for this type of MI, the ECG (empirically interpreted) more often than not shows nonspecific ST-T changes or ischemic T-wave inversion. Even the infrequently found ST-segment depression in all leads (except aV_R, which shows ST-segment elevation) can occur in absence of enzyme changes or in patients with central nervous disease.

Pericarditis

The electrocardiographic pattern of acute pericarditis not due to MI is produced by the associated epicardial myocarditis which, in turn, produces diffuse epicardial injury. The ST segments can be elevated in all leads except aV_R (and rarely in V_1). Symmetrical T-wave inversion (due to epicardial ischemia) usually develops after the ST segments have returned to the base line (but can appear during the injury stage). Neither reciprocal ST-segment changes nor abnormal Q waves are seen.

Normal and Abnormal ST-T Contours

Various types of normal and abnormal ST-segment and T-wave (ST-T) changes are shown in Fig. 15-9.

Conduction Disturbances

The nomenclature of the different types of intraventricular conduction disturbances has produced almost insurmountable difficulties in the understanding of concepts. In view of the multiple names currently in use, it seems that attempts to establish universal nomenclature are practically utopian. Nonetheless, a working classification is necessary,

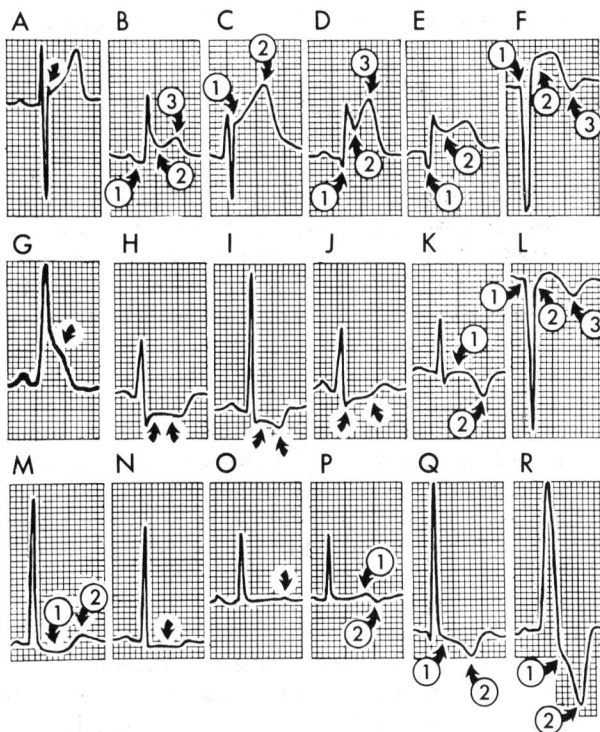

FIGURE 15-9 Normal and abnormal ST-T contours. Arrows in each panel indicate the major features of each complex. *A.* Early repolarization (J-point elevation), normal variant. *B.* Acute pericarditis: (1) depressed T_a, (2) elevated ST, and (3) normal T. *C.* Acute myocardial infarction in lead V_3: (1) elevated ST and (2) tall, peaked T wave. *D.* Acute myocardial infarction in lead V_6: (1) small Q wave, (2) elevated ST segment, and (3) tall peaked T wave with steep $2 \rightarrow 3$ angle. *E.* and *F.* Subacute myocardial infarction with: (1) pathological Q wave, (2) elevated ST segment, and (3) terminal T-wave inversion. *G.* Prinzmetal variant angina with ST elevation during pain. *H.* and *I.* Angina pectoris (usual form) with horizontal or downward-sloping ST segment during pain or exercise. *J.* J-point depression with upsloping ST segment during exercise, normal response. *K.* Ischemic T-wave inversion in ischemia or primary muscle disease. *L.* Ventricular aneurysm: (1) pathological Q, (2) elevated ST segment, and (3) symmetrically inverted T wave. *M.* Digitalis effect: (1) downward coving of ST segment, merging into (2) an upright T wave. *N., O.,* and *P.* "Nonspecific" ST-T wave changes. Left ventricular strain pattern with: (1) downsloping ST segment and (2) asymmetrically inverted (secondary) T wave. *R.* Complete left bundle branch block. *(From R. J. Myerburg, Electrocardiography, in "Harrison's Principles of Internal Medicine," 9th ed., McGraw-Hill Book Company, New York, 1980, p. 999. Reproduced with permission of author and publisher.)*

primarily for didactic reasons, so that the proper concepts can be established.

Left Anterior Hemiblock

In left anterior hemiblock the posteroinferior regions of the left ventricular endocardium are activated abnormally before the anterosuperior left ventricular area. After emerging from the posteroinferior division of the left bundle branch, the impulse first propagates in an inferior, rightward, and usually anterior direction for a short period of time.

EXAMINATION OF THE HEART AND BLOOD VESSELS

This orientation is responsible for the small Q waves in leads I and aV_L and for the R waves in leads II, III, and aV_F (Fig. 15-10A).

Although the posteroinferior division is posterior (dorsal) in reference to the anterosuperior division of the left bundle branch and the anterolateral wall of the left ventricle, it is anterior (ventral) in reference of the posteroinferior wall of the left ventricle. This spatial location of the posteroinferior division explains why in left anterior hemiblock the right chest leads show (as in patients without left anterior hemiblock) a predominantly negative deflection, indicating that the activation front is moving in a posterior direction (away from V_1).

If the posteroinferior division were to end at the posteroinferior (free) wall of the left ventricle, the right chest leads would show predominantly positive deflections since the activation front would be moving toward V_1 and V_2. From the electrocardiographic viewpoint, the divisions of the left branch behave more as if they were superior and inferior rather than anterior and posterior. For this reason the most significant abnormalities produced by left anterior and left posterior hemiblock (in absence of "complete" right bundle branch block) occur in the standard and unipolar extremity leads rather than in the precordial leads (Fig. 15-10A). However, some changes do occur in properly (or improperly) placed precordial leads. Foremost amongst these are the false patterns of anteroseptal MI (which occur when the right chest electrodes are placed too high) and those of anatomical clockwise rotation (which are seen when the left chest leads are placed so low that they record predominantly negative deflections).

Additional points regarding left anterior hemiblock that are noteworthy are (1) the degree of left axis deviation required to make this diagnosis has been a source of debate and speculation—if the EA is between $-30°$ and $-45°$, this conduction disturbance is probably present, but if the axis is between $-45°$ and $-90°$, it is almost certainly present; (2) other processes can also produce abnormal left axis deviation (Fig. 15-10); (3) when left anterior hemiblock coexists with certain types of congenital right ventricular enlargements (Fig. 15-11, bottom) and extensive anterolateral MI (Fig. 15-13C), the EA can be located in the indeterminate (right superior) quadrant. Evidently, the most constant feature of the axis deviation produced by left anterior hemiblock is its *superior* orientation, not necessarily its *superior and leftward* orientation (abnormal left axis deviation); and (4) the differentiation between the indeterminate EA produced by complicated left anterior hemiblock and that resulting exclusively from some atypical types of right ventricular enlargement can best be made by lead aV_L (Fig. 15-11).

Recent experiments using preparations obtained from canine hearts with microelectrode techniques have shown that only a minor delay of activation occurs in the corresponding regions of the left ven-

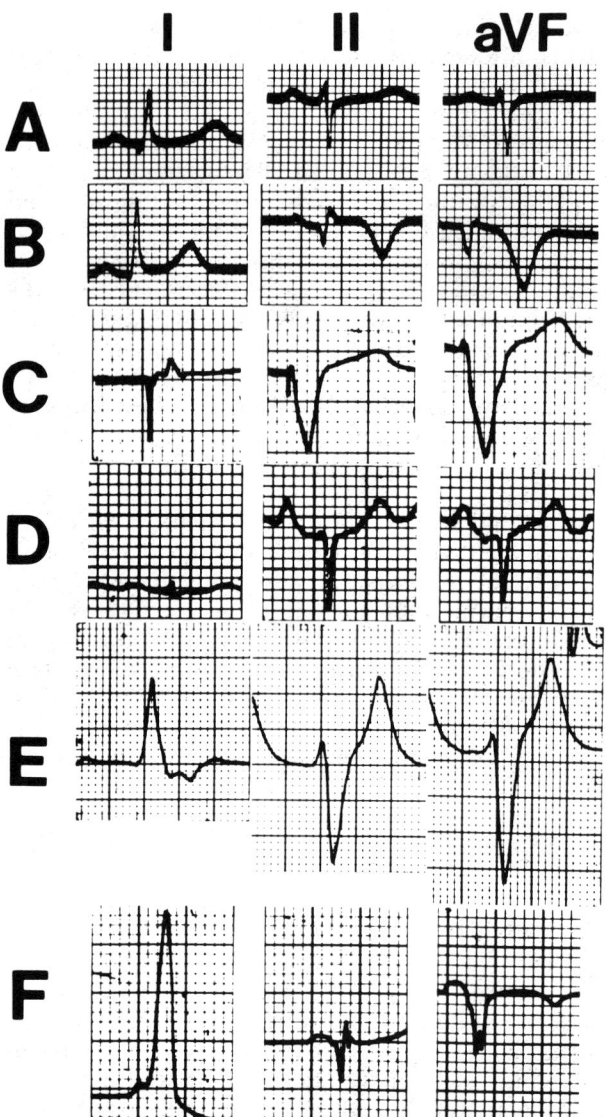

FIGURE 15-10 Causes of abnormal left axis deviation: *A.* left anterior hemiblock. *B.* Extensive inferior myocardial infarction. *C.* Right ventricular apical (or middle cardiac vein) pacing. *D.* Pulmonary emphysema. *E.* Advanced hyperkalemia. *F.* Wolff-Parkinson-White syndrome, usually type B.

tricle after transverse section of the major fascicles or divisions of the left bundle branch.[18] The expected delay was noted only after the section was extended vertically to sever the multiple fibers extending from the intact to the sectioned division. These studies suggest that the hemiblock patterns as seen in the surface 12-lead ECG are due to an extensive rather than to a localized lesion. However, more correlation is required to determine the application of these findings to clinical electrocardiography. For instance, they do not necessarily apply to rate-related, or functional, hemiblocks (produced by premature supraventricular impulses) since in these cases the conduction disturbances can occur more proximally or more distally (within the left bundle system) to the level where the equivalent experimental section was performed.

Because of the multiple interconnections between the divisions of the bundle branch system, the appearance of left anterior hemiblock does not increase QRS duration by more than 0.025 s. A left anterior hemiblock pattern with prolonged QRS duration generally indicates the presence of additional conduction disturbances such as incomplete left bundle branch block, right bundle branch block, focal blocks, or combinations of the above (Fig. 15-12).

The electrocardiographic features of left anterior hemiblock associated with myocardial infarction is shown in Fig. 15-13.

Left Posterior Hemiblock

In "pure" left posterior hemiblock, the impulse, after emerging from the unblocked anterosuperior division, first moves in a superior, leftward, and (somewhat) anterior direction. This produces the small Q waves in leads II, III, and aV_F (Figs. 15-14 and 15-15). Therefore, the general spread of activation occurs through the electrically preponderant left ventricle in an inferior, posterior, and slightly rightward direction. The large magnitude of these

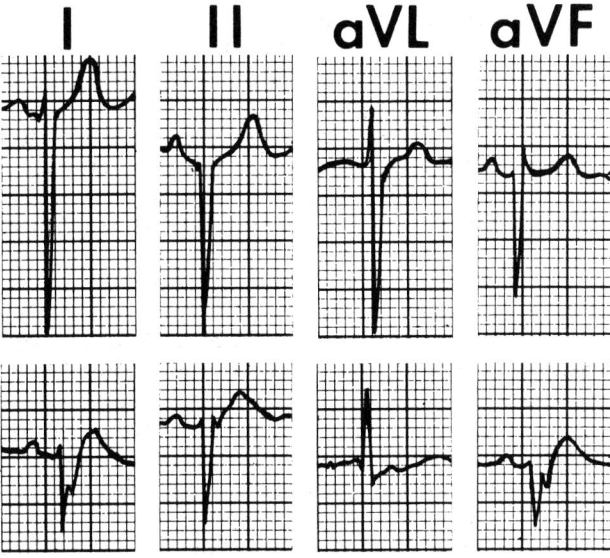

FIGURE 15-11 "Indeterminate," "right superior," or "northwest" electrical axis produced by right ventricular hypertrophy as seen in some patients with congenital heart disease (top) and in left anterior hemiblock (bottom). Lead aV_L is the most important lead to establish the differential diagnosis since in right ventricular hypertrophy this lead shows a predominantly negative deflection, whereas in left anterior hemiblock it shows a predominantly positive deflection.

FIGURE 15-12 A. Left anterior hemiblock with right bundle branch block. B. Left anterior hemiblock with right bundle branch block and left ventricular "focal block," with a pattern of "masquerading" left bundle branch block. C. Left anterior hemiblock with left ventricular focal block due to old anterolateral myocardial infarction—also called periinfarction block.

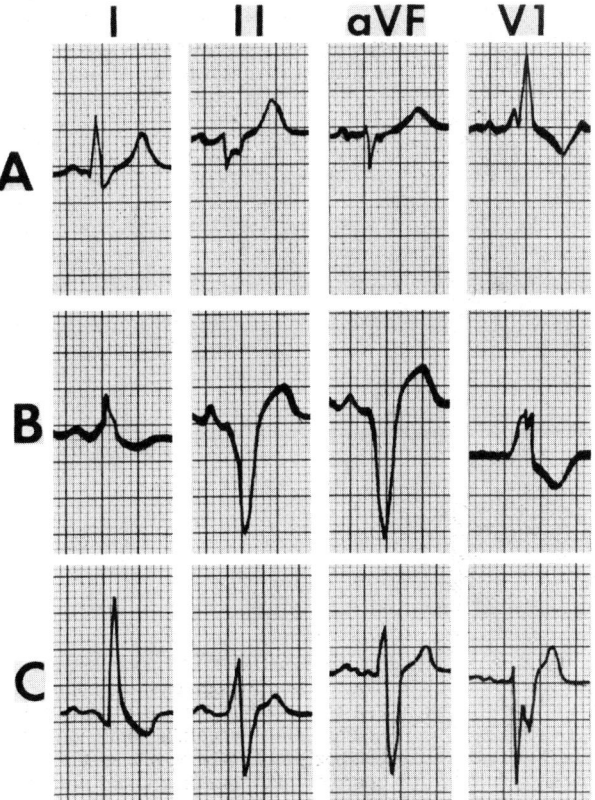

FIGURE 15-13 Diagnosis of left anterior hemiblock associated with myocardial infarction. A. Left anterior hemiblock and anteroseptal myocardial infarction. B. Left anterior hemiblock and anterolateral myocardial infarction. C. Left anterior hemiblock and anterolateral myocardial infarction with electrical axis in right superior ("indeterminate") quadrant. D. Left anterior hemiblock and inferior wall myocardial infarction.

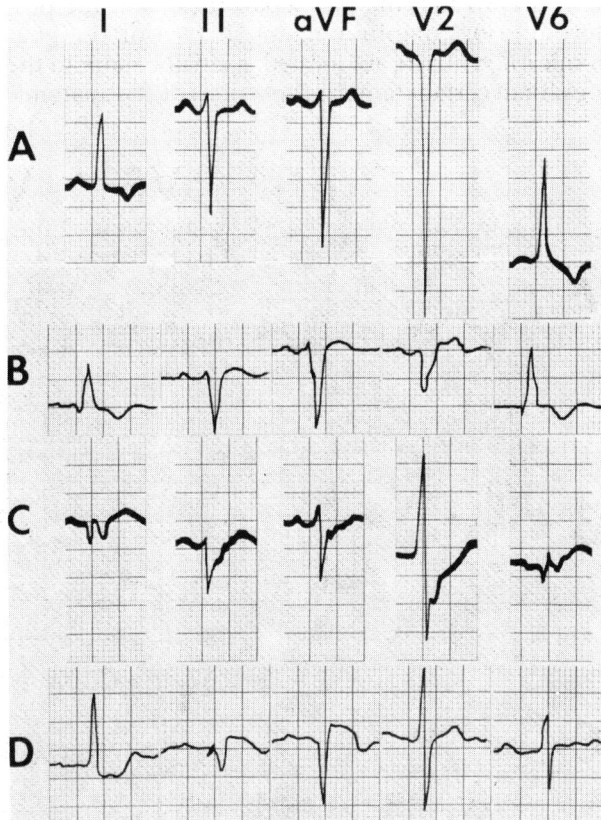

Left Bundle Branch

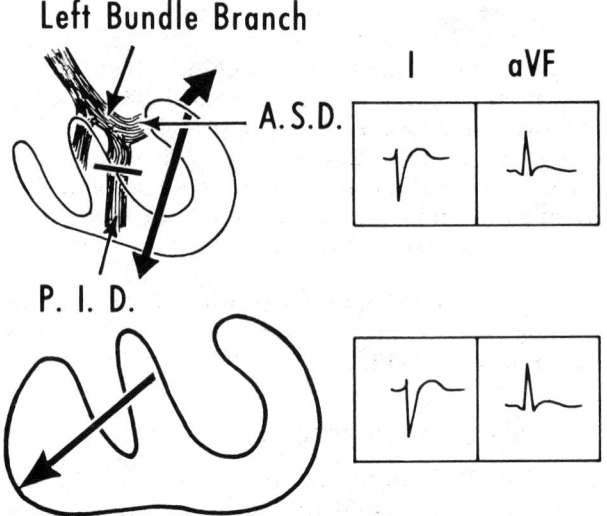

FIGURE 15-14 Electrogenesis of right axis deviation due to left posterior hemiblock (top) and right ventricular hypertrophy (bottom). In the former, right axis deviation due to the hemiblock-related reorientation of electric forces within the anatomically predominant left ventricle. In right ventricular hypertrophy right axis deviation is due to the increase in size of the now anatomically predominant right ventricle. It should be emphasized that the differentation between these two processes cannot be made based on the ECG alone.

forces and the pattern of the intraventricular conduction are responsible for the right axis deviation (at least of $+120°$), large R waves in leads II, III, and aV_F, and the deep S waves in leads I and aV_L.

Radiologic studies of the human heart in situ have shown that the paraseptal regions of the posteroinferior (diaphragmatic) surface of the anatomic *left* ventricle are located, spatially, more to the *right* than certain (anterior) portions of the anatomic

right ventricle. Since the portions of the left ventricle that are spatially located to the right are less significant than those located superiorly, the degree of right axis deviation produced by pure left posterior hemiblock is of lesser magnitude than that of left axis deviation produced by left anterior hemiblock. The hallmark of left posterior hemiblock is, therefore, an *inferior* axis shift as much as *right* axis deviation.

Because a similar sequence of ventricular activation can also occur in right ventricular hypertrophy, pleuropulmonary disease (acute or chronic), and extremely vertical anatomic heart positions due to a slender body build or chest wall deformities, it is evident that the diagnosis of pure left posterior hemiblock cannot be made from the ECG alone. Additional clinical, radiologic, or pathologic information is required for this purpose.

The diagnosis of left posterior hemiblock in presence of MI is shown in Fig. 15-15.

Complete Right Bundle Branch Block

It is now known that a "complete" right bundle branch block pattern (with QRS duration greater than 0.11 s) does not necessarily reflect the existence of a total conduction block in the right branch. This pattern only indicates that the totality, or majority, of both ventricles are activated by the impulse emerging from the left branch. Thus a significant degree of conduction delay (high-grade or incomplete right bundle branch block) can produce a similar pattern. This is best seen when the QRS changes are intermittent, or when spontaneous (or induced) premature atrial beats produce different degrees of functional right bundle branch block. Whereas in

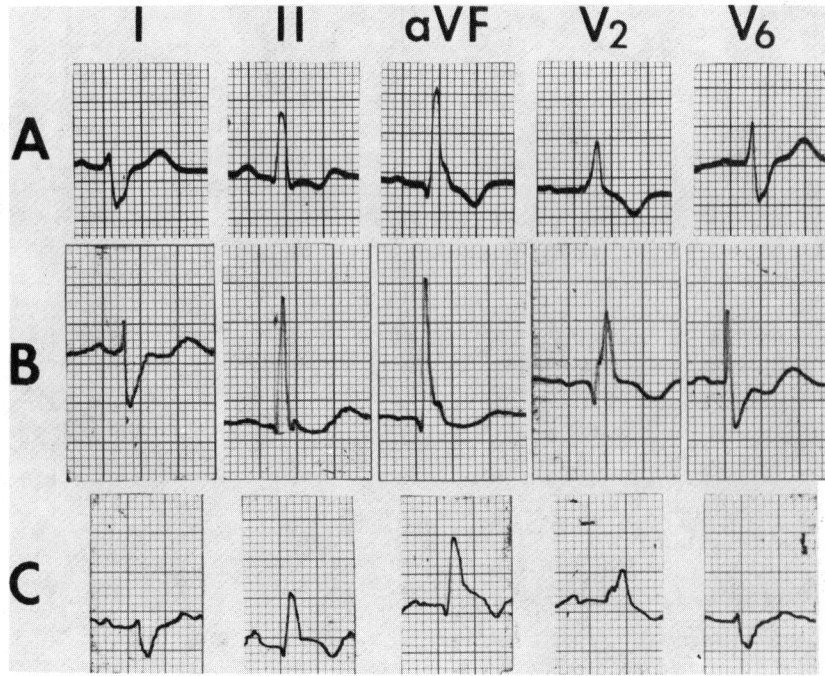

FIGURE 15-15 *A.* Left posterior hemiblock without myocardial infarction. *B.* Left posterior hemiblock coexisting with anteroseptal myocardial infarction. *C.* Left posterior hemiblock with inferior myocardial infarction diagnosed only by evolutionary ST-T changes.

Fig. 15-16 the next-to-last QRS complex has a duration compatible with the diagnosis of complete right bundle branch block, the last ventricular complex is even wider (0.15 s), therefore suggesting that the former was not due to a total conduction block in the right branch.

Some authors have reported that a right ventricular free-wall incision (such as that performed for the complete correction of some congenital heart lesions) can produce a *distal* right bundle branch block pattern by disruption of the terminal (peripheral) ramifications of the right bundle branch.[19]

Incomplete Right Bundle Branch Block Pattern

For many years it has been recognized what has recently been proved with endocardial (catheter) and epicardial mapping, namely that incomplete right bundle branch block patterns can be produced by (1) different degrees of conduction delays through the main trunk of the right bundle branch (Fig. 15-16); (2) an increased conduction time through an elongated right bundle branch, stretched because of a concomitant enlargement of the right septal surface (as in congenital volume overloading of the right ventricle); (3) a diffuse Purkinje-myocardial delay due to right ventricular stretch or dilatation; (4) ventriculotomy- or disease-related interruption of the major ramifications of the right branch (distal right bundle branch block or right hemiblocks); and (5) congenital variations of the distribution of the major distal ramifications resulting in a slight delay in activation of the crista supraventricularis.[19]

Concealed Right Bundle Branch Block

A conduction delay in the main trunk of the right bundle branch or in its major ramifications may not be manifested in the surface ECG when there are coexisting (and of greater degree) conduction disturbances in the main left bundle branch, the anterosuperior division of the left bundle branch and/or in the free left ventricular wall.[13] A right bundle branch block can also be concealed in some patients with Wolff-Parkinson-White syndrome type B provided that the ventricular insertion of the accessory pathway (Kent bundle) causes preexcitation of the right ventricular regions that would be activated late because of the right bundle branch block.[20]

Focal Block

Several names have been applied to the conduction disturbances occurring in the left-sided Purkinje-myocardial junctions, left septal surface, or free walls of the left ventricle: arborization block, diffuse (nonspecific) intraventricular block, periinfarction block, parietal block, etc. Although readers might disagree with what we are hereby considering (in keeping with Rosenbaum's concepts) as focal block, they must nevertheless have a clear understanding of the concept that it implies.[7]

These conduction disturbances have different electrogenetic mechanisms.[7] Thus, the cellular "affectation" due to acute injury resulting from coronary artery disease (Fig. 15-5), hyperkalemia (Fig. 15-10E), drugs (Fig. 15-17G), and intracoronary injections of contrast material occur within (inside) the affected regions. Focal blocks occurring in subacute or chronic MI (Fig. 15-12C), after the appearance of abnormal Q waves (periinfarction block), as well as those occurring in presence of diffuse myocardial fibrosis (of noncoronary etiology) are due to the circuitous and irregular activation of living cells surrounded by (or surrounding) areas of fibrotic tissue.

Complete Left Bundle Branch Block

This conduction disturbance is characterized by wide (greater than 0.11 s) QRS complexes. The diagnostic criteria consists of prolongation of the QRS complexes (over 0.11 s) with neither a Q nor an S wave in leads I and in the properly placed V_6. A wide R wave with a notch on its top (plateau) is seen in these leads. In hearts with an electrical (and anatomic) vertical position a small Q wave may be seen in aV_L in the absence of MI. The right chest leads V_1 and V_2 might or might not show an initial R wave. Unfortunately, as mentioned in reference to complete right bundle branch block, these morphologies can be recorded in patients with high-degree (not necessarily complete) left bundle branch block.

The direction of the EA in patients showing QRS changes typical of complete left bundle branch block has been a widely discussed subject.[11,13] In the majority of the human hearts the site of exit from the right bundle branch does not seem to be at the lowermost right ventricular region (that called in pacemaker nomenclature the *right ventricular apex*). If

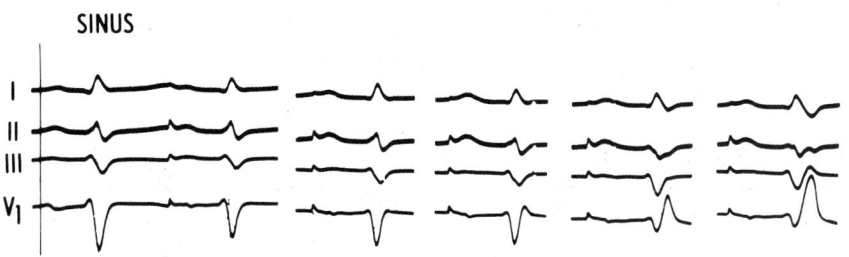

SINUS

I

II

III

V_1

FIGURE 15-16 Right bundle branch block induced by premature right atrial stimulation. Whereas the first beat is of sinus origin, the others show increasing (from left to right) grades of right bundle branch block aberration. Note that the slightest degree of right bundle branch block only produces a decrease in the size of the S wave in V_1 (second ventricular complex).

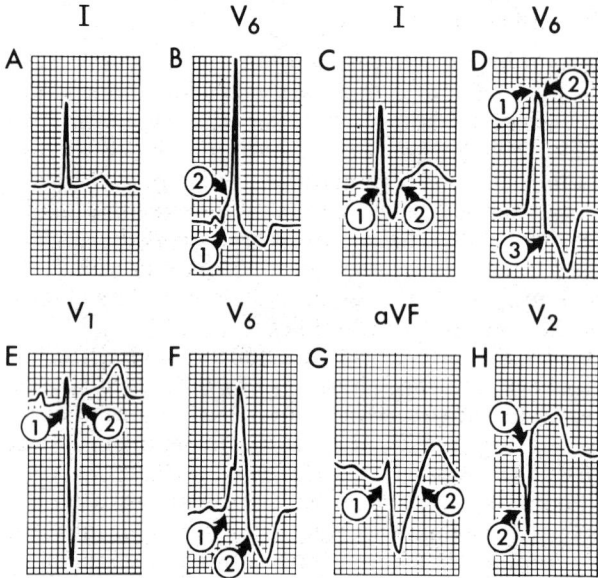

FIGURE 15-17   QRS complexes: *A.* Normal. *B.* Prolongation due to initial QRS delay between (1 → 2) in Wolff-Parkinson-White syndrome. *C.* Prolongation due to terminal delay (1 → 2) in right bundle branch block. *D.* Prolongation due to mid (1 → 2) and late (2 → 3) delay in left bundle branch block. *E.* Minor uniform prolongation (1 → 2) in left ventricular hypertrophy. *F.* Distortion of total QRS pattern (1 → 2) in a cardiomyopathy. *G.* Distortion of total QRS pattern in hyperkalemia or drug toxicity. *H.* Nonspecific initial notchings and slurring in myocardial infarction. The lead is indicated above each example. (*From R. J. Myerburg, Electrocardiography, in Harrison's Principles of Internal Medicine, 9th ed., McGraw-Hill Book Company, New York, 1980, p. 999. Reproduced with permission of author and publisher.*)

this were the case, all complete left bundle branch blocks would show (as when the right ventricular apex is paced) abnormal left axis deviation.

Complete Left Bundle Branch Block Pattern with Abnormal Left Axis Deviation

This surface electrocardiographic morphology has been attributed to (1) the coexistence of an incomplete (high-degree) left bundle branch block with left anterior hemiblock; (2) the association of left anterior hemiblock with an incomplete (high-degree) left posterior hemiblock; (3) the coexistence of complete left bundle branch block with diffuse left ventricular focal block; (4) complete left bundle branch block combined with an extensive MI of the low anterolateral wall; (5) the association of complete left bundle branch block with a block in the superior subdivision of the right bundle branch (right superior hemiblock); and (6) complete left bundle branch block occurring in a patient with abnormal anatomic rotation of the heart as a result of thoracic chest wall deformities or pleuropericardial disease. However, in some cases of complete left bundle branch block with abnormal left axis deviation no cause for the latter can be found (applying presently available knowledge).[13]

Complete Left Bundle Branch Block with Myocardial Infarction

This association is depicted diagrammatically in Fig. 15-18.

Incomplete Left Bundle Branch Block Pattern

An incomplete left bundle branch block pattern can be diagnosed in a heart with an electrically horizontal (or semihorizontal) position when leads I and V_6 show an R wave with a slurring in its upstroke (not on its top as in complete left bundle branch block). However, an S wave may be recorded in lead V_6 when the electrode is placed "too low" or if abnormal left axis deviation is present. Leads V_1 and V_2 may show rS or QS complexes. Although QRS duration usually ranges between 0.08 and 0.11 s, this pattern can be observed with QRS durations of 0.12 and 0.13 s. Not surprisingly, an incomplete left bundle branch block pattern can be produced by various processes, namely, (1) conduction delays in the main trunk of the left bundle branch; (2) conduction delays (of more or less equal degree) in the

FIGURE 15-18   Complete left bundle branch block (CLBBB) and transmural myocardial infarction. Lateral wall myocardial infarction (top row) and inferior myocardial infarction (IMI) (third row) do not produce alterations in the basic (QRS) pattern of CLBBB since the necrotic areas do not affect those in which the onset of depolarization occurs (anterior portions of the right septal surface). However, an anteroseptal myocardial infarction (ASMI) involving the areas where the impulse emerges from the left bundle branch (second row) changes the initial spread of depolarization (toward the right posterior portions of the right ventricular structures). The latter produces a Q wave in lead I as well as in aV_L and V_6 (not shown). The bottom row shows that the Q waves in inferior myocardial infarction (IMI) (in aV_F) will become apparent only when there is an ASMI with total involvement of the interventricular septum.

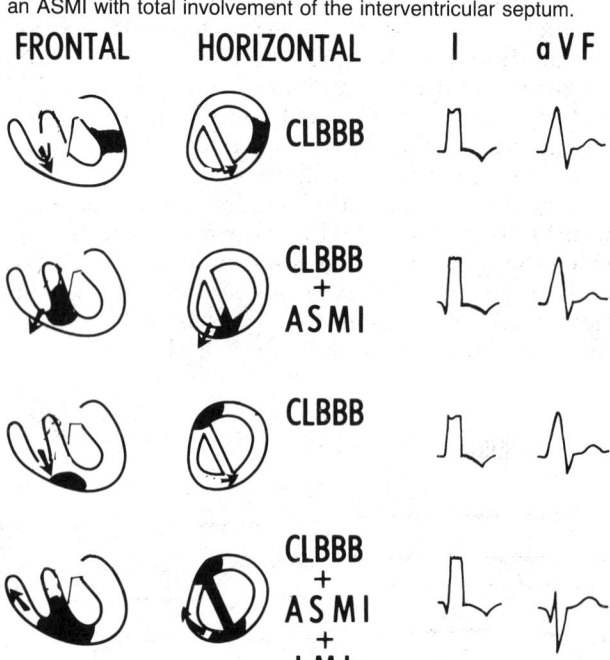

divisions of the left bundle branch; (3) diffuse septal fibrosis; (4) small septal infarctions; (5) left ventricular enlargements (generally pressure overloading in type); and (6) combination of the above.

Ventricular Hypertrophy

The term *ventricular hypertrophy* will be used in reference to ventricular enlargement (either due to an increase in muscle thickness, ventricular dilatation, or both) as it occurs in the adult (over 30 years of age) population. In children with congenital and valvular disease the concept of pressure (systolic) and volume (diastolic) overloading has clinical importance, but in older patients it has no practical value.

The sensitivity and specificity of the various criteria used to diagnose left and right ventricular hypertrophy as well as the corresponding electrocardiographic-anatomic correlations are discussed in the chapter entitled "The Diagnostic Capabilities and Limitations of the Electrocardiogram," which appeared in *The Heart: Update I*, 1979.[21]

Thus, only a few points will be mentioned here:

1. Most *hospitalized* patients with an incomplete left bundle branch block pattern (as defined previously) have, regardless of voltage, left ventricular enlargement by x-ray or echocardiography.
2. Left anterior hemiblock and left posterior hemiblock, by causing reorientation of the activation sequence of the left ventricle, can produce an increase in QRS voltage of sufficient magnitude so as to mimic left or right ventricular hypertrophy.
3. The ST-T wave abnormalities (secondary to depolarization changes) produced by left ventricular hypertrophy (strain pattern) can also be seen (even when left ventricular hypertrophy is absent) in patients with left bundle branch block, left anterior hemiblock, Wolff-Parkinson-White syndrome, and angina pectoris. Thus, in the presence of clinical possibility of left ventricular hypertrophy, the strain pattern corroborates it, but otherwise it is only "compatible" with this diagnosis.
4. In the older literature left axis deviation has been used as a criterion for left ventricular hypertrophy. Yet, recent studies seem to indicate that left ventricular hypertrophy per se does not produce *abnormal* left axis deviation.
5. False patterns of right ventricular hypertrophy can occur in Wolff-Parkinson-White syndrome type A, true posterior wall MI, and certain *atypical* incomplete right bundle branch blocks.

Electrolyte Imbalance

Because multiple factors can affect ventricular repolarization in diseased hearts, the finding characteristic of a specific electrolyte abnormality may be modified, and even mimicked, by various pathologic processes and certain drugs. In practice, the major problem with the electrocardiographic diagnosis of electrolyte imbalance is not the false-negative ECG but the production of similar changes by other conditions.[22]

Hyperkalemia

The initial effect of acute hyperkalemia is the appearance of peaked T waves with a narrow base (Fig. 15-19, left). The diagnosis of hyperkalemia is almost certain when the duration of the base is 0.24 s or less (with rates between 60 and 110 per minute). As the degree of hyperkalemia increases, the QRS widens, the P becomes smaller, and the PR interval prolongs until the P wave disappears (Fig. 15-19, right). Quinidine, procainamide, and disopiramide toxicity as well as ingestion of large doses of tricyclic antidepressants (taken for suicidal purposes) can produce similar degrees (and types) of QRS widening associated with prolonged QT or QU intervals (Fig. 15-22, right). However, wide ventricular complexes followed by narrow-based T waves are almost pathognomonic of hyperkalemia, not of drug toxicity.

Hypocalcemia

The typical electrocardiographic pattern of hypocalcemia consists of QT prolongation at the expense of the ST segment. The T wave is usually of normal width, but can be narrow-based if there is coexistent (moderate) hyperkalemia (Fig. 15-20). A very marked subendocardial ischemia (with the so-called hyperacute ST-T changes) can produce a similar pattern, but in those cases the T wave, though peaked, is not narrow-based as in Fig. 15-9*C*. It has been said that hypocalcemia per se does not produce T-wave inversion. The latter therefore is a reflection of coexisting processes such as left ventricular hypertrophy and incomplete left bundle branch block.

An ECG pattern similar to that of hypocalcemia can be produced by some organic abnormalities of

FIGURE 15-19 Electrocardiographic manifestations of early hyperkalemia (peaked T wave with a narrow base) and advanced hyperkalemia (absent P wave, wide QRS, and peaked T wave).

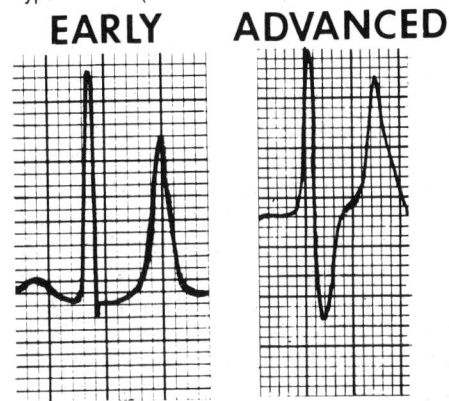

EARLY   ADVANCED

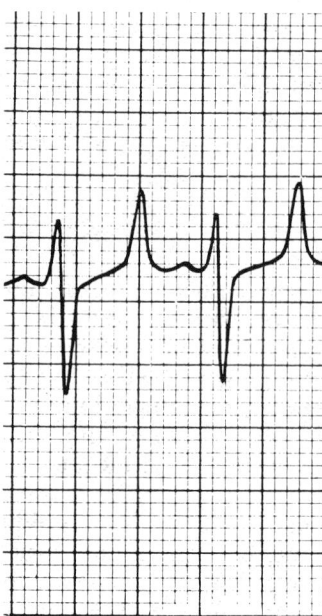

FIGURE 15-20 Hyperkalemia with hypocalcemia producing peaked T waves with a very narrow (0.08 s) base. The T waves start 0.16 s after the beginning of a sloping ST segment.

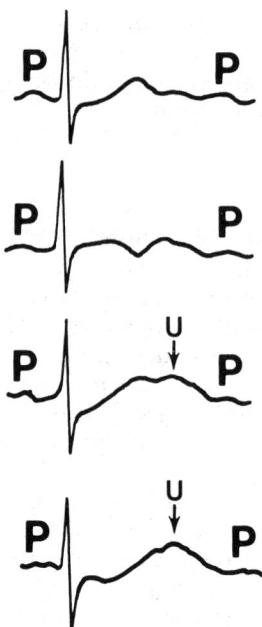

FIGURE 15-21 Electrocardiographic manifestations of hypokalemia (intermediate precordial lead). The top recording is normal control showing a small, but normal U wave. The remaining recordings are arranged to show increasing degrees of hypokalemia.

the central nervous system and by congenitally prolonged QT intervals such as the Jervell-Lange-Nielsen and Romano-Ward syndromes. Prolongation of the QT interval with the T wave starting at the very end of the QRS complex is not characteristic of hypocalcemia. This can occur in complete (infranodal) AV block with slow idioventricular rhythms, after ventricular fibrillation of any etiology, prolonged episodes of sustained ectopic tachycardias, ventricular pacing, and in some patients with organic abnormalities of the central nervous system.

Hypokalemia

The abnormal and delayed repolarization that occurs in hypokalemia is best expressed as QU, rather than QT, prolongation, since at times it can be difficult to differentiate between notching of the T wave and T- and U-wave fusion. The earliest change consists of the U wave being taller than the T wave (Fig. 15-21). As the serum potassium falls, the ST segment becomes more depressed and there is a gradual blending of T waves into what appears to be a tall U wave.

An ECG pattern similar to that of hypokalemia can be produced by some antiarrhythmic drugs, especially quinidine (Fig. 15-22, left). These quinidine-induced repolarization changes need not indicate quinidine toxicity, but can reflect only that the patient is taking the drug. They therefore, are best considered as a quinidine effect. On the other hand, quinidine toxicity is characterized by QRS widening (greater than 25 percent of control values) not due to bundle branch block, generally coexisting with a prolonged QT interval (Fig. 15-22, right).

Hypomagnesemia

Hypomagnesemia does not produce QU prolongation unless the coexisting hypokalemia (with which it is almost invariably associated) is severe. Although long-standing, or severe, magnesium deficiency lowers the amplitude of the T wave and depresses the ST segment, it does not prolong the QT interval.

Hypercalcemia

Hypercalcemia produces a short QT interval but without the upward concavity of the ST segment attributed to digitalis effect.

Other Conditions

As stated earlier, the purpose of the preceding sections was to discuss current views of selected subjects. For further discussion of the ECG of myocardial infarction see Chap. 45. For further discussion of the ECG of left- and right-sided cardiac hypertrophy see Chaps. 36, 38, and 39. For a further discussion of the ECG of pericarditis see Chap. 58. For discussion of the electrocardiographic recognition of cardiac arrhythmias see Chap. 28.

Computer Application

Although the use of the ECG in clinical practice is worldwide, the reading of ECGs is far from uniform. Mejler has stated that "there are almost as many interpretations as there are electrocardiologists."[23]

QUINIDINE "EFFECT"

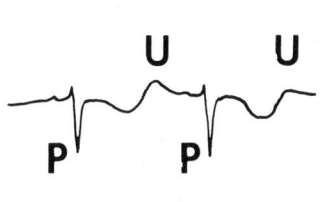

QUINIDINE TOXICITY

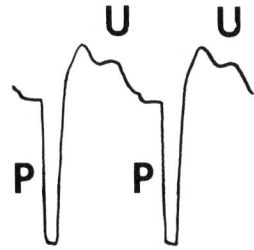

FIGURE 15-22 Electrocardiographic changes, similar to those produced by hypokalemia resulting from the administration of quinidine (quinidine "effect"). Alternation of the U wave is more frequent in quinidine effect than in hypokalemia. On the other hand, quinidine toxicity is manifested by wide QRS complexes and prolonged repolarization due to summation of T and U waves. The latter, as well as the presence of a P wave, are important points to be remembered when attempting to differentiate between QRS widening due to quinidine toxicity and QRS widening due to advanced hyperkalemia (Fig. 15-19).

A thorough understanding of how clinicians approach ECGs explains the reigning empiricism. An electrocardiographic diagnosis can be made in its own dimension; for example, in a heart station, where multiple tracings are dictated, the only information available is more often than not the patient's name, age, and sex and hospital number and location as well as an unreliable ambiguous clinical impression. On the other hand, when treating or evaluating the patient, the ECG usually becomes available after a working clinical diagnosis has already been made.

Some physicians will, at that moment, make a purely electrocardiographic diagnosis, as they would without clinical information, and not modify it. Others will (generally subconsciously) "custom fit" the diagnosis. They thus might try to interpret, i.e., understand, the ECG in the light of the clinical situation. Since the clinical subsettings are innumerable, the ECG interpretations are also multiple. Interpretations (direct or intuitive cognition) are personal, and this explains the significant interreader variability. Because interpretations, thus defined, are also situational (affective-related), it is not surprising that the same physician can interpret the same ECG in a different way at the heart station and in a clinical setting.

The technological advances being more extensively applied to medicine in the United States than in any other country in the world explain why, even though computerization of ECG analysis started in the late 1950s, serious attempts in *clinical* application have been made only recently. This apparent contradiction can be explained by understanding that, as a reaction formation, physicians still tend not to accept computerized reading. Some feel somewhat threatened by machines and are apprehensive about being apparently relegated to a secondary position

by their use. Yet, it is to be expected that in a progress-oriented society the rapid pace of technological advances will result in a gradual increase in the number of computer-processed ECGs. Nevertheless, in our opinion, it appears somewhat premature that ECGs included in Section C of the 1977 and 1979 Board Examination on Cardiovascular Disease had to be interpreted by filling in a computer form (including more than 125 "descriptions") in spite of the fact that this approach is not used to teach electrocardiography in the majority of cardiology training programs nor to interpret ECGs in most private hospitals at the time that this chapter was written.

In general, computerized ECGs are more useful in large county hospitals and in rural areas where there is a fixed supply of qualified interpreters.[24,25] But in any hospital—rural, urban, or suburban—computerization can enhance the efficiency with which a heart station operates. This includes storage of data and consistency of electrocardiographic interpretations. The economics involved—operating costs, payroll, overhead, professional fees, etc.—have to be compared with that of the preexisting system in the same hospital. These factors as well as the alleged more productive utilization of physicians' time and skills vary considerably from hospital to hospital and community to community and must therefore be determined for a particular center's individual requirements.

Computer measurement of amplitudes, duration, and intervals is extremely accurate. Since (as mentioned previously) there is conspicuous lack of uniformity amongst interpreters, evaluation of computer programs should be made in reference to the selected program itself rather than to the interpreter's own concepts.

Unfortunately, as long as standardization does not exist, ECG interpretation will continue to be a highly individualistic, empirical exercise. This should not be a cause of despair. Most physicians still consider that the ECG is a helpful laboratory tool which, when analyzed in the context of the working clinical diagnosis, can give valuable guidelines. Those directly in charge of the patient should interpret the ECG themselves, rather than rely, exclusively, on someone else's diagnosis.

References

1. Waller, A. D.: "The Electrical Action of the Human Heart," University of London Press, Ltd., London, 1922 (preface).
2. Johnston, F. D., and Lepesehkin, E. (eds.): "Selected Papers of Dr. Frank N. Wilson," J. W. Edwards, Publisher, Incorporated, Ann Arbor, Mich., 1955.
3. Barker, J. M.: "The Unipolar Electrocardiogram: A Clinical Interpretation," Appleton-Century-Crofts, Inc., New York, 1952, p. 79 (preface).
4. Sodi-Pallares, D., and Calder, R. M.: "New Bases of Electrocardiography," The C. V. Mosby Company, St. Louis, 1956, pp. 169, 373.

5. Lewis, T., and Rothschild, M. A.: The Excitatory Process in the Dog's Heart. Part II: The Ventricles, *Try. Roy. Soc.*, 206:181, 1915.

6. Sodi-Pallares, D., Medrano, G. A., Bisteni, A., and Ponce de Leon, J.: "Deductive and Polyparametric Electrocardiography," Instituto Nacional de Cardiologia, Mexico, D.F., 1970, pp. 36, 136.

*7. Rosenbaum, M. B., Elizari, M. V., and Lazzari, J. O.: "The Hemiblocks," Tampa Tracings, Oldsmar, Florida, 1970, pp. 31, 71, 138. (Extensively referenced)

*8. Schamroth, L.: "The Electrocardiology of Coronary Artery Disease," Blackwell, London, 1975, pp. 6, 17–23. (Extensively referenced)

9. Lipman, B. S., Massie, E., and Kleiger, R. E.: "Clinical Scalar Electrocardiography," 6th ed., Year Book Medical Publishers, Inc., Chicago, 1972, pp. 210–215.

10. Einthoven, W., Fahr, G., and de Waart, A.: Über die Richtung und die manifeste Grösse der Potential schwankungen im menschlichen Herzen und über den Einfluss der Herzlags auf die Form des Elektrokardiogramms, *Arch. f.d. ges. Physiol.*, 150:275, 1913.

11. Castellanos, A., and Lemberg, L.: "A Programmed Introduction to Electrical Axis and Action Potential," Tampa Tracings, Oldsmar, Florida, 1974, pp. 34, 114–153.

12. Simonson, E.: "Differentiation between Normal and Abnormal in Electrocardiograpy," The C. V. Mosby Company, St. Louis, 1961, p. 262.

*13. Castellanos, A., and Myerburg, R. J.: "The Hemiblocks in Myocardial Infarction," Appleton-Century-Crofts, Inc., New York, 1976, pp. 24, 66, 67. (Extensively referenced)

14. Bayley, R. H.: An Interpretation of Injury and the Ischemic Effects of Myocardial Infarction in Accordance with the Laws Which Determine the Flow of Electric Current in Homogeneous Volume Conductors, and in Accordance with Relevant Pathologic Changes, *Am. Heart J.*, 24:514, 1942.

15. Singer, D. H., Lazzara, R., and Hoffman, B. F.: Interrelationships between Automaticity and Conduction in Purkinje Fibers, *Circ. Res.*, 21:537, 1967.

16. Bruyneel, K. J. J.: Use of Moving Epicardial Electrodes in Defining ST-segment Changes after Acute Coronary Occlusion in the Baboon: Relation to Primary Ventricular Fibrillation, *Am. Heart J.*, 89:731, 1975.

17. The Criteria Committee of the New York Heart Association: "Nomenclature and Criteria for Diagnosis of Diseases of the Heart and Great Vessels," 8th ed., Little, Brown and Company, Boston, 1979, p. 94.

18. Myerburg, R. J., Nelsson, K., and Gelband, H.: Physiology of Canine Intraventricular Conduction and Endocardial Excitation, *Circ. Res.*, 30:217, 1972.

19. Pickoff, A. S., Wolff, G. S., Tamer, D., and Gelband, H.: Arrhythmias and Conduction System Disturbances in Infants and Children—Recent Advances and Contributions of Intracardiac Electrophysiology; in A. Castellanos and A. N. Brest (eds.), "Cardiac Arrhythmias—Mechanisms and Management," *Cardiovasc. Clin.*, 11:203, 1980.

20. Garcia, O. L., Castellanos, A., Sung, R. J., and Gelband, H.: Exposure of Concealed Right Bundle Branch Block in Wolff-Parkinson-White Type B by Pacing from the Vicinity of the A-V Node, *Am. Heart J.*, 96:662, 1978.

21. Silverman, M. E., and Silverman, B. D.: The Diagnostic Capabilities and Limitations of the Electrocardiogram, in Hurst, J. W. (ed.), "The Heart: Update I," McGraw-Hill Book Company, New York, 1979, p. 13.

*22. VanderArk, C. R., Ballantyne, F., and Reynolds, E. W.: Electrolytes and the Electrocardiogram, in C. Fisch and A. N. Brest (eds.), "Complex Electrocardiography." *Cardiovasc. Clin.*, 5:269, 1973. (Extensively referenced).

23. Mejler, F. L.: "A New Coding System for Electrocardiography," Robles de Medina, E. O. Excerpta Medica, Amsterdam, 1972 (preface).

*24. Pipberger, H. J., and Cornfeld, J.: What Computer Programs to Choose for Clinical Application: The Need for Consumer Protection, *Circulation*, 47:918, 1973. (11 references)

*25. Tenth Bethesda Conference on Optimal Electrocardiography, *Am. J. Cardiol.*, 41:111, 1978. (Extensively referenced)

*This article is a review of the literature and contains additional references to the literature.

16

The Chest Roentgenogram

James T. T. Chen, M.D.

The use of a mirror, we submit, is not to be painted upon.
Thomas Babington Macaulay, 1830[1]

A systematic approach to cardiac roentgenology has been found simple and effective. At *first* an objective observation of all roentgen signs is made without the clinical information. This is to prevent the observer from being biased by an opinion which may occasionally be oversimplified or even mistaken. For example, a patient was referred to our pulmonary division because of "bronchial asthma" refractory to therapy for 20 years. The routine chest roentgenograms, however, showed typical signs of severe mitral stenosis. As soon as the appropriate treatment was instituted, the patient's cardiac asthma disappeared for the first time in two decades. Likewise, a secundum atrial septal defect may be misinterpreted as mitral stenosis because of similar physical signs. The split-second sound may be misinterpreted as the opening snap. The diastolic rumble through the tricuspid valve as a result of increased flow may mimic the diastolic murmur of mitral stenosis. The x-ray signs, however, are quite different between the two entities (Figs. 16-1*B* and 16-2*A*).

The *final* radiologic conclusion, however, should be drawn only after correlating the x-ray findings with both the clinical information and the laboratory data.

Major Steps of Roentgenologic Examination

Objective Observation with Clinical Information Purposefully Withheld

Roentgenographic Analysis of Anatomy

A four-view cardiac series should be obtained as a base-line study. For follow-up examinations the standard two-view chest roentgenograms will prove satisfactory in most cases.

To avoid omission of findings which may be essential to the diagnosis, a sequential radiographic analysis is advisable: (1) pulmonary vasculature, (2) size and contour of the heart, (3) size and contour of each chamber, (4) abnormal densities, (5) abnormal lucencies, (6) malpositions of the heart, (7) great vessels, (8) mediastinal structures, (9) lung parenchyma, (10) pleura, (11) bony thorax, (12) soft tissues over the chest, and (13) extrathoracic structures.

Fluoroscopic Observation of Dynamics

Chapter 84 is devoted to the value and limitations of cardiac fluoroscopy.

Statistical Guidance

Statistical information focusing on the most likely diagnoses in the order of frequency should be studied.

Correlation with Other Data

The next step in the radiologic examination is to correlate the roentgenologic findings with the clinical information and other laboratory parameters for the final conclusion.

Pulmonary Vasculature

Since the pulmonary vasculature faithfully reflects the underlying pathophysiology of the heart,[2-4] it would seem advantageous for the observer to start with the pulmonary vessels in order to narrow down the diagnostic possibilities to a manageable level. For example, if uniform dilatation of all pulmonary vessels is present, the diagnosis of a left-to-right shunt (Fig. 16-1*B*) is preferred to a left-sided obstructive lesion. The latter typically shows a cephalad pulmonary blood flow pattern (Fig. 16-2*A*).

The normal roentgen appearance of the pulmonary vasculature is typified by a caudad flow pattern on account of gravity. The pressure differential between the apex and the base of the lung is approximately 22 mmHg in adults in upright position. Therefore, more flow under higher distending pressure is expected in the lower-lobe vessels than in the upper. Normally one sees very little vascularity above the hilum, whereas more and larger vessels are found below the hilum. Since the pulmonary resistance is normal, all vessels taper gradually in a treelike manner from the hilum toward the periphery of the lung. The right descending pulmonary artery measures 10 to 15 mm in diameter in males and 9 to 14 mm in females (Fig. 16-1*A*).[5]

In the evaluation of pulmonary vasculature the caliber of the vessels is more important than the length or the number. In the case of mild to moderate left-to-right shunts, for example, the vessels dilate in proportion to the increased flow with no significant change in pressure, resistance, or flow pattern. This phenomenon is also called *shunt vascularity* or *equalization*. The last expression is based on the fact that the distribution of blood flow tends to be equalized between the upper and lower lung zones; however, this change is not marked, and the lower lobes still receive a great deal more blood than the upper. Mild increase in pulmonary vascularity with slight cardiomegaly is commonly found in pregnant women and trained athletes with greater cardiac output and supranormal performance of the heart.

The pulmonary vascular flow can be assessed by

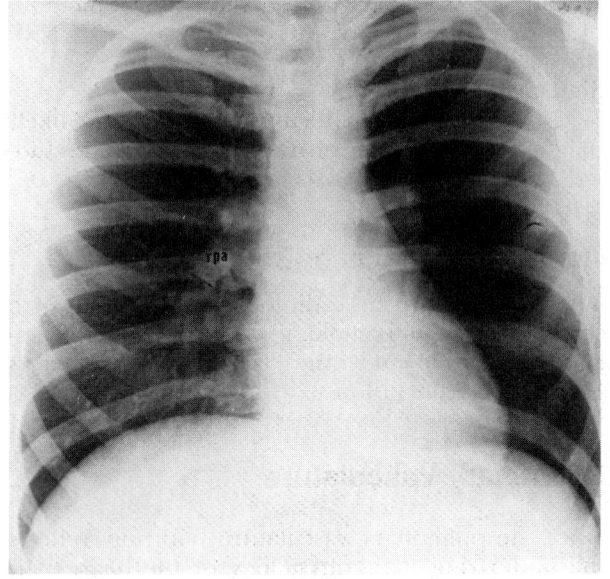

A

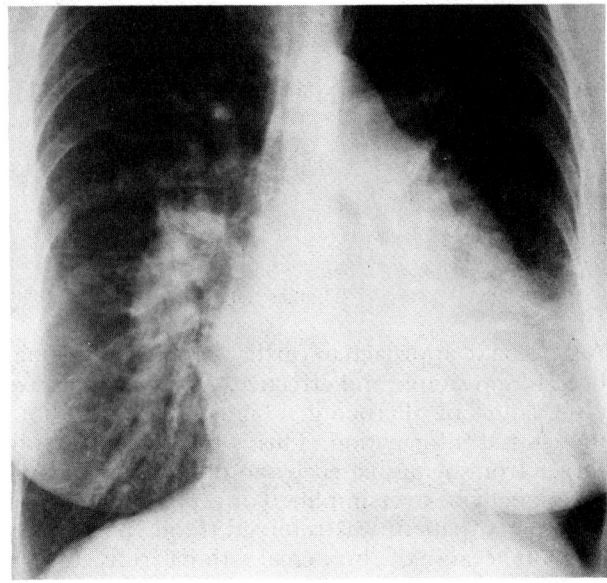

B

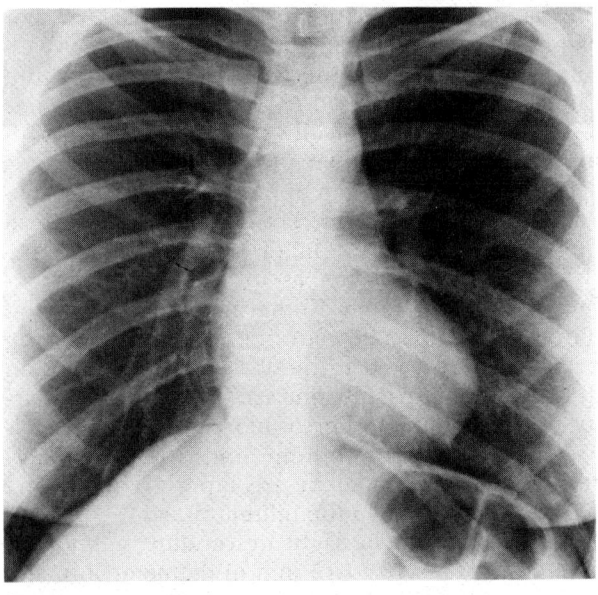

C

FIGURE 16-1 Roentgenographic assessment of the volume of pulmonary blood flow. *A.* Normal: There is caudalization of the pulmonary vascularity due to gravity. The right descending pulmonary artery (rpa) measures (arrows) 13 mm in diameter in this young adult male patient. *B.* Increased: Patient with secundum atrial septal defect showing uniform increase in pulmonary vascularity bilaterally. The right descending pulmonary artery is markedly enlarged, measuring 27 mm. *C.* Decreased: Patient with tetralogy of Fallot showing a boot-shaped heart and uniform decrease in pulmonary vascularity. The right descending pulmonary artery is markedly decreased, measuring 6 mm.

the caliber of the pulmonary arteries (Fig. 16-1). Patients with tetralogy of Fallot frequently show decreased pulmonary vascularity with smaller and shorter pulmonary arteries and more radiolucent lungs (Fig. 16-1C). Marked reduction in pulmonary blood flow is also encountered in patients with right-sided heart failure without a right-to-left shunt (Fig. 16-4D). This is attributed to the significant decrease in cardiac output from both ventricles. A more objective assessment of pulmonary flow can be obtained by comparing the caliber of the pulmonary artery with that of the accompanying bronchus when they are viewed on end. Normally the two structures have an approximately equal diameter. When the artery/bronchus ratio is greater than unity, increased blood flow is suggested. Conversely,

when the ratio is smaller than unity (Fig. 16-1C), decreased flow is likely.

An abnormal flow pattern (or abnormal distribution of flow) always reflects a changed pulmonary vascular resistance, either locally or diffusely.

In the presence of postcapillary pulmonary hypertension the physiological disturbances may begin when the total intravascular pressure exceeds the oncotic pressure of the blood. As a result fluid leaks out of the vessels and collects in the interstitium before pouring into the alveoli.

Pulmonary edema interferes with gas exchange, resulting in a state of hypoxia. Hypoxia has a profound influence on the pulmonary vessels to contract. Since there is a greater pressure increase in the lung bases than in the apices, the basilar vessels

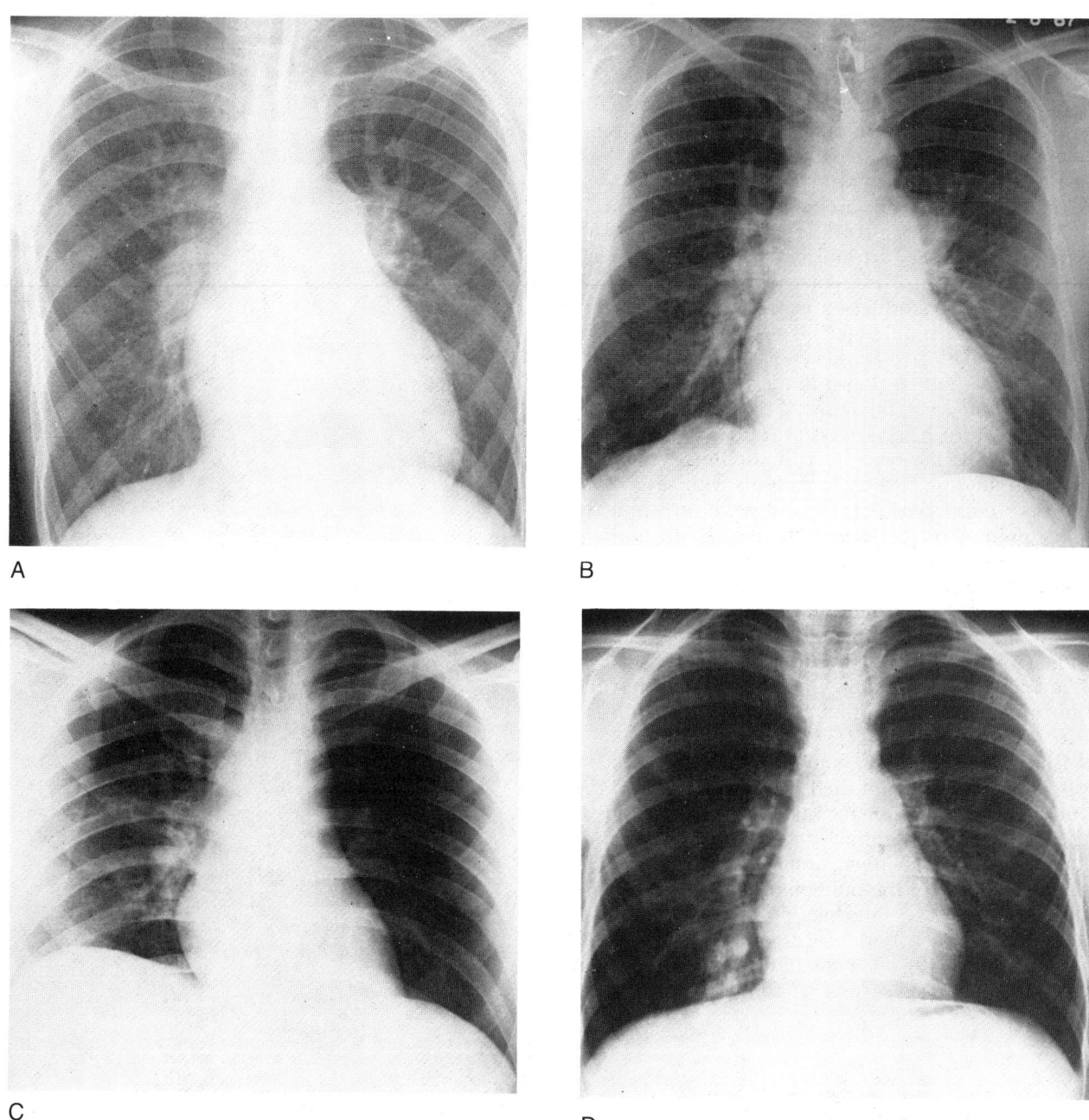

A

B

C

D

FIGURE 16-2   Abnormal pulmonary blood flow patterns. *A.* Cephalization: Patient with severe mitral stenosis showing dilatation of the upper vessels with construction of the lower vessels. *B.* Centralization: Patient with Eisenmenger ASD and VSD showing marked dilatation of the pulmonary trunk and the central segments of both pulmonary arteries with pruning of the peripheral branches. *C.* Lateralization: Patient with massive pulmonary embolism obstructing the left main pulmonary artery. Note the uneven distribution of blood flow between the two lungs in favor of the right. *D.* Localization: A cyanotic child showing localized vascular changes representing a large pulmonary arteriovenous fistula in the right lower lobe. (*A and B from Chen et al.*[3] *Reproduced with permission.*)

begin to constrict, forcing the blood to flow upward. This phenomenon actually represents a reversal of the normal blood flow pattern, redistribution or cephalization of the pulmonary vascularity. Cephalization occurs in one of the three conditions: (1) left-sided obstructive lesions, e.g., mitral stenosis (Fig. 16-2*A*),[5] aortic stenosis; (2) left ventricular failure, e.g., coronary heart disease, cardiomyopathies; (3) severe mitral insufficiency even before pump failure

of the left ventricle occurs. It should be emphasized that unless there is obvious constriction of the lower-lobe vessels the diagnosis of cephalization should not be made. Dilatation of the upper-lobe vessels is of secondary importance and can be found without narrowing of the basilar vessels in a number of entities, most noticeably, left-to-right shunts.

The pulmonary vascular changes associated with acute left ventricular failure are usually not discernible for two reasons: (1) The resultant severe pulmonary edema obscures the pulmonary vasculature. (2) The redistribution of pulmonary blood flow secondary to acute left-sided heart failure is usually relatively mild. The combination of pulmonary edema and a normal-sized heart is the hallmark of acute left-sided heart failure,[3] most commonly seen in acute myocardial infarction (Fig. 16-3A).

In the presence of a large left-to-right shunt, reactive pulmonary arteriolar spasms may cause significant elevation of pulmonary vascular resistance, which in turn produces a centralized pulmonary flow pattern (Eisenmenger's syndrome) (Fig. 16-2B). The pulmonary trunk and central pulmonary arteries now dilate in response to increased pressure in addition to increased volume. The distal pulmonary arteries constrict in a concentric fashion from the hilum toward the periphery of the lung. A similar flow distribution is seen in patients with severe obstructive emphysema, representing severe precapillary pulmonary hypertension (Fig. 16-4A and B). Massive unilateral pulmonary embolism may cause a lateralized flow pattern. Since one major pulmonary artery is obstructed, the blood is forced to flow through the healthy lung only. The paucity of pulmonary vascularity in the diseased lung is termed *Westermark sign* (Fig. 16-2C). A localized abnormal flow pattern is exemplified by the arteriovenous fistula in a cyanotic child (Fig. 16-2D).

In summary, roentgen analysis of the pulmonary vasculature is accomplished in two steps. First, the volume of the pulmonary flow can be estimated by the degree of pulmonary arterial enlargement as long as the flow pattern remains normal. Second, the distribution of the pulmonary flow is assessed by the presence of an abnormal flow pattern. The volume and the distribution of pulmonary blood flow may change singly or in combination depending on the nature and the severity of the underlying heart disease.

Four-View Cardiac Series[6,7,14]

For many years after the discovery of x-rays, fluoroscopy played a greater role than radiography in diagnostic roentgenology. Therefore, traditionally the roentgenogram is viewed on the illuminator in such a fashion as if the viewer were examining the patient under the fluoroscope. The examiner is facing the patient and the oncoming x-rays in the posteroanterior (PA) view. The patient's left lateral aspect of the chest is closest to the examiner (or the fluoroscopic screen) when a left lateral view is taken. Likewise, the right or left anterior aspect is facing the examiner when the right or left anterior oblique view, respectively, is taken. The interrelationships of the cardiovascular structures in the four views and their practical applications are illustrated in Fig. 16-5.

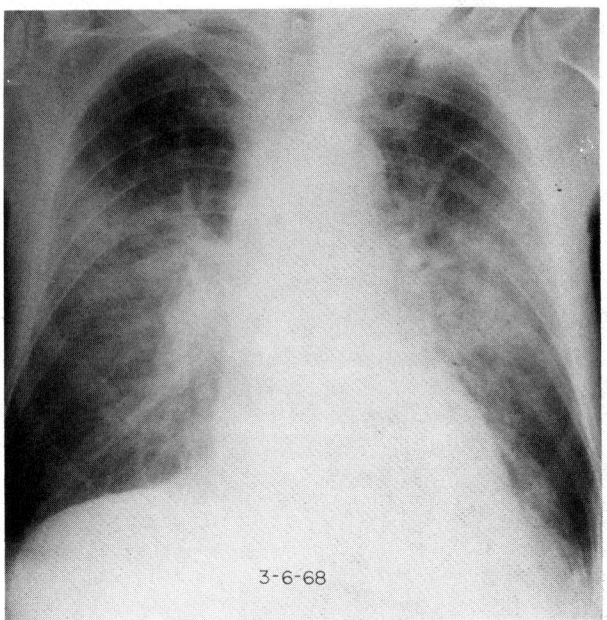

3-6-68

A

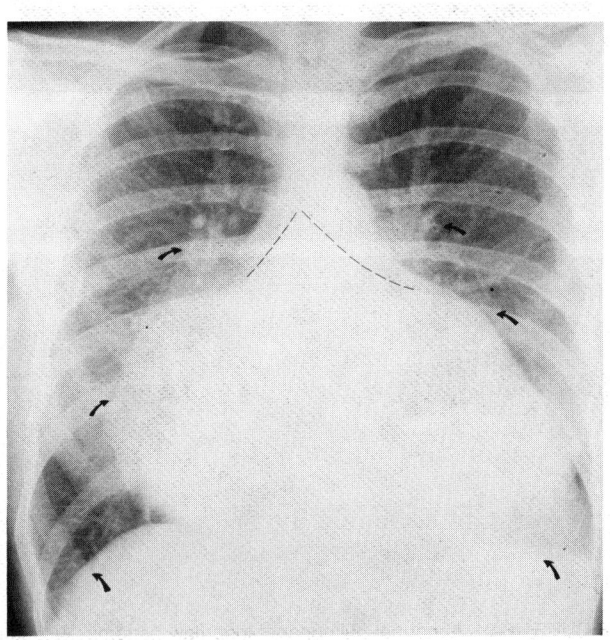

B

FIGURE 16-3 Roentgen appearance of left-sided heart failure. *A.* Acute: Patient with acute myocardial infarction showing "bat wings" appearance of severe alveolar type of pulmonary edema and a normal-sized heart. *B.* Chronic: Patient with severe rheumatic heart disease (severe mitral and tricuspid insufficiency and mild aortic insufficiency). This is a predominantly left-sided failure pattern. Note the giant left atrium forming the right heart border (middle right arrow) and a bulging left atrial appendage along the left heart border (left middle arrow). The peribronchial cuff of edema fluid is indicated by the upper left arrow. The Kerley B lines are marked by the lower right arrow. The upper right arrow points to the markedly dilated right superior pulmonary vein. The lower vessels were constricted. The left ventricle was enlarged with its apex marked by the lower left arrow. The markedly widened subcarinal angle is outlined by the retouched lower margin of both main stem bronchi. (*Part A from Chen et al.*[3] *Reproduced with permission.*)

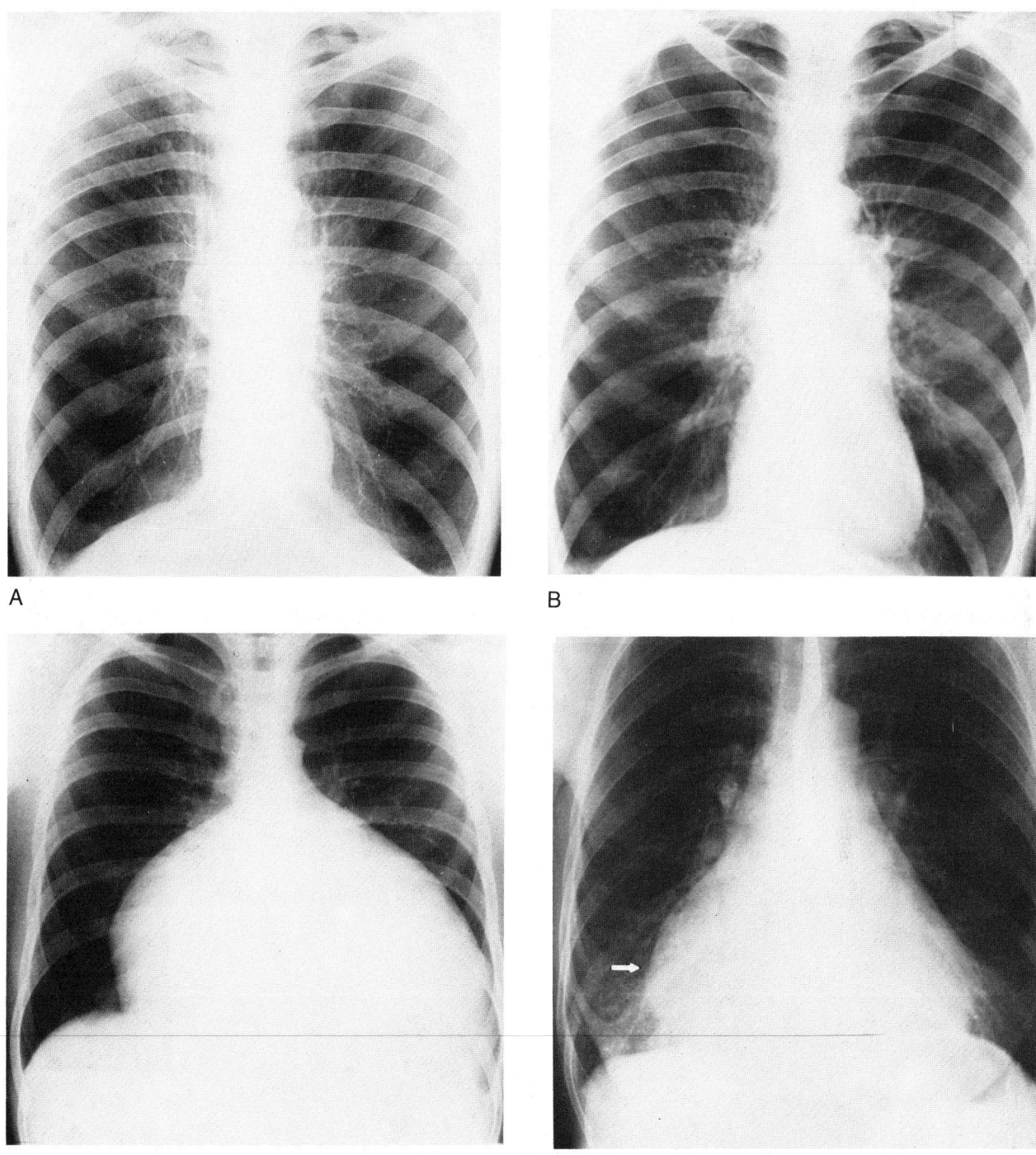

FIGURE 16-4   Roentgen appearance of right-sided heart failure. *A.* Patient with severe obstructive emphysema showing overaeration of the lungs, centralized flow pattern, and a small heart size. *B.* Three years later the patient was in frank right-sided heart failure. Note the heart got bigger as his emphysema got worse. The centralized flow pattern became more severe. *C.* Patient with Ebstein anomaly showing gross cardiomegaly with severe decrease in pulmonary vascularity. The right cardiac border represents the huge right atrium, and the left cardiac border represents the giant right ventricle. *D.* Patient with rheumatic mitral stenosis showing a giant right atrium (arrow) representing severe functional tricuspid insufficiency secondary to unrelenting left-sided failure. The pulmonary venous congestion had improved following the onset of right-sided heart failure.

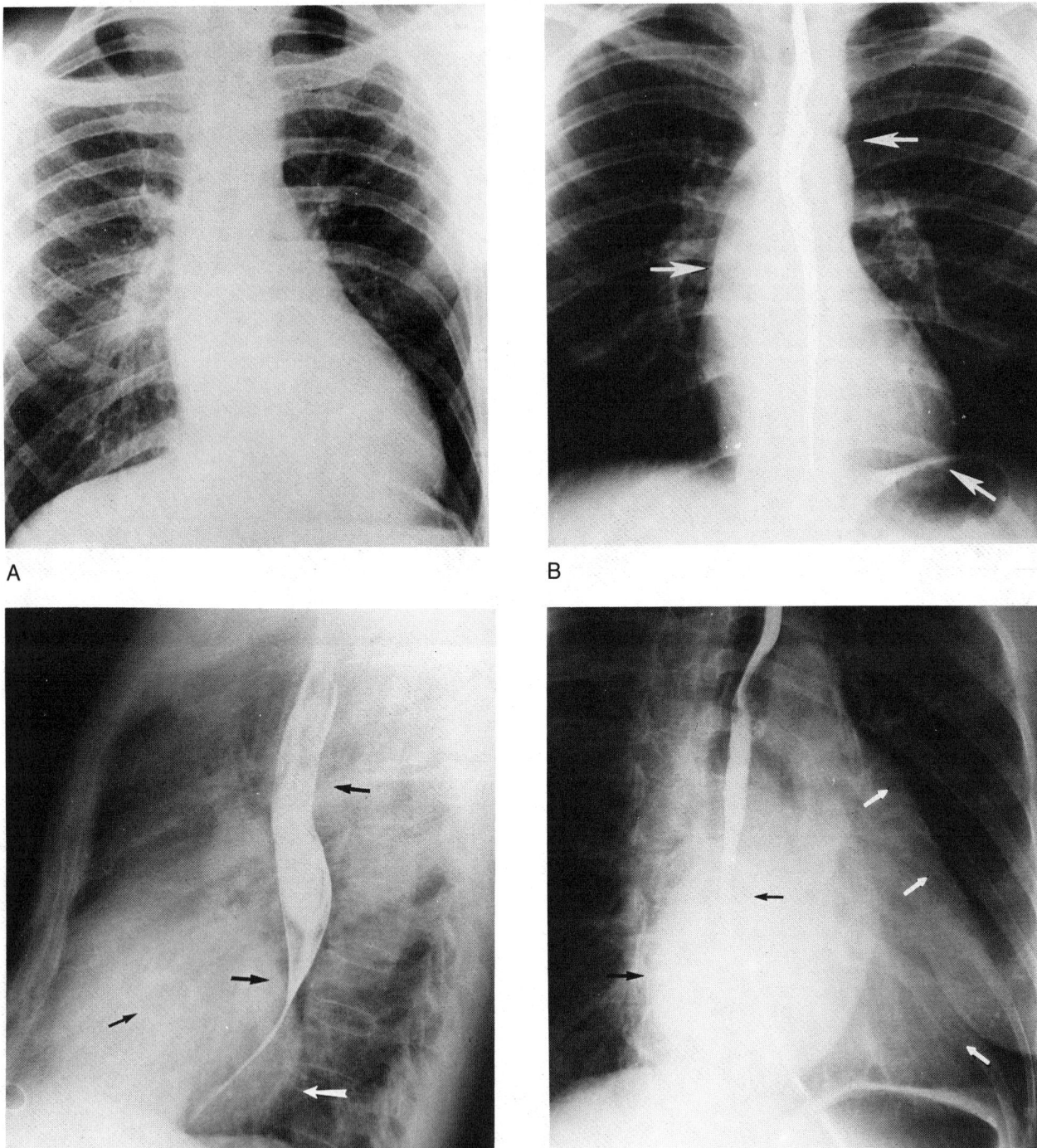

A

B

C

D

Cardiac Size[4,6,7]

A significantly enlarged heart is always abnormal, while mild generalized cardiomegaly may be compatible with a perfectly normal heart with higher than average cardiac output, as seen in an athlete in active training. The cardiothoracic ratio remains the simplest and the most practical yardstick for the assessment of cardiac size. The mean value for adults in deep inspiration is 44 percent. More accurate roentgen measurements of the cardiac size have been well documented[8,9] and are out of the scope of the present discussion. The nature of cardiomegaly can usually be determined by the specific roentgen appearance. As a rule, when the pulmonary blood flow pattern remains normal, cardiac lesions with volume overload tend to present a greater degree of cardiomegaly than lesions with pressure overload alone. For example, patients with aortic stenosis typically show an increase in convexity of the left ventricle but very little cardiac enlargement.

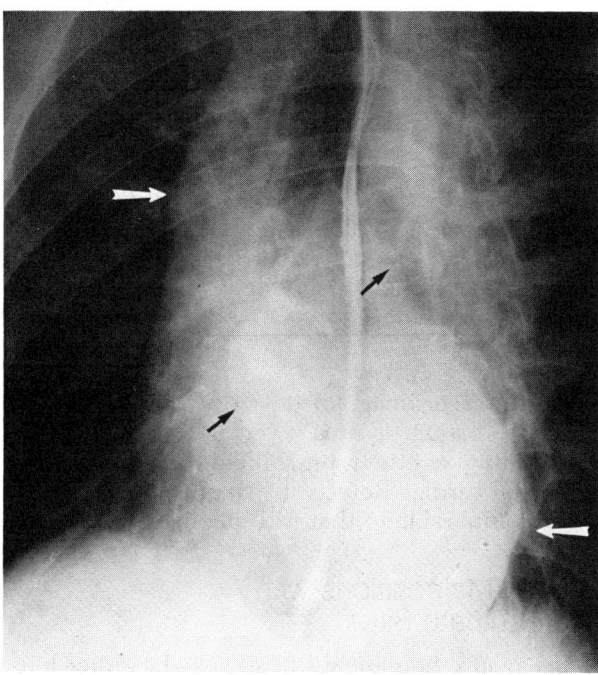

E

FIGURE 16-5   Practical application of four-view cardiac series. *A.* Posteroanterior (PA) view in a patient with coarctation of the aorta showing areas of rib notching bilaterally and left ventricular enlargement in the inferior and leftward direction. *B.* PA view of another patient with coarctation of the aorta following figure-three sign of the deformed descending aorta, and E sign on the barium-filled esophagus. The upper arrow (on the patient's left) points to the level of coarctation. The lower arrow (on the patient's left) marks the apex of the enlarged left ventricle. The arrow on the patient's right indicates the dilated ascending aorta. *C.* Left lateral view of the third patient with coarctation of the aorta showing barium-filled esophagus to be pushed forward (upper arrow) by the poststenotic dilatation of the descending aorta, and pushed backward (middle arrow) by the enlarged left atrium. The very large left ventricle (lower arrow) simply cast a shadow behind the esophagus without displacing the esophagus. The oblique arrow points to the calcium deposits in the stenotic bicuspid aortic valve. *D.* Right anterior oblique view of the same patient whose PA view is shown in Fig. 16-4*D.* Note the huge right atrium casting a triangular density (lower horizontal arrow) behind the esophagus without displacing the esophagus. The esophagus is deviated posteriorly by the enlarged left atrium (upper horizontal arrow). The upper oblique arrows indicate the enlarged pulmonary trunk and the right ventricle in the superior and leftward direction. The lower oblique arrow points to the normal left ventricle. Note that the costophrenic sulcus remains clear and normal. *E.* Left anterior oblique view of a patient with valvular aortic stenosis. The dilated ascending aorta (upper arrow) is found immediately above the flat anterior cardiac border of the normal right ventricle. The lower oblique arrow points to the calcified aortic valve. The upper oblique arrow indicates the elevated left stem bronchus, which is due to left atrial enlargement. The lower left arrow marks the enlarged left ventricle in the inferior, leftward, and posterior direction.

Under such condition, there is only hypertrophy of the myocardium without dilatation of the cardiac lumen. On the other hand, the left ventricle both dilates and hypertrophies in case of aortic insufficiency, producing a much larger heart even before congestive heart failure takes place. Both right-sided and left-sided heart failure can cause gross cardiac enlargement. The associated vascular ab-

normality in each case is, however, drastically different. While decreased flow with increased pulmonary lucency is the hallmark of right-sided failure (Fig. 16-4*B,* and *D*), striking cephalization of the pulmonary vasculature is typical for left-sided decompensation (Figs. 16-2*A,* and 16-3*B*). A heart that is smaller than average size is encountered in patients with chronic obstructive pulmonary disease (Fig. 16-4*A*), Addison's disease, anorexia nervosa, and starvation. However, an abnormally small heart is difficult to define except in a retrospective fashion when the heart has come back to a normal capacity following successful therapy. For example, in patients with Addison's disease, the heart, in response to steroid therapy, may become significantly larger.

Critical assessment of individual cardiac chamber requires a complete cardiac series in four views by aid of fluoroscopy. Left atrial enlargement is the easiest to detect. Basically a barium swallow will show the typical rightward and posterior displacement of the esophagus at the left atrial level in all views except the left anterior oblique. A double density, a bulging left atrial appendage, and an elevated left-stem bronchus are the other manifestations of left atrial enlargement (Figs. 16-3*B,* and 16-5*C*). Left ventricular enlargement is manifested by a leftward inferior and posterior extension of the left lower cardiac border (Fig. 16-5*A* and *E*). Right ventricular enlargement is best appreciated in the lateral and left anterior oblique views as an anterior bulge of the heart. In addition, the anterior cardiac border also gets longer and taller from the level of the diaphragm upward. A large pulmonary trunk is a secondary sign of right ventricular enlargement (Fig. 16-1*B*). Lastly, when the right ventricle enlarges, the left side of the heart is displaced in the superolateral direction, forming a gentle convexity along the left upper cardiac border (Fig. 16-1*B*). Right atrial enlargement is best tested in posteroanterior and right anterior oblique views. In the adult population, greater than 5.5-cm extension of the right heart border from the midline is considered a definite evidence of right atrial enlargement (Fig. 16-4*C* and *D*). In the right anterior view, the enlarged right atrial chamber casts a triangular shadow behind the barium-filled esophagus without displacing it (Fig. 16-5*D*). Occasionally the enlarged right atrial appendage may form a shelflike projection over the upper anterior border of the heart immediately below the ascending aorta in the left anterior oblique view. However, this is a rare sign. When the atrium is huge, it may cast a double density in the lateral view continuous with the dilated inferior vena cava.

Abnormal Densities

Beside the familiar double density cast by an enlarged left atrium, other increased densities may be found within the confine of the heart by a variety of dilated vascular structures, e.g., tortuous descending aorta, aortic aneurysm, coronary artery aneurysm, pulmonary varix, etc. Furthermore, large cardiac calcifications are easily seen, particularly in the lateral and oblique views. If smaller calcific deposits are suspected, they should be promptly verified or ruled out by cardiac fluoroscopy. Any radiologically detectable calcification in the heart is of clinical importance. The heavier the calcification, the more significant it becomes (Fig. 16-5E). As a rule, the extent of valvular calcification is proportionate to the severity of the valve stenosis regardless of the other roentgen signs of the disease. Calcification of the coronary artery is almost always of atherosclerotic nature. Mönckeberg medial calcification of the coronary system is extremely rare. A radiologically detectable coronary calcification is correlated with major-vessel occlusion in 94 percent of patients with chest pain.[10]

Abnormal Lucencies

The abnormal lucencies in and about the heart include (1) the displaced subepicardial fat lines by effusion or thickening of the pericardium (see Chap. 84), (2) the pneumopericardium, and (3) the pneumomediastinum. Pneumomediastinum is differentiated from pneumopericardium by the fact that the former shows a more superior extension of the air strip beyond the confine of the pericardium.

Cardiac Malpositions[11]

Dextrocardia

By definition this is a mirror image of the heart and the abdominal viscera (situs inversus). A ninefold increase in the incidence of congenital cardiac defects is found in patients with dextrocardia (5 percent), as compared with that for the general population (0.6 to 0.8 percent). Also known is the tendency for these patients to develop noncardiac lesions known as Kartagener's triad: dextrocardia, sinusitis, and bronchiectasis.

Dextroversion

Dextroversion represents an anomaly with situs solitus and a right-sided heart (the apex of the ventricles points to the right side and inferiorly). Roentgenographically situs solitus is a certainty when both the aortic knob and the gastric air bubble are on the left side. Situs solitus also means that both the abdominal viscera and the atria are normal. Under these circumstances, if the ventricles fail to swing from their primitive right-sided position to their normal left-sided position, abnormal relationships between the ventricles and the rest of the cardiovascular structures are bound to occur.

The incidence of congenital cardiac defects was estimated at 98 percent in patients with dextroversion. Of these over 80 percent had congenitally corrected transposition (or L-loop transposition) of great arteries. The next commonly associated lesions were a combination of ventricular septal defect and pulmonary stenosis, a tetralogy-like pathophysiology (Fig. 16-6D). Therefore, from the statistical point of view it is important to be able to differentiate dextroversion from dextrocardia, and this is readily accomplished on roentgen grounds alone.

Levoversion

This is a mirror image of dextroversion, consisting of a combination of situs inversus and a left-sided heart. The extremely high incidence of cyanotic congenital cardiac defects in patients with levoversion is comparable to that with dextroversion.

Cardiac Malpositions with Indeterminate Situs

In this group the patient's heart may be either left-sided or right-sided. The situs is ambiguous, with the roentgenogram showing aorticogastric bubble discordance. In other words, the aortic knob and the stomach are not on the same side, and therefore, the situs is unpredictable, though the left atrium tends to be on the side of the aorta. Under these circumstances, interruption of inferior vena cava with azygos continuation is almost always present. The next commonly associated lesions are polysplenia and a left-to-right shunt, most frequently a ventricular septal defect. The only exception to the rule of indeterminate situs is an isolated right-sided arch.

Great Vessels[4,6,7]

The roentgen appearance of the great vessels often provides valuable information for the diagnosis of heart disease. For example, selective dilatation of the ascending aorta is the hallmark of valvular aortic stenosis; generalized dilatation of the entire thoracic aorta, on the other hand, favors the diagnosis of aortic insufficiency and/or systemic hypertension, depending on the size of the left ventricle. A larger left ventricle is associated with aortic insufficiency because of volume overload (see Chap. 84). In atrial septal defect and mitral stenosis the pulmonary trunk is quite large and the aortic knob is usually small (Figs. 16-1B and 16-2A). This is explained on the basis of a leftward cardiac rotation which occurs when an enlarged right ventricle coexists with a normal-sized left ventricle. When the heart rotates to the left, the aorta folds on itself in the midline and becomes inconspicuous. Meanwhile the pulmonary trunk is brought laterad and looks larger than it actually is.

As already mentioned, prominence of the pul-

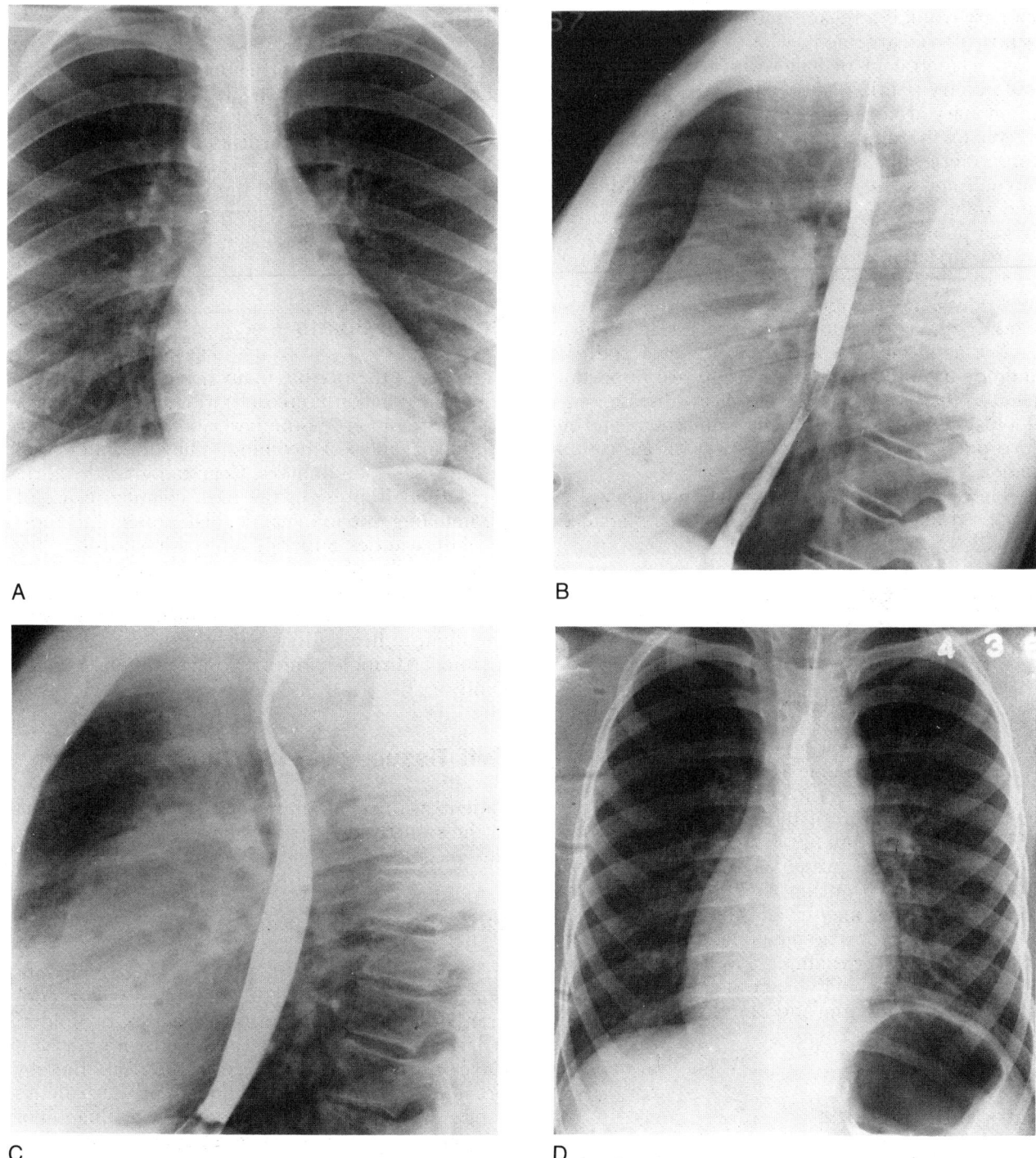

FIGURE 16-6 Statistical guidance focusing on the best diagnostic possibilities. *A.* Posteroanterior view of a patient with tetralogy of Fallot showing a right aortic arch, avian type. Note the esophagus and the trachea are deviated to the left. The cardiovascular structures are otherwise within normal limits. *B.* Lateral view of the same patient showing the aortic arch is normally situated in front of the trachea and esophagus. *C.* Lateral view of a healthy patient with a right aortic arch, common type. Note the esophagus and the trachea are markedly displaced anteriorly by a huge aortic diverticulum from which arises the aberrant left subclavian artery. The posteroanterior view of his chest (not shown) is very similar to that of the first patient shown in *A. D.* Posteroanterior view of a patient with dextroversion. Note the aortic arch and the stomach air bubble are both on the left (situs solitus), and the apex of the ventricles is pointing to the right inferiorly. According to statistics and also proven by cardiac catheterization, this patient had the typical combination of corrected transposition of great arteries, ventricular septal defect, and pulmonary stenosis. He was cyanotic. The pulmonary vascularity appears decreased.

monary trunk is a reliable secondary sign of a right ventricular enlargement, with the following exceptions: (1) tetralogy of Fallot with hypoplasia of the pulmonary trunk, (2) idiopathic dilatation of the pulmonary artery, and (3) straight-back syndrome, pectus excavatum, and scoliosis with narrowed anteroposterior diameter of the chest. Under the latter circumstances the heart is compressed, displaced, and rotated to the left, giving rise to a falsely enlarged pulmonary artery.

In coarctation of aorta, the engorged aortic knob and the poststenotic dilatation of the descending aorta cause an "E" sign on the barium-filled esophagus, outlining the site of coarctation (Fig. 16-5B).

The abnormal size and distribution of both the pulmonary and the systemic veins are important clues to the presence of certain heart diseases, e.g., anomalous pulmonary venous connections and interruption of inferior vena cava with azygos continuation.

The significance of aortic arch anomalies will be discussed under the section on statistical guidance.

Mediastinal Structures[4,6,7,12,13]

The mediastinal organs are frequently affected by the cardiovascular structures because of their close spatial interrelationships. An enlarged left atrium not only displaces the esophagus and the descending aorta but also elevates and compresses the left stem bronchus. A double aortic arch may compress both the trachea and the esophagus. Patients with an anomalous origin of the left pulmonary artery from the right pulmonary artery (the pulmonary artery sling) usually present compression symptoms of the right stem bronchus. On the other hand, malignant processes may invade the heart and great vessels, causing cardiac tamponade, superior vena cava syndrome, for example. More frequently than not, these mediastinal changes are evident on the chest roentgenogram and should be recognized promptly.

Lung Parenchyma[3]

The lung is the mirror of the heart. When the right side of the heart fails, the lung becomes unusually radiolucent on account of decreased pulmonary blood flow. On the other hand, significant left-sided heart failure is easily recognized on the chest roentgenogram by the presence of pulmonary edema and cephalad blood flow pattern. Long-standing severe pulmonary venous hypertension may lead to hemosiderosis and/or ossification of the lung. When right-sided heart failure occurs as a result of severe left-sided heart failure, the preexisting pulmonary congestion will improve because of the decreased pulmonary blood flow (Fig. 16-4D).

Pleura

A right-sided pleural effusion is typically present when the left side of the heart is failing. A bilateral hydrothorax, on the other hand, suggests bilateral heart failure or a noncardiac etiology of the effusion. Congestive heart failure is also known to be associated with a pseudotumor or "vanishing" tumor representing interlobar collection of pleural fluid. As congestive heart failure improves, the "tumor" will disappear.

Bones and Joints

Notching of the ribs has many origins. Basically any of the three major intercostal structures can enlarge, compress, and erode the lower borders of the ribs, producing areas of notching. They are intercostal arteries, veins, and nerves. Coarctation of the aorta (Fig. 16-5A) represents the most common cause of rib notching due to dynamic dilatation and tortuosity of the arteries. Superior vena cava syndrome may cause a similar phenomenon of venous origin. Neurofibromatosis is known to produce rib notching by numerous intercostal neurofibromata. Patients with rheumatoid heart disease may show typical rheumatoid arthritic changes in the acromioclavicular joints.

Soft Tissues over the Chest

Patients with renal failure may show severe edema in the soft tissues over the chest as part of the picture of general anasarca.

Extrathoracic Structures

In Holt-Oram syndrome the upper-extremity abnormalities may be evident in a chest roentgenogram or on other films in the patient's x-ray folder. A large arteriovenous malformation with curvilinear calcifications may be seen in the neck, thereby providing a clue as to the etiology of the patient's congestive heart failure. Radiographic evaluation of the patient's abdominal viscera is an integral part of the workup for cardiac malpositions.[11,14]

Statistical Guidance

In addition to what has been mentioned under the section on cardiac malpositions, other anatomic settings may also provide useful statistical guidance for making a more precise radiographic diagnosis. Different types of aortic arch anomalies are good examples.

When a right-sided aortic arch is present, the incidence of congenital heart disease increased from

TABLE 16-1 Cardiac Defects Associated with Each Type of Right-Sided Aortic Arch

	Type of Anomaly	
	Avian	Common
Anatomic details	With mirror-image branching; the arch is anterior to the trachea	With aberrant left subclavian artery arising from a large aortic diverticulum which is posterior to the esophagus
Patients with cardiac defects, %	98	12
Type of defects, %:		
Tetralogy of Fallot	90	71
Truncus arteriosus	2.5	
Transposition of great arteries	1.5	
ASD and/or VSD	0.5	21
Coarctation of aorta		7
Others	5.5	1

10- to 100-fold, depending on the anatomic details of the anomaly.[12,13] Of practical importance, there are only two types of right-sided aortic arch. The first has been called the *avian type*, implying a normal status for the birds. It is, however, seriously wrong for human beings. The overwhelming majority of humans with this type would be born with cyanotic congenital heart disease. The second may be called the *common type* because of a higher incidence of occurrence. Most patients with this type are physiologically normal, and their arch anomaly is usually discovered incidentally on routine chest x-rays or during a barium meal study. The x-ray findings of the two types are similar in the postero-anterior view but are quite different in the lateral view (Fig. 16-6). The incidence of congenital heart disease in patients with a right-sided aortic arch[13] is shown in Table 16-1. In the presence of the avian type of right aortic arch the patient has only a 2 percent chance of being physiologically normal. The diagnosis of tetralogy of Fallot should be seriously considered under such conditions until proven otherwise.

Patients with a double aortic arch, on the other hand, rarely have congenital heart disease, though they tend to be symptomatic in infancy because of a compressing vascular ring.[12]

References

1. Mr. Robert Montgomery's Poems, *Edinburgh Review*, April 1830.
2. Edwards, J. E., Carey, L. S., Neufeld, H. N., and Lester, R. G.: Congenital Heart Disease, W. B. Saunders Company, Philadelphia, 1965.
*3. Chen, J. T. T., Capp, M. P., Johnsrude, I. S., Goodrich, J. K., and Lester, R. G.: Roentgen Appearance of Pulmonary Vascularity in the Diagnosis of Heart Disease, *Am. J. Roentgenol.*, 112:559, 1971. (20 references)
*4. Swischuck, L. E.: Plain Film Interpretation in Congenital Heart Disease, 2d ed., The Williams & Wilkins Company, Baltimore, 1979. (Extensively referenced)
5. Chen, J. T. T., Behar, V. S., Morris, J. J., McIntosh, H. D., and Lester, R. G.: Correlation of Roentgen Findings with Hemodynamic Data in Pure Mitral Stenosis, *Am. J. Roentgenol.*, 102:280, 1968.
6. Meszaros, W. T.: "Cardiac Roentgenology," Charles C Thomas, Publisher, Springfield, Ill., 1969.
7. Cooley, R. N., "Radiology of the Heart and Great Vessels," 3d ed., The Williams & Wilkins Company, Baltimore, 1978.
*8. Lusted, L. B., and Keats, T. T.: "Atlas of Roentgenographic Measurement," 2d ed., Year Book Medical Publishers, Inc., Chicago, 1967. (Extensively referenced)
9. Chickos, P. M., Figley, M. M., and Fisher, L.: Correlation between Chest Film and Angiographic Assessment of Left Ventricular Size, *Am. J. Roentgenol.*, 128:367, 1977.
*10. Bartel, A. G., Chen, J. T. T., Peter, R. H., Behar, V. S., Kong, Y., and Lester, R. G.: The Significance of Coronary Calcification Detected by Fluoroscopy: A Report of 360 Patients, *Circulation*, 49:1247, 1974. (10 references)
11. Elliott, L. P., Jue, K. L., and Amplatz, K.: A Roentgen Classification of Cardiac Malpositions, *Invest. Radiol.*, 1:17, 1966.
12. Shuford, W. H., and Sybers, R. G.: "The Aortic Arch and Its Malformations," Charles C Thomas, Publisher, Springfield, Ill. 1974.
13. Stewart, J. R., Kincaid, O. W., and Titus, J. L.: Right Aortic Arch: Plain Film Diagnosis and Significance, *Am. J. Roentgenol.*, 97:377, 1966.
14. Elliott, L. P., and Schiebler, G. L.: "X-Ray Diagnosis of Congenital Cardiac Disease," 2d ed, Charles C Thomas Publisher, Springfield, Ill. 1979.

*This article is a review of the literature and contains additional references to the literature.

Section B | Data to Be Collected on Selected Patients

17

Assessment of Structural Abnormalities and Blood Flow

Joseph K. Perloff, M.D.

The prime objectives of clinical examination of the cardiovascular system are to determine whether or not disease is present and to characterize the disease so identified. Information routinely derived from the history, physical examination, electrocardiogram, and chest roentgenograms may provide a sufficient basis for judgment so that additional knowledge is not required, at least at that time. Conversely, there may be important gaps in the information so derived, requiring supplementation from cardiovascular laboratories. Access to such laboratories permits resolution of most, if not all, diagnostic problems confronting the cardiac clinician. In fact, the diagnostic armamentarium is currently so vast and the capabilities so great that the clinician is faced not only with a virtual tyranny of options, but also with the potential for detecting clinically unimportant disease. The physician responsible for patient care remains the ultimate arbiter who must decide whether and which laboratory studies are required. Nothing replaces the judgment of that physician. If questions do not require immediate answer, laboratory study can be deferred, but if such questions can be resolved by safe, painless, and inexpensive investigation, there is often a legitimate inclination to proceed. When important unresolved diagnostic problems cannot or should not be deferred, the clinician must determine which of a number of laboratory options capable of providing answers are most appropriate. The physician has an unassignable obligation to select the safest, most painless, least inconvenient, and least costly study or studies that qualify in answering a given question. The purpose of this chapter is to assist the practitioner in the strategy of making these decisions. Laboratory investigation should be a logical extension of clinical thinking, not a substitute for it. There must be a constant interplay between clinical and laboratory diagnoses, between pragmatic considerations and intellectual curiosity. The important insights gained apart from cardiac diagnostic laboratories must be fostered continually by cultivating the most refined clinical talents, but the complete cardiac physician should be as comfortable and as well versed in dealing with laboratory information as in dealing with clinical information personally secured at the bedside. Laboratory investigations best resolve problems after sound clinical assessment has shown the way. The physician can then ask with confidence, "Are laboratory studies required, and if so, which ones and in what sequence?" In dealing with the practical strategies of laboratory diagnoses, I shall focus on acquired and congenital valvular heart disease, nonvalvular congenital heart disease with expected adult survival, the cardiomyopathies, and pericardial disease. In so doing, my objective will be to foster a point of view, not to be comprehensive. Abnormalities of myocardial contractility, electrical activity, and metabolism (including ischemia) will be considered in Chaps. 18, 19, and 20.

Valvular Heart Disease— Acquired and Congenital

The Aortic Valve

This section deals with the functionally normal bicuspid aortic valve, valvular aortic stenosis (congenital aortic stenosis and acquired nonrheumatic stenosis in the aged), and aortic regurgitation (mild, severe, chronic, acute).

Aortic Stenosis

When a soft, grade I–II/VI midsystolic murmur is most prominent at the right base (especially second right intercostal space) in a child or young adult, suspicion of a functionally normal bicuspid aortic valve arises.[1] Innocent or normal systolic murmurs in the *young* are not heard *maximally* at the right base. The suspicion is heightened if the subject is a male. Auscultation may detect an aortic ejection sound, often loudest at the apex, and a soft, high-frequency, mid-left sternal edge murmur of aortic regurgitation. Identification of the elusive, soft, high-frequency early diastolic murmur is improved with firm pressure of the stethoscopic diaphragm in full exhalation in a quiet room, especially with the subject sitting and leaning forward. Isometric exercise (clenched fist) or squatting further enhances audibility. It is important to suspect and then confirm the presence of a functionally normal bicuspid aortic valve because of the high susceptibility to infective endocarditis[2] and because the subsequent course may culminate in calcific aortic stenosis on the one hand,[1,2] or aortic regurgitation on the other.[3] The problem is most taxing when the suspicion depends on the right basal systolic murmur alone, with the ejection sound in doubt and the murmur of aortic regurgitation undetected. The first laboratory procedure that comes to mind is the echocardiogram, both M-mode and two-dimensional imaging, but the M mode alone usually suffices. The laboratory request should state precisely what is sought so the technician will diligently address the aortic valve, seeking specific diagnostic information. The diastolic closure line of the bicuspid aortic valve on the M-mode echocadiogram lies eccentrically within the aorta (Fig. 17-1A).[4,5] The bicuspid valve may not show abnormal eccentricity of the diastolic closure line in all projections, but recording of distinctly abnormal eccentricity is presumptive evidence that the valve is bicuspid. The technician should also be instructed to record high-quality images of the anterior mitral leaflet, since fine flutter resulting from aortic regurgitation serves to return the clinician to the bedside in search of the faint high-frequency early diastolic murmur.[6] If the M-mode tracing fails to identify the diagnostic eccentricity of the diastolic closure line, a two-dimensional real-time image in the short axis with the transducer directed in a superior fashion records the aortic valve and leaflets and may record individual cusps or two or three leaflets, as the case may be.[7] If the M-mode and two-dimensional echocardiograms are nondiagnostic, the question of further diagnostic pursuit arises. If high-quality echocardiograms were taken by an experienced technician and read by an experienced echocardiographer, the issue need not be pursued further. Thoracic aortography is perhaps an even more sensitive means of identifying a bicuspid aortic valve (Fig. 17-1B), but recourse to this technique is not justified, given the above constraints. On the other hand, if auscultation cannot confidently distinguish a split first heart sound from a first heart sound followed by an aortic ejection sound, then a harmless, inexpensive high-fidelity phonocardiogram recorded with a simultaneous aortic valve echocardiogram usually permits the distinction between a normally split first heart sound which occurs before the valve opens, and an aortic ejection sound which occurs as the leaflets reach their maximum systolic excursion. If suspicion of a bicuspid aortic valve lingers, I suggest clinical reassessment after an interval of approximately a year, including repeat echocardiograms.

For the purpose of the following discussion, let us deal with two forms of congenital valvular aortic stenosis: the valve that is intrinsically stenotic from birth and the fibrocalcific thickening of a bicuspid aortic valve that was functionally normal at birth.

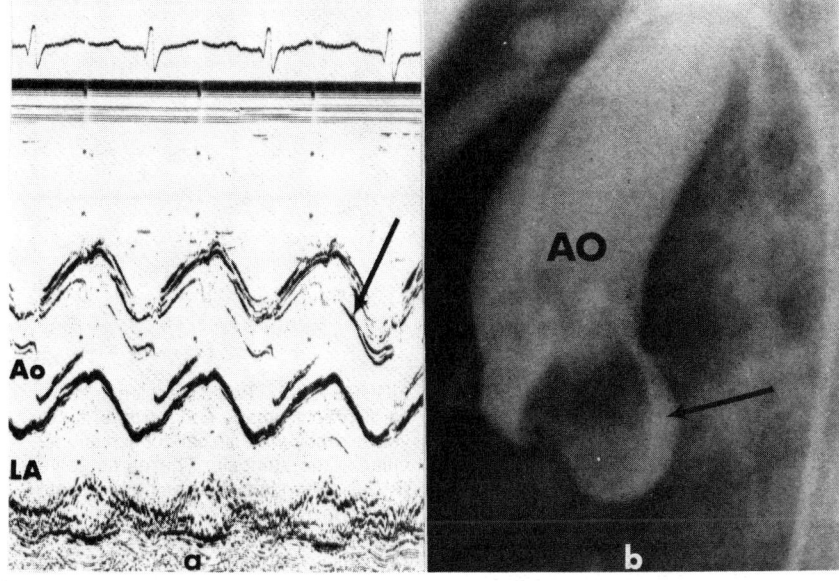

FIGURE 17-1   *a.* The M-mode echocardiogram with ultrasonic beam through the aorta (Ao) records the typical eccentric diastolic closure line (arrow) of a bicuspid aortic valve. The diastolic closure line is close to the anterior aortic wall. LA = left atrium. *b.* Contrast material injected into the aortic root (AO) identifies the typical angiographic image of a bicuspid aortic valve (arrow).

EXAMINATION OF THE HEART AND BLOOD VESSELS

Clinical assessment of severity may pose comparatively little diagnostic difficulties at the far ends of the spectrum—very mild or very severe—but in patients in whom severity is less clear, the clinician is confronted with the taxing problem of the timing, type, and sequence of laboratory investigation. The preadolescent child or teenager with a mobile, intrinsically stenotic congenital aortic valve is typically an asymptomatic, healthy, active male in whom a resting 12-lead electrocardiogram is normal or may exhibit only an ambiguous increase in QRS voltage, and in whom the chest x-ray is normal except for poststenotic dilatation of the aortic root.[1] The first step in laboratory assessment is the M-mode echocardiogram. In assessing severity, the importance of the echocardiogram lies in imaging below the aortic valve, that is, septal/free wall thicknesses and internal dimensions.[8–10] Imaging of the valve per se does not provide reliable insight into severity. If septal/left ventricular free wall thicknesses are greater than normal, it can be assumed that there has been an adaptive increase in left ventricular mass in response to the afterload imposed by valvular obstruction. Furthermore, the M-mode echocardiogram in children is reliable in estimating left ventricular peak systolic pressure, employing a simple wall thickness/cavity dimension ratio.[9,11] Left ventricular peak systolic pressure equals 225 multiplied by systolic thickness of the posterior wall divided by end-systolic dimensions. Given the estimated peak systolic pressure derived from this formulation, the gradient is the difference between that pressure and the cuff manometric systolic pressure. It is important to underscore that in the intrinsically stenotic dome congenital aortic valve, two-dimensional echocardiographic imaging nicely identifies the mobile stenotic valve and dilated aortic root (Fig. 17-2),[7] but competes poorly with the M-mode image in assessing left ventricular mass and severity of obstruction. Exercise electrocardiography can next be selected as a simple, safe, and inexpensive diagnostic tool, shedding light on the capacity of the left ventricle to withstand physical stress.[13,14] Significant depression of the ST segments in an exercising young person with a stenotic aortic valve selects that patient out as one whose ventricular myocardium is in potential jeopardy. Cardiac catheterization remains the definitive means of measuring the transvalvular gradient and estimating orifice size. In young patients with M-mode echocardiographic evidence of an increase in left ventricular mass, a calculated elevation in left ventricular peak systolic pressure,[9] and two-dimensional echocardiographic evidence of the typical, mobile, dome aortic valve, cardiac catheterization and angiocardiography are likely to be largely confirmatory although desirable. However, when the M-mode echocardiogram does not clearly indicate an increase in septal/left ventricular free wall thicknesses or significant calculated elevation in left ventricular peak systolic pressure, and the exercise electrocardiogram exhibits an ischemic response, the next step in resolving the clinical problem is cardiac catheterization.

Refined planning of diagnostic interventions is especially appropriate when dealing with a bicuspid aortic valve that is undergoing progressive obstruction caused by gradual fibrous thickening and calcification. The valve initially may remain sufficiently mobile to preserve the aortic ejection sound, and the electrocardiogram may show few or no repolarization abnormalities of left ventricular hypertrophy or ischemia. In the simplest terms, fluoroscopy (image intensification) should first be used to identify incipient calcification heralding the beginning of progressive obstruction. Valve mobility can be examined further (safely and simply) by two-dimensional echocardiography. Conclusions from these two sources merely indicate that a previously mobile, functionally unobstructed bicuspid aortic valve is beginning to thicken. Abundant aortic valve cal-

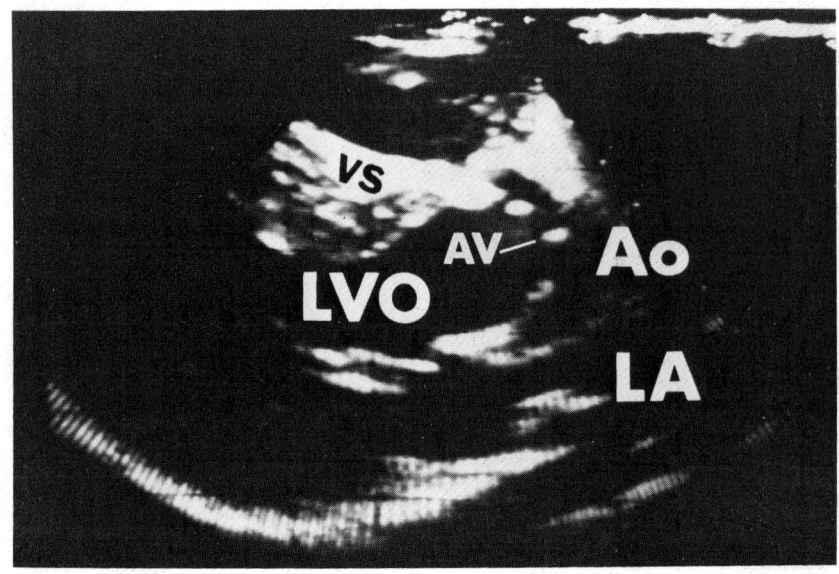

FIGURE 17-2 Two-dimensional echocardiographic image (long axis) in a 15-year-old boy with typical congenital valvular aortic stenosis. The aortic valve (AV) is shown in systole as it domes into the aorta (Ao). LA = left atrium; LVO = left ventricular outflow tract; VS = ventricular septum.

cium at fluoroscopy predicts severe stenosis, but an analogous conclusion cannot be drawn from dense images on echocardiography. Accordingly, inferences regarding the degree of obstruction are difficult if not impossible when either M-mode or two-dimensional echocardiography focuses on the valve alone.[5] Meticulous use of sequential echocardiographic observations (especially M-mode determinations of septal/free wall thicknesses) and exercise electrocardiography are important in determining when cardiac catheterization should be performed with the view toward surgical intervention. It is not uncommon for progression to be represented first by ST-segment depressions in the exercise electrocardiogram rather than by echocardiographic evidence of an increase in ventricular septal/free wall thicknesses or the appearance of symptoms. In applying the echocardiogram, the M mode is preferred, since this technique provides the most refined assessment of the adaptive response of the left ventricle to imposed afterload. Apart from measuring septal/left ventricular free wall thicknesses, the M-mode echocardiogram can be used as described in the above formula, employing the systolic free wall thickness/end-systolic cavity dimension ratio, provided the patient is still a relatively young adult. The presence of symptoms or evidence of progression in the exercise electrocardiogram and echocardiogram set the stage for cardiac catheterization, which remains the ultimate arbiter since, with angiocardiography, the method provides morphologic information as well as more precise physiologic data based upon transvalvular pressure differences and transvalvular flow–calculated aortic stenotic orifice size. Furthermore, aortic valve mobility and left ventricular function (ejection fraction) can be reassessed during aortography and left ventriculography.

A relatively common concomitant of aging in the cardiac and vascular system is the insidious development of firm, ridgelike fibrous thickenings at the base of the aortic cusps as they insert into the sinuses of Valsalva (Fig. 17-3).[1,15] These zones of fibrous thickening often contain small focal deposits of calcium. Early morphologic changes are confined to the base of the cusps, and occur without commissural fusion, without impairment of cusp mobility, and, accordingly, without obstruction.[1] It is appropriate to designate the accompanying murmur *aortic sclerotic*. However, what begins as an innocent aortic systolic murmur represents one end of a continuum that culminates at the other end in severe calcific aortic stenosis as calcium is progressively deposited on the aortic surfaces of previously normal trileaflet valves that stiffen and obstruct even though commissural fusion remains absent.[1,15] The distinction between *aortic sclerosis* and *aortic stenosis* as herein defined and a clinical estimate of the degree of aortic stenosis in this setting can be difficult. The chief auscultatory suspicion is the harsh, right basal midsystolic murmur originating in the aortic root, and the telltale apical high-frequency, musical midsystolic murmur of Gallavardin originating in periodic vibrations of aortic cusps that are thickened but not fused.[1,15] Clinical signs that might shed light on the degree of aortic stenosis in this setting are notoriously unreliable.[15] M-mode imaging of the aortic valve is useful in excluding significant stenosis if mobile leaflets are recorded, but is otherwise of relatively little help, since dense echoes can be reflected from sclerotic but nonstenotic valves.[5] Septal/free wall thickness may be ambiguous. However, a simple but important diagnostic intervention is cardiac fluoroscopy. It is a good rule of thumb that absence of fluoroscopic calcification is presumptive evidence of a sclerotic but nonstenotic valve, while the pres-

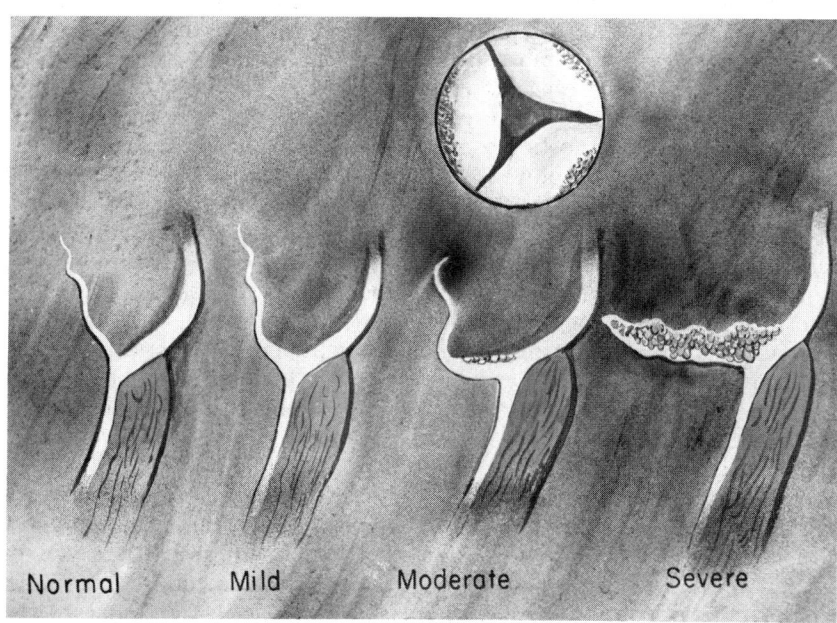

Normal   Mild   Moderate   Severe

FIGURE 17-3 Schematic illustration showing on the left the normal attachment of an aortic cusp to its sinus. The mild alteration consists of fibrous thickening at the base of the cusp as it inserts into the sinus of Valsalva. The ridgelike, fibrous shelf is responsible for an innocent aortic systolic murmur. Moderate progression is represented by calcific deposits on the aortic surface of the fibrous ridge. Severe deformity results from extension of calcium to the free edges of the leaflets, converting a previously normal trileaflet aortic valve into calcific aortic stenosis without commissural fusion. (*From Perloff.*[1] *Reproduced with permission.*)

ence of dense calcification predicts significant stenosis. During fluoroscopy, a special effort should be made to identify calcification of the proximal coronary arteries and mitral annulus, common concomitants of trileaflet calcific aortic stenosis in the aged.[15] Cardiac catheterization remains the means of determining not only the degree of stenosis (gradient and orifice size), but also the presence and degree of atherosclerotic coronary arterial obstruction and the status of left ventricular function. Such patients should be selected for catheterization and angiography only if valve replacement is a viable therapeutic option. This form of aortic stenosis typically occurs above age 65 years and often in the seventies and eighties, so selection for operation requires refined judgment that should precede the decision to catheterize.

Since coronary artery disease is common in this age group, a particularly trying question is the relative effect on left ventricular function and wall motion of coronary arterial obstruction versus aortic valvular obstruction. An M-mode echocardiogram that records a relatively thin, hypokinetic septum or free wall and a significant increase in left ventricular internal dimensions at end diastole does not necessarily identify depressed ventricular function too advanced for salvage, since the areas penetrated by the ultrasonic beam may be segmental and therefore not representative of the ventricle as a whole. Gated cardiac scintigraphy employing technetium 99m as the tracer better quantifies abnormalities of wall motion and ejection fraction. Given an ejection fraction that is moderately depressed (35 to 45 percent), the addition of thallium 201 imaging is unlikely to resolve the relative contributions of coronary arterial and aortic valvular obstruction. However, these radionuclide modalities, together with coronary angiocardiography and left ventriculography usually—but by no means invariably—permit reasoned conclusions.

Aortic Regurgitation

Chronic Severe Aortic Regurgitation In patients with chronic severe aortic regurgitation, the selection of diagnostic studies and the timing of surgical intervention remain unsettled clinical problems. The normal left ventricle adapts to gradual, progressive volume loads by increasing its internal dimensions with proportionate increases in septal/free wall thickness. The purpose of diagnostic investigations in chronic severe aortic regurgitation is to identify the transition beyond a normal adaptive response, that is, to determine when the left ventricle can no longer handle the excess volume as a normal pump. In symptomatic patients, the question is less whether valve replacement is appropriate, but whether the left ventricle can be salvaged. It should be underscored that cardiac catheterization and angiocardiography (thoracic aortography, left ventriculography) are not required to establish that chronic

aortic regurgitation is *severe,* a point that should be clinically evident. Furthermore, critical determinations of left ventricular function can be assessed—and serially reassessed with individual patients as their own controls—at rest and during exercise by relatively safe, inexpensive, noninvasive techniques (see below).[16–19] An important question requiring laboratory resolution in symptomatic patients with chronic severe aortic regurgitation is whether left ventricular performance has deteriorated to a point that precludes an acceptable response to valve replacement at a reasonable operative risk. In answering this pivotal question, two important indexes of left ventricular function—left ventricular end-systolic dimension and percent fractional shortening—are amenable to noninvasive assessment. The standard M-mode echocardiogram is the simplest, safest, and least expensive means of providing this valuable information.[16,17] A second and more refined technique is radionuclide angiography using technetium 99m as noted above.[18] Gated cardiac scintigraphy is more expensive than M-mode echocardiography, but it is safe and provides two-dimensional information on septal and free wall motion, is an accurate means of determining ejection fraction, and permits observations at rest and during graded exercise.[18] As a rule, all necessary information except the anatomy of the coronary arteries can be established by M-mode echocardiography and radionuclide angiography. Accordingly, in *young* patients (third and fourth decades), cardiac catheterization and angiocardiography are not obligatory preoperative procedures. In patients above age 40 years, especially males (who constitute most subjects with chronic severe valvular aortic regurgitation), and especially if left ventricular function is depressed, catheterization is employed chiefly to study the coronary arteries even though in the majority of instances the coronary arteries are large and dilated.

An equally important and perhaps more taxing problem is the *asymptomatic* patient with chronic severe aortic regurgitation. When should such patients undergo aortic valve replacement? Which diagnostic procedures are important in answering this question? It is seldom that clinical assessment fails to establish both the presence and degree of chronic severe aortic regurgitation, but laboratory investigation is required to determine the insidious transition from the normal adaptive response of the volume-loaded left ventricle to incipient, asymptomatic deterioration of left ventricular function. Let us again focus on left ventricular end-systolic dimension and fractional shortening. The first diagnostic technique to be selected is the M-mode echocardiogram. This study not only permits quantification of these indexes of ventricular function,[20] but also provides a base line for safe, simple, convenient reassessment at appropriate intervals.[16,17] A progressive increase in left ventricular end-systolic volume with a reciprocal decrease in fractional shortening selects out even asymptomatic patients with chronic severe aortic regurgitation. A single assessment with no basis for comparison makes interpretation more difficult, but an appreciable increase in end-systolic dimension (in excess of 55 mm) with a reduced ejection fraction warrants careful scrutiny. Two-dimensional echocardiography sheds considerable light on chamber size and wall motion, but technetium radionuclide angiography (see above) provides data on wall motion and ejection fraction both at rest and during exercise.[18] In asymptomatic patients with chronic severe aortic regurgitation, ejection fraction may be normal at rest but abnormal with exercise.[18] In the relatively young (third or fourth decade) asymptomatic patient, cardiac catheterization and angiography provide little or no important information beyond the echocardiogram and radionuclide angiography described above.

Acute Severe Aortic Regurgitation   A common cause of acute severe aortic regurgitation is infective endocarditis on a previously unrecognized, functionally normal bicuspid aortic valve.[3] The clinical manifestations of severe aortic regurgitation of sudden onset are in contrast to the classic manifestations of *chronic* severe regurgitation.[3] Sudden imposition of severe volume load finds the left ventricle unprepared, since time is too short to permit an appropriate adaptive response. Yet time is of the essence since acute severe aortic regurgitation is, by and large, a life-threatening emergency requiring prompt identification and surgical intervention.[3] Given the clinical suspicion, the diagnosis must be confirmed immediately and the etiology established beyond reasonable doubt. The simplest, most important initial study is the M-mode echocardiogram.[3] In the presence of acute severe aortic regurgitation, end-diastolic pressure rises dramatically in response to the increased volume because the unprepared left ventricle is operating on the less compliant portion of its pressure-volume curve.[3,21] The steep rise in left ventricular diastolic pressure exceeds left atrial pressure in latter diastole, prematurely closing the mitral valve, sometimes before the inscription of the P wave of the electrocardiogram.[3] The M-mode echocardiogram recorded with an electrocardiogram as reference tracing permits relatively precise identification of the important sign of premature mitral valve closure. In addition, the M-mode image sheds light on etiology by detecting vegetations on the aortic valve (infective endocarditis) or by suspecting the double aortic wall of a dissecting aneurysm.[3] In identifying vegetations, two-dimensional echocardiography is of even greater value. Urgency requires swift decisions, and the next diagnostic procedure is thoracic aortography to confirm that the acute aortic regurgitation is *severe* and to clarify further the etiology, especially if dissecting aneurysm is suspected. Given the suspicion of acute severe aortic regurgitation due to infective endocarditis, multiple blood cultures should be secured and appropriate antimicrobial therapy begun, but it should be underscored that early surgical intervention is generally obligatory long before a bacteriologic cure.[3,22]

The Mitral Valve

In this section, three major categories of mitral valve disorders will be dealt with. They are prolapse, severe regurgitation (chronic or acute), and obstruction at the mitral orifice.

Mitral Valve Prolapse

The diagnosis of mitral valve prolapse rests securely on the unequivocal identification of typical mid- to late-systolic clicks and a late-systolic murmur.[23] An echocardiogram is not required for purely diagnostic confirmation. It should be underscored that the echocardiogram, despite its high sensitivity, does not always record mitral valve prolapse. A nondiagnostic tracing should *not* weigh against an otherwise secure auscultatory diagnosis. The M-mode echocardiogram is of potentially greater value when auscultation is ambiguous, especially when the clinician is dealing with a patient substrate that arouses suspicion—a young person with palpitations, atypical chest pain, slight pectus excavatum or corinatum, or slight scoliosis.[23] If the M-mode tracing is nondiagnostic in a patient suspected of mitral valve prolapse, there is a tendency to secure a two-dimensional echocardiogram even though strict diagnostic criteria have not been established for real-time imaging. Since mitral valve prolapse with late systolic mitral regurgitation is susceptible to infective endocarditis, it is important to establish the diagnosis. The echocardiogram is a powerful laboratory tool, but its sensitivity is so great that one runs the risk of isolated echocardiographic diagnoses of mitral prolapse in patients who are otherwise entirely normal. It is unwise to draw pathologic conclusions from such echocardiographic observations. It is even more unwise to resort to left ventriculography to identify mitral prolapse. The use of range-gated pulsed Doppler echocardiography in this setting is yet unsettled.[24]

Given a secure auscultatory and echocardiographic diagnosis of mitral valve prolapse, characterization of accompanying arrhythmias may be an important concern.[23,25,26] Ambulatory electrocardiographic monitoring is the most sensitive method of detecting these arrhythmias,[23,26] and is more useful in this regard than exercise testing.[23,25] However, the strategy in applying these techniques is of utmost importance. For example, 24-h ambulatory monitoring should *not* be done in search of asymptomatic arrhythmias. Such application is likely to frighten rather than reassure patients. Study should be reserved chiefly if not exclusively for individuals whose palpitations have not been properly characterized *and* are sufficiently symptomatic to warrant pharmacologic suppression. More often than not, an intelligent, observant patient can describe the palpitations so clearly that accurate diagnostic inferences can be drawn. This is so, for example, with typical reentrant supraventricular tachycardia, the commonest sustained tachyarrhythmia in mitral valve prolapse.[23] Intracardiac electrophysiologic investigations are reserved for the relatively few patients with active bypass tracts (Wolff-Parkinson-White syndrome), and only in a small percentage of those.[23]

Severe Mitral Regurgitation

Chronic Severe Mitral Regurgitation   Insidious progression of mitral regurgitation allows the left ventricle time for adaptation to the augmented volume. In addition, left atrial size usually increases appreciably, sometimes reaching giant proportions, especially in chronic severe rheumatic mitral regurgitation. The larger the left atrium, the more likely that the chamber will handle the regurgitant flow with little or no elevation of its mean pressure.[27] Diagnostic investigation should therefore address left ventricular size and function, left atrial size, and mitral valve structure. The M-mode echocardiogram is the first step, both for accurate confirmation of left atrial size (which can also be inferred with relative accuracy from a cardiac series with barium esophagogram) and more importantly, for left ventricular function and mitral valve structure. Left ventricular internal dimensions can be determined, and excursions as well as thickness of septum/free wall quantified. The M-mode echocardiogram sheds light on when the adaptive response of the volume-loaded left ventricle becomes abnormal, that is, a progressive increase in end-systolic dimensions and a progressive fall in left ventricular ejection fraction (increased E point/septal separation)[23a] and fractional shortening. Echocardiographic assessment of the mitral valve does not, as a rule, clarify the etiology, but occasionally chronic progressive regurgitation can be put into the setting of mitral valve prolapse, especially when chordal rupture and flail leaflets are identified. The two-dimensional echocardiogram yields additional information on wall motion, and is the simplest accurate diagnostic study when "mitral regurgitation" occurs with congenitally corrected transposition of the great arteries (see below) (Fig. 17-4A).[1] The systemic atrioventricular valve is anatomically tricuspid and is incompetent because of Ebstein's anomaly, which can be readily identified on two-dimensional imaging. The degree of mitral regurgitation can also be studied with range-gated pulsed Doppler echocardiography, which is still in its developmental stage.[24] Estimates of regurgitant flow with Doppler echocardiography correlate well with estimates from selective ventriculography.[24] Left ventricular function can be further estimated by the safe, noninvasive technique of radionuclide cineangiography employing technetium 99m (see above).[18-20] The

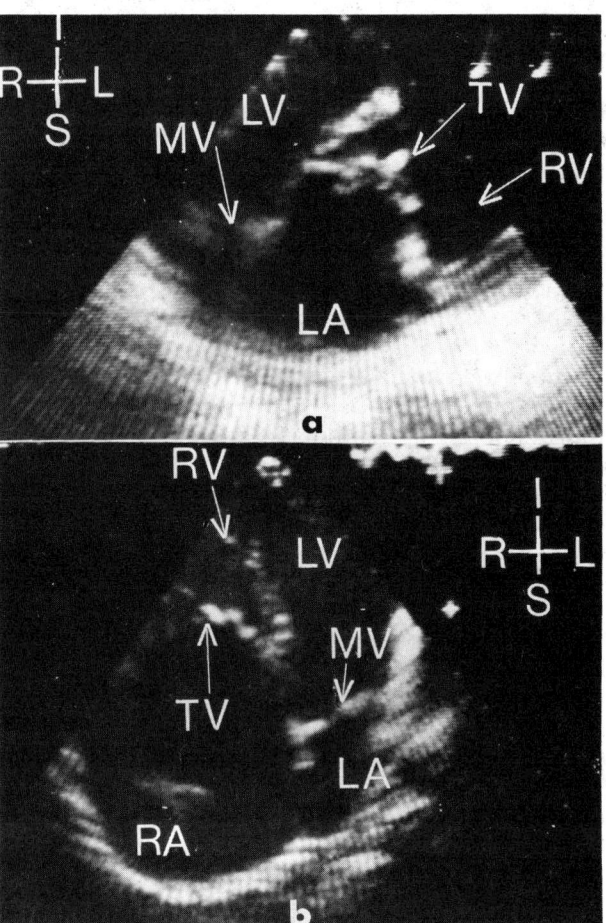

FIGURE 17-4   *a.* Two-dimensional echocardiogram (apical four-chamber view) from a patient with congenitally corrected transposition of the great arteries and systemic AV valve regurgitation. The tricuspid valve (TV) is in the left heart and is dramatically recessed into the cavity of an anatomic systemic right ventricule (RV). This is left-sided Ebstein's anomaly. The left atrium (LA) is enlarged. The mitral valve (MV) and left ventricle (LV) are in the right heart (inverted position). *b.* Similar image in a patient with Ebstein's anomaly of a right-sided (noninverted) tricuspid valve (TV) which is dramatically recessed into the cavity of the right ventricle (RV). The right atrium (RA) is enlarged.

method not only provides accurate quantification of ejection fraction at rest, but also provides important information on response to exercise. Furthermore, preoperative data can be used as a basis for comparison with postoperative ventricular function. Careful assessment using the above modalities reduces the need for cardiac catheterization and angiocardiography, which are best applied when the degree of mitral regurgitation and its structural cause remain unclear, when the presence and magnitude of coexisting aortic valve disease are unsettled, and when older subjects are suspected of coronary artery disease.

Acute Severe Mitral Regurgitation   Severe mitral regurgitation of acute onset due to rupture of primary chordae tendineae or papillary muscle is a fundamentally difficult problem. The hemodynamic response is in contrast to the above descriptions of chronic severe mitral regurgitation.[28] Acute severe mitral regurgitation due to rupture of primary chordae tendineae is a case in point. A previously normal but physiologically unprepared left ventricle and left atrium are suddenly called upon to handle a dramatic increase in volume. Ventricular filling pressure rises steeply while cardiac output generally falls. As the normal-sized left atrium suddenly receives marked regurgitant flow, its pressure rises steeply and is transmitted via the pulmonary veins to the pulmonary artery so that pulmonary hypertension ensues.[28] The diagnostic study that has the virtues of low cost, safety, and high yield is the M-mode echocardiogram, which accurately examines left ventricular internal dimensions and percent fractional shortening, mitral valve structure, and left atrial size. The M-mode echocardiogram is sensitive in detecting ruptured chordae tendineae and is moderately sensitive in identifying elevated pulmonary arterial pressure (pulmonary valve imaging).[5] Normal or relatively normal left atrial size can be confirmed. Two-dimensional echocardiography is not obligatory, but can shed further light on a flail mitral valve, either anterior or posterior leaflet. Since surgical intervention is almost always required, it is appropriate to proceed to cardiac catheterization and angiography, which establish the degree of mitral regurgitation and measure left atrial and pulmonary arterial pressures. Reliance on pulsed Doppler echocardiography for quantifying mitral regurgitation is premature.[24]

Since a secure bedside diagnosis of acute severe mitral regurgitation sets the stage for catheterization, it can be argued that echocardiography is unnecessary. Although echocardiograms are not obligatory, they are desirable because more precise precatheterization information usually permits a shorter, safer, and more informative study in patients who are often acutely ill or at least symptomatic.

Acute severe mitral regurgitation due to chordal rupture is usually spontaneous and only occasionally the result of infective endocarditis. Acute severe mitral regurgitation due to ruptured papillary muscle is more ominous and more urgent, since rupture typically occurs in the setting of recent cardiac infarction, so that sudden severe volume is imposed upon a left ventricle that is suffering from a fresh infarct.[29,30] The clinical distinction between ruptured papillary muscle and perforated ventricular septum is difficult but obligatory. The M-mode echocardiogram points the way by identifying a flail mitral valve; the study can be done at the bedside. At the same time or in immediate sequence, a flotation catheter should be placed in the pulmonary artery[31] to establish that left atrial pressure (wedge) is appreciably elevated (see above), but more importantly to determine the oxygen saturations in the right heart, confirming the absence of a step-up and hence the absence of a perforated ventricular sep-

tum. Salvage is possible if the rupture is due to discontinuity of a head of a papillary muscle rather than of the entire papillary muscle trunk. Cardiac catheterization and angiography are obligatory, not merely to confirm the presence and degree of mitral regurgitation in the absence of perforated ventricular septum, but to establish the anatomy of obstructed coronary arteries which, for all practical purposes, invariably coexist.

Obstruction of the Mitral Orifice

Mitral Stenosis Mitral stenosis is a less complex anatomic and physiological fault than mitral regurgitation and is, as a rule, subject to more precise anatomic and physiological definition.[30] In fact, careful clinical assessment generally discloses most if not all the important information in young subjects with pure isolated rheumatic mitral stenosis (see below). The M-mode echocardiogram is, however, an important extension, giving useful information on mitral valve thickness and mobility, especially the larger anterior cusp.[5] Left atrial size can be measured; right ventricular internal dimensions and ventricular septal motion (normal or paradoxic) provide information on the presence and degree of tricuspid regurgitation (right ventricular volume overload); and the pulmonary valve echo may show evidence of pulmonary hypertension. Simple fluoroscopy remains useful in determining the degree of mitral calcification. The two-dimensional echocardiogram in the short axis permits accurate, direct planimetric measurement of the mitral valve orifice as well as further assessment of individual leaflet mobility and thickness.

The average patient with pure severe rheumatic mitral stenosis is a young (third or early fourth decade) female who does not require cardiac catheterization before operation. This procedure, together with angiography, is best used to establish the coronary arterial anatomy in older subjects, especially males, to refine information on mobility and competence of the valve (reconstruction vs. replacement), and to quantify the degree of pulmonary hypertension and tricuspid regurgitation, thus clarifying the need for tricuspid reconstruction, without which the patient may not survive operation despite ideal relief of the mitral stenosis.

Left Atrial Tumors An additional form of obstruction at the mitral orifice deserves comment, namely, myxoma of the left atrium.[32] When the clinician suspects that the obstruction is not due to rheumatic mitral stenosis, the M-mode echocardiogram emerges as a major step forward in identifying the myxoma, both within the left atrium and as the tumor seats in diastole within the mitral orifice.[5] Two-dimensional imaging provides dramatic confirmation. Cardiac catheterization and left ventriculography remain important, since the presence and degree of mitral regurgitation can be determined, underscoring the important question of integrity of the mitral valve (the "wrecking ball" effect of traumatic impact) that may require replacement. It should be emphasized that clinical suspicion and echocardiographic confirmation of a mobile left atrial mass warn the catheterizer that myxoma is likely to be present so that transseptal left heart catheterization is avoided. The mass is best sought angiographically by injection of contrast material into the pulmonary trunk with left atrial visualization during levophase, or into the left ventricle with left atrial visualization due to mitral regurgitation.

The Tricuspid Valve

Let us first contrast tricuspid regurgitation with or without right ventricular/pulmonary hypertension, and then deal with tricuspid valve obstruction due to rheumatic tricuspid stenosis as opposed to right atrial myxoma.

Tricuspid Regurgitation

Tricuspid Regurgitation with Elevated Right Ventricular Pressure The commonest form of tricuspid regurgitation occurs in patients with morphologically normal tricuspid valves that are rendered incompetent in the face of elevated right ventricular pressure (pulmonary hypertension) and right ventricular failure. Pulmonary hypertensive rheumatic mitral stenosis serves as a useful point of departure. It is important to underscore once again the importance of identifying the presence and degree of tricuspid regurgitation, which, when severe, requires tricuspid reconstruction (seldom replacement) during operation for mitral stenosis (see above). The M-mode echocardiogram is useful in this regard. Registration of the pulmonary valve echo partially addresses the problem of pulmonary hypertension, although atrial fibrillation, by eliminating the *a* wave, compromises the value of the observation.[5] More importantly, the M-mode echocardiogram can measure the internal dimensions of the right ventricle (dilated) and can record ventricular septal motion, which in the presence of tricuspid regurgitation (right ventricular volume overload) exhibits abnormal (paradoxic) anterior movement during systole.[5] Two-dimensional echocardiography is useful in assessing right atrial size. Cardiac catheterization and angiography remain important, however, in establishing the degrees of pulmonary hypertension and tricuspid regurgitation (see above).

Tricuspid Regurgitation with Normal Right Ventricular Pressure "Low-pressure" tricuspid regurgitation (normal right ventricular and pulmonary arterial systolic pressures) stands in contrast to tricuspid regurgitation with pulmonary hypertension. Let us

consider two varieties of low-pressure tricuspid regurgitation: (1) congenital, in the setting of Ebstein's anomaly,[1] and (2) acquired,[34] as a result of tricuspid infective endocarditis. In Ebstein's anomaly, the M-mode echocardiogram is highly revealing, recording the increased excursions of the less involved, mobile anterior leaflet, the delayed tricuspid closure (relative to simultaneously recorded mitral valve closure), the increased internal dimensions of the right ventricle, and paradoxic motion of the ventricular septum in response to volume overload of the right ventricle (tricuspid regurgitation) (Fig. 17-5).[1] These observations are highly specific for Ebstein's anomaly, but two-dimensional echocardiography provides definitive images of the anatomy of the deformed tricuspid valve recessed into the right ventricular cavity (Fig. 17-4*B*). Thus, cardiac catheterization is unnecessary to identify the portion of right heart that is mechanically atrial but electrically ventricular.[1] The degree of tricuspid regurgitation can often be estimated clinically or by right atrial size on two-dimensional echocardiograms, but right ventriculography remains the most definitive means of establishing the degree of tricuspid regurgitant flow. It should be remembered that surgical inter-

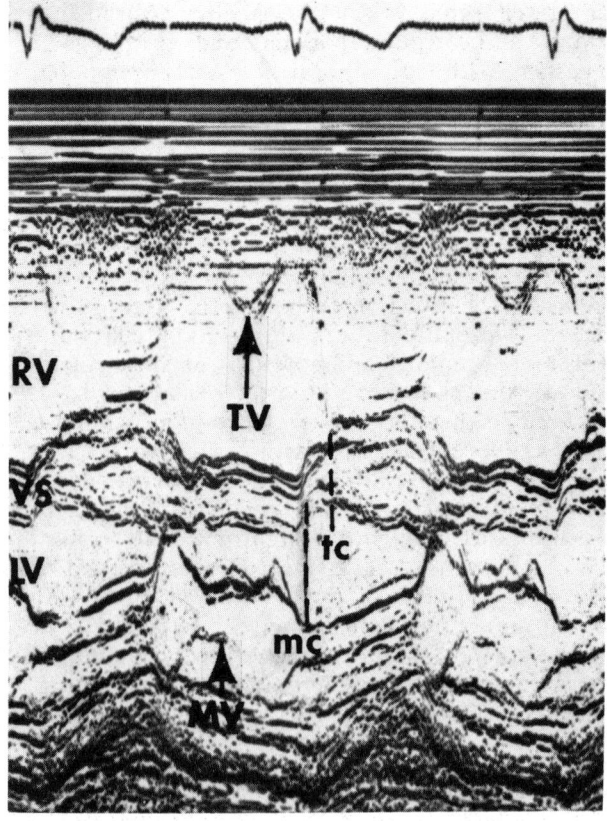

FIGURE 17-5 M-mode echocardiogram from a 9-year-old girl with Ebstein's anomaly of the tricuspid valve. The tricuspid (TV) and mitral valve (MV) were recorded simultaneously. The large, mobile anterior tricuspid leaflet (TV) shows increased excursions, and tricuspid closure (tc) is abnormally delayed relative to mitral closure (mc). There is paradoxical motion of the ventricular septum due to right ventricular (RV) volume overload. LV = left ventricle.

vention in Ebstein's anomaly addresses the morphologic and hemodynamic faults as well as right atrioventricular bypass tracts (Wolff-Parkinson-White). Accordingly, preoperative electrophysiologic investigation is desirable if not obligatory in patients with paroxysmal rapid heart action.[35]

An acquired form of tricuspid regurgitation without right ventricular/pulmonary hypertension is due to tricuspid valve infective endocarditis, generally in intravenous drug abusers. The clinical signs, especially auscultatory, may be subtle, since the murmur is often localized at the left or right lower sternal edge and is soft, medium-frequency, early systolic decrescendo, augmenting or appearing only on inspiration (Fig. 17-6B).[34] The first diagnostic step in a patient suspected of tricuspid infective endocarditis is utilization of the infectious disease laboratory for a series of blood cultures and serial plain film chest roentgenography (septic pulmonary emboli). The M-mode echocardiogram provides important information on both structure and function; the tricuspid valve can often be visualized and vegetations identified (Fig. 17-6A), while right ventricular internal dimensions are measured and septal motion (paradoxic) recorded in the presence of tricuspid regurgitation (volume overload) (Fig. 17-6B). Two-dimensional imaging sometimes confirms tricuspid vegetations when the M-mode does not, and the

two-dimensional record also shows right atrial size, an observation that is useful but not obligatory. The tricuspid regurgitation is generally mild to moderate, but eradication of infection sometimes requires surgical removal of the tricuspid valve followed by further antibiotic therapy. In this setting, the dramatic clinical picture of acute severe low-pressure tricuspid regurgitation emerges. The M-mode echocardiogram allows sequential comparison of right ventricular internal dimensions during the course of therapy. Cardiac catheterization and angiography are not indicated in simple tricuspid infective endocarditis with mild to moderate tricuspid regurgitation and are unnecessary, as a rule, after surgical excision.

Obstruction of the Tricuspid Orifice

Tricuspid Stenosis Rheumatic tricuspid stenosis predicts with virtual certainty the presence of rheumatic mitral stenosis.[36] Despite well-defined clinical diagnostic criteria, tricuspid stenosis is still all too often overlooked. Yet, clinical suspicion is necessary if diagnostic methods for confirmation are to be planned and properly executed. Given the clinical suspicion, the M-mode echocardiogram should deliberately seek high-quality recordings of the tricuspid valve, which can usually be identified as stenotic.

FIGURE 17-6   Tracings from a 28-year-old woman with tricuspid infective endocarditis (heroin abuse). *a.* The transducer beam traverses the right ventricle (RV), imaging the tricuspid valve (TV), upper arrow, which is thickened by vegetations (veg), lower arrow. *b.* Simultaneous electrocardiogram, phonocardiogram, and echocardiogram with superimposed jugular venous pulse. The phonocardiogram shows the typical early systolic murmur (SM) of low-pressure tricuspid regurgitation. The right ventricular (RV) internal dimensions are increased, and there is paradoxical motion of the ventricular septum (arrow) reflecting right ventricular volume overload. The jugular venous pulse shows an (A) wave with obliterated *x* descent, a dominant *v* wave (V) with brisk *y* descent (Y), and the carotid pulse (C).

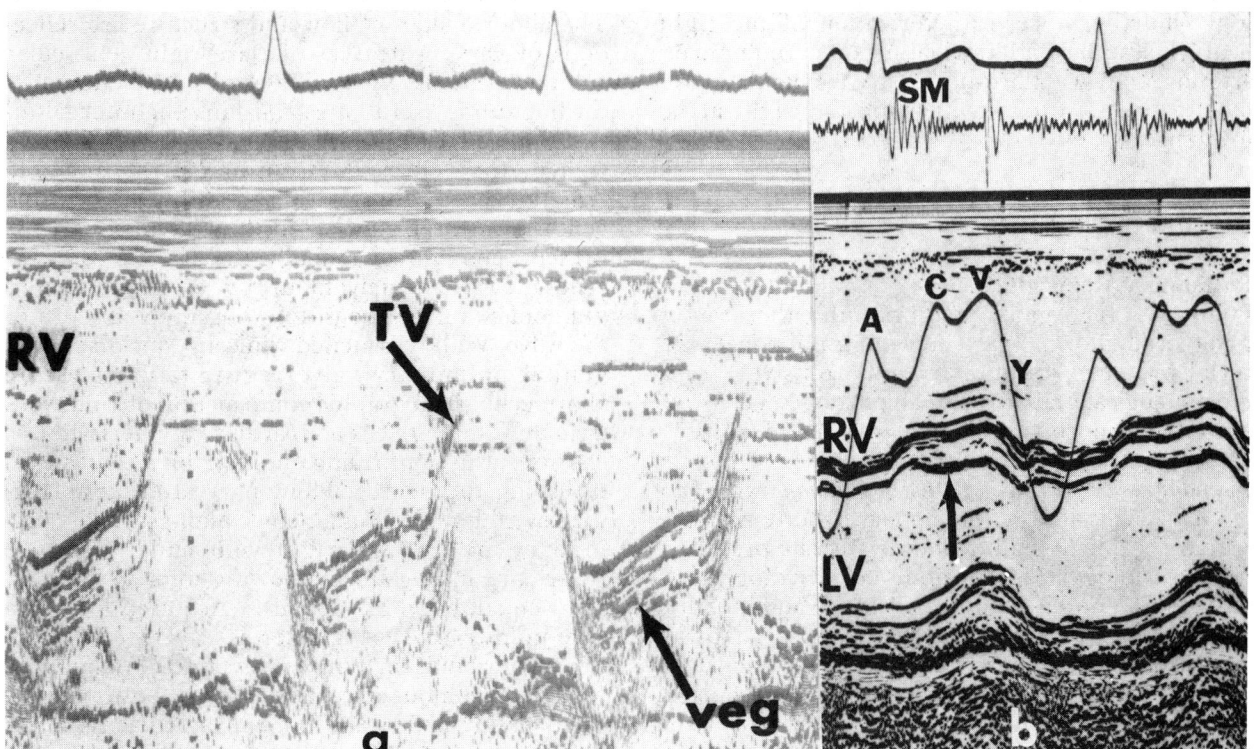

Fortuitous identification of tricuspid stenosis sometimes occurs when M-mode echocardiograms are recorded in patients with rheumatic mitral stenosis. Two-dimensional imaging is of further value in confirming that the tricuspid valve is stenotic and that right atrial size is increased. Cardiac catheterization provides the most refined means of quantifying the degree of tricuspid stenosis. Simultaneous high-sensitivity pressures should be recorded on both sides of the tricuspid valve in the control state, during active respiration, and, if nondiagnostic, during exercise. Tricuspid valve gradients, even in the presence of significant obstruction, are relatively small compared with gradients across a stenotic mitral valve.

Right Atrial Tumor Evidence of tricuspid obstruction in the *absence* of mitral stenosis arouses suspicion of right atrial myxoma.[32] The tumor commonly causes not only obstruction but incompetence of the tricuspid valve (traumatic impact). The M-mode echocardiogram does not image the right atrium, but sometimes records the mobile tumor as it seats in diastole within the tricuspid leaflets. The two-dimensional echocardiogram, however, can be dramatic and diagnostic, identifying the mobile mass within the right atrium in systole and within the tricuspid orifice in diastole. Angiocardiography is not required to confirm the observations of two-dimensional echocardiography, but it should be underscored that myxoma of either right or left atrium can be associated with *biatrial* myxoma. Accordingly, both M-mode and two-dimensional echocardiograms should be recorded and interpreted accordingly. Furthermore, catheterization of the right heart in search of a left atrial myxoma (pulmonary arteriography with levo-phase) may be handicapped by the presence of an unsuspected right atrial myxoma.

The Pulmonic Valve

Pulmonary Regurgitation

Pulmonary regurgitation occurs with either a morphologically normal valve and high pulmonary arterial pressure (pulmonary hypertensive)[37] or a morphologically abnormal valve (congenital or acquired) and normal pulmonary arterial pressure.[1]

Pulmonary Regurgitation Due to Pulmonary Hypertension The causes of pulmonary hypertension are legion,[33,37] but I shall deal only with its presence, not its etiology. The M-mode echocardiogram is useful in identifying the flat EF slope and absent *a* wave in the pulmonary valve tracing, perhaps an increase in right ventricular internal dimensions (regurgitant flow in addition to afterload), abnormal ventricular septal motion (volume overload of the right ventricle), and the fine flutter which is sometimes present on the tricuspid valve.[38] It should be

borne in mind that an increase in right ventricular internal dimensions and abnormal septal motion may be due to right ventricular volume overload of coexisting tricuspid regurgitation. The two-dimensional image adds little to the diagnosis of pulmonary hypertension per se, but can record in the short-axis view the right ventricular outflow tract and pulmonary trunk, which are likely to be enlarged. Cardiac catheterization remains the best method for quantifying the degree of pulmonary hypertension and of determining pulmonary vascular resistance. In the setting of pulmonary hypertensive mitral stenosis, a high-frequency left parasternal early diastolic murmur is more likely to be aortic rather than pulmonary regurgitation (Graham Steell). Thoracic aortography may document incompetence of the aortic valve, leaving the diagnosis of coexisting pulmonary regurgitation in doubt. Pulmonary arteriography is risky and ill-advised in the presence of high pulmonary vascular resistance.

Low-Pressure Pulmonary Regurgitation Low-pressure pulmonary regurgitation, congenital or acquired, stands in contrast to the hypertensive pulmonary regurgitation dealt with above.[1] In congenital pulmonary regurgitation, the morphologic abnormalities of the valve range from mild derangement to virtual or complete absence of valvular tissue, and the degree of pulmonary incompetence varies accordingly. The accompanying murmur is a soft, medium-frequency, middiastolic murmur as opposed to the typical Graham Steell murmur of pulmonary hypertensive regurgitation. The abnormalities of flow and structure are reflections of varying degrees of pure right ventricular volume overload. Accordingly, the M-mode echocardiogram is useful in establishing the internal dimensions of the right ventricle and paradoxic motion of the ventricular septum. If the M-mode tracing records well-defined pulmonary valve echoes, it can be concluded that valvular tissue is present, i.e., not congenitally absent. The converse is not the case; namely, failure to record satisfactory pulmonary valve echoes does not imply absence of the valve. With heightened clinical suspicion of congenital pulmonary valve regurgitation and the above echocardiographic confirmation of right ventricular volume overload, cardiac catheterization is less useful in confirming the diagnosis than in establishing the degree. Pulmonary arteriography is the key, although simultaneous, high-sensitivity pulmonary arterial and right ventricular pressure pulses are important in showing mid- to late diastolic equalization of pressures. Acquired low-pressure pulmonary regurgitation is a feature of infective endocarditis on a previously normal pulmonary valve (intravenous drug abuse) or of postoperative valvular pulmonic stenosis or intracardiac repair of Fallot's tetralogy.[39] In the presence of infective endocarditis, the first diagnostic step lies in the infectious disease laboratory—multiple blood cultures—and in plain film roentgenography—septic pulmonary emboli. The echocardiogram, in addition to identifying features of right ventricular volume overload, occasionally images the pulmonic valve and its vegetations. Two-dimensional echocardiography is of particular value in this regard, sometimes dramatically recording pulmonary valve vegetations.

Obstruction to Right Ventricular Outflow

Obstruction to right ventricular outflow can be acquired or congenital and supravalvular, valvular, or subvalvular, but for the purpose of this discussion, let us focus on congenital valvular pulmonic stenosis.

Congenital Valvular Pulmonic Stenosis The clinical diagnosis can be established with high probability, and quantification relatively accurately assessed.[1] The chief role of the laboratory is the more refined appraisal of severity rather than establishment of a morphologic diagnosis. The M-mode echocardiogram is a useful first step, even though the information may be imprecise. There is a relationship between the degree of pulmonic stenosis, the force of right atrial contraction, and the depth of the *a* wave in the pulmonary valve M-mode image (Fig. 17-7).[40] There is also a relationship between severity and right ventricular free wall and ventricular septal thicknesses. Occasionally the septum is thicker than the posterior left ventricle (disproportionate septal thickness). The two-dimensional echocardiogram records in the short axis the dilated pulmonary trunk and the mobile domed pulmonic valve, but

this merely confirms a relatively secure clinical impression and does not provide information on severity. Cardiac catheterization offers both morphologic information and quantification of severity. However, in patients with a clear clinical diagnosis of *mild* valvular pulmonic stenosis, cardiac catheterization is best deferred, since surgical intervention is not a consideration. The catheterization laboratory serves its most useful purpose in establishing a degree of obstruction sufficient to require pulmonary valvotomy. Since this operation is safe and extracardiac (via an incision in the pulmonary trunk), it is readily applied. Mild postoperative pulmonary regurgitation is a small price to pay for complete relief of obstruction.[39] On the other hand, secondary hypertrophic subpulmonic stenosis is an undesirable concomitant of severe valvular obstruction and may require resection via a right ventriculotomy. Cardiac catheterization and angiography provide information on the presence and degree of hypertrophic subpulmonic stenosis as well as on the degree of obstruction (gradient at rest and with exercise), the presence of isolated valvular pulmonic stenosis, and valve mobility and thickness.

The distinction between mild valvular pulmonic stenosis on the one hand and an innocent or normal pulmonic midsystolic murmur or idiopathic dilatation of the pulmonary trunk on the other sometimes arises. Loss of thoracic kyphosis (straight thoracic spine) is commonly accompanied by a prominent or relatively prominent midsystolic murmur in the second left interspace, so the patient's thoracic configuration should be taken into account.[41] It has been argued that cardiac catheterization is desirable in establishing the presence of mild valvular pulmonic

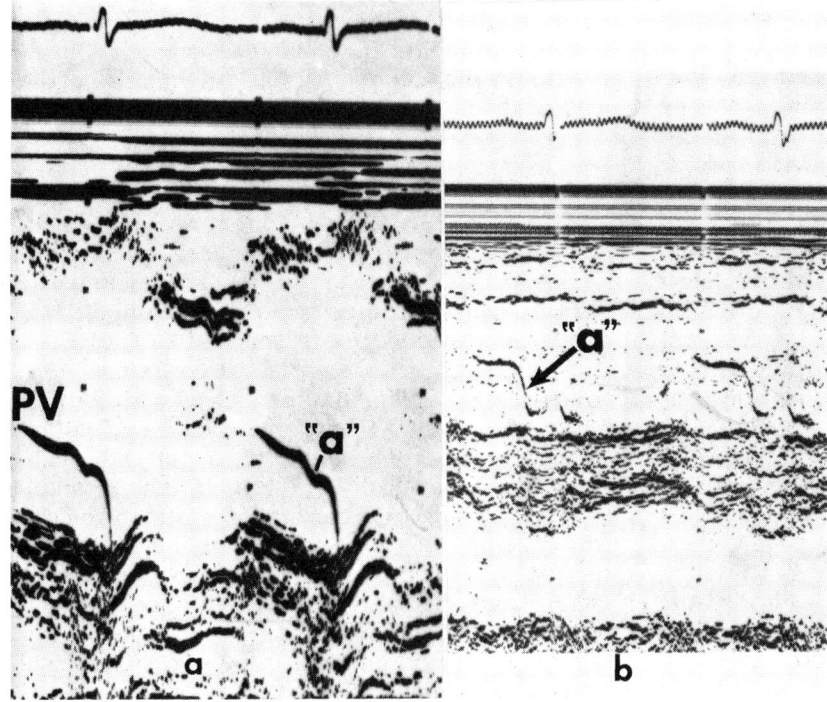

FIGURE 17-7 *a.* M-mode echocardiogram of the pulmonary valve (PV) in a patient with mild congential valvular pulmonic stenosis. The *a* dip is only slightly increased. *b.* M-mode echocardiogram from a patient with severe congenital valvular pulmonic stenosis. The *a* dip is markedly increased as powerful right atrial contraction delivers its force in presystole to the undersurface of the pulmonic valve.

stenosis which is susceptible to infective endocarditis, even though the lesion is functionally benign. As a rule, however, meticulous clinical assessment together with M-mode and two-dimensional echocardiograms make cardiac catheterization unnecessary. The two-dimensional echocardiogram is of special value, since pulmonary trunk dimensions can be measured and pulmonic valve motion recorded.

Nonvalvular Congenital Heart Disease with Expected Adult Survival

Ostium Secundum Atrial Septal Defect

This anomaly, in its uncomplicated state, is readily amenable to clinical diagnosis, especially in children and young adults.[1] However, the diagnostic laboratories provide confirmation and quantification. The first procedure to turn to is the M-mode echocardiogram that confirms the presence of right ventricular volume overload—increased right ventricular internal dimensions and paradoxic motion of the ventricular septum.[5] In addition to a relatively easily imaged tricuspid valve with increased mobility and occasionally fine diastolic vibrations, the mitral valve echogram is important because of the incidence of mitral valve prolapse[23] and because of the occasional presence of mitral stenosis (Lutembacher's syndrome).[1] The two-dimensional echocardiogram is of additional value,[7] since high-resolution images are capable of identifying the presence and location of the anatomic defect in the atrial septum, can often identify one or more normally draining pulmonary veins (eliminating the diagnosis of total anomalous pulmonary venous connection), can confirm the increased internal dimensions of the right ventricle, and can clarify further the abnormal motion of the ventricular septum in response to right ventricular volume overload. The M-mode image of the pulmonary valve sheds light on the absence of pulmonary hypertension, although specificity is not high. Is there need for cardiac catheterization and angiography? Given secure clinical and echocardiographic evidence of an uncomplicated, nonpulmonary hypertensive, low-resistance, high-flow ostium secundum atrial septal defect with normal mitral valve echoes, and given firm identification of one or more pulmonary veins connecting normally to the left atrium, what further data *can* the catheterization laboratory provide prior to surgical intervention? Many would argue that little or no additional information would be forthcoming and cardiac catheterization and angiography are not necessary. If the right superior pulmonary vein connects anomalously to the superior cava, an experienced surgeon can readily identify this variation as soon as the chest is opened, and it makes little difference during surgical repair whether right pulmonary veins connect within the atria on the right atrial side of the septal rim. Although uncompli-

cated ostium secundum atrial septal defects in the young are easily diagnosed, the same defects can be surprisingly difficult to recognize in some adults.[1,42] For example, mitral stenosis with pulmonary hypertension may be considered because of dyspnea, orthopnea, atrial fibrillation, an increased v wave in the jugular venous pulse, a right ventricular impulse, a loud first heart sound, a delayed pulmonary closure sound that is mistaken for an opening snap, a tricuspid flow murmur mistaken for a mitral diastolic murmur, vascular peripheral lung fields believed to represent pulmonary venous congestion, and a cardiac silhouette that exhibits dilatation of the pulmonary trunk and occasionally of both right and left atria. Similarly, mitral regurgitation may seem to be the diagnosis because the holosystolic murmur of tricuspid regurgitation is heard prominently at the apex which is occupied by the right ventricle. A delayed pulmonic component of the second sound followed by a tricuspid flow murmur can be mistaken for the opening snap and middiastolic murmur of coexisting mitral stenosis. At other times, wide splitting of the second heart sound is recognized as such, but incorrectly ascribed to early aortic valve closure associated with mitral regurgitation. The tricuspid flow murmur may be incorrectly attributed to rapid flow across the mitral valve. M-mode and two-dimensional echocardiograms provide the first major clues that one is dealing with an ostium secundum atrial septal defect presenting with the above ambiguities. The stage is then set for cardiac catheterization and angiography, which should be performed in anticipation of surgery. Older subjects with ostium secundum atrial septal defects and pulmonary hypertension can be safely and beneficially operated on, especially if the left-to-right shunt is in excess of 2:1. In such patients, cardiac catheterization is necessary not merely to establish the anatomic diagnosis, but to determine pulmonary vascular resistance and the magnitude of the left-to-right shunt.

Coarctation of the Aorta

The diagnosis of coarctation of the aorta in the adult can almost always be based securely on physical signs and chest x-rays, even though the latter may display surprisingly little or no rib notching despite auscultatory evidence of the murmurs of collateral circulation (Fig. 17-8A).[1,42] Further information from the diagnostic laboratories is not only desirable but often obligatory. The presence of a coexisting bicuspid aortic valve should be sought with deliberate intent, especially in the male. The M-mode echocardiogram, by recording an aortic valve echo with eccentric diastolic closure line, helps confirm that the valve is bicuspid (Fig. 17-1A).[4] Failure to identify an eccentric diastolic closure line does not, however, assure that the valve is tricuspid. In this regard, short-axis imaging using two-dimensional echocardiography can shed further light on the

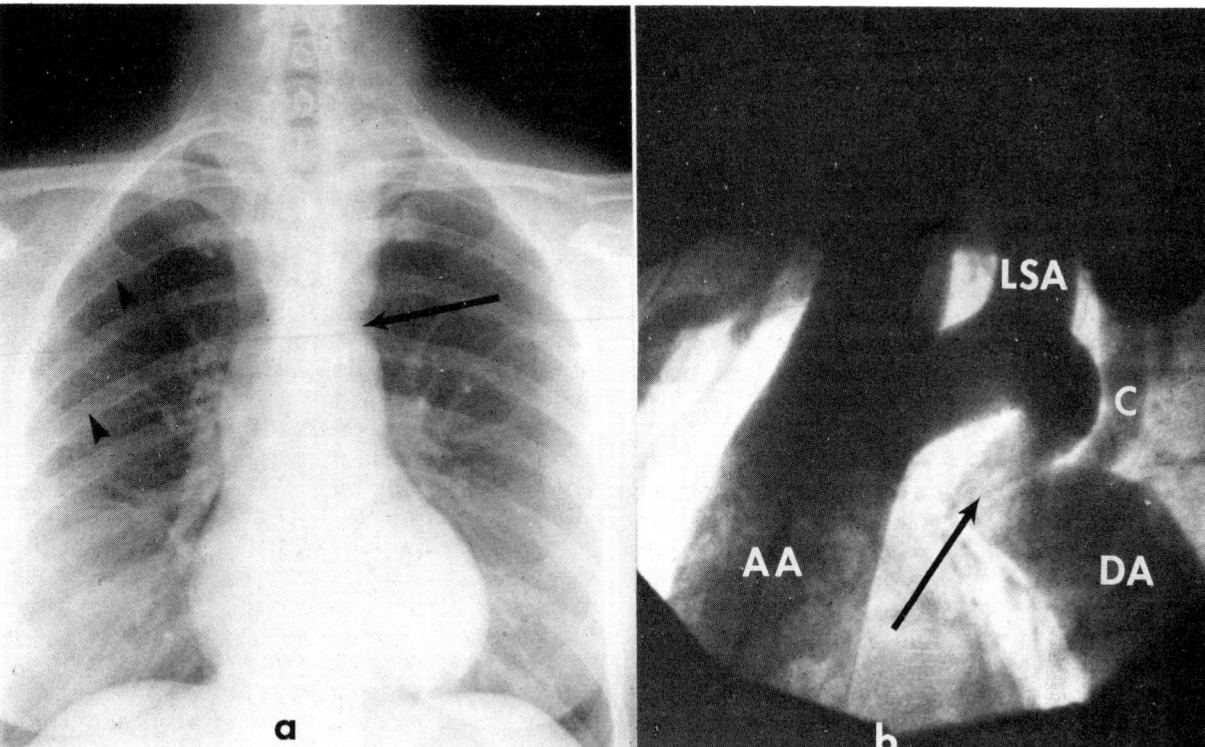

FIGURE 17-8   Thoracic aortogram and x-ray from a 48-year-old woman with coarctation of the aorta. *a.* The arrowheads point to the two areas of rib notching. The arrow on the right points to the zone of coarctation, above which is the convex dilated left subclavian artery, and below which is postcoarctation dilatation of the descending thoracic aorta. The aortic root is dilated. *b.* Contrast material was injected into the ascending arota (AA), visualizing the coarctation (arrow) and a large collateral artery (C) in close proximity. LSA = left subclavian artery; DA = descending aorta. A large internal mammary artery is seen in the upper left corner of the figure.

presence of two or three aortic cusps.[7] Cardiac catheterization is important chiefly for the morphologic details on aortography (Fig. 17-8*B*). A simple end-to-end aortic anastomosis is not always possible in the adult with coarctation, especially older patients in whom large collaterals may be dangerously close to the coarctation (Fig. 17-8*B*), and in whom saccular aneurysms are sometimes found in the poststenotic portion of the descending thoracic aorta. In any event, thoracotomy should not be undertaken in adults with aortic coarctation without careful definition of the collateral circulation in the vicinity of the coarctation and morphologic characterization of the aorta above and below the zone of constriction. It goes without saying that angiographic identification of tubular narrowing as opposed to discrete coarctation is also of major importance to the surgeon.

Patent Ductus Arteriosus

Surprisingly, the presence of a patent ductus arteriosus is sometimes overlooked until adulthood.[1,42] In the small, nonpulmonary hypertensive ductus, diagnosis depends upon detection of the characteristic continuous murmur, which is difficult to distinguish from the murmur of coronary arteriovenous fistula to the pulmonary trunk (Fig. 17-9).[1] Careful two-dimensional echocardiography in the short axis

sometimes identifies the patent ductus as it joins the pulmonary trunk. Given this security, cardiac catheterization is not obligatory. Even patients with large patent ductus and left-to-right shunts sometimes await diagnoses until adulthood, and must be distinguished from aorticopulmonary septal defects. Furthermore, calcification of the ductus complicates repair in an appreciable number of adults. Fluoroscopy should be applied meticulously in search of ductal calcification. The M-mode echocardiogram is useful in identifying left atrial dimensions and left ventricular size and function in the presence of volume overload via the ductus, and sheds light on the presence of pulmonary hypertension reflected in the pulmonary valve M-mode image.[38] Is there an associated aorticopulmonary septal defect? Is the ventricular septum intact? These important questions cannot always be answered securely without recourse to cardiac catheterization and angiography, which are properly applied before surgical intervention. On the other hand, the adult with patent ductus arteriosus, pulmonary hypertension, and suprasystemic pulmonary vascular resistance can be recognized by the differential cyanosis (cyanosed feet and acyanotic hands).[1] This simple physical sign not only makes the anatomic and physiologic diagnosis, but indicates inoperability, since suprasystemic pulmonary vascular resistance directs unoxygenated blood from the pulmonary trunk through

EXAMINATION OF THE HEART AND BLOOD VESSELS

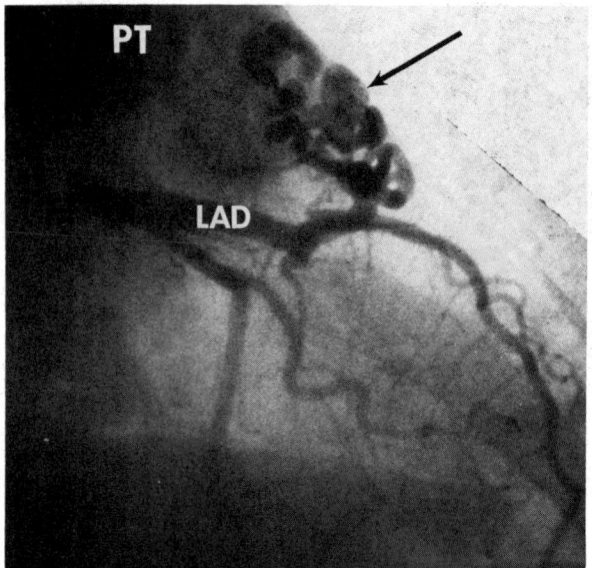

FIGURE 17-9 Selective left coronary arteriogram from a 63-year-old woman with a coronary arteriovenous fistula (arrow) arising from the left anterior descending (LAD) coronary artery and entering the pulmonary trunk (PT).

the ductus into the aorta distal to the left subclavian artery.

Coronary Arteriovenous Fistula

In this anomaly, both coronary arteries arise from the aorta, but a fistulous branch of one or more than one of these vessels communicates directly with a cardiac chamber or with the pulmonary trunk, coronary sinus, or vena cava (Fig. 17-9).[1] A continuous murmur is the hallmark of a coronary arterial fistula, and is distinguished from patent ductus by the site of maximal intensity and by the configuration. It is a good rule of thumb to consider the diagnosis whenever an asymptomatic acyanotic patient exhibits a precordial continuous murmur that does not peak around the second heart sound and that is maximal at an atypical site. The M-mode and two-dimensional echocardiograms are of little diagnostic value. Definitive diagnosis depends upon selective coronary arteriography which not only accurately identifies the vessel or vessels of origin but also the drainage site (Fig. 17-9).

Tetralogy of Fallot

In patients with nonrestrictive ventricular septal defects, the presence of obstruction to right ventricular outflow imposes no greater burden on the already systemic right ventricle, and may serve the useful purpose of regulating pulmonary blood flow so that volume overload of the left heart is avoided while adequate oxygenation prevails. The setting in which this combination usually occurs is tetralogy of Fallot, which remains the commonest cyanotic congenital cardiac anomaly in adults.[1] The clinical diag-

nosis can, as a rule, be made with a high degree of accuracy. Nevertheless, morphologic details require meticulous laboratory study. The first step is the M-mode echocardiogram. A careful sweep of the transducer beam identifies anatomic continuity between posterior aortic wall and anterior mitral leaflet while the anterior aortic wall is anterior to the ventricular septum (biventricular aorta) (Fig. 17-10).[43] The size of the aortic root can be measured; the larger the aortic root, the smaller the outflow tract of the right ventricle. Two-dimensional echocardiography not only confirms the posterior aortic wall–to–mitral valve continuity and the biventricular aorta, but also identifies the ventricular septal defect itself. Contrast echocardiography is useful but not obligatory. When saline solution is injected into an antecubital vein, both M-mode and two-dimensional echocardiography record early appearance of echoes in the aortic root as the right ventricle ejects directly into the biventricular aorta or via the ventricular septal defect into the aorta. Nevertheless, cardiac catheterization with high-quality ventriculography is obligatory before surgical intervention. Much depends upon the morphology of the right ventricular outflow tract from the entrance to the infundibulum through the pulmonic valve to the pulmonary trunk and its branches. In addition, it is important to know whether the subaortic ventricular septal defect identified in the two-dimensional echocardiogram is the *only* defect in the septum, which is usually but not invariably the case.

Situs Inversus

Complete situs inversus of both thoracic and abdominal viscera implies mirror-image dextrocardia. The vast majority of such individuals have no associated congenital cardiac or vascular disease, so that all that is required is simple recognition of the cardiac malposition.[1] This can always be securely accomplished by the physical signs, electrocardiogram, and posteroanterior chest x-ray (Fig. 17-11). No further diagnostic investigations are required, provided the heart is otherwise normal, which is usually the case.

Situs Solitus with Right Thoracic Heart

When the thoracic and abdominal viscera are in the normal or situs solitus position but the cardiac apex is on the right, congenital anomalies coexist, and as a rule, the types are predictable. The commonest associated anomalies are congenitally corrected transposition of the great arteries, pulmonic stenosis, and ventricular or atrial septal defects.[1] These lesions may occur singly or in combination. Although additional diagnostic investigation is seldom necessary to establish the cardiac malposition, assuming that the spleen is present and single, laboratory investigation is required to clarify the presence and degree of complicating anomalies, one or

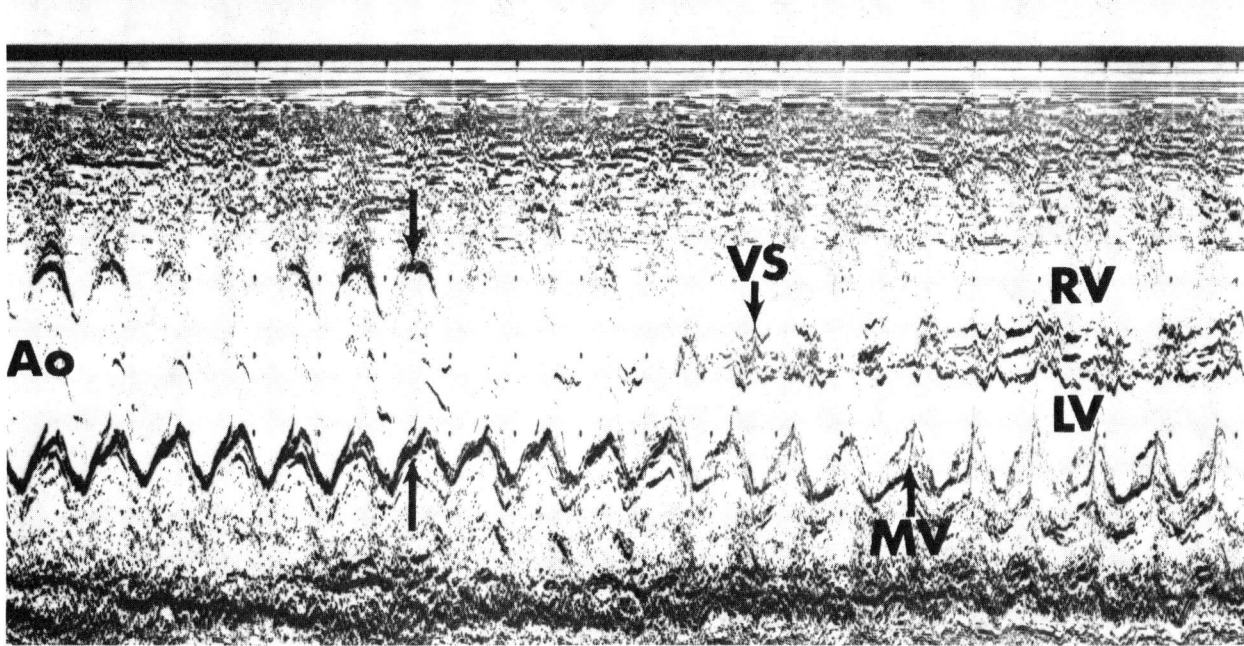

FIGURE 17-10   Typical tetralogy of Fallot with M-mode sweep from dilated aorta (Ao) through mitral valve (MV) and ventricular septum (VS). The anterior aortic wall (left upper arrow) is anterior to the plane of the ventricular septum (right upper arrow); the posterior aortic wall (left lower arrow) is in continuity with the anterior mitral leaflet (right lower arrow). Thus, the dilated aorta takes origin from both left (LV) and right ventricles (RV).

more of which are almost always present. It is worth emphasizing that situs solitus of the lungs and atria and the presence of a single spleen rest securely upon radiographic identification of an anatomic right bronchus and an anatomic left bronchus. A frontal chest x-ray, perhaps deliberately overpenetrated, may be all that is required to visualize the right bronchus (relatively wide and straight) and the morphologic left bronchus (narrower, "sway-backed," and running in a more horizontal course) (Fig. 17-12). The right atrium and the trilobed (right) lung are always concordant with the anatomic right bronchus, while the left atrium and bilobed (anatomic left) lung are always concordant with the anatomic left bronchus.[1] Clear visualization of separate right *and* left bronchi on chest x-ray eliminates the concern that asplenia or polysplenia complicates the cardiac malpositions. Bilateral right bronchi identify asplenia, while bilateral left bronchi identify polysplenia.[1] If doubt remains and the answer is important, two safe, painless, accurate diagnostic tests can resolve the problem. The first and simplest is a smear of peripheral blood to search for the Howell-Jolly bodies and Heinz bodies of asplenia. The second is scanning with an isotope taken up by the spleen and therefore capable of revealing the absence, presence, and type (single, multiple) of splenic tissue. In any case, there is an easy means of determining whether the heart is left or right thoracic: the hemidiaphragm is lower on the side of the

cardiac apex, not higher on the side of the liver as commonly taught.

Diagnostic investigation of the anomalies associated with situs solitus and a right thoracic heart begin with M-mode echocardiography. The technician should be told that the heart is in the right chest so the transducer can be placed and angled appropriately. Cardiac catheterization and angiocardiography are then required, depending upon the complexity of the coexisting anomaly or anomalies.

Congenitally Corrected Transposition of the Great Arteries

This is an anomaly characterized by the presence of a tricuspid valve and morphologic right ventricle in the left heart and a mitral valve and morphologic left ventricle in the right heart.[1] Despite right-to-left interchange of the ventricles and their atrioventricular valves, right atrial blood flows into the pulmonary trunk, albeit across a mitral valve and through an anatomic left ventricle, while left atrial blood flows into the aorta, albeit across a tricuspid valve and through an anatomic right ventricle. There is ventricular great artery discordance, i.e., "transposition," but the transposition is "corrected." Only a small portion of patients with congenitally corrected transposition have hearts that are devoid of coexisting defects. There is a high association with ventricular septal defect, abnormalities of the systemic

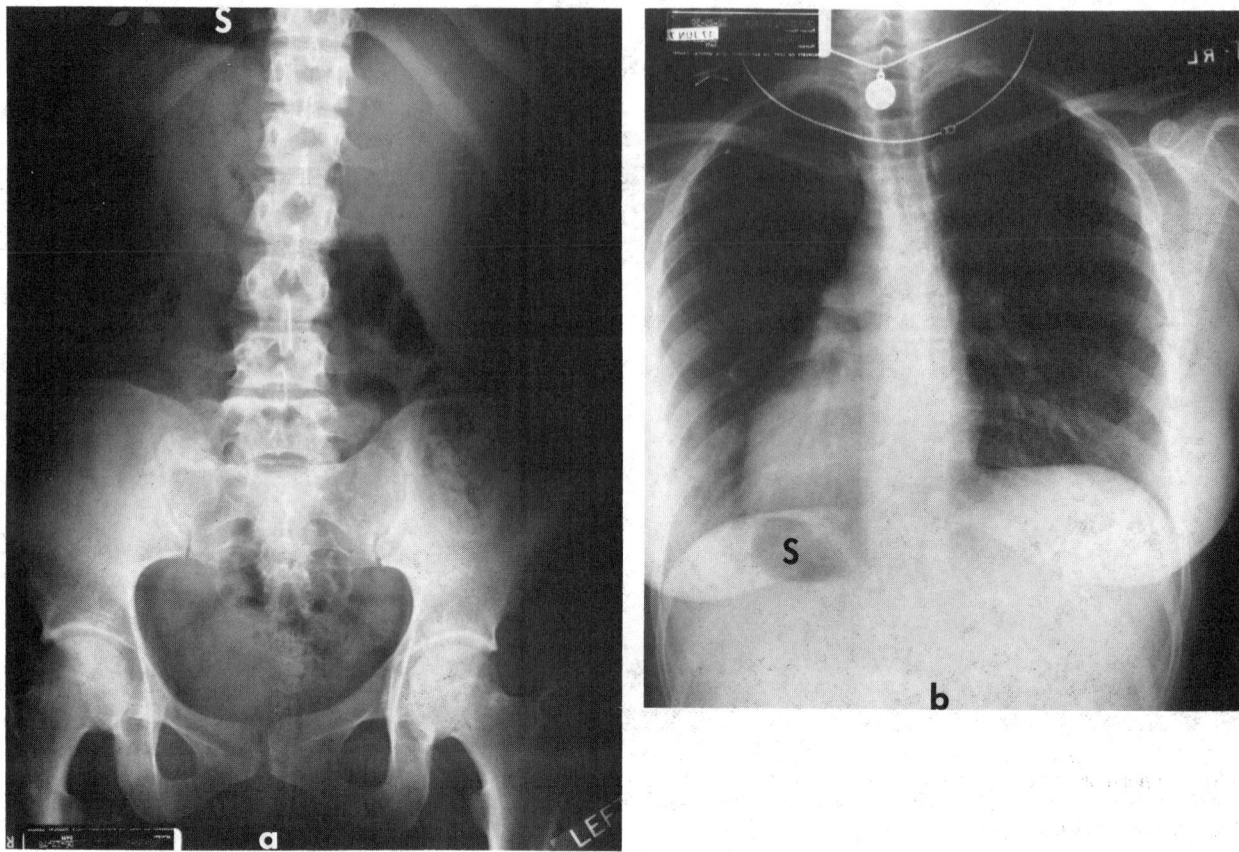

FIGURE 17-11   X-rays from a 32-year-old woman who presented with colicky *left* upper quadrant pain. *a.* The plain film of the abdomen shows the stomach (S) on the right. The liver and gallbladder were on the left, hence the left upper quadrant pain of acute cholecystitis. *b.* Chest x-ray showing typical situs inversus. The stomach (S) is on the right, the descending aorta is seen as a fine line to the right of the vertebral column, and the cardiac apex is on the right.

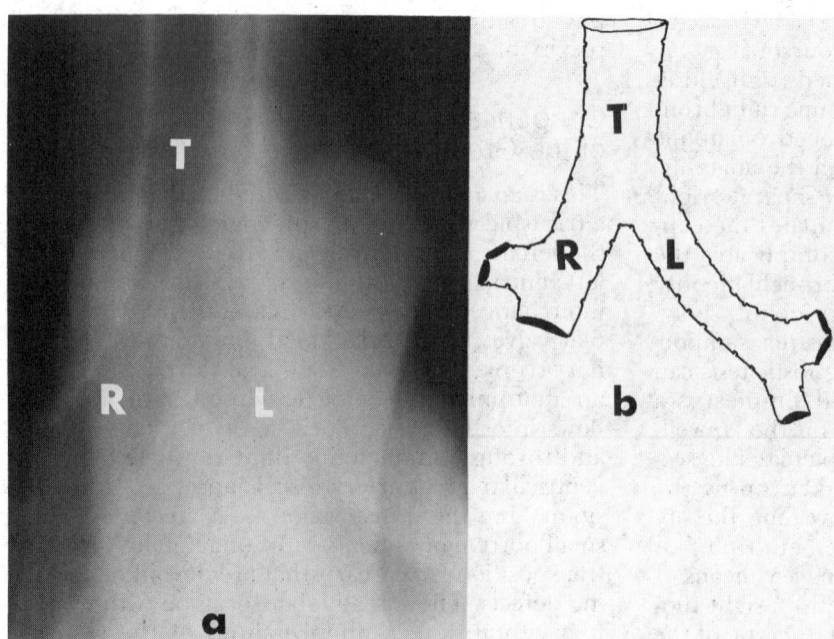

FIGURE 17-12   Posteroanterior chest x-ray (*a*) and (*b*) sketch of the trachea (T) and bronchi in situs solitus (normal position). The anatomic right bronchus (R) is relatively wide and straight; the anatomic left bronchus (L) is relatively narrow and "swaybacked," running in a more horizontal course.

atrioventricular (tricuspid) valve, obstruction to out-flow of the venous (morphologic left) ventricle, and prolonged atrioventricular conduction.[1] In adults, congenitally corrected transposition is often associated with incompetence of the left atrioventricular valve misdiagnosed as "mitral" regurgitation. Careful attention to the chest x-ray (Fig. 17-13) and the electrocardiogram arouses suspicion. The M-mode echocardiogram is useful in identifying the increased left atrial size in response to systemic AV valve incompetence but does not define the morphologic fault of the left atrioventricular valve. However, two-dimensional imaging can be conclusive, since the anatomic derangement that gives rise to left AV valve regurgitation is an Ebstein-like anomaly that is readily identified as recessed tricuspid leaflet tissue into the systemic ventricle (Fig. 17-4A). In fact the morphologic defect is better defined by two-dimensional echocardiography than by systemic ventriculography, which should be applied if quantification of severity of the valvular incompetence is in doubt.

The increased PR interval or prolonged atrioventricular conduction in congenitally corrected transposition can culminate in complete heart block. Occasionally such patients with no other coexisting

FIGURE 17-13 Chest x-ray from a 20-year-old woman with congenitally corrected transposition of the great arteries. The tricuspid valve resides in the systemic ventricle. Epstein's anomaly of that valve resulted in severe systemic atrioventricular valve regurgitation. The thoracic inlet is narrow because the aortic root rises vertically and is directly anterior to the pulmonary trunk. The peculiarly globular shape of the heart is due chiefly to a giant left atrium.

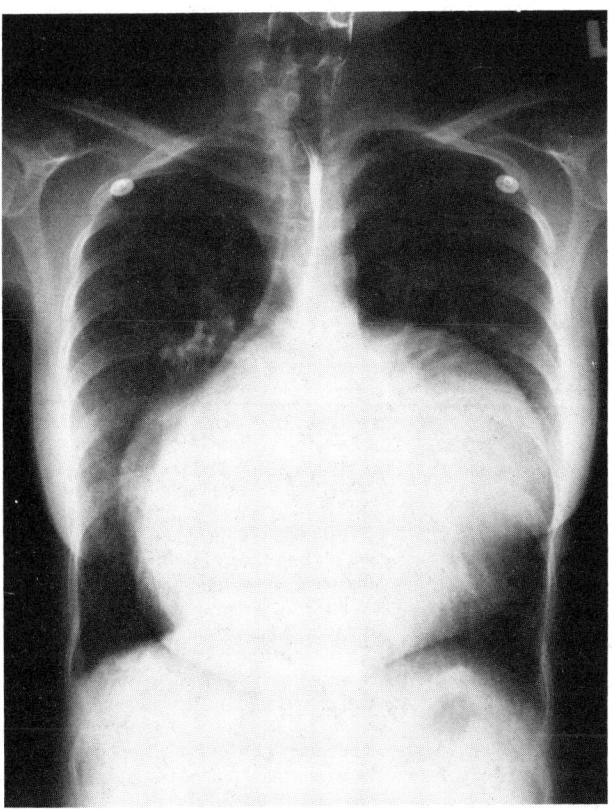

congenital cardiac anomaly present in adulthood with complete atrioventricular block misdiagnosed as "acquired" in the ordinary sense. Even though the QRS configuration is often normal, implying that the block is above the His bundle, the ventricular response may be sufficiently slow to warrant insertion of a right ventricular pacemaker. An important question arises. In patients believed to have isolated, uncomplicated, congenitally corrected transposition (without coexisting anomalies) with prolonged atrioventricular conduction, is the clinical diagnosis sufficiently secure, or is two-dimensional echocardiography or ventriculography required to define a morphologic left ventricle in the venous position and a morphologic right ventricle in the systemic location? A precise anatomic diagnosis is important for two reasons. First, the patient is selected out for more careful observation regarding the potential development of high-degree heart block. Second, an anatomic right ventricle in the systemic location may fail at a relatively early age on those grounds alone.[39] Accordingly, if the index of suspicion is high, and the two-dimensional echocardiogram inconclusive, cardiac catheterization with selective ventriculography is defensible, even in the absence of coexisting anomalies. Ventriculography can almost always establish the internal architecture (trabecular pattern) of anatomic left and right ventricles. In the occasional patient in whom the morphologic distinctions remain in doubt, selective coronary arteriography resolves the problem, since an anatomic right coronary is concordant with an anatomic right ventricle and vice versa. If invasive procedures are undertaken, it may be useful to add electrophysiological investigations to shed light on atrioventricular conduction and the refractory period of the AV node.

Perforated Aortic Sinus of Valsalva Aneurysm

The common form of congenital aortic sinus aneurysm originates from either the right or noncoronary sinus and perforates into the right ventricle or right atrium.[1] The physiological consequences attending these ruptures depend chiefly upon the amount of blood flowing through the abnormal communication, the rapidity with which the perforation develops, and the chamber that receives the shunt. An acute, large rupture is heralded by the dramatic onset of severe retrosternal or upper abdominal pain accompanied by marked dyspnea. At the other end of the spectrum, a small, gradual perforation may go unnoticed and present years later with a soft, continuous murmur at an atypical site. It is well to remember that ruptured sinus of Valsalva aneurysms occur predominantly in males, with a ratio of 4:1. The substantial majority of ruptures develop well after puberty, but before age 30 years. The clinical disorder therefore typically expresses itself in young adult males. The M-mode echocardiogram is useful principally in shedding light on the hemodynamic effects of perforation. Occasionally, the aneurysm can be identified by ultrasound, as it descends from right atrium into the tricuspid orifice in diastole, or if it protrudes into the right ventricular outflow tract.[1] The M-mode echocardiogram defines increased internal dimensions of right ventricle, left atrium, and left ventricle, but paradoxic motion of the ventricular septum is not present, since the left ventricle is also volume-overloaded. Two-dimensional echocardiography sheds light on the morphologic defect per se, identifying the aneurysm itself in the long-axis or short-axis view. Although these preliminary studies are desirable, the ultimate solution lies in cardiac catheterization and angiography. The shunt can then be localized and quantified, while thoracic aortography characterizes the morphologic defect with precision. The stage is then set for surgical intervention, which is generally obligatory for the acute severe perforation. In the rare patient with a small, insidious, asymptomatic perforation and an atypically located continuous murmur, two-dimensional echocardiography may lead the way by identifying the nipple-like protrusion from the aortic sinus into the right atrium or right ventricular outflow tract. Confirmation by thoracic aortography with quantification of the shunt then follows.

The Cardiomyopathies[44]

Three categories of cardiomyopathies will be considered: hypertrophic, dilated, and restrictive.[45] Hypertrophic cardiomyopathy, obstructive or nonobstructive, is a genetic disorder characterized by two anatomic hallmarks, namely, disproportionate ventricular septal thickness and septal cellular disarray.[46] Dilated cardiomyopathy is a pathophysiolog-

ical, not an etiologic, classification, indicating that the primary target site of disease is left ventricular myocardium which responds by dilatation without increase in septal/free wall thicknesses.[47] Right ventricular and atrial myocardium can be target sites, but not necessarily so. Restrictive cardiomyopathy is also a pathophysiological rather than an etiologic classification,[48] implying that left and right ventricular diastolic distensibility and systolic fiber shortening are restricted because of disease of ventricular myocardium.

Hypertrophic Cardiomyopathy

The clinical diagnosis of hypertrophic cardiomyopathy can be firmly established by noninvasive diagnostic means. The presence or absence—though not necessarily the degree—of obstruction to left ventricular outflow can also be determined.[46] The first step is the M-mode echocardiogram, which has been a major step forward in clinical recognition (Fig. 17-14). The M-mode transducer beam is well suited to provide information on three key features of the diagnosis, namely, the absolute increase in ventricular septal thickness with a septal/posterior wall ratio of 1.5:1 or more, hypokinetic or relatively hypokinetic septum that changes its thickness little if at all from diastole or systole probably because of isometric contraction caused by ventricular septal cellular disarray, and systolic anterior motion of the anterior mitral leaflet, implying a left ventricular/aortic systolic gradient. In addition, the M-mode echocardiogram provides accurate information on aortic valve motion (typical midsystolic preclosure), on posterior left ventricular wall endocardial velocity, and on left atrial size.[49] Posterior wall thickness should be meticulously measured just inferior to the mitral annulus. Given an appropriate clinical setting and an absolute increase in ventricular septal thick-

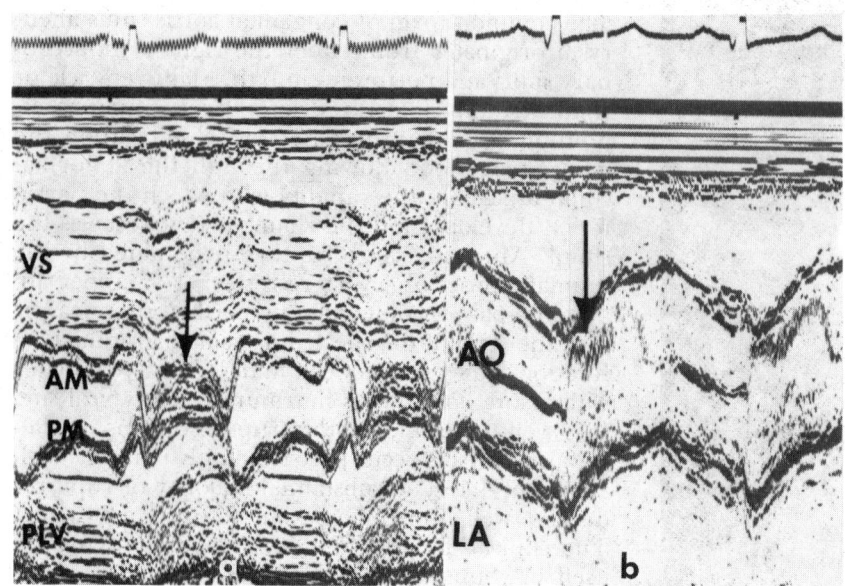

FIGURE 17-14 M-mode echocardiogram from a 9-year-old boy with typical hypertrophic obstructive cardiomyopathy. *a.* The ultrasonic beam is directed through the ventricular septum (VS), which is hypokinetic and dramatically thicker than the posterior left ventricular wall (PLV). The arrow points to systolic anterior motion of the anterior mitral leaflet, which touches the septum during most of systole. AM = anterior mitral leaflet in diastole; PM = posterior mitral leaflet in diastole. *b.* Arrow points to typical aortic valve preclosure accompanied by abnormal vibrations of the aortic leaflets. AO = aorta; LA = left atrium.

ness, a hypokinetic septum, and a septal/posterior wall ratio of 1.5 or more, the diagnosis of hypertrophic cardiomyopathy is relatively secure. Careful observations of the motion of the aortic valve (preclosure) and the anterior mitral leaflet provide information on the presence and approximate degree of obstruction to left ventricular outflow. For routine diagnostic and therapeutic purposes, no further information is needed, but we should not lose sight of other causes of disproportionate septal thickening such as right ventricular hypertension and tumor infiltration, especially metastatic.[50] If clinical suspicion of hypertrophic cardiomyopathy exists but the M-mode echocardiogram fails to identify disproportionate septal thickness when the transducer beam is directed through the base of the septum and through the infraatrial left ventricular free wall, additional information on disproportionate septal thickness is then required. The diagnostic thickening is not always present at the base of the septum, but may be confined to the midportion or apex.[51] The M-mode echocardiogram is useful in sweeping the entire septum, but two-dimensional imaging both in the long and short axes with sweeps from apex to base permits more accurate characterization of septal morphology. If the diagnosis needs further clarification, the next step is a technetium 99m gated blood pool scan. Technetium scans in lateral and left oblique projections dramatically

show in real time (motion) the dynamic contraction of the left ventricular free wall with cavity obliteration, and in the diastolic frames, nicely outlines the ventricular septum (Fig. 17-15A). Thus, in a complex disorder, most if not all necessary information can be secured safely, simply, accurately, and relatively inexpensively by noninvasive means. Noninvasive information on coexisting right ventricular outflow obstruction is, however, imprecise. Furthermore, in symptomatic patients inadequately responsive to propranolol or verapamil, selection for surgical intervention requires the presence of a significant left ventricular/aortic systolic gradient, which is not always securely defined on M-mode and two-dimensional echocardiography. Nor does echocardiography accurately characterize the degree of mitral regurgitation, but instead indirectly implies that an increase in left atrial size may in part be due to regurgitant flow rather than resistance to left atrial contraction (reduced left ventricular compliance). Accordingly, in patients who are potential candidates for operation, catheterization of the right and the left sides of he heart should be done together with left ventriculography. By these means, the presence and degree of right and left ventricular outflow obstruction can be defined, precise determinations of the response to pharmacologic and physical interventions can be measured, and mitral regurgitation can be identified and quantified.

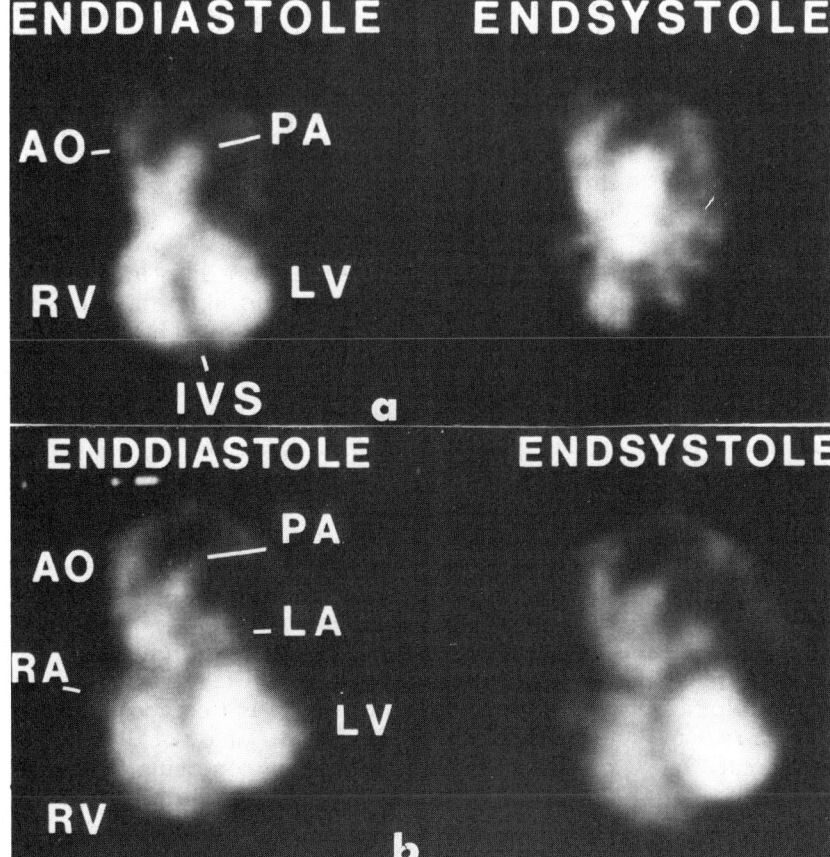

FIGURE 17-15 *a.* Technetium 99m multiple gated acquisition scans from a patient with hypertrophic obstructive cardiomyopathy (left anterior oblique position). The end-systolic frame shows virtual obliteration of the left ventricular (LV) cavity. RV = right ventricle; IVS = interventricular septum; AO = aorta; PA = main pulmonary artery. *b.* Similar study from a patient with chronic dilated cardiomyopathy. From end-diastole to end-systole, there is virtually no change in the dimensions of the dilated hypokinetic left ventricle (LV) and little change in right ventricle (RV). RA = right atrium; LA = left atrium. (*Courtesy of Dr. Gerald Wisenberg, Division of Nuclear Medicine, Center for the Health Sciences, UCLA.*)

Dilated Cardiomyopathy

Dilated cardiomyopathy can be acute, subacute, or chronic and inflammatory or noninflammatory.[47]

Myocarditis

Let us take as a point of departure acute, inflammatory cardiomyopathy (myocarditis) that is believed to be infectious. Virtually all categories of infectious agents have been implicated in inflammatory cardiomyopathy, but for practical clinical purposes in Western Europe and the United States the prevailing causes by far are the enteroviruses (Coxsackie virus A and B, echoviruses and polio viruses).[52–54] Vaccine has dramatically decreased the incidence of polio, and echovirus myocarditis, even types 9, 11, and 22, are now relatively uncommon. Accordingly, the high-order associations for acute infectious (inflammatory) cardiomyopathies in the human host are Coxsackie group A types 4 and 16, and Coxsackie group B types 1 through 5.[54] Thus, despite a wide range of possible infectious etiologies, the practical clinical concerns center on a few enteroviruses, Coxsackie group A and B. The group B Coxsackie is myonecrotic and therefore puts the patient at high risk. The group A is largely interstitial, causing little or no myofiber injury. Initial laboratory studies focus on the erythrocyte sedimentation rate and serum enzymes released by necrotic myocardium [serum glutamic oxaloacetic transaminase (SGOT), lactic acid dehydrogenase (LDH), and creatine phosphokinase (CPK) and their isoenzymes]. If acute inflammatory cardiomyopathy is believed to be due to Coxsackie B, and the patient comes under care during the earliest phases of the disease, throat and stool cultures for virus should be accompanied by serum samples for type-specific antibodies.[54] The initial serum can then be used for comparison with subsequent antibody titers. Acute infectious inflammatory cardiomyopathy puts the patient at high risk on several counts, namely, mechanical failure of the dilated, inflamed left ventricle, electrical instability of that chamber, and systemic emboli from diseased left ventricular endocardium (endocardial clot). Patients are generally ill enough to require hospitalization, and an intensive care setting is appropriate, since surveillance with electrocardiographic monitoring may prove critical. At this stage, M-mode and two-dimensional echocardiography are desirable (their utility is set forth below).

After an initial tissue-invasive phase of acute infectious cardiomyopathy, the causative virus quits the heart,[53,54] and the disease, especially with Coxsackie B, enters a subacute phase of inflammation, which is believed to be autoimmunologic, though there is no firm proof of this. Ventricular electrical instability continues to be a threat, together with further dilatation and failure of the diseased left ventricle, and the risk of systemic emboli persists. If the patient comes under observation at this stage, throat and stool cultures will be negative, serum enzymes lower if not normal, and the erythrocyte sedimentation rate unpredictable. Type-specific antibody titers may still be useful but less so, especially if there is no basis for comparison with acute phase serum. Two important diagnostic steps are now desirable, namely, characterization of ventricular structure and function by echocardiography, and clarification of the presence, type, and degree of arrhythmias by 24-h electrocardiographic monitoring. The first and simplest step in studying the left ventricle in dilated cardiomyopathy in the subacute phase is the M-mode echocardiogram (Fig. 17-16). An increase in internal dimensions at end-diastole can be measured precisely. Septal/free wall thickness (normal or diminished) can be determined and ventricular function assessed (fractional shortening, ejection fraction, etc.).[20,55] Two-dimensional imaging sometimes provides important information on left ventricular endocardial clot, especially when high-resolution images are achieved in the long axis, permitting study of the left ventricular apex. The occasional salutary therapeutic response to steroids is predicated on the assumption that myocardial inflammation persists in the absence of the tissue-invasive virus, and that the inflammation is amenable to immunosuppression. There is tentative evidence that gallium 67 imaging is capable of detecting the active myocardial necrosis that accompanies subacute inflammation.[56] The diagnostic utility of endomyocardial biopsy should now be confronted. Endomyocardial biopsy specimens can be obtained with the Konno or the Olympus catheter via the right ventricle, or with a transthoracic Menghini needle inserted into the left ventricular wall.[57,58] The probability of achieving an etiologic diagnosis in infectious inflammatory cardiomyopathy is by and large confined to the early stages of myocardial tissue invasion by the virus. Once the organism quits the heart, fresh tissue provides, not surprisingly, a paucity of etiologic information; observations are then confined to light and electron microscopy, which are nonspecific.[57] The risk of endomyocardial biopsy in the acute phase of myonecrotic myocarditis is high, and the diagnostic yield in the subacute or chronic phase (see below) is negligible, quite apart from risk. Accordingly, myocardial biopsy is best assigned an investigative role, although in highly selected cases biopsy is believed to assist in monitoring the histologic response to immunosuppressive therapy.[58]

Chronic Dilated Cardiomyopathy

Chronic dilated cardiomyopathy is thought to represent the fibrotic end stage of preexisting acute and subacute infectious myocarditis (see above). Diagnostic information during this phase of the natural history centers on appraisal of ventricular function, potential left ventricular endocardial clot, and the persistent, though perhaps diminished, risk of electrical ventricular instability. The initial step, espe-

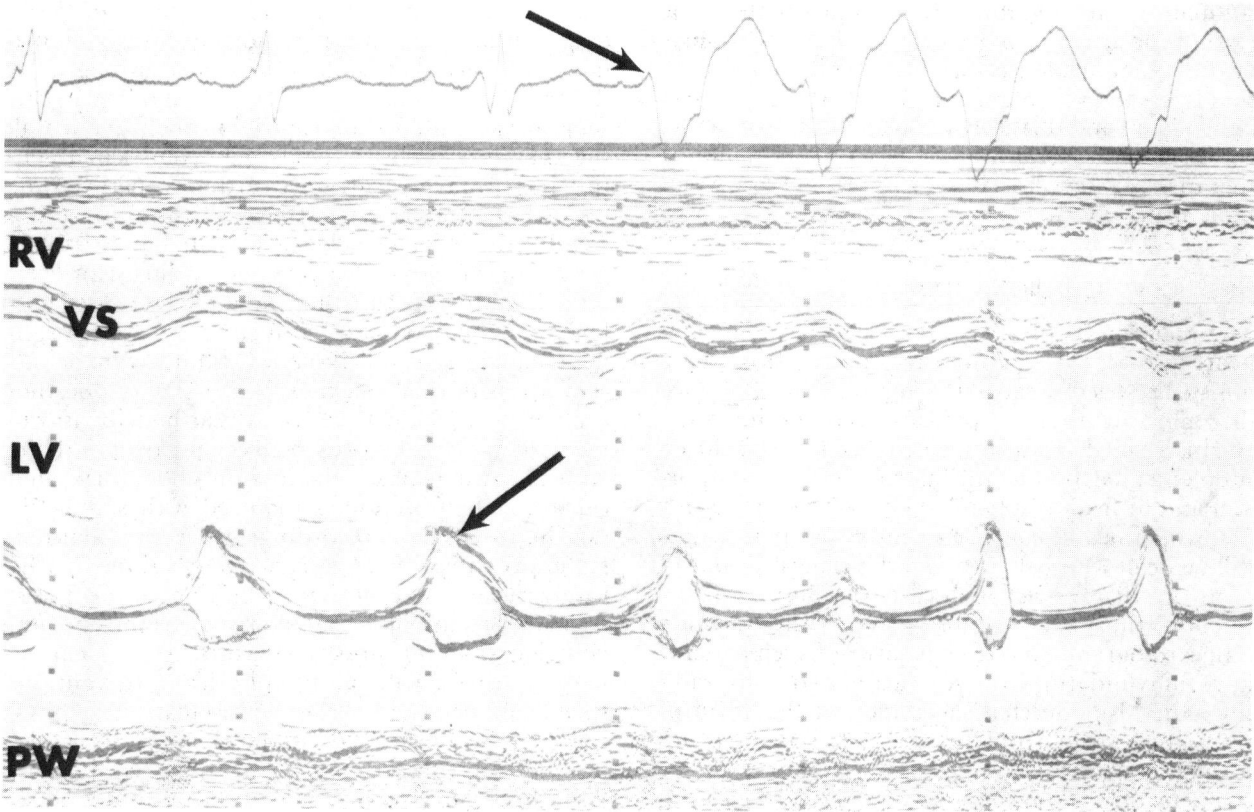

FIGURE 17-16 M-mode echocardiogram from a 20-year-old woman with chronic dilated cardiomyopathy. The ultrasonic beam traversed the right ventricle (RV), ventricular septum (VS), and left ventricle (LV). The mitral valve (lower arrow) is conspicuously displaced from both ventricular septum and posterior wall (PW), which is virtually akinetic. The marked increase in distance from anterior mitral leaflet (E point) to ventricular septum reflects a marked depression in left ventricular ejection fraction. The upper arrow identifies the beginning of ventricular tachycardia, a common complication of dilated cardiomyopathy, especially in the chronic, subacute phase.

cially if the patient comes under study for the first time at this stage, is the M-mode echocardiogram. The increase in left ventricular internal dimensions can be astonishing; septal/posterior wall motion and E point/septal separation (ejection fraction) can be dramatically abnormal (Fig. 17-16).[23a,59] The M-mode echocardiogram as a rule permits accurate pathophysiological characterization of the cardiomyopathy, but the proper etiologic designation becomes *idiopathic dilated cardiomyopathy*. In younger subjects, the distinction between this stage of idiopathic dilated cardiomyopathy and *dilated ischemic cardiomyopathy* is not pressing because of the high improbability of the latter. It should be pointed out, however, that chest pain from myocardial necrosis is common, especially during the acute myonecrotic phase of infectious inflammatory cardiomyopathy. In older subjects, the distinction from dilated ischemic cardiomyopathy is sometimes important.[59] Two-dimensional imaging provides information beyond the M-mode echocardiogram, shedding light on segmental abnormalities of wall motion. In older subjects carrying the clinical and M-mode echocardiographic diagnosis of dilated cardiomyopathy, two-dimensional imaging that reveals segmental abnormalities of left ventricular wall motion select that patient out as a more likely (but not a certain) prod-

uct of ischemic cardiomyopathy due to extramural coronary artery disease. It is chiefly in this setting that coronary arteriography may provide useful diagnostic information. Apart from establishing the presence of obstructive coronary artery disease in older subjects whose ventricular pathophysiology resembles chronic dilated cardiomyopathy, cardiac catheterization and left ventriculography provide little additional information. In subjects with chronic dilated cardiomyopathy, the M-mode and two-dimensional echocardiogram can be supplemented safely by technetium 99m radionuclide cineangiography, which not only refines the information on left ventricular function, but also provides information on right ventricular function and segmental septal/free wall ventricular motion (Fig. 16B).[20] The young patient with a dilated, diffusely hypokinetic left ventricle and no segmental wall abnormalities on two-dimensional imaging and radionuclide gated blood pool scans does not require invasive studies. The older individual with two-dimensional or radionuclide evidence of segmental wall disease is selected out as noted above, but with two important constraints in diagnostic strategy. First, a small portion of patients with ischemic (coronary) heart disease exhibit diffuse hypokinesis of the left ventricle and septum indistinguishable from idiopathic, chronic dilated cardiomyopathy. The second constraint is of greater practical importance. If the radionuclide (technetium 99m) ejection fraction is less than 25 percent in a patient with a markedly dilated and diffusely hypokinetic left ventricle, coronary arteriography becomes unimportant for therapeutic purposes, since bypass surgery provides little or no advantage.

Restrictive Cardiomyopathy

The majority of patients so afflicted have amyloid heart disease.[60,61] The first step in laboratory diagnosis of restrictive cardiomyopathy is the assurance that calcific constrictive pericarditis is not the cause. In this regard, plain films of the chest should be supplemented by careful fluoroscopy. The important and difficult distinction between restrictive cardiomyopathy and *noncalcific* constrictive pericarditis will be dealt with below. Given the clinical suspicion of myocardial restrictive disease without pericardial calcium, the next diagnostic step is the M-mode echocardiogram. Since the majority of such patients have amyloid (infiltrative) cardiomyopathy, and since the M-mode characterization of this form of restrictive cardiomyopathy is now well defined, information from this source is sensitive and relatively characteristic, though not specific. Nevertheless, in an appropriate clinical setting, a symmetric increase in septal/posterior left ventricular wall thicknesses, diffuse hypokinesis of septum and left ventricular free wall, and small to normal left ventricular internal dimensions at end-diastole in conjunction with an increase in right ventricular anterior wall thickness weigh strongly in favor of amyloid restrictive cardiomyopathy and weigh heavily against noncalcific constrictive pericarditis. Two-dimensional echocardiography is useful in dramatizing the structural and functional alterations in right and left ventricular myocardium and ventricular septum, and is therefore desirable though not obligatory. In view of the thickness of right ventricular wall and ventricular septum in amyloid cardiomyopathy,[61] the issue of tissue diagnosis by right ventricular endomyocardial biopsy arises.[57] Of the various types of cardiomyopathy, endomyocardial biopsy of the right ventricle is most likely to be diagnostically useful in restrictive cardiomyopathy due to amyloidosis.[57] Careful search for systematized amyloid often permits an extracardiac tissue diagnosis, which adds considerable weight to the echocardiographic findings described above. Similarly, additional insights on right and left ventricular structure and function provided by technetium 99m gated blood pool scans are interesting but not obligatory.

The distinction between noncalcific constrictive pericarditis and restrictive cardiomyopathy is difficult. The difference is critically important since surgical intervention is indicated in the former but not the latter. Let us assume that the patient under study has evidence of myocardial restrictive disease without systematized amyloid amenable to tissue diagnosis and has on x-ray and fluoroscopy no evidence of pericardial calcium. Is echocardiography definitively diagnostic? As a rule, M-mode echocardiographic evidence of right ventricular free wall thickness *and* a thick, hypokinetic ventricular septum heavily favors restrictive cardiomyopathy, while normal right ventricular free wall thickness and a septum of normal thickness and mobility strongly favor noncalcific constrictive pericarditis. However, a thick, fibrous pericardium potentially causes misleading echocardiographic measurements of right ventricular free wall thickness, and a ventricular septum of normal thickness and mobility does not categorically eliminate restrictive cardiomyopathy in favor of noncalcific constrictive pericarditis. If the clinical setting makes distinction obligatory, then cardiac catheterization is required with simultaneous, high-sensitivity recordings of biventricular diastolic pressures. Since restrictive cardiomyopathy rarely causes identical changes in right and left ventricular distensibility characteristics, right and left ventricular filling pressures will differ, or can be made to differ with simple physical interventions such as induced premature ventricular beats, physical exercise (isotonic or isometric), Valsalva's maneuver, etc. Conversely, since constrictive pericarditis almost invariably results in the *same* degree of restriction of right and left ventricles, the elevated biventricular filling pressures will be identical despite physical interventions.

Other Pericardial Diseases

Calcific Pericarditis

The presence of calcium in the pericardium generally but not invariably restricts ventricular diastolic distension and systolic motion. Careful clinical assessment usually establishes whether or not significant myocardial restriction exists. A first step in confirming restriction of ventricular wall motion is the M-mode echocardiogram, which nicely measures left ventricular posterior wall endocardial velocity and may provide information on right ventricular endocardial movement.[5] Two-dimensional imaging refines these observations, characterizing both the extent and the degree of restricted motion of right and left ventricular walls. If further information on ventricular wall movement and function is required, the next step is technetium 99m gated cardiac blood pool imaging. The technique shows details of right and left ventricular wall motion as well or perhaps better than two-dimensional echocardiography. It can be argued that the radiographic presence of an extensively calcified pericardium together with M-mode and two-dimensional echocardiographic and radionuclide evidence of restricted diastolic and systolic motion of both ventricles suffices in deciding on surgical intervention without the need for additional diagnostic studies. If any doubt on severity remains, however, cardiac catheterization provides secure information based especially on the classic intracardiac pressure pulses. An occasional patient with constrictive pericarditis, atrial fibrillation, and left atrial enlargement carries a mistaken diagnosis of mitral stenosis, but this error is readily prevented with simple echocardiography.

Pericardial Effusion

Let us deal with mild to marked *chronic* pericardial effusion on the one hand,[62] and sudden pericardial effusion with tamponade on the other.[63,64] M-mode echocardiography has been a major step forward in the safe, painless, accurate diagnosis of mild to marked pericardial effusion (Fig. 17-17).[5] When employing the M-mode echocardiogram, attention should focus on both posterior and anterior pericardium, as well as on distortions of motion of intracardiac structures that occur with large effusions. Two echocardiographic features indicate the presence of pericardial effusion, namely, the separation of visceral and parietal pericardium, i.e., a posterior or posterior and anterior echo-free space, and failure of the parietal pericardium to move with the ventricular wall, seen most clearly in the posterior wall echoes (Fig. 17-17). A posterior pericardial effusion is, as a rule, visualized only behind the left ventricle, disappearing as the ultrasonic beam scans upward to include the left atrium. Identification of pericardial fluid from M-mode echocardiographic data permits certain quantitative conclusions. The

FIGURE 17-17 M-mode echocardiogram in a patient with a large pericardial effusion. The ultrasonic beam traverses the right ventricle (RV), ventricular septum (VS), left ventricle (LV), and posterior wall (PW). The posterior pericardial effusion (PE) is represented by an echo-free space behind the posterior wall in both systole and diastole. In addition, there is an anterior pericardial effusion (arrow) represented by an anterior echo-free space.

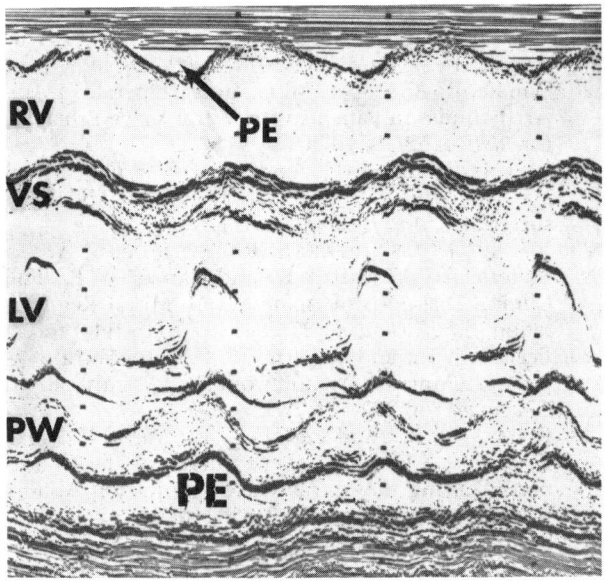

M-mode echocardiogram is sensitive in detecting remarkably small amounts of fluid, so at that end of the spectrum the transition from normal to abnormal is subtle. When the left ventricular posterior wall (epicardium) is never in contact with the parietal pericardium, the effusion is at least moderate. If these features coexist with clear evidence of an obvious anterior effusion, the probability of 500 to 1000 ml of fluid is substantial. A massive effusion permits the heart to "swing" within it, so that conclusions drawn from motion of septum, mitral leaflets, etc., must be deferred. Two-dimensional imaging provides a dramatic visual impact, but as a rule is not required for routine diagnostic purposes. The same holds for gated blood pool imaging.

The principal value of the echocardiogram in patients clinically suspected of cardiac tamponade is the identification of pericardial fluid, as noted above. Tamponade per se is not an echocardiographic diagnosis.[63,64] This is so despite the fact that tamponade can result in markedly diminished motion of anterior and posterior ventricular walls, a derangement amenable to M-mode echocardiographic analysis. In addition, in pericardial tamponade, the M-mode and two-dimensional echocardiograms sometimes identify a selective inspiratory increase in right ventricular internal dimensions with reciprocal decrease in left ventricular internal dimensions. In addition, in experimental cardiac tamponade, serial echocardiograms may show decreasing end-expiratory right and left ventricular internal dimensions and an increasing percentage change in right-to-left ventricular diameters with inspiration.[65] Nevertheless, the diagnosis of pericardial tamponade is secure only when significant M-mode echocardiographic pericardial effusion occurs in the presence of dyspnea, orthopnea, tachycardia, elevated systemic venous pressure, hepatomegaly, decreased systolic arterial pressure, narrow pulse pressure, pulsus paradoxus, normal to diminished heart sounds, etc. In this setting, further diagnostic information is not required before proceeding with removal of the pericardial fluid, be it effusion or blood. An additional diagnostic point is worth making. When large pericardial effusions or pericardial tamponade of unknown cause are treated by pericardial tap, it is wise after removal of most if not all the fluid to inject air and then secure an upright chest x-ray. This simple study sometimes permits identification of pericardial tumor seen in profile in the air-filled pericardial space. Such a procedure can be accomplished with no risk and little additional cost.

References

1. Perloff, J. K.: "The Clinical Recognition of Congenital Heart Disease," 2d ed., W. B. Saunders Company, Philadelphia, 1978, pp. 8, 81, 13, 57, 239, 228, 185, 277, 318, 126, 524, 576, 442, 19, 43, 590.

2. Roberts, W. C.: The Congenitally Bicuspid Aortic Valve: A Study of 85 Autopsy Patients, *Am. J. Cardiol.*, 26:72, 1970.

*3. Morganroth, J., Perloff, J. K., Zeldis, S., and Dunkman, W. B.: Acute Severe Aortic Regurgitation: Pathophysiology, Clinical Recognition and Management, *Ann. Intern. Med.*, 87:223, 1977. (34 references)

4. Nanda, N. C., Gramiak, R., Manning, J., Mahoney, E. B., Sipchick, E. C., and Deweese, J. A.: Echocardiographic Recognition of the Congenital Bicuspid Aortic Valve, *Circulation*, 49:870, 1974.

5. Feigenbaum, H.: "Echocardiography," 2d ed., Lea & Febiger, Philadelphia, 1976, pp. 143, 146, 183, 107, 447, 275, 440, 419.

6. Skorton, D., Child, J. S., and Perloff, J. K.: Accuracy of the Echocardiographic Diagnosis of Aortic Regurgitation, *Am. J. Med.*, 69:377, 1980.

7. Tajik, A. J., Seward, J. B., Hagler, D. J., Mair, D. D., and Lie, J. T.: Two-Dimensional Real-Time Ultrasonic Imaging of the Heart and Great Vessels, *Mayo Clin. Proc.*, 53:271, 1978.

*8. Bennett, D. H., Evans, D. W., and Raj, M. V. J.: Echocardiographic Left Ventricular Dimensions in Pressure and Volume Overload: Their Use in Assessing Aortic Stenosis, *Br. Heart J.*, 37:971, 1975. (32 references)

*9. Blackwood, R. A., Bloom, K. R., and Williams, C. M.: Aortic Stenosis in Children: Experience with Echocardiographic Prediction of Severity, *Circulation*, 57:263, 1978. (26 references)

10. Reichek, N., Devereux, R. B., Perloff, J. K., Klunder, P. J., and Wood, D. C.: Echocardiographic Assessment of Left Ventricular Outflow Obstruction, in M. N. Kotler and B. L. Segal (eds), "Clinical Echocardiography," F. A. Davis Company, Philadelphia, 1978, p. 85.

11. Kirkman, J., Hagen, A. D., DiSessa, T. G., Ti, C., Samtoy, L. M., Friedman, W. F., and Vieweg, W. V. R.: Selection Criteria for Echocardiographic Assessment of Left Ventricular Pressure and Peak Gradient in Patients with Valvular Aortic Stenosis, *Am. J. Cardiol.* 45:471, 1980. (Abstract.)

*12. Hagen, A. D., DiSessa, T. G., Samtoy, L., Friedman, W. F., and Vieweg, W. V. R.: Reliability of Echocardiography in Diagnosing and Quantifying Valvular Aortic Stenosis, *Cardiovasc. Med.*, 4:391, 1980. (33 references)

13. Holloran, K. H.: The Telemetered Exercise Electrocardiogram in Congenital Aortic Stenosis, *Pediatrics*, 47:31, 1971.

14. Patterson, J. A., Naughton, J., Pietras, R. J., and Gunnar, R. M.: Treadmill Exercise in Assessment of the Functional Capacity of Patients with Cardiac Disease, *Am. J. Cardiol.*, 30:757, 1972.

15. Roberts, W. C., Perloff, J. K., and Costantino, T.: Severe Valvular Aortic Stenosis in Patients over 65 Years of Age, *Am. J. Cardiol.*, 27:497, 1971.

16. Henry, W. C., Bonow, R. B., Rosing, D. R., and Epstein, S. E.: Observations on the Optimum Time for Operative Intervention for Aortic Regurgitation. II. Serial Echocardiographic Evaluation of Asymptomatic Patients, *Circulation*, 61:484, 1980.

17. Henry, W. L., Bonow, R. O., Borer, J. S., Ware, J.

H., Kent, K. M., Redwood, D. R., McIntosh, C. L., Morrow, A. G., and Ebstein, S. E.: Observations on the Optimum Time for Operative Intervention for Aortic Regurgitation. I. Evaluation of the Results of Aortic Valve Replacement in Symptomatic Patients, *Circulation*, 61:471, 1980.

18. Borer, J. S., Bacharach, S. L., Green, M. V., Kent, K. M., Henry, W. L., Rosing, D. R., Seides, S. F., Johnston, C. S., and Epstein, S. E.: Exercise-Induced Left Ventricular Dysfunction in Symptomatic and Asymptomatic Patients with Aortic Regurgitation: Assessment with Radionuclide Cineangiography, *Am. J. Cardiol.*, 42:351, 1978.

*19. Burow, R. D., Strauss, H. W., Singleton, R., Pond, M., Terry, R., Bailey, I. K., Griffith, L. C., Nickoloff, E., and Pitt, B.: Analysis of Left Ventricular Function from Multiple Gated Acquisition Cardiac Blood Pool Imaging, *Circulation*, 56:1024, 1977. (7 references)

*20. Shine, K. I., Perloff, J. K., Child, J. S., Marshall, R. C., and Schelbert, H.: Non-invasive Assessment of Myocardial Function, *Ann. Intern. Med.*, 92:78, 1980. (95 references)

21. Welch, G. H., Braunwald, E., and Sarnoff, S. J.: Hemodynamic Effects of Quantitatively Varied Experimental Aortic Regurgitation, *Circ. Res.*, 5:546, 1975.

22. Wilson, W. R., Danielson, G. K., Giuliani, E. R., Washington, J. A., Jaumin, P. M., and Geraci, J. E.: Cardiac Valve Replacement in Congestive Heart Failure Due to Infective Endocarditis, *Mayo Clin. Proc.*, 54:223, 1979.

23. Devereux, R. B., Perloff, J. K., Reichek, N., and Josephson, M. E.: Mitral Valve Prolapse, *Circulation*, 54:3, 1976.

23a. Child, J. S., Perloff, J. K., and Krivokapich, J.: Effect of Left Ventricular Size on Echocardiographic E Point to Ventricular Septal Separation, *Am. Heart J.*, in press.

*24. Abassi, A. S., Allen, M. W., DeCristofaro, D., and Ungar, I.: Detection and Estimation of Degree of Mitral Regurgitation by Range-Gated Pulsed Doppler Echocardiography, *Circulation*, 61:143, 1980. (11 references)

25. Gooch, A. S., Vicencio, F., Maranhao, V., and Goldberg, H.: Arrhythmias and Left Ventricular Asynergy in the Prolapsing Mitral Valve Leaflet Syndrome, *Am. J. Cardiol.*, 29:611, 1972.

26. Winkle, R. A., Lopez, M. G., and Fitzgerald, J. W.: Arrhythmias in Patients with Mitral Valve Prolapse, *Circulation*, 52:73, 1975.

27. Ross, J., Braunwald, E., and Morrow, A. G.: Clinical and Hemodynamic Observations in Pure Mitral Insufficiency, *Am. J. Cardiol.*, 2:11, 1958.

*28. Ronan, J. A., Steelman, R. B., DeLeon, A. C., Waters, T. J., Perloff, J. K., and Harvey, W. P.: The Clinical Diagnosis of Acute Severe Mitral Regurgitation, *Am. J. Cardiol.*, 27:284, 1971. (19 references)

29. Perloff, J. K., and Roberts, W. C.: The Mitral Apparatus: Functinal Anatomy of Mitral Regurgitation, *Circulation*, 46:227, 1972.

30. Roberts, W. C., and Perloff, J. K.: Mitral Valvular Disease. A Clinicopathologic Survey of the Conditions Causing the Mitral Valve to Function Abnormally, *Ann. Intern. Med.*, 77:939, 1972.

31. Swan, H. J. C., Ganz, W., Forrester, J. S., Marcus, H., Diamond, G., and Chonette, D.: Catheterization

*This article is a review of the literature and contains additional references to the literature.

of the Heart in Man with Use of a Flow-Directed Balloon Tipped Catheter, *N. Engl. J. Med.*, 283:447, 1970.

*32. Nasser, W. K., Davis, R. H., Dillon, J. C., Travel, M. E., Helmen, C. H., Feigenbaum, H., and Fisch, C.: Atrial Myxoma: I. Clinical and Pathologic Features in Nine Cases; II. Phonocardiographic, Echocardiographic, Hemodynamic and Angiographic Features in Nine Cases, *Am. Heart J.*, 83:694 and 810, 1972. (76 references)

*33. Perloff, J. K.: Auscultatory and Phonocardiographic Manifestations of Pulmonary Hypertension, *Prog. Cardiovasc. Dis.*, 9:303, 1967. (120 references)

34. Rios, J. C., Massumi, R. A., Breesman, W. T., and Sarin, R. K.: Auscultatory Features of Acute Tricuspid Regurgitation, *Am. J. Cardiol.*, 23:4, 1969.

35. Gallagher, J. J., Pritchett, E. L. C., Sealy, W. C., Kasell, J., and Wallace, A. G.: The Pre-excitation Syndromes, *Prog. Cardiovasc. Dis.*, 20:285, 1978.

*36. Perloff, J. K., and Harvey, W. P.: The Clinical Recognition of Tricuspid Stenosis, *Circulation*, 22:346, 1960. (50 references)

*37. Perloff, J. K., and Szidon, J. P.: Pulmonary Hypertension: Etiologies, Recognition, Consequences, in J. T. Willerson, and C. A. Sanders (eds.), "Clinical Cardiology," Grune & Stratton, Inc., New York, 1977, p. 419. (102 references)

38. Weyman, A. E., Dillon, J. C., Feigenbaum, H., and Chang, S.: Echocardiographic Patterns of Pulmonary Valve Motion with Pulmonary Hypertension, *Circulation*, 50:905, 1974.

39. Perloff, J. K.: Late Postoperative Concerns in Adults with Congenital Heart Disease, in M. A. Engle (ed.) "Pediatric Cardiovascular Disease," F. A. Davis Company, Philadelphia, 1981, p. 431.

40. Weyman, A. E., Dillon, J. C., Feigenbaum, H., and Chang, S.: Echocardiographic Patterns of Pulmonic Valve Motion in Pulmonic Stenosis, *Am. J. Cardiol.*, 34:644, 1974.

41. DeLeon, A. C., Perloff, J. K., Twigg, H., and Majd, M.: The Straight Back Syndrome: Clinical Cardiovascular Manifestations, *Circulation*, 32:193, 1965.

42. Perloff, J. K.: Overlooked Congenital Heart Disease in the Adult, *Cardiovasc. Med.*, 5:535, 548, 1980.

*43. Morris, D. C., Felner, J. M., Schlant, R. C., and Franch, R. H.: Echocardiographic Diagnosis of Tetralogy of Fallot, *Am. J. Cardiol.*, 36:908, 1975. (14 references)

44. Goodwin, J. F., and Oakley, C. M.: The Cardiomyopathies, *Br. Heart J.*, 34:545, 1972.

45. Goodwin, J. F.: Prospects and Predictions for the Cardiomyopathies, *Circulation*, 50:210, 1974.

*46. Maron, B. J., and Epstein, S. E.: Hypertrophic Cardiomyopathy. Recent Observations Regarding the Specificity of Three Hallmarks of the Disease: Asymmetric Septal Hypertrophy, Septal Disorganization and Systolic Anterior Motion of the Anterior Mitral Leaflet, *Am. J. Cardiol.*, 45:141, 1980. (134 references)

47. Roberts, W. C., and Ferrans, V. J.: Pathologic Anatomy of the Cardiomyopathies, *Hum. Pathol.*, 6:287, 1975.

48. Ziady, G. M., Oakley, C. M., Raphael, M. J., and Goodwin, J. F.: Primary Restrictive Cardiomyopathy, *Br. Heart J.*, 37:556, 1975.

49. Shah, P. M., Gramiak, R., Adelman, A. G. and Wigle, E. D.: Role of Echocardiography in Diagnosis and Hemodynamic Assessment of Hypertrophic Subaortic Stenosis, *Circulation*, 44:891, 1971.

50. Stark, R. M., Perloff, J. K., Glick, J. H., Hirshfeld, J. W., and Devereux, R. B.: Clinical Recognition and Management of Cardiac Metastatic Disease, *Am. J. Med.*, 63:653, 1977.

*51. Falicov, R., Resnekov, L., Bharati, S., and Lev, M.: Mid-zone Ventricular Obstruction: A Variant of Obstructive Cardiomyopathy, *Am. J. Cardiol.*, 37:432, 1976. (24 references)

52. Abelmann, W. H.: Virus and the Heart, *Circulation*, 44:950, 1971.

53. Lerner, A. M., Wilson, F. M., and Reyes, M. P.: Enteroviruses and the Heart. I. Epidemiological and Experimental Studies, *Mod. Concepts Cardiovasc. Dis.*, 44:7, 1975.

54. Lerner, A. M., Wilson, F. M., and Reyes, M. P.: Enteroviruses and the Heart. II. Observations in Humans, *Mod. Concepts Cardiovasc. Dis.*, 44:11, 1975.

55. Massie, B. M., Schiller, N. B., Ratshin, R. A., and Parmley, W. W.: Mitral-Septal Separation: A New Echocardiographic Index of Left Ventricular Function, *Am. J. Cardiol.*, 39:1008, 1977.

56. Robinson, J. A., O'Connell, J., Henkin, R. E., and Gunnar, R. M.: Gallium-67 Imaging in Cardiomyopathy, *Ann. Intern. Med.*, 90:198, 1979.

57. Ferrans, V. J., and Roberts, W. C.: Myocardial Biopsy: A Useful Diagnostic Procedure or Only a Research Tool?, *Am. J. Cardiol.*, 41:965, 1978.

*58. Mason, J. W., Billingham, M. E., and Ricci, D. R.: Treatment of Acute Inflammatory Myocarditis Assisted by Endomyocardial Biopsy, *Am. J. Cardiol.*, 45:1037, 1980. (15 references)

*59. Corya, B. C., Feigenbaum, H., Rasmussen, S., and Black, M. J.: Echocardiographic Features of Congestive Cardiomyopathy Compared with Normal Subjects and Patients with Coronary Artery Disease, *Circulation*, 49:1153, 1974. (28 references)

60. Child, J. S., Levisman, J. A., Abbasi, A. S., and MacAlpin, R. N.: Echocardiographic Manifestations of Infiltrative Cardiomyopathy: A Report of Seven Cases Due to Amyloid, *Chest*, 70:726, 1976.

61. Child, J. S., Krivokapich, J., and Abbasi, A. S.: Increased Right Ventricular Wall Thickness on Echocardiography in Amyloid Infiltrative Cardiomyopathy, *Am. J. Cardiol.*, 44:1391, 1979.

62. Brown, A. K.: Chronic Idiopathic Pericardial Effusion, *Br. Heart J.*, 28:609, 1966.

*63. Reddy, P. S., Curtiss, E. I., O'Toole, J. D., and Shaver, J. A.: Cardiac Tamponade: Hemodynamic Observations in Man, *Circulation*, 58:265, 1978. (23 references)

*64. Shabetai, R., Fowler, N. O., and Guntheroth, W. G.: The Hemodynamics of Cardiac Tamponade and Constrictive Pericarditis, *Am. J. Cardiol.*, 26:480, 1970. (32 references)

65. Martins, J. B., and Kerber, R. C.: Can Cardiac Tamponade be Diagnosed by Echocardiography? Experimental Studies, *Circulation*, 60:737, 1979.

18

Assessment of Cardiac Function and Myocardial Contractility

John Ross, Jr., M.D.

Special procedures that can assist in the accurate diagnosis and quantification of cardiac and myocardial dysfunction encompass a broad range and include rather simple examinations such as cardiac fluoroscopy, more complex noninvasive studies such as radionuclide angiography and echocardiography, and cardiac catheterization with radiographic contrast studies of the ventricles and coronary arteries. Whether or not such tests are used at all, as well as the sequence in which they should be applied, must be dictated by the specific problem at hand in each patient. A clear diagnosis may be provided by the patient's history, physical examination, chest roentgenogram, and the electrocardiogram, and proper management can then be decided upon without the need for *any* further tests. In some patients, the addition of a single noninvasive procedure such as echocardiography will adequately characterize cardiac contraction and lead to appropriate therapy. On the other hand, in the patient who has heart failure that is refractory to treatment, full cardiac catheterization is sometimes necessary to completely characterize the pathophysiological process. If a cardiac surgical procedure is under consideration, cardiac catheterization is usually advisable, and it is always necessary to adequately define the anatomy of the coronary arteries.

An enormous amount of information can be obtained from the techniques of clinical examination, and it is essential in selecting an appropriate sequence of additional diagnostic steps that such decisions be grounded on these data (Chaps. 6 to 16). For example, the prominent *v* wave of the jugular venous pulse in atrial septal defect or the inspiratory filling of the neck veins in pericardial constriction may provide the *key observation* in directing the physician toward the next logical step in diagnosis or management. Evidence of cardiac chamber enlargement and gallop rhythm should be carefully sought on physical examination, and supporting evidence for chamber enlargement should be searched for on the chest roentgenogram. The latter is as important to clinical examination of the left side of the heart as study of the jugular venous pulse is to examination of the right side of the heart; left atrial hypertension is reflected by redistribution of pulmonary blood flow with enlargement of the upper-lobe pulmonary veins, while evidence of interstitial pulmo-

nary edema may signify elevation of the mean left atrial pressure to 20 mmHg or more (Chap. 16).

Once the decision is made that an accurate diagnosis and/or proper clinical management depends upon obtaining additional information by special tests, selection of the most appropriate procedure is facilitated by a pathophysiological approach to the clinical problem. In the following sections, we will discuss general definitions of overall cardiac failure and failure of the myocardium, how certain dissociations may occur between cardiac performance and myocardial contractility, methods for assessing contractility using special procedures (Table 18-1), and, finally, the application of these methods in assessing specific cardiac contraction disorders.

Failure of the heart as a pump is not synonymous with myocardial failure, and therefore it will be useful to develop a "black box" definition of overall heart failure. In such a definition, ideally we would like to have two measures of overall cardiac function, both of which determine the effects of heart failure on the tissues of the body: (1) the amount of blood pumped per minute relative to body surface area (the cardiac index) both at rest and during stress, and (2) the pressures behind the two pumping chambers (ventricular filling pressures: the mean atrial pressures or the ventricular end-diastolic pressures) at rest and during stress. The stress employed may consist of muscular exercise, pressure loading by infusion of a vasoconstrictor agent or handgrip, or volume loading by infusion.

Overall Heart Failure

In broad clinical terms, right-sided heart failure at rest is evidenced by the presence of an elevated right heart filling pressure (mean filling pressure over 8 cm H_2O) in the resting state, associated with fluid retention or signs of congestion (peripheral edema, hepatomegaly, ascites). A low cardiac index (less than 2.4 liters/min/m^2) provides supportive evidence. Left-sided heart failure at rest is evidenced by the presence of an abnormally elevated left heart filling pressure sufficient to cause radiographic signs of pulmonary venous congestion on the chest roentgenogram, or pulmonary rales or effusion. A pulmonary artery wedge pressure of 13 mmHg or more and a low cardiac index at rest provide supportive evidence.

Overall heart failure may be further defined as inability of the left heart to produce a normal rise in cardiac output with exercise (less than 600-ml increase in cardiac output per 100-ml increase in V_{O_2})[1] and/or an abnormal increase in the left-sided filling pressure during exercise.[2] The finding of impaired functional capacity, reflected by a reduced maximal oxygen consumption during exercise,[3] may also signify overall cardiac failure since this measure correlates with cardiac output. It has been shown that some patients with poor left ventricular function at rest (ejection fraction below 30 percent)

TABLE 18-1   Special Procedures for Assessing Cardiac Function

Noninvasive Studies	Hemodynamic and Angiographic Studies
Cardiac fluoroscopy	Balloon catheterization of the
Echocardiography:	pulmonary artery:
M-mode	Pulmonary artery wedge
Two-dimensional	pressure
Exercise, handgrip,	Cardiac output
vasopressor agents	Formal cardiac catheterization:
Systolic time intervals	Intracardiac pressures
Treadmill exercise:	Right and left
ECG	ventriculography
Functional capacity	Coronary arteriography
Radionuclide studies:	Exercise, pacing,
Right and left	pharmacologic agents
ventriculography, rest and	
exercise	
Myocardial perfusion, rest	
and exercise	

can exhibit normal exercise capacity and oxygen uptake during a graded treadmill exercise test.[4] Therefore, it should be recognized at the outset that the presence of abnormal ventricular function does not imply that overall heart failure is a necessary consequence, nor does the absence of overall cardiac failure necessarily mean that ventricular function is normal.

The above definitions of overall heart failure say nothing about the *cause* of the failure, and with such broad definitions heart failure may be due to such diverse etiologies as generalized myocardial disease, mitral stenosis, chronic pulmonary disease, or constrictive pericarditis. Nevertheless, these definitions can provide a starting point for the identification of right-sided and left-sided heart failure, or both, from which one may proceed to determine whether or not overall heart failure is due to myocardial disease, mechanical factors, or both. Regardless of its cause, the manifestation of heart failure may be aggravated by other conditions such as fever, dysrhythmia, fluid overload, or metabolic disorders.

Myocardial Failure

Myocardial dysfunction, i.e., depression of the contractility or inotropic state of the ventricular myocardium, constitutes *one cause* of overall heart failure. Myocardial failure can be defined as the inability of each unit of muscle in the resting ventricle to shorten a normal distance at a normal velocity against a normal level of systolic load (afterload); it may also be defined as inability of the left ventricle to develop pressure or tension at a normal velocity during isovolumetric contraction.[5] The direct causes of most forms of myocardial failure remain unknown, but some can be identified. For example, acute depression of contractility can be

produced by certain drugs, including anesthetic agents, and by acidosis and ischemia; chronic depression of contractility can be caused by myocardial scarring or by damage to muscle cells, as in viral and other forms of myocarditis.

In isolated cardiac muscle, depressed contractility (inotropic state) is manifested by shifts of the various curves which describe the muscle's performance over a range of preloading and afterloading conditions. Depressed contractility leads to a parallel shift downward of the inverse force-velocity relation, leading to a reduction of muscle-shortening velocity at zero afterload ($V_{\max}$) and to reduced systolic force development at maximum afterload when the muscle must contract isometrically.[5] There is also downward displacement of the inverse relation between force and active shortening, of the length–active tension curve of the isometrically contracting muscle, and a downward shift of all the positive relations between resting muscle length (preload) and such measures as systolic shortening, work, and velocity of shortening (see Chap. 3).[5,6]

In assessing myocardial function in humans, sometimes the problem is to detect an *acute change in contractility*, which can usually be readily accomplished by a number of noninvasive or invasive techniques.[7–9] More often, the problem is to determine whether or not myocardial *contractility is impaired at rest* in hearts of greatly differing size, or it may be desired to compare the same heart at different points in time under changing loading conditions (as in serial studies after cardiac valve replacement).[8] This poses a more difficult problem; for example, if the absolute extent of systolic shortening of the internal diameter of the left ventricle in the cat were compared with that in the horse, it is obvious that extent of shortening in the cat would be much less, and to compare it is necessary to normalize, or to correct for a given initial heart size. Thus, systolic function is expressed as shortening per unit length (percentage shortening) of a region or diameter of the ventricle (fractional shortening), or as percentage volume change during systole (the ejection fraction). Ideally, systolic loading on the ventricles (afterload) should also be known and should be expressed in normalized terms. Systolic pressure in a great vessel or in the ventricle is often used to provide an index of the afterload, but a variation of the Laplace equation should be applied if possible to define force per unit of cross-sectional area of the ventricular wall (wall stress).[5] Thus, it is generally recognized that a large thin-walled ventricle maintaining a normal systolic pressure in the resting state is carrying a high systolic wall stress, whereas a ventricle that is concentrically hypertrophied may be carrying a very high systolic pressure but have a normal level of systolic wall stress. Such wall stress measurements are not always available, of course, and specific "indexes" of contractility useful for defining both overall and myocardial failure in humans have been developed, as described in a subsequent section.

The Problem of Dissociation between Cardiac and Myocardial Function

Under some circumstances, altered cardiac *loading* conditions can produce failure of the heart as a pump, even though myocardial contractility is not depressed. Under other conditions, favorable loading conditions and/or compensatory events may mask the presence of depressed myocardial contractility. In addition, impaired cardiac *filling* due to a variety of causes can produce changes in overall cardiac performance without impaired myocardial contraction. Finally, severe *segmental contraction* disorders can exist in association with normal overall cardiac function. These general categories of dissociation between cardiac pump function and myocardial contractility are summarized in Table 18-2.

Heart Failure without Myocardial Depression

Mechanical Overload

The level of contractility or inotropic state of the myocardium significantly affects the behavior of the heart, but cardiac *performance* (to be distinguished from myocardial contractility per se) is also importantly influenced by the interplay between the preload and the afterload. For example, severe acute hypertension or sudden mitral regurgitation due to a ruptured chorda can quickly lead to left ventric-

TABLE 18-2 Dissociations between Pump Function and Myocardial Function

1. Overall heart failure without myocardial depression
   - a. Acute mechanical overload
     - (1) Acute cor pulmonale
     - (2) Malignant hypertension
     - (3) Acute volume overload (valvular regurgitation)
   - b. Chronic severe overload
     - (1) High cardiac output states (Paget's disease, beri-beri)
     - (2) Valvular and congenital heart disease
   - c. Impaired cardiac filling
     - (1) Pericardial restriction
     - (2) Restrictive myocardial disease
     - (3) Mechanical obstruction (mitral and tricuspid stenosis, tumor)
     - (4) Tachycardias
   - d. Low cardiac output due to heart block or bradycardia
2. Absence of heart failure with myocardial depression
   - a. Systolic unloading of the ventricle
     - (1) Mitral regurgitation
     - (2) Vasodilator drugs
   - b. Compensated myocardial depression
   - c. Segmental contraction disorders
     - (1) Transient myocardial ischemia
     - (2) Myocardial infarction

ular pump failure, without myocardial depression; this situation can be described within a framework that may be termed *afterload mismatch with limited preload reserve*.[10] That is, when even the normal heart has reached the limit of its preload reserve, a further increase in afterload (as by acute hypertension or acute severe valvular regurgitation, which lead to augmentation of systolic wall stress) can produce a reduction in wall shortening and the stroke volume of the ventricle.[11,12] In heart failure when preload reserve is fully utilized, the situation resembles that in the normal heart under circumstances where the preload is held constant and the afterload is varied,[11] or when aortic pressure is increased when the normal heart is fully distended and cannot compensate by increasing preload;[12] under these conditions the stroke volume is *inversely* related to the afterload, increases in loading leading to decreased performance and vice versa. The increased loading under such circumstances can lead to a "descending limb" of ventricular function, which is due to excess afterload rather than further sarcomere overstretch.[10]

These principles are illustrated using three different schemes for describing cardiac function (the ventricular function curve, the pressure-volume loop and end-systolic pressure-volume points, and force-velocity relations) in Fig. 18-1. Of course, these conditions may then be altered by acute changes in the inotropic state, such as by the administration of a positive inotropic agent. In acute heart failure due to *afterload mismatch*, reduction of the overload by vasodilator therapy or by replacement of a defective valve with a prosthesis will promptly reverse the pump failure since myocardial contractility is basically intact,[10] although sometimes subendocardial ischemia due to high diastolic intracardiac pressures may contribute to heart failure.

In chronic mechanical overload, such as that due to valvular heart disease or a large left-to-right shunt, chronic adaptations initially occur primarily through the development of concentric or eccentric ventricular hypertrophy which prevent overall cardiac failure.[13-15] In these conditions, heart failure generally does not occur until myocardial damage supervenes because of the long-standing hypertrophy and continued mechanical overload.[15] Less is known about heart failure due to the overload of high-output states, such as Paget's disease or beri-beri, although it is likely that in these conditions altered sodium balance with fluid retention can lead to a congested state in the absence of myocardial failure.

Impaired Cardiac Filling

There is much evidence that impaired cardiac filling can lead to heart failure. It has been well documented that decreased forward cardiac output and elevation of cardiac filling pressures are often associated with normal myocardial function in chronic constrictive pericarditis, and in acute cardiac tam-

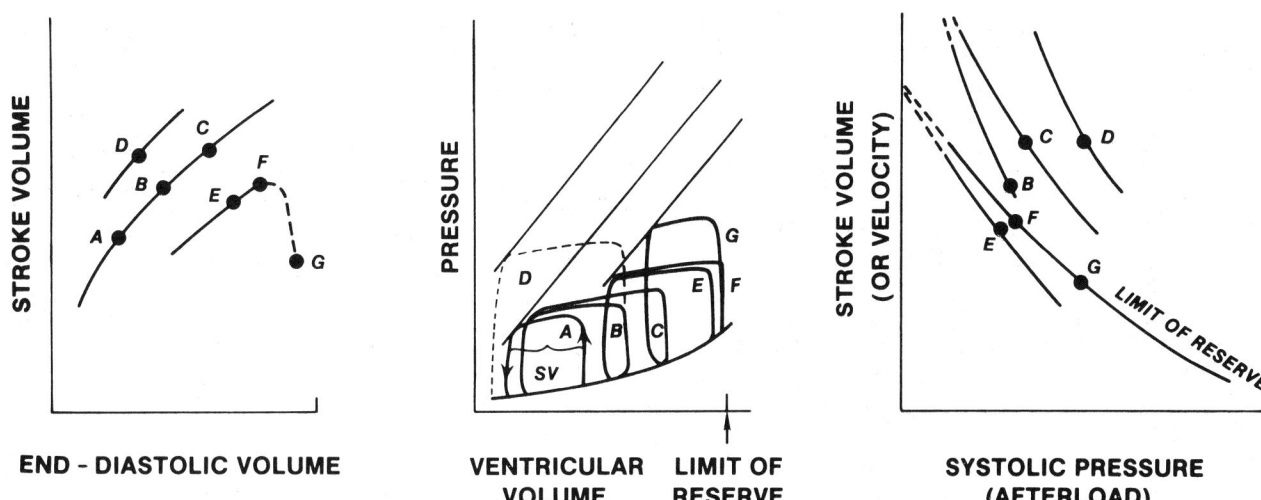

FIGURE 18-1 Three schemata for representing ventricular function and contractility. *Normal contractions: Center.* Pressure-volume loops during normal single cardiac contractions. The stroke volume (SV, bracket) represents the reduction in volume during ventricular ejection, the lower curved line represents the diastolic pressure-volume relation, and the three straight diagonal lines represent end-systolic pressure-volume relations under normal conditions (center line), enhanced inotropic state (left upper line), and depressed contractility (right lower line). Beats A, B, and C show the efects of increasing preload by transfusion in the normal heart; systolic pressure rises only slightly, and they reach almost the same point on the end-systolic pressure-volume relation. *Left.* Beats A, B, and C of the center panel are represented as a function curve relating left ventricular end-diastolic volume to the stroke volume (middle curve). *Right.* Beats B and C are shown as segments of normal force-velocity curves (or stroke volume–afterload relations), in which the curve is shifted to the right without a change in V_{max} by increased preload, at a relatively constant systolic pressure. *Enhanced contractility: Center.* The effects of a positive inotropic intervention are indicated by pressure-volume loop D in which a larger stroke volume is delivered at a higher systolic pressure from the same ventricular end-diastolic volume as beat B; this is represented as a segment of a displaced ventricular function curve in the left-hand panel (beat D), and as an enhanced force-velocity curve in the right-hand panel (beat D). *Myocardial failure: Center.* Beats E and F show pressure-volume loops in the failing heart, a reduced stroke volume being delivered from a large end-diastolic volume (EDV), and a flat, depressed function curve being present (left-hand panel). When the preload reserve is fully utilized (indicated by the arrow, center panel) infusion of a vasopressor such as angiotensin leads to an increased systolic pressure (and wall stress) without a compensatory increase in ventricular diastolic volume, and hence a reduction in the stroke volume ensues (center panel, beat G). Note that this framework illustrates clearly how the ejection fraction (SV/EDV) is dependent on the afterload at a constant level of contractility (beats F and G). This response is represented by a descending limb of function in the left-hand panel (beats F to G); the response would be accompanied by a much larger change in the ventricular end-diastolic pressure than in end-diastolic volume, since the failing ventricle usually operates on a steep diastolic pressure-volume relation (see Fig. 18-2). *Right.* Minimal use of the preload reserve by the failing ventricle is indicated by beats E and F, and when the limit of preload reserve is reached by vasopressor infusion, the further increase in systolic pressure or afterload moves the ventricle downward on a single force-velocity relation (afterload mismatch, beats F to G).

ponade.[16] There is also experimental evidence that acute volume overload, as by overtransfusion, can cause elevated cardiac filling pressures and impaired filling of the left side of the heart because of the limitation of pericardial expansion with right heart overfilling, accompanied by elevation of intrapericardial pressures with *apparent* depression of the ventricular function curve.[17,18] This response can lead to shifts upward of the entire diastolic pressure-volume relation of the left ventricle, which is due largely to changes of intrapericardial pressure, and the shift can be corrected by bleeding or by the use of a vasodilator such as nitroprusside.[17,19,19a] Such responses may explain acute shifts of the left ventricular diastolic pressure-volume relation observed clinically with vasodilators,[19,20] and could play a role in producing the high filling pressures of acute heart failure.

Restrictive disease of the ventricular chambers can lead to elevated diastolic ventricular and atrial pressures despite normal systolic contractile function of the myocardium.[21] Other mechanical obstructions to filling of the ventricles include mitral and tricuspid valve stenosis, cor triatriatum, and intraatrial clots or tumors which lead to pulmonary or systemic venous hypertension. Very rapid ventricular and atrial tachyarrhythmias, including atrial fibrillation, can cause marked reduction of the diastolic ventricular filling time per minute, along with inappropriate timing or loss of atrial systole, which can lead to elevated cardiac filling pressures and a fall in cardiac output. Finally, marked bradyarrhythmias can impair the cardiac output. All of these conditions which impair cardiac filling (Table 18-2) can, of course, produce signs of overall heart failure despite normal function of the ventricular myocardium.

Myocardial Depression without Heart Failure

As might be anticipated, the converse of afterload mismatch can occur when the preload is adequate but the afterload or wall stress on the myocardial fibers is abnormally low. Particularly in chronic mitral regurgitation, the low-impedance leak into the left atrium may result in maintenance of a normal ejection fraction until late in the clinical course, when depression of myocardial function has already occurred.[22] Thus, favorable loading conditions can mask depressed myocardial contractility, which under normal loading conditions would produce a low ejection fraction.

As might be anticipated, the converse of afterload mismatch can occur when the preload is adequate but the afterload or wall stress on the myocardial fibers is abnormally low. Particularly in chronic mitral regurgitation, the low-impedance leak into the left atrium may result in maintenance of a normal ejection fraction until late in the clinical course, when depression of myocardial function has already occurred.[22] Thus, favorable loading conditions can mask depressed myocardial contractility, which under normal loading conditions would produce a low ejection fraction.

Such favorable loading conditions can also be produced by treatment of the failing heart with a vasodilating drug which lowers the afterload on the ventricles during ejection.[23,24] Recent experimental studies indicate that in acute heart failure favorable effects on the cardiac output of a vasodilator such as nitroprusside (which has both arteriolar and venous dilating properties) result *both* from decreased afterload and from increased venous return.[25,26] In this setting, nitroprusside produces a large shift of blood volume from the distended central circulation to the peripheral bed, which is sufficient to counterbalance the peripheral pooling of blood due to venodilatation; this shift of blood volume maintains venous return and, when coupled with the reduced resistance to ventricular ejection, leads to the increase in cardiac output.[26] Conversely, in the normal circulation when nitroprusside produces venodilatation, there is only a small shift of blood volume from the central to the peripheral circulation which fails to counterbalance the dilatation of the veins, and even though the afterload on the normal ventricle is reduced, the venous return falls and the cardiac output is reduced.[26]

With mild forms of myocardial depression, normal overall cardiac function often can be maintained by compensatory mechanisms (Table 18-2). A subtle increase in heart size with a small encroachment on the preload reserve, perhaps accompanied by some reflex sympathetic augmentation of myocardial inotropic state and heart rate, can lead to normal cardiac output and filling pressure despite the mild myocardial dysfunction. Under these conditions, as discussed below, it may be possible to demonstrate limited preload reserve by stressing the heart, such as by raising the blood pressure with a vasoconstrictor agent.[10,27] Nevertheless, it should be emphasized that patients with modest depression of myocardial function (such as in early cardiomyopathy) may exhibit no signs of heart failure, and even patients with considerable myocardial depression may not show clinical signs of heart failure when

they are on therapy with potent diuretics and/or vasodilators.

Overall cardiac function is frequently normal in the presence of segmental contraction disorders. In chronic coronary heart disease, hypertrophy of adjacent normal regions may compensate for areas of myocardial infarction or scar and thereby lead to normal overall ventricular function; during acute transient myocardial ischemia, regional use of the Frank-Starling reserve in normal areas also may allow overall cardiac compensation. Of course, severe transient ischemia or large areas of chronic infarction eventually lead to overall heart failure.

Indexes of Ventricular and Myocardial Function

The reference techniques for evaluating cardiac function have been largely based on hemodynamic and/or angiographic measurements made at cardiac catheterization. It is important that these approaches be understood, since many of them are also amenable to study by noninvasive clinical methods. Broadly, we will first consider evaluation of cardiac pump function, and then more specific approaches for evaluating myocardial contractility.

Cardiac Pump Function

Methods concerned with study of the heart as a pump have usually centered around the Frank-Starling mechanism as expressed by the relation between ventricular diastolic filling and active ventricular performance. In studying cardiac function by means of ventricular function curves,[28] the path of one curve represents primarily the effect of a change in preload, whereas displacement of the entire curve upward or downward signifies a positive or negative inotropic effect (altered myocardial contractility). However, it should be recognized that left ventricular function curves tend to represent a combination of preload and afterload effects, since as preload is augmented, heart size increases, the ventricular wall becomes thinner, and aortic pressure often rises; this, in turn, increases the wall stress and thereby tends to lessen the rise in stroke volume.[5]

Resting Hemodynamics and Ventricular Volumes
In the resting state, when the left or right ventricular end-diastolic pressures are abnormally elevated (over 12 and 7 mmHg, respectively) and the cardiac index and stroke volume are below normal, myocardial contractility is probably depressed. However, either reduction of preload (hypovolemia) or contractility can reduce the stroke volume (or stroke work). In addition, such factors as pericardial disease, restrictive endocardial or myocardial disease, cardiac hypertrophy, or hypervolemia can elevate the ventricular end-diastolic pressures, and in chronic cardiac disease an elevation of ventricular

end-diastolic volume is far more accurate than pressure alone in providing an indication of cardiac dilatation with the encroachment on the Frank-Starling reserve.[29,30]

Ventricular volumes are calculated from angiograms by use of the formula for an ellipsoid of revolution,[31] and in the normal adult man the left ventricular end-diastolic volume averages 70 ± 20 [where 20 is the standard deviation (SD)] ml per square meter of body surface area, the upper limit of normal being 110 ml/m^2 (2 SD).[32] The stroke volume can be calculated by subtracting the end-systolic from the end-diastolic volume, or measured by an independent method for determining the cardiac output. The ejection fraction, the ratio of stroke volume to end-diastolic volume, is discussed subsequently. In the absence of mechanical overload, when the left ventricular end-diastolic volume is clearly elevated, the forward cardiac index or the stroke volume index is low-normal or reduced, and heart rate is normal, cardiac contractility can be defined as depressed.

Ventricular Function in Response to Invoked Stress

In the intact circulation each of the standard measures of cardiac function (such as the stroke work) is influenced by alterations in preload, afterload, and heart rate, and, therefore, they cannot be used alone as simple indexes of contractility. They do, however, provide an approach for defining *directional changes* in contractility (Fig. 18-2).[7,8] For example, a reduction of stroke volume when ventricular end-diastolic pressure (or volume) does not change or increases can be interpreted to reflect an acute depression of the inotropic state, provided aortic pressure and heart rate are unaltered; conversely, an increase in stroke volume when end-diastolic pressure is unchanged or falls would reflect enhanced inotropic state (Fig. 18-2).[7] However, when the stroke volume changes in the *same* direction as the end-diastolic pressure, assessment of directional changes in contractility is not definitive.

Since the basal values for left ventricular end-diastolic pressure and cardiac index are often within the normal range in patients with moderate left ventricular dysfunction, various forms of stress have been used to detect abnormal function or impaired cardiac reserve. For example, supine leg exercise has been employed to evaluate left ventricular performance and reserve during cardiac catheterization. In subjects without left ventricular disease, the left ventricular end-diastolic pressure is less than 12 mmHg at rest and rises slightly (2 to 3 mmHg), remains unchanged, or falls during exercise, whereas the stroke volume usually rises[2] (Fig. 18-2). The failing left ventricle, on the other hand, is characterized by an increase of 4 mmHg or more in end-diastolic pressure during exercise (usually reaching a value over 12 mmHg), with no change or a fall in the stroke volume[2] (Fig. 18-2). A standard isometric exercise stress (4 min of sustained handgrip) has also been reported to separate patients with normal left ventricular function from those with abnormal function.[33,34] The normal left ventricle appears to respond to this stress (increased aortic pressure and heart rate) with little change in left ventricular end-diastolic pressure and an increase in stroke work; in contrast, patients with cardiac disability can exhibit an increase in left ventricular end-diastolic pressure accompanied by little change or a fall in stroke work.[33,34]

Another approach consists of measuring the stroke volume, arterial pressure, and ventricular end-diastolic pressure before and during an increase in left ventricular afterload induced by means of a vasopressor agent such as phenylephrine or angiotensin.[27] Whereas the normal left ventricle responds to this stress with little change in the stroke volume, an increase in stroke work, and a rise in the end-diastolic pressure, in the failing left ventricle the end-diastolic pressure rises markedly but the stroke work either remains constant or declines, while the stroke volume falls[27] (Fig. 18-2). A fluid infusion test has had particular application in the intensive care setting. Segments of curves relating left ventricular filling pressure to stroke volume or stroke work can be constructed,[35] a flat curve or a descending limb indicating impaired left ventricular function.

The responses to these various forms of stress can be helpful not only in the detection of depressed contractility and/or impaired cardiac functional reserve, but also in expressing the severity of this impairment quantitatively. Such stress tests can also be adapted to use with some of the more specific invasive or noninvasive indexes of myocardial performance, described in a subsequent section.

Myocardial Function and Contractility

Often the clinical goal is to assess the basal level of cardiac contractility when the other major determinants of cardiac performance, the preload and afterload, are chronically abnormal. This has led to the development of clinical methods for evaluating *myocardial* function that go beyond hemodynamic measurements of pump function, the goal being to develop "indexes" that can directly define the contractile state of the myocardium.

It might be inferred that when myocardial contractility in the basal state is to be assessed, measures of contraction must be employed that are independent of *acute* alterations in preload and afterload. However, this conclusion is *not necessarily relevant* to the problem of comparing the *basal* level of inotropic state in one individual with that in another, or comparing the level in the same individual after a chronic adaptation has occurred, such as following corrective surgery.[8] Thus, it has been shown that over long periods of time the wall stress (afterload) may remain relatively unchanged because of the

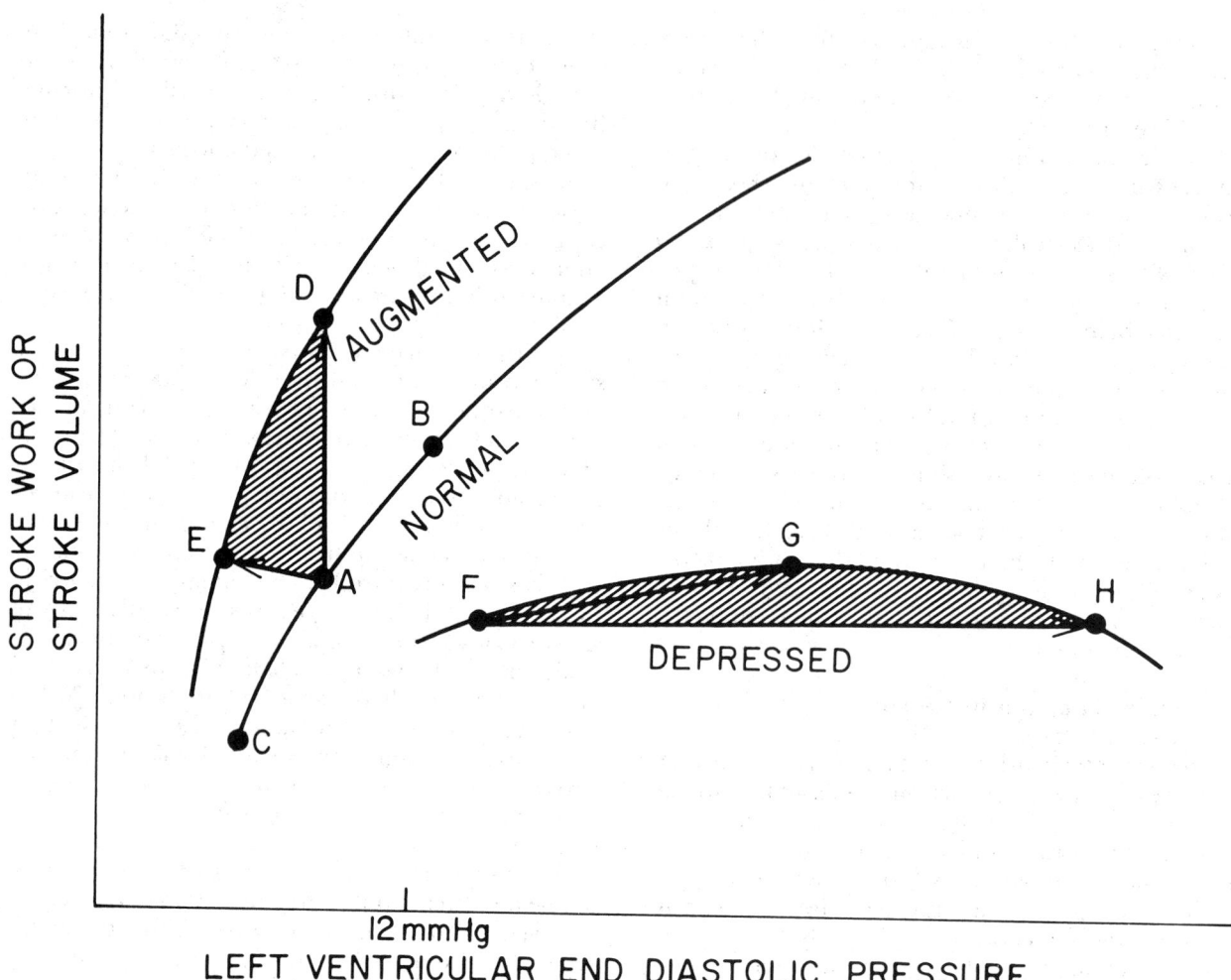

FIGURE 18-2 Ventricular function curves during various interventions in the presence of the normal and depressed myocardial contractility. In the normal ventricle (middle curve) resting conditions are shown at point A, and responses to increased or decreased cardiac filling move the ventricle up and down on this curve (points B and C, respectively); during a vasopressor stress, such as angiotensin infusion, the normal ventricle can compensate by raising the end-diastolic pressure and improving the stroke work (point B). During mild supine exercise, the ventricular end-diastolic pressure often falls in the normal heart as heart rate and contractility increase (augmented function curve), while the stroke volume may show no change or a mild increase (point E and shaded area); with more severe exercise, a substantial rise in stroke volume with little change in end-diastolic pressure may occur (point D). The failing left ventricle is operating on a depressed, flattened curve. Volume loading of the ventricle may result in a large change in end-diastolic pressure with little change in stroke volume (point F to G), or an actual reduction in the stroke volume (point G to H); also, use of a vasopressor such as angiotensin will force the ventricle onto a "descending limb" of function (point G to H) as a result of afterload mismatch[10] rather than diastolic overstretch. With supine exercise, there may be little or no displacement of the ventricular function curve upward, and a large rise in ventricular end-diastolic pressure may occur with little increase (point F to G), no change, or a fall in the stoke volume with a rise in end-diastolic pressure (point G to H).

development of ventricular hypertrophy, as in chronic pressure overloading due to aortic valve disease.[36] Also, in experimental animals subjected to chronic volume overloading, the preload (as reflected by sarcomere length) does not change further as chronic ventricular dilatation slowly occurs, but remains the same as in acute volume overload.[37] Thus, to evaluate *basal contractility* it may not be necessary to use indexes of contractility that are unaffected by acute changes in preload and afterload.[8] In effect, when the preload reserve has been fully utilized, regardless of the chronic level of afterload (wall stress), depressed contractility should usually result in an afterload mismatch expressed by ina-

bility of the ventricle to maintain normal performance *per unit* of its circumference or volume.[10]

Isovolumic Phase Indexes

When the maximum rate of change of left ventricular pressure (peak dP/dt, usually measured with a catheter tip micromanometer) is reduced below about 1400 mmHg/s, myocardial contractility is usually depressed, but this measure is relatively nonspecific and affected by other factors such as the time of aortic valve opening. Because of this problem, simplified methods have been employed to determine indexes of V_{max} using the brief isovolumetric phase of ejecting beats. Values of V_{max} are determined by plotting V_{CE} [contractile element velocity $= (dP/dt)/P$] against the corresponding intraventricular pressure (P) throughout isovolumic systole and extrapolating to zero pressure.[38,39] To avoid difficulties with such extrapolations, some investigators have selected certain points on the curve relating $(dP/dt)/P$ to P; these measures tend to be independent of changes in aortic pressure, since they occur prior to aortic valve opening. One such index—the value of $(dP/dt)/P$ at its maximum point, or V_{pm}—has been reported to be relatively independent of acute changes in loading conditions but sensitive to changes in the inotropic state,[40,41] and it has been advocated as an index of the basal inotropic state in patients.[40]

Many such isovolumic phase indexes are quite useful for detecting acute changes in contractility when the afterload is changing, provided that large alterations in left ventricular end-diastolic pressure do not occur.[42,43] Nevertheless, in support of the view proposed earlier that it may be unnecessary to determine basal contractility by measures that are independent of preload and afterload, it has been found that indexes derived from the isovolumetric phase of left ventricular pressure tracings often are not sensitive for detecting depressed basal levels of contractility.[44,45] For example, while V_{pm} and V_{max} were useful for separating *groups* of patients with clearly normal or depressed left ventricular function,[40,49] they were less reliable than ejection phase indexes in the individual patient, and widely divergent normal and abnormal values have been reported. Their limited usefulness may also relate to theoretical problems, extrapolation techniques, and artifacts in high-fidelity pressure tracings.[46]

Ejecting Phase Indexes

The ejection phase indexes are based on measurements of ventricular volume or dimensions, or their rate of change, during ejection. They have the advantage of being readily measured by noninvasive approaches. Measures of the ejecting phase include the stroke volume, ejection rate, and flow acceleration, all of which are highly sensitive to acute changes in afterload;[43] but the ejection phase indexes are more commonly used to assess *basal* contractility, and therefore they are normalized for heart size. Commonly used indexes include the percentage of the end-diastolic volume ejected (the *ejection fraction* or ratio of stroke volume to end-diastolic volume), the percentage shortening of the ventricular end-diastolic diameter (the *fractional shortening* or extent of systolic diameter change divided by the end-diastolic diameter), and the mean velocity of internal-diameter shortening corrected for end-diastolic diameter (mean V_{CF}).

The ejection fraction is most commonly employed, and a reduced value (below 55 percent) measured in the resting state by left ventriculography has proved useful often for detecting depressed basal myocardial contractility. It has limitations for measuring depressed function when the afterload is low, as in mitral regurgitation, because of the inverse relation between afterload and stroke volume (Fig. 18-1). Because of the known sensitivity of ejecting phase measures to acute changes in afterload,[47] in early studies of basal contractility in humans wall stress was also measured.[48] High-fidelity catheters and cineangiography were used to define the relation between the extent and velocity of shortening of the circumferential fibers and the corresponding wall stress throughout systole,[48] and determination of the relationship between mean wall stress during ejection and mean V_{CF} or fractional shortening can provide a means of assessing basal contractility. Subsequently, however, determinations of mean V_{CF} alone were shown to have a good correlation with these more complex measures.[49] The lower limit of normal for mean V_{CF} in humans, determined angiographically, is 1.2 circumferences per second.[44,49] The mean V_{CF}, the ejection fraction, and the mean systolic ejection rate (corrected for ventricular end-diastolic volume) all effectively separate normal patients from patients with left ventricular myocardial disease who have clearly abnormal ventricular function.[44,45]

Many of the ejection phase measures can also be calculated noninvasively by echocardiography[47,50] or radionuclide angiography,[51] and good agreement with angiographic measurements has generally been found. These noninvasive techniques are also useful for detecting abnormal responses to stress, as, for example, when the radionuclide ejection fraction of the left ventricle fails to rise normally or falls during exercise (see subsequent section).

Analyses of *right ventricular function* have been limited, in part because of the complex shape of this chamber and the difficulty of computing right ventricular volumes angiographically. However, radionuclide techniques have now permitted assessment of the right ventricular ejection fraction at rest and during stress.[52-55] At rest, the lower limit of normal of the right ventricular ejection fraction is lower than that of the left ventricle (approximately 40 to 43 percent) by first-pass and gated techniques.[52-55] Normally the right-sided radionuclide ejection fraction rises during supine exercise by 5 percent or more.[53-55]

End-Systolic Indexes

There has been increasing interest in another approach for assessing cardiac contractility and responses to stress that may avoid some of the problems inherent in the sensitivity of ejection phase indexes to afterload, which can be a particular problem in the presence of valvular heart disease. The points relating end-systolic pressure to the left ventricular volume or diameter at end ejection form a linear relation that is independent of the initial end-diastolic diameter (preload) and the afterload (Fig. 18-1).[56,59] The relation is shifted upward by positive and downward by negative inotropic influences.[57,58,59] In clinical studies the slope also appears linear;[60,61] the slopes as well as the intercepts of these end-systolic pressure-volume relations have been reported to allow separation of groups of patients with and without left ventricular dysfunction.[60] It is also possible to determine the relation noninvasively by measuring peak arterial pressure by the cuff (or intraarterial) method and making an echocardiographic determination of left ventricular end-systolic dimensions while a range of pressures is produced by phenylephrine and/or nitroprusside infusions.[61]

The relation between end-systolic wall stress and volume is also linear.[62] Wall stress can also be calculated by the echocardiographic method,[61] and this approach appears to provide a useful way of studying contractility in humans. It seems likely that for assessing basal contractility in chronic disease, use of wall stress rather than pressure alone may be desirable, since the end-systolic wall stress–ventricular diameter relation at end ejection, rather than the end-systolic pressure–diameter relation, has been found useful for defining basal contractility in experimental animals and in humans with hypertrophy due to pressure overload.[61,63] Since these end-systolic pressure or wall stress versus ventricular dimension (or volume) relations are free of acute effects of preload or afterload, they may find increasing clinical application for invasive and noninvasive studies on myocardial function and contractility at rest and during acute stress.

Types of Special Laboratory Procedures

Before considering the assessment of cardiac function in specific clinical situations, it will be useful to discuss briefly the special procedures currently available (Table 18-1).

Noninvasive Procedures

Whenever possible, the risks and expense of passing a cardiac catheter or performing angiography should be replaced by a suitable noninvasive procedure. In many instances noninvasive studies will provide sufficiently accurate diagnostic information to allow initiation of appropriate management.

Cardiac Fluoroscopy (See Chap. 84)
Under some circumstances, cardiac fluoroscopy can provide valuable information (Chap. 84), although the findings are selective and it cannot be recommended as a routine screening procedure. Cardiac fluoroscopy can confirm the presence or absence of specific chamber or great-vessel enlargement. It is sometimes helpful for confirming the suspicion of a left ventricular aneurysm, detecting left atrial enlargement (particularly in conjunction with barium in the esophagus), defining left ventricular and aortic enlargement, and determining the presence or

absence of hyperdynamic chamber motion. Although echocardiography has replaced fluoroscopy for the quantitative assessment of cardiac chamber size, the method is applicable when the echocardiogram is unsatisfactory or unavailable.

Image-intensification fluoroscopy is uniquely suited to search for cardiac, pericardial, or coronary *calcification,* and it sometimes can thereby help to clarify the etiology of cardiac dysfunction. Fluoroscopy can provide confirmation of the presence of chronic pericarditis or luetic disease of the aortic root; the characteristic motions of the aortic and mitral valves allow the fluoroscopist to localize valvular calcifications, and calcium in the mitral annulus or subvalvular region may clarify the origin of an apical mitral regurgitant murmur; sometimes calcium can be seen in a ventricular aneurysm. Calcification in the aortic valve is an extremely important finding, and it may provide the first clue to the origin of left ventricular failure in an older patient who has a low cardiac output and a soft systolic ejection murmur due to severe aortic stenosis. The detection of coronary artery calcification may provide the first objective evidence of coronary artery disease in the patient with cardiomyopathy.[64]

Echocardiography (See Chap. 95)
In assessing cardiac function, the general applications of M-mode echocardiography (which may be enhanced by two-dimensional studies) can be summarized as follows:[66]

1. Confirmation or exclusion of cardiac chamber and great-vessel enlargement and concentric or asymmetric left ventricular wall hypertrophy.
2. Assessment of overall left ventricular function (Fig. 18-3). The M-mode technique is largely limited to assessing left ventricular wall dynamics in the septal and posterior basal regions, and therefore it can provide accurate estimations of *overall* ventricular function only when ventricular function is normal or uniformly depressed. Determination of the fractional shortening, ejection fraction, V_{CF}, and systolic wall thickening are useful for this purpose.[50,65]
3. Detection of regional myocardial dysfunction, when coronary heart disease is suspected of contributing to overall cardiac dysfunction. The M-mode technique is useful for detecting abnormalities of motion and systolic wall thickening in the interventricular septum and/or posterior wall; however, for locating anterior, lateral, or apical regions of dysfunction, and for detecting left ventricular aneurysm, two-dimensional studies are necessary. Overall function can also be assessed in the presence of regional contraction disorders by two-dimensional echocardiography (Chap. 95).
4. Identification of mechanical cardiac disorders. A variety of valvular lesions can be detected, including rheumatic or congenital lesions, mitral

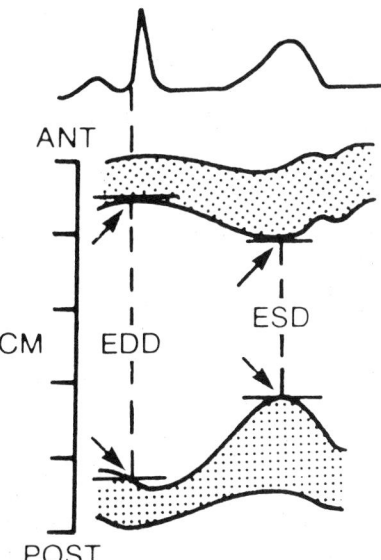

FIGURE 18-3   Diagram of echocardiogram of the normal left ventricle. Upper tracing is the electrocardiogram. The anterior and posterior (ANT and POST) directions are indicated on the echocardiographic scale, which is in centimeters (CM). The septal wall is indicated by a the stippled area anteriorly, and the posterior ventricular wall by the other stippled tracing. Left ventricular end-diastolic diameter (EDD) is measured at the onset of the QRS complex, and the end-systolic diameter (ESD) is also shown. Fractional shortening of the left ventricle is calculated as (EDD − ESD)/EDD, and the ejection fraction can also be estimated based on cube functions. A variety of techniques for measuring the echocardiogram are currently used.[65a] Measurements shown are from the anterior edge of the tracing from each endocardial surface. Either the onset or the peak of the QRS complex can be used to define EDD, and many echocardiographers use the minimum distance between the two walls as the ESD, whether or not they are exactly opposed in time.[65a] With the latter technique the lower limit of normal for fractional shortening is about 28 percent.

valve prolapse, systolic anterior mitral valve motion in hypertrophic obstructive cardiomyopathy, and acute valvular disease such as a flail mitral leaflet. Sometimes, congenital disorders such as atrial septal defect can be detected. Other mechanical problems that can impair cardiac filling or emptying may also be identified. These include pericardial effusion, chronic constrictive pericarditis, restrictive types of cardiomyopathy, and intracardiac tumor or clot.

The finding of entirely normal cardiac chambers on echocardiography can have enormous importance. For example, in the patient with chronic pulmonary disease, a normal echocardiographic study of the left ventricle may permit the exclusion of any contribution of left ventricular dysfunction to dyspnea or to signs of right-sided heart failure. If the echocardiogram shows the left ventricle to be enlarged and to exhibit decreased fractional shortening of the walls (Fig. 18-3), and if mechanical disorders are not identified, intrinsic myocardial disease is likely. If there is left ventricular enlargement with uniformly decreased wall function associated with valvular heart disease, secondary cardiac dys-

function is likely, although one cannot necessarily infer that irreversible depression of myocardial contractility is present.

Echocardiography can be used to study the responses of the left ventricle to various forms of stress. The use of a vasopressor infusion, such as phenylephrine,[47] or handgrip exercise can produce abnormal left ventricular function and serve to detect latent generalized left ventricular dysfunction in valvular or myocardial disease. The two-dimensional technique offers promise of allowing more reliable study of the responses of global ventricular function to stress of various types. For example, two-dimensional techniques have been used to detect regional wall motion abnormalities produced by transient cardiac ischemia during exercise in patients with coronary heart disease.[67]

Certain general limitations of using echocardiography for defining cardiac contraction characteristics should be emphasized (see Chap. 95). Echocardiographic evaluation of overall left ventricular function may be misleading when there is eccentric ventricular hypertrophy with an exaggerated elliptical or spherical shape of the left ventricle, as may occur in aortic regurgitation, leading to under- or overestimation of left ventricular chamber size and function by echocardiography compared with angiography.[68] The M-mode echocardiogram can be misleading in ischemic heart disease;[69] it may not detect significant regional wall motion abnormalities, and the tracing can appear normal even in the presence of severe segmental anterior and apical contraction disorders or aneurysm. Also, in evaluating segmental myocardial disease, it should be recalled that abnormal septal motion is not specific for coronary artery disease and can be produced by right ventricular volume overload, intraventricular conduction defects, and hypertrophic cardiomyopathy. The use of two-dimensional echocardiography, however, allows detection of regional wall motion abnormalities and determination of the ejection fraction in patients with and without ischemic heart disease.[70]

The usefulness of the echocardiogram can be limited in detecting restrictive myocardial disease, particularly if the wall is not greatly thickened and systolic function is normal. Sometimes additional clues to this diagnosis are provided by reduced EF slope of the mitral valve and by left atrial enlargement, both of which can reflect reduced left ventricular compliance. The physiological significance of other mechanical filling problems such as chronic constrictive pericarditis often cannot be determined from the echocardiogram.

Technical limitations of echocardiography include a resolution of about 1 mm under optimum conditions, which limits the precision of measurements of left ventricular wall thickness and wall dynamics, and in some patients it is impossible to adequately image the interventricular septum at the proper region or to clearly define the posterior wall of the left ventricle. The end-diastolic dimension of the right ventricle can usually be ascertained, but systolic function of that chamber often cannot be assessed quantitatively by M-mode echocardiography (see Chap. 95), although two-dimensional studies are finding increasing application.[52]

Radionuclide Angiography (See Chap. 97)

Radionuclide angiography is particularly suitable for determining the ejection fraction of the ventricles,[51] and reliable measurements of absolute ventricular volumes may become possible as well.[71] As indicated in Chap. 97, the ejection fraction can be determined by either the first-pass technique (the initial washout of a radioisotope monitored for maximum and minimum radioactivity during several cardiac cycles) or the gated equilibrium method (multiple cardiac images obtained at selected points in the cardiac cycle).[51] Radionuclide techniques have a potentially important advantage over the M-mode echocardiographic method for determining ventricular function in that the method of calculating the ejection fraction is independent of ventricular geometry; thus, the total number of counts at end-diastole and end-systole within the region of interest are used in calculating the ejection fraction, and regional wall motion abnormalities do not interfere with the evaluation of global function. This advantage does not apply over the two-dimensional echocardiographic method, provided quantitative estimations of ventricular volume in two planes can be obtained.[70] The gated equilibrium technique is also valuable for determining the responses of the left ventricular ejection fraction to various forms of stress such as exercise, vasopressor infusion, or handgrip,[72,73] as well as for studying the performance of the right ventricle at rest and during exercise.[52–55,74] An abnormal decrease in the left ventricular ejection fraction during exercise occurs during regional myocardial ischemia in patients with coronary heart disease,[72] but it can also be observed in patients with severe aortic regurgitation[75] so that such as response is not specific for ischemia.

The limitations of radionuclide angiography for determining ventricular function relate primarily to technical problems, including the method of subtracting background radioactivity and accurate computer recognition of the borders of the cardiac chambers (Chap. 97). Good correlations have been reported between the left ventricular ejection fraction determined by radionuclide techniques and by contrast left ventriculography,[51] although errors of 10 to 15 percent may be encountered in the individual patient (Chap. 97). The lower limit of normal of the radionuclide ejection fraction of the left ventricle (52 to 54 percent)[52–55] is somewhat lower than that determined angiographically. Both the left and right ventricular ejection fractions normally increase by at least 5 percent during supine exercise.[52–55] The reproducibility of left ventricular ejection fraction determinations carried out by equi-

librium radionuclide angiography several weeks apart in the same patient is within about 5 percent, and interobserver variability with this approach usually is low because automated programs are employed to identify the cardiac chambers.[76]

Systolic Time Intervals

Simultaneous measurements of the interval from the onset of the QRS complex to the aortic closure sound and the duration of left ventricular ejection time (LVET) from the carotid pulse tracing allows, by subtraction, measurement of the preejection period (PEP) (Chap. 85). The ratio of these two variables (PEP/LVET) is increased in heart failure primarily as a result of the slow rate of rise of left ventricular pressure (reduced dP/dt, leading to prolongation of PEP) and to reduced stroke volume (leading to shortening of LVET). Although other hemodynamic factors can also influence the systolic time intervals (Chap. 85), making them less reliable than echocardiography for detecting abnormal ventricular function in the individual patient, this ratio has been applied in separating groups of normal subjects from those with heart failure, and it is useful in determining the prognosis of patients with coronary heart disease[77] The upper limit of normal for the PEP/LVET is 0.42 (normal mean = 0.34 + 2 SD).[78]

Invasive Procedures

Techniques of inserting intravascular catheters for measuring right- or left-sided intracardiac pressures and cardiac output, performance of selective angiography, and balloon catheterization for hemodynamic monitoring encompass the so-called invasive techniques described in detail in Chaps. 98 to 100.

Balloon Catheterization of the Pulmonary Artery

Catheterization of the pulmonary artery by the Swan-Ganz technique (Chap. 99) is useful in the evaluation and management of acute and chronic heart failure in several clinical settings. Data that can be obtained by this approach include measurement of pressures in the right atrium, right ventricle, pulmonary artery, and the pulmonary artery wedge positions; determination of the cardiac output; and calculation of systemic and pulmonary vascular resistances. In treating refractory heart failure, such data are highly useful in selecting an appropriate vasodilator and monitoring its initial hemodynamic effects.[79]

Among the acute forms of heart failure appropriate for study by balloon catheterization is acute myocardial infarction complicated by hypotension (see Chap. 100). Sometimes hypovolemia is the problem, and the finding of normal or low right atrial and pulmonary artery wedge pressures can lead to rapid correction of a volume deficit. Acute left ventricular failure can also be produced by complications of acute myocardial infarction, and balloon catheterization of the pulmonary artery is useful in detecting rupture of the interventricular septum, or rupture of the head of a papillary muscle, as well as for monitoring therapeutic responses in cardiogenic shock. In severe power failure, a test of left ventricular function may also be performed by use of a small volume overload (200- to 300-ml dextrose infusion), with determination of the response of the stroke volume or stroke work index relative to the accompanying rise in pulmonary artery wedge pressure.[35] A flat or descending relation indicates that left ventricular function is severely depressed (Fig. 18-2) with maximum use of the Frank-Starling reserve, whereas an increase in the stroke volume indicates some reserve; this test is also useful in prognosis of outcome.[35]

Cardiac Catheterization and Angiography (See Chap. 98)

In the evaluation of cardiac and ventricular dysfunction, because of expense and some risk (Chap. 98) formal cardiac catheterization is undertaken only when a precise diagnosis is critical to the selection of appropriate medical or surgical therapy and when that diagnosis cannot be achieved by noninvasive techniques. For example, cardiac catheterization may be necessary to determine whether or not left ventricular failure is due to restrictive cardiomyopathy or to pericardial disease; it may be valuable in some patients with congestive cardiomyopathy for determining whether or not coronary atherosclerosis is a causative or contributing factor; it may be necessary to determine whether or not a suspected left-to-right shunt is contributing to cardiac failure; and it is often required in the patient with known disease of the heart valves or coronary arteries to quantify severity in considering operation, or to determine whether associated severe myocardial disease may contradict operation.

As described earlier, overall cardiac function can be assessed at cardiac catheterization by determining the right and left ventricular end-diastolic pressures and the cardiac index, as well as from the responses of the stroke volume or stroke work and filling pressures to exercise or vasopressor infusion. Selective ventriculography has long provided the reference standard for accurately quantifying the status of left ventricular function, the standard against which the reliability of noninvasive techniques are tested. As described in Chap. 98, the use of single or biplane left ventriculography allows application of the area-length method for calculation of end-diastolic and end-systolic ventricular volumes and the ejection fraction, mean V_{CF}, the left ventricular wall thickness, and left ventricular mass. As discussed earlier, the ejection phase indexes have served as criteria by which the *basal level* of myocardial contractility can be defined, and high-fidelity measurements of left ventricular pressure by a catheter-tip micromanometer also permit calcula-

tion of isovolumic phase indexes, as well as the diastolic pressure-volume or diastolic stress-strain properties of the heart.

Myocardial Biopsy

This technique (described in Chap. 98) is carried out using a special cardiac catheter which is positioned in the right ventricle, although it can be placed by the retrograde or the transseptal routes into the left ventricle as well. When cardiac catheterization studies fail to reveal a specific cause for unexplained severe cardiac failure, myocardial biopsy can sometimes reveal evidence of an unsuspected infiltrative cardiomyopathy (such as amyloidosis or hemachromatosis), microvascular disease, or inflammation. Unfortunately, however, the diagnostic yield of such myocardial biopsies is relatively low,[80] and the procedure should be undertaken only if it is likely that a tissue diagnosis could significantly affect the selection of proper therapy.

Application of Special Procedures to Specific Clinical Problems

Recognition of Mechanical Factors Sufficient to Cause Heart Failure

In assessing the patient who has clinical signs of acute or chronic overall heart failure, it is important at the outset to consider the possibility that mechanical factors rather than myocardial depression are primarily responsible (see Table 18-2). Impaired cardiac filling due to pericardial disease or some other cause should be carefully excluded, as discussed subsequently in the section on myocardial disease. In some patients, a mechanical cause for secondary heart failure may be relatively obvious, as in severe systemic hypertension, coarctation of the aorta, or arteriovenous fistula due to trauma or other cause. In those settings, extensive evaluation of the associated cardiac dysfunction may not be necessary, since treatment of the primary disorder will correct the cardiac problem. In other patients, a congenital defect or acquired valvular lesion producing an excessive mechanical burden on one or both ventricles may be suspected. It is then necessary to establish whether or not a sufficiently severe mechanical overload, *capable* of causing secondary myocardial dysfunction, is present.

In chronic aortic or mitral regurgitation, cardiac catheterization usually is not necessary to establish the diagnosis of a severe valvular leak. In aortic regurgitation, the physical findings of a widened pulse pressure with low diastolic pressure, coupled with the characteristics of the murmur and the detection of left ventricular enlargement, readily allow the identification of severe regurgitation; echocardiographic measurements of left ventricular size and function should also be carried out (see later section). In mitral regurgitation, the characteristics of the murmur, the presence of a ventricular diastolic gallop and early diastolic mitral flow murmur, and radiographic and echocardiographic measurements of left ventricular and left atrial size usually permit the identification of a severe leak at the mitral valve, although the clinical findings are somewhat less reliable for assessing severity than in aortic regurgitation. When combined obstructive and regurgitant lesions of the mitral and aortic valves are present, hemodynamic and angiographic studies are frequently necessary to characterize the severity of the mechanical overload. Clinical features may be atypical in acute, severe aortic or mitral regurgitation causing heart failure, and special diagnostic studies are often necessary as discussed below.

With congenital or acquired aortic stenosis, mild or moderate obstruction at the aortic valve may be identified by a combination of echocardiographic, electrocardiographic, phonocardiographic, roentgenographic, and physical findings (Chap. 38). However, hemodynamic studies with measurement of the pressure gradient across the outflow tract and aortic valve should be considered in any patient who has symptoms of left ventricular failure that *may* be due to underlying aortic stenosis, since the severity of stenosis can be underestimated from such clinical studies.

The clinical suspicion that cardiac dysfunction is due to the volume overload of a left-to-right shunt at the atrial or ventricular levels can sometimes be confirmed by M-mode and two-dimensional echocardiographic identification of the defect itself, together with evidence of right- or left-sided chamber enlargement. First-pass radionuclide imaging of such shunts, or that due to patent ductus arteriosus, also can provide noninvasive confirmation of their presence. However, in determining the significance of a left-to-right shunt, cardiac catheterization should be carried out to precisely define the magnitude of the shunt, the intracardiac anatomy, and whether or not there is pulmonary hypertension.

Once the presence of mechanical overload is established, it is often possible to exclude or detect the presence of myocardial dysfunction by noninvasive methods. The most useful screening approach is the M-mode echocardiogram, in which direct measurements of the left-sided chamber dimensions, and sometimes right ventricular size, can be made. Alternatively, the left or right ventricular ejection fraction can be determined by radionuclide angiography. In the presence of chronic volume overload, the finding of normal systolic contractile function by echocardiography (normal fractional shortening, V_{CF}, and calculated ejection fraction), or a normal radionuclide ejection fraction, despite the presence of moderately increased ventricular end-diastolic dimension, usually indicates the absence of significant myocardial dysfunction. An important exception occurs in chronic mitral regurgitation, as discussed further below. If coronary artery disease is associated with mechanical overload and produces

regional wall motion abnormalities, the M-mode echocardiogram is often unreliable. Under these circumstances, calculation of left ventricular volumes by the two-dimensional echo technique may be feasible, or the ejection fraction may be determined by the radionuclide technique. The details of follow-up in the patient with chronic pressure or volume overload due to valvular heart disease are discussed further in the next section.

In heart failure due to sudden, severe volume overload consequent to infective endocarditis of the aortic or mitral valves, ruptured chordae, infarction of a papillary muscle, or ruptured interventricular septum after myocardial infarction, noninvasive studies should be used initially and may provide clues to the diagnosis as well as to the presence of severe ventricular dysfunction. M-mode echocardiographic studies when associated with two-dimensional studies may allow the identification of a flail mitral valve leaflet, ventricular septal defect, or vegetations on the aortic, mitral, or tricuspid valves. Diastolic fluttering of the anterior mitral valve leaflet may be noted in aortic valve regurgitation, and with acute severe aortic regurgitation preclosure of the mitral valve in middiastole, indicative of a severe acute leak, may be identified on the M-mode echocardiogram (Chap. 38). The echocardiogram will also allow identification of the reduction in fractional shortening and ejection fraction of the left ventricle that usually accompanies severe acute overload, which may be due to full utilization of the preload reserve with acute afterload mismatch rather than significant depression of myocardial contractility.[10] In the further diagnosis and treatment of heart failure due to sudden cardiac overload in the intensive care setting, insertion of a balloon catheter usually is advisable to measure the wedge pressure, search for a left-to-right shunt, and guide vasodilator and other therapy. Prior to considering surgical treatment, full cardiac catheterization should usually be performed to characterize the severity of the mechanical lesion and the state of the left ventricle, and to examine the coronary arteries.

Recognition of Myocardial Depression in Chronic Valvular Heart Disease

Those valvular lesions that overload the left ventricle (aortic stenosis, aortic regurgitation, and mitral regurgitation) can, over time, produce severe left ventricular hypertrophy, which eventually is associated with myocardial fibrosis and irreversible left ventricular dysfunction. Such dysfunction may persist following surgical correction of the valve defect, and in the clinical management of patients with chronic valvular heart disease it is important that objective methods be used in follow-up in order to prevent this occurrence.[80a] Types of special studies on the left ventricle and the frequencies with which they should be performed vary somewhat among the three valvular lesions.

Valvular Aortic Stenosis

In the young patient suspected of having severe aortic stenosis, cardiac catheterization studies are generally carried out early, and operation is undertaken if the suspicion of severe stenosis is confirmed, since the risk of surgery is less than the risk of sudden death in such individuals.[81] In these patients, the question of myocardial dysfunction does not usually pose a significant problem. In the adult patient with clinical features of significant aortic stenosis who develops symptoms of left ventricular dysfunction, syncope, or angina pectoris, prompt cardiac catheterization is indicated. Sometimes, particularly in older individuals, the aortic systolic murmur may not be loud and the pulse pressure may be normal, even in the presence of severe stenosis (Chap. 38). In such individuals, echocardiography, phonocardiography, and fluoroscopy for aortic calcification may be contributory, but if there is unexplained left ventricular dysfunction clinically, hemodynamic studies should usually be done. The cardiac catheterization should document whether or not the aortic valve narrowing is significant (valve orifice area less than 0.75 cm^2 or 0.6 cm/m^2 are approximate guidelines),[82] whether associated coronary atherosclerosis is contributing to the patient's symptoms, and whether or not there is depressed contractile function. Generally, if the stenosis is severe, operation is undertaken since the outlook with medical therapy is poor.[81,83]

In the older patient with no symptoms but with physical findings of aortic stenosis, the chest roentgenogram will typically reveal a normal heart size, and the electrocardiogram may be nonspecific. A base-line M-mode echocardiogram should ordinarily be obtained to document thickening of the aortic valve, to determine the degree of thickening of the left ventricular walls, and to assure that the left ventricular end-diastolic dimension, the fractional shortening, and the ejection fraction are all within the normal range. In following such patients, the characteristics of the left ventricle can usually be identified satisfactorily by sequential echocardiographic studies. The development of mild dilatation of the ventricular chamber at end-diastole, with relative thinning of the ventricular wall, and reduced fractional shortening can identify increasing severity of stenosis or early left ventricular decompensation.

Serial echocardiographic or catheterization studies carried out after aortic valve replacement for aortic stenosis indicate that hypertrophy regresses and left ventricular function remains normal in most patients, or even if moderately depressed preoperatively, it tends to return toward normal during the first 6 months postoperatively.[84,85,85a] Even in patients with severely depressed ventricular function preoperatively, the average ejection fraction returned to normal, although in a few patients it remained below normal.[86] These findings suggest that mechanical overload per se, rather than irreversibly depressed myocardial contractility, was often responsible for reduced left ventricular function. The mechanisms of reduced function when present preoperatively are not entirely clear. In some patients, marked hypertrophy may result in impaired ventricular filling due to reduced ventricular compliance, so that the preload reserve is not fully utilized[10] to counterbalance the excessive afterload posed by the narrowed aortic valve. It has also been suggested that sometimes the degree of hypertrophy may be inadequate for the level of afterload.[87] In other patients, myocardial contractility is depressed.[87a] In any case, aortic valve replacement allows the ventricle to eject normally in most instances, and irreversible myocardial changes postoperatively are now relatively uncommon.

Such findings suggest that serial echocardiographic studies of left ventricular function are not as important in patients with aortic stenosis as in patients with chronic volume overload (see below) in reaching a decision concerning operation, and that the current criteria for surgical treatment based largely on the development of significant symptoms remain appropriate. Thus, it would appear that in aortic stenosis operation need not be considered *solely* to protect the left ventricle from irreversible myocardial damage. In addition, the data suggest that even in the patient with severe left ventricular dysfunction and an ejection fraction as low as 18 to 20 percent, operation should *not* be denied, since ventricular function frequently will improve postoperatively.

Aortic Regurgitation

In following the asymptomatic patient with chronic aortic regurgitation (Chap. 38) who has only a mild to moderate leak, as assessed from the heart murmur and pulse pressure, and in whom the heart is only slightly enlarged, as assessed by physical examination and the chest roentgenogram, serial clinical examinations can be done relatively infrequently. On the other hand, when the patient has clinically severe aortic regurgitation with symptoms suggestive of early left ventricular failure (or other limiting symptoms), provided the symptoms persist after ordinary therapy with digitalis and diuretics, it is generally advisable to proceed directly with cardiac catheterization to assess the appropriateness of surgical treatment. Such studies will characterize the severity of the regurgitation, the status of left ventricular function, and the presence or absence of coronary artery disease. Echocardiographic or radionuclide studies prior to cardiac catheterization in such individuals may help to confirm the need for catheterization studies, if the criteria discussed below are met.

In the patient without significant symptoms who has severe aortic regurgitation and whose heart size is increased, as assessed by the chest roentgenogram and by physical examination, a base-line M-mode echocardiogram should be obtained for measurement of the left ventricular dimensions. If moderate enlargement of the left ventricular with normal fractional shortening (Fig. 18-3) and calculated ejection fraction are found, and the patient remains asymptomatic, serial echocardiographic studies about every 2 years can be recommended to assure that progressive cardiac enlargement and deterioration of left ventricular function do not occur. If the left ventricular enlargement is marked (end-diastolic diameter of the ventricle 70 mm or more), annual follow-up should probably be advised.

Studies in which angiographic or echocardiographic analyses have been made before and after aortic valve replacement for severe aortic regurgitation indicate that in patients with marked cardiomegaly and very severely depressed function, irreversible left ventricular dysfunction can persist postoperatively;[88] when there is only moderate cardiomegaly and normal or mild depression of left ventricular function, by 6 months to 1 year after aortic valve replacement the heart size has diminished, hypertrophy has regressed,[85,89,90] and left ventricular function has returned to normal.[89,90] However, when there is more marked cardiomegaly and left ventricular function is moderately impaired (ejection fraction is 25 to 40 percent) there is less improvement, and in some patients left ventricular function remains abnormal in the postoperative period.[91,92] It would clearly be desirable to avoid the latter occurrence, and there is a growing tendency to consider operation even in patients with relatively few symptoms if there is evidence of considerable left ventricular dysfunction or progression toward given limits on echocardiography.[90,92,93] These limits may be summarized in general as follows: if the left ventricular end-diastolic diameter in severe aortic regurgitation approaches 75 mm, the end-systolic diameter is 55 mm or greater, the fractional shortening falls below 25 percent, the calculated ejection fraction falls below 40 percent, and the ratio of ventricular radius to wall thickness exceeds 3.8,[93] confirmation of these findings by cardiac catheterization[68] and consideration of operation are advisable.

At cardiac catheterization in aortic regurgitation, the possibility of detecting myocardial dysfunction by infusion of a vasopressor agent has been explored.[94] A fall in forward stroke volume during this stress in the face of a rise in end-diastolic pressure has been considered to indicate depression of myocardial contractility, but the role of increased valvular regurgitation in the face of enhanced systemic arterial pressure, the importance of the pericardium in contributing to elevated filling pressures in this setting, and the possibility of limited preload reserve with acute afterload mismatch during the stress may prohibit direct determination of whether or not myocardial contractility is chronically depressed. Moreover, the status of left ventricular function after valve replacement in patients with abnormal responses to pressor stress have not yet been reported. The significance of a fall in the radionuclide ejection fraction during exercise[73] in some patients also deserves further study.

Mitral Regurgitation

In the asymptomatic patient with clinical evidence of only moderate chronic mitral regurgitation (Chap. 39) and in whom the left ventricle is only mildly enlarged based on physical examination and the chest roentgenogram, relatively infrequent examinations are required. If the patient has severe symptoms of left ventricular failure that are refractory to medical treatment, cardiac catheterization should be carried out to confirm the severity of the regurgitation, to determine the degree of left ventricular dysfunction, and to assess whether or not associated disease of other valves or the coronary arteries is contributory. In such patients, if left ventricular function is normal or only mildly depressed, replacement or surgical repair of the mitral valve is usually undertaken.

In the relatively asymptomatic patient with severe mitral regurgitation, the possibility of developing "silent" irreversible myocardial dysfunction poses an important problem. As discussed earlier, mitral regurgitation places relatively favorable systolic loading conditions on the left ventricle, and eccentric hypertrophy coupled with low wall stress due to the low-impedance leak early and late in systole allows maintenance of a high normal ejection fraction when contractility is normal (Fig. 18-4A). Even when contractility is depressed, a relatively normal ejection fraction can be maintained (Fig. 18-4B), although mean V_{CF} is sometimes reduced.[95] Thus, if significant cardiomegaly is seen on the chest roentgenogram or found on physical examination in such patients, a base-line M-mode echocardiographic study should be obtained. It may also be advisable to confirm the M-mode echocardiographic study by a two-dimensional echocardiogram or by a radionuclide ejection fraction determination, particularly if associated coronary disease with wall motion abnormality is suspected.

In contrast to aortic regurgitation, studies before and after mitral valve replacement indicate that left ventricular function tends to be somewhat reduced following operation even if it was within the normal range preoperatively,[22] but when cardiomegaly is moderate, there is nevertheless a progressive reduction in ventricular size and mass after valve replacement.[22] However, when there was a marked increase in left ventricular size preoperatively, even if the ejection fraction was low normal, ventricular function deteriorated further at 6 months to 1 year following mitral valve repair or replacement and ventricular hypertrophy and dilatation failed to regress.[22] The marked fall in the ejection fraction following valve replacement in the latter patients suggests that the ejection fraction was maintained at

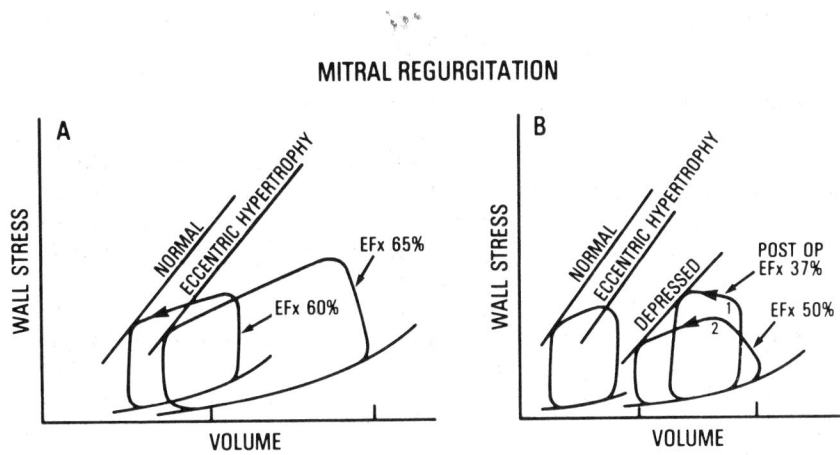

MITRAL REGURGITATION

FIGURE 18-4 Diagrammatic representation of left ventricular function in mitral regurgitation. *A.* Volume overload hypertrophy (eccentric hypertrophy) causes a displacement of the loop of left ventricular contraction (volume versus wall stress) well to the right of normal, and with normal contractility both the curved diastolic relation and the linear end-systolic volume–wall stress relation are shifted to the right. Because of the low-impedance leak into the left atrium, the ejection fraction can be maintained at a high-normal level (65 percent). *B.* The development of depressed myocardial function shifts the linear end-systolic volume–wall stress relation to the right. In this setting, prior to mitral valve replacement, the ventricle can still maintain a relatively low average wall stress during ejection because of the regurgitant leak, and therefore the ejection fraction is only mildly reduced (beat 2). Following mitral valve replacement, despite some reduction in end-diastolic volume, the ventricle must now face the higher impedance of the aorta, the wall stress throughout ejection rises substantially, and the ejection falls (beat 1).

an artificially high value preoperatively, despite depression of myocardial function (Fig. 18-4*B*). Following correction of the low-impedance leak, the depression of ventricular function then became manifest, since all of the ventricular ejection was now into the relatively high impedance of the aorta, and the ejection fraction fell (Fig. 18-4*B*). Additional studies are needed to confirm these findings.

In the follow-up of the patient with severe mitral regurgitation who has cardiomegaly but relatively few symptoms, serial echocardiographic studies should be performed annually. If on initial or serial studies the left ventricular end-diastolic diameter approaches 8.0 cm, the end-systolic diameter exceeds 5.0 cm, the fractional shortening falls below 30 percent, or the calculated ejection fraction drops below 55 percent, cardiac catheterization should be undertaken to confirm the degree of mitral regurgitation and the status of left ventricular function.[22] If the echocardiographic findings are confirmed, operative intervention to protect myocardial function should then be considered.[80a] However, in contrast to aortic valve disease, since severe further deterioration of ventricular function can occur postoperatively in patients with depressed left ventricular function, it is probably not advisable to recommend operation if the ejection fraction is markedly reduced.

Recognition of Myocardial Depression Following Heart Surgery

Signs of left or right ventricular failure in the early or late postoperative period after aortic or mitral valve replacement can be due to irreversible myocardial disease existing preoperatively. Occasionally,

it is due to intraoperative myocardial infarction or damage due to inadequate myocardial preservation of the hypertrophied heart, although the advent of hypothermic cardioplegia has made this occurrence less common.[96] Heart failure in this setting can also be due to a paravalvular leak causing severe valvular regurgitation,[97] or to prosthetic valve dysfunction due to clotting or fibrosis[97a] producing obstruction or regurgitation.

It is very important to identify a mechanical cause of the heart failure, if present, so that reoperation can be considered. However, in the postoperative setting physical findings are often not definitive; for example, a severe paravalvular leak around a prosthetic mitral valve can occur with little or no systolic murmur.[97] Echocardiography may be useful for detecting severe left ventricular dysfunction, and radionuclide techniques may also reveal a depressed ejection fraction, but these approaches are less satisfactory for excluding a mechanical abnormality of the prosthetic valve. Therefore, it is usually advisable to proceed promptly with diagnostic cardiac catherization and ventriculography, together with coronary arteriography, to definitively establish the cause of postoperative heart failure.

Recognition and Evaluation of Primary Myocardial Disease

In suspected myocardial disease, the initial goal should be to establish, by the simplest possible methods, whether or not myocardial dysfunction is present. The physiological pattern of the disease and its cause should then be sought, although complete information may not be necessary to decide upon appropriate treatment.

Is Myocardial Disease Present?

The most useful and inexpensive initial screening test is the M-mode echocardiogram, supplemented if necessary by a two-dimensional study. If these are technically unsatisfactory, or inconclusive, a radionuclide angiogram can be performed.

If the left ventricular end-diastolic chamber diameter is increased on the echocardiogram without a significant increase in wall thickness and the fractional shortening or calculated ejection fraction is reduced (Fig. 18-3), it is likely that a cardiomyopathy (or myocarditis) of the dilated type is present (see Chap. 56); the right ventricular internal diameter may also be increased in this condition. This diagnosis is particularly likely in the absence of a heart murmur, hypertension, or other cause for secondary ventricular enlargement and dysfunction. Identification of a depressed ejection fraction of either the left or right sides of the heart also may be established by radionuclide angiography, and this approach can sometimes clarify equivocal changes on echocardiography.

In some endurance-trained athletes, the internal chamber diameter of the right or left ventricle, or both, may be abnormally large and associated with electrocardiographic evidence of ventricular hypertrophy. However, measures of systolic contractile function (fractional shortening, calculated ejection fraction, and V_{CF}) are normal in such individuals.[98–100]

If the echocardiogram shows an abnormally thickened left ventricular wall, but the end-diastolic chamber diameter and systolic function are normal, hypertrophic cardiomyopathy is likely, provided hypertension or aortic stenosis are absent (Chap. 56). The echocardiogram will usually allow further differentiation into the symmetric or asymmetric type of hypertrophy, and if systolic anterior motion of the mitral valve is associated with a heart murmur, subaortic hypertrophic obstruction to left ventricular outflow should be considered. If there is a significantly reduced EF slope of an otherwise normal mitral valve, together with significant left atrial enlargement, a restrictive pathophysiology of the hypertrophic cardiomyopathy is suggested. Echocardiography may also detect a thickened pericardium or pericardial effusion, valvular abnormalities, or unexpected wall motion disorders.

Occasionally, in detecting subtle forms of myocardial dysfunction, the use of handgrip or pressor stress during echocardiography may be useful in revealing an abnormal decrease in fractional shortening,[50] and in some patients with cardiomyopathy radionuclide angiography during excerise can produce an abnormal decrease in the ejection fraction, even when coronary heart disease is absent.[73] Thus, for simply establishing the presence or absence of significant myocardial disease, cardiac catheterization is rarely necessary.

When Should Cardiac Catheterization Be Done?

Whenever the patient with myocardial disease is refractory to therapy or there is a deteriorating clinical course, a pathophysiological diagnosis which is as complete as possible should be reached by cardiac catheterization. When diagnostic cardiac catheterization is undertaken, catheterization of both the right and left sides of the heart, left ventriculography, and coronary arteriography should generally be done since, even if a specific etiology is not identified, such studies often assist in management. In a few patients, endomyocardial biopsy of either the right or the left ventricles may be performed to search for a specific diagnosis, such as an infiltrative process or the endomyocardial type of idiopathic cardiomyopathy.[80]

One major goal of the cardiac catheterization study is to exclude the presence of surgically treatable disease, such as unsuspected congenital heart disease with a left-to-right shunt (atrial septal defect is often missed clinically), unexpectedly severe valvular aortic stenosis or mitral regurgitation, an obstructive component of hypertrophic cardiomyopathy, constrictive pericarditis, or a significant contribution from unsuspected coronary atherosclerosis. Another major goal is to establish the pathophysiological pattern of the myocardial disease in order to allow more rational selection of therapy. Basically, there are three patterns: the congestive, restrictive, and obstructive types; several of these patterns may coexist (Chap. 56). The congestive type is most common, and the pure restrictive type is quite rare. A restrictive pattern can be mimicked by constrictive pericarditis, and the latter condition should be carefully excluded (Chap. 56).[16]

Selective ventriculography and analysis of pressure tracings from the right and left ventricles and atria will generally establish whether the disorder is primarily due to congestive cardiomyopathy with dilatation of the chambers, wall thinning, and reduced systolic function, or to restrictive disease. In the latter condition, the chamber size and systolic function may be normal, although this is not always the case.[20,100a] There may be a thickened left ventricular wall, and there is evidence of reduced ventricular diastolic compliance with impaired filling of the left ventricle; characteristically, there is an early diastolic dip followed by a rapid rise and then a plateau of pressure during diastasis, a prominent *a* wave with an elevated end-diastolic pressure, and a delayed *y* descent on the pulmonary artery wedge pressure or left atrial tracing, indicating impaired atrial emptying into the diseased ventricle.[21,100a] The right ventricle may also exhibit these features. In congestive cardiomyopathy, typically these features are absent, although the ventricular end-diastolic pressure is usually elevated and the early diastolic pressure is also high. Thus, the dominant physiological pattern, congestive or restrictive, can usually be identified.[16] The pattern carries important implications for therapy since vigorous use of diuretics and positive inotropic stimuli are appropriate for the congestive pattern, whereas such therapy in the patient with restrictive pathophysiology can lead to decreased ventricular filling pressures and volumes, with further impairment of the filling of the stiffened ventricle, and a reduction of the cardiac output.[21] Likewise, afterload reduction therapy by vasodilators is more appropriate in the congestive setting, since in restrictive cardiomyopathy ventricular systolic emptying may already be near maximum; venodilator properties of these agents may also lead to reduced diastolic filling in the restrictive setting.

The restrictive type of pathophysiology may blend with that due to outflow tract obstruction in hypertrophic cardiomyopathy, and surgical relief of a severe resting outflow gradient identified at cardiac catheterization may become necessary in some patients who are refractory to medical therapy.[101] Also, there is now evidence that calcium antagonists (such as verapamil) may be effective in relieving obstruction in hypertrophic obstructive cardiomyopathy, and they may alter the diastolic properties of the hypertrophied ventricle is well.[102]

Coronary arteriography should accompany diagnostic studies to exclude the possibility of silent ischemia in the patient with cardiomyopathy. Thus, ischemic cardiomyopathy sometimes cannot be distinguished from other types of cardiomyopathy without such studies, as discussed further below.

There are some settings in which limited cardiac catheterization should be considered. In the patient with established myocardial disease associated with heart failure that is refractory to treatment, if vasodilator therapy is being considered it may be advisable to undertake balloon catheterization of the right side of the heart in order to characterize the hemodynamic setting. Moreover, serial measurements following single oral doses of the proposed therapeutic regimen (e.g., a balanced arteriolar dilator and venodilator such as prazosin, a venodilator such as isosorbide dinitrate, or combination therapy with isosorbide dinitrate and the arteriolar dilator hydralazine) can allow selection of the most appropriate drugs.[79] Alternatively, the finding of an unexpectedly low cardiac filling pressure with a normal cardiac output, together with lack of response to a therapeutic test, may contraindicate the use of chronic vasodilator therapy.

Recognition and Evaluation of Ischemic Myocardial Dysfunction

Ischemic Cardiomyopathy
In the patient with cardiomyopathy, the clinical symptoms and the electrocardiogram may not suggest prior myocardial infarction or recurrent ischemia, yet coronary heart disease is occasionally the underlying process.[65,103,104] In some patients, attacks of dyspnea without pain or atypical pain may reflect recurrent myocardial ischemia or subendocardial infarction, and "silent" ischemia is being recognized with increasing frequency[105] even in the absence of diabetes mellitus, which is known to be associated with silent ischemia and infarction.[106]

The finding of coronary artery calcification on image-intensification fluoroscopy may be very helpful in suggesting the diagnosis, and among a group of younger patients with cardiomyopathy those shown on coronary arteriography to have an ischemic type invariably showed calcification of either two or three coronary arteries.[65] Thallium perfusion imaging during and after exercise may also indicate the presence of myocardial scar at rest, or show transient exercise-induced perfusion defects. Generally, however, if this diagnosis is suspected, cardiac catheterization with coronary arteriography will be required to fully characterize the degree of coronary atherosclerosis. In the more typical patient with "ischemic cardiomyopathy," a clear history of several previous myocardial infarctions and angina pectoris will be obtained. Such patients should usually undergo cardiac catheterization as well, even if heart failure without angina pectoris is the presenting picture, since myocardial revascularization has resulted in improvement of dyspnea and heart failure, or transient attacks of myocardial ischemia, in a few patients with ischemic cardiomyopathy.[107] Generally, however, the surgical results have not been satisfactory.[108]

In the patient with established coronary heart disease who has angina pectoris and cardiomegaly, noninvasive studies of left ventricular size and function may be important in selecting medical therapy. For example, if there is left ventricular enlargement, the use of propranolol combined with digoxin may reduce heart size and diminish the severity of anginal attacks.[109]

Ventricular Aneurysm
Sometimes, heart failure or low cardiac output due to a left ventricular aneurysm is suggested by the electrocardiogram, or the chest roentgenogram. The M-mode echocardiogram may exhibit relatively normal septal and posterior wall systolic shortening in the presence of an apical aneurysm, but the use of two-dimensional echocardiography has proved much more reliable in detecting the presence of an aneurysm.[110] The radionuclide angiogram is also useful for this purpose.[110a] If a ventricular aneurysm is seriously suspected in a patient who has significant symptoms due to heart failure, cardiac catheterization should be carried out to define the extent of the aneurysm and to assess the degree of coronary artery disease prior to considering corrective operation (Chap. 45).

Regional Left Ventricular Dysfunction and Its Reversibility
It has been established in experimental animals that transient ischemia during exercise produces regional myocardial dysfunction which impairs overall cardiac function,[111,112] and in patients with coronary heart disease the ejection fraction falls during exercise-induced ischemia.[72,73,113] Therefore, the assessment of regional left ventricular function and the detection of abnormal myocardial perfusion by

noninvasive techniques during exercise stress has become important in detecting the presence of latent coronary stenosis and in evaluating the patient with chest pain (Chaps. 45, 87, and 95).

When there are signs or symptoms of persistent left ventricular dysfunction in the resting state, the degree to which dysfunction is due to coronary atherosclerosis with previous myocardial infarction or to potentially reversible sustained ischemic dysfunction continues to constitute an important and difficult question. In general, the ejection fraction has been useful for detecting global left ventricular dysfunction in coronary heart disease, and this can be determined noninvasively by radionuclide ventriculography[51] or by special two-dimensional echocardiographic studies.[70] Regional wall motion abnormalities at rest can also be identified by both of these techniques. Some studies suggest that analysis of the first one-third of systole may improve the sensitivity of the ejection fraction for detecting left ventricular dysfunction in coronary heart disease,[113a] and this approach is also feasible using radionuclide ventriculography.[113b] In the patient who is found to have persistent regional or global myocardial dysfunction at rest by noninvasive studies or as determined by left ventriculography, operation not only for the relief of angina pectoris but also for a possible beneficial effect on ventricular function must be considered.

Studies at about 6 months following myocardial revascularization indicate that many zones of regional dysfunction fail to show improvement after operation, some exhibit enhanced shortening, and a few show decreased function. Although average ventricular function (as assessed by the ejection fraction) usually does not change significantly following myocardial revascularization,[114–119] some more recent studies do show overall improvement.[119a] There appears to be a correlation between the adequacy of revascularization and recovery of resting function[114,116] and improvement of the ejection fraction during exercise.[119] In some patients with unstable angina pectoris without infarction, marked improvement in regional wall motion and the ejection fraction has been noted within 2 weeks of operation, even when extensive regional wall motion abnormalities existed preoperatively.[120]

There is some experimental and clinical evidence suggesting that it may be possible to identify preoperatively those zones which will show improvement following coronary artery bypass operations.[121–126] In the experimental setting, the administration of nitroglycerin or postextrasystolic potentiation[121,122] results in improved regional systolic shortening in zones that are hypokinetic due to ischemia or partial scar; such regions tend to be on the border zone between an area of severe ischemia or scar and normal regions, but whether the response is due to potentiation of a population of myocardial cells which are partially ischemic or to an admixture of fully ischemic or scarred cells and nor-

mal cells (only the normal cells being potentiated) is unclear. Nevertheless, regions which are fully ischemic acutely and which exhibit holosystolic expansion do not tend to show increased function with nitroglycerin or postextrasystolic potentiation.

Myocardial biopsies taken at the time of operation in patients with coronary heart disease indicate that regions which showed improved wall motion following nitroglycerin at preoperative study exhibit only a small amount of scar, and such regions may show improved function on later ventriculographic studies.[127] Whether or not such improved function several months after operation reflects correction of "chronic ischemia," as may be seen in patients with the unstable anginal syndromes, or whether improved regional oxygen supply/demand relations due to the revascularization allow compensatory hypertrophy of adjacent regions of myocardium, or both,[128] remains to be established.

References

1. Harvey, R. M., Ferrer, M. I., Samet, P., Bader, R. A., Bader, M. E., Cournand, A., and Richards, D. W.: Mechanical and Myocardial Factors in Rheumatic Heart Disease with Mitral Stenosis, *Circulation*, 11:531, 1955.
2. Ross, J., Jr., Gault, J. H., Mason, D. T., Linhart, J. W., and Braunwald, E.: Left Ventricular Performance during Muscular Exercise in Patients with and without Cardiac Dysfunction, *Circulation*, 34:597, 1966.
3. Bruce, R. A.: Exercise Testing for Evaluation of Ventricular Function, *N. Engl. J. Med.*, 296:671, 1977.
4. Benge, W., Litchfield, R. L., and Marcus, M. L.: Exercise Capacity in Patients with Severe Left Ventricular Dysfunction, *Circulation*, 61:955, 1980.
5. Braunwald, E., Ross, J., Jr., and Sonnenblick, E. H.: "Mechanisms of Contraction of the Normal and Failing Heart," 2d ed., Little, Brown and Company, Boston, 1976.
6. Karliner, J. S., Peterson, K. L., and Ross, J., Jr.: Left Ventricular Myocardial Mechanics: Assessment of Isovolumic and Ejection Phase Indices of Performance and Diastolic Indices of Distensibility, in W. Grossman (ed.), "Cardiac Catheterization and Angiography," 2d ed., Lea & Febiger, Philadelphia, in press.
7. Ross, J., Jr.: The Assessment of Myocardial Performance in Man by Hemodynamic and Cineangiographic Techniques, *Am. J. Cardiol.*, 23:511, 1969.
8. Ross, J., Jr., and Peterson, K. L.: On the Assessment of Cardiac Inotropic State: An Editorial, *Circulation*, 47:435, 1973.
9. Braunwald, E., and Ross, J., Jr.: Control of Cardiac Performance, in R. M. Berne, N. Sperelakis, and S. R. Geiger (eds.), "Handbook of Physiology," Waverly Press, Inc., Baltimore, 1979, p. 533.
10. Ross, J., Jr.: Afterload Mismatch and Preload Reserve: A Conceptual Framework for the Analysis of Ventricular Function, *Prog. Cardiovasc. Dis.*, 18:255, 1976.

11. Ross, J., Jr., Covell, J. W., Sonnenblick, E. H., and Braunwald, E.: Contractile State of the Heart Characterized by Force-Velocity Relations in Variably Afterloaded and Isovolumic Beats, *Circ. Res.*, 18:149, 1966.

12. MacGregor, D. C., Covell, J. W., Mahler, F., Dilley, R. B., and Ross, J., Jr.: Relations between Afterload, Stroke Volume, and Descending Limb of Starling's Curve, *Am. J. Physiol.*, 227:884, 1974.

13. Ross, J., Jr.: Adaptation of the Left Ventricle to Chronic Volume Overload, *Circ. Res.*, 35(suppl. 2):64, 1974.

14. Sasayama, S., Ross, J., Jr., Franklin, D., Bloor, C. M., Bishop, S., and Dilley, R. B.: Adaptations of the Left Ventricle to Chronic Pressure Overload, *Circ. Res.*, 38:172, 1976.

*15. Ross, J., Jr.: Pathophysiology of the Human Heart: Function of the Heart under Abnormal Loading Conditions, in H. P. Krayenbuehl and W. Kuebler (eds.), "Kardiologie in Klinik und Praxis," Georg Thieme Verlag, Stuttgart, in press. (70 references)

*16. Shabetai, R., Mangiardi, L., Bhargava, V., Ross, J., Jr., and Higgins, C. B.: The Pericardium and Cardiac Function, *Prog. Cardiovasc. Dis.*, 22:107, 1979. (128 references)

17. Shirato, K., Shabetai, R., Bhargava, V., Franklin, D., and Ross, J., Jr.: Alteration of the Left Ventricular Diastolic Pressure-Segment Relation Produced by the Pericardium: Effects of Cardiac Distension and Afterload Reduction in Conscious Dogs, *Circulation*, 57:1191, 1978.

18. Stokland, O., Miller, M. M., Lekven, J., and Ilebekk, A.: The Significance of the Intact Pericardium for Cardiac Performance in the Dog, *Circ. Res.*, 47:27, 1980.

19. Alderman, E. L., and Glantz, S. A.: Acute Hemodynamic Interventions Shift the Diastolic Pressure-Volume Curve in Man, *Circulation*, 54:662, 1976.

19a. Glantz, S. A., Misbach, G. A., Moores, W. Y., Mathey, D. G., Lekven, J., Stowe, D. F., Parmley, W. W., and Tyberg, J. V.: The Pericardium Substantially Affects the Left Ventricular Diastolic Pressure-Volume Relationship in the Dog, *Circ. Res.*, 42:443, 1978.

20. Brodie, B. R., Gross, W., Mann, T., and McLaurin, L. P.: Effects of Sodium Nitroprusside on Left Ventricular Diastolic Pressure-Volume Relations, *J. Clin. Invest.*, 59:59, 1977.

21. Meaney, E., Shabetai, R., Bhargava, V., Shearer, M., Weidner, C., Mangiardi, L., Smalling, R., and Peterson, K.: Cardiac Amyloidosis, Constrictive Pericarditis and Restrictive Cardiomyopathy, *Am. J. Cardiol.*, 38:547, 1976.

22. Schuler, G., Peterson, K., Johnson, A., Francis, G., Dennish, G., Utley, J., Daily, P., Ashburn, W., and Ross, J., Jr.: Temporal Response of Left Ventricular Performance to Mitral Valve Surgery, *Circulation*, 59:1218, 1979.

23. Franciosa, J. A., and Cohn, J. N.: Hemodynamic Responsiveness to Short and Long Acting Vasodilators in Left Ventricular Failure, *Am. J. Med.*, 65:126, 1978.

*24. Ross, J., Jr.: Role of Vasodilator Therapy, in J. Karliner and G. Gregoratos (eds.), "Coronary Care," Churchill Livingstone Publishers, New York, 1980. (69 references)

25. Pouleur, H., Covell, J. W., and Ross, J., Jr.: Effects of Alterations in Aortic Input Impedance on the Force-Velocity-Length Relationship in the Intact Canine Heart, *Circ. Res.*, 45:126, 1979.

26. Pouleur, H., Covell, J. W., and Ross, J., Jr.: Effects of Nitroprusside on Venous Return and Central Blood Volume in the Absence and Presence of Acute Heart Failure, *Circulation*, 61:328, 1980.

27. Ross, J., Jr., and Braunwald, E.: The Study of Left Ventricular Function in Man by Increasing Resistance to Ventricular Ejection with Angiotensin, *Circulation*, 29:739, 1964.

28. Sarnoff, S. J., and Mitchell, J. H.: Control of Function of Heart, in W. F. Hamilton and P. Dow (eds.), "Handbook of Physiology," American Physiological Society, Washington, 1962, p. 489.

28a. Sonnenblick, E. H., and Downing, S. E.: Afterload as a Primary Determinant of Ventricular Performance, *Am. J. Physiol.*, 204:604, 1963.

29. Braunwald, E., and Ross, J., Jr.: Editorial. The Ventricular End-Diastolic Pressure: An Appraisal of Its Value in the Recognition of Ventricular Failure in Man, *Am. J. Med.*, 34:147, 1963.

30. Rackley, C. E., Dalldorf, F. G., Hood, W. P., Jr., and Wilcox, B. R.: Sarcomere Length and Left Ventricular Function in Chronic Heart Disease, *Am. J. Med. Sci.*, 259:90, 1970.

31. Dodge, H. T., and Tanenbaum, H. L.: Left Ventricular Volume in Normal Man and Alterations with Disease, *Circulation*, 14:927, 1956.

32. Kennedy, J. W., Baxley, W. A., Figley, M. M., Dodge, H. T., and Blackmon, J. R.: Quantitative Angiocardiography. I. The Normal Left Ventricle in Man, *Circulation*, 34:272, 1966.

33. Kivowitz, C., Parmley, W. W., Donoso, R., Marcus, H., Ganz, W., Swan, H. J. C.: Effects of Isometric Exercise on Cardiac Performance: The Grip Test, *Circulation*, 44:994, 1971.

34. Helfant, R. H., deVilla, M., and Meister, S. G.: Effect of Sustained Isometric Handgrip Exercise on Left Ventricular Performance, *Circulation*, 44:982, 1971.

35. Raphael, L. D., Mantle, J. A., Moraski, R. E., Rogers, W. J., Russell, R. O., and Rackley, C. E.: Quantitative Assessment of Ventricular Performance in Unstable Ischemic Heart Disease by Dextran Function Curves, *Circulation*, 55:858, 1977.

36. Dodge, H. T., and Baxley, W. A.: Left Ventricular Volume and Mass and Their Significance in Heart Disease, *Am. J. Cardiol.*, 23:528, 1969.

37. Ross, J., Jr., Sonnenblick, E. H., Taylor, R. R., Spotnitz, H. M., and Covell, J. W.: Diastolic Geometry and Sarcomere Lengths in the Chronically Dilated Canine Left Ventricle, *Circ. Res.*, 28:49, 1971.

38. Wolk, M. J., Keefe, J. F., Bing, O. H. L., Finkelstein, L. J., and Levine, H. J.: Estimation of V_{max} in Auxotonic Systoles from the Rate of Relative Increase of Isovolumic (dP/dt)dP, *J. Clin. Invest.*, 50:1276, 1971.

39. Mirsky, I., and Parmley, W. W.: Force-Velocity Studies in Isolated and Intact Heart Muscle, in I. Mirsky, D. N. Ghista, and H. Sandler (eds.), "Cardiac Mechanics: Physiological, Clinical, and Math-

*This article is a review of the literature and contains additional references to the literature.

ematical Considerations," John Wiley & Sons, Inc., New York, 1974, p. 87.

40. Nejad, N. S., Klein, M. D., Mirsky, E., and Lown, B.: Assessment of Myocardial Contractility from Ventricular Pressure Recordings, *Cardiovasc. Res.,* 5:15, 1971.

41. Mehmel, H., Krayenbuehl, H., and Rutishauser, W.: Peak Measured Velocity of Shortening in the Canine Left Ventricle, *J. Appl. Physiol.,* 29:637, 1970.

42. Grossman, W., Haynes, F., Paraskos, J. A., Saltz, S., Dalen, J. E., and Dexter, L.: Alterations in Preload and Myocardial Mechanics in the Dog and in Man, *Circ. Res.,* 31:83, 1972.

43. Mahler, F., Covell, J. W., O'Rourke, R. A., and Ross, J., Jr.: Effects of Acute Changes in Loading and Inotropic State on Left Ventricular Performance and Contractility Measures in the Conscious Dog, *Am. J. Cardiol.,* 35:626, 1975.

44. Peterson, K. L., Sklovan, D., Ludbrook, P., Uther, J. B., and Ross, J., Jr.: Comparison of Isovolumetric and Ejection Phase Indices of Myocardial Performance in Man, *Circulation,* 49:1088, 1974.

45. Kreulen, T., Bove, A. A., McDonough, M. T., Sands, M. J., and Spann, J. F.: The Evaluation of Left Ventricular Function in Man: A Comparison of Methods, *Circulation,* 51:677, 1975.

46. Ross, J., Jr., and Sobel, B. E.: Regulation of Cardiac Contraction, *Ann. Rev. Physiol.,* 34:47, 1972.

47. Hirshleifer, J., Crawford, M., O'Rourke, R. A., and Karliner, J. S.: Influence of Acute Alterations in Heart Rate and Systemic Arterial Pressure on Echocardiographic Measures of Left Ventricular Performance in Normal Human Subjects, *Circulation,* 52:835, 1975.

48. Gault, J. H., Ross, J., Jr., and Braunwald, E.: Contractile State of the Left Ventricle in Man: Instantaneous Tension-Velocity-Length Relations in Patients with and without Disease of the Left Ventricular Myocardium, *Circ. Res.,* 22:451, 1968.

49. Karliner, J. S., Gault, J. H., Eckberg, D. L., Mullins, C. B., and Ross, J., Jr.: Mean Velocity of Fiber Shortening: A Simplified Measure of Left Ventricular Myocardial Contractility, *Circulation,* 44:323, 1971.

*50. Mason, S. J., and Fortuin, N. J.: The Use of Echocardiography for Quantitative Evaluation of Left Ventricular Function, *Prog. Cardiovasc. Dis.,* 21:119, 1978. (78 references)

*51. Ashburn, W. L., Schelbert, H. R., and Verba, J. W.: Left Ventricular Ejection Fraction—A Review of Several Radionuclide Angiographic Approaches Using the Scintillation Camera, *Prog. Cardiovasc. Dis.,* 20:267, 1978. (54 references)

52. Bommer, W., Weinert, L., Neumann, A., Neef, J., Mason, D. T., and DeMaria, A.: Determination of Right Atrial and Right Ventricular Size by Two-Dimensional Echocardiography, *Circulation,* 60:91, 1979.

53. Maddahi, J., Berman, D. S., Matsuoka, D. T., Waxman, A. D., Stankus, K. E., Forrester, J. S., and Swan, H. J. C.: A New Technique for Assessing Right Ventricular Ejection Fraction Using Rapid Multiple-Gated Equilibrium Cardiac Blood Pool Scintigraphy: Description, Validation and Findings in Chronic Coronary Disease, *Circulation,* 60:581, 1979.

54. Johnson, L. L., McCarthy, D. M., Sciacca, R. R., and Cannon, P. J.: Right Ventricular Ejection Fraction during Exercise in Patients with Coronary Artery Disease, *Circulation,* 60:1284, 1979.

55. Berger, H. J., Johnstone, D. E., Sands, J. M., Gottschalk, A., and Zaret, B. L.: Response of Right Ventricular Ejection Fraction to Upright Bicycle Exercise in Coronary Artery Disease, *Circulation,* 60:1292, 1979.

56. Suga, H., Sagawa, K., and Shoukas, A. A.: Load Independence of the Instantaneous Pressure-Volume Ratio of the Canine Left Ventricle and Effects of Epinephrine and Heart Rate on the Ratio, *Circ. Res.,* 32:314, 1973.

*57. Sagawa, K.: The Ventricular Pressure-Volume Diagram Revisited, *Circ. Res.,* 43:677, 1978. (63 references)

58. Suga, H., Yamakoshi, K.: Effects of Stroke Volume and Velocity of Ejection on End-Systolic Pressure of Canine Left Ventricle. End-Systolic Volume Clamping, *Circ. Res.,* 40:445, 1977.

59. Mahler, F., Covell, J. W., and Ross, J., Jr.: Systolic Pressure-Diameter Relations in the Normal Conscious Dog, *Cardiovasc. Res.,* 9:447, 1975.

60. Grossman, W., Braunwald, E., Mann, T., McLaurin, L. P., and Green, L. H.: Contractile State of the Left Ventricle in Man as Evaluated from End-Systolic Pressure-Volume Relations, *Circulation,* 56:845, 1977.

61. Takahashi, M., Sasayama, S., Kawai, C., and Kotoura, H.: Contractile Performance of the Hypertrophied Ventricle in Patients with Systemic Hypertension, *Circulation,* 62:116, 1980.

62. Taylor, R. R., Covell, J. W., and Ross, J., Jr.: Volume-Tension Diagrams of Ejection and Isovolumic Contractions in Left Ventricle, *Am. J. Physiol.,* 216:1097, 1969.

63. Sasayama, S., Franklin, D., and Ross, J., Jr.: Hyperfunction with Normal Inotropic State of the Hypertrophied Left Ventricle, *Am. J. Physiol.,* 232(4):H418, 1977.

64. Johnson, A. D., Laiken, S. L., and Shabetai, R.: Noninvasive Diagnosis of Ischemic Cardiomyopathy by Fluoroscopic Detection of Coronary Artery Calcification, *Am. Heart J.,* 96:521, 1978.

65. Crawford, M. H., Grant, D., O'Rourke, R. A., Starling, M. R., and Groves, B. M.: Accuracy and Reproducibility of New M-Mode Echocardiographic Recommendations for Measuring Left Ventricular Dimensions, *Circulation,* 61:137, 1980.

66. Cooper, R. H., O'Rourke, R. A., Karliner, J. S., Peterson, K. L., and Leopold, G. R.: Comparison of Ultrasound and Cineangiographic Measurements of the Mean Rate of Circumferential Fiber Shortening in Man, *Circulation,* 46:914, 1972.

67. Wann, L. S., Faris, J. V., Childress, R. H., Dillon, J. C., Weyman, A. E., and Feigenbaum, H.: Exercise Cross-Sectional Echocardiography in Ischemic Heart Disease, *Circulation,* 60:1300, 1979.

68. Abdulla, A. M., Frank, M. J., Canedo, M. I., and Stafadouros, M. A.: Limitations of Echocardiography in the Assessment of Left Ventricular Size and Function in Aortic Regurgitation, *Circulation,* 61:148, 1980.

69. Teichholz, L. E., Kreulen, T., Herman, M. V., and Gorlin, R.: Problems in Echocardiographic Volume Determinations: Echocardiographic-Angio-

graphic Correlations in the Presence or Absence of Asynergy, *Am. J. Cardiol.,* 37:7, 1976.

70. Schiller, N. B., Acquatella, H., Ports, T. A., Drew, D., Goerke, J., Ringertz, H., Silverman, N. H., Brundage, B., Botvinick, E. H., Boswell, R., Carlsson, E., and Parmley, W. W.: Left Ventricular Volume from Paired Biplane Two-Dimensional Echocardiography, *Circulation,* 60:547, 1979.

71. Slutsky, R., Karliner, J., Ricci, D., Kaiser, R., Pfisterer, M., Gordon, D., Peterson, K., and Ashburn, W.: Left Ventricular Volumes by Gated Equilibrium Radionuclide Angiography: A New Method, *Circulation,* 61:556, 1980.

72. Borer, J., Bachrach, S. L., and Green, M. V.: Real-Time Radionuclide Cineangiography in the Noninvasive Evaluation of Global and Regional Left Ventricular Function at Rest and during Exercise in Patients with Coronary Artery Disease, *N. Engl. J. Med.,* 296:839, 1977.

*73. Bodenheimer, M. M., Banka, V. S., and Helfant, R. H.: Nuclear Cardiology. I. Radionuclide Angiographic Assessment of Left Ventricular Contraction: Uses, Limitations and Future Directions, *Am. J. Cardiol.,* 45:661, 1980. (81 references)

74. Tobinick, E. H., Schelbert, R., Henning, H., LeWinter, M., Taylor, A., Ashburn, W. L., and Karliner, J. S.: Right Ventricular Ejection Fraction in Patients with Acute Anterior and Inferior Myocardial Infarction Assessed by Radionuclide Angiography, *Circulation,* 57:1078, 1978.

75. Borer, J. S., Bachrach, S. L., Green, M. V., Kent, K. M., Henry, W. L., Rosing, D. R., Seides, S. F., Johnston, G. S., and Epstein, S. E.: Exercise-Induced Left Ventricular Dysfunction in Symptomatic and Asymptomatic Patients with Aortic Regurgitation: Assessment with Radionuclide Cineangiography, *Am. J. Cardiol.,* 42:351, 1978.

76. Slutsky, R., Karliner, J., Battler, A., Pfisterer, M., Swanson, S., and Ashburn, W.: Reproducibility of Ejection Fraction and Ventricular Volume by Gated Radionuclide Angiography after Myocardial Infarction, *Radiology,* 132:155, 1979.

77. Gillian, R. E., Parnes, W. P., Khan, M. A., Bouchard, R. J., and Warbasse, J. R.: The Prognostic Value of Systolic Time Intervals in Angina Pectoris Patients, *Circulation,* 60:268, 1979.

78. Garrard, C. L., Jr., Weissler, A. M., and Dodge, H. T.: Relationship of Alterations in Systolic Time Intervals to Ejection Fraction in Patients with Cardiac Disease, *Circulation,* 42:455, 1970.

*79. Chatterjee, K., and Parmley, W. W.: The Role of Vasodilator Therapy in Heart Failure, *Prog. Cardiovasc. Dis.,* 19:301, 1977. (133 references)

80. Olsen, E. G. J.: Endomyocardial Biopsy, *Br. Heart J.,* 40:95, 1978.

80a. Ross, J., Jr.: Left Ventricular Function and the Timing of Surgical Treatment in Valvular Heart Disease, *Ann. Int. Med.,* in press.

81. Ross, J., Jr., and Braunwald, E.: Aortic Stenosis, *Circulation,* 37(suppl. 5):61, 1968.

82. Tobin, J. R., Jr., Rahimtoola, S. H., Blundell, P. E., and Swan, H. J. C.: Percentage of Left Ventricular Stroke Work Loss, A Simple Hemodynamic Concept for Estimation of Severity in Valvular Aortic Stenosis, *Circulation,* 35:868, 1967.

83. Frank, S., Johnson, A., and Ross, J., Jr.: Natural History of Valvular Aortic Stenosis, *Br. Heart J.,* 35:41, 1973.

84. Kennedy, J. W., Doces, J., and Stewart, D. K.: Left Ventricular Function before and following Aortic Valve Replacement, *Circulation,* 56:944, 1977.

85. Pantely, G., Morton, M., and Rahimtoola, S. H.: Effects of Successful, Uncomplicated Valve Replacement on Ventricular Hypertrophy, Volume, and Performance in Aortic Stenosis and in Aortic Incompetence, *J. Thorac. Cardiovasc. Surg.,* 75:383, 1978.

85a. Henry, W. L., Bonow, R. O., Borer, J. S., Kent, K. M., Ware, J. H., Redwood, D. R., Itscoitz, S. B., McIntosh, C. L., Morrow, A. G., and Epstein, S. E.: Evaluation of Aortic Valve Replacement in Patients with Valvular Aortic Stenosis, *Circulation,* 61:814, 1980.

86. Smith, N., McAnulty, J. H., and Rahimtoola, S. H.: Severe Aortic Stenosis with Impaired Left Ventricular Function and Clinical Heart Failure, Results of Valve Replacement, *Circulation,* 58:255, 1978.

87. Gunther, S., and Grossman, W.: Determinants of Ventricular Function in Pressure-Overload Hypertrophy in Man, *Circulation,* 59:679, 1979.

87a. Peterson, K. L.: Instantaneous Force-Velocity-Length Relations of the Left Ventricle: Methods, Limitations, and Applications in Humans, in A. P. Fishman (ed.), "Heart Failure," Hemisphere Publishing Corporation, Washington, 1978.

88. Gault, J. H., Covell, J. W., Braunwald, E., and Ross, J., Jr.: Left Ventricular Performance Following Correction of Free Aortic Regurgitation, *Circulation,* 42:773, 1970.

89. Schwarz, F., Flameng, W., Thormann, J., Sesto, M., Langebartels, F., Hehrlein, F., and Schlepper, M.: Recovery from Myocardial Failure after Aortic Valve Replacement, *J. Thorac. Cardiovasc. Surg.,* 75:854, 1978.

90. Schuler, G., Peterson, K. L., Johnson, A. D., Francis, G., Ashburn, W., Dennish, G., Daily, P. O., and Ross, J., Jr.: Serial Non-invasive Assessment of Left Ventricular Hypertrophy and Function after Surgical Correction of Aortic Regurgitation, *Am. J. Cardiol.,* 44:585, 1979.

91. Clark, D. G., McAnulty, J. H., and Rahimtoola, S. H.: Valve Replacement in Aortic Insufficiency with Left Ventricular Dysfunction, *Circulation,* 61:411, 1980.

92. Henry, W. L., Bonow, R. O., Borer, J. S., Ware, J. H., Kent, K. M., Redwood, D. R., McIntosh, C. L., Morrow, A. G., and Epstein, S. E.: Observations on the Optimum Time for Operative Intervention for Aortic Regurgitation. I. Evaluation of the Results of Aortic Valve Replacement in Symptomatic Patients, *Circulation,* 61:471, 1980.

93. Gaasch, W. H., Andrias, C. W., and Levine, H. J.: The Effect of Aortic Valve Replacement on Left Ventricular Volume, Mass and Function, *Circulation,* 58:825, 1978.

94. Bolen, J. L., Holloway, E. L., Zener, J. C., Harrison, D. C., and Alderman, E. L.: Evaluation of Left Ventricular Function in Patients with Aortic Regurgitation Using Afterload Stress, *Circulation,* 53:132, 1976.

95. Eckberg, D. L., Gault, J. H., Bouchard, R. L., Karliner, J. S., and Ross, J., Jr.: Mechanics of Left

Ventricular Contraction in Chronic Severe Mitral Regurgitation, *Circulation*, 47:1252, 1973.

96. Ellis, R. J., Pryor, W., and Ebert, P. A.: Advantages of Potassium Cardioplegia and Perfusion Hypothermia in Left Ventricular Hypertrophy, *Ann. Thorac. Surg.*, 24:299, 1977.

97. Rockoff, S. D., Ross, J., Jr., Oldham, N. H., Mason, D. T., Morrow, A. G., and Braunwald, E.: Left Ventricular Performance during Muscular Exercise in Patients with and without Cardiac Dysfunction, *Circulation*, 34:597, 1966.

97a. Copans, H., Lakier, J. B., Kinsley, R. H., Colsen, P. R., Fritz, V. U., and Barlow, J. B.: Thrombosed Bjork-Shiley Mitral Prostheses, *Circulation*, 61:169, 1980.

98. Morganroth, J., Maron, B. J., Henry, W. L., and Epstein, S. E.: Comparative Left Ventricular Dimensions in Trained Athletes, *Ann. Intern. Med.*, 82:521, 1975.

99. Roeske, W. R., O'Rourke, R. A., Klein, A., Leopold, G., and Karliner, J. S.: Noninvasive Evaluation of Ventricular Hypertrophy in Professional Athletes, *Circulation*, 53:286, 1976.

100. Gilbert, C. A., Nutter, D. O., Felner, J. M., Perkins, J. B., Heymsfield, S. B., and Schlant, R. C.: Echocardiographic Study of Cardiac Dimensions and Function in the Endurance-Trained Athlete, *Am. J. Cardiol.*, 40:528, 1977.

100a. Benotti, J. R., Grossman, W., and Cohn, P. F.: Clinical Profile of Restrictive Cardiomyopathy, *Circulation*, 57:1205, 1978.

101. Maron, B. J., Merrill, W. H., Freier, P. A., Kent, K. M., Epstein, S. E., and Morrow, A. G.: Long-Term Clinical Course and Symptomatic Status of Patients after Operation for Hypertrophic Subaortic Stenosis, *Circulation*, 57:1205, 1978.

102. Rosing, D. R., Kent, K. M., Borer, J. S., Seides, S. F., Maron, B. J., and Epstein, S. E.: Verapamil Therapy: A New Approach to the Pharmacologic Treatment of Hypertrophic Cardiomyopathy. I. Hemodynamic Effects, *Circulation*, 60:1201, 1979.

103. Burch, G. E., Giles, T. D., and Colcolough, H. L.: Ischemic Cardiomyopathy, *Am. Heart J.*, 79:291, 1970.

104. Dash, H., Johnson, R. A., Dinsmore, R. E., and Harthorne, J. W.: Cardiomyopathic Syndrome Due to Coronary Artery Disease. I. Relation to Angiographic Extent of Coronary Disease and to Remote Myocardial Infarction, *Br. Heart J.*, 39:733, 1977.

105. Maseri, A., Pesola, A., Marzilli, M., Severi, S., Parodi, O., L'Abbate, A., Ballestra, A. M., Maltinti, G., Denes, D. M., and Biagini, A.: Coronary Vasospasm in Angina Pectoris, *Lancet*, 1:713, 1977.

106. Lloyd-Mostyn, R. H., and Watkins, P. J.: Defective Innervation of Heart in Diabetic Autonomic Neuropathy, *Br. Med. J.*, 3:15, 1975.

107. Mundth, E. D., Hawthorne, J. W., and Buckley, M. J.: Direct Coronary Arterial Revascularization: Treatment of Cardiac Failure Associated with Coronary Artery Disease, *Arch. Surg.*, 103:529, 1971.

108. Yatteau, R. F., Peter, R. H., Behar, V. S., Bartel, A. G., Rosati, R. A., and Kong, Y.: Ischemic Cardiomyopathy: The Myopathy of Coronary Artery Disease, Natural History and Results of Medical Versus Surgical Treatment, *Am. J. Cardiol.*, 34:520, 1974.

109. Crawford, M. H., LeWinter, M. M., O'Rourke, R. A., Karliner, J. S., and Ross, J., Jr.: Combined Propranolol and Digoxin Therapy in Angina Pectoris, *Ann. Intern. Med.*, 83:449, 1975.

*110. Kotler, M. N., Mintz, G. S., Segal, B. L., and Parry, W. R.: Clinical Uses of Two-Dimensional Echocardiography, *Am. J. Cardiol.*, 45:1061, 1980. (104 references)

110a. Froehlich, R. T., Falsetti, H. L., Doty, D. B., and Marcus, M. L.: Prospective Study of Surgery for Left Ventricular Aneurysm, *Am. J. Cardiol.*, 45:923, 1980.

111. Tomoike, H., Franklin, D., McKown, D., Kemper, W. S., Guberek, M., and Ross, J., Jr.: Regional Myocardial Dysfunction and Hemodynamic Abnormalities during Strenuous Exercise in Dogs with Limited Coronary Flow, *Circ. Res.*, 42:487, 1978.

112. Kumada, T., Gallagher, K., Shirato, K., McKown, D., Miller, M., Kemper, W. S., White, F., and Ross, J., Jr.: Reduction of Exercise-Induced Regional Myocardial Dysfunction by Propranolol: Studies in a Canine Model of Chronic Coronary Artery Stenosis, *Circ. Res.*, 46:190, 1980.

113a. Slutsky, R., Karliner, J. S., Battler, A., Peterson, K., and Ross, J., Jr.: Comparison of Early Systolic and Holosystolic Ejection Phase Indexes by Contrast Ventriculography in Patients with Coronary Artery Disease, *Circulation*, 61:1083, 1980.

113b. Slutsky, R., Gordon, D., Karliner, J., Battler, A., Walaski, S., Verba, J., Pfisterer, M., Peterson, K., and Ashburn, W.: Assessment of Early Ventricular Systole by First Pass Radionuclide Angiography: Useful Method for Detection of Left Ventricular Dysfunction at Rest in Patients with Coronary Artery Disease, *Am. J. Cardiol.*, 44:459, 1979.

114. Arbogast, R., Solignac, A., and Bourassa, M. G.: Influence of Aortocoronary Saphenous Vein Bypass Surgery on Left Ventricular Volumes and Ejection Fraction: Comparison before and One Year after Surgery in 51 Patients, *Am. J. Med.*, 54:290, 1973.

115. Achuff, S. C., Griffith, L. S. C., Conti, C. R., Humphries, J. O., Brawley, R. K., Gott, V. L., and Ross, R. S.: The "Angina-Producing" Myocardial Segment: An Approach to the Interpretation of Results of Coronary Bypass Surgery, *Am. J. Cardiol.*, 36:723, 1975.

116. Levine, J. A., Bechtel, D. J., Cohn, P. F., Herman, M. V., Gorlin, R., Cohn, L. H., and Colins, J. J., Jr.: Ventricular Function before and after Direct Revascularization Surgery, A Proposal for an Index of Vascularization to Correlate Angiographic and Ventriculographic Findings, *Circulation*, 51:1071, 1975.

117. Righetti, A., Crawford, M. H., O'Rourke, R. A., Schelbert, H., Daily, P. O., Ross, J., Jr.: Interventricular Septal Motion and Left Ventricular Function after Coronary Bypass Surgery, *Am. J. Cardiol.*, 39:372, 1977.

118. Zir, L. M., Dinsmore, R., Vexeridis, M., Singh, J. B., Harthorne, J. W., Daggett, W. M.: Effects of Coronary Bypass Grafting on Resting Left Ventricular Contraction in Patients Studied 1 to 2

Years after Operation, *Am. J. Cardiol.*, 44:601, 1979.

119. Kent, K. M., Borer, J. S., Green, M. V., Bachrach, S. L., McIntosh, C. L., Conkle, D. M., and Epstein, S. E.: Effects of Coronary-Artery Bypass on Global and Regional Left Ventricular Function during Exercise, *N. Engl. J. Med.*, 298:1434, 1978.

119a. Hellman, C., Schmidt, D. H., Kamath, L., Anholm, J., Balu, F., and Johnson, W. D.: Bypass Graft Surgery in Severe Left Ventricular Dysfunction, *Circulation*, 62(suppl. 1):I-103, 1980.

120. Chatterjee, K., Swan, H. J. C., Parmley, W. W., Sustaita, H., Marcus, H. S., and Matloff, J.: Influence of Direct Myocardial Revascularization on Left Ventricular Asynergy and Function in Patients with Coronary Heart Disease, *Circulation*, 47:276, 1973.

121. Theroux, P., Franklin, D., Ross, J., Jr., Kemper, W. S.: Regional Myocardial Function during Acute Coronary Artery Occlusion and Its Modification by Pharmacologic Agents in the Dog, *Circ. Res.*, 35:896, 1974.

122. Crozatier, B., Franklin, D., Theroux, P., Tomoike, H., Sasayama, S., and Ross, J., Jr.: Loss of Regional Ventricular Postextrasystolic Potentiation after Coronary Occlusion in Dogs, *Am. J. Physiol.*, 23:H392, 1977.

123. Helfant, R. H., Pine, R., Meister, S. G., Feldman, M. S., Trout, R. G., and Banka, V. S.: Nitroglycerin to Unmask Reversible Asynergy: Correlation with Post Coronary Bypass Ventriculography, *Circulation*, 50:108, 1974.

124. McAnulty, J. H., Hattenbauer, M. T., Rosch, J., Kloster, F. E., and Rahimtoola, S. H.: Improvement in Left Ventricular Wall Motion Abnormalities after Nitroglycerin, *Circulation*, 51:140, 1975.

125. Banka, V. S., Bodenheimer, M. M., Shah, R., and Helfant, R. H.: Intervention Ventriculography, Comparative Value of Nitroglycerin, Post-extrasystolic Potentiation and Nitroglycerin plus Post-extrasystolic Potentiation, *Circulation*, 53:632, 1976.

126. Komer, R. R., Edalji, A., and Hood, W. B.: Effects of Nitroglycerin on Echocardiographic Measurements of Left Ventricular Wall Thickness and Regional Myocardial Performance during Acute Coronary Ischemia, *Circulation*, 59:926, 1979.

127. Bodenheimer, M. M., Banka, V. S., Hermann, G. A., Trout, R. G., Pasdar, H., and Helfant, R. H.: Reversible Asynergy, *Circulation*, 53:792, 1976.

128. Theroux, P., Ross, J., Jr., Franklin, D., Kemper, W. S., and Sasayama, S.: Coronary Arterial Reperfusion. III. Early and Late Effects on Regional Myocardial Function and Dimensions in Conscious Dogs, *Am. J. Cardiol.*, 38:599, 1976.

19

Assessment of Electrical Abnormalities

Douglas P. Zipes, M.D.
R. Joe Noble, M.D.

As always, the initial evaluation of the patient begins with obtaining a careful history of the problem and performing a physical examination. Routine tests, including a 12-lead electrocardiogram and chest x-ray, provide information that dictates the subsequent approach. For example, the evaluation of a young patient who complains of palpitations and has no evidence of organic heart disease should follow a different course and tempo than the evaluation of a patient who has had a myocardial infarc-

Supported in part by the Herman C. Krannert Fund, by Grants HL-06308, HL-07182, and HL-18795 from the National Heart, Lung, and Blood Institute of the National Institutes of Health, Bethesda, Maryland, and by the American Heart Association, Indiana Affiliate, Inc.

tion and complains of presyncopal spells, or a patient with the physical findings of aortic stenosis and complaints of syncope. Thus, the nature of the rhythm disturbance viewed in the context of the individual patient and the effect of the rhythm disturbance on the individual patient determine the approach. It is important to remember that the physician evaluates a patient who has a rhythm disturbance and does not evaluate a rhythm disturbance in isolation. Some rhythm disturbances are hazardous to the patient regardless of the clinical setting, while others are only hazardous *because* of the clinical setting.

In general, the physician should seek to use the simplest, most noninvasive, least expensive tests that will enable him or her to define the problem and outline a therapeutic regimen, always asking whether the information provided by the test is sufficiently important to justify the risk and expense to the patient. The sequence of tests usually should follow an order that progresses from the simplest to the most complex, from the least invasive and safest to the most invasive and risky, and from the most inexpensive out-of-hospital evaluations to those that require hospitalization and sophisticated, costly procedures. When possible, the physician should choose tests that have a great deal of sensitivity and specificity. Occasionally, depending on the clinical circumstances, the physician may wish to proceed directly to a high-risk, expensive procedure, such as an electrophysiological study, prior to obtaining a 24-h electrocardiographic (ECG) recording, for example.

Information Provided by the History

Patients who have cardiac rhythm disturbances may present with a variety of complaints, but commonly palpitations, syncope, or presyncope bring them to the physician. Sometimes, they may profess symptoms of heart failure such as fatigue or shortness of breath.

Patients' awareness of regular or irregular cardiac action varies greatly. Some patients may perceive slight variations in their heart rhythm with uncommmon accuracy, while others are oblivious even to sustained episodes of ventricular tachycardia; still others complain of palpitations when they actually have a regular sinus rhythm.

The physician should always inquire about the rate, rhythm (regular or irregular), and nature of onset and termination of the rhythm disturbance. Patients should be instructed to recognize and record these parameters. Tapping on the patient's knee or chest or on a desk top is a useful way to illustrate a regular or irregular rhythm. A brief demonstration of how to determine heart rate is also helpful. Answers by the patient to key questions may provide clues to the nature of the rhythm disturbance, particularly if the physician has some information about the patient, such as physical findings and a 12-lead electrocardiogram. For example, a young man with a presyncope, normal physical findings, and ECG changes indicating Wolff-Parkinson-White syndrome should be asked whether the palpitations are regular or irregular, how fast they are, and how they start or stop. If the rhythm of the tachycardia is regular, with a rate of approximately 200 per minute and sudden onset and termination, it is likely that he is experiencing a reciprocating tachycardia (paroxysmal supraventricular tachycardia). If the rhythm is irregular, he probably has atrial fibrillation. In an elderly patient with presyncope, the physician should suspect ventricular tachycardia if the rate is fast and atrioventricular (AV) heart block if the rate is slow. Either rhythm may be regular or irregular. Probably the most common arrhythmia is premature atrial or ventricular beats, perceived as dropped or skipped beats by the patient.

Transtelephonic Electrocardiographic Transmission

The transmitters that patients with pacemakers use to send their electrocardiographic signal transtelephonically to their physician's office may be used equally well to transmit any electrocardiographic information.[1] Such an instrument converts the patient's electrocardiogram to an audiotone, which, when transmitted to a recorder-receiver, is converted back to an electrocardiographic signal for interpretation. By having patients transmit their electrocardiogram whenever they experience symptoms, it may be possible to establish which rhythm disturbance correlates with the symptoms, and perhaps even to learn something of its electrophysiological mechanism.

Such information is quite helpful from a therapeutic point of view. On the one hand, the "forceful" beats that the patient describes may be of sinus origin, in which case antiarrhythmic therapy is not required. Alternately, any variety of tachycardia or bradycardia may be uncovered.

This means of detecting an abnormality in rhythm or conduction is indicated when the rhythm disturbance is sufficiently infrequent that continuous ECG recording is impractical, is of sufficient duration (several minutes) to permit the transmission, and is not associated with syncope or other symptoms that would prevent the patient from transmitting. A disadvantage to this approach is that it relies on the patient's perception of a cardiac rhythm disturbance, and many patients may be unaware of significant or serious bradyarrhythmias and tachyarrhythmias. In addition, the technique requires access to a receiver and technician, which might not be available 24 h a day.

This technique does not permit as detailed an analysis of the ECG as a continuous recording, yet it does correlate the rhythm with the moment of symptoms. It is more practical than long-term ECG recording when the arrhythmia is infrequent; and it is much less expensive than 24-h ECG recording, costing no more than a standard 12-lead electrocardiogram.

The sensitivity and specificity of the technique depends totally upon the frequency of the arrhythmia, its duration, and the dependability and "detectability" of the patient. It imposes no risk and is inexpensive. In short, when provided to patients with appropriate symptoms, the telephone transmitter unit is a practical, inexpensive, and useful way to correlate symptoms with specific rhythm disturbances.

Exercise Testing

Exercise testing can document suspected rhythm disturbances as well as expose potentially serious, though previously unsuspected, arrhythmias. The therapeutic and prognostic significance of most exercise-induced arrhythmias, however, is poorly understood. In this discussion, we will review what is known about exercise-induced arrhythmias in groups of patients sufficiently well studied to permit generalizations (normal patients and patients with ischemic heart disease, idiopathic hypertrophic subaortic stenosis, or mitral valve prolapse) in order to consider the indications for stress testing in the detection of arrhythmias.

Information Provided by Exercise Testing in Arrhythmia Detection

In response to exercise testing, about one-third of normal subjects develop ventricular ectopy, usually in the form of occasional, uniform premature ventricular complexes (PVCs).[2–8] These are more likely to occur at higher heart rates and are not reproducible. [2,4–6] Even pairs of PVCs may be recorded in the normal population. In normal patients with known ventricular ectopy, most PVCs that develop during exercise are of right ventricular origin as determined by the scalar ECG.[9] Multiform PVCs and ventricular tachycardia usually do not develop in response to exercise in normal patients; however, since they may be recorded in normal patients, their presence does not establish the existence of ischemia or other heart disease. Supraventricular premature complexes are more common during exercise than at rest, and they increase with age; their occurrence does not suggest the presence of structural heart disease.[2]

Perhaps 50 to 60 percent [5–8,10] of patients with coronary disease develop PVCs in response to exercise testing. Ventricular ectopy appears at lower heart rates (less than 130 per minute) than in the normal population, and often occurs in the early recovery period as well. The ectopy is more reproducible from one test to the next.[5–8] Frequent PVCs (greater than 10 per minute), multiform PVCs, and ventricular tachycardia are more likely to occur in patients with coronary disease than in normal patients. PVCs that are documented at rest may be suppressed by exercise in patients with coronary disease, so this observation does not necessarily imply a benign prognosis or absence of underlying structural heart disease.[10] The incidence of sudden cardiac death is increased in patients with coronary disease who develop ventricular ectopy at heart rates less than 130 per minute with exercise,[6] and in whom the ectopy is associated with ST-segment changes, presumably as a manifestation of the relationship between ventricular ectopy and ischemia.[11]

Patients with more extensive coronary disease and more significant impairment of left ventricular function have more frequent and complex forms of ventricular ectopy.[5,10]

In patients with idiopathic hypertrophic subaortic stenosis (IHSS), previously undetected arrhythmias may be elicited by exercise. In studies reported thus far, however, long-term ECG recording has detected all of the serious arrhythmias recorded during exercise.[12,13]

Exercise may induce arrhythmias in as many as 75 percent of patients with mitral valve prolapse. Complex and previously unsuspected arrhythmias

may be found. For instance, atrial fibrillation or ventricular tachycardia, not previously recorded on resting ECG, may be elicited by exercise.[14] Most of these arrhythmias would be detected by long-term ECG recording.[15]

Indications for Exercise Testing in Arrhythmia Detection (Table 19-1)

Patients with symptoms consistent with an arrhythmia induced by exercise (syncope, sustained palpitations, etc.) should be considered for stress testing. Even if an arrhythmia has been detected by other means (prolonged ECG recording, ECG fortuitously recorded during symptoms, etc.), the stress test may relate the arrhythmia to heart rate and degree of stress and hence aid in antiarrhythmic management.

When a ventricular arrhythmia is suspected on the basis of symptoms in patients with ischemic heart disease, or even when it is detected by prolonged ECG recording or other techniques, stress testing may be indicated. More complex grades of ventricular ectopy may be detected by stress testing than by other means.[4,14] The response to stress testing may also be used to judge a therapeutic response.

Stress testing may be indicated in many patients recovering from myocardial infarction, including either a low-level exercise test prior to hospital discharge, or a 3-month postinfarction stress test, or both.[16–18] The test is not performed expressly to detect ventricular arrhythmias, but their occurrence suggests continued myocardial ischemia; and they are also a separate risk factor. The exact frequency and complexity of ventricular ectopy that might benefit from antiarrhythmic therapy is unknown; however, ventricular tachycardia in response to stress would clearly indicate further diagnostic and therapeutic considerations.

Stress testing need not be performed routinely on all patients with IHSS or mitral valve prolapse since long-term ECG recording appears to be more sensitive and probably should be accomplished first, when indicated.[12,15] However, if serious arrhythmias are detected by prolonged recording or resting

Table 19-1 Indications for Exercise Testing in the Detection of Arrhythmias

Exercise testing may be indicated to detect arrhythmias in patients who have:

1. Suspected exercise-induced arrhythmia
2. Coronary artery disease, with suspected ventricular arrhythmia
3. Postmyocardial infarction
4. Hypertropohic subaortic stenosis (selected patients)
5. Mitral valve prolapse (selected patients)
6. Any complex ventricular arrhythmia detected by any other means
7. Pre- and postantiarrhythmic therapy for ventricular ectopy

has occurred in patients with no documented arrhythmia on prolonged monitoring.[46]

Syncope and Transient Cerebral Symptoms

In a substantial proportion of patients with otherwise unexplained syncope or transient diffuse cerebrovascular symptoms, rhythm disturbances are found by long-term ECG recording to be responsible for the symptoms; these rhythm disturbances are potentially remediable.[47–49]

Bradycardia-Tachycardia Syndrome

Long-term ECG recording may permit the correlation of symptoms in patients with known bradycardia-tachycardia syndrome with periods of bradycardia (due to sinus bradycardia, sinus exit block, sinus arrest, or AV conduction disturbances) or tachycardia (atrial fibrillation, atrial flutter, or paroxysmal supraventricular tachycardia).[50] Should therapy for tachycardia be initiated, long-term recording may be helpful in detecting any potentiation of the bradycardia by the therapy.

Wolff-Parkinson-White Syndrome

The ability of long-term recording to detect supraventricular tachycardia in patients with Wolff-Parkinson-White syndrome (WPW syndrome) depends upon each patient's symptomatology. In patients with only electrocardiographic evidence of preexcitation, supraventricular tachycardia is rarely recorded;[51] in symptomatic patients, supraventricular tachycardia is much more frequently recorded.[52] Should a recording expose an episode of supraventricular tachycardia, the information may be of therapeutic significance by displaying the mode of onset of the tachycardia and suggesting the anatomic pathway the reentrant circuit employs.

Conduction Disturbances

For symptomatic patients with conduction disturbances, such as right bundle branch block and left axis deviation, invasive electrophysiological (His bundle) studies may be useful if distal His conduction delay or, more importantly, distal His block can be demonstrated. Unfortunately, finding a normal HV interval at the time of electrophysiological study does not eliminate the possibility of heart block. Clinical documentation of intermittent heart block in some of these patients can be obtained by long-term ECG recording (Fig. 19-1).

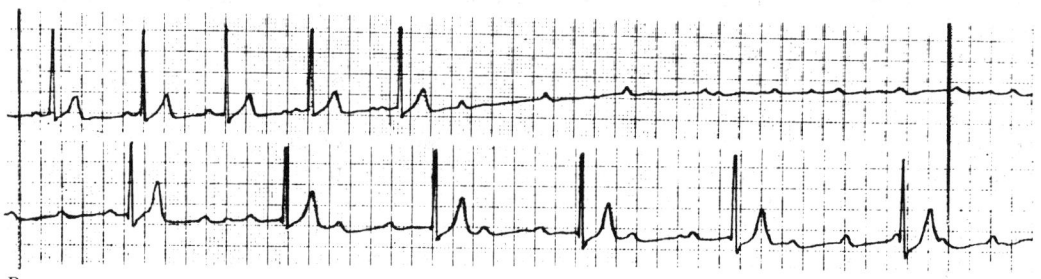

FIGURE 19-1 Paroxysmal complete atrioventricular (AV) block. His bundle study and ECG recorded during Holter monitoring in a 25-year-old male with syncope for 7 years. Physical examination, chest x-ray, treadmill exercise test, echocardiogram, 12-lead ECG, and response to carotid massage were normal, and no clinical evidence of manifest heart disease could be found. The tracings recorded during electrophysiological (His bundle) study (2A, top panel) reveal a normal AH (100 ms) and HV (40 ms) interval, and slight functional aberration of the QRS when the right atrium was stimulated prematurely at an interval (A_1-A_2) of 280 ms. Normal 1:1 AV conduction occurred at a cycle length of 350 ms (171 beats per minute) (2A, bottom panel). The PR (stimulus-R) interval prolonged as expected during rapid atrial pacing. In spite of the completely normal electrophysiological study, Holter recording documented intermittent complete AV block (2B). In this continuous tracing, complete AV block occurred suddenly, without significant change in the initial PP intervals. Complete ventricular asystole was terminated by a junctional escape rhythm, with continuation of the AV block. The importance of the apparent "fractionation" of the P wave, as well as the electrophysiological mechanism giving rise to the AV block, is unknown. BAE, bipolar recording from the upper portion of the right atrium; BHE, bipolar recording of low right atrium (A), His bundle (H), and ventricle (V). AH interval is a measure of AV nodal conduction; HV interval is a measure of His-Purkinje conduction. I, II, III, V_1 represent surface tracings; S, stimulus channel during right atrial pacing. In 1A, top, only the last regular cycle (700 ms) and the premature cycle (280 ms) are shown. In 1A, bottom, continuous right atrial pacing (350 ms) is presented. Paper speed, 100 mm/s; time lines at 1-s intervals.

Antiarrhythmic Therapy

In normal patients and in patients with serious rhythm disturbances, the cardiac rhythm may vary markedly from one recording period to the next. To prove the efficacy of antiarrhythmic therapy, it is essential to demonstrate that the frequency of the abnormal rhythm disturbance is reduced more by the agent than by chance alone. Spontaneous reductions in the frequency of PVCs of up to 90 percent have been demonstrated between two recording periods.[25,53] It has been suggested that an antiarrhythmic agent must reduce the frequency of premature ventricular complexes by about 80 percent, and the frequency of complex ventricular complexes 70 percent, from one 24-h recording period to another in order to be considered effective.[54]

Clinical Indications for Prolonged Monitoring (Table 19-2)

Recording the cardiac rhythm in patients with a suspected rhythm disturbance is essential to rational management. The first step in evaluation is to determine if the rhythm disturbance is of supraventricular or ventricular origin and if it is a tachycardia or bradycardia. It is equally important to correlate symptoms with the rhythm disturbance. Thus, syncope that cannot otherwise be explained may owe its origin to unexpected cardiac arrhythmias; angina pectoris may occur subsequent to a supraventricular tachycardia, and paroxysmal dyspnea or even idiopathic pulmonary edema may develop as a result of a cardiac arrhythmia. Palpitations may be quite bothersome to some patients, and appropriate management depends upon documentation of the responsible rhythm disturbance, which can range

TABLE 19-2 Indications for Prolonged ECG Recording

1. Recording of cardiac rhythm
   a. Documentation of suspected rhythm disturbance
   b. Correlation of rhythm disturbance with symptoms
      (1) Syncope
      (2) Palpitations
      (3) Chest pain
      (4) Unexplained dyspnea
   c. Mechanism of rhythm disturbance
   d. Efficacy of antiarrhythmic therapy
   e. Pacemaker function
   f. Specific patients with:
      (1) Ischemic heart disease
      (2) Idiopathic hypertrophic subaortic stenosis
      (3) Mitral valve prolapse
      (4) Bradycardia-tachycardia syndrome
      (5) Wolff-Parkinson-White syndrome
      (6) Conduction disturbances
2. Recording of QRS-ST-T pattern
   a. Prinzmetal's variant angina
   b. Correlation of symptoms with ST-T changes
   c. Effort tolerance

from sinus arrhythmia to a complex ventricular arrhythmia. In each example, the documentation of a rhythm disturbance and resultant symptoms establishes the need for therapy as well as the clinical therapeutic approach.

Recording the onset and termination of a rhythm disturbance may provide insight into the electrophysiological mechanisms responsible for the arrhythmia, and this information may be of therapeutic value. Such data may be particularly useful when the arrhythmia proves refractory to conventional therapy and more unusual modalities must be considered, such as overdrive pacing or experimental antiarrhythmic medication.

Once therapy is deemed essential and an agent is administered, the efficacy of the agent should be established. Prolonged ECG recording provides an ideal method for accurately and quantitatively documenting the efficacy and lack of toxicity of a drug (Fig. 19-2). The cardiac rhythm can also be correlated with serum concentrations and time of administration of an antiarrhythmic agent. For example, if ventricular ectopy increases markedly just prior to the next due dose of an antiarrhythmic agent and the serum concentration falls to a subtherapeutic level at the same time, then perhaps the drug should be administered more often.

When pacemaker surveillance clinics fail to document pacemaker dysfunction or other arrhythmias that are clinically suspected to be intermittent, long-term recording is the preferable diagnostic technique, both to evaluate pacemaker function and to detect pacemaker-induced arrhythmias. Care must be taken in placing leads to optimally visualize the pacemaker artifact.[55]

Whereas it is clear that recording frequent and complex ventricular ectopy in patients with ischemic heart disease implies a worse prognosis, it is not clear precisely which frequency and degree of complexity require therapy. The optimal duration of recording required to detect these abnormalities and the optimal times for recording (immediately prior to discharge from the hospital or at some interval posthospitalization) are unknown. The efficacy of antiarrhythmic therapy in altering the ultimate prognosis has not yet been established. Although it may seem likely that ventricular ectopy in these patients is etiologically related to the pathogenesis of ventricular fibrillation, it has not been demonstrated that suppression of the ventricular ectopy reduces the likelihood of sudden death. Consequently, though prolonged recording provides a means of detecting arrhythmias in patients with coronary heart disease, this detection cannot yet be equated with specific therapeutic recommendations. Hence, routine recording, though informative, cannot be advised for all such patients.

In patients with mitral valve prolapse, arrhythmias are common, yet are not clearly related to prognosis.[15,43–45] Hence, prolonged recording as a routine does not appear justified in these patients. In those patients with symptoms suggestive of an

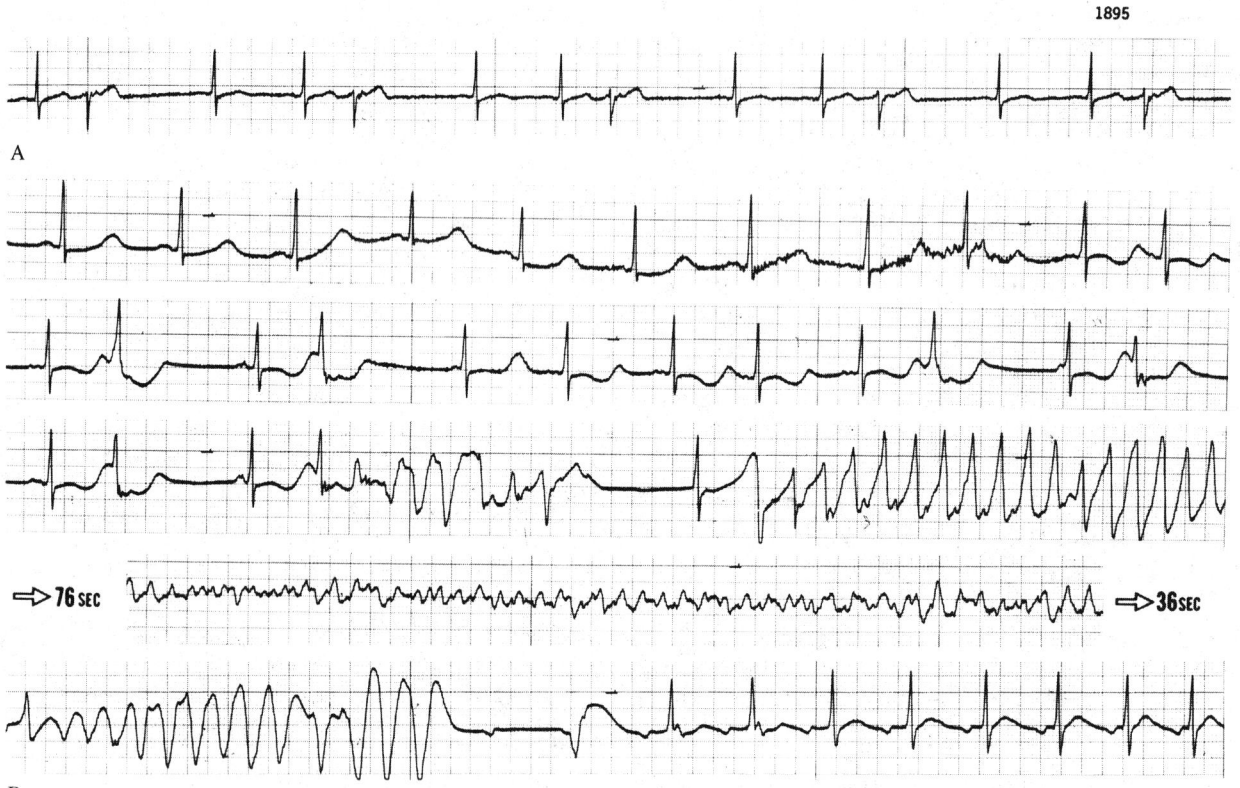

FIGURE 19-2 Quinidine-related ventricular tachyarrhythmia recorded on Holter monitor during sleep. During the control period (A), ventricular premature systoles (VPS) are coupled to the dominant rhythm with an RR′ interval of 480 to 560 ms, producing a trigeminal pattern. After quinidine administration (B) the VPS persist, but at a longer coupling interval (RR′ = 620 to 640 ms). However, quinidine has also lengthened the QT interval from 400 to 680 ms. Consequently, the VPS occur near the peak of the T wave, during the vulnerable period, and elicit ventricular flutter-fibrillation, which in this instance spontaneously reverted. The patient dreamed she died at this precise time. *(This interesting and informative tracing was recorded in a patient of Drs. A. Fasola and C. Fisch.)*

arrhythmia, such as syncope, prolonged recording may be indicated.

Prolonged recording is indicated for symptomatic patients with bradycardia-tachycardia syndrome,[50] Wolff-Parkinson-White syndrome,[52] conduction abnormalities, and other known or suspected abnormalities in rhythm or conduction, when it has not been possible to establish a cause-effect relation between the symptoms and the arrhythmia. Documentation of this correlation may verify a need for therapy.

The indications for long-term recording of the ECG pattern are more limited. Prinzmetal's variant angina may be diagnosed by recording marked ST-segment elevation simultaneously with pain during prolonged recording even when exercise testing fails to reveal evidence of ischemia. Similarly, it is possible to correlate a patient's symptoms, as recorded in the diary, with ST-T alterations, and to determine tolerance to everyday activity and emotional state. However, as discussed in Chap. 88, long-term recording of the QRS-T pattern is usually not essential to the diagnosis of latent ischemic heart disease, and the records must be interpreted with caution unless the test is properly standardized and validated.

Comparison of Prolonged ECG Recording with ECG, Exercise Testing, and Invasive Electrophysiological Studies in the Detection of Paroxysmal Arrhythmias

Intermittent ECG sampling is unreliable in detecting and quantitating arrhythmias, and either over- or underestimates the occurrence of the arrhythmia.[56] Prolonged recording is much more sensitive than the standard 12-lead electrocardiogram for detecting abnormal rhythms and displaying their frequency and character. Though prolonged monitoring may be 8 to 10 times more expensive, it records more than a 1000-fold more complexes for analysis.[48]

Prolonged recording may also be compared with exercise testing to detect arrhythmias. Some investigators have recorded a greater frequency of ventricular arrhythmias and potentially more serious ventricular arrhythmias during an exercise test than during a 24-h recording period with normal activity,[57] while others have reported the opposite.[20] Clearly, the choice of the best method for detecting arrhythmias depends on the individual. If symptoms of a rhythm disturbance develop during exertion, or are related to ischemia, then exercise testing would probably be preferable; conversely, if the arrhythmia develops at rest and is unprovoked by exertion, then long-term ECG recording would be the logical first choice. Each technique complements the other, so that both may occasionally be required to detect a rhythm disturbance.

Electrophysiological studies employing programmed stimulation of the heart, though extremely informative and useful in selected patients, are invasive and provide data during a circumscribed time period. Detection by long-term ECG recording of a spontaneously occurring rhythm disturbance that elicits simultaneous symptoms is of considerable help to the clinician in selecting therapy. As with exercise testing, electrophysiological studies and prolonged ECG recording also supplement each other in attaining this goal, and the choice for a specific patient must be individualized. Patients in whom invasive electrophysiology would be superior to long-term recording include those whose rhythm disturbance occurs so infrequently that prolonged recording would be impractical and patients in whom knowledge of the electrophysiological mechanism responsible for the arrhythmia would be therapeutically helpful. In still other patients with serious ventricular arrhythmias it may be essential to establish the efficacy of current antiarrhythmic management expeditiously; in such patients, electrophysiological studies may provide this information quickly. The comparable sensitivity of the two tests has not yet been established with certainty and may depend on the individual patient and nature of the arrhythmia.

Sensitivity and Specificity

Arrhythmias often are evanescent, occurring with marked variability anywhere from once in a lifetime to very frequently or even continuously. Consequently, it is impossible to know the absolute sensitivity of long-term ECG recording. The technique is usually more sensitive than other techniques in documenting rhythm disturbances, and its sensitivity can thus be contrasted with other techniques, but not with the actual frequency of arrhythmias.

When rhythm disturbances are recorded, they are specific, assuming proper interpretation and lack of artifact. However, when long-term recording is performed to explain a symptom, only the simultaneous recording of the arrhythmia and the patient's sensation of the symptom are of diagnostic value. Thus, it is extraordinarily important to correlate the patient's symptoms and the cardiac rhythm.

It is possible, however, to assess the accuracy of a given long-term recording system in detecting rhythm disturbances during a specific monitoring period by comparing the results of the recorder-scanner–interpreting system with the direct write-out and real-time interpretation of the same record.

Accuracy varies from one system to another. When technologists interpret the tape without semiautomated computer systems, an excellent qualitative analysis may be provided, i.e., detection of PVCs, ventricular tachycardia, asystolic intervals, etc., but not a quantitative account of the actual number of each event (see Chap. 88). With semiautomated interpreting systems, the error rate is 5 to 10 percent of ectopic complexes. Recently developed, fully automated computers reportedly miscount or misinterpret less than 3 percent of ectopic complexes.[58,59] Real-time analysis by microcomputers may prove even more accurate.

The clinical utility of such accuracy is open to question. All systems already record more information than modern-day cardiology knows how to interpret. Does it really matter whether a patient demonstrates 97 or 100 PVCs over a 24-h period? So long as the monitoring system detects some ectopy, or ventricular tachycardia, or whenever asystolic intervals occur and semiquantitates those abnormalities, the physician is provided all the clinical information that is needed. In fact, though the investigator of experimental antiarrhythmic agents requests information on the actual number of PVCs, until it is clearly demonstrated that reducing the number of PVCs to a certain level improves prognosis, even the necessity for this sort of quantitation is equivocal.

Risks and Costs

There are no patient risks inherent in continuous ambulatory recording. Out-of-hospital recording for a potentially lethal arrhythmia is contraindicated. Overconfidence in a negative result, and overtreatment of a benign disturbance, could also pose risks to the patient. Long-term recording is expensive, as a result of costly recorders, scanners, and either personnel or computer technology used to interpret rhythm disturbances. Patient costs vary from about $150 to $250, depending upon the duration of recording, equipment employed, and region. It is likely that the indications for long-term recording will increase as the prognosis of specific rhythm disturbances is clarified, as the electrophysiological mechanisms of various arrhythmias are established, and as a wider variety of antiarrhythmic drugs with more specific electrophysiological effects become available. Prolonged recording of the ECG represents a significant addition to the physician's diagnostic tools.

Continuous In-Hospital Electrocardiographic Monitoring

Continuous electrocardiographic monitoring may be accomplished in the hospital with bedside recorders, telemetry, or portable magnetic tape recorders. In-hospital monitoring is indicated for many of the same reasons outlined in Table 19-2 in patients who have had or are at high risk for developing potentially serious or life-threatening arrhythmias. Patients who have acute myocardial infarction, have undergone major surgery, have a critical illness, or have drug intoxication or conduction system disease are some who require in-hospital monitoring.

Telemetry is used mainly in progressive care units where patients are not restricted to bed. Some computer programs are available for automatic detection, diagnosis, and quantification of arrhythmias, but reliance is placed primarily on human surveillance of the continuous recording and on simple alarms based on rate changes. These approaches fail to detect many transient arrhythmias.

The advent of microprocessor and minicomputer technology may drastically improve the usefulness of in-hospital monitoring systems, but these latter systems are not widely available and their accuracy and reliability have not been validated. Programmed therapeutic intervention could be coupled to arrhythmia detection, employing continuous in-hosptal monitoring. Also, greater capacity for receiving and storing data would allow the recording of more leads and offer some of the advantages of body surface mapping.

Invasive Electrophysiological Studies

Invasive electrophysiological procedures are performed in human beings for diagnostic and therapeutic purposes. Diagnostically, the procedure provides information on the type of rhythm disturbance, for example, differentiating a supraventricular tachycardia with aberration from a ventricular tachycardia. It also provides insight into the electrophysiological mechanism responsible for the dysrhythmia, for example, detecting a supraventricular tachycardia utilizing an accessory pathway and the AV node for reentrant conduction. The procedure can be used therapeutically to terminate a tachycardia by electrical stimulation and to evaluate effects of therapy by determining whether a particular intervention prevents electrical induction of a tachycardia or can be used to terminate it. In this section, we shall consider when such testing is useful in patients who have AV block, intraventricular conduction defects, sinus node dysfunction, tachyarrhythmias, unexplained syncope, or palpitations.

Indications for Invasive Electrophysiological Studies

Patients with AV Block
Generally, the site of AV block can be determined from an analysis of the scalar ECG (Table 19-3). The site of block usually dictates the clinical course of the patient and whether or not a pacemaker is needed.[60,61] When the site of block is not known

TABLE 19-3   Site of Second-Degree Atrioventricular Block*

Type of Block	Normal QRS	BBB
First degree	AVN>>>>HPS	AVN>HPS
Second degree:		
Type I	AVN>>>>HPS	AVN>HPS
Type II	HPS>AVN	HPS>>>>AVN
1:1→2:1; fixed 2:1 or greater	HPS=AVN	HPS>>AVN
Third degree	AVN>>>>HPS	AVN<<<HPS

*Except for the location of type I atrioventricular block with a normal QRS, type II atrioventricular block with a bundle branch block, and third-degree AV block, quantitative data regarding the other sites of block are not available, and these statements must be regarded as the authors' impressions.

Note: AVN = atrioventricular node; HPS = His-Purkinje system; BBB = bundle branch block. Arrows (>) indicate relative frequency of atrioventricular block at different sites, with one arrow meaning slightly more frequent, and four arrows meaning far more frequent.

from an analysis of scalar electrocardiograms,[62] and when knowing the site of block will determine the management of the patient, an invasive electrophysiological study is indicated. Conversely, if the clinical evaluation accurately and adequately supports the decision to implant a permanent pacemaker on the basis of standard electrocardiography, symptoms, and other tests, invasive electrophysiological studies usually provide only confirmatory information.

The response of AV block to either spontaneous or induced changes of autonomic nerve activity may be used to establish the site of block based on the premise that His-Purkinje conduction time remains fairly fixed while AV nodal conduction time shortens in response to atropine or isoproterenol and prolongs following vagomimetic maneuvers. Thus, exercise may shorten the PR interval or increase the number of conducted P waves during type I second-degree AV block when the conduction disturbance is within the AV node. However, during type II second-degree AV block, the number of blocked P waves may increase during exercise or following atropine because the atrial rate increases and the conduction disturbance within the His-Purkinje system remains unchanged. At times, the response to autonomic manipulations may be misleading. Though it is considered that vagal stimulation generally increases and atropine decreases the extent of type I AV block, such conclusions are based on the assumption that the intervention acts primarily on AV conduction and fail to consider rate changes. For example, an injection of atropine that minimally improves conduction in the AV node, but markedly increases the heart rate, can increase AV nodal conduction time and the degree of block as a result of the faster atrial rate. Conversely, if an increase in vagal tone, produced pharmacologically or by carotid sinus massage, minimally prolongs AV nodal

Patients with Tachycardias

Information Provided by Electrophysiological Testing An electrophysiological study may provide useful information to help differentiate aberrant supraventricular conduction from QRS complexes that originate in the ventricle. Since all of the electrocardiographic manifestations of ventricular tachycardia may be mimicked, under certain circumstances, by aberrantly conducted supraventricular tachycardia, exceptions exist to the criteria that help to differentiate supraventricular tachyarrhythmias with abnormal QRS complex from ventricular tachyarrhythmias.[94,95] Often, a wide QRS tachycardia simply lacks distinctive features that may characterize it as supraventricular or ventricular, or it may share features of both supraventricular and ventricular tachyarrhythmias.

A supraventricular tachycardia is recognized electrophysiologically by the presence of an HV interval that equals or exceeds the HV interval recorded during normal sinus rhythm (Fig. 19-8). In contrast, the HV interval during ventricular tachycardia is shorter than normal. A short HV interval occurs in only two situations: during retrograde activation of the His bundle when the prolonged QRS complex originated in the ventricle or during conduction over an accessory pathway (Wolff-Parkinson-White syndrome).

Atrial pacing at rates faster than the rate of the tachycardia can be used to demonstrate a ventricular origin of the wide QRS tachycardia by producing fusion and capture beats and normalization of the HV interval (Fig. 19-9).[96] Such a response would not be expected by a tachycardia conducting with functional aberrancy. In some patients atropine administration to improve AV nodal conduction may facilitate atrial capture. During aberrantly conducted supraventricular tachycardia, premature ventricular stimulation can be used to "peel back" the refractory period of the blocked bundle branch and restore normal ventricular conduction (Fig. 19-10).[97]

In patients in whom supraventricular or ventricular tachycardia can be reproducibly initiated and/or terminated with programmed electrical stimulation or by provocative techniques, the potential ef-

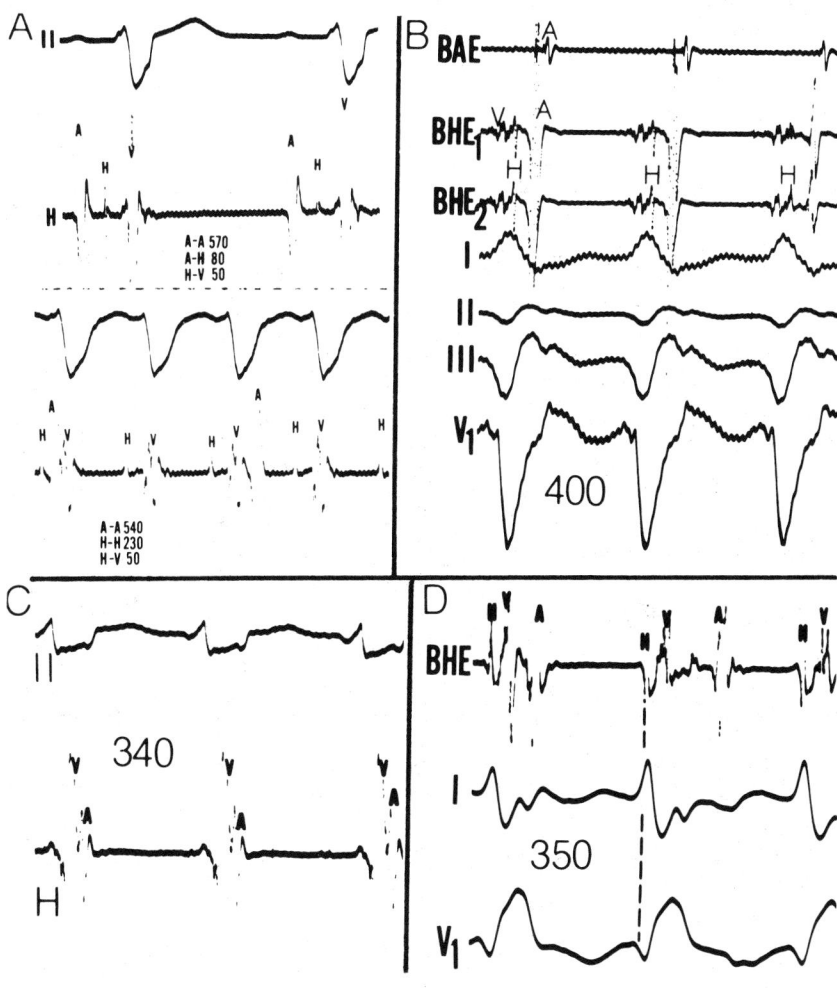

FIGURE 19-8 His bundle recordings in four different patients with tachycardias. *A.* Top portion of the tracing illustrates His-bundle recording during sinus rhythm. The HV interval is 50 ms. The bottom portion of *A* illustrates His bundle recording during tachycardia. The QRS complex and HV interval are unchanged from those recorded during sinus rhythm. Therefore, this is clearly a supraventricular tachycardia. Of note is the fact that the atria discharged at a different rate (not a multiple) than the ventricular rate. Therefore, AV dissociation is present during a junctional supraventricular tachycardia. *B.* His bundle activity occurred after the onset of the QRS complex, during ventricular septal depolarization, which assured the diagnosis of ventricular tachycardia. The RP interval remained fixed and atria were captured retrogradely from the ventricles. Therefore, AV dissociation is not present during this ventricular tachycardia. *C.* His bundle activity was not recorded in spite of careful exploration of the His bundle area with the catheter electrode tip. This most likely represents a ventricular tachycardia with 1:1 retrograde atrial capture, but one cannot be as certain as for *B* and *D*. *D.* His bundle activity preceded the onset of ventricular septal depolarization (interrupted line) but followed the onset of the QRS complex. Therefore, this must be a ventricular tachycardia. The retrograde (VA) Wenckebach was also present and is not shown in its entirety. In *B* and *D*, Wolff-Parkinson-White syndrome with anterograde conduction over an accessory pathway is unlikely in view of the long VA interval and was excluded by data obtained during the rest of the study.

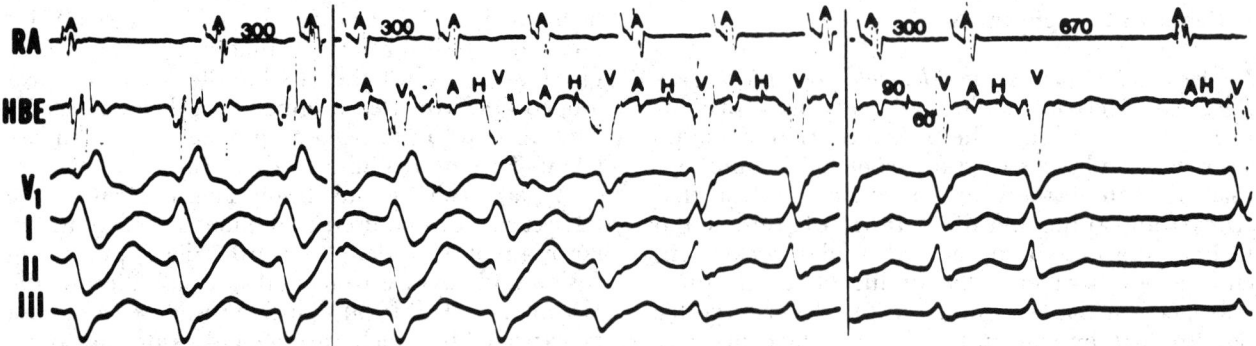

FIGURE 19-9 Right atrial pacing (left panel) at a cycle length of 300 ms in a patient with ventricular tachycardia captured the ventricular tachycardia (middle panel) and normalized the QRS complex and HV interval. Following cessation of right atrial pacing (right panel), normal sinus rhythm resumed.

ficacy of pharmacologic and/or pacemaker therapy can be evaluated.[98-101] One can compare the ability to initiate tachycardia after acute and after chronic administration of a drug or combination of drugs. Such an approach is particularly well suited to the patient who has infrequent spontaneous episodes of tachycardia, with little ectopy between episodes.

The site of origin and/or the pathways involved in maintenance of some tachycardias can be localized by endocardial mapping. This technique has proved to be efficacious in patients with Wolff-Par-

kinson-White syndrome or its variants[102] and in selected patients with ventricular tachycardia.[103,104]

Finally, an electrophysiological study may provide some insight into the electrophysiological mechanisms responsible for the tachycardia.[105] Although it is difficult in many instances to differentiate reentry from automaticity,[96] evidence in favor of one or the other mechanism may be obtained. In selected patients, a differentiation between reentry and automaticity may influence the selection of therapy, particularly as new antiarrhythmic agents or

FIGURE 19-10 A wide QRS tachycardia was initiated in this patient. Despite numerous changes in catheters and in catheter positions, an adequate His bundle electrogram could not be recorded, raising the possible diagnosis of ventricular tachycardia. The diagnosis of supraventricular tachycardia with aberrancy was made by prematurely stimulating the ventricles (S_1-S_2), which "peeled" back the refractory period and restored normal QRS complexes at the identical tachycardia rate. CS_p and CS_d, proximal and distal coronary sinus electrograms; RV, right ventricular electrogram. Major time lines = 50 ms.

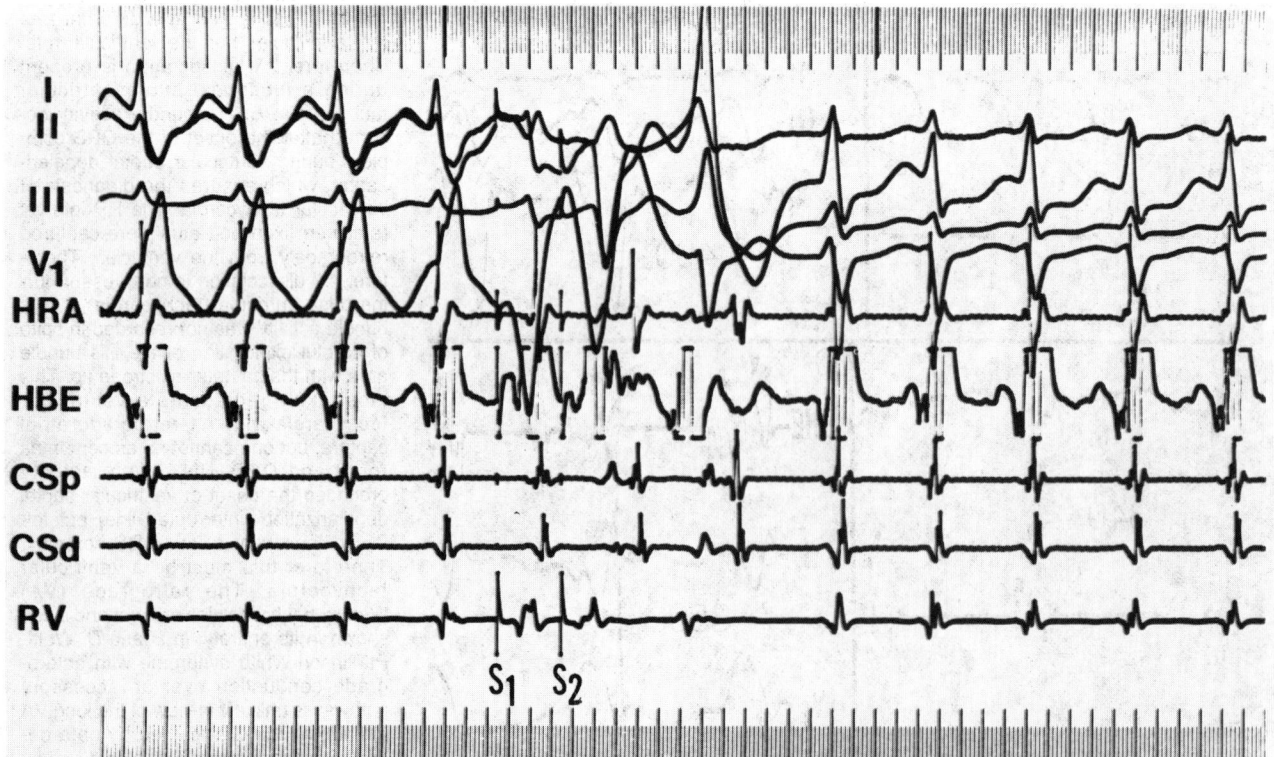

pacing or surgical approaches are developed that may preferentially affect one or the other mechanism.

Indications for Electrophysiological Study in Patients with Tachycardia An electrophysiological study should be considered in patients who have life-threatening tachyarrhythmias, such as ventricular tachyarrhythmias, or atrial flutter or fibrillation with a very rapid ventricular response (often, though not always, associated with the Wolff-Parkinson-White syndrome) and in patients who have symptomatic recurrent supraventricular tachyarrhythmias that appear to be resistant to conventional drug therapy.

Studies are indicated to obtain the following information:

1. To differentiate ventricular tachycardia from supraventricular tachycardia with aberrant ventricular conduction
2. To evaluate electrophysiological mechanisms and site of origin responsible for hard-to-control tachyarrhythmias in order to help establish a therapeutic approach
3. To evaluate conduction and refractoriness of various cardiac tissues since such data may provide prognostic or therapeutic information
4. To initiate the tachyarrhythmia in order to evaluate the ventricular rate and the patient's hemodynamic response, such as precipitation of atrial fibrillation in patients who have WPW syndrome
5. To evaluate response to medical, surgical, or pacemaker therapy

In general, patients with atrial flutter or atrial fibrillation are not candidates for electrophysiological studies. However, if atrial flutter is difficult to control, an electrophysiological study may be performed to determine whether pacing modalities can be used to terminate the atrial flutter.[106,107]

Recently, it has been suggested that electrophysiological testing could be used to identify patients at risk for the subsequent development of ventricular tachycardia or sudden death by eliciting a repetitive ventricular response following premature ventricular stimulation.[108] This initial observation has not been confirmed by several groups, and further studies must be done to establish the usefulness of this test.[109–111]

Patients with Unexplained Palpitations or Syncope

Information Provided by Electrophysiological Study in Patients with Unexplained Palpitations or Syncope The three common arrhythmic causes of syncope or palpitations in humans include sinus node dysfunction, tachyarrhythmias, and AV block. Of the three, tachyarrhythmias are probably most reliably initiated in the electrophysiology laboratory, followed by sinus node abnormalities and then His-Purkinje AV block.

Initiation of sustained supraventricular[112] or ventricular[113] tachyarrhythmia during an electrophysiological study provides relatively trustworthy information that the induced tachyarrhythmia is clinically significant and may be responsible for the patient's symptoms. Induction of sustained tachyarrhythmia during an electrophysiological study in patients who are not subject to the spontaneous development of the tachyarrhythmia appears to be uncommon although appropriate control groups have not yet been studied. On the other hand, failure to initiate the tachyarrhythmia does not exclude it as a possible cause of the patient's palpitations. Similar conclusions apply to patients with sinus node dysfunction. Initiation of an abnormally long pause following overdrive pacing, for example, is uncommon in patients without abnormal sinus node function. However, as many as 50 percent of patients with sinus bradycardia and 20 percent of those with sinus pauses or sinus exit block may have a normal response to overdrive pacing.[87–89] His-Purkinje block of a spontaneous or electrically induced premature atrial complex may occur in totally normal patients, particularly when the basic cycle length is long and the patient has fairly rapid AV node propagation. But development of block in the His-Purkinje system during sinus rhythm, at atrial-paced rates less than 130 to 150 per minute,[66] or at premature intervals (H_1-H_2) longer than 450 ms[67] indicates abnormal refractoriness and/or conduction in the His-Purkinje system.

The electrophysiological study may fail to explain the patient's symptoms if the dysrhythmia cannot be induced or if an abnormal rhythm is induced and the patient remains asymptomatic. If the arrhythmia is induced and replicates the patient's symptoms, important information has been obtained to explain the cause of the palpitations or syncope.

Indications for Electrophysiological Study in Patients with Unexplained Palpitations or Syncope Electrophysiological study is indicated in patients with syncope when noninvasive approaches do not reveal a cause of the syncope. Palpitations alone are not an indication for electrophysiological study. If, however, the patient complains of symptoms such as angina, shortness of breath, or lightheadedness during the palpitations, if there is evidence that the palpitations may represent a significant rhythm disturbance, and if noninvasive studies fail to reveal a cause of the palpitations, an electrophysiological study may be indicated.

Sensitivity and Specificity

Invasive electrophysiological studies provide important information when a particular abnormality can be demonstrated. However, if an abnormality does not occur or cannot be precipitated during the study, the negative result does not exclude the possibility that an abnormality may be present on another occasion. Thus, the sensitivity of an electrophysiological study may be low depending on the nature of the rhythm disturbance.

Generally, abnormalities such as sustained tachycardia, prolonged pauses following overdrive right atrial pacing, or type II AV block cannot be induced in patients who do not or may not experience these abnormalities spontaneously. Thus electrophysiological studies have a high level of specificity.

Comparison with Stress Testing and Prolonged ECG Recording

It is difficult to compare the sensitivity of a single electrophysiological study with techniques such as stress testing or prolonged ECG recording. The likelihood of recording a significant rhythm disturbance with the latter studies, for example, is influenced by many variables such as the nature of the underlying heart disease and dysrhythmia, how often the dysrhythmia occurs, and the duration of the recording. However, certain judgments are possible.

In patients who have infrequent, spontaneous episodes of sustained tachyarrhythmias, a single electrophysiological study is often more revealing than stress testing or prolonged ECG recording. Generally, the success rate of producing tachyarrhythmias by stress testing is low, particularly tachyarrhythmias not related to ischemia. Similarly, many days or months of ECG recordings may be required to capture the tachycardia in patients with widely spaced episodes.

Electrophysiological testing initiates paroxysmal supraventricular tachycardia due to Wolff-Parkinson-White syndrome or AV node reentry in over 90 percent of patients who have spontaneously occurring tachycardias. The ability to precipitate ventricular tachycardia in patients who have spontaneous, sustained episodes varies with the etiology of the heart disease. In our experience, during right ventricular pacing the yield is probably in excess of 90 percent in patients with coronary artery disease, but 40 to 60 percent in patients without coronary artery disease. Administration of drugs or left ventricular pacing may increase the success rate.

Risks and Costs

The risks of an electrophysiological study are small, yet considerably greater than those associated with noninvasive tests used to assess electrical abnormalities. The morbidity of the study includes vascular complications such as bleeding, thrombosis, thrombophlebitis, pulmonary embolus, inadvertent puncture of the femoral artery, development of arteriovenous fistula, and cardiac perforation. If the left ventricle is mapped or stimulated, morbidity increases, including problems associated with an arterial puncture and left heart catheterization. If the subclavian approach is used, development of a pneumothorax is possible. Finally, since precipitation of AV block or a tachyarrhythmia is often a desirable goal of the study, symptoms from such rhythm disturbances may result, adding to the morbidity. Mortality from the study should be almost zero, although it depends on the extent of the illness of the patients being studied. In patients with significant myocardial dysfunction, it may be possible to precipitate a ventricular tachyarrhythmia that cannot be terminated by direct-current cardioversion or that results in cerebral, renal, or cardiac ischemia or infarction before termination.

The cost of the procedure varies greatly throughout the country but may range between $300 and $500 for a laboratory charge and $350 and $600 for professional charge. Since many repeat studies performed to evaluate a drug response are shorter than the initial study, employ a catheter electrode left in place from the first study, or introduce only one or two catheter electrodes, they may cost less than the first study. Often, the test is cost-efficient if compared with the many days of 24-h ECG recording or in-hospital monitoring required to document the presence of an electrical abnormality.

Electrophysiological studies require experienced personnel who are willing to devote many hours to the interpretation of recordings of the more complex electrical disorders. One or preferably two physicians and a nurse/technician are required for the actual study. These factors plus the specialized recordings and stimulating equipment required limit the general availability and applicability of electrophysiological studies.

Other Techniques for Assessing Electrical Abnormalities

Esophageal Electrocardiography

Esophageal electrocardiography is a useful noninvasive technique to diagnose arrhythmias.[114–116] The esophagus is adjacent to the posterior atria, and an electrode inserted into the esophagus can record atrial potentials.[117] In adults, optimum atrial recordings are obtained when the distal electrode on the esophageal lead is positioned approximately 40 cm from the patient's nares.[116] Recently, a capsule electrode that is easily swallowed has been used to record continuous atrial electrograms from the esophagus.[115]

The esophageal atrial electrogram is useful in differentiating supraventricular tachycardia with aberrancy from ventricular tachycardia. During a wide QRS tachycardia when the ventricular rate exceeds the atrial rate, AV dissociation is often present and the most likely diagnosis is ventricular tachycardia. If each ventricular depolarization is coupled to an atrial depolarization, either supraventricular tachycardia or ventricular tachycardia with 1:1 ventriculoatrial conduction may be present. Uncommonly, junctional tachycardia with aberrancy may mimic ventricular tachycardia, and His bundle recordings are needed for a definitive diagnosis. When the same number of atrial and ventricular depolarizations occur, the autonomic nervous system may be manipulated to evoke AV nodal block or to slow the supraventricular rate to differentiate ventricular tachycardia from supraventricular tachycardia.

Esophageal atrial electrograms are also helpful to define the mechanism of supraventricular tachycardias. For example, a narrow QRS tachycardia with a ventricular rate of 150 beats per minute may be due to atrial flutter with a 2:1 ventricular response; finding an atrial rate of 300 beats per minute allows one to make this diagnosis. If atrial and ventricular depolarization occur simultaneously during paroxysmal supraventricular tachycardia, reentry utilizing an accessory AV pathway (WPW) is excluded, and AV nodal reentry is the most likely mechanism for the tachycardia.

Vectorcardiography

Vectorcardiography is discussed extensively elsewhere (Chap. 86). Though extremely helpful as a teaching aid to enable the student of electrocardiography to understand the genesis of the scalar ECG, the technique is limited in detecting or appraising abnormalities of rhythm and conduction.[118–121]

Vectorcardiography may be indicated to assess conduction abnormalities in several instances.

1. It may provide evidence of myocardial infarction that is camouflaged by left bundle branch block. Though the sensitivity of vectorcardiography in this differential is equivocal, a distortion in the loop with more posteriorly directed vector than expected often suggests coexistent anterior wall myocardial infarction.[122]
2. Vectorcardiography may explain prolonged QRS duration in the presence of myocardial infarction, specific bundle branch block patterns, distal Purkinje block (peri-infarction), or hemiblock patterns.
3. It also may confirm suspected left anterior hemiblock accompanying right bundle branch block. An abnormal leftward axis in the frontal loop of the vectorcardiogram will confirm left anterior hemiblock when its presence is equivocal on scalar ECG.
4. It may confirm suspected preexcitation and help localize the site of the accessory pathway. Slurring of initial electrical forces in the scalar ECG may be explained by conditions other than preexcitation, such as left ventricular conduction delay, left ventricular hypertrophy, and even myocardial infarction. Only if the vectorcardiogram records distinctive initial forces in all three planes can preexcitation be confirmed. The

vector of the delta wave may help establish the site of the bypass tract.
5. It may provide an explanation for a relatively tall R in lead V_1. The causes of an increase in the R/S ratio in V_1—right ventricular conduction delay, right ventricular hypertrophy, counterclockwise rotation, preexcitation, and true posterior infarction—can be easily differentiated with the horizontal loop of the vectorcardiogram.[123]

Although the vectorcardiogram is more accurate than scalar electrocardiography in distinguishing between the above situations, most often the information is not clinically essential. There is no risk to the patient in performing vectorcardiographic studies. They are, however, three to four times more expensive than scalar electrocardiography, and rarely prove cost-effective in analyzing rhythm and conduction abnormalities.

Body Surface Mapping

Isopotential body surface maps are used to provide a complete picture of the effects of the currents from the heart on the body surface.[124] The potential distributions are represented by contour lines of equal potential, and each distribution is displayed instant by instant throughout activation or recovery, or both.

At present, body surface maps provide a standard for testing and comparing the ability of lead systems to reproduce accurately all available body surface electrocardiographic information. Another use is to evaluate conditions that produce localized changes in the ventricle (ischemia), conditions with the simultaneous presence of prominent repolarization and depolarization potentials (ventricular extrasystoles), and conditions with anomalous sites of excitation (Wolff-Parkinson-White syndrome).

Body surface maps have been used primarily for research purposes; however, there has been preliminary clinical application in the following areas: localization and sizing of myocardial infarction,[125,126] detection of areas of ischemia (especially those apparent only with exercise), localization of ectopic foci or accessory pathways, and differentiation of aberrant supraventricular conduction from ventricular origin.

Direct Cardiac Mapping—Recording of Potentials Directly from the Heart

Cardiac mapping is a method whereby potentials recorded directly from the heart are spatially depicted as a function of time in an integrated manner. The location of recording electrodes (epicardial, intramural, or endocardial) and the recording mode used (unipolar versus bipolar), as well as the method of display (isopotential versus isochrone maps), depend upon the problem under consideration.

The most successful application of direct cardiac mapping has been in localizing accessory pathways associated with the Wolff-Parkinson-White syndrome.[127,128] Experience to date has attested to the value of surgical interruption of the accessory pathway in managing selected patients with life-threatening or medically refractory arrhythmias associated with the preexcitation syndrome. The ability to map the sequence of atrial and ventricular activation is of pivotal significance in the new frontier of electrophysiological surgery.[102–104]

Endocardial mapping has been used to delineate the anatomic course of the His bundle during open heart surgery to avoid injury during procedures to correct congenital heart defects.[129] More recently, direct cardiac mapping has been used to identify the site of rhythm disturbances in patients with ventricular arrhythmias refractory to medical therapy and has fostered surgical approaches for their extirpation.[102–104] Similarly, atrial mapping has been used to define the origin of rhythm disturbances in the atria for purposes of surgical ablation.

Another clinical application of cardiac mapping has been to identify areas of myocardial ischemia or infarction for purposes of revascularization or to define margins for surgical resection in the treatment of ischemic heart disease.[130,131]

Direct cardiac mapping is presently restricted to those few patients who have life-threatening or incapacitative supra- or ventricular tachyarrhythmias that are recurrent and drug-resistant. Such patients must be acceptable surgical candidates with adequate hemodynamic ventricular function. The technique is restricted to institutions capable of the combined electrophysiological-surgical approach.

Signal-Averaging Techniques

Signal averaging is a method to improve signal-to-noise ratio applicable to recurrent signals if the noise is random, that is, not synchronous with the signal. In conjunction with other methods of noise reduction, signal averaging can detect cardiac signals of a few microvolts.

With this method, potentials generated by the His bundle and bundle branches are detectable at the body surface.[132–136] The duration of the His-Purkinje waveform corresponds to the HV interval recorded by the catheter technique.

Signal averaging also has been applied to improve resolution of potentials that are detectable by standard recording techniques. Examples of such application include recording fetal electrocardiograms[137] as well as P waves and ST-T waves during exercise.[138,139] In the last instance, the problem entails reduction of a high noise level introduced by exercise.

At present, the technique must be regarded as an experimental research tool. It may become indicated when long-term recording of the HV time is useful. Recording His-Purkinje waveforms would allow not only the temporal analysis (HV time) now provided by the electrode catheter technique but also vectoral analysis. Abnormalities of the His-Purkinje waveform might aid in detecting conduction system disease earlier, anticipating development of heart block, and differentiating conduction system disease from other causes of electrocardiographic abnormalities. The detection of late ventricular activation (after completion of the manifest QRS complex) in patients who have intraventricular conduction delay and ventricular tachyarrhythmias may become clinically useful.[140] The application of signal averaging to ST-T waves or the TP segment might help to detect delayed activation of abnormal ventricular myocardium. Delayed activation potentials might serve as a portent of serious ventricular arrhythmias, a guide to antiarrhythmic therapy, a diagnostic aid in detecting heart disease, or a means of differentiating between reentrant and automatic ectopic beats.

Magnetocardiography

Magnetocardiography is the measurement of the weak magnetic field around the torso that is generated by the heart.[141] Recording these fields requires sophisticated equipment and is facilitated by an environment shielded from the earth's and urban electromagnetic fields.

Magnetocardiography seems particularly well suited to the measurements of "currents of injury," which are manifested by ST- and TP-segment shifts in the electrocardiogram. These shifts have been correlated with reduction of the resting membrane potentials and shortening of the action potential in an ischemic region.[142,143] The measurement of direct-current magnetic fields during ST and TP segments in experimental myocardial infarction[144] is worthy of future study.[145]

At present, the techniques of body surface mapping, direct cardiac mapping, signal averaging, and magnetocardiography must be considered research tools and are restricted to certain specialized institutions; the sensitivity, specificity, cost, and clinical indications of the techniques remain to be determined.

References

1. Furman, S., Parker, B., and Escher, D. J. W.: Transtelephonic Pacemaker Clinic, *J. Thorac. Cardiovasc. Surg.*, 61:287, 1971.
2. McHenry, P. L., Fisch, C., Jordan, J. W., and Corya, B. R.: Cardiac Arrhythmias Observed during Maximal Treadmill Exercise Testing in Clinically Normal Men, *Am J. Cardiol.*, 29:331, 1972.
3. Blackburn, H., Taylor, H., Hamrell, B., Buskirk, E., Nicholas, W. C., Thorsen, R. D.: Premature Ventricular Complexes Induced by Stress Testing.

Their Frequency and Response to Physical Conditioning, *Am. J. Cardiol.*, 31:441, 1973.

4. Faris, J. V., McHenry, P. L., Jordan, J. W., and Morris, S. N.: Prevalence and Reproducibility of Exercise-Induced Ventricular Arrhythmias during Maximal Exercise Testing in Normal Men, *Am. J. Cardiol.*, 37:617, 1976.

5. McHenry, P. L., Morris, S. N., Kavalier, M., and Jordan, J. W.: Comparative Study of Exercise-Induced Ventricular Arrhythmias in Normal Subjects and Patients with Documented Coronary Artery Disease, *Am J. Cardiol.*, 37:609, 1976.

*6. Morris, S. N., and McHenry, P. L.: Cardiac Arrhythmias during Exercise Testing and Exercise Conditioning, *Cardiovasc. Clin.*, 9:57, 1978. (27 references)

*7. McHenry, P. L., Morris, S. N., and Kavalier, M.: Exercise-Induced Arrhythmias—Recognition, Classification, and Clinical Significance, *Cardiovasc. Clin.*, 6:245, 1974. (12 references)

*8. Goldschlager, N., Cohn, K., and Goldschlager, A.: Exercise-Related Ventricular Arrhythmias, *Mod. Concepts Cardiovasc. Dis.*, 48:67, 1979. (39 references)

9. Kennedy, H. L., and Underhill, S. J.: Frequent or Complex Ventricular Ectopy in Apparently Healthy Subjects, *Am J. Cardiol.*, 38:141, 1976.

10. Goldschlager, N., Cake, D., and Cohn, K.: Exercise-Induced Ventricular Arrhythmias in Patients with Coronary Artery Disease: Their Relation to Angiographic Findings, *Am. J. Cardiol.*, 31:434, 1973.

11. Helfant, R. H., Pine, R., Kabde, V., and Banka, V. S.: Exercise-Related Ventricular Premature Complexes in Coronary Heart Disease, *Ann. Intern. Med.*, 80:589, 1974.

12. McKenna, W. J., Chetty, S., Oakley, C. M., and Goodwin, J. F.: Arrhythmia in Hypertrophic Cardiomyopathy: Exercise and 48 Hour Ambulatory Electro-Cardiographic Assessment with and without Beta Adrenergic Blocking Therapy, *Am J. Cardiol.*, 45:1, 1980.

13. Savage, D. D., Seides, S. F., Maron, B. J., Myers, D. H., and Epstein, S. E.: Prevalence of Arrhythmias during 24-Hour Electrocardiographic Monitoring and Exercise Testing in Patients with Obstructive and Nonobstructive Hypertrophic Cardiomyopathy, *Circulation*, 59:866, 1979.

14. Gooch, A. S., Vicencio, F., Maranhao, V., and Goldberg, H.: Arrhythmias and Left Ventricular Asynergy in the Prolapsing Mitral Leaflet Syndrome, *Am J. Cardiol.*, 29:611, 1972.

15. Winkle, R. A., Lopes, M. G., Fitzgerald, J. W., Goodman, D. J., Schroeder, J. S., and Harrison, D. C.: Arrhythmias in Patients with Mitral Valve Prolapse, *Circulation*, 52:73, 1975.

*16. Goldschlager, N.: Exercise Testing in Patients with Recent Myocardial Infarction, *Counc. Clin. Cardiol. Newsl.*, 5:1, 1980. (12 references)

17. Erricson, M., Granath, A., Ohlsen, P., Sodermark, T., and Volpe, U.: Arrhythmias and Symptoms during Treadmill Testing Three Weeks after Myocardial Infarction in 100 Patients, *Br. Heart J.*, 37:787, 1973.

18. Markiewicz, W., Houston, N., and DeBusk, R. F.: Exercise Testing Soon after Myocardial Infarction, *Circulation*, 56:26, 1977.

19. Sheps, D. S., Ernst, J. C., Briese, F. R., Lopez, L. V., Conde, C. A., Castellanos, A., and Myerburg, R. J.: Decreased Frequency of Exercise-Induced Ventricular Ectopic Activity in the Second of Two Consecutive Treadmill Tests, *Circulation*, 55:891, 1977.

20. Crawford, M., O'Rourke, R. A., Ramakrishna, N., Henning, H., and Ross, J., Jr.: Comparative Effectiveness of Exercise Testing and Continuous Monitoring for Detecting Arrhythmias in Patients with Previous Myocardial Infarction, *Circulation*, 50:301, 1974.

21. Stuart, R. J., Jr., and Ellestad, M. H.: A National Survey of Exercise Testing Facilities, *Chest*, 77:94, 1980.

22. Holter, N. J.: New Method for Heart Studies: Continuous Electrocardiography of Active Subjects over Long Periods is Now Practical, *Science*, 134:1214, 1961.

23. Gibson, J. S., Holter, N. J., and Glasscock, W. R.: Clinical Observations Using This Electrocardiocorder—AVSEP Continuous Electrocardiographic System, *Am J. Cardiol.*, 14:204, 1964.

*24. Harrison, D. C., Fitzgerald, J. W., and Winkle, R. A.: Ambulatory Electrocardiography for Diagnosis and Treatment of Cardiac Arrhythmias, *N. Engl. J. Med.*, 294:373, 1976. (53 references)

*25. Harrison, D. C., Fitzgerald, J. W., and Winkle, R. A.: Contribution of Ambulatory Electrocardiographic Monitoring to Antiarrhythmic Management, *Am. J. Cardiol.*, 41:996, 1978. (46 references)

26. Brodsky, M., Wu, D., Denes, P., Kanakis, C., and Rosen, K. M.: Arrhythmias Documented by 24 Hour Continuous Electrocardiographic Monitoring in 50 Male Medical Students without Apparent Heart Disease, *Am. J. Cardiol.*, 39:390, 1977.

27. Hinkle, L. E., Carver, S. T., and Stevens, M.: The Frequency of Asymptomatic Disturbances of Cardiac Rhythm and Conduction in Middle-Aged Men, *Am J. Cardiol.*, 24:629, 1969.

28. Kostis, J. B., Moreyra, A. E., Natarajan, N., Gotzoyannis, S., Hosler, M., McCrone, K., and Kuo, P. T.: Ambulatory Electrocardiography: What is Normal? *Am J. Cardiol.*, 43:420, 1969.

29. Lown, B., and Wolf, M.: Approaches to Sudden Death from Coronary Heart Disease, *Circulation*, 44:130, 1971.

30. Fisher, F. D., and Tyroler, H. A.: Relationship between Ventricular Premature Contractions on Routine Electrocardiography and Subsequent Sudden Death from Coronary Heart Disease, *Circulation*, 47:712, 1973.

31. Kennedy, H. L., Chandra, V., Sayther, K. L., and Caralis, D. G.: Effectiveness of Increasing Hours of Continuous Ambulatory Electrocardiography in Detecting Maximal Ventricular Ectopy, *Am. J. Cardiol.*, 42:925, 1978.

32. Kotler, M. N., Tabatznik, M., Mower, M. M., and Tominaga, S.: Prognostic Significance of Ventricular Ectopic Beats with Respect to Sudden Death in the Late Post-infarction Period, *Circulation*, 47:959, 1973.

33. Moss, A. J., DeCamilla, J., Engstrom, F., Hoffman, W., Odoroff, C., and Davis, H.: The Post-hospital

*This article is a review of the literature and contains additional references to the literature.

Phase of Myocardial Infarction: Identification of Patients with Increased Mortality Risk, *Circulation*, 49:460, 1974.

34. Moss, A. J., DeCamilla, J., Mietlowski, W., Greene, W. A., Goldstein, S., and Locksley, R.: Prognostic Grading and Significance of Ventricular Premature Beats after Recovery from Myocardial Infarction, *Circulation*, 51, 52(suppl. 3):204, 1975.

35. Vismara, L. A., Amsterdam, E. A., and Mason, D. T.: Relation of Ventricular Arrhythmias in the Late Hospital Phase of Acute Myocardial Infarction to Sudden Death after Hospital Discharge, *Am J. Med.*, 59:6, 1975.

36. Ruberman, W., Weinblatt, E., Goldberg, J. D., Frank, C. W., and Shapiro, S.: Ventricular Premature Beats and Mortality after Myocardial Infarction, *N. Engl. J. Med.*, 297:750, 1977.

37. Anderson, K. P., DeCamilla, J., and Moss, A. J.: Clinical Significance of Ventricular Tachycardia (3 Beats or Longer) Detected during Ambulatory Monitoring after Myocardial Infarction, *Circulation*, 57:890, 1978.

38. Vismara, L. A., Vera, Z., Forester, J. M., Amsterdam, E. A., and Mason, D. T.: Identification of Sudden Death Risk Factors in Acute and Chronic Coronary Artery Disease, *Am J. Cardiol.*, 39:821, 1977.

39. Fitzgerald, J. W., and DeBusk, R. F.: Early Post-infarction Ambulatory Monitoring and Exercise Testing in Detection of Arrhythmias, *Am. J. Cardiol.*, 35:136, 1975.

40. Schulze, R. A., Jr., Strauss, H. W., and Pitt, B.: Sudden Death in the Year Following Myocardial Infarction, *Am J. Cardiol.*, 62:192, 1977.

41. Vismara, L. A., Amsterdam, E. A., and Mason, D. T.: Relation of Ventricular Arrhythmias in the Late Hospital Phase of Acute Myocardial Infarction to Sudden Death after Hospital Discharge, *Am J. Med.*, 59:6, 1975.

42. Frank, M. J., Abdulla, A. M., Canedo, M. I., and Saylors, R. E.: Long-Term Medical Management of Hypertrophic Obstructive Cardiomyopathy, *Am. J. Cardiol.*, 42:993, 1978.

43. DeMaria, A. N., Amsterdam, E. A., Vismara, L. A., Neumann, A., and Mason, D. T.: Arrhythmias in the Mitral Valve Prolapse Syndrome, *Ann. Intern. Med.*, 84:656, 1976.

44. Leichtman, D., Nelson, R., Gobel, F. L., Alexander, C. A., and Cohn, J. N.: Bradycardia with Mitral Valve Prolapse, *Ann. Intern. Med.*, 85:453, 1976.

45. Winkle, R. A., Lopes, M. G., Popp, R. L., and Hancock, E. W.: Life-Threatening Arrhythmias in the Mitral Valve Prolapse Syndrome, *Am. J. Med.*, 60:961, 1976.

46. Shappell, S. D., Marshall, C. E., Brown, R. E., and Bruce, T. A.: Sudden Death and the Familial Occurrence of Mid Systolic Click, Late Systolic Murmur Syndrome, *Circulation*, 48:1128, 1973.

47. Walter, P. F., Reid, S. D., Jr., and Wenger, N. K.: Transient Cerebral Ischemia Due to Arrhythmia, *Ann. Intern. Med.*, 72:471, 1970.

48. Lipski, J., Cohen, L., Espinoza, J., Motro, M., Dack, S., and Donoso, E.: Value of Holter Monitoring in Assessing Cardiac Arrhythmias in Symptomatic Patients, *Am J. Cardiol.*, 37:102, 1976.

49. Tzivoni, D., and Stern, S.: Pacemaker Implantation Based on Ambulatory ECG Monitoring in Patients with Cerebral Symptoms, *Chest*, 67:274, 1975.

50. Crook, B. R. M., Cashman, P. M. M., Stott, F. D., and Raftery, E. B.: Tape Monitoring of the Electrocardiogram in Ambulant Patients with Sino-atrial Disease, *Br. Heart J.*, 35:1009, 1973.

51. Hindman, M. C., Last, J. H., and Rosen, R. M.: Wolff-Parkinson-White Syndrome Observed by Portable Monitoring, *Ann. Intern. Med.*, 79:654, 1973.

52. Isaeff, D. M., Gaston, J. H., and Harrison, D. C.: Wolff-Parkinson-White Syndrome: Long-Term Monitoring for Arrhythmias, *J. Am. Med. Assoc.*, 222:449, 1972.

53. Winkle, R. A.: Antiarrhythmic Drug Effect Mimicked by Spontaneous Variability of Ventricular Ectopy, *Circulation*, 57:1116, 1978.

54. Morganroth, J., Michelson, E., Horowitz, L. N., Josephson, M. E., Pearlman, A. S., and Dunkman, W. B.: Limitations of Routine Long-Term Ambulatory Electrocardiographic Monitoring to Assess Ventricular Ectopy Frequency, *Circulation*, 58:408, 1978.

*55. Bleifer, S. B., Bleifer, D. J., Hansmann, D. R., Sheppard, J. J., and Karpman, H. I.: Diagnosis of Occult Arrhythmias by Holter Electrocardiography, *Prog. Cardiovasc. Dis.*, 16:569, 1974. (68 references)

56. Ryden, L., Waldenstrom, A., and Holmberg, S.: The Reliability of Intermittent ECG Sampling in Arrhythmia Detection, *Circulation*, 51:540, 1975.

57. Kosowsky, B. D., Lown, B., Whiting, R., and Guiney, T.: Occurrence of Ventricular Arrhythmias with Exercise as Compared to Monitoring, *Circulation*, 44:826, 1971.

*58. Michelson, E. L., and Morganroth, J.: How to Use Holter Monitoring to Your Patient's Best Advantage, *J. Cardiovasc. Med.*, 5:119, 1980. (14 references)

59. Knoebel, S. B., Lovelace, D. E., Rasmussen, S., and Wash, S. E.: Computer Detection of Premature Ventricular Complexes: A Modified Approach, *Am. J. Cardiol.*, 38:440, 1976.

60. Dreifus, L. S.: Clinical Judgment is Sufficient for the Management of Conduction Defects, *Cardiovasc. Clin.*, 8:195, 1977.

61. Wu, D., and Rosen, K. M.: Clinical Judgment is Not Sufficient for the Management of Conduction Defects. Indications for Diagnostic Electrophysiologic Studies, *Cardiovasc. Clin.*, 8:203:1977.

62. Zipes, D. P.: Second Degree Atrioventricular Block, *Circulation*, 60:465, 1979.

63. Donoso, E., Adler, L. N., and Friedberg, C. K.: Unusual Forms of Second Degree Atrioventricular Block, Including Mobitz Type II Block, Associated with the Morgagni-Adams-Stokes Syndrome, *Am. Heart J.* 67:150, 1964.

64. Langendorf, R., and Pick, A.: Atrioventricular Block, Type II (Mobitz). Its Nature and Clinical Significance, *Circulation*, 38:819, 1968.

65. Dhingra, R. C., Denes, P., Wu, D., Chuquimia, R., and Rosen, K. M.: The Significance of Second-Degree Atrioventricular Block and Bundle Branch Block. Observations Regarding Site and Type of Block, *Circulation*, 49:638, 1978.

66. Dhingra, R. C., Wyndham, C., Bauernfeind, R.,

Swiryns, S., Deedwania, P. C., Smith, T., Denes, P., and Rosen, K. M.: Significance of Block Distal to the His Bundle Induced by Atrial Pacing in Patients with Chronic Bifascicular Block, *Circulation*, 60:1455, 1979.

67. Damato, A. N., Varghese, P. J., Caracta, A. R., Akhtar, M., Lau, S. H.: Functional 2:1 Block within the His-Purkinje System: Simulation of Type II AV Block, *Circulation*, 47:534, 1973.

68. Narula, O. S., and Narula, J. T.: Junctional Pacemakers in Man. Response to Overdrive Suppression with and without Parasympathetic Blockade, *Circulation*, 57:880, 1978.

69. Puech, P., Grolleau, R., and Guimond, L.: Incidence of Different Types of AV Block and Their Localization by His Bundle Recordings, in H. J. J. Wellens, K. I. Lie, and M. J. Janse (eds.), "The Conduction System of the Heart," Lea & Febiger, Philadelphia, 1976, p. 467.

*70. McAnnulty, J. H.: Chronic Bundle Branch Block, *Counc. Clin. Cardiol. Newsl., Am. Heart J.*, 5:1, 1980. (15 references)

71. Lie, K. I., Wellens, H. J. J., Schuilenburg, R. M., Becker, A. E., and Durrer, D.: Factors Influencing Prognosis of Bundle Branch Block Complicating Acute Anteroseptal Infarction. The Value of His Bundle Recordings, *Circulation*, 50:935, 1974.

72. Hindman, M. C., Wagner, G. S., JaRo, M., Atkins, J. M., Scheinman, M. M., DeSanctis, R., Hutter, A. H., Jr., Yeatman, L., Rubenfire, M., Pujura, C., Rubin, M., and Morris, J. J.: The Clinical Significance of Bundle Branch Block Complicating Acute Myocardial Infarction. I. Clinical Characteristics, Determinants of Mortality and One-Year Follow-Up, *Circulation*, 58:679, 1978.

73. Hindman, M. C., Wagner, G. S., JaRo, M., Atkins, J. M., Scheinman, M. M., DeSanctis, R., Hutter, A. H., Jr., Yeatman, L., Rubenfire, M., Pujura, C., Rubin, M., and Morris, J. J.: The Clinical Significance of Bundle Branch Block Complicating Acute Myocardial Infarction. II. Indications for Temporary and Permanent Pacemaker Insertion, *Circulation*, 58:789, 1978.

74. Holden, W., McAnnulty, J. H., and Rahimtoola, S. H.: Characterization of Heart Rate Response to Exercise in the Sick Sinus Syndrome, *B. Heart J.*, 40:923, 1978.

75. Morton, H. J. V., and Thomas, E. T.: Effect of Atropine on the Heart Rate, *Lancet*, 2:1313, 1958.

76. Jose, A. D.: Effect of Combined Sympathetic and Parasympathetic Blockage on Heart Rate and Cardiac Function in Man, *Am. J. Cardiol.*, 18:476, 1966.

77. Jordan, J. A., Yamaguchi, I., and Mandel, W. J.: Studies on the Mechanism of Sinus Node Dysfunction in a Sick Sinus Syndrome, *Circulation*, 57:217, 1978.

78. Eckberg, D. L., Drabinsky, M., and Braunwald, E.: Defective Cardiac Parasympathetic Control in Patients with Heart Disease, *N. Engl. J. Med.*, 285:877, 1971.

79. Cleaveland, C. R., Rangno, R. E., and Shand, D. G.: A Standardized Isoproterenol Sensitivity Test: The Effects of Sinus Arrhythmia, Atropine and Propranolol, *Arch. Intern. Med.*, 130:147, 1972.

80. Stern, S., and Eisenberg, S.: The Effect of Propranolol (Inderal) on the Electrocardiogram of Normal Subjects, *Am. Heart J.*, 77:192, 1969.

81. Mandel, W. J., Hayakawa, H., Danzig, R., and Marcus, H . S.: Evaluation of Sinoatrial Node Function in Man by Overdrive Suppression, *Circulation*, 44:59, 1971.

82. Narula, O. S., Samet, P., and Javier, R. P.: Significance of the Sinus Node Recovery Time, *Circulation*, 45:140, 1972.

83. Breithardt, G., Seipel, L., and Loogen, F.: Sinus Node Recovery Time and Calculated Sinoatrial Conduction Time in Normal Subjects and Patients with Sinus Node Dysfunction, *Circulation*, 56:43, 1977.

84. Benditt, D. G., Strauss, H. C., Scheinmann, M. M., Behar, V. S., and Wallace, A. G.: Analysis of Secondary Pauses Following Termination of Rapid Atrial Pacing in Man, *Circulation*, 54:436, 1976.

85. Steinbeck, G., and Luderitz, B.: Comparative Study of Sinoatrial Conduction Time and Sinus Node Recovery Time, *Br. Heart, J.*, 37:956, 1975.

86. Bigger, J. T., Jr., Cramer, M., and Reid, S.: Ability of Holter Electrocardiographic Recording and Atrial Stimulation to Detect Sinus Node Dysfunction in Symptomatic and Asymptomatic Patients with Sinus Bradycardia, *Am. J. Cardiol.*, 40:189, 1977.

*87. Josephson, M. E., and Seides, S. F.: "Clinical Cardiac Electrophysiology," Lea & Febiger, Philadelphia, 1979, p. 68. (56 references)

*88. Prystowsky, E. N.: The Sick Sinus Syndrome—Diagnosis and Treatment, in F. Donoso (ed.), "Advances and Controversies in Cardiology," Grune & Stratton, Inc., New York, in press. (140 references)

89. Rosen, K. M., Loeb, H. S., Sinno, M. Z., Rahimtoola, S. H., and Gunnar, R.: Cardiac Conduction in Patients with Symptomatic Sinus Node Disease, *Circulation*, 43:836, 1971.

90. Narula, O. S.: Atrioventricular Conduction Disturbances in Patients with Sinus Bradycardia, *Circulation*, 44:1096, 1971.

91. Narula, O. S., Shanto, N., Vasquez, M., Towne, W. D., and Linhart, J. W.: A New Method for Measurement of Sinoatrial Conduction Time, *Circulation*, 58:706, 1978.

92. Breithardt, G., and Seipel, L.: Comparative Study of Two Methods of Estimating Sinoatrial Conduction Time in Man, *Am. J. Cardiol.*, 42:965, 1978.

93. Hariman, R. J., Krongrad, E., Boxer, R. A., Weiss, M. B., Steeg, C. N., and Hoffman, B. N.: Method for Recording Electrical Activity of the Sinoatrial Node and Automatic Atrial Foci during Cardiac Catheterization in Human Subjects, *Am. J. Cardiol.*, 45:775, 1980.

*94. Zipes, D. P., and Fisch, C.: Supraventricular Tachycardia with Abnormal QRS Complex, *Arch. Intern. Med.*, 129:993, 1972; 130:129, 1972; 130:426, 1972, 130:781, 1972, 130:950, 1972. (34 references)

95. Wellens, H. J. J., Bar, F. W. H. M., and Lie, K. I.: The Value of the Electrocardiogram in the Differential Diagnosis of a Tachycardia with a Widened QRS Complex, *Am. J. Med.*, 64:27, 1978.

96. Zipes, D. P., Foster, P. R., Troup, P. J., and Pedersen, D. H.: Atrial Induction of Ventricular Tachycardia: Reentry versus Triggered Automaticity, *Am. J. Cardiol.*, 44:1, 1979.

97. Wellens, H. J. J., and Durrer, D.: Supraventricular

Tachycardia with Left Aberrant Conduction Due to Retrograde Invasion into the Left Bundle Branch, *Circulation*, 38:474, 1968.

98. Wu, D., Amat-Y-Leon, F., Simpson, R. J., Jr., Latif, P., Wyndham, C. R. C., Denes, P., and Rosen, K. M.: Electrophysiologic Studies with Multiple Drugs in Patients with Atrioventricular Reentrant Tachycardia Utilizing an Extranodal Pathway, *Circulation*, 56:727, 1977.

99. Fisher, J. D., Cohen, H. L., Mehra, R., Altschuler, H., Escher, D. J. W., and Furman, S.: Cardiac Pacing and Pacemakers. II. Serial Electrophysiologic-Pharmacologic Testing for Control of Recurrent Tachyarrhythmias, *Am. Heart J.*, 93:658, 1977.

100. Mason, J. W., and Winkle, R. A.: Electrode-Catheter Arrhythmia Induction in the Selection and Assessment of Antiarrhythmic Drug Therapy for Antiarrhythmic Recurrent Ventricular Tachycardia, *Circulation*, 58:971, 1978.

101. Horowitz, L. N., Josephson, M. E., Farshidi, A., Spielman, S. R., Michelson, E. L., and Greenspan, A. M.: Recurrent Sustained Ventricular Tachycardia. 3. Role of the Electrophysiologic Study in Selection of Antiarrhythmic Regimens, *Circulation*, 58:986, 1978.

*102. Gallagher, J. J., Kasell, J., Sealy, W. C., Pritchett, E. L. C., and Wallace, A. G.: Epicardial Mapping in the Wolff-Parkinson-White Syndrome, *Circulation*, 57:854, 1978. (42 references)

103. Josephson, M. E., Harken, A. H., and Horowitz, L. N.: Endocardial Excision: A New Surgical Technique for the Treatment of Recurrent Ventricular Tachycardia, *Circulation*, 60:1430, 1979.

104. Fontaine, G., Guiraudon, G., Frank, R., Vedel, J., Grosgogeat, Y., Cabrol, C., and Facquet, J.: Stimulation Studies and Epicardial Mapping in Ventricular Tachycardia: Study of Mechanisms and Selection for Surgery, in H. E. Kulbertus (ed.), "Reentrant Arrhythmias," MTP Press, Lancaster, England, p. 334, 1977.

105. Josephson, M. E., Horowitz, L. N., Farshidi, A., and Kastor, J. A.: Recurrent Sustained Ventricular Tachycardia. I. Mechanisms, *Circulation*, 57:431, 1978.

106. Zipes, D. P., and DeJoseph, R. L.: Dissimilar Atrial Rhythms in Man and Dog, *Am. J. Cardiol.*, 32:618, 1973.

107. Wells, J. L., Jr., MacLean, W. A. H., James, T. N., and Waldo, A. L.: Characterization of Atrial Flutter. Studies in Man after Open Heart Surgery Using Fixed Atrial Electrodes, *Circulation*, 60:665, 1979.

108. Greene, L. H., Reid, P. R., and Schaeffer, A. H.: The Repetitive Ventricular Response in Man: A Predictor of Sudden Death, *N. Engl. J. Med.*, 299:729, 1978.

109. Naccarelli, G. V., Prystowsky, E. N., Jackman, W. M., Heger, J. J., Rinkenberger, R. L., Zipes, D. P.: The Repetitive Ventricular Response: Prevalence and Prognostic Significance, *Br. Heart J.*, in press.

110. Mason, J. W.: Repetitive Beating after Single Ventricular Extrastimuli: Incidence and Prognostic Significance in Patients with Recurrent Ventricular Tachycardia, *Am. J. Cardiol.*, 45:1126, 1980.

111. Farshidi, A., Michelson, E. L., Greenspan, A. M., Spielman, S. R., Horowitz, L. N., and Josephson,

M. E.: Repetitive Responses to Ventricular Extrastimuli: Incidence, Mechanism and Significance, *Am. Heart J.*, 100:59, 1980.

112. Wu, D., Denes, P., Amat-y-Leon, F., Dhingra, R., Wyndham, C. R. C., Bauernfeind, R., Latif, P., and Rosen, K. M.: Clinical Electrocardiographic and Electrophysiologic Observations in Patients with Paroxysmal Supraventricular Tachycardia, *Am. J. Cardiol.*, 41:1045, 1978.

113. Vandepol, C. J., Farshidi, A., Spielman, S. R., Greenspan, A. M., Horowitz, L. N., and Josephson, M. E.: Incidence and Clinical Significance of Induced Ventricular Tachycardia, *Am. J. Cardiol.*, 45:725, 1980.

114. Zipes, D. P., and DeJoseph, R. L.: Dissimilar Atrial Rhythms in Man and Dog, *Am. J. Cardiol.*, 32:618, 1973.

115. Jenkins, J. M., Wu, D., and Arzbacher, R. C.: Computer Diagnosis of Supraventricular and Ventricular Arrhythmias. A New Esophageal Technique, *Circulation*, 60:977, 1979.

116. Prystowsky, E. N., Pritchett, E. L. C., and Gallagher, J. J.: Origin of the Atrial Electrogram Recorded from the Esophagus, *Circulation*, 61:1017, 1980.

117. Barold, S. S.: Filtered Bipolar Esophageal Electrocardiography, *Am. Heart J.*, 83:431, 1972.

118. Frank. E.: An Accurate, Clinically Practical System for Spatial Vectorcardiography, *Circulation*, 13:737, 1956.

119. McFee, R., and Parungao, A.: An Orthazonal Lead System for Clinical Electrocardiography, *Am. Heart J.*, 62:93, 1961.

*120. Benchimol, A., and Desser, K. B.: Advances in Clinical Vectorcardiography, *Am. J. Cardiol.*, 36:76, 1975. (72 references)

121. Witham, A. C.: Vectorcardiography, in J. W. Hurst, R. B. Logue, R. C. Schlant, and N. K. Wenger (eds.), "The Heart," McGraw-Hill Book Company, New York, 1978, p. 373.

122. Benchimol, A., Bartall, H., Desser, K. B., and Massey, B. J.: Vectorcardiographic Study of Initial QRS Forces in Left Bundle Branch Block Associated with Myocardial Infarction, Primary Myocardial Disease and Valvular Heart Disease, *J. Electrocardiol.*, 11:307, 1978.

*123. Benchimol, A., and Desser, K. B.: The Electrovectorcardiographic Diagnosis of Posterior Wall Myocardial Infarction, *Cardiovasc. Clin.*, 5:183, 1974. (6 references)

124. Zipes, D. P., Spach, M. S., Holt, J. H., Gallagher, J. J., Lazzara, R., and Boineau, J. P.: Task Force VI: Future Directions in Electrocardiography, Tenth Bethesda Conference on Optimal Electrocardiography, *Am. J. Cardiol.*, 41:184, 1978.

125. Flowers, N. C., Horan, L. B., Sohi, G. S., et al.: New Evidence for Inferoposterior Myocardial Infarction on Surface Potential Maps, *Am. J. Cardiol.*, 38:576, 1976.

126. Holt, H. J., Jr., Barnard, A. C. L., and Kramer, J. O.: Body Surface Potentials in Ventricular Hypertrophy: Analysis Using a Multiple Dipole Model of the Heart, in T. Alper (ed.),"Cardiac Hypertrophy," Academic Press, Inc., New York, 1971, p. 611.

127. Durrer, D., and Roos, J. P.: Epicardial Excitation

of the Ventricles in a Patient with Wolff-Parkinson-White Syndrome (Type B), *Circulation*, 35:15, 1967.

128. Boineau, J. P., Moore, E. N., Sealy, W. C., et al.: Epicardial Mapping in Wolff-Parkinson-White Syndrome, *Arch. Intern. Med.*, 135:422, 1975.

129. Waldo, A. L., and James T. N.: The Cardiac Conduction System: Electrophysiological Studies during Open Heart Surgery. *Arch. Intern. Med.*, 135:411, 1975.

130. Kaiser, G. A., Waldo, A. L., Bowman, F. O., et al.: The Use of Ventricular Electrograms in Operation for Coronary Artery Disease and Its Complications, *Ann. Thorac. Surg.*, 10:153, 1970.

131. Fontaine, G., Frank, R., Bonnet, M., et al.: Methode d'etude experimentale et clinique des syndromes de Wolff-Parkinson-White et d'ischemie myocardique par cartographie de la depolarisation ventriculaire epicardique, *Coeur Med. Interne.*, 12:105, 1973.

132. Berbari, E. J., Lazzara, R., Samet, P., et al.: Noninvasive Technique for Detection of Electrical Activity during the PR Segment, *Circulation*, 48:1005, 1973.

133. Flowers, N. C., Hand, R. C., Orander, P. C., et al.: Surface Recording of Electrical Activity from the Region of the Bundle of His, *Am. J. Cardiol.*, 33:384, 1974.

134. Furness, A., Sharratt, G. P., and Carson, P.: The Feasibility of Detecting His Bundle Activity from the Body Surface, *Cardiovasc. Res.*, 9:390, 1975.

135. Hishimoto, Y., and Toshitami, S.: Noninvasive Recording of His Bundle Potential in Man: Simplified Method, *Br. Heart J.* 37:635, 1975.

136. Berbari, E. J., Scherlag, B. J., El-Sherif, N., et al.: The His-Purkinje Electrocardiogram in Man: An Initial Assessment of Its Uses and Limitations, *Circulation*, 54:219, 1976.

137. Hon, E. H., and Lee, S. T.: Noise Reduction in Fetal Electrocardiography, *Am. J. Obstet. Gynecol.*, 87:1086, 1963.

138. Irisawa, H., and Seyama, I.: Configuration of the P Wave During Mild Exercise, *Am. Heart J.*, 71:467, 1966.

139. Brody, D., Arzbaecher, R. C., Woolsey, M. D., et al.: The Normal Atrial Electrocardiogram: Morphologic and Quantitative Variability in Bipolar Extremity Leads, *Am. Heart J.*, 74:4, 1967.

140. Rozanski, J. J., Myerburg, R. J., and Castellanos, A.: A New ECG Wave Form Identified by Signal Averaging in Patients with Recurrent Ventricular Tachycardia, *Circulation*, 49–50(suppl. II):22, 1979.

141. Baule, G., and McFee, R.: Detection of the Magnetic Field of the Heart, *Am. Heart J.*, 66:95, 1963.

142. Samson, W. E., and Scher, A. M.: Mechanism of ST Segment Alteration during Acute Myocardial Injury, *Circ. Res.*, 8:780, 1960.

143. Prinzmetal, M., Toyoshima, H., Ekmekci, A., et al.: Angina Pectoris. VI. Nature of ST-Segment Elevation and Other ECG Changes in Acute Severe Myocardial Ischemia, *Clin. Sci.*, 23:489, 1962.

144. Cohen, D., and Kaufman, L. A.: Magnetic Determination of the Relationship between the ST Segment Shift and the Injury Current Produced by Coronary Artery Occlusion, *Circ. Res.*, 36:414, 1975.

145. Fozzard, H. A., and DasGupta, D. S.: ST-Segment Potentials and Mapping: Theory and Experiments, *Circulation*, 54:533, 1976.

20

Assessment of Myocardial Ischemia and Infarction

Richard M. Steingart, M.D.
James Scheuer, M.D.

Ischemic heart disease is defined by the World Health Organization as "myocardial impairment due to imbalance between coronary blood flow and myocardial requirements caused by changes in the coronary circulation."[1] This definition emphasizes that atherosclerotic coronary artery obstruction is the major, but not the only, pathophysiological cause of ischemia.

The prevalence of symptomatic atherosclerotic coronary artery disease in the United States is estimated at 4,240,000.[2] In the total population within the United States there are approximately 30,000,000 middle-aged men without symptoms of heart disease. Of these, it is estimated that between 3 and 12 percent have occult coronary artery disease.[3,4] The clinician's role is to determine whether or not coronary artery disease is present and its severity, whether or not myocardial damage has occurred and its severity, and the basis for a logical approach to treatment. He or she may be called on to answer these questions at any point in the continuum of coronary artery disease, extending from an asymptomatic patient with minimal disease to the patient with extensive three-vessel disease, infarction of a majority of the left side of the heart, and shock.

Approach to the Patient

The evaluation of the patient suspected of having atherosclerotic coronary artery disease must begin with appreciation of the population from which he or she presents.[5,6] The prevalence of atherosclerotic coronary artery disease in asymptomatic individuals is approximately 5 percent.[7–10] This asymptomatic group is composed of patients with divergent risks for coronary artery disease, and can be subcategorized in terms of the prevalence of disease by using "risk factors" for atherosclerotic coronary artery disease (see Chaps. 41, 43, and 45).[4,11] The prevalence of coronary disease in symptomatic populations can be further defined using analysis of symptoms such as nonanginal chest pain, atypical angina, typical angina, and myocardial infarction (Table 20-1).[5,12,13]

By reviewing the literature, Diamond and Forrester[4] have estimated prevalence of coronary artery disease based on age and sex. The symptomatic state can then be applied as the test, and a posttest probability based on age, sex, and symptomatic status can be determined using Bayesian analysis (Table 20-1). A new probability has not been created by this process; rather, extent probabilities have been ordered in a useful format.[14]

Decision Making: Bayes' Theorem

Bayes' Theorem

Fundamental to any discussion of decision making following the acquisition of a clinical and laboratory data base is an understanding of the ability of a test to establish the probability of the presence or absence of a disease. This is commonly defined as a given test's *sensitivity, specificity*, and *predictive value*. These characteristics can be considered to reflect the test's accuracy (defined here as the fraction of the test results that are correct).[14] Sensitivity describes the fraction of a population with a specific disease who have a positive test result for that disease. Specificity describes the fraction of a population without the disease who have a negative test. Bayes' theorem states that the fraction of the positive tests that are false positives is inversely proportional to the prevalence of the disease in the study population and that the fraction of negative tests that are false negatives is directly proportional to the prevalence of the disease in the study population. This relationship of disease prevalence and false-positive and false-negative tests becomes critical when the clinician attempts to evaluate the importance of a positive or negative test in patients with high or low likelihood of disease. This intellectual process may be mathematically described as the predictive value of a positive test, which is the number of patients with a truly positive test divided by all true-positive and false-positive tests, i.e., how many patients with a positive test have the disease; conversely, the predictive value of a negative test is the fraction of patients with a negative test who do not have the disease.

Once a test has been performed the question of its predictive value is most relevant. For example, if a patient gives a history of angina, what are the chances that ischemic heart disease is present? That is, what is the predictive value of the history of angina?

In studies constructed to find the sensitivity, specificity, and predictive value of a test the test must be carefully standardized, and it must be administered to a large and representative patient population. Sample spectrum and bias can markedly influence the defined accuracy of diagnostic tests.[15] Many of the studies on the accuracy of diagnostic tests in ischemic heart disease employ unique testing methods and are conducted in truncated and possibly unrepresentative patient populations.[16–20]

All the diagnostic tests to be discussed in this section have less-than-perfect sensitivity and specificity. Predictions of the presence or absence of disease in a patient are thus probability statements. For instance, if a perfectly sensitive test is used to detect a disease with a prevalence of 1:1000 and there is a false-positive rate of 5 percent, only 1 in 1000 persons with a positive test will have the disease but 5 percent of 999, or approximately 50 people, would have a falsely positive test.[21] Thus, only 1 of 51 positive tests would accurately reflect the presence of disease. The predictive value of this positive test would only be 2 percent. This illustration also points out how disease prevalence (pretest probability of disease) can influence the predictive value of a diagnostic test. *The coronary arteriogram provides our most accurate test for determining the presence or absence of anatomical coronary artery disease.* However, every patient with chest pain cannot and should not

---

TABLE 20-1 Pretest Likelihood of Coronary-Artery Disease According to Age and Sex*

Age, years	Asymptomatic		Nonanginal Chest Pain		Atypical Angina		Typical Angina	
	Men	Women	Men	Women	Men	Women	Men	Women
30–39	1.9 ± 0.3	0.3 ± 0.1	5.2 ± 0.8	0.8 ± 0.3	21.8 ± 2.4	4.2 ± 1.3	69.7 ± 3.2	25.8 ± 6.6
40–49	5.5 ± 0.3	1.0 ± 0.2	14.1 ± 1.3	2.8 ± 0.7	46.1 ± 1.8	13.3 ± 2.9	87.3 ± 1.0	55.2 ± 6.5
50–59	9.7 ± 0.4	3.2 ± 0.4	21.5 ± 1.7	8.4 ± 1.2	58.9 ± 1.5	32.4 ± 3.0	92.0 ± 0.6	79.4 ± 2.4
60–69	12.3 ± 0.5	7.5 ± 0.6	28.1 ± 1.9	18.6 ± 1.9	67.1 ± 1.3	54.4 ± 2.4	94.3 ± 0.4	90.6 ± 1.0

*Each value represents the percent ± 1 standard error of the percent of symptomatic groups who had proven coronary disease.
Source: Adapted from G. A. Diamond and J. S. Forrester.[4] Reprinted with permission.

matic limitations in the patient with documented coronary disease. Because of the reproducibility of the treadmill test, it is ideally suited to objectively assess the adequacy of drug therapy.[65] Recently, maximal treadmill testing has been shown to aid in patient selection for coronary artery bypass grafting[61] and to document symptomatic and functional changes[66] and their relation to graft patency.[67]

The considerations noted above have the following implications regarding the role of exercise electrocardiography in assessing myocardial ischemia. *The exercise test is of little additional diagnostic value in patients with known angina, and its predictive accuracy is low and therefore of limited value in screening normal persons.* A positive test is useful, especially in men with chest pain of uncertain cause, and the work load and heart rate at which positive results are observed in those with coronary disease are useful in assessing prognosis. Thus, exercise testing can contribute to the decision-making process regarding catheterization and surgery. Finally, perhaps its major value is a reproducible test of cardiovascular performance which can be used to objectively and inexpensively assess the benefit of pharmacological and surgical therapy.

Thallium Scintigraphy (See Chap. 97)

Experimental work in animals[68] has shown that after an intravenous injection of thallium 201 the distribution in the myocardium is linearly related to myocardial blood flow. Thus, when inequalities of regional flow are present, myocardial imaging with a gamma camera reveals defects in the corresponding zone (cold-spot imaging). This relative flow reduction must be in the range of 50 percent to permit optimal resolution of defects.[69] Since resting coronary blood flow will be maintained at a normal level in the presence of obstructions even as severe as 80 to 85 percent of the vessel's diameter,[70] a stimulus is necessary to increase the demand for flow and to provoke measurable regional perfusion inequalities. Although pharmacological maneuvers have been used to induce this flow differential,[69,71] exercise testing remains the procedure of choice. Defects present upon exercise but not present at rest indicate flow deficits that may represent cellular ischemia, while resting defects usually,[72] but not invariably, represent infarction.[73,74] Although quantitative techniques are presently being developed[75-78] to improve the accuracy of this technique, most laboratories currently rely on qualitative methods with the inherent problems of intra- and interobserver variability[79] and varying standards for interpretation.[80-82]

Since thallium is injected at or near peak exercise, data are available on the comparative efficacy of electrocardiographic stress testing versus thallium radionuclide techniques in the diagnosis of coronary artery disease. The important effects of exercise protocol, electrocardiogram lead systems, exclusion criteria, and standards employed for the determination of positivity in electrocardiogram stress testing must be carefully considered when comparing the results of exercise electrocardiogram testing and thallium scanning. In addition, technical considerations involving data acquisition and processing will greatly influence the apparent usefulness of thallium scans.

In general, rest-exercise thallium scans are more sensitive than exercise electrocardiography for the detection of coronary disease. Specificity of the thallium scan is very high. When patients with inadequate or uninterpretable exercise electrocardiographic tests are excluded from the accuracy calculations, thallium and electrocardiogram tests have comparable sensitivity.[83-85] In a large collaborative experience[86] the combined sensitivity of rest and exercise electrocardiogram and thallium was 91 percent, greater than either test alone, and the combination did not produce a significant fall in specificity. Again, in this study thallium scintigraphy was of greatest value in patients with uninterpretable or inadequate electrocardiographic stress tests, but the precise sensitivity and specificity of thallium scanning at submaximal levels of exercise remains unclear.

The sensitivity of stress electrocardiography and of thallium scanning increases the extent of coronary artery disease.[40,43,51,52,87] To evaluate whether thallium would enhance the diagnostic accuracy for multivessel coronary disease, Dash et al.[87] compared patients with a markedly positive electrocardiogram stress test (greater than 2 mm horizontal or downsloping ST depression at less than stage 3 of a Bruce protocol) with patients having a markedly positive thallium scan (exercise-induced perfusion defects in distributions that would correspond to three-vessel or left main coronary artery disease). The electrocardiogram and thallium tests had sensitivities for left main or three-vessel disease of 34 percent and 43 percent, respectively, with corresponding specificity of 95 percent and 86 percent (not significantly different in either case). If either test was markedly positive, the combined sensitivity of 68 percent was significantly higher than for either test alone. Unfortunately, a test with this level of accuracy would be impractical in a population of patients with a low prevalence of multivessel coronary artery disease. Nevertheless, such an approach could be of value in patients with typical angina and therefore a greater likelihood of coronary artery disease.

Exercise thallium scintigraphy lends itself well to the study of patients undergoing myocardial revascularization. Detection of graft closure and/or incomplete revascularization has been reported to be 67 percent with a specificity of 100 percent. Knowledge of preoperative coronary anatomy can aid in differentiating and localizing an area of incompletely revascularized myocardium from one with an occluded graft, although the distinction can be difficult if coronary artery disease is extensive and defects are seen in scintigraphic regions where the vascular supply may be overlapping (inferoapex).[88] Unfortunately, although the predictive value of a positive perioperative thallium scan is excellent, little diagnostic insight can be gained from a negative result.

Thallium scanning as a single test would appear to be of greatest value in the diagnosis of coronary artery disease in patients with inadequate (less than 85 percent maximal predicted heart rate achieved) or uninterpretable electrocardiogram stress tests, as in the presence of an abnormal resting electrocardiogram (left bundle branch block, digitalis effect, and left ventricular hypertrophy). This is a major advantage when one considers that in some studies one-third of patients tested have ST-segment responses that are not diagnostic.[52] In addition a positive exercise thallium scan postoperatively is highly predictive of myocardial ischemia, but a negative test does not exclude ischemia.

Exercise Radionuclide Angiography (See Chap. 97)

Assessment of left ventricular function by contrast ventriculography during cardiac catheterization has provided invaluable information regarding prognosis[62,89–91] and the pathophysiology of systolic functional abnormalities[92] in medically[89,90] and surgically[62,91] treated patients. Much attention has also been directed to the questions of reversible myocardial asynergy[93,94] and how it affects prognosis and therapy.[95,96] Several noninvasive approaches[97,98] are now being applied to detecting asynergy, but depressed regional or global myocardial function may not be present at rest even in the presence of significant coronary stenosis.[90] Radionuclide cineangiography[99] using technetium provides a method to examine myocardial contractile function at rest and with exercise. Exercise-induced abnormalities in regional wall motion can also be detected.[100–102] As might be anticipated, technological,[103] procedural,[104] and population variables influence the sensitivity, specificity, and predictive value of the test. In evaluating ventricular function during exercise, ejection fraction and regional wall motion have been studied in an attempt to identify patients with myocardial ischemia. The normal variability and reproducibility of ejection fraction[101,105] and regional wall motion at rest and during exercise are now being defined.[106,107] An abnormal response to exercise in the ejection fraction is observed in approximately 80 to 90 percent of patients with atherosclerotic coronary disease, but is not specific for coronary artery disease.[108,109] Focusing on new regional abnormalities of wall motion during exercise can be anticipated to enhance the specificity of the test, but how much it does so remains uncertain. One of the major values of the radionuclide angiogram is its simplicity and accuracy in providing a noninvasive way to assess

ventricular function. Since resting left ventricular function is an important prognostic factor in patients with coronary disease and is also an important factor in estimating surgical risk, the ability to obtain the information with the scan will surely play an important role in guiding selection of appropriate candidates for catheterization.

Invasive Tests (Chaps. 45 and 98)

Invasive studies are the only current methods by which the anatomical extent and severity of coronary artery disease can be evaluated. Since invasive procedures carry certain risks to the patient, and the cost of the procedures to the medical care system is appreciable, the cardiologist should have clear reasons for performing these tests. In general, cardiac catheterization and angiography should be carried out in patients in the coronary age group who are being evaluated for any type of heart surgery, whenever coronary artery surgery is being considered, when noninvasive evaluations continue to leave serious uncertainty about a diagnosis of coronary disease in a patient with unexplained chest pain, and in certain asymptomatic patients with an electrocardiographic or hemodynamic response to exercise compatible with severe coronary disease.

The invasive tests primarily define the anatomy and structural concomitants of ischemic heart disease. They generally do not identify the presence or absence of ischemia at the time of the study, and they do not lend themselves to rest-exercise comparisons.

The Resting Ventriculogram (See Chap. 98)

Cardiac catheterization and angiography performed with the patient at rest are unlikely to provide information regarding the presence of ischemia, but angiography during certain interventions can provide evidence that is compatible with the presence of the ischemic state. The resting ventriculogram does provide important information that helps estimate the prognosis of the patient if treated medically and can assist in a decision regarding surgical therapy. It also helps the surgeon plan the optimal procedure. The ejection fraction is a simple measurement which provides useful information on prognosis and the choice of therapy.[90,110]

$$\text{Ejection fraction} = \frac{(\text{end-diastolic volume}) - (\text{end-systolic volume})}{\text{end-diastolic volume}}$$

The ejection fraction is derived from planimetric measurements, with the assumption that the ventricle is ellipsoidal in shape. In symmetrical ventricles, volume and therefore ejection fraction are quite accurate by this technique. Distortion introduced by ventricular asymmetry with coronary disease and infarction can result in erroneous estimates.[111] In addition to measuring the ejection fraction, it is also useful to assess regional wall motion from the ventriculogram. The wall motion may be normal or show decreased inward movement (hypokinesis), absent movement (akinesis), or paradoxical movement (dyskinesis).[112] Patient survival with medical therapy varies inversely with the resting ejection fraction[89] and is reduced in the presence of hemodynamic compromise or ventriculographic evidence of previous infarction. The mortality associated with coronary artery bypass surgery in the presence of severely depressed ventricular function is also increased.

In addition to the detection of the various types of ventricular asynergy described above, the ventriculogram may also demonstrate the presence of a discrete left ventricular aneurysm which may be clinically manifest as congestive heart failure, arrhythmias, or systemic emboli. This is important because the surgical removal of the aneurysm and the ectopic electrical foci may be indicated.[113]

Finally in patients with coronary artery disease the resting ventriculogram will provide information regarding the presence and extent of structural abnormalities of the heart, such as mitral regurgitation and ventricular septal defect. These evaluations are particularly important in patients who are being evaluated because of hemodynamic deterioration soon after myocardial infarction.

Intervention Ventriculography (See Chap. 98)

The presence of a hypokinetic or akinetic segment on the resting ventriculogram does not necessarily indicate the presence of myocardial scar tissue. Regional wall motion may show improvement either after the preload is acutely reduced by administration of sublingual nitroglycerin or during the positive inotropic state of extrasystolic potentiation. This postintervention improvement has been taken as evidence that the affected myocardium is viable but may be functioning in a depressed state because of inadequate myocardial blood flow.[114] It has recently been demonstrated that patients with reversible asynergy are more likely to show improvement in wall motion following coronary artery bypass surgery.[115]

Contrast Coronary Angiography (See Chap. 98)

When coronary angiograms are analyzed, the narrowing is frequently expressed as percent decrease in the diameter of the vessels. The corresponding reduction in cross-sectional area of the lumen is proportional to the square of the decrease in diameter. Studies in experimental animals indicate that there must be approximately an 85 percent decrease in the diameter of a coronary vessel (98 percent cross-sectional narrowing) before resting coronary flow declines.[70] When the myocardial demand for oxygen is increased three- or fourfold in the experimental animal, a luminal diameter narrowing of 60 percent (84 percent cross-sectional) will produce myocardial ischemia. In humans, 72 percent luminal diameter–narrowing stenosis (92 percent cross-sectional decrease) has been estimated to result in myocardial ischemia at rest.[117,118] Long segments of stenosis or multiple lesions appear to reduce coronary flow more markedly than do discrete single, short lesions.[117,118] The complexity of these relationships makes it difficult to predict the precise physiological effect of many lesions observed on routine angiograms. It is important for the angiographer to state if he or she implies diameter narrowing or cross-sectional narrowing.

Several studies have demonstrated significant intraobserver and interobserver variability in assessing the severity of lesions and in defining the number of coronary vessels involved in any one patient.[119–121] Agreement has been greater in reading right coronary than left coronary lesions. In one study the standard deviation for any one reader in repeatedly estimating the severity of a lesion was 8 percent, and there was disagreement among different readers in 31 percent of cases on the number of vessels narrowed by 70 percent or more.[121]

It has recently been reported that both the area of the lesion and the reference area with which the narrowed segment is being compared can dilate with verapamil infusion.[122] This observation suggests yet another source of error other than observer error that must be appreciated when evaluating coronary angiograms. The fact that this may be a clinically significant problem has been demonstrated by Arnett et al.[123] and by Roberts and Jones,[124] who showed that the large proximal segments of the coronary vessel may be significantly narrowed by atheromatous plaque at autopsy, yet not appear narrowed on angiography.

Studies have been done that attempt to compare angiographically estimated stenoses with measurements made on the vessels at postmortem examination.[125–128] In general, the angiographer underestimates the severity of the obstruction. On the other hand, experienced readers were found to overestimate the amount of narrowing caused by relatively severe lesions compared with a quantitative computer reading of the lesion.[129] Despite the above problems, subjective and angiographic readings have provided important prognostic information related to survival from single-, double-, and triple-vessel and main left coronary involvement.[130–133]

Coronary artery spasm may contribute to the ischemic syndrome when angina pectoris occurs at rest (see Chaps. 45 and 47). The variant anginal syndrome, or Prinzmetal's angina, is of major interest in this regard. Patients with this condition may have coronary arteries that appear normal at the time of angiography, but coronary spasm may be demonstrated following the intravenous administration of ergonovine (see Chap. 98). Ergonovine may be most useful in patients with a characteristic pain pattern but in whom electrocardiograms have not been recorded during pain. The ergonovine provocative test is also useful in evaluating the effectiveness of therapeutic agents.[134,135] Failure to induce spasm with ergonovine in a patient on therapy who had previously been demonstrated to have spasm is an indication of the efficacy of the therapy. Although ergonovine tests are generally safe,[134–138] there is a risk of producing nitrate-resistant spasm and subsequent infarction.[139] Vasodilating agents should be immediately available to reverse the spasm by intracoronary injection if sublingual nitroglycerin initially fails. It is recommended that ergonovine not be given outside the catheterization laboratory.

The Role of Hemodynamic Evaluation

It has been demonstrated that groups of patients with coronary artery disease and impaired hemodynamics have poorer medical prognoses than groups of patients with normal hemodynamics.[89,140,141] Also, patients with depressed cardiac output tend to have more prolonged survival after surgical therapy than after medical treatment.[141] This suggests that hemodynamic measurements can provide prognostic information that may be helpful in selecting medical versus surgical therapy. It has also been observed that patients with high left ventricular end-diastolic pressures tend to show more extensive coronary involvement and more severe wall motion abnormalities on the ventriculogram than patients with normal end-diastolic pressure, although this has not been a reliable index of the severity of coronary disease.[142]

Although all of the above hemodynamic abnormalities can be correlated with ventriculographic abnormalities that are of prognostic value, they do not appear to add independently to the power of the ventriculogram in evaluating patients with ischemic heart disease, except in patients with congestive heart failure due to mitral regurgitation, ventricular aneurysm, or ventricular septal defect. In these subsets of patients with complications, hemodynamic evaluation is important in determining the degree of impairment in order to provide base-line information against which improvement with medical therapy, such as unloading, or surgical therapy can be measured.

Coronary Sinus Studies (See Chap. 98)

Cardiac metabolic abnormalities reported during myocardial ischemia have been outlined in Chaps. 5 and 44. The main method of evaluating myocardial metabolism in patients has been the insertion of a catheter in the coronary sinus and the measurement of coronary blood flow and metabolites, including oxygen, lactate, pyruvate, free fatty acids, and other substances.

Coronary blood flow is measured by the washout of foreign materials from the myocardium that are delivered to the heart by intravenous injection, by direct intracoronary injection, or after inhalation of a reference gas. Thermal dilution measurements of cold solution injected into the coronary sinus can also be employed. Although early studies did not show consistent abnormalities in coronary blood flow at rest in patients with ischemic heart disease, more recent work has demonstrated diminished flow in areas distal to an obstructed vessel when energy demands are increased.[117]

The most frequently employed measure of myocardial ischemia in humans has been the determination of lactate extraction/production across the myocardium. Lactate is normally extracted by the heart. Decreased extraction or net lactate production has been regarded as indicating myocardial ischemia.[143] Earlier studies in patients with documented coronary artery disease indicate that lactate extraction of 10 percent or less is indicative of ischemia. Recent studies in men with no clinical evidence of coronary artery disease have demonstrated that at rest or during rapid pacing lactate extraction by the human heart may fall below 10 percent but lactate is not produced.[144] Thus lactate production by the myocardium is probably abnormal, but low or diminishing levels of lactate extraction during stress are not necessarily diagnostic of ischemia in humans. Lactate metabolism is also affected by a variety of other factors, particularly free fatty acid metabolism by the heart.[145] Thus the nutritional state, levels of circulating catecholamines, and many other factors may alter lactate metabolism in any individual.

Other metabolites released from the myocardium during ischemia include potassium, phosphate, adenosine, and inosine. Although tests involving the determination of some of these have been used in humans for the detection of ischemia, they have not proved to be more sensitive than determination of lactate alone.

One of the problems with coronary sinus studies in ischemic heart disease is that coronary disease is a regional condition and therefore myocardial metabolism is heterogeneous. If there is disease of the right coronary artery alone, ischemia might not be detected in coronary sinus studies because much of the sampled blood emanates from the normal left coronary artery bed and dilutes the abnormal venous drainage from the right coronary bed. Detection of ischemia in the area perfused by the left anterior descending coronary artery is more accurate. Attempts have been made to demonstrate this phenomenon by regional sampling of the effluent with catheters inserted into different areas of the coronary venous system.[146]

Although metabolic and flow studies are not generally used clinically, they may be helpful in some patients with chest pain and angiographically normal coronary arteries. Kemp et al. have demonstrated that some of these patients may have myocardial lactate production induced by atrial pacing.[147] Also of interest in this regard is the finding that patients with Prinzmetal's angina decrease coronary blood flow and produce lactate during ergonovine-induced spasm.[137,138] At the present time coronary sinus technique for measuring myocardial blood flow and metabolism remain an investigational method for demonstrating myocardial ischemia and are of limited usefulness as a clinical tool.

Risks of Catheterization and Coronary Angiography (See Chap. 98)

Numerous complications may arise from coronary arteriography, and the risk of these must be weighed against the risk of avoiding the procedure and not knowing the extent of the patient's disease. A recent collaborative study demonstrated a 0.2 percent mortality rate within 24 h of catheterization among patients with coronary artery disease and an 0.25 percent nonfatal myocardial infarction rate within 48 h.[148] In patients with greater than 50 percent narrowing of the left main coronary artery, the mortality plus infarction rate was almost seven times as great as in other cases. Patients with congestive heart failure, hypertension, ejection fractions less than 30 percent, and arrhythmias prior to catheterization also had an increased risk for the procedure. Thus, patients with the greatest risk from the natural history of their disease have the highest risk from cardiac catheterization and angiography. As stated, the figures just quoted were derived from a collaborative study. It must be emphasized that many laboratories have far less complications than this study indicates (see Chap. 98). The clinician must therefore decide whether or not the risk of the procedure is outweighed by the potential benefit to be gained from the information.

Summary

In patients with classic angina pectoris (particularly men), presently available noninvasive diagnostic tests cannot efficiently alter the strong probability of disease presence. Rather, the tests should be used to determine the extent of functional impairment,[64] presence of multivessel disease,[55,87] adequacy of medical or surgical therapy, and risk for a morbid event.[66,67,149–152] In patients with typical angina, cardiac catheterization is undertaken whenever symptoms dictate that a surgical approach to treatment is indicated, or if the noninvasive tests indicate that information gained from catheterization may contribute significantly to estimating prognosis or may identify an anatomical situation in which surgical therapy is warranted on the basis of survival data even though symptoms may not be severe.

Assessment of Myocardial Infarction

The question of whether or not there has been a change in the state of the coronary circulation that warrants hospitalization is based on the history and physical examination. Electrocardiographic evidence of acute ischemia, infarction, or life-threatening arrhythmias would support a decision to admit a patient for observation or treatment, but the absence of these findings does not justify a decision that no significant change in the coronary system is occurring. *It is not possible to exclude a diagnosis of acute infarction by physical examination or electrocardiogram in the emergency room in a patient with chest pain.* Therefore, if there is a reasonable suspicion that the patient has coronary artery disease and an unstable clinical picture, he or she should be admitted to the coronary care facility. Questions will then arise regarding (1) the presence or absence of infarction, (2) the location and size of the infarct, (3) whether or not there is continuing ischemia and progressive infarction, (4) the hemodynamic consequences of infarction, (5) whether or not structural abnormalities that may warrant surgical consideration have occurred, and finally (6) the immediate and long-range prognosis.

A full discussion of myocardial infarction, its natural history, complications, treatment, and prognosis is developed in Chap. 45. When a question persists regarding myocardial infarction even after a history, physical examination, electrocardiogram, and chest x-ray have been obtained, what does the physician do next and what is the role of various laboratory tests that may contribute to answering the question? We will consider this in the following discussion.

The Release of Enzymes (See Chap. 45)

Loss of membrane control of cell osmolality and disruption of membrane integrity constitute major factors leading to irreversible cell damage from ischemia. Therefore, on a theoretical basis, the release of cell proteins should signify the presence of irreversibly damaged cells. Although some loss of enzyme has been observed in a few experiments without unequivocal evidence of necrosis[153,154] most work supports the view that when myocardial proteins are detected in the serum irreversibly damaged cells will be found.[155,156] The major use of serum enzyme measurements has been to answer the question of whether myocardial infarction is present or absent.[157] The enzymes that have been employed include serum glutamic oxaloacetic transaminase (SGOT), lactate dehydrogenase (LDH), and creatine kinase (CK or CPK).

Creatine kinase is a dimer made up of isomeric subunits, M for muscle and B for brain. Three isoenzyme forms are found in the cytoplasm: MM in muscle, BB in brain and gastrointestinal tract, and MB in myocardium. Even though MB-CK constitutes a minority of the myocardial CK (about 14 percent), its appearance in the blood is highly specific for myocardial damage.

LDH has two types of subunits, H for hepatic and M for muscle. Since these subunits form tetrameric combinations, there are five isomeric isoenzyme combinations. All of the isoenzymes exist in the myocardium, but there is a greater proportion of LDH_1. Therefore after myocardial damage LDH_1 will predominate in the serum.[157] However, since erythrocytes also contain large amounts of LDH_1, small amounts of hemolysis may obscure the diagnosis of myocardial necrosis. LDH_1 is resistant to heating, so that a rise in heat-stable LDH provides a tool for measuring serum LDH that can be identified with cardiac damage.

Creatine kinase rises to a peak at about 24 h, SGOT at 24 to 48 h, and LDH at 36 to 64 h. Serum MB-CK rises earlier and declines faster than the total CK.[158] These characteristics of timing have led to the use of various serum enzyme patterns at different times after the onset of chest pain to provide evidence about the presence or absence of infarction.

SGOT is quite sensitive to infarction but is also elevated in some patients with pulmonary embolism, myocarditis, pericarditis, hepatic congestion, or skeletal muscle disease, and in some patients using oral contraceptives.[157] Elevated SGOT levels are also observed after surgery and cardioversion. LDH is also a sensitive indicator of infarction and is more specific than SGOT, although LDH elevations are found in megaloblastic anemia, liver disease, pulmonary infarction, myxedema, and hemolysis.[157] Total CK elevations are very sensitive for infarction but are seen with skeletal muscle, brain, or gastrointestinal damage.[157] The early rise in the serum MB-CK after infarction is thought to be the most sensitive and specific enzyme indicator of the presence or absence of infarction.[159-162] Table 20-3 demonstrates the predictability of the ECG, SGOT, heat-stable LDH, total LDH, total CK, and MB-CK tests in defining the presence or absence of myocardial infarctions. It shows that MB-CK is as accurate for including or excluding myocardial damage as all the other tests. If patients are seen within 24 h of the onset of chest pain, MB-CK obtained twice a day for the next 2 days yields diagnostic information that is as accurate as the electrocardiogram and combinations of the other enzyme tests.[159]

A failure of MB-CK levels to become elevated in the first 17 h after admission effectively excludes acute myocardial infarction. *It does not exclude prolonged ischemia without infarction.* Thus, in patients who are seen early, the use of MB-CK may obviate the need for other enzyme tests. LDH isoenzymes would have to be relied upon for patients seen later, after the onset of pain. Because tissues containing any of the enzymes may be damaged in the shock syndrome, rises in the serum level of these proteins are not diagnostic of acute infarction in the presence of shock.

Analysis of serum enzymes are of great value in patients with accelerated angina or intermediate syndromes. A certain number of patients with these clinical conditions do not respond to medical intervention and will require early angiography and perhaps surgery. Assurance that myocardial infarction is absent is of considerable clinical importance. Also, in patients with a recent myocardial infarction and recurrent pain, it is necessary to know if the infarct has extended or whether ischemia without infarction is present. In these cases serum enzymes, especially MB-CK, are the major basis upon which the diagnosis of extension is made.

Isoenzymes are important in evaluating the presence or absence of myocardial infarction after noncardiac surgery. MB-CK has proved to be extremely useful in these situations for documenting the presence or absence of infarction.[162,163] It has also been of use following cardiac surgery when ST-segment and T-wave alterations are frequent and raise the question of myocardial damage, although its sensitivity and specificity following cardiac surgery are diminished.

The misuse and limitations of cardiac enzymes in determining the presence of infarction is discussed in Chap. 45.

Enzyme Estimation of Infarct Size

Creatine kinase (CK) has been the primary enzyme employed experimentally for the estimation of infarct size.[157,164] An inverse correlation has been found between the size of an infarct and total CK content measured in the tissue following experimental myocardial infarction.[165] There is a direct correlation between serum CK levels drawn serially after myocardial infarction in dogs, CK depletion from the myocardium at 24 h, and the size of the infarct observed at postmortem examination.[166] Prediction of the amount of myocardial necrosis found 24 h after infarction can be made from the serial CK blood levels measured during the first few hours after infarction.[164,167] Use of this predictive approach clinically depends upon the patient reaching the hospital early during infarction.

There are several variables that may alter these predictive relationships.[157,164] These include the slow rate of washout of the enzymes from unperfused portions of the myocardium, possible destruction of the enzyme in the cardiac lymph and venous blood, and variability in the rate of removal of CK from the serum by the reticuloendothelial system. Homogeneous infarctions appear to provide a better quantitative CK-release curve than scattered areas of infarction. The clinical situation in humans

TABLE 20-3 Predictability of Positive and Negative Results of Various Test Parameters for the Diagnosis of Acute Myocardial Infarction[159]

Test	Positive	Negative
ECG	1.00	0.88
GOT	0.75	1.00
LDH (heat stable)	0.75	0.99
LDH	0.83	1.00
CK	0.73	1.00
MB-CK	1.00	0.98

is obviously different from studies in the experimental model in that the onset of the infarct cannot be precisely timed in humans and in fact may not be a discrete event in time.[164,168] Furthermore, CK elevations may be due to damage to skeletal muscle by intramuscular injections or cardioversion trauma, or diverse in origin as seen in the shock syndrome resulting in misleading CK elevations from noncardiac tissue. Thus, CK curves for the prediction of infarct size are probably less accurate in humans, although good correlations have been claimed by some workers.[169] CK levels during infarction have been found to correlate with the occurrence of severe ventricular arrhythmias[170] and mortality.[164] MB-CK curves have not been widely used clinically to predict infarct size; however, they may hold greater potential in humans than the total CK curves to predict infarct size in humans.

Myoglobin and Myosin Light Chains (See Chap. 45)

A recent development in the quest for a biochemical marker of infarction is the finding that myoglobin is released from the myocardium during infarction. A specific radioimmunoassay for myoglobin has been developed for use in patients with myocardial infarction.[171] These studies have demonstrated that myoglobin peaks in the serum rapidly after discrete infarction, and its detection can be a sensitive indicator of tissue necrosis. Since serum myoglobin falls rapidly, it has been used to follow the course of infarction, particularly when necrosis has continued for several days.[172,173] Myoglobin levels correlate well with CK levels[174] and theoretically should have the same power as MB-CK for detecting necrosis.

Cardiac myosin contains two small subunits of approximately 27,000 and 20,000 MW, which are designated as light chains. The cardiac light chains are immunologically and structurally distinct from those of skeletal muscle. As myosin degrades in necrotic cells, these subunits may be released into the serum, where they can be detected by radioimmunoassay.[175] The appearance of light chains from the heart in the serum has been found to be sensitive and specific for myocardial infarction in humans.[176] This approach has been employed to a limited degree in patients, but has not been demonstrated to be superior to standard enzymatic analyses for the diagnosis of myocardial damage.

The Radionuclide Detection of Infarction (See Chaps. 45 and 97)

Technetium pyrophosphate is infarct-avid and accumulates in regions of acute myocardial necrosis.[177,178] Scanning with this agent has been reported to be highly sensitive (up to 100 percent) for the diagnosis and localization of acute transmural myocardial infarction,[177–180] particularly if scanning is performed within 3 to 5 days[178–180] of the onset of symptoms. However, the sensitivity for nontransmural myocardial infarction[179,181] and the specificity of acute myocardial infarction in general have been challenged by a number of investigators.[179,182–185] Positive technetium scans have been noted in patients with angina pectoris[181] with ventricular asynergy (especially if dyskinesis is present)[183] and in patients without prior history of myocardial infarction who were undergoing a bone scan.[186] Much of the disagreement stems from interpretation of a diffuse pattern of uptake, which is a frequent finding in nontransmural myocardial infarction[181,185,187,188] but also may be a false-positive pattern. Diffuse pyrophosphate positivity can persist in as many as 54 percent of patients for months following myocardial infarction, thereby limiting the usefulness of this test during subsequent clinical events.[188,189]

Thallium scintigrams are highly sensitive (82 to 100 percent) but not adequately specific for the diagnosis of acute myocardial infarction.[190,191] The lack of specificity is due to resting defects that occur with scar tissue secondary to prior myocardial infarction.[72,76,80,192] Early scanning in myocardial infarction is important for diagnostic accuracy, as sensitivity falls if scans are performed more than 24 h after the clinical event.[191] Time is also important because the size of the defect decreases with time,[181,191] perhaps due to regression of periinfarction ischemia. Therefore the late thallium image corresonds more closely to other measures of infarct size.[81] Accurate infarct localization by thallium scanning has been confirmed by electrocardiogram,[191,192] ventriculography,[192] and postmortem studies.[72]

Most patients have right-dominant coronary systems so that the right coronary artery provides the blood supply to a major portion of the posterior and inferior left ventricle. Infarctions due to disease of the right coronary artery may be associated not only with involvement of the left ventricle but also posterior septal and right ventricular infarction and dysfunction. If the infarction is extensive, marked elevation of the right ventricular end-diastolic pressure may be observed.[192a,192b] These patients may have physical signs of right heart failure and depressed cardiac outputs, but the cause may not be obvious on clinical examination or when only the pulmonary artery or pulmonary wedge pressures are monitored.[193]

Scintigraphic techniques have also been proved to be of value in the diagnosis of right ventricular infarction. Clinical recognition of this entity is difficult, especially in the absence of hemodynamic compromise.[193] Combined thallium and pyrophosphate scanning of patients with documented inferior wall infarctions have demonstrated a 38 percent incidence of right ventricular involvement.[194] Radionuclide ventriculography has been of particular value in this clinical setting because the presence of a dilated, hypokinetic right ventricle in a patient who is hemodynamically compromised[194,195] has important diagnostic and therapeutic implications.[193,195]

Assessment of Infarct Size

Thallium and pyrophosphate scanning have been used to estimate infarct size,[177,192] and to stratify risk[183,189,190] for morbid events in patients with acute myocardial infarction. Although pyrophosphate uptake is not simply related to infarct size,[196] it has been shown to correlate fairly well with the size of anterior infarcts estimated by CK-curve analysis.[190] Patients with acute myocardial infarction and large areas of technetium pyrophosphate uptake tend to have a complicated clinical course, usually secondary to myocardial failure.[182,197] The "doughnut" pattern (large rim of technetium pyrophosphate activity with a central clear zone) carries an ominous prognosis.[197,198] On the other hand, a falsely negative pyrophosphate scan has been associated with an uncomplicated course[182] and in general is associated with small infarcts.[196] The prevalence of angina, congestive heart failure, and persistent ST-segment elevation is higher in patients with persistently positive pyrophosphate scans.[188]

The size of thallium defects in patients with acute myocardial infarction correlates with infarct size at postmortem examination.[72] However, the inability to distinguish acute ischemia and old infarct from acute necrosis limits its utility for this purpose. The size of a thallium defect at rest has been shown to correlate with the magnitude of ventricular asynergy in patients studied late after myocardial infarction.[192] Since thallium defects reflect both old and new infarction as well as ischemia, thallium scanning in acute myocardial infarction may serve as an excellent prognostic indicator for short-term mortality.[199]

Radionuclide studies to assess ejection fraction and to analyze segmental wall motion have important therapeutic and prognostic value. The location of akinesis by radionuclide ventriculography corresponds closely with the location of Q waves on the electrocardiogram.[200,201] Radionuclide ventriculography has also been shown to be sensitive and specific for the detection of discrete left ventricular aneurysm.[202,203] Global[200,201,204,205] and regional ejection fractions have been found to be depressed in the majority of patients with acute transmural myocardial infarction. Early improvement in ejection fraction in such patients is associated with a better prognosis, although the absolute level of ejection fraction is a relatively poor predictor of prognosis in clinically uncomplicated infarcts.[204]

Vectorcardiography and Body Surface Electrocardiographic Mapping (See Chaps. 45 and 86)

The detailed description of vectorcardiographic analysis in patients with myocardial infarction is discussed in Chap. 86. The vectorcardiogram (VCG) has a low false-positive rate[206] and appears to be more sensitive than the standard electrocardiogram for the diagnosis of infarction.[207,208] However, if the scalar electrocardiogram is used in combination with serum enzymes and infarct-avid radionuclide techniques in ambiguous cases, it is likely that their combination will be more sensitive for detecting acute infarction than the VCG alone.

The importance of being able to evaluate the initial size of a myocardial infarct and to follow the course of the infarction has led to other electrocardiographic techniques that are currently of *research interest*. ST-segment shifts in the precordial electrocardiogram have been used to estimate the extent of myocardial ischemia and its progression to infarction[209] in animal models of acute coronary artery occlusion. The technique employs the summed magnitude of ST-segment elevation recorded by multiple epicardial or precordial electrodes with observations throughout the course of ischemia and infarction. Soon after the onset of transmural ischemic injury the ST segments become elevated, reach a peak, and gradually decline toward base line over the next 12 to 24 h. Good correlations have been observed in experimental animals between the magnitude of ST-segment elevations, and the area over which they occur, and blood flow to an ischemic region, subsequent creatine kinase depletion, and histological evidence of infarction.[166,210,211] However, other experimental and theoretical work has raised serious questions about the validity of the ST-segment approach.[212,213]

QRS mapping has also been used to try to determine the extent of myocardial injury and subsequent infarction. This approach is based on observations in dogs that the degree of ST-segment elevation 15 min after coronary occlusion correlates with the extent of R-wave loss (and Q-wave development) at 6 and 24 h after occlusion.[166] As with ST-segment mapping, R-wave changes and the development of Q waves have been shown to correlate with tissue CK depletion and histologic changes after experimental myocardial infarction.

Both ST-segment and QRS-complex changes have been employed in patients with precordial mapping techniques to predict the extent of ischemic injury and myocardial infarction.[166,214] These methods use multiple precordial electrodes in a grid and depend upon the calculation of changes in ST segments or changes in R-wave height. However, there may be a considerable amount of variability in these measurements within any one patient, and the technique may be more useful for comparing groups of patients in which different treatment modalities are being investigated. A number of investigations of therapy have been performed in humans using this technique, but the approach has not been validated or used enough to provide information useful in the clinical care of individual patients.

There are several limitations to precordial mapping. At present, its use must be restricted to patients with anterior or anterolateral infarctions where the area of infarct can be entirely encompassed within the field of the multiple electrode grid. Maps cannot be employed when a change occurs in the ventricular conduction pattern, since alterations in conduction can affect the depth of Q waves, the height of R waves, and the ST segments independent of the amount of necrosis. Precordial maps are likely to provide information related mainly to the subepicardial half of the myocardium and are altered in an unknown way by infarctions of the subendocardium or infarction in the posterior or diaphragmatic walls of the heart.

Echocardiography in Myocardial Infarction (See Chap. 95)

Notwithstanding the limited view M-mode echocardiography provides of the left ventricle, abnormalities in systolic function have been reported in acute myocardial infarction.[215] During acute infarction or ischemia, systolic thinning can be seen in involved segments,[216] and with healing, scar tissue can be identified echocardiographically.[217] Although ventricular asynergy can be detected using M-mode echocardiography,[218] two-dimensional echocardiographic techniques have been shown to be better suited for this purpose.[219,220] Preliminary results indicate that the correlation of wall motion changes between two-dimensional echocardiograms and contrast angiography is good. As with radionuclide ventriculographic techniques, echocardiographically defined systolic abnormalities are not specific for acute events, nor for infarction. In assessing global left ventricular function (e.g., ejection fraction) M-mode echocardiography is unreliable in the presence of ventricular asynergy.[221] On the other hand, two-dimensional echocardiography correlates well with angiographic ejection fraction even when asynergy is present.[222,223]

Two-dimensional echocardiography has also been shown to be helpful in differentiating papillary muscle dysfunction[222] from a ruptured interventricular septum[224] in the infarct patient who develops a new systolic murmur.

Hemodynamic Monitoring in Myocardial Infarction (See Chap. 45)

When the patient with myocardial infarction is normotensive or hypertensive, the arterial blood pressure is satisfactorily monitored via the cuff technique in most situations. Direct intraarterial pressure monitoring is advantageous in the following situations: when blood pressure is low and difficult to detect by cuff; when agents are employed that may cause rapid shifts in blood pressure; and when blood pressure is being used to guide therapy with such agents.

The hemodynamic indications for Swan-Ganz catheterization are outlined in Chap. 45. The catheter and techniques are fully described in Chap. 99. The measurements made with the Swan-Ganz cath-

eter include (1) pulmonary occlusive pressure (POP); (2) pulmonary artery pressure (PAP); (3) right atrial pressure (RAP); (4) thermodilution cardiac output (CO) or cardiac index (CI); and (5) oxygen contents in right atrial and pulmonary artery blood.

Cardiac output measured with thermodilution techniques have been reported to be quite compatible with values obtained by dye-dilution techniques, with differences of 16 to 17 percent between the techniques and repeatability of about 5 percent.[225] It is prudent to simultaneously measure systemic and pulmonary arterial oxygen content because the difference between the two (arteriovenous oxygen difference) varies inversely with properly performed thermodilution cardiac outputs.

Use of the Swan-Ganz catheter is usually reserved for patients with some degree of pump failure or cardiogenic shock. The catheter is also employed to determine whether ventricular septal defect or acute mitral regurgitation are present and whether signs of right ventricular infarction is present as evidenced by disproportionately elevated right ventricular end-diastolic or right atrial pressure. Swan-Ganz catheterization is used more generally to follow the course of left ventricular filling pressure and cardiac output as fluid therapy or diuretics are administered, or as agents are administered to unload the heart or improve the inotropic state; it is also used to follow the progress of patients being treated with the intraaortic balloon pump.

The risks of Swan-Ganz catheterization include (1) pulmonary infarction with prolonged monitoring; (2) ruptured pulmonary artery; (3) knotting of the catheter in the heart; (4) infection related to the catheter; and (5) pulmonic or tricuspid regurgitation.[226-228] These are rare events and relate mainly to either prolonged use or less than rigorous attention to catheter position and balloon deflation.[229]

Angiographic Studies during Acute Myocardial Infarction (See Chap. 45)

Angiographic studies during the acute stage of myocardial infarction are used mainly for those patients in whom urgent surgery is being considered because of persistent ischemia or an unstable hemodynamic state. Generally this will include patients with congestive heart failure, cardiogenic shock, acute mitral regurgitation, or acute ventricular septal defect, and those unable to be removed from inotropic agents or the intraaortic balloon pump (IABP).

In order to obtain the most accurate information concerning left ventricular function and anatomy, a biplane ventriculogram should be performed. Although satisfactory for most purposes, single-plane left ventriculography may not reveal the true extent of asynergy and may not be as accurate for the determination of ventricular volume data and ejection fraction. Coronary angiograms should be performed with sufficient views to define all the lesions so that the proper decisions concerning surgical intervention can be made.

The success of surgical treatment in these hemodynamically unstable infarct patients has not yet been defined. The surgical mortality is high,[230,231] and the salvage rate is relatively low. The surgeon must deal with friable necrotic tissue, and the technical problems posed in this setting are formidable. Despite these problems, there are many surgical successes in these patients who would have extremely low survival rates with medical therapy. In the future, both short-term and long-term survival rates must be evaluated in matched medical and surgical series.

Summary

Serial enzyme determinations, especially the isoenzymes of CK, are recommended in patients with suspected acute infarction. Characteristic changes of these enzymes are the most sensitive and specific signs of acute myocardial necrosis in humans. Nuclear scanning after injection of either technetium pyrophosphate or thallium[201] is a highly sensitive method for detecting recent infarction, but these methods *lack the desired level of specificity*. Electrocardiography, vectorcardiography, and pyrophosphate scanning can each be used to locate regions of infarction with reasonable precision. The size of an infarct is probably assessed best by the physician using a combination of electrocardiographic, enzymatic, and hemodynamic observations. Hemodynamic monitoring is probably best reserved for patients with complicated infarctions who require therapy with agents that require hemodynamic assessment to judge effectiveness and optimal dose. Cardiac catheterization with ventriculography and coronary arteriography is used only in patients who are considered to be surgical candidates. Patients become surgical candidates because of either persistent ischemic pain or an unstable hemodynamic state that seems likely to have resulted from surgically treatable complication of acute infarction such as acute mitral regurgitation or ruptured interventricular septum.

References

*1. Report of the Joint International Society and Federation of Cardiology, World Health Organization Task Force on Standardization of Clinical Nomenclature and Criteria for Diagnosis of Ischemic Heart Disease, *Circulation*, 59:607, 1979. (Extensively referenced)
 2. "Heart Facts, 1980," American Heart Association, New York, 1979.
*3. Epstein, S. E.: Value and Limitations of the Elec-

trocardiographic Response to Exercise in the Assessment of Patients with Coronary Artery Disease, *Am. J. Cardiol.*, 42:667, 1978. (35 references)
 4. Diamond, G. A., and Forrester, J. S.: Analysis of Probability as an Aid in the Clinical Diagnosis of Coronary Artery Disease, *N. Engl. J. Med.*, 300:1350, 1979.
 5. Friesinger, G. C., and Smith, R. F.: Correlation of Electrocardiographic Studies and Arteriographic Findings with Angina Pectoris, *Circulation*, 46:1173, 1972.
*6. Chaitman, B. R., Waters, D. D., Bourassa, M. G., Tuban, J. F., Wagniart, P., and Ferguson, R. J.: The Importance of Clinical Subsets in Interpreting Maximal Treadmill Test Results: The Role of Multiple Lead ECG Systems, *Circulation*, 59:560, 1979. (45 references)
 7. Spain, D. M., and Bradiss, V. A.: Occupational Physical Activity and the Degree of Coronary Atherosclerosis in Normal Men: A Postmortem Study, *Circulation*, 22:239, 1960.
 8. White, N. K., Edwards, J. E., and Dry, T. J.: The Relationship of the Degree of Coronary Atherosclerosis with Age, in Men, *Circulation*, 1:645, 1950.
 9. Erikssen, J., Enge, I., Forfang, K., and Storstein, O.: False Positive Diagnostic Tests and Coronary Angiographic Findings in 105 Presumably Healthy Males, *Circulation*, 54:371, 1976.
 10. Gensini, G. G., and Kelley, A. E.: Incidence and Progression of Coronary Artery Disease: An Angiographic Correlation in 1263 Patients, *Arch. Intern. Med.*, 129:814, 1972.
 11. "Coronary Risk Handbook," American Heart Association, New York, 1973.
 12. Proudfit, W. L., Shirey, E. K., and Sones, F. M.: Selective Cine Coronary Arteriography Correlation with Clinical Findings in 1000 Patients, *Circulation*, 33:901, 1966.
*13. Weiner, D. A., Regan, T. J., McCabe, C. H., Kennedy, J. W., Schloss, M., Tristani, F., Chaitman, B. R., and Fisher, L. D.: Exercise Stress Testing. Correlations among History of Angina, ST-Segment Response and Prevalence of Coronary Artery Disease in the Coronary Artery Surgery Study (CASS), *N. Engl. J. Med.*, 301:230, 1979. (22 references)
 14. Patton, D. D.: Introduction to Clinical Decision Making, *Semin. Nucl. Med.*, 8:273, 1978.
 15. Ransohoff, D. F., and Feinstein, A. R.: Problems of Spectrum and Bias in Evaluating the Efficacy of Diagnostic Tests, *N. Engl. J. Med.*, 299:926, 1978.
 16. Redwood, D. R., and Epstein, S. E.: Uses and Limitations of Stress Testing in the Evaluation of Ischemic Heart Disease, *Circulation*, 46:1115, 1972.
 17. Selzer, A., Cohn, K., and Goldschlager, N.: On the Interpretation of the Exercise Test, *Circulation*, 58:193, 1978.
 18. McHenry, P. L.: The Actual Prevalence of False Positive ST-Segment Responses to Exercise in Clinically Normal Subjects Remains Undefined, *Circulation*, 55:683, 1977.
 19. Morris, S. N., and McHenry, P. L.: Role of Exercise Stress Testing in Healthy Subjects and Patients with Coronary Heart Disease, *Am. J. Cardiol.*, 42:659, 1978.
 20. Sheffield, L. T., Reeves, T. J., Blackburn, H., Ellisted, M. H., Froelicher, V. F., Roitman, D., and

*This article is a review of the literature and contains additional references to the literature.

Kansal, S.: The Exercise Test in Perspective, *Circulation*, 55:681, 1977.

21. Casscells, W., Schoenberger, A., and Graboys, T. B.: Interpretation by Physicians of Clinical Laboratory Results, *N. Engl. J. Med.*, 299:999, 1978.

22. Gorlin, R.: Pathophysiology of Cardiac Pain, *Circulation*, 32:138, 1965.

23. Scheuer, J., and Brachfeld, N.: Coronary Insufficiency: Relations between Hemodynamic, Electrical, and Biochemical Parameters, *Circ. Res.*, 18:178, 1966.

24. Tennant, R., and Wiggers, C. J.: The Effect of Coronary Occlusion on Myocardial Contraction, *Am. J. Physiol.*, 112:351, 1935.

25. Vincent, W. R., and Rapaport, E.: Serum Creatine Phosphokinase in the Diagnosis of Acute Myocardial Infarction, *Am. J. Cardiol.*, 15:17, 1965.

26. Parkey, R. W., Bonte, F. J., Meyer, S. L., Atkins, J. M., Curry, G. L., Stokely, E. M., and Willerson, J. T.: A New Method for Radionuclide Imaging of Acute Myocardial Infarction in Humans, *Circulation*, 50:540, 1974.

27. Holman, B. L., DeWanjee, M. K., Idoine, J., Fliegel, C. P., Davis, M. A., Treves, S., and Eldh, P.: Detection and Localization of Experimental Myocardial Infarction with ^{99M}Tc-Tetracycline, *J. Nucl. Med.*, 14:595, 1973.

28. Holmberg, S.: Effect of Severe Muscular Work on Total and Coronary Circulation in Men in Relation to Findings in the Coronary Arteriogram, in G. Marchetti and B. Taccardi (eds.), "Coronary Circulation and Energetics of the Myocardium," Karger, New York, 1967.

29. Braunwald, E., Ross, J., and Sonnenblick, E. H.: "Mechanisms of Contraction of the Normal and Failing Heart," 2d ed., Little, Brown and Company, Boston, 1976.

30. Fortuin, N. J., and Weiss, J. L.: Exercise Stress Testing, *Circulation*, 56:699, 1977.

31. Nelson, R. R., Gobel, F. L., Jorgensen, C. R., Wang, K., Wang, Y., and Taylor, H. L.: Hemodynamic Predictors of Myocardial Oxygen Consumption during Static and Dynamic Exercise, *Circulation*, 50:1179, 1974.

32. Robinson, B. F.: Relation of Heart Rate and Systolic Blood Pressure to the Onset of Pain in Angina Pectoris, *Circulation*, 35:1073, 1967.

33. Fabian, J., Stoly, I., Janota, M., and Rohac, J.: Reproducibility of Exercise Tests in Patients with Symptomatic Ischemic Heart Disease, *Br. Heart J.*, 37:785, 1975.

34. Master, A. M.: The Two Step Test of Myocardial Function, *Am. Heart J.*, 10:495, 1935.

35. Aronow, W. S., and Cassidy, J.: Five Year Follow Up of Double Master's Test, Maximal Treadmill Stress Test and Resting and Post Exercise Apexcardiogram in Asymptomatic Persons, *Circulation*, 52:616, 1975.

36. Doyle, J. T., and Kinch, S. H.: The Prognosis of an Abnormal Electrocardiographic Stress Test, *Circulation*, 41:545, 1970.

37. Martin, C. M., and McConahay, D. R.: Maximal Treadmill Exercise Electrocardiography, *Circulation*, 46:956, 1972.

38. Bruce, R. A.: Methods of Exercise Testing, *Am. J. Cardiol.*, 33:715, 1974.

*39. McNeer, J. F., Margolis, J. R., Lee, K. L., Kisslo, J. A., Peter, R. H., Kong, Y., Behar, V. S., Wallace, A. G., McCants, C. B., and Rosati, R. A.: The Role of the Exercise Test in the Evaluation of Patients for Ischemic Heart Disease, *Circulation*, 57:64, 1978. (18 references)

40. Goldschlager, N., Selzer, A., and Cohn, K.: Treadmill Stress Tests as Indicators of Presence and Severity of Coronary Artery Disease, *Ann. Intern. Med.*, 85:277, 1976.

41. Rochmis, P., and Blackburn, H.: Exercise Tests. A Survey of Procedures, Safety and Litigation Experience in Approximately 170,000 Tests, *J. Am. Med. Assoc.*, 217:1061, 1971.

42. Irving, J. B., and Bruce, R. A.: Exertional Hypotension and Postexertional Ventricular Fibrillation in Stress Testing, *Am. J. Cardiol.*, 39:849, 1977.

43. Kaplan, M. A., Harris, C. N., Aronow, W. S., Parker, D. P., and Ellestad, M. H.: Inability of the Submaximal Treadmill Stress Test to Predict the Location of Coronary Disease, *Circulation*, 47:250, 1973.

*44. Cohn, K., Kamm, B., Feteih, N., Brand, R., and Goldschlager, N.: Use of Treadmill Score to Quantify Ischemic Response and Predict Extent of Coronary Disease, *Circulation*, 59:286, 1979. (25 references)

45. Rifkin, R. D., and Hood, W. B.: Bayesian Analysis of Electrocardiographic Exercise Stress Testing, *N. Engl. J. Med.*, 297:681, 1977.

46. Redwood, D. R., Borer, J. S., and Epstein, S. E.: Whither the ST Segment during Exercise?, *Circulation*, 54:703, 1976.

47. Surawicz, B., and Saito, S.: Exercise Testing for Detection of Myocardial Ischemia in Patients with Abnormal Electrocardiograms at Rest, *Am. J. Cardiol.*, 41:943, 1978.

48. Kattus, A. A.: Exercise Electrocardiography: Recognition of the Ischemic Response, False Positive and Negative Patterns, *Am. J. Cardiol.*, 33:721, 1974.

49. Lary, D., and Goldschlager, N.: Electrocardiographic Changes during Hyperventilation Resembling Myocardial Ischemia in Patients with Normal Coronary Arteriograms, *Am. Heart J.*, 87:383, 1974.

50. Whinnery, J. E., Froelicher, V. F., Jr., Stewart, A. J., Longo, M. R., Jr., Triebwasser, J. H., and Lancaster, M. C.: The Electrocardiographic Response to Maximal Treadmill Exercise of Asymptomatic Men with Left Bundle Branch Block, *Am. Heart J.*, 94:316, 1977.

*51. Berman, J. L., Wynne, J., and Cohn, P. F.: A Multivariate Approach for Interpreting Treadmill Exercise Tests in Coronary Artery Disease, *Circulation*, 58:505, 1978. (46 references)

52. Bartel, A. G., Behar, V. S., Peter, R. H., Orgain, E. S., and Kong, Y.: Graded Exercise Stress Tests in Angiographically Documented Coronary Artery Disease, *Circulation*, 49:348, 1974.

53. Linhart, J. W., and Turnoff, H. B.: Maximum Treadmill Exercise Test in Patients with Abnormal Control Electrocardiograms, *Circulation*, 49:667, 1974.

54. Harris, F. J., Mason, D. T., Lee, G., Amsterdam, E. A., and DeMaria, A.: Value and Limitations of Exercise Testing in Detecting Coronary Disease in the Presence of ST-T Abnormalities on Standard

12 Lead Electrocardiogram, *Am. J. Cardiol.*, 37:141, 1976.

*55. San Marco, M. E., Pontius, S., and Silvester, R. H.: Abnormal Blood Pressure Response and Marked Ischemic ST-Segment Depression as Predictors of Severe Coronary Artery Disease, *Circulation*, 61:572, 1980. (15 references)

56. Hollenberg, M., Budge, W. R., Wisneski, J. A., and Gertz, E. W.: Treadmill Score Quantifies Electrocardiographic Response to Exercise and Improves Test Accuracy of Reproducibility, *Circulation*, 61:276, 1980.

57. Zohman, L. R., and Kattus, A. A.: Exercise Testing in the Diagnosis of Coronary Heart Disease: A Perspective, *Am. J. Cardiol.*, 40:243, 1977.

58. Robb, G. P., and Seltzer, F.: Appraisal of the Double Two Step Exercise Test, *J. Am. Med. Assoc.*, 234:722, 1975.

59. Froelicher, V. F., Thomas, M. M., Pillow, C., and Lancaster, M. C.: Epidemiologic Study of Asymptomatic Men Screened by Maximal Treadmill Testing for Latent Coronary Artery Disease, *Am. J. Cardiol.*, 34:770, 1974.

60. Froelicher, V. F., Yunowitz, F. G., Thompson, A. J., and Lancaster, M. C.: The Correlation of Coronary Arteriography and the Electrocardiographic Response to Maximal Treadmill Testing in 76 Asymptomatic Men, *Circulation*, 48:597, 1973.

61. Borer, J. S., Brensike, J. F., Redwood, D. R., Itscoitz, S. B., Parsamani, E. R., Stone, N. J., Richardson, J. M., Levy, R. I., and Epstein, S. E.: Limitations of the Electrocardiographic Response to Exercise in Predicting Coronary Artery Disease, *N. Engl. J. Med.*, 293:367, 1975.

*62. Hammermeister, K. E., DeRouen, A., and Dodge, H. T.: Variables Predictive of Survival in Patients with Coronary Disease, *Circulation*, 59:421, 1979. (19 references)

63. Ellestad, M. H., and Wan, M. K. C.: Predictive Implications of Stress Testing. Follow Up of 2700 Subjects after Maximum Treadmill Stress Testing, *Circulation*, 51:363, 1975.

64. Bruce, R. A.: Exercise Testing for Evaluation of Ventricular Function, *N. Engl. J. Med.*, 296:671, 1977.

65. Battock, D. J., Alarez, H., and Chidsey, C. A.: Effects of Propranolol and Isosorbide Dinitrate on Exercise Performance in Patients with Angina Pectoris, *Circulation*, 39:157, 1969.

66. Bartel, A. G., Behar, V. S., Peter, R. H., Orgain, E. S., and Kong, Y.: Exercise Testing in Evaluation of Aortocoronary Bypass Surgery, *Circulation*, 48:141, 1973.

67. Lawrie, G. M., Morris, G. C., Howell, J. F., Ogura, J. W., Spencer, W. H., Cashion, W. R., Winters, W. L., Beazley, H. L., Chapman, D. W., Peterson, P. K., and Lie, J. T.: Results of Coronary Bypass More than 5 Years after Operation in 434 Patients, *Am. J. Cardiol.*, 40:665, 1977.

68. Strauss, H. W., Harrison, K., Langen, J. K., Lebowitz, E., and Pitt, B.: Thallium-201 for Myocardial Imaging: Relation of Thallium-201 to Regional Myocardial Perfusion, *Circulation*, 51:641, 1975.

69. Gould, K. L.: Noninvasive Assessment of Coronary Stenoses by Myocardial Imaging during Pharma-cologic Coronary Vasodilation. I. Physiologic Basis and Experimental Validation, *Am. J. Cardiol.*, 41:267, 1978.

70. Gould, K. L., Lipscomb, K., and Hamilton, G. W.: Physiological Basis for Assessing Critical Coronary Stenosis, *Am. J. Cardiol.*, 33:87, 1974.

71. Gould, K. L., Westcott, R. J., Albro, P. C., and Hamilton, G. W.: Non Invasive Assessment of Coronary Stenoses by Myocardial Imaging during Pharmacologic Coronary Vasodilation. II. Clinical Methodology and Feasibility, *Am. J. Cardiol.*, 41:279, 1978.

72. Wackers, F. J. T., Becker, A. E., Samson, G., Sokole, E. B., Van Der Schoot, J. B., Andreas, J. T. M., Lie, K. I., Durrer, D., and Wellens, H.: Location and Size of Acute Transmural Myocardial Infarction Estimated from Thallium-201 Scintiscans. A Clinicopathological Study, *Circulation*, 56:72, 1977.

73. Gewirtz, H., Beller, G. A., Strauss, H. W., Dinsmore, R. E., Zir, L. M., McKusick, K. A., and Pohost, G. M.: Transient Defects of Resting Thallium Scans in Patients with Coronary Artery Disease, *Circulation*, 59:707, 1979.

74. Maseri, A., Parodi, O., Severi, S., and Pesola, A.: Transient Transmural Reduction of Myocardial Blood Flow Demonstrated by Thallium 201 Scintigraphy, as a Cause of Variant Angina, *Circulation*, 54:280, 1976.

*75. Verani, M. S., Jhingran, S., Attar, M., Rizk, A., Quinones, M. A., and Miller, R. R.: Poststress Redistribution of Thallium-201 in Patients with Coronary Artery Disease, with and without Prior Myocardial Infarction, *Am. J. Cardiol.*, 43:1114, 1979. (24 references)

76. Berger, B. C., Watson, D. D., Burwell, L. R., Crosby, I. K., Wellons, H. A., Teates, C. D., and Beller, G. A.: Redistribution of Thallium at Rest in Patients with Stable and Unstable Angina and the Effect of Coronary Artery Bypass Surgery, *Circulation*, 60:1114, 1979.

77. Burow, R. D., Pond, M., Schafer, A. W., and Becker, L.: "Circumferential Profiles." A New Method for Computer Analysis of Thallium-201 Myocardial Perfusion Images, *J. Nucl. Med.*, 20:771, 1979.

78. Goris, M. L., Daspit, S. G., McLaughlin, P., and Kriss, J. P.: Interpolative Background Subtraction, *J. Nucl. Med.*, 17:744, 1976.

79. Hamilton, G. W., Trobaugh, G. B., Ritchie, J. L., Williams, D. L., Weaver, W. D., and Gould, K. L.: Myocardial Imaging with Intravenously Injected Thallium-201 in Patients with Suspected Coronary Artery Disease, *Am. J. Cardiol.*, 39:347, 1977.

80. Wackers, F. J. T., Lie, K. I., Liem, K. L., Sokole, E. B., Samson, G., Van Der Schoot, J. B., and Durrer, D.: Thallium-201 Scintigraphy in Unstable Angina Pectoris, *Circulation*, 57:738, 1978.

81. Smitherman, T. C., Osborn, R. C., Jr., and Narahara, K. A.: Serial Myocardial Scintigraphy after a Single Dose of Thallium-201 in Men after Acute Myocardial Infarction, *Am. J. Cardiol.*, 42:177, 1978.

82. Verani, M. S., Marcus, M. L., Razzak, M. A., and Ehrhardt, J. C.: Sensitivity and Specificity of Thallium 201 Perfusion Scintigrams under Exercise in the Diagnosis of Coronary Artery Disease, *J. Nucl. Med.*, 19:773, 1978.

83. Bailey, I. K., Griffith, L. S. C., Rouleau, J. R., Strauss, H. W., and Pitt, B.: Thallium-201 Myocardial Perfusion Imaging at Rest and during Exercise, *Circulation*, 55:79, 1977.

84. Botvinick, E. H., Taradash, M. R., Shames, D. M., and Parmley, W. W.: Thallium 201 Myocardial Perfusion Scintigraphy for the Clinical Clarification of Normal, Abnormal, and Equivocal Electrocardiographic Stress Tests, *Am. J. Cardiol.*, 41:34, 1978.

85. McCarthy, D. M., Blood, D. K., Sciacca, R. R., and Cannon, P. J.: Single Dose Myocardial Perfusion Imaging with Thallium-201: Application in Patients with Non Diagnostic Electrocardiographic Stress Tests, *Am. J. Cardiol.*, 43:899, 1979.

86. Ritchie, J. L., Zaret, B. L., Strauss, W. B., Pitt, B., Berman, D. S., Schelbert, H. R., Ashburn, W. L., Berger, H. J., and Hamilton, G. W.: Myocardial Imaging with Thallium 201: A Multicenter Study in Patients with Angina Pectoris or Acute Myocardial Infarction, *Am. J. Cardiol.*, 42:345, 1978.

87. Dash, H., Massie, B. M., Botvinick, E. H., and Brundage, B. H.: The Noninvasive Identification of Left Main and Three Vessel Coronary Artery Disease by Myocardial Stress Perfusion Scintigraphy and Treadmill Exercise Electrocardiography, *Circulation*, 60:276, 1979.

88. Leppo, J., Yipintsoi, T., Blankstein, R., Bontemps, R., Freeman, L. M., Zohman, L., and Scheuer, J.: Thallium-201 Myocardial Scintigraphy in Patients with Triple Vessel Disease and Ischemic Exercise Stress Tests, *Circulation*, 59:714, 1979.

89. Bruschke, A. V. G., Proudfit, W. L., and Sones, F. M., Jr.: Progress Study of 590 Consecutive Nonsurgical Cases of Coronary Disease Followed 5–9 Years. II. Ventriculographic and Other Correlations, *Circulation*, 47:1154, 1973.

90. Nelson, G. R., Cohn, P. F., and Gorlin, R.: Prognosis in Medically Treated Coronary Artery Disease. Influence of Ejection Fraction Compared to Other Parameters, *Circulation*, 52:408, 1975.

91. Cohn, P. F., Gorlin, R., Cohn, L. H., and Collins, J. J.: Left Ventricular Ejection Fraction as a Prognostic Guide in Surgical Treatment of Coronary and Valvular Heart Disease, *Am. J. Cardiol.*, 34:136, 1974.

92. Herman, M. V., Heinle, R. A., Klein, M. D., and Gorlin, R.: Localized Disorders in Myocardial Contraction: Asynergy and Its Role in Congestive Heart Failure, *N. Engl. J. Med.*, 227:222, 1967.

93. Helfant, R. H., Bodenheimer, M. M., and Banka, V. S.: Asynergy in Coronary Heart Disease, *Ann. Intern. Med.*, 87:475, 1977.

94. See, J. R., Cohn, P. F., Holman, B. L., Adams, D. F., and Maddox, D. E.: Significance of Reduced Regional Myocardial Blood Flow in Asynergic Areas Evaluated with Intervention Ventriculography, *Am. J. Cardiol.*, 43:179, 1979.

95. Helfant, R. H., Pine, R., Meister, S. G., Feldman, M. S., Trout, R. G., and Banka, V. S.: Nitroglycerine to Unmask Reversible Asynergy, *Circulation*, 50:108, 1974.

96. Popio, K. A., Gorlin, R., Bechtel, D., and Levine, J. A.: Postextrasystolic Potentiation as a Predictor of Potential Myocardial Viability: Preoperative Analyses Compared with Studies after Coronary Bypass Surgery, *Am. J. Cardiol.*, 39:944, 1977.

97. Salel, A. F., Berman, D. S., De Nardo, G. L., and Mason, D. T.: Radionuclide Assessment of Nitroglycerin Influence on Abnormal Left Ventricular Segmental Contraction in Patients with Coronary Heart Disease, *Circulation*, 53:975, 1976.

98. Cohn, P. F., Angoff, G. H., Zoll, P. M., Sloss, L. J., Markis, J. E., Graboys, T. B., Green, L. H., and Braunwald, E.: A New, Noninvasive Technique for Inducing Post-extrasystolic Potentiation during Echocardiography, *Circulation*, 56:598, 1977.

99. Borer, J. S., Bacharach, S. L., Green, M. V., Kent, K. M., Apstein, S. E., and Johnston, G. S.: Real Time Radionuclide Cineangiography in the Non Invasive Evaluation of Global and Regional Left Ventricular Function at Rest and during Exercise in Patients with Coronary Artery Disease, *N. Engl. J. Med.*, 296:839, 1977.

*100. Bodenheimer, M. M., Banka, V. S., Fooshee, C. M., and Helfant, R. H.: Comparative Sensitivity of the Exercise Electrocardiogram, Thallium Imaging and Stress Radionuclide Angiography to Detect the Presence and Severity of Coronary Heart Disease, *Circulation*, 60:1270, 1979. (30 references)

101. Caldwell, J. H., Hamilton, G. W., Sorensen, S. G., Ritchie, J. L., Williams, D. L., and Kennedy, J. W.: The Detection of Coronary Artery Disease with Radionuclide Techniques: A Comparison of Rest-Exercise Thallium Imaging and Ejection Fraction Response, *Circulation*, 61:610, 1980.

*102. Borer, J. S., Kent, K. M., Bacharach, S. L., Green, M. V., Rosing, D. R., Seides, S. F., Epstein, S. E., and Johnston, G. S.: Sensitivity, Specificity and Predictive Accuracy of Radionuclide Cineangiography during Exercise in Patients with Coronary Artery Disease, *Circulation*, 60:572, 1979. (25 references)

103. Bacharach, S. L., Green, M. V., Borer, J. S., Douglas, M. A., Ostrow, H. G., and Johnston, G. S.: A Real Time System for Multi-image Gated Cardiac Studies, *J. Nucl. Med.*, 18:79, 1977.

*104. Brady, T. J., Thrall, J. H., Clare, J. M., Rogers, W. L., Lo, K., and Pitt, B.: Exercise Radionuclide Ventriculography: Practical Considerations and Sensitivity of Coronary Artery Disease Detection, *Radiology*, 132:697, 1979. (14 references)

105. Marshall, R. C., Berger, H. J., Reduto, L. A., Gottschalk, A., and Zaret, B. L.: Variability in Sequential Measures of Left Ventricular Performance Assessed with Radionuclide Angiocardiography, *Am. J. Cardiol.*, 41:531, 1978.

*106. Okada, R. D., Kirshenbaum, H. D., Kushner, F. G., Strauss, H. W., Dinsmore, R. E., Newell, J. B., Boucher, C. A., Block, P. C., and Pohost, G. M.: Observer Variance in the Qualitative Evaluation of Left Ventricular Wall Motion and the Quantitation of Left Ventricular Ejection Fraction Using Rest and Exercise Multigated Blood Pool Imaging, *Circulation*, 61:128, 1980. (24 references)

107. Maddox, D. E., Wynne, J., Uren, R., Parker, J. A., Idoine, J., Siegel, L. C., Neill, J. M., Cohn, P. F., and Holman, B. L.: Regional Ejection Fraction: A Quantitative Radionuclide Index of Regional Left Ventricular Performance, *Circulation*, 59:1001, 1979.

108. Borer, J. S., Bacharach, S. L., Green, M. V., Kent, K. M., Henry, W. L., Rosing, D. R., Seides, S. F.,

Johnston, G. S., Epstein, S. E., and Mack, B.: Exercise-Induced Left Ventricular Dysfunction in Symptomatic and Asymptomatic Patients with Aortic Regurgitation: Assessment with Radionuclide Cineangiography, *Am. J. Cardiol.*, 42:351, 1978.

109. Borer, J. S., Rosing, D. R., Kent, K. M., Bacharach, S. L., Green, M. V., McIntosh, C. J., Morrow, A. G., and Epstein, S. E.: Left Ventricular Function at Rest and during Exercise after Aortic Valve Replacement in Patients with Aortic Regurgitation, *Am. J. Cardiol.*, 44:1297, 1979.

110. Gross, H., Vaid, A., and Cohen, M. V.: Prognosis in Patients Rejected for Coronary Revascularization Surgery, *Am. J. Med.*, 64:9, 1978.

111. Hamilton, G. W., Murray, J. A., and Kennedy, J. W.: Quantitative Angiography in Ischemic Heart Disease: The Spectrum of Abnormal Left Ventricular Function and the Role of Abnormally Contracting Segments, *Circulation*, 45:1065, 1972.

112. Herman, M. V., and Gorlin, R.: Implications of Left Ventricular Asynergy, *Am. J. Cardiol.*, 23:538, 1969.

113. Horowitz, L. N., Harken, A. H., Kastor, J. A., and Josephson, M. E.: Ventricular Resection Guided by Epicardial and Endocardial Mapping for Treatment of Recurrent Ventricular Tachycardia, *N. Engl. J. Med.*, 302:589, 1980.

114. Banka, V. S., Bodenheimer, M. M., Shah, R., and Helfant, R. H.: Intervention Ventriculography: Comparative Value of Nitroglycerin, Post-extrasystolic Potentiation and Nitroglycerin plus Post-extrasystolic Potentiation, *Circulation*, 53:632, 1976.

115. Stadius, M., McAnulty, J. H., Cutler, J., Rosch, J., and Rahimtoola, S. H.: Specificity, Sensitivity and Accuracy of the Nitroglycerin Ventriculogram as a Predictor of Surgically Reversible Wall Motion Abnormalities, *Am. J. Cardiol.*, 45:399, 1980. (Abstract.)

116. McMahon, M. M., Brown, G., Cukingnan, R., Rolett, E. L., Bolsin, E., Frimer, M., and Dodge, H. T.: Quantitative Coronary Angiography: Measurement of the "Critical" Stenosis in Patients with Unstable Angina and Single-Vessel Disease without Collaterals, *Circulation*, 60:106, 1979.

117. Klocke, F. J.: Coronary Blood Flow in Man, *Prog. Cardiovasc. Dis.*, 19:117, 1976.

118. Gould, K. L., and Lipscomb, K.: Effect of Coronary Stenoses on Coronary Flow Reserve and Resistance, *Am. J. Cardiol.*, 34:48, 1974.

119. Detre, K. M., Wright, E., Murphy, M. L., and Takaro, T.: Observer Agreement in Evaluating Coronary Angiograms, *Circulation*, 52:979, 1975.

120. Zir, L. M., Miller, S. W., Dinsmore, R. E., Gilbert, J. P., and Harthorne, J. W.: Interobserver Variability in Coronary Angiography, *Circulation*, 53:627, 1970.

121. DeRouen, T. A., Murray, J. A., and Owen, W.: Variability in the Analysis of Coronary Arteriograms, *Circulation*, 55:324, 1977.

122. Dhew, C. Y. C., Brown, G. B., Wong, M., Shah, P. M., and Singh, B. N.: The Effects of Verapamil on Coronary Hemodynamics and Vasomobility in Patients with Coronary Artery Disease, *Am. J. Cardiol.*, 45:389, 1980. (Abstract.)

123. Arnett, E. N., Isner, J. M., Redwood, D. R., Kemt, K. M., Baker, W. P., Ackerstein, H., and Roberts, W. C.: Coronary Artery Narrowing in Coronary Heart Disease: Comparison of Cineangiographic and Necropsy Findings, *Ann. Intern. Med.*, 91:350, 1979.

*124. Roberts, W. C., and Jones, A. A.: Quantification of Coronary Arterial Narrowing and Necropsy in Acute Transmural Myocardial Infarction. Analysis and Comparison of Findings in 27 Patients and 22 Controls, *Circulation*, 61:786, 1980. (4 references)

125. Vlodaver, Z., Frech, R., Van Tassel, R. A., and Edwards, J. E.: Correlation of the Antemortem Coronary Arteriogram and the Postmortem Specimen, *Circulation*, 47:162, 1973.

126. Grondin, C. M., Dyrda, I., Pasternac, A., Campeau, L., Bourassa, M. G., and Lesperance, J.: Discrepancies between Cineangiographic and Postmortem Findings in Patients with Coronary Artery Disease and Recent Myocardial Revascularization, *Circulation*, 49:703, 1974.

127. Schwartz, J. N., Kong, Y., Hackel, D. B., and Bartel, A. G.: Comparison of Angiographic and Postmortem Findings in Patients with Coronary Artery Disease, *Am. J. Cardiol.*, 36:174, 1975.

128. Hutchins, G. M., Bulkley, B. H., Ridolfi, R. L., Griffith, L. S. C., Lohr, F. T., and Piasio, M. A.: Correlation of Coronary Arteriograms and Left Ventriculograms with Postmortem Studies, *Circulation*, 56:32, 1977.

129. Brown, B. G., Bolson, E., Frimer, M., and Dodge, H. T.: Quantitative Coronary Arteriography: Estimation of Dimensions, Hemodynamic Resistance, and Atheroma Mass of Coronary Artery Lesions Using the Arteriogram and Digital Computation, *Circulation*, 55:329, 1977.

130. Bruschke, A. V. G., Proudfit, W. L., and Sones, F. M., Jr.: Progress Study of 590 Consecutive Nonsurgical Cases of Coronary Disease Followed 5–9 Years. I. Arteriographic Correlations, *Circulation*, 47:1147, 1973.

131. Webster, J. S., Moberg, C., and Rincon, G.: Natural History of Severe Proximal Coronary Artery Disease as Documented by Coronary Cineangiography, *Am. J. Cardiol.*, 33:195, 1974.

132. Conley, M. J., Ely, R. L., Kisslo, J., Lee, K. L., McNeer, J. F., and Rosati, R. A.: The Prognostic Spectrum of Left Main Stenosis, *Circulation*, 57:947, 1978.

133. Takaro, T., Hultgren, H. N., Lipton, M. J., Detre, K. M., and participants in the study group: The VA Cooperative Randomized Study of Surgery for Coronary Occlusive Disease. II. Subgroup with Significant Left Main Lesions, *Circulation*, 54:III-107, 1976.

134. Curry, R. C., Jr., Pepine, C. J., Sabom, M. B., Feldman, R. L., Christie, L. G., and Conti, C. R.: Effects of Ergonovine in Patients with and without Coronary Artery Disease, *Circulation*, 56:803, 1977.

135. Schroeder, J. S., Bolen, J. L., Quint, R. A., Clark, D. A., Hayden, W. G., Higgins, C. R., and Wexler, L.: Provocation of Coronary Spasm with Ergonovine Maleate. New Test with Results in 57 Patients Undergoing Coronary Arteriography, *Am. J. Cardiol.*, 40:487, 1977.

136. Ricci, D. R., Orlick, A. E., Doherty, P. W., Cipri-

ano, P. R., and Harrison, D. C.: Reduction of Coronary Blood Flow during Coronary Artery Spasm Occurring Spontaneously and after Provocation by Ergonovine Maleate, *Circulation,* 57:392, 1978.

137. Curry, R. C., Jr., Pepine, C. J., Sabom, M. B., Feldman, R. L., Christie, L. G., Varnell, J. H., and Conti, C. R.: Hemodynamic and Myocardial Metabolic Effects of Ergonovine in Patients with Chest Pain, *Circulation,* 58:648, 1978.
138. Goldberg, S., Lam, W., Mudge, G., Green, L. H., Kushner, F., Hirshfeld, J. W., and Kastor, J. A.: Coronary Hemodynamic and Myocardial Metabolic Alterations Accompanying Coronary Spasm, *Am. J. Cardiol.,* 43:481, 1979.
139. Buxton, A., Goldberg, S., Hirshfeld, J. W., Wilson, J., Mann, T., Williams, D. O., Oliva, P., and Kastor, J. A.: Refractory Ergonovine Induced Coronary Vasospasm: Importance of Intracoronary Nitroglycerin, *Am. J. Cardiol.,* 45:390, 1980. (Abstract.)
140. Burggraf, G. W., and Parker, J. O.: Prognosis in Coronary Artery Disease: Angiographic, Hemodynamic, and Clinical Factors, *Circulation,* 51:146, 1975.
141. McNeer, J. F., Starmer, C. F., Bartel, A. G., Behar, V. S., Kong, Y., Peter, R. H., and Rosati, R. A.: The Nature of Treatment Selection in Coronary Artery Disease: Experience with Medical and Surgical Treatment of a Chronic Disease, *Circulation,* 49:606, 1974.
142. Moraski, R. E., Russell, R. O., Jr., Smith, M., and Rackley, C. E.: Left Ventricular Function in Patients with and without Myocardial Infarction and One, Two or Three Vessel Coronary Artery Disease, *Am. J. Cardiol.,* 35:1, 1975.
143. Krasnow, N., and Gorlin, R.: Myocardial Lactate Metabolism in Coronary Insufficiency, *Ann. Intern. Med.,* 59:781, 1963.
*144. Gertz, E. W., Wisneski, J. A., Neese, R., Houser, A., Korte, R., and Bristow, J. D.: Myocardial Lactate Extraction: Multi-determined Metabolic Function, *Circulation,* 61:256, 1980. (30 references)
145. Olson, R. E.: "Excess Lactate" and Anaerobiosis, *Ann. Intern. Med.,* 59:960, 1963.
146. Herman, M. V., Elliott, W. C., and Gorlin, R.: An Electrocardiographic, Anatomic, and Metabolic Study of Zonal Myocardial Ischemia in Coronary Heart Disease, *Circulation,* 35:834, 1967.
147. Kemp, H. G., Elliott, W. C., and Gorlin, R.: The Anginal Syndrome with Normal Coronary Arteriography, *Trans. Assoc. Am. Physicians,* 80:59, 1967.
148. Davis, K., Kennedy, J. W., Kemp, H. G. Jr., Judkins, M. P., Gosselin, A. J., and Killip, T.: Complications of Coronary Arteriography from the Collaborative Study of Coronary Artery Surgery (CASS), *Circulation,* 59:1105, 1979.
149. Ritchie, J. L., Narahara, K. A., Trobaugh, G. B., Williams, D. L., and Hamilton, G. W.: Thallium-201 Myocardial Imaging before and after Coronary Revascularization, *Circulation,* 56:830, 1977.
150. Verani, M. S., Marcus, M. L., Spoto, G., Rossi, N. P., Ehrhardt, J. C., and Razzak, M. A.: Thallium-201 Myocardial Perfusion Scintigrams in the Evaluation of Aorto-Coronary Saphenous Bypass Surgery, *J. Nucl. Med.,* 19:765, 1978.
151. Battock, D. J., Alvarez, H., and Chidsey, C. A.: Effects of Propranolol and Isosorbide Dinitrate on Exercise Performance and Adrenergic Activity in Patients with Angina Pectoris, *Circulation,* 39:157, 1969.
152. Bruce, R. A., DeRouen, T., Peterson, D. R., Irving, J. B., Chinn, N., Blake, B., and Hofer, V.: Noninvasive Predictors of Sudden Cardiac Death in Men with Coronary Heart Disease, *Am. J. Cardiol.,* 39:833, 1977.
153. Sakai, K., Gebhard, M. M., Spieckermann, P. G., and Bretschneider, J. H.: Enzyme Release Resulting from Total Ischemia and Reperfusion in the Isolated, Perfused Guinea Pig Heart, *J. Mol. Cell. Cardiol.,* 7:827, 1975.
154. Chiong, M. A., West, R., and Parker, J. O.: Myocardial Balance of Inorganic Phosphate and Enzymes in Man: Effects of Tachycardia and Ischemia, *Circulation,* 49:283, 1974.
155. Ahmed, S. A., Williamson, J. R., Roberts, R., Clark, R. E., and Sobel, B. E.: The Association of Increased Plasma MB CPK Activity and Irreversible Ischemic Myocardial Injury in the Dog, *Circulation,* 54:187, 1976.
156. Conrad, G. L., Rau, E. E., and Shine, K. I.: Creatine Kinase Release, Potassium-42 Content, and Mechanical Performance in Anoxic Rabbit Myocardium, *J. Clin. Invest.,* 64:155, 1979.
157. Ahumada, G., Roberts, R., and Sobel, B. E.: Evaluation of Myocardial Infarction with Enzymatic Indices, *Prog. Cardiovasc. Dis.,*18:405, 1976.
*158. Grande, P., Christiansen, C., Pedersen, A., and Christensen, M. S.: Optimal Diagnosis in Acute Myocardial Infarction. A Cost-Effectiveness Study, *Circulation,* 61:723, 1980. (29 references)
159. Blomberg, D. J., Kimber, W. D., and Burke, M. D.: Creatine Kinase Isoenzymes, Predictive Value in the Early Diagnosis of Acute Myocardial Infarction, *Am. J. Med.,* 59:464, 1975.
160. Wagner, G. S., Roe, C. R., Limbird, L. E., Rosati, R. A., and Wallace, A. G.: The Importance of Identification of the Myocardial-Specific Isoenzyme of Creatine Phosphokinase (MB Form) in the Diagnosis of Acute Myocardial Infarction, *Circulation,* 47:263, 1973.
161. Roberts, R., Henry, P. D., and Sobel, B. E.: An Improved Basis for Enzymatic Estimation of Infarct Size, *Circulation,* 52:743, 1975.
162. Klein, M. S., Shell, W. E., and Sobel, B. E.: Serum Creatine Phosphokinase (CPK) Isoenzymes after Intramuscular Injections, Surgery, and Myocardial Infarction, *Cardiovasc. Res.,* 7:412, 1973.
163. Alderman, E. L., Matlof, H. J., Shumway, N. E., and Harrison, D. C.: Evaluation of Enzyme Testing for the Detection of Myocardial Infarction Following Direct Coronary Surgery, *Circulation,* 48:135, 1973.
164. Shell, W. E., and Sobel, B. E.: Biochemical Markers of Ischemic Injury, *Circulation,* 53/54:I-98, 1976.
165. Kjekshus, J. K., and Sobel, B. E.: Depressed Myocardial Creatine Phosphokinase Activity Following Experimental Myocardial Infarction in Rabbit, *Circ. Res.,* 27:403, 1970.
166. Kjekshus, J. K., Maroko, P. R., and Sobel, B. E.: Distribution of Myocardial Injury and Its Relation to Epicardial ST-Segment Changes after Coronary

Artery Occlusion in the Dog, *Cardiovasc. Res.,* 6:490, 1972.

167. Armstrong, P. W., Watts, D. G., Hamilton, D. C., Chiong, M. A., and Parker, J. O.: Quantification of Myocardial Infarction: Template Model for Serial Creatine Kinase Analysis, *Circulation,* 60:856, 1979.

168. Roe, C. R., and Starmer, C. F.: A Sensitivity Analysis of Enzymatic Estimation of Infarct Size, *Circulation,* 52:1, 1975.

169. Bleifeld, W., Mathey, D., Hanrath, P., Buss, H., and Effert, S.: Infarct Size Estimated from Serial Serum Creatine Phosphokinase in Relation to Left Ventricular Hemodynamics, *Circulation,* 55:303, 1977.

170. Roberts, R., Husain, A., Ambos, H. D., Oliver, G. C., Cox, J. R., Jr., and Sobel, B. E.: Relation between Infarct Size and Ventricular Arrhythmia, *Br. Heart J.,* 37:1169, 1975.

171. Stone, M. J., Willerson, J. T., Gomez-Sanchez, C. E., and Waterman, M. R.: Radioimmunoassay of Myoglobin and Human Serum: Results in Patients with Acute Myocardial Infarction, *J. Clin. Invest.,* 56:1334, 1975.

172. Kagen, L., Scheidt, S., and Butt, A.: Serum Myoglobin in Myocardial Infarction: The "Staccato Phenomenon." Is Acute Myocardial Infarction in Man an Intermittent Event? *Am. J. Med.,* 62:86, 1977.

173. Gilkeson, G., Stone, M. J., Waterman, M., Ting, R., Gomez-Sanchez, C. E., Hull, A., and Willerson, J. T.: Detection of Myoglobin by Radioimmunoassay in Human Sera: Its Usefulness and Limitations as an Emergency Room Screening Test for Acute Myocardial Infarction, *Am. Heart J.,* 95:70, 1978.

174. Tommaso, C. L., Salzeider, K., Arif, M., and Klutz, W.: Serial Myoglobin vs. CPK Analysis as an Indicator of Uncomplicated Myocardial Infarction Size and Its Use in Assessing Early Infarct Extension, *Am Heart J.,* 99:149, 1980.

175. Khaw, B. A., Gold, H. K., Fallon, J. T., and Haber, E.: Detection of Serum Cardiac Myosin Light Chains in Acute Experimental Myocardial Infarction: Radioimmunoassay of Cardiac Myosin Light Chains, *Circulation,* 58:1130, 1978.

176. Trahern, C. A., Gere, J. B., Krauth, G. H., and Bigham, D. A.: Clinical Assessment of Serum Myosin Light Chains in the Diagnosis of Acute Myocardial Infarction, *Am. J. Cardiol.,* 41:641, 1978.

177. Parkey, R. W., Bonte, F. J., Meyer, S. L., Atkins, J. M., Curry, G. L., Stokely, E. M., and Willerson, J. T.: A New Method for Radionuclide Imaging of Acute Myocardial Infarction in Humans, *Circulation,* 50:540, 1974.

178. McLaughlin, P., Coates, G., Wood, D., Cradduck, T., and Morch, J.: Detection of Acute Myocardial Infarction by Technetium-99m Polyphosphate, *Am. J. Cardiol.,* 35:390, 1975.

179. Berman, D. S., Amsterdam, E. A., Hines, H. H., Salel, A. F., Bailey, G. J., DeNardo, G. L., and Mason, D. T.: New Approach to Interpretation of Technetium-99m Pyrophosphate Scintigraphy in Detection of Acute Myocardial Infarction, *Am. J. Cardiol.,* 39:341, 1977.

180. Poliner, L. R., Buja, L. M., Parkey, R. W., Bonte, F. J., and Willerson, J. T.: Clinicopathologic Findings in 52 Patients Studied by Technetium-99m Stannous Pyrophosphate Myocardial Scintigraphy, *Circulation,* 59:257, 1979.

181. Massie, B. M., Botvinick, E. H., Werner, J. A., Chatterjee, K., and Parmley, W. W.: Myocardial Scintigraphy with Technetium-99m Stannous Pyrophosphate: An Insensitive Test for Nontransmural Myocardial Infarction, *Am. J. Cardiol.,* 43:186, 1979.

182. Holman, B. L., Chisholm, R. J., and Braunwald, E.: The Prognostic Implications of Acute Myocardial Infarct Scintigraphy with ^{99m}Tc-Pyrophosphate, *Circulation,* 57:320, 1978.

183. Ahmad, M., Dubiel, J. P., Verdon, T. A., and Martin, R. H.: Technetium-99m Stannous Pyrophosphate Myocardial Imaging in Patients with or without Left Ventricular Aneursym, *Circulation,* 53:833, 1976.

184. Mason, J. W., Myers, R. W., Alderman, E. L., Stinson, E. B., Goris, M. L., and Kriss, J. P.: Technetium-99m Pyrophosphate Myocardial Uptake in Patients with Stable Angina Pectoris, *Am. J. Cardiol.,* 40:1, 1977.

185. Ahmad, M., Dubiel, J. P., Logan, K. W., Verdon, T. A., and Martin, R. H.: Limited Clinical Diagnostic Specificity of Technetium-99m Stannous Pyrophosphate Myocardial Imaging in Acute Myocardial Infarction, *Am. J. Cardiol.,* 39:50, 1977.

186. Prasquier, R., Taradash, M. R., Botvinick, E. H., Shames, D. M., and Parmley, W. W.: The Specificity of the Diffuse Pattern of Cardiac Uptake in Myocardial Infarction Imaging with Technetium-99m Stannous Pyrophosphates, *Circulation,* 55:61, 1977.

187. Willerson, J. T., Parkey, R. W., Bonte, F. J., Meyer, S. L., and Stokely, E. M.: Acute Subendocardial Myocardial Infarction in Patients, *Circulation,* 51:436, 1975.

188. Olson, H. G., Lyons, K. P., Aronow, W. S., Kuperus, J., Orlando, J., and Hughes, D.: Prognostic Value of a Persistently Positive Technetium-99m Stannous Pyrophosphate Myocardial Scintigram after Myocardial Infarction, *Am. J. Cardiol.,* 43:889, 1979.

189. Olson, H. G., Lyons, K. P., Aronow, W. S., Brown, W. T., and Greenfield, R. S.: Follow-Up Technetium-99m Stannous Pyrophosphate Myocardial Scintigrams after Acute Myocardial Infarction, *Circulation,* 56:181, 1977.

190. Henning, H., Schelbert, H. R., Righetti, A., Ashburn, W. L., and O'Rourke, R. A.: Dual Myocardial Imaging with Technetium-99m Pyrophosphate and Thallium-201 for Detecting, Localizing and Sizing Acute Myocardial Infarction, *Am. J. Cardiol.,* 40:147, 1977.

191. Wackers, F. J. T., Sokole, E. B., Samson, G., Van der Schoot, J. B., Lie, K. I., Liem, K. L., and Wellens, H. J. J.: Value and Limitations of Thallium-201 Scintigraphy in the Acute Phase of Myocardial Infarction, *N. Engl. J. Med.,* 295:1, 1976.

192. Niess, G. S., Logic, J. R., Russell, R. O., Rackley, C. E., and Rogers, W. J.: Usefulness and Limitations of Thallium-201 Myocardial Scintigraphy in Delineating Location and Size of Prior Myocardial Infarction, *Circulation,* 59:1010, 1979.

192a. Cohn, J. N., Guiha, N. H., Broder, M. I., and Limas, C. J.: Right Ventricular Infarction: Clinical and Hemodynamic Features, *Am. J. Cardiol.*, 33:209, 1974.

192b. Rotman, M., Ratliff, N. B., and Hawley, J.: Right Ventricular Infarction: A Haemodynamic Diagnosis, *Br. Heart J.*, 36:941, 1974.

*193. Cohn, J. N.: Right Ventricular Infarction Re-visited, *Am. J. Cardiol.*, 43:666, 1979. (11 references)

194. Wackers, F. J. T., Lie, K. I., Sokole, E. B., Res, J., Van der Schoot, J. B., and Durrer, D.: Prevalence of Right Ventricular Involvement in Inferior Wall Infarction Assessed with Myocardial Imaging with Thallium-201 and Technetium-99m Pyrophosphate, *Am. J. Cardiol.*, 42: 358, 1978.

*195. Lorell, B., Leinbach, R. C., Pohost, G. M., Gold, H. K., Dinsmore, R. E., Hutter, A. M., Jr., Pastore, J. O., and DeSanctis, R. W.: Right Ventricular Infarction, Clinical Diagnosis and Differentiation from Cardiac Tamponade and Pericardial Constriction, *Am. J. Cardiol.*, 43:465, 1979. (22 references)

196. Marcus, M. L., Tomanek, R. J., Ehrhardt, J. C., Kerber, R. E., Brown, D. D., and Abboud, F. M.: Relationships between Myocardial Perfusion, Myocardial Necrosis, and Technetium-99m Pyrophosphate Uptake in Dogs Subjected to Sudden Coronary Occlusion, *Circulation*, 54:647, 1976.

197. Ahmad, M., Logan, K. W., and Martin, R. H.: Doughnut Pattern of Technetium-99m Pyrophosphate Myocardial Uptake in Patients with Acute Myocardial Infarction: A Sign of Poor Long-Term Prognosis, *Am. J. Cardiol.*, 44:13, 1979.

198. Rude, R. E., Parkey, R. W., Bonte, F. J., Lewis, S. E., Twieg, D., Buja, L. M., and Willerson, J. T.: Clinical Implications of the Technetium-99m Stannous Pyrophosphate Myocardial Scintigraphic "Doughnut" Pattern in Patients with Acute Myocardial Infarct, *Circulation*, 59:721, 1979.

199. Silverman, K. J., Becker, L. C., Bulkley, B. H., Burow, R. D., Mellits, E. D., Kallman, C. H., and Weisfeldt, M. L.: Value of Early Thallium-201 Scintigraphy for Predicting Mortality in Patients with Acute Myocardial Infarction, *Circulation*, 61:996, 1980.

200. Schelbert, H. R., Henning, H., Ashburn, W. L., Verba, J. W., Karliner, J. S., and O'Rourke, R. A.: Serial Measurements of Left Ventricular Ejection Fraction by Radionuclide Angiography Early and Late after Myocardial Infarction, *Am. J. Cardiol.*, 38:407, 1976.

201. Kostuk, W. J., Ehsani, A. A., Karliner, J. S., Ashburn, W. L., Peterson, K. L., Ross, J., Jr., and Sobel, B. E.: Left Ventricular Performance after Myocardial Infarction Assessed by Radioisotope Angiocardiography, *Circulation*, 47:242, 1973.

202. Rigo, P., Murray, M., Strauss, H. W., and Pitt, B.: Scintiphotographic Evaluation of Patients with Suspected Left Ventricular Aneurysm, *Circulation*, 50:985, 1974.

203. Friedman, M. L., and Cantor, R. E.: Reliability of Gated Heart Scintigrams for Detection of Left Ventricular Aneurysm: Concise Communication, *J. Nucl. Med.*, 20:720, 1979.

204. Rigo, P., Murray, M., Strauss, H. W., Taylor, D., Kelly, D., Weisfeldt, M., and Pitt, B.: Left Ventricular Function in Acute Myocardial Infarction Evaluated by Gated Scintiphotography, *Circulation*, 50:678, 1974.

205. Battler, A., Slutsky, R., Karliner, J., Froelicher, V., Ashburn, W., and Ross, J., Jr.: Left Ventricular Ejection Fraction and First Third Ejection Fraction Early after Acute Myocardial Infarction: Value for Predicting Mortality and Morbidity, *Am. J. Cardiol.*, 45:197, 1980.

206. Starr, J. W., Wagner, G. S., Behar, V. S., Walston, A., II, and Greenfield, J. C., Jr.: Vectorcardiographic Criteria for the Diagnosis of Inferior Myocardial Infarction, *Circulation*, 49:829, 1974.

207. Benchimol, A., and Desser, K. B.: The Electrovectorcardiographic Diagnosis of Posterior Wall Myocardial Infarction, *Cardiovasc. Clin.*, 5:183, 1974.

208. Benchimol, A., and Desser, K. B.: Advances in Clinical Vectorcardiography, *Am. J. Cardiol.*, 36:76, 1975.

*209. Muller, J. E., Maroko, P. R., and Braunwald, E.: Precordial Electrocardiographic Mapping: A Technique to Assess the Efficacy of Interventions Designed to Limit Infarct Size, *Circulation*, 57:1, 1978. (169 references)

210. Maroko, P. R., Kjekshus, J. K., Sobel, B. E., Watanabe, T., Covell, J. W., Ross, J., Jr., and Braunwald, E.: Factors Influencing Infarct Size Following Experimental Coronary Occlusions, *Circulation*, 43:67, 1971.

211. Hillis, L. D., and Braunwald, E.: Myocardial Ischemia, *N. Engl. J. Med.*, 296:971, 1977.

212. Irvin, R. G., and Cobb, F. R.: Relationship between Epicardial ST-Segment Elevation, Regional Myocardial Blood Flow, and Extent of Myocardial Infarction in Awake Dogs, *Circulation*, 55:825, 1977.

213. Holland, R. P., and Brooks, H.: Precordial and Epicardial Surface Potentials during Myocardial Ischemia in the Pig: A Theoretical and Experimental Analysis of the TQ and ST Segments, *Circulation*, 37:471, 1975.

*214. Inoue, M., Hori, M., Fukunami, M., Fukushima, M., Tada, M., Abe, H., Minamino, T., and Fukui, S.: Evaluation of Precordial ST Segment Mapping as an Index of Infarct Size in Patients with Acute Myocardial Infarction, *Br. Heart J.*, 42:726, 1979. (16 references)

215. Corya, B. C., Rasmussen, S., Knoebel, S. B., and Feigenbaum, H.: Echocardiography in Acute Myocardial Infarction, *Am. J. Cardiol.*, 36:1, 1975.

216. Corya, B. C., Rasmussen, S., Feigenbaum, H., Knoebel, S. B., and Black, M. J.: Systolic Thickening and Thinning of the Septum and Posterior Wall in Patients with Coronary Artery Disease, Congestive Cardiomyopathy and Atrial, Septal Defects, *Circulation*, 55:109, 1977.

217. Rasmussen, S., Corya, B. C., Feigenbaum, H., and Knoebel, S. B.: Detection of Myocardial Scar Tissue by M-Mode Echocardiography, *Circulation*, 57:230, 1978.

218. Jacobs, J. J., Feigenbaum, H., Corya, B. C., and Phillips, J. F.: Detection of Left Ventricular Asynergy by Echocardiography, *Circulation*, 48:263, 1973.

219. Weyman, A. E., Peskoe, S. M., Williams, E. S., Dillon, J. C., and Feigenbaum, H.: Detection of Left Ventricular Aneurysms by Cross-Sectional Echocardiography, *Circulation*, 54:936, 1976.

220. Kisslo, J. A., Robertson, D., Gilbert, B. W., Von Ramm, O., and Behar, V. S.: A Comparison of Real-Time, Two-Dimensional Echocardiography

and Cineangiography in Detecting Left Ventricular Asynergy, *Circulation*, 55:134, 1977.

221. Teichholz, L. E., Kreulen, T., Herman, M. V., and Gorlin, R.: Problems in Echocardiographic Volume Determinations: Echocardiographic-Angiographic Correlations in the Presence or Absence of Asynergy, *Am. J. Cardiol.*, 137:7, 1976.

*222. Kotler, N. M., Mintz, G. S., Segal, B. L., and Parry, W. R.: Clinical Uses of Two Dimensional Echocardiography, *Am. J. Cardiol.*, 45:1061, 1980. (104 references)

223. Carr, K. W., Engler, R. L., Forsythe, J. R., Johnson, A. D., and Gosink, B.: Measurement of Left Ventricular Ejection Fraction by Mechanical Cross-Sectional Echocardiography, *Circulation*, 59:1196, 1979.

224. Farcot, J.-C., Boisante, L., Rigaud, M., Bardet, J., and Bourdarias, J.-P.: Two-Dimensional Echo Sector Angiographic Diagnosis of Ventricular Septal Defect Following Acute Myocardial Infarction, *Am. J. Cardiol.*, 45:436, 1980. (Abstract.)

225. Ganz, W., Donoso, R., Marcus, H. S., Forrester, J. S., and Swan, H. J. C.: A New Technique for Measurement of Cardiac Output by Thermodilution in Man, *Am. J. Cardiol.*, 27:392, 1971.

226. Foote, G. A., Schabel, S. I., and Hodges, M.: Pulmonary Complications of the Flow-Directed Balloon-Tipped Catheter, *N. Engl. J. Med.*, 290:927, 1974.

227. Page, D. W., Teres, D., and Hartshorn, J. W.: Fatal Hemorrhage from Swan-Ganz Catheter, *N. Engl. J. Med.*, 291:260, 1974.

228. Lipp, H., O'Donoghue, K., and Resnekov, L.: Intracardiac Knotting of a Flow-Directed Balloon Catheter, *N. Engl. J. Med.*, 284:220, 1971.

229. Swan, H. J. C., and Ganz, W.: Guidelines for Use of Balloon-Tipped Catheter, *Am. J. Cardiol.*, 34:119, 1974.

230. McEnany, M. T., Kay, H. R., Buckley, M. J., Daggett, W. M., Erdmann, A. J., Mundth, E. D., Rao, R. S., De Toeuf, J., and Austen, W. G.: Clinical Experience with Intraaortic Balloon Pump Support in 728 Patients, *Circulation*, 58:I-124, 1978.

*231. Fox, A. C., Glassman, E., and Isom, O. W.,: Surgically Remediable Complications of Myocardial Infarction, *Prog. Cardiovasc. Dis.*, 21:461, 1979. (148 references)

PART III Disorders of the Cardiovascular System

The purpose of Part III—"*Disorders* of the Cardiovascular System"—is to present a group of conditions that represent, for the most part, the consequences of heart disease.

Many hours were spent trying to identify a word or words that would indicate the difference between a disease process and the consequences of the disease. There are no words that will satisfy the purist because it is not possible to create pigeonholes by which one can categorize all conditions. The following discussion points out how we view the difference in the words *disorder* and *disease*.

The term *disorder* implies that the duties assigned to the heart are not being implemented properly. The heart and circulation have the following duties: to cause no pain; to pump blood properly (not too much and not too little); to maintain a proper arterial blood pressure; to maintain normal rhythm; to prevent transient unconsciousness; and to continue beating. A disorder is the result of a derangement of function. A derangement of function may be the consequence of one or several different disease processes. A patient becomes ill because of the derangement of cardiovascular mechanisms that has resulted from the disease process. The pathologist cannot determine whether the patient had chest pain, ventricular dysfunction, shock, a hyperdynamic circulation, arrhythmia, or syncope by examining the heart and blood vessels, although indirect evidence of these disorders may be found in other organs. *Accordingly, when-ever a physician identifies a disorder of the cardiovascular system, he or she must ask the following question: What cardiovascular disease caused this set of abnormalities?* This question is mandatory because the management of the disease process itself may be quite different from the management of the derangement of function that the disease produces.

The word *disease* implies the presence of a basic abnormality of the heart or blood vessels. The pathologist can usually identify the process when he or she examines the heart and vessels. Heart disease may be present without the patient knowing it. The disease process must develop to a certain point before cardiovascular mechanisms become deranged and make the patient ill. The word *disease* also has a deeper meaning. It implies that a basic abnormality exists in the tissue. The condition may be due to a congenital defect or inflammatory disease, or it may be the result of atheroma or a myriad of other causes. On the other hand, the exact cause of the cardiovascular abnormality may be unknown (as it is in many arrhythmias). The basic abnormality of the tissue is designated as heart *disease* or vascular *disease*. The derangements of the cardiovascular mechanisms that are eventually produced by the disease are called *disorders. Accordingly, whenever a physician identifies a disease process, he or she must ask the following question: Are any of the known consequences (disorders) of the disease present in my patient?*

Section A

Chest Pain Secondary to Cardiovascular Disease

21

Chest Pain Secondary to Cardiovascular Disease

J. Willis Hurst, M.D.

If a disorder is defined as being a consequence of a disease process, then chest pain due to cardiovascular disease can be classified as a disorder. Accordingly, a discussion of chest pain should be included in this part of the book. Since the details of chest pain are discussed elsewhere in the book, the purpose of this short discussion is to emphasize the importance and frequency of the disorder. Each physician must become expert in recognizing chest pain due to cardiovascular disease and in identifying all diseases that mimic the pain of cardiovascular origin.

There are multiple cardiovascular causes of chest pain. These are discussed in Chaps. 7, 45, 58, and 62. A common cardiac cause of chest pain is myocardial ischemia, and there are multiple causes of it. The chest pain due to ischemic heart disease is discussed in Chaps. 38, 45, 47, and 56. Myocardial ischemia may be due to coronary atherosclerosis; nonatherosclerotic coronary disease, including spasm; noncoronary disease such as aortic valve disease; and cardiomyopathy. Chest pain due to noncardiovascular causes that simulates pain due to myocardial ischemia is discussed in Chaps. 7, 45, and 78. The strategy used to identify the presence and cause of myocardial ischemia is discussed in Chap. 20.

The analysis of chest pain challenges the physician's ability. It requires many years to learn to take an accurate history. It takes even longer to learn the *predictive value* of the history that is obtained. We now know that diagnostic errors are commonly made when the predictive value of a particular symptom is poor (see Chap. 7). *Accordingly, when the etiology of chest pain is obscure and a cardiac cause is in the differentiated diagnosis, the physician may need to use a laboratory procedure that yields a result that has a high predictive value so that a definitive decision can be made regarding the patient* (see Chaps. 20, 45, 95, and 98).

One might ask why other symptoms due to heart disease, such as dyspnea, palpitation, syncope, fatigue, etc., are not highlighted here. The answer is that at this point in time there is a great deal of new information related to chest pain, and we have included this brief discussion to emphasize this fact. The reader should refer to Chaps. 7, 23, 28, and 30 for a discussion of other symptoms due to heart disease.

Section B Heart Failure

22

Pathophysiology of Heart Failure

Robert C. Schlant, M.D.
Edmund H. Sonnenblick, M.D.

Definitions

In clinical medicine there is an increasing appreciation of the need for precise physiologic definitions. Nevertheless, at times there is still a considerable difference between the physiologic and clinical use of similar terms. This situation is particularly common in considerations of patients with heart failure. The following definitions and classification (Table 22-1) are presented with the realization that future research will allow a much more precise analysis and classification of different types of heart failure based upon differences in their biochemistry and biophysics.[1-5]

Circulatory failure is a general term that refers to an inadequacy of the cardiovascular system in performing its basic functions of providing nutrition to the cells of the body and removing metabolic products from the cells. It may be caused primarily by either cardiac or peripheral (noncardiac) conditions. Noncardiac conditions that can cause circulatory failure include inadequate blood volume, decreased venous return, increased capacity of the vascular system, peripheral vascular abnormalities or disease, and inadequate oxyhemoglobin.

Circulatory overload or congestion is a general term referring to excess blood volume from either car-

diac or noncardiac causes.[6] *Noncardiac circulatory overload* may be divided into two categories: (1) those conditions in which the primary defect appears to be an increase in blood volume (the accumulation of excess salt and water due to salt-retaining steroids, excess blood or fluid administration, acute glomerulonephritis, oliguria, or anuria); and (2) those conditions in which the primary defect appears to be an increased venous return and/or decreased peripheral resistance (arteriovenous fistulas, beriberi, cirrhosis, severe anemia, etc.). Many patients with noncardiac circulatory overload eventually develop secondary "high-output" heart failure. (See Chap. 26.)

Heart failure or cardiac failure is that condition in which the heart is no longer able to pump an adequate supply of blood for the metabolic needs of the body, provided there is adequate venous return to the heart. In addition to this primary "pump" failure, there is often an abnormally high diastolic pressure within the ventricle. In patients with mild heart failure, the ventricular end-diastolic pressure and the cardiac output may be normal at rest, but the former often becomes elevated to abnormal levels during stress such as exercise, and the increase in cardiac output demanded by exercise becomes limited. In patients with more severe ventricular failure, the early- and end-diastolic pressures may be elevated even at rest. The elevated left ventricular diastolic pressure is reflected in an elevation of pulmonary venous and capillary pressures and in dyspnea that results from changes in pulmonary compliance and/or pulmonary congestion and edema. Since the basic fundamental of heart failure is an inability of the heart as a pump to supply adequately the demands of the body, it is apparent that this term could be applicable in a very general sense whenever the demands are not met as a result of cardiac limitations. This implies that any heart would eventually "fail" if the demands were increased sufficiently. In fact, this might occur in persons with apparently normal hearts during extreme exertion. In most individ-

TABLE 22-1 Classification of Circulatory Failure and Circulatory Overload

1. Circulatory failure
   a. Heart (cardiac) failure
   b. Noncardiac (peripheral) circulatory failure
      (1) Decreased return of blood to heart, inadequate blood volume
      (2) Increased capacity of vascular bed
      (3) Peripheral vascular abnormalities or disease
      (4) Inadequate oxyhemoglobin
2. Circulatory congestion
   a. Cardiac circulatory overload
      (1) Heart (cardiac) failure
   b. Noncardiac circulatory overload
      (1) Increase in blood volume
      (2) Increase in venous return and/or decrease in peripheral vascular resistance

uals, however, exertion is stopped prior to heart failure by fatigue or breathlessness. In most patients with the clinical syndrome of heart failure, the cardiac output is decreased somewhat at rest and becomes progressively decreased during exercise.

As noted in Table 22-2, the causes of overall heart pump failure may be classified into three main categories: (1) failure primarily related to work overloads or mechanical abnormalities, (2) failure primarily related to myocardial abnormalities, and (3) failure related to abnormal cardiac rhythm or

TABLE 22-2 Causes of Overall Heart Pump Failure

1. Mechanical abnormalities
   a. Increased pressure load
      (1) Central (aortic stenosis, etc.)
      (2) Peripheral (systemic hypertension, etc.)
   b. Increased volume load (valvular regurgitation, shunts, increased "preload," etc.)
   c. Obstruction to ventricular filling (mitral or tricuspid stenosis)
   d. Pericardial construction, tamponade
   e. Endocardial or myocardial restriction
   f. Ventricular aneurysm
   g. Ventricular dyssynergy
2. Myocardial (muscular) abnormalities
   a. Primary
      (1) Cardiomyopathy
      (2) Myocarditis
      (3) Metabolic
      (4) Toxic (alcohol, cobalt, etc.)
      (5) Presbycardia
   b. Secondary
      (1) Dysdynamic (secondary to mechanical abnormalities)
      (2) Oxygen deprivation (coronary heart disease)
      (3) Metabolic
      (4) Inflammatory
      (5) Systemic disease
      (6) Chronic obstructive lung disease
3. Altered cardiac rhythm or conduction sequence
   a. Standstill
   b. Fibrillation
   c. Extreme tachycardia or bradycardia
   d. Electrical asynchrony, conduction disturbances

conduction sequence. Although heart failure is usually considered as being due to ventricular failure, atrial failure (see below) can contribute significantly.

Clinically, the term *congestive heart failure* is used to describe a complicated and variable symptom complex that usually, but not necessarily, includes dyspnea and increased fatigability, tachypnea and tachycardia, pulmonary rales, cardiomegaly, ventricular gallop sound, and peripheral edema. More precisely, however, congestive heart failure is that state in which abnormal circulatory congestion occurs as the result of heart failure and the peripheral circulatory and sympathetic-renal compensatory mechanisms that are brought into play. When intravascular circulatory congestion is present for any length of time, there is usually increased transudation of fluid from the capillaries into the interstitial spaces. In the pulmonary circulation, if the rate of transudation exceeds the rate of lymphatic drainage, pulmonary edema develops. Initially, this may be detected by x-ray examination, and only later may audible rales be detected on physical examination. In the systemic venous system, venous congestion may be visible and may result in the development of peripheral edema or hepatomegaly. In the majority of patients, congestive heart failure develops chronically and is associated with the retention of sodium and water by the kidneys. In most patients with clinical congestive heart failure due to mechanical or myocardial abnormalities, the heart failure is preceded by periods of *myocardial* dysfunction and of *myocardial* failure, during which overall cardiac pump function and cardiac output may be maintained by compensatory mechanisms (at least while at rest). *Acute congestive heart failure* can develop following a myocardial infarction of the left ventricle or following the rupture of a cardiac valve structure. In this situation an acute shift of blood from the systemic circulation to the pulmonary circulation may occur before the retention of significant sodium or water. It should be emphasized that the term *congestive heart failure* should not be used unless the congestion is of cardiac origin. When the cause of the pulmonary or peripheral congestion is not clear, however, it is usually preferable to describe the symptoms or signs, which are nonspecific, and to avoid improperly diagnosing heart failure.

Myocardial dysfunction and *myocardial failure* are terms used to refer to mild and to more marked decreased systolic performance of the myocardium, respectively. In some patients with more marked myocardial dysfunction, or myocardial failure, the decreased myocardial function can be detected by studies of total cardiac pump function, whereas in patients with milder dysfunction the decreased myocardial function may be detected only by more specific indexes of myocardial contractility. In many patients with myocardial "dysfunction," and even more advanced myocardial "failure," the overall cardiac pump function (and cardiac output at rest) may be maintained reasonably well by compensatory mechanisms such as increased ventricular filling or preload (dilatation) and/or cardiac hypertrophy. Myocardial failure may occur as a result of an initial loss of cells, i.e., acute myocardial infarction with segmental loss or a myocarditis with diffuse loss. Scarring occurs, along with hypertrophy of the remaining myocardium. As compensatory hypertrophy becomes severe, contractility of the myocardium declines. Ultimately, however, the myocardial failure (plus mechanical abnormalities) often leads to a decrease in pump function and to overall pump or heart failure. In most patients, significant dysfunction and failure of the myocardium occur before the clinical stages of heart (pump) dysfunction or failure, and before the clinical syndrome of congestive heart failure. (See Chap. 18.)

In some patients it is also useful to consider separately the *systolic* and the *diastolic* properties of the ventricle.[7] Thus, some patients may have marked *systolic ventricular dysfunction* or *failure* at a time when they do not have significant, if any, elevation of diastolic pressures. On the other hand, some patients may have marked elevation of left ventricular diastolic pressure and pulmonary congestion (*diastolic failure of the ventricle*) at a time when the systolic or pumping function of the ventricle is well maintained or even greater than normal. The latter situation may occur in some patients with aortic stenosis, in whom the elevated diastolic pressure may be present because of a combination of the effects of the marked ventricular hypertrophy and myocardial diastolic dysfunction at a time when the systolic function or cardiac output is normal or even slightly elevated. Similarly, some patients with high-output states or primary noncardiac circulatory overload may develop pulmonary congestion and edema secondary to an abnormal elevation or ventricular diastolic pressure at a time when the cardiac output (systolic function) is normal or even markedly increased. The latter syndrome can occur in conditions associated with an increase in blood volume from the accumulation of excess salt and water due to salt-retaining steroids, excess blood or fluid administration, acute glomerulonephritis, oliguria, or anuria. It may occur in patients with an abnormally increased venous return and/or decreased peripheral resistance, as might occur in patients with arteriovenous fistulas, beriberi, cirrhosis, severe anemia, etc. In these conditions the chronic volume and/or pressure load upon the ventricle may eventually produce myocardial and ventricular systolic dysfunction or failure. Ultimately, this can result in the cardiac output falling to abnormally low levels. When symptoms of pulmonary congestion or pulmonary edema occur while the cardiac output is still normal or elevated, the syndrome is referred to as *high-output failure*. (See also Chap. 26.)

As noted in Table 22-2, there are several causes of both primary and secondary myocardial failure. Myocardial failure is said to be *primary* when it is caused by (1) idiopathic cardiomyopathy or cardiomyopathy due to a primary disease of muscle dystrophy (Chap. 56); (2) myocarditis (Chap. 55); (3) metabolic deficiencies of the myocardium, such as beriberi and possibly hyper- or hypothyroidism (Chaps. 26 and 70); or (4) inadequate quantity of myocardium, such as might result from myocardial infarction, hypoplasia, or replacement of fibrosis, tumor, or other masses. Myocardial failure is said to be *secondary* (Table 22-2) when it is produced by (1) dysdynamic myocardial failure (see below); (2) metabolic factors such as ischemia, chronic shock, or depression by drugs or toxins; (3) myocardial inflammation (Chap. 55); or (4) presbycardia, senile heart disease, or senile cardiomyopathy (see below). The cause of left ventricular dysfunction in patients with chronic obstructive lung disease is unknown, although the combination of hypoxia and hypercapnia may be important.

Dysdynamic myocardial failure is a nonspecific term used to refer to the common forms of secondary myocardial failure that commonly develop after a period of increased ventricular preload or afterload. A designation of dysdynamic (i.e., "with impaired force or power") myocardial failure implies that the mechanical performance of myocardial contractility per unit mass is significantly decreased; however, overall cardiac (pump) function may be compensated, and the cardiac output may not be abnormally decreased.

Forward failure and *backward failure* are expressions that have been used at times with somewhat different meanings. In oversimplified terms, a designation of forward failure has been used to imply that most of the patient's symptoms resulted from a low cardiac output with resultant symptoms of easy fatigability, weakness, or even shock, whereas backward failure has been used to imply that most of the patient's symptoms resulted from elevation of venous pressure behind the failing ventricle(s). This elevation of venous pressure was usually thought to be caused by obstruction to ventricular filling (mitral or tricuspid stenosis) or by the inability of the ventricle to empty itself properly. The two expressions have also been used in reference to concepts of the pathogenesis of the retention of salt and water. Thus, according to some early investigators, in backward failure, it was postulated that most of the patient's symptoms and signs of congestion resulted from an elevation of venous pressure upstream from the failing ventricle. The cardiac output might be increased or might be returned to normal by the increased venous pressure behind the ventricle and the resultant increase in diastolic filling or stretch of the ventricle. When right ventricle failure developed, systemic venous and capillary pressures became elevated and edema developed, producing a decrease in effective circulating blood volume. An increase in tubular reabsorption of salt and water was thought to occur as a result of renal vasoconstriction secondary to the change in *effective* blood volume or as a result of an elevation of renal venous pressure. In forward failure the decreased cardiac output was postulated at one time to produce tissue edema by an increase in capillary permeability secondary to tissue hypoxia. Later, when this theory became untenable, it was postulated that the decreased cardiac output altered renal plasma flow and glomerular filtration, thereby contributing to the retention of salt and water and producing a secondary increase in blood volume, elevation of venous pressure, and edema formation. Subsequent studies have demonstrated that both the forward-failure and the backward-failure theories are oversimplifications of the pathogenesis of salt and water retention and edema formation in heart failure. Accordingly, even though the expressions are no longer completely applicable in this regard, they may possibly have a very limited usefulness as a form of shorthand to describe the clinical symptom-sign complex. Thus, when the symptoms are predominantly related to pulmonary or systemic venous congestion, backward failure may be said to exist. If the symptoms are due to a marked decrease in cardiac output, forward cardiac failure, which is often acute, may be said to exist.

Left-heart (left-sided) failure and *right-heart (right-sided) failure* are clinical terms used to refer to conditions in which the primary impairment is of the left side of the heart or of the right side of the heart, respectively. Since both sides of the heart are in a circuit, it is apparent that one side cannot pump significantly more blood for any length of time in the absence of abnormal shunts, communications, or regurgitation, Furthermore, there is evidence that experimentally produced pure failure of one ventricle may produce significant hemodynamic and biochemical abnormalities of the other ventricle, even without the usual hemodynamic manifestations of ventricular failure. Accordingly, even though the pumping ability of one side may be primarily impaired, the output of the other side is secondarily decreased, and the biochemistry and hemodynamics of the contralateral ventricle can be abnormal in "pure" one-sided failure. The most common cause of clinical right-sided heart failure is, of course, left-sided heart failure. Though this is usually ascribed to failure secondary to elevation of the pulmonary artery pressure, it is possible that the biochemical changes which may occur in the opposite ventricle in experimental pure unilateral failure may play a significant role. In most situations, the expression *left-sided heart failure* is used in reference to symptoms and signs of elevated pressure and congestion in the pulmonary veins and capillaries, whereas *right-sided heart failure* is used in reference to symptoms and signs of elevated pressures and congestion in the systemic veins and capillaries. Actually, significant amounts of sodium and water retention, with subsequent peripheral edema formation, may occur with pure left-sided heart failure without clinical evidence of right-sided heart failure.

Latent heart failure is that state in which heart failure is not present at rest but is apparent during periods of increased stress, such as during exercise, emotional stress, episodes of fever, or surgical operations, or after an increase in blood volume.

Compensated heart failure is that condition in which heart failure was previously present, but in which cardiac output is returned to (or maintained at) a normal level by compensatory mechanisms or by therapy. The usual compensatory mechanisms include increased sympathetic adrenergic stimulation of the heart, fluid retention by the kidney with increased venous return and increased ventricular preload, and cardiac dilatation and hypertrophy. Clinically, compensation may be produced by an increase in myocardial contractility by digitalis glycosides or by the use of vasodilator drugs. The term *compensated heart failure* is also used, often less appropriately, in reference to patients with congestive heart failure whose symptoms and signs of pulmonary or peripheral congestion are relieved by diuretic therapy. In such patients, the cardiac function and cardiac output are usually not truly compensated (and cardiac output may actually be further decreased by diuretic therapy), even though the diuretic therapy may produce relief from the clinical symptoms due to congestion.

Atrial failure is that condition in which the atrium fails to provide adequate filling of the ventricle in relation to the venous return to the atrium. Although isolated atrial failure rarely, if ever, produces failure of the entire heart, the development of atrial fibrillation or flutter can produce heart failure in patients with compensated heart failure, particularly when marked ventricular hypertrophy is present and when an "atrial kick" is important to maintaining cardiac output.

Compensatory Mechanisms in Heart Failure

Many of the adjustments to heart failure are similar to the homeostatic mechanisms utilized by the body in response to circulatory failure from any cause, such as acute blood loss and acute myocardial infarction. Many of these cardiac reserve mechanisms (Table 22-3) are also utilized by normal subjects during exercise or during periods of increased stress. In human beings with heart failure, it is often impossible to separate the many different complex mechanisms of adjustment, many of which affect and modify each other. It should also be emphasized that with mild heart failure these compensatory mechanisms are often able to restore to normal or near-normal the arterial blood pressure, organ perfusion, and cardiac output at rest and perhaps even during moderate exercise. When the failure is mild, there may be few if any symptoms or organ dysfunctions resulting from these compensatory mechanisms. Eventually, however, many of the

TABLE 22-3   Compensatory Mechanisms in Heart Failure

1. Autonomic nervous system
   a. Heart
   b. Peripheral circulation
2. Kidney: renin-angiotensin-aldosterone
   a. Arterial vasoconstriction (increased afterload)
   b. Sodium and water retention (increased preload)
3. Frank-Starling law of the heart
   a. Increased end-diastolic fiber length, volume, and pressure (increased preload)
4. Hypertrophy
5. Peripheral oxygen delivery
   a. Oxygen-hemoglobin dissociation curve
   b. Increased oxygen extraction
6. Anaerobic metabolism

symptoms and organ dysfunctions that occur in patients with heart failure are the result of overcompensation by these same mechanisms. (See also Chap. 23.)

Autonomic Nervous System

One of the more important acute adjustments to heart failure is a reflex increase in autonomic sympathetic excitation to the heart and to most of the arteries and veins.[8–10] In general, the increased sympathetic activity, in combination with increased plasma concentrations of norepinephrine and angiotensin II, produces generalized arterial vasoconstriction and an increase in venous tone. The increased sympathetic adrenergic stimulation of the heart is associated with inhibition of cardiac parasympathetic activity.[9] An acute increase in sympathetic impulses to the heart normally stimulates the local release of norepinephrine and thereby produces beta stimulation with an increase in heart rate and an increase in myocardial contractility. Norepinephrine also increases the rate of ventricular relaxation, which further contributes to increased ventricular filling. In addition, the generalized increased sympathetic activity and the release of norepinephrine from the adrenal medulla and the peripheral blood vessels contribute toward increasing myocardial contractility.

Patients with chronic congestive heart failure have a significant decrease in the myocardial concentration of norepinephrine.[1,2,11–15] This is associated with decreased activity of tyrosine hydroxylase, which is the rate-limiting enzyme in the synthesis of norepinephrine.[16] Interestingly, when right ventricular hypertrophy and failure is experimentally produced, the myocardial norepinephrine concentration is decreased in both the right and left ventricles.[17] In experimental chronic heart failure, there also is a decrease in the amount of myocardial norepinephrine released per nerve impulse as well as defects in the uptake and the binding of norepinephrine.[15,18] In contrast, the arterial concentration

of norepinephrine in patients with congestive heart failure is elevated at rest and it increases to more than normal during exercise; both of these findings are presumably due to an increased synthesis of norepinephrine in the peripheral vasculature and the adrenal medulla.[19] Although the myocardial synthesis of norepinephrine is impaired in congestive heart failure, the myocardium is normally responsive to exogenous norepinephrine and may even be supersensitive.[17] In general, the failing heart appears to become progressively dependent upon extracardiac, circulating norepinephrine. As a result, congestive heart failure is occasionally made worse by drugs such as propranolol, guanethidine, or reserpine, all of which may interfere with the myocardial sympathicoadrenergic system. Overall, however, the defective synthesis and the depletion of myocardial norepinephrine does not appear to be a major, primary cause of myocardial failure, although it is an important contributing mechanism. Patients with chronic congestive heart failure also have a significant depression of the normal parasympathetic nervous control of the heart.[12]

The complex reflex actions of the autonomic nervous system and local autoregulatory mechanisms tend to preserve circulation to the brain and heart in patients with heart failure, while decreasing blood flow to the skin, skeletal muscles, splanchnic organs, and kidneys.[20–26] The increased sympathicoadrenergic stimulation of the peripheral arteries and the increased concentrations of circulating norepinephrine and angiotensin II contribute to the arteriolar vasoconstriction and the maintenance of arterial pressure, while the sympathetic stimulation of the veins contributes to an increase in venous tone, which helps to maintain venous return and ventricular filling and to support cardiac performance by Starling's law of the heart. The increased systemic arteriolar vasoconstriction associated with heart failure is an example of a compensatory mechanism that may have evolved in response to an inadequate cardiac output from other causes, such as hemorrhage or an inadequate blood volume. In such an acute situation, the reflex has obvious advantages in maintaining arterial pressure, whereas in the patient with chronic heart failure, the compensatory increase in arteriolar resistance may actually make it more difficult for the failing heart to eject blood. One of the major cornerstones of the modern therapy of heart failure is the reduction of peripheral vascular resistance by vasodilator drugs (see below).

Kidney: Renin, Angiotensin, and Aldosterone

The compensatory, homeostatic adjustments that occur when the heart fails tend to restore normal ventricular systolic pump function, although often at the price of increased diastolic pressures within the involved ventricle and in the venous system fill-

387

ing the ventricle. One important compensatory mechanism is the increase in ventricular filling pressures produced by an increase in plasma volume as the result of salt and water retention by the kidneys. As indicated in Fig. 22-1, the mechanisms leading to an increase in plasma volume may ultimately contribute to the formation of interstitial edema. The precise mechanisms or stimuli for the initial changes in the kidneys that produce salt and water retention in heart failure are still not clear.[27-30] Possible mechanisms include a decrease in the effective arterial blood volume, decreased distending pressure in the carotid sinus, inadequate organ perfusion during exercise, failure of the arterial systolic pressure to increase normally during exercise, or even reflexes from the heart itself. If there is an increase in renal venous pressure, this may also contribute to sodium retention by the kidneys.

During the phase of edema formation, patients with heart failure have a significantly reduced ability to excrete a load of either sodium chloride or water. If normal renal perfusion is restored by the expansion of blood volume in patients with mild heart failure, the handling of additional small amounts of sodium may return toward normal; however, patients with severe failure remain unable to excrete

FIGURE 22-1 Schema of the major events in heart failure that lead to the release of renin by the kidney, the increased secretion of aldosterone, the increased tubular reabsorption of sodium and water, and the production of edema. (*From Cannon.*[30] *Reproduced with permission of the author and publisher.*)

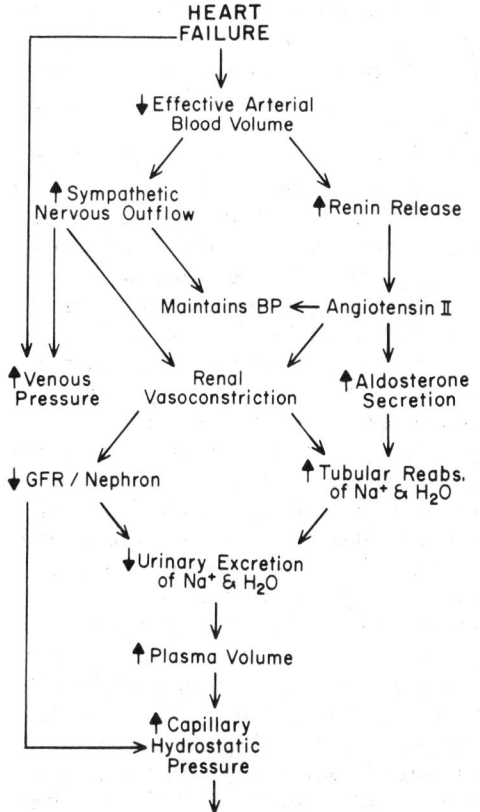

solute and water normally despite a marked expansion of blood volume and interstitial fluid volume.

The renal vasoconstriction of patients with congestive heart failure is thought to result primarily from increased activity of both the sympathetic nervous system and the renin-angiotensin system. In addition to a reduction in total renal blood flow, there is a redistribution of flow that produces a greater reduction of flow in the outer renal cortex with a relative maintenance of perfusion in the juxtamedullary areas.[28,31-33]

Patients with mild heart failure have a normal glomerular filtration rate despite the reduced renal blood flow. This is a result of an increased filtration fraction due to a marked efferent renal arteriolar vasoconstriction and decreased hydrostatic pressure in the peritubular capillaries. In patients with more severe heart failure, total renal blood flow is even more decreased, and the glomerular filtration rate may be significantly decreased even though the filtration fraction may increase further. In this situation, *prerenal azotemia* is often present with an increase in the blood urea concentration.

The sympathetic nervous system, which can be activated by lowering of the arterial blood pressure or by direct stimulation of the renal nerves, plays a facilitative role in the renal retention of sodium and water in heart failure. The increased tubular reabsorption of sodium and water in heart failure is aided by the marked redistribution of renal blood flow described above.[28,32,33] In addition, the uptake of fluid from the interstitium into the peritubular capillaries is enhanced by the efferent renal arteriolar vasoconstriction which increases colloid osmotic pressure in the peritubular capillaries. These hemodynamic mechanisms work synergistically to increase sodium and water reabsorption.[31,34]

Patients with heart failure have significantly decreased excretion rates of sodium chloride as a result of increased tubular reabsorption, even when the glomerular filtration rate is normal. Most of the glomerular filtrate is normally reabsorbed in the proximal convoluted tubules. Sodium appears to diffuse into proximal tubular cells, from which it is pumped into the lateral and basal intercellular spaces, with chloride and water following passively.[28,30,35,36] At present, it is uncertain whether or not proximal tubular reabsorption is increased in heart failure.[28,37]

About 25 percent of sodium reabsorption normally occurs in the ascending limb in the loop of Henle. In the thick ascending limb, the absorption of chloride is active, with sodium following passively.[28] Again, however, it is uncertain whether or not there is increased reabsorption of sodium and water in the thick ascending limb in heart failure.[33,34,37] Normally, the remaining 10 percent of filtered sodium is reabsorbed in the distal convoluted tubules and collecting ducts by active sodium transport[33] which is linked to the excretion of potassium or hydrogen ions. There is strong evidence that experimental heart failure very significantly increases sodium reabsorption in the collecting ducts.[28,33,35] It has been suggested that the sensitivity of the cells of the distal tubules and collecting ducts to aldosterone may be increased by an unidentified factor.[30]

Within hours after the production of heart failure, the kidneys secrete increased amounts of *renin*.[29,38-42] The secretion of renin is controlled by at least the following four mechanisms: (1) changes in wall tensions in renal afferent arterioles, (2) a macula densa receptor that detects changes in the rate of delivery of sodium and/or chloride to the distal tubule, (3) a negative-feedback effect of circulating angiotensin, and (4) the central nervous system, which influences renin secretion by the renal nerves, adrenal medulla, and the posterior pituitary.[41] Carotid sinus or atrial distension may also influence renin secretion.[29,43]

Renin acts upon angiotensinogen, which is produced mainly in the liver, to produce angiotensin I, which is converted in the lungs and to a lesser extent in the kidney and blood vessels to *angiotensin II*.[39-43] Angiotensin II has strong arterial vasoconstrictor properties and contributes to the increase in peripheral vascular resistance and the maintenance of blood pressure in heart failure when "effective" filling of arterial circulation decreases.[30,38,40,44] Angiotensin II further constricts renal arterioles; in the brain, it also stimulates thirst; while in the adrenal gland, it stimulates secretion of *aldosterone,* which very strongly promotes the reabsorption of sodium and chloride in the distal tubules and collecting ducts of the kidney and which is metabolized in the liver. There is evidence that in mild experimental heart failure, the secretion of renin and the plasma concentrations of angiotensin II and aldosterone may return to or toward normal after the retention of sodium and water has produced expansion of the blood volume and interstitial fluid volume.

In severe heart failure there is also evidence of increased secretion of antidiuretic hormone. Although this may contribute to the decreased ability of some patients to secrete a water load, it is not felt to play a major role in edema formation.[30] There is also suggestive evidence that there may exist a *natriuretic* hormone whose absence in heart failure might contribute to edema formation; however, its chemical nature and sites of action are not established.[28,42] The kidneys synthesize prostaglandins E_2 and $F_{2\alpha}$ in the interstitial and collecting duct cells of the medulla. These are released into the renal interstitial fluid and renal venous blood, and are metabolized both in the renal cortex and the lungs. Their precise role in the maintenance of normal sodium balance or in heart failure is still unclear.[42,45] There is also suggestive evidence that bradykinin and perhaps other members of the kallikrein-kinin system may be involved in the intrarenal distribution of blood flow and the excretion of sodium,[42,46]

but their importance in heart failure is also unknown.

Frank-Starling Law of the Heart

The Frank-Starling law of the heart is immediately brought into play following acute failure of the heart. When the ventricle fails to eject a normal quantity of blood during one beat, its end-systolic volume increases. Consequently, this increased volume remains and is added to the blood entering the ventricle during the next diastole. The net result is an increased end-diastolic volume for the next beat. By the Frank-Starling law of the heart (Chap. 3) this increased "preload" produces an increased amount of stroke work and a larger stroke volume during the next contraction. Over a period of time, the ventricle may become compensated and may be able to maintain normal or nearly normal stroke volume and work at an increased end-diastolic fiber length and volume (see Fig. 3-10). In many patients with a chronic increase in preload as a result of aortic or mitral regurgitation, the ventricle dilates markedly and increases its end-diastolic volume strikingly without an increase in pressure. Later, with the onset of diastolic failure of the ventricle, the diastolic pressure becomes progressively elevated. Theoretically, an increase in cardiac output with increased preload would not occur if the heart were operating on the "descending limb" of its function curve. It appears, however, that the heart can function on a descending limb for only brief periods.[47,48] Of great interest are recent studies which suggest that the chronically dilated left ventricle subjected to additional volume load may not utilize the Frank-Starling mechanism to a significant degree at the ultrastructural level.[50-55]

In patients with congestive heart failure the retention of salt and water by the kidneys increases effective blood volume, which tends to increase ventricular filling volume and to return stroke output toward normal. This compensatory mechanism may return stroke output to normal or near normal, but at the expense of increased venous pressure in the pulmonary venous or the systemic venous systems. In some patients this increased filling pressure appears to be chronically necessary for a reasonable cardiac output. Such patients may develop symptoms of decreased cardiac output if the ventricular filling pressure is excessively decreased by diuretics. This is particularly likely to occur in patients with pericardial constriction, aortic stenosis, or hypertrophic cardiomyopathy (see Chap. 56).

Another characteristic of the failing heart is that it becomes pressure-dependent. The normal heart can sustain large changes in systolic loading with little change in cardiac output through minor changes in diastolic volume. When muscle failure is present and diastolic volume is augmented, an increase in pressure leads to substantial falls in cardiac output. Alternatively, a fall in pressure loads in this circumstance yields substantial increase in the cardiac output (Figs. 22-2 and 22-3).

Hypertrophy and Dilatation of the Heart

Hypertrophy is one of the major adjustments of the heart to chronically increased stress. Experimentally, there is metabolic evidence of hypertrophy within a few hours after an increase in cardiac work.[56-62] Hyperplasia, or an actual increase in the total number of myocardial cells, is thought to occur in human beings only if the increased stress occurs within a few months of age. On the other hand, cardiac hypertrophy is associated with a significant increase in the number or size of sarcomeres within each myocardial cell.

Two classic types of left ventricular hypertrophy are recognized: concentric and eccentric. In pure *concentric hypertrophy* of the left ventricle, there is an increase in the thickness of the ventricular wall, but the ventricular chamber does not increase in diameter. In some instances, the ventricular chamber may actually decrease in size. This type is classically

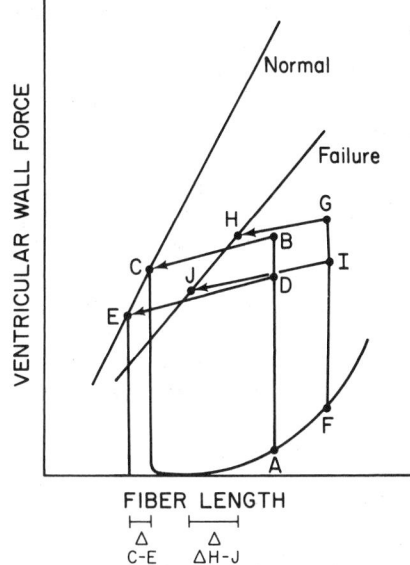

FIGURE 22-3 Relation between ventricular wall force and fiber length. Hypothetical contractile cycles have been portrayed for the normal and failing ventricle. In the normal heart, contraction starts at point A; wall force rises until the aortic valve is opened (point B); the ventricle empties (point B to C); and relaxation ensues. If arterial pressure (afterload) is reduced, e.g., to point D, ejection then starts at point D and proceeds to point E. In the presence of ventricular failure, the fiber length in diastole is increased and ventricular contraction starts at point F. With systolic contraction, ventricular wall force rises to point G, and during ventricular emptying, fiber length decreases to point H. If the afterload is decreased, wall force only needs to reach point I when ventricular emptying occurs to point J. Note that, for the same relative change in afterload, the increase in shortening is greater in the failing ventricle (ΔH to J) than in the normal heart (ΔC to E) because of the relative flattening of the systolic curve in the former case.

FIGURE 22-2 Relation between stroke volume and left ventricular end-diastolic pressure (LVEDP). *Right.* Relation between stroke volume and blood pressure. Normally, the ventricle operates on a sharply rising Frank-Starling curve with an LVEDP less than 12 mmHg (point A), where small changes in filling pressure yield large changes in stroke volume. Further, stroke volume is largely independent of the arterial blood pressure. When failure occurs, ventricular function is characterized by a shift of the curve relating stroke volume to LVEDP to the right and downward. Low output may ensue if the curve is depressed to a great enough extent while pulmonary congestion occurs as the LVEDP is increased. At the same time, this failing ventricle is now highly pressure-dependent (point D) so that small changes in blood pressure produce large changes in stroke volume. When arterial pressure is reduced in the normal circulation (i.e., point A to B), stroke volume rises very slightly. If venodilatation occurs at the same time, stroke volume falls to point C. The net result is a decrease in stroke volume. On the contrary, when arterial pressure is reduced in the presence of severe ventricular failure, stroke volume is increased (point D to C). Since the Frank-Starling curve is relatively flattened, a simultaneous decrease in venous tone leads to a decrease in LVEDP with only a small decrease in stroke volume (point E to F). The net result is an increase in stroke volume. These results are observed clinically when nitroprusside is administered as an "unloading" agent for treating the failing ventricle.

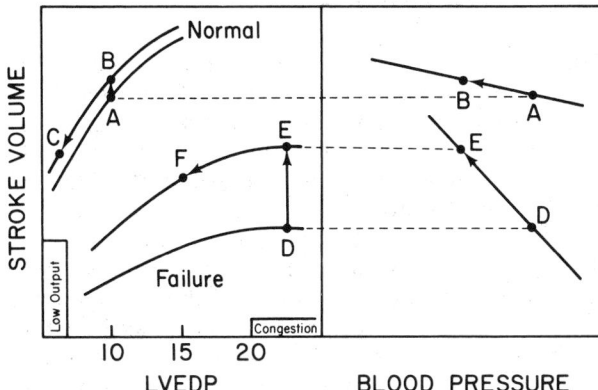

present in patients with isolated valvular aortic stenosis. In pure *eccentric hypertrophy,* the thickness of the left ventricular wall and the internal diameter of the ventricle increase proportionately. This may be seen in normal growth or in patients with volume overload of the left ventricle, as in isolated mitral regurgitation.[62-66] Although the exact myocardial stimulus for hypertrophy is unknown,[56-62] it has been suggested that an increase in systolic wall tension of the ventricle in conditions associated with increased afterload stimulates the synthesis of sarcomeres in parallel to existing sarcomeres and thereby produces concentric hypertrophy.[62-66] Conversely, it has been suggested that an increase in diastolic wall tension in conditions with increased preload primarily stimulates the synthesis of sarcomeres in series with preexisting sarcomeres and produces eccentric hypertrophy. In compensated hypertrophy, the increase in wall thickness is such that the tension in the wall is maintained in a normal range.

It is significant that the increase in the length of individual myocardial cells in patients with chronically dilated hearts is not adequate to explain the increase in heart size frequently encountered. In such patients, there is also significant myocardial "slippage" or rearrangement at the level of myofibrils, myocardial fibers, and muscle bundles.[2,63,67–79]

In general, most studies have indicated that the compensatory hypertrophy in many patients with chronic pressure or volume overload can be adequate to return the calculated systolic wall stress to normal, although diastolic wall stress may remain abnormal in patients with volume overload.[1,2,55,63–66,70–74]

Uncompensated failure is commonly characterized by an increase in systolic wall stress despite the compensatory hypertrophy. Growth hormone and other hormones appear to be necessary for normal cardiac hypertrophy to develop in response to stress.[75]

Effect of Cardiac Hypertrophy on Diastolic Compliance

The diastolic compliance or distensibility of ventricles with concentric hypertrophy due to pressure overload is typically much less than that present in patients with eccentric hypertrophy due to volume overload in the absence of severe myocardial failure. Thus, the extremely thick hypertrophied ventricle of a patient with concentric hypertrophy from aortic stenosis may require a high left ventricular end-diastolic pressure for normal filling as a result of the hypertrophy itself. In such patients an elevation of ventricular diastolic pressure is not necessarily due to myocardial failure. In contrast, many patients with eccentric hypertrophy from mitral or aortic regurgitation may have markedly increased end-diastolic volumes with relatively normal diastolic pressures, often in the presence of significant myocardial and ventricular systolic dysfunction. These findings limit the value of ventricular end-diastolic pressure as an index of left ventricular performance, especially if the diastolic pressure is not correlated with other data.[76–82] (See Chap. 18.)

Effects of Experimental Cardiac Hypertrophy on Indexes of Myocardial Contractility

When the heart is caused to become hypertrophied experimentally by increasing ventricular preload (volume overload), it is generally agreed that the myocardial contractility per unit mass is not decreased until shortly before the onset of failure.[2,51,53–55,83,84] In contrast, there is lack of agreement as to whether or not myocardial contractility per unit mass is decreased soon after the development of hypertrophy that is experimentally produced by increased ventricular afterload (pressure overload), i.e., the experimental production of aortic or pulmonic stenosis. A number of studies of this type of hypertrophy have found that myocardial contractility per unit mass is decreased prior to the development of failure and have suggested that ventricular compensation is maintained by an increase in total myocardial mass.[1,2,17,85–87] It has also been found that this decreased contractility may be

reversible if the experimental hypertrophy is reversed by unbanding before the onset of failure.[88] Other studies of pressure-induced hypertrophy have found that myocardial contractility per unit mass may also return to normal if the elevated pressure load is maintained for 24 weeks,[89] while other investigators found normal ventricular function at rest in animals with stable hypertrophy from either volume or pressure overload.[90] It appears that alterations in myocardial contractility with associated cardiac hypertrophy are variable and depend upon the inciting stimulus.[84–91] For example, left ventricular hypertrophy induced by high-altitude hypoxia is not associated with a decrease in the indexes of contractility, but there is a decrease in the indexes with chronic experimental coarctation of the aorta.[54] Part of these discrepancies may depend on the acuteness of the overload, its severity, the extent of resultant hypertrophy, and the age of the individual when it occurs.

Peripheral Oxygen Delivery

The usual decrease in blood flow to the peripheral tissues in heart failure is associated with a progressive decline in the affinity of hemoglobin for oxygen, which is caused by an increase in 2,3-diphosphoglycerate (DPG).[92] This change in affinity, which is reflected in a rightward shift in the oxygen-hemoglobin dissociation curve, facilitates the release of oxygen in the peripheral capillaries of underperfused tissues.

The peripheral tissues in heart failure extract more oxygen per unit of blood flow with a resultant increase in the body's arteriovenous oxygen difference. This venous oxygen reserve is potentially less useful to the mycoardium, which even normally extracts about 65 to 75 percent of the oxygen coming to it.

Some tissues also utilize anaerobic metabolism during transient periods of increased stress such as exercise. Unfortunately, this reserve mechanism is of only very limited value to the myocardium. (See Chap. 5.)

The Law of Laplace

The law of Laplace and the effects of ventricular dilatation upon the mechanics and energetics of myocardial contraction are important factors in heart failure. On first thought, it might seem that ventricular dilatation is advantageous. With an increased end-diastolic ventricular volume and sarcomere length, each sarcomere would have to shorten less to eject a given volume of blood, and each myocardial fiber would be able to perform more work by virtue of greater preload and the law of the heart. In many situations, however, these seeming advantages are negated by several important hemodynamic consequences of dilatation. The more important of these is the need for the myocardial fibers in the wall of a dilated ventricle to develop greater tension in order to produce a given pressure within the ventricle. In general, ventricular myocardial wall tension is calculated by employing the law of Laplace, which actually applies to a distensible membrane with a spherical or cylindrical shape, and by assuming that the ventricle has a spherical cavity. Figure 22-4 illustrates three definitions of contractile tension in the ventricular myocardium, as used by different authors. Badeer[70] has recommended that calculations of myocardial tension be expressed in terms of force per unit of cross-sectional area (formula shown on right in Fig. 22-4). By all three formulas, it is apparent that as the radius acutely increases, more tension must be developed by each fiber to produce or maintain a given intraventricular pressure. In formula 3, an increased thickness of the ventricular wall tends to decrease the required systolic tension per cross-sectional area. The law of Laplace expresses an additional disadvantage of the dilated ventricle. In a normal ventricle during ejection, the decrease in average radius of the ventricle is relatively large; consequently, the effect of this decrease in diameter upon instantaneous wall tension is normally greater than the opposite effect of the increasing pressure in the ventricle. As a result, the myocardial fiber tension, or force, may actually *decrease* soon after the beginning of ejection from a normal-sized ventricle, and the tension is usually less at the moment of peak systolic pressure in the ventricle than at the beginning of ejection. On the other hand, if the ventricle is markedly dilated, both the relative and the absolute decrease in average radius is much less during the ejection of an equal volume. In a markedly dilated ventricle, therefore, the average tension in the myocardial fibers may continue to increase from the beginning of ejection up to the peak systolic pressure.[70,92–97] In a sense, this is an additional type of "afterload" encountered during ejection by ventricles that are significantly dilated by increased "preload." A further disadvantage of dilatation is that the increased force, or tension, in the myocardial fibers required to develop a given pressure inside a dilated ventricle results in a decrease in the *rate* of

myocardial fiber shortening (see Chap. 3), thereby decreasing the ability of the ventricle to eject blood.[2,50,52,70,98,99] In mitral regurgitation, the early reduction in afterload (impedance) produced by the relatively rapid emptying of the left ventricle into both the low-pressure left atrium and the aorta helps to maintain left ventricular function for many years.[5,100]

Basic Mechanisms of Heart Failure

Chronic heart failure is characterized by ventricular hypertrophy and dilatation. One hallmark of the end stage is irreversible cell loss. This may be segmental, secondary to coronary artery disease, or diffuse and focal, due to microvascular obstruction with local necrosis, again with local fibrosis. Cell loss, whether segmental or diffuse, then provides a further load for the remaining heart, and additional compensatory hypertrophy ensues. Severe hypertrophy, in and of itself, decreases performance of each remaining cell. Thus, conceptually, the chronically failing heart may be thought of as akin to cirrhosis of the liver or chronic glomerulonephritis. This concept is very helpful in explaining some of the early reversibility and the late irreversibility in patients with heart failure.

The basic biochemical-biophysical mechanisms of myocardial failure remain a very active area of investigation. It is unlikely that a single mechanism is present in all cases; it is more likely that different mechanisms (Table 22-4) exist and contribute under different circumstances.

Energy Production and Utilization

Myocardial Oxygen Consumption in Heart Failure

Most patients with heart failure have a normal coronary blood flow at rest and a normal or elevated myocardial oxygen consumption per 100 g of tissue.[101] Because of the increased total mass and the increase in myocardial systolic wall tension due to the Laplace relation in patients with heart failure,

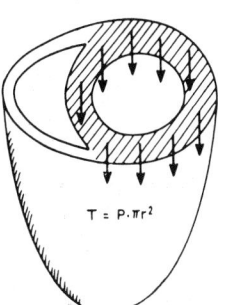

T = Force across the total cross-sectional area of muscle.

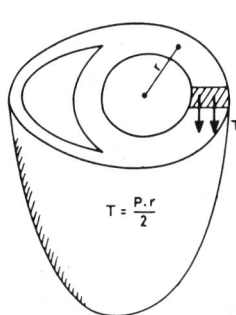

T = Force per unit length of circumference and the entire thickness of wall.

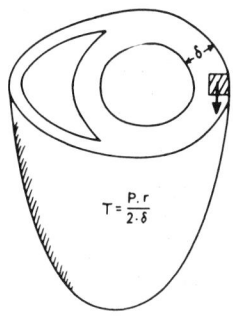

T = Force per unit cross-sectional area of muscle.

FIGURE 22-4 Three definitions of contractile force in the myocardium and the formulas based on the law of Laplace used to calculate each. *T* = contractile tangential tension or force in the wall of the ventricle; *P* = transmural pressure across the wall of the ventricle; *r* = average radius of the ventricle, assuming it to be spherical; and δ = ventricular wall thickness. (*From Badeer.[70] Reprinted with the permission of the author and the C. V. Mosby Company.*)

TABLE 22-4 Possible Mechanisms of Myocardial Failure

1. Loss of myocytes
2. Energy production and utilization
   a. Energy supply
   b. Substrate utilization and energy storage
   c. Inadequate mitochondria mass and function
3. Contractile proteins
   a. Sarcomere "overstretch"
   b. Abnormal myocardial proteins
   c. Defective protein synthesis
   d. Abnormal myosin ATPase
4. Activation of contractile elements
   a. Sarcolemma ATPase
   b. Sarcoplasmic reticulum (SR)
      (1) Ca^{2+} sequestration rate
      (2) Concentration of SR
5. Autonomic nervous system
   a. Depletion of myocardial norepinephrine
6. Presbycardia

the total amount of oxygen consumed by the heart may be significantly increased. This may result in a greater amount of oxygen being extracted from each unit of coronary blood flow and a widening of the coronary arteriovenous oxygen difference. Many patients with heart failure are able to increase coronary blood flow during exercise; however, some patients with a dilated ventricle that increases in diameter during exercise may have a further widening of the coronary arteriovenous oxygen difference during exercise (Chap. 3). In one study of a group of patients with left ventricular failure, the left ventricular oxygen consumption averaged 16 percent of the total oxygen consumed by the body compared with 5 percent in normal subjects.[102] In one patient with severe aortic valve disease, the left ventricle accounted for 27 percent of the total amount of oxygen consumed by the body.

Substrate Utilization and Energy Storage

Although the myocardial uptake of fatty acids and glucose per 100 g of myocardium in heart failure is normal,[101] there is conflicting evidence on whether or not there is a primary decrease in energy liberation by mitochondrial oxidative phosphorylation.[1,2,84,101–111] Although reductions in store of myocardial high-energy phosphate, creatine phosphate (CP), and/or adenosine triphosphate (ATP) have often been found in heart failure, these changes are usually thought to be a secondary and not a primary cause of the failure.[1,2,82,103–105,112,113]

Inadequate Mitochondria Mass and Function

Several workers have found a significant decrease in the mass of mitochondria relative to the mass of myofibrils in experimental cardiac hypertrophy.[114,115] As noted below, there may also be defects in mitochondrial oxidative phosphorylation and in mitochondrial calcium metabolism associated with myocardial failure.

Contractile Proteins

Sarcomere "Overstretch"

As noted in Chap. 3, when myocardial sarcomeres function at lengths up to the L_{max} at about 2.2 μm, they operate on the *ascending limb* of the length-tension curve and develop more active tension with increasing length. When the sarcomeres are stretched beyond the length at which maximal active tension is developed (L_{max}), however, the amount of active tension decreases and the sarcomeres are said to be operating on the *descending limb* of the length-tension curve.[1,2,50–52,67–69,116,117] The existence of a descending limb of cardiac function for the entire ventricle is uncertain, however, and some of the apparent decrease in function may be due to increased afterload.[47–49] At one time it was thought that sarcomere overstretch might be responsible for the decreased myocardial contractility characteristic of many patients with ventricular dilatation and heart failure. Subsequent studies have shown, however, that acute volume loading is associated with an increase in left ventricular midwall mean sarcomere length to about L_{max} (2.2 to 2.4 μm after fixation) and that with chronic volume loading there is additional recruitment of subendocardial and subepicardial sarcomere length to L_{max} but no sarcomere overstretch.[50–55] Other changes that contribute to the marked ventricular dilatation that is frequently present with volume overload include the synthesis of sarcomeres in series with preexisting sarcomeres, slippage of myofibrils and myocardial fibers, and rearrangement of myocardial fibers along cleavage planes of the left ventricle.[1,2,50–53,55,63,67–69,118] Thus, although overstretch of sarcomeres may occasionally be present transiently, it does not appear to be an important primary mechanism of chronic heart failure. The effect of ventricular dilatation and the law of Laplace have been noted above.

Myosin ATPase

There is substantial evidence of significantly decreased activity of myofibrillar and myosin adenosine triphosphatase (ATPase) both in patients and experimental animals with heart failure.[103,119–127] These changes could significantly interfere with the liberation of energy for myocardial contraction. It has been suggested that the changes in activity of myosin ATPase may be related to associated changes in the number of light chains of myosin.[103,125–127]

Defective Protein Synthesis

In most patients with heart failure, there are preceding phases of increased protein synthesis and of stable hyperfunction and hypertrophy, which are thought to be initiated by a chronic increase in myocardial stress.[56–62,71,128] Meerson has concluded that the subsequent onset of myocardial failure is causally related to a decrease in the synthesis of normal protein due to "wear and tear."[62,128] As noted above, experimental hypertrophy may be associated with changes in the number of light chains of myosin.[1,125–127]

Activation of Contractile Elements

Sarcolemma ATPase

Heart failure may also be associated with defects in the activity of the membrane transport enzyme Na^+-K^+-ATPase,[2,129–131] although the role of this enzyme in the pathogenesis of myocardial failure is less definite.[103]

Sarcoplasmic Reticulum (SR)

Calcium (Ca^{2+}) Sequestration Rate   There is also substantial evidence of reduced Ca^{2+} rates of uptake and of binding by sarcoplasmic reticulum in association with increased mitochondrial Ca^{2+} in many types of clinical or experimental heart failure.[103,132–144] These abnormalities of calcium metabolism appear to be of primary importance in some types of failure, whereas they may be secondary changes in other types. Intracellular acidosis decreases the affinity of troponin-C for Ca^{2+} and may contribute to some forms of heart failure, especially those associated with ischemia.[145] The amount of activator Ca^{2+} available for contraction can also be reduced by elevation of intracellular Na^+.[2,137,142–148]

Autonomic Nervous System

As noted above, there is good evidence of defects both in cardiac sympathetic neurotransmitter and in the cardiac parasympathetic control system in congestive heart failure.[11–19] These changes are not thought to be primary causes of the myocardial failure, although they may contribute significantly.

Senile Cardiomyopathy (Presbycardia or Senile Heart Disease)

In some elderly individuals there may be involutional changes of the myocardium associated with decreased elasticity of the skeleton of the heart and with mild fibrotic changes of the valves. The chemical basis of these aging changes and of the associated pigmentation of the heart is not known. This condition, known as *presbycardia, senile heart disease,* or *senile cardiomyopathy*, probably only rarely produces heart failure by itself; however, it decreases the adaptive capacity of reserves of the heart.[149–151] Accordingly, patients with this condition more readily develop heart failure in the presence of other forms of heart disease or, occasionally, even from the increased demands of fever, moderate anemia, mild hyperthyroidism, excess fluid administration, etc. Aged myocardium has also been shown to have a diminished inotropic response to catecholamines.[152]

Heart Failure Due to Pressure Overload and Volume Overload

Most types of congenital and acquired heart disease result in a mechanical stress upon the heart and myocardium. The two most common general types of mechanical cardiac stress are (1) that resulting from an increased resistance to ventricular emptying of increased afterload (i.e., aortic stenosis, systemic hypertension, etc.) and (2) that resulting from an increased preload or increased ventricular filling (i.e., aortic or mitral regurgitation, ventricular septal defect, etc.). The hemodynamics of several other specific types of mechanical abnormalities are described elsewhere: mitral stenosis (Chap. 39), pericardial tamponade or constriction (Chap. 57), endocardial restriction (Chap. 56), and the several varieties of ventricular dyssynergy and aneurysm (Chap. 45).

In some patients with acute mechanical abnormalities, such as the acute rupture of a mitral chordae tendineae or of an aortic valve leaflet, the overall function of the heart may fail even though the contractility of the myocardium may be relatively normal. Some chronic mechanical abnormalities by themselves can also prevent the heart from pumping an adequate amount of blood without the development of myocardial failure. In the majority of patients with a chronic pressure load (afterload) or a chronic volume load on the left ventricle, however, the development of clinical congestive heart failure is preceded by the development of myocardial dysfunction and then myocardial failure, which significantly limits overall cardiac performance.

Compensatory Mechanisms in Heart Failure Due to Increased Afterload (Pressure Overload)

Isolated increased afterload (pressure overload) of the left ventricle is classically seen in patients with systemic hypertension, coarctation of the aorta, or aortic stenosis. The basic reaction of isolated myocardium to an increased afterload is to contract more forcefully but more slowly. In addition, when the heart is acutely subjected to increased afterload, there is metabolic evidence of hypertrophy within a few hours.[56–62] The precise biochemical signal is unknown, but may be related to a chronic increase in systolic wall tension.[62–66] As noted above, the classic type of cardiac hypertrophy associated with aortic stenosis is *concentric hypertrophy*, in which there is marked thickening of the left ventricular walls (including the interventricular septum), but there is no increase in the size of the left ventricular cavity, which may even get smaller.[66] It has been suggested that the increased afterload stimulates myocardial thickening by replication of sarcomeres in parallel.[66] Although the contractility of the myocardium subjected to pressure overload may be decreased per unit mass (see above), overall ventricular compensation is maintained by the increase in myocardial mass (Fig. 22-5). Systolic wall tension may be returned to normal by the concentric hypertrophy and the spherical shape, although diastolic wall stress may remain abnormal.[1,2,62–66,70–74,104,113,116] Eventually, however, myocardial dysfunction and myocardial failure develop, followed by cardiac pump dysfunction and failure. Some of the possible structural and biochemical mechanisms responsible for myocardial failure are discussed above. In Fig. 22-5, the dotted line represents the hypothetical changes in myocardial contractility following an increase in ventricular afterload (assuming that the contractility per unit mass in this form of hypertrophy is decreased from the onset of hypertrophy) (see above). Overall cardiac (pump) function may be reasonably maintained by the concentric hypertrophy until the myocardial failure becomes marked.

In aortic stenosis there may be special difficulties with the delivery of adequate amounts of oxygen to the myocardial cells, particularly in the endocardium. Some of the particular factors responsible for this in aortic stenosis include the elevated myocardial oxygen requirements and the very high intramyocardial pressure, which throttles systolic coronary blood flow even more than usual, especially with tachycardia.[153–155] An elevated ventricular diastolic pressure may be necessary to fill the hypertrophied ventricle but will also impede diastolic coronary blood flow to the endocardium.[156] In addition,

FIGURE 22-5 Hypothetical curves of ventricular hypertrophy, overall cardiac or ventricular pump performance, and myocardial contractility following the onset of a significant increase in ventricular preload or ventricular afterload. Three levels of overall cardiac pump function and myocardial function (contractility) are shown: normal; "dysfunction," or slightly to moderately decreased; and "failure," or markedly decreased. In general, myocardial function or contractility decreases prior to a decrease in overall cardiac pump function because of compensatory mechanisms, particularly ventricular hypertrophy. The solid line of myocardial contractility represents the hypothetical curve following the onset of an increased preload (volume load). The dotted line of myocardial contractility represents the hypothetical curve following the onset of an increased afterload (pressure load); it is drawn as if this form of hypertrophy is associated with a decrease in contractility per unit mass from the onset of hypertrophy, although this is uncertain. See text for discussion.

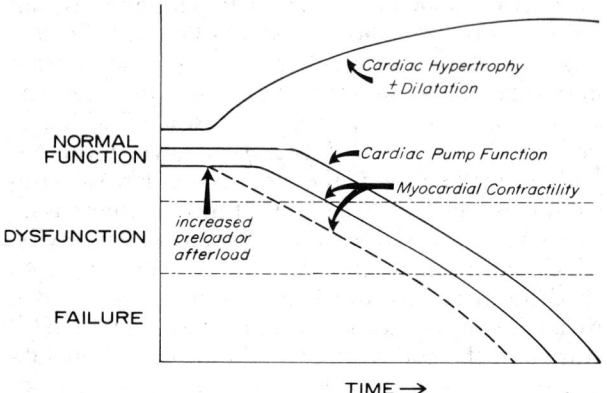

the diffusion distance from myocardial capillaries to the center of the hypertrophied myocardial cells may be significantly increased.[157] Patients with marked concentric hypertrophy from aortic stenosis or other causes frequently have an elevation of left ventricular diastolic filling pressure (and decreased left ventricular compliance or distensibility) that is due to the hypertrophy itself, rather than to cardiac failure.[73,74,76–81] (See "Hemodynamic Characteristics of Heart Failure," below.)

Compensatory Mechanisms with Increased Left Ventricular Preload (Volume Overload)

The classic type of ventricular hypertrophy that develops in patients with increased left ventricular preload (volume overload) is *eccentric hypertrophy* in which the ventricular chamber and the left ventricular wall increase in size proportionately.[56–65] It has been suggested that this type of hypertrophy is produced by a chronic increase in diastolic wall stress and is associated with the synthesis of additional sarcomeres, predominantly in series.[66] Since increased preload also increases systolic wall stress and afterload by the law of Laplace, some replication in parallel also occurs and helps to normalize systolic stress.

When the ventricle is acutely subjected to an increased preload, the ventricle acutely dilates and functions on the ascending limb of its length-tension function curve with an increase in the sarcomere length to about 2.2 µm in the midwall of the left ventricle. This length approximates L_{max}, the sarcomere length at which the maximal performance is achieved on the sarcomere length-tension function curve.[68,69] In experimental animals subjected to chronic left ventricular volume loading, the left ventricle may continue to appear to work on a slightly ascending limb of a function curve. In this situation, however, there does not appear to be any additional increase in sarcomere length in the midwall of the left ventricle beyond about 2.2 µm when the ventricle is subjected to increased preload, although there is some additional recruitment in sarcomere length up to about 2.2 µm in the left ventricular endocardial and epicardial area.[50,52,55,68,69,117] Normally, the functioning sarcomere lengths are somewhat less in the endocardium and the epicardium than in the midwall of the left ventricle.[50] The marked ventricular dilatation of chronic volume loading is produced by several mechanisms, including the increase in individual sarcomere length, the synthesis of new sarcomeres in series and parallel with previous sarcomeres, slippage between and within myofibrils and fibers, and the rearrangement of myocardial fibers along the normal cleavage planes of the ventricle.[2,50–54,63,67–69,118]

The performance of the ventricle with mitral regurgitation is somewhat aided by the fact that during systole the left ventricle is emptied relatively rapidly by both aortic ejection and by regurgitation into the left atrium. This rapid decrease in the mean left ventricular diameter has the effect of rapidly decreasing the systolic wall tension and afterload (impedance) and thus increasing the velocity of contraction.[53,55,99,158] The diastolic capacity of the ventricle with chronically increased volume loads is often markedly increased so that it may accommodate a large volume without excess elevation of diastolic pressure,[55,58] although additional volume loading may produce a precipitous elevation of diastolic pressure, indicative of reduced compliance.[51] When the myocardial contractility eventually becomes markedly decreased in patients with chronic volume overload, ventricular dilatation and hypertrophy are no longer able to compensate adequately, and overall heart pump function decreases and may eventually fail (Fig. 22-3).

Atrial Failure and Heart Failure[159–162]

The two major functions of the atria are pumping and serving as a reservoir. Normally, the atria contribute approximately 15 to 20 percent of ventricular filling, but the relative contribution increases markedly with tachycardia. In normal individuals or patients with mild heart disease, loss of the atrial pumping function may result in no change in cardiac output at rest, although the response to exercise may be diminished. On the other hand, in patients with heart disease and limited cardiac reserve, atrial fibrillation or atrial flutter can produce *atrial failure* with severe detrimental effects on ventricular filling and on the overall pump function of the heart.

The more common forms of atrial failure are due to arrhythmia (e.g., atrial fibrillation), mechanical abnormalities (e.g., mitral or tricuspid stenosis), or dysdynamic failure of the atrial myocardium. In some patients with compensated heart disease, congestive heart failure may at times be precipitated by the onset of atrial fibrillation even when the ventricular response rate is controlled by digitalis. In these patients the restoration of normal sinus rhythm may result in a marked improvement in their hemodynamics, presumably by restoration of the normal "booster-pump" function of the atria. Interestingly, in some patients following cardioversion and the restoration of normal sinus rhythm, atrial contraction may not occur for several days.[163] Very rarely, atrial fibrillation may produce heart failure in patients with otherwise apparently normal hearts.[164]

Left Atrial Compliance and Heart Failure

The compliance of the left atrium is of great importance in determining the level of left atrial pressure produced by disease of the left side of the heart and especially mitral regurgitation. Thus, a given volume of mitral regurgitation in a patient with a lax, capacious left atrium may produce only slight elevation of left atrial pressure, whereas the same volume regurgitated into a smaller left atrium with less distensibility may produce marked elevation of left atrial pressure and severe pulmonary congestion.[55,162] (See Chap. 39.)

Hemodynamic Characteristics of Heart Failure

The major hemodynamic alterations and several of the major compensatory mechanisms that are produced by myocardial and pump failure are shown in Fig. 22-6. Also indicated are the sites of action of three major therapeutic interventions.

As described in Chaps. 3 and 18, the performance of the intact heart should generally be assessed at two levels. The first type of analysis is an evaluation of the overall *cardiac pump function* as indicated by the relation between stroke work (or cardiac output) and ventricular end-diastolic volume (or pressure). Ideally, these or other systolic indexes of pump performance are measured at rest and again after induced changes in preload in order to construct a function curve, although this is seldom done clinically. The second type of assessment is of *myocardial function* (*myocardial contractility* or *inotropic state*). Although decreases in myocardial contractility can sometimes be inferred from studies of overall cardiac function (i.e., when the cardiac output and stroke volume are significantly decreased despite a markedly increased end-diastolic ventricular volume greater than 110 ml/m^2 and in the presence of normal afterload and heart rate), more specific and more sensitive quantitative evidence of changes in myocardial contractility in patients are obtained from two types of analyses: (1) isovolumic phase indexes utilizing the rate of rise of ventricular pressure (dP/dt) or a derivative, and (2) ejection phase indexes of contractility utilizing circumferential fiber shortening rate (V_{cf}). The techniques used clinically for evaluation of cardiac function and of myocardial contractility are reviewed in Chap. 18.

Changes in the Contralateral Ventricle

In evaluating left ventricular performance, it is important to keep in mind that experimental right ventricular hypertrophy may be associated with changes in left ventricular end-diastolic pressure or compliance that are probably due in part to a "reversed" Bernheim effect.[165–168] In addition, the contralateral left ventricle may have decreased norepinephrine concentration,[17,169] decreased myofibrillar adenosine triphosphatase activity,[120] and increased amounts of collagen.[170] In general, any time there is moderate or marked ventricular hypertrophy, the diastolic pressure-volume relationships of the opposite ventricle may be altered.

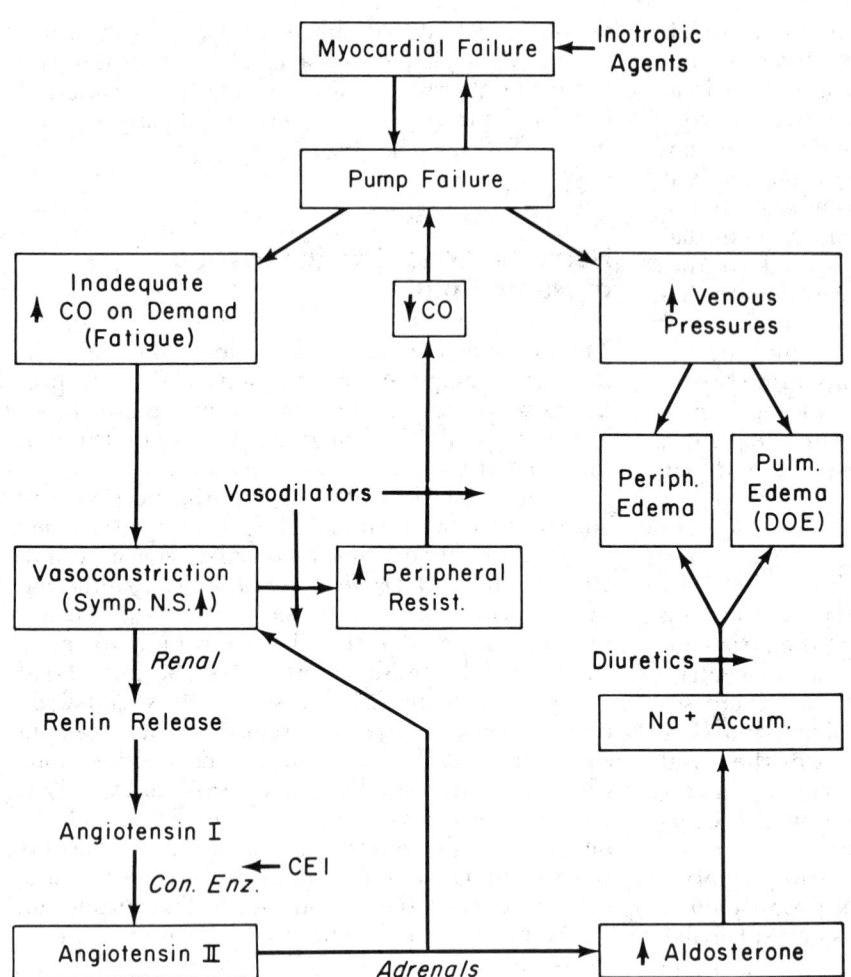

FIGURE 22-6 Schematic diagram of the major hemodynamic alterations and several of the major compensatory mechanisms that result from the development of myocardial failure and pump (heart) failure. Also shown are the sites of action of three major therapeutic interventions: administration of ionotropic agents, diuretics, and vasodilators.

Secondary Mitral or Tricuspid Regurgitation

"Functional" mitral valve regurgitation may develop secondary to left ventricular myocardial failure, and a similar form of tricuspid regurgitation occurs secondary to right ventricular failure. In both instances the regurgitation is principally the result of failure of the papillary muscles and chordae tendineae of the dilated ventricle to anchor or constrain the atrioventricular valve leaflets. A secondary mechanism, which is present in chronic lesions, is dilatation and failure of the valve annulus to constrict properly during systole. If the regurgitation is moderate or severe, the atrial pressure tracings may have a large regurgitant r wave (giant v wave).

Pulsus Alternans

Pulsus alternans may occur in patients with heart failure, particularly from aortic stenosis. It is usually associated with an alteration of end-diastolic volume or fiber length, though not necessarily with an alteration of end-diastolic pressure. Some instances appear to be associated primarily with an alteration of myocardial contractility with no detectable alteration of end-diastolic volume. Pulsus alternans is probably related to a defect in the Ca^{2+} release-binding systems involved in excitation-contraction coupling. It may occur briefly in some apparently normal hearts during or following marked tachycardia.

Pulmonary Circulation in Heart Failure

In moderate or severe left ventricular failure, elevated left ventricular diastolic pressure is reflected in an elevation of left atrial, pulmonary capillary, and pulmonary artery diastolic pressures. Initially, the pulmonary artery pressure and right ventricular systolic pressure are abnormally elevated only during exercise, although later they may be chronically elevated to systemic levels at rest, particularly in patients with mitral valve disease (see Chap. 39). In the absence of significant pulmonary vascular disease or tachycardia, the pulmonary artery diastolic pressure can be used as a reasonably good reflection of mean left atrial pressure.

Right Ventricle in Heart Failure

Right ventricular dilatation and failure, with a decreased ejection fraction and rate of ejection, may occur secondary to the chronic pressure load produced by left ventricular failure and, perhaps, secondary to biochemical changes in the contralateral right ventricular myocardium.[1,2,17,112,120,169,170] Right ventricular failure may be reflected in a decreased right ventricular stroke volume and ejection fraction, despite an abnormal elevation of the right ventricular end-diastolic volume pressure, the mean right atrial pressure, and the mean systemic venous pressure. If the failure is mild, these abnormalities may be absent at rest but apparent during exercise. Failure of the right ventricle may also be associated with development of right ventricular pulsus alternans, auscultatory alternans, and a right ventricular diastolic gallop sound. The sequence of severe right ventricular failure secondary to left ventricular failure is frequently associated with the development of tricuspid regurgitation or occasionally with the development of functional pulmonary regurgitation due to dilatation of the pulmonary valve ring. Severe pulmonary regurgitation can produce an equalization of the pulmonary artery and right ventricular pressures during mid- or late diastole, although functional pulmonary regurgitation is rarely this marked. Secondary, or so-called functional, tricuspid regurgitation is caused by the inability of the papillary muscles and chordae tendineae of the dilated right ventricle to anchor and to maintain adequate closure of the tricuspid valve; dilatation, or overstretch, of the tricuspid valve ring also contributes to the regurgitation when the ventricular dilatation is severe and chronic. Tricuspid regurgitation may produce large regurgitant r waves during systole in the right atrium and systemic veins (see Chap. 10). Clinically, the development of marked right ventricular failure in association with tricuspid regurgitation in a patient with severe left-sided heart failure may occasionally be associated with a significant decrease in the clinical symptoms of pulmonary congestion.

Effects of Exercise in Patients with Myocardial Failure

During exercise in the supine position, the normal ventricle increases its cardiac output predominantly by an increase in rate, although the stroke volume may increase 10 to 20 percent.[171] The increased stroke volume occurs from an unchanged or slightly smaller end-diastolic volume;[172,173] consequently the ejection fraction may increase and the end-systolic volume decrease. The ventricular end-diastolic pressure normally stays the same or decreases slightly, whereas the systolic ejection period shortens and the mean systolic ejection rate increases.[2,171–183] In contrast, during exercise in the upright position, the stroke volume may double,[184,185] and during maximal exercise the end-diastolic volume may increase.[2] The calculated efficiency (ratio of external work to oxygen consumed by the heart) increases during exercise in normal individuals, perhaps in part as the result of the de-

creased average ventricular radius throughout systole.

Conversely, in patients with heart failure due to dysdynamic myocardial failure, exercise may result in the following changes: an elevation of the end-diastolic pressure above 12 mmHg; only a slight increase or an actual decrease in stroke volume despite an increased end-diastolic volume; a decreased ejection fraction;[186] an increased end-systolic volume; and a prolonged preejection phase.[2,97,98,171,174,175,178–180,186] The calculated ventricular efficiency decreases as the result of no increase (or an actual decrease) in stroke volume despite an increased ventricular end-diastolic volume. The latter increases the mean radius of the ventricle and, by the Laplace relation, increases the sarcomere tension necessary to produce a given intraventricular pressure. Not only does the increased tension required by the dilated ventricle increase the myocardial oxygen consumption (MV_{O_2}), it also decreases the velocity of shortening, further limiting the performance of the ventricle.[2,63,70,71,72,93–98,187] Exercise may also increase functional atrioventricular valvular regurgitation. (See Chap. 18.)

In patients with heart failure during dynamic exercise, the cardiac output either does not increase or does not increase adequately relative to the increased oxygen requirements of the body. Usually, the increase in blood flow to the exercising limb or limbs is less than normal in heart failure, while there are marked decreases in the already diminished flow to skin, kidneys, and splanchnic organs. Coronary flow usually increases, whereas cerebral flow remains unchanged. The excessive increase in venous tone and central venous pressure during exercise in heart failure may be partially related to a reflex with the afferent limb in the exercising muscle and the efferent limb in the sympathetic nervous system.[1] In addition, the plasma concentration of norepinephrine, which is already increased in congestive heart failure, is further increased. High concentrations of angiotensin may also contribute.

The fact that the peripheral blood vessels of patients with heart failure are relatively stiff and relatively unresponsive to local metabolic vasodilator influences during exercise may have a protective influence. For example, if the cardiac output did not increase or even decreased during extensive exercise, the vasodilatation of large skeletal muscle groups could produce an excess fall in the mean arterial pressure.

Effects of Heart Failure on the Peripheral Circulation[20,23,25]

In heart failure, there is evidence of a generalized state of arteriolar constriction and venoconstriction, resulting in an elevation of total peripheral vascular resistance and an increase in venous tone (i.e., the venous bed is less distensible than normal).[20,23,25] These changes tend to maintain arterial blood pressure in the face of a decrease in cardiac output at rest or a decrease in the normal increase in organ blood flow during exercise. They are mediated in part by sympathetic vasoconstrictor impulses, related to the generalized increase in sympathetic activity of the body, and, perhaps, by mechanical alterations in the distensibility of the resistance (arteriolar) vessels, with increased "stiffness" due to increased sodium and water content.[20,21,23,25] In addition, the concentrations of both norepinephrine and angiotensin II are elevated and contribute to both arterial vasoconstriction and the increase in venous tone.[19,44] Increased plasma concentration of antidiuretic hormone may also contribute. In some active organs with high oxygen requirements, these vasoconstrictor tendencies may be partially overridden by local metabolic vasodilators or local changes in P_{O_2}, P_{CO_2}, pH, or K^+. In general, however, the usual markedly increased blood flow to exercising muscles is significantly attenuated.

In heart failure associated with a diminished cardiac output, there is a significant redistribution of blood flow which in part resembles the normal redistribution occurring during exercise (Chap. 3). Thus, in heart failure, the renal and skin blood flows are disproportionately reduced early, whereas the decreases in blood flow to the cerebral, splanchnic, and skeletal muscle areas are approximately proportional to the decrease in total cardiac output until the failure is severe. Coronary blood flow per 100 g of tissue tends to remain normal or nearly normal in most patients in heart failure (see Chap. 3). The decreased skin circulation contributes to the heat intolerance and even mild temperature elevations that occur during heart failure, while the decreased flow to the brain and kidneys contributes significantly to the deranged functions of these organs.

As noted above, the increased sympathetic impulses to the kidney and the high levels of norepinephrine and angiotensin produce a redistribution of intrarenal blood flow and lead to increased blood levels of renin and angiotensin.

In addition to a redistribution of blood flow in heart failure, the tissues extract more oxygen per unit of blood flow and utilize anaerobic metabolism to a greater extent than normal, particularly during acute exertion. The increased oxygen extraction results in a widening of the arteriovenous oxygen differences for most organs and for the body as a whole. The pulmonary arteriovenous oxygen difference, which indicates the average of the whole body, is one of the better parameters for judging the adequacy of the heart as a pump to provide oxygen to the tissues.

Physiologic Basis of the Therapy of Heart Failure

Heart failure and the resulting compensatory mechanisms described above result in abnormalities in each of the major determinants of myocardial performance: preload, afterload, and contractility. In the selection of therapy for a patient with heart failure it is useful to consider each of these determinants separately. The three hemodynamic abnormalities usually present and the corresponding major therapeutic interventions currently available are listed in the following table. In general, an excessive increase in preload is treated with either diuretics or venous vasodilators. The relative increase in afterload associated with heart failure is treated with vasodilators or angiotensin II inhibitors. Figure 22-7 illustrates schematically the mechanism of action of vasodilator therapy in heart failure. Myocardial failure is present in most patients with pump (heart) failure, either as a primary or as a secondary event. Therapy for a decrease in myocardial contractility includes the administration of inotropic agents (Fig. 22-8). (See Chap. 23 for further details of the treatment of heart failure.)

Abnormalities	Therapy
Preload	Diuretics
	Vasodilators
Afterload	Vasodilators
	Angiotensin II inhibitors
Contractility	Inotropic agents

Pulmonary Function and Pulmonary Edema in Congestive Heart Failure

Pulmonary Function in Congestive Heart Failure

The ventilatory functions of the lungs are frequently impaired because of pulmonary congestion from left ventricular failure or mechanical obstruction at the mitral valve.[188-190] The amount of intrathoracic space available for ventilation may be decreased by fluid in the interstitial, perivascular, and alveolar spaces; by hydrothorax; or, in some patients, by an increase in pulmonary blood volume.[192,193] The increased amount of fluid and congestion in the lungs decreases the compliance (increases the stiffness) of the lungs and increases the work and oxygen cost of breathing. Alveolar fluid decreases pulmonary compliance by altering the normal surface tension characteristics, while pericapillary thickening and interstitial edema interfere with alveolar-capillary diffusion of oxygen. The respiratory muscles, which have an increased work load because of the decreased pulmonary compliance, may suffer from relative ischemia and, rarely, may produce pain difficult to distinguish from pain of myocardial origin.

Many patients with moderate pulmonary congestion have compensatory hyperventilation with respiratory alkalosis, although some patients with severe pulmonary edema may have metabolic and respiratory acidosis.[194,195] Pulmonary congestion alters many pulmonary function tests, and it is often

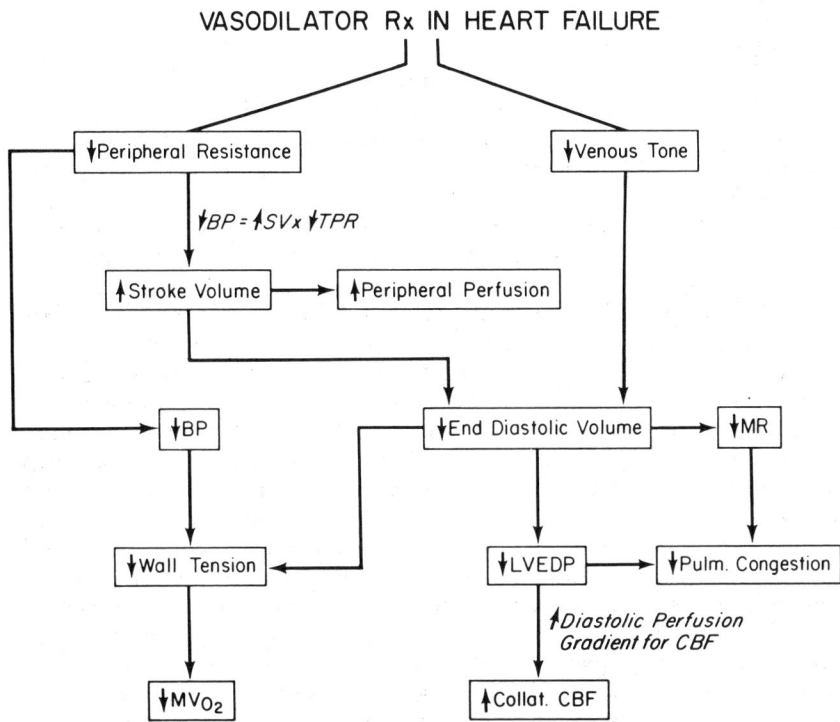

VASODILATOR Rx IN HEART FAILURE

FIGURE 22-7 Schematic diagram of the major actions of vasodilator therapy in heart failure. The decrease in arterial resistance (decreased afterload) leads to an increase in stroke volume and improved peripheral perfusion. The decrease in arterial pressure combined with a decrease in end-diastolic volume (resulting from the decrease in venous tone) decrease systolic wall tension and myocardial oxygen requirements. The left ventricular end-diastolic volume is decreased as a result of both the improved stroke volume and the decreased venous return. It produces a decrease in left ventricular end-diastolic pressure. The latter reduction may significantly improve coronary blood flow and collateral blood flow to the left ventricle, particularly the subendocardium.

difficult to distinguish between dyspnea due to cardiac causes and dyspnea due to pulmonary causes by such tests. In clear-cut instances, however, such a separation is often possible.[190,191] (See Chaps. 52 and 53.)

Pulmonary Edema[196–203]

The hydrostatic pressure in the pulmonary capillaries is normally 7 to 12 mmHg at rest in the supine position. When this pressure exceeds plasma oncotic pressure, which is normally 25 to 30 mmHg, net transudation of fluid from the pulmonary capillaries occurs. Pulmonary edema occurs when this rate of transudation exceeds the rate of lymphatic drainage from the tissues. If the plasma oncotic pressure is low because of a decreased serum protein concentration, transudation of fluid across the pulmonary capillaries occurs at even lower pressure.[204] There is little evidence that altered capillary permeability due to central nervous system influences or hypoxia is ordinarily an important factor in the production of pulmonary edema in most patients, although changes in capillary permeability can be important in some specialized forms of pulmonary edema due to the *capillary leak syndrome*[205] or in some patients with virus infections of the respiratory tract. The major factor in cardiac pulmonary edema is the pulmonary capillary pressure.[196,197] The pulmonary capillaries have a significant "reserve" compared with systemic capillaries, since the pulmonary capillary pressure can ordinarily increase by 10 to 20 mmHg before significant transudation occurs.

An important consideration in the pulmonary circulation is the normal increase in hydrostatic pressure in both the arteries and veins in the de-

pendent areas of the lungs. This increased pressure accounts, in part, for the initial appearance of pulmonary edema in the lower lobes in many patients with congestive failure. In normal persons in the upright position, relatively little pulmonary blood flow goes to the upper areas of the lungs. In patients with severe mitral stenosis or with severe left ven-

1. CALCIUM

2. DIGITALIS GLYCOSIDES   Na–K ATPase inhib.

3. CATECHOLAMINES

I.V. {
Norepinephrine
Epinephrine
Isoproterenol
Dopamine
Dobutamine
} β_1 stim. → ↑Cyclic AMP

Oral {
Prenalterol (Astra)
Butopamine (Lilly)
H 80/62 (CIBA-Geigy)
} β_1 stim.

{
Pirbuterol (Pfizer)
Salbutamol
} β_2 a(?) β_1 stim.

4. XANTHINES
   Aminophylline   phosphodiesterase
   BDPU   inhib. → ↑cyclic AMP

5. GLUCAGON   ↑ cyclic AMP

6. AMRINONE   ↑ Ca⁺⁺ movement (?)

7. OTHER
   RMI 82,249 (Merrell)   ↑ Ca⁺⁺ flux (?)

FIGURE 22-8 The major inotropic agents that are currently available or that are under investigation and their probable mechanism of action.

tricular failure, however, the relative blood flow to the upper lobes may equal or even exceed that to the lower lobes. It is as yet uncertain whether this change in distribution of pulmonary blood flow is caused by local vasoconstriction produced by alveolar hypoxia, by a reactive hypertrophy and increased vascular tone of small arteries secondary to the elevation of pulmonary arterial pressure, or by reflexes from the left atrium or pulmonary veins.

Patients with marked elevation of left atrial pressure for long periods of time may often withstand elevations of pulmonary capillary pressure reasonably well, whereas the same level of pulmonary capillary pressure can produce severe, fulminating pulmonary edema in 5 to 10 min in a patient whose pulmonary circulation is not accustomed to the high pressure levels. The explanation for this difference may be that patients with chronic transudation of fluid from pulmonary capillaries often develop capacious lymphatic channels which are capable of removing large quantities of fluid from the pulmonary interstitial spaces. In addition, the pericapillary thickening and the perivascular edema associated with chronic pulmonary capillary hypertension tend to decrease the rate of fluid transudation. Since pulmonary lymphatic drainage empties into systemic veins, any elevation of central systemic venous pressure tends to decrease pulmonary lymphatic drainage and to worsen pulmonary edema. The importance of pulmonary lymphatic vessels in pulmonary edema has been emphasized by Uhley et al.[206]

It is probable that the occurrence of localized pulmonary edema in areas of acute infection or of previous infection is partially related to permanent alterations in local lymphatic drainage. It is also possible that the relative rareness of pulmonary rales in infants with left ventricular failure is, in part, related to the presence of a pulmonary lymphatic system unscarred by respiratory tract infection. Patients with severe pulmonary disease may have such marked destruction of their pulmonary lymphatics that they develop interstitial pulmonary edema much more readily than normal.

Morphine in Pulmonary Edema[207–210]
The beneficial effects of morphine in acute pulmonary edema are in part produced by decreased arterial resistance and pressure, which decrease ventricular afterload; by a decrease in venous return, perhaps aided by depression of the respiratory pump; and by "pharmacologic phlebotomy" resulting from an increase in the capacity of the peripheral vascular beds with perfusion of unperfused areas and venous pooling.

Noncardiac Pulmonary Edema[211]

High-Altitude Pulmonary Edema
High-altitude pulmonary edema (HAPE) is apparently associated with marked pulmonary artery hypertension and pulmonary arteriolar vasoconstriction but with normal pulmonary artery wedge ("pulmonary capillary") pressure.[212–217] The mechanism of pulmonary edema in this rare syndrome is uncertain, although it is possible that the development of HAPE is related to an unusually marked, nonuniform vasoconstriction of the terminal pulmonary arterioles in response to decreased partial pressure of oxygen in the alveoli. As a consequence, there is excessive blood flow in the other areas of the lung, and the capillary bed may be relatively "unprotected" from the high pulmonary arterial pressure. An additional factor that may be important is the presence of preterminal arterioles, which are short, nonmuscular vessels that arise at right angles from small and medium-sized pulmonary arteries, bypass the pulmonary arterioles, and empty directly into the venous side of the pulmonary capillary bed.[218] These may be important in transmitting the strikingly elevated pulmonary artery pressure directly to the capillary bed in subjects with HAPE. Acute pulmonary hypertension may also damage the arterial walls and lead to direct transarterial leakage of plasma or even blood and allow the formation of microthrombi that may shower the distal capillary bed.[211] Postmortem studies have also suggested that pulmonary vascular obstruction by thrombi may occur in some cases. (See Chap. 80.)

Miscellaneous Forms of Pulmonary Edema
The occasional occurrence of pulmonary edema secondary to pulmonary emboli may be related to acute left ventricular failure or to an "overperfusion edema,"[219] similar to that described for high-altitude pulmonary edema. The mechanism of pulmonary edema in patients with opiate-induced pulmonary edema (OPE) or heroin intoxication is uncertain, though it may be due to acute apnea with hypoxic pulmonary edema from high-pressure damage to the pulmonary vascular endothelium.[211,220] Acute cardiomyopathy may also occur.[221] Changes in pulmonary capillary permeability appear to occur in some forms of pulmonary edema associated with infection, inhalation of toxic gases, or with chemicals such as ethchlorvynol or ingested paraquat.[194,211] Vasoconstriction of the pulmonary veins may also be an important factor in the pulmonary edema produced by certain endotoxins.[222] Neurogenic pulmonary edema appears to be associated with intensive elevations in systemic arterial and venous pressures and pulmonary arterial, capillary, and venous pressures. The abrupt elevation of pulmonary vascular pressure and volume may damage the vascular endothelium, altering permeability and allowing pulmonary edema to develop.[211,223]

References

*1. Mason, D. T. (ed.): "Congestive Heart Failure: Mechanisms, Evaluation and Treatment," Yorke Medical Books, New York, 1976, p. 448. (Extensively referenced)

*This article is a review of the literature and contains additional references to the literature.

*2. Braunwald, E., Ross, J., Jr., and Sonnenblick, E. H.: "Mechanisms of Contraction of the Normal and Failing Heart," 2d ed., Little, Brown and Company, Boston, 1976, p. 417. (Extensively referenced)

3. Levine, H. J.: Congestive Heart Failure, in H. J. Levine (ed.), "Clinical Cardiovascular Physiology," Grune & Stratton, Inc., New York, 1976, p. 367.

4. Braunwald, E. (ed.): "The Myocardium: Failure and Infarction," H. P. Publishing Co., New York, 1974, p. 409.

5. Schlant, R. C., and Nutter, D. O.: Heart Failure in Valvular Heart Disease, *Medicine*, 50:421, 1971.

6. Eichna, L.: Circulatory Congestion and Heart Failure, *Circulation*, 22:864, 1960.

7. Weber, K. T., and Janicki, J. S.: The Heart as a Muscle-Pump System and the Concept of Heart Failure, *Am. Heart J.*, 98:371, 1979.

8. Korner, P. L.: Integrative Neural Cardiovascular Control, *Physiol. Rev.*, 51:312, 1971.

9. Higgins, C. B., Vatner, S. F., and Braunwald, E.: Parasympathetic Control of the Heart, *Pharmacol. Rev.*, 25:119, 1973.

10. Braunwald, E.: Regulation of the Circulation, *N. Engl. J. Med.*, 290:1124, 1420, 1974.

11. Chidsey, C. A., and Braunwald, E.: Sympathetic Activity and Neurotransmitter Depletion in Congestive Heart Failure, *Pharmacol. Rev.*, 18:685, 1966.

12. Eckberg, D. L., Drabinsky, M., and Braunwald, E.: Defective Cardiac Parasympathetic Control in Patients with Heart Disease, *N. Engl. J. Med.*, 285:877, 1971.

13. Rutenberg, H. L., and Spann, J. F., Jr.: Alterations of Cardiac Sympathetic Neurotransmitter Activity in Congestive Heart Failure, *Am. J. Cardiol.*, 32:427, 1973.

14. Goldstein, R. E., Beiser, G. D., Stampfer, M., and Epstein, S. E.: Impairment of Autonomically Mediated Heart Rate Control in Patients with Cardiac Dysfunction, *Circ. Res.*, 36:571, 1975.

15. Rutenberg, H. L., and Spann, J. F., Jr.: Alterations of Cardiac Sympathetic Neurotransmitter Activity in Congestive Heart Failure, in D. T. Mason (ed.), "Congestive Heart Failure: Mechanisms, Evaluation and Treatment," Yorke Medical Books, New York, 1976, p. 85.

16. Pool, P. E., Covell, J. W., Levitt, M., Gibb, J., and Braunwald, E.: Reduction of Cardiac Tyrosine Hydroxylase Activity in Experimental Congestive Heart Failure: Its Role in the Depletion of Cardiac Norepinephrine Stores, *Circ. Res.*, 20:349, 1967.

17. Spann, J. F., Jr., Buccino, R. A., Sonnenblick, E. H., and Braunwald, E.: Contractile State of Cardiac Muscle Obtained from Cats with Experimentally Produced Ventricular Hypertrophy and Heart Failure, *Circ. Res.*, 21:341, 1967.

18. Covell, J. W., Chidsey, C. A., and Braunwald, E.: Reduction of the Cardiac Response to Postganglionic Sympathetic Nerve Stimulation in Experimental Heart Failure, *Circ. Res.*, 19:51, 1966.

19. Thomas, J. A., and Marks, B. H.: Plasma Norepinephrine in Congestive Heart Failure, *Am. J. Cardiol.*, 41:233, 1978.

20. Zelis, R., Longhurst, J., Capone, R. J., and Lee, G.: Peripheral Circulatory Control Mechanisms in Congestive Heart Failure, *Am. J. Cardiol.*, 32:481, 1973.

21. Zelis, R.: The Contribution of Local Factors to the Elevated Venous Tone of Congestive Heart Failure, *J. Clin. Invest.*, 54:219, 1974.

22. Korner, P. I.: Control of Blood Flow to Special Vascular Areas: Brain, Kidney, Muscle, Skin, Liver, and Intestine, in A. C. Guyton and C. E. Jones (eds.), "Cardiovascular Physiology," Physiology Series I, vol. I, University Park Press, Baltimore, 1974, p. 123.

*23. Zelis, R., Nellis, S. H., Longhurst, J., Lee, G., and Mason, D. T.: Abnormalities in the Regional Circulations Accompanying Congestive Heart Failure, *Prog. Cardiovasc. Dis.*, 18:181, 1975. (75 references)

24. Abboud, F. M., Heistad, D. D., Mark, A. L., and Schmid, P. G.: Reflex Control of the Peripheral Circulation, *Prog. Cardiovasc. Dis.*, 18:371, 1976.

25. Zelis, R., Longhurst, J., Capone, R. J., Lee, G., and Mason, D. T.: Peripheral Circulatory Control Mechanisms in Congestive Heart Failure, in D. T. Mason (ed.), "Congestive Heart Failure: Mechanisms, Evaluation and Treatment," Yorke Medical Books, New York, 1976, p. 129.

26. Oberg, B.: Overall Cardiovascular Regulation, *Ann. Rev. Physiol.*, 38:537, 1976.

*27. Davis, J. O.: The Physiology of Congestive Heart Failure, in W. F. Hamilton and P. Dow (eds.), "Handbook of Physiology," sec. 2: "Circulation," vol. 3, American Physiological Society, Washington, D.C., 1965, p. 2071. (341 references)

*28. deWardener, H.: The Control of Sodium Excretion, in J. Orloff and R. W. Berliner (eds.), "Handbook of Physiology," sec. 8: "Renal Physiology," American Physiological Society, Washington, D.C., 1973, p. 677. (266 references)

*29. Laragh, J. H., Sealey, J. E.: The Renin-Angiotensin-Aldosterone Hormonal System and Regulation of Sodium, Potassium, and Blood Pressure Homeostasis, in J. Orloff and R. W. Berliner (eds.), "Handbook of Physiology," sec. 8: "Renal Physiology," American Physiological Society, Washington, D.C., 1973, p. 831. (625 references)

*30. Cannon, P. J.: The Kidney in Heart Failure, *N. Engl. J. Med.*, 296:26, 1977. (19 references)

31. Barger, A. C.: Renal Hemodynamics in Congestive Heart Failure, *Ann. N.Y. Acad. Sci.*, 139:786, 1973.

32. Kilcoyne, M. M., Schmidt, D. H., and Cannon, P. J.: Intrarenal Blood Flow in Congestive Heart Failure, *Circulation*, 47:786, 1973.

33. Stein, J. H., Boinjarern, S., Wilson, C. B., and Ferris, T. F.: Alterations in Intrarenal Blood Flow Distribution, *Circ. Res.*, 32–33:61, 1973.

34. Lewy, J. E., Windhager, E. E.: Peritubular Control of Proximal Tubular Fluid Reabsorption in the Rat Kidney, *Am. J. Physiol.*, 214:943, 1968.

*35. deWardener, H. E.: Mechanisms Influencing Urinary Sodium Excretion, in C. J. Dickinson and J. Marks (eds.), "Developments in Cardiovascular Medicine," University Park Press, Baltimore, 1978, p. 179. (56 references)

36. Windhager, E. E., and Giebisch, G.: Proximal Sodium and Fluid Transport, *Kidney Int.*, 9:121, 1976.

37. Stumpe, K. O., Solle, H., Klein, H., and Kruch, F.: Mechanism of Sodium and Water Retention in Rats with Experimental Heart Failure, *Kidney Int.*, 4:309, 1973.

38. Vandongen, R., and Gordon, R. D.: Plasma Renin

in Congestive Heart Failure in Man, *Med. J. Aust.,* 1:215, 1970.

39. Haber, E.: The Role of Renin in Normal and Pathological Cardiovascular Homeostasis, *Circulation,* 54:849, 1976.

40. Watkins, L., Jr., Burton, J. A., Haber, E., Cart, J. R., Smith, F. W., and Barger, A. C.: The Renin-Angiotensin-Aldosterone System in Congestive Failure in Conscious Dogs, *J. Clin. Invest.,* 57:1606, 1976.

*41. Reid, I. A., Morris, B. J., and Ganong, W. F.: The Renin-Angiotensin System, *Ann. Rev. Physiol.,* 40:377, 1978. (233 references)

*42. Baer, P. G., and McGiff, J. C.: Hormonal Systems and Renal Hemodynamics, *Ann. Rev. Physiol.,* 42:589, 1980. (55 references)

*43. Linden, R. J.: Neurocirculatory Control of Sodium and Water Excretion, in C. J. Dickinson and J. Marks (eds.), "Developments in Cardiovascular Medicine," University Park Press, Baltimore, 1978, p. 191. (56 references)

44. Curtiss, C., Cohn, J. N., Vrobel, T., and Franciosa, J. A.: Role of the Renin-Angiotensin System in the Systemic Vasoconstriction of Chronic Congestive Heart Failure, *Circulation,* 58:763, 1978.

45. McGiff, J., and Itskovitz, H. D.: Prostaglandins and the Kidney, *Circ. Res.,* 33:479, 1973.

46. Margolius, H. S., Horwitz, D., Pisano, J. J., and Keiser, H. R.: Relationships among Urinary Kallikrein, Mineralocorticoids and Human Hypertensive Disease, *Fed. Proc.,* 35:203, 1976.

47. Katz, A. M.: The Descending Limb of the Starling Curve and the Failing Heart, *Circulation,* 32:871, 1965.

48. Rader, B., Smith, W. W., Berger, A. R., and Eichna, L. W.: Comparison of the Hemodynamic Effects of Mercurial Diuretics and Digitalis in Congestive Heart Failure, *Circulation,* 29:328, 1964.

49. MacGregor, D. C., Covell, J. W., Mahler, F., Dilley, R. B., and Ross, J., Jr.: Relations between Afterload, Stroke Volume, and the Descending Limb of Starling's Curves, *Am. J. Physiol.,* 227:884, 1974.

50. Ross, J., Jr., Sonnenblick, E. H., Taylor, R. R., Spotnitz, H. M., and Covell, J. W.: Diastolic Geometry and Sarcomere Lengths in the Chronically Dilated Left Ventricle, *Circ. Res.,* 28:49, 1971.

51. McCullagh, W. H., Covell, J. W., and Ross, J., Jr.: Left Ventricular Dilatation and Diastolic Compliance Changes during Chronic Volume Overload, *Circulation,* 45:943, 1972.

52. Spotnitz, H. M., Leyton, R. A., Kelly, D. T., et al.: "Outstretched" Sarcomere in Subacute Volume-Pressure Loading of Dog Right Ventricle, *Circulation,* 46(suppl. 2):44, 1972.

53. Ross, J., Jr., and McCullagh, W. H.: The Nature of Enhanced Performance of Dilated Left Ventricle during Chronic Volume Overloading, *Circ. Res.,* 30:549, 1972.

54. Meerson, F. Z., and Kapelko, V. I.: The Contractile Function of the Myocardium in Two Types of Cardiac Adaptation to a Chronic Load, *Cardiology,* 57:183, 1972.

55. Ross, J., Jr.: Adaptations of the Left Ventricle to Chronic Volume Overload, *Circ. Res.,* 35(suppl. 2):64, 1974.

56. Alpert, N. R. (ed.): "Cardiac Hypertrophy," Academic Press, Inc., New York, 1971, p. 641.

57. Rabinowitz, M., and Zak, R.: Biochemical and Cellular Changes in Cardiac Hypertrophy, *Ann. Rev. Med.,* 23:245, 1972.

58. Meerson, F. Z., Javitz, M. P., Breger, A. M., and Lerman, M. I.: The Mechanism of the Heart's Adaptation to Prolonged Load and Dynamics of RNA Synthesis in the Myocardium, *Basic Res. Cardiol.,* 69:484, 1974.

59. Cohen, J., and Shah, P. M. (eds.): Cardiac Hypertrophy and Cardiomyopathy, *Circ. Res.,* 35(suppl. 2):1, 1974.

60. Rabinowitz, M.: Overview on Pathogenesis of Cardiac Hypertrophy, *Circ. Res.,* 35(suppl. 2):3, 1974.

61. Morkin, E.: Activation of Synthetic Processes in Cardiac Hypertrophy, *Circ. Res.,* 35(suppl. 2):37, 1974.

62. Meerson, F. Z.: Development of Modern Components of the Mechanism of Cardiac Hypertrophy, *Circ. Res.,* 35(suppl. 2):58, 1974.

*63. Linzbach, A. J.: Heart Failure from the Point of View of Quantitative Anatomy, *Am. J. Cardiol.,* 5:370, 1960. (53 references)

64. Badeer, H. S.: Biological Significance of Cardiac Hypertrophy, *Am. J. Cardiol.,* 14:133, 1964.

65. Grant, C. D., Greene, G., and Bunnell, I. L.: Left Ventricular Enlargement and Hypertrophy: A Clinical Angiographic Study, *Am. J. Med.,* 39:895, 1965.

66. Grossman, W., Jones, D., and McLaurin, L. P.: Wall Stress and Patterns of Hypertrophy in the Human Left Ventricle, *J. Clin. Invest.,* 56:56, 1975.

67. Rackley, C. E., Dalldorf, F. G., Hood, W. P., Jr., and Wilcox, B. R.: Sarcomere Length and Left Ventricular Function in Chronic Heart Disease, *Am. J. Med. Sci.,* 259:90, 1970.

68. Spotnitz, H. M., and Sonnenblick, E. H.: Structural Conditions in the Hypertrophied and Failing Heart, *Am. J. Cardiol.,* 32:398, 1973.

69. Sonnenblick, E. H., and Skelton, C. L.: Reconsideration of the Ultrastructural Basis of Cardiac Length-Tension Relations, *Circ. Res.,* 35:517, 1974.

70. Badeer, H. S.: Contractile Tension in the Myocardium, *Am. Heart J.,* 66:432, 1963.

71. Sandler, H., and Dodge, H. T.: Left Ventricular Tension and Stress in Man, *Circ. Res.,* 13:91, 1963.

72. Hood, W. P., Jr., Rackley, C. E., and Rolett, E. L.: Wall Stress in the Normal and Hypertrophied Human Left Ventricle, *Am. J. Cardiol.,* 22:550, 1968.

73. Grossman, W., McLaurin, L. P., Moos, S. P., Stefandouros, M. A., and Young, D. T.: Wall Thickness and Diastolic Properties of the Left Ventricle, *Circulation,* 49:129, 1974.

74. Sasayama, S., Ross, J., Jr., Franklin, D., Bloor, C. M., Bishop, S., and Dilley, R. B.: Adaptations of the Left Ventricle to Chronic Pressure Overload, *Circ. Res.,* 38:172, 1976.

75. Cohen, J.: Role of Endocrine Factors in the Pathogenesis of Cardiac Hypertrophy, *Circ. Res.,* 35(suppl. 2):49, 1974.

76. Braunwald, E., and Ross, J., Jr.: The Ventricular End-Diastolic Pressure: Appraisal of Its Value in the Recognition of Ventricular Failure in Man, *Am. J. Med.,* 34:147, 1963.

77. Rackley, C. E., Hood, W. P., Jr., Rolett, E. L., and Young, D. T.: Left Ventricular End-Diastolic Pres-

sure in Chronic Heart Disease, *Am. J. Med.,* 48:310, 1970.

78. Levine, H. J.: Compliance of the Left Ventricle, *Circulation,* 46:423, 1972.

79. Covell, J. W., and Ross, J., Jr.: Nature and Significance of Alterations in Myocardial Compliance, *Am. J. Cardiol.,* 32:449, 1973.

80. Grossman, W., and McLaurin, L. P.: Diastolic Properties of the Left Ventricle, *Ann. Int. Med.,* 84:316, 1976.

81. Wisneski, J. A., and Bristow, J. D.: Left Ventricular Stiffness, *Ann. Rev. Med.,* 29:475, 1978.

*82. Lewis, B. S., and Gotsman, M. S.: Current Concepts of Ventricular Relaxation and Compliance, *Am. Heart J.,* 99:101, 1980. (74 references)

83. Taylor, R. R., and Hopkins, B. E.: Left Ventricular Response to Experimentally Induced Chronic Aortic Regurgitation, *Cardiovasc. Res.,* 6:404, 1972.

84. Cooper, G., IV, Puga, F. J., Zujko, K. J., Harrison, C. E., and Coleman, H. N., III: Normal Myocardial Function and Energetics in Volume-Overload Hypertrophy in the Cat, *Circ. Res.,* 32:140, 1973.

85. Spann, J. F., Jr.: Heart Failure and Ventricular Hypertrophy: Altered Cardiac Contractility and Compensatory Mechanisms, *Am. J. Cardiol.,* 23:504, 1969.

86. Spann, J. F., Jr., Covell, J. W., Eckberg, D. L., Sonnenblick, E. H., Ross, J., Jr., and Braunwald, E.: Contractile Performance of the Hypertrophied and Chronically Failing Cat Ventricle, *Am. J. Physiol.,* 223:1150, 1972.

87. Pool, P. E., Chandler, B. M., Spann, J. F., Jr., Sonnenblick, E. H., and Braunwald, E.: Mechanochemistry of Cardiac Muscle. IV. Utilization of High-Energy Phosphates in Experimental Heart Failure in Cats, *Circ. Res.,* 24:313, 1969.

88. Cooper, G., IV, Satava, R. M., Harrison, C. E., and Coleman, H. N., III: Normal Myocardial Function and Energetics after Reversing Pressure-Overload Hypertrophy, *Am. J. Physiol.,* 226:1158, 1974.

89. Williams, J. F., Jr., and Potter, R. D.: Normal Contractile State of Hypertrophied Myocardium Following Pulmonary Artery Constriction in the Cat, *J. Clin. Invest.,* 54:1266, 1974.

90. Malik, A. B., Abe, T., O'Kane, H. O., and Geha, A. S.: Cardiac Performance in Ventricular Hypertrophy Induced by Pressure and Volume Overloading, *J. Appl. Physiol.,* 37:867, 1974.

91. Skelton, C. L., and Sonnenblick, E. H.: Heterogeneity of Contractile Function in Cardiac Hypertrophy, *Circ. Res.,* 35(suppl. 2):83, 1974.

92. Valeri, C. R., and Fortier, N. L.: Red-Cell 2,3-Diphosphoglycerate and Creatine Levels in Patients with Red-Cell Mass Deficiency or with Cardiopulmonary Insufficiency, *N. Engl. J. Med.,* 281:1452, 1969.

93. Burch, G. E., Ray, C. T., and Cronvich, J. A.: Certain Mechanical Peculiarities of the Human Cardiac Pump in Normal and Diseased States, *Circulation,* 5:504, 1952.

94. Burch, G. E.: Theoretic Considerations of the Time Course of Pressure Developed and Volume Ejected by the Normal and Dilated Left Ventricle during Systole, *Am. Heart J.,* 50:352, 1955.

95. Burton, A. C.: Physical Principles of Circulatory Phenomena: The Physical Equilibria of the Heart and Blood Vessels, in W. F. Hamilton and P. Dow (eds.), "Handbook of Physiology," sec. 2: "Circulation," vol. 1, American Physiological Society, Washington, D.C., 1962, p. 85.

96. Gorlin, R.: Recent Conceptual Advances in Congestive Heart Failure, *J. Am. Med. Assoc.,* 179:441, 1962.

97. Burch, G. E., DePasquale, N. P., and Cronvich, J. A.: Influence of Ventricular Size on the Relationship between Contractile and Manifest Tension, *Am. Heart J.,* 69:624, 1965.

98. Mason, D. T., Spann, J. F., Jr., Zelis, R., and Amsterdam, E. A.: Alterations of Hemodynamics and Myocardial Mechanics in Patients with Congestive Heart Failure: Pathophysiologic Mechanisms and Assessment of Cardiac Function and Ventricular Contractility, *Prog. Cardiovasc. Dis.,* 12:507, 1970.

99. Brutsaert, D. L., and Sonnenblick, E. H.: Cardiac Muscle Mechanics in the Evaluation of Myocardial Contractility and Pump Function: Problems, Concepts and Directions, *Prog. Cardiovasc. Dis.,* 16:337, 1973.

100. Urschel, C. W., Covell, J. W., Sonnenblick, E. H., Ross, J., Jr., and Braunwald, E.: Myocardial Mechanics in Aortic and Mitral Valvular Regurgitation: The Concept of Instantaneous Impedance as a Determinant of the Performance of the Intact Heart, *J. Clin. Invest.,* 47:867, 1968.

101. Scheuer, J.: Metabolism of the Heart in Heart Failure, *Prog. Cardiovasc. Dis.,* 13:24, 1970.

102. Levine, H. J., and Wagman, R. J.: Energetics of the Human Heart, *Am. J. Cardiol.,* 9:372, 1962.

103. Schwartz, A., Sordahl, L. A., Entman, M. L., et al.: Abnormal Biochemistry in Myocardial Failure, in D. T. Mason (ed.), "Congestive Heart Failure: Mechanisms, Evaluation and Treatment," Yorke Medical Books, New York, 1976, p. 25.

104. Alpert, N. R., Hamrell, B. B., and Halpern, W.: Mechanical and Biochemical Correlates of Cardiac Hypertrophy, *Circ. Res.,* 35(suppl. 2):71, 1974.

105. Sobel, B. E., Spann, J. F., Jr., Pool, P. E., Sonnenblick, E. H., and Braunwald, E.: Normal Oxidative Phosphorylation in Mitochondria from the Failing Heart, *Circ. Res.,* 21:355, 1967.

106. Walker, J. G., and Bishop, S. P.: Mitochondrial Function and Structure in Experimental Canine Congestive Heart Failure, *Cardiovasc. Res.,* 5:444, 1971.

107. Sordahl, L. A., McCollum, W. B., Wood, W. B., and Schwartz, A.: Mitochondria and Sarcoplasmic Reticulum Function in Cardiac Hypertrophy and Failure, *Am. J. Physiol.,* 224:497, 1973.

108. Henry, P. D., Eckberg, D., Gault, J. H., and Ross, J., Jr.: Depressed Inotropic State and Reduced Myocardial Oxygen Consumption in the Human Heart, *Am. J. Cardiol.,* 31:300, 1973.

109. Gunning, J. F., and Coleman, H. N., III: Myocardial Oxygen Consumption during Experimental Hypertrophy and Congestive Heart Failure, *J. Mol. Cell. Cardiol.,* 5:25, 1973.

110. Cooper, G., Satava, R. M., Harrison, C. E., and Coleman, H. N., III: Mechanism for the Abnormal Energetics of Pressure-Induced Hypertrophy of Cat Myocardium, *Circ. Res.,* 33:213, 1973.

111. Katz, A. M.: "Physiology of the Heart," Raven Press, New York, 1977, p. 450.

112. Pool, P. E., Spann, J. F., Buccino, R. A., Sonnenblick, E. H., and Braunwald, E.: Myocardial High

Energy Phosphate Stores in Cardiac Hypertrophy and Heart Failure, *Circ. Res.,* 21:365, 1967.

113. Alpert, N. R., and Hamrell, B. B.: Cardiac Hypertrophy: A Compensatory and Anticompensatory Response to Stress, in M. Vassalle (ed.), "Cardiac Physiology for the Clinician," Academic Press, Inc., New York, 1976, p. 173.

114. Goldstein, M. A., Sordahl, L. A., and Schwartz, A.: Ultrastructural Analysis of Left Ventricular Hypertrophy in Rabbits, *J. Mol. Cell. Cardiol.,* 6:265, 1974.

115. Rabinowitz, M., and Zak, R.: Mitochondria and Cardiac Hypertrophy, *Circ. Res.,* 36:367, 1975.

116. Spotnitz, H. M., and Sonnenblick, E. H.: Structural Conditions in the Hypertrophied and Failing Heart, in D. T. Mason (ed.), "Congestive Heart Failure: Mechanisms, Evaluation and Treatment," Yorke Medical Books, New York, 1976, p. 13.

117. Yoran, C., Covell, J. W., and Ross, J., Jr.: Structural Basis for the Ascending Limb of Left Ventricular Function, *Circ. Res.,* 32:297, 1973.

118. Spotnitz, H. M., Spotnitz, W. D., Cottrell, T. S., Spiro, D., and Sonnenblick, E. H.: Cellular Basis for Volume Related Wall Thickness Changes in the Rat Left Ventricle, *J. Mol. Cell. Cardiol.,* 6:317, 1974.

119. Alpert, N. R., and Gordon, M. S.: Myofibrillar Adenosine Triphosphate Activity in Congestive Heart Failure, *Am. J. Physiol.,* 202:940, 1962.

120. Chandler, B. M., Sonnenblick, E. H., Spann, J. F., Jr., and Pool, P. E.: Association of Depressed Myofibrillar Adenosine Triphosphatase and Reduced Contractility in Experimental Heart Failure, *Circ. Res.,* 21:717, 1967.

121. Luchi, R. J., Kritcher, E. M., and Thyrum, P. T.: Reduced Cardiac Myosin Adenosine-Triphosphatase Activity in Dogs with Spontaneously Occurring Heart Failure, *Circ. Res.,* 24:513, 1969.

122. Henry, P. D., Ahumada, G. G., Friedman, W. F., and Sobel, B. E.: Simultaneously Measured Isometric Tension and ATP Hydrolysis in Glycerinated Fibers from Normal and Hypertrophied Rabbit Heart, *Circ. Res.,* 31:740, 1972.

123. Conway, G., Heazlitt, R. A., Montag, J., and Mattingley, S. F.: The ATPase Activity of Cardiac Myosin from Failing and Hypertrophied Hearts, *J. Mol. Cell. Cardiol.,* 7:827, 1975.

124. Wikman-Coffelt, J., McPherson, J., Salel, A. F., Kamiyama, T., and Mason, D. T.: Mechanism of Impaired Contractile Protein Function in Aortic Stenosis: Alterations in Myosin ATPase Activity in the Chronically Pressure Overload Canine Left Ventricle, *Am. J. Cardiol.,* 35:177, 1975.

125. Wikman-Coffelt, J., Walsh, R., Fenner, C., Kamiyama, T., Salel, A., and Mason, D. T.: Effects of Severe Hemodynamic Pressure Overload on the Properties of Canine Left Ventricular Myosin: Mechanisms by Which Myosin ATPase Activity Is Lowered during Chronic Increased Hemodynamic Stress, *J. Mol. Cell. Cardiol.,* 8:263, 1976.

126. Wikman-Coffelt, J., Fenner, C., Salel, A. F., Kamiyama, T., and Mason, D. T.: Myofibrillar Proteins and the Contractile Mechanism in the Normal and Failing Heart, in D. T. Mason (ed.), "Congestive Heart Failure: Mechanisms, Evaluation and Treatment," Yorke Medical Books, New York, 1976, p. 53.

127. Wikman-Coffelt, J., and Mason, D. T.: Mechanism of Decreased Contractility in Chronic Hemodynamic Overload, in D. T. Mason (ed.), "Advances in Heart Diseases," Grune & Stratton, New York, 1977, vol. 1, p. 491.

128. Meerson, F. Z.: The Myocardium in Hyperfunction, Hypertrophy and Heart Failure, *Circ. Res.,* 15(suppl. 2):11, 1969.

129. Mead, R. J., Peterson, M. D., and Welty, J. D.: Sarcolemmal and Sarcoplasmic Reticular ATPase Activities in the Failing Canine Heart, *Circ. Res.,* 29:14, 1971.

130. Dhalla, N. S., Singh, J. N., Fedelesova, M., Balasubramanian, V., and McNamara, D. B.: Biochemical Basis of Heart Function. XII. Sodium-Potassium Stimulated Adenosine Triphosphatase Activity in the Perfused Rat Heart Made to Fail by Substrate-Lack, *Cardiovasc. Res.,* 8:227, 1974.

131. Beller, G. A., Conroy, J., and Smith, T. W.: Ischemia-Induced Alterations in Myocardial (Na^+ and K^+) ATPase and Cardiac Glycoside Binding, *J. Clin. Invest.,* 57:341, 1976.

132. Harigaya, S., and Schwartz, A.: Fate of Calcium Binding and Uptake in Normal Animals and Failing Human Cardiac Muscle: Membrane Vesicles (Relaxing System) and Mitochondria, *Circ. Res.,* 25:781, 1969.

133. Gertz, E. W., Stam, A. C., Jr., and Sonnenblick, E. H.: A Quantitative and Qualitative Defect in the Sarcoplasmic Reticulum in the Hereditary Cardiomyopathy of the Syrian Hamster, *Biochem. Biophys. Res. Commun.,* 40:746, 1970.

134. McCollum, W. B., Crow, C., Harigaya, S., Bajusz, E., and Schwartz, A.: Calcium Binding by Cardiac Relaxing System Isolated from Myopathic Syrian Hamsters, *J. Mol. Cell. Cardiol.,* 1:445, 1970.

135. Suko, J., Vogel, J. H. K., and Chidsey, C. A.: Intracellular Calcium and Myocardial Contractility. III. Reduced Calcium Intake and ATPase of the Sarcoplasmic Reticular Fraction Prepared from Chronically Failing Calf Hearts, *Circ. Res.,* 27:235, 1970.

136. Ueba, Y., Ito, Y., and Chidsey, C. A.: Intracellular Calcium and Myocardial Contractility, *Am. J. Physiol.,* 220:1553, 1971.

137. Harris, P., and Opie, L. (eds.): "Calcium and the Heart," Academic Press, Inc., New York, 1971, p. 198.

138. Kaufmann, R. L., Homburger, H., and Wirth, H.: Disorder in Excitation-Contraction Coupling of Cardiac Muscle from Cats with Experimentally Produced Right Ventricular Hypertrophy, *Circ. Res.,* 28:346, 1971.

139. Sulakhe, P. V., and Dhalla, N. S.: Excitation-Contraction Coupling in Heart. VII. Calcium Accumulation in Subcellular Particles in Congestive Heart Failure, *J. Clin. Invest.,* 50:1019, 1971.

140. Katz, A. M., and Repke, D. I.: Calcium-Membrane Interactions in the Myocardium: Effects of Ouabain, Epinephrine and 3′,5′-Cyclic Adenosine Monophosphate, *Am. J. Cardiol.,* 31:193, 1973.

141. Ito, Y., Suko, J., and Chidsey, C. A.: Intracellular Calcium and Myocardial Contractility. V. Calcium Uptake of Sarcoplasmic Reticulum Fraction in Hypertrophied and Failing Rabbit Hearts, *J. Mol. Cell. Cardiol.,* 6:237, 1974.

142. Reuter, H.: Exchange of Calcium Ions in the

Mammalian Myocardium: Mechanisms and Physiological Significance, *Circ. Res.*, 34:599, 1974.

*143. Katz, A. M.: Congestive Heart Failure: Role of Altered Myocardial Cellular Control, *N. Engl. J. Med.*, 293:1184, 1975. (9 references)

144. Dhalla, N. S., Tomlinson, C. W., Yates, J. C., et al.: Role of Mitochondrial Calcium Transport in Failing Heart, in N. S. Dhalla (ed.), "Recent Advances on Cardiac Structure and Metabolism," University Park Press, Baltimore, 1975, vol. 5, p. 177.

145. Katz, A. M., and Hecht, H. E.: The Early "Pump" Failure of the Ischemic Heart, *Am. J. Med.*, 47:497, 1969.

146. Langer, G. A.: Ionic Movements and the Control of Contraction, in G. A. Langer and A. J. Brady (eds.), "The Mammalian Myocardium," John Wiley & Sons, Inc., New York, 1974, p. 193.

147. Carafoli, E., Tiozzo, R., Lugli, G., Crovetti, F., and Kratzing, C.: The Release of Calcium from Heart Mitochondria by Sodium, *J. Mol. Cell. Cardiol.*, 6:361, 1974.

148. Van Winkle, W. B., and Schwartz, A.: Ions and Inotropy, *Annu. Rev. Physiol.*, 38:247, 1976.

149. Dock, W.: How Some Hearts Age, *J. Am. Med. Assoc.*, 195:442, 1966.

150. Burch, G., and Giles, T.: Senile Cardiomyopathy, *J. Chronic Dis.*, 24:1, 1971.

151. Dock, W.: Cardiomyopathies of the Senescent and Senile, in G. E. Burch (ed.), "Cardiomyopathy," F. A. Davis Company, Philadelphia, 1972, p. 361.

152. Lakatta, E. G., Gerstenblith, G., Angell, C. S., Shock, N. W., and Weisfeldt, M. L.: Diminished Inotropic Response of Aged Myocardium to Catecholamines, *Circ. Res.*, 36:262, 1975.

153. Vincent, W. R., Buckberg, G. D., and Hoffman, J. E.: Left Ventricular Subendocardial Ischemia in Severe Valvular and Supravalvular Aortic Stenosis: A Common Mechanism, *Circulation*, 49:326, 1974.

154. Brazier, J. R., and Buckberg, G. D.: Effects of Tachycardia on the Adequacy of Subendocardial Oxygen Delivery in Experimental Aortic Stenosis, *Am. Heart J.*, 90:222, 1975.

155. Downey, J. M., and Kirk, E. S.: Inhibition of Coronary Blood Flow by a Vascular Waterfall Mechanism, *Circ. Res.*, 36:753, 1975.

156. Brazier, J., Cooper, M., and Buckberg, G.: The Adequacy of Subendocardial Oxygen Delivery: The Interaction of Determinants of Flow, Arterial Oxygen Content, and Myocardial Oxygen Need, *Circulation*, 49:968, 1974.

157. Honig, C. R., and Bourdeau-Martini, J.: Extravascular Component of Oxygen Transport in Normal and Hypertrophied Hearts with Special Reference to Oxygen Therapy, *Circ. Res.*, 35(suppl. 2):97, 1974.

158. Eckberg, D. L., Gault, J. H., Bouchard, R. L., Karliner, J. S., and Ross, J., Jr.: Mechanics of Left Ventricular Contraction in Chronic Severe Mitral Regurgitation, *Circulation*, 47:1252, 1973.

159. Mitchell, J. H., Gilmore, J. P., and Sarnoff, S. J.: The Transport Function of the Atrium: Factors Influencing the Relation between Mean Left Atrial Pressure and Left Ventricular End Diastolic Pressure, *Am. J. Cardiol.*, 9:237, 1962.

160. Braunwald, E.: Hemodynamic Significance of Atrial Systole, *Am. J. Med.*, 37:665, 1964.

161. Burchell, H. B.: A Clinical Appraisal of Atrial Transport Function, *Lancet*, 1:775, 1964.

162. Suga, H.: Importance of Atrial Compliance in Cardiac Performance, *Circ. Res.*, 35:39, 1974.

163. Ikram, H., Nixon, P. G. F., and Arcan, T.: Left Atrial Function after Electrical Conversion to Sinus Rhythm, *Br. Heart J.*, 30:80, 1968.

164. Brill, I. C., Rosenbaum, E. E., and Flanery, J. R.: Congestive Failure Due to Auricular Fibrillation in an Otherwise Normal Heart, *J. Am. Med. Assoc.*, 173:784, 1960.

165. Dexter, L.: Atrial Septal Defect, *Br. Heart J.*, 203:18, 1956.

166. Taylor, R. R., Covell, J. W., Sonnenblick, E. H., and Ross, J., Jr.: Dependence of Ventricular Distensibility on Filling of the Opposite Ventricle, *Am. J. Physiol.*, 213:711, 1967.

167. Kelly, D. T., Spotnitz, H. M., Beiser, G. D., Pierce, J. E., and Epstein, S. E.: Effects of Chronic Right Ventricular Volume and Pressure Loading on Left Ventricular Performance, *Circulation*, 44:403, 1971.

168. Bemis, C. E., Serur, J. R., Borkenhagen, D., Sonnenblick, E. H., and Urschel, C.: Influence of Right Ventricular Filling Pressure on Left Ventricular Pressure and Dimension, *Circ. Res.*, 34:498, 1974.

169. Chidsey, C. A., Kaiser, G. A., Sonnenblick, E. H., Spann, J. F., Jr., and Braunwald, E.: Cardiac Norepinephrine Stores in Experimental Heart Failure in the Dog, *J. Clin. Invest.*, 43:2386, 1964.

170. Buccino, R. A., Harris, E., Spann, J. F., Jr., and Sonnenblick, E. H.: Response of Myocardial Connective Tissue to Development of Experimental Hypertrophy, *Am. J. Physiol.*, 216:425, 1969.

171. Ross, J., Jr., Gault, J. H., Mason, D. T., Linhart, J. W., and Braunwald, E.: Left Ventricular Performance during Muscular Exercise in Patients with and without Cardiac Dysfunction, *Circulation*, 34:597, 1966.

172. Braunwald, E., Goldblatt, A., Harrison, D. C., and Mason, D. T.: Studies on Cardiac Dimensions in Intact, Unanesthetized Man. III. Effects of Muscular Exercise, *Circ. Res.*, 13:460, 1963.

173. Gorlin, R., Cohen, L. S., Elliott, W. C., Klein, M. D., and Lane, F. J.: Effect of Supine Exercise on Left Ventricular Volume and Oxygen Consumption in Man, *Circulation*, 32:361, 1965.

174. Gorlin, R., Krasnow, N., Levine, H. J., and Messer, J. V.: Effect of Exercise on Cardiac Performance in Human Subjects with Minimal Heart Disease, *Am. J. Cardiol.*, 13:293, 1964.

175. Braunwald, E.: The Control of Ventricular Function in Man, *Br. Heart J.*, 27:1, 1965.

176. Chapman, C. B. (ed.): Physiology of Muscular Exercise, *Circ. Res.*, 20(suppl. 2):1, 1967.

177. Bevegard, B. S., and Shepherd, J. T.: Regulation of the Circulation during Exercise in Man, *Physiol. Rev.*, 47:178, 1967.

178. Weissler, A. M., Harris, W. S., and Schoenfeld, C. D.: Systolic Time Intervals in Heart Failure in Man, *Circulation*, 37:149, 1968.

179. Ostrand, P.-O., and Rodahl, K.: "Textbook of Work Physiology," McGraw-Hill Book Company, New York, 1970, p. 669.

180. Weissler, A. M., Lewis, R. P., and Leighton, R. F.: The Systolic Time Intervals as a Measure of Left

Ventricular Performance in Man, in P. N. Yu and J. F. Goodwin (eds.), "Progress in Cardiology," Lea & Febiger, Philadelphia, 1972, vol. 1, p. 155.

181. Vatner, S. F., Franklin, D., Higgins, C. B., Patrick, T., and Braunwald, E.: Left Ventricular Response to Severe Exertion in Untethered Dogs, *J. Clin. Invest.*, 51:3052, 1972.

182. Horwitz, L. D., Atkins, J. M., and Leshin, S. J.: Role of the Frank-Starling Mechanism in Exercise, *Circ. Res.*, 31:868, 1972.

183. Guyton, A. C., Jones, C. E., and Coleman, T. G.: Cardiac Output in Muscular Exercise, in "Circulatory Physiology: Cardiac Output and Its Regulation," 2d ed., W. B. Saunders Company, Philadelphia, 1973, p. 436.

184. Epstein, S. E., Robinson, B. F., Kahler, R. L., and Braunwald, E.: Effects of Beta-Adrenergic Blockage on the Cardiac Response to Maximal and Submaximal Exercise in Man, *J. Clin. Invest.*, 44:1745, 1965.

185. Robinson, B. F., Epstein, S. E., Kahler, R. L., and Braunwald, E.: Circulatory Effects of Acute Expansion of Blood Volume: Studies during Maximal Exercise and at Rest, *Circ. Res.*, 19:26, 1966.

186. Bristow, J. D., Kloster, F. E., Farrehi, C., Brodeur, M. T. H., Lewis, R. P., and Griswold, H. E.: The Effects of Supine Exercise on Left Ventricular Volume in Heart Disease, *Am. Heart J.*, 71:319, 1966.

187. Skelton, C. L., and Sonnenblick, E. H.: Physiology of Cardiac Muscle, in H. J. Levine (ed.), "Clinical Cardiovascular Physiology," Grune & Stratton, Inc., New York, 1976, p. 57.

188. Wilhelmsen, L.: Lung Mechanics in Rheumatic Valvular Disease, *Acta Med. Scand.*, 184(suppl. 489):1, 1968.

189. Fishman, A. P., and Hecht, H. H.: "The Pulmonary Circulation and Interstitial Space," The University of Chicago Press, Chicago, 1969.

190. Bates, D. V., MacKlem, P. T., and Christie, R. V.: "Respiratory Function in Disease," 2d ed., W. B. Saunders Company, Philadelphia, 1971, p. 585.

191. Rapaport, E.: Dyspnea: Pathophysiology and Differential Diagnosis, *Prog. Cardiovasc. Dis.*, 13:532, 1971.

192. Yu, P. N.: "Pulmonary Blood Volume in Health and Disease," Lea & Febiger, Philadelphia, 1969, p. 328.

193. Luepker, R., Liander, B., Korsgren, M., and Varnauskas, E.: Pulmonary Intravascular and Extravascular Fluid Volumes in Exercising Cardiac Patients, *Circulation*, 44:626, 1971.

194. Avery, W. G., Samet, P., and Sackner, M. A.: The Acidosis of Pulmonary Edema, *Am. J. Med.*, 48:320, 1970.

195. Aberman, A., and Fulop, M.: The Metabolic and Respiratory Acidosis of Acute Pulmonary Edema, *Ann. Intern. Med.*, 76:173, 1972.

196. Visscher, M. B., Haddy, F. J., and Stephens, G.: The Physiology and Pharmacology of Lung Edema, *Pharmacol. Rev.*, 8:389, 1956.

197. Greene, D. G.: Pulmonary Edema, in W. O. Fenn and H. Rahn (eds.), "Handbook of Physiology," sec. 3: "Respiration," vol. 2, American Physiological Society, Washington, 1965, p. 1585.

198. Staub, N. C., Nagano, H., and Pearce, M. L.: Pulmonary Edema in Dogs, Especially the Sequence of Fluid Accumulation in Lungs, *J. Appl. Physiol.*, 22:227, 1967.

*199. Lee, G. de J.: Pulmonary Oedema, in P. N. Yu and J. F. Goodwin (eds.), "Progress in Cardiology," Lea & Febiger, Philadelphia, 1972, vol. 1, p. 261. (85 references)

200. Fishman, A. P.: Pulmonary Edema: The Water-Exchanging Function of the Lung, *Circulation*, 46:390, 1972.

*201. Robin, E. D., Cross, C. E., and Zelis, R.: Pulmonary Edema, *N. Engl. J. Med.*, 288:239, 292, 1973. (102 references)

*202. Staub, N. C.: Pulmonary Edema, *Physiol. Rev.*, 54:678, 1974. (547 references)

203. Schreiner, B. F., and Yu, P. N.: Pulmonary Circulation and Edema: Anatomic and Physiologic Considerations, in H. J. Levine (ed.), "Clinical Cardiovascular Physiology," Grune & Stratton, Inc., New York, 1976, p. 635.

204. Gaar, K. A., Jr., Taylor, A. E., Owens, L. J., and Guyton, A. C.: Development of Pulmonary Edema, *Am. J. Physiol.*, 213:79, 1967.

205. Robin, E. D., Carey, L. C., Grenvik, A., Glauser, F., and Gaudio, R.: Capillary Leak Syndrome with Pulmonary Edema, *Arch. Intern. Med.*, 130:66, 1972.

206. Uhley, H. N., Leeds, S. E., Sampson, J. J., and Friedman, M.: Right Duct Lymph Flow in Experimental Heart Failure Following Acute Elevation of Left Atrial Pressure, *Circ. Res.*, 20:306, 1967.

207. Vasko, J. S., Henney, P., Oldham, H. N., Brawley, R. K., and Morrow, A. G.: Mechanisms of Action of Morphine in the Treatment of Experimental Pulmonary Edema, *Am. J. Cardiol.*, 18:876, 1966.

208. Ward, J. M., McGrath, R. L., and Weil, J. V.: Effects of Morphine on the Peripheral Vascular Response to Sympathetic Stimulation, *Am. J. Cardiol.*, 29:659, 1972.

209. Zelis, R., Mansour, E. J., Capone, R. J., and Mason, D. T.: The Cardiovascular Effects of Morphine: The Peripheral Capacitance and Resistance Vessels in Human Subjects, *J. Clin. Invest.*, 54:1247, 1974.

210. Vismara, L. A., Leaman, D. M., and Zelis, R.: Effects of Morphine on Venous Tone in Patients with Acute Pulmonary Edema, *Circulation*, 54:335, 1976.

*211. Overland, E. S., and Severinghaus, J. W.: Noncardiac Pulmonary Edema, *Ann. Rev. Med.*, 23:307, 1978. (55 references)

212. Hultgren, H. N., and Grover, R. F.: Circulation Adaptation to High Altitude, *Annu. Rev. Med.*, 19:119, 1968.

213. Roy, S. B., Guleria, J. S., Khanna, P. K., Manchanda, S. C., Pande, J. N., and Subba, P. S.: Haemodynamic Studies in High Altitude Pulmonary Oedema, *Br. Heart J.*, 31:52, 1969.

214. Viswanathan, R., Jain, S. K., and Subramanian, S.: Pulmonary Edema of High Altitude. III. Pathogenesis, *Am. Rev. Respir. Dis.*, 100:342, 1969.

215. Vogen, J. H. D. (ed.): Hypoxia, High Altitude and the Heart, in "Advance in Cardiology," S. Karger, Basel, 1970, vol. 5.

216. Severinghaus, J. W.: Transarterial Leakage: A Possible Mechanism of High Altitude Pulmonary

Edema, in R. Porter and J. Knight (eds.), "High Altitude Physiology: Cardiac and Pulmonary Aspects," Churchill Livingston, London, 1971, p. 61.

217. Kleiner, J. P., and Nelson, W. P.: High Altitude Pulmonary Edema: A Rare Disease?, *J. Am. Med. Assoc.*, 234:491, 1975.

218. Recavarren, S.: The Preterminal Arterioles in the Pulmonary Circulation of High Altitude Natives, *Circulation*, 33:177, 1966.

219. Hultgren, H., Robinson, M., and Wuerflein, R.: Over-Perfusion Pulmonary Edema, *Circulation*, 34(suppl. 3):132, 1966. (Abstract.)

220. Duberstein, J. L., and Kaufman, D. M.: A Clinical Study of an Epidemic of Heroin Intoxication and Heroin-Induced Pulmonary Edema, *Am. J. Med.*, 51:704, 1971.

221. Paranthaman, S. K., and Khan, F.: Acute Cardiomyopathy with Recurrent Pulmonary Edema and Hypotension Following Heroin Overdosage, *Chest*, 69:117, 1976.

222. Kuida, H., Hinshaw, L. B., Bilbert, R. P., and Visscher, M.: Effect of Gram-Negative Endotoxin on Pulmonary Circulation, *Am. J. Physiol.*, 192:335, 1958.

223. Theodore, J., and Robin, E. D.: Pathogenesis of Neurogenic Pulmonary Edema, *Lancet*, 2:749, 1975.

23

The Recognition and Management of Heart Failure

James F. Spann, M.D.
J. Willis Hurst, M.D.

When the patient thinks there is something amiss with his heart, he fears it may fail. It is therefore necessary that the doctor should understand what heart failure is, and the signs by which it is made manifest.

Sir James Mackenzie, 1916[1]

Heart failure is said to be present when the heart fails to function properly as a pump. The compensatory mechanisms of the body which ordinarily aid the failing heart are only useful up to a point, because they can, and often do, lead to the derangement of the function of other organs. In fact, it is the derangement of the function of other organs that causes many of the troublesome signs and symptoms that are associated with heart failure.

The *clinical description* of heart failure and its treatment will be discussed in this chapter. The details of the altered physiology that is responsible for heart failure and its signs and symptoms are discussed in Chap. 22 and later in this chapter.

The clinical recognition of heart failure is based on a constellation—a cluster—of clinical abnormalities occurring in a patient with heart disease.[2]

Definition of Terms

The use of the term *heart failure* is not adequate. It is important to recognize the various subsets of heart failure since each subset may require a different therapeutic approach. The subsets of heart failure should be viewed by the clinician as a continuum which progresses in severity from normal → ventricular overload or damage → ventricular dysfunction with or without continued overload → ventricular dysfunction and compensation with symptoms and signs of congestion with a normal cardiac output at rest → persistence of signs and symptoms of congestion with a low cardiac output at rest.

In practice we identify the following subsets of heart failure.

Ventricular Dysfunction

The patient exhibits signs of ventricular dysfunction such as a ventricular gallop rhythm but presents no evidence of pulmonary congestion such as dyspnea, rales, radiographic evidence of congestion, abnormal neck vein pulsation, or peripheral edema.

Congestive Heart Failure

The patient experiences dyspnea on effort and has evidence of ventricular dysfunction and pulmonary congestion on the chest x-ray and may have bilateral edema of the extremities. This subset of heart failure may be divided into mild, moderate, and severe by determining the degree of dyspnea the patient experiences, for example, as a result of activity. The New York Heart Association established the system of grading the degree of heart failure. This system was used until 1973 when the *functional capacity* category was replaced by the *cardiac status* definition.[3] (See Chap. 8.) Since the functional capacity category is no longer used by the New York Heart Association, the degree of congestive heart failure should be described. Mild congestive heart failure implies that moderate activity produces dyspnea (formerly labeled class II). Moderate congestive heart failure implies that mild activity produces dyspnea (formerly labeled class III). Severe congestive heart failure implies that the patient is dyspneic at rest (formerly labeled class IV). We agree with the New York Heart Association's attempt to change the *functional classification* to the *new cardiac status classification* since it is wise to utilize all the available data to determine the clinical status of a patient rather than to use symptoms alone.

Compensated Congestive Heart Failure

This term should imply that the heart and circulation utilize compensatory mechanisms (mechanisms which frequently result in the signs and symptoms that we recognize as the congestive syndrome) *to prevent a fall in cardiac output below systemic requirements at rest and to optimally distribute the limited cardiac output during exercise.* In practice, however, physicians refer to patients as having compensated congestive heart failure when, by appropriate treatment, they are able to eliminate the congestion that troubled the patient.

Intractable Heart Failure

There are many definitions of this form of heart failure. The term should imply that heart failure persists despite adequate therapy. The problem then becomes, What is adequate therapy? The purpose of this chapter is to discuss the adequate treatment of heart failure. *Intractable heart failure* is said to exist when the failure persists after the physician has made every effort to control all four components of the management plan. These include control of the heart rate, improvement in myocardial contractility, control of the preload, and control of the afterload (see later in this chapter).

Modern drug therapy is very powerful. Therefore, one can convert a patient who has severe congestive heart failure into a patient who has the low-cardiac-output syndrome. The physician may trade dyspnea for signs of poor output, which include weakness, postural hypotension, poor urine output, and mental confusion. The modern physician learns to attain a middle ground and avoid the extremes of the condition.

There was a time when the terms *left-sided heart failure* and *right-sided heart failure* were used to designate certain clinical syndromes. The attribute of the failure that permitted the physician to designate a patient as having left-sided failure was the presence of dyspnea. The attribute of the failure that permitted the physician to designate a patient as having right-sided failure was the presence of edema and abnormal neck vein pulsation. While such terms may be useful clinical "shorthand," they do not accurately depict the abnormal physiology that is responsible for heart failure. Accordingly, we do not recommend their use.

The terms *forward failure* and *backward failure* do not assist the clinician in recognizing or treating heart failure, and for this reason we do not recommend their use.

The Clinical Setting

The Context in Which Heart Failure Occurs

It is not wise to diagnose heart failure in a patient unless there is evidence of heart disease. It is also not wise to diagnose heart failure just because heart disease is present. Assuming that evidence for heart disease has been established, the clinician must then make an etiologic diagnosis.[4] The data needed to make an etiologic diagnosis of the heart disease are usually collected when the data needed to establish the presence of heart disease are collected. It is useful to realize, however, that the thought process used to identify the presence of heart disease is different from the thought process that is used to establish the etiology of heart disease. Heart failure should be viewed as a marker of the severity of heart disease rather than the disease process itself.

Questions the Clinician Must Ask

The physician concerned with the problem of heart failure must ask and answer the following questions regarding the patient:

- Is there evidence of heart disease?
- What is the exact nature of the heart disease?
- Is there evidence of heart failure?
- Are there any conditions present, in addition to the primary heart disease, that may precipitate or aggravate heart failure?
- Is there any specific therapy, either medical or surgical, that should be considered?
- Can specific therapy be offered for the precipitating and aggravating factors?
- Has the treatment created any new problems for the patient?

Words That Alarm the Patient

Patients do not like to be told that they have heart failure. They are often terrified by the term because they believe it signifies that death from cessation of the heartbeat must be imminent. The wise physician avoids using the words *heart failure* and discusses the patient's condition using positive terms such as, "The drug you are taking will strengthen your heart muscle" or "The treatment should clear up the congestion causing your shortness of breath."

Factors That Precipitate and Aggravate Heart Failure

Although congestive heart failure may occur as part of the natural history of organic heart disease, it is prudent to look for certain additional factors which may either precipitate or aggravate heart failure. Such factors include myocardial infarction (which may be painless), abnormal cardiac rhythms, pulmonary emboli, rupture of chordae tendineae, pulmonary infection in children or adults with cor pulmonale, renal failure, rheumatic fever, infective endocarditis, prostatic obstruction, thyrotoxicosis, anemia, obesity, liver disease, pregnancy, corticosteroid or estrogen administration, increased workload, recent dietary sodium excess, propranolol therapy, and emotional stress.

The implication of discovering the factors that may precipitate or aggravate heart failure is self-evident. The treatment of such factors is quite different from the treatment of heart failure itself.

Abnormal Physiology

The details of the altered physiology that is responsible for heart failure are discussed in Chap. 22. The altered physiology that is essential for the understanding of the recognition and management of heart failure is discussed below.

In the more common forms of heart failure, the basic lesion is a depression of myocardial contractility with or without a continuing overload on the heart.[5–8] The myocardial lesion can result from direct damage, as in cardiomyopathy or coronary heart disease,[9] or can be related to chronic overload on the heart, as in valve disease[8] or systemic hypertension.[10,11] However, even when extensive depression of myocardial contractility is present, the heart's compensatory mechanisms can usually maintain a relatively normal resting cardiac output.[6,8] Not until relatively late in the usual clinical course of congestive failure are the patient's symptoms caused by reduced resting cardiac output. Before that time, the disturbing symptoms of heart failure

are caused by the compensatory mechanisms which are striving to maintain cardiac output. These undesirable secondary effects unfortunately limit the utility of compensatory mechanisms.

Since much heart failure therapy involves selective manipulation of these compensatory mechanisms, thorough understanding of these mechanisms and how they work is essential.

The Frank-Starling mechanism, whereby diastolic cardiac dilatation causes increased force and volume of the subsequent systolic contraction and ejection, is vital for the maintenance of cardiac output but is also responsible for many congestive heart failure symptoms.[4,8,12] Figure 23-1 shows this principle. In these diagrams systolic events are shown as solid curves, while the corresponding diastolic events are shown as dashed curves. The vertical axis for systolic events (cardiac output) is on the left, and the vertical axis for diastolic events (left ventricular end-diastolic pressure, [LVEDP]) is on the right. When the heart muscle is damaged, the systolic muscle function falls from the upper systolic curve (solid line), at point A, to the lower systolic curve (solid line), at point B. However, at point B the systolic cardiac output would be too low to support systemic needs, and low-output symptoms such as fatigue, weakness, renal failure, and even confusion and stupor or death would ensue. Fortunately, the end-diastolic volume (shown in the dashed curve) increases, and this diastolic change results in improvement in the subsequent systole. Cardiac residual volume increases as a result of the low ejection fraction, venous constriction occurs, and salt and water are retained, which increases left ventricular end-diastolic volume from point A' to point C' along the diastolic curve (dashed line). At diastolic C', the associated subsequent systole C is improved and ejects a greater stroke volume, resulting in a better cardiac output. However, as the heart in-

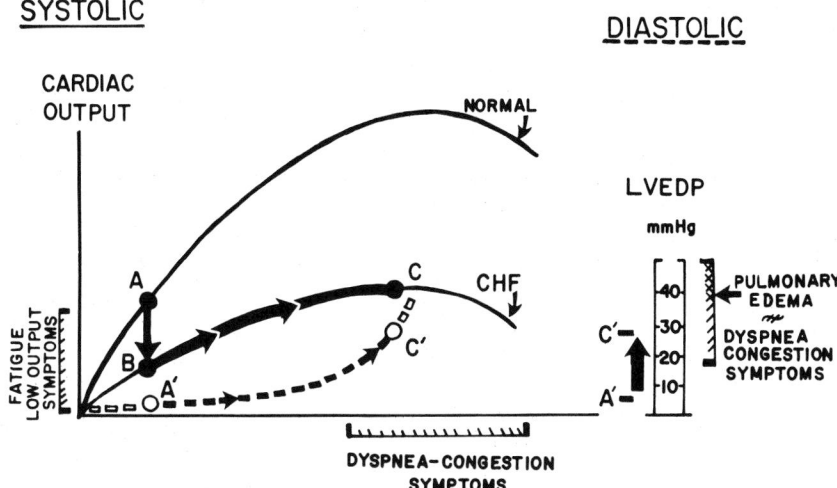

FIGURE 23-1 Compensated heart failure. Frank-Starling compensation for heart failure and how it causes congestive symptoms. (See text for explanation.) LV = left ventricle; LVEDP = left ventricular end-diastolic pressure.

creases its diastolic volume from point A′ to point C′, it has moved to the right and upward along the dashed curve relating passive ventricular diastolic distension to left ventricular end-diastolic pressure (LVEDP); LVEDP becomes elevated, and dyspnea and other congestive symptoms are caused. Thus, the symptoms of pulmonary congestion with dyspnea, orthopnea, and even pulmonary edema may occur as unfortunate side effects of the Frank-Starling mechanism which has maintained cardiac output.

Other compensatory mechanisms include changes in peripheral venous and arterial circulation and in the sympathetic nervous system. In congestive heart failure there is an increase in total sympathetic discharge and an abnormal augmentation of the norepinephrine blood level with exercise.[13,14] The failing heart has improved support of contractility and an increase in heart rate due to increased circulating catecholamines despite a reduction of intrinsic cardiac norepinephrine[13,15] and impairment of direct cardiac sympathetic nerve function.[16] The patient with heart failure has increased venous pressure and venous tone at rest, which is due to increased blood volume, venous tone, and tissue pressure.[17,18] The increased blood volume is caused by the renal retention of salt and water. With exercise the venous pressure and tone are further exaggerated by a sympathetically mediated constriction of the veins,[19] which aids the return of blood to the heart when heart failure is present. This increased venous return provides part of the increased preload which could be used by the Frank-Starling compensation, but it heightens congestive symptoms such as dyspnea and edema. Increased peripheral resistance and altered flow distribution are compensation mechanisms provided by the systemic arterial system.[20] Three major factors appear to cause the increased peripheral resistance: first, increased sympathetic tone and circulating catecholamines to the peripheral resistance vessels;[14,21] second, increased local stiffness of resistance vessels that is thought to be caused by increased arterial sodium content and increased tissue pressure;[20,22] and third, increased angiotensin level. The resistance vessels demonstrate an abnormal response to exercise, resulting in intense visceral vasoconstriction and subnormal dilatation of the arteries to the exercising muscles.[23,24] In severe cases, this altered flow distribution is present at rest.[23] When the heart is severely failing and unable to maintain cardiac output, these changes in arterial resistance maintain central blood pressure and allocate the limited cardiac output, providing flow to vital areas such as the brain and heart while reducing flow to less essential areas such as the skin, renal system, and viscera and maintaining an intermediate level of flow to the exercising muscles.[25–28]

These arterial and venous compensations are diagramed in Figs. 23-2A and B. Figure 23-2A shows the normal circulation, in which preload is normal because venous capacitance and diastolic ventricular size are normal and, therefore, ventricular end-diastolic pressure is normal and there are no congestive symptoms. Cardiac contractility is normal. The heart contracts from a normal end-diastolic volume (the outer concentric circle) to a normal end-systolic volume (the inner concentric circle). The ejection fraction, which is the ratio of end-systolic volume to end-diastolic volume, is normal at 0.60. Stroke volume, which is the volume of the shell of blood extruded when the outer diastolic circle constricts to the inner systolic circle, is also normal and moves as blood flow into the arteries, shown by the arrows in the figure. Systemic resistance and blood pressure (flow times resistance) are normal, cardiac output is normal, and there are no low-output symptoms. Figure 23-2B shows severe overt heart failure. Cardiac contractility is low, so less systolic contraction occurs from any diastolic volume and the ejection fraction is low. Venous constriction helps increase venous return thus dilating the heart and allowing utilization of Frank-Starling compensation (also see Fig. 23-1).[18,19] However, the increased ventricular volume causes increased diastolic pressure with resultant congestive symptoms. Despite this venous compensation, stroke volume continues to be low and less blood flows into the arteries. With inadequate blood flow, the only way that blood pressure can be maintained is by increased peripheral arterial resistance.[20,21]

Here again, the compensation which is essential to life causes adverse symptoms and signs. Decreased skin flow is accompanied by an increase of arteriovenous oxygen extraction and produces cool, bluish extremities and, in advanced situations, impairs the ability of the body to rid itself of heat. Decreased flow to the exercising muscles, while preventing hypotension, also causes fatigue and muscle weakness, which are prominent symptoms in advanced heart failure. The chronic increase in general arteriolar tone is an increased afterload on the heart that may result in a "vicious circle" or positive-feedback loop. The increased afterload further decreases the diminished ejection fraction of the failing heart, which in turn further reduces cardiac output.[29] The natural history of severe congestive heart failure is to worsen, whether or not the inciting cause is worsening, because of this positive-feedback loop. Arterial vasodilators attempt to break this vicious circle. The use of vasodilators will be discussed in detail later in this chapter

The principles described above are the basic mechanisms of heart failure. Understanding them is of practical bedside use to the treating physician. It will help you understand the cause of your patients' symptoms. It will help you select and apply specific effective therapy and avoid undesirable side effects of therapy.

Therapy is often the selective removal of a portion of a compensation that has "gone too far" and is causing symptoms or has become part of a posi-

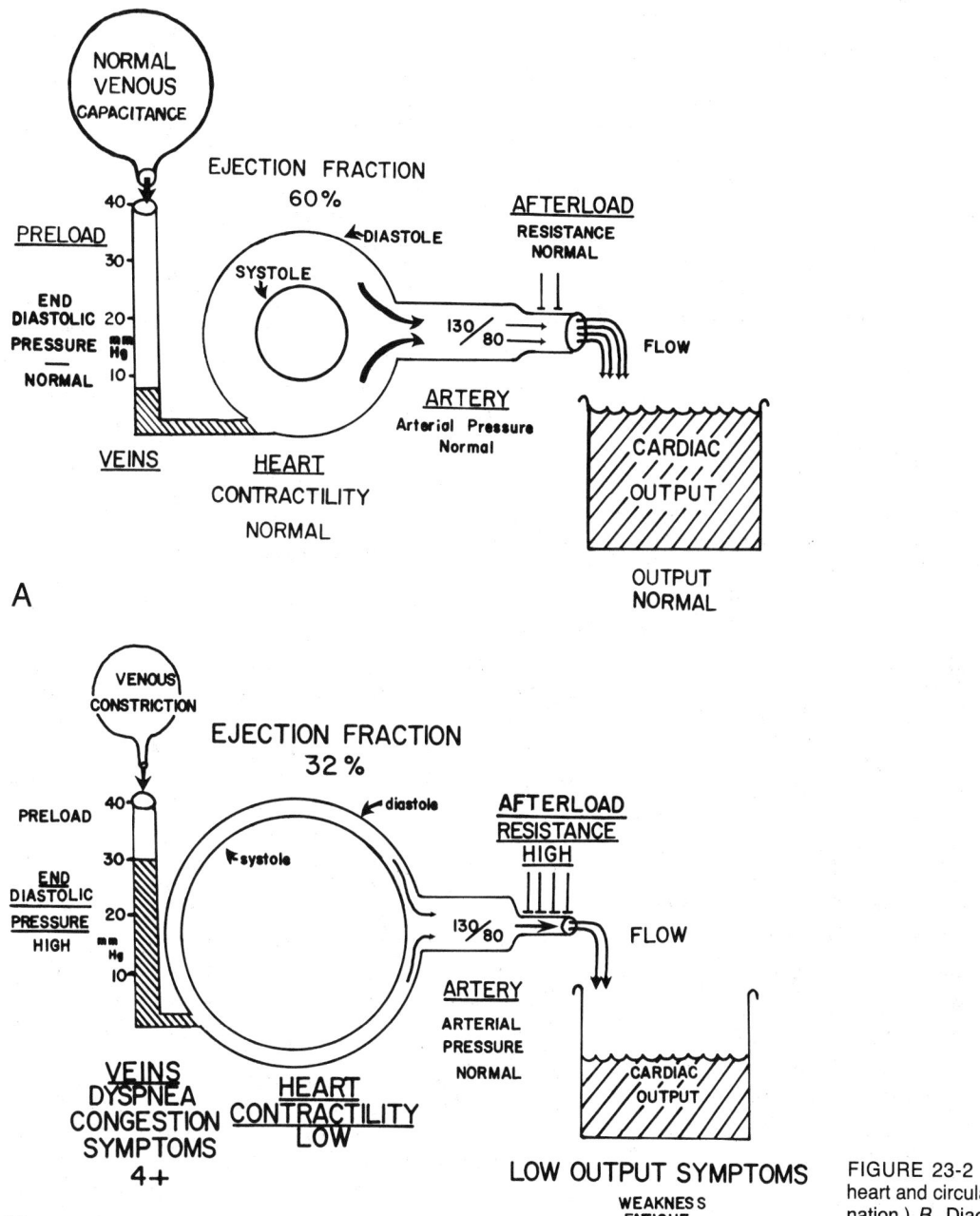

FIGURE 23-2 *A.* Diagram of normal heart and circulation. (See text for explanation.) *B.* Diagram of failing heart and circulation. (See text for explanation.)

tive-feedback loop. For example, dyspnea is the symptom caused by overuse of the Frank-Starling mechanism as it supports the cardiac output. Diuretics selectively remove some of the Frank-Starling mechanism and relieve dyspnea. In addition, excessive removal of a compensation by therapy often causes undesirable side effects. For example, too extensive a diuresis removes too much of the Frank-Starling compensation, thus causing the cardiac output to fall. Thus, excessive use of diuretics relieves the patient's dyspnea but causes new symptoms of low cardiac output such as fatigue and weakness. The discussion of therapy in this chapter is based on these pathophysiological concepts. Figures

23-10, 23-11, and 23-12, which show therapy, will be based on Figs. 23-1 and 23-2*A* and *B*.

Clinical Manifestations

The heart itself produces no symptoms when it fails to function as a pump. Symptoms are the result of the physiological derangement of the lungs, kidneys, liver, muscles, and other organ systems. The physical signs of heart disease and heart failure may be detected by examining the heart, arteries and veins, lungs, liver, and subcutaneous tissue. The purpose of this discussion is to describe the symptoms, physical signs, and laboratory abnormalities associated with heart failure. The abnormalities with the highest predictive value will be emphasized.

Symptoms (See Chap. 7)

Dyspnea

Most types of heart disease affect primarily and initially the left side of the heart. The output from the left atrium may be impeded by mitral stenosis, or the left ventricle may function abnormally as a result of atherosclerotic coronary heart disease, myocardial disease, systemic hypertension, or disease of the aortic or mitral valve.

The patient with heart failure may complain of "breathlessness" or "shortness of breath." The medical term for this unpleasant subjective sensation is *dyspnea*. Dyspnea may or may not be associated with an increase in respiratory rate in adult patients. Infants with heart failure cannot complain of dyspnea but exhibit a marked increase in respiratory rate. Dyspnea occurs when ventricular contractile performance becomes impaired and the Frank-Starling mechanism is required to maintain cardiac output by compensating for this impairment through increased ventricular end-diastolic volume and pressure. In turn, the left atrial, pulmonary venous, and pulmonary capillary pressures become elevated (see Fig. 23-1). When the hydrostatic pressure in the pulmonary capillary bed exceeds the oncotic pressure of plasma proteins, transudation of fluid into surrounding lung tissue occurs. The increased turgidity and decreased compliance of the congested lungs increase the work of breathing, which is, in part, responsible for the subjective symptom of dyspnea. Dyspnea may also be related to an inadequate blood flow to the respiratory muscles. This latter mechanism may be partly responsible for the dyspnea associated with cardiac lesions which are not associated with pulmonary congestion, e.g., severe pulmonary valve stenosis.

The dyspnea associated with cor pulmonale is, for the most part, due to parenchymal lung disease.

Dyspnea on Effort Dyspnea on effort is a common and relatively early symptom of heart failure. The most common cause of this symptom is disease of the left ventricle or mitral stenosis. Dyspnea on effort may not be noted by the following groups of patients:

- Patients with congenital heart disease may limit their activities so that symptoms may not occur. They may recognize their limitations and dyspnea only in retrospect after corrective surgery.
- Patients with acquired heart disease may gradually decrease their activities so that dyspnea does not occur. The surprising aspect of this accomplishment is that it can be done without the patient

being conscious of it, and family members often describe the true limitations that patients impose upon themselves.

- Sedentary persons may have such limited activity for other reasons that respiratory symptoms do not develop.
- Chronically ill or bedridden patients may not be aware of any dyspnea on effort.
- Patients who are phlegmatic or stoical may not appreciate the symptom of dyspnea as early as anxious patients. This fact makes it difficult to determine the severity of heart failure by estimating the severity of dyspnea.
- Patients with cerebral disease whose mental acuity is dulled may be completely unaware of symptoms.
- Rarely, patients with severe heart failure do not complain of shortness of breath when all other evidence indicates that they should. The cause of this phenomenon is not known.

The symptom of dyspnea on effort is not specific for congestive heart failure. Patients with chronic lung disease, those who are obese, and those in poor physical condition may also have this complaint. The latter two conditions are usually obvious, but the diagnosis of chronic lung disease is not so easily detected, especially when heart disease and lung disease coexist. When there has been a rather definite change in exercise tolerance over a short period of time, heart failure rather than lung disease should be suspected. As a rule, the dyspnea associated with chronic lung disease develops more gradually, and the patient learns to live within certain limits in order to avoid the unpleasant symptoms. On the other hand, when pulmonary infection, increased bronchospasm, or pneumothorax become superimposed on the basic lung disease, abrupt changes in effort tolerance may develop, and the dyspnea may closely mimic that of congestive heart failure. *Effort asthma* should be considered in physically fit individuals without evidence of heart disease who become abnormally dyspneic during excessive exercise. Bronchospasm may be detected on physical examination at that point but may not be detected when the patient is at rest. The response of a patient to a trial treatment for heart failure may be useful in determining the presence of heart failure in patients who have both lung disease and disease of the left side of the heart.

The dyspnea of *anxiety* is quite different from the dyspnea of heart failure, but despite the differences the two conditions are often confused (see Chaps. 7 and 78). The patient with anxiety exhibits deep, sighing respiration and a feeling that the "breath does not go down." Hyperventilation, fatigue, and other symptoms of anxiety are often present. The complaint of dyspnea at rest but not during exercise favors anxiety as the cause.

Patients with *diabetic acidosis* or *renal acidosis* may

breathe deeply and rapidly and may appear to have respiratory distress; however, these patients seldom complain of breathing difficulty.

During the late stage of *pregnancy* a woman may complain of "huffing and puffing," but she is rarely concerned about it.

Patients with *severe anemia* may become dyspneic with effort. On the other hand, it is surprising how a phlegmatic patient may experience neither dyspnea nor fatigue despite a hematocrit of 10 percent. Patients with thyrotoxicosis may have dyspnea on effort because of the increased metabolic demand and, at times, associated myopathy.

Orthopnea Orthopnea is present when a patient breathes more comfortably when his or her trunk is elevated. The patient experiences dyspnea in the recumbent position and has less dyspnea in the upright position. Relief occurs in the upright position because of a decrease in venous return, a decrease in hydrostatic pressure in the upper portion of the lungs, and an increase in vital capacity. At times, patients may go to sleep lying flat but later awaken because of breathlessness, which requires them to sit upright for relief (see discussion of paroxysmal nocturnal dyspnea below).

Patients with mitral stenosis may lose the symptom of orthopnea as the disease progresses. This phenomenon is not well understood but has been attributed to the development of relative tricuspid regurgitation. It also may be due to the development of increased pulmonary arteriolar resistance, which tends to "protect" the pulmonary capillaries. In exceptional cases of mitral stenosis, increased pulmonary arteriolar resistance may develop so rapidly and to such a marked degree that orthopnea and paroxysmal nocturnal dyspnea do not occur. In such patients fatigue and edema may dominate the clinical picture, although dyspnea on exertion is still experienced. In these patients a marked elevation of left atrial pressure may not occur even on effort or excitement. Orthopnea may also diminish in patients who have progressive heart failure due to other causes. This may be because of the development of tricuspid regurgitation, although other factors may be present.

The symptom of orthopnea is not specific for heart failure. The patient with *chronic lung disease,* such as pulmonary emphysema, may choose to sleep with his or her head and trunk elevated because the abdominal organs crowd the lung space in the recumbent position, the bronchi may become smaller when the patient lies down, and the work of breathing may be greater in the recumbent position. In such patients, other clues usually indicate that lung disease is present, but it may be difficult to exclude associated disease of the left side of the heart. Clues which are useful in distinguishing the dyspnea of heart failure from lung disease are discussed in Chap. 53. A therapeutic trial for heart failure is oc-

casionally justified in order to identify the contribution of heart failure to the dyspnea that occurs in patients with lung disease. Whenever there is doubt about the possible pulmonary cause of severe dyspnea, morphine should not be given and oxygen administration restricted to low flow rates.

Paroxysmal Nocturnal Dyspnea A patient with heart failure associated with left-sided heart disease is said to have paroxysmal nocturnal dyspnea when he or she suddenly awakens with dyspnea a few hours after retiring. Such patients often sit on the side of the bed or get up for a drink of water. Occasionally the patient will go to the window for a "breath of fresh air." The symptoms subside and the patient returns to bed and usually sleeps the remainder of the night. If the symptoms recur it usually is 2 to 3 h later. When the patient is examined by a physician some hours later, there may be no rales or venous distension, and there may or may not be a ventricular diastolic gallop rhythm or sound. The chest roentgenogram may reveal evidence of interstitial pulmonary edema.

This unique type of breathing difficulty is considered to be a very specific symptom of heart failure related to disease of the left side of the heart. Even this symptom complex, however, may be due to other causes.

Patients with *advanced pulmonary emphysema* and *chronic bronchitis* may have paroxysmal nocturnal dyspnea because of increased wheezing associated with the recumbent position and because of the accumulation of bronchial secretions when lying flat. *Pulmonary emboli* may of course occur at night and produce paroxysmal nocturnal dyspnea, but it is unlikely that a patient would have repeated pulmonary emboli for several nights in succession.

Anxious patients may awaken from sleep, with or without recalling a nightmare, sit on the side of the bed, and have an episode of extreme hyperventilation. They may go to the window, searching for air, and finally return to bed. Such an episode is rarely as "paroxysmal" as the type related to heart failure, and it is just as likely to occur soon after patients drop off to sleep as it is to awaken them later in the night. A history of anxiety and the absence of signs of heart disease serve to identify this rather common problem. The diagnostic difficulty arises in the anxious patient with known heart disease.

Cardiac Asthma Cardiac asthma may be the dominant complaint in patients with heart failure. The wheezing is due to bronchospasm secondary to heart failure. Individuals with pulmonary edema vary in their tendency to bronchospasm. Patients with heart failure who have a tendency to bronchospasm from other causes, such as chronic bronchitis or allergy, are more likely to wheeze than those without such a condition; however, wheezing due to heart failure may occur without associated lung disease. When there is no evidence of pulmonary disease in the patient above the age of 40, it is proper to consider the possibility that newly developed "asthma" is due to heart failure associated with disease of the left side of the heart. Cardiac asthma is usually precipitated by effort or occurs during the night. Patients may or may not be aware of their wheezing, and occasionally such patients may complain only of a cough.

Patients with *bronchial asthma,* with or without significant chronic lung disease or associated heart disease, experience increasing wheezing and coughing with effort. As a rule, the long history of these symptoms will aid in identifying the nature of the problem. The clinical distinction between these two causes of wheezing becomes more difficult when chronic lung disease is associated with left-sided heart disease. Additional clues found on physical examination and roentgenogram of the chest may aid in determining the relative contribution of lung disease and heart failure to the clinical picture. Pulmonary function studies rarely help. Occasionally, the response of the patient to a trial treatment for heart failure may be necessary to clarify the problem.

Severe Dyspnea of Acute Pulmonary Edema The sudden onset of suffocation due to acute pulmonary edema is terrifying to the patient. It may occur in patients with known symptomatic heart disease, but often it is the presenting symptom of a patient whose heart disease has not previously been recognized. It is due to disease of the left side of the heart such as acute myocardial infarction, acute ischemia, tight mitral stenosis, advanced aortic stenosis or regurgitation, severe hypertension, or rupture of the chordae tendineae. In the infant it may occur with ectopic tachycardia.

Acute fulminating pulmonary edema is uncommon with predominant mitral regurgitation unless the latter is due to rupture of the chordae tendineae or is precipitated by an uncontrolled arrhythmia. In patients with tight mitral stenosis, severe acute pulmonary edema is less common when there is marked pulmonary arteriolar disease. Acute pulmonary edema rarely occurs secondary to left-to-right shunts except in infants with large ventricular septal defects or ductus arteriosus. In general, acute pulmonary edema does not occur with cor pulmonale, pulmonic stenosis, tetralogy of Fallot, or constrictive pericarditis. The patient with chronic heart failure due to coronary atherosclerosis and old infarcts may develop acute pulmonary edema as the result of further acute myocardial infarction (which may be painless), the onset of ectopic tachycardia, or pulmonary embolism. Ectopic tachycardia or pulmonary embolism may also precipitate acute pulmonary edema in a person with a normal heart.

The circumstances in which an episode of acute pulmonary edema may occur are varied. A middle-aged man with acute myocardial infarction may be awakened from sleep or may develop the symptoms during the course of a normal day's activities; a young woman with tight mitral stenosis may develop pulmonary edema for the first time during a bout of atrial fibrillation.

Patients with pulmonary edema may sit or may stand in the upright position. Frequently they are anxious, agitated, pale, and drenched with sweat. The skin may be cyanotic, cold, and clammy. The respiratory rate is rapid; the depth of respiration may be deep or shallow. Quite often, infants have a respiratory rate of 100 per minute; adults commonly have rates of 30 to 40 per minute. The alae nasi may be dilated, and the accessory muscles of respiration may be used prominently. Retraction of intercostal spaces and supraclavicular areas is often present. There may be coughing, prolonged expiratory wheezing, and rattling sounds in the trachea. The sputum may be profuse, frothy, watery, or blood-tinged. The pulse rate is rapid. If the pulse is not rapid in a patient with pulmonary edema, it is wise to suspect an associated heart block, often complete arterioventricular (AV) dissociation. The systolic and diastolic blood pressures may be elevated to high levels, but this may not necessarily mean that there is true chronic systemic hypertension. If there is profound pulmonary edema, however, the systemic blood pressure may drop to shock levels. The systemic venous pressure may be elevated as a result of systemic venous constriction or failure of the right ventricle. Bubbling rales, wheezing, and rhonchi may be heard throughout the lungs and may obscure the auscultatory finding of underlying valvular heart disease or ventricular diastolic gallop rhythm. The chest roentgenogram may show the characteristic pattern of pulmonary edema. The symptoms of acute pulmonary edema may subside after an interval of 15 min to several hours. In the absence of primary heart disease, pulmonary edema may occur also with acute glomerulonephritis, with cerebral disease such as stroke or brain tumor, after inhalation of noxious gas, in acute heroin poisoning, with viral pneumonia, with drowning, or at high altitudes.

Acute pulmonary edema is unmistakable in its classic form. When the sputum is not frothy and pink-tinged, acute pulmonary edema may resemble acute bronchial asthma, although other evidence of heart failure can be found. On the other hand, when the patient is too sick to give a history and the heart is not audible because of chest wheezing, it may be difficult to distinguish pulmonary edema from acute bronchial asthma. If it is not possible to distinguish acute pulmonary edema from bronchial asthma, it is wise to avoid administering morphine, which is ordinarily used for pulmonary edema, or epinephrine, which is often used for bronchial asthma, until the situation is clarified. Aminophylline and oxygen are useful in both pulmonary edema and acute asthma. Reduction in venous return by rotating tourniquets and/or the use of sublingual nitroglycerin will not usually harm a patient with asthma and will greatly relieve the patient with pulmonary edema. The use of these measures may bring enough relief to enable one to obtain a chest x-ray, which usually clarifies the problem.

Cough
Patients with acute pulmonary edema may cough up frothy blood-tinged sputum. Cough due to chronic heart failure may produce no sputum. The cough usually appears when the patient first lies down, or it may bother the patient throughout the night. Its cardiac origin is frequently overlooked, particularly when the cough first appears after a respiratory infection. Cough is common in children with congenital heart disease due to left-to-right shunts. The recurrent attacks of coughing, which are frequent in patients with mitral stenosis, are occasionally mistaken for "winter bronchitis." Cough due to heart failure may be present with or without rales, and the cardiac origin of the cough may be revealed by the pattern of interstitial pulmonary edema seen on the chest roentgenogram. In patients with left-sided heart disease it may be difficult to distinguish chronic bronchial infection from heart failure. The diagnostic strategy may entail the use of therapy for bronchitis and heart failure which has been organized so that a clinical response assists in the diagnosis of the problem.

Insomnia
Patients with heart failure due to left-sided heart disease may complain of restlessness and inability to sleep. In some patients the insomnia is due to pulmonary congestion that, for some unknown reason, has not progressed to the point where dyspnea occurs. In others the insomnia is due to Cheyne-Stokes breathing, which may be the dominant symptom of heart failure secondary to left ventricular disease.

Cheyne-Stokes Respiration[30,31]
Cheyne-Stokes breathing tends to occur soon after the patient goes to sleep. The patient may awaken during the rapid, deep-breathing phase which follows a period of apnea and sleep. Cheyne-Stokes respiration is more likely to occur in association with central venous system disease. When Cheyne-Stokes breathing is caused by heart disease, it appears to be partially due to a prolonged lung-to-brain circulation time which disturbs the feedback mechanism regulating respiration. The complete explanation for this distinctive type of breathing remains obscure, even though the condition has been studied extensively. Clinically significant Cheyne-Stokes respiration rarely occurs in children and is seldom observed in patients with cor pulmonale. The breathing abnormality is increased by opiates and sedatives and may be prevented or relieved by aminophylline. Cardiac arrhythmias may occur in patients with Cheyne-Stokes respiration, and may be related to rapid changes in blood gases or to altered hemodynamics occurring during the extreme respiratory excursions.

History of Weight Gain and Peripheral Edema
Although pulmonary edema due to acute left ventricular failure may occur without weight gain, patients with severe chronic heart failure usually gain weight because of abnormal retention of salt and water by the kidneys. This, of course, may produce edema. Although patients may detect "swelling of the ankles," a patient with chronic heart failure may gain 10 lb or more without the development of pitting edema of the feet and ankles. Peripheral edema is therefore a late sign of heart failure. During the period of fluid retention the patient may have decreased urinary frequency and volume during the day but increased urinary frequency and volume at night (nocturia). The patient may note swelling of the feet and ankles at the end of the day. This swelling subsides at night with recumbency. At times, a weight loss of 5 lb or more in the 24 to 36 h following a potent diuretic is helpful as a therapeutic test for the presence of chronic congestive heart failure. The noncardiac causes of edema are varicose veins, obesity, phlebitis, pregnancy, liver disease, renal disease, cyclical edema, lymphedema, corticosteroid administration, retroperitoneal tumor, or even prolonged periods of standing or sitting. The distinction of heart failure from renal disease may be difficult since patients with either condition may have oliguria, nocturia, facial edema, albuminuria, elevated blood urea nitrogen level, decreased creatinine clearance, or occasional microscopic hematuria. In the elderly male with heart failure, these findings may be wrongly attributed to prostatism.

History of Increasing Body Girth
An increase in body girth as a result of ascites is another type of localized accumulation of extracellular fluid. Ascites is more likely to occur in patients with heart failure who have cirrhosis than in patients with heart failure who do not have primary liver disease. Ascites occurs in patients with constrictive pericarditis, restrictive cardiomyopathy, or tricuspid valve disease. Ascites occurs in infants more readily than in adults.

Weakness
Weakness due to heart failure may be produced by a variety of mechanisms. The symptoms may not be noted by some patients because of their preoccupation with dyspnea, but in some patients weakness is a major complaint. It may occur in the following circumstances:

1. Some patients complain of weakness on effort along with the sensation of dyspnea. Presumably this is related to inadequate blood flow to the skeletal muscles during exertion (see Fig. 23-2B).
2. Patients with far-advanced heart failure and marked cardiac enlargement who undergo suc-

DISORDERS OF THE CARDIOVASCULAR SYSTEM

cessful diuresis may complain of profound weakness following the diuresis (see Fig. 23-11). In this situation the reduced blood volume, although still greater than normal, may not permit an adequate ventricular filling pressure and the cardiac output may fall. The weakness is due to excessive reversal of the Starling mechanism of compensation. This reversal, while eliminating congestive symptoms, simultaneously deprives the heart of the capacity for maintaining the cardiac output which was being supported by the high filling pressure. This clinical state may be associated with a feeling of exhaustion and postural hypotension. The patient may complain of profound weakness and may faint when he or she stands to go to the bathroom. The hypotension may provoke a dangerous cardiac arrhythmia in some patients.

3. Some patients may verbalize a complaint of weakness in a dramatic way. For example, patients who have struggled to breathe for days and nights, who have been unable to sleep, who are never comfortable as a result of unrelenting heart failure, may actually say, "I can't fight it any more—I am too tired to go on," and simply stop fighting to live. Such patients seem to voluntarily stop breathing, as if they are overpowered by exhaustion. This state occurs when the cardiac output is low and there is marked pulmonary congestion, which is associated with an increase in the work of breathing over a prolonged period of time.

4. The symptom of weakness may be associated with electrolyte depletion, especially potassium ion depletion. At times weakness thought to be due to electrolyte depletion is in reality related to a state of relative hypovolemia.

5. Weakness may be accentuated because of poor appetite and poor food intake. The anorexia may be related to drug toxicity or may be part of the natural history of progressive congestive heart failure.

Mental Confusion

The majority of patients with congestive heart failure do not demonstrate symptoms associated with cerebral dysfunction. However, certain patients may have emotional disorders, including psychotic behavior, related to the chronic condition. This is likely to occur when patients find that, despite optimum therapy, they must limit their activity and modify their life considerably. In addition, many patients develop cerebral symptoms as a complication of therapy with drugs, including barbiturates and tranquilizers. When heart failure is severe, there may be a decrease in cerebral blood flow and metabolism of sufficient magnitude to evoke cerebral symptoms in some patients. The cerebral symptoms associated with heart failure include dizziness, somnolence, and confusion. On rare occasions it is possible to document more dramatic symptoms. For example a patient with severe congestive heart failure and atrial fibrillation may exhibit stupor. A dramatic improvement in cerebral function may become apparent after the atrial fibrillation reverts to normal. Patients with partial occlusion of the carotid artery may develop cerebral ischemic attacks and hemiparesis associated with atrial tachycardia or some other arrhythmia. Obviously, this is more likely to occur when the cardiac output is already compromised by heart failure. A previously alert elderly patient with heart failure may have a personality change and become confused or somnolent when diuresis produces relative hypovolemia.

Gastrointestinal Symptoms

Patients with heart failure may exhibit gastrointestinal symptoms, including anorexia, nausea, vomiting, abdominal distension, "fullness" after meals, and abdominal pain. These complaints may be due to venous engorgement and to congestion of the gastrointestinal tract but are often due to digitalis toxicity. Many patients with congestive heart failure have constipation; this is due in part to inactivity. An old clinical rule has been to consider thyrotoxicosis in a patient with chronic heart failure when constipation is not present. Actually this rule is not too useful, since drugs—especially digitalis and quinidine—may produce diarrhea. When diarrhea occurs, the physician may be prompted to carry out a number of exhausting procedures in an effort to explain the condition. On occasion anorexia may be so pronounced because of poor diet and digitalis toxicity, that food intake may become very inadequate. Weight loss may become so marked in such patients that carcinoma of the bowel may be suspected.

Bleeding from the gastrointestinal tract may be observed in patients with heart failure. This may be from an associated lesion or as a part of the heart failure syndrome and its treatment. Enteric-coated ammonium or potassium chloride tablets plus chlorothiazide medication may produce ulcerations of the small bowel. Gangrene of the intestine may occur as a result of heart failure. This may occur without intrinsic disease of the mesenteric arteries and appears to be due to intense splanchnic vasoconstriction.

Protein-losing enteropathy may occur in some patients with severe chronic heart failure.[32]

Liver Pain

Congestion of the liver is a common feature of heart failure. It causes tension on the liver capsule, which produces pain and tenderness. A few patients may notice hepatic pain on effort.

Symptoms Related to Renal Dysfunction

During the period of salt and water retention, patients with heart failure may have a decreased urine volume during the day when they are active and may have an increase in urine volume during the night. Men with heart failure may also have an enlarged prostate. The fluid retention of heart failure may cause additional enlargement of the prostate, which may produce more symptoms, such as nocturia and difficulty in starting and maintaining a stream of urine. In addition, moderate obstructive uropathy may aggravate or precipitate heart failure.

History of Cyanosis

Patients with severe heart failure may complain of a "dusky" appearance of their face. Arterial oxygen saturation is usually normal in patients with severe chronic heart failure. The cyanosis occurs because the oxygen content of the venous blood is decreased as a result of an increase in oxygen extraction by the tissues. Arterial oxygen saturation may be decreased and cyanosis may be obvious in patients with heart failure who have pulmonary disease. This is especially true when the heart failure is due to cor pulmonale, but it may be true when acute pulmonary edema, pulmonary embolism, or pulmonary infection occurs in a patient with heart failure. Cyanosis may also be noted in patients with heart failure who have right-to-left shunts, such as may occur with congenital heart disease.

History of Fever

It has been said that a temperature elevation of 1 to 2 degrees may occur in heart failure because of cutaneous vasoconstriction and diminished heat loss. Though this may be true, it is prudent to assume that there should be *no* elevation of body temperature in patients with heart failure because the slightest temperature rise should stimulate the physician to search for pulmonary infarction, pulmonary infection, renal infection, thrombophlebitis, infective endocarditis, and silent myocardial infection.

History of Sweating

Some patients with heart failure complain of excessive sweating; this is thought to be due to a need to lose body heat through sweating since it cannot be dissipated properly through the constricted skin circulation. This increased sweating may be quite noticeable in the infant with heart failure. Some observers believe that patients with heart failure due to aortic regurgitation sweat more than other patients with heart failure.

Cardiac Cachexia

Cardiac cachexia may occur in the very late stages of chronic severe heart failure.[33] This condition occurs because cellular hypoxia develops with severe heart failure. Hypermetabolism, protein-losing enteropathy, poor appetite as a result of congestion, drug toxicity, and mental depression all contribute to this condition. Severe malnutrition may, in turn, have an adverse effect on the heart itself.

Physical Examination

The physical signs of heart failure may be found by examining the heart itself, the arteries and veins, and the organs and tissues that are affected by heart failure. The latter include the lungs, liver, spleen, subcutaneous tissue, and eyes.

Physical Examination of the Heart (See Chaps. 10 to 12)

Ventricular Gallop Sound (Chap. 12) A ventricular gallop sound (protodiastolic gallop, third heart sound gallop, S_3 gallop) is the hallmark of ventricular failure (see Chap. 12). This low-pitched sound is heard best when the bell of the stethoscope is applied with light pressure. This sound occurs in early diastole and is the result of rapid ventricular filling into a noncompliant or distended ventricle. A left ventricular gallop sound is heard best at the apex, and a right ventricular gallop sound is heard best over the right ventricle. The normal third sound of the child or adolescent is identical to the abnormal gallop sound. Therefore the finding of a ventricle gallop (S_3) does not indicate heart failure in the child or in the young adult. The normal adult rarely has a ventricular gallop sound. Patients with mitral regurgitation, aortic regurgitation, patent ductus arteriosus, interventricular septal defect, or interatrial septal defect may also exhibit a ventricular gallop sound, but this does not always indicate ventricular failure. Young women who are pregnant or young adults who have thyrotoxicosis or anemia may also develop a third heart sound that is not necessarily an indication of heart failure. Since AV valve stenosis prevents rapid ventricular filling of the involved ventricle, a patient with tricuspid stenosis cannot exhibit a right ventricular gallop sound, nor can a patient with pure tight mitral stenosis exhibit a left ventricular gallop sound. The patient with tight mitral stenosis and right-sided heart failure due to pulmonary hypertension can, of course, have a right ventricular gallop.

In years past, the term *gallop rhythm* was applied to the heart sounds when a third sound was heard in a patient with tachycardia. It is now clear that this extra sound has the same significance regardless of the heart rate. The ventricular gallop sound becomes a reliable sign of early myocardial failure when its appearance is documented in a patient with heart disease. For example, a ventricular gallop at the apex that is heard for the first time the day after a myocardial infarction is a definite sign of left ventricular myocardial failure. As a rule, therapy for heart failure should be started if the onset of a ventricular gallop sound is noted in a patient with heart disease due to cardiomyopathy, aortic valve disease, hypertension, or atherosclerotic heart disease.

Both heart sounds and systolic murmurs may alternate in intensity when there is alternating strength of ventricular contraction. Patients with this abnormality always have pulsus alternans (see discussion below).

Atrial Gallop Sound (Chap. 12) An atrial gallop sound (presystolic gallop, fourth heart sound gallop, S_4 gallop) may occur in patients with a long PR interval, in patients with hypertension, aortic stenosis, cardiomyopathy, or atherosclerotic coronary heart disease and may occur in some individuals for unknown reasons (see Chap. 12). The atrial gallop sound is often associated with a thick-walled ventricle and is not a specific indicator of congestive heart failure.

Abnormal Precordial Movements The precordial movements associated with audible or subaudible ventricular or atrial gallop sounds may be seen or felt (see Chap. 11). In order to identify the precordial movements associated with audible atrial or ventricular gallop sounds, it is necessary to listen to the heart, to identify the first and second sounds, and to determine whether the abnormal movement occurs just before the first heart sound (atrial gallop) or shortly after the second heart sound (ventricular gallop).

In a patient with disease of the left side of the heart, a sustained systolic lift of the sternum as a result of right ventricular enlargement suggests heart failure, since it is unlikely that left ventricular enlargement alone will displace the right ventricle anteriorly. In such cases the right ventricle is large secondary to the elevation of pressure in the pulmonary circuit produced by prolonged failure to the left ventricle. The pulmonic component of the second sound may become louder as pulmonary hypertension develops. Right ventricular enlargement due to disease of the right side of the heart may force the left ventricle posteriorly, and the normal left ventricular impulse may be replaced with a right ventricular impulse. This finding does not indicate heart failure.

Pulsus Alternans Pulsus alternans of the peripheral arteries indicates heart failure due to disease of the left ventricle (see Chap. 10). It may be associated with alteration of other cardiac events which depend on left ventricular contraction. For example, the intensity of the heart sounds may be faint one cycle and louder the next cycle. Heart murmurs, especially the murmur of aortic stenosis, may alternate in intensity from cycle to cycle. Most patients with pulsus alternans have a left ventricular gallop sound associated with left ventricular disease and failure.

Abnormalities of the Neck Veins (See Chap. 10)
Abnormalities of the neck veins are frequently overlooked during physical examination. Signs of heart failure which may be detected from examination of the neck veins include the following: pulsations of the deep jugular veins when the trunk of the body is elevated approximately 45°, a prominent early *v* wave, prominent sustained *a* and *v* waves with a rapid and deep *y* descent, and an abnormal hepatojugular reflux test. The deep jugular veins can be thought of as valveless tubes filled with blood and connected to the right atrium. They should be viewed as fairly good manometers. Measurement of the vertical distance from the upper level of pulsation of the deep jugular veins to a horizontal line projected through the center of the right atrium is a very useful indicator of mean central venous pressure and, more importantly, right ventricular end-diastolic pressure. Severe distension of the neck veins can be difficult to detect. The veins can be distended to such a degree that the pulsations at 45° body elevation cannot be detected. Thus, it is important to routinely examine the neck veins with the patient sitting up at 90° in addition to the more usual semirecumbent positions.

Physical Examination of the Lungs (See Chap. 14)
Heart failure may be associated with *moist rales* which may be heard at the lung bases or over the entire lung field. It is not generally appreciated that the rales of heart failure may be heard only on the dependent side, and that they may shift to the opposite side when the patient turns. Heart failure is often present without rales, and rales may be due to noncardiac disease. Accordingly, rales are not considered to have the predictive value they were once assigned.

Bronchial wheezing is often caused by heart failure and is frequently misinterpreted as being produced by bronchial asthma.

Hydrothorax may develop in patients with heart failure. It may occur on either side but is more frequently located predominantly or solely on the right side. The finding of hydrothorax on the left side with little fluid on the right side suggests the diagnosis of pulmonary infarction. Hydrothorax rarely occurs in patients with cor pulmonale.

Physical Examination of the Subcutaneous Tissues (See Chap. 14)
Edema, a late sign of heart failure, occurs in the dependent parts of the body, usually the feet and ankles. The location of edema is determined by local factors, the most important of which is increased hydrostatic pressure. The erect position favors collection of the fluid in the feet, ankles, and lower portion of the legs, whereas the recumbent position favors the accumulation of the fluid in the sacral region. A search for presacral edema is an important part of the physical examination of patients who spend a considerable portion of their time in bed. Thrombophlebitis or varicose veins may lead to unilateral edema of the extremities, although unilateral edema from heart failure may occur if the patient spends long periods of time with one leg in a dependent position. Periorbital edema is common in children with heart failure or acute glomerular nephritis. The common denominator is that there is an increase in extracellular fluid in both conditions, and the periorbital tissue pressure is lower in children than it is in adults. In comparison with adults, infants with heart failure tend to have less peripheral edema but more ascites. *Anasarca* is a

term denoting generalized edema. In such patients hydrothorax and ascites are often present.

Physical Examination of the Abdomen (See Chap. 14)

The *liver may become large and tender* in some patients with severe heart failure. Movement of the liver occurs in association with the large venous *v* waves which occur in severe tricuspid regurgitation. The liver also expands slightly with each systole in such patients. When there is a large aortic pulsation, the liver will be displaced anteriorly with each heartbeat. Such displacement of the liver must be distinguished from true expansion of the liver.

Ascites may be due to chronic heart failure and always represents advanced disease. Young patients and adult patients with chronic constrictive pericarditis, restrictive cardiomyopathy, or tricuspid valve disease tend to develop ascites. Patients with heart failure and separate liver disease also tend to develop ascites.

The *spleen may become enlarged* as a result of chronic, passive congestion related to heart failure. Splenomegaly is usually encountered in patients who have hepatomegaly, and it may be associated with cardiac cirrhosis. It has been said that the spleen is enlarged in about 20 percent of patients with chronic heart failure. The significance of this figure is difficult to interpret because the incidence of splenomegaly would depend on duration of chronic congestion and the management of the patient.

Physical Examination of the Eyes

Patients with long-standing severe heart failure may have a *stare* and *slight exophthalmos* because of an increase in venous pressure. This finding must be differentiated from the exophthalmos due to thyrotoxicosis.[34] *Systolic movement of the ears, systolic propulsion of the eyes,* and *systolic lateral motion of the head* may be due to severe tricuspid regurgitation.[34]

Jaundice may be detected in a small percentage of patients, but the level of bilirubin is seldom greater than 2 mg/dl. Jaundice in patients with heart failure should provoke the clinician to consider pulmonary infarction as well as centrilobular necrosis of the liver.

Chest Roentgenogram (See Chap. 16)

The abnormalities due to heart failure which can be identified on chest x-ray have considerable predictive value.

An early hemodynamic change characteristic of failure of the left ventricle is pulmonary venous hypertension, which may occur without auscultatory abnormalities. When the pulmonary venous pressure becomes raised over the normal value (about 5 to 13 mmHg) and approaches and exceeds the oncotic pressure of plasma protein (25 to 30 mmHg), fluid may move from the capillary into the interstitial tissue of the lungs. This engorgement may lead to stiffening of the lung and decreased compliance. The concentration of plasma proteins, the efficiency of lymphatic drainage, the character of the alveolar membrane, and the interstitial tissue pressure determine the level of oncotic pressure at which transudation occurs. When most physicians think of pulmonary edema, they think in terms of the alveolar variety, which represents a more advanced state than the more common interstitial type. The interstitial type of pulmonary edema is often overlooked.

Interstitial pulmonary edema occurs when an excess amount of fluid enters the tissue which surrounds the pulmonary capillaries. This stage of pulmonary edema can often be detected by x-ray examination before it becomes clinically apparent. In a study of 114 patients with radiographic evidence of interstitial pulmonary edema at Emory University Hospital, heart failure was previously unrecognized by the clinicians in 24 percent of the patients.[35] The transverse diameter of the heart was less than half the transverse diameter of the chest (cardiothoracic ratio) in 28 percent of the patients. This was undoubtedly due to the fact that most of the patients in this study had heart failure due to myocardial infarction. The heart size is often normal when acute heart failure is secondary to acute myocardial infarction, mitral stenosis, aortic stenosis, or acute aortic regurgitation.

Dilatation of the Pulmonary Veins (Fig. 23-3)

In the normal lung the veins to the lower portion of the lungs are more prominent when the individual is in the upright posture because of the effects of hydrostatic pressure. Thus, on an upright chest radiogram in the normal person there is relative prominence of the inferior vessels in relation to the vessels of the superior aspects of the lung. This relationship is altered in pulmonary venous hypertension as a result of the generalized dilatation of the pulmonary veins, so that in heart failure there is unusual prominence of the superior pulmonary veins. This can be seen on routine upright chest radiographs in patients with heart failure and may give rise to the "antler" appearance. Patients with mitral stenosis commonly exhibit this abnormality (Fig. 23-3).

Dilatation of the Central Right and Left Pulmonary Arteries

Shortly after the pulmonary venous pressure becomes elevated in heart failure due to disease of the left side of the heart, the pulmonary artery pressure becomes elevated. On x-ray examination this may be noted as a dilatation of the central right and left pulmonary artery shadows. The right descending pulmonary artery, which forms the major vascular structure in the right hilum, normally measures 9 to 16 mm at its greatest diameter. When it measures 17 mm or more, it is a good sign of elevation of the

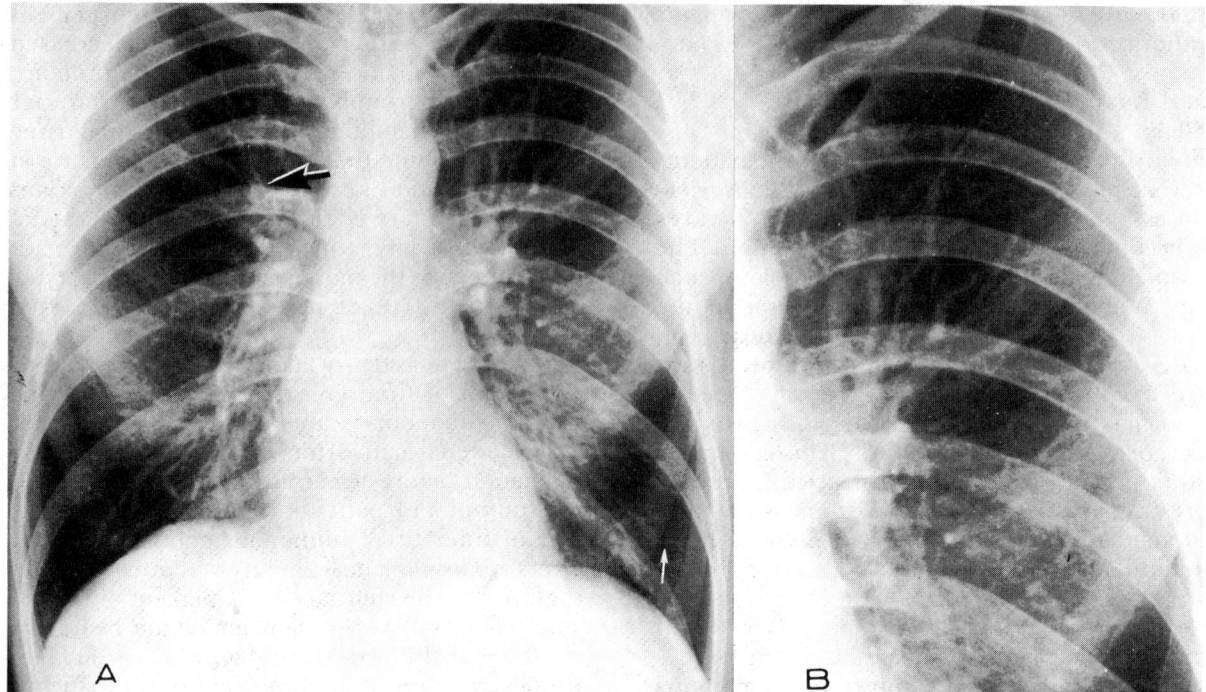

FIGURE 23-3   T. S., a 41-year-old male with mild mitral stenosis. The cause of his hemoptysis was initially diagnosed as bronchiectasis. *A.* Note the distension of superior pulmonary veins (large arrow) and costophrenic septal lines (small arrow). *B.* The antler-like appearance of the superior pulmonary veins.

pulmonary artery pressure if pulmonary blood flow is not increased (Fig. 23-3). At times both the major arteries and the veins are obscured by the pulmonary clouding of interstitial edema.

Pulmonary Clouding and Interstitial Pulmonary Edema (Figs. 23-4 to 23-6)

Pulmonary clouding with increased interstitial density of the central lung markings occurs early in the course of interstitial pulmonary edema. This x-ray finding is often attributed by the unsophisticated radiologist to "poor technique." The arteries and veins are surrounded by connective tissue. The accumulation of edema fluid in the perivascular tissues causes haziness and loss of the sharp outline of the arteries and veins (Figs. 23-4 and 23-5).

Interlobar Fissure "Thickening" (Fig. 23-6)

The accumulation of fluid in the septal planes and in the interlobar fissures causes a "thickening," which may be visible on the radiograph.

The secondary lobules of the lungs are separated by fine interlobular septa, and, at the periphery of the lungs, these septa lie perpendicular to the pleural surface. These interlobular septa near the periphery of the lung are normally microscopic in size, and therefore they are not seen in the chest roentgenogram. When they are thickened by edema fluid or fibrosis, however, they become apparent as sharp linear densities. These linear densities are more commonly seen in the lower portions of the lungs for two reasons: (1) the fibrous connective tis-

FIGURE 23-4   H. P., a 57-year-old male, suffered an acute myocardial infarction. Note A lines (large arrows) and B lines (small arrow), pulmonary clouding, and hilar engorgement.

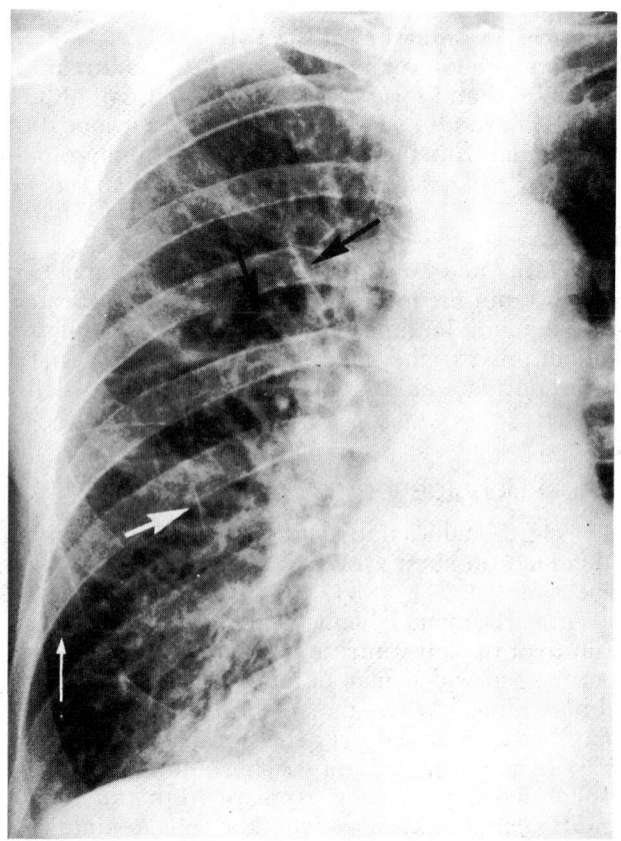

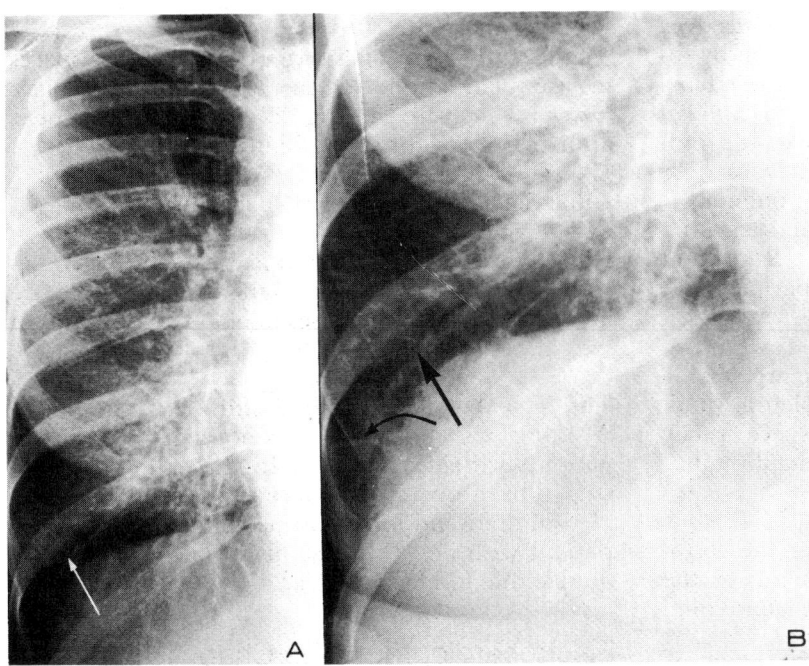

FIGURE 23-5 A. O., a 43-year-old male, had mitral stenosis. Note costophrenic septal lines, dilated superior pulmonary veins, and increased interstitial density (clouding) of the lungs.

sue septa in the lingula and middle lobes are well developed, vertically stacked, and located anteriorly and laterally in a visible area; and (2) the hydrostatic pressure is greater in the lower lungs, and consequently edema fluid accumulates early. These thickened septa are usually horizontal, and they may extend to the pleural surface. They are rarely longer than 3 cm or wider than 0.2 cm. Occasionally they are vertical and project perpendicular to the pleural surface over the diaphragm. These peripheral markings were termed *B lines* by Kerley (Fig. 23-5B). Similar longer lines extending peripherally from the hilum in the upper and midportions of the lungs have been termed *A lines*. The A lines correspond to the anatomic arrangement of long unbroken interlobular connective tissue septa in the upper and midportions of the lungs. Both types of septal lines may result from any condition which thickens

FIGURE 23-6 T. G., a 74-year-old male, had coronary atherosclerotic heart disease with old myocardial infarctions. *A.* Typical changes of interstitial pulmonary edema. *B.* In the lateral film fluid is seen in the posterior costophrenic sulcus, which cannot be seen well in the posteroanterior view. There is also thickening of the interlobar fissures, which is usually more apparent in the lateral views.

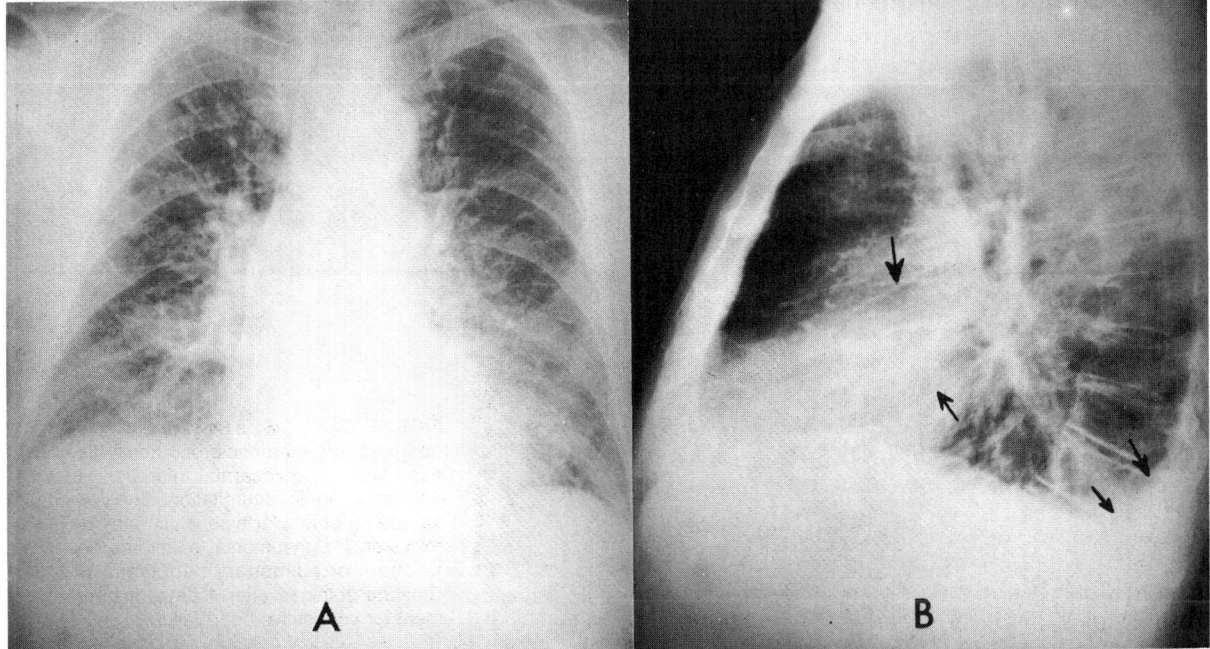

the septa—inflammation such as that produced by viral infection, hemochromatosis, infiltration by tumor, or fibrosis. When they are due to the edema fluid of heart failure, however, the left atrial mean pressure, pulmonary capillary pressure, and pulmonary artery diastolic pressure usually exceed 18 mmHg. When the lines result from brief pulmonary congestion, they are often transitory and leave no trace after the heart failure improves. Recurrent failure may cause the lines to become permanent.

Subpleural Fluid

Subpleural fluid may accumulate in the area of the costophrenic sulci and simulate free pleural fluid. When localized in the basal subpleural space, it may simulate the elevation of a leaf of the diaphragm.

Free Pleural Fluid

Free pleural fluid produces blunting of the costophrenic angles. This occurs more frequently on the right side and is usually seen best in the lateral film.

Alveolar Pulmonary Edema (Figs. 23-7 and 23-8)

Advanced pulmonary alveolar edema is recognized without difficulty. Edema fluid fills alveolar spaces in the central area of the chest, giving a "butterfly" appearance to the chest roentgenogram. The heart makes the body of the butterfly, and the edema makes the wings. Pulmonary edema may also occur from noncardiac causes such as circulatory overload, viral infection of the lungs, renal failure, increase in cerebrospinal fluid pressure, drowning, inhalation of toxic substance, injection of heroin, high altitude, etc.

All or any of the above findings may be present in any patient with heart failure, and, in addition, at times there may be localized areas of alveolar pulmonary edema. When these areas are large or confluent, they may simulate pneumonia, tumor, or infarction.

Pseudotumor

The accumulation of fluid in the interlobar spaces may simulate a tumor. Such a *pseudotumor* or *phantom tumor* is illustrated in Fig. 23-9. It may disappear after treatment for heart failure.

Dilatation of the Superior Vena Cava and Azygos Veins

The superior vena cava and azygos veins often become dilated when there is right-sided heart failure in association with increases in blood volume and in systemic vasoconstriction.

The Absence of Mediastinal Shift

A shift of the mediastinum is not likely to occur in patients with heart failure because the lungs are stiff. Therefore, when there is a large amount of pleural fluid and a mediastinal shift is present in a patient with heart disease, it is not likely that the fluid is due to heart failure.

Electrocardiogram (See Chap. 15)

The electrocardiogram of patients with heart failure is usually abnormal. This is true because heart failure is a consequence of severe heart disease, which, as a rule, is associated with an abnormal electrocardiogram. There are, however, no electrocardiographic findings of heart failure itself.

An electrocardiogram should be obtained in patients who are suspected of having heart failure. When correlated with other findings, it may give information regarding the cause of the condition. For example, unsuspected myocardial infarction may be detected or the characteristic changes of mitral stenosis may be suggested by the presence of right axis deviation of the QRS complex and atrial fibrillation or by abnormal M-shaped P waves. It serves as a base line to evaluate further changes regarding digitalis toxicity, electrolyte disturbance,

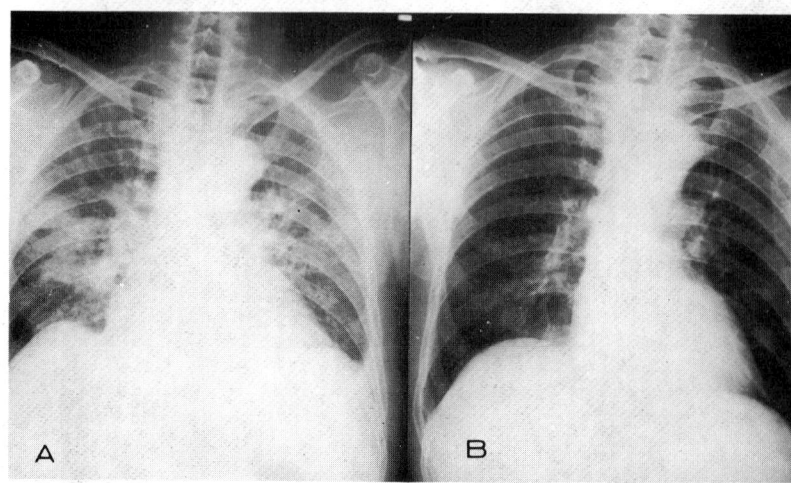

FIGURE 23-7   L. S., a 64-year-old male, had coronary atherosclerotic heart disease with old myocardial infarction, in addition to aortic regurgitation. *A.* Alveolar edema of lobular type which may be mistaken for pneumonia, pulmonary infarction, or pulmonary neoplasm. *B.* Clearing obtained after 4 days of treatment for congestive heart failure.

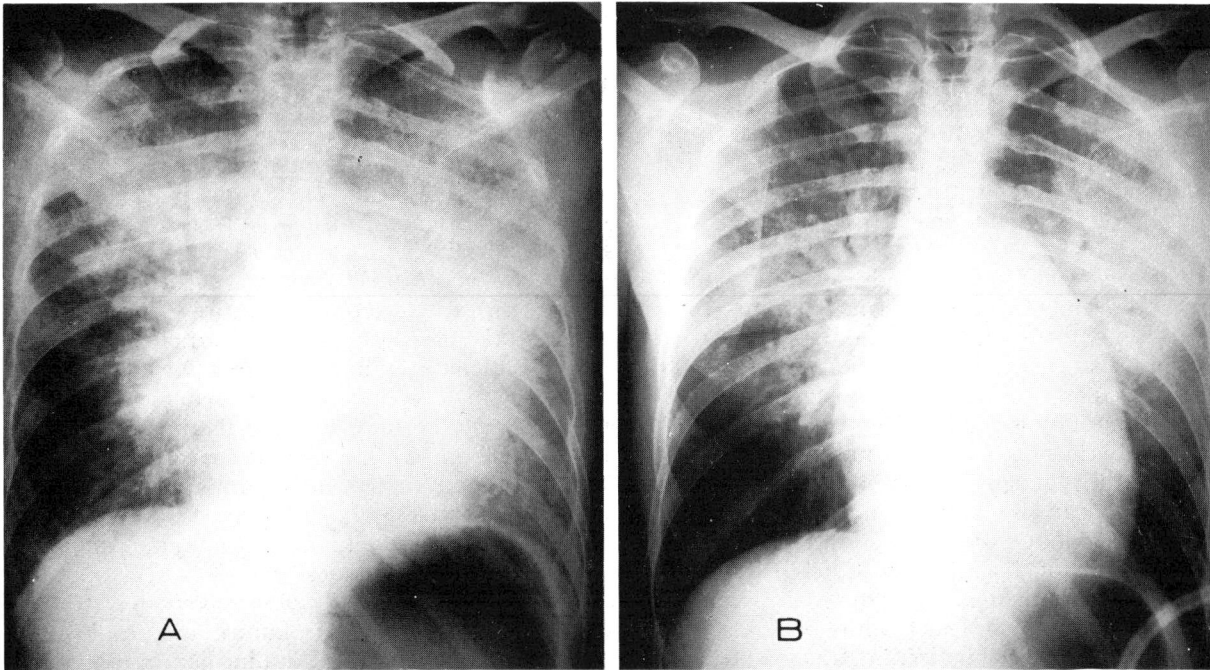

FIGURE 23-8 Roentgenogram of a 24-year-old male with tight mitral stenosis. *A.* Intraalveolar pulmonary edema. *B.* 24 h later. Partial clearing of the intraalveolar edema on the right side with persistent interstitial edema on the left side.

acute myocardial infarction, unrecognized arrhythmias, or changes in atrioventricular or intraventricular conduction.

Special Laboratory Studies

The special laboratory studies which may be useful in some patients with congestive heart failure include Swan-Ganz catheterization, radionuclide an-

giograms, echocardiography, cardiac catheterization, and exercise stress testing. These special studies are discussed in detail in Chaps. 87, 95, and 97 to 99.

Exercise testing is rarely necessary to document the degree of heart failure. In an occasional patient this test will help quantitate the degree of functional impairment and the patient's tolerance (Chap. 87).

Swan-Ganz catheterization is not usually necessary to determine that a patient has heart failure. This

FIGURE 23-9 R. R., a 76-year-old male, had coronary atherosclerotic heart disease with old myocardial infarction and pulmonary emphysema. *A.* Changes of interstitial pulmonary edema and the "pseudotumor" due to loculated interlobar pleural effusion. *B.* Considerable clearing, obtained after 4 days of treatment for congestive heart failure.

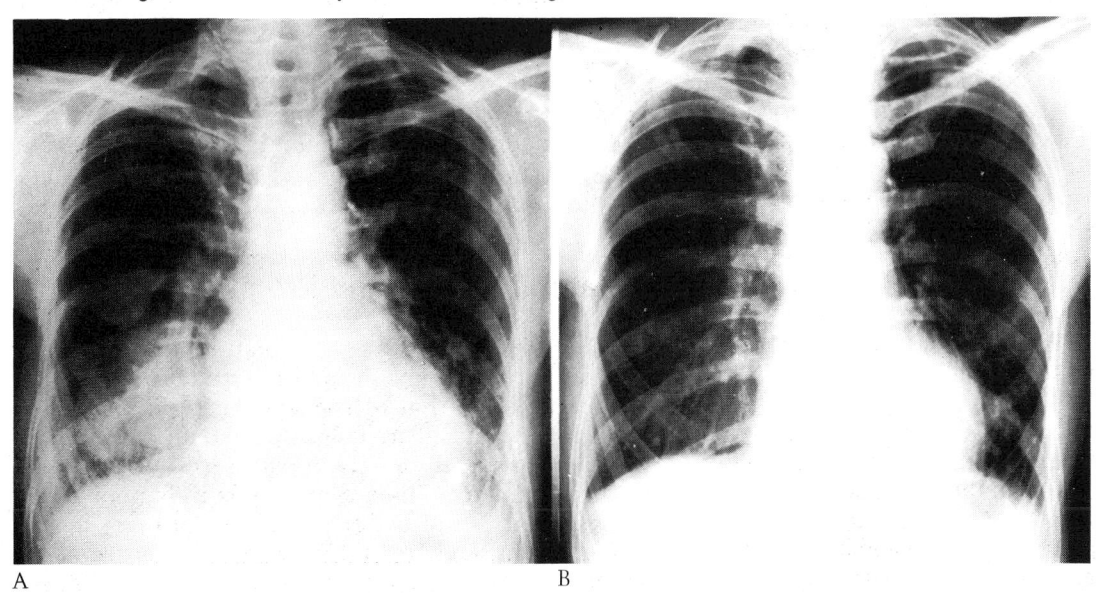

A   B

study can be helpful in documenting the presence of congestive heart failure by measurement of central venous, right ventricular end-diastolic, and pulmonary wedge pressures as well as cardiac output. These determinations can be especially helpful in some patients in the acute phase of a myocardial infarction and in some patients who may need vasodilator therapy for late-stage heart failure (Chap. 99).

Radionuclide angiograms provide accurate, noninvasive measurement of ejection fraction. This study is helpful in determining the etiology of congestive heart failure since a reduced ejection fraction indicates ventricular dysfunction. For example, if the diagnostic question is whether the patient has a cardiomyopathy causing both heart failure and a murmur of mitral regurgitation or has primary mitral valve disease causing both the heart failure and murmur, knowledge of the ejection fraction may help. The ejection fraction, an indicator of poor ventricular function, must be reduced if a cardiomyopathy is the cause of heart failure, whereas ventricular function and the ejection fraction may be preserved in mitral regurgitation due to primary mitral valve disease. Radionuclide angiography may be useful in a patient with severe or end-stage heart failure due to known coronary artery disease by detecting a surgically resectable ventricular aneurysm (Chap. 97).

Echocardiography also can determine the ejection fraction, although limited areas of regional ventricular wall dysfunction can be misleading. Echocardiography is of major use in determining the etiology of heart failure. This is especially true in mitral stenosis, aortic stenosis, idiopathic hypertrophic subaortic stenosis, ruptured mitral chordae, valvular endocardial vegetations, and left atrial myxoma (Chap. 95).

As with clinical evidence of heart failure, there is no single finding at *cardiac catheterization* which indicates heart failure. In the patient with heart failure one or more of the following may be found on cardiac catheterization: an elevated end-diastolic pressure in the involved ventricle; a lower resting cardiac output as compared with that prior to the onset of failure; an inability to increase cardiac output in response to exercise; an abnormally high arteriovenous oxygen difference at rest or during exercise; or a reduced ventricular ejection fraction determined during angiography. One does not subject a patient to cardiac catheterization to determine the presence or absence of heart failure; rather, this procedure is used to determine the cause or to grade the severity of the underlying heart disease.[36,37]

Since the *circulation time* is in part a reflection of the volume of the pulmonary vascular bed and of the volume of the heart in addition to the cardiac output, patients with acute heart failure induced by myocardial infarction may occasionally have normal circulation time.[38] The circulation time may not be significantly prolonged with mild degrees of heart failure. This measurement does have value in the identification of patients with high-output heart failure, in whom the circulation time is shorter than expected.

The value of measurements of *vital capacity* in assessing the presence of heart failure is greatest when managing patients with heart disease during pregnancy. Normally the vital capacity increases or remains the same during pregnancy, whereas it decreases with the onset of congestive heart failure.

The total *blood volume* may be normal or increased in the patient with heart failure. Obviously, when the problem is one of acute redistribution of blood, the total volume may be normal whereas the pulmonary blood volume may be increased. Patients with acute pulmonary edema and shock due to myocardial infarct may have a decrease in their total blood volume. (Fluid apparently goes into the interstitial spaces of the tissues.)

Dysfunction of the liver, kidney, or brain may develop in the late stages of heart failure as a result of altered cardiac output and diminished organ perfusion, or as a result of increased venous pressure. Such dysfunction causes no permanent structural changes in the kidney and brain; however, permanent changes due to chronic passive congestion may be produced in the liver. Urinalysis may reveal moderate proteinuria. The specific gravity of the urine may be high during the phases of salt and water retention and low during periods of diuresis. The blood urea nitrogen level may be moderately elevated, usually no higher than 50 mg/dl, secondary to heart failure (prerenal azotemia).

Hepatic dysfunction, often with structural damage to the liver, may result in moderate retention of Bromsulphalein or indocyanine green, an abnormal cephalin flocculation test, and slight elevations of serum bilirubin and serum glutamic oxaloacetic transaminase (SGOT) levels.[39] Hepatic necrosis may be associated with marked elevation of the serum SGOT. The serum lactic dehydrogenase level may also become elevated in patients with congestive heart failure with secondary liver dysfunction.[40]

The *erythrocyte sedimentation* rate may be retarded during congestive heart failure. This occurs because the fibrinogen level is decreased secondary to impaired liver function.

Natural History and Prognosis

There is little definitive work on the long-term prognosis. In patients with mild heart failure the prognosis is often that of the underlying disease. For example, mild heart failure due to an old myocardial infarction in a patient with severe triple-vessel coronary artery disease has a relatively poor prognosis because of the triple-vessel coronary artery disease rather than the history of myocardial infarction. By the same principle, mild heart failure due to rheumatic mitral regurgitation has a relatively favorable and predictable long-term prognosis. Mild heart failure in patients with aortic stenosis is an ominous sign.

In thin-walled cardiomyopathy the prognosis appears related to depression of ventricular function measured by the ejection fraction; patients with ejection fractions below 20 percent have a poor prognosis and generally do not live 5 years.

In patients with very severe chronic heart failure of any cause, the prognosis is not good, although the first carefully controlled statistical study is just now being conducted. Due to the vicious circle or positive-feedback loops discussed earlier in this chapter, severe heart failure usually gets worse whether or not the inciting condition gets worse. Interrupting the positive-feedback loops by therapy may stabilize a patient's condition and improve the patient's quality of life, but statistical proof of increased longevity resulting from such therapeutic intervention is not yet available.

Management of Patients with Heart Failure

Prevention of Heart Failure

Since heart failure results from heart disease, preventing heart disease should be the first step in our effort to prevent heart failure. At present, we do know how to modify or prevent certain types of heart disease, including the following, which are discussed in later chapters: congenital heart disease (Chap. 36), rheumatic heart disease (Chap. 37), atherosclerotic coronary heart disease (Chap. 43), hypertensive heart disease (Chap. 50), pulmonary heart disease, (Chap. 53), infective endocarditis (Chap. 54), constrictive pericarditis (Chap. 58), traumatic heart disease (Chap. 59), syphilitic heart disease (Chap. 61), high-cardiac-output states (Chap. 26), and obesity heart disease (Chap. 73). Hypertension may produce heart disease and heart failure in the absence of other heart diseases. In such cases, control of the hypertension is of utmost importance in preventing heart failure.

Unfortunately, these and other forms of heart disease cannot always be prevented, so our next step in preventing heart failure is to prevent or delay the onset of heart failure in patients with heart disease. There are no easily applied formulas or rules, but many rules of caution have evolved. From our experience, physical and mental activities of patients with heart disease must be considered. Too often in the past, physicians have imposed general rules on patients rather than evaluating specific patient activities. For some patients, it may be appropriate to suggest ways to reduce the effort expended in performing their job activities. For others, programs of increased activity may be best. For instance, many patients with moderately severe heart disease without overt failure can and should regularly participate in a reasonable exercise program, such as walking, bowling, or golf, coupled with periodic rest during daily activities. By the same token, we should beware of urging too much activity. Jogging, for example, a commonly prescribed exercise, is not useful for patients with latent heart failure.

Infections should be treated promptly. Pulmonary infections are common precipitating causes of heart failure in small children with congenital heart disease (Chap. 36). Streptococcal pharyngitis must be prevented or promptly treated to eliminate heart failure secondary to rheumatic carditis and rheumatic heart disease (Chap. 37). Infective endocarditis likewise must be prevented or treated promptly (Chap. 54). Viral diseases that involve the lungs are especially difficult for heart disease patients. The Asian influenza epidemic of 1958 taught us that patients with mitral stenosis or congestive heart failure may develop pulmonary edema when they are stricken with Asian flu. Since the effectiveness of immunization to prevent viral diseases such as Asian flu varies at least annually, it is necessary to be alert to current programs and to keep abreast of current information by contacting the Center for Disease Control in Atlanta, Georgia.

Excessive ingestion of salt should be avoided. Many patients with compensated heart disease eat more than average amounts of salt and may go on salt sprees by eating salted ham, or fish, or the like. Such patients may retain sufficient salt and water to precipitate heart failure. Similarly, sodium-retaining hormones should be used with caution, and intravenous fluid should be administered with great care. In patients with tight mitral stenosis, for instance, even a small amount of fluid given rapidly may precipitate heart failure. Remember, also, that sodium administered with the fluid may contribute to the problem.

Obese patients with heart disease must lose weight (Chap. 73). An effective program of weight reduction may enable such patients to enjoy months or years of activity and may even prevent heart failure entirely. Patients with significant heart disease who could eventually develop heart failure must not smoke (Chap. 53). Among environmental factors, high temperature, high humidity, and high altitude should be avoided by patients with heart disease (Chap. 80). Hypertension, when present, should also be controlled.

Many other conditions in heart disease patients contribute greatly to heart failure but can be controlled or prevented if diagnosed. If thrombophlebitis, pulmonary emboli, or cardiac arrhythmias occur, it is proper to apply the available preventive measures (Chaps. 23 and 59). Similar prompt treatment should be instituted for renal disease or lower urinary tract obstructions, although circulatory overload may develop in patients with these diseases even when heart disease is not present. Anemia and thyrotoxicosis may produce heart failure even in some patients who do not have heart disease. More often, however, heart failure related to these conditions occurs in patients with additional heart disease (Chaps. 26 and 70). Special consideration must be given to patients with heart disease who undergo surgical procedures (Chaps. 76 and 77).

An issue of continuing concern is whether administering digitalis is effective to delay the onset of heart failure in heart disease patients. Though digitalis increases the contractile force of both the failing and nonfailing myocardium, it does not increase the cardiac output of the nonfailing heart[41] except when used to control the ventricular rate of a patient with atrial fibrillation. In rapid atrial fibrillation, digitalis may increase the cardiac output of a nonfailing heart because it slows the ventricular rate rather than increasing myocardial contractility. In theory, digitalis might delay the onset of failure in patients who have heart disease, and recent animal experiments raise further interest in this possibility.[42] In these short-term animal studies, prophylactic digitalis therapy in one group prevented the loss of ventricular contractility which occurred in the non-digitalis-protected group subjected to similar severe pressure overload. Until additional experimental and clinical investigations extend these preliminary results, however, digitalis may be given to patients with heart disease who have subtle signs of failure, but we do not recommend that it be routinely given to patients who have heart disease without evidence of heart failure. Nevertheless, digitalis should be given to patients with known heart disease or moderate to marked cardiomegaly who have even minimal symptoms and signs of failure when they must undergo known stresses such as major surgical procedures. In such cases, the risk of toxicity can be reduced by giving only two-thirds of the usual doses, because toxicity usually occurs with higher doses,[43] although improvement in cardiac contraction is proportional to the size of the dosage. With respect to elderly patients, Dock and others have pointed out that they are more likely than younger persons to suffer heart failure during stressful situations such as surgical procedures, infusions of fluid, pneumonia, etc., with or without preexisting heart disease.[44] Some physicians have recommended the use of digitalis for elderly patients in such cases, but we do not routinely prescribe digitalis for such patients unless there is evidence of heart disease such as cardiomegaly. Rather, we urge that they be watched carefully and treated promptly. Indications for the use of digitalis in cardiac surgery patients are discussed in Chap. 76.

Management Components

In this section, eight management components will be discussed in detail. In the next section, these components will be arranged in various combinations to describe the appropriate practical therapy for various degrees of heart failure. The management components will be related to the pathophysiology described earlier in this chapter and in Chap. 22. The specific overused compensation which is causing symptoms and which can be selectively withdrawn by the therapy will be identified. New symptoms which may be expected if the therapy is overapplied will be outlined, with suggestions for avoiding them. In-depth discussion of clinical pharmacology of digitalis, diuretics, and vasodilators will be provided.

The eight management components for treatment of heart failure are:

1. Determine and manage specific etiology.
2. Discover and manage precipitating causes so as to decrease workload of the heart.
3. Control heart rate.
4. Increase myocardial contractility and increase cardiac output.
5. Decrease congestion by reducing preload.
6. Decrease afterload and increase cardiac output.
7. Decrease workload by agents who alter preload and afterload.
8. Manage surgically.

Determine and Manage Specific Etiology
Identification of a specific etiology is the first step in heart failure treatment and one which is often overlooked. Certain relatively infrequent lesions such as masked thyrotoxicosis, an unrecognized patent ductus arteriosus, a large systemic arteriovenous fistula, and obscure mitral stenosis can be cured, while many more common lesions as yet receive only palliative treatment. Unfortunately, the instances of heart failure caused by specifically curable forms of heart disease are much rarer than instances of heart failure caused by atherosclerotic coronary disease with repetitive myocardial infarction or diffuse myocardial fibrosis. The more experienced a physician becomes, the more discouraged he or she may feel in the nonproductive search for specific curable lesions causing heart failure. A way to avoid this is to recall that the diagnosis "congestive heart failure" is never complete; it must always be followed by "due to..." or a set of problems to be explored in the search for etiology. Discouraging though the odds may be, identification of the occasional curable patient justifies a reasonable search for a specific etiology in all patients. Further, specific diagnosis may aid selection of the proper drugs and procedures to improve the incurable patient.

To provide a clinically practical framework for the diagnostic search, we divide the possible etiologies into the following categories:

1. Direct myocardial damage: myocardial infarction, viral myocarditis, etc.
2. Ventricular overload
   a. Volume overload including mitral regurgitation, systemic arteriovenous fistula, etc.
   b. Pressure overload including systemic hypertension, aortic stenosis, etc.

3. Restriction to diastolic filling: mitral stenosis, constrictive pericarditis, etc.

This framework, albeit arbitrary and somewhat incomplete, is recommended because it is simple to remember and use at the bedside. On physical examination and chest x-ray, patients who fit into the categories of direct myocardial damage and ventricular overload usually have enlarged hearts, while patients who fit into the category of restriction to diastolic filling generally have small hearts unless there is complication by pericardial fluid. Patients with heart disease due to direct myocardial damage often have a weak apex impulse, low-amplitude carotid pulses, and, almost always, a low ejection fraction. Many patients with direct myocardial damage do not have diagnostic heart murmurs. Patients in the subcategory of disease due to ventricular pressure overload often have diagnostic physical findings such as high systemic blood pressure, a diagnostic murmur of aortic stenosis, and a forceful apex impulse. Patients in the volume overload subcategory may have increased amplitude carotid pulses; a dynamic, large displacement apical impulse; and diagnostic murmurs of a shunt lesion or valvular regurgitation. Patients with ventricular overload who have not sustained extensive cardiac muscle damage may have a normal ejection fraction. In patients who have direct myocardial damage, the ejection fraction will be reduced. Now that the ejection fraction can be obtained very accurately and noninvasively by gated radionuclide scintigraphy and often by echocardiography, measurement of the ejection fraction is of practical diagnostic value.

These three etiologic categories are also helpful in selecting therapy. Patients with ventricular myocardial weakness in the direct myocardial damage category need the increase in ventricular contractility provided by digitalis. Patients in the category of restriction to diastolic filling due to chronic constrictive pericarditis or pure mitral stenosis with normal sinus rhythm may receive little or no benefit from this drug. Patients with ventricular dysfunction and congestive symptoms caused by chronic ventricular pressure overload of systemic hypertension may lose all symptoms of congestive failure when blood pressure is reduced by antihypertensive medication.[11]

Discover and Manage Precipitating Causes So as to Decrease the Work Load on the Heart

The treatment of factors which precipitate and aggravate heart failure vary with the factor. Pulmonary emboli may require anticoagulation, thyrotoxicosis may require radioactive iodine or surgery, obesity may require weight loss, recent dietary sodium excess may require diet education and modification, etc. Some extracardiac factors require specific therapy, and others may be eliminated. Such factors include excessive activity; excessive salt and water intake, including intravenous fluid administration; pulmonary infection; pulmonary embolism; cardiac arrhythmias; myocardial infarction; prostatic enlargement with lower genitourinary tract obstruction; renal disease; obesity; anemia; and thyrotoxicosis.

Pulmonary emboli are so common as a complication, aggravating factor, or precipitating cause of heart failure in patients with congestive heart failure that they seem to be part of the clinical syndrome. Long-term anticoagulant therapy has been used in an effort to decrease the thromboembolic complications in such patients. The procedure has not been generally adopted as a routine prophylactic measure in the management of such cases, perhaps because hepatic congestion often leads to difficulties in controlling prothrombin levels. Anticoagulants are clearly indicated when the pulmonary emboli are obvious, but since only 10 percent of pulmonary emboli produce the clinical picture of pulmonary infarction, the majority of emboli go unrecognized. Anticoagulation may be indicated for a limited time in the hospitalized patient confined to bed during therapy for severe congestive failure, since pulmonary emboli are more common in such patients. Low-dose heparin therapy also may be of benefit in such patients.[45] Anticoagulation may also help prevent pulmonary emboli in patients with cor pulmonale who have high hematocrit levels and in whom a vigorous diuresis is expected.

Ligation of the inferior vena cava has been used in patients with chronic congestive heart failure. This procedure seems to decrease the number of pulmonary microemboli, and in addition, it has a long-term tourniquet effect. However, because of its unfortunate side effects, it has not been adopted as a routine measure and is reserved for situations in which the definite diagnosis is recurrent pulmonary emboli despite full anticoagulation. It may temporarily decrease the filling pressure of the heart in some patients (especially those with poor cardiac compliance) and cause hypotension, poor cardiac output, and oliguria, as well as aggravate dependent edema. It is obvious that we have not as yet solved the serious problem of thromboembolism in patients with heart failure.

The work load of the heart may be diminished by decreasing physical activity and reducing emotional turmoil. The desired level of physical activity of the patient with heart failure must be calculated to cause as little harm as possible while providing what the patient needs for a meaningful, happy life. Also, from a practical standpoint, most patients with heart failure must continue to earn a living. Therefore, it is usually economically necessary as well as psychologically valuable to keep patients "on the job" as long as possible. The maximum degree of safe rehabilitation should be foremost in the physician's mind.

The initial guidelines to the degree of restriction of activity are determined by the severity of the patient's heart failure. The physician's therapeutic approach to a patient with advanced heart failure is very different from the approach to a patient with slight heart failure. However, symptoms do not always parallel the degree of heart failure. An elderly patient with moderate heart failure who prefers a very sedentary life may volunteer minimal complaints; a patient with long-standing disease and gradually decreasing cardiac reserve may unknowingly modify his or her lifestyle to avoid symptoms.

Some patients have advanced symptoms when they first seek medical help. They may be exhausted from nights of orthopnea and sleeplessness. Such patients require hospitalization. They require the trunk up–legs down position, and for patients who have severe orthopnea, a large chair may be more comfortable than a bed. If so, the chair should be used several times a day. For those patients, dyspnea may be relieved by elevating the head of the bed, using blocks under the two legs at the head of the bed if necessary. The condition of some of these patients may be vastly improved by careful use of opiates for a day or two, unless there are definite contraindications to their use.

Other patients do not seek help until even minimal activity causes symptoms. The activity of these patients should be greatly restricted until effective therapy has been established, diuresis has occurred, and symptoms have been relieved. These patients should be encouraged to sit in comfortable chairs and, while in bed, should utilize the trunk up–legs down position, which aids in the relief of dyspnea. The decreased venous return achieved by this position may improve congestive symptoms, and edema fluid may be transferred from the lungs to the subcutaneous portion of the dependent parts. For those patients, care must be taken to eliminate the harmful effects of bed and chair rest. Passive exercises of the extremities, especially the legs, should be carried out several times each day in an effort to prevent venous stasis, which predisposes to pulmonary emboli. Elastic stockings may also help decrease venous stasis by increasing the velocity of blood flow in the veins. As a rule, the period of rest should be continued for a few days or even weeks after the failure has been controlled. Thereafter, the patient may gradually assume more activity and then return to work, although working adjustments and other restrictions may be indicated.

Congestive heart failure occurring under certain conditions such as pregnancy or acute rheumatic myocarditis may require more prolonged rest or complete inactivity until the pregnancy is terminated or the acute rheumatic myocarditis subsides (Chaps. 37 and 67). A number of complications may result from prolonged bed rest, including poor muscle tone, poor cardiovascular reactivity (including postural hypotension and decreased cardiac output), venous stasis with predisposition to thromboembolism, mental depression, and anxiety on resuming activity. Complications are especially likely to occur in elderly patients. The physician must carefully assess the need for long periods of rest, and brief periods of mobilization and change in posture are desirable throughout any extended inactivity.

A simple, commonsense approach to prescribing the appropriate degree of activity is quite satisfactory in most cases. Many patients with slight degree of heart failure require little or no change in their activities. Others may need adjustments in hours of work and manner of work, as well as curtailment of nonessential activities. For example, the person in business may benefit by being driven to work, and might break the work routine by an hour of rest in the middle of the day. The person who does housework may need domestic help, or may need to reorganize the housework to require the smallest expenditure of energy and to allow appropriate periods of rest. Shopping trips may need to be restricted. Unfortunately, the natural course of the disease is such that patients may eventually be unable to work, and their activity becomes more and more restricted until they must be confined to a bed or chair to avoid symptoms.

Tolerance testing is becoming popular to determine the patient's cardiac performance capacity (see Chap. 87). It may be used when a patient's history is thought to be inaccurate or when a patient's performance has not been tested, such as during convalescence following a myocardial infarction or following surgical correction of a cardiac abnormality. The tolerance test may be simple or sophisticated. A safe, simple, and inexpensive test can be performed by the physician with very little specialized equipment by accompanying the patient as he or she walks rapidly up and down stairs or down a hallway. Such a test may disclose vital information which is not otherwise readily apparent; extreme breathlessness may be evident in a relatively complaint-free, stoic, chronically ill patient; no breathlessness may be evident in the overreactive, emotional patient who has been distracted by conversation. During and after the test the physician should observe the development of symptoms, including dyspnea and chest pain, the general appearance of the patient; the appearance of a ventricular gallop sound, atrial gallop sound, abnormal apex or ectopic precordial impulse, pulsus alternans, or rales; change in blood pressure; and electrocardiographic abnormalities, including the development of arrhythmias and abnormal ST-segment changes. From this information, the physician may gain insight into the degree of activity that may properly be prescribed for the patient. A more sophisticated tolerance test utilizes a motor-driven treadmill, continuous electrocardiographic monitoring during the test period, and determination of the blood pressure before, during, and after the test (see Chap. 87). This more sophisticated test permits physiological monitoring for safety during the course of the testing. Its objective is to determine the maximum degree of exercise that can be achieved by the patient, together with the physiological correlates of blood pressure and heart rate, to enable the physician to predict those activities in which the patient can safely take part. In the controlled setting of the treadmill test, the physician observes the maximum level of exercise a patient can perform without overt symptoms or occult arrhythmias or ischemic electrocardiographic changes. This individually determined level of exercise is then compared with the expected level of exercise for various activities and occupations, available from standard reference sources. In spite of tolerance testing, the final arbiter of the permissible degree of activity is and should remain the commonsense judgment of the treating physician.

Relief from emotional trauma is more difficult to achieve than physical rest. It is more difficult to judge the patient's existing degree of emotional turmoil, and it is more difficult to determine the effect of this turmoil on the patient's cardiovascular system. When a patient has hungry children to feed, the emotional impact of requiring him or her to cease all activity may be more devastating than the physical strain of performing light work. In some patients, rest may not be possible until an important document has been read or difficult decisions made. Slight sedation at night and during the day may be needed for some patients, but should not be routinely prescribed nor used over a prolonged period unless absolutely necessary.

Control Heart Rate

Abnormalities of heart rate or rhythm can precipitate or aggravate heart failure in certain heart diseases. In congestive heart failure of any etiology these abnormalities are distinct from the standard compensatory sinus tachycardia mediated by increased sympathetic activity.

Intermittent ectopic tachyarrhythmias or severe sinus tachycardia can increase ventricular dysfunctions in heart failure due to ischemic heart disease by increasing cardiac oxygen consumption and aggravating myocardial ischemia. The same is true for dilated cardiomyopathy. Such tachyarrhythmias are often so subtle that the patient is unaware of them. The therapy of tachyarrhythmias is discussed in Chap. 29. Frequent premature ventricular beats can enhance mitral regurgitation. If one suspects such occult arrhythmia as a contributing factor in the worsening of heart failure, continuous 24-h ambulatory monitoring should be done to make the diagnosis (Chap. 88). When the patient has severe heart failure, ventricular contractile depressant effects of many antiarrhythmic drugs must be considered and are discussed in Chap. 29. From a practical standpoint, if cessation of the arrhythmia is a major benefit, any negative inotropic effect of the necessary antiarrhythmia drug is usually well tolerated. The potential for worsening latent heart failure by beta-blocking drugs is not as real as was previously thought, and the use of such drugs for angina or arrhythmias in patients with latent or mild congestive failure is now believed to be reasonably safe. Increases in diuretic drugs may be required to allow addition of beta-blocking drugs.

The appearance of atrial fibrillation intermittently or continuously where sinus rhythm was present previously may suddenly and severely aggravate or precipitate heart failure in patients with idiopathic hypertrophic subaortic stenosis (see Chap. 56). This symptomatic worsening is believed to be due to the loss of the atrial contraction as a contributor to late ventricular filling in a ventricle which has reduced compliance. Beta-blocking drugs may be useful in this condition. Atrial antiarrhythmic drugs may be used when sinus rhythm has been restored.

In mitral stenosis, the natural history includes sudden appearance of intermittent atrial fibrillation, usually followed by persistence of this arrhythmia. When there is sudden atrial fibrillation with a rapid ventricular response, severe worsening of the degree of heart failure and even pulmonary edema is not infrequent. The problem is the decreased time left for diastolic filling when tachycardia increases the portion of time per minute that the heart must spend in systole. If total cardiac output is to be maintained, the flow per diastolic second across the mitral valve must increase. Such increase requires increased left atrial pressure and causes increased dyspnea or even pulmonary edema. Control of the heart rate is the important goal of treatment for this condition. Digitalis is the usual therapy. It increases the atrioventricular refractory time, thereby decreasing the number of atrial impulses per minute which can get through to the ventricle. Propranolol may also be used in this situation to decrease the ventricular response to the atrial rate.

In mitral stenosis patients with intermittent rapid atrial fibrillation in a background of sinus rhythm with no heart failure, the rapid ventricular rate often causes intermittent heart failure. Such patients should be placed on regular digitalis dosage to prevent atrial fibrillation from causing rapid ventricular responses. Conversely, digitalis has been proved to be of no use in patients with left-sided heart failure symptoms due to pure mitral stenosis with sinus rhythm and no intermittent atrial fibrillation.

A very slow heart rate due to complete heart block can initiate or precipitate heart failure, especially in patients with preexisting heart disease. In order to maintain cardiac output despite a very low number of beats per minute, stroke volume per beat must be excessive. Such excessive stroke volume usually requires large end-diastolic volume, especially if coexisting primary myocardial disease limits the ejection fraction. As shown in Fig. 23-1, increased end-diastolic volume can cause congestive symptoms, and pacemaker therapy may be required, as described in Chap. 29.

Increase Myocardial Contractility and Increase Cardiac Output

The effect of administering a positive inotropic drug such as digitalis is shown in Fig. 23-10. An increase in myocardial contractility results, and the

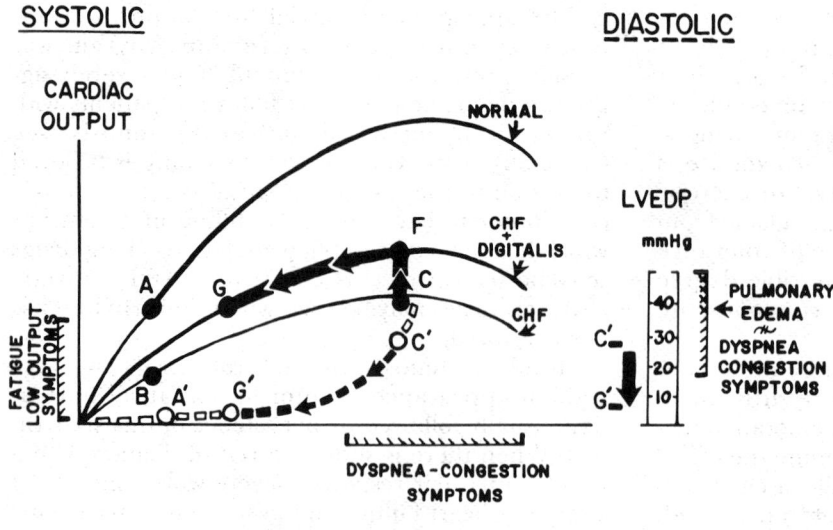

SYSTOLIC   DIASTOLIC

LV DIASTOLIC VOLUME

FIGURE 23-10 Heart failure and digitalis. Effect of digitalis on the Frank-Starling compensation, the cardiac output, and the congestive symptoms of heart failure. (See text for explanation.)

solid lower systolic curve of congestive heart failure (CHF) is increased to the intermediate solid curve of increased contractility with congestive heart failure at point F. On this improved curve, the required cardiac output can be achieved at point G. As the ejection fraction increases, cardiac size decreases and the stimulus to retain salt and water decreases. The ventricle then has moved from C′ to G′ on the dashed diastolic pressure curve with resultant lower left ventricular end-diastolic pressure (LVEDP), and there is relief of congestive symptoms with maintenance of cardiac output. If the original cardiac output had been low, then the positive inotropic drug would increase the cardiac output by this mechanism. All of the positive inotropic drugs, including digitalis, dopamine, dobutamine, and amrinone, affect the failing heart in this way, although the mechanism by which each works may vary.

Digitalis has the following actions: the drug increases myocardial contractility; increases the cardiac output in the failing heart; decreases conduction velocity of the AV node and Purkinje fibers; may increase the conduction velocity in the atrium; decreases the refractory period in the atrium and ventricle; increases the refractory period in the AV node and Purkinje fibers; increases the excitability of the Purkinje fibers, has little effect on the excitability of the atrium, and has a variable effect on the excitability of the ventricles; increases the pacemaker automaticity of the Purkinje fibers and has little effect on the pacemaker automaticity of the SA node; produces arrhythmias in toxic doses which include AV block, atrial arrhythmias, especially atrial tachycardia with block, and ventricular arrhythmias; and shortens the QT interval in the electrocardiogram, prolongs the PR interval, and produces displacement of the ST segment (mean ST vector becomes opposite to mean QRS vector).

The description of the observations by William Withering,[47] who first used digitalis, is reproduced below since it is such an important contribution to the history of medicine.

In the month of November 1777, in consequence of an application from that very celebrated surgeon, Mr. Russel of Worcester I sent him the following account, which I choose to introduce here, as showing the ideas I then entertained of the medicine, and how much I was mistaken as to its real dose: "I generally order it in decoction. Three drams of the dried leaves, collected at the time of the blossoms expanding, boiling in twelve to eight ounces of water. Two spoonfuls of this medicine, given every two hours, will sooner or later excite a nausea. I have sometimes used the green leaves gathered in winter, but then I order three times the weight; and in one instance I used three ounces to a pint decoction, before the desired effect took place. I considered the Foxglove thus given, as the most certain diuretic I know, nor do its diuretic effects depend merely upon the nausea it produces, for in cases where squill and ipecac have been so given as to keep up a nausea several days together, and the flow of urine not taken place, I have found the Foxglove to succeed; and I have, in more than one instance, given the Foxglove in small and more distant doses, so that the flow of urine has taken place without any sensible affection of the stomach; but in general I give it in the manner first mentioned, and order one dose to be taken after the sickness commences. I then omit all medicine, except those of the cordial kind are wanted, during the space of three, four, or five days. By this time the nausea abates, and the appetite becomes better than it was before. Sometimes the brain is considerably affected by medicine, and indistinct vision ensues; but I have never yet found any permanent bad effects from it."

Digitalis is the most important of the positive inotropic drugs (Fig. 23-10). The discussion here concerns the use of digitalis in patients with heart failure. In particular the positive inotropic effect of digitalis will be explored, and certain aspects of its pharmacology and toxic manifestations will be discussed. Digitalis also has a second, separate thera-

produce profound weakness and induce cardiac arrhythmias. Other diuretics do not produce a kaluresis and may under certain circumstances cause potassium toxicity.

2. In some patients the hypovolemia produced by a vigorous diuresis may cause considerable harm or even death.

A diuretic is used to provide a selective reduction of a portion of an excessively used compensation in order to relieve congestive symptoms. Use of the Frank-Starling mechanism to increase the force of systolic cardiac contraction by increased diastolic ventricular filling is one of the major compensatory mechanisms which maintain cardiac output in the failing heart (see Fig. 23-1). If too much of this compensation is removed by overvigorous diuresis, cardiac output will fall to levels which cause symptoms shown as moving too far to the left on the lower solid-line curve in Fig. 23-11. The Frank-Starling compensatory mechanism is lost and cardiac output and tissue perfusion suffer, producing complaints of weakness and even confusion and oliguria. The extreme effectiveness of diuretics makes it possible to "overdiurese" even the most severe cases of congestive heart failure, and, in fact, the most common mistake in using diuretics is using them excessively. In general, it is far wiser to err on the side of going too slowly with diuresis than to proceed too quickly.

To maximize effectiveness and minimize possible harm, diuretics should be used in the following manner. Note the importance of collecting data to assist in avoiding some of the complications of diuresis.

1. Determination of accurate daily body weight is the best way to monitor a diuresis. Since each liter of lost fluid weighs 1 kg and since daily weight changes in excess of 0.25 kg are all due to loss or gain of body water, a daily weight determination is always desirable and at times indispensable. It enables the physician to appraise the effect of treatment on fluid loss on a daily basis. Whether the fluid loss itself is beneficial or harmful is determined by other clinical observations. In patients with chronic heart failure who must attempt to maintain their weight at a "dry" level, daily weighing may help greatly in determining the appropriate diuretic dosage. Weight gain of 1 or 2 kg in a few days would indicate that additional diuretic drugs should be used. Weight gain or loss can also be indicative of the need to adjust the interval of time between doses.

2. Many diuretics produce electrolyte depletion. Therefore, the serum level of these ions should be measured. To minimize electrolyte depletion, it is frequently necessary to supplement the diuretic with potassium chloride or to use combinations of potassium-wasting with potassium-sparing diuretics. Primary renal failure or a ris-

ing blood urea nitrogen (BUN) level indicates that the potassium supplementation and any potassium-sparing drug must be decreased or eliminated.

3. Accurate measurement of the intake of fluid and output of urine is essential during the early days of treatment. Along with accurate recording of body weight and hematocrit determination, these will enable the physician to estimate the amount of diuresis and its effect on the patient.

4. To assess the effect of the altered blood volume on the circulation, specific measurements must be made. Since we cannot predict the exact amount of diuresis that will occur, nor the location of the heart's function on the ventricular function curve, nor the degree of cardiac compliance present on an individual patient, we must monitor certain features of the clinical response to diuresis. The pulse rate should be recorded frequently, because an increased pulse rate is a sign that the patient's response is not ideal. Hypotension recorded while the patient is in the recumbent position is a clear sign that the patient is not tolerating the diuresis well. A moderate increase in pulse rate and reduction of systolic pressure occurring after the patient stands for a few minutes may be a signal that excessive overdiuresis has occurred. Cardiac arrhythmias may occur after the patient stands for a few minutes. Some patients will complain of thirst, dizziness, fatigue, and weakness as they are relieved of their dyspnea. In the advanced state, overdiuresis may be followed by oliguria and progressive renal failure. Older patients may become confused or have a personality change.

5. To ensure that these drugs will reach the renal tubule certain diuretics should be given when the patient is at rest, because patients with heart failure may have greater cardiac output and renal blood flow at rest than when they are walking around. Similarly, it may be necessary for a drug to be given intravenously to assure that it will reach the renal tubule, because severe heart failure may impair the absorption of a drug from the intestinal tract or from an intramuscular depot.

Certain patients with heart failure may need no diuretics; some will require mild diuretics given several times a week; other will require more potent diuretics, alone or in combination with others. The physician must manage each patient as an individual and modify the rest, diet, digitalis, and diuretics in order to achieve the optimum state of rehabilitation. While this is being done, the patient must be watched carefully to ensure that no harm is caused by the therapy.

Specific Diuretic Agents Diuretic drugs may be divided into the following groups: thiazide and related sulfonamide compounds, mercurial compounds, potassium-retaining drugs, very potent diuretics, and osmotic diuretics (see Table 23-1).

Since they may be taken orally, *thiazide* and related sulfonamide compounds have largely replaced mercurial diuretics. These drugs are absorbed rapidly from the gastrointestinal tract, and the onset of action on the kidney occurs within 1 h. The duration of action varies with the compound, but the effect of most thiazide drugs lasts for 12 to 24 h. Thiazide drugs act predominantly on the distal tubule of the kidney, producing an increase in urinary excretion of sodium, potassium, chloride, and water. All of the thiazide diuretics listed in Table 23-1 are equally effective.

The toxic effects of thiazide diuretics include agranulocytosis, thrombocytopenia, pancreatitis, glomerulonephritis, necrotizing vasculitis, intrahepatic cholestasis, skin rashes, and yellow vision. The newborn child of a mother receiving thiazide diuretics may have thrombocytopenia, neutropenia, and agranulocytosis. Azotemia may develop, most often in patients with subnormal renal function or as a result of reduced plasma volume and renal blood flow. Thiazide diuretics may induce hyperuricemia and precipitate an acute attack of gout. In gouty patients, such attacks may be prevented by the use of uricosuric agents, and attacks may be treated with colchicine. Hyperglycemia may also develop as a result of thiazide therapy, but it is rarely severe and does not substantially alter the diabetic state. Potassium chloride supplementation or the use of a potassium-retaining diuretic may prevent this hyperglycemia effect.

The most common complications of thiazide di-

TABLE 23-1 Classification and Dosage of Diuretic Drugs

Generic Name	Trade Name	Usual Daily Dosage, mg
Thiazides and related drugs:		
Chlorothiazide	Diuril	500–1.500
Hydrochlorothiazide	Esidrix, HydroDiuril, Orctic	50–150
Methyclothiazide	Enduron	5–10
Polythiazide	Renese	2–8
Chlorthalidone	Hygroton	50–100
Quinethazone	Hydromox	50–150
Mercurials:		
Meralluride	Mercuhydrin	2 (ml)
Mercaptomerin	Thiomerin	2 (ml)
Potassium-retaining drugs:		
Spironolactone	Aldactone	100
Triamterene	Dyrenium	200
Very potent diuretics:		
Ethacrynic acid	Edecrin	50–200
Furosemide	Lasix	40–200

*The daily dosage listed does not imply that the drug is given daily. The frequency of administration is determined by many factors. See text.

Source: Modified from Brest et al.[71a]; reprinted with permission of authors and publisher.

uretics are hypokalemia and hypochloremic alkalosis. Severe degrees of potassium loss caused by these drugs may result in hyporeflexia, flaccid paralysis, respiratory arrest, ileus, renal tubular dysfunction, and degenerative changes in the heart and skeletal muscle. The single most common problem, however, relates to the cardiac arrhythmias that may be precipitated by hypokalemia. To relieve or prevent hypokalemia in a mildly failing patient who does not require daily diuretics, one should give the diuretic for 5 days out of 7 and be sure the patient eats potassium-containing foods such as orange juice or bananas daily. The normal kidney can then retain potassium 2 of every 7 days.

Since many patients who receive thiazide diuretics require oral potassium supplementation, many preparations of potassium salts are available. If a preparation does not contain chloride, the diet or some acceptable non-sodium-containing source must provide it. The enteric-coated tablets of potassium chloride may produce stenosing small-bowel ulcers, so a solution of potassium chloride in tomato juice should be used. Unfortunately, it has long-lasting bad taste. Slow-release potassium chloride tablets without enteric coating have recently been proposed instead, but the safety of these slow-release preparations have been controversial. The alternatives to oral potassium supplementation are dietary supplementation with high potassium-containing foods, intermittent therapy allowing natural repletion of potassium, or combination therapy with an aldosterone antagonist. Potassium supplements or aldosterone antagonists should not be given to patients with renal failure. If a potassium-retaining diuretic is given at the same time as a thiazide diuretic, all potassium chloride medication must be discontinued to avoid any potassium intoxication. The physician must also be alert to the possibility of potassium intoxication in any patient whose renal function is deteriorating, even among patients receiving potassium-losing diuretics where no supplemental potassium is being used.

Oral and parenteral *mercurial diuretics* are not used today. They have been replaced by the new oral diuretics and the group of very potent diuretics which can be given orally or intravenously.

The potassium-retaining drugs, *spironolactone* and *triamterene,* are more effective when combined with other diuretics than when used alone. Spironolactone (Aldactone) begins to act within 24 to 48 h after oral administration, and its maximum effect may not be attained for 3 days. Spironolactone acts on the distal tubules, offsetting the effects of aldosterone and deoxycorticosterone. It increases the excretion of sodium, promotes the retention of potassium, and decreases the excretion of hydrogen ion. Triamterene (Dyrenium) also acts on the renal tubule, promoting potassium retention. This drug is not an aldosterone antagonist. Both these drugs may produce hyperkalemia, so potassium supplementation must be discontinued if either drug is administered. Spironolactone may cause mental confusion, drowsiness, skin rash, and gynecomastia. Triamterene may cause nausea, diarrhea, vomiting, headache, and weakness. These drugs are not the agents of choice in patients with renal failure of any degree. They are most effective in patients with marked secondary aldosteronism.

Ethacrynic acid (Edecrin) and furosemide (Lasix) (see Table 23-1) are the most potent diuretic agents in existence today. They are excellent but expensive drugs that can be used orally and intravenously.[72] They have become the favorites of many physicians and are often the first diuretics to be given. We believe they should be used in patients with heart failure only if the patients do not respond to thiazide compounds. These drugs prevent the reabsorption of sodium in the ascending limb of the loop of Henle. The excretion of potassium and hydrogen is increased, but to a lesser degree than the excretion of sodium and chloride. Diuretic action begins within an hour (probably in about 30 min) after oral administration of either drug and lasts for 6 to 8 h. When injected intravenously, diuretic action begins a few minutes after injection and reaches its peak effect in 1 h, and the effects last for several hours. The drugs produce an increased venous capacitance which is useful in the relief of acute pulmonary edema. When the prescribed dose of either drug does not cause a diuresis, the dosage must be increased rather than giving the same dose more often.

These two drugs are very effective; they are also potentially very harmful if not properly used. The dangers include low cardiac output, hyponatremia, hypokalemia, hypochloremia, and alkalosis. An excessive diuresis is always a potential problem. It may so reduce the circulatory blood volume that circulatory collapse may develop. Both the potassium loss and hypovolemia may precipitate a cardiac arrhythmia in patients receiving digitalis. Vascular thrombosis and embolism may also occur after excessive diuresis. These drugs may produce hyperglycemia, hyperuricemia, agranulocytosis, and acute hearing loss, although there is suggestive evidence that hearing loss is more likely to occur when both drugs plus kanamycin are used together than when either drug is used separately. Ethacrynic acid and furosemide are effective even when renal function is impaired. They may be useful in the treatment of acute pulmonary edema occurring in patients with chronic heart failure, but they may be harmful in patients with pulmonary edema occurring with normal blood volume and a normal-sized heart.

It is customary to use a thiazide diuretic plus ethacrynic acid or furosemide in patients with severe congestive heart failure.

The osmotic diuretics, *mannitol* and *urea*, are rarely used today. When heart failure is present, either may produce further cardiocirculatory overload by increasing plasma volume. In addition, urea has an unpleasant taste.

Potassium Depletion Potassium depletion in patients with heart failure is usually due to the effects of diuretics. The thiazides, ethacrynic acid, and furosemide may produce severe potassium depletion. The depletion is accentuated when the patient has diarrhea, is given intravenous fluid without potassium, or has inadequate dietary potassium intake. The excessive loss of potassium may produce alkalosis, because the hydrogen ions may enter the cells, leaving the plasma alkaline. Potassium depletion may cause weakness and diminished reflexes and may also precipitate cardiac dysrhythmias in the patient who is receiving digitalis.

The electrocardiographic changes typical of potassium depletion may be the first diagnostic clue to this disorder. The serum potassium level in such patients may be normal or slightly low, although weakness and diminished reflexes may occur with a normal serum potassium level.

When potassium depletion requires prompt therapy, 40 meq of potassium chloride (3 g) dissolved in 250 ml of 5% glucose in water may be given intravenously in 4 h, and it may be necessary to repeat the dose in 12 to 24 h. Great care must be exercised when potassium chloride is given intravenously: a large vein or central venous catheter should be used; the serum potassium level should be known before potassium is given; the urine output should be adequate; and the heart rhythm should be continuously monitored with the electrocardiograph during the infusion. When oral medication is acceptable, 1 g of potassium chloride (13.4 meq) may be given in tomato juice three times a day. Preparations such as Kaon or Triplex, which contain potassium salts, may be used if the chloride ion is supplied from other sources. Some believe that chloride must be available in such patients. In the usual case when the thiazides or ethacrynic acid or furosemide must be continued, potassium chloride must be given continuously in order to prevent potassium depletion. Potassium-retaining diuretics such as triamterene (Dyrenium) or spironolactone (Aldactone) may be used in conjunction with the potassium-losing group, to offset the potassium depletion. Potassium supplements should not be used while potassium-retaining diuretics are being given, since dangerous hyperkalemia may develop.

Potassium excess and toxicity may develop in the following circumstances in patients with heart failure who are receiving potassium chloride supplementation: when potassium chloride supplementation is continued in a patient who no longer receives a potassium-losing diuretic or has been started on a potassium-sparing diuretic; when potassium is given to a patient with renal failure (i.e., with a blood urea nitrogen level above 60 mg/dl); when potassium is given to a patient who has less than 500 to 600 ml of urine output daily; and when potassium is given to a patient with metabolic acidosis.

Hyponatremia may be a problem—often of ominous significance—which exists when the serum sodium level is below 130 meq/liter. In congestive heart failure cases, hyponatremia is almost always associated with excess body water and is often called *dilutional hyponatremia.* The body stores of sodium are usually increased but, because of low-salt diets and diuretics, not as much as the total body water is increased. Accordingly, the ratio of body content of sodium to body water (i.e., the serum sodium concentration) may be low as a result of excess body water. Whenever hyponatremia is present in congestive heart failure, it is desirable to try to reduce body water content relative to sodium content by reducing the patient's fluid intake to 500 ml daily. This reduction may be aided by the cautious use of diuretics, and potassium supplements should also be given if not previously supplied. Sodium should not be given since total body sodium is already increased. Hypertonic sodium chloride should never be used except to combat acute water intoxication.

Hyperchloremic acidosis may develop in patients with heart failure who are given ammonium chloride, L-lysine, L-arginine monohydrochloride, or acetazolamide (Diamox) in excessive amounts over a long period of time. These drugs are contraindicated in patients with renal disease, hepatic failure, and respiratory acidosis. The symptoms are hyperventilation (which may be confused with the respiratory distress of heart failure), anorexia, nausea, vomiting, drowsiness, and even stupor. The serum electrolytes show elevation of the chloride level and a decrease in pH. The condition is treated with an intravenous infusion of 5% sodium bicarbonate solution.

Management of Excessive Diuresis As discussed above, diuretics may be used in patients to the point where the reduction of venous filling pressure reduces cardiac output (see Fig. 23-11). This is a very frequent complication of diuretics. This point is often detected by observing muscle weakness and fatigue or by a rising blood urea nitrogen or a drop in arterial blood pressure when the patient stands up. In some patients with very severely reduced myocardial contractility, constrictive pericarditis, cor pulmonale, or poor cardiac compliance, the cardiac output may fall even with venous pressure above normal and with some edema present. Patients at this stage complain of an extreme degree of muscular weakness, lassitude, and inability to get up from bed.

The elderly patient with marginal cerebral blood flow may become confused or have a subtle negative personality change. The level of the blood urea nitrogen may become elevated under these circumstances because of reduced renal blood flow. Treatment requires removal of diuretics and, if that does not work, removal of dietary sodium restriction for a day or two.

Venous-Vasodilating Drugs Congestive heart failure can be treated by altering the preload with drugs that dilate the venous system. There are three major categories of vasodilator drugs: those that act principally on the veins to increase venous pooling, those that act principally on the arteries to decrease systemic arterial resistance, and those that have combined venous-pooling and arterial dilatation effects.[4] These drugs vary in method of administration, onset of action, duration of action, and specific toxic side effects summarized in Table 23-2. The venous-pooling drugs will be discussed here. The arterial-dilating drugs and the mixed venous-pooling and arterial-dilating drugs will be discussed later in the section on afterload reduction.

When a drug works directly only to reduce venous tone and thereby increase venous pooling, it only reduces preload.[73] The effect of preload reduction is shown in Figs. 23-11 and 23-12. As venous pooling occurs, diastolic ventricular volume falls, just as it does with a diuretic along the diastolic curve (dashed line) from C' to D' in Fig. 23-11. There is a large reduction in end-diastolic pressure and in congestive symptoms. Cardiac output falls from C to D along the systolic curve (solid lower curve) as preload is reduced. However, this output reduction may be small or may not be perceived at all in severe heart failure because of the flat systolic curve (solid lower curve) relating output to ventricular volume.

From the above description, it is clear that overuse of venous-vasodilating drugs can cause low-output symptoms or even shock in an improperly selected patient. For example, if cardiac output is very low and end-diastolic pressure is not high, perhaps as a result of previous extensive use of diuretics, then cardiac output may further deteriorate with venous vasodilatation.[12,70] It is therefore important to estimate reliably or actually measure ventricular filling pressure before administering vasodilator drugs.

Generally, the patient with both high diastolic ventricular pressure and low cardiac output is most benefited by vasodilator therapy.[74] Other patients will benefit most from a mixture of venous and arterial vasodilatation (see Figs. 23-2B and 23-12). A patient with advanced heart failure who suffers weakness on exertion during the day and dyspnea at night may be improved by arterial dilators to increase cardiac output during the day and by venous dilators at bedtime to further reduce preload and resultant nocturnal dyspnea.

Two of the major venous vasodilator drugs are *nitroglycerin* and *isosorbide dinitrate.*

Nitroglycerin causes a direct relaxation of the smooth muscle in the systemic veins, which increases the capacitance of this reservoir. As blood pools in the veins, cardiac size is reduced and there is a direct reduction of ventricular preload. Nitroglycerin is usually given sublingually. When given by this route it is rapidly absorbed, has a peak hemodynamic effect in 5 min, and lasts for 30 min. The average sublingual dose in treating chronic heart failure is

TABLE 23-2 Summary of the Action of Major Vasodilator Drugs

Predominant Action in Heart Failure	Drug	Usual Route of Administration	Peak Effect	Duration of Action	Average Dose	Major Side Effects and Comments	Mechanism of action
Venous pooling	Nitroglycerin	Sublingual	5 min	30 min	0.4–2.4 mg	Occasional headache limited to first weeks of therapy with all nitrates	Direct effect to relax smooth muscle of veins
		Topical	60 min	5 h	1½ in	Messy	Direct effect to relax smooth muscle of veins
	Isosorbide dinitrate (Isordil)	Sublingual	20 min	1 h	10 mg		Direct effect to relax smooth muscle of veins
		Oral	60 min	5 h	20 mg		
Arterial dilation	Hydralazine (Apresoline)	Oral	60 min	6 h	50–75 mg	Fluid retention, LE-like syndrome, tolerance	Direct effect to relax smooth muscle of arteries
	Minoxidil	Oral	? in CHF	? in CHF	? in CHF	Minimal experience in heart failure, possible salt and water retention, hypertrichosis	Direct effect to relax smooth muscle of arteries
	Phenoxybenzamine (Dibenzyline)	Oral	1 h	3–4 days	10–30 mg	Orthostatic hypotension, sexual impotence, nasal congestion	Alpha-adrenergic blockade
	Phentolamine (Regitine)	IV	5 min	12–24 h	1–2 mg/min titrated		Alpha-adrenergic blockade
Mixed venous pooling and arterial dilation	Nitroprusside (Nipride)	IV	1 min	5 min	By titration of effect— 40–60 µg/min	Degraded by exposure to light; prolonged infusion produces toxic levels of cyanide	Direct relaxation of smooth muscle of arteries and veins
	Prazosin (Minipress)	Oral	60 min	6 h	2–7 mg	Occasional mild nausea; attenuation of effect develops requiring increased dose; salt and water retention	Blocks phosphodiesterase in vascular smooth muscle and also causes postsynaptic alpha-adrenergic receptor blockade, causing balanced dilation of arteries and veins
	Captopril	Oral	1½ h	6 h	25 mg	Hypotension; bradycardia	Inhibits the conversion of angiotensin I to angiotensin II; causes decreased systemic vascular resistance and may decrease venous tone in heart failure

Note: CHF = congestive heart failure.

0.3 to 0.6 mg, but much larger doses have been used as emergency therapy for pulmonary edema.

Nitroglycerin in ointment form is also easily absorbed through the skin with a hemodynamic effect which reaches its peak in 1 h and has a duration of 5 h.[73] The average topical dose is 1.5 in of ointment containing 12.5 mg/in. In one recent report pulmonary capillary wedge pressure was decreased from an average of 30 to 19 mmHg in 10 patients with severe chronic congestive heart failure who were treated with 1.5 to 4 in of topical nitroglycerin.[73] The ointment is rather messy for daytime use in the ambulatory patient, but it is especially useful as a therapy at bedtime. Patients who are particularly troubled by orthopnea, sleeplessness, nightmares, or paroxysmal nocturnal dyspnea may achieve significant relief with the application of 1 or 2 in of topical nitroglycerin ointment at bedtime. The use of sublingually administered nitroglycerin, 0.4 mg, may quickly relieve episodes of nocturnal dyspnea.

Nitroglycerin can be given intravenously as well, with rapid onset of action and brief duration (Chap. 45).

The effect of nitroglycerin on cardiac output is variable, depending on the severity of the heart failure condition. In general, the higher the initial wedge pressure and the lower the initial cardiac output, the more likely it is that nitroglycerin will achieve a moderate increase in cardiac output. However, Massie et al., in an excellent study of 12 patients suffering refractory heart failure, reported no change in an initial cardiac index of 2.1 liters/min/m² with a fall in wedge pressure from 28 to 17 mmHg under nitroglycerin therapy.[75] Accordingly, nitroglycerin can be thought of as a major preload-reducing agent which changes points C and C′ to points D and D′ on the systolic and diastolic curves of the Frank-Starling relationship in the failing ventricle, shown in Fig. 23-12. These changes are similar to those produced by diuretics, dietary salt restriction, and tourniquets.

DISORDERS OF THE CARDIOVASCULAR SYSTEM

Sublingual nitroglycerin has also been used for treatment of acute pulmonary edema.[4] A moderate fall of pulmonary wedge pressure has been seen in patients with acute pulmonary edema who were treated with 0.3 mg of nitroglycerin administered sublingually. Pulmonary edema has also been treated experimentally by 0.8 to 2.4 mg of nitroglycerin sublingually given at intervals of 5 to 10 min as the only treatment, with excellent clinical results.

Isosorbide dinitrate (Isordil) is another currently available venous-pooling drug. Its major effect, like that of nitroglycerin, is direct relaxation of the systemic venous smooth muscle, which results in venous pooling and reduction of ventricular preload. When given sublingually, its peak effect occurs in 20 min and the duration of the effect is 1 to 1½ h. The usual sublingual dose is 5 to 10 mg. Despite early controversy about hepatic degradation, oral administration has now been established as an effective method of achieving relatively long-lasting, hemodynamically effective nitrate medication. The peak effect occurs in 1 h, and a significant effect lasts for 5 h. The usual oral dose of isosorbide dinitrate is 10 to 30 mg every 4 to 6 h. Rarely, dosage of 40 to 60 mg every 4 to 6 h is required.

Long-term tolerance to nitrates has been questioned, but, in a study by Kovick, each patient showed a further reduction in pulmonary wedge pressure when sublingual isosorbide dinitrate was given as a single dose upon recatheterization after an average of 7 months of chronic isosorbide dinitrate therapy.[76] Side effects of chronic isosorbide dinitrate use do not appear to be significant; Williams et al. observed no adverse reactions from nitrates over an average of 7 months.[74] One relatively minor side effect of nitrate therapy is the occurrence of headaches in some patients at the onset of the treatment. The headaches are usually of limited duration, however, so that if the patient can tolerate the discomfort for 1 to 2 weeks at the outset, the headaches generally resolve and do not give further trouble. The reduction of preload by any means in improperly selected patients who do not have initially excessive diastolic ventricular volume and pressure can lead to low cardiac output, hypotension, and syncope.

Decrease Afterload and Increase Cardiac Output

As discussed earlier, the chronic increase in arteriolar tone results in a vicious circle or positive-feedback loop which worsens the heart failure (see Fig. 23-2B). While the increased arteriolar tone provides compensation by maintaining blood pressure and redistributing the limited cardiac output, it also results in an increased cardiac afterload which itself further compromises the failing heart. Arterial vasodilator therapy of heart failure consists of selective, controlled reduction of afterload by drugs, often done in conjunction with preload reduction.

The effects of both arterial and venous vasodilators on heart failure are diagramed in Fig. 23-12, and the effects of afterload are shown in Figs. 23-2A, 23-2B, and 23-12. These figures depict car-

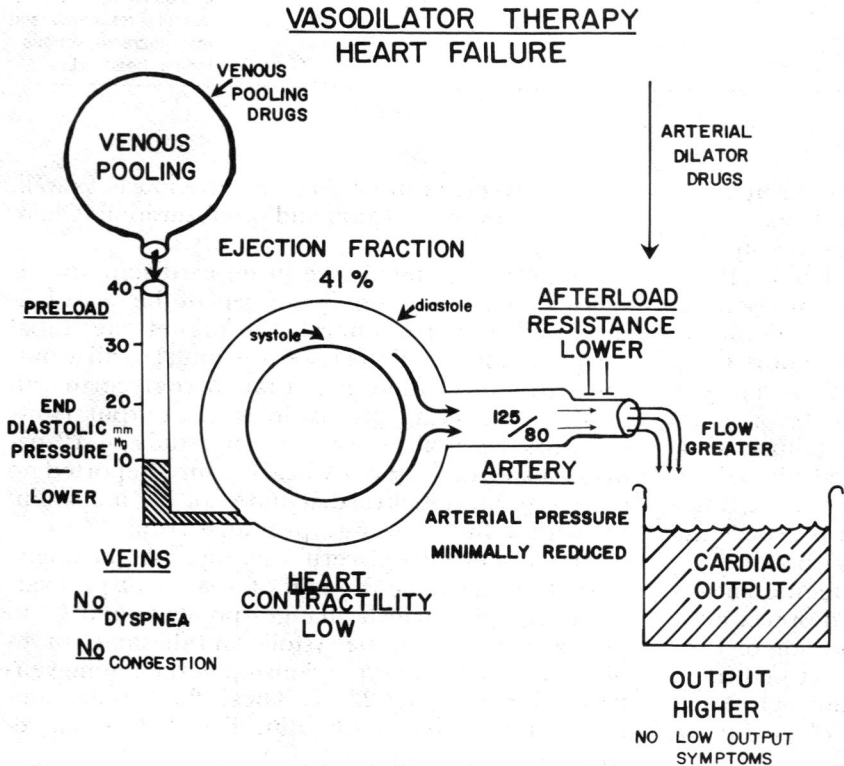

FIGURE 23-12 Diagram of effects of arterial dilatation and venous pooling drugs on the failing heart and circulation. (See text for explanation.)

diac output and three of the four major factors which determine it: preload, contractility, and afterload. The fourth major factor, heart rate, is not of major importance to this topic.

As the vasodilator drug causes a reduction in peripheral arterial resistance, peripheral flow increases. If stroke volume did not increase, there would be depletion of central arterial volume and central blood pressure would fall, resulting in disastrous syncope and shock. Fortunately, as resistance falls, afterload is reduced and, even though contractility remains low, stroke volume and ejection fraction are increased because it is easier for the heart to eject blood against a decreased afterload. Since blood pressure is the product of resistance times flow, the central blood pressure falls little, despite the decreased resistance, because the flow increases simultaneously. Cardiac output is increased and low-output symptoms are ameliorated. Congestive symptoms are also improved by the arterial vasodilators, because the end-systolic residual volume and consequently the end-diastolic volume both fall as the afterload falls (compare the size of the concentric circles in Fig. 23-12 with those in Fig. 23-2B). The fall in end-diastolic volume also lowers end-diastolic pressure [see also diastolic curve (dashed line) of Fig. 23-11], further relieving congestive symptoms.

Arterial vasodilator therapy has additional beneficial effects on severe heart failure patients with mitral or aortic regurgitation. Systolic regurgitation of blood across the mitral valve is enhanced by increases in afterload which oppose antegrade ejection from the left ventricle. Therefore, in patients with severe mitral regurgitation, the vasodilator therapy reduces the extent of regurgitation. Similarly, in patients with aortic regurgitation, the amount of aortic regurgitation is reduced by decreasing the diastolic arterial resistance.

Vasodilator therapy in heart failure patients with ischemic coronary artery disease has unique advantages. Nitroprusside administration has been shown to reduce pressure time per minute and stress-time index, two of the determinants of oxygen consumption, with no fall in cardiac output or any increase in heart rate. Angina may be relieved and contractile function of ischemic ventricular muscle improved by such an improvement in the relation between myocardial oxygen demand and supply.

The effects of arterial vasodilator therapy on the heart rate and blood pressure are of special interest. One would expect reflex tachycardia with even moderate decreases in mean arterial pressure, and even greater tachycardia with the use of hydralazine (Apresoline), which has a sympathetically mediated direct effect to increase heart rate. Surprisingly and fortunately, no significant change in heart rate occurs when any of the current vasodilators are properly used to treat severe congestive heart failure. Instead, withdrawal of the excessive sympathetic stimulation of advanced heart failure decreases the heart rate, counterbalancing any tendency of the therapy to increase heart rate.

Initial experimental results with captopril, the angiotensin-converting enzyme inhibitor, show that this new drug lowers both blood pressure and heart rate.

Specific Arterial Dilator Drugs Four major arterial dilator drugs are currently in use, three of which may be given orally and one intravenously (see Table 23-2).

Hydralazine (Apresoline), which has been used for a number of years to treat systemic hypertension, is also widely used for arterial vasodilator therapy in heart failure.[77] It directly relaxes the smooth muscle of the arterial wall and has little or no effect on the veins. It is given orally and has a peak action in 1 h and a duration of 6 h. The usual dosage in treatment of congestive heart failure is 50 to 75 mg every 6 h, a smaller dosage than is used in the treatment of systemic hypertension. Hydralazine acts to reduce afterload and to allow increased cardiac output (Fig. 23-12) with little or no venous-pooling effect. The complication of tachycardia which occurs when hydralazine is used for treatment of hypertension does not occur when it is used to treat heart failure. Hydralazine causes a lupus erythematosus–like (LE) syndrome in 2 to 3 percent of hypertensive patients taking 200 to 400 mg of hydralazine per day for prolonged periods, but this syndrome appears to be dose-related and is rapidly reversed by putting a stop to hydralazine therapy. Since antinuclear antibody usually appears in the plasma 3 to 6 months before toxic symptoms develop, regular testing for antinuclear antibody is advised, so that the therapy may be discontinued before the LE syndrome occurs. Fluid retention is a known side effect of hydralazine use in the treatment of hypertension, and this may also occur in heart failure therapy. If it occurs, diuretics should be increased. Hydralazine should be useful when decreased kidney function complicates heart failure, because it increases renal blood flow.

Minoxidil is a new agent which has had moderate trial in treatment of hypertension but has not yet been approved by the FDA for clinical trial in treatment of heart failure. It appears to be of potential use in heart failure because it is a potent, direct arterial smooth-muscle relaxant, requiring only once-a-day dosage, and it is not associated with an LE syndrome. It has no effect on venous capacitance. Like hydralazine, minoxidil increases the cardiac output as it drops peripheral resistance in hypertensive patients. Fluid retention and hypertrichosis are side effects of minoxidil use in some patients.

Phenoxybenzamine (Dibenzyline) is an alpha-adrenergic blocking agent which has its predominant effect on the arterial resistance vessels. It can be given orally, it has a peak action in 1 h, and its duration of action is 3 to 4 days. Kovick et al. recently used phenoxybenzamine in combination with sublingually administered isosorbide dinitrate in a study of chronic therapy of refractory heart failure in 15 patients.[76] While all patients were classified as having severe heart failure and were refractory to conventional therapy before vasodilator treatment, all improved following therapy, and five returned to work. The only side effects attributed to the alpha blockage were as follows: two patients developed sexual impotency, one developed orthostatic hypotension, and three developed mild nasal congestion. While it is impossible to tell how much of the improvement resulted from the phenoxybenzamine and how much from the isosorbide dinitrate, this study was the first to establish that arterial dilators combined with venous-pooling drugs have a sustained effect in chronic heart failure cases.

Phentolamine (Regitine), an alpha-receptor blocking drug, has been used as an intravenous infusion as treatment for congestive heart failure. An increase in cardiac index and a fall in systemic vascular resistance occur, but the limitation to intravenous use is the major problem with this drug. An oral preparation of this drug is now being developed.

Drugs with Mixed Arterial-Dilating and Venous-Pooling Effects (See Table 23-2)

Some patients respond either to selected venous pooling or to arterial dilatation; others respond best to a combination of arterial dilatation and venous pooling. The combined effect is often achieved by administering both hydralazine and nitrates, but also may be provided in some cases by a single drug.[75] There are currently two such combination drugs: nitroprusside, which must be given intravenously, and prazosin, which may be given orally. A third experimental drug, captopril, which inhibits angiotensin-converting enzyme, can be taken orally and appears to affect both arteries and veins.

Nitroprusside relaxes the smooth muscle of arteries and veins. It has no direct effect on nonvascular smooth muscle or on the heart. It can only be given intravenously. When given by this route, its peak effect occurs almost instantly and the effect is gone 5 min after cessation of the drug. Nitroprusside has been widely used as therapy for cardiogenic shock resulting from myocardial infarction, but more recently, it has been used extensively in the acute therapy of severe refractory congestive heart failure.[78] It usually causes a substantial decrease in left ventricular end-diastolic pressure and a decrease in both systemic vascular resistance and venous tone. Its effect on cardiac output is variable and depends on the left ventricular filling pressure achieved. If the filling pressure falls below 10 mmHg, there is little increase in cardiac output, whereas if the filling pressure does not fall below 10 mmHg, there may be an increase in cardiac output. This variable effect of nitroprusside on cardiac output represents an interplay between the venous-pooling and arterial dilator effects of this drug (see Fig. 23-12). The arterial dilatation decreases afterload, increases

ejection fraction, and tends to increase cardiac output. The venous pooling reduces filling pressure to low levels, reducing use of the Frank-Starling mechanism (see Fig. 23-11) and either preventing an increase or causing a net reduction in cardiac output. Using nitroprusside to treat a patient with relatively low filling pressure may cause a reduction in cardiac output, so it is very important to know that left ventricular filling pressure is elevated before administration of this drug. The metabolic degradation of nitroprusside produces cyanide, and cyanide toxicity and even death may result from long periods of nitroprusside infusion. To prevent cyanide toxicity, the dose of nitroprusside should be limited, and hydroxocobalamin may be useful in the management of this problem.

Prazosin is an oral agent with combined arterial-dilating and venous-pooling effects and has recently been the topic of considerable interest, research, and controversy. Initially, it was thought to have great promise in the treatment of heart failure, but subsequent studies showed that its effect lessened after the first few doses. More recent studies have shown objectively measured useful effects for 2 and 8 weeks. The current state of research on this potentially useful drug is as follows: This quinazoline derivative has a balanced dilator effect on both systemic arteriolar and venous systems. It works by blocking phosphodiesterase in vascular smooth muscle and also by producing a postsynaptic, alpha-adrenergic receptor blockage. It has a peak effect in 1 h and lasts for 6 h when given orally. Awan and coworkers have found that the effect of oral prazosin is very similar to that of intravenous nitroprusside in patients with refractory heart failure.[79] Prazosin, 3 mg, caused a rise in cardiac index from 2 to 3 liters/min/m² and a fall in left ventricular filling pressure from 30 to 17 mmHg. Nitroprusside increased cardiac index from 2.2 to 3 liters/min/m² and reduced filling pressure from 28 to 17 mmHg in these same patients. Neither drug changed the heart rate, and each drug lowered mean arterial pressure 20 percent. The extent of arterial dilatation was similar to the extent of venous pooling with each drug. Forearm arterial resistance fell about 50 percent, while forearm venous tone decreased about 65 percent. Awan and coworkers have extended these observations to the use of prazosin as ambulatory therapy in nine patients for an average of 3 months.[80] They obtained excellent results with 2 to 7 mg of prazosin administered orally every 6 h in addition to continuation of previous digitalis and diuretics. The dose of prazosin for each patient was determined by its effect on cardiac output, left ventricular filling pressure, and systemic blood pressure, determined by Swan-Ganz catheterization at the start of therapy. From the initial dose of prazosin, cardiac output rose from 1.9 to 2.9 liters/min/m², filling pressure decreased from 32 to 19 mmHg, and mean systemic blood pressure was reduced from 100 to 88 mmHg. After 2 weeks of therapy, there was an increase in maximum treadmill exercise duration to 315 S (compared with the predrug value of 209 S) and there was a decrease in echocardiographic ventricular dimensions. Symptoms of fatigue and dyspnea were improved in all patients over an average follow-up period of 3 months. The average New York Heart Association (NYHA) function class was 3.7 before prazosin and 2.2 after adding this medication to continued administration of digitalis and diuretics. Orthostatic hypotension did not occur in any patient. Transient headache and mild nausea were seen in two patients. No side effects required the prazosin therapy to be stopped. Five of the nine patients noted substantial reduction in the frequency of angina pectoris while taking prazosin. This additional beneficial effect is not surprising since several of the major determinants of myocardial oxygen consumption were found to have been reduced in this study.

Subsequent study by Packer et al. noted a large increase in cardiac output and fall in filling pressure of the left ventricle after the first dose of 5 mg of prazosin but a significant attenuation of the effects by the third dose, with doses given at 12- to 24-h intervals.[81] Other groups of researchers observed similar attenuation of response by the fifth dose of prazosin, compared with the initial dose. These studies have cast doubt on the usefulness of prazosin, but very recent studies have indicated continued useful effects of prazosin for 2 and 8 weeks in severe congestive heart failure. In one carefully conducted double-blind trial, prazosin therapy for 8 weeks caused clear improvement in symptoms and objective measures of exercise duration, ejection fraction by radionuclide angiography, and ventricular dimension by echocardiography.[82] The dose was titrated up to initial effectiveness and a maximum of 16 mg/day. After 4 weeks, the dose of prazosin was again titrated up to effectiveness and a new maximum of 24 mg/day. As therapy continued, the patients retained more sodium, which required increased doses of diuretics. The plasma renin activity was increased on prazosin, and this was thought to cause sodium retention by stimulation of aldosterone secretion. These researchers conclude that decreased responsiveness to prazosin can be overcome by increased dosage but that increased diuretics are also necessary. While much research must still be done, prazosin or some similar drug which has yet to be developed may have a useful place in clinical therapy of chronic congestive heart failure.

Agents which *oppose the renin-angiotensin system* in heart failure are now being studied. It is thought that in heart failure there is a stimulation of the renin-angiotensin system and that the increased angiotensin promotes increased systemic vascular resistance.[83] *Saralasin* and *teprotide*, which must be given intravenously, have been investigated[84] and found effective. *Captopril* is an oral agent which inhibits the conversion of inactive angiotensin I and angiotensin II; in a short-duration study, this drug increased cardiac output 28 percent and decreased pulmonary capillary wedge pressure 48 percent.[85] Seven patients were kept on the drug for 8 weeks; six of the seven had clinical improvement and increased duration of exercise capacity by treadmill or supine bicycle testing, but mean arterial pressure fell an average of 20 percent and heart rate declined by 13 percent. The most troubling problem in this early study was the development of severe hypotension and bradycardia in two patients and postural hypotension in another. It is evident that captopril's place in therapy of heart failure needs further research.

Surgical Management

As indicated earlier, the prevention of heart disease is our primary goal, but to the extent that this primary goal is not attainable, elimination or modification of heart disease becomes our next priority. Eliminating heart disease may eliminate or delay the development of heart failure or eliminate or decrease existing heart failure. If surgery is selected, the procedure employed must be safe compared with the untreated condition. Certain procedures carry such small risks that they are performed routinely to prevent later development of heart failure or other complications. An example of this is the surgical correction of patent ductus arteriosus. Commissurotomy for noncalcified pure mitral stenosis has a slightly greater risk but should be considered for patients who have symptoms of heart failure. Replacement of a chronically diseased valve with a prosthesis has a greater risk and therefore is usually reserved for patients who have mild to moderate symptoms despite medical therapy.

On the other hand, patients with severe heart failure may choose to undergo a high-risk surgical procedure because their condition is otherwise intractable. The surgical removal of a ventricular aneurysm that was caused by myocardial infarction secondary to atherosclerotic coronary heart disease falls in this category. The following are some of the abnormalities that may produce heart failure, each of which may be partially or completely corrected by surgical treatment: patent ductus arteriosus; atrial septal defect; ventricular septal defect; congenital pulmonic stenosis; coarctation of the aorta; aortic valve disease of many types; mitral valve disease of many types; rupture of the papillary muscle; rupture of chordae tendineae; removal of a ventricular aneurysm; and traumatic heart disease, including peripheral arteriovenous fistulas. (See chapters related to these subjects.)

Three conditions in this area deserve special comment:

1. Rupture of chordae tendineae of the mitral valve may produce heart failure in the absence of additional heart disease or may precipitate or aggravate heart failure in a patient with rheumatic

mitral valve disease. In either event, surgical treatment may be helpful (see Chap. 39).

2. The aortic valve may be abruptly destroyed by infective endocarditis, and the resulting aortic regurgitation usually produces severe heart failure, including pulmonary edema. The aortic valve of such a patient must be repaired or replaced by a prosthetic valve at the earliest time despite the severe heart failure and active endocarditis (the latter being treated with appropriate antibiotic therapy). The risk of such surgery is high but is acceptable because the alternative is death. (see Chap. 54).

3. A rare patient with severe coronary artery disease but without extensive previous myocardial infarction may have episodes of exercise-induced failure with little or no angina. Such episodes involve intermittent, severe generalized ischemia with resultant intermittent ventricular dysfunction. Such a patient may be relieved by coronary bypass surgery.

Cardiac transplantation has been used for certain patients who are dying of severe, intractable heart failure (Chap. 108). The surgical technique of transplantation has been highly developed, but tissue rejection has occurred in the majority of cases and scarcity of suitable donors also limits the use of this procedure. Bold, creative men and women continue to investigate other techniques, such as use of non-human hearts and mechanical devices.

Practical Application of Management Components

In this section, we will discuss practical outlines for organizing the eight management components into combinations suitable for various types of patients.

Management of Mild Heart Failure

1. Search for curable etiology.
2. Decrease the physical activity of the patient to such a degree that the work load placed on the heart is decreased but the patient continues to live a satisfactory life.
3. Give an average loading dose of digitalis followed by an average maintenance dose, or start with an average maintenance dose.
4. Decrease salt in the diet by having the patient omit obviously salty foods and omit any salt during cooking or eating.

Management of Moderately Severe Heart Failure

1. Search for curable etiology.
2. Decrease physical activity to a moderate degree, increasing permitted activity after improvement occurs.

3. Give an average loading dose of digitalis followed by an average maintenance dose, or start with an average maintenance dose.
4. Give a thiazide diuretic 5 days per week.
5. Give 1 g of liquid potassium chloride in tomato juice twice a day to prevent potassium depletion.
6. If the above therapy does not produce the desired results, give the thiazide diuretic more often or change to furosemide or ethacrynic acid. Also, start a venous vasodilator if there is congestion and an arterial vasodilator if weakness or other low-output symptoms are present. If this does not produce the desired effect, the therapy suggested in the following list for severe chronic heart failure may be employed. If class II or class III heart failure symptoms are caused by severe mitral stenosis where there is no valvular calcification and no mitral regurgitation, mitral commissurotomy is recommended.

Management of Severe Chronic Heart Failure

1. Search for curable etiology.
2. The physical activity of the patient should be severely restricted, but total bed rest should be avoided if possible and the patient's legs should be exercised to prevent thromboembolic episodes.
3. The patient with a history of severe nocturnal orthopnea should be given topical nitroglycerin at bedtime. If that does not relieve the nocturnal orthopnea, then small amounts of morphine sulfate may be given in the muscle 2 or 3 h before the expected episode. After the other therapeutic measures have had some effect (ordinarily 2 to 3 days), the narcotic may be discontinued and topical nitroglycerin used.
4. A loading dose of digitalis should be given, followed by an average maintenance dose. After the other therapeutic measures have become effective, it may be necessary to increase the dosage of digitalis if the patient's condition requires further treatment.
5. Furosemide or ethacrynic acid should be given. If this does not produce the desired results, a potassium-sparing diuretic may be added. If this combination of diuretics does not work, a thiazide diuretic may be added. *Warning:* When three diuretics are required to produce diuresis, if and when diuresis does occur, the patient will probably develop secondary complications such as cardiovascular collapse or progressive renal failure. Although complications do not always occur, they are more likely to occur in patients who do not achieve diuresis easily.
6. Vasodilator therapy should be given. If congestive symptoms predominate, use venous vasodilators. If low-output symptoms predominate, use arterial vasodilators. Many patients have both congestive and low-output symptoms and benefit

from either a combination of drugs or a drug with mixed arterial- and venous-dilating effects. Certain patients do not respond to initial vasodilator therapy; in others you cannot be certain whether the left ventricular end-diastolic pressure is high or low or the cardiac output is reduced or not. Both groups should have cardiac catheterization with vasodilator trial. This can be done in many cases by Swan-Ganz technique or at the time of a regular diagnostic cardiac catheterization. While the data are not yet conclusive, it appears that certain patients receiving long-term arterial or mixed arterial and venous vasodilators may require increased doses of diuretics or, perhaps, addition of aldosterone antagonists.

7. Surgical therapy may be considered. If a patient's heart failure is due to a correctable valvular dysfunction and if symptoms persist despite medical therapy, it is appropriate to consider valve-replacement surgery. Such surgery may also be considered for the patient who has a surgically resectable ventricular aneurysm, although patient selection is more difficult and risk of surgery is higher.

Management of Acute Heart Failure and Acute Pulmonary Edema

Acute pulmonary edema is life-threatening and requires prompt measures. The physician should be prepared to act in a decisive, rapid, and confident manner. Many of the following management steps are carried out simultaneously.

1. The majority of patients are more comfortable in the trunk up–legs down position and assume it spontaneously. When shock is present, this position may need to be modified.

2. From 5 to 10 mg of morphine sulfate should be given slowly intravenously, with close scrutiny for respiratory depression. Morphine antagonists, nalorphine hydrochloride (Nalline) or naloxone (Narcan), should be available. Hypotension may be induced by morphine and nalorphine hydrochloride, and with advanced pulmonary edema, shock may be present prior to treatment. If it is not possible to be sure that pulmonary edema due to heart failure rather than primary respiratory failure is the patient's problem, morphine should not be used until the heart failure diagnosis is certain. Morphine is contraindicated in the presence of pulmonary disease, myxedema, or severe kyphoscoliosis.

3. Oxygen should be given by mask or intranasal catheter. The proper administration of oxygen by positive pressure may be helpful, but care must be taken not to decrease cardiac output by excessive impairment of venous return or to produce gastric dilatation. An oxygen tent is ineffective and impractical.

4. It is important to reduce preload so as to decrease dyspnea and pulmonary congestion, but the potentially deleterious effects of preload reduction must be considered. Sublingual nitroglycerin, 0.4 to 1.2 mg, may be given, or tourniquets (sufficiently tight to occlude venous return but not to impair arterial flow) may be applied to three extremities and rotated every 15 min. Tourniquets have the advantage of being immediately reversible. The withdrawal of 500 ml of blood by phlebotomy may help an occasional patient with known preexisting chronic congestive heart failure, increased blood volume, and normal or increased hematocrit. Preload reduction will substantially help relieve dyspnea in patients with a large blood volume and a large heart due to an elevated left ventricular end-diastolic volume and pressure. Such therapy is used in most patients. On the other hand, administration of large doses of nitroglycerin, the application of tourniquets, or a phlebotomy may occasionally precipitate hypotension in patients who develop acute pulmonary edema with a normal blood volume and normal or near-normal heart size. This latter clinical situation results relatively frequently from myocardial infarction. Where doubt exists and whenever an adverse reaction occurs, Swan-Ganz cardiac catheterization may be helpful (Chap. 99). Similarly, the slower reduction of preload brought about by furosemide or ethacrynic acid may also cause a more gradual onset of hypotension. Although most heart failure patients can tolerate altered preload or blood volume, some cannot. When the preload is altered, it is vital to monitor the blood pressure, urine output, and BUN level and to utilize Swan-Ganz catheterization in some patients to monitor filling pressure and cardiac output.

5. If response to other measures is not prompt or if bronchospasm and wheezing are prominent, aminophylline may be given intravenously—250 mg diluted in 50 ml of dextrose and water is administered in a 30-min infusion. This drug should be used cautiously in patients in shock.

6. When the patient is not receiving digitalis, 0.75 mg digoxin may be given intravenously, followed by additional doses as indicated. This drug is usually of secondary importance in comparison with morphine, oxygen, and tourniquets unless there is an ectopic tachycardia which is responsive to it. Such rhythms as supraventricular tachycardia, atrial flutter, and atrial fibrillation with uncontrolled ventricular rate may respond dramatically to rapid digitalization.

7. When supraventricular ectopic tachycardia and ventricular tachycardia do not respond to the usual therapy, the rhythm may be reverted electrically with a dc synchronized cardioverter. The cardioverter may be used at the bedside with the patient under the influence of morphine. In urgent cases it may be used as the initial mode of treatment, especially when mitral stenosis is the underlying disease.

8. Diuretics, especially ethacrynic acid and furosemide, have been used extensively in the treat-

ment of pulmonary edema. It appears that some diuretics may have acute vasodilator effects as well as renal effects. The exact place of diuretics in the treatment of pulmonary edema is not clear.

There should be a difference between the therapeutic response to diuretics in a patient with chronic heart failure, a large heart, and acute pulmonary edema and the response of a patient with no previous heart failure, a heart of normal size, and pulmonary edema. The former patient probably has a greater than normal blood volume and has suddenly partitioned a large amount of fluid in the lungs, such as in the case of a patient with longstanding heart failure due to old myocardial infarcts who has a new myocardial infarct. On the other hand, a patient with pulmonary edema who has a normal blood volume but has redistributed too much fluid in the lungs is obviously in a different group. This latter situation may occur in a patient with fresh myocardial infarction but a heart that was "normal" just a few minutes earlier, in which instance the heart will not be as large.

Since pulmonary edema may be self-limited, responding to old, tested measures, and since not all pulmonary edema occurs in the same clinical setting, we may properly ask whether diuretics, including ethacrynic acid, are always beneficial to, or merely tolerated by or even harmful to, patients with pulmonary edema. The study done at Johns Hopkins Hospital answers some of these questions. In a controlled study comparing the therapeutic effectiveness of intravenous ethacrynic acid with that of intramuscular mercaptomerin in patients with acute pulmonary edema, all 39 patients were treated by the usual methods except that 19 received ethacrynic acid and 20 received mercaptomerin.[85] Although ethacrynic acid induced a noticeably greater diuresis and natriuresis in the first 3 h, differences in this respect were not significant at the end of 6 h. The diuretic response to mercaptomerin was evenly distributed around a mean of 1239 ml per 6 h, whereas the response to ethacrynic acid was biphasic, with six patients failing to respond (mean diuresis of 287 ml per 6 h) and the remaining 13 voiding an average of 2506 ml per 6 h. The rate of clinical improvement was independent of the rapidity of diuresis, thus casting doubt on the necessity for the use of the most rapidly acting diuretics in the treatment of pulmonary edema. This study suggests that a vigorous diuresis is not necessary for clinical improvement in patients with pulmonary edema. The increase in tachycardia in some of these patients was interpreted as suggesting a relatively hypovolemic state. They stress that diuretics should be given because of serious chronic underlying cardiovascular disease, but the choice of a diuretic agent should not be predicated upon the expected short-term benefits of a rapid diuresis. No reported study as yet deals exclusively with pulmonary edema occurring in an individual who had a normally functioning heart a few minutes earlier and in whom the heart size is normal and the lungs are full of fluid merely because of redistribution of the normal blood volume. It seems unlikely that a vigorous diuresis could decrease the total blood volume and promote a redistribution of blood in such a patient so that the pulmonary edema would clear up. On the basis of theoretical considerations and the studies mentioned earlier, the lungs might clear up, but at the same time effective blood volume might reach a critical level, causing serious hypotension or shock. This risk might be justifiable, for the clearing of pulmonary edema would allow better oxygenation of the blood, but serious arrhythmia might accompany the hypovolemia. Therefore, diuretic drugs should be used with caution under these unique circumstances. Falling blood pressure, increasing heart rate, and decreasing blood flow may indicate that the total circulation is not tolerating the diuresis. In addition, some patients with myocardial infarction may have normal blood pressure with decreased blood volume, presumably because of fluid lost into the tissues from the capillaries, which in turn is thought to be due to arteriolar constriction. In these circumstances, it is possible for a vigorous diuresis to trigger shock or hypotension. Recent studies have defined 15 to 18 mmHg as the optimal ventricular filling pressure in patients with shock complicating acute myocardial infarction.

9. Normotensive patients often develop paroxysmal hypertension early in an attack of pulmonary edema, presumably because of fear and apprehension and an increased liberation of catecholamines, but the blood pressure returns to normal when the symptoms are controlled. Acute pulmonary edema that is causally related to severe systemic hypertension may respond to trimethaphan (Arfonad) or nitroprusside intravenously. Routine use of arterial vasodilators in pulmonary edema is not recommended. The usual measures for treating pulmonary edema are generally successful; therefore, the potential risk of precipitating hypotension in certain patients does not appear justified.

Management of Intractable Heart Failure

In practice there are two definitions of intractable heart failure:

1. There is heart failure that is not responsive to the simple methods of treatment, including the proper use of rest, diet, digitalis, diuretics, and vasodilators. Under these circumstances the physician must survey the patient's condition and treatment in an attempt to develop a new approach to the seemingly intractable heart failure. The physician must ask questions such as, Is the diagnosis correct? Does the patient really have heart disease, or is it some other condition that mimics heart disease? Is there any clue to a correctable form of heart disease? Have any factors that might aggravate heart failure been over-

looked? Has the proper combination of rest, diet, digitalis, diuretics, and vasodilators been used? Is this a suitable patient for vigorous vasodilator therapy? Have all the complications of treatment been identified and corrected? Should open heart surgery be undertaken for valve replacement or resection of a ventricular aneurysm? Should the new approach produce results, the patient's condition may be reclassified; it is no longer intractable heart failure.

2. There is unrelenting heart failure in which every known form of therapy has been tried without success. The physician has considered all the points listed above and has modified the therapy to the utmost, but heart failure persists. This second definition of heart failure has a very personal meaning for each physician. It implies that the responsible physician has done all that he or she knows how to do, without success. Another opinion may yet be sought; a new observer may possibly identify an overlooked factor. Even so, there comes a time when no one can help, and perhaps the term *absolute refractory heart failure* should be applied to this clinical state. At this point, the wise physician's foremost concern is the comfort of the patient, justifying use of morphine in small doses, even on a daily basis, to relieve dyspnea, or using very powerful diuretics to reduce preload, so that the patient has more comfort and less dyspnea even though cardiac output and renal function are further reduced.

References

1. Mackenzie, J.: "Principles of Diagnosis and Treatment in Heart Affections," Henry Frowde and Hadder and Storighton, London, 1916, p. 38.
2. Feinstein, A. R.: "Clinical Judgment," The Williams & Wilkins Company, Baltimore, 1967.
3. The Criteria Committee of the New York Heart Association: "Diseases of the Heart and Blood Vessels (Nomenclature and Criteria for Diagnosis)," 7th ed., Little, Brown and Company, Boston, 1973.
*4. Spann, J. F., and Hurst, J. W.: Vasodilator Therapy of Congestive Heart Failure, in J. W. Hurst (ed.), "Update I: The Heart," McGraw-Hill Book Company, New York, 1979, p. 167. (88 references)
5. Spann, J. F., Jr., Bucciono, R. A., Sonnenblick, E. H., and Braunwald, E.: Contractile State of Cardiac Muscle Obtained from Cats with Experimentally Produced Ventricular Hypertrophy and Heart Failure, *Circ. Res.*, 21:341, 1967.
6. Spann, J. F., Jr., Covell, J. W., Eckberg, D. L., Sonnenblick, E. H., Ross, J., Jr., and Braunwald, E.: Contractile Performance of the Hypertrophied and Chronically Failing Cat Ventricle, *Am. J. Physiol.*, 223:1150, 1972.
7. Newman, W. H., and Webb, J. G.: Pressure Overload Cardiac Hypertrophy: Length-Tension Curves, and Responses to Isoproterenol, Ca^{2+}, and Ouabain, *Am. J. Physiol.*, 238(*Heart and Circ. Phys.* 7):134, 1980.
*8. Spann, J. F., Bove, A. A., Natarajan, G., and Kreulen, T.: Ventricular Performance, Pump Function and Compensatory Mechanisms in Patients with Aortic Stenosis, *Circulation*, 62:576, 1980. (34 references)
9. Gorlin, R.: "Coronary Artery Disease," W. B. Saunders Company, Philadelphia, 1976.
10. Kannel, W. B., Castelli, W. P., McNarmara, P. M., McKee, P. A., and Feinleib, M.: Role of Blood Pressure in the Development of Congestive Heart Failure, The Framingham Study, *N. Engl. J. Med.*, 287:781, 1972.
11. Veterans Administration Cooperative Study Group on Antihypertensive Agents: Effects of Treatment on Morbidity in Hypertension, *J. Am. Med. Assoc.*, 202:1028, 1967.
12. Spann, J. F., Jr., Mason, D. T., and Zelis, R. F.: Recent Advances in the Understanding of Congestive Heart Failure, Parts I and II, *Mod. Concepts Cardiovasc. Dis.*, 39:73, 1970.
13. Chidsey, C. A., Braunwald, E., and Morrow, A. G.: Catecholamine Excretion and Cardiac Stores of Norepinephrine in Congestive Heart Failure, *Am. J. Med.*, 39:442, 1965.
14. Chidsey, C. A., Harrison, D. C., and Braunwald, E.: Augmentation of the Plasma Norepinephrine Response to Exercise in Patients with Congestive Heart Failure, *N. Engl. J. Med.*, 267:650, 1962.
15. Spann, J. F., Chidsey, C. A., Pool, P. E., and Braunwald, E.: Mechanisms of Norepinephrine Depletion in Experimental Heart Failure Produced by Aortic Constriction in the Guinea Pig, *Circ. Res.*, 17:312, 1965.
16. Covell, J. W., Chidsey, C. A., and Braunwald, E.: Reduction of Cardiac Response to Postganglionic Sympathetic Nerve Stimulation in Experimental Heart Failure, *Circ. Res.*, 19:51, 1966.
17. Wood, J. E., Litter, J., and Wilkins, R. W.: Peripheral Venoconstriction in Human Congestive Heart Failure, *Circulation*, 13:524, 1956.
18. Zelis, R.: The Contribution of Local Factors to the Elevated Venous Tone of Congestive Heart Failure, *J. Clin. Invest.*, 54:219, 1974.
19. Wood, J. E.: The Mechanism of the Increased Venous Pressure with Exercise in Congestive Heart Failure, *J. Clin. Invest.*, 41:2020, 1962.
20. Zelis, R., and Mason, D. T.: Compensatory Mechanisms in Congestive Heart Failure—The Role of the Peripheral Resistance Vessels, *N. Engl. J. Med.*, 282:962, 1970.
21. Zelis, R., Mason, D. T., and Braunwald, E.: A Comparison of the Effects of Vasodilator Stimuli on Peripheral Resistance Vessels in Normal Subjects and in Patients with Congestive Heart Failure, *J. Clin. Invest.*, 47:960, 1968.
22. Zelis, R., Longhurst, J., Capone, R. J., Lee, G., and Mason, D. T.: Peripheral Circulatory Control Mechanisms in Congestive Heart Failure, in Dean T. Mason (ed.), "Congestive Heart Failure," Yorke Medical Books, New York, 1976, p. 129.
23. Zelis, R., Mason, D. T., and Braunwald, E.: Partition of Blood Flow to the Cutaneous and Muscular Beds of the Forearm at Rest and during Leg Exercise in Normal Subjects and in Patients with Heart Failure, *Circ. Res.*, 24:799, 1969.

*This article is a review of the literature and contains additional references to the literature.

24. Higgins, C. B., Vatner, S. F., Franklin, D., and Braunwald, E.: Effects of Experimentally Produced Heart Failure on the Peripheral Vascular Response to Severe Exercise in Conscious Dogs, *Circ. Res.,* 31:196, 1972.

25. Zelis, R., Mason, D. T., and Braunwald, E.: Partition of Blood Flow to the Cutaneous and Muscular Beds of the Forearm at Rest and during Leg Exercise in Normal Subjects and in Patients with Heart Failure, *Circ. Res.,* 24:799, 1969.

26. Epstein, S. E., Beiser, G. D., Stampfer, M., et al.: Characterization of the Circulatory Response to Maximal Upright Exercise in Normal Subjects and Patients with Heart Disease, *Circulation,* 35:1049, 1967.

27. Sparks, H. V., Kopald, H. H., Carrière, S., Chimoskey, J. E., Kinoshita, M., and Barger, A. C.: Intrarenal Distribution of Blood Flow with Chronic Congestive Heart Failure, *Am. J. Physiol.,* 223:840, 1972.

28. Cannon, P. J.: The Kidney in Heart Failure, *N. Engl. J. Med.,* 296:26, 1977.

29. Reeve, R., Sakai, F. J., Kennedy, J. W., Hood, W. P., Jr., Rackley, C. E., Alderman, E. L., and Lawson, W.: Ejection Fraction in Man. A Comparison of Methods, *Circulation,* 51:677, 1975.

30. Cheyne, J.: A Case of Apoplexy in Which the Fleshy Part of the Heart was Converted to Fat, Dublin Hospital Reports and Communications, *Med. Surg.,* 11:216, 1818.

31. Lange, R. L., and Hecht, H. H.: The Mechanisms of Cheyne-Stokes Respiration, *J. Clin. Invest.,* 41:42, 1962.

32. Davidson, J. D., Waldmann, T. A., Goodman, D. G., and Gordon, R. S., Jr.: Protein-Losing Enteropathy in Congestive Heart Failure, *Lancet,* 1:899, 1961.

33. Pittman, J. G., and Cohen, P.: The Pathogenesis of Cardiac Cachexia, *N. Engl. J. Med.,* 271(9):403, 1964.

34. Earnest, D. L., and Hurst, J. W.: Exophthalmos, Stare, Increase in Intraocular Pressure and Systolic Propulsion of the Eyeballs Due to Congestive Heart Failure, *Am. J. Cardiol.,* 26:351, 1970.

*35. Logue, R. B., Rogers, J. V., Jr., and Gay, B. B., Jr.: Subtle Roentgenographic Signs of Left Heart Failure, *Am. Heart J.,* 65:464, 1963. (14 references)

36. Grossman, W.: "Cardiac Catheterization and Angiography," Lea & Febiger, Philadelphia, 1974.

37. Kreulen, T. H., Bove, A. A., McDonough, M. T., Sands, M. J., and Spann, J. F.: The Evaluation of Left Ventricular Function in Man: A Comparison of Methods, *Circulation,* 51:677, 1975.

38. Knott, D. H., and Barlow, G.: The Comparison of Fluorescein and Decholin Circulation Times, *Am. J. Med. Sci.,* 247:304, 1964.

39. Fragge, R. G., Kopel, F. B., and Iglauer, A.: Serum Glutamic Oxalacetic Transaminase (SGOT) in Congestive Heart Failure: Clinical Study and Review of the Literature, *Ann. Intern. Med.,* 52:1042, 1960.

40. West, M., Pilz, C. G., and Zimmerman, H. J.: Serum Enzymes in Disease. III. Significance of Abnormal Serum Enzyme Levels in Cardiac Failure, *Am. J. Med. Sci.,* 241:350, 1960.

41. Mason, D. T., and Braunwald, E.: Digitalis: New Facts about an Old Drug, *Am. J. Cardiol.,* 22:151, 1968.

42. Carey, R. A., Bove, A. A., Coulson, R. L., and Spann, J. F., Jr.: Normal Cardiac Myosin ATPase and Mechanics in Pressure Overload with Digitalis Treatment, *Am. J. Physiol.,* 243:253, 1978.

43. Williams, J. F., Jr., Klocke, F. J., and Braunwald, E.: Studies on Digitalis. XIII. Comparison of the Effects of Potassium on the Inotropic and Arrhythmia-Producing Actions of Ouabain, *J. Clin. Invest.,* 45:346, 1966.

44. Dock, W.: How Some Hearts Age, *J. Am. Med. Assoc.,* 195:442, 1966.

45. Rogers, P. H., and Sherry, S.: Current Status of Antithrombotic Therapy in Cardiovascular Disease, *Prog. Cardiovasc. Dis.,* 19:235, 1976.

46. Brenner, O.: The Management of Heart Failure, in A. M. Jones (ed.), "Cardiology," Hoeber Medical Division, Harper & Row, Publishers, Inc., New York, 1964.

46a. Morrison, J., Coromilas, J., Robbins, M., et al.: Digitalis and Myocardial Infarction in Man, *Circulation,* 62:8, 1980.

47. Withering, W.: "An Account of the Foxglove, and Some of Its Medical Uses: With Practical Remarks on Dropsy, and Other Diseases," C. G. J. and J. Robinson, London, 1785.

48. Mason, D. T., Zelis, R., Lee, G., Hughes, J. L., Spann, J. F., and Amsterdam, E. A.: Current Concepts and Treatment of Digitalis Toxicity, *Am. J. Cardiol.,* 27:546, 1971.

48a. Doering, W.: Quinidine-Digoxin Interaction: Pharmacokinetics, Underlying Mechanism and Clinical Implication, *N. Engl. J. Med.,* 301:400, 1979.

49. Smith, T. W., and Hager, T.: Digitalis (Third of Four Parts), *N. Engl. J. Med.,* 289:1063, 1973.

*50. Kim, Y. I., Noble, R. J., and Zipes, D. P.: Dissociation of the Inotropic Effect of Digitalis from its Effect on Atrioventricular Conduction, *Am. J. Cardiol.,* 36:459, 1975. (31 references)

51. Smith, T. W.: Drug Therapy (First of Two Parts), *N. Engl. J. Med.,* 288:719, 1973.

52. Marcus, F. I., Kapadia, G. G., and Goldsmith, C.: Inhibition of Myocardial Uptake of Tritiated Digoxin by Acute Hyperkalemia in the Dog, *Clin. Res.,* 15:28, 1967.

53. Marcus, F. I.: Current Concepts of Digoxin Therapy, *Mod. Concepts Cardiovasc. Dis.,* 45:77, 1976.

54. Doherty, J. R., Flanigan, W. J., Perkins, W. H., and Ackerman, G. L: Studies with Tritiated Digoxin in Anephric Human Subjects, *Circulation,* 35:298, 1967.

55. Weissler, A. M., Schoenfeld, C. G., and Harris, W. S.: Cardiac Response to Digitalis in Heart Failure, *Circulation,* 36(suppl. 1):166, 1967.

56. Doherty, J. E., Perkins, W. H., and Mitchell, G. K.: Tritiated Digoxin Studies in Human Subjects, *Arch. Intern. Med.,* 108:531, 1961.

57. Marcus, F. I., Kapadia, G. G.: The Metabolism of Tritiated Digoxin in Cirrhotic Patients, *Gastroenterology,* 47:517, 1964.

*58. Marcus, F. I., Kapadia, G. J., and Kapadia, G. G.: The Metabolism of Digoxin in Normal Subjects, *J. Pharmacol. Exp. Ther.,* 145:203, 1964. (17 references)

59. Mason, D. T., Spann, J. F., Jr., and Zelis, R.: New Developments in the Understanding of the Actions of the Digitalis Glycosides, *Prog. Cardiovasc. Dis.,* 11:443, 1969.

60. Doherty, J. E., and Perkins, W. H.: Digoxin Metabolism in Hypo- and Hyperthyroidism—Studies with Tritiated Digoxin, *Ann. Intern. Med.,* 64:489, 1966.

61. Doherty, J. E., and Perkins, W. H.: Tritiated Digoxin Turnover in Pulmonary Heart Disease and Congestive Heart Failure, *Clin. Res.*, 15:54, 1967.

62. Doherty, J. E., Perkins, W. H., and Flanigan, W. J.: The Distribution and Concentration of Tritiated Digoxin in Human Tissues, *Ann. Intern. Med.*, 66:116, 1967.

63. Marcus, F. I., Burhalter, L., Cuccia, C., Pavlovich, J., and Kapadia, G. G.: Administration of Titriated Digoxin with and without a Loading Dose, *Circulation*, 34:865, 1966.

*64. Smith, T. W., Butler, V. P., Jr., and Haber, E.: Determination of Therapeutic and Toxic Serum Digoxin Concentrations by Radioimmunoassay, *N. Engl. J. Med.*, 281:1212, 1969. (23 references)

*65. Ingelfinger, J. A., and Goldman, P.: The Serum Digitalis Concentration—Does It Diagnose Digitalis Toxicity? *N. Engl. J. Med.*, 294:867, 1976. (28 references)

66. Smith, T. W., and Haber, E.: Digitalis Intoxication: The Relationship of Clinical Presentation to Serum Digoxin Concentration, *J. Clin. Invest.*, 49:2377, 1971.

67. Corwin, N. D., Klein, M. J., and Friedberg, C. K.: Countershock Conversion of Digitalis-Associated Paroxysmal Atrial Tachycardia with Block, *Am. Heart J.*, 22:251, 1968.

*68. Smith, T. W., Haber, E., Yeatman, L., and Butler, V. P.: Reversal of Advanced Digoxin Intoxication with Fab Fragments of Digoxin-Specific Antibodies, *N. Engl. J. Med.*, 294:797, 1976. (30 references)

69. LeJemtel, T. H., Keung, E., Ribner, H. S., Davis, R., Wexler, J., Beaufox, M. D., Sonnenblick, E. H.: Sustained Beneficial Effects of Oral Amrinone on Cardiac and Renal Function in Patients with Severe Congestive Heart Failure, *Am. J. Cardiol.*, 45:123, 1980.

70. Stamfer, M., Epstein, S. E., Beiser, G. D., and Braunwald, E.: Hemodynamic Effects of Diuresis at Rest and during Upright Exercise in Patients with Impaired Cardiac Function, *Circulation*, 37:900, 1968.

71. Laragh, J. H.: Diuretics in the Treatment of Congestive Heart Failure, in E. Braunwald (ed.), "The Myocardium: Failure and Infarction," H. P. Publishing Company, New York, 1974.

71a. Brest, A. N., Seller, R., Onesti, G., Ramirez, O., Swarts, C., and Moyer, J. H.: Clinical Selection of Diuretic Drugs in the Management of Cardiac Edema, *Am. J. Cardiol.*, 22:168, 1968.

*72. Kirkendall, W. M., and Stein, J. H.: Clinical Pharmacology of Furosemide and Ethacrynic Acid, *Am. J. Cardiol.*, 22:162, 1968. (52 references)

*73. Taylor, W. R., Forrester, J. S., Magnusson, P., Chatterjee, K., and Swan, H. J. C.: Hemodynamic Effects of Nitroglycerin Ointment in Congestive Heart Failure, *Am. J. Cardiol.*, 38:469, 1976. (26 references)

74. Williams, D. O., Bommer, W. J., Miller, R. R., Amsterdam, E. A., and Mason, D. T.: Hemodynamic Assessment of Oral Peripheral Vasodilator Therapy in Chronic Congestive Heart Failure: Prolonged Effectiveness of Isosorbide Dinitrate, *Am. J. Cardiol.*, 39:84, 1977.

*75. Massie, B., Chatterjee, K., Werner, J., Greenberg, B., Hart, R., Parmley, W. W.: Hemodynamic Advantage of Combined Administration of Hydralazine Orally and Nitrates Nonparenterally in the Vasodilator Therapy of Chronic Heart Failure, *Am. J. Cardiol.*, 40:794, 1977. (39 references)

76. Kovick, R. B., Tillisch, J. H., Berens, S. C., Bramowitz, A. D., and Shine, K. I.: Vasodilator Therapy of Chronic Left Ventricular Failure, *Circulation*, 53:322, 1976.

77. Franciosa, J. A., Pierpont, G., and Cohn, J. N.: Hemodynamic Improvement after Oral Hydralazine in Left Ventricular Failure, *Ann. Intern. Med.*, 86:388, 1977.

78. Guiha, N. H., Cohn, J. N., Mikulic, E., Franciosa, J. A., and Limas, C. J.: Treatment of Refractory Heart Failure with Infusion of Nitroprusside, *N. Engl. J. Med.*, 291:587, 1974.

79. Awan, N. A., Miller, R. R., and Mason, D. T.: Comparison of Effects of Nitroprusside and Prazosin on Left Ventricular Function and the Peripheral Circulation in Chronic Refractory Congestive Heart Failure, *Circulation*, 57:152, 1978.

80. Awan, N. A., Miller, R. R., DeMaria, A. N., Maxwell, K. S., Neumann, A., and Mason, D. T.: Efficacy of Ambulatory Systemic Vasodilator Therapy with Oral Prazosin in Chronic Refractory Heart Failure, *Circulation*, 56:346, 1977.

81. Packer, M. D., Meller, J., Gorlin, R., Herman, M. V.: Hemodynamic and Clinical Tachyphylaxis to Prazosin-Mediated Afterload Reduction in Severe Chronic Congestive Heart Failure, *Circulation*, 59:531, 1979.

*82. Colucci, W. S., Wynne, J., Holman, B. L., and Braunwald, E.: Long-Term Therapy of Heart Failure with Prazosin: A Randomized Double Blind Trial, *Am. J. Cardiol.*, 45:337, 1980. (45 references)

83. Curtiss, C., Cohn, J. N., Vrobel, T., and Franciosa, J. A.: Role of Renin-Angiotensin System in the Systemic Vasoconstriction of Chronic Congestive Heart Failure, *Circulation*, 58:763, 1978.

84. Faxon, D. P., Creager, M. A., Halperin, J. L., Gavras, H., Coffman, J. D., and Ryan, T. J.: Central and Peripheral Hemodynamic Effects of Angiotensin Inhibition in Patients with Refractory Congestive Heart Failure, *Circulation*, 61:925, 1980.

85. Ader, R., Chatterjee, K., Ports, T., Brundage, B., Hiramatsu, B., and Parmley, W.: Immediate and Sustained Hemodynamic and Clinical Improvement in Chronic Heart Failure by an Oral Angiotensin-Converting Enzyme Inhibitor, *Circulation*, 61:931, 1980.

Section C Hypotension and Shock

24

Pathophysiology of Hypotension and Shock

Francois M. Abboud, M.D.

The clinical picture of shock (see Chap. 25) is easy to recognize, but its pathophysiology is complex. This chapter includes a description of the mechanisms involved in the pathogenesis of shock and the compensatory adjustments in the circulation that tend to restore arterial blood pressure, cardiac output, and tissue perfusion. Early treatment and correction of the abnormal circulatory state before cellular membranes are damaged is essential for the reversal of shock. This requires an understanding of circulatory physiology and the pharmacology of vasoactive drugs. Some of the basic concepts related to the physiology and pharmacology of shock are reviewed. Lastly, the cellular and biochemical events leading to cellular death and irreversibility are described.

Physiological Definition

Shock is a defect in tissue perfusion or a failure of the circulatory system to deliver the necessary substrates and to remove the waste products of cellular metabolism. This hemodynamic abnormality results in cellular damage and eventually cellular death.

Stages of Shock

The progress of the syndrome and its pathogenesis seem to occur in three stages that reflect the severity of the defect in tissue perfusion and the intensity of cellular damage. (See Table 24-1.)

Stage I: Compensated Hypotension
The fall in blood pressure may be caused either by a fall in cardiac output or by vasodilatation. In the majority of situations, a fall in cardiac output rather than vasodilatation is responsible for the hypotension, except in septic shock, where cardiac output may be normal or increased but the increase is insufficient to meet the metabolic demands of tissues. As soon as arterial blood pressure falls, there are compensatory mechanisms triggered by activation of baroreceptor reflexes that result in restoration of arterial blood pressure through an increase in cardiac output and in peripheral resistance. Blood flow to vital organs such as the brain and heart is preserved, and the symptoms and signs of this compensated state are minimal.[1]

Stage II: Decreased Tissue Perfusion
The compensatory mechanisms in this phase are insufficient to maintain arterial blood pressure or perfusion of vital organs. There is evidence of cerebral, renal, and myocardial ischemia. There are signs of excessive sympathetic discharge, and the majority of patients in this stage should be treated aggressively to restore cardiac output and tissue perfusion and reverse the syndrome.[2]

Stage III: Microcirculatory Failure and Cellular Membrane Injury
In this stage, severe ischemia, toxins, antigen-antibody reactions, or complement activation damages cellular membranes. The damage may involve the blood cellular elements, the capillary endothelium, the kidneys, the liver, the lungs, etc. Vasoconstriction, which takes place initially as a compensatory response to the hypotension, is intense and may result in aggregation and sludging of blood corpuscles in the capillaries and venules. A progressive fall in arterial blood pressure below critical levels results in

452

TABLE 24-1   Pathogenesis and Stages of Shock

Stage	Description
I	Compensated hypotension; redistribution of blood flow
II	Decreased tissue perfusion; ischemia
III	Microcirculatory failure; endothelial damage
	Cellular membrane injury; cellular death

ischemia of all organs. Necrotic damage of the gastrointestinal mucosa leads to absorption of bacteria and toxins into the circulation, which, in turn, may have detrimental effects on other organs and may contribute to a generalized endothelial damage with potentially disseminated intravascular coagulation. Renal ischemia and hypotension may lead to acute tubular necrosis. Coronary ischemia in patients with coronary artery disease would lead to a depression of myocardial contractility, further hypotension, and a vicious cycle. Damage to the capillary endothelium increases permeability and transudation of fluids and proteins into the extracellular space, exacerbating the hypovolemia and hypotension. Neutrophils may release vasodilator peptides. Severe acidosis causes myocardial depression and vasodilatation. Finally, the release of lysosomal enzymes and the depletion of high-energy phosphates are associated with cellular destruction.

The types and causes of shock are shown in Table 24-2.

TABLE 24-2   Types and Causes of Shock

1. Hemorrhagic, hypovolemic
   a. Acute hemorrhage, e.g., GI bleeding, retroperitoneal bleeding, trauma
   b. Excessive fluid loss, e.g., vomiting, intestinal or pyloric obstruction, diarrhea, peritonitis, splanchnic ischemia, extensive muscle injury, burns
   c. Relative hypovolemia, vasodilatation
      (1) Neurogenic vasodilatation, e.g., spinal anesthesia, adrenergic blockers, spinal cord injury, poisons
      (2) Metabolic, toxic, hormonal causes, e.g., septicemia, adrenal insufficiency, hypoglycemia, poisons
2. Cardiogenic
   a. Myocardial infarction or myocarditis
   b. Myocardial depression, e.g., hypoxia, acidosis, myocardial depressant factors, septic shock, drugs, hypoglycemia
   c. Arrhythmias, e.g., severe bradycardia or tachycardia
   d. Mechanical compression or obstruction, e.g., pericardial tamponade, positive-pressure breathing, pulmonary embolism, atrial myxoma
3. Microcirculatory: endothelial injury and cellular aggregation
   a. Anaphylaxis
   b. Disseminated intravascular coagulation
   c. Burns, sepsis, trauma
4. Cellular membrane damage
   a. Sepsis
   b. Anaphylaxis
   c. Ischemia, prolonged hypoxia, tissue injury, pancreatitis

Hemodynamic Abnormalities in Shock

The perfusion of any organ depends on systemic arterial pressure and resistance of that particular organ. Systemic arterial pressure is determined by cardiac output and total vascular resistance. Vascular resistance is predominantly related to the radius of the blood vessels, and the radius is influenced by the structure of the vessel wall and the degree of encroachment on the lumen as well as the tone of vascular smooth muscle. The tone of vascular muscle is regulated by neurogenic impulses, humoral factors, and intrinsic myogenic factors. Thus, the amount of blood flow to an organ depends on cardiac performance as well as total vascular resistance and local resistance in that organ. The exchange of substrates and metabolites is dependent not only upon the amount of blood flow reaching an organ, but also upon whether that flow perfuses the nutritional capillaries in the microcirculation. The capillary network is the critical interface between the blood and the cells.

Major Determinants of Tissue Perfusion

Cardiac Output

The cardiac output is the product of heart rate and stroke volume. A normal output of approximately 5 liters/min delivers 250 ml of oxygen to the tissues, which meets our metabolic demands at rest. A drop in cardiac output below 2 liters per square meter of body surface area per minute is an indication of severe shock.

A fall in blood pressure may result from a fall in cardiac output, and the latter may be caused by an abnormal heart rate or a low stroke volume.

Heart Rate   Bradycardia may cause a fall in output. Sinus bradycardia and atrioventricular block are often seen immediately following infarction and may cause hypotension. Severe bradycardia is also seen in the common faint syndrome or vasovagal syncope. Tachycardia may decrease cardiac output significantly, because a rapid heart rate may limit cardiac filling time and lower stroke volume, particularly in patients with limited myocardial reserve. Failure to correct the tachycardia may result in cardiogenic shock, whereas early treatment could restore heart rate and normal blood pressure. One has to be aware of the possibility that an increase in rate may be compensatory in some patients with anemia, fever, sepsis, or hemorrhage, and under such circumstances tachycardia is an appropriate reflex response to maintain cardiac output.

Stroke Volume   A decrease in stroke volume may occur because of a fall in cardiac filling pressure or end-diastolic pressure, a decrease in myocardial contractility, or a mechanical obstruction to blood flow.

The amount of blood *filling the ventricles* at the end of diastole regulates the subsequent contraction and stroke volume in accordance with Starling's law of the heart. There are many factors that determine filling pressure, such as the heart rate, duration of filling, ventricular compliance, venous tone, and total blood volume as well as the posture of the patient. A reduction in total blood volume may be apparent as a result of external or internal bleeding, vomiting, diarrhea, diuretics, burns, or excessive perspiration without fluid replacement. It may also be relative as a result of loss of vascular tone, which might occur with administration of anesthetics, ganglion blockers, or venodilators; after spinal cord injury; and in patients with autonomic insufficiency. Excessive pooling of blood in the lower extremities may also cause a significant reduction in filling pressure.

Compression of the heart may also prevent its filling. This may be seen with pericardial tamponade, tension pneumothorax and positive-pressure breathing, particularly in hypovolemic individuals.[3]

Reduction in *myocardial contractility* is the major cause of shock in myocardial infarction and a contributing factor in many different types of shock, including septic and hemorrhagic shock. There are important reversible factors that depress contractility.

A *fall in arterial* P_{O_2} results from ventilation-perfusion abnormalities of the lung which occur early in shock. In late shock malignant hypoxia is associated with the pathologic entity of shock lung. Hypoxia has a direct vascular effect, causing vasodilatation, particularly in the heart and brain, and an indirect effect (through activation of chemoreceptors) that causes reflex vasoconstriction in vessels of skeletal muscle, skin, and splanchnic bed. The combination of a direct dilator effect and an indirect vasoconstrictor effect allows redistribution of blood flow to the organs that depend on aerobic metabolism. Despite the compensatory mechanisms that permit delivery of oxygen to the vital organs, myocardial contractility may be impaired as arterial P_{O_2} declines. Often the severity of the decline in arterial P_{O_2} reflects the extent of myocardial infarction. Hypoxia is one of the reversible causes of myocardial depression that should be treated aggressively.

Acidosis[4] may result from anaerobic metabolism and decreased tissue perfusion with release of lactate or from accumulation of organic acids because of renal failure. Severe hypoventilation may contribute to both hypoxia and respiratory acidosis. The reduction in arterial and intracellular pH causes a depression of myocardial contractility, vasodilatation, and a decreased responsiveness to sympathomimetic amines. Correction of acidosis may restore arterial blood pressure in hypotensive patients and eliminate the need for more aggressive therapy.

It has often been stated that the main goal of therapy is to restore perfusion of the organs without being too concerned about the level of arterial blood pressure. It is important to realize that myocardial performance in acute myocardial infarction depends on *perfusion of the ischemic myocardium and the latter is determined to a great extent by the level of arterial diastolic pressure.*[5,6] A fall in arterial pressure during hemorrhagic or hypovolemic shock in patients with coronary artery disease may complicate the syndrome by causing myocardial ischemia. Although it is true that restoration of perfusion is the main goal of therapy, the restoration of arterial pressure is essential to maintain myocardial function, cardiac output, and, consequently, also perfusion pressure. In myocardial infarction the resistance to blood flow through the coronary vessels is caused by structural changes in the vessel wall, and the degree of vasomotor tone is minimal because of excessive accumulation of vasodilator metabolites downstream from the site of coronary narrowing in the region of ischemia. Delivery of collateral blood flow to the ischemic region depends on the level of arterial pressure. Unfortunately, the optimum level of arterial pressure is difficult to define and may vary from patient to patient, depending on the severity and degree of vascular narrowing in the coronary vessels or the cerebral vessels. The pressure necessary to drive flow across an arterial narrowing or through collateral vessels in each patient is difficult to determine. For this reason, judicious restoration of arterial pressure to reasonable levels between 100 and 120 mmHg, guided by the clinical picture of the patient, should be the goal of therapy, assuming that the patients are normotensive before they go into shock.

Oxygen requirement of the myocardium varies and can influence cardiac performance since an *increase in oxygen requirement without increase in oxygen supply means deterioration of function.*[7] The factors that increase myocardial demand are increases in rate, arterial blood pressure, cardiac size, and myocardial wall tension. Hypertension, therefore, is detrimental in patients with myocardial ischemia because it increases myocardial oxygen work and demand. Hypotension, bradycardia, and reduced cardiac size decrease oxygen demand. A significant reduction in arterial pressure, however, may be detrimental, as it reduces myocardial perfusion. Increased cardiac size is associated with increased myocardial wall tension and oxygen consumption; thus reduction in preload reduces oxygen demand and can be achieved by appropriate venodilator and diuretic therapy. Excessive reduction in preload, however, reduces cardiac output. Major dilator drugs, such as isoproterenol, might, in addition to lowering arterial blood pressure, increase myocardial oxygen demand because of the associated tachycardia, and the lowering of arterial pressure may have a detrimental effect on the perfusion of ischemic myocardial segments. Conversely, propranolol, which will decrease myocardial oxygen demand through its effect on heart rate, would be protective, but its myocardial-depressant action in patients with cardiogenic shock may be a hazardous complication.

Depression of contractility may result from administration of barbiturates; from suppression of adrenergic drive to the myocardium, such as seen after the administration of ganglion-blocking drugs, reserpine, guanethidine, propranolol, or high spinal anesthetics; and from spinal cord injury or intracranial lesions involving the medullary centers. Severe hypoglycemia may also interfere with adrenergic drive and may have a direct depressing effect on cardiac or vascular muscle.

All these factors not only depress contractility and vascular tone, but they create a state of relative hypovolemia with a reduction of effective blood volume, filling pressure, and consequently cardiac output.

Cellular damage in various organs may be associated with the release of factors that have a myocardial-depressant effect.[8] Myocardial-depressant factors may appear not only in cardiogenic shock, but also in burns, septicemia, hemorrhage, and the shock syndrome.

Mechanical Obstruction to Blood Flow Extensive pulmonary embolism or occlusion of the large pulmonary vessels will result in severe shock. Early recognition of the presence of a large pulmonary embolus may be lifesaving if emergency surgery is performed. Compression of the heart from cardiac tamponade, left atrial myxoma, or a ball-valve thrombus may all contribute to progressive hypotension.

Vascular Factors

Blood vessels have five different functions which may be altered during shock:[9]

Large Arteries These provide an impedance function that dampens pulsatile flow and contributes to cardiac afterload. In shock, increased impedance may cause a significant afterload. In addition, marked constriction of large arteries may prevent the accurate estimation of arterial blood pressure by sphygmomanometry. This may result in undetectable blood pressure by sphygmomanometry when intraarterial pressure may be normal.[10] The effectiveness of vasodilator therapy may depend, in large part, on the reduction in impedance and associated decrease in afterload rather than on decreased arterial pressure.

Arterioles These vessels develop the critical resistance to blood flow. The tone of vascular muscle in the arteriole is controlled by neurogenic, humoral, and local metabolic factors, and the relative degree of vascular resistance in different organs determines the amount of blood flow reaching that organ. Intense constriction in the splanchnic or renal circulation and relaxation of coronary arterioles allow a redistribution of flow to favor the coronary circulation. The effects of the sympathetic nervous system, vasoactive humoral agents, and drugs on arterioles in various vascular beds are not uniform, and this selectivity determines the blood flow between organs and is an important determinant of our choice of vasoactive drug to use.[1,9,11]

Arterioles are also important in determining the distribution of flow *within* an organ. Adequate perfusion of any organ depends not only on the amount of blood reaching that organ but on the patency of the nutritional capillaries and vascular channels in which diffusion between blood and tissue occurs. Nonnutritional channels such as arteriovenous shunts, either anatomic or functional, reduce tissue perfusion. An example of the importance of intraorgan redistribution of blood flow is observed in myocardial infarction when an increase in total coronary blood flow may not necessarily increase the perfusion of an ischemic or infarcted segment. Under some circumstances a coronary vasodilator might be detrimental in redistributing the flow away from an ischemic region toward a nonischemic region, a phenomenon referred to as a *vascular steal*.

Intraorgan redistribution of blood flow occurs in acute tubular necrosis associated with shock and reflects a reduction in glomerular filtration in the outer cortex because of localized increase in vascular resistance in this region. Conversely, renal vasodilatation with furosemide may shunt blood toward the outer cortical nephrons.

Precapillary Sphincters These determine the patency of exchange capillaries and capillary surface area. Their tone may be modulated by neurohumoral factors as well as local metabolites. Exchange of fluids between the intravascular compartment and the extracellular space depends on the hydrostatic pressure, the oncotic pressure, capillary surface area, and capillary permeability. In hypovolemic or hemorrhagic shock, the fall in arterial pressure causes activation of the sympathoadrenal system, constriction of arterioles and precapillary sphincters, and a fall in capillary hydrostatic pressure, facilitating the movement of fluids from the extracellular space to the intravascular compartment. This tends to restore blood volume. Hematocrit, viscosity of blood, and plasma oncotic pressure fall. The decline in plasma oncotic pressure may be partially corrected by rapid synthesis of new proteins. As hypotension persists and ischemia is prolonged, arteriolar vasoconstriction becomes less pronounced because of metabolic acidosis, and the precapillary sphincters dilate, capillary surface area increases, and fluid may shift back to the extracellular space.

Capillaries and Venules The *venules* are postcapillary resistance vessels. They are a major determinant of capillary hydrostatic pressure and filtration, and intravascular volume. The reactivity of venules to neurohumoral factors involved in the shock syndrome is important. Venules may constrict *relatively* more than precapillary resistance vessels in response to catecholamines.[11,12] Late in shock, when acidosis prevails, the tone of precapillary sphincters is reduced, but venular resistance may remain elevated. The resulting increase in the ratio of post- over precapillary resistance compounds the hypovolemic state by increasing capillary hydrostatic pressure and filtration. The ratio of post- over precapillary resistance may vary significantly from organ to organ as well as during the various stages of shock, and it is difficult to direct a specific treatment for that particular state. One may consider administration of a venodilating agent in late stages of shock in which failure of the microcirculation is a predominant feature and venular sludging is suspected. The administration of an alpha-adrenergic receptor blocker, such as phentolamine, might reverse the detrimental imbalance between post- and precapillary resistance and facilitate perfusion of the microcirculation.

Albumin, with a molecular weight of 69,000, is the main osmotically active protein in plasma, and the balance between transcapillary *colloidal osmotic pressure* and transcapillary hydrostatic pressure determines fluid flux across the capillaries. *Capillary permeability* may increase in shock because of endothelial injury or the formation of vasoactive peptides. Protein leaks out, plasma oncotic pressure drops, and capillary filtration increases.[13] In addition to the fall in oncotic pressure, severe hypoproteinemia causes an increase in hydraulic conductivity across the capillary endothelium, exaggerating the loss of intravascular fluid.[14]

The balance between oncotic and hydrostatic pressure is a determinant of the level of pulmonary edema and is critical in the management of the shock lung syndrome.[15] Plasma oncotic pressure of normal adults is approximately 25 mmHg, whereas the pulmonary wedge pressure which parallels the pulmonary hydrostatic capillary pressure is 10 to 12 mmHg. Despite this imbalance, capillary filtration takes place because of the high interstitial oncotic pressure in the lung. Plasma oncotic pressure may fluctuate drastically. After 12 h of bed rest, for example, it declines markedly, and this may be a factor in the pulmonary edema after bed rest. If oncotic pressure remains significantly higher than pulmonary capillary hydrostatic pressure (by approximately 8 mmHg or more), the risk of pulmonary edema is negligible; but if oncotic pressure is only 1 to 3 mmHg above pulmonary wedge pressure, the patient is at high risk of pulmonary edema. This has implications concerning the choice of fluid for treatment of hypovolemia. Although the administration of saline solution or Ringer's lactate may be appropriate in many hypovolemic states, a more effective treatment, if there is protein loss, is the use of colloids such as human serum albumin, purified plasma protein, dextran, or hydroxyethyl starch. Colloids that stay longer in the circulation and increase oncotic pressure are necessary when patients have manifestations of extensive endothelial damage and interstitial or pulmonary edema, or when they are chronically ill or malnourished and have hypoalbuminemia.[16] When given intravenously, dextran and mannitol are excreted by the kidney and increase oncotic pressure in Bowman's capsule, creating a pressure gradient across the glomerulus that facilitates filtration even at low arterial pressure.[17] If, after dextran administration, arterial pressure is not restored and oliguria persists, despite administration of diuretics such as furosemide, then there might be danger of overexpansion of plasma volume and accentuation of pulmonary edema with further administration of colloids.

Shock resulting from increased capillary permeability, such as anaphylactic shock or snake venom poisoning, is characterized by a dramatic reduction in plasma volume. The increased capillary permeability may be caused by the release of histamine from macrophages or the release of other metabolites or humoral factors which alter endothelial function.[18] A similar capillary abnormality may complicate shock from sepsis or prolonged hypovolemic or cardiogenic shock. Hematocrit rises sharply and oncotic pressure drops.

Thus, loss of intravascular volume may result from several factors: increased ratio of post- to precapillary resistance, dilatation of precapillary sphincters, excessive capillary permeability, and loss of intravascular proteins. There may also be an increase in cellular permeability and a shift of fluids from extracellular to intracellular spaces.

The erythrocytes, leukocytes, and platelets undergo agglutination to a variable degree in association with the shock syndrome. These aggregates obstruct capillaries and venules. Precipitating events may include platelet aggregation by catecholamines; damage to the endothelial lining of small blood vessels; damage to capillaries with fibrin deposition and formation of microthrombi; hypoxia, which increases the rigidity of red cells. The release of vasoactive peptides and anaphylatoxins as a result of complement activation may cause cellular aggregation and in addition alter capillary permeability and the tone of precapillary sphincters, leading to fluid loss and reduction in tissue perfusion and tissue damage. A state of disseminated intravascular coagulation is often seen in shock, particularly in gram-negative septicemia. The syndrome causes necrosis of several organs and consumption of coagulation factors with complicating hemorrhage; it contributes to the pathogenesis of the shock lung syndrome.[18]

The Large Veins These subserve a capacity function that can influence cardiac filling pressure and cardiac output.[19] In hypotension high levels of circulating catecholamines or vasopressin cause intense venoconstriction that maintains cardiac filling pressure and cardiac output. Conversely, the administration of a spinal anesthetic, sympathetic blockers, or a venodilator such as phentolamine or nitroprusside might precipitate a serious reduction in cardiac filling pressure if blood volume is reduced. For this reason, adequate replacement of blood volume is necessary before the administration of a venodilator.[2,19]

Mechanisms of Cardiovascular Adjustments in Shock

The stress of shock triggers circulatory adjustments. The mechanisms by which these adjustments come into play to restore cardiac output, filling pressure, and arterial blood pressure may be discussed under three headings: (1) neural and reflex adjustments, (2) humoral and metabolic factors, and (3) autoregulatory adjustments of blood vessels.

Neural and Reflex Mechanisms The autonomic control of the circulatory system is regulated by neurons in the medulla. The activity of these neurons is modulated by afferent neural impulses originating in various receptor regions located in strategic areas around the body.[1,20] Some of these receptors trigger impulses that suppress the sympathoadrenal drive and are called *inhibitory receptors,* e.g., arterial baroreceptors and left ventricular receptors. Other receptors generate impulses that stimulate the sympathoadrenal system and are called *excitatory receptors,* e.g., chemoreceptors.

Arterial baroreceptors are located in the adventitia and media of the arch of the aorta and in the adventitia of the carotid arteries in the carotid sinus regions. Increases in receptor activity are caused by their stretch or deformation during the rise in arterial pressure, and conversely, a fall in pressure results in decreased activity. When their activity decreases in shock, the number of "inhibitory" nerve impulses reaching the vasomotor center decreases, resulting in an excessive sympathetic discharge. Increased sympathetic discharge causes arteriolar constriction that is more predominant in the splanchnic and renal than in skeletal muscle beds and is negligible in the coronary and cerebral vascular beds. This preferential effect favors the distribution of blood flow to the vital organs.

There is also a reflex splanchnic constriction that mobilizes a large amount of blood from the splanchnic bed to the central veins, increases central venous pressure and cardiac filling pressure, and tends to restore cardiac output during hypotension.

Increased sympathetic drive to the heart causes tachycardia and increased contractility that may help to restore cardiac output. Increased sympathetic drive to the kidneys causes the release of renin and formation of angiotensin, which raises arterial blood pressure.

The integrity of this reflex may not be preserved in certain types of shock. We have recently found that after coronary occlusion the gain of the arterial baroreceptor reflex may be suppressed significantly. It has also been shown that after endotoxin administration in dogs there is a shift in the baroreceptor discharge frequency of the carotid sinus nerve to the left so that there is a greater discharge frequency for the same level of distending pressure.[21] A higher level of carotid sinus nerve activity suppresses sympathetic drive and contributes to endotoxic shock.

Cardiac receptors are cardiac sensory nerve endings, mostly in the left ventricle, which initiate impulses that travel predominantly along unmyelinated fibers in the vagus, reach the vasomotor centers, and inhibit the sympathetic discharge.[1] These sensory endings may be activated either mechanically, by distension of the left ventricle, or chemically, through the release, in the myocardium, of metabolites and chemicals such as bradykinin or prostaglandin. Their activity is reduced when cardiac filling pressure falls (e.g., hemorrhage or hypovolemia), and this triggers an increased sympathoadrenal drive.[22] The well-known cardiocirculatory inhibition with bradycardia, vasodilatation, and hypotension, described as the Bezold-Jarisch reflex, is ascribed to activation of these cardiac nerve endings with veratridine or other chemicals. The clinical counterpart of this chemical activation may be the bradycardia and hypotension seen following intracoronary injection of contrast medium. During myocardial infarction the release of metabolites or chemicals within the myocardium, such as prostaglandin and bradykinin, may activate these nerve endings. They may also be activated as a result of the dyskinesis and stretch of the ischemic region, and the reflex response is an inhibition of sympathoadrenal drive. Thus, in shock cardiac receptors may have decreased activity during hypovolemia or increased activity during myocardial infarction.

Activation of these cardiac afferents may cause the bradyarrhythmia and hypotension frequently seen immediately following myocardial infarction. The greater incidence of bradyarrhythmia and hypotension in posterior-inferior myocardial infarction in contrast to anterior myocardial infarction may be caused by a greater density of these nerve endings in the region of the posterior-inferior wall of the left ventricle.[20] It has been known that the hypotension associated with acute myocardial infarction in humans is rarely accompanied by acute renal failure, whereas the hypotension from hemorrhagic shock frequently causes acute renal failure. It is possible to ascribe the preservation of renal perfusion during myocardial infarction to activation of these cardiac nerve endings, which inhibit the sympathoadrenal drive, particularly to the renal circulation.[23] Because these receptors are sensitive to changes in cardiac size and blood volume, their regulatory effect on the renal sympathetic nerves is important in modulating urinary sodium and water excretion and thereby regulating blood volume.

The chemoreceptors[1] provide a control system for oxygen conservation and for increasing oxygen delivery during hypoxic states. The sensors are present in the carotid and aortic bodies and they are particularly sensitive to reductions in arterial P_{O_2}, increases in P_{CO_2}, and decreases in pH. During shock, the hypoxia and acidosis activate the reflex that consists primarily of arteriolar constriction in the muscle and splanchnic circulation and arteriolar dilatation in the coronary vessels without a significant change in cerebral vascular resistance. This selective effect on the arterioles of various vascular beds favors a distribution of blood flow and oxygen delivery to the coronary and cerebral circulations. The reflex also includes venous constriction, primarily of the splanchnic veins, favoring a central shift of blood volume to increase cardiac filling pressure and cardiac output. If the hyperventilatory response to chemoreceptor stimulation is prevented, a pronounced reflex bradycardia may be seen. The bradycardia is beneficial in that it reduces myocardial oxygen demand, but if the ventilatory drive is suppressed and apnea and asphyxia coexist, the bradycardia may be excessive and lead to cardiac arrest.

In a patient in shock, *several reflexes*[20] may be activated simultaneously because of hypovolemia, hypotension, and hypoxia. The net effect on the cardiovascular system is the result of a complex central integration of the various afferent signals. This may result in one set of afferent impulses overriding the effects of another. For example, during cardiogenic hypotension following myocardial infarction, the fall in arterial pressure unloads the arterial baroreceptors and triggers a reflex increase in sympathetic activity to the kidneys, but the cardiac sensory endings are activated simultaneously and cause a reflex inhibition of the sympathetic efferents to the kidneys. The net result of this interaction is generally a reduction in the sympathetic efferent impulses to the kidneys. In some situations, activation of two reflex mechanisms may be synergistic: for example, unloading of the arterial baroreceptors during hypotension augments the reflex response to chemoreceptor stimulation.

Humoral and Metabolic Factors The release of hormones such as renin, vasopressin, steroids, prostaglandins, and kinins is partly mediated through the sympathoadrenal system and cardiovascular mechanoreceptors and partly through direct and indirect cellular effects of toxins, ischemia, and antigens in various organs. These hormones have direct cardiovascular and renal effects and indirect effects on central and peripheral adrenergic transmission that allow circulatory adjustments to take place. There are vasodilator factors and vasoconstrictor factors.

Vasodilator factors include hypoxia, acidosis, and the various metabolites resulting from ischemia. The vasodilator effects of these metabolites in the coronary and cerebral circulations are potent and override the vasoconstricting effect of the sympa-

thoadrenal system to maintain perfusion of these vital organs.

The *kinins* are vasodilator polypeptides that are formed by the action of certain proteolytic enzymes on plasma protein precursors. The substance bradykinin serves as the prototype for this class of endogenous peptides. Their major physiological role may be the local regulation of blood flow and function of such organs as the salivary gland, pancreas, kidney, and possibly the heart. In pathophysiological states, kinins are believed to play a part in the hyperemia associated with inflammation and as vasodilators in the hypotension produced by anaphylactic reactions. Renal kinins may increase sodium and water excretion, and cardiac kinins may participate in the activation of cardiac receptors and may cause the perception of anginal pain by activation of sympathetic afferents.

Prostacyclin is an extremely potent vasodilator prostaglandin which is released in various organs during periods of ischemia and which contributes to reactive hyperemia. Prostaglandin precursors, the endoperoxides, are formed in blood vessels from arachidonic acid and are pivotal in the synthesis of prostacyclin, mostly in the endothelial layers of blood vessels, where they may cause vasodilatation and inhibit platelet aggregation. The prostaglandin endoperoxides have opposite effects in platelets, where they are converted to thromboxane A2, a compound which has vasoconstrictive properties and induces platelet aggregation. In shock, the damaged endothelial cells do not synthesize prostacyclin, and the thromboxane A2 released from platelets enhances platelet aggregation, clumping, and vasoconstriction, causing additional endothelial damage.

Beta endorphins are vasodilator peptides that appear to be released from the pituitary gland along with the adrenocorticotropic hormones during periods of stress. Recently it has been shown that the administration of naloxone, a beta-endorphin antagonist, is beneficial in the management of endotoxic shock in rats and dogs and hypovolemic shock in dogs. The effectiveness of naloxone raised the possibility that part of the hemodynamic failure in shock may be related to the release of endorphins.[24] Furthermore, endorphin receptors have been identified not only in brain, but also in heart, gastrointestinal tract, and various other organs. It is not known, however, whether the hypotensive effects of endorphins in shock is related to a central or a peripheral action of the compounds or some of their metabolites.

Vasoconstrictor factors include norepinephrine, epinephrine, dopamine, vasopressin, and angiotensin.[25]

Catecholamines such as norepinephrine and epinephrine are released from the sympathetic terminals and from the adrenal medulla as a result of excessive sympathetic discharge during hypotension. Their effects on the circulation are mediated through adrenergic receptors. The adrenergic receptors may be classified as alpha or beta receptors with respect to their cardiovascular action. The alpha receptors are predominantly in blood vessels and mediate vasoconstriction. The beta receptors are present in blood vessels as well as in myocardium. Activation of the $beta_1$ receptors in myocardium causes an increase in myocardial contractility and heart rate, whereas activation of $beta_2$ receptors in blood vessels causes vasodilatation. The same catecholamine may activate both alpha and beta receptors, depending on the dose and the organ on which it is acting.

Norepinephrine increases myocardial contractility by activating $beta_1$ receptors and increases cardiac output in shock. In blood vessels it activates primarily alpha or vasoconstricting receptors.[26] The magnitude of its effect on alpha receptors varies from one organ to another. It is a potent vasoconstrictor in skin, muscle, and splanchnic beds, whereas in the coronaries it activates $beta_2$ receptors as well as alpha receptors; but because there is a paucity of alpha receptors in the coronary vessels (in contrast to other vascular beds), the drug causes predominantly vasodilatation in the coronaries. It offers several distinct advantages in the treatment of shock because it increases cardiac output and redistributes blood flow away from the extremities and toward the heart and brain and increases arterial pressure, which, in turn, increases coronary flow to the ischemic myocardium.

Epinephrine released from the adrenal gland activates primarily myocardial $beta_1$ receptors and vasoconstrictor alpha receptors in most vessels except in skeletal muscle and coronary vessels, where it activates $beta_2$ receptors when administered in low doses. It increases cardiac output, but redistributes blood flow away from kidney and splanchnic circulation towards skeletal muscle. Its effect on redistribution of blood flow is not optimal, and its effect on arterial pressure is only modest because of its dilator influence in skeletal muscle.

Dopamine is another naturally occurring catecholamine.[27] It is the precursor of norepinephrine and has a different cardiovascular effect, depending on its dose level. When it is given in a low concentration, its dilator effect, mediated through $beta_2$ receptors and through specific dopaminergic receptors, is most apparent in the renal and mesenteric circulations. It also has a slight dilator effect in the cerebral and coronary circulations. When given in larger doses, it increases myocardial contractility and cardiac output through activation of $beta_1$ receptors, but in very large doses it causes vasoconstriction by activation of alpha receptors in both arterioles and veins. The drug may redistribute blood flow away from the extremities and towards the kidneys, gut, heart, and brain. However, it may be necessary to give large doses to maintain arterial pressure and coronary flow, particularly following myocardial infarction, and these large doses will

then tend to oppose to some degree the advantageous vasodilator effect seen in some vascular beds.

Circulating levels of *renin-angiotensin* are too small to cause significant circulatory effects in physiological states, but angiotensin may traverse the blood-brain barrier in the area postrema where it affects medullary cardiovascular centers and causes the release of vasopressin. A fall in arterial pressure and an increase in sympathoadrenal discharge to the kidneys cause the release of renin, the formation of angiotensin and peripheral vasoconstriction, as well as sodium and water retention. Angiotensin constricts the coronary vessels as well as other vascular beds. This is in contrast to the catecholamines, which have a minimal constricting effect on the coronary vessels.

Vasopressin, an important constrictor hormone, is released from the posterior pituitary gland primarily in response to changes in osmolality, and its release may be inhibited by neurogenic afferent impulses originating in the left atrium or arterial baroreceptors. Increased arterial pressure and stretch of the left atrium inhibit the release of vasopressin and, conversely, during hemorrhage and systemic hypotension and in patients on cardiopulmonary bypass, vasopressin levels increase significantly because of a reduction in the cardiac and arterial baroreceptor afferent impulses. Recent observations suggest that thirst and the release of vasopressin may be induced by a central nervous system action of angiotensin. Vasopressin is a vasoconstricting hormone with potent effects in the coronary circulation as well as several other vascular beds. This coronary vasoconstriction may explain in part the negative inotropic effect occasionally seen during its infusion. It is also an antidiuretic hormone that contributes to the retention of water and the compensation for hypovolemia and shock.

Local Autoregulatory Adjustments of Blood Vessels Blood vessels have an intrinsic ability to regulate vascular tone and thereby maintain blood flow to the organ over a wide range of perfusion pressure. This property is known as the *autoregulatory capacity* for blood flow. It is independent of neurogenic influences or humoral factors. Different vascular beds vary with respect to their ability to maintain blood flow. The cerebral, coronary, and renal circulations are most potent. Thus, during a fall in arterial pressure, vasodilatation of the cerebral, coronary, and renal vasculatures maintains blood flow and oxygen delivery to the brain and heart and also maintains sodium and water balance. Although a myogenic response intrinsic to smooth muscle may explain the phenomenon, accumulation of tissue metabolites following a transient period of ischemia may also cause vasodilatation and restore blood flow. The specific mediator of this vasodilatation is not known, but it is likely that a combination of changes contributes to adjustments in tone, i.e., oxygen, carbon dioxide, hydrogen ion and other cations, osmolality, the amount of adenosine compounds, the Kreb's cycle intermediates, and other metabolites released in the immediate environment of the blood vessels.

Cellular and Biochemical Factors in Shock

Oxygen-Hemoglobin Affinity

The extraction of oxygen from hemoglobin by the tissues is not complete and depends to a large extent on the affinity of hemoglobin for oxygen. This affinity varies with the change in hydrogen ion (the Bohr effect), carbon dioxide, and the accumulation of 2,3-diphosphoglyceric acid (2,3-DPG), which causes a greater dissociation of oxygen from hemoglobin because of its preferential affinity for reduced hemoglobin. The 2,3-DPG concentration in red blood cells results from a side reaction of glycolysis and increases during anemia, hypoxia, and acidosis.[28] The shift of the oxygen dissociation curve to the right during these conditions favors greater delivery of oxygen to the tissues at the same P_{O_2}.[29] In certain tissues, however, such as the myocardium, extraction of oxygen at rest is already large, and any additional oxygen demand and a decrease in oxygen-hemoglobin dissociation, such as seen in alkalosis, requires greater delivery of oxygen, i.e., higher coronary blood flow. In shock, the pH, carbon dioxide, and 2,3-DPG levels are changing, and one cannot calculate oxygen extraction from values of P_{O_2} because the shape of the oxygen dissociation curb cannot be predicted accurately. It is preferable to measure oxygen content or saturation of venous and arterial blood. If saturation is lower than predicted from values of P_{O_2}, one can deduce that there has been a shift of the dissociation curve to the right, and vice versa. One should caution against overzealous correction of acidosis with bicarbonate because the hemoglobin affinity for oxygen increases through the Bohr effect and oxygen delivery to the tissues is reduced.

Cellular Structure and Function in Shock[30,31]

Synthesis of adenosine triphosphate (ATP) from adenosine diphosphate (ADP) is associated with the most active state of respiration in mitochondria (state III respiration) and is determined by the cell energy demands. In addition to oxidative phosphorylation and ATP synthesis, the mitochondria bind and accumulate calcium. This function determines calcium availability for other intracellular organelles and thereby regulates biochemical processes or contractile events, as in cardiac or vascular muscle. Cellular death may be caused by two processes. One is a marked inhibition of the electron transport system because of severe ischemia and anoxia. This process leads to depletion of ATP and early suppression of membrane transport function including calcium transport mechanisms. Another type of cell death is initiated by an injury to the cell membrane caused by activation of complement, an antigen-antibody reaction, or certain bacterial products such as phospholipases or antitoxins. In this type of cellular damage, ATP synthesis is preserved and membrane activity is maintained so that calcium may be transported into the cell and is precipitated in mitochondria. Thus, the two types of cellular death may be differentiated from the appearance of the mitochondria. In one situation, because of inhibition of the energy-dependent calcium transport mechanism, there is no calcium in the mitochondria, and in the other the preservation of these membrane transport mechanisms allows the precipitation of calcium in the mitochondria.

The earliest manifestation of the cellular damage consists of swelling of the cells, associated with an increase in intracellular sodium and clumping of nuclear chromatin, followed by dilatation of endoplasmic reticulum.[32] In this phase the cell membrane is unstable, and "blebs" may appear on the surface. The mitochondria then begin to swell, and flocculent material appears within them. As the swelling of the mitochondria continues, calcium may or may not accumulate depending on the type of cellular damage. The process of cellular death becomes irreversible at that stage, and lysosomes begin to disappear from the cell; finally the cell is converted to a mass of debris with large inclusions resembling myelin.

The initial cellular membrane damage results in increased cellular permeability for sodium and water, causing cellular swelling. This may contribute to the hypovolemia of shock. The increased intracellular sodium activates sodium potassium ATPase in an attempt to drive sodium out of the cell. Increased membrane ATPase activity might eventually lead to depletion of ATP and cyclic adenosine monophosphate (AMP), resulting in an alteration in the cellular response to various hormones which exert their cellular effect through activation of cyclase and cyclic AMP. For example, the effect of insulin on glucose uptake by muscle in animals that have been subjected to hemorrhagic shock is reduced. This unresponsiveness to insulin may be one of the reasons for the hyperglycemia of injured individuals and may result from cellular membrane damage. Similarly, reduced responsiveness to catecholamines may be caused by reduced cyclic AMP and ATP. There is also significant reduction in ATP, particularly in the liver early in shock and in most organs in late shock. One does not know the necessary level of ATP for cellular function, but it is believed that as long as ADP and oxygen become available and substrate is provided, ATP generation can be resumed within minutes as long as mitochondrial structure has not been damaged. In fact, it has been shown that after a period of hypoxia, the rate of

ATP generation is increased as soon as oxygen is made available.

Mitochondrial Damage[33,34]

Hypoxia may reduce the rate of ATP synthesis by mitochondria, but it does not cause significant damage to the mitochondrial membrane function unless it is severe, sustained, or associated with ischemia, which reduces the availability of substrates. In contrast to hypoxia, hemorrhagic and endotoxic shock, as well as ischemia, reduce calcium transport by mitochondrial membranes, reduce state III respiration, reduce ATP synthesis as well as mitochondrial ATPase activity, and finally cause mitochondrial damage.[34] The mechanism by which endotoxins and ischemia cause mitochondrial damage is not known. Whether such mitochondrial damage is the result of deprivation of substrates, the release of lysosomal enzymes, changes in intracellular pH, or other changes in cellular ionic environment with accumulation of metabolites is not apparent. It is of interest that glucocorticoids may exert a protective effect on mitochondrial function in endotoxemia in rats.

Lysosomal Theory[35]

Lysosomes are cytoplasmic granules that contain a variety of potent hydrolytic enzymes bound in a latent form in a relatively impermeable membrane. These enzymes are capable of hydrolyzing a wide variety of both natural and synthetic substances and can digest all intra- and extracellular macromolecules if they are released from their membranes. When released from the organelles, either inside or outside the cell, as a consequence of certain forms of cellular injury, they may contribute to the pathogenesis or the propagation and perpetuation of shock. They are most active at an acid pH, which would make them potentially most destructive in the setting of hypoxia and shock.

Numerous morphologic and biochemical observations implicate the lysosomal enzymes in the perpetuation of shock, but at this time the evidence for their primary involvement is not convincing. In organs such as the liver, spleen, and intestine, the lysosomes enlarge and lose their granules during the early phases of shock. This is associated with a decrease in the total activity of lysosomal hydrolases in tissues and a corresponding increase in the activity in the soluble fraction of the tissue homogenate. The loss of lysosomal membrane integrity in vivo is suggested from these findings; furthermore, the lysosomes obtained from animals in shock demonstrate an enhanced release of enzymes in vitro. Administration of endotoxin to animals causes a reduction in lysosomal membrane integrity, and in several studies the level of hydrolases in blood, lymph, and serum correlate with the severity of shock.

The appearance of a *myocardial-depressant factor* (MDF) in shock,[8] although still controversial, may be an indirect manifestation of the effect of lysosomal enzymes. Experimentally induced pancreatitis and a variety of other shock states are associated with plasma MDF activity that parallels lysosomal hydrolases in the plasma. It has been suggested that pancreatic ischemia associated with shock results in the release of lysosomal and other enzymes within the pancreas and these act on an endogenous substrate to yield a peptide with low molecular weight and MDF activity, which is then released into the circulation. The resulting myocardial depression maintains the state of low cardiac output and sustains shock.

Another indication of the involvement of MDF has been the reproducibility of the shock syndrome with infusion of lysosomal hydrolases in animals. The animals demonstrate the hypotension, collapse, and pathologic changes in tissues that are seen in experimental forms of shock.

Other indirect suggestive evidence of the involvement of MDF has been the responsiveness of certain animals in shock to large amounts of corticosteroids.[36,37] In vitro corticosteroids stabilize the lysosomal membranes and prevent their lysis. Treatment with steroids has been shown to suppress circulating serum levels of lysosomal hydrolases in a variety of shock states.

Endotoxemia is associated with increased levels of serum hydrolases, but in vitro the endotoxins do not increase the lysis of lysosome. This led to the suggestion that endotoxins may cause the formation of the lysosomal-releasing factor (LRF) through activation of the alternative as well as the classic complement pathways. Activation of complement in fresh human serum has been found to generate a factor (LRF) that stimulates human polymorphonuclear leukocytes to release their lysosomal enzymes.[38] This factor has many of the properties of human C5a, a complement component known to have chemotactic and anaphylatoxin activities.

Complement Activation in Shock[39,40]

The activity of the immune system may depend on *complements*, which may be the primary humoral mediators of antigen-antibody reactions. The complement system consists of a series of discrete plasma proteins that are present as inactive precursors until they are activated by highly specific biochemical reactions which involve limited proteolytic cleavage. Many antigen-antibody reactions, particularly those involving the IgG and IgM immunoglobulins, which can also evoke acute anaphylactic reactions, depend on complement as the primary humoral mediator of that reaction. The complement, when activated, promotes certain specialized functions by the cells but could eventually impair membrane functions and cause cellular death. There are some antigen-antibody reactions, such as in anaphylactic shock seen after penicillin or pollen antigens involving IgE antibodies, that do not require complement.

Complement has a recognition function that allows the macromolecules to attach themselves to the membrane surface of a target cell with the appropriate antibody. Activation of complements is then triggered either with the antigen-antibody complex (classic pathway) or by bacterial or fungal mucopolysaccharides without the participation of any immunoglobulins (alternative pathway). Such activation releases several low-molecular-weight vasoactive peptides from the complement molecules by cleavage, and these in turn have significant biologic effects, including beneficial actions as phagocytosis, the inflammatory response to local infection, neutralization of viruses, or modulation of immune response. They also have detrimental effects that lead to destruction of cellular membranes and cellular death. For example, during the activation of C2, a cleavage product occurs which has kinin-like activity and which can significantly increase capillary permeability. Two other activation peptides, C3a and C5a, release histamine from mast cells, have chemotactic activity, and constrict vascular smooth muscle. Another fragment, C3b, acts as an opsonin and facilitates phagocytosis. Polymorphonuclear leukocytes may be attracted chemotactically through activation of esterases on their surface and may release their lysosomal enzymes if the concentration of the complement reaction product C5a is large enough. Platelets may have an increase in their procoagulant activity, and endothelial cells may contract. In addition to the direct and indirect effects of the fragments of activated complements on cells, their aggregation as decamolecular complexes on the surface of the cell membrane may cause cellular destruction. The expression of all these effects is increased permeability; increased leukocyte accumulation, such as is observed in glomerulitis; the release of lysosomal enzymes, which may cause necrotizing vasculitis; intravascular coagulation factors, which could induce a Schwartzman reaction; and thrombocytopenia and other manifestations of microcirculatory collapse and intravascular plugging seen in prolonged shock and in endotoxemia.

References

*1. Abboud, F. M., Heistad, D. D., Mark, A. L., and Schmid, P. G.: Reflex Control of the Peripheral Circulation, *Prog. Cardiovasc. Dis.*, 18:371, 1976. (182 references)

2. Abboud, F. M.: The Sympathetic Nervous System and Alpha Adrenergic Blocking Agents in Shock, *Med. Clin. North Am.*, 52:1049, 1968.

3. Feisal, K. A., Abboud, F. M., and Eckstein, J. W.: Effect of Adrenergic Blockade on Cardiovascular Responses to Increased Airway Pressure, *Am J. Physiol.*, 213:127, 1967.

4. Williamson, J. R., Schaffer, S. W., Ford, C., and Safer, B.: Contribution of Tissue Acidosis to Ischemic Injury in the Perfused Rat Heart, *Circulation*, 53(suppl. 1):3, 1976.

5. Mueller, H., Ayres, S. M., Gregory, J. J., Giannelli, S., Jr., and Grace, W. J.: Hemodynamics, Coronary Blood Flow, and Myocardial Metabolism in Coronary Shock; Response to *l*-Norepinephrine and Isoproterenol, *J. Clin. Invest.*, 49:1885, 1970.

6. Mueller, H., Ayers, S. M., Giannelli, S., Jr., Conklin, E. F., Mozzara, J. T., and Grace, W. J.: Effect of Isoproterenol, *l*-Norepinephrine and Intraaortic Counterpulsation on Hemodynamics and Myocardial Metabolism in Shock Following Acute Myocardial Infarction, *Circulation*, 45:335, 1972.

7. Maroko, P. R., and Braunwald, E.: Effects of Metabolic and Pharmacologic Interventions of Myocardial Infarct Size Following Coronary Occlusion, *Circulation*, 53(suppl. 1):162, 1976.

8. Lefer, A. M., and Martin, J.: Origin of Myocardial Depressant Factor in Shock, *Am. J. Physiol.*, 218:1423, 1970.

9. Abboud, F. M.: Control of the Various Components of the Peripheral Vasculature, *Fed. Proc.*, 31:1226, 1972.

10. Cohn, J. N.: Blood Pressure Measurement in Shock, *J. Am. Med. Assoc.*, 199:972, 1967.

11. Abboud, F. M., and Eckstein, J. W.: Comparative Changes in Segmental Vascular Resistance in Response to Nerve Stimulation and to Norepinephrine, *Circ. Res.*, 18:263, 1966.

12. Abdel-Sayed, W. A., Abboud, F. M., and Ballard, D. R.: Contribution of Venous Resistance to Total Vascular Resistance in Skeletal Muscle, *Am. J. Physiol.*, 218:1291, 1970.

13. Brigham, K. L., Woolverton, W. C., Blake, L. H., and Staub, N. C.: Increased Sheep-Lung Vascular Permeability Caused by *Pseudomonas* Bacteremia, *J. Clin. Invest.*, 54:792, 1974.

14. Mason, J. C., Curry, F. E., and Michel, C. C.: The Effects of Proteins upon the Filtration Coefficient of Individually Perfused Frog Mesenteric Capillaries, *Microvasc. Res.*, 13:185, 1977.

15. Guyton, A. C., and Lindsey, A. W.: Effect of Elevated Left Atrial Pressure and Decreased Plasma Protein Concentration in the Development of Pulmonary Edema, *Circ. Res.*, 7:649, 1959.

16. Dawidson, I., Hadling, E., and Gelin, L. E.: Hemodilution and Oxygen Transport to Tissue in Shock, *Acta Chir. Scand.*, 489(suppl.):245, 1979.

17. Wendling, M. G., Eckstein, J. W., and Abboud, F. M.: Effects of Mannitol on the Renal Circulation, *J. Lab. Clin. Med.*, 74:541, 1969.

18. Ayres, S. M.: The Shock Lung, in "The Organ in Shock," The Upjohn Company, Kalamazoo, Mich., April 1977, pp. 24–31.

19. Abboud, F. M., Schmid, P. G., and Eckstein, J. W.: Vascular Responses after Alpha Adrenergic Receptor Blockade. I. Responses of Capacitance and Resistance Vessels to Norepinephrine in Man, *J. Clin. Invest.*, 47:1, 1968.

*20. Abboud, F. M.: Integration of Reflex Responses in the Control of Blood Pressure and Vascular Resistance, *Am. J. Cardiol.*, 44:903, 1979. (31 references)

*This article is a review of the literature and contains additional references to the literature.

21. Trank, J. W., and Visscher, M. B.: Carotid Sinus Baroreceptor Modifications Associated with Endotoxin Shock, *Am. J. Physiol.*, 202:971, 1962.

22. Abboud, F. M., and Mark, A. L.: Cardiac Baroreceptors in Circulatory Control in Humans, in R. Hainsworth and R. Linden (eds.), "Cardiac Receptors," Cambridge University Press, Oxford, 1979, pp. 437–462.

23. Thames, M. D., and Abboud, F. M.: Reflex Inhibition of Renal Sympathetic Nerve Activity during Myocardial Ischemia Mediated by Left Ventricular Receptors with Vagal Afferents in Dogs, *J. Clin. Invest.*, 63:395, 1979.

24. Holaday, J. W., and Faden, A. I.: Naloxone Reversal of Endotoxin Hypotension Suggests Role of Endorphins in Shock, *Nature*, 275:450, 1978.

25. Abboud, F. M.: Vascular Responses to Norepinephrine, Angiotensin, Vasopressin and Serotonin, *Fed. Proc.*, 27:1391, 1968.

26. Abboud, F. M., and Eckstein, J. W.: Vascular Responses after Alpha Adrenergic Receptor Blockade. II. Responses of Venous and Arterial Segments to Adrenergic Stimulation in the Forelimb of Dog, *J. Clin. Invest.*, 47:10, 1968.

27. Goldberg, L. I.: Dopamine—Clinical Uses of an Endogenous Catecholamine, *N. Engl. J. Med.*, 291:707, 1974.

28. Lecompte, F., Aberkane, H., Azoulay, C., Muffat-Joly, M., and Pocidalo, J. J.: Blood Affinity for Oxygen in Experimental Hemorrhagic Shock with Metabolic Acidosis, *Pfluegers Arch.*, 359(1–2):147, 1975.

29. Thomas, H. M., 3d, Lefrak, S. S., Irwin, R. S., Fritts, H. W., Jr., and Coldwell, P. R. B.: The Oxyhemoglobin Dissociation Curve in Health and Disease. Role of 2,3-Diphosphoglycerate, *Am. J. Med.*, 37:331, 1974.

30. Baue, A. E., Chaudry, I. H., Wurth, M. A., and Sayeed, M. M.: Cellular Alterations with Shock and Ischemia, *Angiology*, 25:31, 1974.

31. Trump, B. F.: The Role of Cellular Membrane Systems in Shock, in "The Cell in Shock," The Upjohn Company, Kalamazoo, Mich., April 1976, pp. 16–29.

32. Laiho, K. U., and Trump, B.: Relationship of Ionic, Water, and Cell Volume Changes in Cellular Injury of Ehrlich Ascites Tumor Cells, *Lab. Invest.*, 31:207, 1974.

33. Trump, B. F., Mergner, W. J., Kahng, M. W., and Saladino, A. J.: Studies on the Subcellular Pathophysiology of Ischemia, *Circulation*, 53(suppl. 1):17, 1976.

34. Mela, L., Bacalzo, L. V., Jr., and Miller, L. D.: Defective Oxidative Metabolism of Rat Liver Mitochondria in Hemorrhagic and Endotoxin Shock, *Am. J. Physiol.*, 220:571, 1971.

35. deDuve, C., and Wattiaux, R.: Functions of Lysosomes, *Ann. Rev. Physiol.*, 28:435, 1966.

36. Nishijima, H., Weil, M. H., Shubin, H., and Cavanilles, J.; Hemodynamic and Metabolic Studies on Shock Associated with Gram Negative Bacteremia, *Medicine*, 52:287–294, 1973.

37. Altura, B. M., and Bella, T.: Peripheral Vascular Actions of Glucocorticoids and Their Relationship to Protection in Circulatory Shock, *J. Pharmacol. Exp. Ther.*, 190:300, 1974.

38. Goldstein, I., Hoffstein, S., Gallin, J., and Weissmann, G.: Mechanisms of Lysosomal Enzyme Release from Human Leukocytes: Microtubule Assembly and Membrane Fusion Induced by a Component of Complement (C5a/Chemotaxis Cytochalasin B/cAMP:cGMP Antagonism), *Proc. Nat. Acad. Sci. U.S.A.*, 70:2916, 1973.

39. Muller-Eberhard, H. J.: "Complement. Annual Review of Biochemistry," Annual Reviews, Inc., Palo Alto, Calif., 1975, pp. 607–724.

40. Muller-Eberhard, H. J.: The Significance of Complement Activity in Shock, in "The Cell in Shock," The Upjohn Company, Kalamazoo, Mich., April 1976, pp. 16–29.

25

Recognition and Management of Shock and Acute Pump Failure*

Jay N. Cohn, M.D.

Clinical Definitions

Shock is a term applied to that state of the circulation in which a functional deficit of tissue perfusion in one or more vital organs is so severe that organ

*The pathophysiology of hypotension and shock is discussed in Chap. 24.

function is impaired and/or an unstable state of progressively more severe blood flow deficiency develops. The regional flow abnormality results from some combination of reduced perfusion pressure and increased regional vascular resistance.

Precise criteria for the diagnosis of shock applicable to all situations are not available, primarily because the term *shock* itself has not been rigidly defined. In experimental animals diagnosis of the shock state usually is based upon specific hemodynamic abnormalities, including a specific percent reduction in arterial pressure and in cardiac output.[1] In the clinical setting, however, criteria for the diagnosis of shock have usually depended more upon evidence of impaired organ function relating to impaired flow. Since the degree of abnormality of organ function may not necessarily correspond directly with quantitative reductions in flow, the severity of the flow deficiency may vary widely in patients in whom the clinical diagnosis of shock is made.

Clinical Shock

Medical personnel are usually alerted to the possibility of shock because of a fall in auscultatory blood pressure. However, blood pressure is a poor criterion for the diagnosis of clinical shock for several reasons: (1) cuff pressure may be an unreliable guide to true intraarterial pressure;[2] (2) inadequate regional perfusion and progressive circulatory deterioration may proceed in the presence of a normal arterial pressure;[3] and (3) low arterial pressure may be well tolerated in some clinical situations with no evidence of impaired organ perfusion. The clinical diagnosis of shock therefore should be based upon evidence of impaired regional perfusion. At least two of the signs listed in Table 25-1 should be present before the diagnosis of shock is made.

Preshock

In recent years, less emphasis has been placed upon the precision of the diagnosis of shock and more emphasis upon the early recognition of signs of reduced perfusion that may allow therapy to be initiated early enough to prevent the development of shock. This change in emphasis has resulted from an awareness that in the fully developed shock state organ impairment has already occurred and vicious cycles have been initiated so that mortality may be high despite the most aggressive therapy. It is becoming increasingly apparent that the earlier therapy is instituted the more likely there will be a successful result. This emphasis upon early treatment means that therapy may be instituted at a time before the circulatory impairment can be precisely diagnosed as shock. These states have been referred to by a variety of terms, including *preshock, pseudoshock*, and *low-flow* or *low-output states*. The condition may be suspected when a high-risk patient exhibits an unexplained change in pulse rate, pulse volume, blood pressure, urine output, or skin temperature even though the findings do not fulfill the criteria listed in Table 25-1.

Pump Failure

The term *pump failure* refers to that subgroup of patients with shock or preshock in whom the circulatory insufficiency is directly related to impaired pumping ability of the left ventricle. Acute myocardial infarction is the most common cause of this syndrome, and the term is sometimes employed specifically for severe left ventricular failure in that group of patients. Hemodynamically, pump failure may be defined as a low cardiac output usually with an inappropriately high left ventricular filling pressure (left ventricular end-diastolic pressure or pulmonary wedge pressure). Clinically, the syndrome is recognized by evidence of left ventricular failure associated with signs of a reduced cardiac output, although the reduction in regional perfusion need not necessarily be so severe that the criteria for clinical shock shown in Table 25-1 are met. Some degree of clinically detectable pump failure probably always precedes the development of cardiogenic shock. Because of the current emphasis on early treatment of pump failure in acute myocardial infarction, cardiogenic shock may be viewed as a syndrome which should be prevented rather than treated.

Hemodynamic Mechanisms in Shock

A reduction in regional blood flow implies that total cardiac output is inadequate to maintain perfusion to all organs. Although most states of shock or preshock are associated with a cardiac output below the normal range, some patients exhibit a cardiac output which under normal circumstances should be adequate to maintain perfusion; in other patients the cardiac output may actually be higher than the normal range. The syndrome of clinical shock in the presence of a normal or high cardiac output can represent an occurrence in either (1) a patient whose premorbid cardiac output is higher than normal and in whom the output during shock is thus reduced from the patient's normal even though it is still within the normal population mean, or (2) a situation in which the disease state is associated with a high cardiac output and the increase in output occurring in the individual is inadequate to maintain the increased perfusion required by the underlying disease process. The former abnormality is characteristic of patients with Laennec's cirrhosis or other high-output states who develop shock. In these situations normal resting cardiac output may be over 10 liters/min, and a state of inadequate regional perfusion may exist when the cardiac output is as high as 6 or 7 liters/min.[4] Patients with severe infections, particularly those with chronic suppurative processes involving a large organ system such as the splanchnic viscera, may require an extremely high cardiac output in order to maintain normal tissue perfusion.[5] A limitation in the rise in cardiac output thus may be associated with inadequate regional flow.

Only two mechanisms may be responsible for an inadequate cardiac output: (1) inadequate cardiac filling, or (2) impairment of pump function. Distinction between these two factors is the first responsibility of the physician whose goal is prompt restoration of tissue perfusion. These two abnormalities may coexist in the patient with well-established shock.

The most common cause of shock in medical and

TABLE 25-1   Signs of Clinical Shock

1. Urine output < 20 ml/h with urine Na$^+$ concentration < 30 meq/ liter
2. Cool, moist skin
3. Auscultatory systolic blood pressure less than 90 mmHg
4. Impaired state of consciousness: agitation, somnolence, confusion, coma
5. Metabolic acidosis (lactic acidosis)

surgical patients is an inadequacy in circulating blood volume leading to inadequate cardiac filling. While this circulatory state is characteristic of trauma, hemorrhage, or burns in which there may be external loss of circulating volume, it also is a common occurrence in patients who have not sustained obvious local injuries. In some situations an internal redistribution of body fluids may result in depletion of the intravascular compartment despite the fact that total body fluids and the extracellular fluid volume may be normal. Whether this occurs as a primary event initiating shock or as a secondary event perpetuating shock once vasoconstriction has already occurred has not been well established. Rapid plasma volume expansion usually results in prompt clinical improvement.[6] This phenomenon can be recognized in patients with a wide variety of medical illnesses not necessarily associated with primary shifts of intravascular volume. The common denominator of many of these illnesses is a heightened sympathoadrenal discharge, which may result in venoconstriction, a rise in capillary hydrostatic pressure, and an increased rate of transudation of plasma out of the vascular space.[7]

Although the term *hypovolemic shock* is often applied to these clinical situations, measured circulating volume is not always reduced. Indeed, the correlation between measured circulating volume, cardiac filling pressure, and cardiac output is so variable in patients with low-output states that it is not possible to use the term *hypovolemia* accurately to represent all such patients.[8] Some have preferred the term *functional hypovolemia* to reflect that there is a deficit of circulating volume even though the total measured volume in the vascular space may be normal. The term *circulatory torpor* has also been employed to allude to the fact that the circulation is slowed even though the volume is normal. An appropriate term may be *volume-responsive shock*, because the common denominator of patients with this form of circulatory embarrassment is that rapid expansion of the intravascular volume has a markedly salutary effect on regional perfusion.[9] The beneficial effect of the volume expansion may be related more to "pump priming" than to volume expansion; that is, if end-diastolic myocardial fiber length is acutely increased by a rapid intravenous infusion, then the resultant increase in cardiac output will itself increase venous return to the heart (*vis a tergo*) and produce a new steady state in which output may be higher with little change in circulating volume.

When volume expansion precipitates a rise in cardiac filling pressure to abnormal levels without demonstrable improvement in regional perfusion, it may be assumed that an abnormality of pump function is a critical factor in the genesis of the impaired perfusion. This abnormality may be nonspecific or may reside primarily in the performance of the right ventricle or left ventricle. The cause of the abnormal functional and metabolic state of the myocardium are important in the selection of appropriate therapy.

Peripheral Vascular Factors

Systemic Vascular Resistance
When cardiac output falls, a reflex increase in systemic vascular resistance usually is observed. The rise in resistance is not homogeneous throughout the vascular tree and is dependent on the intensity of neural, humoral, and local factors affecting vascular tone. In some situations resistance may not rise and the arterial pressure falls *pari passu* with the fall in cardiac output.[10] Inhibition of the expected reflex vasoconstriction has been described, particularly in experimental myocardial ischemia or infarction, and has been attributed to activation of left ventricular receptors.[11] These appear to be more numerous in the inferior wall of the left ventricle,[12] and thus hypotension and bradycardia due to stimulation of these vagal afferent receptors (a Bezold-Jarisch-type reflex) may be more common in inferior wall infarcts.[13]

An increase in peripheral vascular resistance supports the arterial pressure, but it also alters the regional distribution of cardiac output and may further depress cardiac output. Since cardiac output is inversely related to aortic impedance (or outflow resistance), particularly when cardiac function is impaired, a preponderant constriction of large and small arteries and arterioles will result in a further reduction of what may already be a reduced cardiac output.[14] The potential for a vicious circle (positive-feedback system) leading to progressive circulatory deterioration is evident.

Some increase in vascular resistance is necessary to support life when cardiac output falls, since a very low aortic pressure may result in a critical reduction of cerebral and coronary perfusion. Frequently, however, the rise in systemic vascular resistance is so intense that arterial pressure is supported at normal or even frankly elevated levels. The adverse systemic hemodynamic effect of heightened impedance is most apparent in this clinical situation.

Regional Vascular Resistance
Regional perfusion is critically dependent upon the state of the microvasculature. The large conduit arteries and veins play a relatively minor role in controlling circulation to regional vascular beds; however the smaller arteries, arterioles, capillaries, and postcapillary venules all are critical in the control of regional flow and of microcirculatory pressures that determine capillary filtration rates.[15] Activation of the sympathetic nervous system with release of norepinephrine and of the renin-angiotensin system with the formation of angiotensin II are the best understood factors leading to constriction of small arteries, arterioles, and venules. Intense constriction may markedly reduce perfusion of a vascular bed even in the presence of an adequate arterial perfusion pressure. Such arteriolar constriction may occur, particularly in certain regional beds (e.g., renal, cutaneous, skeletal muscle), resulting in signs

of tissue underperfusion even though arterial pressure may still be within the normal range.

In some regional beds preferential arteriovenous shunt vessels may also influence the adequacy of tissue perfusion. While their presence has not been demonstrated in all vascular beds, it is apparent that in certain states of advanced shock arterial and venous flow may persist in the absence of functional tissue perfusion. This situation may result either from the opening up of potential collateral channels or from the maintenance of flow through anatomically normal channels that perfuse areas in which cellular metabolism has ceased.

Capillary Pressure

The relative constriction of the precapillary and post-capillary vessels is an important determinant of the capillary pressure. An increase in arteriolar resistance would normally be expected to reduce capillary pressure, but if this is balanced by an increase in postcapillary venular resistance, capillary pressure may be supported. Indeed, if venular resistance rises to a greater extent than precapillary arteriolar resistance, capillary pressure may rise, and thus capillary filtration may increase at the same time that regional perfusion is reduced. Such a series of events may lead to a reduction of circulating volume that may aggravate and perpetuate a low-flow state and eventuate in what has been called *irreversibility*.[16] The persistence of venular constriction out of proportion to arteriolar constriction has been attributed to the ability of the venules to maintain high vascular tone in the face of a falling blood pH as reduction in regional perfusion leads to lactic acidosis. In contrast, arterioles are thought to be more sensitive to a falling pH and may lose their ability to constrict under these circumstances.[17]

Cardiac Factors

Although impairment of cardiac performance may not necessarily be a precipitating factor in shock, metabolic changes in the myocardium may alter its performance once shock has developed. A fall in aortic pressure may reduce myocardial oxygen delivery, particularly to the subendocardium,[18] at the same time that myocardial oxygen demand is increased by a reflex increase in heart rate. Furthermore, a humoral substance (myocardial-depressant factor) that some investigators have found accumulating in the blood during low-flow states may have a direct deleterious effect on myocardial function,[19] and lactic acidosis may impair myocardial contractility.[20] Consequently, once shock has existed for any period of time, cardiac function is rarely normal, and impairment of this cardiac performance may play a role in the perpetuation or aggravation of the shock state. This positive-feedback system is an important reason to recommend early therapy for preshock states so that circulation can be restored before a cardiac component impairs the response to therapy.

Determinants of Cardiac Output

End-Diastolic Fiber Length The Frank-Starling mechanism is an important determinant of moment-to-moment changes in stroke volume in normal individuals as well as an important factor in the level of cardiac output achieved during disease states. In volume-depleted states a marked reduction in end-diastolic fiber length leads to a reduction in force of ventricular contraction and a fall in stroke volume that, despite reflex attempts at compensation, may lead to a fall in cardiac output. When pump function is abnormal, changes in cardiac filling may not produce as much effect on stroke volume. Even in this situation, however, cardiac output may be lower than it could be because the end-diastolic fiber is not at its optimal length. Therefore, attempts to challenge the heart with volume in an effort to increase end-diastolic fiber length to optimal levels has served as a cornerstone of the therapy of shock.

It must be recognized that the end-diastolic filling pressure of the ventricular chamber is only an indirect assessment of end-diastolic fiber length. Changes in the distensibility or compliance of the ventricle may have an important impact on the relationship between its filling pressure and fiber length.[21] Since accurate measurement of ventricular volume is difficult to obtain in acutely ill patients and no sensitive and practical means presently exist for sequential monitoring of ventricular volume, the importance of compliance changes as a factor in the genesis of shock and as a contributing factor to changes in cardiac filling pressures is only conjectural.

Contractility Alterations in the rate of fiber shortening independent of initial fiber length provide a measure of the intrinsic contractile properties of myocardial muscle. The normal myocardium responds to sympathoadrenal discharge with a marked increase in contractility. When cardiac output falls and the sympathetic nervous system is activated, as in most patients with shock, an increase in myocardial contractility would be expected. Even in the presence of intense sympathetic discharge, however, this reflex increase in contractility is not maximal, and administration of potent inotropic drugs can further augment contractile force. When a depression of myocardial function is an important factor in the precipitation of shock, the depression of contractility may be the major cause of the low stroke volume and cardiac output. In these circumstances inotropic agents might be particularly useful, unless the myocardium (because of inadequate nutrition or intrinsic muscle disease) cannot respond appropriately to the administration of these agents.

Heart Rate Alterations in heart rate within the physiological range usually do not markedly alter cardiac output when the heart is normal and the peripheral circulation is compensated; however, in the presence of myocardial dysfunction, alterations in heart rate may play an important role in limiting the cardiac output. Only when the heart rate appears to be inappropriate for the general circulatory state of the patient should primary attempts be made to alter heart rate in the management of shock.

Afterload The afterload represents the ventricular wall stress during ejection and is influenced by outflow resistance (impedance), ventricular chamber size and shape, wall thickness, stroke volume, and the rate of ejection. Since a number of these factors may be altered in varying directions in shock states, the systolic, diastolic, or mean arterial pressure (which are functions of only some of these factors) do not serve as a reliable guide to afterload. Increases in afterload tend to reduce stroke volume, particularly when pump function is abnormal. Furthermore, afterload is directly related to myocardial oxygen consumption. The importance of alterations in systemic vascular resistance on cardiac output in shock was considered in a previous section.

Right versus Left Ventricular Function
Shock results from an inadequate left ventricular output. When the pulmonary vascular bed is normal and no disease affecting specifically the left or right ventricle is present, the right ventricle serves as a simple conduit assisting in maintenance of left ventricular filling. Under these circumstances the right ventricular filling pressure and the left ventricular filling pressure bear a relatively constant and normal relationship to each other (the left ventricular filling pressure being slightly higher than the right), and cardiac function can be evaluated as a whole.[22] In disease states, however, a discrepancy between right and left ventricular function may appear. In acute myocardial infarction left ventricular dysfunction usually predominates and the left ventricular filling pressure is considerably higher than the right ventricular filling pressure because the disease usually is more severe in the left ventricular myocardium. When the pulmonary vascular bed is partially obliterated by obstruction or vasoconstriction, the fall in systemic output may relate in large part to inability of the right ventricle to maintain left ventricular filling. In this situation the right ventricular filling pressure may be as high or even higher than left ventricular filling pressure, and a knowledge of both may be necessary to understand the relationship between right and left ventricular function. A generalized depression of myocardial function, as may be observed in patients with septic shock, pancreatitis, and exposure to myocardial-depressant drugs, usually does not distort the normal relationship between right and left ventricular function, and both ventricles may therefore exhibit rather comparable depression of pump performance.[22]

Monitoring the Patient in Shock

Central Venous Pressure

The adequacy of the heart as a pump can best be evaluated clinically by relating the cardiac filling pressure to the stroke volume or cardiac output. When the heart or pulmonary vascular bed is not directly involved in the etiology of the low-flow state, the adequacy of cardiac filling can be assessed by measurement of the central venous pressure. This pressure approximates the right ventricular end-diastolic pressure or the mean right atrial pressure. It is a measure of the filling pressure of the right heart and provides a useful assessment of left ventricular filling pressure only when the pulmonary vascular bed is normal and the left ventricle is not primarily involved by a disease process. The normal right ventricular filling pressure may range from a mean of 0 to 8 mmHg. The peak of the venous pressure recorded in the right atrium or central veins is often somewhat higher than that figure because of an *a* wave of atrial contraction. When venous pressure is monitored with a highly damped water manometer system or an electronically meaned strain gauge transducer, a pressure above 8 mmHg, using the midaxillary line at the nipple level as a rough estimate of the position of the right atrium, is usually considered abnormal. If the venous pressure is measured visually by observing the peak of the undulating wave in the deep venous circulation of the neck or by measuring the peak of pulsatile pressure monitored with an electronic transducer, a peak of 10 or 12 mmHg may be considered normal. The importance, however, of the venous pressure is not in the use of a single measurement to make an assessment of normalcy, but rather the response of this venous pressure when a volume challenge is given to the patient who has shock or preshock. Response to a fluid load, preferably an intravascular substance such as albumin or dextran, provides the most precise guide as to whether the low-flow state is related to an inadequate venous return to the heart or to an abnormality of heart function.[6] The test may be performed by rapid infusion of volume in increments of 50 to 100 ml given as bolus injections. A rise in venous pressure of more than 3 mmHg without any associated improvement in the signs of reduced tissue perfusion may be taken as evidence that the shock is not volume-responsive. In contrast, an improvement in evidences of regional hypoperfusion associated with little or no increase in venous pressure is evidence of a volume-responsive state and an indication for further infusion of volume until the abnormal circulatory state is corrected. Since cardiac dysfunction is such a common component of shock, even when the shock is primarily volume-responsive, a higher than normal central venous pressure often is required in order to maintain an adequate cardiac output; that is, the cardiac function curve (Frank-Starling curve) is shifted somewhat downward and to the right, indicating a higher than normal cardiac filling pressure needed for the same cardiac output. Consequently, the filling pressure of the heart must often be increased to levels above those generally considered to be normal in order to reverse shock. After the shock has been corrected, the venous pressure may again fall while the circulatory improvement persists, probably because restoration of tissue perfusion results in an improvement in pump function. The height to which venous pressure may be safely raised cannot be categorically stated in every situation. In general, however, a mean right atrial pressure as high as 12 mmHg, assuming normal pulmonary vascular bed and no specific abnormalities of the left ventricle, is usually well tolerated and may be the most effective way of treating volume-responsive shock even in the presence of mild abnormalities of cardiac function.

Left Ventricular Filling Pressure

When acute volume expansion is ineffective in restoring the circulation, it must be assumed that cardiac dysfunction (pump failure) is playing an important role in the low-flow state. Under these circumstances it is usually mandatory to identify whether the disturbance resides predominantly in the right ventricle, the pulmonary vascular bed, or the left ventricle, and some measure of left ventricular filling pressure usually is necessary. Two approaches may be utilized:

1. Direct catheterization of the left ventricle may be accomplished by advancing a precurved catheter inserted percutaneously into a femoral artery up the aorta and into the left ventricle.[23] This procedure can usually be safely accomplished at the bedside without fluoroscopy, although the availability of a portable fluoroscopic unit is preferred by most physicians. Since catheters advanced into the aorta, particularly into the root of the aorta, may be the source of emboli to vital vascular beds, and since the catheter entering the left ventricle may induce transient arrhythmias, this procedure should be undertaken only in an intensive care setting where life-support systems are available and knowledgeable personnel are at the bedside to deal with any untoward complications. Meticulous care to avoid introducing clot through the catheter and to avoid inadvertent injections of air is of extreme importance. With careful attention to detail this procedure can be accomplished quickly and with a high degree of safety. A strain gauge transducer then is attached to the end of the catheter, and the pressure in the left ventricle is recorded directly, allowing assessment not only of the systolic pressure in the left ventricle but of the end-diastolic pressure, which provides an index of the adequacy of ventricular filling.
2. A more commonly used clinical procedure is

catheterization of the pulmonary artery, preferably with a balloon flotation catheter which can be introduced percutaneously through a sheath introduced into an antecubital vein. The catheter is designed so that a terminal balloon can be filled with approximately 1 ml of air, allowing the catheter to float from a central vein through the right atrium and right ventricle into the pulmonary artery.[24] The catheter can be advanced somewhat into the pulmonary artery after the balloon is deflated so that reinflation of the balloon provides temporary occlusion of a branch of the pulmonary artery and thus a stagnant column of blood from the end of the catheter into the left atrium. This pressure, the pulmonary capillary or wedge pressure, approximates the left ventricular diastolic pressure and provides a satisfactory index of left ventricular filling pressure. A proximal port on the catheter allows simultaneous monitoring of right atrial pressure. (See Chaps. 99 and 100.)

Mean left ventricular filling pressure normally is less than 12 mmHg. In the presence of mild left ventricular dysfunction in patients with volume-responsive shock a filling pressure as high as 20 mmHg may sometimes be required in order to provide an adequate cardiac output to maintain normal tissue perfusion. On the other hand, certain deleterious effects may result from even modest elevations in filling pressure. A rise in pulmonary capillary pressure may favor transudation of fluid into the lung, particularly if pulmonary capillary permeability is increased, and a rise in left ventricular diastolic pressure may impair subendocardial perfusion, especially if aortic diastolic pressure is reduced. Pressures above 20 mmHg may commonly be associated with pulmonary congestive symptoms, and left ventricular filling pressures above this level should generally be regarded as indicating that a low-flow state is not volume-responsive. Normally, left ventricular filling pressure ranges from 3 to 7 mmHg higher than right ventricular filling pressure. In the presence of disease confined predominantly to the left ventricle, the left ventricular filling pressure surpasses right ventricular filling pressure by more than the normal gradient, whereas when right ventricular filling pressure surpasses left ventricular filling pressure, a disease confined predominantly to the right ventricle or to the pulmonary vascular bed should be suspected. This latter phenomenon is most frequently observed in acute and chronic cor pulmonale and in the syndrome of right ventricular infarction.[25]

Arterial Pressure

Although shock is often recognized clinically by a fall in auscultatory blood pressure, it is now recognized that this reduced cuff pressure does not necessarily correspond to a reduction in intraarterial pressure. The advent of intraarterial pressure monitoring in acutely ill patients has made it clear that the clinical syndrome of shock may exist in the absence of hypotension. Therefore, a low arterial pressure no longer should be considered a prerequisite for the diagnosis of shock.

Since the level of arterial pressure is often an important factor in selecting therapy, knowledge of pressure is important in patient management. In patients with warm extremities, easily palpable pulses, and easily auscultable Korotkov sounds, intraarterial pressure usually corresponds quite closely with cuff pressure, even when the pressures are at hypotensive levels. In the patient who is peripherally vasoconstricted with cool upper extremities and thready brachial and radial pulses, the indirect pressure measured by deflating an arm cuff while palpating or auscultating over the brachial artery may be unreliable.[2] The only way to accurately assess arterial pressure in this setting is to directly cannulate an artery. This can be accomplished very simply in most patients with shock by inserting a plastic needle into either the femoral or brachial artery and connecting it directly to a pressure transducer and oscilloscope or recorder. The electronic measurement of arterial pulsatile pressure represents the only accurate way to assess true arterial pressure in the patient with shock.

Cardiac Output

The measurement of cardiac output at the bedside of acutely ill patients has previously been limited to research units. In recent years, however, the introduction of simplified instrumentation for performing and analyzing indicator-dilution cardiac outputs has brought this technique within the reach of most well-organized intensive care units. (See Chap. 100.) The thermal method employing a bolus injection of iced fluid provides the simplest means of performing sequential measurements of cardiac output in sick patients.[26] This technique requires the insertion into the pulmonary artery of a balloon-tipped catheter with a thermistor probe and a proximal injection lumen. Dye-dilution curves utilizing indocyanine green have been in use for many years and can be obtained by injecting into a central venous catheter while sampling from a peripheral artery, but in patients with severe shock the resultant dye-dilution curves may be so long and distorted that an accurate measurement of cardiac output is not possible. Monitoring of pulmonary arterial oxygen saturation can serve as a rough guide to the level of cardiac output.

In most patients with shock the actual measurement of cardiac output is not necessary, for the physician is better served by monitoring the adequacy of cardiac output as reflected in tissue perfusion and organ function as defined in Table 25-1. Actual measurements of output become useful only in situations where a therapeutic decision may be based upon the absolute level of cardiac index or where it seems important to monitor the patient's output in order to determine whether therapy is producing a salutary effect.

Blood Gases

Metabolic acidosis may develop because of inadequate tissue perfusion in shock and may even be aggravated when therapy is instituted because of the washout of accumulated lactate from areas of stasis;[27] therefore, frequent assessment of arterial blood pH and P_{CO_2} are important in the management of shock. Lactate levels might provide a more precise guide to the severity of tissue underperfusion, but frequent measurements of lactate are not practical in most institutions and reliance on the arterial blood pH and P_{CO_2} usually provides adequate information. The need for adequate oxygenation also makes it mandatory that P_{O_2} be monitored.

Therapeutic Approaches

The purpose of therapy in shock is to restore adequate tissue perfusion as quickly as possible. Since shock is an unsteady state characterized by positive-feedback mechanisms, therapy involves not only correction of the precipitating factors but also correction of those factors that may have been aggravating the shock state.

General Measures

Maintenance of oxygenation, correction of acid-base disorders, and relief of pain are necessary in all patients. High fever should be treated by skin cooling, and ventilatory function should be assisted if necessary. The use of corticosteroids has been advocated by some because in certain animal studies it has been demonstrated to reduce the mortality rate of shock.[28] Steroids do appear to have a protective effect on lysosomal membranes and therefore may reduce the rate of release of lysosomal enzymes that may contribute to circulatory deterioration.[29] High-dose steroids in the form of 30 mg/kg of methylprednisolone or its equivalent may therefore be employed, but the rationale for its use appears to be most appropriate in patients with shock whose circulatory inadequacy cannot be promptly restored by aggressive hemodynamic manipulation. Furthermore, it must be recognized that the safety of large-dose steroids in the setting of acute myocardial infarction has not yet been demonstrated.[30]

Adjustment of Cardiac Filling Pressure

Left and/or right ventricular filling pressure may be adjusted to its optimal level by volume expansion with the use of albumin, dextran, or saline solution or by volume depletion with the use of diuretics, phlebotomy, or tourniquets. When volume depletion is the major factor in the precipitation of the shock state, rapid expansion of volume will result in prompt and dramatic improvement. When cardiac factors predominate, adjustment of filling pressure will usually result in no remarkable change in the peripheral circulation. Because of the discrepancy between right and left ventricular function in some disease states, the absolute level of cardiac filling pressure which should be achieved varies. In pulmonary embolism, for instance, a central venous pressure as high as 15 to 20 mmHg may be required to achieve adequate left ventricular filling. In acute myocardial infarction, however, a venous pressure within the normal range may be associated with severe left ventricular failure, and left ventricular filling pressure must therefore be measured.[22]

Adjustment of Outflow Resistance

When left ventricular pump function is impaired, the outflow resistance becomes an important determinant of stroke volume and cardiac output. Vasodilator therapy may therefore markedly augment cardiac output and improve tissue perfusion. The limiting factor in the use of vasodilator drugs in the treatment of low-output states with left ventricular failure is the level of the arterial pressure. If therapy is instituted at a time that intraarterial pressure is still within the normal range or when systolic arterial pressure is at least 90 mmHg, cautious infusion of a vasodilator drug may be rewarded by marked improvement of the circulation.[31] The most useful agent for this purpose has been sodium nitroprusside (Nipride), which can be titrated in increasing doses (20 to 400 μg/min) while arterial pressure, ventricular filling pressure, and the signs of peripheral perfusion are closely monitored. Use of this approach to therapy in patients with shock usually requires an indwelling arterial needle and a catheter in the pulmonary artery as well as continuous monitoring of the drug infusion rate.

Since severe hypotension may result in rapid deterioration of the heart and peripheral circulation, it must be dealt with promptly. Although drugs which increase systemic vascular resistance by constricting peripheral arterioles might further reduce cardiac output by increasing outflow resistance, such drugs may be lifesaving in patients with severe hypotension. Indeed, the restoration of arterial pressure in such a hypotensive patient may immediately improve myocardial function and result in a rise rather than a fall in cardiac output.[32] In these selected instances it may be necessary to employ such drugs, and the vasoconstrictor agents of choice usually have inotropic as well as vasoconstrictor properties (e.g., norepinephrine, metaraminol). These drugs, however, do constrict the renal and splanchnic visceral vascular beds, and their prolonged use may be associated with progressive impairment of regional perfusion.

Drugs with a predominant inotropic effect, such as dopamine, may be effective in acutely raising arterial pressure in a hypotensive patient without impairing regional perfusion. These drugs, however, are not as reliable as norepinephrine in supporting arterial pressure.

The effect of vasoactive drugs on left ventricular filling pressure is dependent not only upon their effects on outflow resistance but also upon their effects on venous capacitance vessels. Venodilator drugs will lead to redistribution of volume into the periphery and a fall in filling pressures, whereas venoconstrictor drugs may shift blood centrally and augment filling pressure. Since nitroprusside is a potent venodilator, it produces a marked fall in left ventricular filling pressure by virtue of its effect on both resistance and capacitance.

Increase in Contractility

Inotropic agents (Table 25-2) increase myocardial contractile force and may result in a rise in cardiac output in patients with shock. These drugs also augment myocardial oxygen consumption and therefore should be used cautiously in the setting of ischemic heart disease (see below).

Each of these inotropic drugs has, in addition, distinct peripheral vascular actions. Therefore the choice of agent may depend as much on the state of the peripheral circulation as it does upon the myocardium. In general, those drugs that produce the greatest peripheral vasodilatation, such as isoproterenol, produce the greatest increase in cardiac output; but an increase in heart rate usually also occurs, and the distribution of the cardiac output may not necessarily be to the vascular beds in most desperate need. Dopamine (Intropin) has become a popular agent in the management of shock because its peripheral actions are not as prominent and in the usual therapeutic doses it does not redistribute regional flow in an adverse way. A newer analogue of dopamine, dobutamine, has even less peripheral vascular action and a more prominent inotropic effect. This drug also produces little change in heart rate and thus may not augment myocardial oxygen consumption as much as the

TABLE 25-2 Agents That Exert Inotropic Effect in Patients with Shock or Pump Failure

1. Drugs that have a net vasoconstrictor effect on the periphery
   a. Norepinephrine
   b. Metaraminol
   c. Epinephrine
   d. Digitalis
   e. Dopamine (high dose)
2. Drugs that have a net vasodilator effect on the periphery
   a. Isoproterenol
   b. Dobutamine
   c. Glucagon
   d. Dopamine (low dose)

other inotropic sympathomimetic agents. The virtue of these drugs is that they can be titrated and the response of the patient observed to determine whether the net effect is beneficial or deleterious.

Digitalis is not the inotropic drug of choice in shock, because its effect on contractility is not as great as that of the sympathomimetic amines, it does not usually produce much increase in cardiac output,[33] and dosage titration is more difficult and more dangerous. If a sustained inotropic effect is needed after the patient has stabilized, however, initiation of digitalis therapy may be indicated.

The effect of inotropic drugs on left ventricular filling pressure in pump failure is somewhat variable. Although a modest reduction might be anticipated because of better left ventricular emptying, vascular effects (arterial or venoconstrictor) may predominate and actually lead to an increase in filling pressure.

Combined Use of Inotropic and Vasodilator Drugs

Combined administration of an inotropic drug, such as dobutamine or dopamine, with a vasodilator drug, such as nitroprusside, provides the opportunity to optimize contractility and outflow resistance in patients with severe pump failure. In practice the inotropic drug is administered in a dosage of from 5 to 15 μg/kg/min, while the vasodilator is titrated on the basis of left ventricular filling pressure, peripheral perfusion, and arterial pressure. Combined therapy results in a greater augmentation of left ventricular function than can be achieved with either agent alone.[34]

Adjustment of Heart Rate

If shock exists in the presence of heart block with a bradycardia, emergency pacing should be initiated with a transvenous or transthoracic wire. Rapid supraventricular or ventricular tachycardias may necessitate prompt electrical cardioversion. In general antiarrhythmic drugs should be avoided as much as possible in pump failure because of their potential depressive effect on myocardial function.

Pump Failure in Acute Myocardial Infarction

When shock develops in the setting of acute myocardial infarction, the prognosis is extremely poor, even with the most aggressive medical therapy. The mortality rate in such patients is generally accepted to be between 80 and 95 percent,[35] although some variation in this figure may be due to differing clinical criteria for the diagnosis of shock. Patients who have lived long enough to arrive in the hospital after suffering an acute myocardial infarction have prob-

ably already demonstrated that the initial destruction of functioning myocardial mass was not so great to make pump function inadequate to sustain life. This concept has led to the suggestion that shock after acute myocardial infarction frequently represents a progressive process in which pump function may become gradually worse because of changes in the heart and/or the peripheral circulation occurring after the initial myocardial insult. It is therefore appropriate to assume that all patients who are destined to develop the shock syndrome pass through a phase of less severe impairment of pump function before the full-blown syndrome develops.

The management of the patient with pump failure after acute myocardial infarction requires an understanding of a variety of hemodynamic and metabolic events. These are discussed in the following sections.

Hemodynamics of Acute Myocardial Infarction

Some degree of pump dysfunction is common after acute myocardial infarction. In the majority of patients the infarct is confined to the left ventricle, and the left ventricular dysfunction is characterized by an elevated left ventricular filling pressure and a low stroke volume.[36] Cardiac output may in part be compensated by an increase in heart rate; but when the infarct is severe, cardiac output is usually depressed. Despite the low cardiac output, arterial pressure is usually normal and sometimes elevated.

In some instances, the infarction affects predominantly the right ventricle. This syndrome presents with electrocardiographic evidence of inferior wall myocardial infarction, usually accompanied by heart block and hypotension.[25] The venous pressure is elevated out of proportion to any elevation of left ventricular filling pressure, accounting for the coexistence of distended neck veins and clear lung fields. The hemodynamic picture therefore is that of acute right ventricular failure, but some degree of left ventricular dysfunction is also often evident. Indeed, the low-output shock which may accompany this syndrome appears to be related in large part to the inability of the damaged right ventricle to generate enough pressure to fill the left ventricle in the face of a modestly elevated left ventricular filling pressure.[37] Both anatomically and functionally this syndrome involves infarct in both the right and left ventricles.

Periinfarction Zone

Recent experimental evidence suggests that the area of the myocardial infarct may not necessarily be determined at the time of infarction. Since necrosis of myocardium occurs because of an imbalance between myocardial oxygen supply and oxygen requirement, it is likely that the area of myocardium in which oxygen delivery is jeopardized is larger than the area of necrosis. Thus a zone of relative ischemia may exist around or near the area that has already become infarcted.[38] Furthermore, it is possible that this area of ischemia may either eventually recover, perhaps because of the development of a more effective collateral circulation, or eventually go on to necrosis, particularly if, during the period this myocardium is jeopardized, its oxygen consumption is increased or its oxygen delivery is further reduced. In experimental models of myocardial infarction it has been demonstrated that the eventual size of myocardial infarcts may be altered by pharmacologic or mechanical interventions after the coronary arterial supply has been obstructed.[39] If this thesis also holds for human myocardial infarcts, therapy initiated to treat pump failure in the early phases of acute myocardial infarction must be carefully selected to avoid further aggravation of the myocardial imbalance between oxygen delivery and oxygen consumption.

Dynamics of Infarcted Zone

Myocardial contraction ceases soon after the acute event in the central area of myocardial necrosis.[40] Loss of contractile function in this area, however, is not the only potential adverse effect of the myocardial infarction. Changes in compliance also may occur in this infarct zone. If compliance increases, as it may in the early phase after infarction, a bulge in this area during systole would further aggravate the low cardiac output in this syndrome. In contrast, an increase in stiffness of the infarcted zone, a phenomenon which has been described,[41] would inhibit left ventricular filling and lead to a rise in left ventricular filling pressure and a high pulmonary capillary pressure. In addition, changes in electrical depolarization leading to some delay in depolarization in the areas immediately surrounding the infarct might also depress pump function by producing dyssynergy of contraction and/or delayed relaxation.

Coronary Blood Flow

Total coronary blood flow is dependent on the perfusion pressure and the coronary vascular resistance. When an atherosclerotic plaque in a proximal coronary artery produces significant obstruction, the reduced coronary arterial pressure beyond the obstruction becomes the driving pressure for coronary flow. Minor changes in caliber of these coronary arteries, either by virtue of active vasomotor changes or passive changes resulting from alterations in transmural pressure, could produce striking effects on the proximal resistance and therefore on the pressure gradient from the proximal to the distal coronary arterial segment.[42] In addition, arteriolar dilatation induced by ischemia may further decrease distal pressure in the presence of a proximal stenosis.[43]

Perfusion of the subendocardium is particularly dependent as well upon the level of intracavitary pressure during diastole. A rise in left ventricular diastolic pressure, which is characteristic of angina or myocardial infarction, will inhibit subendocardial perfusion during diastole by virtue of the high extravascular pressure transmitted into the subendocardium.[44] When perfusion pressure is already reduced because of a proximal stenotic lesion, the superimposition of a high left ventricular diastolic pressure may reduce the effective coronary perfusion pressure and lead to marked reductions of subendocardial perfusion. Since total coronary blood flow measurements do not provide information about transmural distribution of flow and since transmural flow patterns cannot be measured in human beings, the importance of these phenomena in affecting the course of left ventricular damage after acute myocardial infarction is not known.

Myocardial Oxygen Consumption

The oxygen consumption of myocardium is dependent upon the wall tension, which relates to chamber pressure and radius, the cardiac rate, and myocardial contractility.[45] Shortening itself is only a minor factor in myocardial oxygen consumption. It may therefore be assumed that any intervention which increases heart size, raises systolic blood pressure, or increases contractility will result in an increase in myocardial oxygen consumption. If this increase occurs in an area which has a jeopardized blood flow, it is possible that ischemia would be aggravated and the infarct extended.

Causes of Low Cardiac Output

In addition to the loss of functioning myocardium in the area of necrosis, and perhaps in the periinfarct ischemic zone as well, and to the effect of changes in wall characteristics in the area of damage, a number of other factors may be operating that could eventuate in a fall in cardiac output and the syndrome of pump failure or shock.

Hypovolemia
Circulating plasma volume may be reduced after acute myocardial infarction because of release of catecholamines, sweating, reduced fluid intake, or administration of diuretics. When myocardial function is impaired, the left ventricle requires a higher-than-normal end-diastolic volume in order to maintain an adequate cardiac output. If venous return is impaired because of this hypovolemia, the left ventricular filling may fall below its optimal level and cardiac output may be correspondingly reduced. Hypovolemia is rarely the major factor in development of shock after acute myocardial infarction, but it may contribute often enough that it must be kept in mind and evaluated by measuring left ventricular filling pressure.

Arrhythmias

Both bradyarrhythmias and tachyarrhythmias may significantly impair cardiac output, particularly when pump function is abnormal. Heart rates below 60 per minute may be associated with hypotensive states that are corrected when the rate is increased by administration of atropine or by ventricular pacing. Rapid heart rates may not only reduce cardiac output, but since they also markedly augment myocardial oxygen consumption, they may initiate a vicious circle in which ischemic injury is aggravated and pump function gradually deteriorates. Therefore electrical control of rapid tachyarrhythmias is often an important factor in correcting the circulation. Although isolated premature ventricular beats probably do not significantly alter cardiac function, these premature beats may consume oxygen without doing useful work. Therefore when premature beats become frequent, they may indeed adversely affect pump performance. The relationship between depolarization pathway and pump function has not been well defined, but delayed intraventricular conduction by altering the pathway of depolarization and therefore the sequence of contraction could well result in some dyssynergy of contraction and a further impairment of cardiac performance.

Drugs

The ischemic ventricle may be very sensitive to the deleterious effects of drugs that normally produce little or no depression of cardiac function. Antiarrhythmic drugs are frequently used in the setting of acute myocardial infarction and may occasionally precipitate or aggravate left ventricular failure. These drugs should be used with caution in the setting of pump failure; the dose should be kept low, and care should be taken that indication for treatment is clear. Propranolol particularly may depress left ventricular function, and its use in the setting of pump failure is extremely hazardous. It must be recognized that the physiological effect of cardiac-depressant drugs may long outlast the biological half-life of the agent, since positive-feedback mechanisms initiated during the period of drug action may continue and become self-perpetuating even though the drug is withdrawn.

Structural Factors

Depending on the location of the myocardial necrosis, alterations in function of the mitral valve apparatus may allow for mitral regurgitation and a depression of left ventricular output on that basis. Interventricular septal rupture may produce a similar syndrome. These sometimes severe complications of acute myocardial infarction usually can be recognized at the bedside.

Treatment of Pump Failure

Optimal management of the patient with pump failure after acute myocardial infarction is best accomplished with invasive monitoring of left ventricular filling pressure (pulmonary wedge pressure) and arterial pressure. Under circumstances when it is not possible or not desirable to utilize these invasive techniques, it may be possible to estimate the left ventricular filling pressure and the arterial pressure on the basis of bedside observations. Although these gross estimates may frequently be reliable enough to allow proper selection of therapy, in as many as 25 percent of cases these clinical estimates are in error and may lead to inappropriate treatment.

General Treatment

As in other forms of shock, relief of pain, maintenance of normal oxygenation, and correction of acid-base abnormalities should be accomplished before specific therapy is initiated. If hypotension or signs of pump failure coexist with a heart rate below 60 beats per minute, atropine should be administered. If a supraventricular tachycardia with a rate of over 150 beats per minute coexists with hypotension, consideration may be given to an attempt at cardioversion. More modest degrees of tachycardia are common in the setting of pump failure and usually reflect sympathoadrenal discharge consequent to the low stroke volume. A therapy that is effective in improving pump function will usually result in a reduction in the increased heart rate.

Diuretics in the form of intravenous furosemide (40 to 400 mg) should be administered to maintain urine flow in the face of poor renal perfusion. Administration of large doses of steroids in the form of 30 mg/kg of prednisolone or its equivalent may be considered if it is anticipated that the period of pump failure will be prolonged. A single dose of steroids probably has no deleterious effect, although repetitive doses may delay the rate of healing if the patient survives the acute episode of pump failure.[30]

Volume Manipulation

If the initial left ventricular filling pressure is less than 15 mmHg (using the midchest as the zero level), a therapeutic trial with acute plasma volume expansion is indicated. This is best accomplished by administering albumin, plasma protein, or dextran in 50-ml bolus injections while the left ventricular filling pressure is closely monitored. The volume expansion may be continued until the left ventricular filling pressure rises to 20 mmHg. If this therapy results in evidence of improved peripheral circulation, maintenance of left ventricular filling pressure at this level should be accomplished by continuous monitoring of the pressure and further volume expansion if needed. If the initial left ventricular filling pressure is over 25 mmHg and there is clinical evidence of pulmonary edema, consideration may be given to application of tourniquets or phlebotomy to acutely reduce pulmonary capillary pressure; however, therapy with vasodilator drugs, as described in the next section, usually is preferable.

Vasodilator Drugs

An elevated left ventricular filling pressure with signs of a low cardiac output is an indication for a therapeutic trial with vasodilator drugs if the systolic arterial pressure is over 90 mmHg. Even in the presence of hypotension, with arterial systolic pressures in the range of 80 to 90 mmHg, a beneficial effect of vasodilator therapy is occasionally observed. Nitroprusside (Nipride) is the agent of choice and should be administered in increasing doses starting at an infusion rate of 15 g/min until either the left ventricular filling pressure is reduced by about 50 percent, the arterial pressure falls to dangerously low levels, or the patient becomes symptomatic from induced hypotension. If the vasodilator infusion results in evidence of improved peripheral blood flow, the drug should be continued at a stable infusion rate until it can be weaned. The period of infusion may range from 12 to 72 h without any significant risk of nitroprusside toxicity.

Nitrate therapy in the form of nitroglycerin ointment or isosorbide dinitrate administered sublingually or orally may be substituted for nitroprusside. Nitrates, however, do not result in as much improvement in cardiac output as does nitroprusside, and the titration of dosage is considerably more difficult. Other intravenous agents such as phentolamine and trimethaphan are more difficult to use than nitroprusside and appear to have no advantages.

Inotropic Drugs

If vasodilator drugs alone are unable to restore peripheral perfusion, or if the initial arterial pressure is dangerously low, the administration of an inotropic drug is appropriate. The best tolerated agents are dopamine and dobutamine. These drugs should be given intravenously in a dose of from 5 to 15 μg/kg/min. An effect is characterized by a rise in systolic blood pressure, a slight but often insignificant increase in heart rate, and evidence of improved peripheral blood flow.

Norepinephrine and metaraminol, inotropic agents with potent peripheral vasoconstrictor effects, may be employed specifically in the patient with severe hypotension and pump failure. It should be recognized, however, that these drugs will support arterial pressure in part by an increase in systemic vascular resistance and that the improvement in regional perfusion may therefore be less than with the other inotropic agents. Therefore, therapy with these vasoconstrictor drugs should be considered emergency treatment to support arterial pressure and preserve life while more effective means of therapy are being considered.

Digitalis does not have an important place in the management of pump failure after acute myocardial infarction. Previous studies have not demonstrated much rise in cardiac output after digitalis administration in this setting,[33] and the drug is difficult to titrate and prone to produce dangerous arrhythmias. In addition, its peripheral vasoconstrictor effect may further limit the improvement in peripheral blood flow that otherwise might occur.

Mechanical Cardiac Assistance

Intraaortic balloon counterpulsation is now widely employed to support left ventricular function in the failing heart.[46] This technique is accomplished by advancing from the femoral artery into the descending thoracic aorta a catheter with a terminal balloon that holds approximately 30 ml. This balloon is then sequentially inflated with carbon dioxide, utilizing the R wave of the electrocardiogram for automatic timing. The balloon is deflated immediately prior to left ventricular systole so that the left ventricle ejects against a low outflow resistance. The balloon is then reinflated immediately after the aortic valve closes in order to raise aortic pressure during diastole, when the pressure load will not affect myocardial oxygen consumption. The net effect of this mechanical assistance is that left ventricular stroke volume is increased, aortic diastolic pressure is elevated, coronary blood flow is increased, and peripheral perfusion should be improved. (See Chap. 102.)

Intraaortic balloon pumping frequently results in prompt clinical improvement in the patient with pump failure. Sometimes the beneficial effect persists, but often the improvement is either short-lived or the patient deteriorates as soon as the mechanical assistance is discontinued. When this occurs, it is assumed that the left ventricular damage was so severe that temporary support of the circulation was inadequate to reestablish adequate cardiac function. Some experts have recommended intervention with mechanical assistance at an earlier stage of the disease, hopefully before such severe and irreversible myocardial damage has occurred. No controlled studies have been carried out to evaluate the efficacy of mechanical assistance as a means of temporary circulatory support in patients with milder degrees of pump failure.

Emergency Surgery

Surgery designed to improve perfusion of ischemic myocardium has been employed with limited success in patients with acute myocardial infarction. Some patients who have exhibited temporary response to balloon counterpulsation have been salvaged when coronary bypass surgery is carried out during the period of mechanical assistance.[47] Experience to date suggests that if such bypass surgery is to be effective it should be performed as soon as possible after the onset of acute myocardial infarction, preferably within the first 12 h. This is probably due to the likelihood that reversibly ischemic areas are playing a role in the pump failure in this early stage of the disease but that these ischemic areas become progressively more necrotic as the shock state persists.

Surgery to correct other structural abnormalities contributing to pump failure may also be effective. Repair of ruptured septum, ruptured papillary muscle, or perforation of the ventricle all have resulted in dramatic improvement. Removal of a portion of the infarcted myocardium has been attempted in several centers but has not resulted in uniform improvement, unless the area of infarction dilated aneurysmally during systole.[47] (See Chap. 104.)

References

1. Bloch, J. H., Pierce, C. H., Manax, W. G., Lyons, G. W., and Lillehei, R. C.: Experimental Cardiogenic Shock, *Arch. Surg.*, 91:77, 1965.
2. Cohn, J. N.: Blood Pressure Measurement in Shock: Mechanism of Inaccuracy in Auscultatory and Palpatory Methods, *J. Am. Med. Assoc.*, 199:972, 1967.
3. Cohn, J. N., and Luria, M. H.: Studies in Clinical Shock and Hypotension. The Value of Bedside Hemodynamic Observations, *J. Am. Med. Assoc.*, 190:891, 1964.
4. Udhoji, V. N., and Weil, M. H.: Hemodynamic and Metabolic Studies on Shock Associated with Bacteremia: Observations on Sixteen Patients, *Ann. Intern. Med.*, 62:966, 1965.
5. Wilson, R. F., Thal, A. P., Kindling, P. H., Grifka, T., and Ackerman, E.: Hemodynamic Measurements in Septic Shock, *Arch. Surg.*, 91:121, 1965.
6. Cohn, J. N., Luria, M. H., Daddario, R. C., and Tristani, F. E.: Studies in Clinical Shock and Hypotension. V. Hemodynamic Effects of Dextran, *Circulation*, 35:316, 1967.
7. Cohn, J. N.: Relationship of Plasma Volume Changes to Resistance and Capacitance Vessel Effects of Sympathomimetic Amines and Angiotensin in Man, *Clin. Sci.*, 30:267, 1966.
8. Cohn, J. N.: Central Venous Pressure as a Guide to Volume Expansion, *Ann. Intern. Med.*, 66:1283, 1967.
9. Tristani, F. E., and Cohn, J. N.: Studies in Clinical Shock and Hypotension. VII. Renal Hemodynamics before and during Treatment, *Circulation*, 42:839, 1970.
10. Cohn, J. N., and Luria, M. H.: Studies in Clinical Shock and Hypotension. IV. Variations in Reflex Vasoconstriction and Cardiac Stimulation, *Circulation*, 34:823, 1966.
11. Constantin, L.: Extracardiac Factors Contributing to Hypotension during Coronary Occlusion, *Am. J. Cardiol.*, 11:205, 1963.
12. Thames, M. D., Klopfenstein, H. S., Abboud, F. M., Mark, A. L., and Walker, J. L.: Preferential Distribution of Inhibitory Cardiac Receptors with Vagal Afferents to the Inferoposterior Wall of the Left Ventricle Activated during Coronary Occlusion in the Dog, *Circ. Res.*, 43:512, 1978.
13. Webb, S. W., Adgey, A. A., and Pantridge, J. F.: Autonomic Disturbance at Onset of Acute Myocardial Infarction, *Br. Med. J.*, 3:89, 1972.
14. Cohn, J. N.: Vasodilator Therapy for Heart Failure: The Influence of Impedance on Left Ventricular Performance, *Circulation*, 48:5, 1973.
15. Haddy, F. J., Fleishman, M., and Emanuel, D. A.: Effect of Epinephrine, Norepinephrine and Serotonin upon Systemic Small and Large Vessel Resistance, *Circ. Res.*, 5:247, 1957.
16. Mellaner, S., and Lewis, D. H.: Effect of Hemorrhagic Shock on the Reactivity of Resistance and Capacitance Vessels and on Capillary Filtration Transfer in Cat Skeletal Muscle, *Circ. Res.*, 13:105, 1963.
17. Cobbold, A., Folkow, B., Kjellmer, I., and Mellander, S.: Nervous and Local Chemical Control of Precapillary Sphincters in Skeletal Muscle as Measured by Changes in Filtration Coefficient, *Acta. Physiol. Scand.*, 57:180, 1963.
18. Kjekshus, J. K.: Mechanism for Flow Distribution in Normal and Ischemic Myocardium during Increased Ventricular Preload in the Dog, *Circ. Res.*, 33:489, 1973.
19. Lefer, A. M.: Role of a Myocardial Depressant Factor in the Pathogenesis of Hemorrhagic Shock, *Fed. Proc.*, 29:1836, 1970.
20. Wiedanthal, K., Mierzwiak, D. S., Meyers, R. W., and Mitchell, J. H.: Effects of Acute Lactic Acidosis on Left Ventricular Performance, *Am. J. Physiol.*, 214:1352, 1968.
21. Gaasch, W. H., Levine, H. J., Quinones, M. A., and Alexander, J. K.: Left Ventricular Compliance: Mechanisms and Clinical Implications, *Am. J. Cardiol.*, 38:645, 1976.
22. Cohn, J. N., and Tristani, F. E.: Studies in Clinical Shock and Hypotension. VI. Relationship between Left and Right Ventricular Function, *J. Clin. Invest.*, 48:2008, 1969.
23. Cohn, J. N., Khatri, I. M., and Hamosh, P.: Bedside Catheterization of the Left Ventricle, *Am. J. Cardiol.*, 25:66, 1970.
24. Swan, H. J. C., Ganz, W., Forrester, J., Marcus, H., Diamond, G., and Chonette, D.: Catheterization of the Heart in Man with the Use of a Flow-Directed Balloon-Tipped Catheter, *N. Engl. J. Med.*, 283:447, 1970.
25. Cohn, J. N., Guiha, N. H., Broder, M. I., and Limas, C. J.: Right Ventricular Infarction: Clinical and Hemodynamic Features, *Am. J. Cardiol.*, 33:209, 1974.
26. Ganz, W., and Swan, H. J. C.: Measurement of Blood Flow by Thermodilution, *Am. J. Cardiol.*, 29:241, 1972.
27. Sriussadaporn, S., and Cohn, J. N.: Lactate Metabolism in Clinical and Experimental Shock, *Clin. Res.*, 16:519, 1968.
28. Spath, J. A., Jr., Goreynski, R. J., and Lefer, A. M.: Possible Mechanisms of the Beneficial Action of Glucocorticoids in Circulatory Shock, *Surg. Gynecol. Obst.*, 137:597, 1973.
29. Weissman, G.: Corticosteroids and Membrane Stabilization, *Circulation*, 53:I-171, 1976.
30. Bulkley, B. H., and Roberts, W. C.: Steroid Therapy during Acute Myocardial Infarction—A Cause of Delayed Healing and of Ventricular Aneurysm, *Am. J. Med.*, 56:244, 1974.

31. Cohn, J. N., Mathew, K. J., Franciosa, J. A., and Snow, J. A.: Chronic Vasodilator Therapy in the Management of Cardiogenic Shock and Intractable Left Ventricular Failure, *Ann. Intern. Med.*, 81:777, 1974.

32. Cohn, J. N., and Luria, M. H.: Studies in Clinical Shock and Hypotension. II. Hemodynamic Effects of Norepinephrine and Angiotensin, *J. Clin. Invest.*, 44:1494, 1965.

33. Cohn, J. N., Tristani, F. E., and Khatri, I. M.: Cardiac and Peripheral Vascular Effects of Digitalis in Clinical Cardiogenic Shock, *Am. Heart J.*, 78:318, 1969.

34. Mikulic, E., Cohn, J. N., and Franciosa, J. A.: Comparative Hemodynamic Effects of Inotropic and Vasodilator Drugs in Severe Heart Failure, *Circulation*, 56:528, 1977.

*35. Scheidt, S., Ascheim, R., and Killip, T.: Shock after Acute Myocardial Infarction, *Am. J. Cardiol.*, 26:556, 1970. (20 references)

36. Hamosh, P., and Cohn, J. N.: Left Ventricular Function in Acute Myocardial Infarction, *J. Clin. Invest.*, 50:523, 1971.

37. Cohn, J. N.: Right Ventricular Infarction Revisited, *Am. J. Cardiol.*, 43:666, 1979.

38. Cox, J. L., McLaughlin, V. W., Flowers, N. C., and Horan, L. G.: The Ischemic Zone Surrounding Acute Myocardial Infarction. Its Morphology as Detected by Dehydrogenase Staining, *Am. Heart J.*, 76:650, 1968.

*This article is a review of the literature and contains additional references to the literature.

39. Maroko, P. R., Kjekshus, J. K., Sobel, B. E., Watanaber, T., Covell, J. W., Ross, J ., Jr., and Braunwald, E.: Factors Influencing Infarct Size Following Experimental Coronary Artery Occlusion, *Circulation*, 43:67, 1971.

40. Tennant, R., and Wiggers, C. J.: Effect of Coronary Occlusion on Myocardial Contraction, *Am. J. Physiol.*, 112:351, 1935.

41. Weisse, A. B., Saffa, R. S., Levinson, G. E., Jacobson, W. W., and Regan, T. J.: Left Ventricular Function during the Early and Late Stages of Scar Formation Following Experimental Myocardial Infarction, *Am. Heart J.*, 79:370, 1970.

42. Schwartz, J. S., Carlyle, P. F., and Cohn, J. N.: Effect of Dilation of the Distal Coronary Bed on Flow and Resistance in Severely Stenotic Coronary Arteries in the Dog, *Am. J. Cardiol.*, 43:219, 1979.

43. Schwartz, J. S., Carlyle, P. F., and Cohn, J. N.: Effect of Coronary Arterial Pressure on Coronary Stenosis Resistance, *Circulation*, 61:70, 1980.

44. Salisbury, P. F., Cross, C. E., and Rieban, P. A.: Acute Ischemia of Inner Layers of Ventricular Wall, *Am. Heart J.*, 66:650, 1963.

45. Sonnenblick, E. H., and Skelton, C. L.: Myocardial Energetics: Basic Principles and Clinical Implications, *N. Engl. J. Med.*, 285:668, 1971.

46. Kuhn, L. A.: Current Status of Diastolic Augmentation for Circulatory Support, *Am. Heart J.*, 81:281, 1971.

47. Mundth, E. D., Mechanical and Surgical Interventions for the Reduction of Myocardial Ischemia, *Circulation*, 53:I-176, 1976.

Section D High Cardiac Output

26

High-Cardiac-Output States

Noble O. Fowler, M.D.

In 1947, Burwell and Dexter[1] first demonstrated by the direct Fick method that the cardiac output was increased in a patient with acute beriberi and congestive heart failure. They stated:

> These observations supplement and confirm those of Hayasaka and Inawashiro, Weiss and Wilkins, and Porter and Downs in showing that cardiac failure in patients with beri-beri is associated with a cardiac output that is *increased*. They supplement previous observations of peripheral arterial and venous pressures. They are the first reported measurements of the pressure in the pulmonary artery and the right ventricle in beri-beri disease.
>
> This man had congestive heart failure which would have been recognized as such by any member of this Association. Since this method is preferable to those previously used, these are the most reliable measurements so far available of the cardiac output in heart failure due to beri-beri heart disease.
>
> The conclusion, therefore, is that in heart failure due to beri-beri the cardiac output may be elevated both absolutely and in relation to the oxygen consumption.

The disorders discussed in this chapter are those in which the resting cardiac output is increased in human adults beyond the normal range of 2.3 to 3.9 liters/min/m^2. The cardiac output may be raised by increasing either the heart rate, the stroke volume, or both. In the pathologic high-output states, usually both heart rate and stroke volume are increased.

Braunwald emphasized that the contraction of ventricular muscle is controlled by four major factors.[2]

1. Preload (ventricular end-diastolic fiber tension, usually estimated from atrial pressure or ventricular end-diastolic pressure)
2. Myocardial contractility
3. Afterload
4. Heart rate

Variations in cardiac filling pressure are not usually responsible for increasing cardiac output beyond normal values in resting human beings. In the non-failing heart, the cardiac output is not limited by the myocardial contractile state, and augmentation of the contractile state, i.e., by digitalis or paired electrical stimulation, does not increase the output of the heart. Hence, although neurohumoral mechanisms are important in controlling the output of the heart, the increased cardiac output of the hyperdynamic states usually does not result from increased cardiac contractility alone.

In most of the hyperdynamic states, which may be exemplified by anemia or thyrotoxicosis, the increased cardiac output results from a rise in both heart rate and stroke volume, although the heart rate is seldom greatly above 100 beats per minute.

It is probable that a reduced afterload is a major mechanism in many human hyperdynamic states. Left ventricular afterload is defined as the resistance to ejection and further shortening encountered by the contracting muscle fibers at the end of isovolumic systole. Reduced left ventricular afterload may occur when there is peripheral shunting of blood (systemic arteriovenous fistula), central shunting (patent ductus arteriosus), peripheral vasodilatation (thyrotoxicosis), or reduced blood viscosity (anemia). Reduced afterload is important in the increased cardiac output of anemia. Reduction of blood viscosity can be shown to increase the cardiac output in the heart-lung preparation and in intact animals.[3] Restoration of normal mean blood pressure by α-adrenergic agents reduces the elevated cardiac output in people with anemia[4] or thyrotoxicosis,[5] suggesting the importance of reduced ventricular afterload in these two disorders.

Physical Findings in the Hyperdynamic States

When there is an increase of the cardiac output at rest, certain physical findings tend to appear. Thyrotoxicosis, liver disease, and severe anemia are by far the commonest clinical disorders associated with an increase of cardiac output at rest, if one excepts pregnancy, fever, and emotional excitement. The physical findings commonly associated with the hyperdynamic state in these disorders may be taken as a model for the physical findings to be expected when the resting cardiac output is increased. These physical findings are related to the following areas: the heart rate, the systemic veins, the systemic arteries, the blood pressure, and auscultation of the precordium.

Heart Rate

The heart rate and stroke volume are each usually increased in the high-cardiac-output states. The tachycardia is usually moderate, however, and the heart rate at rest is likely to be in the range of 85 to 105 beats per minutes. Anemic patients with hyperdynamic states usually have a resting heart rate below 100 beats per minute unless there is acute blood loss.[6] In hyperthyroidism, the heart rate is seldom above 110 beats per minute unless there is severe thyrotoxicosis, bordering on thyroid storm, or complicating atrial fibrillation.

Systemic Veins

The ventricular preload is usually normal in the hyperdynamic states, and thus the systemic venous pressure is normal and the cervical veins are not abnormally distended unless there is a complicating systemic congestive state with "heart failure." However, the systemic veins may display useful signs of an accelerated circulation. A cervical venous hum, heard over the deep internal jugular veins, more often on the right side, is a common finding in the hyperdynamic states. This continuous murmur with diastolic accentuation can be heard as a normal finding in children in the sitting posture. When a cervical venous hum is readily heard in an adult, however, especially in the recumbent posture, a hyperdynamic state is likely. Uncommonly, there may be a venous hum over the femoral veins, especially in patients with sickle-cell anemia.

Systemic Arteries

The systemic arteries may display signs related to the increased left ventricular stroke volume, to the increased rate of ejection, and to the decreased peripheral resistance. Consequently the pulse tends to be bounding with a quick upstroke. The pulse pressure typically is wide, with a decrease of diastolic pressure and an increase of systolic blood pressure. Pistol-shot sounds, and Duroziez's murmur may be heard over the femoral arteries. A systolic bruit may be heard over the carotid arteries. In the absence of aortic regurgitation or patent ductus arteriosus, or other left-to-right extracardiac shunt, these signs are highly suggestive of an elevated left ventricular stroke volume and, if the heart rate is normal or rapid, of an increased cardiac output. It should be recalled that the pulse pressure may be high with a normal diastolic pressure where there is increased sclerosis of the thoracic aorta—a finding usually restricted to the elderly. Further, the left ventricular stroke volume may be high but the cardiac output normal or low when there is complete AV block with a slow ventricular rate; this is especially true in congenital complete AV block.

Precordial Auscultation

The increased rate of ventricular ejection commonly produces turbulence and causes a midsystolic murmur in the second and third left intercostal spaces. Decreased blood viscosity may contribute to increased turbulence of blood flow. Increased rate of ventricular filling may cause a third heart sound to be audible at the cardiac apex. An apical fourth heart sound is common in thyrotoxicosis if there is sinus rhythm, but its mechanism is uncertain. Diastolic aortic murmurs have been described in occasional patients with severe anemia or thyrotoxicosis, but are rare in the absence of associated aortic valvular disease except in uremic patients. Mitral diastolic murmurs are occasionally heard in patients with sickle-cell anemia.

Systemic and Pulmonary Congestion in the Hyperdynamic States

Patients with one of the many high-cardiac-output states may develop the signs, symptoms, and physiologic evidence of pulmonary or systemic congestion or both. Systemic and pulmonary venous hypertension and water and sodium retention may occur much as in other varieties of cardiac decompensation, even though in these patients the cardiac output, although lower than before the onset of congestion, remains above normal. The appropriate label for the congestive state accompanying the hyperdynamic states is controversial. Eichna suggested that these patients be designated by the term *noncardiac circulatory congestion*[7] rather than heart failure, since the cardiac output is above normal and these patients often have little or no response to digitalis. Since the symptoms and physical findings are similar to those of patients with the more common "low-output" congestive failure syndrome, however, we have used the more common label of *congestive failure* for the congestive state accompanying the hyperdynamic disorders. (See Chap. 22.)

Thyrotoxicosis

Abnormal Physiology

Thyrotoxicosis, which has several different causes, is characterized by an increased cardiac output. The increased oxygen consumption raises the cardiac output to supply the metabolic needs of the body, yet in many patients there is an increase in cardiac output beyond this requirement. Tachycardia, which is usually found in this disorder, serves to increase the output of the heart while cardiac stroke volume is maintained. In addition, there is often an increased cardiac stroke volume.[8] There are at least three major factors for consideration in the increased cardiac stroke volume of thyrotoxicosis. There is probably a direct action of thyroid hormone upon the heart that causes it to beat more rapidly, even when devoid of adrenergic and cholinergic influences. Increased sensitivity to circulating epinephrine and norepinephrine has been demonstrated in thyrotoxicosis. This tends to increase cardiac stroke volume. Studies of subjects with spontaneous hyperthyroidism demonstrated that β-sympathetic receptor blockade reduced oxygen consumption and heart rate and lengthened the circulation time. The left ventricular preejection period and ejection times remained abbreviated, however, as is characteristic of hyperthyroidism. The left ventricular preejection period/ejection time ratio (PEP/LVET) is decreased in hyperthyroidism and returns to normal when the patient becomes euthyroid.[9] Administration of reserpine to hyperthyroid patients failed to alter the circulatory dynamics toward normal. Hence the concept that the circulatory effects of thyrotoxicosis are mediated by the sympathetic nervous system was not supported. In thyrotoxicosis there is evidence of decreased peripheral vascular resistance, which tends to increase cardiac output. When the systemic vascular resistance was increased in thyrotoxic subjects by infusion of phenylephrine, cardiac output was decreased.[5] This observation suggests that peripheral vasodilatation with decreased left ventricular afterload is important in the increased cardiac output of thyrotoxicosis.

Clinical Manifestations

Physical Findings
Most patients with thyrotoxicosis have evidence of increased cardiac output without congestive heart failure. Congestive heart failure is said to be uncommon in hyperthyroidism without underlying heart disease unless the patient is in the older age group. It is postulated that most patients who have congestive heart failure with thyrotoxicosis have additional underlying heart disease, but in many instances nei-

ther the heart disease nor its nature can be clearly established. In patients under the age of 35 one occasionally observes cardiac decompensation without evident additional heart disease.[8] Most patients with thyrotoxicosis demonstrate the usual physical findings of stare; exophthalmos; enlarged and firm thyroid gland with or without nodule formation; fine tremor of the outstretched hands; warm, moist skin of salmon hue; and tachycardia. If the metabolic rate is considerably increased, there is usually a loud cervical venous hum. In this writer's experience, continuous murmurs over the thyroid gland in thyrotoxic patients have almost always been caused by a cervical venous hum rather than by dilated arteries within the gland. In thyrotoxicosis without heart failure, the cardiac rhythm is usually of normal sinus origin; approximately 10 percent of patients have atrial fibrillation, which is often paroxysmal. On the other hand, in patients with heart failure, and here we are referring primarily to the older age groups, atrial fibrillation is found in over 50 percent of instances. There is characteristically an increase of systolic blood pressure with a modest decrease of diastolic pressure, and thus the pulse pressure is increased and the peripheral arterial pulse may be bounding. The heart is usually of normal size, unless there is complicating heart disease or congestive heart failure. The first heart sound is often of increased intensity and may at times suggest an incorrect diagnosis of mitral stenosis. Both presystolic and diastolic apical gallop sounds are common in hyperthyroidism.[10] In older patients with thyrotoxicosis and heart disease, the thyrotoxicosis may be masked; namely, the eye signs may be minimal or absent, and the thyroid enlargement and tachycardia may be inconspicuous. The possibility of thyrotoxic heart disease is often suggested by the observation of atrial fibrillation without obvious cause, some widening of the arterial pulse pressure, and an unusually alert patient with congestive heart failure. Studies for thyrotoxicosis should be made in patients with unexplained atrial fibrillation or atrial flutter. Thyrotoxicosis should be more strongly considered as a possibility in patients with atrial fibrillation whose ventricular rate fails to respond with an adequate decrease with adequate amounts of digitalis. Persistent unexplained sinus tachycardia, especially in elderly patients, should suggest the possibility of thyrotoxicosis. Generalized lymphadenopathy and splenomegaly are found in about 10 percent of instances.

Special Laboratory Studies
The diagnosis of thyrotoxicosis is made by demonstrating a raised plasma total (protein-bound and unbound) thyroxine (total T_4), together with a raised radioactive triiodothyronine uptake (rT_3U). The latter test is a measure of protein binding. It is necessary to obtain both tests, since the total T_4 may be elevated by increased levels of thyroxine-binding globulin in the absence of thyroid dysfunction, as in

pregnancy, estrogen administration (including oral contraceptives), etc. The free T_4 level (FT_4) is calculated from the total T_4 and the rT_3U, and gives the approximate level of unbound T_4. An elevated FT_4, therefore, also indicates thyrotoxicosis. The total plasma triiodothyronine (T_3) measures circulating T_3, and should not be confused with the rT_3U. The T_3 level is a sensitive indicator of thyrotoxicosis. In rare instances it may be elevated in the presence of a normal total T_4 and FT_4 (T_3 toxicosis). It is also affected somewhat by protein binding. Radioactive iodine uptake by the thyroid is now less commonly used for the diagnosis of thyrotoxicosis.

Catheterization   Hemodynamic studies characteristically reveal an increase of the resting cardiac output and at times an increase of cardiac stroke volume with an arteriovenous oxygen difference decreased below the normal value of 4.5 ± 0.7* ml/dl of blood. The circulation time characteristically is shortened in the absence of heart failure. The heart rate is increased. The central venous pressure and right atrial pressure are normal in the absence of congestive heart failure. When heart failure develops, the circulation time usually lies within the normal arm-to-tongue time of 9 to 16 s measured with Decholin. The cardiac output is lower than before, but usually is still elevated above the normal range.[8]

Echocardiogram   An echocardiographic study was made of 11 patients with hyperthyroidism.[9] Left ventricular end-diastolic diameter was not significantly altered. The mean velocity of circumferential fiber shortening and the maximum velocity of posterior wall motion were increased; these variables did not change with propranolol therapy, but became normal when the patients became euthyroid. The left ventricular systolic time intervals showed a decreased PEP/LVET ratio that was not changed with propranolol therapy.

Management
The diagnosis of thyrotoxicosis is based upon the characteristic physical findings and laboratory data. Treatment of younger patients under the age of 25 years usually consists of subtotal thyroidectomy preceded by adequate preparation with the combination of methimazole and Lugol's solution. In older patients, and especially in those with congestive heart failure or recurrent thyrotoxicosis after surgical treatment, the oral administration of radioactive iodine is usually preferred. In patients with a history of heart failure, oral antithyroid drugs, e.g., propylthiouracil, should be given before radioiodine treatment.[11] If there is severe thyrotoxicosis, propranolol may mitigate some of the adverse effects upon the heart until the thyrotoxicosis can be controlled. Guanethidine decreases the cardiac output in induced hyperthyroidism, but it is not generally employed in the therapy of thyrocardiacs. The use of guanethidine may aggravate the manifestations of heart failure in euthyroid patients with cardiac decompensation. Propranolol, a β-adrenergic blocking agent, is often used in dosages of 10 to 40 mg orally four times daily. This agent decreases the heart rate and may decrease the oxygen consumption in thyrotoxic patients, and thus appears useful until the effects of thyroidectomy or radioactive iodine can be assessed. The preejection period is not affected and the stroke volume remains elevated, however, and there is some risk of a deleterious effect upon left ventricular function. In patients with hyperthyroidism and congestive failure, propranolol should probably not be used until digitalis and diuretics have been administered.[11]

Beriberi Heart Disease

Abnormal Physiology

Beriberi heart disease is a rare disorder in the United States and is apparently now even less common than it was 20 years ago. Blankenhorn collected 12 cases from 1940 to 1948 at the Cincinnati General Hospital,[12] and Akbarian and associates reported four instances from the Boston City Hospital.[13]

The mechanisms of increased cardiac output in beriberi is obscure. Some patients with beriberi have lesions of the sympathetic nuclei[13] that may decrease peripheral arterial resistance, thus increasing cardiac work and leading to congestive failure. In addition, thiamine deficiency interferes with myocardial metabolism of pyruvate to active acetate.

Clinical Manifestations

Physical Examination
In Blankenhorn's study made at a large city general hospital,[12] patients with beriberi heart disease were almost invariably chronic alcoholics. They demonstrated evidence of either (1) peripheral neuritis, with calf tenderness, decreased or absent vibratory sense in the lower extremities, and loss of knee or ankle reflexes, or (2) pellagra, with a red, smooth tongue, and perhaps skin changes over the face, neck, upper chest, hands, and elbows. Patients with advanced beriberi heart disease display the usual findings of biventricular congestive failure. These findings include elevation of the systemic venous pressure and pulmonary wedge pressure, edema, and hepatic engorgement. Characteristically, there are widening of the arterial pulse pressure and bounding peripheral arterial pulses. Pistol-shot sounds may be heard over the peripheral arteries. The heart is usually dilated, and apical diastolic gallop rhythm is characteristic.

*Standard deviation.

Electrocardiogram

The electrocardiogram in patients with beriberi heart disease is usually normal except for sinus tachycardia and perhaps minor nonspecific ST-segment and T-wave changes.

Special Laboratory Studies

Catheterization

The circulation time is usually within normal limits. On occasion it is shorter than normal. Hemodynamic studies in patients with heart failure due to beriberi have shown elevations of the right atrial and pulmonary wedge pressures, an increase in cardiac index,[1,13] and a decrease in arteriovenous oxygen difference. These abnormalities can be returned to normal after treatment with thiamine and other vitamins of the B-complex group.

Natural History and Prognosis

An example of clinical and hemodynamic data in beriberi heart disease is given in the following case description:

The patient was a 28-year-old barmaid, who was admitted to the Cincinnati General Hospital on September 18, 1950. There was a history of alcoholism for 3 years. The diet was considered deficient in bread and meat. She complained of dependent edema and numbness of the hands and legs for 4 days before admission.

On examination, her blood pressure was 150/70 mmHg; heart rate, 106 beats per minute; temperature, 37.1°C (98.8°F). The neck veins were abnormally distended. The skin was warm. The heart was enlarged with a ventricular gallop. There were fine rales at the lung bases, and signs of peripheral neuritis were detected.

Laboratory Data Hemoglobin was 10.2 g. Arm-to-tongue Decholin circulation times were 9.5, 7.5, and 10 s on three occasions. The electrocardiogram was normal except for very slight decrease of T-wave amplitude. The results of catheterizations of the right side of the heart are as follows:

	Dates of Catheterization		
	9/22	**11/17**	**12/29**
Pressures, mmHg:			
Right atrium	10	5*	3
Pulmonary artery	36/25(32)	25/8(17)	21/7(14)
Pulmonary wedge	22	8.5	8
Systemic arterial O_2 saturation, percent of capacity	87	93	94
Arteriovenous O_2 difference, ml/dl	3.4	4.5	3.1
Cardiac index, liter/min/m²	6.1	4.9	4.5

*Right ventricular end-diastolic pressure.

Comment This patient was first studied 4 days after admission to the hospital while still in clinical heart failure. The catheterization data from the right side of the heart were consistent with biventricular failure. There was elevation of both right atrial and pulmonary wedge pressures, and the cardiac output was twice the average normal cardiac index of 3.1 liters/min/m². The arteriovenous oxygen difference was decreased. After the patient was treated with rest and thiamine and other vitamins of the B complex, clinical and hemodynamic evidence of congestive heart failure was no longer present when she was studied on November 17 and December 29, 1950. The right atrial and pulmonary wedge pressures were normal at the time of the second and third studies. The cardiac output had decreased but remained above the normal range (cardiac index, 3.1 ± 0.4* liters/min/m²).

Burwell and Dexter[1] showed that recovery from acute beriberi heart disease was associated with a decrease in cardiac output, heart rate, and oxygen consumption, a return of arteriovenous oxygen difference to normal, and a rise of diastolic blood pressure. Another report described an abnormally great increase in cardiac output with exercise in a patient with beriberi heart disease.

Diagnosis

The criteria for the diagnosis of beriberi heart disease were listed by Blankenhorn.[12] They include a history of a thiamine-deficient diet for 3 months or longer, absence of another cause of heart disease, elevation of systemic venous pressure, edema, enlarged heart, minor electrocardiographic changes, evidence of peripheral neuritis or pellagra, and a response to thiamine with a decrease in heart size, or autopsy findings consistent with the diagnosis. Akbarian and associates reported that elevation of the serum transketolase values was a useful laboratory test.[13] Nutritional cirrhosis is found at autopsy in many instances. At the University of Cincinnati Hospitals, it is doubted that beriberi leads to a specific anatomic form of chronic myocardial disease or intractable congestive failure. In our experience patients with beriberi heart disease either died suddenly in the acute stage or made a complete recovery. One report, however, described a patient with low-output cardiac failure following in the wake of acute beriberi with high-output heart failure.

Management

These patients should be treated with bed rest. Because there is a tendency to syncope and sudden death, it is important that they receive treatment early. The optimum treatment is thiamine along with the remainder of the vitamin B complex. Thiamine may be given parenterally in doses of 50 mg daily.

Digitalis has been thought to be of little use,[7] but Akbarian and associates showed that ouabain might be beneficial.[13] Sodium restriction and diuretics are of some value. Lactic acidosis has been described, and cautious bicarbonate infusion may be of merit.[14]

*Standard deviation.

Anemia

Abnormal Physiology

Despite many studies of the mechanism of increased cardiac output in chronic anemia, the exact pathologic physiology is not completely understood. The circulatory effects of anemia were reviewed.[6] Possible factors involved in the elevated cardiac output of anemia, like other hyperdynamic states, include variations in ventricular preload, ventricular contractility, and ventricular afterload. It has been shown that the adrenal glands are not necessary for the increase in cardiac output, nor is the sympathetic nervous system. Blockade of β-adrenergic nerves does not prevent the increase of left ventricular performance with anemia.[15] The possibility of an unidentified humoral agent has not been excluded.[15] Increased preload is not likely to be the major factor but may contribute to some degree. Decreased left ventricular afterload seems to be the most important mechanism,[15] but the manner in which this decreased peripheral resistance is mediated remains uncertain. Peripheral vasodilatation, arteriovenous shunts, and decreased blood viscosity may be important. Cardiac output did not rise in dogs when blood oxygen transport was reduced without lowering blood viscosity by means of transfusion of red blood cells containing methemoglobin. Fowler and Holmes showed that experimental anemia increased the cardiac output much less when blood viscosity was not allowed to fall.[3] These observations supported the concept that reduction of blood viscosity is an important mechanism in the increased cardiac output of anemia. In patients with chronic anemia, administration of methoxamine decreased the cardiac output an average of 20 percent.[4] This study is consistent with the concept that decreased peripheral resistance is important in the high cardiac output of anemia. Brannon and associates[16] found that the cardiac output was usually not increased by anemia until the hemoglobin is below 7 g/dl of blood, or about one-half the normal value. Fowler and Holmes[15] found improved left ventricular performance in dogs with anemia. Anemic patients with angina pectoris usually have associated coronary artery disease. Patients who are anemic may develop congestive heart failure. As in thyrotoxicosis, most patients who develop congestive heart failure with anemia have underlying heart disease, and the anemia serves as an aggravating factor which increases the work of the heart.[6] On the other hand, congestive heart failure may occur from very severe anemia alone. This event is uncommon in the United States but apparently is more common in tropical countries. As a rule, it may be said that cardiac enlargement of congestive heart failure caused solely by chronic blood loss anemia is unlikely unless the hemoglobin is below 5 g/dl of blood. When anemia results from sickle-cell disease or from thalassemia, cardiac enlargement may occur

with lesser degrees of anemia. In sickle-cell anemia this is perhaps a reflection of myocardial and pulmonary arterial disease and an altered oxyhemoglobin dissociation curve. An echocardiographic study of 44 children with sickle-cell anemia (average age 8.6 years) showed significantly depressed left ventricular performance.[17] The increased cardiac output of anemia is produced by both tachycardia and increased cardiac stroke volume. In many patients there is an increase in the systemic arterial pulse pressure. Dyspnea, dependent edema, and reduction in vital capacity may result from anemia alone without added congestive heart failure.

Clinical Manifestations

Physical Examination

In patients with severe anemia (hemoglobin below 7 g/dl of blood) there is pallor of the skin and mucous membranes. Tachycardia is usually present. There is often an increase in systemic arterial pulse pressure which reflects the increase in cardiac stroke volume. The peripheral arterial pulses may be bounding, and there may be a Duroziez's sign and pistol-shot sounds over the femoral artery. There may be "capillary" pulsations in the lips and nail beds. Cervical venous hums are common in these patients, and were described in the majority of patients receiving hemodialysis for renal failure.[18] Systolic bruits are often found over both carotid arteries. These bruits are usually rather short, occupying little more than the first half of ventricular systole. There is commonly a pulmonary midsystolic murmur, presumably reflecting the increased blood flow and turbulence in this area. With severe anemia, there may be cardiac dilatation with resulting murmurs of mitral and tricuspid regurgitation. Murmurs of aortic regurgitation have been described in patients with severe anemia. This finding is extremely unusual in our experience at the University of Cincinnati Hospitals unless the patient is uremic, where hypertension may be a factor. Anemia may be associated with a vibratory or musical systolic Still's murmur. Patients with sickle-cell anemia may display a wider variety of cardiac murmurs. A diastolic apical murmur may suggest mitral stenosis, and as a rule the diagnosis of mitral stenosis should be made with great caution in patients with sickle-cell anemia. In children with sickle-cell anemia, systolic murmurs are found almost invariably.[19] Most commonly these are loudest in the second left intercostal space and presumably are related to increased pulmonary arterial blood flow. A prominent third heart sound in middiastole is common in sickle-cell anemia. There is a tendency to some exaggeration of the expiratory splitting of the second heart sound,[19] and the auscultatory findings of atrial septal defect may be closely simulated. In sickle-cell anemia, cor pulmonale may develop because of pulmonary arterial thrombosis, but this complication is uncommon.

Special Laboratory Studies

Catheterization

In patients with anemia, the circulation time is usually normal or decreased, and this finding may persist during congestive heart failure.[6] Studies made by catheterization of the right side of the heart show an increase of resting cardiac output which is partly the result of tachycardia. There is usually an additional increase of cardiac stroke volume.[20] Graettinger and associates found that in patients with mild anemia (average hemoglobin 9.4 g) the cardiac output was normal at rest, but with exercise it rose more than normally.[20] With maximal treadmill exercise, the peak cardiac output and the exercise level achieved were little affected by anemia, but the oxygen debt was increased. In patients with anemia who develop congestive failure the cardiac output may fall from the peak value but tends to remain above the normal resting value.[20] When studied by echocardiography, patients with sickle-cell anemia have increased left ventricular systolic and diastolic dimensions; evidence of ventricular dysfunction may be found.[17,21] In chronic anemia, systolic time intervals were generally normal when blood hemoglobin was above 7 g/dl. In severe anemia without heart failure, PEP was decreased and LVET was increased, with a decrease of PEP/LVET ratio. With severe anemia and heart failure, PEP/LVET ratio was increased.[22]

Management

The treatment of anemia depends on the underlying cause, whether this be iron deficiency, pernicious anemia, sickle-cell anemia, related to bone marrow replacement, hemolysis, or blood loss. In patients who have anemia associated with congestive heart failure, it may be necessary to correct the anemia before optimal response of the heart failure can occur. It is generally believed that digitalis is of little or no benefit in congestive heart failure accompanied by severe anemia.[7] On the other hand, we found that ouabain was effective in anemia heart failure produced in the heart-lung preparation, since it lowered elevated atrial pressures and increased cardiac output. Anemia alone is seldom the cause of heart failure; hence it seems logical to use digitalis when heart failure occurs in an anemic patient. Bed rest, sodium restriction, and diuretics may be desirable. The anemia should be corrected gradually. In chronic anemia,[23] expansion of plasma volume tends to correct total blood volume almost to normal; hence rapid infusion of whole blood in the severely anemic patient may precipitate heart failure with pulmonary edema. When rapid improvement in anemia is necessary, slow infusions of one-half unit of packed red blood cells (125 ml) may be carried out over a period of 3 or 4 h, with careful examination of the patient for dyspnea and auscultation of the lungs for evidence of pulmonary edema. Monitoring of the central venous pressure during transfusion is an added precaution, but it may not necessarily warn of pulmonary edema. Hence monitoring pulmonary wedge pressure with the Swan-Ganz flow-directed catheter technique as a guide to sudden increments to left ventricular diastolic pressure should prove more useful. At times it may be necessary to correct anemia quickly in this way in order to obtain satisfactory improvement in congestive heart failure. Too rapid correction of anemia by transfusing 1000 to 2000 ml of whole blood within 24 h is observed to cause pulmonary edema; this occurs in our institution several times a year. It may be necessary to employ diuretics simultaneously with transfusion, or to use phlebotomy along with transfusion, to prevent a rise of pulmonary wedge pressure.

Systemic Arteriovenous Fistula

Abnormal Physiology

The decreased systemic vascular resistance (decreased left ventricular afterload) associated with large systemic arteriovenous fistulae usually evokes an increase of cardiac output to maintain adequate blood pressure and adequate blood supply to the tissues. As a rule, increased cardiac output can be demonstrated only when there is a large fistula that involves a major artery such as the aorta, or such arteries as the subclavian artery, the femoral artery, the common carotid arteries, and the iliac vessels. Multiple small arteriovenous fistulae may cause a rise of cardiac output. Pulmonary arteriovenous fistulae involve the low-resistance lesser circulation and seldom, if ever, lead to increased cardiac output, cardiac enlargement, or congestive heart failure. Congenital systemic arteriovenous fistulae are usually not of sufficient size to produce generalized circulatory signs. The mechanism of increased cardiac output in systemic arteriovenous fistula apparently does not involve an increase in cardiac filling pressure. When there is an arteriovenous fistula, arterialized blood from a high-pressure artery is shunted into a low-pressure vein, thus decreasing the arterial blood flow to the tissue beyond the fistula and increasing the venous pressure distal to the fistula. The venous pressure proximal to the fistula and pressures in the right side of the heart are usually normal unless there is congestive heart failure. As a compensatory mechanism for the low systemic vascular resistance, the heart rate and stroke volume increase. The diastolic blood pressure falls, and the cardiac output rises. Circulatory reflexes were not essential to the increase of cardiac output in experimental systemic arteriovenous fistula. Obliteration of the arteriovenous fistula by compression results in a fall in cardiac output. There tends to be an increase of plasma volume in patients with systemic arteriovenous fistulae. Catheterization of the right side of the heart in patients with large systemic arteriovenous fistulae reveals increased oxygenation of venous blood at the site of the communication.

Physical Findings

If the examiner finds an increased systemic arterial pulse pressure when there is no evidence of aortic regurgitation, the possibility of a systemic arteriovenous fistula should be considered. If the patient has had an injury or a surgical operation, careful auscultation should be carried out over the site in order to look for the typical continuous murmur of arteriovenous fistula with a systolic accentuation. Manual compression of the fistula tends to produce slowing of the heart. This response is known as Branham's sign. We have studied a patient who acquired a large arteriovenous fistula as a complication of nephrectomy. Hepatic arteriovenous fistula was reported in two patients with hereditary hemorrhagic telangiectasia,[24] and we have studied two similar patients, each of whom had an elevated cardiac output. Patients with large arteriovenous fistulae may develop congestive heart failure. The onset of heart failure may be quite delayed. In one instance a 30-year-old man who was studied at the Cardiac Laboratory of the Cincinnati General Hospital developed congestive heart failure in 1951, 7 years following a gunshot wound involving the internal iliac artery and vein. In another instance, a 68-year-old patient developed congestive heart failure 57 years after a gunshot wound involving the femoral artery and vein. Presumably, in patients like the latter there is additional underlying heart disease; however, in such patients repair of the fistula may result in the return of heart size and function to normal.

Hepatic Hemangiomatosis
This rare condition has been studied by de Lorimer et al.[25] Of 27 patients with hepatic hemangioendothelioma, 23 had cutaneous capillary hemangiomas and all but 2 had heart failure.[25] This lesion acts as an arteriovenous fistula between hepatic artery and veins. The congestive failure responds to hepatic artery ligation; however, in adults hepatic artery ligation might cause fatal hepatic necrosis.

Hemodialysis
Striking increases of cardiac output may be found in patients with subcutaneous arteriovenous fistulae for hemodialysis.[26] Anemia accompanying uremia usually contributes to the high cardiac output in such patients.

Special Laboratory Studies

Catheterization
Intracardiac pressures are ordinarily normal unless congestive heart failure develops. If right-sided heart failure develops, right atrial and peripheral venous pressures rise. The cardiac output is above normal resting levels,[27] and may show a greater than normal increase with mild exercise in the absence of heart failure. Heart failure may develop in patients with hearts that are apparently normal otherwise.[27] When clinical signs of congestive failure have developed, the cardiac output may fall with exercise.[27] We have observed, however, that exercise evoked an above normal increase in cardiac output in such patients when the heart was previously normal. The following description illustrates some of the hemodynamic features of a large systemic arteriovenous fistula:

The patient, a 57-year-old man, was admitted to the hospital because of the symptoms of congestive heart failure which had been present for 4 years. Twenty-two years before admission, he had sustained a gunshot wound of the right supraclavicular area. Physical examination revealed signs of a right subclavian arteriovenous fistula. Hemoglobin was 14.5 g per deciliter of blood. The results of catheterization of the right side of the heart during exercise and at rest are as follows:

	Rest	Exercise
Pressures, mmHg:		
Right atrium	7	
Pulmonary artery	56/18(31)	64/28(43)
Pulmonary wedge	24	
Systemic arterial O$_2$ saturation, percent of capacity	92.5	94.4
Arteriovenous O$_2$ difference, ml/dl	3.3	4.4
O$_2$ consumption, ml/min	246	386
Cardiac index, liter/min/m^2	4.1	5.1

Comment The cardiac catheterization data were consistent with biventricular failure with an elevated resting cardiac output. Both right atrial and pulmonary wedge pressures were above normal. The cardiac index was well above the normal range of 3.1 ± 0.4 liter/min/m^2. The increased cardiac output was associated with a narrow arteriovenous oxygen difference. Venous blood proximal to the fistula showed a step-up in oxygen content of 3.4 volumes per deciliter of blood. With exercise, there was a relatively normal increase of total cardiac output from 7.6 to 8.8 liters/min with an exercise-induced increment of oxygen consumption of 140 ml/min. Such response of cardiac output to exercise would be very unusual for patients with "low-output" heart failure.

Diagnosis and Treatment

The possibility of a systemic arteriovenous fistula should be considered in all patients who have an increase in systemic arterial pulse pressure with bounding arterial pulses. When there is no obvious cause of heart failure or for a wide arterial pulse pressure, such as aortic regurgitation, patent ductus arteriosus, severe anemia, or thyrotoxicosis, careful auscultation should be carried out over all scars and major arteries. If the characteristic continuous murmur with systolic accentuation is found in an area of trauma or surgical operation, no further studies should be required to establish the diagnosis. When there is doubt, arteriography may be employed to demonstrate the lesion. In some instances the systemic arteriovenous fistula may become infected so that there is endarteritis. This complication in turn may lead to aortic valve involvement with aortic infective endocarditis. In dogs with large experimental arteriovenous fistulae, aortic, mitral or tricuspid endocarditis may develop with or without infection of the fistula. The treatment of a systemic arteriovenous fistula, when it is large enough to produce increased arterial pulse pressure, cardiac enlargement, or congestive heart failure, should be surgical repair or excision of the fistula.

Hepatic Disease

It is known that the resting cardiac output may be increased in patients with liver disease, especially in those with nutritional cirrhosis or infectious hepatitis. The increase in cardiac output in patients with nutritional cirrhosis is usually moderate and occurs in approximately one-third of the patients. The mechanism is uncertain but has been attributed to increased blood volume, intrahepatic arteriovenous shunts, mesenteric arteriovenous shunts, and defects in inactivation of a circulating vasodilator.[27a] Some patients with nutritional cirrhosis have anemia or coexisting beriberi. In a few patients with nutritional cirrhosis or infectious hepatitis, the cardiac output may be considerably elevated and accompanied by the clinical evidence of a bounding pulse and wide pulse pressure. Congestive heart failure may develop,[28] but most patients in this group probably die of hepatic failure before heart failure can develop. One authority has described a cardiac output as high as 15 liters/min, or at least twice the normal, in a patient with infectious hepatitis.[28]

Paget's Disease of Bone

In Paget's disease of the bone the more common circulatory effects are increased systemic arterial pulse pressure and increased cardiac output. Cor pulmonale and atrioventricular (AV) block may occasionally occur. In most patients with Paget's disease this is not a prominent finding. Lequime and Denolin found evidence of increased blood flow to limbs involved by Paget's disease, but increase of resting cardiac output was unusual.[29] The cardiac output in patients with extensive bone involvement showed a greater than normal increase with exercise. The increased cardiac output is presumably related to multiple, small systemic arteriovenous fistulas in the bones involved by this disorder, especially in the lower extremities. Injection of radioactive albumin microspheres 15 to 30 μm in diameter was made into the femoral arteries of nine patients with Paget's disease of the bone. No evidence of increased AV shunting in the lower extremities was found.[30] The possibility of Paget's disease of the bone as a cause of an increased systemic arterial pulse pressure must be considered in a middle-aged or older patient who has enlargement of the skull, decreased stature, and bowing of the tibias. Radiologic studies of the skull, pelvis, and bones of the lower extremities will usually confirm the diagnosis. As a rule, serum alkaline phosphatase is increased. Calcitonin therapy may decrease the elevated cardiac output.

Hyperdynamic Heart Syndrome

Gorlin and associates[31] described a hyperkinetic syndrome of unknown cause which they found principally in young patients and in those of early middle age. In their report 24 patients were described. The majority of the patients had an increased cardiac output at rest. Others did not but had an increased rate of ventricular ejection. Bounding peripheral pulses were common. Heart failure developed in some patients observed for as long as 16 years. Electrocardiograms usually showed evidence of left ventricular enlargement. Systolic ejection clicks were common. Ejection and apical pansystolic murmurs were found. Gorlin's description of some of these patients is very similar to that of patients who have idiopathic muscular obstruction of the left ventricular outflow tract. The possibility that a common denominator of increased activity of the sympathetic nervous system exists in these two groups of patients must not be overlooked, since β-adrenergic receptor blockade may be of value in therapy.[32]

Cor Pulmonale (See Chap. 53)

The resting cardiac output may be above normal in some patients with chronic cor pulmonale associated with chronic obstructive airway disease. This finding apparently is most common when the patient has an acute pulmonary infection and may be in part related to acute hypoxia and hypermetabolism associated with fever and infection. In our own experience, and in that of others, increased cardiac output in cor pulmonale associated with obstructive airway disease was not found in the majority of patients.[33] In some a tendency to increased cardiac output may be overcome because the pulmonary vascular resistance is greatly elevated or because heart failure is too advanced. In our study, the cardiac output in patients with cor pulmonale caused by chronic obstructive lung disease was on the average higher during heart failure than in patients with hypertensive or coronary artery disease accompanied by congestive heart failure.[33]

Polyostotic Fibrous Dysplasia (Albright's Syndrome)

In patients with polyostotic fibrous dysplasia the cardiac output may be increased above normal. The cardiac index was 3.9 liters/min/m² or greater in five of six patients studied by McIntosh and associates.[34] The authors thought that anxiety or increased metabolic demands were not responsible. Biopsy material from involved bones showed numerous thin-walled sinusoidal capillaries. The authors postulated that the lesions of polyostotic fibrous dysplasia act as minute arteriovenous fistulae, thus increasing cardiac output by lowering peripheral resistance.

Carcinoid Syndrome

The resting cardiac output may be increased in patients with metastatic carcinoid tumors.[35] The patients may have a lowered arteriovenous oxygen difference and decreased peripheral vascular resistance. Serotonin, known to be elaborated by carcinoid tumors, increases myocardial contractility by direct action. It seems likely that the increased cardiac output combined with tricuspid or pulmonary valve deformity, often found in patients with the carcinoid syndrome, may explain the high incidence of heart failure in this disease.

Warm and Humid Environment (See Chap. 80)

Burch and associates[36] studied 10 subjects in New Orleans during the summers of 1957 and 1958. The mean of their cardiac outputs when in an air-conditioned ward was 4.0 liters/min. When the subjects were exposed to environmental conditions with the room temperature of 30.5 to 33.3°C (87 to 92°F) and relative humidity 58 to 93 percent, the mean cardiac output rose 43 percent to 5.7 liters/min. Calculated ventricular work rose in some subjects, suggesting that an air-conditioned ward may reduce the workload of the heart in some patients with heart disease. Short periods of exposure to dry heat apparently had little effect on cardiac output. When whole-body hyperthermia was used to treat malignant neoplasms, however, a body temperature of 41.8°C was associated with doubling of cardiac output.[37]

Cold Environment (See Chap. 80)

In healthy young men exposed to 5°C ambient temperature, cardiac output and total body oxygen consumption were increased.[38] Since the arteriovenous oxygen difference was also increased, the rise of cardiac output can be explained by the increased metabolic demands of the tissues.

Renal Disease

In acute glomerulonephritis, the cardiac output at rest may be normal (in other words, relatively high) when the right atrial pressure is elevated, and there are clinical features usually found in heart disease.[39] Some patients have hypervolemia, increased systemic venous pressure, enlargement of the heart, and pulmonary edema. Systemic arterial hypertension is common but is not invariably present. The decreased glomerular filtration and increased aldosterone secretion lead to retention of sodium and water with resultant hypervolemia. Some such patients, when treated with intravenous digoxin, show no decrease of right atrial or venous pressure, no increase of cardiac output, and no sodium or water diuresis.[7] The authors concluded that some patients with edema and increased venous pressure with acute glomerulonephritis do not have heart failure; these patients can be recognized clinically by demonstrating that they have a normal circulation time.

An increase of resting cardiac index, not explained by fever or anemia, may be found in patients with acute renal failure associated with tubular necrosis. With chronic renal failure and anemia, the cardiac output is usually increased.[40] The cardiac output was found to return to normal when the anemia was corrected. Patients undergoing hemodialysis for the treatment of uremia tend to have an elevated cardiac output. In addition to anemia, the shunt used for dialysis and a uremic hypermetabolic state may contribute to the elevated cardiac output.[26]

Polycythemia Vera

The cardiac output and cardiac stroke index may be increased in patients with polycythemia vera.[41] The mechanism of increased cardiac output is uncertain but appears to be correlated with the degree of hypervolemia. Right atrial and pulmonary wedge pressures are not increased.

Pregnancy (See Chap. 67)

During normal pregnancy the cardiac output increases progressively until the seventh or eighth month. The increase averages 30 to 50 percent. Until recently it was believed that the cardiac output declines considerably from its peak elevation during the last 6 weeks of pregnancy. The observations responsible for these conclusions were made while the pregnant woman was in the supine position, however, so that the enlarged uterus compromised venous return through the inferior vena cava. When the cardiac output is measured with the pregnant woman lying on her side, a significant decline in cardiac output during the last 6 weeks of pregnancy is not observed.

Certain Cutaneous Diseases

A significant increase in the resting cardiac output may occur in patients with "erythrodermic" skin disease. It is believed that increased blood flow to the skin might be at least partly responsible for the elevated cardiac output. Hecht and coworkers found high resting cardiac output in psoriasis and in exfoliative dermatitis and also demonstrated a hyperdynamic state in patients with Kaposi's sarcoma.[42]

Obesity (See Chap. 73)

In extreme obesity, the cardiac output tends to be increased, but only in proportion to the increased weight and oxygen consumption. The arteriovenous oxygen difference is not decreased.[43]

Systemic Arterial Hypertension (See Chap. 48)

The resting cardiac index has been found to be elevated in some patients with labile hypertension or borderline blood pressure elevation. The cardiac output tends to be higher in those patients with labile hypertension than in those with established hypertension. An increased cardiac output, however, may be found in some patients with severe hypertension.[44]

References

1. Burwell, C. S., and Dexter, L.: Beri-Beri Heart Disease, *Trans. Assoc. Am. Physicians*, 60:59, 1957.
2. Braunwald, E.: On the Difference between the Heart's Output and Its Contractile State, *Circulation*, 43:171, 1971 (editorial).
3. Fowler, N. O., and Holmes, J. C.: Blood Viscosity and Cardiac Output in Acute Experimental Anemia, *J. Appl. Physiol.*, 39:453, 1975.
4. Duke, M., and Abelmann, W. H.: The Hemodynamic Response to Chronic Anemia, *Circulation*, 39:503, 1969.
5. Theilen, E. O., and Wilson, W. R.: Hemodynamic Effects of Peripheral Vasoconstriction in Normal and Thyrotoxic Subjects, *J. Appl. Physiol.*, 22:207, 1967.
*6. Varat, M. A., Adolph, R. J., and Fowler, N. O.: Cardiovascular Effects of Anemia, *Am. Heart J.*, 83:415, 1972. (91 references)
7. Eichna, L. W., Farber, S. J., Berger, A. R., Rader, R., Smith, W. W., and Albert, R. E.: Non-cardiac Circulatory Congestion Simulating Congestive Heart Failure, *Trans. Assoc. Am. Physicians*, 68:72, 1954.
8. Graettinger, J. S., Muenster, J. J., Selverstone, L. A., and Campbell, J. A.: A Correlation of Clinical and Hemodynamic Studies in Patients with Hyperthyroidism with and without Congestive Heart Failure, *J. Clin. Invest.*, 38:1316, 1959.
9. Lewis, B. S., Ehrenfeld, E. N., and Lewis, N.: Echocardiographic LV Function in Thyrotoxicosis, *Am. Heart J.*, 97:460, 1979.
10. Leonard, J. J., and deGroot, W. J.: The Thyroid State and the Cardiovascular System, *Mod. Concepts Cardiovasc. Dis.*, 38:23, 1969.
11. Blonde, L., and Skelton, C. L.: Hyperthyroidism and Cardiovascular Disease: Concepts and Management, *Cardiovasc. Med.*, 1145, 1978.
12. Blankenhorn, M. A.: Effect of Vitamin Deficiency on the Heart and Circulation, *Circulation*, 11:288, 1955.
13. Akbarian, M., Yankopoulos, N. A., and Abelmann, W. H.: Hemodynamic Studies in Beriberi Heart Disease, *Am. J. Med.*, 41:197, 1966.
14. Attas, M., Hanley, H. G., Stultz, D., Jones, M. R., and McAllister, R. G.: Fulminant Beriberi Heart Disease with Lactic Acidosis: Presentation of a Case with Evaluation of Left Ventricular Function and Review of Pathophysiologic Mechanisms, *Circulation*, 58:566, 1978.
15. Fowler, N. O., and Holmes, J. C.: Ventricular Function in Anemia, *J. Appl. Physiol.*, 31:260, 1971.
16. Brannon, E. S., Merrill, A. J., Warren, J. V., and Stead, E. A., Jr.: The Cardiac Output in Patients with Chronic Anemia as Measured by the Techniques of Right Atrial Catheterization, *J. Clin. Invest.*, 24:332, 1945.
17. Rees, A. H., Stefadouros, M. A., Strong, W. B., Miller, M. D., Gilman, P., Rigby, J. A., and McFarlane, J.: Left Ventricular Performance in Children with Homozygous Sickle Cell Anaemia, *Br. Heart J.*, 40:690, 1978.
18. Danaly, D. T., and Ronan, J. A., Jr.: Cervical Venous Hums in Patients on Chronic Hemodialysis, *N. Engl. J. Med.*, 291:237, 1974.
19. Shubin, H., Kaufman, R., Shapiro, M., and Levinson, D. C.: Cardiovascular Findings in Children with Sickle Cell Anemia, *Am. J. Cardiol.*, 6:875, 1960.
20. Graettinger, J. S., Parsons, R. L., and Campbell, J. A.: A Correlation of Clinical and Hemodynamic Studies in Patients with Mild and Severe Anemia with and without Congestive Failure, *Ann. Intern. Med.*, 58:617, 1963.
21. Val-Mejias, J., Lee, W. K., Weisse, A. B., and Regan, T. J.: Left Ventricular Performance during

*This article is a review of the literature and contains additional references to the literature.

and after Sickle Cell Crisis, *Am. Heart J.*, 97:585, 1979.

22. Abdullah, A. K., Siddiqui, M. A., and Tajuddin, M.: Systolic Time Intervals in Chronic Anemia, *Am. Heart J.*, 94:287, 1977.

23. Duke, M., Herbert, V. D., and Abelmann, W. H.: Hemodynamic Effects of Blood Transfusion in Chronic Anemia, *N. Engl. J. Med.*, 271:975, 1964.

24. Razi, B., Beller, B. M., Ghidoni, J., Linhart, J. W., Talley, R. C., and Urban, E.: Hyperdynamic States due to Intrahepatic Fistula in Osler-Weber-Rendu Disease, *Am. J. Med.*, 50:809, 1971.

25. deLorimier, A. A., Simpson, E. B., Baum, R. S., and Carlsson, E.: Hepatic Artery Ligation for Hepatic Hemangiomatosis, *N. Engl. J. Med.*, 277:333, 1967.

26. McMillan, R., and Evans, D. B.: Experience with Three Brescia-Cimino Shunts, *Br. Med. J.*, 3:781, 1968.

27. Muenster, J. J., Graettinger, J. S., and Campbell, A. J.: Correlation of Clinical and Hemodynamic Findings in Patients with Systemic Arteriovenous Fistulas, *Circulation*, 20:1079, 1959.

*27a. Schlant, R. C.: Cardiovascular Effects of Hepatic Cirrhosis, in J. W. Hurst (ed.), "Update III: The Heart," McGraw-Hill Book Company, New York, 1980, p. 129. (171 references)

28. Murray, J. F., Dawson, A. M., and Sherlock, S.: Circulatory Changes in Chronic Liver Disease, *Am. J. Med.*, 24:358, 1958.

29. Lequime, J., and Denolin, H.: Circulatory Dynamics in Osteitis Deformans, *Circulation*, 12:215, 1955.

30. Rhodes, B. A., Grayson, N. D., Hamilton, C. R., Jr., White, R. I., Jr., Giargiana, F. A., Jr., and Wagner, H. N., Jr.: Absence of Arteriovenous Shunts in Paget's Disease of Bone, *N. Engl. J. Med.*, 287:686, 1972.

31. Gorlin, R.: The Hyperkinetic Heart Syndrome, *J. Am. Med. Assoc.*, 182:823, 1962.

32. Frolich, E. D.: Beta Adrenergic Blockade in the Circulatory Regulation of Hyperkinetic States, *Am. J. Cardiol.*, 27:195, 1971.

33. Fowler, N. O., Westcott, R. N., Scott, R. C., and Hess, E.: The Cardiac Output in Chronic Cor Pulmonale, *Circulation*, 6:888, 1952.

34. McIntosh, H. D., Miller, D. E., Gleason, W. L., and Goldner, J. L.: The Circulatory Dynamics of Polyostotic Fibrous Dyplasia, *Am. J. Med.*, 32:393, 1962.

35. Schwaber, J. R., and Lukas, D. S.: Hyperkinemia and Cardiac Failure in the Carcinoid Syndrome, *Am. J. Med.*, 32:846, 1962.

36. Burch, G. E., dePasquale, N., Hyman, A., and DeGraff, A. C.: Influence of Tropical Weather on Cardiac Output, Work, and Power of Right and Left Ventricles of Man Resting in Hospital, *A.M.A. Arch. Intern. Med.*, 104:553, 1959.

37. Bull, J. M., Lees, D., Schuette, W., Whang-Peng, J., Smith, R., Bynum, G., Atkinson, E. R., Gottdiener, J. A., Gralnick, H. R., Shawker, T. H., and DeVita, V. T., Jr.: Whole Body Hyperthermia. A Phase-1 Trial of a Potential Adjuvant to Chemotherapy, *Ann. Intern. Med.*, 90:137, 1979.

38. Raven, P. B., Niki, I., Dahms, T. E., and Horvath, S. M.: Compensatory Cardiovascular Responses during Environmental Cold Stress, 5°C, *J. Appl. Physiol.*, 29:417, 1970.

39. Farber, S. J.: Physiologic Aspects of Glomerulonephritis, *J. Chronic Dis.*, 5:87, 1957.

40. Neff, M. S., Kim, K. E., Persoff, M., Onesti, G., and Swartz, C.: Hemodynamics of Uremic Anemia, *Circulation*, 43:876, 1971.

41. Cobb, L. A., Kramer, R. J., and Finch, C. A.: Circulatory Effects of Chronic Hypervolemia in Polycythemia Vera, *J. Clin. Invest.*, 39:1722, 1960.

42. Hecht, H. H. (by invitation), Candiolo, B. M., Malkinson, F. D., Nair, K. G., and Saqueton, A. C.: On Cardio-cutaneous Syndromes, *Trans. Assoc. Am. Physicians*, 80:91, 1967.

43. White, R. I., Jr., and Alexander, J. K.: Body Oxygen Consumption and Pulmonary Ventilation in Obese Subjects, *J. Appl. Physiol.*, 20:197, 1965.

44. Ibrahim, M. M., Tarazi, R. C., and Dustan, H. P.: Hyperkinetic Heart in Severe Hypertension: A Separate Clinical Hemodynamic Entity, *Am. J. Cardiol.*, 35:667, 1975.

Section E

Disturbances of Rhythm and Conduction

27

Mechanisms of Arrhythmias and Conduction Abnormalities

John J. Gallagher, M.D., F.A.C.C.

No fact is better established concerning the histological structure of cardiac muscle than that there exist connexions between the various portions or columns of cells. There exist therefore closed circuits in the myocardium. Supposing an excitation to be started in such a closed circuit and supposing that for some reason it travels in one direction but not in the other. If the rate of propagation is rapid as compared with the duration of the wave, the whole circuit will be in the excited state at the same time, and the excitation will die out. . . . But if, on the other hand, the wave is slower and shorter (and it is made slower and shorter by the conditions which produce fibrillation) the excited state will have passed off at the region where the excitation started before the wave of excitation reaches this point on the circle at the completion of its revolution. Not only so, but there will have been time for the excitability of the muscle to return to something near the value it had at the time of the first excitation. Under these circumstances, the wave of excitation may spread a second time over the same tract of tissue; once started in this way it will continue unless interfered with by some external stimulus arriving during that part of the cycle when the portion of the muscle stimulated is neither in the excited state nor in the condition of depressed excitability which outlasts it.

G. R. Mines, 1913[1]

The sinoatrial node is the normal cardiac pacemaker since it has the fastest inherent rate (i.e., the highest degree of automaticity). Normally, impulses arise in the sinus node at a rate of 60 to 100 per minute and result in atrial contraction followed shortly by ventricular contraction. The physiologic basis of normal activation was developed in Chap. 4. Broadly speaking, any significant deviation from normal cardiac rhythm can be defined as an *arrhythmia*. These deviations may be due to an abnormality in rate or regularity of the heartbeat. The term *arrhythmia* also encompasses any disturbance in the sequence of a normal atrial activation coupled at a physiologic interval to a normal ventricular activation. Rhythm disturbances may be classified in a variety of ways: rate, site of origin, and site of conduction delay or block.

In the early 1900s, Mines, Lewis, and other investigators of the day[1-8] attempted to identify the role of automaticity and reentry in cardiac arrhythmias. To this day we are faced with a similar dilemma. With the advent of direct microelectrode recordings of cellular activity[9,10] and the voltage clamp technique,[11,12] a gap began to develop between our knowledge of in vitro cellular events and our comprehension of clinically observed arrhythmias. Clinically, the development of multiple catheter-electrode recordings from the atria, ventricles, and specialized conducting tissues (Chaps. 19, 89, and 90), together with the use of programmed stimulation, led to remarkable advances. Unfortunately, present methodology does not yet permit us to define precisely the mechanisms responsible for many clinical arrhythmias. Nevertheless the ability to reproduce disorders experimentally that resemble clinical arrhythmias often has led to hypotheses regarding the pathogenesis of these abnormalities in humans. It remains difficult to get a total representation of any arrhythmia at the cellular level alone; comprehension usually follows only when arrhythmias are viewed in terms of an integrated cellular system. Nor are we yet at the point where knowledge of a specific mechanism can be equated with specific therapy.

489

Despite all these limitations, knowledge of basic electrophysiologic mechanisms provides a setting in which discussion of potential mechanisms of arrhythmias and their response to therapy can take place. For didactic purposes, these basic mechanisms have been arbitrarily divided into abnormalities of impulse formation (including automaticity), impulse conduction (including reentry), combinations of both these mechanisms, and finally repolarization.[13-25]

Mechanisms of Arrhythmias

Impulse Formation

In this section we will describe (1) normal automaticity, (2) abnormal automaticity, and (3) triggered activity. These phenomena can all be demonstrated at a cellular level and are all the result of impulse formation due to diastolic depolarization occurring during phase 4 of the action potential.[13,18–20,22,24–37]

Normal Automaticity

The ability to develop slow diastolic depolarization allows some cells in the heart to spontaneously reach threshold, initiating action potentials. The property of *self*-initiation of excitation in the absence of an external stimulus is properly termed *automaticity,* as exemplified by the sinus node. In addition, some specialized cells in the atria, distal atrioventricular node, bundle of His, bundle branches, and Purkinje network possess latent ability to become pacemakers, especially if the sinus node ceases to be dominant. When *enhanced* automaticity is discussed, this usually refers to automaticity arising in cells outside the sinus node but at high levels of maximum diastolic potential (i.e., greater than -60 mV) and capable of being suppressed by overdrive pacing. Such enhanced automaticity is not observed in ordinary atrium or ventricle (Fig. 27-1).

There is almost certainly more than one ionic mechanism for spontaneous diastolic depolarization. The most obvious example is the difference in automaticity exhibited by fibers capable of the so-called fast response compared with fibers with a slow response (see Chap. 4).

Fast response fibers in the atrium and specialized conduction system are capable of spontaneous depolarization that begins *after* repolarization to a maximum diastolic potential of greater than -60 mV and results from a time- and voltage-dependent decrease in membrane potassium (K^+) conductance and a coexisting steady inward sodium (Na^+) current. When the rate of spontaneous diastolic depolarization is rapid and the threshold is normal, the resulting action potential will have a *fast* Na^+-dependent depolarization phase or a so-called fast response (Fig. 27-1A). Under certain conditions, part of the fast-fiber action potential, i.e., the upstroke and repolarization phases, can be converted to the slow response while the mechanism for spontaneous

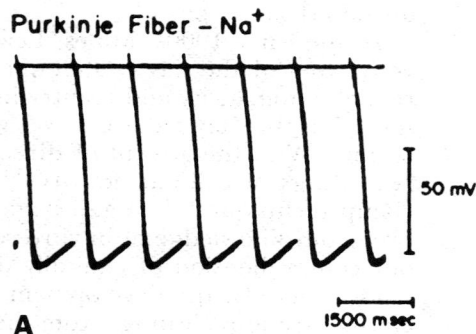

Purkinje Fiber – Na⁺

50 mV

A

1500 msec

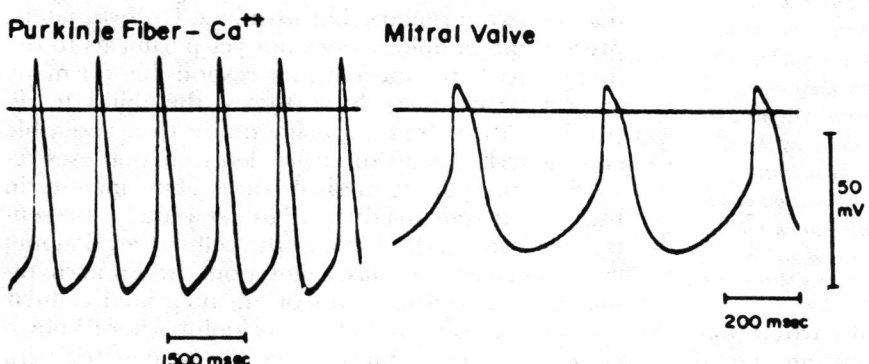

Purkinje Fiber – Ca⁺⁺   **Mitral Valve**

50 mV

1500 msec

200 msec

B

FIGURE 27-1 Automatic activity associated with the "fast" and "slow" response. *A.* Spontaneous diastolic depolarization and fast-response activity recorded from a canine Purkinje fiber with a maximum diastolic potential of -90 mV. *B.* On the left is shown a slow response recorded from a canine Purkinje fiber perfused with a sodium-free medium. Spontaneous diastolic depolarization is prominent, and the maximum diastolic potential is -65 mV. On the right is shown slow-response potentials recorded from a cardiac fiber in the mitral valve leaflet of a monkey. Prominent phase 4 depolarization is present. The maximum diastolic potential in this fiber is -58 mV. (*From Wit et al.*[21] *Reproduced with permission of author and publisher.*)

diastolic depolarization remains characteristic for fast fibers.[20] This occurs if maximum diastolic potential remains high but the rate of spontaneous diastolic depolarization is slow and threshold potential is shifted toward zero.

Since the spontaneous diastolic depolarization that occurs in fast response fibers is the result of a time- and voltage-dependent *decrease* in membrane K^+ conductance, its slope is enhanced by lowering extracellular K^+; the slope is suppressed by raising extracellular K^+.

A second mechanism of spontaneous diastolic depolarization probably exists only in slow response fibers. This spontaneous diastolic depolarization occurs at low maximum diastolic potentials of -60 mV or less (Fig. 27-1*B*); the fast response is thus inactivated. The prototype for spontaneous diastolic depolarization in slow fibers is the sinus node, although this type of automaticity probably occurs in cardiac fibers of the mitral and tricuspid valves as well as the lower AV node (Fig. 27-1*B*).

Two major features determine the rate of firing of automatic cells (see Fig. 4-9): the slope of diastolic depolarization, which is more important, and the difference between maximum diastolic potential and threshold potential. A normal hierarchy of pacemaker dominance ranging from the sinus node to the peripheral Purkinje network exists because the slope of phase 4 depolarization gradually decreases as one moves down the conducting system. The dominant pacemaker also suppresses the rate of firing of subsidiary pacemakers by overdrive[25] as well as underdrive[38] suppression.

The sinus node is under the tonal influence of the autonomic nervous system and can increase its rate of firing, resulting in a disturbance of rhythm. Enhanced vagal activity can inhibit sinus node automaticity but may have minimal effect on the automaticity of latent pacemakers in the atrium or His-Purkinje system, allowing a passive shift in the site of impulse formation to ectopic sites. Clinically, this phenomenon may be observed with sinus node dysfunction or atrioventricular block. Local influences that increase the rate of firing of latent pacemakers (enhanced automaticity) or agents, such as catecholamines, which differentially augment the rate of firing of latent pacemakers may lead to active usurpation of the normal dominance of the sinus node. Such enhanced automaticity may arise in fibers exhibiting either a fast or a slow response.

Abnormal Automaticity

Diseased cardiac tissue with *partially* depolarized cells exhibits automaticity that appears to differ from the mechanism of spontaneous depolarizations seen in normal automatic cells.[39–43] In contrast to normal mechanisms of automaticity, impulses arising from abnormal automatic mechanisms in the diseased heart can originate from ordinary atrial or ventricular muscle cells as well as from specialized conducting tissue. Thus, the number of potential sites of disturbance due to impulse formation outside the sinus node is greatly expanded in the setting of disease. This type of automaticity does not necessarily suppress and in fact may be accelerated by overdrive pacing. Abnormal automaticity occurs at low resting membrane potentials of -60 mV or less and is probably related to the slow response.

Afterdepolarization and Triggered Activity

In addition to the normal and abnormal mechanism of automaticity, in which a cell or group of cells undergoes repetitive *spontaneous* diastolic depolarization, there is another mechanism of impulse formation in abnormal cells referred to as *triggered activity*. This mechanism can be elicited in cells that are quiescent in the absence of an excitatory stimulus (in contrast to automatic cells), but once excited, give rise to two or more action potentials or a long run of repetitive responses. Triggered activity results from depolarizing *afterpotentials*, which may be of two types: *early* and *delayed* afterdepolarization.[26–36]

If the action potential of a cardiac cell fails to return to the normal level along its normal time course, so that repolarization is interrupted or delayed, that interruption or delay is referred to as an *early afterdepolarization* (Fig. 27-2). A second action potential may arise from an early afterdepolarization (see Fig. 27-3) *before* the membrane potential returns to the level it had prior to the initiating beat. Aconitine-induced extrasystoles studied by Scherf are one example; early afterdepolarizations are also seen experimentally during severe hypoxia and in tissue that is stretched or damaged, and may appear in digitalis-toxic tissues. Early afterdepolarizations appear at slow rates and are not more rapidly provoked by increases in rate or premature stimulation. It is not known whether any extrasystoles observed clinically arise from early afterdepolarizations.

In 1973, Cranefield and Aronson[26] described another cause of impulse initiation. Working with Na^+-free solutions exposed to ouabain, they recorded delayed afterdepolarizations: transient low-amplitude depolarizations occurring at membrane potentials of -70 to -80 mV following full

FIGURE 27-2 Various types of afterpotentials. The delay in repolarization shown in *A* is an early afterdepolarization; the swing in membrane potential during repolarization to a level more negative than the resting potential shown in *B* and *C* is an early afterhyperpolarization; in *C*, the early afterhyperpolarization is followed by a delayed afterdepolarization. (*From Cranefield.*[22] *Reproduced with permission of author and publisher.*)

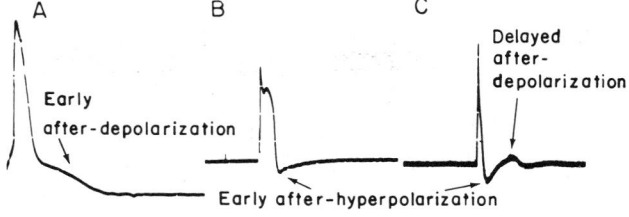

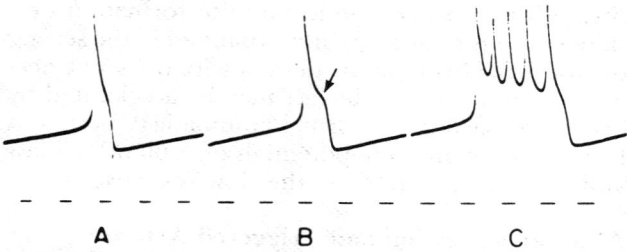

FIGURE 27-3 Early afterdepolarization. The action potentials shown were obtained by a rhythmically active canine Purkinje fiber exposed to normal Tyrode's solution. *A.* A normal action potential. *B.* An early afterdepolarization (arrow). *C.* Four nondriven action potentials occur at a membrane potential corresponding to that of the early afterdepolarization. Behavior of the kind seen in *B* and *C* is often seen in vitro in fibers usually regarded as having been slightly damaged during dissection or during mapping of the tissue bath. Time marks appear at 1-s intervals. (*From Cranefield.*[28] *Reproduced with permission of author and publisher.*)

repolarization (and often preceded by an afterhyperpolarization). The transient nature of these depolarizations distinguishes them from normal spontaneous depolarization (Fig. 27-4). Normally, the fibers in these preparations were quiescent. However, with a shortening of cycle length (at times even a single cycle length) or with the introduction of a premature depolarization, it was found that the low-amplitude depolarization was augmented and occurred earlier in diastole. If the depolarization achieved a sufficiently large amplitude, threshold was reached, resulting in a nondriven response; the latter was followed by a delayed afterdepolarization which could give rise to yet another nondriven response. It was also noted that the amplitude of the

delayed afterdepolarization could be increased by catecholamines. The triggered sustained rhythmic activity caused by this mechanism differs importantly from automaticity: with automaticity, there is spontaneous initiation of each impulse, whereas with triggered activity the cell remains quiescent until driven.

Another characteristic of triggered activity due to delayed afterdepolarization is that the first extrasystole may be middiastolic with reference to the driven impulse that triggered it, but the subsequent nondriven impulses appear *earlier and earlier* with respect to their predecessors until a stable rate is reached which may exceed the original driven rate.

Triggerable activity has been described in fibers from the atrial surface of the mitral and tricuspid valves of the normal dog and monkey,[26,30] the canine coronary sinus,[31] and the human mitral valve.[32] Ouabain and acetyl strophanthidin have been noted to cause afterdepolarizations and triggered activity in specialized atrial fibers and in isolated Purkinje fibers.

Triggered activity thus exhibits behavior formally reserved for reentry (see below); sustained rhythmic activity due to this mechanism can be induced and terminated by stimulation. Nonetheless, other distinctive features are also present: (1) there is a tendency toward a gradual increasing rate, or so-called warm-up effect; (2) the phenomenon is usually observed at fast basic rates (in contrast to reentry, which is more common at slow rates); (3) overdrive pacing results in acceleration of the rate of activity (in contrast to reentry, which in general terminates or is unaffected by overdrive); (4) the number of triggered responses appears directly related to the

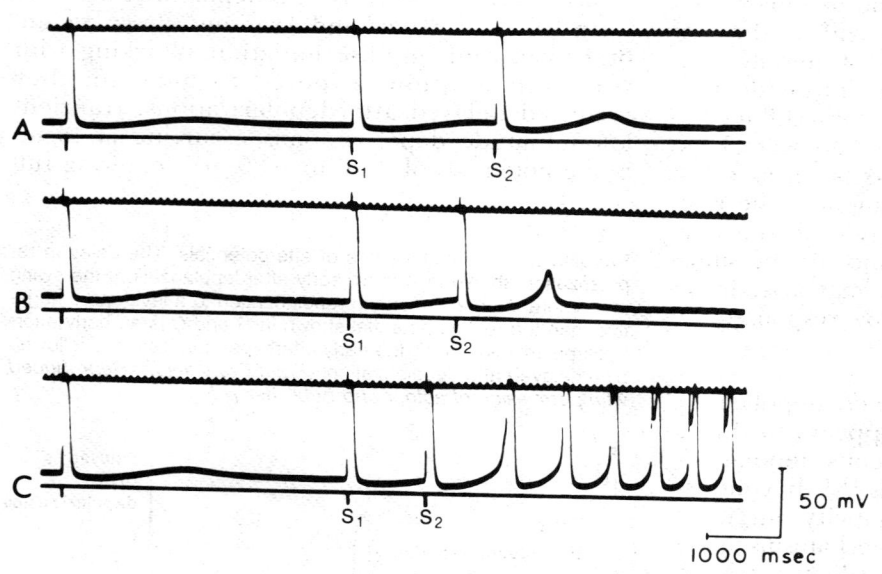

50 mV

1000 msec

FIGURE 27-4 Afterdepolarization and triggered activity. The potentials shown were recorded from a canine coronary sinus. The transmembrane recording is shown on the middle trace of each panel, and the time of stimulation is indicated by a vertical marker on the bottom trace. The fiber is stimulated at a cycle length of 4000 ms for 10 cycles and is then stimulated prematurely; in each panel, the last cycle of the basic drive train is shown followed by a premature stimulus (S₂), which is delivered at increasing prematurity from *A* to *C. A.* At a coupling interval of 2000 ms, the afterdepolarization is 11 mV in amplitude and occurs long after the premature response. *B.* The coupling interval is decreased to 1400 ms. The afterdepolarization increases to 31 mV in amplitude and peaks relatively soon after the premature response. *C.* The coupling interval is 1000 ms. Triggered activity now arises from the peak of the afterdepolarization and is sustained. In addition note the "warm-up" in the rate of triggered activity. (*From A. L. Wit and P. F. Cranefield, Triggered Automatic Activity in the Canine Coronary Sinus, Circ. Res., 41:435, 1977. Reproduced with permission of author and publisher and the American Heart Association, Inc.*)

basic cycle length of pacing (no such direct relationship is seen with reentry); and (5) triggered activity can be promptly suppressed by verapamil, whereas reentry (at least that confined to small regions in the ventricle) seems resistant to verapamil.

At present, the role of triggered activity in the genesis of clinically observed arrhythmias is unknown, although some reports have alluded to this mechanism.[36,37]

Other less well studied and defined mechanisms of abnormal automaticity have been recorded,[22,27,33] including oscillatory changes (prepotentials) in membrane potential which gradually increase until an action potential is evoked, as well as slow and very gradual depolarization (in contrast to the usual phase 4 depolarization) in markedly abnormal fibers.[27]

Impulse Conduction

Abnormalities of impulse propagation or conduction are probably more common as a basis for arrhythmias than abnormal impulse formation. In this section, the basis of conduction *delay* and *block* will be examined, followed by some consideration of reentry.

The determinants of conduction velocity (presented in Chap. 4) are (1) the action potential amplitude; (2) the rate of rise of the action potential in phase 0; (3) the threshold potential; and (4) the internal and external resistance. As previously noted, the cardiac fibers constitute a syncytium and may be likened to cylindrical conductors surrounded by an insulating membrane. This membrane has properties of *capacitance* and a high electrical *resistance;* in contrast, the intercalating disks that connect fibers end to end present a pathway of low resistance. These anatomic and electrophysiologic properties liken cardiac fibers to a cable conductor, favoring longitudinal progression of current, although the complexities of fiber dimension and geometry of cells must be taken into account.[44]

Action potential amplitude, by its influence on the flow of depolarizing current, determines the distance ahead that already depolarized tissue can initiate a propagated action potential. Increasing the magnitude of this depolarizing current allows excitation of quiescent tissue at a greater distance ahead. Similarly, increasing the rate of depolarization accelerates conduction because threshold can be reached more rapidly in more distant excitable tissues. Decreasing thresholds can enhance conduction velocity by decreasing the amount of current needed to initiate propagated action potential ahead of a wave front. Finally, a lower resistance to axial flow made possible by the presence of more numerous "tight" junctions favors longitudinal flow of current in the direction of the wave front, while an increase in sarcolemma resistance also favors longitudinal current flow by reducing the loss of depolarizing current across the sarcolemma perpen-

dicular to the wave front of activation.[24] Changes in *local* properties along the route of conduction can influence conduction velocity, accounting for *decremental* conduction. This phenomenon, which was first recognized by Erlanger[6,7] during his study of conduction disorders caused by pressure and local application of potassium in the canine His bundle, occurs when a normal action potential encounters a region of myocardium with slow conduction velocity. In this situation, the amplitude of the propagating impulse progressively decreases, thus serving as an increasingly less adequate stimulus to unexcited tissues in its path; successful conduction thus depends on the length of the abnormal segment, the amplitude and upstroke velocity of the action potential that penetrates the segment, and the threshold or responsiveness of the fibers beyond the abnormal segment. The activation process may fail, and impulse spread will then be in accordance with the passive electrical properties of the zone (electronic spread). If severe decremental conduction occurs, block results. Slow decremental conduction can be mediated by either a depressed fast-fiber response or a true slow-fiber response.

The presence of a slow response gives rise to another mechanism of decremental conduction leading to delay and block. With depolarization of cardiac fibers to -50 mV, current is carried by slow inward current channels. In this situation, long abnormal segments without the fast response exist, and the success of propagation is not as critically dependent on the length of the abnormal segment or on the rate of rise of the action potential that entered the abnormal segment. Nevertheless, the safety factor for conduction is low, and block is not uncommon.

Decremental conduction occurs in certain regions of the normal heart, such as the AV node; here a decreased resting membrane potential, a low upstroke velocity in phase 0 (due to the absence of a fast inward Na^+ channel), a relative paucity of gap junctions, the presence of small-diameter fibers, and a loosely arranged architecture all contribute to the appearance of decremental conduction. Impulse propagation is therefore exceedingly slow. In the atrioventricular mode, normal delay may be exaggerated by cholinergic influences which further depress the rate of rise of phase 0 and result in block; early premature beats may also invade the AV node before recovery is complete, leading to delay and block. Recovery of full excitability typically outlasts the duration of the action potential in the AV node, resulting in a time and voltage dependence of refractoriness. These features account for the protective behavior of the AV node in preventing rapid impulse transmission from the atrium to the ventricle.

Under abnormal conditions of ischemia and hypoxia, cells such as Purkinje fibers can lose their fast response and revert to a slow-response mechanism similar to that in the AV node, resulting in delay and block in vivo.[45–47] For example, slow responses are typically obtained in Purkinje fibers by increasing extracellular potassium and adding norepinephrine; similar responses are found under experimental conditions of acute ischemia. A correlation of the presence or absence of slow responses has been found between in vitro cells removed from diseased human atria and atrial arrhythmias in vivo.[39,40,43]

Unidirectional block is one variety of conduction delay and block that deserves further emphasis. This unique disorder underlies most varieties of reentry (see below). The term implies impulse propagation in one direction but not the other. *Structural* conditions may permit only unidirectional conduction along cardiac fibers because of impedance mismatch;[48,49] alternatively, a *functional* state of unidirectional block may result when a premature beat encounters temporary inequality of excitability in a tissue, resulting in a dissociation of two potential routes for impulse propagation. Unidirectional block is especially common in tissues that exhibit slow responses.[18]

Reentry

In certain situations, conduction delay and block paradoxically lead to tachyarrhythmias by the mechanism of reentry, which might be defined as reexcitation caused by continuous propagation of the same impulse for one or more cycles. This group of arrhythmias differs from automaticity in that an initiating beat is required (although as we have seen, triggered activity also requires an initiating beat).

During normal conduction, a variety of potential routes of divergence of the cardiac impulse exists at all levels of the heart. The ability of many cardiac fibers to conduct in both directions and the presence of many cross connections between cardiac fibers create situations in which conduction can occur in a functionally closed loop. Fortunately there is uniformity of conduction and refractoriness at each "level" of the heart (i.e., atria, atrioventricular node, His-Purkinje system), resulting in uniform direction of impulse propagation. This normal sequence of events is schematically represented in Fig. 27-5A, where an impulse conducting through a proximal common pathway meets two divergent pathways (alpha and beta) converging upon a distal common pathway. Uniform depolarization results in synchronous activation of both divergent pathways and is followed by uniform recovery. This pattern of uniform activation may be distributed by pathological processes as well as by functional abnormalities that accompany premature beats. In Fig. 27-5B the propagating impulse encounters two divergent pathways with different properties. The impulse is blocked in the beta pathway, which contains an area of depressed conduction, and passes sufficiently slowly through the alpha pathway that it not only reaches the distal common pathway but is also transmitted retrogradely through the beta pathway. In Fig. 27-5C, the impulse has arrived in the previously

depolarized proximal portion of the beta pathway, which has recovered from its state of refractoriness; the impulse may reexcite or reenter this area, giving rise to a new impulse. In a similar manner a sustained reentry can occur (Fig. 27-5D). If a circulating wave front exits from the closed loop with each cycle, the surrounding cardiac tissue will also be excited.

The closed loop of reentry may be formed by anatomic or functional elements in normal cardiac structures or may be comprised in part by an accessory pathway. The latter situation is encountered in a group of disorders known as the preexcitation syndromes (see below). Regardless of the location of the closed loop, the requirements for reentry are in general the same as those depicted in Fig. 27-5B: a closed loop, conduction delay, and an area of unidirectional block. In the setting of an anatomic accessory pathway or in the presence of an anatomic obstacle, reentry of this type is easy to visualize. In the absence of an anatomic substrate, perpetuation of reentry can be explained on a functional basis which involves alteration of refractoriness. This latter mechanism has been described as the *leading circle* concept by Allessie.[50]

Before the discovery of the slow response, many investigators felt that it was unlikely that conduction which was sufficiently slow to allow a reentrant rhythm could occur outside the AV node. Considering the normal velocity of conduction and cardiac fibers, a large macroreentry loop appeared to be a requirement for such a mechanism. This objection has been overcome by the knowledge that very depressed fast responses or the so-called slow responses can permit reentry to occur in a very small area.

Reflection

Reentry usually implies a circuit. Another kind of reentry, called *reflection*,[22,51] can be readily demonstrated in isolated bundles of cardiac tissue. Thus a driven response can cross a depressed or depolarized portion of the linear strand (possibly by electrotonic spread), and, if there is sufficient delay so that recovery of excitability occurs on the driven side, a recurrent response or reentry occurs. This model of ectopic impulse formation has been used to explain some of the behavior of parasystolic pacemaker activity.

Concealed Conduction

The disorders of conduction described thus far all result in some manifest behavior of the propagating impulse, i.e., either conduction delay or obvious block. In 1948, Langendorf introduced the important concept of concealed conduction; this concept was derived from electrocardiographic studies[52] and subsequently verified by microelectrode techniques and His bundle electrocardiography in humans.[53,54] Concealed conduction occurs whenever depolarization of fibers of the AV transmission system is not

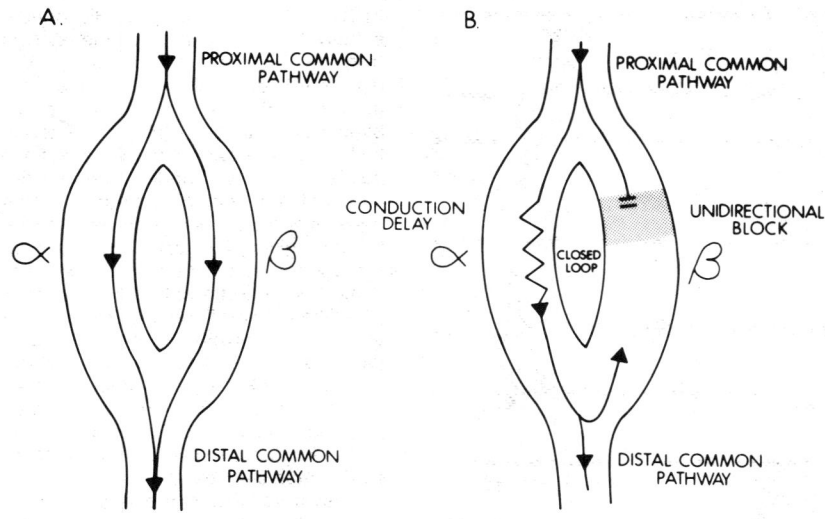

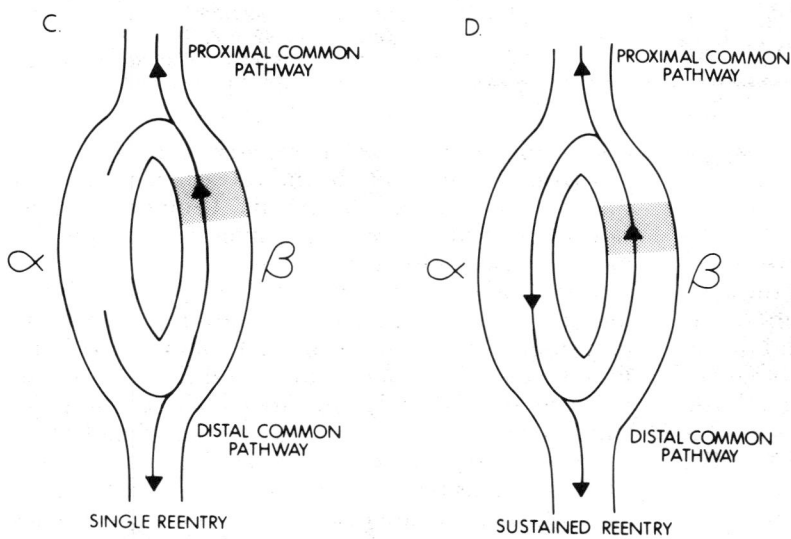

FIGURE 27-5   Mechanism of reentry. A hypothetical reentry circuit is demonstrated in which a proximal common pathway divides into two divergent paths, the alpha and beta pathways, before reuniting in the distal common pathway. *A.* Conduction proceeds equally in both the alpha and beta pathways under normal circumstances. *B.* A premature beat encounters an area of unidirectional block in the beta pathway. Conduction succeeds in the alpha pathway, but with considerable delay. *C.* The excitability of the beta pathway has recovered, allowing the impulse traveling down the alpha pathway to return up the beta pathway, resulting in reentry. *D.* Sustained reentry is present.

accompanied by identifiable events on the surface electrocardiogram. Such phenomena are not readily recognized (hence "concealed"), but are inferred from their effect on subsequent impulse formation and conduction (Fig. 27-6).

Combinations of Abnormal Impulse Formation and Conduction

It is not uncommon for conditions of abnormal impulse formation to coexist with abnormal impulse conduction. Thus as we have seen, under various abnormal conditions resulting in partial depolarization of cells with attendant slow conduction, pacemaker activity of abnormal cells is enhanced. Similarly, phase 4 depolarization can reduce transmembrane potential, resulting in diminished ability of a fiber to generate a normal action potential. If phase 4 depolarization is enhanced in some

part of the specialized conducting system or if it proceeds for an unusually long period of time, the response to a propagated impulse will be abnormal. The latter is the most likely cause of abnormal impulse propagation observed with long diastolic intervals (so-called phase 4 block).[55–57]

The association of abnormal impulse formation and conduction is particularly important in the phenomenon of parasystole,[58,59] in which abnormal automaticity coexists with abnormal conduction into (entrance block) and/or out of (exit block) an automatic focus.

Abnormalities of Repolarization

The role of nonuniform recovery of tissue in the genesis of reentry has previously been mentioned. We will now expand on this topic to elucidate the

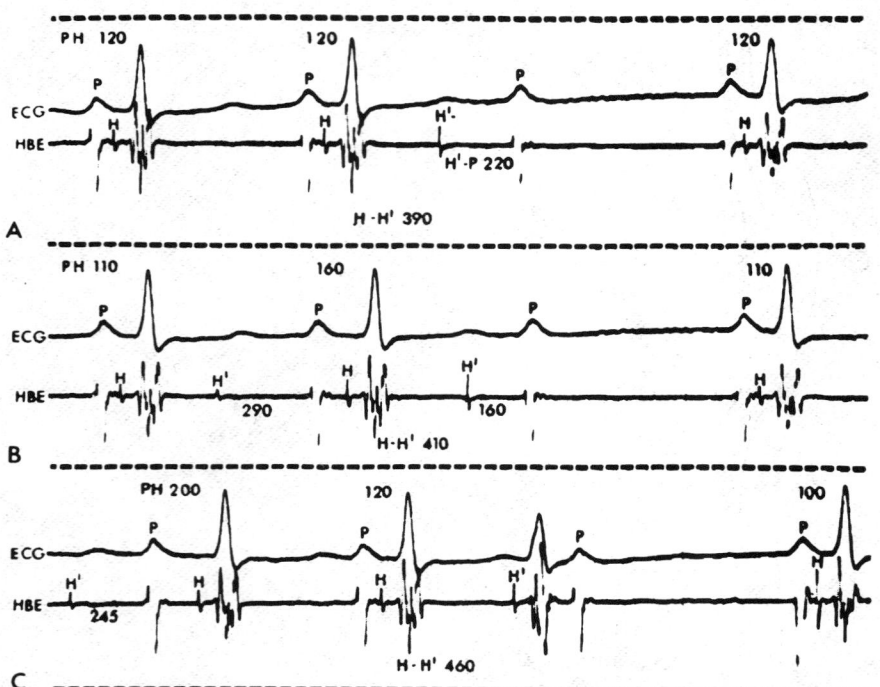

FIGURE 27-6 Concealed His bundle extrasystoles. In each panel, the tracings from the top down are standard ECG lead II recorded with a His bundle electrogram (HBE). *A.* The premature His bundle depolarization (H') is blocked in both antegrade and retrograde directions but leaves the AV node refractory because of "concealed" conduction. This causes the next sinus P wave to be blocked, giving the appearance of type II second-degree AV block. *B.* Two concealed His bundle extrasystoles occur with different H'P intervals, producing an electrocardiographic pattern of type I (Wenckebach) second-degree AV block. *C.* The first H'P interval produces sudden PR prolongation. The second H' wave propagates to the ventricle but is blocked in the AV node, resulting in the electrocardiographic appearance of a junctional extrasystole. Again the next sinus P wave is blocked because of concealed conduction of the second H' extrasystole. (*From K. M. Rosen et al., Pseudo A-V Block Secondary to Premature Nonpropagated His Bundle Depolarizations, Circulation, 42:367, 1970. Reproduced with permission of author and the American Heart Association, Inc.*)

phenomenon of aberrant conduction and reentry related to differential refractoriness.

Aberration

The duration of the action potential and recovery of excitability are nonuniform throughout the His-Purkinje system and ventricular myocardium so that a certain heterogeneity of repolarization and of the refractory periods of cardiac cells is physiologic in fibers that exhibit the fast response. In general, the action potential duration and refractoriness gradually increase from the proximal to the distal His-Purkinje system until an area of maximum refractoriness or "gate" is encountered near the junction of the Purkinje network with muscle; just beyond this gate, the refractoriness markedly decreases at the level of the myocardium.[60] The values of the gate for the conducting tissues in the right ventricle exceed those for the left ventricle. Thus a premature beat entering the conduction system tends to delay or block on the right side, so that clinically, right bundle branch block is the most common variety of aberration encountered.

The duration of the action potential and refractoriness is directly related to cycle length; thus longer cycle lengths augment subsequent refractoriness and shorter cycle lengths abbreviate refractoriness. Clinically, aberration is therefore probable when long cycle lengths are followed by short cycle lengths, as often occurs during atrial fibrillation.

Reentry Due to Nonhomogeneous Repolarization

The mechanism of reentry does not require the presence of abnormal conduction in depolarized fibers to achieve conduction delay or block; dissociation of the elements of the reentry pathway can result from an inequality in the refractory periods of different portions of the circuit. Temporal dispersion of myocardial recovery times may be physiologic or due to disease.

Local factors can influence the duration of cardiac action potentials, so that following the passage of a single wave front of depolarization, excitability may recover in one region of the heart *before* an adjacent area has fully repolarized. Under these circumstances, current may pass from the depolarized tissue to the recovered tissue, resulting in focal reexcitation.[61] This type of reentry can be observed, for example, when acute ischemia suddenly abbreviates the action potential duration in a focal area of the ventricles; the same mechanism can obviously occur when disease regionally prolongs the duration of the action potential or repolarization.

Inequality of refractory periods favors the appearance of reentry following premature beats by enhancing the likelihood that such beats will encounter an area of functional unidirectional block. A common example of this phenomenon is the initiation of reciprocating tachycardia by block of a premature beat in the accessory pathway of patients with a preexcitation syndrome (see below).

Long QT syndromes

This group of arrhythmias[62] is related to a more global disorder of repolarization due to imbalance in the sympathetic innervation of the heart. This imbalance allows asynchronous recovery of large portions of the ventricles to occur, setting the stage for electrical instability and susceptibility to ventricular fibrillation. The resulting abnormality of repolarization is reflected in a prolonged QT interval on the electrocardiogram.

Basis of Determination of Mechanisms of Arrhythmias in Humans

In the following section, some of the more common *tachyarrhythmias* and *bradyarrhythmias* will be discussed, with emphasis on those situations in which interrelationships between clinical electrophysiologic findings and basic electrophysiologic mechanisms are most apparent. Unfortunately, the exact mechanism of many clinical arrhythmias is not known with certainty; in some instances, multiple mechanisms may play a role. Our information concerning abnormal impulse formation, for example, is based almost entirely on concepts derived from microelectrode studies of single cardiac cells. Our knowledge of abnormal impulse conduction, on the other hand, is derived for the most part from studies of the intact heart.

The use of programmed stimulation of the heart (see Chaps. 19 and 90) in concert with multiple electrode-catheter recordings of activity from the atria, ventricles, and specialized conduction system (see Chap. 89) has greatly advanced our understanding of many clinical arrhythmias, permitting us to tentatively classify them based on the role of abnormal impulse formation (including automaticity), abnormal impulse conduction (including reentry), a combination of disordered impulse formation and conduction, and abnormal repolarization. Thus reentry is said to be strongly favored when clinical electrophysiologic study finds the following: ability to initiate and terminate tachycardia by premature stimulation delivered within well-defined, reproducible coupling intervals; ability to demonstrate continuous excitation of elements of the proposed reentry circuit; ability to terminate tachycardia abruptly by overdrive pacing; inverse relationship between the coupling interval of a premature beat that initiates tachycardia and the interval between the premature beat and the first beat of tachycardia. In contrast, the mechanism of automaticity is suggested by: *inability* to induce and terminate tachycardia with programmed stimulation; and overdrive pacing resulting in a pause followed by reappearance of the tachycardia with a progressive increase in rate (warm-up). Thus, automaticity is largely a diagnosis of exclusion.[63] The most recently discovered mechanism—triggered activity—remains a problem in terms of diagnostic criteria. In vitro it can be induced and terminated with stimulation (like reentry), but appears to have other particularities: it tends to occur only at fast basic rates; discontinuation of overdrive pacing may result in a transient acceleration of the triggered activity to the rate of pacing; there is an apparent direct relationship between the coupling interval of the premature beat that initiates triggered activity and the interval from the premature beat to the first beat of triggered activity; triggered activity appears highly sensitive to verapamil.

Tachyarrhythmias

Sinus Tachycardia, Sinus Node Reentry

Excessive sympathetic drive is by far the most common cause of sinus tachycardia and is mediated by an increased rate of diastolic depolarization resulting from an increased inward current. This usually occurs clinically with a gradual onset and offset and is a result of altered activity of the autonomic nervous system, rather than a primary disorder in the function of the sinus node.

Using multiple microelectrode recordings of the sinus node in an isolated preparation, Allessie[64] recently demonstrated the ability of the sinus node to sustain reentry (Fig. 27-7).

Clinical reports[65–68] have described episodes of supraventricular tachycardia with P-wave morphology identical to sinus rhythm that can be initiated and terminated by programmed stimulation in humans. These tachycardias are infrequent and unstable, and rarely present a clinical problem. A promising method has been described recently that permits recording of the sinus node potential in humans using catheter-electrode technique.[68,69]

Atrial Tachycardias

Atrial tachycardias may result from automaticity or reentry. Those resulting from digitalis excess appear to be caused by abnormal impulse formation, perhaps related to afterdepolarizations. The multifocal atrial tachycardias observed in patients with chronic lung disease are probably also related to abnormal automaticity. Goldreyer[70] first proposed the criteria that have come to be regarded as strongly suggestive of automaticity in the study of atrial tachycardia in humans. These included the following observations:

1. The P-wave morphology of tachycardia differed from that of the sinus P wave.
2. Atrial tachycardia was induced by premature atrial beats that did not result in conduction delay in the AV node.
3. During atrial tachycardia, the cycle length of tachycardia was not a function of conduction in the AV node.
4. A gradual acceleration of the rate of tachycardia, or warm-up, was observed following overdrive pacing or premature atrial stimulation.
5. The introduction of premature atrial beats during tachycardia resulted in reset of the tachycardia.
6. The tachycardia could not be terminated by pacing nor could it be initiated by programmed stimulation during periods of quiescence.

SINUS RHYTHM ECTOPIC BEAT SINUS ECHO

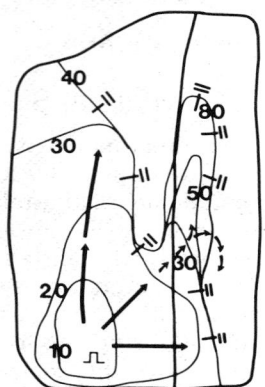
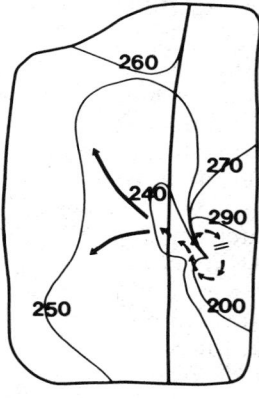

FIGURE 27-7 Sinus node reentry. Excitation patterns of a sinoatrial preparation during sinus rhythm, ectopic atrial beats, and resulting sinus node echo. In sinus rhythm there is a completely normal spread of activation from the center of the sinus node to the atrium. During the ectopic beat, intraatrial conduction block occurred at the higher part of the crista terminalis, resulting in an exclusive invasion of the sinus node at the lower part of the sinoatrial border. From this site of entrance, the impulse moved upward, then returned around in a clockwise direction within the node to reexcite the atrium 240 ms after the stimulus (sinus echo). (*From M. A. Allessie et al., Reentry within the Sino-Atrial Node, in F. I. M. Bonke (ed.), "The Sinus Node," Martinus Nijhoff, The Hague, 1978, p. 420. Reproduced with permission of author and publisher.*)

Evidence of atrial reentry as a mechanism for supraventricular tachycardia in humans has recently been summarized by Coumel.[71] Experimentally it has been demonstrated that reentry in the atrium can be determined by anatomically defined circuits as originally suggested by Mines[1] or solely by the functional properties of atrial tissue[72] (see "Atrial Flutter," below). The characteristics of these two types of circus movement are summarized in Fig. 27-8. The ability of the atrium to sustain reentry in the absence of an anatomically defined obstacle was recently shown by Allessie using the *leading circle concept.*[72] In this model, a premature stimulus was used to initiate a tachycardia in isolated left atrial tissue (Fig. 27-9). Recordings were made from approximately 100 sites, demonstrating a clockwise circus movement with a revolution time of 105 ms. In this model, the circus movement is the smallest possible circuit in which the stimulating efficacy of the circulating wave front is sufficient to excite the relatively refractory tissue ahead. Thus the head of the circulating wave is continually traveling in the wake of its own refractoriness. From this leading circle, centripetal wavelets activate the area in the center of the circle but collide with each other. On the other hand, centrifugal wavelets readily activate the surrounding atrial tissues. Allessie was able to demonstrate sustained reentry in pieces of atrial muscle with a radius of 5 to 6 mm. Because the dimensions are so small, it would obviously be difficult to distinguish such a leading circle from a focus of spontaneously discharging atrial fibers.[73]

Atrial Flutter

The majority of available studies support the mechanism of circus rhythm and reentry as the most common basis for atrial flutter.[74] The idea that a circuitous activation process was responsible for atrial flutter was first popularized by Lewis in 1920 based on experiments in the dog, although he himself found it very difficult to reproducibly initiate atrial flutter.[75] Later, Rosenbluth and Garcia Ramos[76] developed a model based on the concept introduced by Mines, namely that the conduction time around the reentry circuit must exceed the longest refractory period in the circuit in order to permit self-sustained reexcitation to proceed. These workers crushed a band of atrial tissue adjacent to the natural orifice of the inferior vena cava to provide a large anatomic obstacle. Following stimulation of the atria, a regular tachycardia developed during which sequential activation could be recorded around the borders of the lesion. It was generally

FIGURE 27-8 Circus movement. See text for discussion.

ANATOMIC OBSTACLE

(MINES, 1913)

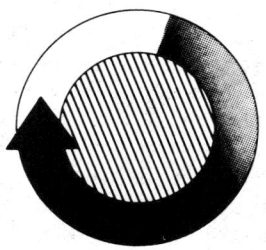

LEADING CIRCLE WITHOUT OBSTACLE

(ALLESSIE, 1977)

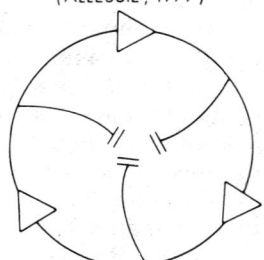

1. FIXED PATHWAY LENGTH DETERMINED BY OBSTACLE

2. USUALLY EXCITABLE GAP BETWEEN HEAD AND TAIL OF IMPULSE

3. INVERSE RELATION BETWEEN REVOLUTION TIME AND CONDUCTION VELOCITY

1. VARIABLE PATHWAY LENGTH DETERMINED BY ELECTROPHYSIOLOGIC PARAMETERS

2. NO GAP OF FULL EXCITABILITY

3. REVOLUTION TIME PROPORTIONAL TO LENGTH OF REFRACTORY PERIOD

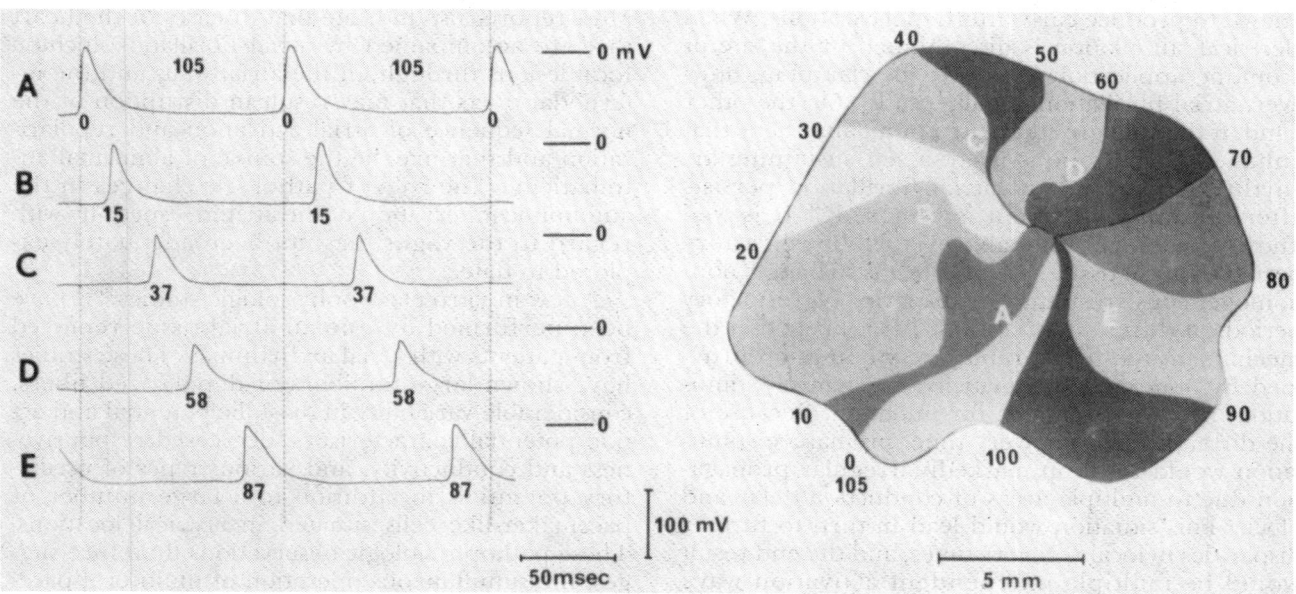

FIGURE 27-9   Atrial reentry in isolated left atrial muscle. *A to E*. The transmembrane potentials of five fibers which lie along the circular path. To the right, the isochronous map derived from recordings of action potentials from 94 different fibers is shown. The moments of depolarization in milliseconds are given together with the action potentials and the isochronic lines of the map. (*From M. A. Allessie, Circulating Excitation in the Heart, doctoral thesis, University of Limburg, Maastricht, 1977, p. 101. Reproduced with permission of author and publisher.*)

assumed that some degree of asymmetry at the site of initiation resulting in unidirectional block was necessary to initiate reentry in this model, a hypothesis later proved by a mathematical model.[73] Pastelin[77] postulated that the circus movement during atrial flutter may involve the preferential atrial pathways, and Boineau[78] pointed to the possible role of atrial hypoplasia and discontinuity of preferential atrial conduction pathways as the basis of flutter.

There has been a general consensus that atrial flutter would be impossible in a truly homogeneous tissue unless some asymmetry was present at least at the moment of initiation. However, it has been clearly demonstrated that a physical obstruction is not necessary for atrial flutter to ensue. The refractory period of the atrium itself, serving as a functional obstacle, can permit circus movement, as demonstrated mathematically by Moe.[79] More recently, Allessie extended his observations of atrial reentry in isolated pieces of atrial tissue to the study of sustained atrial flutter in the intact canine heart. Using simultaneous recordings from 192 locations, he was able to demonstrate sustained reentry on the basis of the leading circle mechanism with no requirement for an anatomic obstacle.[80]

Almost all studies of atrial flutter to date emphasize the ability to induce flutter with premature stimulation as well as the important role of conduction delay and areas of unidirectional block due to nonuniformity of refractory periods, regardless of the presence or absence of an anatomic obstacle. These features suggest a reentry basis for flutter. Some microelectrode studies have suggested a potential role for automaticity.[81] In addition, Scherf[82] dem-

onstrated the ability of aconitine to induce flutter via the mechanism of abnormal impulse formation, but again it is difficult to exclude the possibility that the rapid impulse formation set up functional reentry pathways as a result of rate-related conduction delay and block. Clinical studies of atrial flutter in humans[83–89] have confirmed the ease with which atrial flutter can be induced with premature beats in susceptible patients. Termination of flutter has been achieved by overdrive pacing at 115 to 125 percent of the basic flutter rate. It has also been noted that termination is associated with *entrainment*,[88] whereby at critical rates of overdrive atrial pacing, the P-wave morphology changes from that present in flutter, suggesting that the reentry pathway has been engaged. The fact that the "entrained" P-wave morphology is not identical to that obtained by pacing at the same site during sinus rhythm suggests that atrial fusion or rate-related atrial conduction disturbances are present during the period of entrainment.

Despite many observations in favor of reentry, it is still impossible to exclude a role of abnormal automaticity in some clinical cases of flutter.

Atrial Fibrillation

The physiologic mechanism of atrial fibrillation has not been conclusively established,[90] but experimental findings strongly suggest that while it can be induced by pacemaker activity, it is sustained by a reentrant process. In dogs anesthetized by barbiturates, fibrillation can be induced by rapid atrial pacing or the local application of aconitine,[82] which is known to produce early afterdepolarizations. When electrical stimulation is discontinued or the site of aconitine application is isolated by clamping, however, atrial fibrillation usually ceases. On the other hand, if the vagi are stimulated or an anesthetic that enhances vagal tone is used, a self-sustaining arrhythmia suggestive of atrial fibrillation persists after the initiating agent is removed.[91] It is well known that vagal tone abbreviates the refractory period of atrial tissue.[92] This effect is strikingly nonhomogeneous, resulting in disparity of refractory periods at different atrial sites.[93] It is likely that the mechanism requires premature stimulation provided by abnormal automaticity, mechanical stimulation, rapid pacing, etc., for initiation. Because of the differences in recovery time, premature stimulation would result in markedly irregular propagation due to multiple areas of conduction delay and block. This situation would lead in turn to further disparities in local recovery times, and the end result would be multiple independent activation wave fronts or wavelets due to reentry. A mathematical model incorporating features of nonuniform refractory periods (subject to the effect of cycle length) in addition to an effect of incomplete recovery or conduction velocity confirmed the feasibility of this mechanism.[73,94]

A number of features strongly support the mechanism of reentry in the genesis of sustained atrial fibrillation. Atrial fibrillation occasionally terminates spontaneously, which would be unlikely if it were caused by multiple ectopic pacemakers. A reentry mechanism would explain the so-called vulnerable period, that is, the limited period of time in a cardiac cycle during which atrial fibrillation can be induced by premature atrial stimulation. The necessary degree of nonhomogeneity of recovery would only exist at such a critical interval. The multiple wavelet reentry hypothesis is also most compatible with the fact that a single electric shock is able to terminate atrial fibrillation. Finally, in 1914 Garrey established that a critical mass of atrial tissue was necessary for atrial fibrillation, an observation again most compatible with a reentrant mechanism. Nevertheless, it is still impossible to exclude some role of pacemaker activity in the mechanism of sustained atrial fibrillation. For example, Nadeau[95] has found that experimentally induced atrial fibrillation persists longer in the presence of an intact sinus node.

Despite the wealth of information concerning experimental atrial fibrillation, relatively little information is available on atrial fibrillation in humans. A wide variety of anatomic abnormalities[96] have been found in patients with atrial fibrillation, including abnormalities of the sinus node, the atrioventricular node, and other areas. The diversity of findings has led some workers to conclude that no special abnormality is characteristic of atrial fibrillation. In general, however, it should be noted that pathologic involvement of the sinus node is a fairly consistent finding in the published anatomic studies.

Most reports also indicate that diseases of the heart that are accompanied by atrial fibrillation include focal lesions throughout the atrial walls and the internodal tracts that may result in disruption of the normal sequence of atrial activation and repolarization and that may be the source of abnormal automaticity. The role of pathologic changes in the autonomic innervation of the atrium, especially with regard to the vagus, has not been adequately explored to date.

A few in vitro electrophysiologic studies[39,43] have been performed on human atrial tissue removed from patients with atrial arrhythmias. These studies have shown large numbers of depolarized fibers, considerable variability in diastolic potential and action potential characteristics, decreased responsiveness and conductivity, and various types of oscillatory potentials in addition to a large number of pacemaker-like cells situated in atypical locations. These pathophysiologic observations therefore suggest the simultaneous operation of multifocal pacemaker activity, reentry, and abnormal automaticity in the pathogenesis of atrial fibrillation.

The Preexcitation Syndromes

Ventricular preexcitation[97] is said to be present when, in relation to atrial events, the whole or part of the ventricular myocardium is activated by the impulse originating in the atrium *earlier* than would be expected if the impulse reached the ventricles by way of the normal specialized conducting system. This classic definition, of course, refers only to phenomena occurring during *antegrade* conduction. It is now well established that the accessory pathway underlying preexcitation syndromes can exhibit unidirectional block in the antegrade *or* retrograde direction. Thus a more liberal definition is necessary: Preexcitation is present when one cardiac chamber is activated in whole or part by an impulse originating in the other chamber *earlier* than would be expected if the impulse had proceeded over the normal conducting system.

The term *syndrome* is applied when electrocardiographic or electrophysiologic evidence of preexcitation is accompanied by clinical arrhythmias. A variety of potential anatomic substrates exist for which a new nomenclature has been suggested (Fig. 27-10).[98] These include fibers coursing directly from atrium to ventricle (accessory atrioventricular pathways or Kent bundles); fibers coursing from atrium to His bundle, bypassing the physiological delay of the AV node (atrio-Hisian fibers); and two varieties of Mahaim fibers: those passing from the AV node to the ventricle (nodoventricular fibers) and those arising in the His bundle–bundle branches and inserting in the ventricular myocardium (fasciculoventricular fibers).

The most common variety of preexcitation is the accessory atrioventricular pathway that makes up the anatomic substrate for the Wolff-Parkinson-

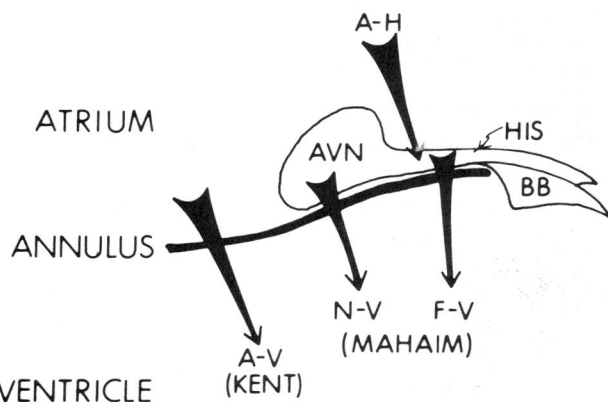

FIGURE 27-10 Substrates of preexcitation. A schematic representation of the atrioventricular junction in the region of the normal conduction system is shown. Atrio-Hisian (A-H) fibers insert directly into the His bundle, thus bypassing the area of physiological delay; atrioventricular (A-V) pathways or Kent bundles pass directly from atrium to ventricle; nodoventricular (NV) fibers (Mahaim fibers) pass directly from the AV node to the ventricle; fasciculoventricular (FV) fibers pass from the His bundle or bundle branches directly to the ventricle. AVN = atrioventricular node; BB = bundle branch.

White (WPW) syndrome and some of its variants (Fig. 27-11). If it is assumed that the accessory pathway linking atrium to ventricle is capable of antegrade conduction, two parallel routes of conduction are possible, one subject to physiologic delay over the AV node and the other passing directly from atrium to ventricle. In general, ventricular activation in sinus rhythm will be the result of fusion of these two ventricular inputs, resulting in abbreviations of the PR interval and an anomalous QRS complex due to the abnormal sequence of ventricular activation that results from eccentric depolarization of the ventricles by the accessory pathway (Fig. 27-12).

The most common arrhythmia associated with the WPW syndrome is a reciprocating supraventricular tachycardia, which has become the model of reentrant rhythms. Initiation of a typical paroxysm of tachycardia (Fig. 27-12) results from a premature beat that blocks in the accessory pathway and conducts with delay down the normal conducting system (resulting in a normal QRS complex). Activation spreading through the ventricles finds the accessory pathway excitable in the retrograde direction (as a result of functional unidirectional block), allowing impulse propagation back to the atrium. Circus movement is then established by antegrade conduction over the normal conducting system and retrograde conduction over the accessory pathway. The typical conditions for reentry illustrated in Fig. 27-5 are thus all present: closed circuit, conduction delay, and unidirectional block. Detailed recordings

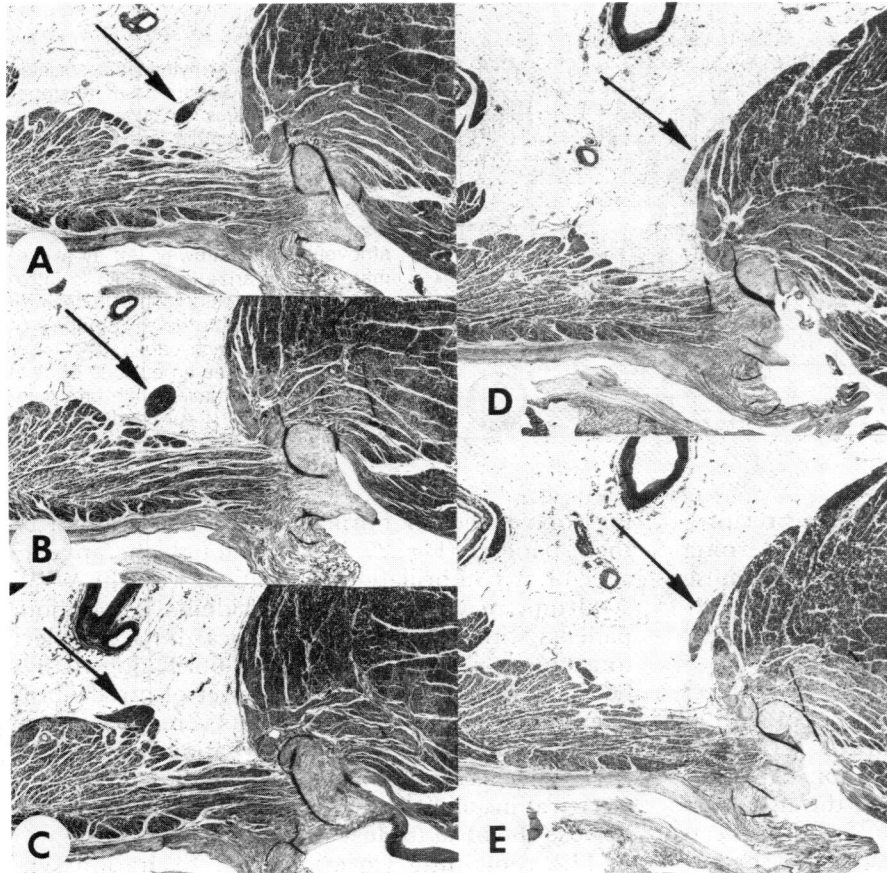

FIGURE 27-11 Accessory atrioventricular pathway (Kent bundle). *A* to *E*. Sequential steps taken from the left atrioventricular junction of a patient with WPW syndrome. Note the bridge passing from left atrium in *A* across epicardial fat in *B, C,* and *D* and joining the left ventricle in *E*. Epicardial fat is to the right; left atrial and left ventricular cavities are to the left. Masson's stain; × 9.5.' (*From G. J. Klein et al., Anatomic Substrate of Impaired Antegrade Conduction over an Accessory Atrioventricular Pathway in the Wolff-Parkinson-White Syndrome, Circulation, 61:1249, 1980. Reproduced with permission of the author and the American Heart Association, Inc.*)

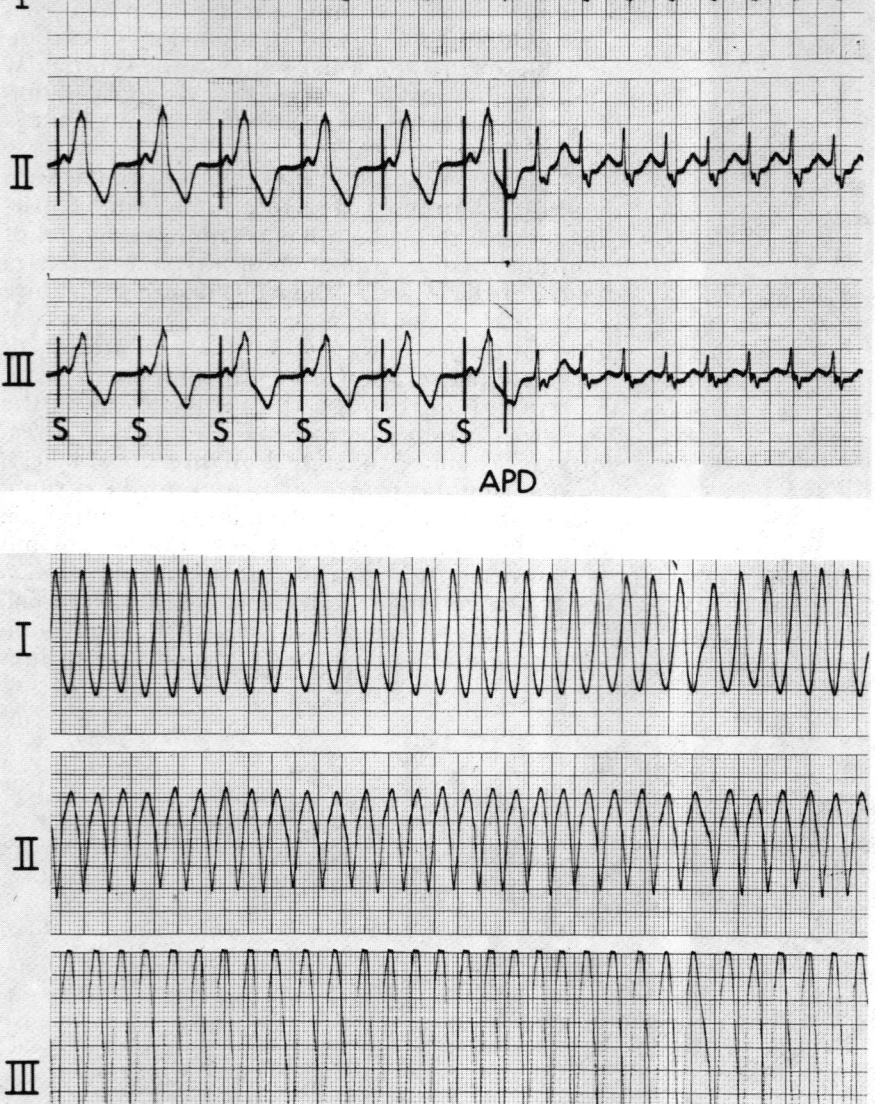

FIGURE 27-12 Arrhythmias associated with the WPW syndrome. The upper panel demonstrates induction of a supraventricular tachycardia in a patient with WPW syndrome. The atria are initially being paced, resulting in a short PR interval, wide QRS complex due to ventricular preexcitation over an accessory atrioventricular pathway. An atrial premature depolarization (APD) is introduced which blocks in the accessory pathway and initiates an episode of supraventricular tachycardia. The lower panel demonstrates an episode of atrial flutter in another patient with preexcitation, resulting in 1:1 AV conduction with an anomalous QRS complex.

of the sequence of atrial activation during reciprocating tachycardia provide information concerning the point in the atria where the retrograde impulse first penetrates and thus can be used to localize accessory pathways by electrode-catheter techniques (Fig. 27-13).

Patients with the WPW syndrome are also subject to a second symptomatic arrhythmia, that of a rapid ventricular response occurring in the setting of atrial fibrillation. During atrial fibrillation, rapid impulses in the atria are not subject to the usual decremental conduction of the AV node and thus can result in a malignant ventricular response, account-

ing for ventricular fibrillation in a small subset of these patients (Fig. 27-14).[99] Although the appearance of atrial fibrillation in a patient with the WPW syndrome may represent a coincidental association, patients with reciprocating tachycardia are subject to a unique mechanism of atrial fibrillation. It has been demonstrated[97] that the onset of atrial fibrillation in a subset of these patients is invariably due to a preceding period of reciprocating tachycardia. Atrial distension during tachycardia, together with electrical instability due to the rapid rate, may predispose the atria to develop fibrillation.

The remaining varieties of preexcitation syn-

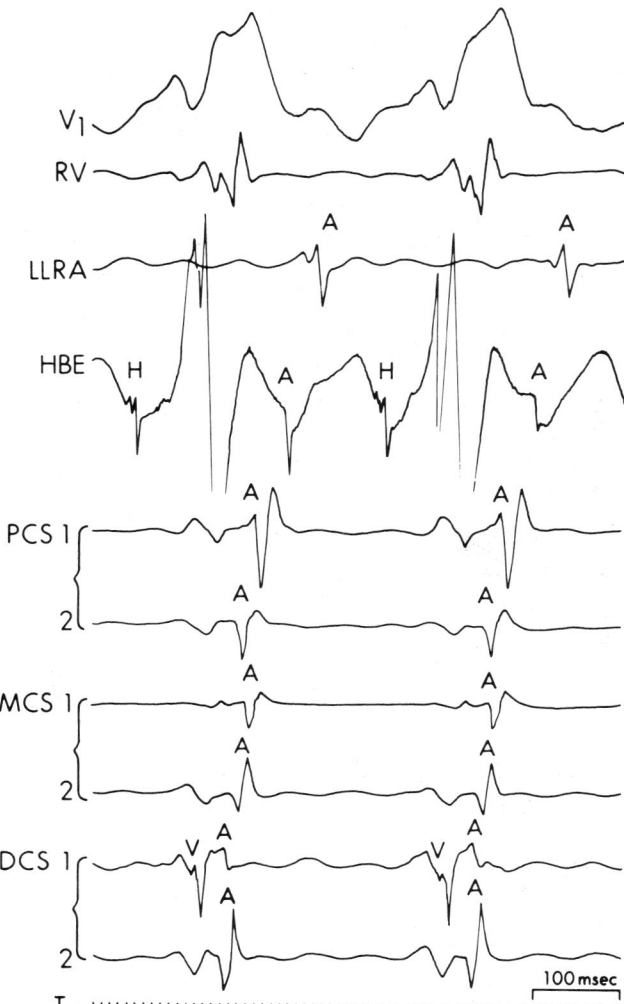

FIGURE 27-13 Atrial mapping during reciprocating tachycardia in a patient with WPW syndrome. The recordings from the top down include standard ECG leads V_1 and bipolar electrograms from the right ventricle (RV), the low lateral right atrium (LLRA), the region of the His bundle (HBE), and the proximal coronary sinus (PCS), midcoronary sinus, (MCS) and distal coronary sinus (DCS). The recordings were obtained during reciprocating tachycardia using the normal atrioventricular conduction system as the antegrade limb and the accessory pathway as the retrograde limb of a reentrant circuit. The QRS complex demonstrates right bundle branch block. The sequence of retrograde atrial activation is eccentric, with earliest atrial activity recorded in the distal coronary sinus tracing, reflecting early activity of the lateral left atrium. (*From G. J. Klein et al., Anatomic Substrate of Impaired Antegrade Conduction over an Accessory Atrioventricular Pathway in the Wolff-Parkinson-White Syndrome, Circulation, 61:1249, 1980. Reproduced with permission of the author and the American Heart Association, Inc.*)

dromes are considerably less common (Fig. 27-25).[97,100–103] As demonstrated in Fig. 27-15, all of these can sustain a normal QRS supraventricular tachycardia by providing a return limb for the reentry circuit, comparable to the situation described for Kent bundles. Atrio-Hisian fibers can result in a short PR interval and normal QRS complex, which in association with clinical arrhythmias has been

termed the *Lown-Ganong-Levine syndrome.*[100] Patients with this syndrome are subject to a variety of mechanisms of tachycardia. Thus in addition to a reciprocating supraventricular tachycardia, they may be subject to a rapid ventricular response in the setting of atrial fibrillation because of the bypass of their AV node. In some instances, it appears that the mechanism of arrhythmia may be unrelated to the abnormality of the AV node. Recently, studies have been undertaken in patients with Mahaim fibers in an attempt to define a role for these ubiquitous structures in the genesis of cardiac arrhythmias in humans.[101–103] It has been demonstrated that in addition to a supraventricular tachycardia with a narrow QRS complex, nodoventricular fibers are capable of sustaining a wide QRS tachycardia indistinguishable from ventricular tachycardia (see below). Thus far, it has been impossible to incriminate fasciculoventricular fibers in any demonstrable arrhythmia. However, they could form the substrate for certain varieties of ventricular tachycardia.

AV Junctional Tachycardia

In this section, the topic of narrow QRS supraventricular tachycardia (SVT) occurring in patients *without* overt evidence of preexcitation will be discussed. A variety of potential mechanisms exist which in general can be subdivided into paroxysmal and nonparoxysmal, with or without 1:1 association of atrial and ventricular activity.

Paroxysmal AV Junctional Tachycardia with 1:1 AV Association

This descriptor identifies a subset of patients with SVT most commonly due to three potential mechanisms: reentry utilizing a concealed accessory pathway of the atrioventricular type (Kent bundle), reentry confined to the AV node, and atrial tachycardia. This undoubtedly accounts for the variety of terms that have been used to describe the electrocardiographic entity (Fig. 27-16). Atrial tachycardia has already been discussed and is suggested by the contour of the P wave and the ability of the tachycardia to continue despite block in the AV node.

Reentry Utilizing a Concealed Accessory Pathway The mechanism of this tachycardia is identical to that described for SVT in classic WPW syndrome, with the exception that the accessory pathway is incapable of conducting antegradely (unidirectional block). One wonders why such patients are not in a constant state of tachycardia. One explanation is that the atrium near the accessory pathway is still refractory from the sinus impulse when the retrograde impulse attempts to reexcite the atrium over the accessory pathway. With sinus tachycardia (resulting in decreased atrial refractoriness) or with a premature atrial beat (which results in AV conduction delay), recovery of the accessory pathway occurs, resulting in reentry. In our experience this

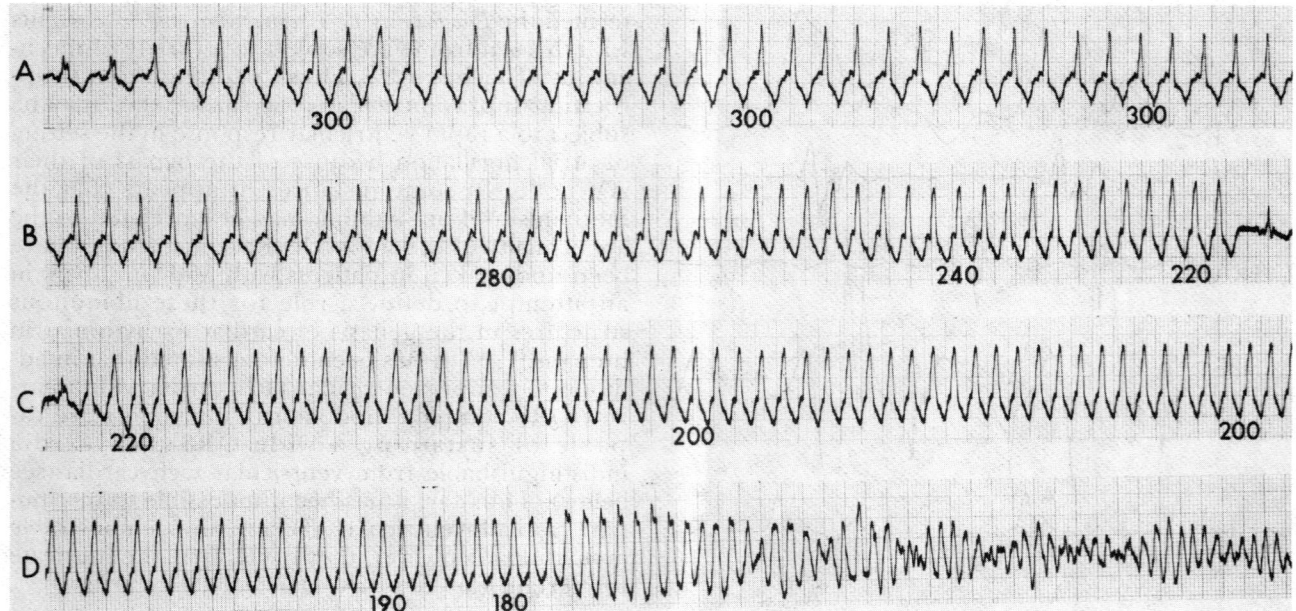

FIGURE 27-14 Induction of ventricular fibrillation in a patient with WPW syndrome by atrial pacing. *A* and *B*. These are continuous and demonstrate 1:1 AV conduction during rapid atrial pacing from cycle length 300 ms to 220 ms. *C*. After a resting period of sinus rhythm, pacing was reinstituted at a cycle length of 220 ms. *D*. Ventricular fibrillation appeared shortly after reaching a cycle length of 180 ms. The patient had a history of spontaneous ventricular fibrillation.

mechanism accounts for 40 percent of SVT in patients with no overt evidence of preexcitation.

Reentry Confined to the AV Node SVT due to reentry confined to the AV node is a common cause of AV junctional tachycardia, accounting for 40 to 50 percent of cases in most series. Evidence for this mechanism was provided by Moe,[104,105] who demonstrated that SVT could be produced by longitudinal dissociation of the AV node into two functional pathways designated alpha and beta. The mechanism he proposed is essentially that shown in Fig. 27-5. He originally suggested that the alpha pathway was the slower conducting pathway but had

FIGURE 27-15 Extranodal mechanisms of supraventricular tachycardia. A schematic ladder diagram depicts some theoretical representations of reentry circuits involving accessory pathways. The return limb of the reentry circuit can be provided by retrograde conduction over a pathway between ventricle and atrium (Kent bundle), between the His bundle and atrium (atrio-Hisian fiber), or a fiber between the ventricle and the AV node (nodoventricular or Mahaim fiber).

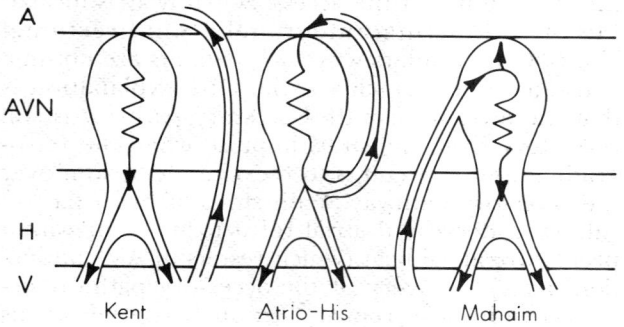

the shorter refractory period, while the beta pathway conducted faster but had a longer refractory period. Thus a premature atrial beat might tend to block in the beta pathway and conduct slowly down the alpha pathway. If sufficient conduction delay occurred, the beta pathway would recover, permitting reentry from the alpha pathway. The mechanism was subsequently confirmed using multiple microelectrode recordings in AV nodal preparations from rabbits demonstrating SVT.[106,107] The interrelationship of conduction and refractoriness has been validated in humans as well through the use of programmed premature stimulation.[14,63,108,109] Although a number of potential configurations for the reentry circuit in the AV node can be imagined (Fig. 27-17), in most cases atrial and ventricular activation occur almost simultaneously. This provides an easy method to differentiate SVT due to a concealed accessory pathway from reentry confined to the AV node (Fig. 27-18):[110] with a concealed accessory pathway, the propagating impulse must depolarize the ventricle *before* it can return to the atrium, resulting in an obligatory relationship of these events during tachycardia; with reentry in the AV node, the QRS complex and P wave can occur simultaneously. A simple examination of the relationship of the P wave and QRS complex during SVT by electrocardiographic or esophageal lead recordings allows exclusion of a concealed accessory pathway if the P wave during tachycardia does not *follow* the QRS complex.

Recently, yet another mechanism of SVT has been discovered in which tachycardia occurs almost incessantly and the RP interval is long, exceeding

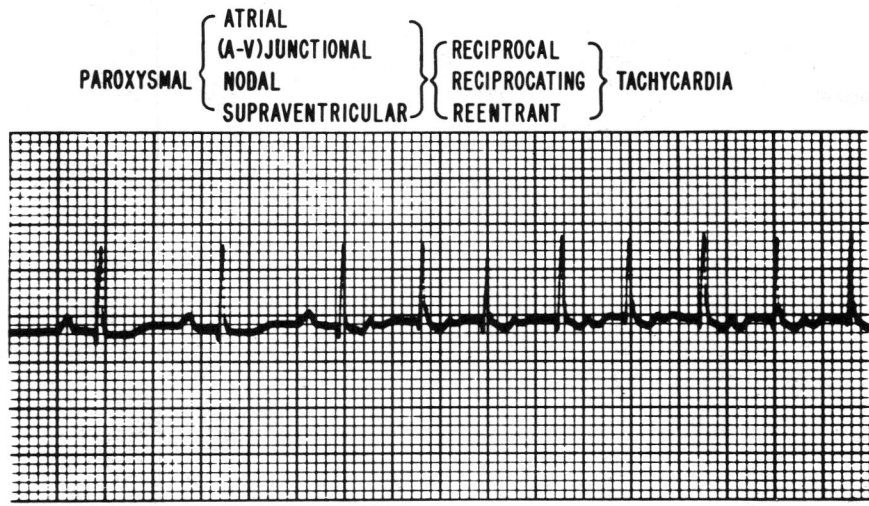

FIGURE 27-16 AV junctional tachycardia. A representative rhythm strip demonstrating the onset of AV junctional tachycardia is shown along with the variety of terms that have been used to describe this arrhythmia. After three sinus beats associated with a normal PR interval and normal QRS complex, there is sudden onset of a narrow QRS tachycardia.

the PR interval. This has been demonstrated to be due to either an accessory AV node,[111] a "fast-slow" configuration of the functional pathways in the AV node, or ectopic atrial tachycardia (Fig. 27-19).

Paroxysmal AV Junctional Tachycardia with AV Dissociation

This is an uncommon variety of AV junctional tachycardia in which the atrium is not required for perpetuation of tachycardia. As shown in Fig. 27-16 and demonstrated by Mignone and Wallace,[112] the atrium is not necessarily required for reentry in the AV node to ensue, although this possibility is considered rare.

Mahaim fibers of the nodoventricular variety[101] have been demonstrated to produce this type of arrhythmia, again on the basis of reentry.

Brechenmacher[113] has described pathologic findings in a child who died from rapid AV junctional tachycardia with AV dissociation: the His bundle was split into several thin and longitudinally oriented strands, suggesting the possibility of reentry due to longitudinal dissociation.

Nonparoxysmal AV Junctional Tachycardia with AV Dissociation (Accelerated Junctional Rhythm)

This type of arrhythmia[114] generally occurs at relatively slow rates with gradual onset and offset and is likely to be observed in the setting of an acute diaphragmatic myocardial infarction or digitalis toxicity. Most reports suggest that this rhythm is due to abnormally enhanced automaticity of a pacemaker in the junctional region.

Ventricular Tachycardia

A variety of mechanisms of premature ventricular beats and sustained ventricular tachycardia have been proposed, including automaticity,[58,115–117] triggered activity,[36] microreentry circuits in the ventricle,[118–128] macroreentry circuits confined to the specialized conduction system,[129–134] and Mahaim fibers.[101–103] Even in the same disease model (i.e., ischemia), the mechanism of the arrhythmia dem-

FIGURE 27-17 Mechanisms of reentry confined to the atrioventricular node. A schematic ladder diagram depicts theoretical representations of reentry circuits in the AV node. Areas of delay can be postulated either in one limb of the so-called dual-pathway model or in the initial or final common pathway issuing from a smaller microreentrant circuit. Depending on the location and magnitude of delay, a variety of relationships between atrial (P waves) and ventricular (R waves) depolarization is possible. Thus atrial depolarization may precede, occur simultaneously with, or follow ventricular depolarizations. A = atrium; N = node; V = ventricle. (*From J. J. Gallagher et al.*[110] *Reproduced with permission of the author and publishers.*)

FIGURE 27-18 Comparison of reentry confined to the AV node with reentry utilizing a Kent bundle. The most common variety of reentry confined to the AV node has been schematically depicted, with atrial and ventricular depolarization occurring almost simultaneously. In contrast, reentry utilizing an accessory pathway (Kent bundle) requires that ventricular depolarization precede retrograde atrial depolarization. (*From J. J. Gallagher et al.*[110] *Reproduced with permission of author and publisher.*)

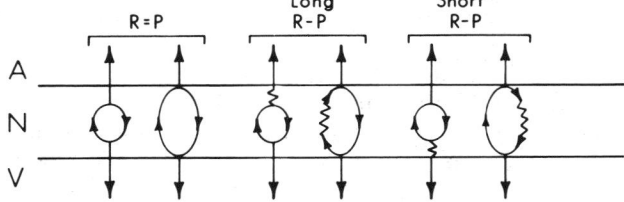

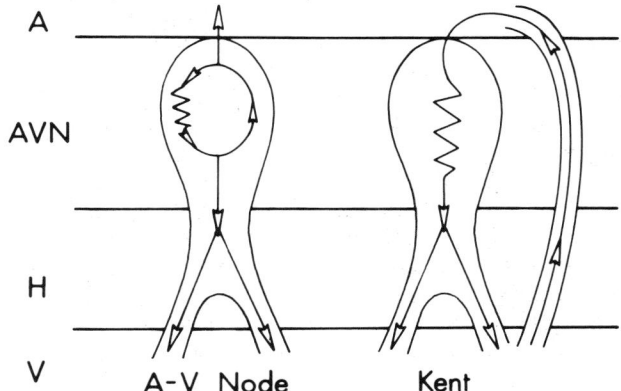

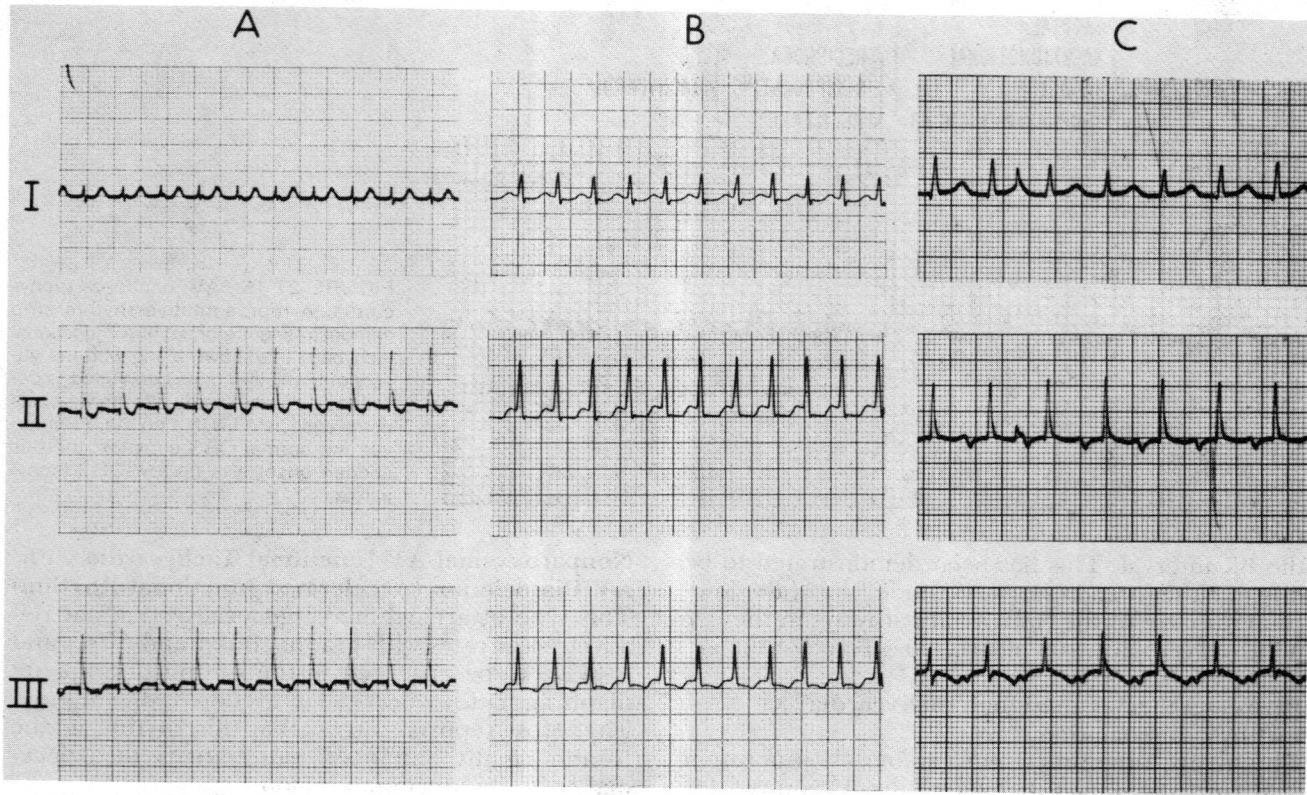

FIGURE 27-19   Three varieties of supraventricular tachycardia. *A*. Examination of lead III demonstrates that a P wave deforms the IST segment, which is compatible with tachycardia utilizing a Kent bundle. *B*. No P wave is visible because the P wave occurs simultaneously with the QRS complex, which is compatible with reentry in the AV node. *C*. P waves occur just after the T wave, and in fact are situated closer to the following QRS complex. This latter configuration is compatible with reentry utilizing an accessory AV node, with atrial tachycardia, or with an atypical form of reentry in the AV node. See text for discussion.

onstrated in any given stage may vary, depending on the experimental conditions.[135,136] Immediately following coronary occlusion there is an initial arrhythmogenic period which appears to be related to conduction delay and reentry. This is followed shortly by quiescence due to block of the early-appearing reentry pathways. Reperfusion at this time will result in reappearance of ventricular arrhythmias due to reentry. If, however, the occlusion is maintained, or reperfusion is gradual or delayed, automatic rhythms appear to predominate during the first 24 h. After several days to weeks, ventricular arrhythmias can again be initiated by programmed stimulation of the ventricle, suggesting that a mechanism of reentry is again present.

The first studies that provided direct evidence of unidirectional block and circus movement in ventricular muscle were carried out by Schmitt and Erlanger in 1929.[7] These workers used a multicompartmented model of turtle ventricle in which segmental areas of depressed function were induced by local pressure and the application of potassium chloride. Unidirectional block was frequently observed in this preparation, and multiple responses to a single stimulus could be elicited. Schmitt and Erlanger speculated that the special arrangement of the specialized conducting tissues in the mammalian heart might favor reentry. The hypothetical micro-

circuit of a Purkinje twig anastomosing with ventricular muscle that they proposed had essentially the same features as the diagrammatic representation of reentry shown in Fig. 27-5. For some time, however, there was reluctance to accept reentry as a mechanism of microreentry in the ventricles because of hypothetical considerations concerning the size of the reentry loop. For example, assuming an area of unidirectional block in a tissue exhibiting a conduction velocity of 3 m/s and a refractory period of 300 ms, a reentry pathway of 1 m would be required to allow reexcitation. However, if conduction velocity could proceed at 0.01 m/s, a 3-mm pathway would satisfy the conditions for reentry. The subsequent discovery of the slow response or depressed fast response provided the low conduction velocity required for hypothesizing this type of microreentry.

The mechanism of the ubiquitous premature ventricular contraction has not been defined with certainty, although many workers favor the presence of fixed coupling as strongly suggestive of reentry. Moe has demonstrated, however, that a parasystolic focus operating under electrotonic influences could produce the same pattern of coupling.[58] The mechanism of chronic sustained tachyarrhythmias has been more thoroughly studied, and in the majority of instances a reentrant mechanism

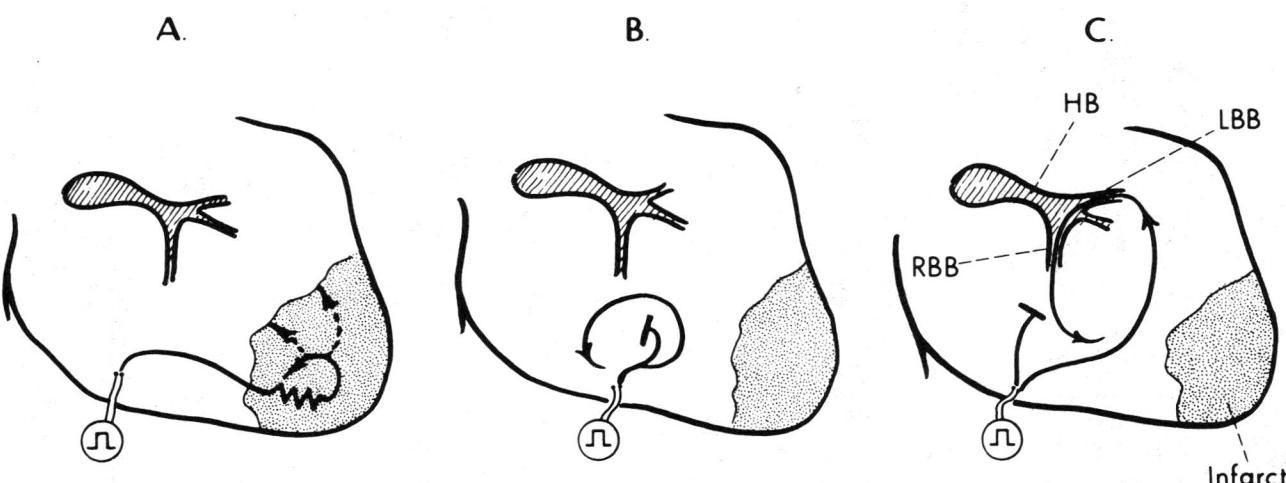

FIGURE 27-20 Mechanisms of ventricular arrhythmias induced by programmed stimulation. The figures demonstrate a stippled zone representing a theoretical area of infarction. *A.* Stimulation results in the creation of a reentrant arrhythmia in the area of infarction. *B.* Programmed stimulation results in reentry adjacent to the site of stimulation in nonpathological myocardium. *C.* Programmed stimulation results in the induction of a macroreentrant ventricular tachycardia which utilizes the bundle branches of the specialized conduction tissues for its perpetuation.

has been favored. To date, however, no three-dimensional representation of the reentry circuit has been possible in either animals or human beings. Clinical investigation of ventricular arrhythmias in humans is limited by the complex architecture of the ventricle. Insights into potential mechanisms underlying ventricular tachycardia have been largely gleaned from observations using catheter-electrode recordings in concert with programmed stimulation. As previously mentioned, the implicit hypothesis of this technique is that a reentry mechanism can be equated with the ability to initiate and terminate the tachycardia by programmed stimulation. Unfortunately, no criteria exist for the diagnosis of triggered activity in the ventricle; in addition, the technique of programmed stimulation has limitations which have recently been reviewed.[63] A representative example of this technique is shown in Figs. 27-20 and 27-21. Programmed stimulation may result in an initiation of reentry in an area of pathology, local reentry in nonpathological myocardium, or macroreentry involving conduction in portions of the specialized conducting tissues. However, the technique has intrinsic false-positive and false-negative results. For example, with aggressive stimulation it is possible to induce so-called nonclinical ventricular tachycardias in patients who have not previously experienced such arrhythmias; this emphasizes the need to correlate the morphology and characteristics of arrhythmias induced by programmed stimulation with those occurring spontaneously (Fig. 27-21). Most investigators have found that in the setting of chronic ventricular tachycardia, the tachycardia can be reproduced by programmed stimulation in the laboratory in as many as 70 percent of cases. The results of catheter-electrode studies together with cardiac-mapping studies at the time of surgery suggest that in a majority of instances, the reentrant process is confined to a rela-

tively small area, although macroreentry has been observed (Fig. 27-22).[129–134] In general, it has not been possible to reproducibly initiate ventricular arrhythmias due to acute ischemia, mitral valve prolapse, long QT syndrome, and exercise-induced ventricular tachycardia.

Although definitive three-dimensional localization of ventricular tachycardia has not yet been realized, the development of multiple-electrode recording systems and the facility for online computer analysis suggest that this will soon be possible.[137,138] Some insight into the site of origin of ventricular tachycardia has been obtained by the use of catheter-electrode recording techniques as well as intraoperative cardiac mapping. It has been assumed for some time that ventricular tachycardia arising in the right ventricle has a benign prognosis and is unlikely to be associated with obvious cardiac pathology.[139] Recent investigations of ventricular tachycardia associated with a left bundle branch block morphology have shed new light on a variety of substrates: thus Josephson[140] found that ventricular tachycardia with a left bundle branch block morphology in patients with ischemic heart disease often arose in the septum; Fontaine[141] has demonstrated a new entity, arrhythmogenic right ventricular dysplasia, emphasizing the need to perform right ventricular angiography in patients with a left bundle branch block morphology during ventricular tachycardia (Fig. 27-23); finally, the nodoventricular variety of Mahaim fibers has been found to sustain a tachycardia with left bundle branch block morphology that is indistinguishable from ventricular tachycardia (Figs. 27-24 and 27-25).[101,142]

The role of the autonomic nervous system in the initiation and maintenance of ventricular tachycardia as well as other arrhythmias deserves emphasis. There has been an unfortunate tendency to view the substrate of most arrhythmias as static rather

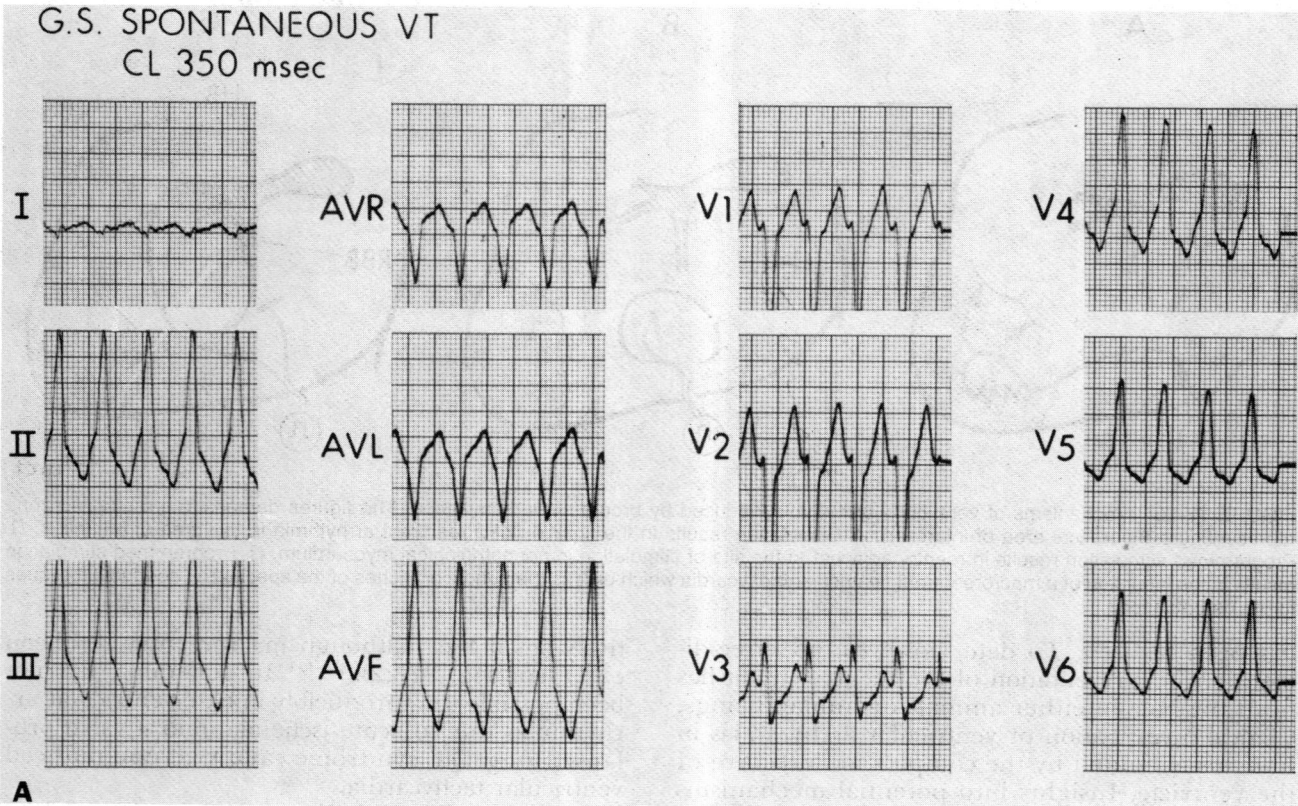

G.S. SPONTANEOUS VT
CL 350 msec

A

than dynamic and subject to varying autonomic influences, stretch, hypoxia, etc.[143–145] For example, Waxman[146,147] recently showed that, contrary to popular opinion, enhanced vagal tone is capable of terminating ventricular tachycardia in some cases, presumably due to reflex sympathetic withdrawal.

Ventricular Fibrillation

No single mechanism can be proposed to explain all types of spontaneous or induced ventricular fibrillation. As in the case of atrial fibrillation, however, the features of (1) critical mass of tissue, (2) critical interrelationship between conduction velocity and refractoriness required to initiate and maintain ventricular fibrillation, and (3) the ability to terminate the arrhythmia with a single shock all favor the role of multiple wavelets due to random reentry as the mechanism for sustaining this arrhythmia.[148]

Very few clinical investigations of ventricular fibrillation have been reported to date.[149,150] In general, there appears to be a correlation between the ease of induction of ventricular fibrillation in laboratory studies and its clinical occurrence. Of particular interest has been the ability to induce a sustained ventricular tachycardia which subsequently deteriorates into ventricular fibrillation during laboratory investigation of patients resuscitated from out-of-hospital ventricular fibrillation. This suggests that in some patients a prodromal period of ven-

tricular tachycardia may be the initiating cause of ventricular fibrillation.[150] Recent interest in coronary spasm has increased the appeal of the concept that transient spasm[136] resulting in reperfusion arrhythmias may be a cause of spontaneous ventricular fibrillation associated with ischemia in humans (Fig. 27-26).

Finally, the important role that the autonomic nervous sytem and neuropathology[145,151] play in the genesis of ventricular fibrillation in humans remains to be adequately defined.

Bradyarrhythmias

Sinus Node Dysfunction

Abnormalities of the sinus node may be caused by abnormal impulse formation within the sinus node itself or abnormal conduction of impulses propagating out of the sinus node. In many instances it is difficult to distinguish between abnormal automaticity and varying degrees of sinus node exit block. This is because our information concerning the sinus node is derived only indirectly from the surface electrocardiogram (see Chap. 28).

There are many similarities between the sinus node and the AV node: the sinus node lacks "fast" channels and thus sinus node cells have a low resting membrane potential and a contour suggestive of a

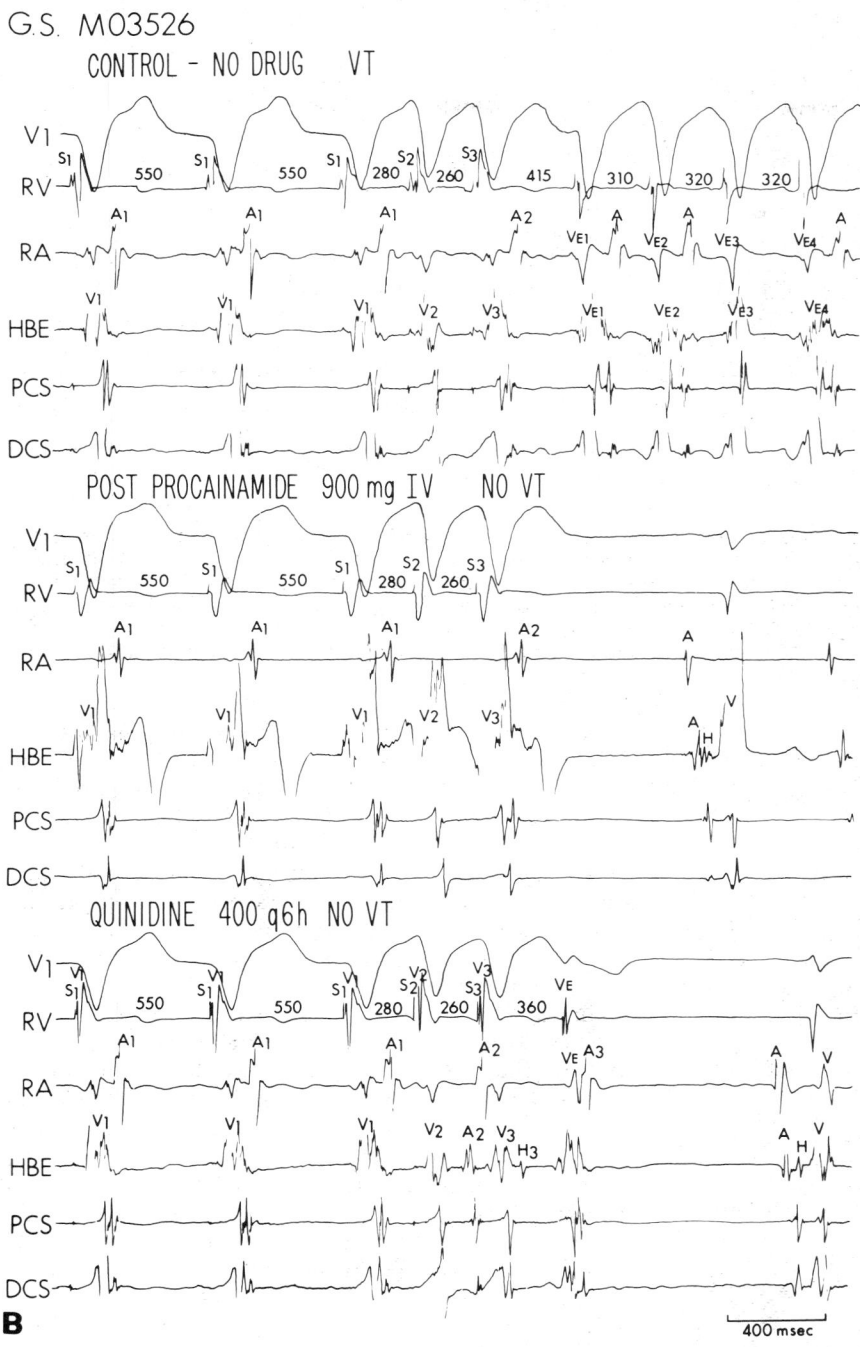

G.S. M03526

FIGURE 27-21 Induction of ventricular tachycardia in a patient with chronic recurrent ventricular tachycardia. *A* (opposite). 12-lead ECG obtained in a patient during a spontaneous episode of ventricular tachycardia at a rate of 171 per minute. *B.* Recordings during serial electrophysiologic studies. From top to bottom in each panel are surface ECG lead V_1, and intracardiac electrocardiograms from the right ventricular apex (RV), the high lateral right atrium (RA), the His bundle (HBE), and the proximal and distal coronary sinus (PCS and DCS). In each panel, the ventricles are being paced at a basic cycle length of 550 ms and two successive premature beats are introduced (S_2 and S_3). In the top panel recording in the absence of drug, ventricular tachycardia is induced. Using the same coupling intervals, the administration of procainamide (middle panel) and quinidine (bottom panel) abolishes the ability to induce ventricular tachycardia. (*From D. G. Benditt et al., Recurrent Ventricular Tachycardia in Man: Evaluation of Antiarrhythmic Drug Therapy by Programmed Intracardiac Stimulation, in E. Sandoe (ed.), "Management of Ventricular Tachycardia—Role of Mexiletine," Excerpta Medica, Amsterdam, 1978, p. 507. Reproduced with permission of author and publisher.*)

slow response. The sinus node is surrounded by perinodal fibers which have a normal resting membrane potential and upstroke velocity but which also have a refractory period that is greater than cells of the sinus node or atrium; we have previously seen that the safety margin with the slow response is low and that block may appear at boundaries of dissimilar refractoriness. It is therefore not surprising that disorders of impulse formation in the sinus node as well as disorders due to delay and block at the sinoatrial junction (exit block) are observed.[152–154]

Very few cases of sinus node dysfunction have been studied from a histological viewpoint; in most reported cases[96,155–157] alterations are generally found in the sinus node, the atrial wall, and the perinodal nervous structures, although the sinus node artery itself is rarely involved.

In a recent report dealing with sinus node dysfunction in adolescence,[157] fibrosis and fatty infiltration were noted in the atrial approaches to the sinus node and AV node as well as the preferential atrial pathways, but no involvement was present in the sinus node itself. Histopathologic findings indicate that the sclerodegenerative processes observed in patients with sinus node dysfunction are not generally limited to the sinus node and the atria but sometimes also involve the AV node and the His-Purkinje system. These observations correlate with

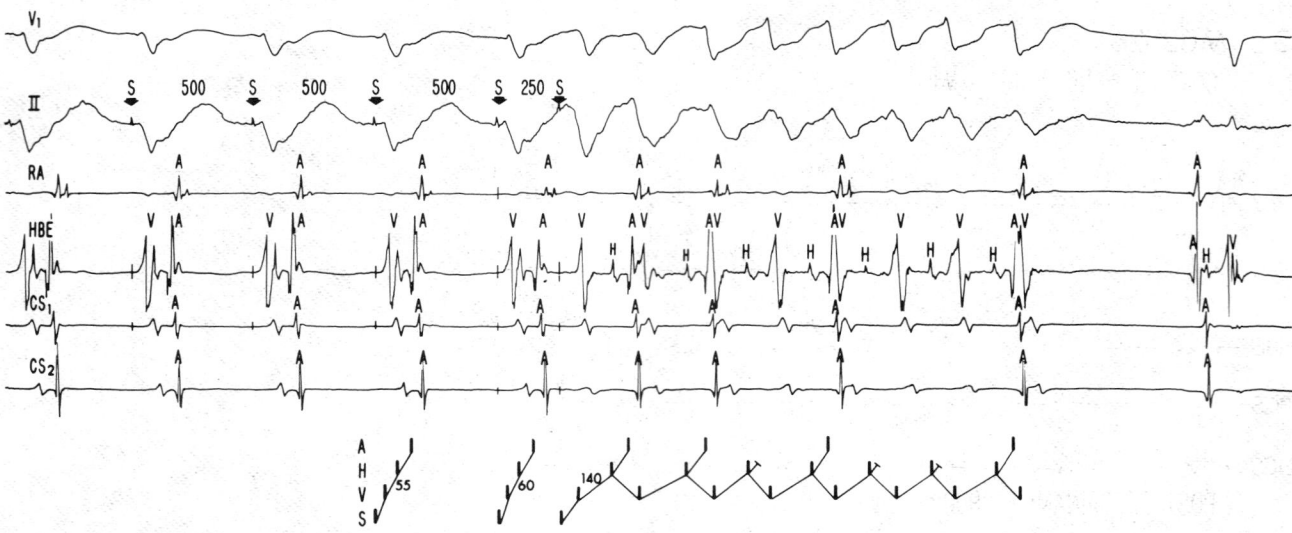

FIGURE 27-22 Induction of a macroreentrant ventricular tachycardia. This tracing was taken from the study of a patient with recurrent palpitations following a diaphragmatic myocardial infarction. The ventricles are being paced at a basic cycle length of 500 ms. During ventricular pacing, a retrograde His deflection is observed in the ventricular electrogram. The sequence of events is diagrammatically shown in a ladder diagram below the electrograms. Following a premature ventricular beat at a coupling interval of 250 ms, the interval between ventricular depolarization and the retrograde His bundle lengthens from 60 ms to 140 ms, initiating a rapid ventricular tachycardia with ventriculoatrial dissociation. Note that in this macroreentrant ventricular tachycardia, a His deflection precedes each QRS complex. This finding is typical of macroreentry in the ventricles.

the multiple functional abnormalities of the conduction system demonstrated in patients with sick sinus node.[158,159]

Atrioventricular Block (Including Bundle Branch Block)

A variety of factors may affect propagation of cardiac impulses, particularly in depressed tissues. Thus decremental conduction is likely to develop in the presence of a lower level of membrane potential

FIGURE 27-23 Angiogram of a patient with arrhythmogenic right ventricular dysplasia. A selected frame from a cineangiogram of the right ventricle is shown. An electrode catheter is present in the coronary sinus and an angiographic catheter has been positioned near the apex of the right ventricle. Note the abnormal appearance of the right ventricle with numerous thin-walled areas. These abnormal areas constitute the anatomic substrate of ventricular tachycardia in patients with this disorder. The disorder is notably marked at the apex, where stagnated for 10 cardiac cycles.

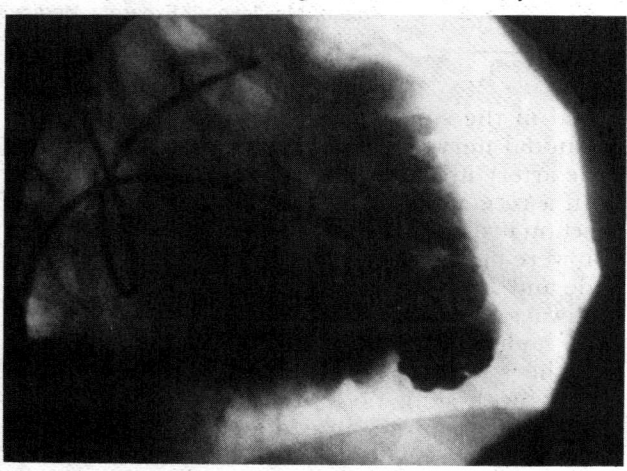

and a slower rate of rise of phase 0 depolarization. These conditions can be seen in any fibers showing either incomplete repolarization, significant diastolic depolarization, or partial depolarization caused by various pathophysiologic factors.[160,161] Since the fibers in the N region of the AV node show the above characteristics even under physiologic conditions, decremental conduction is more commonly seen in this tissue than in other portions of the AV conduction system. Many factors known to impair AV conduction, such as acetylcholine, cardiac glycosides, low potassium, or ischemia, enhance the degree of decrement and usually result in conduction delay and block in the AV node. Disorders of conduction in the His-Purkinje system on the other hand appear more "all or none" in keeping with the low safety factor observed in fibers from the His-Purkinje system during experimental study of the slow response in these tissues. It is entirely possible that the pathophysiologic mechanisms of conduction delay and block are the same in the AV node and His-Purkinje system and the observed functional differences in these two sites of conduction disorders relate more to other factors such as tissue architecture, nature of intercellular connections, nervous innervation, etc.

Most of our information concerning the functional behavior of conduction disorders in humans is derived from catheter-electrode recordings of the specialized conducting tissues performed during stimulation of the heart (see Chap. 89). Only a few studies have been published that attempt to correlate these electrophysiologic studies with pathologic findings.[162,163] In general, there is good correlation between electrophysiologic and pathologic findings in the setting of chronic atrioventricular and bundle

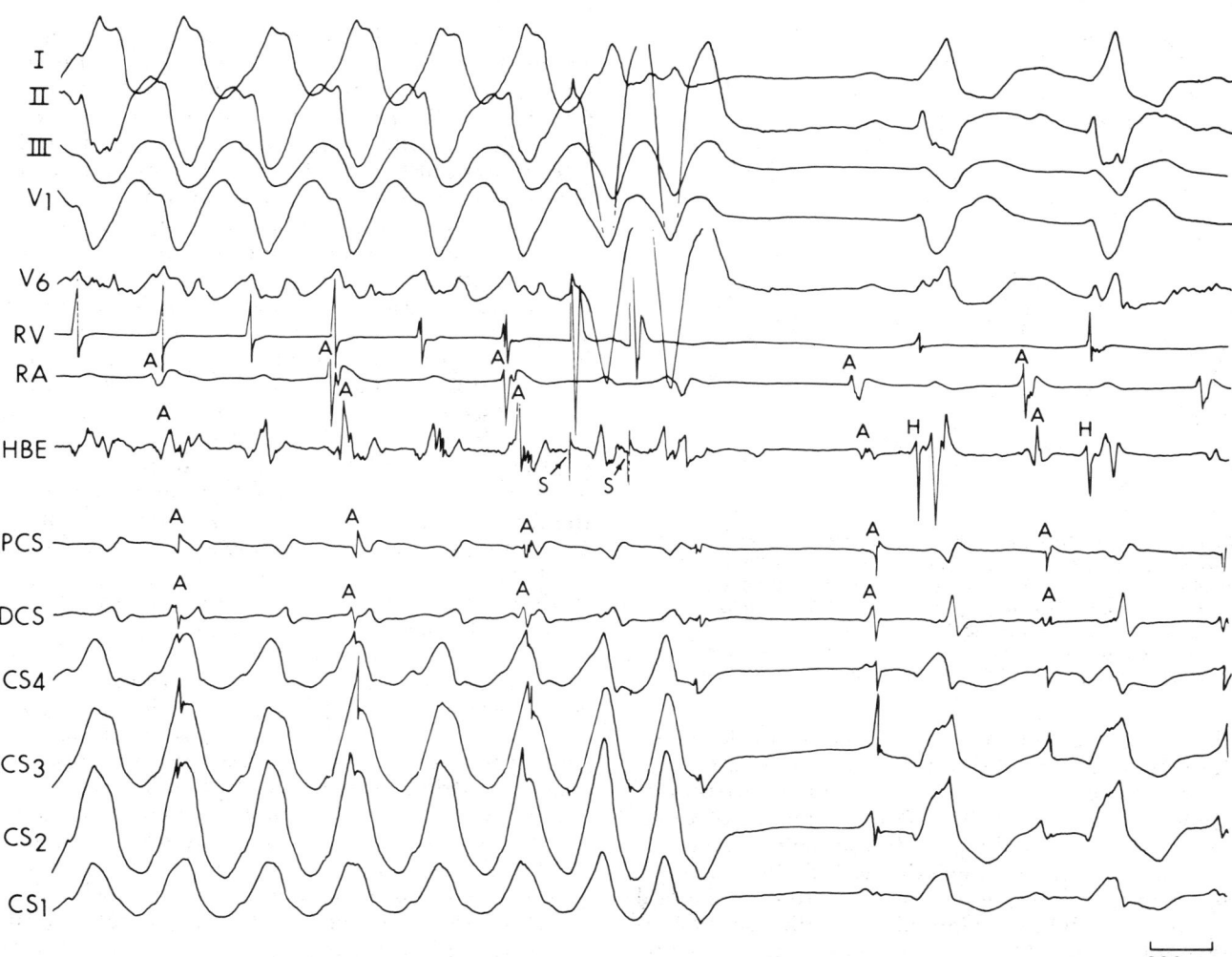

FIGURE 27-24 Ventricular tachycardia due to a nodoventricular fiber. The recordings from top down are standard ECG leads I, II, V$_1$, V$_6$, bipolar electrograms from the right ventricle (RV), the right atrium (RA), the region of the His bundle (HBE), the proximal coronary sinus (PCS) and distal (DCS) coronary sinus, and unipolar electrograms recorded from the same coronary sinus catheter going from proximal (CS$_4$) to distal (CS$_1$) coronary sinus. Initially a tachycardia with left bundle branch block morphology is present. Ventriculoatrial dissociation is apparent. No His deflections can be observed preceding the onset of the QRS complex. Following six beats of tachycardia, two successive premature depolarizations are introduced to the right ventricular apex during tachycardia, resulting in termination of tachycardia. Following the return to sinus rhythm, a normal PR interval is present associated with QRS complexes with left bundle branch block morphology. Note however that the His deflection occurs at the onset of the QRS complex. The latter combination of events was proved to be due to a nodoventricular fiber.

branch block. The extent of pathologic change is often more diffuse than might have been predicted on clinical grounds. It is impossible to predict function completely from structural changes since it is not known how much structure must be retained for proper function. This is especially true of structures with wide cross-sectional areas, such as approaches to the AV node.

The electrocardiogram has frequently been used to suggest the presence of block in localized areas of the specialized conducting tissues. It must be stressed however that the electrocardiogram merely represents the summation of electric forces derived from myocardium. Thus intramural delay distal to the Purkinje-myocardial junction can conceivably result in patterns of conduction delay and block normally attributable to lesions in the specialized con-

ducting tissues.[164] Furthermore, although the term *block* is liberally applied, the same pattern can result from simple delay in a localized segment of the conduction system. Thus a pattern of bundle branch block can result from a 40-ms delay in a bundle branch; similarly, a pattern of hemiblock can result from a delay of 20 ms in a fascicle. Finally it should be recalled that the appearance of bundle branch block can likewise result from preexcitation in the distribution of a contralateral bundle.

Electrode-catheter recordings have confirmed that complete atrioventricular block can result from interruption of conduction at the level of the AV node or the His bundle, or can be due to bilateral bundle branch block (see Chap. 89). The most common cause of chronic complete heart block appears to be bilateral bundle branch block. Pathologically,

DISORDERS OF THE CARDIOVASCULAR SYSTEM

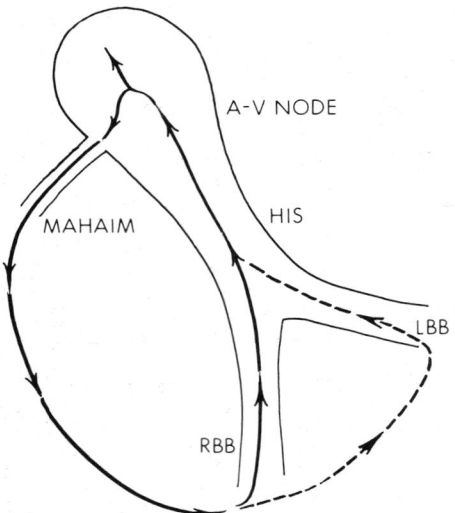

FIGURE 27-25 Schematic diagram of reentry utilizing a nodo-ventricular fiber. The proposed mechanism of arrhythmia demonstrated in Fig. 27-24 is illustrated. Conduction proceeds antegradely over a nodoventricular fiber from the AV node to the right ventricle and returns retrogradely up the right bundle (or left bundle branch) retrogradely over the His bundle. The reentrant loop is completed by a portion of the circuit located in the AV node.

the most frequent cause of this entity is idiopathic fibrosis of the His-Purkinje system (Lenègre's disease),[165] the etiology of which remains disputed; some cases appear to be the consequence of exaggerated aging resulting in fibrocalcific changes in the cardiac skeleton (Lev's disease). Pathologic studies of chronic complete heart block due to bilateral bundle branch block generally show diffuse changes throughout the His-Purkinje system, undoubtedly accounting for the slow, capricious behavior of subsidiary pacemaker function in these cases.[166]

Disturbances of conduction accompanying ischemic heart disease can best be understood by referring to the vascular supply of the conduction system (Fig. 27-27). In 90 percent of cases the AV node is supplied by the posterior descending coronary artery, accounting for the frequent association of conduction disturbance in the AV node with diaphragmatic myocardial infarction. The His bundle derives its blood supply from two sources: the AV nodal artery and the first septal perforator of the left anterior descending branch of the left coronary artery. In 50 percent of cases, the right bundle branch has a twofold blood supply: the AV nodal artery and the first septal perforator of the left anterior descending artery, in the other 50 percent, it derives its blood supply only from the first septal perforator of the left anterior descending artery. The anterior fascicle of the left bundle branch has the same blood supply as the right bundle branch, accounting for the frequent association of right bundle branch block with left anterior fascicular block during acute myocardial infarction. Finally, the left posterior fascicle derives its blood supply from the AV nodal artery in 50 percent of cases, while in the remaining cases it has a dual blood supply: the first septal perforator of the left anterior descending artery and the AV nodal artery.[167] From the vascular distribution to the conduction system, it is apparent that conduction disturbances in the AV node and, rarely, in the His bundle might be expected following diaphragmatic myocardial infarction; right bundle branch block and left anterior fascicular block, possibly progressing to complete heart block, might be expected in the setting of anteroseptal myocardial infarction (Fig. 27-28). Functional block may also result from local hyperkalemia secondary to potassium efflux from the infarcted myocardium.

FIGURE 27-26 Ventricular fibrillation due to reperfusion. This tracing demonstrates femoral artery pressure and standard electrographic monitoring lead in a dog in whom the left anterior descending coronary artery was temporarily ligated. At the beginning of the tracing, the coronary was released, resulting within seconds in the onset of ventricular fibrillation and loss of blood pressure.

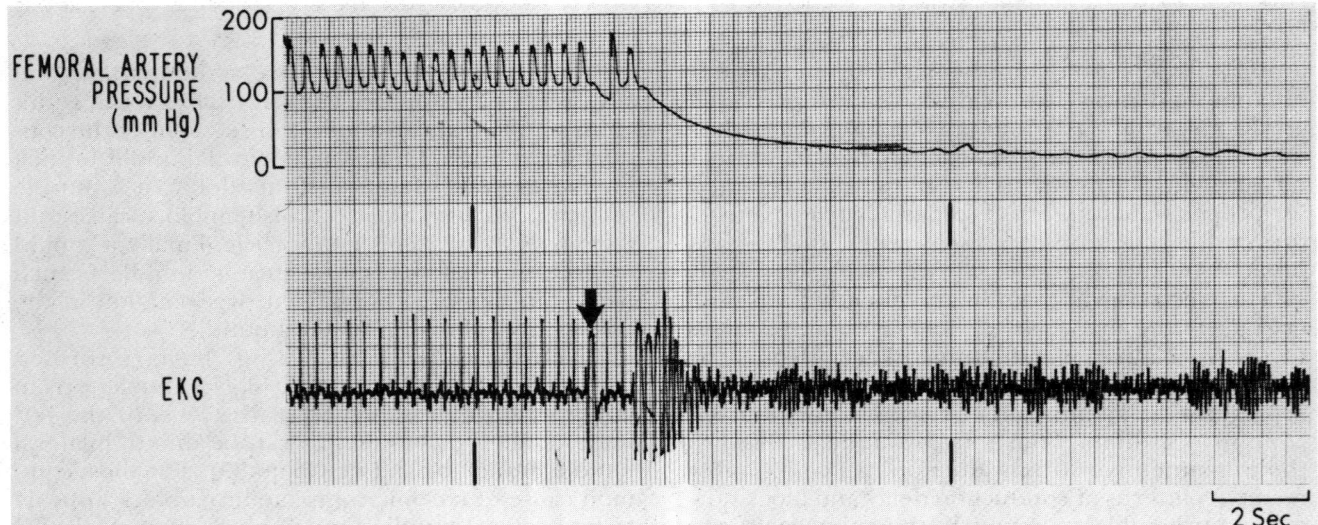

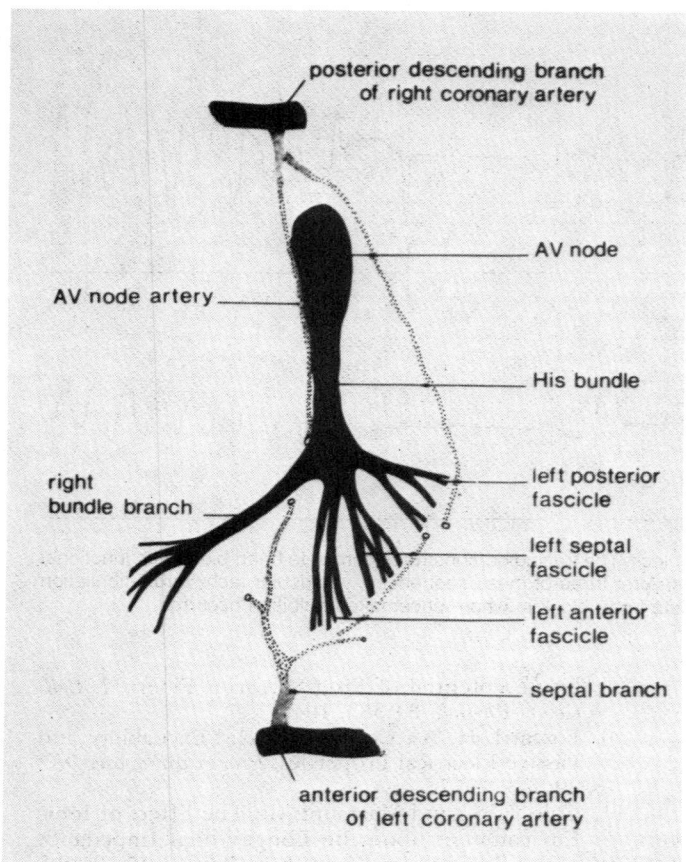

FIGURE 27-27 Schematic representation of blood supply in the AV node, His bundle, and bundle branches. See text for discussion. (*From Roos et al.*[167] *Reproduced with permission of author and publisher.*)

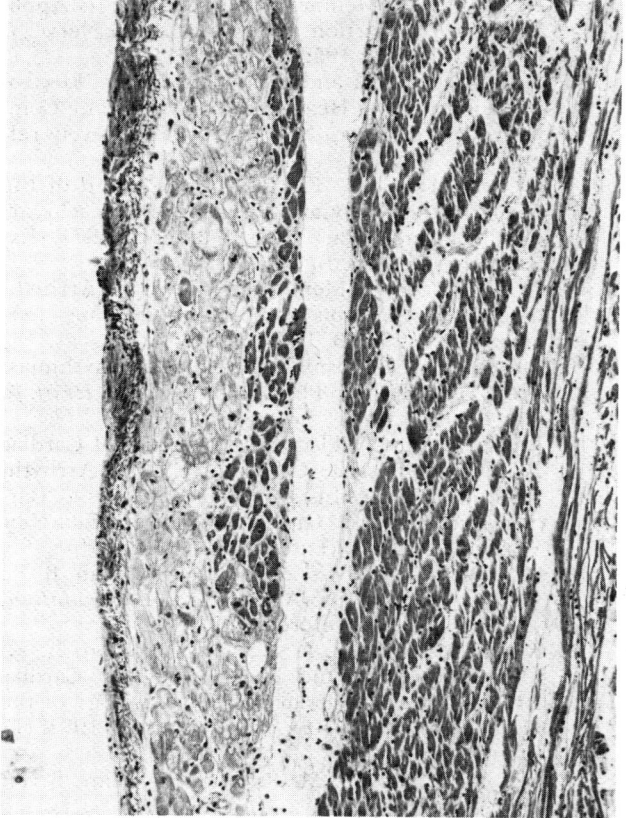

FIGURE 27-28 Necrosis of the left bundle branch in a patient dying 5 days after the onset of an acute anteroseptal myocardial infarction. The dark fibers to the right of the figure represent the necrotic muscle of the interventricular septum. The light-staining fibers on the left side of the figure are conducting fibers of the left bundle. Note that the inner fibers of the left bundle adjacent to the necrotic muscle of the interventricular septum are also necrotic. [*From D. B. Hackel, Anatomy and Pathology of the Cardiac Conducting System, in J. E. Edwards, M. Lev, and M. R. Abell (eds.), "The Heart," The Williams & Wilkins Company, Baltimore, 1974, p. 245, and the United States-Canadian Division of the International Academy of Pathology. Reproduced with permission of author and publisher.*]

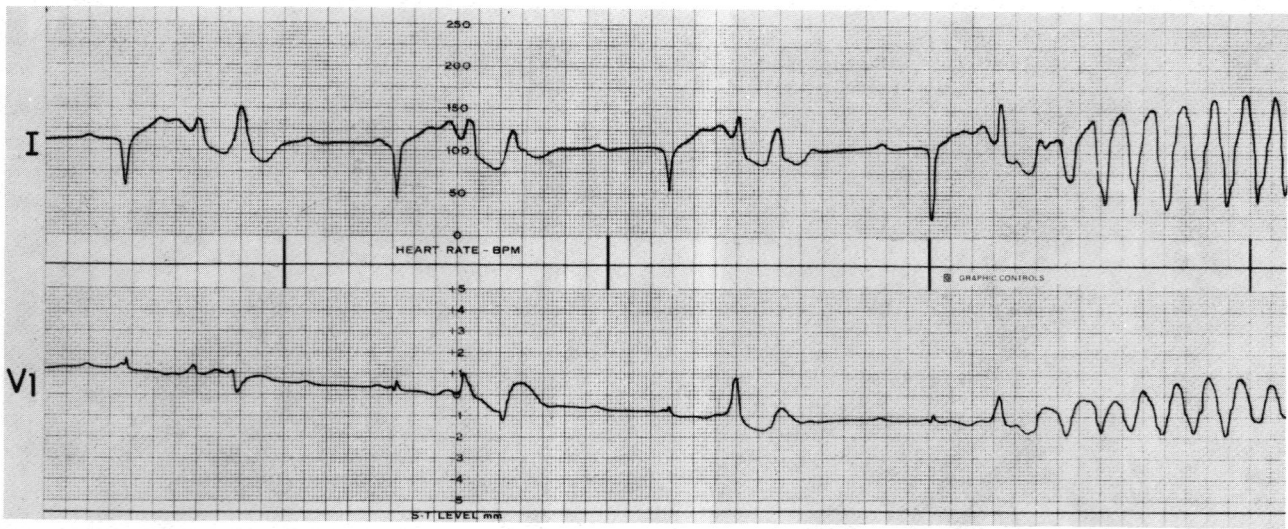

FIGURE 27-29   Ventricular fibrillation precipitated by complete heart block. The tracing demonstrates complete heart block with junctional escape beats followed initially by pairs of ventricular premature beats. After three of these sequences, ventricular tachycardia-fibrillation occurs. This sequence was observed in a patient with chronic complete heart block in whom pacemaker inhibition occurred.

Although one might logically expect that the cause of fatality in cases of complete heart block might be the appearance of asystole, it is well known that ventricular tachycardia and fibrillation constitute the fatal arrhythmia in approximately 50 percent of cases, emphasizing the importance of non-homogeneous depolarization and repolarization that occurs at slow heart rates (Fig. 27-29).

References

1. Mines, G. R.: On Dynamic Equilibrium in the Heart, *J. Physiol.*, 46:349, 1913.
2. Mines, G. R.: On Circulating Excitations in Heart Muscles and Their Possible Relation to Tachycardia and Fibrillation, *Trans. R. Soc. Can.*, IV:43, 1914.
3. Lewis, T.: "The Mechanism and Graphic Registration of the Heart Beat," Shaw and Sons, London, 1925.
4. Mayer, A. G.: Rhythmical Pulsation in Scyphomedusae, Publication No. 47, The Carnegie Institution of Washington, 1906.
5. Mayer, A. G.: Rhythmical Pulsation in Scyphomedusae. II. Papers from the Marine Biological Laboratory at Tortugas, Washington, 1908, p. 115.
6. Erlanger, J.: Further Studies on the Physiology of Heart Block: The Effect of Extrasystoles upon the Dog's Heart and upon Strips of Terrapin's Ventricle in the Various Stages of Block, *Am. J. Physiol.*, 16:160, 1906.
7. Schmitt, F. O., and Erlanger, J.: Directional Differences in the Conduction of the Impulse through Heart Muscle and Their Possible Relation to Extrasystolic and Fibrillary Contractions, *Am. J. Physiol.*, 87:326, 1928–29.
8. Garrey, W. E.: The Nature of Fibrillary Contraction of the Heart: Its Relation to Tissue Mass and Form, *Am. J. Physiol.*, 33:397, 1914.
9. Ling, G., and Gerard, R. W..: The Normal Membrane Potential of Frog Sartorius Fibers, *J. Cell. Comp. Physiol.*, 34:383, 1949.
10. Fozzard, H. A.: Cardiac Muscle: Excitability and Passive Electrical Properties, *Prog. Cardiovasc. Dis.*, 29:343, 1977.
11. Cole, K. S., and Marmont, G.: The Effect of Ionic Environment upon the Longitudinal Impedance of the Squid Giant Axon, *Fed.. Proc.*, 1:15, 1942.
12. Hodgkin, A. L., and Huxley, A. F.: A Quantitative Description of Membrane Current and Its Application to Conduction and Excitation in Nerve, *J. Physiol.*, 117:500, 1952.
*13. Hoffmann, B. F., and Cranefield, P. F.: "Electrophysiology of the Heart," Futura Publishing Company, Mount Kisco, N.Y., 1976. (Extensively referenced)
*14. Wellens, H. J. J.: "Electrical Stimulation of the Heart in the Study and Treatment of Tachycardias," University Park Press, Baltimore, 1971. (Extensively referenced)
15. Arnsdorf, M. F.: Membrane Factors in Arrhythmogenesis: Concepts and Definitions, *Prog. Cardiovasc. Dis.*, 29:413, 1977.
16. Pick, A.: Mechanisms of Cardiac Arrhythmias: From Hypothesis to Physiologic Fact, *Am. Heart. J.*, 86:249, 1973.
*17. Bigger, J. T., Jr.: Electrical Properties of Cardiac Muscle and Possible Causes of Cardiac Arrhythmias, in L. S. Dreifus and W. Lidoff (eds.), "Cardiac Arrhythmias," Grune & Stratton, Inc., New York, 1973. p. 13. (Extensively referenced)
*18. Cranefield, P. F., Wit, A. L., and Hoffman, B. F.: Genesis of Cardiac Arrhythmias, *Circulation*, 47:190, 1973. (48 references)
*19. Rosen, M. R., Wit, A. L., and Hoffman, B. F.: Electrophysiology and Pharmacology of Cardiac Arrhythmias. I. Cellular Electrophysiology of the Mammalian Heart, *Am. Heart J.*, 88:380, 1974. (17 references)
*20. Wit, A. L., Rosen, M. R., and Hoffman, B. F.:

*This article is a review of the literature and contains additional references to the literature.

Electrophysiology and Pharmacology of Cardiac Arrhythmias. II. Relationship of Normal and Abnormal Electrical Activity of Cardiac Fibers to the Genesis of Arrhythmias. A. Automaticity, *Am. Heart J.*, 88:515, 1974. (38 references)

*21. Wit, A. L., Rosen, M. R., and Hoffman, B. F.: Electrophysiology and Pharmacology of Cardiac Arrhythmias. II. Relationship of Normal and Abnormal Electrical Activity of Cardiac Fibers to the Genesis of Arrhythmias. B. Reentry, *Am. Heart J.*, 88:798, 1974. (38 references)

*22. Cranefield, P. F.: "The Conduction of the Cardiac Impulse," Futura Publishing Company, Mount Kisco, New York, 1975, p. 199. (Extensively referenced)

23. Hoffman, B. F., Rosen, M. R., and Wit, A. L.: Electrophysiology and Pharmacology of Cardiac Arrhythmias. III. Causes and Treatment of Cardiac Arrhythmias. Part A, *Am. Heart J.*, 89:115, 1975.

24. Katz, A. M.: "Physiology of the Heart," Raven Press, New York, 1977.

25. Vassalle, M.: Cardiac Automaticity and Its Control, *Am. J. Physiol.*, 223:H625, 1977.

26. Cranefield, P. F., and Aronson, R. S.: Initiation of Sustained Rhythmic Activity by Single Propagated Action Potentials in Canine Purkinje Fibers Exposed to Sodium Free Solution or to Ouabain, *Circ. Res.*, 34:477, 1974.

27. Cranefield, P. F.: Does Spontaneous Activity Arise from Phase 4 Depolarization or from Triggering?, in F. Bonke (ed.), "The Sinus Node: Structure, Function and Clinical Relevance," Martinus Nijhoff, The Hague, 1978, p. 348.

28. Cranefield, P. F.: Action Potentials, After-Potentials and Arrhythmias, *Circ. Res.*, 41:415,, 1977.

*29. Wit, A. L., Boyden, P. A., Gadsby, D. C., and Cranefield, P. F.: Triggered Activity as a Cause of Atrial Arrhythmias, in O. S. Narula (ed.), "Cardiac Arrhythmias. Electrophysiology, Diagnosis and Management," The Williams & Wilkins Company, Baltimore, 1979, p. 14. (Extensively referenced)

30. Wit, A. L., and Cranefield, P. F.: Triggered Activity in Cardiac Muscle Fibers of the Simian Mitral Valve, *Circ. Res.*, 38:85, 1976.

31. Wit, A. L., and Cranefield, P. F., Triggered and Automatic Activity in the Canine Coronary Sinus, *Circ. Res.*, 38:85, 1976.

32. Fenoglio, J. J., Reemtsma, K., Hordof, A. J., and Wit, A. L.: The Human Anterior Mitral Valve Leaflet as a Possible Site of Origin of Atrial Arrhythmias, *Am. J. Cardiol.*, 4:386, 1978.

33. Hauswirth, O., Noble, D., and Tsien, R. W.: The Mechanism of Oscillatory Activity at Low Membrane Potentials in Cardiac Purkinje Fibers, *J. Physiol.*, 200:255, 1969.

*34. Ferrier, G. R.: Digitalis Arrhythmias: Role of Oscillatory Potentials, *Prog. Cardiovasc. Dis.*, 29:459, 1977. (72 references)

35. Ferrier, G. R., and Moe, G. K.: Effect of Calcium on Acetyl-strophanthidin-Induced Transient Depolarization in Canine Purkinje Tissue, *Circ. Res.*, 33:508, 1973.

36. Zipes, D. P., Foster, P. R., Troup, J., and Pedersen, D. H.: Atrial Induction of Ventricular Tachycardia: Reentry versus Triggered Automaticity, *Am. J. Cardiol.*, 44:1, 1979.

37. Rosen, M. R., Fisch, C., Hoffman, B., Danilo, P.,

Lovelace, E., and Knoebel, S. B.: Can Accelerated Atrioventricular Junctional Escape Rhythms Be Explained by Delayed After Depolarizations?, *Am. J. Cardiol.*, 45:1272, 1980.

38. Loeb, J. M., Murdock, D. K., Randall, W. C., and Euler, D. E.: Supraventricular Pacemaker Underdrive in the Absence of Sinus Nodal Influences in the Conscious Dog, *Circ. Res.*, 44:329, 1979.

39. Ten Eick, R. E., and Singer, D. H.: Electrophysiological Properties of Diseased Human Atrium. I. Low Diastolic Potential and Altered Cellular Response to Potassium, *Circ. Res.*, 44:545, 1979.

*40. Hordof, A. J., Edie, E. R., Malm, J. R., Hoffman, B. F., and Rosen, M. R.: Electrophysiologic Properties and Response to Pharmacologic Agents of Fibers from Diseased Human Atria, *Circulation*, 54:774, 1976. (16 references)

41. Friedman, P. L., Stewart, J. R., Fenoglio, J. J., Jr., and Wit, A. L.: Survival of Subendocardial Purkinje Fibers after Extensive Myocardial Infarction in Dogs, *Circ. Res.*, 33:597, 1973.

42. Lazzara, R., El-Sherif, N., and Scherlag, B. J.: Electrophysiological Properties of Canine Purkinje Cells in One Day Old Myocardial Infarction, *Circ. Res.*, 33:722, 1973.

43. Singer, D. H., Ten Eick, R. E., and DeBoer, A. A.: Electrophysiologic Correlates of Human Atrial Tachyarrhythmias, in L. S. Dreifus and W. Lidoff (eds.), "Cardiac Arrhythmias," Grune & Stratton, Inc., New York, 1973, p. 97.

44. Roberts, D. E., Hersh, L. T., and Scher, A. M.: Influence of Cardiac Fiber Orientation Velocity and Tissue Restivity in the Dog, *Circ. Res.*, 44:701, 1979.

45. Cranefield, P. F., Klein, H. O., and Hoffman, B. F.: Conduction of the Cardiac Impulse. I. Delay, Block, and One-Way Block in Depressed Purkinje Fibers, *Circ. Res.*, 28:199, 1971.

46. Cranefield, P. F., and Hoffman, B. F.: Conduction of the Cardiac Impulse. II. Summation and Inhibition, *Circ. Res.*, 28:220, 1971.

47. Wit, A. L., Cranefield, P. F., and Hoffman, B. F.: Slow Conduction and Reentry in the Ventricular Conducting System. II. Single and Sustained Circus Movement in Networks of Canine and Bovine Purkinje Fibers, *Circ. Res.*, 30:11, 1972.

48. De la Fuente, D., Sasyniuk, B., and Moe, G. K.: Conduction through a Narrow Isthmus in Isolated Canine Atrial Tissue: A Model of the WPW Syndrome, *Circulation*, 44:803, 1971.

*49. Downar, E., and Waxman, M. B..: Depressed Conduction and Unidirectional Block in Purkinje Fibers, in H. J. J. Wellens, K. I. Lie, and M. J. Janse (eds.), "The Conduction System of the Heart," Lea & Febiger, Philadelphia, 1976, p. 393. (Extensively referenced)

50. Allessie, M. A., Bonke, F. M., and Schopman, F. J. G.: Circus Movement in Rabbit Atrial Muscle as a Mechanism of Tachycardia. III. The "Leading Circle" Concept, *Circ. Res.*, 41:9, 1977.

51. Antzelevitch, C., Jalife, J., and Moe, G. K.: Characteristics of Reflection as a Mechanism of Reentrant Arrhythmias and Its Relationship to Parasystole, *Circulation*, 61:182, 1980.

52. Langendorf, R.: Concealed AV Conduction: The Effect of Blocked Impulses on the Formation and Conduction of Subsequent Impulses, *Am. Heart J.*, 35:542, 1948.

53. Watanabe, Y.: Terminology and Electrophysiologic Concepts in Cardiac Arrhythmias. II. Concealed Conduction, *PACE*, 1:345, 1978.

54. Moore, E. N., Knoebel, S. B., and Spear, J. F.: Concealed Conduction, *Am. J. Cardiol.*, 28:406, 1971.

*55. Rosenbaum, M. B., Lazzari, J. O., and Elinzari, M. V.: The Role of Phase 3 and Phase 4 Block in Clinical Electrocardiography, in H. J. J. Wellens, K. I. Lie, and M. J. Janse (eds.), "The Conduction System of the Heart," Lea & Febiger, Philadelphia, 1976. p. 126. (Extensively referenced)

56. Watanabe, Y., and Nishimura, M.: Terminology and Electrophysiologic Concepts in Cardiac Arrhythmias. VI. Phase 3 Block and Phase 4 Block. Part II, *PACE*, 2:624, 1979.

57. Watanabe, Y., and Nishimura, M.: Terminology and Electrophysiologic Concepts in Cardiac Arrhythmias. V. Phase 3 Block and Phase 4 Block. Part I, *PACE*, 2:335, 1979.

58. Moe, G. K., Jalife, J., Mueller, W. J., and Moe, B.: A Mathematical Model of Parasystole and Its Application to Clinical Arrhythmias, *Circulation*, 56:968, 1977.

59. Pick, A.: The Electrophysiologic Basis of Parasystole and Its Variants, in H. J. J. Wellens, K. I. Lie, and M. J. Janse (eds.), "The Conduction System of the Heart," Lea & Febiger, Philadelphia, 1976, p. 143.

60. Myerburg, R. J., Stewart, J. W., and Hoffman, B. F.: Electrophysiological Properties of the Canine Peripheral AV Conducting System, *Circ. Res.*, 26:361, 1970.

61. Janse, M. J., Cinca, J., Morena, H., Fiolet, J. W. T., Kléber, A. G., de Vries, G. P., Becker, A. E., and Durrer, D.: The "Border Zone" in Myocardial Ischemia: An Electrophysiological, Metabolic and Histochemical Correlation in the Pig Heart, *Circ. Res.*, 44:576, 1979.

62. Smith, W. M., and Gallagher, J. J.: Les Torsades de Points, *Ann. Intern. Med.*, 93:578, 1980.

*63. Wellens, H. J. J.: Value and Limitations of Programmed Electrical Stimulation of the Heart in the Study and Treatment of Tachycardias, *Circulation*, 57:845, 1978. (95 references)

64. Allessie, M. A., and Bonke, F. I. M.: Direct Demonstration of Sinus Node Reentry in the Rabbit Heart, *Circ. Res.*, 44:557, 1979.

*65. Wu, D., Amat-y-Leon, F., Denes, P., Dhingra, R., Pietras, R. J., and Rosen, K. M.: Demonstration of Sustained Sinus and Atrial Re-entry as a Mechanism of Paroxysmal Supraventricular Tachycardia, *Circulation*, 51:234, 1975. (36 references)

66. Damato, A. N.: Clinical Evidence of Sinus Node Reentry, in F. I. M. Bonke (ed.), "The Sinus Node," Martinus Nijhoff, The Hague, 1978, p. 379.

*67. Wellens, H. J. J.: Role of Sinus Node Reentry in the Genesis of Sustained Cardiac Arrhythmias, in F. I. M. Bonke (ed.), "The Sinus Node," Martinus-Nijhoff, The Hague, 1978, p. 422. (Extensively referenced)

68. Hariman, R. J., Krongrad, E., Boxer, R. A., Weiss, M. B., Steeg, C. N., and Hoffman, B. F.: Method for Recording Electrical Activity of the Sinoatrial Node and Automatic Atrial Foci during Cardiac Catheterization in Human Subjects, *Am. J. Cardiol.*, 45:775, 1980.

69. Cramer, M., Hariman, R. J., Boxer, R., and Hoffman, B. F.: Electrograms from the Canine Sinoatrial Pacemaker Recorded in Vitro and in Situ, *Am. J. Cardiol.*, 42:939, 1978.

70. Goldreyer, B. N., Gallagher, J. J., and Damato, A. N.: The Electrophysiological Demonstration of Atrial Ectopic Tachycardia in Man, *Am. Heart J.*, 88:202, 1973.

71. Coumel, P., Flammang, D., and Attuel, P.: Intra-atrial Reentry Tachycardia, in P. Puech and R. Slama (eds.), "The Cardiac Arrhythmias," The Arrhythmia Working Group of the French Cardiac Society, Roussel UCLAF, Paris, 1979, p. 108.

72. Allessie, M. A., Bonke, F. I. M., and Schopman, F. J. G.: Circus Movement in Rabbit Atrial Muscle as a Mechanism of Tachycardia. III. The "Leading Circle" Concept: A New Model of Circus Movement in Cardiac Tissue without the Involvement of an Anatomical Obstacle, *Circ. Res.*, 41:9, 1977.

*73. Moe, G. K., Pastelin, G., and Mendez, R.: Circus Movement Excitation of the Atria, in R. C. Little (ed.), "Physiology of Atrial Pacemakers and Conductive Tissues," Futura Publishing Company, Mount Kisco, New York, 1980, p. 207. (Extensively referenced)

74. Rytand, D. A.: Circus Movement (Entrapped Circuit Wave) Hypothesis and Atrial Flutter, *Ann. Intern. Med.*, 65:125, 1966.

75. Lewis, T., Feil, H. S., and Stroud, W. D.: Observations on Flutter and Fibrillation. Part II: The Nature of Auricular Flutter, *Heart*, 7:191, 1920.

76. Rosenblueth, A., and Garcia-Ramos, J.: Studies on Flutter and Fibrillation, *Am. Heart J.*, 33:677, 1947.

77. Pastelin, G., Mendez, G. R., and Moe, G. K.: Participation of Atrial Specialized Conduction Pathways in Atrial Flutter, *Circ. Res.*, 42:386, 1978.

78. Boineau, J. P., Schuessler, R. B., Mooney, C. R., Miller, C. B., Wylds, A. C., Hudson, R. D., Borremans, J. M., and Brockus, C. W.: Natural and Evoked Atrial Flutter Due to Circus Movement in Dogs: Role of Abnormal Atrial Pathways, Slow Conduction, Nonuniform Refractory Period Distribution and Premature Beats, *Am. J. Cardiol.*, 45:1167, 1980.

79. Moe, G. K., Rheinboldt, W. C., and Abildskov, J. A.: A Computer Model of Atrial Fibrillation, *Am. Heart J.*, 67:200, 1964.

80. Allessie, M. A.: Mechanism of Atrial Flutter in the Isolated Canine Heart, in "European Congress of Cardiology 1980 (Abstracts)," S. Karger A. G., Basel, 1980, p. 255.

81. Hogan, P. M., and Davis, L. D.: Evidence for Specialized Fibers in the Canine Right Atrium, *Circ. Res.*, 23:387, 1968.

82. Scherf, D.: Studies on Auricular Tachycardia Caused by Aconitine Administration, *Proc. Soc. Exp. Biol. Med.*, 64:233, 1967.

83. Puech, P.., Latour, H., and Grolleau, R..: Le Flutter et ses limites, *Arch. Mal. Coeur*, 63:116, 1970.

84. Josephson, M. E., and Seides, S. F.: "Clinical Cardiac Electrophysiology: Techniques and Interpretations," Lea & Febiger, Philadelphia, 1979, p. 191.

85. Wellens, H. J. J., Janse, M. J., van Dam, R. T., and Durrer, D.: Epicardial Excitation of the Atria in a Patient with Atrial Flutter, *Br. Heart J.*, 33:233, 1971.

86. Watson, R. M., and Josephson, M. E.: Atrial Flutter. 1. Electrophysiological Substrates and Modes

of Initiation and Termination, *Am. J. Cardiol.*, 45:732, 1980.

*87. Wells, J. L., MacLean, W. A. H., James, T. N., and Waldo, A.: Characterization of Atrial Flutter: Studies in Man after Open Heart Surgery Using Fixed Atrial Electrodes, *Circulation*, 60:665, 1979. (19 references)

*88. Waldo, A. L., MacLean, W. A. H., Karp, R. B., Kouchoukos, N. T., and James, T. N.: Entrainment and Interruption of Atrial Flutter with Atrial Pacing: Studies in Man Following Open Heart Surgery, *Circulation*, 56:737, 1977. (32 references)

*89. Waldo, A. L., Wells, J. L., Plumb, J. V., Cooper, T. B., and MacLean, W. A. H.: Characterization of Atrial Flutter: Studies in Patients Following Open Heart Surgery, in O. S. Narula (ed.), "Cardiac Arrhythmias, Electrophysiology, Diagnosis and Management," The Williams & Wilkins Company, Baltimore, 1979, p. 257. (Extensively referenced)

90. Abildskov, J. A., Miller, K., and Burgess, M. J.: Atrial Fibrillation, *Am. J. Cardiol.*, 28:263, 1971.

91. Moe, G. K., and Abildskov, J. A.: Atrial Fibrillation as a Self-sustaining Arrhythmia Independent of Focal Discharge, *Am. Heart J.*, 58:59, 1959.

92. Rothberger, C. J., and Winterberg, H.: Uber Vorhofflimmern und Verhofflatten, *Pfügers Arch.*, 160:42, 1914.

93. Allessi, R., Nusynowitz, M., Abildskov, J. A., and Moe, G. K.: Nonuniform Distribution of Vagal Effects on the Atrial Refractory Period, *Am. J. Physiol.*, 194:406, 1958.

94. Moe, G. K.: On the Multiple Wavelet Hypothesis of Atrial Fibrillation, *Arch. Int. Pharmacodyn.*, 140:183, 1962.

95. Nadeau, R. A., Roberge, F. A., and Billette, J.: Role of Sinus Node in the Mechanism of Cholinergic Atrial Fibrillation, *Circ. Res.*, 27:129, 1970.

96. James, T. N.: Interpretation of Pathologic Anatomy Associated with Arrhythmias and Conduction Disturbances, in J. W. Hurst, R. B. Logue, R. C. Schlant, and N. K. Wenger (eds.), "The Heart," 4th ed., McGraw-Hill Book Company, New York, 1978, p. 607.

*97. Gallagher, J. J., Pritchett, E. L. C., Sealy, W. C., Kasell, J., and Wallace, A. G.: The Preexcitation Syndromes, *Prog. Cardiovasc. Dis.*, 20:285, 1978. (166 references)

98. Anderson, R. H., Becker, A. E., Brechenmacher, C., Davies, M. J., and Rossi, L.: Ventricular Preexcitation Nomenclature for Its Substrates, *Eur. J. Cardiol.*, 3:27, 1975.

*99. Klein, G. J., Bashore, T. M., Seller, T. D., Pritchett, E. L. C., and Gallagher, J. J.: Ventricular Fibrillation in the Wolff-Parkinson-White Syndrome, *N. Engl. J. Med.*, 301:1080, 1979. (29 references)

*100. Benditt, D. G., Pritchett, E. L. C., Smith, W. M., Wallace, A. G., and Gallagher, J. J.: Characteristics of Atrioventricular Conduction and the Spectrum of Arrhythmias in Lown-Ganong-Levine Syndrome, *Circulation*, 57:454, 1978. (43 references)

101. Gallagher, J. J., Smith, W. M., Kasell, J. H., Benson, D. W., Sterba, R., and Grant, A. O.: Role of Mahaim Fibers in Cardiac Arrhythmias in Man, *Circulation*, July 1981.

102. Motte, G., Brechenmacher, C., Davy, J. M., and Belhassen, B.: Association de fibres nodoventriculaires et atrio-ventriculaires à l'origine de tach-

ycardies réciproques: Confrontation électrophysiologique et anatomo-pathologique, *Arch. Mal. Coeur*, 73:737, 1980.

103. Bharati, S., Bauernfiend, R., Scheinman, M., Massie, B., Cheitlin, M., Denes, P., Wu, D., Lev, M., Rosen, K. M.: Congenital Abnormalities in the Conduction System of Two Patients with Tachyarrhythmias, *Circulation*, 59:593, 1979.

104. Moe, G. K., Preston, J. B., Burlington, H.: Physiologic Evidence for a Dual A-V Transmission System, *Circ. Res.*, 4:357, 1956.

105. Moe, G. K., and Mendez, C.: The Physiological Basis of Reciprocal Rhythm, *Prog. Cardiovasc. Dis.*, 8:461, 1966.

106. Janse, M. J., van Capelle, F. J. L., Freud, G. E., and Durrer, D.: Circus Movement within the AV Node as a Basis for Supraventricular Tachycardia as Shown by Multiple Microelectrode Recordings in the Isolated Rabbit Heart, *Circ. Res.*, 28:403, 1971.

107. Wit, A. L., Goldreyer, B. N., and Damato, A. N.: An in Vitro Model of Paroxysmal Supraventricular Tachycardia, *Circulation*, 43:862, 1971.

108. Akhtar, M.: Paroxysmal Atrioventricular Nodal Reentrant Tachycardia, in O. S. Narula (ed.), "Cardiac Arrhythmias," The Williams & Wilkins Company, Baltimore, 1979, p. 294.

109. Denes, P., Dhingra, R. C., Chuquima, R., and Rosen, K. M.: Demonstration of Dual A-V Nodal Pathways in Patients with Paroxysmal Supraventricular Tachycardia, *Circulation*, 43:549, 1973.

110. Gallagher, J. J., Smith, W. M., Kasell, J., Smith, W. M., Grant, A. O., and Benson, D. Woodrow: Use of Esophageal Lead in the Diagnosis of Mechanisms of Reciprocating Supraventricular Tachycardia, *PACE*, 3:440, 1980.

111. Gallagher, J. J., and Sealy, W. C.: The Permanent Form of Junctional Reciprocating Tachycardia: Further Elucidation of the Underlying Mechanism, *Eur. J. Cardiol.*, 8:413, 1978.

112. Mignone, R. J., and Wallace, A. G.: Ventricular Echoes: Evidence for Dissociation of Conduction and Reentry within the AV Node, *Circ. Res.*, 19:638, 1966.

113. Brechenmacher, C., Coumel, P., and James, T. N.: De Subitanis Mortibus, *Circulation*, 53:377, 1976.

114. Rosen, K. M.: Junctional Tachycardia: Mechanism, Diagnosis, Differential Diagnosis and Management, *Circulation*, 47:654, 1973.

115. Gallagher, J. J., Damato, A. N., Lau, S. H.: Electrophysiologic Studies during Accelerated Idioventricular Rhythm, *Circulation*, 44:671, 1971.

116. Coumel, P., Fidelle, J., Lucet, V., Attuel, P., and Bouvrain, Y.: Catecholamine-Induced Severe Ventricular Arrhythmias with Adams-Stokes Syndrome in Children: Report of Four Cases, *Br. Heart J.*, 15(suppl.):28, 1978.

117. Benson, D. W., Gallagher, J. J., Sterba, R., Klein, G. J., and Armstrong, B. E.: Catecholamine Induced Double Tachycardia: Case Report in a Child, *PACE*, 3:96, 1980.

118. Wellens, H. J. J., Schuilenburg, R.M., and Durrer, D.: Electrical Stimulation of the Heart in Patients with Ventricular Tachycardia, *Circulation*, 46:216, 1972.

*119. Wellens, H. J. J., Lie, K. I., and Durrer, D.: Further Observations on Ventricular Tachycardia as Studied by Electrical Stimulation of the Heart:

Chronic Recurrent Ventricular Tachycardia and Ventricular Tachycardia during Acute Myocardial Infarction, *Circulation,* 49:647, 1974. (22 references)

120. Wellens, H. J. J., Durrer, D., and Lie, K. I.: Observations on Mechanisms of Ventricular Tachycardia in Man, *Circulation,* 54:237, 1976.

121. Boineau, J. P., and Cox, J. L.: Slow Ventricular Activation in Acute Myocardial Infarction: A Source of Re-entrant Premature Ventricular Contractions, *Circulation,* 43:702, 1973.

122. Wellens, H. J. J., Farre, J., and Bar, F. W.: Ventricular Tachycardia: Value and Limitations of Stimulation Studies, in O. S. Narula (ed.), "Cardiac Arrhythmias," The Williams & Wilkins Company, Baltimore, 1979, p. 436.

*123. Hope, R. R., Scherlag, B. J., and Lazzara, R.: Excitation of Ischemic Myocardium: Altered Properties of Conduction, Refractoriness and Excitability, *Am. Heart J.,* 99:753, 1980. (39 references)

124. Karagueuzian, H. S., Fenoglio, J. J., Weiss, M. B., and Wit, A. L.: Protracted Ventricular Tachycardia Induced by Premature Stimulation of the Canine Heart after Coronary Artery Occlusion and Reperfusion, *Circ. Res.,* 44:833, 1979.

125. Josephson, M. D., Horowitz, L. N., and Farshidi, A.: Continuous Local Electrical Activity: A Mechanism of Recurrent Ventricular Tachycardia, *Circulation,* 57:659, 1978.

126. Josephson, M. D.: Recurrent Sustained Ventricular Tachycardia: Mechanisms, *Circulation,* 57:431, 1978.

127. Touboul, P., Clavyrolas, R., Huerta, F., Porte, J., and Delahaye, J. P.: Tachycardie ventriculaire induite par des battements supraventriculaires prematures à complex QRS normal: Analyse d'une cas, *Arch. Mal. Coeur,* 68:969, 1975.

128. Vandepol, C., Farshidi, A., Spielman, S. R., Greenspan, A. M., Horowitz, L. N., and Josephson, M. E.: Incidence of Clinical Significance of Induced Ventricular Tachycardia, *Am. J. Cardiol.,* 45:725, 1980.

129. Reddy, Pratap, C., and Khoraschian, A.: Intraventricular Reentry with Narrow QRS Complex, *Circulation,* 61:641, 1980.

130. Lozano, J., Mandel, W. J., Hayakawa, H., Shine, K. I., and Eber, L. M.: Reentrant Tachycardia: Participation of the Distal A-V Conduction System, *Chest,* 63:23, 1972.

131. Reddy, Pratap, C., and Slack, J. D.: Recurrent Sustained Ventricular: A Report of a Case with His-Bundle Branches Reentry as the Mechanism, *Eur. J. Cardiol.,* 11:23, 1980.

132. Spurrell, R. A. J., Sowton, E., and Deuchar, D. C.: Ventricular Tachycardia in 4 Patients Evaluated by Programmed Electrical Stimulation of the Heart and Treated in 2 Patients by Surgical Division of the Anterior Radiation of the Left Bundle Branch, *Br. Heart J.,* 35:1014, 1973.

133. Akhtar, M., Damato, A. N., Batsford, W. P., Ruskin, J. N., Ogunkelu, J. B., and Vargas, G.: Demonstration of Reentry within the His-Purkinje System in Man, *Circulation,* 50:1150, 1974.

134. Guerot, C. L., Vateri, P. A., Castello-Fenoy, A., and Tricot, R.: Tachycardie par réentre de branche à branche, *Arch. Mal. Coeur,* 67:1, 1975.

*135. Karagueuzian, H. S., and Wit, A. L.: Studies on Ventricular Arrhythmias in Animal Models of Ischemic Heart Disease: What can we learn?, in H. E. Kulbertus and H. J. J. Wellens (eds.), "Sudden Death," Martinus Nijhoff, The Hague, 1980, p. 69. (Extensively referenced)

136. Murdock, D. K., Loeb, J. M., Euler, D. E., and Randall, W. C.: Electrophysiology of Coronary Reperfusion: A Mechanism for Reperfusion Arrhythmias, *Circulation,* 61:175, 1980.

*137. Ideker, R. E., Klein, G. J., Smith, W. M., Harrison, L., Kasell, J., Wallace, A. G., and Gallagher, J. J.: Epicardial Activation Sequences during the Onset of Ventricular Tachycardia and Ventricular Fibrillation, in H. E. Kulbertus and H. J. J. Wellens (eds.), "Sudden Death," Martinus Nijhoff, The Hague, 1980, p. 165. (Extensively referenced)

138. Harumi, K., Wyatt, R., Lux, R., Abildskov, J. A., and Smith, C. R.: Initiating Mechanisms of Ventricular Fibrillation, *Am. J. Cardiol.,* 43:374, 1979.

139. Pietras, R. J., Mautner, R., Denes, P., Wu, D., Dhingra, R., Towne, W., and Rosen, K. M.: Chronic Recurrent Right and Left Ventricular Tachycardia: A Comparison of Clinical, Hemodynamic and Angiographic Findings, *Am. J. Cardiol.,* 40:32, 1977.

140. Josephson, M. E., Seides, S. F.: Clinical Cardiac Electrophysiology, Lea & Febiger, Philadelphia, p. 247.

*141. Fontaine, G. F., Guiraudon, G., and Frank, R.: Mechanism of Ventricular Tachycardia with and without Chronic Myocardial Ischemia: Surgical Management Based on Epicardial Mapping, in O. S. Narula (ed.), "Cardiac Arrhythmias," The Williams & Wilkins Company, Baltimore, 1979, p. 516. (Extensively referenced)

142. Reiter, M. J., Smith, W. M., Benson, D. W., and Gallagher, J. J.: Right Ventricular Tachycardia: Uncommon, Benign and Idiopathic?, *Circulation,* 62:321, 1980. (Abstracts.)

143. Verrier, R. L.: Neural Factors and Ventricular Electrical Instability, in H. E. Kulbertus and H. J. J. Wellens (eds.), "Sudden Death," Martinus Nijhoff, The Hague, 1980, p. 137.

144. Coumel, P., Leclercq, J. F., Attuel, P., Levallee, J. P., and Flammang, D.: Autonomic Influences and the Genesis of Ventricular Arrhythmias, in O. S. Narula (ed.), "Cardiac Arrhythmias," The Williams & Wilkins Company, Baltimore, 1979, p. 457.

*145. Lown, B., DeSilva, R. A., and Lenson, R.: Roles of Psychologic Stress and Autonomic Nervous System Changes in Provocation of Ventricular Premature Beats, *Am. J. Cardiol.,* 41:979, 1978. (29 references)

146. Waxman, M. B., Downar, E., Berman, N. D., and Felderhof, C. H.: Phenylephrine (Neo-Synephrine) Terminated Ventricular Tachycardia, *Circulation,* 50:656, 1974.

147. Waxman, M. B., and Wald, R. W.: Termination of Ventricular Tachycardia by an Increase in Vagal Drive, *Circulation,* 56:385, 1977.

148. Surawicz B.: Ventricular Fibrillation, *Am. J. Cardiol.,* 28:268, 1971.

149. Spielman, S. R., Farshidi, A., Horowitz, L. W., and Josephson, M. E.: Ventricular Fibrillation during Programmed Ventricular Stimulation: Incidence, and Clinical Implications, *Am. J. Cardiol.,* 42:913, 1978.

*150. Ruskin, J., DiMarco, J. P., and Garan, H.: Out-of-Hospital Cardiac Arrest: Electrophysiologic Observations and Selection of Long-Term Antiarrhythmic Therapy, *N. Engl. J. Med.*, 303:607, 1980. (17 references)

*151. James, T. N.: Neural Pathology of the Heart in Sudden Death, in H. E. Kulbertus and H. J. J. Wellens (eds.), "Sudden Death," Martinus Nijhoff, The Hague, 1980, p. 49. (Extensively referenced)

152. Strauss, H. C., Prystowsky, E. N., and Scheinman, M.: Sino-Atrial Electrogenesis, *Prog. Cardiovasc. Dis.*, 29:385, 1977.

153. Brooks, McC. C., and Lu, H. H.: The Sino-Atrial Pacemaker of the Heart, Charles C Thomas, Springfield, Ill. 1972.

154. Bonke, F. I. M.: "The Sinus Node," Martinus Nijhoff, The Hague, 1978.

155. Lev, M.: The Conduction System, in S. E. Gould (ed.), "Pathology of the Heart and Blood Vessels," 3d ed., Charles C Thomas, Springfield, Ill., 1968.

156. Kulertus, H. E., DeLeval-Rutten, F., and Demoulin, J. C.: Sinoatrial Disease: A Report on 13 Cases, *J. Electrocardiol.*, 6:303, 1973.

*157. Bharati, S., Nordenberg, A., Bauernfiend, R., Varghese, J. P., Carvalho, A. G., Rosen, K., and Lev, M.: The Anatomic Substrate for the Sick Sinus Syndrome in Adolescence, *Am. J. Cardiol.*, 46:163, 1980. (42 references)

158. Rosen, J. M., Loeb, H. S., Sinno, M. Z., Rahimtoola, S. H., Gunnar, R. M.: Cardiac Conduction in Patients with Symptomatic Sinus Node Disease, *Circulation*, 43:836, 1971.

*159. Kaplan, B. M., Langendorf, R., Lev, M., and Pick, A.: Tachycardia-Bradycardia Syndrome (So-Called "Sick Sinus Syndrome"): Pathology, Mechanisms and Treatment, *Am. J. Cardiol.*, 31:497, 1973. (72 references)

160. Childers, R.: The A-V Node: Normal and Abnormal Physiology, *Prog. Cardiovasc. Dis.*, 29:361, 1977.

*161. Watanabe, Y., and Dreifus, L. S.: Arrhythmias: Mechanisms and Pathogenesis, in L. S. Dreifus and W. Likoff, "Cardiac Arrhythmias," Grune & Stratton, Inc., New York, 1973, p. 35. (Extensively referenced)

*162. Bharati, S., and Lev, M.: Histological and Electrophysiological Correlations in Atrioventricular Block and Bundle Branch Block, in O. S. Narula (ed.), "Cardiac Arrhythmias," The Williams & Wilkins Company, Baltimore, 1979, p. 164. (Extensively referenced)

163. Rossi, Lino: His Bundle in Electrocardiographic Semantics of AV Block: Anatomicoclinical Considerations, *PACE*, 3:275, 1980.

164. Uhley, H. N.: The Concept of Trifascicular Introventricular Conduction: Historical Aspects and Influence on Contemporary Cardiology, *Am. J. Cardiol.*, 43:643, 1979.

165. Lenègre, J.: The Pathology of Complete Atrioventricular Block, *Prog. Cardiovasc. Dis.*, 6:317, 1964.

*166. Kulbertus, H. E., and Demoulin, J. C.: The Conduction System: Anatomical and Pathological Aspects, in D. M. Krikler and J. F. Goodwin, "Cardiac Arrhythmias, the Modern Electrophysiological Approach," W. B. Saunders Company, Philadelphia, 1975, p. 25. (Extensively referenced)

167. Roos, J. C., and Dunning, A. J.: Bundle Branch Block in Acute Myocardial Infarction, *Eur. J. Cardiol.*, 6:403, 1978.

28

Recognition of Arrhythmias and Conduction Abnormalities

Henry J. L. Marriott, M.D.
Robert J. Myerburg, M.D.

Glossary

atrial capture Retrograde conduction to the atria following a period of AV dissociation.

automatic beat A beat arising in an automatic focus, independent of the dominant rhythm.

automaticity The property of spontaneously generating impulses.

AV dissociation The independent beating of atria and ventricles.

block A pathologic delay or interruption of impulse conduction.

bradyarrhythmia Any disturbance of rhythm resulting in a heart (or chamber) rate under 60 beats per minute.

bradycardia A heart (or chamber) rate under 60 beats per minute.

capture(d) beat A conducted beat following a period of AV dissociation.

coupling The relation of a premature beat to its preceding "forcing" beat.

coupling interval The interval between a premature beat and the beat preceding it.

ectopic beat A beat arising in any focus other than the normal sinus pacemaker.

escape beat An automatic beat occurring after an interval longer than the dominant cycle length.

extrasystole An ectopic beat, dependent on and coupled to the preceding beat, occurring before the next dominant beat.

idionodal rhythm An independent, relatively slow rhythm arising in the AV junction and controlling only the ventricles.

idioventricular rhythm A relatively slow rhythm arising in and controlling only the ventricles.

parasystole An independent, ectopic rhythm operating alongside the dominant rhythm; its pacemaking center is "protected" so that it cannot be discharged by the dominant pacemaker's impulses.

premature beat See extrasystole.

tachyarrhythmia Any disturbance of rhythm resulting in a heart (or chamber) rate over 100 beats per minute.

tachycardia A heart (or chamber) rate over 100 beats per minute.

ventricular capture Conduction to the ventricles following a period of AV dissociation.

Graphic Methods

Standard Electrocardiogram

The easiest test, and frequently the only one necessary, for the evaluation of a disturbance of rhythm or conduction remains the standard electrocardiogram. A long strip of leads carefully selected to yield the most informative QRS complexes and discrete P waves and which reflect direction of atrial propagation as well (usually leads II and V_1) will yield sufficient information in most instances to make the proper diagnosis.

The analysis of a rhythm strip may be facilitated by the use of *ladder diagrams*. These diagrams are useful for illustrating the mechanism of any rhythm, but they are especially valuable in elucidating complex arrhythmias. Sir Thomas Lewis used them freely; they are sometimes called *Lewis lines*. For most purposes they are constructed with only three tiers—A, AV, and V (Fig. 28-1A)—but for special arrhythmias an additional tier must be added: one above (Fig. 28-1B) to depict the mechanism of sinoatrial (SA) block, or one below (Fig. 28-1C) for the finer points of some ectopic ventricular rhythms.

The three main tiers, A, AV, and V, represent conduction through the atria, the AV junction, and the ventricles. The lines representing conduction are diagramed under the actual tracing and are accurately drawn so that the A line begins at the beginning of the P wave, and the V line at the beginning of the QRS. Passage of time is indicated by the slope of the line, and arrowheads are sometimes added to clarify direction of spread, but these are not necessary since the direction of the slope im-

mediately tells which way the impulse is traveling. (Many authors use only vertical lines in A and V tiers, reserving the sloping lines to depict conduction in the AV junction.) The site of impulse formation may or may not be represented by a black dot. When an impulse is blocked, the block is indicated by a short bar at a right angle to the main line (Fig. 28-2C and D). A symbol we have adopted to indicate aberrant ventricular conduction is a pair of slightly divergent lines (Fig. 28-2A). A variety of arrhythmic mechanisms are diagramed in Fig. 28-2.

In using the diagram for unraveling a difficult arrhythmia, the first rule is draw in only what you can see—do not fill the AV tier with guesses. Only after you have represented the atrial impulses in the A tier and the ventricular impulses in the V tier should you start trying to join them. These stages are illustrated in Fig. 28-3.

Special Leads

When standard surface electrocardiography fails to yield sufficient information to make a diagnosis, special systems may be employed. Since failure of the standard techniques sometimes results from failure to identify atrial activity, some special systems are designed to amplify atrial activity in relation to ventricular activity. The unipolar or bipolar esophageal lead to record atrial activity and the unipolar or bipolar intraatrial lead to record right atrial activity are two systems commonly used. In either case, a surface electrocardiographic lead should be used

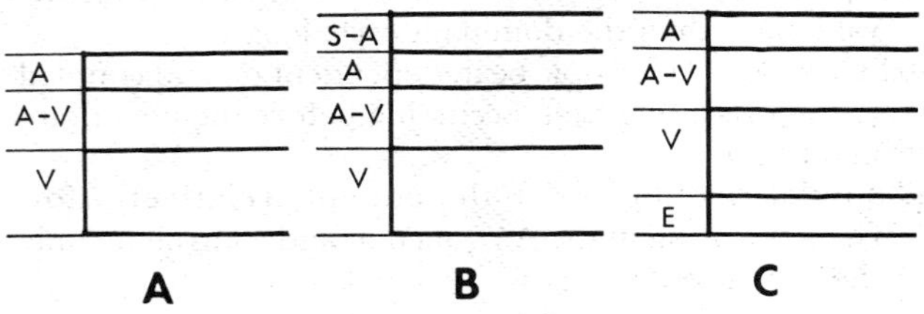

FIGURE 28-2 The following mechanisms are diagrammed: *A.* Sinus beat with normal conduction (a); sinus beat with prolonged AV conduction (b); atrial premature beat with prolonged AV and aberrant ventricular conduction (c). *B.* AV beat with atrial-before-ventricular activation (a); AV beat with ventricular-before-atrial activation (b); AV beat with retrograde delay and reciprocal beating (c). *C.* Ventricular ectopic beat without retrograde conduction (a); ventricular ectopic beat with penetration into AV junction (b); ventricular ectopic beat with retrograde conduction to atria (c). *D.* AV dissociation between sinus and ventricular pacemakers (a); ventricular fusion beat (b); atrial fusion beat (c).

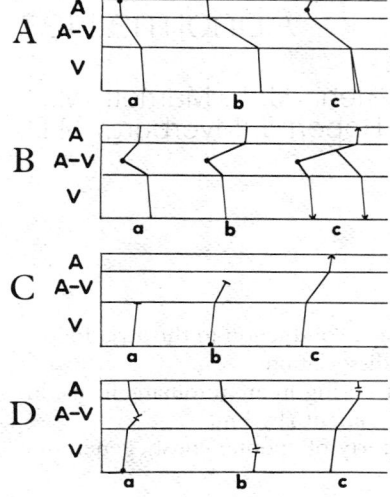

FIGURE 28-1 Skeletons of ladder diagrams used for illustrating the mechanisms of rhythm and conduction.

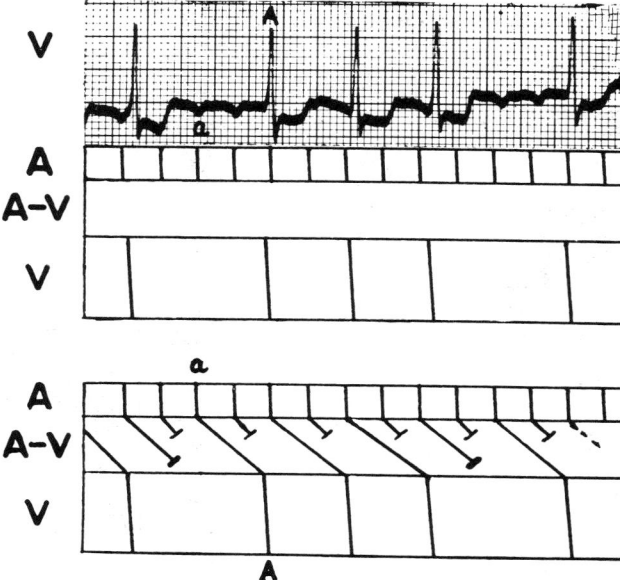

FIGURE 28-3 The proper use of ladder diagrams involves two stages. *Stage 1*: Draw in lines to represent the atrial flutter waves (seen and inferred by measurement) and the ventricular complexes. *Stage 2*: Since in flutter the FR interval usually ranges between 0.26 and 0.45 s, we start by connecting F wave *a* to the QRS A. As we proceed to diagram successive impulses, it quickly becomes plain that we have a basic 2:1 AV conduction with a Wenckebach period of the alternate cycles.[1]

simultaneously with the special lead if a two-channel recorder is available.

For constant monitoring in special care units, a right-sided chest lead takes advantage of precordial QRS morphology and is superior to the formerly popular modified lead II. Of right-sided bipolar leads, MCL_1 (modified CL_1)—in which the positive electrode is situated at the C_1 (V_1) position with the negative electrode at the left shoulder—has proved most satisfactory.

Intracardiac Electrography

Although in the great majority of cases, surface electrocardiography is adequate to make an accurate diagnosis of rhythm and conduction disturbances, in difficult cases intracardiac electrograms constitute the final court of appeal (Chap. 89). Together with intracardiac pacing techniques, they may be indispensable for determining the origin of wide QRS complexes, especially in differentiating ventricular tachycardia from supraventricular tachycardia with ventricular aberration; for identifying the precise pathways of reciprocating tachycardias, ventricular and supraventricular; for establishing the site of accessory pathways in the Wolff-Parkinson-White (WPW) syndrome; for ascertaining the level of AV block, whether above or below the bundle of His; for distinguishing genuine AV block from pseudo block caused by concealed junctional extrasystoles; and for evaluating sinus nodal function.

Sinus Rhythms

Sinus or sinoatrial (SA) rhythm is the heart's normal mechanism, the controlling impulses arising regularly or almost regularly in the sinus node and driving the heart at a rate between 60 and 100 beats per minute. The node possesses inherent automaticity, but its rate of impulse formation is influenced by vagal and sympathetic tone. If the regularity of rate deviates from the defined standard, the sinus mechanism becomes arrhythmia, tachycardia, or bradycardia.

Sinus Arrhythmia

Slight variation in the cycle length is a feature of normal sinus rhythm; if the variation exceeds 0.12 s between the longest and shortest cycles, sinus arrhythmia is present (Fig. 28-4*A*). A normal finding in children and young adults, it tends to diminish and disappear with advancing years. Its presence does *not* rule out organic heart disease.

Sinus arrhythmia occurs in two forms: phasic (respiratory) and nonphasic (nonrespiratory). In the more common phasic form, the heart accelerates with inspiration and slows with expiration; this is mainly owing to rhythmic fluctuations in vagal tone mediated through Bainbridge's reflex. In the nonphasic variety, the irregularity is unrelated to the phases of respiration. Either form may be induced or exaggerated by factors that increase vagal tone. Electrocardiographic features include a variation of at least 0.12 s between the longest and shortest PP intervals with normal and constant P wave configuration and PR intervals.

Sinus Bradycardia

By the generally accepted definition, sinus bradycardia implies a rate of less than 60 beats per minute (Fig. 28-4*C*). In adult life, under basal conditions, *physiologic* sinus bradycardia occurs much more often than tachycardia and is frequently associated with arrhythmia. As already mentioned, sinus bradycardia was found in 38 percent of 1000 healthy aviators in their twenties;[2] it also appeared in 15 to 28 percent of 6014 asymptomatic Air Force personnel.[3] Its frequency decreased with advancing age: it was present in 22 to 28 percent of subjects between the ages of 20 and 30, but in only 15 or 16 percent between the ages of 35 and 58. Nevertheless, in old age it is not uncommon to find a significant sinus bradycardia in persons with no signs of heart disease. Physiologic sinus bradycardia is often found in well-trained athletes, especially those whose activities involve sustained effort (e.g., long-distance runners), and it may develop in other persons during sleep. It is part of the normal reaction to vagal stimulation, as by carotid sinus pressure or eyeball compression, or following Valsalva's maneuver. *Pharmacologic* sinus bradycardia may result from digitalis, morphine, reserpine, pressor amines, or propranolol. *Pathologic* sinus bradycardia may accompany the vagal stimulation produced by vomiting; it is also seen in convalescence from febrile illnesses (notably typhoid and influenza). It accompanies the hypometabolic state, including hypothermia and myxedema. It may be part of the clinical picture of obstructive jaundice, increased intracranial pressure, and depressed mental states. Sinus bradycardia may be the earliest or only manifestation of a "sick sinus." It is common in acute myocardial infarction, averaging 12.5 percent in several series. The incidence of sinus bradycardia is higher when the patient is seen in the early hours of infarction, and it is seen much more often in inferior than in anterior infarctions. The incidence of sinus bradycardia in patients with inferior infarction seen within 1 h of the onset was 41 percent.[4]

The development of sinus bradycardia in acute myocardial infarction, unless it is hemodynamically devastating, appears to presage a favorable outcome: pooled series indicate that the mortality rate among patients with infarctions and untreated sinus bradycardia was 13 percent compared with 28 percent in patients who developed no sinus bradycardia. In another series of 735 patients, the mortality among those with normal sinus rates between 60 and 100 beats per minute was 15 percent, in contrast with a mortality of only 6 percent in patients with sinus bradycardia.[5]

Sinus Tachycardia (Fig. 28-4B)

Although the range of normal sinus rates is generally set at 60 to 100 beats per minute, this does not imply that rates outside this range are abnormal. Graybiel found that 96 percent of 1000 healthy airmen between 20 and 30 years of age had basal heart rates between 40 and 85; only 3 (0.3 percent) had rates over 100, whereas 38 percent had rates below 60 beats per minute. Again, analysis of 6014 normal electrocardiograms recorded from asymptomatic Air Force personnel between the ages of 16 and 58 years disclosed a rate range from 39 to 129 beats per minute. Accepted ranges of normal rates in infancy and childhood are indicated in Table 28-1.

The word *tachycardia* itself sometimes evokes argument. It is one of our basic arrhythmic terms and as such should be clearly defined; it usually is defined as a heart or chamber rate over 100 beats per minute. Though a heart rate of 140 beats per minute with a sinus mechanism is normal for an infant, it is nonetheless a tachycardia—a physiological tachycardia. Physiological sinus tachycardia also occurs during and after exercise and as a result of anxiety or other emotional stress. It is an integral part of the "fight-or-flight" adaptive response mediated through the sympathetic nervous system.

By definition, the lower limit of sinus tachycardia is 100 beats per minute. The upper reaches of the rate range vary. In infants, the sinus tachycardia rate may exceed 200 beats per minute; well-trained

TABLE 28-1   Normal Heart Rate in Infancy and Childhood

Age	Minimum	Mean	Maximum
30 h	95	126	155
1 month	110	152	200
2–3 months	95	147	180
4–5 months	115	139	170
6–8 months	110	136	160
9–11 months	95	127	150
12–19 months	95	121	140
2–5 years	70	98	130
6–14 years	65	86	120

Source: Based on data of E. P. Namin, in B. M. Gasul, R. A. Arcilla, and M. Lev (eds.), "Heart Disease in Children: Diagnosis and Treatment." J. B. Lippincott Company, Philadelphia, 1966. With permission of author and publisher.

young athletes, driving themselves to the maximal effort, may sometimes attain a rate of 190 to 200. The maximum attainable with extreme exertion tends to decrease with advancing age and poorer conditioning. Most tachycardias induced by exercise or emotional stress in adults fall in the range of 100 to 150 beats per minute.

It is not always easy to distinguish between physiological, pharmacological, and pathological sinus tachycardia. Nevertheless, these three categories provide a useful framework. *Physiological* sinus tachycardia characterizes infancy and early childhood, occurs during and after exercise, and is produced by excitement, anxiety, and other everyday emotions. *Pharmacological* sinus tachycardia can result from medications such as atropine, epinephrine, ephedrine, amyl nitrite, isoproterenol, and thyroid extract, and from such social drugs as alcohol, nicotine, and caffeine. *Pathological* sinus tachycardia occurs with abnormal states such as fever, hypoxia, hemorrhage, hypotension, shock, infections, hyperthyroidism, anemia, beriberi, pulmonary embolism, and heart failure.

Diagnosis

Clinically, sinus rhythms are assumed to be present when the regularity or pattern of irregularity is appropriate, with normally shaped and directed P waves preceding every ventricular complex by an adequate PR interval. Minor variations in the shape and size of the P waves do not exclude a consistent sinus mechanism, since normal P waves may be influenced by respiration and by fluctuations in autonomic tone. The rate and regularity obviously determine whether the mechanism is classified as sinus rhythm or as sinus arrhythmia (Fig. 28-4A), tachycardia (Fig. 28-4B), or bradycardia (Fig. 28-4C).

Atrial Extrasystoles

Premature beats (extrasystoles) arising in ectopic foci in the atria are common. They may or may not be conducted to the ventricles, depending on (1)

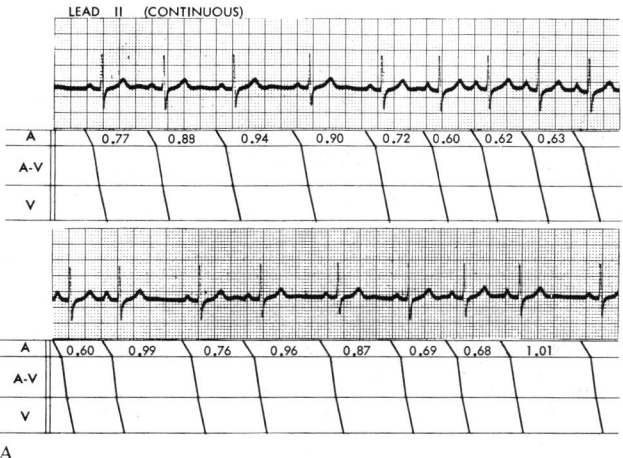

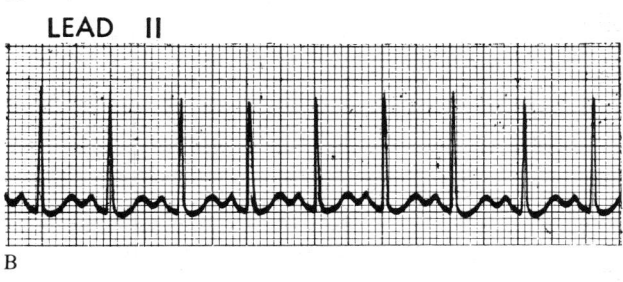

B

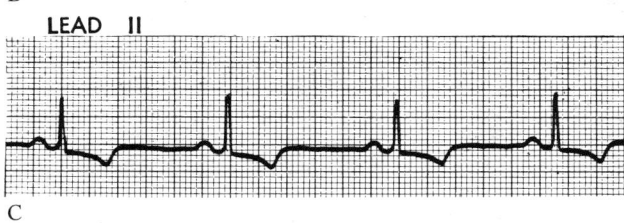

C

FIGURE 28-4   *A.* Sinus arrhythmia. The sinus cycles are indicated in seconds in the atrial (A) tier; they range from 0.60 to 1.01 s. Notice that as the sinus pacemaker accelerates, the P waves become more prominent. *B.* Sinus tachycardia. Note normally shaped and directed P waves, normal PQ (PR) interval, and a rate of almost 150. *C.* Sinus bradycardia. Note normally directed (but abnormally wide) P waves, normal PQ interval, and a rate of slightly more than 50.

their degree of prematurity and (2) the state of AV conduction. They occur at all ages and are often seen in the absence of heart disease; they were found in 0.4 percent of 122,000 apparently healthy male Air Force personnel between the ages of 16 and 50 years.[6] However, atrial disease obviously predisposes to them, and they in turn undoubtedly predispose to atrial tachyarrhythmias (tachycardia, flutter, and fibrillation).

Emotion, fatigue, alcohol, tobacco, or coffee may precipitate atrial premature beats in normal persons. They may result from digitalis, atrial distension (as in congestive failure), or ischemia. They are reported in up to 50 percent of myocardial infarctions and are sometimes a sign of atrial infarction. When atrial extrasystoles are due to digitalis intoxication, they may forerun the development of atrial tachycardia with block.

The hallmark of the atrial premature beat is a premature abnormal P wave (P′). When followed by

a ventricular complex, the P′R interval is usually normal and often somewhat prolonged. The P′ wave is often difficult to find when it is superimposed on the preceding T wave. Most atrial premature beats are conducted to the ventricles with a QRS-T configuration identical with that of the surrounding conducted sinus beats (Fig. 28-5A); but many are conducted with ventricular aberration (Fig. 28-5B), and then may closely simulate ventricular premature beats. The cycle following the atrial extrasystole is usually slightly longer than the dominant sinus cycle (Fig. 28-5A) but less than fully compensatory. At times it is exactly the same as the sinus

FIGURE 28-5   *A.* The fifth beat is an atrial premature beat: there is a premature P′ wave followed by a normal QRS-T complex, and the postextrasystolic pause is longer than the sinus cycle but less than compensatory. *B.* The fourth beat is an atrial premature beat with aberrant ventricular conduction: there is a premature P′ wave followed by an anomalous QRS-T complex; the postextrasystolic pause is less than compensatory. *C.* Nonconducted atrial premature beat. Following the third ventricular complex, a P′ wave negatively deforms the ST segment and is not followed by a ventricular response.

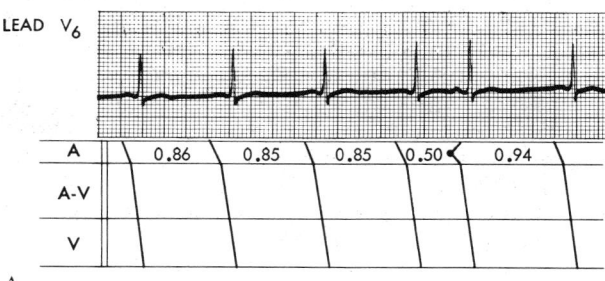

A

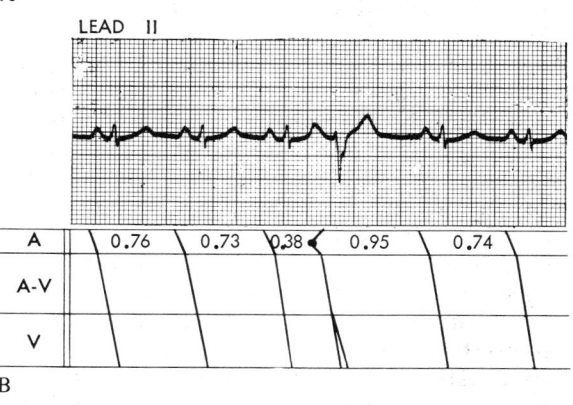

B

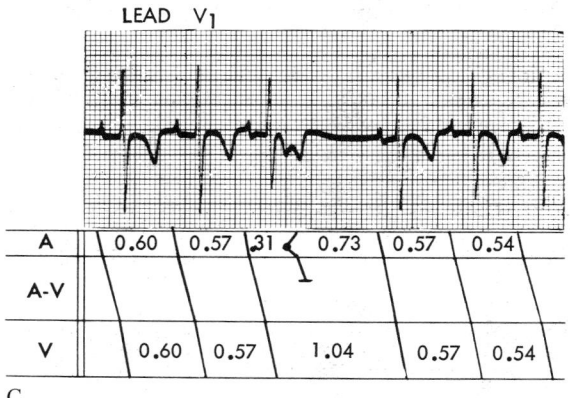

C

cycle, and at other times the ectopic atrial impulse may so suppress the sinus pacemaker that the pause is fully compensatory or even longer. Nonconducted atrial extrasystoles are quite common (Fig. 28-5C) and are often overlooked if the premature P′ wave is inconspicuous. In fact, the nonconducted atrial premature beat is easily the most common cause of an abruptly lengthened cycle for which the reason is not apparent at first sight. Careful comparison of the T wave of the ventricular complex immediately preceding the pause with another nearby T wave will often reveal subtle distortion owing to the superimposition of an ectopic P wave. Nonconducted atrial bigeminy is of importance because, if the P′ waves are overlooked, it can simulate sinus bradycardia (Fig. 28-6) and invite erroneous treatment.

AV Junctional Extrasystoles

Physiologists have been unable to find pacemaking cells in the AV node of the experimental animal, though they have found them at its junction with the His bundle and in the bundle itself. For this reason it has become the vogue to refer to beats arising in the AV junction as *junctional*. However, there is no conclusive evidence that the human AV node lacks automaticity,[7] and, so long as the matter remains unsettled, we have no objection to the terms *AV nodal* or, simply, *nodal*. We shall here use the more noncommittal terms *junctional* or *AV* as used by Frank Wilson 60 years ago.

Impulses arising in the AV junction spread simultaneously upward to the atria and downward to the ventricles. Depending on the rate of spread in each direction, and perhaps to some extent on the level of origin within the AV junction, the atria may be activated before, after, or simultaneously with the ventricles.

AV premature beats are much less common than atrial or ventricular premature beats, both in health and disease. They were found in 0.2 percent of 122,000 apparently healthy Air Force personnel ranging in age from 16 to over 50 years.[6]

The "retrograde" P waves characteristic of AV rhythm are typified in Fig. 28-7. They are inverted in leads II, III, and aV_F and upright in leads aV_R and aV_L. They are nearly isoelectric in lead I (unless

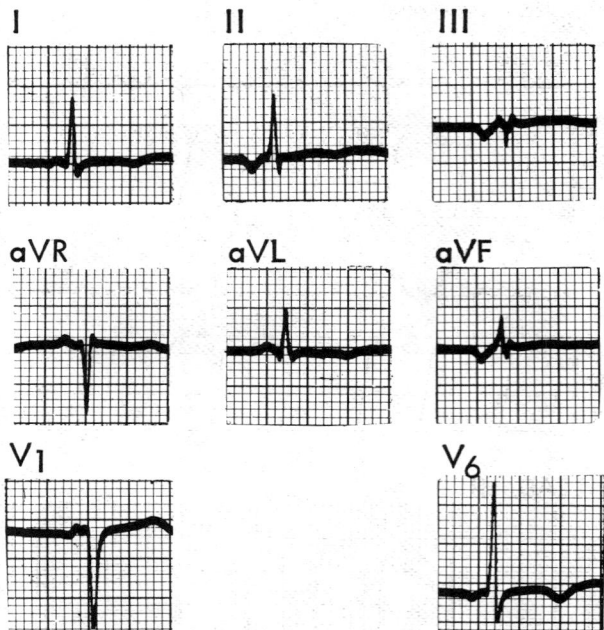

FIGURE 28-7   The short PQ (PR) interval and the polarity of retrograde P waves in key leads in AV (nodal) rhythms: inverted in leads II, III, aV_F, and V_6; upright in leads aV_R, aV_L, and V_1; almost isoelectric in lead I.

there is atrial hypertrophy); i.e., their frontal-plane axis is close to −90°. They are usually upright, or diphasic, in right precordial leads and shallowly inverted in left precordial leads. These P waves precede the QRS complex by less than 0.12 s, coincide with the QRS complex, or follow it.

The retrograde P′ waves of AV extrasystoles are usually associated with normal QRS-T complexes, but, as with atrial premature beats, ventricular aberration may complicate the picture (Fig. 28-8A). At times, no retrograde conduction to the atria occurs, so that the sinus rhythm is undisturbed and the postextrasystolic pause is fully compensatory (Fig. 28-8B). When the typical retrograde P-wave pattern is associated with a normal—rather than short—PR interval, the rhythm may arise in the junction and be conducted with delay below the junctional pacemaker; or it may arise in an ectopic atrial focus.

Supraventricular Tachycardia

The supraventricular tachycardias (SVT) include all the tachyarrhythmias whose site of impulse formation or reentry circuit is above the bifurcation of the His bundle. By strict definition this group includes sinus, atrial, and AV tachycardias as well as the tachycardias associated with atrial flutter and fibrillation. Sinus tachycardia, atrial flutter, and atrial fibrillation are dealt with elsewhere; this section deals with atrial and junctional tachycardia due either to reentry or to enhanced ectopic automaticity.

Up to about 1970, it was generally thought that the supraventricular tachycardias were due to en-

FIGURE 28-6   Atrial bigeminy, nonconducted. The strips are continuous. After three sinus beats, five nonconducted atrial bigeminal sequences simulate sinus bradycardia.

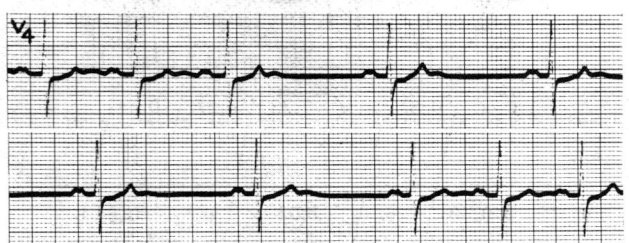

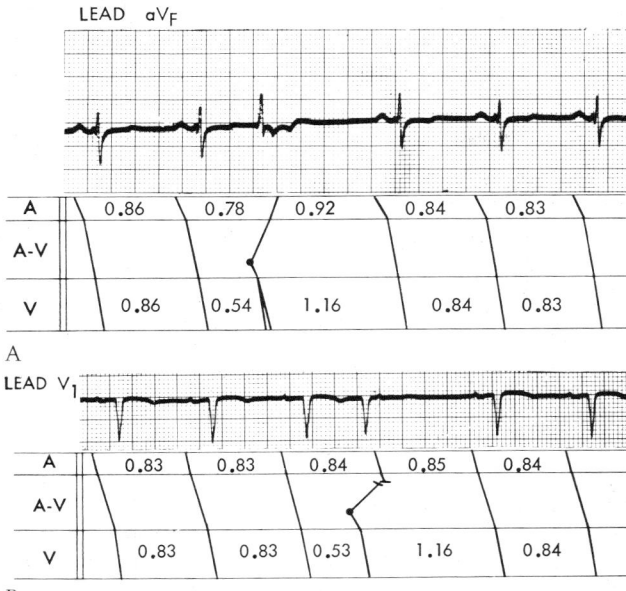

FIGURE 28-8 *A.* "Lower" AV extrasystole; the retrograde P wave follows the premature QRS complex, which shows some degree of ventricular aberration. *B.* The fourth beat is an AV premature beat without retroconduction to the atria, so that the sinus rhythm is undisturbed.

hanced automaticity, i.e., rapid discharge from an ectopic pacemaking center; since then, the electrophysiologists have demonstrated that the majority of such tachycardias are in fact due to a circulating wave front (reentrant, reciprocating, or circus-movement tachycardia). The majority of these reciprocating tachycardias (RT) occupy a circuit within the AV junction. However, there are many other available circuits, and the SVTs have been reclassified as indicated in Table 28-2.

Ectopic Supraventricular Tachycardia
Ectopic atrial or junctional tachycardia may complicate such conditions as acute myocardial infarction, chronic or acute cor pulmonale, pneumonia, and pharmacological intoxications (alcohol, catechols, digitalis, etc.). Ectopic atrial tachycardia is commonly caused by digitalis intoxication, and then it is often associated with AV block, usually 2:1 but sometimes in varying ratios so that the ventricular rhythm is quite irregular. Occasionally the AV block is latent, becoming manifest only with carotid sinus

TABLE 28-2   The Supraventricular Tachycardias

1. Ectopic
   a. Atrial
   b. AV junctional
2. Reentrant
   a. AV junctional
   b. AV junctional bypass
   c. SA nodal
   d. Intraatrial
   e. Kent bundle (WPW)

stimulation. Atrial tachycardia with AV block has long been recognized as a common manifestation of digitalis toxicity. Although in the experience of some investigators as much as 75 percent of atrial tachycardias with AV block were due to digitalis toxicity,[8] others have found that only a small percentage of such atrial tachycardias were so caused and that most resulted from underlying heart disease which required digitalis in therapy.[9] The simultaneous occurrence of atrial and AV tachycardia is highly suggestive of digitalis intoxication.

Multifocal atrial tachycardia (also called "chaotic" atrial tachycardia) is unquestionably of ectopic origin, and, although it may complicate any disease of the myocardium, it is most often found in chronic lung disease. Multifocal atrial tachycardia with AV block is illustrated in Fig. 28-9.

Ectopic junctional tachycardia can be a devastating occurrence in children, in whom heredity and the trauma of nearby surgery appear to play causative roles.[10]

Reentrant Supraventricular Tachycardias
These constitute the great majority of the SVTs; and of them, approximately two-thirds are due to reentry within the AV node and almost another third to reentry involving a bypass tract.[11] The percentage of SVTs that are due to reentry within the AV node as reported from three centers are listed in Table 28-3. A small number result from reentry within the sinus node or from atrial myocardium. Reentrant supraventricular tachycardias occur in both the normal and diseased heart. If they are paroxysmal and not chronic or persistent, they are usually well tolerated. The healthy heart may tolerate them well for hours, days, or even weeks. On the other hand, the extremely rapid ventricular rates (300 to 400) sometimes achieved in infancy may cause even the normal heart to fail. Rarely, a paroxysm of supraventricular tachycardia precipitates shock or heart failure in an otherwise healthy youth. Even in the presence of myocardial infarction, short paroxysms of supraventricular tachycardia often require little or no therapy; on the other hand, when such a paroxysm attacks an already disabled heart, it may rapidly induce congestive heart failure, pulmonary edema, or shock. Supraventricular tachycardia has been reported in 6 percent of patients with mitral valve prolapse.[12] Reentrant SVT can be precipitated by atropine.[13]

Differentiation between Reentry and Ectopic Tachycardias
Since the mechanism and therapy differ, it is clearly desirable to distinguish between the SVT that is due to reentry and the SVT that is due to ectopic automaticity. Although their precise mechanisms can be identified only by invasive methods (Chap. 89), they can often be separated with a high degree of probability from features in the clinical (surface) tracing.[14–16]

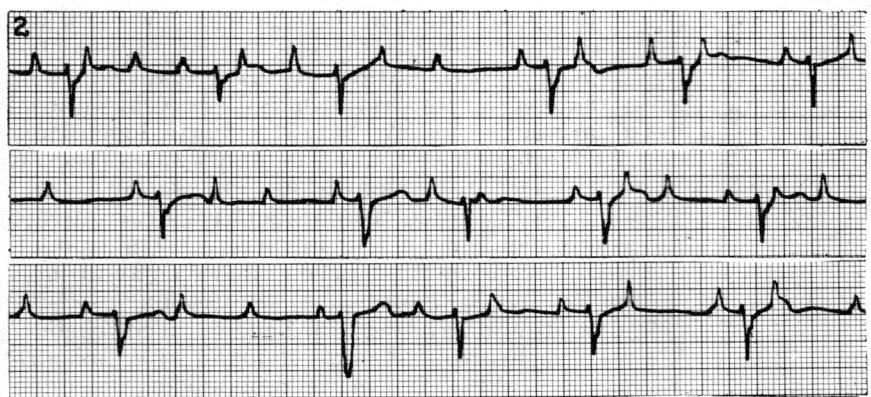

FIGURE 28-9 Multifocal (or "chaotic") atrial tachycardia with varying AV block (from a patient with chronic cor pulmonale).

The following features are suggestive of an ectopic mechanism: (1) the presence of "warm-up" (progressive acceleration for the first few beats) (Fig. 28-10A); (2) sameness of all the P′ waves, including the first (Fig. 28-10A); and (3) the "resetting" of the tachycardia by a premature stimulus (Fig. 28-10C), just as an atrial premature beat resets the sinus. On the other hand, in a reentering tachycardia: (1) warm-up is absent; (2) the initial (ectopic) P′ wave differs from the subsequent (retrograde) P′ waves (Fig. 28-10B); (3) a premature stimulus does not reset but may terminate the tachycardia (Fig. 28-10D); and (4) prolongation of the first P′R interval is the rule (Fig. 28-10B).

Several other clues point to specific mechanisms: If the P′ wave during the paroxysm is similar to the sinus P waves, there is a likelihood of sinus nodal reentry. If the P′ waves are neither of retrograde form and polarity nor like the sinus P waves, an ectopic atrial or reentrant atrial tachycardia is likely. The presence of AV dissociation or AV block rules out AV nodal bypass reentry; on the other hand, the presence of ventricular aberration tends to confirm the presence of an AV nodal bypass; and when the cycle length of the tachycardia increases (rate decreases) with the development of bundle branch block (BBB), it indicates that the bypass tract is on the same side as the BBB. A negative P′ in lead I indicates a probably left-sided bypass.

Electrocardiographic Features of Supraventricular Tachycardias

Supraventricular tachycardia is recognizable in the electrocardiogram (1) if the ventricular complexes are normal or (2) if, in the presence of widened QRS complexes, an ectopic P wave that is clearly not of

retrograde form is related to each ventricular complex. If the P′ waves are of retrograde form, ventricular tachycardia with 1:1 retrograde conduction may not be excludable. But P′ waves are often not distinguishable with certainty; if they are, one may be able to distinguish between atrial and AV junctional tachycardia (Fig. 28-11A). AV junctional tachycardia (Fig. 28-11B) can be recognized with certainty only if either of the following occurs:

1. The beginning or end of a paroxysm is recorded and the first or last beat of the paroxysm is associated with an appropriately directed retrograde P′ wave that either follows or shortly precedes the QRS complex.
2. Independent atrial activity (independent P waves or atrial fibrillation) is evident (Fig. 28-11C).

Atrial tachycardia can be diagnosed with certainty only if abnormal P waves, not appropriately directed for retrograde impulses, are seen in recognizable relation to the QRS complexes. If in the presence of rapid normal ventricular complexes, P waves are not discernible or are of retrograde or uncertain form, one cannot usually tell whether the mechanism is atrial, AV, or reciprocating. The retrograde P wave that is closely associated with a QRS complex may "belong" to it (AV junctional tachycardia) or may represent the ectopic atrial impulse that is responsible for the next ventricular complex (atrial tachycardia). Complete invisibility of the P waves may mean that they are "lost" in the T wave or QRS complex; if lost in the QRS, they may be retrograde P waves of junctional origin, or, since PR intervals are frequently prolonged in atrial tachycardia, they may be ectopic atrial P waves responsible for the following QRS complex. When the P′ waves of atrial tachycardia are plainly visible, their important feature is that they are different from the dominant P of the sinus rhythm. Ectopic rhythms may have P waves with polarity similar to that of sinus P waves but different in shape, or they may be indistinguishable from retrograde P waves of AV origin. The P waves of atrial tachycardia caused by digitalis toxicity tend to be normally directed but of small amplitude (Fig. 28-12A) (unlike the sturdy P

TABLE 28-3 Proportion of SVTs Due to AV Nodal Reentry (AVNR)

Authors	Total SVTs	AVNR	Percent
Wellens and Durrer (1975)	54	47	87
Wu et al. (1978)	79	50	63
Farshidi et al. (1978)	60	40	67

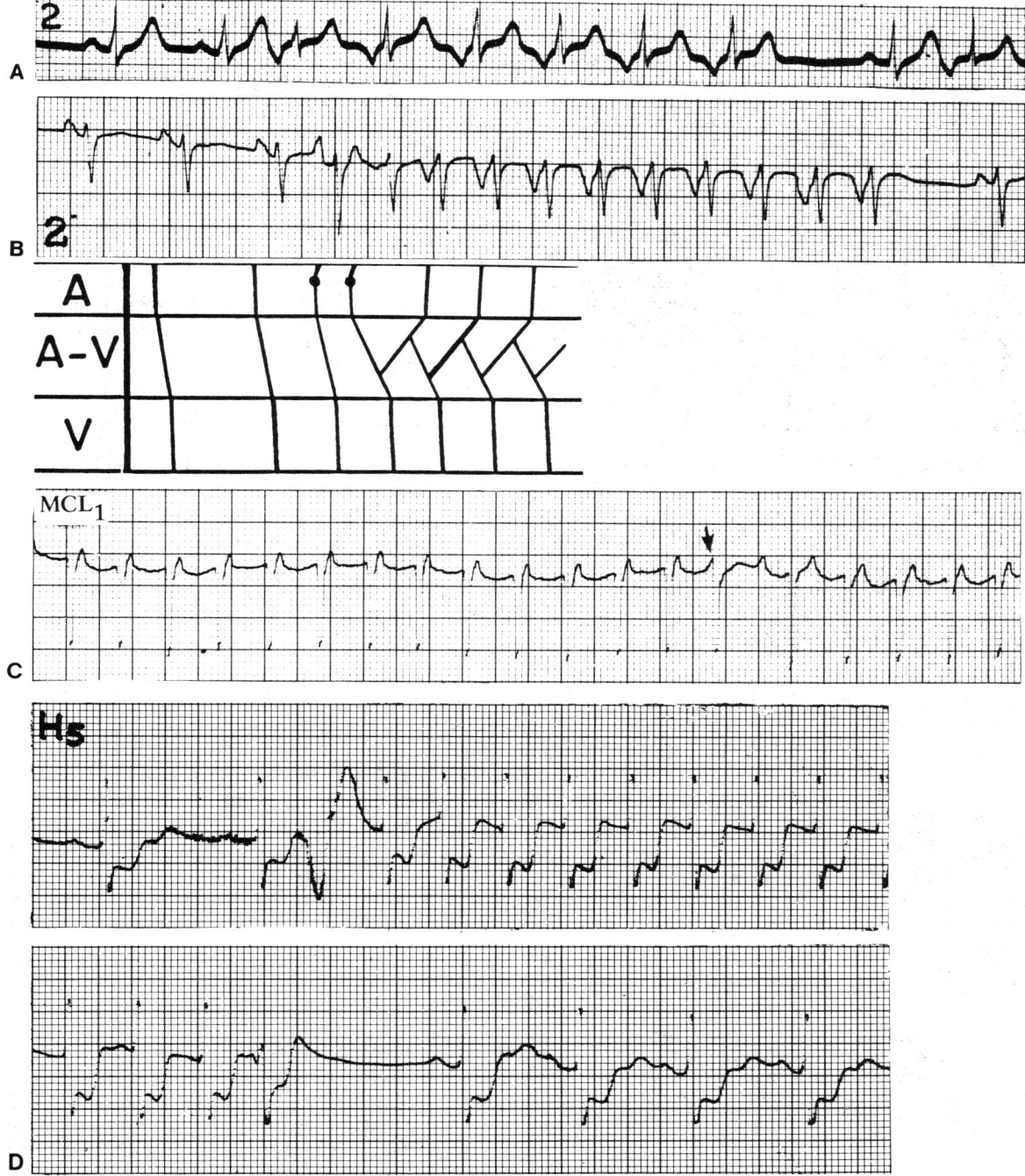

FIGURE 28-10   *A.* Ectopic atrial tachycardia: the inverted P′ waves are all identical and the first few atrial beats show gradual acceleration. *B.* Reciprocating tachycardia: the tachycardia is initiated by the second of two atrial extrasystoles (upright P′ wave) while all subsequent P′ waves are inverted (retrograde). *C.* Ectopic atrial tachycardia: the regular tachycardia is interrupted by a premature P′ wave (arrow) which "resets" the ectopic atrial pacemaker. *D.* Reciprocating tachycardia initiated by a ventricular extrasystole and terminated by another premature beat (from a Holter recording).

waves of sinus tachycardia) and somewhat variable in form from beat to beat; the P′P′ intervals are often slightly irregular. Multifocal atrial tachycardia (also called chaotic atrial tachycardia) is diagnosed when the ectopic P waves vary in shape and the P′P′ intervals also vary (Fig. 28-12*B*).[17]

Atrial Flutter

Atrial flutter has never been satisfactorily defined. When an elderly person with heart disease develops an atrial rate of about 320 impulses per minute, with typical "sawtooth" waves in the electrocardiogram

HOLTER MONITOR LEAD

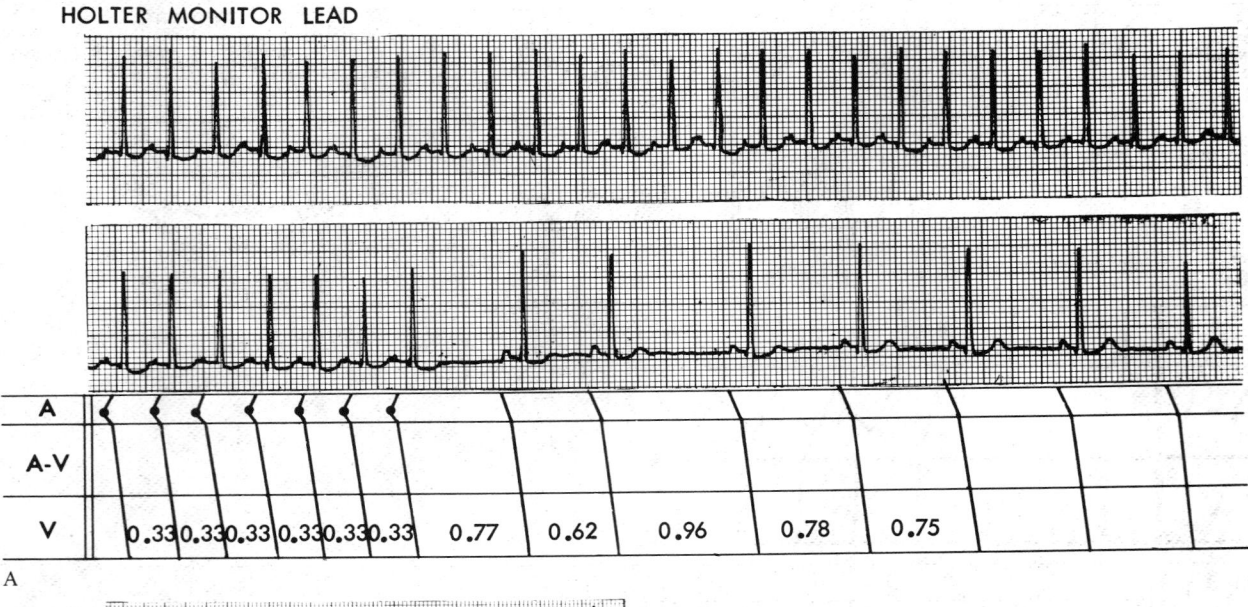

A

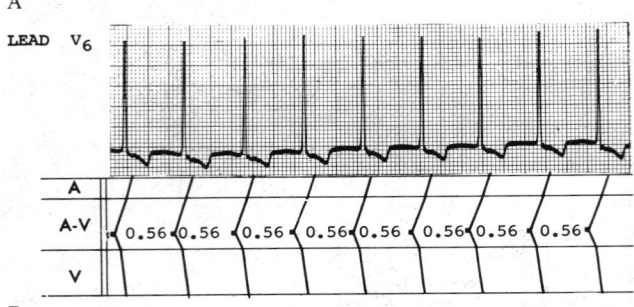

B

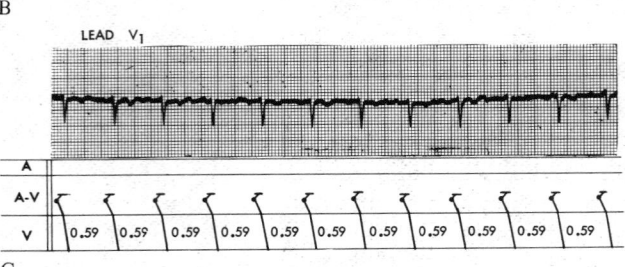

C

FIGURE 28-11   *A.* Atrial tachycardia. End of typical paroxysm. Note P′ wave preceding each normal QRS complex at the rate of 190; paroxysm abruptly stops in lower strip. *B.* AV tachycardia. Note retrograde P wave shortly following each QRS complex at the rate of 105. *C.* AV tachycardia at the rate of 102 in the presence of atrial fibrillation.

and 2:1 AV conduction, the term *flutter* is universally applied. When a healthy adolescent develops an atrial rate of about 180 beats per minute with abnormal P waves and 1:1 AV conduction, everyone calls it atrial tachycardia. But between these two classic pictures there is a shadowland of imprecision in which there are no sure signposts, and it is a moot point whether the boundaries between tachycardia and flutter can be set.

Mindful of the overlap with tachycardia, one can say that the typical example of atrial flutter occurs in a patient with heart disease, that the atrial rate is usually between 280 and 320 beats per minute, and

that there is usually a 2:1 conduction ratio. It is wrong to call this 2:1 "block" because, at rates around 300, physiological refractoriness—not pathological block—prevents the 1:1 ventricular response.

Atrial flutter is rarely seen in normal subjects. It was found only once among the 67,000 Air Force personnel screened by Fosmoe.[18] It may occur at all ages, even in infancy, and in fact is more common than atrial fibrillation in the first few years of life.[19] However, flutter is most commonly encountered in persons with ischemic heart disease over the age of 40 years, and paroxysms complicate 2 to 5 percent of cases of acute myocardial infarction. It may rarely be caused by digitalis intoxication, and sometimes results from treatment of atrial fibrillation with quinidine or procainamide. Paroxysms of flutter may complicate any form of heart disease or be precipitated by many acute illnesses.

Electrocardiographic Features

The waves of flutter in the ECG are labeled F waves, and their rate is usually between 280 and 320 per minute. Their pattern is variable, but the most common one presents the typical sawtooth waves in leads II, III, and aV_F, more discrete waves separated by isoelectric intervals in V_1 and other precordial leads, and poorly registered activity in lead I (Fig. 28-13). When the rate is slow enough, a definite isoelectric "shelf" appears even in the limb leads. Less commonly, atrial activity may not show up at all in the limb leads but may be evident only in right precordial leads; or again, it may be obvious in limb leads but relatively inconspicuous in right chest leads. Rarely the F waves may be notched or undulating, rather than serrated.

The commonest AV conduction ratio is 2:1; at this ratio it often happens that alternate F waves are lost in or merge with the QRS complex, so that the

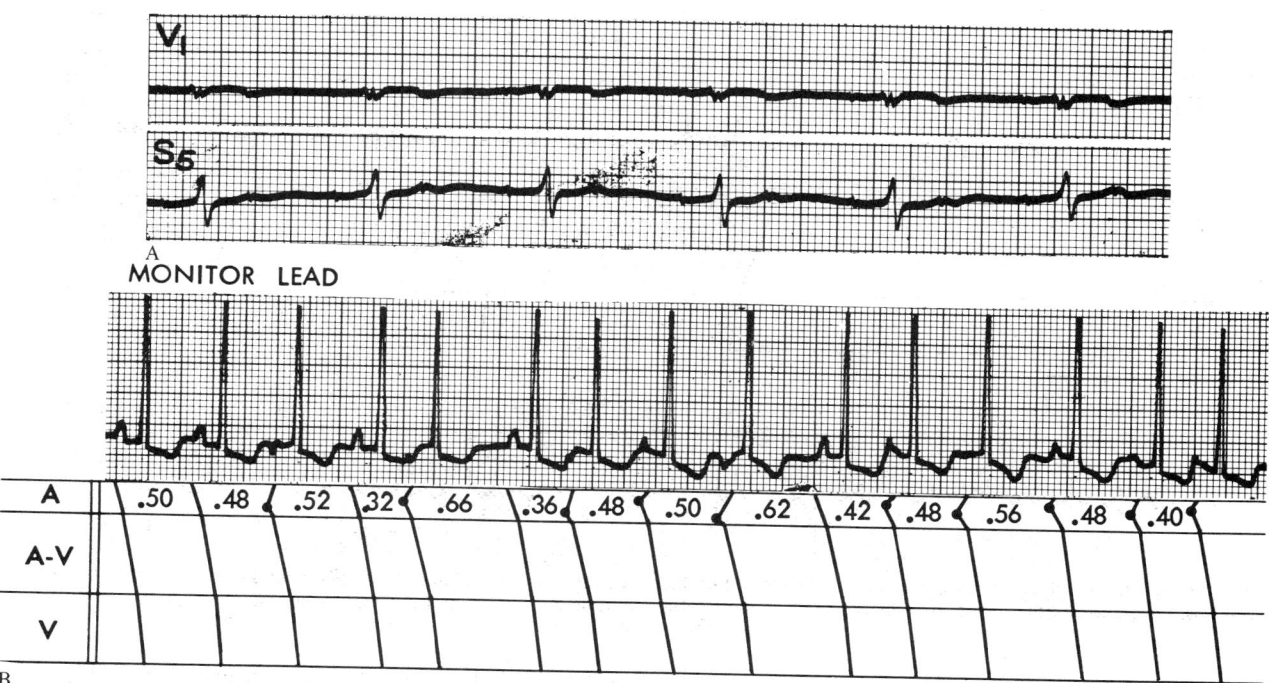

FIGURE 28-12 *A.* Atrial tachycardia with 2:1 AV block due to digitalis intoxication. Note the diminutive P waves, barely visible even in V₁. *B.* Multifocal (chaotic) atrial tachycardia. Note the constantly changing form of the ectopic P waves and the irregular rhythm at the rate of 122.

underlying mechanism may be overlooked. In this situation, when flutter is suspected, carotid sinus stimulation may prove the point by momentarily increasing AV blockade and so uncovering the lurking F waves (Fig. 28-14). The next most common ratio is 4:1, especially after therapy with digitalis or propranolol. Ratios of 5:1, 3:1, and 1:1 are rare. Atrial flutter with 1:1 AV conduction should always be sus-

FIGURE 28-13 Atrial flutter. Note the "sawtooth" pattern in leads II and III with poorly registered atrial activity in leads I and V₆.

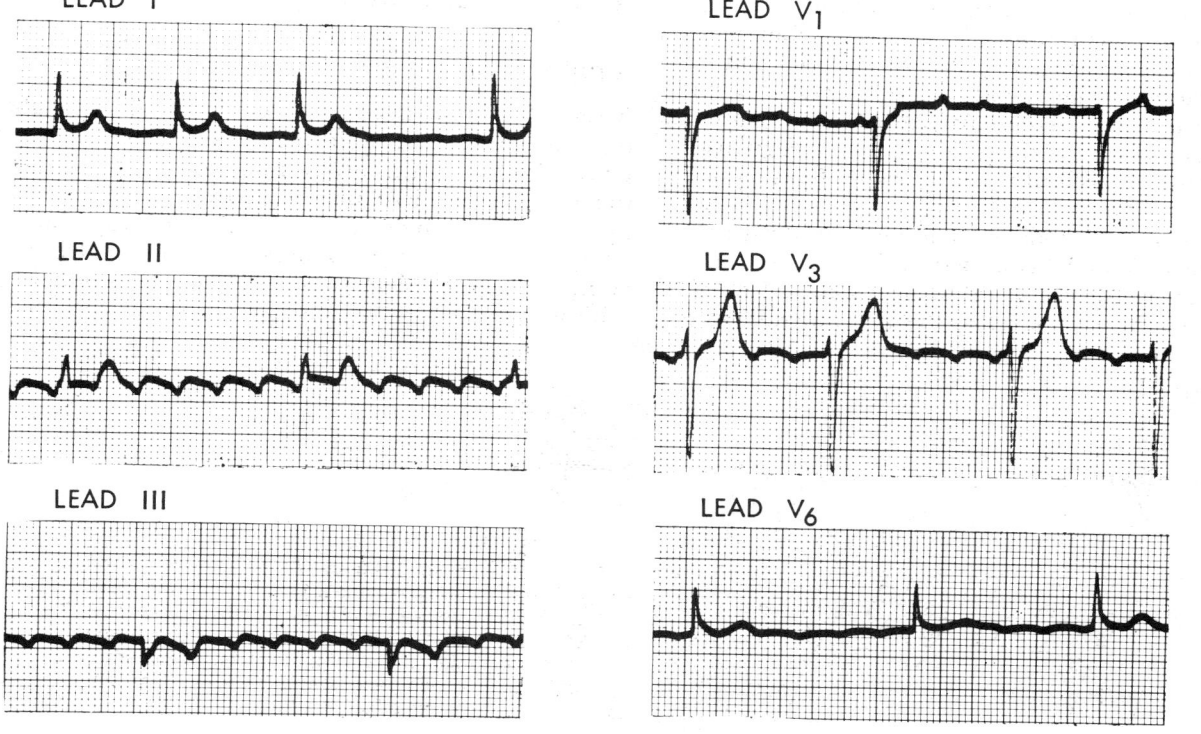

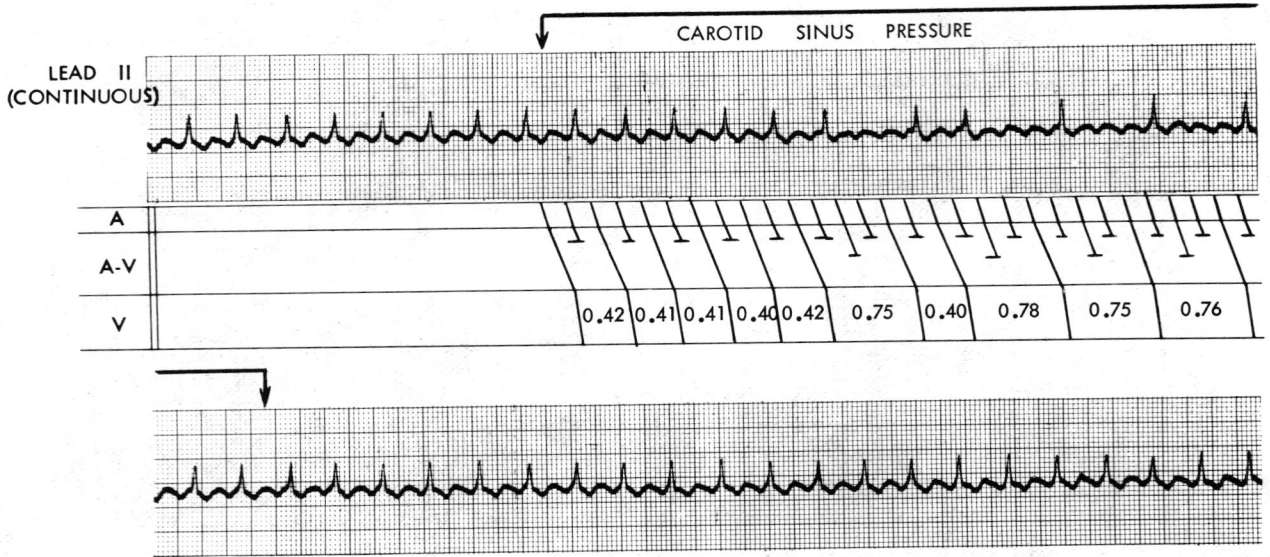

FIGURE 28-14   Atrial flutter. At the beginning of the strip there is the common 2:1 ratio, and flutter (F) waves can be suspected but not proved; however, after carotid sinus stimulation, the conduction ratio increases to 4:1 and the F waves are clearly exposed.

pected when a tachycardia with a rate in the neighborhood of 300 beats per minute is seen.

Atrial flutter with alternating 4:1 and 2:1 conduction is quite common and is a significant cause of bigeminal rhythm (Fig. 28-15). At times the ventricular complex ending the shorter RR interval shows aberration, and then ventricular bigeminy is simulated. This can be a dangerous situation if the patient is receiving digitalis to control the ventricular rate; often the simulation of ventricular bigeminy is thought to be due to digitalis intoxication and the drug is stopped, when, in fact, more digitalis may be indicated to increase the conduction ratio still further to a constant 4:1. A less common cause of bigeminal grouping is 3:2 conduction. Sometimes the AV ratio is variable (e.g., 2:1, 4:1, 5:1, 3:1, etc.), and then the utter irregularity of atrial fibrillation is mimicked (Fig. 28-16A). Such bizarre irregularity is probably due to "multilevel" block in the AV junction.[20]

Wenckebach periods are common in atrial flutter. When 4:1 and 2:1 conduction alternate, the condition is generally attributed to a constant 2:1 transmission at an upper level in the AV junction with 3:2 Wenckebach periods at a lower level (Fig. 28-15).[1]

Atrial flutter may be associated with complete AV block, in which case the slow but regular ventricular complexes are seen to vary their relation to the preceding F wave (Fig. 28-16B).

Because of "concealed conduction" of the atrial impulses that are constantly bombarding and penetrating the AV junction to varying levels, the FR interval of conducted beats (measured from the nadir of the F wave to the beginning of the QRS complex) is believed to be constantly prolonged, ranging between 0.26 and 0.46 s.[1]

Atrial Fibrillation

Atrial fibrillation exacts two hemodynamic penalties: the ineffective writhing of atrial muscle deprives the heart of its atrial transport function, and the incessant and irregular bombardment of the AV junction with numerous impulses excites rapid and irregular ventricular responses. In the heart already compromised by disease, these handicaps may be critical. Atrial fibrillation also predisposes to periph-

MONITOR   LEAD II

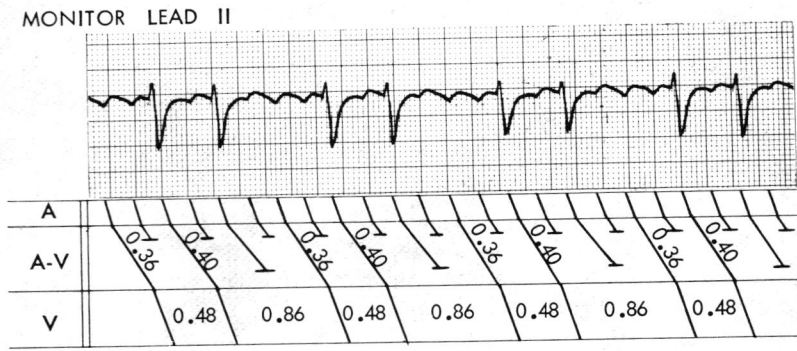

FIGURE 28-15   Atrial flutter with alternating 4:1 and 2:1 conduction. This common cause of bigeminal rhythm is almost always due to a basic 2:1 AV conduction high in the AV junction with 3:2 Wenckebach periods at a lower level (as diagrammed).

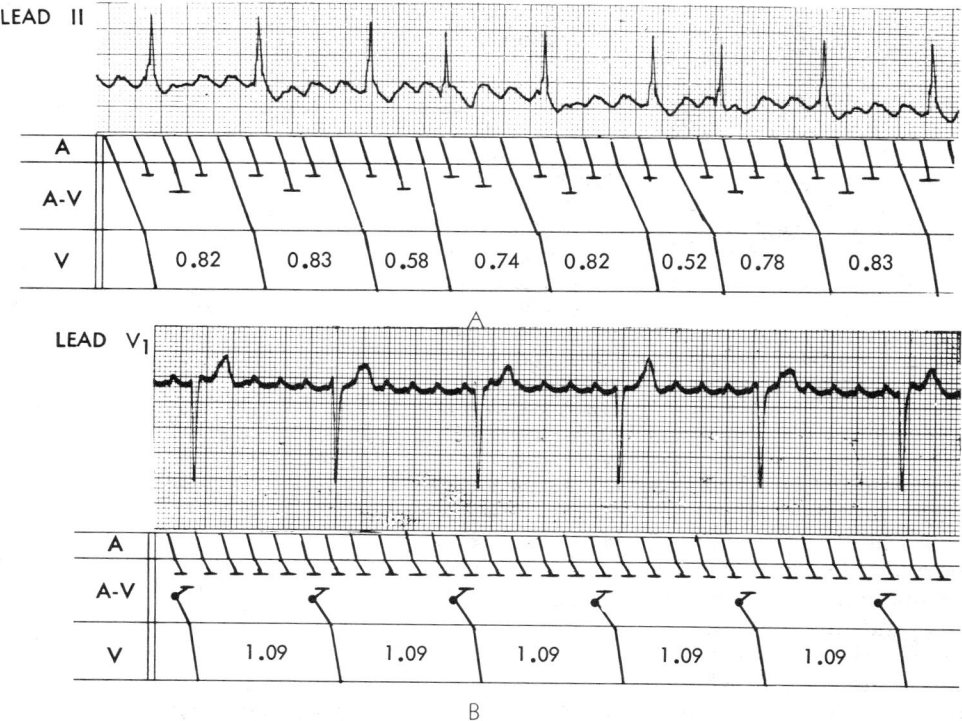

FIGURE 28-16 *A.* Atrial flutter with varying AV conduction, resulting in an irregular ventricular rhythm that mimics atrial fibrillation. *B.* Atrial flutter with high-grade AV block and resulting AV dissociation; note that the ventricular rhythm remains perfectly regular while the relation of the ventricular complexes to the F waves varies.

eral or pulmonary emboli. Approximately 30 percent of all persons with long-standing chronic atrial fibrillation experience at least one embolic episode during the course of the fibrillation. Some studies have indicated that atrial fibrillation is present in 90 percent of patients with mitral stenosis who have peripheral emboli.

Atrial fibrillation is a relatively common arrhythmia and is much more common than the other atrial tachyarrhythmias. It may occur in sustained or paroxysmal form. Atrial fibrillation usually draws attention to one of four diseases: rheumatic mitral disease, hypertension, ischemic heart disease, or thyrotoxicosis. It has a less common but well-recognized association with atrial septal defect, chronic lung disease, and constrictive pericarditis. The arrhythmia is reported in from 7 to 16 percent of continuously monitored patients with myocardial infarction. In susceptible persons with otherwise apparently normal hearts, the arrhythmia is occasionally precipitated by an alcoholic spree ("holiday heart").[21] Heart failure from any cause may initiate atrial fibrillation; on the other hand, the recent onset of fibrillation may precipitate failure in the diseased but otherwise well-compensated heart. It is occasionally found in apparently healthy persons, when it is called *lone fibrillation;* some of these may be due to occult thyrotoxicosis.[22]

Atrial fibrillation may be precipitated by an atrial extrasystole occurring in the vulnerable period of the atrial cycle; this is likely when the ectopic atrial

impulse is so early that the PP' cycle is less than half the preceding PP cycle. Factors which favor the development or perpetuation of fibrillation include an adequately increased mass of atrial muscle, increased vagal tone, and asynchrony (temporal dispersion) in the recovery curves of adjacent myocardial fibers.

Electrocardiographic Features

The cardinal features of atrial fibrillation in the ECG are (1) fibrillatory (f) waves of atrial activity and (2) an irregular ventricular response. Of the routine 12 leads, the best for identifying atrial activity is V_1; next best are leads II, III, and aV_F, and leads I, aV_L, and the left chest leads often show little sign of atrial activity. The fibrillatory waves may vary in amplitude from nothingness (Fig. 28-17A) to irregular waves the size of respectable flutter waves (Fig. 28-17B). Contrary to previous opinion, it is now believed that the f-wave amplitude does not correlate with either left atrial size or the type of heart disease.[23] When there is no sign of atrial activity, even in right precordial leads, yet the ventricular response is characteristically irregular, one may reasonably infer the diagnosis of ("straight-line") atrial fibrillation.

In uncomplicated atrial fibrillation, the QRS complexes are of normal configuration, though irregular, testifying to normal intraventricular conduction. It is important, however, to appreciate the fre-

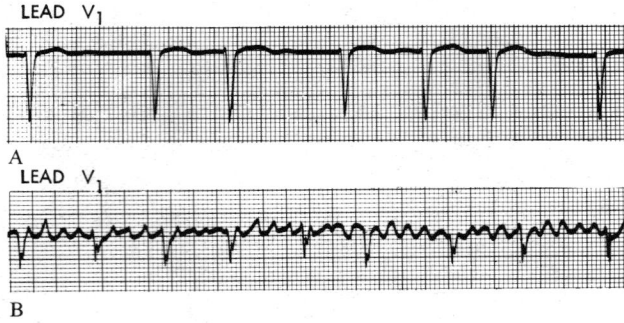

LEAD V₁

A

LEAD V₁

B

FIGURE 28-17 *A.* Atrial fibrillation leaving virtually no imprint on the base line ("straight-line" fibrillation). *B.* Coarse atrial fibrillation; the fibrillatory (f) waves are the size of respectable flutter waves but irregular.

quency of aberrant ventricular conduction. This is more difficult to identify in the presence of atrial fibrillation, since the diagnostic value of preceding atrial activity is lost. Its importance lies in the fact that aberrantly conducted beats may be mistaken for ectopic ventricular activity, and this may influence the physician to withhold digitalis when it is sorely needed or to give antiarrhythmic drugs when they are not needed and may even be contraindicated. Aberration is particularly likely to develop when a lengthening of the ventricular cycle is immediately followed by a short cycle; the beat ending the short cycle shows aberrant conduction (Fig. 28-18). This long cycle–short cycle sequence promoting aberration is often called *Ashman's phenomenon.*[24] Runs of consecutive aberrant beats may imitate ventricular tachycardia and so create a real therapeutic dilemma. Because the diagnostic assistance of a preceding P wave is obviated by fibrillating atria, in separating the aberration from ventricular ectopy special reliance has to be placed on the shape of the anomalous complexes.[25] Criteria that may be employed in differentiation, with their approximate relative values in differentiation, are summarized in Table 28-4.

FIGURE 28-18 Ashman's phenomenon. During atrial fibrillation, the beat ending a short cycle preceded by a relatively long cycle manifests aberrant ventricular conduction. In this example the aberrant beat shows typical RBBB-type aberration with rsR′ pattern and the initial deflection identical with that of the flanking conducted beats.

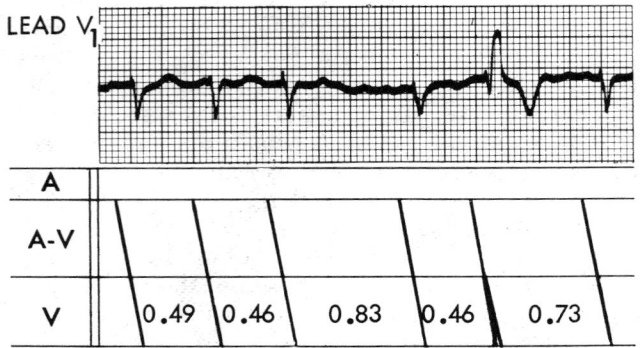

LEAD V₁

A				
A-V				
V	0.49	0.46	0.83	0.46	0.73

TABLE 28-4 Specificity Rating of Criteria for Aberration or Ectopy*

Criterion	Likelihood of Aberration	Likelihood of Ectopy
Right bundle branch block:		
rsR′ in V₁	4+	1+
R or qR in V₁		
With taller left peak	1+	4+
With taller right peak	2+	3+
qRs in V₆	3+	–
Left bundle branch block	2+	2+
Fixed coupling	1+	3+
Identical initial vector	3+	–
Long-short cycle sequence	4+	4+
Short-long cycle sequence	–	3+
Wide r in V₁	–	3+
Concordant positivity (V₁ to V₆)	+ (WPW)	3+
Concordant negativity (V₁ to V₆)	–	3+
Frontal axis −95 to −175	–	3+

*Notes: 4+, highly likely; 3+, often seen; 2+, not uncommon; 1+, not characteristic, but seen; −, unlikely.

Arrhythmias Complicating the Wolff-Parkinson-White (Preexcitation) Syndrome[26]

The predisposition of people with the Wolff-Parkinson-White syndrome to supraventricular arrhythmias is well known. There is evidence that atrial premature beats are seen more frequently in patients with WPW syndrome than in the general population, and there is no doubt that atrial fibrillation and atrial flutter affect a significant minority of these patients. Atrial flutter occurs in 5 percent, while atrial fibrillation has been found in 11 to 20 percent.[27] But the most common tachyarrhythmia to complicate the syndrome is a supraventricular tachycardia initiated by a premature beat and perpetuated by a circulating (reentering, reciprocating, circus-movement) wave front using both the accessory or bypass pathway and the AV junction—going down one and up the other.[28] Whether the QRS-T complex during the tachycardia is normal or wide and bizarre depends on which limb of the circuit is used as the downward pathway, the AV junction or the accessory bundle. The majority (85 percent) use the AV junction for the downward journey and consequently have narrow QRS complexes. Although most tachycardias make use of the anomalous pathway in one direction or the other, some reciprocal mechanisms are confined to the AV junction,[29] the atria, or the ventricle.[30] If surgical intervention is entertained, identification of the prevailing circuit obviously becomes crucial.

Some individuals have accessory pathways that will not conduct anterogradely so that they never manifest preexcitation during sinus rhythm; yet the accessory bundle may conduct retrogradely and provide a tailor-made circuit for a reentering tachycardia.

This situation has been called *concealed WPW* syndrome and is being reported with increasing frequency.[31–33] Again, if surgery is considered, the implications are obvious. Occasionally an unsuspected, underlying WPW syndrome may be unmasked by vagal stimulation or isoproterenol.[34]

When the QRS is wide, ventricular tachycardia may be closely simulated. During atrial fibrillation the accessory bundle may be used as the downward pathway, and the resulting wide, irregular ventricular complexes (Fig. 28-19) have often been mistaken for and published as ventricular tachycardia.

Ventricular premature beats are no more frequently seen in WPW patients than in the general population. True ventricular tachycardia has rarely been reported but is probably unrelated to the presence of the preexcitation syndrome. Ventricular fibrillation sometimes eventuates and may be the cause of death in some cases; it may develop because a descending impulse invades the ventricles during their vulnerable period, or it may be secondary to the hypoxia engendered by a frenetic ventricular rate approaching 300 beats per minute.

Since the anatomic matrix for preexcitation and its arrhythmias is congenital, it follows that its manifestations may affect all ages. Fortunately, most infants with the anatomic trait "outgrow" their tendency to develop tachyarrhythmias;[35] in one series[36] only 4 of 46 infants retained their predisposition to tachyarrhythmias into childhood and adolescence.

Sick-Sinus Syndrome

Under this catchy heading many authorities include any form of sinus nodal depression, including marked sinus bradycardia, prolonged sinus pauses, sinus arrest, or sinoatrial (SA) block (see next section), but the term is most often applied—although this application has been criticized as "inaccurate and inappropriate"[37]—to the tachycardia-bradycardia syndrome, in which bursts of an ectopic atrial tachyarrhythmia, often atrial fibrillation, alternate with prolonged periods of sinus nodal inertia and often AV junctional inertia as well. Apart from these florid signs of dysfunction, the syndrome may initially manifest itself as paroxysmal atrial fibrillation, as prolonged sinus inactivity following cardioversion or spontaneous reversion of atrial fibrillation, or as an inappropriate sinus rate, for instance in failure to develop adequate sinus acceleration with exercise or fever. Lone atrial fibrillation, at any age but particularly in youth, is most likely due to a sick sinus node, and intraatrial block or shifting atrial pacemaker may precede symptomatic sinus nodal disease by years. Although much more common in older age groups, the syndrome spares no decade, and it may be the cause of sudden death in young athletes.

Temporary and reversible manifestations of the syndrome may be induced by vagotonia, including that due to digitalis or subarachnoid hemorrhage, or by thyrotoxicosis, hyperpotassemia, quinidine, nicotine, beta blockers, or aerosol propellants. Such influences must always be excluded before diagnosing the chronic progressive syndrome, which may result from ischemic, rheumatic, or inflammatory disease; from involvement of the sinus node by pericarditis, one of the cardiomyopathies (especially amyloidosis), Friedreich's progressive muscular dystrophy, collagen disease, or metastatic disease; or from surgical injury. Apathy of the sinus node is sometimes familial and may accompany the prolonged QT syndrome. When it results from acute myocardial infarction, it is usually associated with occlusion of the right coronary or left circumflex artery. Some degree of dysfunction, usually an asymptomatic sinus bradycardia, complicates at least 50 percent of acute inferior infarctions. It is said that patients who develop serious sinus nodal dysfunction during myocardial infarction, despite complete recovery, should be followed indefinitely since later recurrence is not uncommon.[38]

Nevertheless, sinoatrial dysfunction appears to be a relatively benign malady. Shaw and coworkers[39] in a 10-year prospective survey found no significant difference in survival rates of patients with established or potential sick-sinus syndromes, whether paced or not, when compared with the normal population.

FIGURE 28-19 Atrial fibrillation with Wolff-Parkinson-White (WPW) conduction. Left, sinus rhythm with a typical preexcitation pattern. Right, persistence of the preexcitation pattern, the QRS axis having shifted to the left (as it often does with the development of tachycardia); the ventricular rhythm is now irregular at a rate well over 200. (*Courtesy of Dr. Arland A. Adams.*)

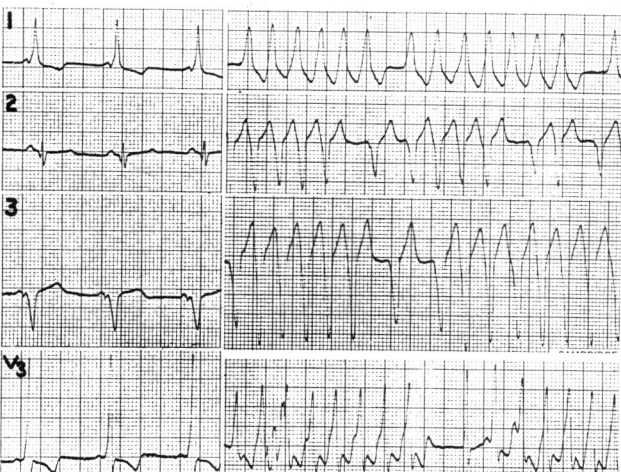

Electrocardiographic Features

At the time of examination, the tracing may be entirely normal or may show signs of the associated ischemic or other cardiac disease. The rhythm may be normal, or there may be evidence of sinus bradycardia, intraatrial block, or shifting atrial pace-maker. Sinus bradycardia or prolonged sinus pauses may alternate with runs of atrial tachycardia, flutter, or fibrillation. Sinus arrest or patterns of SA block may be recognized, and coexisting AV and interventricular blocks complicate the picture in a significant proportion of patients.

It is important to appreciate the fact that quite marked sinus bradycardia and prolonged sinus pauses (more than 1.75 s) are common occurrences in apparently healthy young adults.[40]

Diagnosis

Although the diagnosis of an ailing sinus node is sometimes easily made from the history, physical findings, and routine electrocardiogram, it often requires more sophisticated investigation. Continuous tape recording for 24 h by Holter monitor may be necessary, but this may also fail to record diagnostic stretches of sinus nodal dysfunction. At times the syndrome may be recognized only when evoked by provocative tests, such as failure to accelerate appropriately after an intravenous dose of 1 to 2 mg atropine or during titration with an intravenous drip of isoproterenol (1 to 2 mg per 500 ml). Atrial pacing at a rate of 120 to 140 beats per minute for 2 to 4 min may be necessary to demonstrate that the sinus node recovery time (SNRT), that is, the interval from the last paced P wave to the first returning sinus P wave, is inappropriately long.[41] A prolonged SNRT is good evidence of sinus dysfunction, but a normal SNRT by no means excludes a sick sinus. Sinoatrial conduction time (SACT) is an adjunctive but less sensitive test of sinus dysfunction.

Ventricular Arrhythmias

Ventricular Extrasystoles

The mechanisms of production of premature (extrasystolic) beats are not certainly known; theories of their genesis are discussed in Chap. 27. Since they bear a more or less constant time relation (coupling interval) to the preceding beat, it is assumed that they are in some way "forced" by it; when the coupling interval is almost unvaried, the relation is called *fixed coupling*. The allowable variation is about 0.04 s, although some authors are much more lenient and permit—erroneously, we think—much greater variation (up to 0.12 s)[42] to qualify as "fixed."

Ventricular extrasystoles are the most common form of rhythm disturbance, both in health and in disease. Hiss[7] found them in 0.8 percent of 122,000 asymptomatic Air Force personnel ranging in age from 16 to over 50 years; they are recorded in the majority of continuously monitored patients with acute myocardial infarction, but they were also found in the majority (62 percent) of 300 actively

employed middle-aged men monitored for a period of 6 h.[43] In some apparently normal persons, ventricular extrasystoles may persist, even in the form of bigeminy, for many years. On the other hand, they may result from any form of heart disease and are frequently due to overdigitalization. They commonly accompany heart failure; in this situation digitalis may eliminate them. Since potassium depletion also favors them, digitalis-induced extrasystoles are especially likely to appear after diuresis with kaliuretic preparations. They may result from hypocalcemia and from caffeine, tobacco, alcohol, and any of the sympathomimetic drugs—epinephrine, isoproterenol, and amphetamine (even in the form of nose drops, sprays, or inhalers). Hypoxia is a potent cause of ventricular extrasystoles, as in anesthesia, especially with cyclopropane. They may develop as a result of infectious diseases, visceral reflexes (e.g., from a diseased gallbladder), or psychic stimuli. Vagal stimulation and exercise, even in some normal persons,[44] may elicit them. Ventricular extrasystoles are claimed to develop in about 33 percent of apparently healthy men and in about 15 percent of normal women with exercise.[45] Although ventricular premature beats may be evoked by exercise in the normal subject, it has been claimed that if the axis of the extrasystole is markedly superior it may furnish evidence of ischemic heart disease.[46] They have been reported in 45 percent of patients with

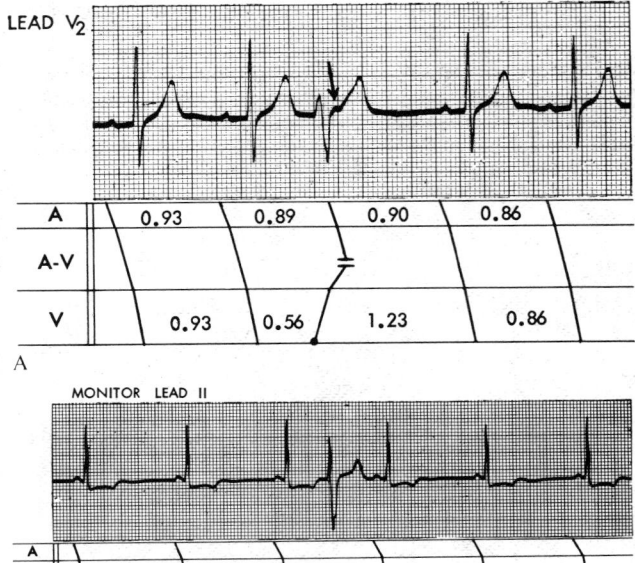

FIGURE 28-20 *A.* Ventricular premature beat. The third beat is wide and bizarre—quite unlike the QRS-T pattern of the sinus beats—and, since the sinus rhythm is undisturbed (next sinus P wave indicated by arrow), the postextrasystolic pause is compensatory. *B.* The fourth beat is an interpolated ventricular premature beat; it is sandwiched between two consecutive sinus beats.

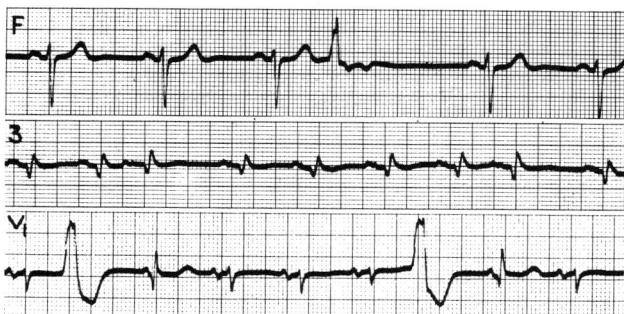

FIGURE 28-21 Exceptions to the rules for compensatory pauses. *Top.* Ventricular extrasystole with less-than-compensatory pause. Retrograde conduction to the atria (retrograde P wave deforms first part of ST segment) discharges the sinus pacemaker early and so shortens the postextrasystolic cycle. *Middle.* Atrial premature beat followed by fully compensatory pause. The third and eighth beats are atrial extrasystoles but, presumably because they suppress the sinus pacemaker, are followed by compensatory pauses. *Bottom.* Ventricular extrasystoles with less-than-compensatory pauses. Each postextrasystolic cycle ends in an escape beat and so is slightly less than compensatory.

mitral valve prolapse.[13] Total abstinence from smoking and caffeine with a reduction in alcohol intake and a program of physical conditioning failed to affect the frequency or occurrence of ventricular extrasystoles in apparently healthy men with persistent and frequent premature beats.[47]

Ventricular extrasystoles have prognostic implications for patients who have recovered from acute myocardial infarction. Of more than 2000 patients who had survived infarction by 3 months or more, 11.5 percent had ventricular premature beats in a resting electrocardiogram containing 50 beats.[48] The 3-year mortality was twice as great (22 percent) in those who had *any* ventricular extrasystoles as in those with none (11 percent). In another study[49] sudden cardiac death was six times more common in coronary patients who had frequent ventricular premature beats as in those who had few or none.

Electrocardiographic Features

Since the impulse of a ventricular extrasystole originates in one of the ventricles and spreads anomalously, the QRS complex is wide and bizarre as well as premature. If the focus of origin is in the septum near the bifurcation of the bundle, the QRS may be little widened and only slightly deformed. Rosenbaum postulates that such beats arise from proximal segments of the main intraventricular conduction fascicles (fascicular beats).[50] The ST-T segment usually points in a direction opposite to the terminal portion of the QRS. Most ventricular premature beats do not disturb the rhythm of the sinus node and are therefore followed by a compensatory pause or cycle (Fig. 28-20A); or they may be interpolated between two consecutive sinus beats (Fig. 28-20B). On the other hand, it is quite common for the ectopic impulse to be conducted retrogradely into the atria and to inscribe a retrograde P' wave on the ST segment (Fig. 28-21), usually 0.12 to 0.20 s after the

beginning of the QRS complex.[51] If the sinus node is discharged ahead of schedule by the retrograde impulse, the following pause may be less than compensatory. Most ventricular extrasystoles maintain a constant coupling interval (fixed coupling), not varying by more than 0.04 s, in contrast with parasystolic beats, whose coupling intervals typically vary. Some ventricular premature beats, however, manifest marked variation in coupling, yet do not conform with the criteria for parasystole. Although ventricular extrasystoles are commonly found in normal hearts, when the ectopic QRS complex is unduly wide (more than 0.16 s) or splintered, it is presumptive evidence of heart disease.

In the majority of ventricular ectopic beats, the ventricle of origin can be inferred from the polarity of the ectopic complex in a right chest lead such as V_1 (predominantly positive = *left* ventricular, predominantly negative = *right* ventricular). It is claimed that organic heart disease is the rule in people with left ventricular extrasystoles, and that when extrasystoles affect persons without heart disease, they are almost invariably right ventricular.[52]

If an impulse arises in the Purkinje network of, say, the anterior fascicle of the left bundle branch, it presumably reaches the myocardium supplied by that fascicle sooner than it can spread retrogradely to and down the posterior fascicle and the right bundle branch. Depending upon the respective distances involved and the rates of propagation anterogradely and retrogradely, it writes a QRS pattern resembling less or more complete right bundle branch block with left posterior hemiblock. Similarly, an impulse arising in the territory of the posterior fascicle writes a pattern resembling less or more complete right bundle branch block with left anterior hemiblock.[53] Such beats, usually somewhat narrower than full-fledged ectopic ventricular beats, are now often alluded to as *fascicular* beats.[54]

The dangerous potential of early ventricular extrasystoles (R on T) has been frequently stressed. But in one series of 20 consecutive patients with ventricular fibrillation complicating acute myocardial infarction, 11 were initiated by "late" extrasystoles.[55] Moreover, it was found that pairs and runs of ventricular ectopic beats after myocardial infarction were initiated more often by late than by early beats.[56]

Ventricular Tachycardia

Three or more ectopic ventricular beats, occurring at a rate equivalent to more than 100 per minute, constitute a run of ventricular tachycardia (VT). Paroxysms of VT usually begin with a coupled (forced) ventricular premature beat—*extrasystolic* VT. Some of these may be perpetuated by rapid firing of a single ectopic focus; others, by a circulating wave front using a microscopic Purkinje circuit (microreentry) of a wider sweep involving fascicular pathways (macroreentry). The paroxysm may begin with an ectopic beat that is or is not closely coupled to the preceding beat; if there are repeated paroxysms beginning with variation in the initial coupling interval, and if the interectopic interval between the last beat of a paroxysm and the first beat of the next paroxysm is a multiple of the ventricular cycle during the tachycardia, it is a *parasystolic* VT.

It is well established, both experimentally and clinically, that an impulse reaching the ventricles in their "vulnerable" period can initiate a repetitive response in the form of VT, flutter, or fibrillation. The initiating impulse may be an endogenous ectopic ventricular impulse, a descending supraventricular impulse, or an artificial, extrinsic electric impulse of sufficient magnitude. Nevertheless, more recent studies have documented the fact that many, if not most, paroxysms of VT are initiated by late-coupled ventricular extrasystoles.[57] In one series, only 6 of 44 (14 percent) paroxysms began with R on T.[58] Others noted that many late-coupled extrasystoles that initiated VT fell on the P wave, suggesting that atrial contraction producing myocardial stretch might be the trigger.[59]

VT almost always affects a diseased heart, although it has rarely been described in apparently normal ones. Lesch was able to collect 34 such cases.[60] Only one three-beat burst was found among the more than 67,000 asymptomatic Air Force personnel screened by Hiss.[61] Six of seventeen young patients with VT had no recognizable heart disease.[62] In another small series, 10 percent of the patients had no demonstrable heart disease, while ischemia (71 percent) and rheumatic disorders (12 percent) were the most common pathologic associations. VT has been reported in 6 percent of patients with mitral valve prolapse,[12] and indeed malignant refractory ventricular tachyarrhythmias have complicated this "syndrome."[63] Among contin-

uously monitored patients with acute myocardial infarction, the reported incidence ranges from 6 to 28 percent. On the other hand, among 52 men Holter-monitored for 24 h during the first 2 days of an acute infarction, VT was detected in 24 (46 percent).[64]

Intractable VT sometimes complicates a ventricular aneurysm resulting from myocardial infarction. Undoubtedly the arrhythmia can complicate any form of heart disease; examples have been reported in sarcoidosis, hypertrophic cardiomyopathy,[65] and myxedema coma undergoing treatment. Numerous drugs, including digitalis, quinidine, procainamide, sympathetic amines, papaverine, potassium, intravenous mercurials, chloroform, and cyclopropane, have been incriminated. Runs of VT are frequently induced at cardiac catheterization and often follow in the wake of countershock; less often the arrhythmia may be caused by a malfunctioning ("runaway") artificial pacemaker or by one delivering its stimulus in the vulnerable phase of a competitive natural beat.

Runs of VT are sometimes initiated by a simple change of posture—standing up (orthostatic tachycardia) or lying down. Exercise or emotional excitement may bring one on. Vagal stimulation sometimes evokes a run of ectopic ventricular beats.

Electrocardiographic Features
The ventricular complex is wide and bizarre, recurs regularly at a rate of over 100 beats per minute (usually between 150 and 200 but may approach 300), and gives the appearance of a run of ventricular premature beats. If the onset is observed, the paroxysm may be seen to begin with a coupled ventricular extrasystole. In perhaps 20 percent of cases, independent P waves will be discernible (Fig. 28-22A), and in a smaller percentage retrograde P waves (Fig. 28-22B) may be found in the surface

FIGURE 28-22 *A.* Ventricular tachycardia with regular independent P waves (indicated by arrows). *B.* Ventricular tachycardia with retroconduction to atria (retrograde P waves indicated by arrows). *C.* Ventricular tachycardia with fusion (Dressler's) beats—indicated by arrows. Note the sinus P wave preceding each fusion beat.

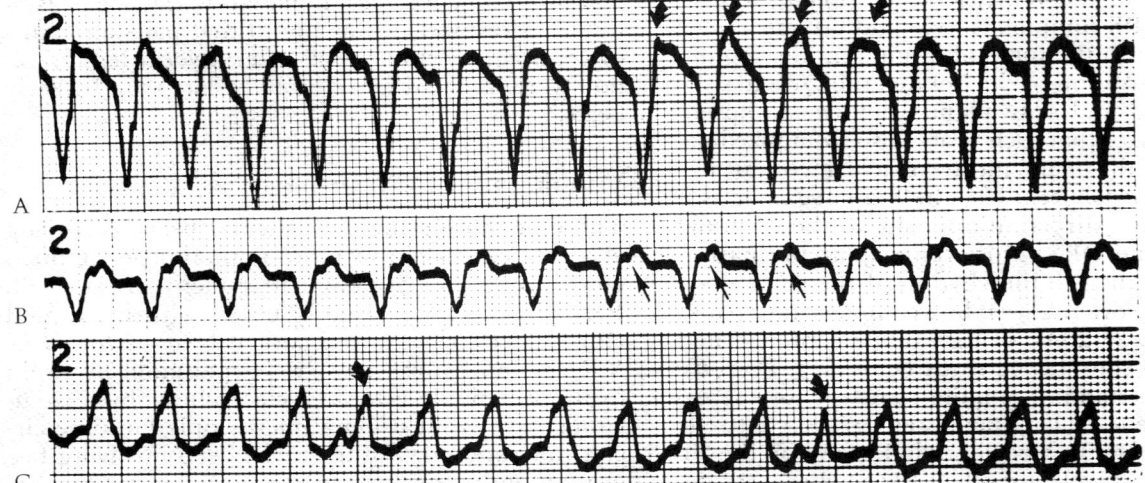

tracing. Occasionally retrograde conduction occurs with Wenckebach periodicity or in a 2:1 ratio. If it is important to record atrial activity, an esophageal or intracardiac electrode will invariably capture it. With intracardiac recordings, independent atrial activity and retrograde conduction to the atria were each found in about half of 70 cases studied.[66] One should stress that independent atrial activity does *not* prove that the tachycardia is of ventricular origin, but it increases the probability.

The presence of fusion beats is helpful, but they are likely to be seen only if the rate is relatively slow (i.e., 150 or less). They are due to partial capture of the ventricles by an opportunistic sinus impulse (Fig. 28-22C). Such beats are always on time or slightly early—never late.

In recognition of the VT, the shape of the ventricular complexes is often helpful; the morphologic probabilities are, of course, the same as for ventricular premature beats, which were described earlier in this chapter and are summarized in Table 28-5. If an rsR′ variant is present in V_1, the rhythm is probably not VT. On the other hand, a dominant monophasic R in all chest leads (Fig. 28-23A)—provided preexcitation can be excluded—or a totally negative (QS) complex in all chest leads (Fig. 28-23B) is much more likely to indicate an ectopic ventricular rather than an aberrant mechanism.

Until 1978, the morphologic clues in use for more than a decade were based only upon clinical observation and deduction. Wellens and coworkers[66] retrospectively examined the morphology of the ventricular complex in 140 patients with wide-QRS tachycardias (70 with VT and 70 with supraventricular tachycardia with ventricular aberration proven by intracardiac recordings) and confirmed the validity of the clues just described. In an ongoing prospective study,[67] they have since been able to diagnose over 90 percent of wide-QRS tachycardias correctly from the clinical surface tracing *before* establishing the diagnosis with intracardiac recordings.

Several variants of VT are worth noting. When the rate is unusually rapid and the pattern a continuous regular zigzag without clear definition of QRS

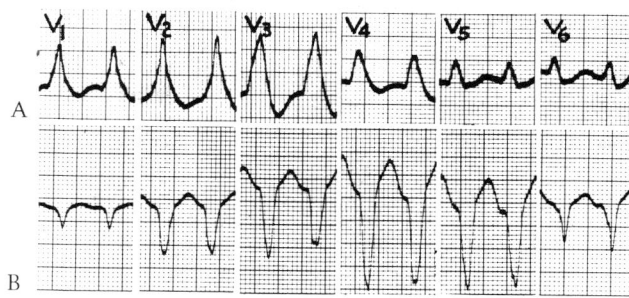

FIGURE 28-23 Ventricular tachycardia with concordant QRS complexes across precordium: all upright in *A;* all negative in *B.*

complexes and T waves (Fig. 28-24), the term *ventricular flutter* is sometimes applied; it is frequently an intermediary between tachycardia and fibrillation. Sometimes relatively brief runs of tachycardia (Fig. 28-25) are separated by one or two sinus beats, and the term *repetitive tachycardia* applies. This is usually a relatively benign form of the arrhythmia and is sometimes found in hearts without evident disease. *Bidirectional tachycardia* is the term used when the ventricular complexes alternate in polarity (Fig. 28-26A). It usually carries an ominous prognosis and is often associated with digitalis intoxication. When the ventricular complexes alternate in height but have the same polarity, some call it *alternating tachycardia*. The distinction between bidirectional and alternating tachycardia is far from complete, since in the same paroxysm in the same patient the contour is often "bidirectional" in one lead but "alternating" in another.

Torsade de pointes ("twisting of the points") is a term used for the "swinging" pattern when the polarity of the ectopic QRS complex swings from positive to negative and vice versa (Fig. 28-26B). It is of importance because it may presage ventricular fibrillation, and type I drugs such as quinidine are reportedly dangerous.[68] When the QRS complex in VT manifests many shapes, the terms *pleomorphic*[69] and *polymorphous*[70] have both been applied. Such paroxysms are most likely to develop in the presence of severe myocardial disease when the QT interval has been prolonged by drugs.[70] Despite their variegation, pleomorphic beats may be shown to arise from a single center.[69]

Accelerated Idioventricular Rhythm

When an ectopic ventricular pacemaker discharges at a rate of less than 100 beats per minute and con-

TABLE 28-5 Electrocardiographic Recognition of Ventricular Tachycardia*

V_1	V_6	Probability†
rsR′	Rs or qRs	AVC
rsR′	rS	AVC
qR or R	Rs or qRs	AVC
qR or R	rS or QS	Ect
qR or R	R	Ect (unless WPW)
QS	QS	Ect
QS or rS	R	Either

*Morphologic probabilities in V_1/V_6.
†*Notes:* AVC = aberrant ventricular conduction; Ect = ectopic ventricular.

FIGURE 28-24 Ventricular flutter. Note the regular zigzag pattern without definite QRS-T formation at a rate of 172.

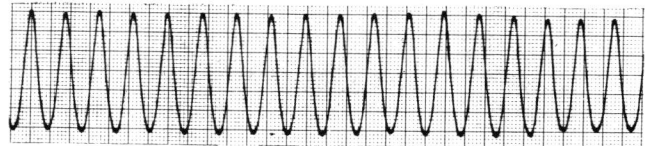

DISORDERS OF THE CARDIOVASCULAR SYSTEM

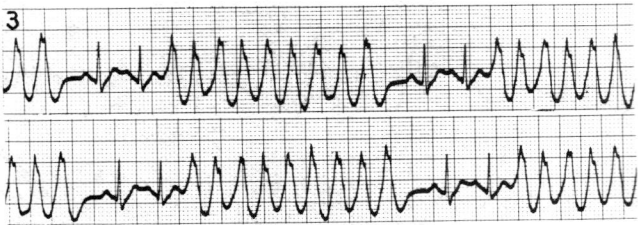

FIGURE 28-25 Repetitive ventricular tachycardia. The strips are continuous. Note that the tachycardia recurs in short nine-beat bursts separated by pairs of sinus beats.

trols only the ventricles, it is called *idioventricular.* When the idioventricular rate exceeds 45 to 50 but is less than 100 beats per minute (Fig. 28-27), it must be considered abnormal for that site of impulse formation. By definition, it is not a tachycardia and is best referred to as *accelerated idioventricular rhythm,* though such terms as *idioventricular tachycardia, nonparoxysmal ventricular tachycardia,* and *slow ventricular tachycardia* have been applied. Such rhythms received scant attention before the coronary care era, but are now recorded with surprising frequency in series of patients with acute myocardial infarction who are continuously monitored. These slower ventricular rhythms are, in fact, as common as true ventricular tachycardia, being recognized in 15 to 20 percent of patients after acute myocardial infarction, especially of the inferior wall.

The ectopic rate is often similar to the prevailing sinus rate, and these rhythms therefore usually appear because of slight slowing of the sinus pacemaker or slight acceleration of the ectopic center. They often begin with a fusion beat or two, produce a short run of isorhythmic dissociation,[71] and then surrender control once more to the sinus pacemaker. Occasionally, instead of dissociation, retrograde conduction to the atria develops. A few of

these rhythms are parasystolic, but most are not. Some possibly represent an underlying ventricular tachycardia with exit block. Most runs are short-lived, lasting for only 3 to 30 beats.

As a rule, these accelerated idioventricular rhythms are benign and have been found even in healthy children.[72] They usually require no treatment, even after myocardial infarction, unless the loss of atrial transport function consequent to the AV dissociation compromises the patient's hemodynamic status. Rarely, accelerated idioventricular rhythm is associated with more serious ventricular arrhythmias.[73,74]

Parasystole

Parasystole (from the Greek *para,* "beside") is an independent, ectopic rhythm that operates alongside the primary rhythm and whose pacemaker enjoys neighborhood protection from invasion by outside impulses; its behavior is analogous to that of a fixed-rate artificial pacemaker. Because the ectopic pace-making center is "protected," it is able to maintain its rhythm without interruption.

Parasystole is not as uncommon as used to be thought. In 1963 Scherf was able to collect only 51 examples of the arrhythmia, but many more cases have been reported since then. Most of the reported cases have been found in diseased hearts, but it is probable that parasystole, particularly the supraventricular varieties, may occur in normal persons. The parasystolic center is usually ventricular; it is atrial or AV junctional much less commonly.

Electrocardiographic Features

There are two cardinal features of the ectopic beats of parasystole: (1) variation in coupling intervals and (2) a common denominator in the interectopic

LEAD V6

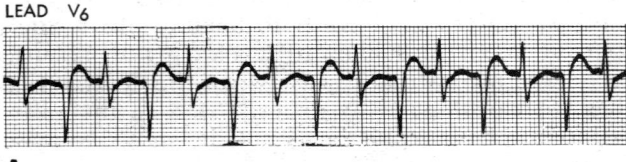

A

FIGURE 28-26 Bidirectional or alternating tachycardia. The tachycardia is regular at a rate of 160, but the form of the QRS-T complexes alternates. *B.* Torsade de pointes, a dangerous form of ventricular tachycardia in which the polarity of the ventricular complexes swings between positive and negative.

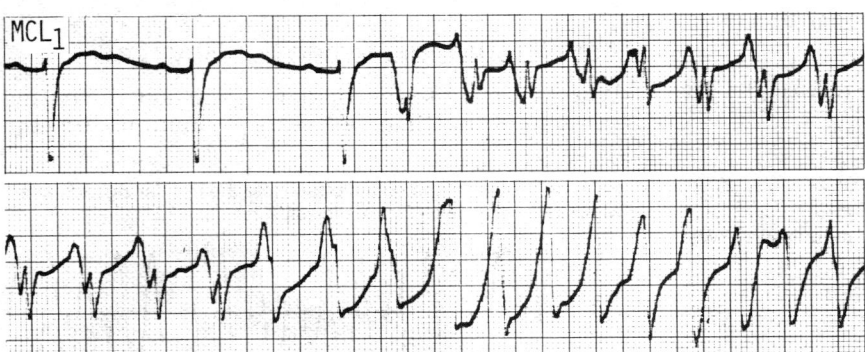

B

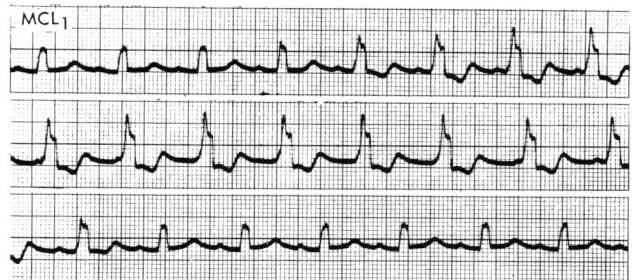

FIGURE 28-27 Accelerated idioventricular rhythm, rate 85. After three sinus beats conducted with right bundle branch block, an ectopic left ventricular pacemaker gradually takes over—via three fusion beats—gaining full control of the ventricles by the end of the top strip. Note that the ectopic beats have a tall left peak ("rabbit ear") characteristic of left ventricular ectopy. In the bottom strip, the sinus pacemaker regains control. (The strips are continuous.)

intervals (Fig. 28-28). The variation in coupling is a sign that the beats represent an independent mechanism, i.e., they are not dependent beats; the mathematic relation of the interectopic intervals testifies to the protection, which prevents their rhythm from being interrupted. The steps in diagnosis are usually (1) noticing that the coupling interval is variable and (2) measuring the interectopic intervals

and disclosing a common denominator. Fusion beats are commonly seen (Fig. 28-28). The *manifest* rate of most parasystolic pacemakers is slow, usually in the neighborhood of 20 to 60 beats per minute, but much faster rates are sometimes seen.

Because the manifest rate of parasystolic rhythms is often about half that of most sinus rhythms, parasystole may produce a form of ventricular bigeminy in which the coupling intervals progressively shorten or lengthen for a few couplets. On rare occasions a true extrasystolic ventricular bigeminy may alternate with runs of parasystolic rhythm from the same ectopic center.

In supraventricular parasystole, the P waves, or unchanged QRS complex manifest a changing relationship to the beats of the dominant rhythm; and the interectopic intervals between consecutive parasystolic complexes demonstrate a common denominator.

Aberrant Ventricular Conduction

Aberrant ventricular conduction (ventricular aberration or aberrancy), first described by Lewis in 1910, is the *temporary* abnormal intraventricular con-

FIGURE 28-28 Ventricular parasystole. The strips are continuous. Note (1) that the interval between an ectopic beat and the preceding sinus beat varies; (2) that the interectopic intervals all have a common denominator of 0.95 s; and (3) occasional fusion beats (third beat in top strip; fourth beat in second strip; last beat in bottom strip). (*From J. W. Hurst and R. Myerburg, "Introduction to Electrocardiography," McGraw-Hill Book Company, New York, 1973. Reproduced with permission.*)

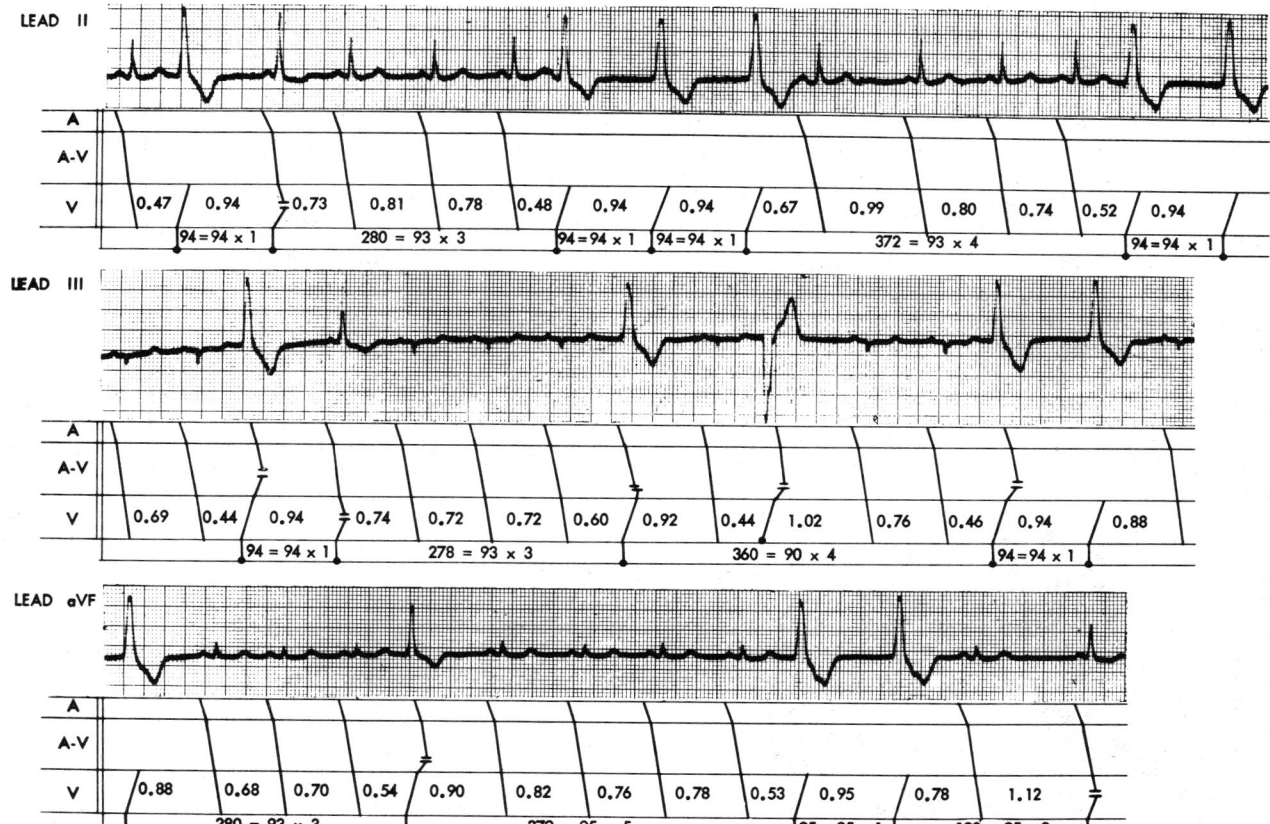

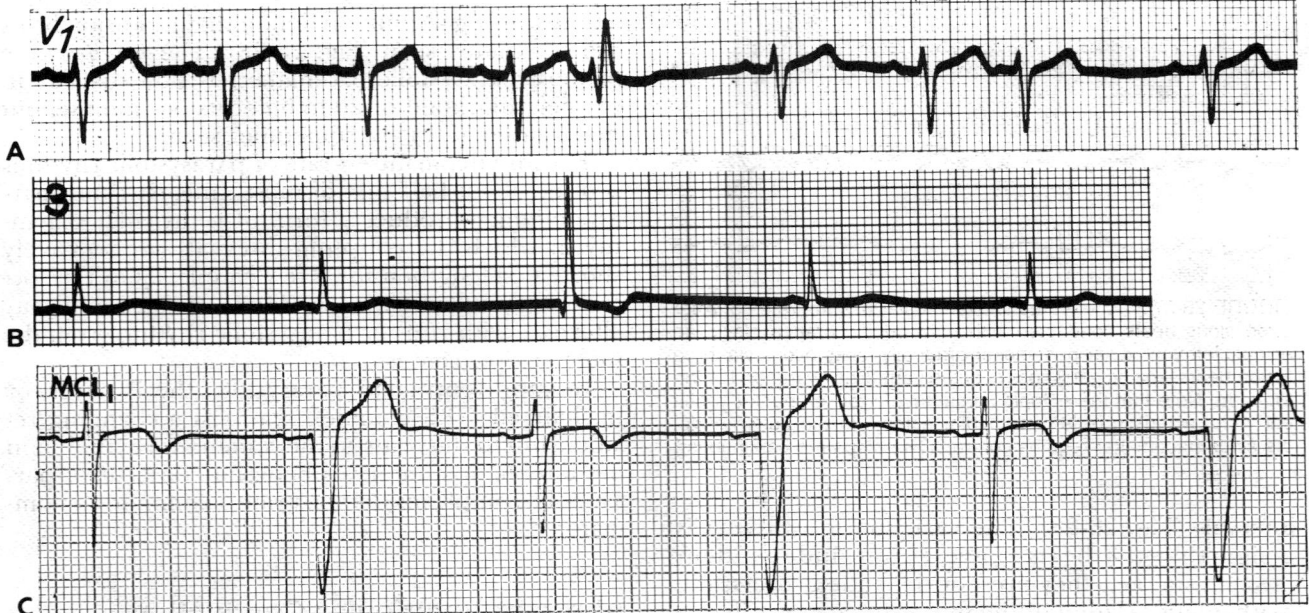

FIGURE 28-29 The three forms of ventricular aberration. *A.* The fifth beat is an atrial extrasystole with RBBB aberration. This is the common form due to an early impulse finding a fascicle still refractory. *B.* The third beat, although one cannot exclude a "fascicular" origin, is probably a junctional beat conducted aberrantly because it arises from an eccentric focus. *C.* Paradoxical critical rate (?phase 4) aberration: only the beats that end the slightly *longer* cycles are conducted with LBBB.

duction of supraventricular impulses. There are three forms of aberration: the common form develops when a supraventricular impulse arrives at some point in the ventricular conduction system that is still refractory. This form is therefore associated with early impulses and is the form we are most concerned with in differentiating aberration from ventricular ectopy (Fig. 28-29*A*). It complicates supraventricular extrasystoles (and other causes of early beats, such as ventricular captures and reciprocal beats) and supraventricular tachycardias (Fig. 28-30); it can be a particularly treacherous mimic during atrial fibrillation (Fig. 28-31), when it is often called Ashman's phenomenon. This form occasionally occurs, not because the aberrant beat is early, but because the *previous* cycle has unexpectedly lengthened, thereby prolonging the ensuing refrac-

tory period of the conduction system. The most common form of aberration is right bundle branch block (RBBB). By experimentally producing ventricular aberration with progressively premature atrial stimulations, Kulbertus[75] obtained the patterns listed in Table 28-6.

The second form of aberration is due to anomalous conduction above the ventricles, leading to maldistribution within the ventricles (Fig. 28-29*B*). Since this form of aberration is not dependent upon refractoriness, it is independent of cycle length and may be found in early, late, or punctual beats. The most obvious example of this form of aberration results from preexcitation in which the ventricular complex is distorted because anomalous conduction at a supraventricular level (accessory pathway) produces an unorthodox sequence of activation in the

FIGURE 28-30 The beginning of two paroxysms of atrial tachycardia with aberrant ventricular conduction simulating ventricular tachycardia. Each paroxysm starts with a telltale premature P′ wave (arrow).

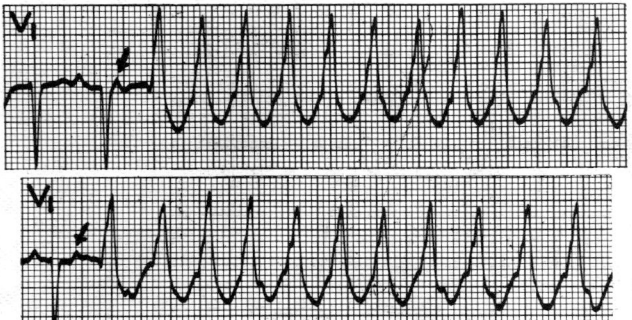

FIGURE 28-31 Atrial fibrillation complicated by aberrant ventricular conduction. The beats that end the shortest ventricular cycles (0.28 to 0.32 s) present anomalous, widened complexes. These almost certainly represent a right bundle branch block (RBBB) type of ventricular aberration rather than ventricular ectopy. Note that the cycle preceding the onset of the salvos of anomalous beats is relatively long (0.54 and 0.50 s) in accordance with Ashman's phenomenon (see Fig. 28-18).

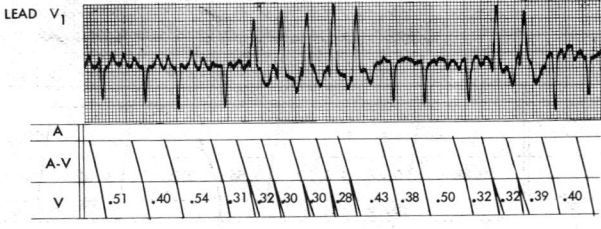

TABLE 28-6   Patterns of Induced Aberration*[75]

RBBB alone	28
RBBB + LAHB	21
RBBB + LPHB	12
LAHB alone	17
LPHB alone	10
LBBB	10
ILBBB	6
Unclassified	12
	116

i.e:	RBBB	= 53%
	LAHB	= 32%
	LPHB	= 19%
	LBBB	= 15 %
	Unclassified	= 10%

*Note: RBBB = right bundle branch block; LAHB = left anterior hemiblock; LPHB = left posterior hemiblock; LBBB = left bundle branch block; ILBBB = incomplete left bundle branch block.

ventricles. This second form of aberration is frequently seen in AV junctional beats when they arise eccentrically in the junction and spread "preferentially," either via a Mahaim tract or asynchronously down the bundle branches.

The third form of aberration results from lengthening of the ventricular cycle and may be due to (phase 4) spontaneous depolarization of a conducting fascicle. In this form, only late beats are aberrant (Fig. 28-29C), and the term *paradoxical critical rate* or *bradycardia-dependent bundle branch block* may be applicable.

Differentiation of Ventricular Premature Beats from Supraventricular Beats with Aberrant Ventricular Conduction

The ventricular extrasystole is often morphologically indistinguishable from an aberrant beat, but there are a number of clues that may help us to separate them.

Preceding Ectopic P Wave

The presence of a preceding ectopic P (P') wave (Figs. 28-29A, 28-30, and 28-32A) is excellent evidence favoring conduction with aberration, although one cannot always exclude the coincidence of simultaneous atrial ventricular premature beats.

Postextrasystolic Pause

More often than not the postextrasystolic pause is fully compensatory after a ventricular premature beat (Fig. 28-20A) and less than compensatory after a supraventricular beat (Figs. 28-29A and 28-32A); but the postextrasystolic cycle length is not entirely reliable (see exceptions below).

Second in the Row

When only the second in a row of rapidly consecutive beats is anomalous (Fig. 28-32B), it is more likely aberrant than an isolated ventricular ectopic beat.

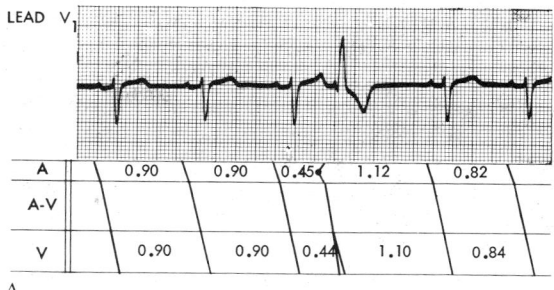

A

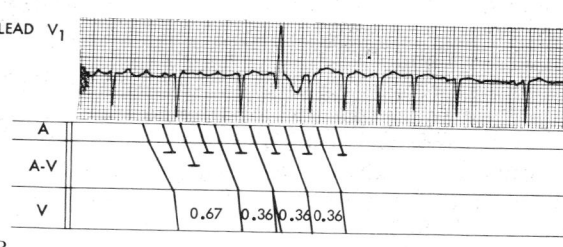

B

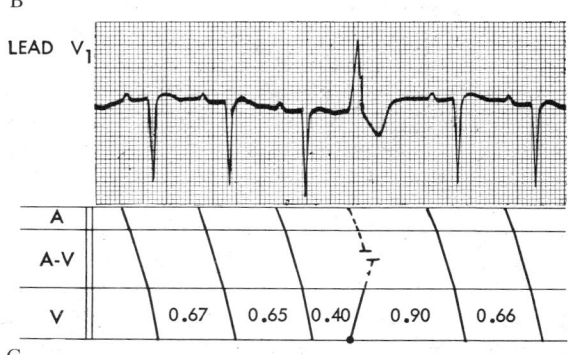

C

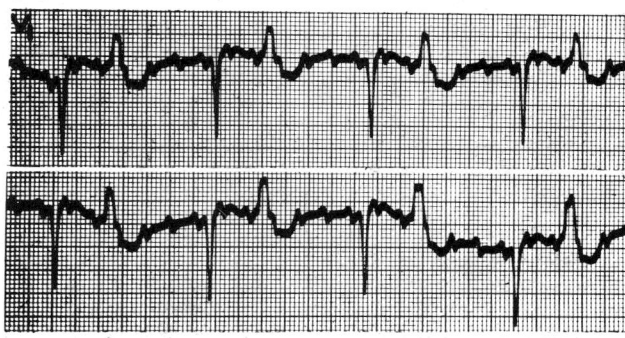

D

FIGURE 28-32   A. Atrial premature beat with ventricular aberration. Note the premature P' wave peaking the T wave of the third beat and followed by a wide, triphasic (rsR') complex; the ensuing cycle is less than compensatory. B. The fourth beat looks like a ventricular premature beat; but, since it is the second of a group of rapid beats, it is more likely aberrantly conducted than ectopic ventricular. (The basic rhythm is as diagrammed: atrial flutter with 4:1 conduction changing to 2:1, with aberration of the beat that ends the first short cycle.) C. Ventricular premature beat. Note the monophasic R-wave pattern and compensatory pause. D. Atrial flutter with alternating 4:1 and 2:1 conduction; the beats ending the shorter cycles show ventricular aberration and so simulate ventricular bigeminy.

QRS Morphology

Right ventricular ectopic beats simulate a *left* bundle branch block (LBBB) pattern, and indeed these two mutual mimics may be indistinguishable. However, there are a few clues that sometimes help: It is rare for supraventricular beats with LBBB to be associated with right axis deviation, whereas right ventricular ectopic beats frequently have right axis deviation. In LBBB, if there is an initial r wave in V_1, it is almost invariably narrow, whereas in right ventricular ectopic beats such an initial r wave is often wide (0.04 s or more). Finally, the deepest negative QRS complex in the precordial leads in LBBB is almost always found between V_1 and V_3, whereas in right ventricular ectopic beats the deepest negative complex is frequently in V_4 or V_5.[76]

Left ventricular ectopic beats simulate a *right* BBB pattern, but there are several points that help to distinguish them.[77,78] In lead V_1 the ventricular ectopic beats are usually diphasic (qR) or monophasic (R), whereas the aberrant beat of RBBB type is often triphasic and of rsR' form (Fig. 28-32A). Moreover, when the aberrant beat *is* diphasic or monophasic, it almost always reaches its peak relatively late, whereas the ectopic beat often (in about 55 percent of cases) reaches an early peak (Fig. 28-32C).

The great majority of ventricular ectopic beats have an initial deflection that obviously differs from that of the conducted beats (Fig. 28-32C).

Varying Degrees of the Same BBB Pattern

Differing degrees of the same BBB pattern correlated with variations in the coupling intervals (the shorter the coupling, the greater the degree of block) undoubtedly favor aberration over ectopy.

Cycle Sequences

In the presence of atrial fibrillation, or other causes of ventricular irregularity, a study of cycle sequences[25] may be revealing: an anomalous beat that ends a cycle *longer* than cycles ending in normally conducted beats is more likely to be ectopic than aberrant.

Bigeminy in Atrial Flutter

Whenever apparent ventricular bigeminy complicates atrial flutter, one should always suspect that one of the conduction ratios that produce pairing of the ventricular complexes (3:2, or alternating 4:1 and 2:1) has developed and that there is aberrant ventricular conduction of the beats ending the shorter ventricular cycles (Fig. 28-32D). Proper distinction of this form of aberration from true bigeminy is important and may be lifesaving.

The Compensatory Pause

Since it begins and ends in the ventricles the ventricular extrasystole does not disturb the sinus rhythm, and therefore the next sinus beat falls when expected and the pause is *compensatory*. On the other hand, if the premature beat arises in the atrium, it depolarizes the sinus node ahead of schedule, so that the next sinus beat is also ahead of schedule and the cycle is *less than compensatory*.

Unfortunately there are so many exceptions that the compensatory pause is rather a broken reed: ventricular ectopic impulses are often conducted backward to the atria;[51] these retrograde impulses may discharge the sinus node ahead of schedule and so result in a pause that is less than compensatory (Fig. 28-21, top). Because of the propensity of ectopic impulses to suppress pacemakers, an ectopic atrial impulse may so suppress the sinus pacemaker that the postextrasystolic cycle is fully compensatory (Fig. 28-21, middle). Two further situations in which a ventricular extrasystole is followed by a less than compensatory pause are when the postectopic cycle ends with an escape beat (Fig. 28-21, bottom) and when the premature beat interrupts a Wenckebach sequence.

Differentiation of Ventricular Tachycardia from Supraventricular Tachyarrhythmias with Aberration

Many of the points of differentiation between ventricular tachycardia and supraventricular tachyarrhythmias with aberrant ventricular conduction (Fig. 28-30) have already been touched upon. It remains to outline a systematic approach to the distinction.

When a rapid run of anomalous beats is seen, one should never take it for granted that it represents an ectopic ventricular mechanism. Instead, one should develop the habit of immediately recognizing the possibility that the mechanism is *either* ventricular ectopic *or* ventricular aberration, and then seek confirmation of one or the other.

1. Morphologic features of the QRS complexes may be most helpful and are the same as for premature beats.
2. Fusion (Dressler) beats are strong evidence in favor of an ectopic ventricular origin, although fusion has been demonstrated to occur between two supraventricular impulses provided one of them travels aberrantly via a preferential pathway.
3. If independent atrial activity is discernible, atrial tachycardia with aberration is excluded; but the possibility of AV junctional tachycardia with aberration but without retroconduction (thus permitting independent atrial activity) remains (Fig. 28-33).

As indicated earlier, the differentiation between the various supraventricular tachycardias is often difficult, as is the distinction between ventricular tachycardia and supraventricular tachycardia with aberration. At times the diagnosis rests on uncovering causative atrial waves that are buried invisibly in the ventricular complexes. When the underlying mechanism is supraventricular with conduction to the ventricles, inhibiting AV conduction temporarily may bring the latent P waves to light and so reveal the true mechanism. Carotid sinus pressure or other

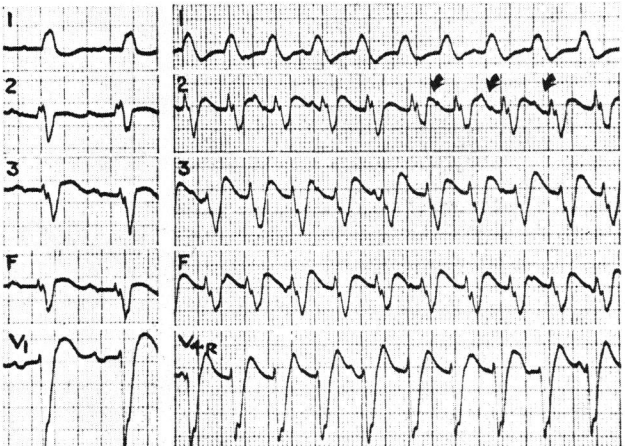

FIGURE 28-33   AV (nodal) tachycardia with left bundle branch block (LBBB) and without retrograde conduction to the atria. The strips on the right simulate ventricular tachycardia with their wide QRS complexes and independent P waves (arrows); but the pattern on another occasion during sinus rhythm (strips on left) shows that the ventricular pattern is not ectopic but represents a fixed LBBB. The tachycardia therefore must have arisen above the bifurcation of the common bundle.

means of vagal stimulation is the first maneuver to try. If this fails, intravenous edrophonium or acetylcholine may be successful. In the presence of widened QRS complexes that may represent either ventricular tachycardia or ventricular aberration, intravenous procainamide may be tried; if the arrhythmia is a ventricular tachycardia, this drug is appropriate treatment, and if the underlying mechanism is supraventricular, the drug may induce AV block and so reveal the culpable atrial waves.

In the presence of atrial fibrillation, a run of aberrant beats simulating ventricular tachycardia can create a clinical problem of great importance. Differentiation may be difficult (Fig. 28-31), and considerable reliance must be placed on the structure of the anomalous complexes[77] if these are of the RBBB type. Additional pointers of modest assistance are (1) the very presence of an RBBB pattern gives a statistical edge in favor of aberrant conduction (but unfortunately a majority of ectopic beats arise in the left ventricle, which narrows this edge); (2) the presence of a longer cycle preceding the short cycle that initiates the run of anomalous beats favors aberrancy (but by the rule of bigeminy, a similar cycle sequence also favors the development of ventricular ectopy); (3) the presence of a considerably longer cycle immediately following the run of anomalous beats suggests an abortive compensatory pause and favors an ectopic ventricular mechanism (but it is not uncommon for aberrant conduction to be fortuitously followed by abrupt cycle lengthening); (4) obviously the presence in previous tracings of single beats of similar contour that can be identified with reasonable certainty as ectopic or aberrant may be of crucial aid in differentiation; (5) the persistence of the anomalous pattern despite

adequate lengthening of the ventricular cycle obviously speaks against aberration; but even this is not foolproof since aberration, once established, sometimes persists in the face of cycle lengthening well beyond the measure of previous cycles that ended with normal intraventricular conduction.[25]

Another situation that requires special consideration is the presence of a supraventricular tachyarrhythmia complicated by Wolff-Parkinson-White (WPW) conduction. The error of mistaking atrial fibrillation with WPW conduction for ventricular tachycardia, and then investing the error with the sanctity of print, is one of the main reasons that ventricular tachycardia has acquired its undeserved reputation for irregularity. There are several clues that help us to avoid this mistake: (1) If the patient is known to have a WPW syndrome, even if the complexes during the tachycardia are different from his or her usual preexcitation pattern, the tachyarrhythmia is likely to be supraventricular; (2) an irregular tachycardia with bizarre complexes at a rate of 240 beats or more (Fig. 28-19) is said to be virtually diagnostic of atrial fibrillation with WPW conduction; and (3) the presence of slurred initial components (delta waves or equivalents) in the bizarre tachycardial complexes (Fig. 28-19) suggests, but does not prove, a WPW mechanism. Care must be taken not to mistake T waves "buttressing" the next QRS complex for delta waves.

Heart Block

Sinoatrial (SA) Block

If impulses fail to emerge or emerge tardily from the sinus node, SA block is present. If the impulse merely takes an undue length of time to enter the atrial muscle, first-degree SA block is present, but it cannot be recognized in the clinical electrocardiogram. If one or more impulses fail to emerge, second-degree block exists. If no impulses emerge, complete SA block is present.

SA block is relatively uncommon. Vagal stimulation can suppress SA nodal function in sensitive subjects, but most instances of SA block are due to structural disease or drug toxicity. Digitalis is a potent cause of SA block, often producing Wenckebach periods (see below). Quinidine, atropine, and salicylates are all reported to cause SA block. Block may result from myocardial ischemia or infarction; rheumatic fever, diphtheria, and other acute infections have produced SA block.

Electrocardiographic Features

SA block is recognized by the absence of an expected P wave. Since the sinus impulse is wanting, no ventricular response is provoked, and so the entire P-QRS-T sequence is missing—unless the sinus cycle is replaced by an escaped beat from a lower center. When a sinus beat is dropped, the resulting

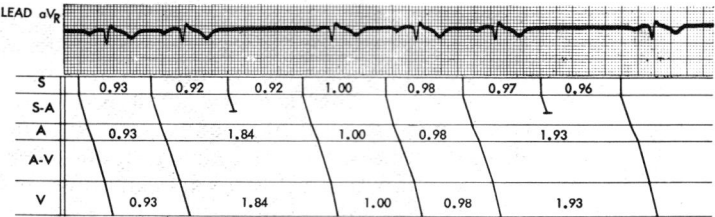

FIGURE 28-34 SA block. In each pause the entire P-QRS-T sequence is missing, and the long cycle is approximately equal to two of the sinus cycles.

pause is equal to two sinus cycles (Fig. 28-34); if an existing sinus rate exactly halves, 2:1 SA block is diagnosed.

It is important to recognize SA Wenckebach periods because they invariably indicate an abnormality of the sinus node, yet they are usually overlooked and called sinus arrhythmia—a normal mechanism. Their recognition is discussed further on in this chapter. If P waves are entirely absent, complete SA block may be diagnosed, but it is well to keep in mind that there are four possible explanations for absent P waves: (1) failure of the sinus node to form impulses (generator failure); (2) failure of the impulse to emerge from the node (exit block); (3) atrial paralysis, as in potassium intoxication; and (4) a sinus impulse that is too weak to activate normally responsive atria (inadequate stimulus). Block should be diagnosed only when a mathematical relationship can be demonstrated between the P waves, or when the cycle sequence of Wenckebach conduction is recognized.

Any abrupt pause produced by failure of one or more sinus impulses to occur on time, and failure to satisfy the mathematic relations of recognizable block, may be called *sinus pause* and its duration specified.

Atrioventricular (AV) Block

AV block is usually classified into three degrees (Table 28-7). In *first-degree*, AV conduction time is prolonged, but all impulses are conducted to the ventricles. *Second-degree* means that more or less frequent impulses are blocked and fail to reach the ventricles. This is usually subdivided into type I, type II, and high grade (or advanced). *Third-degree* is complete block, in which no impulses can reach the ventricles.

The current classification of AV block has serious shortcomings because its categories fail to correlate with prognosis or with indicated therapy. This is because two decades ago there was no consistently effective treatment for AV block, and consequently it mattered little how blocks were graded. Pacemakers then entered the picture and revolutionized the therapy of block, while nothing was done to renovate its taxonomy. It is regrettable that, in the days before pacemakers muddied the prognostic waters, a careful assessment of the many and various patterns of AV conduction disturbance was not attempted. There is no doubt that, to correlate realistically with prognosis and the need for therapy, a

classification expanded by several additions and subcategories is needed (Table 28-7, bottom).

One of the many factors that have helped to maintain the unsatisfactory status quo is the consistent failure of almost all authors to define terms such as complete, high-grade (or advanced), and type II AV block. An extreme example of the unfortunate result of not defining these terms is that disturbances as different as spontaneous ventricular asystole and AV dissociation, at least partly due to block but in the company of an independent junctional rhythm at a rate of 45 per minute or more—a combination which, for want of a better term, we have called *block/acceleration dissociation*—are often lumped under the heading of "complete AV block." Yet, in acute myocardial infarction transient spontaneous ventricular asystole (Fig. 28-35A) is associated with a mortality (whether paced or not) of about 90 percent, while block/acceleration dissociation (Fig. 28-35B) in our experience is associated with a mortality of less than 10 percent.

Another factor is that "degrees" as they are cur-

TABLE 28-7 Classification of AV Block

Common Classification of AV Block

First degree (prolonged PR interval)
Second degree:
    Type I (Wenckebach periodicity)
    Type II
    High grade (advanced)
Third degree (complete)

Categories of AV Block Requiring Consideration

Prolonged PR interval
Block/acceleration dissociation
Occasional "dropped" beats:
    Type I (Wenckebach periodicity)
    Type II
2:1 AV block:
    Type I
    Type II
High-grade block:
    Type I
    Type II
Complete block:
    Junctional escape
    Ventricular escape
Transient ventricular asystole:
    Spontaneous
    Phase 4 (?)
    Vagal

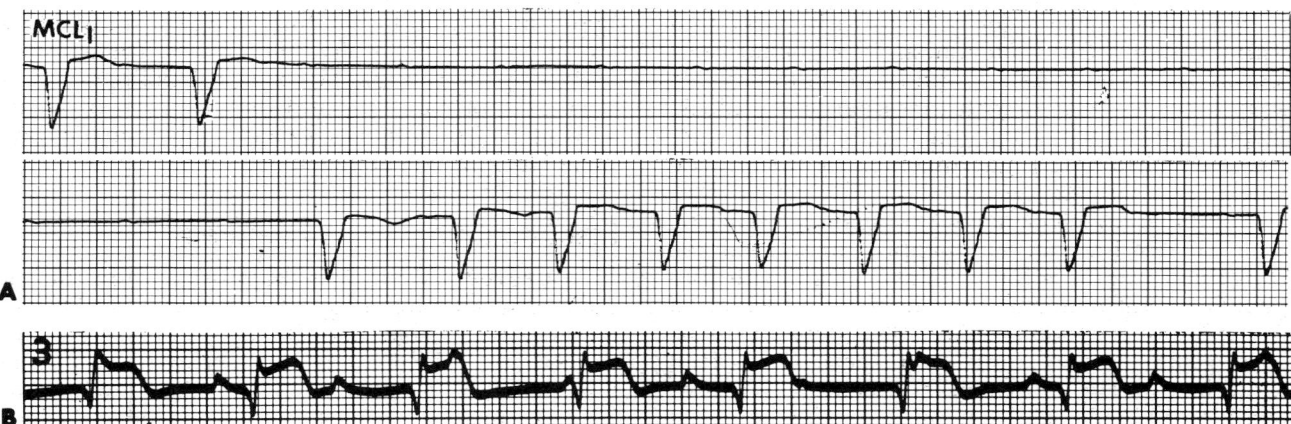

FIGURE 28-35   *A.* Spontaneous ventricular asystole lasting for over 7 s and due to the abrupt development of AV block at a time when no escaping pacemaker is active. From a patient with acute anteroseptal infarction. *B.* Complete AV dissociation due to a combination of *some* degree of AV block with an accelerated junctional rhythm (rate 68 per minute). From a patient with acute inferior infarction.

rently defined do not necessarily correlate with the severity of the conduction disturbance—definitions are predicated mainly on conduction ratios to the neglect of atrial rate. Thus 2:1 block, which some classify as high grade, may represent anything from a disaster (2:1 block at an atrial rate of 60) to a blessing (2:1 block at an atrial rate of 140). Again, if the sinus rate is 70 and, despite a slow independent ventricular rate of 30, no impulses are conducted to the ventricles, complete AV block can be diagnosed; but if the rate of an independent accelerated AV junctional pacemaker is 85, complete absence of AV conduction in these circumstances may represent only a minor degree of block. In fact, mere delayed AV conduction (prolonged PR interval) associated with an accelerated subsidiary pacemaker may be responsible for this form of complete AV dissociation. It is therefore obvious that in any meaningful consideration of AV block the respective rates of the involved pacemakers must be taken into account.

In fact, with definitions and misconceptions as they presently exist, a patient with "first-degree block" may have a worse conduction disturbance than another erroneously labeled as having "high-grade block."

The recipe for confusion is complete if we add the following widespread misconceptions to the lack of precise definitions and the fact that "degrees" are not really degrees: 2:1 AV block is necessarily high-grade;[79] 2:1 AV block is necessarily type II block;[80,81] the block is necessarily high-grade when most, but not all, atrial impulses are not conducted to the ventricles;[82] and total absence of conduction, as in Fig. 28-35*B*, is necessarily evidence for complete block.[83] In view of these deficiencies in current usage, it seems desirable that the following three remedial measures be implemented: (1) "degrees," as presently used, should be eliminated or at least deemphasized; (2) the inclusion of stated atrial and ventricular rates should be an integral part of all

diagnoses of AV conduction disorders; and (3) the AV blocks should be reclassified into a realistic set of sufficient and *defined* categories, including at least those listed in Table 28-7. Only then will the current confusion be remedied and indications for therapy clearly limned.

Since most reports concerned with AV block fail to define their terms, and since basic terms are variably used, some of the following observations on etiology and incidence must be accepted with appropriate reservation.

Prolonged PR intervals are occasionally found in apparently normal subjects.[40] In their survey of over 67,000 asymptomatic Air Force personnel, Johnson et al.[84] found 350 examples of first-degree block (5.2 per 1000). Twenty percent of them had PR intervals that were over 0.24 s. Of 19,000 young aircrew applicants, 59 had PR intervals of 0.24 s or greater.[85]

In both normal and diseased hearts, atropine, standing, exercise, and isoproterenol tend to shorten the lengthened PR interval. There is a widespread belief that the PR interval tends always to shorten with an increase in heart rate. Though this is true in normal hearts with natural acceleration, when the rate is increased with artificial atrial pacing, the PR lengthens even in normal hearts; in diseased hearts a natural increase in rate is frequently associated with lengthening of the PR interval. AV block with Wenckebach periods may occur in normal hearts[40] and was found in 3 of the 67,000 Air Force personnel screened by Johnson.[84]

Prolonged AV conduction (PR interval) and dropped beats can be caused by vagal stimulation and by a variety of drugs, including digitalis, quinidine sulfate, procainamide, propranolol, and potassium. Diseases that most commonly produce AV block are rheumatic fever, chronic ischemic heart disease, and myocardial infarction, especially inferior infarction. Any infectious disease that produces myocarditis may have this effect. Some patients with hyperthyroidism have prolonged PR intervals.

Adrenocortical insufficiency tends to be associated with a prolonged PR interval, and congenital heart lesions, atrial septal defect, and Ebstein's disease are sometimes associated with first-degree AV block. Hypoxia from any cause (e.g., anesthesia, pulmonary embolism, etc.) may produce significant AV block.

Complete AV block may be congenital, occurring as an isolated finding; but in approximately half the congenital cases it is found in association with congenital malformations of the heart, viz., corrected transposition and ventricular septal defect (usually as part of a more complex defect). It is often thought that the most common cause of chronic complete AV block is ischemic heart disease, but there are a surprising number of cases with no clear-cut evidence of ischemic or any other sort of myocardial disease. Some authorities postulate that these are due to "primary" disease of the specialized conducting tissues; in one series,[86] these cases constituted the majority (59 percent against 23 percent ischemic).

Two lesions that involve the conduction fascicles and produce AV and intraventricular blocks in the absence of associated myocardial disease are Lenègre's disease and Lev's disease. Lenègre's disease[87] is an obscure sclerodegenerative process involving only the conduction system and is one of the most common causes of right bundle branch block and left anterior hemiblock in persons over the age of 50 years. The natural course of this disease is a slow progression toward complete heart block several years later.

Lev's disease,[88] on the other hand, is caused by an invasion of the conduction system from without—an involvement of the fascicles by fibrosis or calcification spreading from any of the fibrous structures adjacent to the conducting system. One of the common causes of right bundle branch block with left anterior hemiblock in elderly subjects is fibrosis of the summit of the muscular septum. Calcification of the aortic valve may cause right bundle branch block, left bundle branch block, bilateral bundle branch block, left anterior hemiblock, or complete AV block. Fibrosis or calcification of the central fibrous body or mitral ring is the most common cause of complete heart block with narrow QRS complex in the elderly. Among patients whose conduction is continuously monitored after myocardial infarction, 4.2 to 8.6 percent are said to develop complete block. In a series of personally observed 1001 consecutive acute myocardial infarctions, the incidence of complete block was only 2.1 percent. Most of these blocks complicate inferior infarction. Occasional cases are associated with calcific aortic stenosis, diphtheria, or syphilitic involvement of the His bundle. Digitalis and potassium intoxication may produce complete AV block. Rare causes of complete AV block include sarcoidosis, Hodgkin's disease, myeloma and other tumors of the heart, rheumatoid disease, dermatomyositis, Paget's disease,

hyperthyroidism, myxedema, amyloidosis, progressive muscular dystrophy, and trauma (penetrating and nonpenetrating). The surgical closure of ventricular septal defects and implantation of aortic valves have furnished new causes of traumatic complete block in recent years.

Electrocardiographic Features

First-degree AV block is diagnosed when the PR interval is prolonged to 0.21 s or beyond. The interval may be constant, or it may vary inversely with the RP interval during a sinus arrhythmia, a situation that the French have aptly called *floating PR*. Though most examples of first-degree AV block have PR intervals between 0.21 and 0.35 s (Fig. 28-36), occasional intervals have been recorded up to 1.0 s or slightly greater.

In second-degree AV block, some P waves are not followed by QRS complexes (dropped beats). The most common form, type I, is the Wenckebach period, in which, after progressively lengthening PR intervals, the final P wave is not followed by a ventricular response. The sequence of PR lengthening usually follows a recognizable pattern, at least for the first few beats: although the lengthening is progressive, the amount by which the PR interval increases over the previous PR interval (the increment) decreases (Fig. 28-37A). Since each ventricular cycle is determined by the basic sinus cycle and the current increment, an apparent paradox results, provided the sinus rhythm is regular: as the PR interval lengthens, the RR interval shortens. Thus the pause of the dropped beat is followed by slight but measurable ventricular acceleration (Fig. 28-37A). Since the pause of the dropped beat contains the shortest PR interval, it is always equal to less than two of the shortest cycles. These features enable one to recognize the Wenckebach type of conduction even when no conduction intervals are available for measurement. An example of such conduction out of the sinus node is illustrated in Fig. 28-37B. In this tracing the P waves show the same type of periodicity that the QRS complexes showed in Fig. 28-37A: the longest PP interval is less than twice the shortest PP interval, and after the long interval

FIGURE 28-36 First-degree AV block. The PR interval is prolonged to 0.35 s.

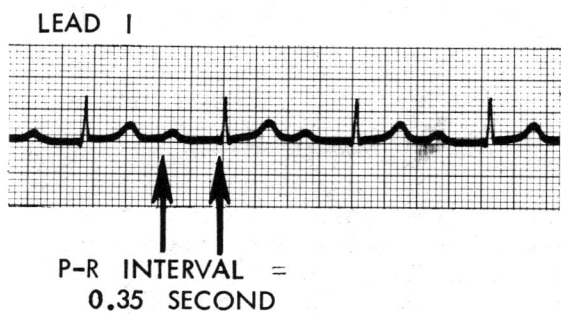

LEAD I

P–R INTERVAL = 0.35 SECOND

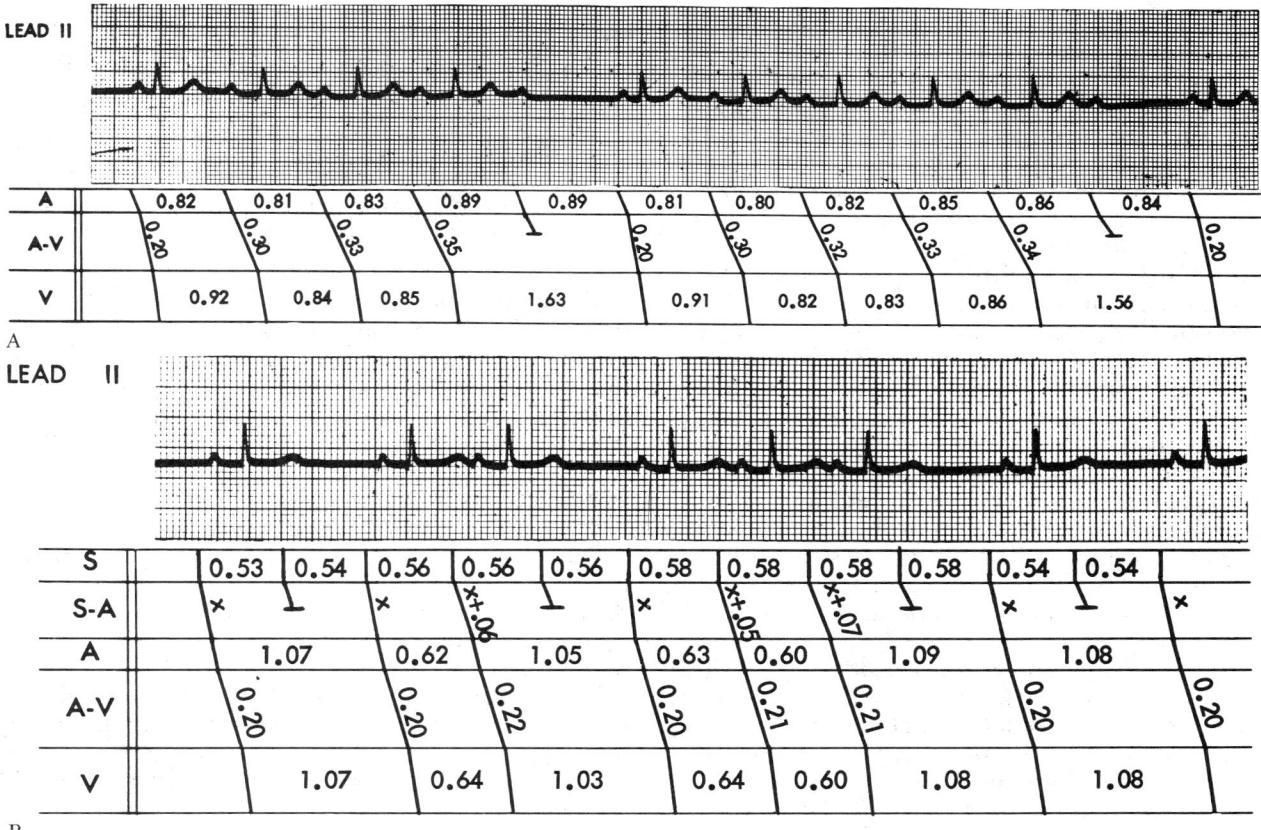

FIGURE 28-37 Wenckebach phenomenon. *A.* A 5:4 and 6:5 AV Wenckebach period. Note that the PQ interval progressively lengthens, but by a decreasing increment; therefore the ventricular cycle tends to shorten (at least for the first two cycles following the dropped beat). *B.* A 3:2 and 4:3 sinus Wenckebach period with 2:1 SA block at beginning and end of strip. (*From J. W. Hurst and R. Myerburg, "Introduction to Electrocardiography," McGraw-Hill Book Company, New York, 1973. Reproduced with permission.*)

there is measurable acceleration of the sinus P waves. It is important not to overlook sinus Wenckebach periods and mistake them for sinus arrhythmia, because sinus arrhythmia is a normal mechanism whereas the sinus Wenckebach period is almost invariably a sign of drug effect or disease.

The most common Wenckebach ratio is 3:2, leaving the ventricular complexes grouped in pairs, but any $(x + 1):x$ ratio (e.g., 4:3, 7:6, etc.) may be seen. In type II block, a beat is dropped after *consecutive* preceding atrial impulses have been conducted with a constant, usually normal, PR interval and with bundle branch block. His bundle electrography has demonstrated that type I AV block is almost always due to conduction delay in the AV node proper, whereas type II block occurs in or below the bundle of His;[89] in fact, Damato regards type II block as a manifestation of bilateral bundle branch block.[90] Type I block with Wenckebach periods usually develops in acute situations (myocardial infarction, rheumatic fever, or digitalis intoxication), is therefore temporary, and carries a relatively good prognosis. Type II block is usually permanent and often progresses to complete AV block.

In second-degree AV block, either type I or type II, every alternate beat may be dropped so that there are two P waves to each QRS complex (2:1 block) (Fig. 28-38); or there may be several P waves to each QRS complex (3:1, 4:1, etc.), in which case, provided the atrial rate is reasonable, a diagnosis of high-grade (or advanced) block is justified.

In complete (third-degree) AV block the ventricular complexes occur independently at a slow rate, usually between 30 to 45 beats per minute, except in congenital heart block, in which the rate is somewhat faster. Usually regular but independent P waves constantly change their relation to the QRS

FIGURE 28-38 Second-degree AV block. There are two P waves to each QRS—2:1 AV block (every alternate sinus impulse is blocked).

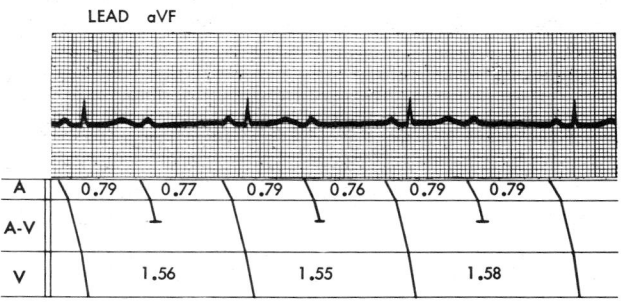

complexes (Fig. 28-39). Despite complete antero-grade block, retroconduction to the atria may occasionally produce retrograde P waves after the ventricular complex occurs. In a more recent series of 42 patients with "complete" block investigated with sophisticated electrophysiologic techniques, retrograde conduction to the atria was detected in 36 percent, with concealed conduction as far as the AV junction in an additional 17 percent.[91]

The ventricular complex may be normal or anomalous. If the site of block is high in the AV junction (monofascicular) and the pacemaker is situated above the bifurcation of the AV bundle, the QRS complex will be normal unless there is an associated BBB. An abnormal QRS complex will also be written if the pacemaker is ectopic ventricular (idioventricular). The distinction between an AV (junctional) pacemaker with BBB and an idioventricular mechanism is often impossible, but the same distinguishing morphologic characteristics outlined earlier for ventricular ectopy and for aberration may be helpful. At times two or more ventricular pacemakers operate simultaneously or in sequence, often at remarkably similar rates, producing varying patterns of fusion beats. The picture of complete AV block is often preceded, sometimes for years, by a pattern of BBB; and indeed many cases of complete block are in fact due to bilateral BBB (bifascicular) or to multifascicular block.[92] The slow ventricular rates in complete AV block frequently favor the development of ventricular extrasystoles, in accordance with the rule of bigeminy.

In conclusion, one must remember that first-degree AV block, second-degree type I and type II block, and high-grade AV block can all be imitated by concealed junctional[93] or fascicular[94] extrasystoles or parasystole.[95]

Group Beating

This term is applied when bursts of similar ventricular complexes are separated by pauses. The most common cause is undoubtedly repetitive Wenckebach periods in the presence of atrial tachycardia (Fig. 28-40). The P waves often are difficult or impossible to discern, but the diagnosis can be confi-

FIGURE 28-39 Complete (third-degree) AV block. There is a regular idioventricular rhythm at rate 36, and the P waves indicate their independence by changing their relation to the QRS complexes.

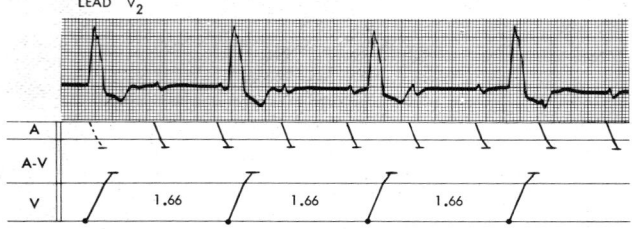

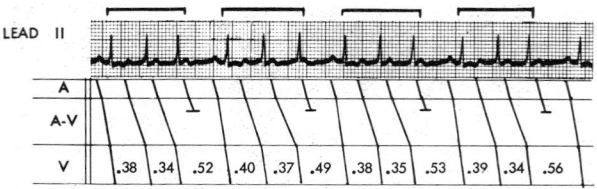

FIGURE 28-40 Group beating during atrial (sinus?) tachycardia as a result of 4:3 Wenckebach periods.

dently made from the cycle sequences (see "Wenckebach Phenomenon," above).

Other, less common causes are bursts of repetitive ventricular tachycardia and groups of agonal beats in the dying heart.

AV Dissociation

AV dissociation, like jaundice, is not in itself a diagnosis. It is always a secondary result of a primary disturbance. Like jaundice, it may be the first sign that catches the eye, but the underlying cause must then be uncovered.

The terminology of the subject has been unnecessarily confused. *AV dissociation* is commonly used in three different ways: as a synonym for complete AV block; in a quasi-specific sense for an arrhythmic sequence that was called *interference dissociation;* and simply to describe the state of independence between atria and ventricles whenever the normal AV sequence has been interrupted. This third sense—to characterize the independent state of affairs—is its legitimate usage.

The word *interference* has been so sinned against that, to avoid confusion, we prefer not to use it. For those who wish to pursue the semantic problems further, we draw your attention to an earlier review[96] and the pertinent references.

Disregarding the momentary dissociation occasioned by single ectopic beats and the dissociation secondary to complete AV block, AV dissociation may result from atrial slowing (*default* of primary pacemaker) (Fig. 28-41A); from AV nodal or ventricular acceleration (*usurpation* by secondary pacemaker) (Fig. 28-41B); from reduction in the number of atrial impulses reaching the AV junction or ventricles because of SA or AV block (Fig. 28-41C); from the opportunism of an escaping pacemaker taking advantage of the pause provided by a premature beat; or from a combination of any of these conditions.

AV dissociation may affect the normal heart, as when it results from sinus bradycardia in an athlete. It may also result from sinus bradycardia induced by unnatural stimuli such as anesthesia or eye operations. Among its many other causes are (1) drugs, including digitalis, atropine, quinidine, and procainamide; (2) infections; (3) rheumatic fever; and (4) ischemic heart disease, especially acute inferior infarction.

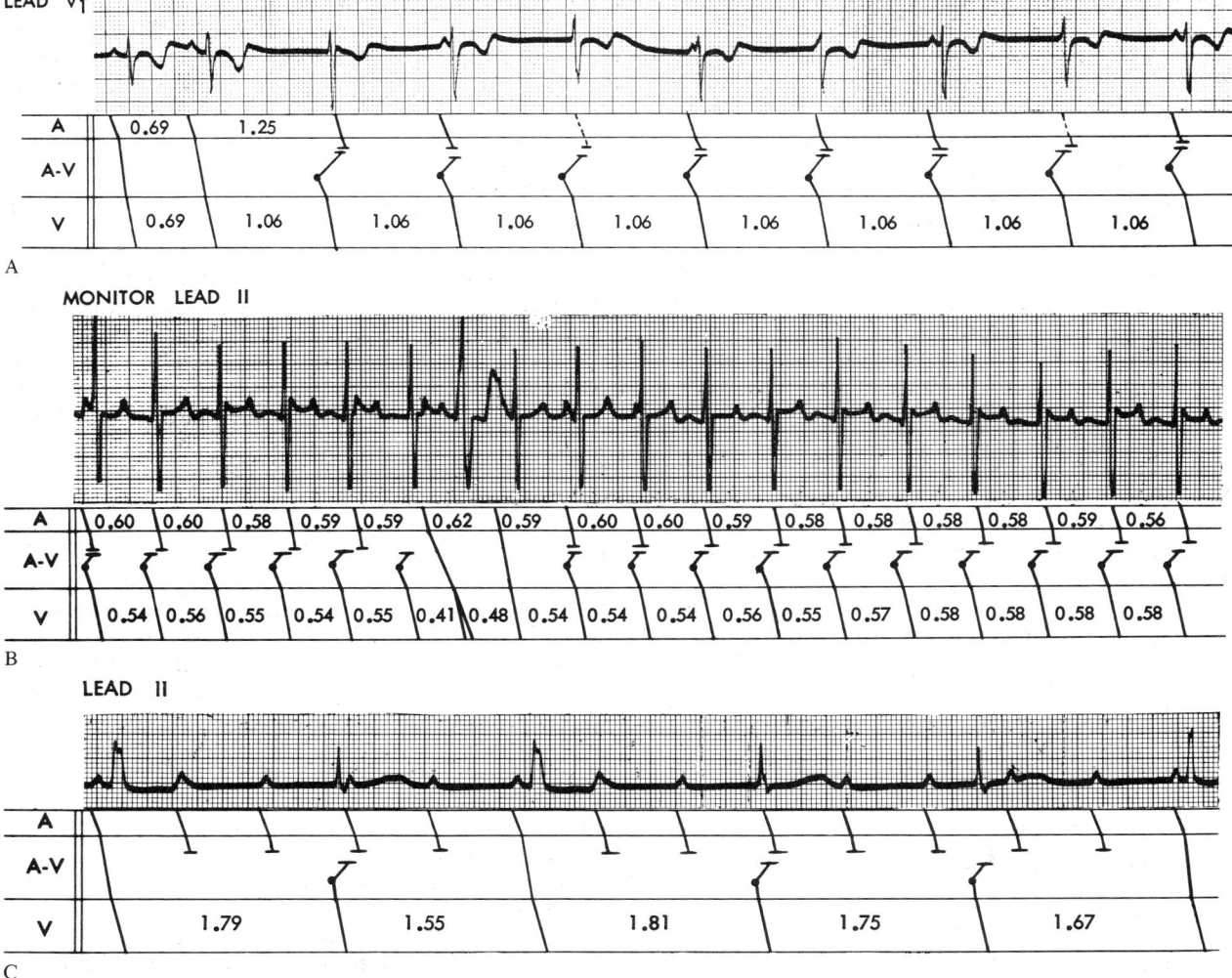

FIGURE 28-41 AV dissociation. *A.* Sinus arrhythmia: the bradycrotic phase enables the AV node to escape, with resulting dissociation. *B.* AV tachycardia: the tachycardia enables the AV pacemaker to usurp control of the ventricles, with resulting dissociation; the seventh and eighth beats are ventricular captures, the seventh, ending the shorter cycle, showing ventricular aberration. *C.* High-grade AV block permits the AV node to escape (second, fourth, and fifth beats), with resulting dissociation.

Electrocardiographic Features

Since there are so many and such varied circumstances in which AV dissociation can arise, one cannot give a unified description of its electrocardiographic findings. But one cardinal electrocardiographic sign is common to all conditions in which dissociation in any form is sustained: a changing relation between atrial and ventricular complexes.

The dissociated sequence that earned the name *interference dissociation* from Mobitz in 1923 is illustrated in Fig. 28-41*B.* Because the automatic AV pacemaker is beating faster than the SA node, the P waves "overtake" and pass the QRS complex. Since there may be little or no disturbance in AV conduction, when the P wave has emerged far enough beyond the QRS complex, the atrial impulse is conducted to the ventricles to effect "capture" (captured beat, ventricular capture).

Dissociation does not necessarily occur between

sinus and AV pacemakers; two AV junctional pacemakers may dissociate, the upper one controlling the atria, and the lower the ventricles. Or the ventricles may be controlled by a dissociated idioventricular pacemaker (Fig. 28-27). In such cases ventricular fusion beats frequently intervene between the runs of dissociation and the captured beats.

It is quite common for a heart to harbor two independent pacemakers with identical or nearly identical rates. It therefore sometimes happens that dissociated pacemakers may beat at similar rates for longer or shorter periods without the occurrence of conduction (capture). In the tracing, the P waves are seen to flirt with the QRS complexes, never leaving them far in front or behind, until a sufficient change in the rate of one of them restores AV conduction. This situation was called *isorhythmic dissociation* by French authors. The isorhythmicity may be the result of fortuitous identity of rates; or at times there may be evidence that the two pacemakers are held in phase by electrical or mechanical influences, a phenomenon called *synchronization* or *accrochage*.

Sometimes, when two pacemakers with similar rates are operative, the dissociated P wave approaches the QRS complex, disappears within it for several beats, then reappears again and recedes from the QRS complex until a normal PR interval is achieved and maintained for a few beats. It then once again approaches the QRS complex and repeats this sequence again and again (Fig. 28-42). Such behavior has been attributed to fluctuations in arterial blood pressure conditioned by changes in atrial transport function secondary to changes in the relationship of atrial to ventricular contraction.

Just as ventricular fusion beats may occur between runs of dissociation and capture beats when the lower pacemaker is idioventricular, so atrial fusion beats can occur between runs of AV rhythm and dissociation if the atria are not protected by retrograde block from ascending AV impulses. Both forms of fusion represent *partial* dissociation: in the one case only a part of the ventricular moiety is dissociated from the atria, and in the other only part of the atria is dissociated. Thus, although AV dissociation can occur in the presence of normal anterograde and retrograde conduction, impairment of conduction in either direction favors the development and maintenance of dissociation.

AV Junctional Variants

Accelerated Junctional Rhythm

Depending at least to some extent upon the level of the pacemaker,[7] junctional rhythms have an inherent rate between 30 and 60 beats per minute. If the rate exceeds 60 beats per minute, the rhythm is *accelerated*. Accelerated junctional rhythms may control both ventricles and atria, or the atria may continue to beat independently. Accelerated junctional rhythm is most commonly seen as a complication of

FIGURE 28-42   Accelerated idionodal rhythm with resulting isorhythmic AV dissociation. After four sinus beats, the sinus rate slows slightly, enabling the accelerated junctional pacemaker to escape at a rate of 94. After several seconds the sinus pacemaker accelerates and recaptures the ventricles. The same sequence is then repeated. (The strips are continuous.)

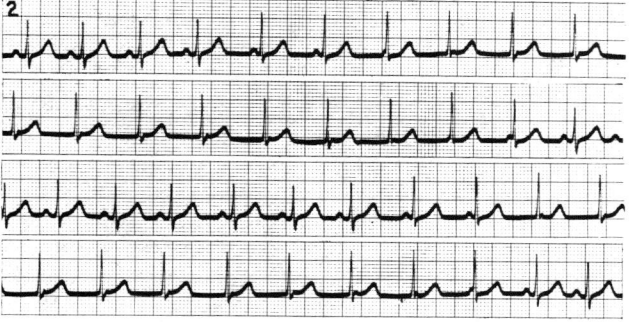

acute inferior infarction, acute rheumatic fever, or digitalis intoxication. Figure 28-35*B* illustrates accelerated junctional rhythm complicating an acute inferior infarction, and Fig. 28-43 shows an accelerated junctional rhythm due to digitalis toxicity.

Reciprocal Rhythm

Reciprocal rhythms require the assumption of at least two functioning pathways in the AV junction with unequal refractory periods. In a reciprocal beat the impulse arises in the AV junction and travels both downward to the ventricles and upward into the atria. The impulse on its upward journey encounters a refractory path which it cannot penetrate and proceeds upward by another path to reach the atria. Higher in the AV junction, the impulse may find a level in the hitherto refractory path at which it is no longer refractory, "spill over" into it, and descend to reach and activate the ventricles. Such spillover and downward descent are favored by delay in retrograde conduction, since such delay affords the descending path more time for recovery. The phenomenon of the retrograde impulse reentering an anterograde path and reactivating the ventricles is known as *reciprocal rhythm* or *beating*, and the beat so produced is a *reciprocal* or *echo beat*. The point in the AV junction at which the impulse spills over and turns down is the *reflecting level*.

There are several variations on the reciprocal theme, as is indicated in the diagrams in Figs. 28-44 and 28-45. When the impulse begins in the ventricle as an ectopic beat and returns to reactivate the ventricles, it has been called a *return extrasystole*. When the impulse circulates rapidly around the AV junction, giving off daughter impulses to atria and ventricles at two reflecting levels, a *reciprocating tachycardia* results.

A reciprocal beat usually occurs at the end of a run of AV junctional rhythm with progressively lengthening retrograde conduction. Any of the factors that can produce AV junctional rhythm can contribute to the production of reciprocal beating; undoubtedly one of the commonest causes is digitalis excess.

Wandering or Shifting Pacemaker

These terms are applied when, as a result of suppression of one pacemaker, usually the sinus node, another center takes over the role of pacemaking. Most commonly, pacemaking activity shifts back and forth between the sinus node and AV junction. The terms should not be applied when the pacemaking changes are due to premature beats. The mechanism may appear in normal hearts and may be a manifestation of fluctuating vagal tone; it obviously can be encouraged by any influence that enhances vagal activity.

In the electrocardiogram, a changing contour of the P waves is associated with changes in cycle length

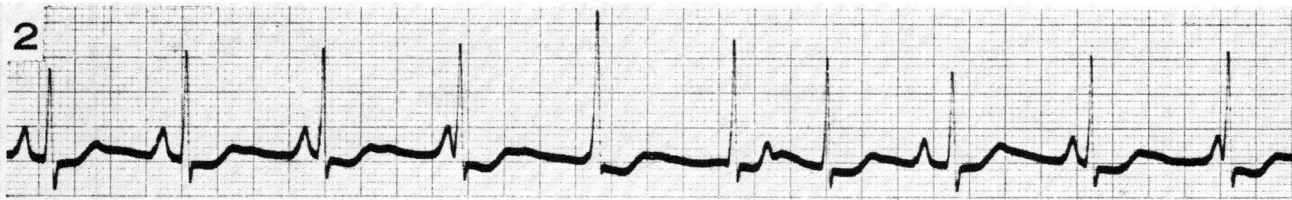

FIGURE 28-43 Accelerated idionodal rhythm producing AV dissociation. From a girl of 10 years with rheumatic heart disease and digitalis intoxication developing after mitral valvotomy. The seventh beat is a ventricular capture.

and in the PR interval. In the most typical case, sinus P waves are replaced after several beats by retrograde P' waves, often with intermediate fusion P waves (Fig. 28-46A); then, after a few AV beats, pacemaking reverts to the sinus node. The characteristic feature of wandering pacemaker is that changes in the P waves occur, at least part of the time, with cycle *lengthening,* never with abrupt decrease in cycle length. A momentary shift of pacemaker is often occasioned by a postextrasystolic pause, the beat ending the lengthened cycle (atrial escape) showing an altered P wave (Fig. 28-46B).

Escape Rhythms

When a higher pacemaker defaults, a lower pacemaker may come to the rescue and "escape." Thus by definition an escape (or escaped) beat is a *late* beat occurring only after an interval longer than the dominant cycle. If the sinus pacemaker unduly slows or otherwise defaults, the most likely pacemaker to take over and escape is the AV junction. Less often, an ectopic ventricular pacemaker escapes. When the sinus pacemaker is suppressed by an atrial extrasystole or other ectopic atrial activity, the returning beat is often an atrial escape. If several junctional escape beats occur in succession, with the AV pacemaker controlling both atria and ventricles, a *junctional escape rhythm* is present. If a series of escape beats occurs but the atria continue to be controlled by their own sinus pacemaker, we have *AV dissociation.* If pacemaking switches back and forth between sinus and junctional pacemakers, the rhythm is called *shifting* or *wandering pacemaker.* If a junctional rhythm shows considerable retrograde delay of conduction to the atria, *reciprocal beating* may occur. There is thus an intimate interplay between escape, junctional rhythm, shifting pacemaker, reciprocal rhythm, and AV dissociation, so that to some extent they must be considered together.

FIGURE 28-44 Diagram of reciprocal mechanisms.

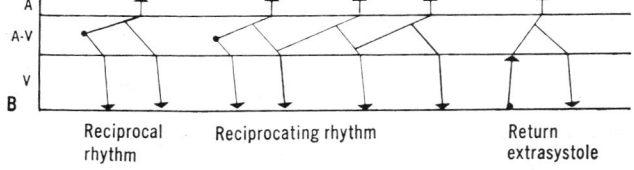

Escape Beats

Escape occurs after an interval longer than the dominant cycle. It represents a safety mechanism; escape beats therefore should never be suppressed. Anything that provides a pause longer than the prevailing cycle may permit escape to occur: the slow phase of sinus arrhythmia, SA block, AV block, extrasystoles, and the ending of a paroxysm of tachycardia each may provide an adequate pause to release an escaping beat.

In the electrocardiogram the junctional escape beat usually shows a QRS-T contour similar to that of the sinus beats, but it sometimes shows a slight variation from the dominant beats (Fig. 28-47A). Less often it can show quite marked distortion and widening (aberration) of the QRS complex and simulate an ectopic ventricular beat. This is contrary to what one would expect, since aberration classically develops with shortening of the cycle, not lengthening. This seeming paradox is explained by assuming that such escaping impulses travel by preferential pathways provided by paraspecific (Mahaim) fibers and so enter the ventricles by an unorthodox path. Or such AV impulses may arise from an eccentric focus in the AV junction and therefore spread asymmetrically down the bundle of His to enter one bundle branch before the other, and thus result in an anomalous ventricular complex.[97]

Junctional escape beats in the presence of atrial fibrillation present a special problem because there is no dominant cycle. Escape is usually diagnosed when the longest ventricular cycles are all equal in length.

Ventricular escapes are characterized by the late rather than early occurrence of the usual patterns of ectopic ventricular beats (Fig. 28-47B).

Atrial escape beats are seldom described and yet are common; they are often seen when there is suppression of the sinus node by atrial extrasystoles, by runs of atrial tachycardia, or by retrograde atrial activation (Fig. 28-11).

AV Junctional Rhythm

In AV junctional rhythm a junctional pacemaker controls both ventricles and atria. This rhythm can result from anything that suppresses sinus node activity—physiological sinus bradycardia, any form of vagal stimulation, digitalis, the initial phase of atro-

DISORDERS OF THE CARDIOVASCULAR SYSTEM

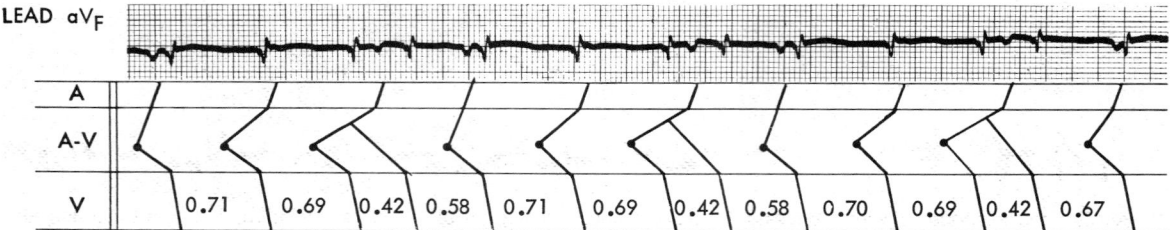

FIGURE 28-45 Reciprocal rhythm. AV nodal rhythm with progressively lengthening retrograde conduction until, with the third beat, there is enough retrograde delay for the impulse to find a nonrefractory downward path and be "reflected" back to the ventricles—the reciprocal beat.

pine action, SA block, or congenital absence of the SA node; or from anything that enhances AV automaticity—digitalis intoxication, rheumatic fever, inferior myocardial infarction, etc. When the rhythm is due to default of the sinus pacemaker, the rate is usually between 30 and 60 beats per minute, and it is referred to as a *junctional escape rhythm*. When it results from enhanced junctional automaticity, the rate is faster (60 to 100) and the rhythm is best termed *accelerated junctional rhythm*. This is the preferred term because the rate is faster than the normal rate for this pacemaker site (30 to 60 per minute) but less than the necessary rate of more than 100 to meet the criterion for a tachycardia. When the rate exceeds 100, the term *junctional tachycardia* is appropriately employed.

In the electrocardiogram the P′ wave of retrograde atrial activation may be seen in front of the QRS complex (with short P′R interval) or following the QRS complex, or it may be lost within the ventricular complex. When the P′ waves are visible, they are narrow and usually inverted in leads II, III, aV_F, and often in the left chest leads; they are upright in aV_R and aV_L and often in V_1. The QRS-T pattern is usually normal but may be somewhat aberrant as a result of preferential pathway conduction or eccentric impulse origin.

Idioventricular Rhythm

When the ventricles operate independently under control of an ectopic ventricular pacemaker at slow or normal rates (20 to 100 beats per minute), the rhythm is called *idioventricular*. Three consecutive ventricular escape beats constitute the shortest run of idioventricular rhythm, and they may result from any of the causes of escape enumerated above. However, idioventricular rhythm is usually a manifestation of complete AV block, and the subject has been dealt with under that heading. Rarely it may result from complete SA block. If the idioventricular rate is between 50 and 100 beats per minute, the appropriate term is *accelerated idioventricular rhythm* (see earlier in this chapter).

Cardiac Arrest

Cardiac arrest includes all conditions in which effective ventricular contraction has ceased. Thus it embraces (1) ventricular fibrillation (VF), the ultimate arrhythmia, in which the ventricular myocardium writhes in uncoordinated activity; (2) ventricular standstill or asystole, in which there is no mechanical or electrical ventricular activity; and (3) agonal

FIGURE 28-46 *A.* Wandering pacemaker. The first four beats are AV junctional, the next is an atrial fusion beat, and the next three are sinus. *B.* Shift of pacemaker induced by an atrial extrasystole (arrow); immediately following the premature beat, pacemaking shifts to the AV node and then returns, via several atrial fusion beats, to sinus rhythm.

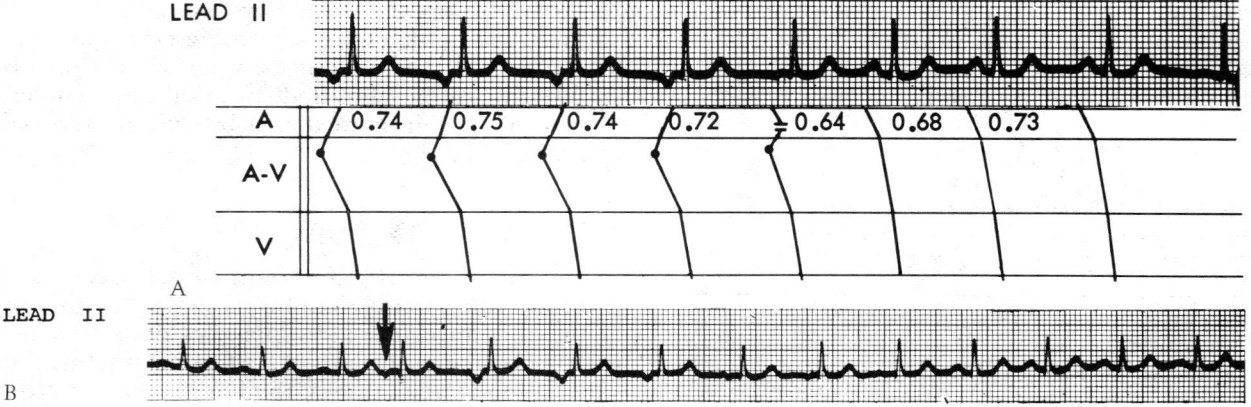

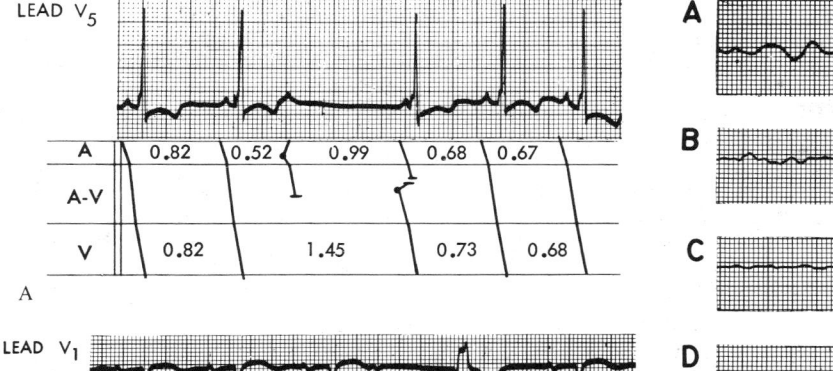

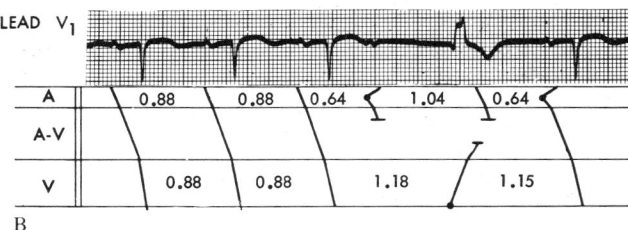

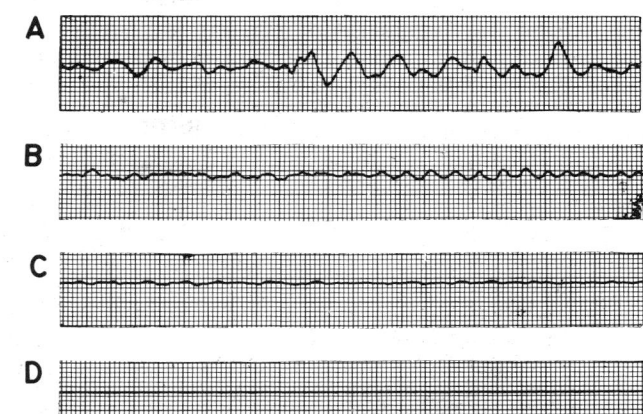

FIGURE 28-48 *A, B,* and *C.* Deteriorating ventricular fibrillation. *D.* Ventricular standstill.

FIGURE 28-47 *A.* AV (nodal) escape beat. After two sinus beats there is a nonconducted atrial premature beat; the pause that follows this ends with an escape beat whose QRS-T pattern is similar to that of the sinus beats. *B.* Ventricular escape beat. After three sinus beats there is a nonconducted atrial premature beat; the pause that follows this ends with a bizarre beat of typical ectopic ventricular contour.

rhythm, in which there are wide, distorted ventricular complexes but no associated mechanical activity.

Factors that may contribute to the development of cardiac arrest include hypotension, shock, anoxia, metabolic acidosis, bradycardia, or tachycardia. Autonomic influences, both vagal and sympathetic, may play a role. Fibrillation may be initiated by potassium depletion; drugs, such as digitalis, quinidine sulfate, procainamide and disopyramide;[98] and anesthetic agents, such as chloroform and cyclopropane. Atropine, administered intravenously for sinus bradycardia in acute myocardial infarction, has precipitated ventricular fibrillation.[99] An electric shock of appropriate voltage—as from household ac

outlets or from lightning—will induce fibrillation. Other causes of arrest include anaphylaxis and drowning. Rarely, paroxysms of VF, starting and stopping spontaneously, may occur in otherwise apparently normal hearts.

In VF there are no formed ventricular complexes in the tracing; instead, there is an irregular zigzag pattern of variable amplitude (Fig. 28-48*A* to *C*). The pattern of fibrillation is of some importance, since the larger and better formed the zigzag contours, the easier is defibrillation. Ventricular standstill (Fig. 28-48*D*) is recognized by the complete absence of any sign of ventricular activity in the electrocardiogram. Agonal rhythm, which may appear in any heart approaching death, results in wide, bizarre complexes on the tracing (Fig. 28-49); these are usually irregular and are often recorded at an extremely slow rate.

References

1. Besoin-Santander, M., Pick, A., and Langendorf, R.: A-V Conduction in Auricular Flutter, *Circulation,* 2:604, 1950.

FIGURE 28-49 Agonal rhythm (continuous strips). Grossly widened and distorted ventricular complexes occur irregularly and slow to a standstill.

MONITOR LEAD II (CONTINUOUS)

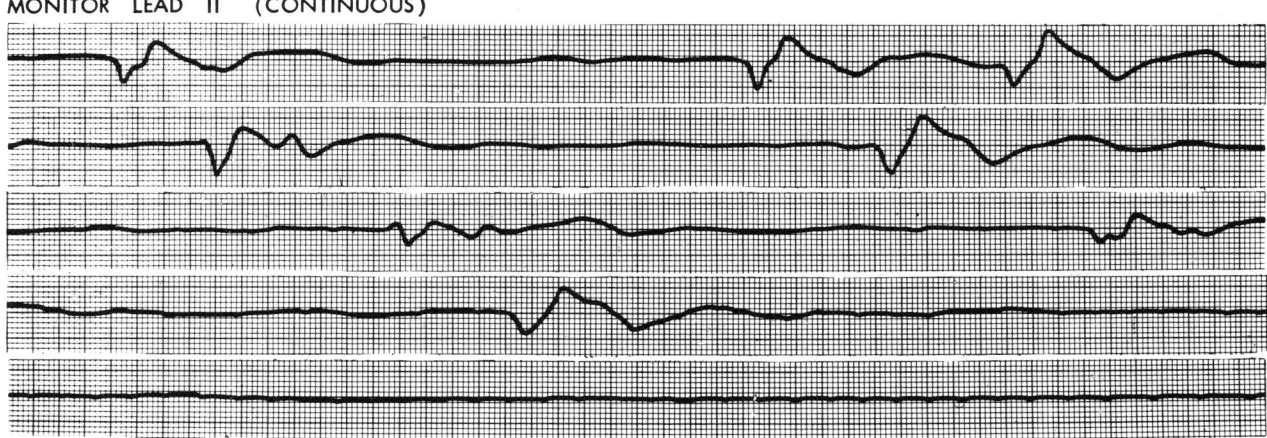

2. Graybiel, A., McFarland, F. A., Gates, D. C., and Webster, F. A.: Analysis of the Electrocardiograms Obtained from 1000 Young Healthy Aviators, *Am. Heart J.,* 27:524, 1944.

3. Hiss, R. G., Lamb, L. E., and Allen, M. F.: Electrocardiographic Findings in 67,375 Asymptomatic Subjects. X. Normal Values, *Am. J. Cardiol.,* 6:200, 1960.

4. Adgey, A. A. J., Geddes, J. S., Mulholland, H. C., Keegan, D. A. J., and Pantridge, J. F.: Incidence, Significance, and Management of Early Bradyarrhythmia Complicating Acute Myocardial Infarction, *Lancet,* 2:1097, 1968.

5. Norris, R. M., Mercer, C. J., and Yeates, S. E.: Sinus Rate in Acute Myocardial Infarction, *Br. Heart J.,* 34:901, 1972.

6. Hiss, R. G., and Lamb, L. E.: Electrocardiographic Findings in 122,043 Individuals, *Circulation,* 25:947, 1962.

7. Scherlag, B. J., Lazzara, R., and Helfant, R. H.: Differentiation of "A-V Junctional Rhythms," *Circulation,* 48:304, 1973.

8. Lown, B., Wyatt, N. F., and Levine, H. D.: Paroxysmal Atrial Tachycardia with Block, *Circulation,* 21:129, 1960.

9. Morgan, W. L., and Breneman, G. M.: Atrial Tachycardia with Block Treated with Digitalis, *Circulation,* 25:787, 1962.

10. Garson, A., and Gilette, P. C., Junctional Ectopic Tachycardia in Children: Electrocardiography, Electrophysiology and Pharmacologic Response, *Am. J. Cardiol.,* 44:298, 1979.

11. Josephson, M. E., and Seides, S. F.: "Clinical Cardiac Electrophysiology: Techniques and Interpretations," Lea & Febiger, Philadelphia, 1979, pp. 148–176.

12. Swartz, M. H., Teichholz, L. E., and Donoso, E.: Mitral Valve Prolapse: A Review of Associated Arrhythmias, *Am. J. Med.,* 62:377, 1977.

13. Akhtar, M., Damato, A. N., Batsford, W. P., Caracta, A. R., Ruskin, J. N., Weisfogel, G. M., and Lau, S. H.: Induction of AV Nodal Reentrant Tachycardia after Atropine, *Am. J. Cardiol.,* 36:286, 1975.

14. Josephson, M. E.: Paroxysmal Supraventricular Tachycardia: An Electrophysiologic Approach, *Am. J. Cardiol.,* 41:1123, 1978.

15. Wu, D., Denes, P., and Amat-y-Leon, F.: Clinical, Electrocardiographic and Electrophysiologic Observations in Patients with Paroxysmal Supraventricular Tachycardia, *Am. J. Cardiol.,* 41:1045, 1978.

16. Benditt, D. G., Pritchett, E. L. C., Smith, W. M., and Gallagher, J. J.: Ventriculo-atrial Intervals: Diagnostic Use in Paroxysmal Supraventricular Tachycardia, *Ann. Intern. Med.,* 91:161, 1979.

17. Shine, K. I., Kastor, J. A., and Yurchak, P. M.: Multifocal Atrial Tachycardia: Clinical and Electrocardiographic Features in Thirty-two Cases, *Circulation,* 36(suppl. 2): 236, 1967.

18. Fosmoe, R. J., Averill, K. H., and Lamb, L. E.: Electrocardiographic Findings in 67,375 Asymptomatic Subjects. II. Supraventricular Arrhythmias, *Am. J. Cardiol.,* 6:84, 1960.

19. Langendorf, R., and Pick, A.: Cardiac Arrhythmias in Infants and Children, in B. M. Gasul, R. A. Arcilla, and M. Lev (eds.), "Heart Disease in Children," J. B. Lippincott Company, Philadelphia, 1966, p. 121.

20. Slama, R., Leclercq, J. F., Rosengarten, M., Coumel, P., and Bouvrain, Y.: Multilevel Block in the Atrioventricular Node during Atrial Tachycardia and Flutter Alternating with Wenckebach Phenomenon, *Br. Heart J.,* 42:463, 1979.

21. Ettinger, P. O., Wu, D. F., De La Cruz, C., Weisse, A. B., Ahmed, S. S., and Regan, T. J.: Arrhythmias and the "Holiday Heart": Alcohol-Associated Cardiac Rhythm Disorders, *Am. Heart J.,* 95:555, 1978.

22. Forfar, J. C., Miller, H. C., and Toft, A. D.: Occult Thyrotoxicosis: A Correctable Cause of "Idiopathic" Atrial Fibrillation, *Am. J. Cardiol.,* 44:9, 1979.

23. Morganroth, J., Horowitz, L. N., Josephson, M. E., and Kastor, J. A.: Relationship of Atrial Fibrillatory Wave Amplitude to Left Atrial Size and Etiology of Heart Disease. An Old Generalization Re-examined, *Am. Heart J.,* 97:194, 1979.

24. Gouaux, J. L., and Ashman, R.: Auricular Fibrillation with Aberration Simulating Ventricular Paroxysmal Tachycardia, *Am. Heart J.,* 34:366, 1947.

25. Marriott, H. J. L., and Sandler, I. A.: Criteria, Old and New, for Differentiating between Ectopic Ventricular Beats and Aberrant Ventricular Conduction in the Presence of Atrial Fibrillation, *Prog. Cardiovasc. Dis.,* 9:18, 1966.

*26. Gallagher, J. J., Pritchett, E. L. C., Sealty, W. C., Kasell, J., and Wallace, A. G.: The Preexcitation Syndromes. *Prog. Cardiovasc. Dis.,* 20:285, 1978. (166 references)

27. Wellens, H. J., and Durrer, D.: Wolff-Parkinson-White Syndrome and Atrial Fibrillation, *Am. J. Cardiol.,* 34:777, 1974.

28. Durrer, D., Schoo, L., Schuilenburg, R. M., and Wellens, H. J. J.: The Role of Premature Beats in the Initiation and the Termination of Supraventricular Tachycardia in the Wolff-Parkinson-White Syndrome, *Circulation,* 36:644, 1967.

29. Rosen, K. M.: A-V Nodal Reentrance: An Unexpected Mechanism of Paroxysmal Tachycardia in a Patient with Preexcitation, *Circulation,* 47:1267, 1973.

30. Wellens, H. J. J.: Contribution of Cardiac Pacing to Our Understanding of the Wolff-Parkinson-White Syndrome, *Br. Heart J.,* 37:231, 1975.

31. Sung, R. J., et al.: Mechanisms of Reciprocating Tachycardia during Sinus Rhythm in Concealed Wolff-Parkinson-White Syndrome, *Circulation,* 54:338, 1976.

32. Barold, S. S., and Coumel, P.: Mechanisms of Atrioventricular Tachycardia: Role of Reentry and Concealed Accessory Bypass Tracts, *Am. J. Cardiol.,* 39:97, 1977.

33. Gillette, P. C.: Concealed Anomalous Cardiac Conduction Pathways: A Frequent Cause of Supraventricular Tachycardia, *Am. J. Cardiol.,* 40:848, 1977.

34. Przybylski, J., Chiale, P. A., Halpern, M. S., Nau, G. J., Elizari, M. V., and Rosenbaum, M. B.: Unmasking of Ventricular Preexcitation by Vagal Stimulation or Isoproterenol Administration, *Circulation,* 61:1030, 1980.

35. Giardina, A. C. V., Ehlers, K. H., and Engle, M. A.: Wolff-Parkinson-White Syndrome in Infants and Children: A Long-Term Follow-Up Study, *Br. Heart J.,* 34:839, 1972.

36. Wolff, G. S., Han, J., and Curran, J.: Wolff-Parkin-

*This article is a review of the literature and contains additional references to the literature.

son-White Syndrome in the Neonate, *Am. J. Cardiol.*, 41:559, 1978.

37. Kaplan, B. M., Langendorf, R., Lev, M., and Pick, A.: Tachycardia-Bradycardia Syndrome (So-Called "Sick Sinus Syndrome"), *Am. J. Cardiol.*, 31:497, 1973.

38. Ferrer, M. I.: "The Sick Sinus Syndrome," Futura Publishing Company, Mt. Kisco, N.Y., 1974.

39. Shaw, D. B., Holman, R. R., and Gowers, J. I.: Survival in Sinoatrial Disorder (Sick-Sinus Syndrome), *Br. Med. J.*, 1:139, 1980.

40. Brodsky, M., Wu, D., Denes, P., Kanakis, C., and Rosen, K. M.: Arrhythmias Documented by 24-Hour Continuous Electrocardiographic Monitoring in 50 Male Medical Students without Apparent Heart Disease, *Am. J. Cardiol.*, 39:390, 1977.

41. Strauss, H. C., Bigger, J. T., Jr., Saroff, A. L., and Giardina, E. G. V.: Electrophysiologic Evaluation of Sinus Node Function in Patients with Sinus Node Dysfunction, *Circulation*, 53:763, 1976.

42. Surawicz, B., and MacDonald, M. G.: Ventricular Ectopic Beats with Fixed Variable Coupling: Incidence, Clinical Significance and Factors Influencing the Coupling Interval, *Am. J. Cardiol.*, 13:198, 1964.

43. Hinkle, L. E., Carver, S. T., and Stevens, M.: The Frequency of Asymptomatic Disturbances of Cardiac Rhythm and Conduction in Middle-Aged Men, *Am. J. Cardiol.*, 24:629, 1969.

44. Faris, J. V., McHenry, P. L., Jordan, J. W., and Morris, S. N.: Prevalence and Reproducibility of Exercise-Induced Ventricular Arrhythmias during Maximal Exercise Testing in Normal Man, *Am. J. Cardiol.*, 37:617, 1976.

45. Ekblom, B., Hartley, L. H., and Day, W. C.: Occurrence and Reproducibility of Exercise-Induced Ventricular Ectopy in Normal Subjects, *Am. J. Cardiol.*, 43:35, 1979.

46. Mardelli, T. J., Morganroth, J., and Dreifus, L. S.: Superior QRS Axis of Ventricular Premature Complexes: An Additional Criterion to Enhance the Sensitivity of Exercise Stress Testing, *Am. J. Cardiol.*, 45:236, 1980.

47. DeBacker, G., Jacobs, D., Prineas, R., Crow, R., Vilandre, J., Kennedy, H., and Blackburn, H.: Ventricular Premature Contractions: A Randomized Non-drug Intervention Trial in Normal Men, *Circulation*, 59:762, 1979.

48. Coronary Drug Project Research Group: The Prognostic Importance of Premature Beats Following Myocardial Infarction: Experience in the Coronary Drug Project, *J. Am. Med. Assoc.*, 223:1116, 1973.

49. Kotler, M. N., Tabatsnik, B., Mower, M. M., and Tominaga, S.: Prognostic Significance of Ventricular Ectopic Beats with Respect to Sudden Death in the Late Postinfarction Period, *Circulation*. 47:959, 1973.

50. Rosenbaum, M. B., Halpern, M. S., Nau, G. J., Elizari, M. V., and Lazzari, J. O.: The Mechanism of Narrow Ventricular Ectopic Beats, in "Symposium of Cardiac Arrhythmias," AB Astra, Sodertalje, Sweden, 1970, p. 223

51. Kistin, A., and Landowne, M.: Retrograde Conduction from Premature Ventricular Contractions, a Common Occurrence in the Human Heart, *Circulation*, 3:738, 1951.

52. Lewis, S., Kanakis, C., Rosen, K. M., and Denes, P.: Significance of Site of Origin of Premature Ventricular Contractions, *Am. Heart J.*, 97:159, 1979.

53. Rosenbaum, M. B.: Classification of Ventricular Extrasystoles According to Form, *J. Electrocardiol.*, 2:289, 1969.

54. Massumi, R. A., Hilliard, G., DeMaria, A., Fabregas, R., Lindsay, A. E., Amsterdam, E., and Mason, D. T.: Paradoxic Phenomenon of Premature Beats with Narrow QRS in the Presence of Bundle Branch Block, *Circulation*, 47:543, 1973.

55. Lie, K. I., Wellens, H. J. J., Downar, E., and Durrer, D.: Observations on Patients with Primary Ventricular Fibrillation (A Double-Blind Randomized Study of 212 Consecutive Patients), *N. Engl. J. Med.*, 291:1324, 1974.

56. Roberts, R., Ambos, H. D., Loh, C. W., and Sobel, B. E.: Initiation of Repetitive Ventricular Depolarizations by Relatively Late Premature Complexes in Patients with Acute Myocardial Infarction, *Am. J. Cardiol.*, 41:678, 1978.

57. Winkle, R. A., Derrington, D. C., and Schroeder, J. S.: Characteristics of Ventricular Tachycardia in Ambulatory Patients, *Am. J. Cardiol.*, 39:487, 1977.

58. Chou, T-C, and Wenzke, F.: The Importance of R on T Phenomenon, *Am. Heart J.*, 96:191, 1978.

59. Tye, K-H, Samant, A., Desser, K. B., and Benchimol, A.: R on T or R on P Phenomenon? Relation to the Genesis of Ventricular Tachycardia, *Am. J. Cardiol.*, 44:632, 1979.

60. Lesch, M., Lewis, E., Humphries, J. O., and Ross, R. S.: Paroxysmal Ventricular Tachycardia in the Absence of Organic Heart Disease: Report of a Case and Review of the Literature, *Ann. Intern. Med.*, 66:950, 1967.

61. Hiss, R. G., Averill, K. H., and Lamb, L. E.: Electrocardiographic Findings in 67,375 Asymptomatic Subjects. III. Ventricular Rhythms, *Am. J. Cardiol.*, 6:96, 1960.

62. Pedersen, D. H., Zipes, D. P., Foster, P. R., and Troup, P. J.: Ventricular Tachycardia and Ventricular Fibrillation in a Young Population, *Circulation*, 60:988, 1979.

63. Wei, J. Y., Bulkley, B. H., Schaeffer, A. H., Greene, H. L., and Reid, P. R.: Mitral-Valve Prolapse Syndrome and Recurrent Ventricular Tachyarrhythmias: A Malignant Variant Refractory to Conventional Drug Therapy, *Ann. Intern. Med.*, 89:6, 1978.

64. de Soyza, N., Meacham, D., Murphy, M. L., Kane, J. J., Doherty, J. E., and Bissett, J. K.: Evaluation of Warning Arrhythmias before Paroxysmal Ventricular Tachycardia during Acute Myocardial Infarction in Man, *Circulation*, 60:814, 1979.

65. McKenna, W. J., Chetty, S., Oakley, C. M., and Goodwin, J. F.: Arrhythmia in Hypertrophic Cardiomyopathy. Exercise and 48-Hour Ambulatory Electrocardiographic Assessment with and without Beta Adrenergic Blocking Therapy, *Am. J. Cardiol.*, 45:1, 1980.

66. Wellens, H. J. J., Bar, F. W. H. M., and Lie, K. I.: The Value of the Electrocardiogram in the Differential Diagnosis of a Tachycardia with a Widened QRS Complex, *Am. J. Med.*, 64:27, 1978.

67. Wellens, H. J. J.: Personal communication.

68. Kossman, C. E.: Torsade de Pointes: An Addition to the Nosography of Ventricular Tachycardia, *Am. J. Cardiol.*, 42:1054, 1978.

69. Josephson, M. E., Horowitz, L. N., Farshidi, A., Spielman, S. R., Michelson, E. L., and Greenspan, A. M.: Recurrent Sustained Ventricular Tachycardia. 4. Pleomorphism, *Circulation*, 59:459, 1979.

70. Sclarovsky, S., Strasberg, B., Lewin, R. F., and Ag-

mon, J.: Polymorphous Ventricular Tachycardia: Clinical Features and Treatment, *Am. J. Cardiol.,* 44:339, 1979.

71. Massumi, R. A., and Ali, A.: Accelerated Isorhythmic Ventricular Rhythms, *Am. J. Cardiol.,* 26:170, 1970.

72. Gaum, W. E., Biancaniello, T., and Kaplan, S.: Accelerated Ventricular Rhythm in Childhood, *Am. J. Cardiol.,* 43:162, 1979.

73. DeSoyza, N., Bissett, J. K., Kane, J. J., Murphy, M. L., and Doherty, J. E.: Ectopic Ventricular Prematurity and Its Relation to Ventricular Tachycardia in Acute Myocardial Infarction in Man, *Circulation,* 50:529, 1974.

74. Lichstein, E., Ribas-Meneclier, C., Gupta, P. K., and Chadda, D. K.: Incidence and Description of Accelerated Ventricular Rhythm Complicating Acute Myocardial Infarction, *Am. J. Med.,* 58:192, 1975.

75. Kulbertus, H. E., de Leval-Ruten, F., and Casters, P.: Vectorcardiographic Study of Aberrant Conduction. Anterior Displacement of QRS: Another Form of Intraventricular Block, *Br. Heart J.,* 38:549, 1976.

76. Swanick, E. J., LaCamera, F., and Marriott, H. J. L.: Morphologic Features of Right Ventricular Ectopic Beats, *Am. J. Cardiol.,* 30:888, 1972.

77. Marriott, H. J. L.: Differential Diagnosis of Supraventricular and Ventricular Tachycardia, *Geriatrics,* 25:91, 1970.

78. Sandler, I. A., and Marriott, H. J. L.: The Differential Morphology of Anomalous Ventricular Complexes of RBBB-Type in Lead V1: Ventricular Ectopy versus Aberration, *Circulation,* 31:551, 1965.

79. WHO/ISC Task Force: Definition of Terms Related to Cardiac Rhythm, *Am. Heart J.,* 95:796, 1978.

80. DePasquale, N. P.: The Electrocardiogram in Complicated Acute Myocardial Infarction, *Prog. Cardiovasc. Dis.,* 13:72, 1970.

81. Stock, R. J., and Macken, D. L.: Observations on Heart Block during Continuous Electrocardiographic Monitoring in Myocardial Infarction, *Circulation,* 38:993, 1968.

82. Scheinman, M., and Brenman, B.: Clinical and Anatomic Implications of Intraventricular Conduction Blocks in Acute Myocardial Infarction, *Circulation,* 46:753, 1972.

83. Beregovich, J., Fenig, S., Lasser, J., and Allen, D.: Management of Acute Myocardial Infarction Complicated by Advanced Atrioventricular Block: Role of Artificial Pacing, *Am. J. Cardiol.,* 23:54, 1969.

84. Johnson, R. L., Averill, K. H., and Lamb, L. E.: Electrocardiographic Findings in 67,375 Asymptomatic Subjects. VII. Atrioventricular Block, *Am. J. Cardiol.,* 6:153, 1960.

85. Manning, G. W., and Sears, G. A.: Postural Heart Block, *Am. J. Cardiol.,* 9:558, 1962.

86. Zoob, M., and Smith, K. S.: The Aetiology of Complete Heart-Block, *Br. Med. J.,* 2:1149, 1963.

87. Rosenbaun, M. B.: Intraventricular Trifascicular Block, *Heart Lung,* 1:216, 1972.

88. Lev, M.: Anatomic Basis for Atrioventricular Block, *Am. J. Med.,* 37:742, 1964.

89. Damato, A. N., Lau, S. H., Helfant, R. H., Stein, E., Berkowitz, W. D., and Cohen, S. I.: A Study of Heart Block in Man Using His Bundle Recordings, *Circulation,* 39:297, 1969.

90. Damato, A. N., and Lau, S. H.: Clinical Value of the Electrocardiogram of the Conducting System, *Prog. Cardiovasc. Dis.,* 13:119, 1970.

91. Khalilullah, M., Singhal, N., Gupta, U., and Padmavati, S.: Unidirectional Complete Heart Block, *Am. Heart J.,* 97:608, 1979.

92. Rosenbaum, M. B.: Intraventricular Trifascicular Block, *Heart Lung,* 1:216, 1976.

93. Fisch, C., Zipes, D. P., and McHenry, P. L.: Electrocardiographic Manifestations of Concealed Junctional Ectopic Impulses, *Circulation,* 53:217, 1976.

94. Castellanso, A., Befeler, B., and Myerburg, R. J.: Pseudo AV Block Produced by Concealed Extrasystoles Arising below the Bifurcation of His Bundle, *Br. Heart J.,* 36:457, 1974.

95. Lindsay, A. E., and Schamroth, L.: Atrioventricular Junctional Parasystole with Concealed Conduction Simulating Second Degree AV Block, *Am. J. Cardiol.,* 31:397, 1973.

*96. Marriott, H. J. L., and Menendez, M. M.: A-V Dissociation Revisited, *Prog. Cardiovasc. Dis.,* 8:522, 1966. (28 references)

97. Sherf, L., and James. T. N.: A New Electrocardiographic Concept: Synchronized Sinoventricular Conduction, *Dis. Chest,* 55:127, 1969.

98. Nicholson, W. J., Martin, C. E., Gracey, J. G., and Knoch, H. R.: Disopyramide-Induced Ventricular Fibrillation, *Am. J. Cardiol.,* 43:1053, 1979.

99. Cooper, M. J., and Abinader, E. G.: Atropine-Induced Ventricular Fibrillation: Case Report and Review of the Literature, *Am. Heart J.,* 97:225, 1979.

29

Management of Arrhythmias and Conduction Abnormalities

Warren M. Smith, M.B., Ch.B., F.R.A.C.P.
John J. Gallagher, M.D., F.A.C.C.

I do not know what I may appear to the world: but to myself I seemed to have been only like a boy, playing on the seashore, and diverting myself and now and then finding a smoother pebble, or a prettier shell than ordinary, while the great ocean of truth lay all undiscovered before me.

Sir Isaac Newton[1]

The last decade has seen further progress in our ability to treat arrhythmias. More antiarrhythmic drugs are available to the physician, and they are being used more effectively through a better appreciation of drug pharmacokinetics. Advances in electrophysiology have made valuable contributions, especially to the mechanisms and control of reentrant arrhythmias, while increasingly sophisticated pacemakers are becoming available, together with effective surgical procedures, for a widening spectrum of arrhythmias refractory to medical management. And yet, Newton's perceptive humility has contemporary relevance (see quotation above). Despite well-documented effects of the common antiarrhythmic drugs upon normal cardiac tissues, their actions in the pathological environment of diseased heart tissue are less certain. The treatment of most arrhythmias is still largely empirical.

Treatment is generally recommended for sustained arrhythmias because symptoms are frequently present and there is often the potential for sudden death. It remains the responsibility of the treating physician to perform the clinical titration of the possible harmful effects of any given arrhythmia against the known toxicity and hazards of present modes of treatment. Although it is often assumed that ventricular arrhythmias are intrinsically more serious than supraventricular rhythms, the clinical import of any given arrhythmia is more a function of the rate of the ventricular response and the presence and severity of coexistent cardiovascular disease. Thus, rapid supraventricular tachycardia in the presence of impaired left ventricular function may precipitate left ventricular failure and ventricular fibrillation (VF), whereas slower ventricular tachycardia (VT) in the presence of apparently normal myocardium may be well tolerated for several days.

The elective treatment of a symptomatic arrhythmia begins with a careful assessment of the patient by history and physical examination, evaluation of the serum electrolytes, and examination of a chest x-ray and 12-lead ECG. Many factors may be relevant to the expression of an arrhythmia, including associated heart disease, concurrent drug therapy, QT prolongation, pulmonary disease, endocrine or autonomic imbalance, psychologic stress, excessive dieting, and undue dependence on cigarettes, caffeine, or alcohol.[2–5] Electrolyte imbalance should always be excluded, especially hypokalemia, which not only exacerbates many arrhythmias but also impairs the effectiveness of many standard drugs. If specific antiarrhythmic therapy is required, the physician must be familiar with the side effects, correct dosage, and appropriate intervals of administration. If a patient appears refractory to a particular drug, the plasma concentration (before a dose) should be measured. Careful documentation of the response to each drug given is essential, particularly if surgery or pacemaker therapy is being considered.

In this chapter, the principal antiarrhythmic agents presently available will be reviewed, with briefer accounts of some newer drugs, followed by the treatment of certain categories of clinical arrhythmias, and concluding with the consideration of the various modes of electrical control of arrhythmias, including cardioversion. Many promising investigational drugs that are not discussed have recently been reviewed elsewhere.[6]

Classification of Antiarrhythmic Drugs

There is, unfortunately, no generally accepted classification of antiarrhythmic drugs available.[7] The four classes of drug action proposed by Vaughn Williams constitute perhaps the most popular classification used clinically.[8] Under this scheme (Table 29-1) drugs with a class I action interfere directly with depolarization, class II drugs produce antisympathetic effects, and class III drugs markedly prolong the duration of the action potential. A fourth class of action appears to relate to blockade of the slow inward depolarizing current. Some drugs possess more than one class of action.

Recently, a tentative classification has been proposed on the basis of the ionic currents associated with depolarization and repolarization. Drugs are

TABLE 29-1   Classification of Antiarrhythmic Drugs[8]

Class I	Quinidine, procainamide, disopyramide, lidocaine, diphenylhydantoin
Class II	Beta-adrenergic blocking drugs
Class III	Bretylium
Class IV	Verapamil,* Nifedipine*

*This drug has not been approved by the Food and Drug Administration of the United States at the time of publication.

classified according to their principal actions on the fast inward sodium current, the slow inward calcium current, and repolarization currents, and finally the relationship between membrane currents and adrenergic receptor excitation and inhibition.[9] At the present level of knowledge, quinidine, procainamide, lidocaine, and probably the newer "class I" drugs reduce the fast inward current by reducing the number of sodium channels available. Diphenylhydantoin affects both fast and slow inward currents while the latter is selectively blocked by verapamil.* Both lidocaine and propranolol affect potassium repolarization currents. Thus some correlation between the two classifications (Vaughan Williams and ionic) exists, although the ionic basis underlying class III actions is not presently known.

Quinidine

Quinidine is one of the alkaloids obtained by chemical extraction of cinchona bark and is the optical isomer of quinine. It was prepared and named by Pasteur in 1853 but was not introduced into Western medicine until its antiarrhythmic effects were reported by Wenckebach (1914) and Frey (1918).

Pharmacokinetic Properties (Table 29-2)

Quinidine sulfate is rapidly and almost completely absorbed, with peak levels occurring about 1.5 h after ingestion. About 80 percent (range 60 to 100 percent) of the dose is available to the systemic circulation, in contrast to the gluconate salt, which is more slowly absorbed, with peak levels at 4 h and 71 percent systemic availability (range 40 to 93 percent).[10] Eighty percent of the drug is bound to plasma albumin, and the half-life averages 5 to 7 h. Quinidine is partly excreted unchanged and partly

*This drug has not been approved by the Food and Drug Administration at the time of publication.

metabolized by the liver, with the metabolites having little or no antiarrhythmic activity. Therapeutic levels range from 2.3 to 5 μg/ml.[11] Toxic effects are common with levels greater than 10 μg/ml.

Pharmacodynamic Properties

Electrophysiologic Effects Quinidine is principally concentrated in the cell membrane, where it decreases transmembrane permeability to sodium influx during phase 0 of the action potential. It depresses the maximum rate of depolarization (MRD) of the action potential and reduces the amplitude of the overshoot potential in all cardiac tissues.[12] These membrane effects are markedly lessened by hypokalemia and appear to be rate-related.[13] Quinidine also reduces phase IV depolarization and elevates the diastolic threshold of excitability. The effective refractory period (ERP) is markedly increased without a comparable increase in duration of the action potential. In awake dogs, serum concentrations of 5 to 10 mg/liter had little effect on AV node conduction but slowed conduction in Purkinje tissue and prolonged ventricular activation.[14] Similar results have been reported in human beings, with decreased conduction and increased refractoriness of the atrium and His-Purkinje system[15] without significant effect on AV nodal conduction during sinus rhythm. However, shortening of the AH interval during atrial pacing was noted, together with shortening of the ERP of the AV node, these effects being consistent with an indirect (antivagal) action. The effects of quinidine on the ECG include prolongation of both the QRS complex and QT intervals.

Hemodynamic and Cardiovascular Effects Intravenous quinidine markedly depresses myocardial contractility and decreases systemic vascular resistance, primarily by alpha-adrenergic receptor block-

TABLE 29-2 Pharmacokinetics of Antiarrhythmic Drugs

	Quinidine (Sulfate)	Procainamide	Disopyramide	Lidocaine	Diphenylhydantoin	Propranolol	Verapamil*
Percent systemic availability	80	75–90	85	Low	95 (variable)	40 (variable)	10–22
Percent plasma protein bound	80	15	35–95†	60	70–95	90–96	90
Therapeutic range	2.3–5 μg/ml	4–10 μg/ml	2–5 μg/ml	1.5–5 μg/ml	10–20 μg/ml	40–100 ng/ml	?
Half-life, h	5–7	2.5–4.7	4.5 (IV)	1.2–2	6–32	4–6 (chronic dosage)	3–7
Route of excretion	Hepatic/renal	Hepatic/renal	Renal	Hepatic	Hepatic	Hepatic	Renal
Dosage:							
Oral	300–600 mg q 6 h	250–750 mg q 4 h	100–300 mg q 6 h		200–500 mg daily	10–100 mg q 6 h	30–180 mg q 6 h
IV	5–10 mg/kg‡	10–15 mg/kg‡		15–50 μg/kg/min infusion	10–15 mg/kg‡	0.1 mg/kg‡	0.145 mg/kg

*This drug has not been approved by the Food and Drug Administration at the time of publication.
†Concentration dependent.
‡Must be given very slowly. See text for details.

ade.[16] Although severe hypotension is a feature in reports from the older literature, more recent studies[17,18] with slow infusion rates have shown only minor falls in systolic blood pressure (5 to 15 mmHg).

Clinical Application and Toxicity
Quinidine may be used to suppress atrial and ventricular premature beats, which are often the initiating mechanism of paroxysmal tachycardia. It is also used to maintain sinus rhythm after successful reversion of atrial flutter and atrial fibrillation (AF) to sinus rhythm. Because quinidine is capable of slowing the rate of atrial flutter while enhancing conduction of the AV node, quinidine alone may result in atrial flutter with 1:1 AV conduction, thereby dangerously accelerating the ventricular rate. Most patients with atrial flutter/fibrillation should be given quinidine only after prior digitalization. The one exception to this rule is patients with the Wolff-Parkinson-White (WPW) syndrome in whom quinidine prolongs refractoriness and slows conduction in the accessory pathways mediating the ventricular response to AF. The usual oral dosage is 300 to 600 mg every 6 h; intravenous administration is also possible, provided the infusion rate is slow.[17,18] Quinidine is contraindicated in the treatment of digitalis intoxication and relatively contraindicated in partial AV block because of the danger of asystole if progression to complete AV block occurs.

Unfortunately, side effects are frequent with quinidine, with gastrointestinal intolerance, particularly diarrhea, being the most common.[19] Large doses may cause cinchonism, a constellation of symptoms including tinnitus, blurred vision, and headache with gastrointestinal and cardiac toxicity in more advanced cases. Widening of the QRS complex is an indication of cardiac toxicity. Idiosyncratic reactions may result in thrombocytopenic purpura, and quinidine syncope,[20] commonly due to torsades de pointes, appears to occur as a result of both individual susceptibility and excessive plasma concentration.[21] In the older literature fatalities from this complication were reported to occur in 2 to 4 percent of patients, although 0.5 percent has been cited in the more recent reports.[19] Excessive prolongation of the QT interval may herald susceptibility to this complication. Because the normal range of QT prolongation with therapeutic quinidine levels has never been established, the actual values that constitute "excessive prolongation" are uncertain: we presently regard a QT_c greater than 0.55 as undesirable and a value of 0.60 or more as an indication to discontinue therapy. The addition of quinidine may increase the plasma digoxin concentration by displacing digoxin from its tissue-binding sites.[22]

Procainamide (Pronestyl)

Procainamide, introduced in 1951, was a result of a systematic study of congeners of procaine, an agent with known local antiarrhythmic actions on cardiac tissue but whose short half-life and central nervous system toxicity precluded clinical application. Procainamide differs from procaine by the substitution of an amide structure for an ester linkage, a change conferring resistance to plasma esterases and reducing the central excitatory effect.

Pharmacokinetic Properties
Absorption of procainamide is from 75 to 95 percent[23] in most subjects, with maximal plasma concentrations occurring about 60 min after ingestion. Procainamide is extensively localized in body tissues, but its apparent volume of distribution varies among individual patients and is lower in patients with heart failure. At therapeutic concentrations, 15 percent of the drug is bound to plasma proteins. The biologic half-life is short, 3.5 h, with a range of 2.5 to 4.7 h. Procainamide is partly eliminated by the kidneys and partly acetylated by the liver to N-acetyl procainamide, which has antiarrhythmic actions in its own right and is almost entirely excreted by the kidneys. The half-life of this metabolite in patients with normal renal function is 6 to 8 h, and effective plasma levels range from 2 to 22 µg/ml.[24]

Pharmacodynamic Properties

Electrophysiologic Effects Procainamide has effects similar to quinidine, namely decreasing the amplitude and the MRD of phase 0 of the action potential. Unlike with other class I drugs, these effects are independent of the external potassium concentration.[25] The ERP of Purkinje fibers is prolonged more than the duration of the action potential, diastolic threshold is increased, and phase IV depolarization is depressed. In Purkinje fibers with conduction disturbances due to enhanced phase IV depolarization, a biphasic effect of procainamide has been noted;[26] low procainamide concentrations (10 to 30 mg/liter) restored the diastolic membrane potential toward normal and improved conduction, whereas higher concentrations (60 to 120 mg/liter) usually further increased the conduction disturbance and actually enhanced automaticity. In studies on Purkinje fibers perfused with arterial blood from donor dogs in which therapeutic levels of procainamide had been attained, a rapid decrease in Purkinje fiber automaticity was seen, whereas slowing of conduction occurred later simultaneously with changes in the duration of the QRS complex.[27] Membrane responsiveness was not significantly depressed until toxic plasma concentrations were reached.

Studies in humans have confirmed animal experiments, with minimal prolongation of atrioventricular nodal conduction, prolongation of His-Purkinje conduction and the relative refractory period of the His-Purkinje system, and increases in the atrial ERP being observed.[28] The ERP of the AV node was also noted to decrease, possibly through an anticholinergic effect of the drug. With therapeutic levels of procainamide, the QRS complex may be prolonged 5 to 10 percent, but usually remains within the normal range unless prior abnormality was present. The PR and QT intervals are also prolonged.

Hemodynamic and Cardiovascular Effects Procainamide decreases cardiac contractility and causes hypotension via peripheral vasodilatation, probably mainly as a result of ganglionic blockade.[16] Cardiac toxicity is manifest by progressive QRS widening, ventricular arrhythmias, or electrical asystole and may be reversed by intravenous molar sodium lactate, while hypotension and impaired conduction may be improved by catecholamine infusion.[29]

Clinical Application and Toxicity

Procainamide is effective against a wide range of ventricular and supraventricular arrhythmias[30] but is probably best avoided in arrhythmias secondary to digitalis toxicity, where intensification of digitalis-related AV block may occur, together with enhancement of reentrant ventricular arrhythmias because of conduction delay. Procainamide may revert AF of recent onset to sinus rhythm, but acceleration of the ventricular response during atrial flutter, similar to quinidine, has been documented.[30]

Severe hypotension and fatalities have been recorded following intravenous procainamide.[31] The rate of intravenous administration should therefore be no greater than 50 mg/min;[23] in one study with administration of 100 mg every 5 min, hypotension and toxicity were not observed.[32] If an arrhythmia fails to revert after a total of 1 g intravenously, an alternative strategy, such as cardioversion, is preferable to the risk of inducing cardiovascular depression.

The short biologic half-life has required that procainamide be administered orally every 3 h if fluctuations greater than 50 percent in plasma concentration are to be avoided.[23] However, sustained-release preparations are now available that allow a 6-h dosage schedule. Oral dosages vary widely, largely because of variable absorption; plasma levels have a good relation to clinical effects. Initial therapy with 50 mg/kg divided into three hourly doses is a reasonable starting regimen, with recourse to estimation of the plasma levels if the desired therapeutic effect is not attained. Concentrations of 4 to 10 μg/ml are now accepted as therapeutic.[29,32] Toxic manifestations are common with levels greater than 12 μg/ml, and usual if levels exceed 16 μg/ml. Although procainamide prolongs the QT interval, in contrast to quinidine, torsade de pointe has only rarely been reported. Gastrointestinal intolerance is common. With prolonged therapy a syndrome resembling systemic lupus erythematosus (LE) may develop in patients who are slow acetylators of the drug. Fifty to seventy percent of patients can be expected to develop positive antinuclear factor titers or the LE cell phenomenon within weeks to months

of therapy, although only one-third of these will develop a systemic lupus erythematosus–like syndrome. This acquired syndrome does not usually include renal and cerebral involvement, and there is no female predilection.

Lidocaine (Lignocaine)

Lidocaine is a local anesthetic synthesized in 1946 and was first used successfully as an antiarrhythmic drug in 1950.

Pharmacokinetic Properties (Table 29-2)

Lidocaine is 60 percent bound to plasma proteins and metabolized by the liver to monoethylglycine and xylidine, which necessitates parenteral administration. Because the clearance of lidocaine approaches hepatic blood flow, drugs that reduce blood flow, such as propranolol and norepinephrine, will decrease lidocaine clearance and drugs that increase blood flow, such as isoproterenol, will increase lidocaine clearance.[33] Lidocaine clearance is also increased by phenobarbital, presumably by microsomal enzyme induction. Toxic accumulation of the drug may also occur in patients with severe liver disease. Plasma concentrations of lidocaine after bolus administration reflect a distribution phase and an elimination phase. Studies in monkeys have shown that within half a minute of bolus administration, 70 percent of the drug has left the blood and entered the lung, viscera, and muscle, while less than 1 percent has been metabolized.[34] Thereafter, as plasma levels fall, redistribution from tissues to plasma occurs, and elimination is determined by the hepatic clearance; the drug has a metabolic half-life of approximately 1.5 h (range 1.2 to 2.0 h). The duration of the antiarrhythmic effect following bolus injection approximates that of the distribution phase (10 to 20 min).

Pharmacodynamic Properties

Electrophysiologic Effects The effects of lidocaine on cardiac tissues vary according to the external potassium concentration. Initial studies performed using Tyrodes solution containing 2.7 to 3.0 meq of potassium per liter suggested that although lidocaine did reduce the MRD in canine Purkinje fibers, the required concentrations were so high as to be unlikely to contribute to the drug's antiarrhythmic action.[35] Subsequent experiments, however, showed that lidocaine at a concentration of 3 mg/liter produced a marked reduction in the MRD of atrial and ventricular potentials in 5.6 mmol KCL, whereas higher concentrations of lidocaine (5 mg/liter) had no effect in 3 mmol KCL.[36] Lidocaine also shortens the action potential duration (APD) in ventricular muscle and Purkinje tissue, with the ratio of APD/ERP being less than unity. The magnitude of this effect varies with Purkinje fiber location within the specialized conduction system,[37] being greatest in those fibers with the longest action potential durations situated in the "gate" region. Lidocaine depresses automaticity in Purkinje fibers by decreasing the slope of phase IV depolarization, an effect apparently due to an increase in membrane potassium conductance.[38]

In awake dogs, the administration of lidocaine produced no change in spontaneous heart rate or atrioventricular conduction time, although the conduction time in Purkinje tissue and the total ventricular activation time were slightly prolonged.[39] In dogs with heart block, a dose-dependent marked decrease in the ventricular escape rate was observed.

Therapeutic doses of lidocaine in patients with normal AV conduction produce minimal effects on heart rate and atrioventricular and intraventricular conduction[40] with no consistent effect on the ERP of the atria or the AV node. However, significant shortening of the ERP of the AV node does occur in some individuals, and probably explains the acceleration of ventricular rate documented in some patients given lidocaine for atrial flutter.[41] Shortening of the ERP and relative refractory period of the His-Purkinje system has also been noted.[42] In contrast, in patients with impaired atrioventricular conduction, lidocaine has precipitated complete heart block,[43,44] usually localized to the His-Purkinje system rather than the AV node. Similarly, in patients with sinus node dysfunction, sinus arrest has occurred following intravenous administration of the drug.[45,46] Lidocaine has no significant effect upon the QT interval.

Hemodynamic and Cardiovascular Effects Therapeutic doses of lidocaine cause little hemodynamic effect, although transient depression of myocardial function has been noted in patients with heart disease.[47] Animal studies suggest it is a mild cardiac depressant.

Clinical Application and Toxicity
The effectiveness of lidocaine, together with its rapid metabolism and limited toxicity, have resulted in its general use for the emergency treatment of ventricular arrhythmias complicating myocardial infarction and cardiac surgery. It also appears to be effective in controlling ventricular arrhythmias secondary to digitalis intoxication. It is less effective against atrial arrhythmias and should be avoided in atrial flutter, where enhancement of AV node conduction and slowing of the flutter rate may result in 1:1 atrioventricular conduction.

Therapeutic plasma levels are from 1.5 to 5 μg/ml. In patients with normal hepatic blood flow and function, plasma clearance is about 10 ml/kg/min.[24] As drug plasma concentration at a steady-state level equals the infusion rate divided by the plasma clearance, infusion rates of 15 to 50 μg/kg/min are appropriate. Toxic effects may occur if the infusion rate exceeds 50 μg/kg/min and blood levels exceed 5 μg/ml,[48] although the levels with serious toxicity

are usually around 9 to 10 μg/ml. In patients with heart failure, the volume of distribution is lower and hepatic clearance reduced, so that lower dosages should be used and serum levels carefully followed during maintenance infusion therapy. There also appears to be a progressive reduction in clearance with prolonged infusion, with the expected half-life of 100 min being prolonged up to 4 h in some patients receiving lidocaine after uncomplicated myocardial infarction.[49] The mechanism is unclear, but titration of the infusion rate to the antiarrhythmic effect rather than maintenance of constant rates seems prudent.

Although the common clinical practice is to administer a bolus injection of lidocaine, a single loading dose is unsatisfactory because the volume of distribution of lidocaine at equilibrium exceeds the initial volume of distribution by a factor of 3. This disadvantage may be avoided by giving either a series of smaller loading doses at approximately 8-min intervals (the half-life of the distribution phase) or a more rapid infusion (e.g., 120 μg/kg/min) for a short time preceding the standard maintenance infusion.[24] The maximum permissible bolus dosage is not clearly established, although it seems unwise to exceed 300 mg.[50] Certainly the usual clinical dose is considerably less, of the order of 1 to 2 mg/kg. With overdosage, central nervous system symptoms occur, including drowsiness, disorientation, hearing loss, paresthesia, and convulsions.[29] Rarely hypotension, sinus arrest, and death have been reported.

Diphenylhydantoin

Diphenylhydantoin was introduced as a treatment for convulsive disorders in 1938 and advocated for the treatment of acute ventricular arrhythmias in 1950. The drug was first used intravenously in 1956.

Pharmacokinetic Properties (Table 29-2)
Absorption of diphenylhydantoin may be variable, but is usually almost complete. It is 70 to 95 percent bound to plasma proteins, mainly albumin, and less than 5 percent is excreted unchanged in the urine. Most of the drug is parahydroxylated in the liver to an inactive metabolite and excreted as a glucuronic acid conjugate. The plasma half-life is approximately 24 h, but may vary enormously.[51] Furthermore, the relationship of serum level to dose in any given patient is not linear because the half-life increases with increasing drug concentration. Effective plasma levels are between 10 and 20 μg/ml, with toxic effects usually seen at levels greater than 25 μg/ml. In patients with hypoalbuminemia (e.g., nephrotic syndrome) the therapeutic level of the free drug will be associated with lower total plasma levels, which cannot therefore be used for accurate monitoring.[24] Toxic accumulation of the drug may occur in patients with severe hepatic disease; conversely, phenobarbital accelerates the rate of metabolism by induction of the hepatic microsomal

enzymes that effect parahydroxylation. Drug interactions may occur with the warfarin anticoagulants and isonicotinic acid hydrazide when administered with *para*-aminosalicylic acid, both of which decrease diphenylhydantoin's metabolism, and with quinidine sulfate, whose half-life may be shortened by 50 percent.

Pharmacodynamic Properties

Electrophysiologic Effects The electrophysiologic effects of diphenylhydantoin depend upon the extracellular potassium concentration, the drug concentration, and state of the cardiac fiber being tested. Thus experimentally, with low potassium (3.0 mg/liter) and drug (1 μg/ml) concentrations, no depressant effect upon ordinary atrial fibers has been noted,[52] whereas depression of membrane depolarization does occur with higher potassium and drug concentrations. In atrial fibers depressed by ouabain, enhancement of the rate of rise of phase 0 of the action potential is seen, and ouabain-induced SA block may be relieved.

In normal Purkinje fibers, diphenylhydantoin appears to have little or no effect upon the rate of the rise of the action potential or the size of the overshoot potential.[53] Accordingly, conduction velocity is not affected, and diastolic threshold is also unchanged. Repolarization in Purkinje fibers is accelerated, and shortening of the ERP occurs, with recovery of excitation shortened to a lesser extent than the time for repolarization. Diphenylhydantoin moderately decreases the slope of phase IV depolarization but seldom abolishes automaticity.

Some of the effects of diphenylhydantoin are consistent with an increase in potassium conductance. The drug's ability to increase membrane responsiveness requires a different explanation, however; it may also increase the activity of the sodium-carrying system or increase the electrochemical gradient for sodium by enhancing diastolic ion pumping.[54]

Studies in intact, awake dogs[55] have shown some shortening of the AV conduction time, although in cardiac denervated dogs, AV conduction time was prolonged by diphenylhydantoin, suggesting a direct depressant effect. Studies in humans have shown diphenylhydantoin to have no consistent effect on His-Purkinje or AV nodal conduction times.[56] Effects on the ECG include slight reduction of the PR interval and significant shortening of the QT interval.

Hemodynamic and Cardiovascular Effects Diphenylhydantoin appears well tolerated, although a slight fall in systolic blood pressure is usually seen with slow intravenous administration. With rapid administration cardiovascular collapse and death may occur. In patients with heart disease, 250 mg of intravenous diphenylhydantoin has been reported to transiently elevate left ventricular end-diastolic pressure without altering the cardiac index or systemic arterial pressure.[57]

Clinical Application and Toxicity

Diphenylhydantoin is a second-line drug rarely used alone. It is effective in controlling arrhythmias consequent to digoxin toxicity,[58] and this is its main current use. It is reported to be variably effective against ventricular arrhythmias unrelated to digoxin toxicity, although failure to obtain adequate plasma levels may in part explain the conflict in published reports of its efficacy.[59,60] Atrial arrhythmias respond rather poorly, and it is uniformly unsuccessful in reverting atrial flutter or fibrillation to sinus rhythm. Contraindications to its use include severe bradycardia and high-grade AV block.

The recommended intravenous dosage is 100 mg given every 5 min until the desired therapeutic effect occurs, or a total of 1000 mg has been given, or signs of toxicity (nystagmus) supervene.[61] If oral loading is desired, a reasonably rapid effect (24 h) may be achieved by administering 1000 mg on day 1, 500 mg on days 2 and 3, and thereafter maintenance doses of 300 to 500 mg daily. Acute oral overdose produces central nervous system toxicity, predominantly referable to the cerebellum and vestibular system (nystagmus, ataxia, diplopia, and vertigo), although numerous other effects, including macrocytic anemia, systemic lupus erythematosus, and pseudolymphoma, are well documented with long-term therapy.

Beta-Adrenergic Receptor Antagonists

Propranolol

The synthesis in 1957 of dichloroisoproterenol, followed by pronethalol in 1962 and propranolol in 1964, drugs capable of blocking beta adrenoreceptors, finally vindicated Alquist's concept of two types of adrenergic receptors, alpha and beta.[62] Although many newer agents have been developed, including some with partial selectivity for cardiac beta receptors, the widest experience has been with propranolol, which will be used as the index drug for the group.

Pharmacokinetic Properties (Table 29-2)

Propranolol is well absorbed from the alimentary tract, but the systemic availability of an oral dose may be less than 30 percent because of high-affinity binding by the liver and subsequent metabolism before the drug enters the systemic circulation (first-pass effect).[63] This results in a high degree of variability in plasma concentration of propranolol, so that a sevenfold range in plasma concentration has been documented in patients taking a single 80-mg dose.[64] Peak levels occur 1 to 2 h after oral administration, and the drug is 90 to 96 percent protein-bound. The half-life is 2 to 4 h, although with chronic oral administration this increases to 4 to 6 h because of some saturation of the excretion pathway. Therapeutic plasma levels range from 40 to 100 ng/ml.

Pharmacodynamic Properties

Electrophysiologic Effects The only electrophysiologic effect of propranolol in concentrations that inhibit cardiac beta adrenoreceptors is a reduction in the slope of the pacemaker potential of the sinus node, especially when this has been increased by catecholamines.[65] A second property of propranolol, completely unrelated to beta-adrenergic blockade, is a local anesthetic action, characterized by reduction in the MRD of the action potential and reduction in the overshoot potential. These changes are best explained by inhibition of the depolarizing inward sodium current, and considerable controversy has arisen over their relevance to the clinical antiarrhythmic effectiveness of propranolol and similar drugs. However, present evidence favors beta-adrenergic blockade as the mechanism of propranolol's antiarrhythmic actions when used in clinically realistic dosages. Arrhythmias have been shown to be suppressed by plasma propranolol concentrations one-fiftieth to one-hundredth of the level necessary to achieve membrane-depressant effects in isolated cardiac muscle while the dextro (+) isomer of propranolol, which has little beta-adrenergic blocking activity, is a weak antiarrhythmic drug even when patients receive 5 to 10 times the effective dose of racemic (±) propranolol. In humans, intravenous propranolol given at a dosage of 0.1 mg/kg slowed the sinus rate, increased the AH interval, and prolonged both the functional and effective refractory periods of the AV node.[66,67] No significant effects were noted on conduction or refractoriness of the normal ventricular specialized conducting system. On the ECG the corrected QT interval is slightly shortened.

Hemodynamic and Cardiovascular Effects Propranolol decreases heart rate and stroke index in both normal subjects and patients with heart disease, some of whom have shown a significant rise in the left ventricular end-diastolic pressure,[68] and indexes of myocardial contractility are also reduced. Blood flow to all tissues except the brain is reduced, and peripheral resistance is increased, probably as a reflex adjustment.

Clinical Application and Toxicity
Propranolol has proved more useful in treating supraventricular than ventricular arrhythmias. It slows the ventricular response in AF, particularly when combined with digoxin, and it often terminates acute reentrant supraventricular tachycardia when given intravenously. It may suppress ventricular premature beats and VT and is particularly indicated for exercise-induced arrhythmias. Propran-

olol has been recommended for treating some digitalis intoxication arrhythmias, but diphenylhydantoin or lidocaine are preferable if partial AV block is present.

Propranolol may be given as an intravenous bolus at a dosage of 0.1 mg/kg with the injection rate not exceeding 1 mg/min. In patients with impaired left ventricular function, the drug should be given more slowly and atropine and isoproterenol should be available to treat AV block or excessive sinus bradycardia should they occur. The oral dosage of propranolol may range from 40 to 400 mg or more daily, in part due to the variable systemic availability. Side effects mainly relate to unwanted aspects of beta blockade. Heart failure may be precipitated but is reportedly uncommon.[69] Other side effects include excessive bradycardia, bronchoconstriction, hypoglycemia, and disturbed sleep. In patients with intermittent claudication or Raynaud's phenomenon, worsening of symptoms may occur, but sudden withdrawal in patients with ischemic heart disease has (rarely) led to increasing angina and acute myocardial infarction.

Disopyramide (Norpace)

The antiarrhythmic activity of disopyramide was described in 1962 by Mokler and Van Arman. The drug was first marketed in France in 1969, and it was approved for use in the United States in 1977.

Pharmacokinetic Properties (Table 29-2)
Absorption is almost complete, with peak serum levels occurring 2 to 3 h after administration. However, absorption may be lower in patients recovering from myocardial infarction. The major route of elimination is via urinary excretion, with 60 percent of the drug being recovered unchanged within 48 h. The protein binding of disopyramide is concentration-dependent in the therapeutic range, with the free fraction ranging from 0.05 to 0.65 at concentrations between 0.1 and 10 mg/ml.[70] The half-life is 4.5 h after intravenous disopyramide and 7 h after oral administration, with therapeutic plasma levels said to be from 2 to 5 μg/ml.[71]

Pharmacodynamic Properties

Electrophysiologic Effects Disopyramide's electrophysiologic properties resemble those of quinidine and procainamide so that the amplitude and MRD of phase 0 of the action potential are reduced, and there is a concentration-dependent decrease in the slope of phase IV depolarization.[72] Repolarization is altered so that action potentials with dissimilar durations recorded from the gate region and proximal and distal sites in the Purkinje fibers become equalized. In canine Purkinje fibers surviving experimental myocardial infarction, the duration of the action potential was augmented most in fibers with originally shorter action potentials, resulting in more homogeneous repolarization within the infarcted areas.[73] Studies in humans have shown no significant effect upon AV nodal or His-Purkinje conduction, although shortening of the ERP of the AV node has been noted, possibly as an indirect anticholinergic effect.[74]

Hemodynamic and Cardiovascular Effects In intact dogs, disopyramide decreases cardiac output, coronary blood flow, and myocardial contractility. In patients, rapid intravenous injection can transiently decrease myocardial contractility and cardiac output, but associated hypotension is rare.[75] With oral dosage the negative inotropic effects of 100 mg of disopyramide and 80 mg of propranolol have been shown to be comparable, although chronic disopyramide therapy (200 mg every 6 h for 1 week) had a greater negative inotropic effect than chronic propranolol therapy (80 mg every 8 h for 1 week).[76]

Clinical Application and Toxicity

Disopyramide appears effective against both ventricular and supraventricular arrhythmias and is useful in maintaining sinus rhythm after conversion from atrial fibrillation. The usual oral dosage is 100 to 200 mg every 6 h with a maximum dose of 300 mg every 6 h. Because of the marked negative inotropic effect, extreme caution is necessary when prescribing the drug to patients with impaired left ventricular function, in whom a precipitous fall in cardiac output may occur. The most common side effects reflect the drug's anticholinergic action and are dose-dependent. Thus dryness of the mouth, blurred vision, and urinary hesitancy are common but usually transient. In patients at risk, glaucoma and acute urinary retention may be precipitated. Delayed repolarization arrhythmias (torsades de pointes) may occur with this drug as with quinidine and procainamide, usually when marked QT prolongation has occurred.

Bretylium

Bretylium, originally introduced as a hypotensive agent in 1959, was subsequently found to have antiarrhythmic properties.

Pharmacokinetic Properties

Oral absorption is unreliable, and the drug is usually given intramuscularly or intravenously. It is excreted without metabolic alteration, and the average half-life is 9.8 h (range 4 to 17 h). Therapeutic levels are stated to be 0.5 to 1.5 mg/liter.

Pharmacodynamic Properties

Electrophysiologic Effects Bretylium differs from most antiarrhythmic agents in that it fails to significantly depress automaticity. Although increased Purkinje fiber automaticity has been noted in normal dogs, this is most likely due to the release of

catecholamines into the perfusing fluid from postganglionic sympathetic nerve endings, and is not seen in reserpine-pretreated animals. Bretylium does not appear to have class I effects. Further, the membrane response curve was not shifted in one group of experiments except at the highest concentration of bretylium studied (4.8×10^{-5} mol).[77] Bretylium does however exhibit a class III effect: it prolongs the action potential duration and ERP of canine Purkinje fibers in both normal and reserpine-pretreated dogs, which suggests that this is a direct effect. Bretylium also has marked antisympathetic actions, which include initial release of norepinephrine from adrenergic nerve endings with blockade of uptake of norepinephrine and epinephrine back into the nerve terminals and decreased release of norepinephrine by subsequent sympathetic nerve activity. Bretylium appears to have an important antifibrillatory action. Dogs pretreated with bretylium are substantially protected against electrically induced VF, and spontaneous defibrillation after drug administration has been observed.[78]

Hemodynamic and Cardiovascular Effects Bretylium is said to increase contractility acutely and thus have a positive inotropic effect. However this action is absent in animals treated with reserpine and can be abolished by beta-adrenergic receptor blockade with propranolol.[79] Given acutely in patients, bretylium may cause an initial rise in blood pressure accompanied by tachycardia, with later hypotension and bradycardia.[80]

Clinical Application and Toxicity

Preliminary reports of the use of bretylium in refractory VT and VF are encouraging.[80,81] There is some uncertainty as to the optimal dose and treatment intervals, although parenteral doses of 5 to 10 mg/kg given every 6 to 8 h have been most commonly used. Toxicity to date appears largely restricted to postural hypotension. Potentiation of concomitant catecholamine infusions can occur, and parotid pain has been reported in patients with chronic oral therapy.[80]

Verapamil*

Verapamil is derived from papaverine and was first introduced as a smooth-muscle relaxant with peripheral and coronary vasodilator properties. Subsequently, it was found to also have antiarrhythmic effects.[82] In the United States it is presently an investigational drug.

Pharmacokinetic Properties (Table 29-2)

Although gastrointestinal absorption is almost complete, systemic availability is low, being only 10 to 22 percent, suggesting substantial first-pass metabolism

*This drug has not been approved by the Food and Drug Administration at the time of publication.

in the liver. Following both oral and intravenous administration, there is a bi-exponential decline in plasma levels with an initial rapid distribution phase lasting 18 to 35 min and a slower elimination phase lasting 3 to 7 h. The drug is 90 percent protein-bound, and up to 70 percent of an oral or intravenous dose is excreted via the kidneys.

Pharmacodynamic Properties

Electrophysiologic Effects Verapamil is thought to exert its antiarrhythmic effect by depressing the slow response.[83] It principally acts on the superficially located membrane storage sites for calcium and does not modify calcium uptake or binding or affect calcium-activated ATPase. Studies in humans show that verapamil exerts a selective effect upon conduction through the AV node, prolonging the AH interval, an effect only partly reversible with atropine.[84]

Hemodynamic and Cardiovascular Effects The hemodynamic effects in humans to date suggest that the negative inotropic action of verapamil is substantially lessened by the concomitant reduction of afterload via peripheral dilatation, so that the cardiac index remains unchanged.[82] However few data are available on its effect in severely compromised patients, in whom the drug may be contraindicated. Verapamil is also a powerful coronary vasodilator.

Clinical Application and Toxicity

Verapamil appears to have a narrow antiarrhythmic spectrum. Given intravenously, it reliably terminates paroxysmal atrial tachycardia on the basis of reentry within the AV node or orthodromic reciprocating tachycardia (in which activation proceeds over the AV node–His bundle and return via an accessory pathway). The ventricular response in AF and flutter is slowed.[85] Verapamil appears to have negligible effects on antegrade and retrograde conduction in accessory atrioventricular pathways,[86] and is ineffective against VT. The usual intravenous dose is 10 mg (or 0.145 mg per kilogram of body weight) given over 15 to 60 s, which may be safely repeated after 30 min. Oral dosages are considerably higher because of the low systemic availability and range from 120 to 720 mg daily. Serious side effects are uncommon, but severe hypotension, bradycardia, and asystole have been reported following intravenous use, especially when the patient was receiving concurrent beta-adrenergic blocking drugs.[87]

Management of Bradyarrhythmias and Conduction Defects

The management of chronic conduction disturbances is largely a question of the indications for permanent cardiac pacing.

Sinus Bradycardia

Sinus bradycardia generally does not require treatment unless congestive heart failure, cerebral hypoperfusion, or exercise intolerance ensues. In such circumstances, a trial of temporary pacing is indicated, with permanent pacing if unequivocal benefit is observed. In occasional patients with myocardial infarction and bradycardia-related suboptimal cardiac output, temporary pacing to speed the heart rate may improve the circulatory status during the early recovery phase.

The Sick-Sinus Syndrome

Although sanctioned by common usage, the term *sick-sinus syndrome* (SSS) focuses attention on only one aspect of what is now appreciated as a more pervasive disorder, with frequently associated impairment of atrioventricular conduction, atrial tachyarrhythmias, and suppression of subsidiary pacemakers.[88] Most patients require permanent cardiac pacing either for symptomatic bradyarrhythmias or to enable effective drug treatment of associated atrial tachyarrhythmias regardless of possible aggravation of AV block or sinus arrest. Usually a ventricular or synchronous atrioventricular pacing mode is chosen because of the possible development of complete AV block in predisposed patients.[89] However in some patients with intact VA conduction, ventricular pacing alone may be associated with decreased hemodynamic efficiency. Atrial pacing is therefore not unreasonable in selected patients without evidence of AV conduction impairment. In patients with the bradycardia-tachycardia syndrome, the development of permanent AF in one-half of the group may result in spontaneous "cure."

The role of digitalis in SSS is slightly controversial. Although digitalis has been shown not to exacerbate resting bradycardia or prolong the duration of overdrive suppression in some patients with SSS,[90] other patients definitely appear sensitive to the drug, with marked aggravation of postpacing asystole. Therefore pacemaker implantation is recommended *before* digitalization in symptomatic patients with SSS. Similarly, propranolol, quinidine, and disopyramide for the treatment of paroxysmal AF or atrial flutter usually require the presence of a pacemaker. Patients with the brady-tachy syndrome appear to have a substantial risk of thromboembolism, and anticoagulation should be considered if paroxysmal AF or atrial flutter are not suppressed by drug medication. With treatment, the prognosis of SSS appears to be that of any associated coronary artery disease or congestive heart failure.

Atrioventricular Block

As discussed in Chap. 28, conduction disturbances are most usefully divided into those occurring proximal to the His bundle (usually in the AV node) and those occurring distal to the His bundle, intra-

Hisian conduction disorders being uncommon. Thus escape pacemakers associated with a proximal level of block are situated in the region of the AV node–His bundle and result in stable, reliable rhythms of 40 to 60 per minute. In contrast, when block occurs below the His bundle, escape pacemakers arise in the distal His-Purkinje tissue and result in unstable rhythms of 20 to 40 per minute. Thus cardiac pacing is likely to be much more important for distal than for proximal conduction disturbances.

First-Degree Heart Block

This is virtually never an indication for permanent pacing, unless the prolongation is entirely at the expense of the HV interval and the patient is symptomatic, a situation discussed below.

Second-Degree Heart Block

Type I second-degree AV block (Wenckebach) is generally benign, reflecting its usual localization to the AV node, although decremental responses may occur in severely diseased His-Purkinje tissue. It is the anticipated response to rapid atrial pacing and has been observed during resting sinus rhythm in some athletes. Progression to complete AV block is unusual, and escape of a stable subsidiary rhythm may be anticipated. Therapy is therefore usually conservative and guided by the ventricular response.

In contrast, type II second-degree AV block (Mobitz) is uncommon, is almost invariably localized to the His-Purkinje system, and frequently progresses to complete heart block with anticipated escape of a slow, unstable, idioventricular pacemaker. It is therefore almost always an indication for permanent cardiac pacing. An exception is the "pseudo" type II block that has been demonstrated in the laboratory in patients with enhanced AV node conduction when atrial pacing is begun early in diastole.[91] In these artificial circumstances, block is physiological and without prognostic significance.

AV block with a fixed conduction ratio (e.g., 2:1) cannot immediately be characterized as either a type I or type II response, but the probable site of block may be judged by the attendant circumstances. Thus, if the QRS complex is wide and periods of sustained conduction are followed by sudden block, a distal site of block is probable and suggests that permanent pacing will be required. Conversely, if 2:1 block is interrupted by periods of typical type I Wenckebach cycles with narrow QRS complexes, block at the level of the AV node is probable with a favorable prognosis, although temporary pacing may be necessary if the ventricular rate is unduly slow. If doubt persists, recourse to direct recording of the His bundle deflection may be necessary (see Chap. 89).

Third-Degree (Complete) Heart Block

Complete heart block, whether arising from chronic conduction tissue disease or complicating normal sinus rhythm following acute myocardial infarction, is a medical emergency. Although the prompt institution of cardiac pacing is the anticipated response to acute heart block, considerable time may elapse before reliable ventricular capture is ensured with an electrode catheter. In the interim, the intrinsic rate of the escape pacemaker distal to the site of block may or may not be adequate to support the circulation. In the latter circumstance, and in the absence of acute myocardial infarction, an isoproterenol infusion should be started to accelerate the idioventricular pacemaker while arrangements for cardiac pacing are being made. An initial infusion rate of 0.5 μg/min is appropriate, increasing as necessary to a maximum rate of 4 μg/min providing hypotension or enhanced ventricular ectopy do not first supervene. In the presence of acute myocardial infarction, the threshold for this intervention will be higher because of the deleterious effects of catecholamines upon the survival of injured myocardium. Nevertheless, if circulatory collapse is present in this setting, an isoproterenol infusion may be lifesaving until emergency cardiac pacing is achieved.

In the majority of patients, temporary cardiac pacing will be succeeded by implantation of a permanent unit (see section on pacemakers later in this chapter). However, some children in whom congenital block apparently occurs at the level of the AV node have a sufficiently reliable junctional pacemaker to at least postpone the need for permanent pacing.

AV Dissociation

AV dissociation is never a primary diagnosis, and treatment depends upon the underlying cause. When AV dissociation arises by "default" (as a result of slowing of a primary pacemaker) or because of AV block, with emergence of a subsidiary escape rhythm, treatment should never be directed toward suppression of the escape rhythm itself, which may be life-supporting. Temporary pacing may be required, depending upon the patient's hemodynamic status. Specific therapy should aim at counteracting factors responsible for depressing sinus node function and/or AV conduction, such as stopping beta-adrenergic blocking drugs or giving atropine. When AV dissociation is due to an enhanced subsidiary pacemaker, treatment should again be directed to the underlying cause, such as digitalis toxicity or hypokalemia. Suppression of the focus with antiarrhythmic therapy should be considered only if the tachycardia rate is rapid.

Indications for Prophylactic Cardiac Pacing (See Chaps. 92 and 93)

Temporary Pacing

Complete AV block as a complication of myocardial infarction occurs in about 5 percent of patients, and opinions differ as to the indications for prophylactic pacing. In the majority of cases of inferior (posterior) infarction there is no significant conduction tissue damage and block is apparently due to a reversible process affecting the AV node.[92] Occasionally, inferior infarction alone, if it extends well forward into the interventricular septum, may involve both bundle branches at their origins, although the overall infarct size need not be large to achieve this result. In contrast, anterior infarction causes block by necrosis and destruction of the bundle branches in the middle and lower thirds of the septum and is usually very extensive. Thus prognosis for complete AV block due to anterior infarction is poor irrespective of cardiac pacing.

At present prophylactic pacing seems reasonable in patients with newly acquired right bundle branch block (RBBB) complicating acute myocardial infarction. Some authors require the additional presence of axis deviation greater than -60 to $+90°$ (i.e., associated hemiblock) and advocate frequent 12-lead electrocardiograms in the remaining patients with RBBB in whom the cardiac axis has not exceeded these limits.[93] Prophylactic pacing is not recommended for acquired left bundle branch block (LBBB) or for preexisting LBBB or RBBB. Some evidence suggests that patients with transient complete heart block associated with anterior infarction warrant long-term pacing.

Permanent Pacing
The indications for permanent pacing in patients with bundle branch block and marked prolongation of the HV interval have been much debated and remain unresolved. For the present many, but not all, authorities would agree that symptomatic patients in whom a markedly prolonged HV interval is recorded (HV interval ≥ 100 ms) should be offered permanent cardiac pacing, even though AV block has not been documented. This seems particularly reasonable in elderly patients. No consensus has been reached on whether asymptomatic patients with HV prolongation are at increased risk of sudden death from complete heart block.

Management of Tachyarrhythmias

The management of tachyarrhythmias includes pharmacologic, electronic, and surgical modes of therapy. This section will emphasize the former two approaches, while surgical therapies and indications are discussed in greater detail in Chap. 94.

Supraventricular Arrhythmias

Atrial Flutter
Paroxysmal atrial flutter is usually associated with the presence of heart disease and not infrequently follows acute myocardial infarction or open heart surgery. The aims of treatment are to control the

ventricular rate and to restore sinus rhythm and prevent recurrences. When urgent control of the ventricular rate is required, direct-current (dc) cardioversion using low energies (50 to 100 W·s) is often most appropriate, although carotid sinus massage may be temporarily effective by increasing the conduction ratio of the flutter waves over the AV node. Alternatively, either intravenous verapamil or propranolol is effective if given slowly. Verapamil may be preferable in the presence of myocardial infarction, as initial experience suggests it is well tolerated and may restore sinus rhythm.[94] In less urgent situations, oral digitalization will usually adequately control the ventricular rate.

Previously, persistent flutter was an indication for quinidine and/or elective cardioversion. However, the termination of atrial flutter by rapid atrial pacing has met with considerable success. This is certainly the most convenient approach for postoperative cardiac patients in whom temporary atrial-pacing wires are usually available, and the large majority may be converted to sinus rhythm.[95] For atrial flutter arising in other circumstances, reversion is achieved in only 50 to 75 percent of the patients.[96] A pacing rate slightly faster than the atrial flutter rate is usually required, and after atrial entrainment is attained, cessation of pacing may be followed by sinus rhythm directly or following transient atrial fibrillation. If atrial fibrillation persists as the predominant rhythm, slowing of the ventricular rate is usually observed because of concealed conduction into the AV node. Recently, termination of atrial flutter has been successful with pacing from an esophageal catheter. Quinidine and disopyramide remain the most useful drugs for long-term prophylaxis.

Atrial Fibrillation
Atrial fibrillation is usually managed in similar fashion to atrial flutter, although termination of the arrhythmia by rapid atrial pacing is not possible. Neither atrial flutter nor atrial fibrillation should be treated with quinidine without previous digitalization of the patient. Direct-current cardioversion is usually effective in restoring sinus rhythm, although if atrial fibrillation is of long duration, maintenance of sinus rhythm is usually very brief. Treatment in such cases must therefore be directed to controlling the ventricular rate with digitalis, propranolol, or verapamil. In a minority of patients, a satisfactory ventricular rate cannot be attained without toxic drug effects, and surgical section of the His bundle with pacemaker implantation is necessary.

Paroxysmal Atrial Tachycardia
Most patients with paroxysmal atrial tachycardia have either reentry within the AV node or an atrioventricular bypass tract (concealed or overt) as the basis of their arrhythmia. Uncommon causes include sinus node reentry, intraatrial reentry, and ectopic atrial tachycardia. For the treatment of acute

paroxysms where the AV node is part of the tachycardia circuit, carotid sinus massage either before or after drug therapy may terminate tachycardia. Intravenous verapamil is the drug of choice,[86] although intravenous propranolol[65] is also effective. Although a majority of patients may be reverted without complication, intravenous drug therapy should be given in a hospital setting. Persistent rhythms may require cardioversion or overdrive pacing for termination.

Prophylaxis may be achieved with drug therapy or implantation of a radio-frequency overdrive pacemaker. The aim of drug therapy is to slow conduction in the AV node (digoxin, propranolol, verapamil) or to suppress supraventricular or ventricular premature beats that initiate tachycardia (quinidine, disopyramide). Patients in whom a radio-frequency pacemaker is considered should have relatively infrequent episodes of tachycardia, and overdrive pacing should consistently interrupt tachycardia without induction of either atrial fibrillation or flutter. If the rate of tachycardia is very fast, concurrent treatment with digoxin or propranolol may slow the rate to a range more suitable for overdrive termination. Patients who fail to respond to aggressive drug therapy and are not suitable pacemaker candidates may require surgical section of an atrioventricular accessory pathway and/or ablation of the His bundle. A rare subgroup of patients in whom tachycardia is virtually continuous appears to have an accessory AV node.[97] Such patients are characteristically refractory to medical management and usually require surgery.

Ventricular Arrhythmias

Ventricular Premature Beats
Ventricular premature beats are extremely common and increase in frequency with age. Identification of patients most likely to benefit from antiarrhythmic therapy however remains at present unsatisfactory. The Lown criteria are an attempt to quantify degrees of risk associated with ventricular premature beats,[98] but the classification is open to substantial criticism.[99] Even when the presence of ventricular premature beats is known to be predictive of an increased risk of sudden death (e.g., exercise related), there remains doubt as to the degree of protection conferred by antiarrhythmic treatment. In our present state of uncertainty, it seems reasonable to treat patients whose premature beats are multifocal or demonstrate short coupling intervals (R on T phenomenon). Quinidine is still perhaps the drug of choice, although disopyramide and propranolol are good alternatives provided ventricular function is not substantially impaired. Sustained-release procainamide is also satisfactory, although its use long term is less desirable because of the possible development of a lupus erythematosus–like syndrome (see section on procainamide).

Whenever treatment is prescribed for ventricular premature beats, however, the physician carries a responsibility to carefully monitor the effects of therapy, as drug-induced rhythms are not so uncommon and when unrecognized may lead to an inappropriate and potentially fatal intensification of therapy.[21]

Ventricular Tachycardia
The treatment of VT may be divided into treatment of a spontaneous episode and the strategy for determining the best prophylactic drug regimen in patients susceptible to recurrences. In the setting of acute myocardial infarction with important LV dysfunction, immediate cardioversion of a wide QRS tachycardia, presumed to be ventricular, is very appropriate. In other settings a wide QRS tachycardia which is hemodynamically and symptomatically well tolerated is not an indication for immediate cardioversion. Accurate diagnosis of the rhythm is essential. A satisfactory and quick method is to pass an esophageal catheter to record atrial activity and look for evidence for VA dissociation.

Once the diagnosis of VT is established, intravenous lidocaine is the treatment of choice, with recourse to intravenous procainamide if conversion is not obtained. However, if neither drug reverts the tachycardia, elective cardioversion is often more appropriate than subjecting the patient to the risks of drug-induced myocardial depression and/or hypotension with further pharmacologic therapy. Alternatively, where facilities exist, the passage of a pacing electrode to the RV apex will usually allow termination by overdrive pacing or programmed stimulation.

The treatment of chronic VT has been substantially improved by the development of electrophysiologic techniques, allowing serial testing of antiarrhythmic drug regimens. All patients do not necessarily require a full electrophysiologic study. Empirical treatment may be successful if episodes of tachycardia recur frequently and drugs are administered according to their pharmacokinetic properties so that therapeutic plasma levels are achieved.[100] Experience has shown that patients whose tachycardias are self-limited or related to acute myocardial infarction or mitral valve prolapse, or in whom QT prolongation appears etiologic, are unlikely to profit by electrophysiologic study as initiation of the arrhythmia during catheterization is very uncommon. For the remainder, an electrophysiologic study is desirable to plan management.[101] Serial testing of individual or combinations of drugs can be performed by administering sequential intravenous doses, but it is usually more convenient to leave a catheter positioned in the RV apex for up to 6 days to allow testing of different oral regimens. Quinidine, disopyramide, propranolol, and procainamide are the most commonly effective drugs, although second-line drugs such as diphenylhydantoin may be very effective in individual patients. Patients refractory to conventional antiarrhythmic drugs can often be controlled by newer investigational drugs such as amiodarone.*[6] A minority may prove suitable for either pacemaker therapy or surgery provided VT is unifocal and responsive to programmed stimulation.

Arrhythmias Associated with Digitalis Intoxication

Digitalis toxicity may be associated with bradyarrhythmias due to impaired AV conduction and/or tachyarrhythmias due to either reentry or enhanced automaticity. The decision whether a given arrhythmia requires more digitalis or signifies that toxicity is already present is not always obvious. Although serum digoxin levels may be very helpful, they are not always immediately available and there is a substantial overlap between therapeutic and toxic values.[102] The serum potassium should be promptly checked, as associated hypokalemia markedly increases the likelihood of toxicity being present. Once the diagnosis of digitalis toxicity has been made, the first step is to withhold further digitalis.

In the absence of digitalis-related AV block, hypokalemia should be promptly corrected (intravenous potassium may be given up to 0.5 to 0.75 meq/min with ECG monitoring) and plasma concentrations maintained in the high-normal range.[103] Special care is necessary when administering potassium to patients with atrial flutter and a fixed AV conduction ratio, as conduction may be improved, resulting in acceleration of the ventricular response. If drug therapy for digitalis-induced arrhythmias is required, diphenylhydantoin is effective for both supraventricular and ventricular arrhythmias, and lidocaine is effective for ventricular arrhythmias. Beta-adrenergic blocking drugs have also been recommended[104] and are theoretically attractive because the sympathetic nervous system appears to at least partly mediate the effects of digitalis toxicity. Cardioversion should be avoided if at all possible, because of the increased incidence of postreversion arrhythmias, including refractory VF.[105] If cardioversion becomes essential after failure of all other measures, hypokalemia should first be corrected and a preliminary infusion of diphenylhydantoin given. Initially, very low energy levels (e.g., 10 W·s) should be used with subsequent gradual increases as necessary.

In the presence of digitalis-induced AV block, potassium and any antiarrhythmic drugs should be given very cautiously. If progression to complete AV block occurs, asystole may ensue because of drug-related suppression of subsidiary pacemakers. Therefore, if impairment of AV conduction beyond first-degree block is present, placement of a temporary-demand ventricular pacemaker is desirable before proceeding with drug therapy.

*This drug has not been approved by the Food and Drug Administration at the time of publication.

Recently several new approaches to treating digitalis toxicity have been reported. Most promising is the rapid reversal of digoxin toxicity following intravenous infusion of purified Fab fragments of digoxin-specific antibodies.[106] Potassium canrenoate, a specific aldosterone antagonist, has been reported to be effective against ouabain-induced arrhythmias in animals, with preliminary reports of successful use in small groups of patients.[107]

Arrhythmias Associated with Preexcitation Syndromes

Wolff-Parkinson-White Syndrome

The principal arrhythmias requiring treatment in patients with WPW syndrome are atrial flutter/fibrillation and orthodromic reciprocating tachycardia (RT). Atrial fibrillation is a particularly dangerous rhythm in patients whose accessory pathway has a short antegrade ERP, as VF may occur.[108] Rapid atrial fibrillation or flutter with 1:1 atrioventricular conduction is therefore usually best treated by cardioversion. Alternatively, agents blocking antegrade conduction over the accessory pathway, such as intravenous procainamide or ajmaline,* may be tried. Lidocaine appears to be variably effective, while propranolol, which does not affect antegrade conduction or refractoriness in the accessory pathway, is not appropriate in this setting. Digitalis is contraindicated in rapid atrial fibrillation, as it may increase the rate of the ventricular response.[109]

Orthodromic reciprocating tachycardia may often be terminated by simple vagal maneuvers such as carotid sinus massage or the Valsalva maneuver, combined if necessary with intravenous Tensilon or Neo-Synephrine. If these measures fail, intravenous propranolol or procainamide may be tried, although in countries where they are available verapamil and ajmaline are the drugs of choice. Pharmacologically resistant tachycardias require atrial or esophageal overdrive pacing or elective cardioversion.

Prophylaxis against Recurrent Arrhythmias
Quinidine and disopyramide are the main drugs used to prevent recurrences of atrial flutter/fibrillation, although in countries outside the United States, amiodarone has proved very effective. Failure to medically control the ventricular response during atrial fibrillation (AF) is one indication for surgical section of the accessory pathway or pathways. The long-term treatment of RT seeks both to reduce the number of premature beats that may initiate tachycardia and to lessen the disparity between the respective refractory periods of the normal and accessory pathways, and thereby diminish the probability of reentry occurring. The role of surgery is discussed in Chap. 94.

Other Forms of Preexcitation

A rapid ventricular response during AF is also encountered with the Lown-Ganong-Levine syndrome and its variants, which have in common the presence of enhanced AV node conduction.[108] Such patients are not uncommonly refractory to medical therapy and may require surgical ablation of the His bundle. RT may also occur in patients with nodoventricular Mahaim fibers, though the limited experience to date suggests that satisfactory control may be achieved with conventional medication.

Delayed Repolarization Arrhythmias

Over the last decade, considerable progress has been made in understanding the relationship between delayed repolarization, usually manifest on the surface ECG by QT prolongation and vulnerability to ventricular arrhythmias.[2] These arrhythmias include VF and torsades de pointes, whose characteristic association with QT prolongation has been well described in the French literature.[110]

The treatment of delayed repolarization arrhythmias consists of correction of the underlying cause, where this is possible, and cardiac pacing. Hypokalemia, even of mild degree, is an important aggravating factor and should always be promptly corrected. All drugs known to cause QT prolongation should be withheld, especially antiarrhythmic agents such as quinidine or procainamide, which may seriously aggravate the frequency and severity of associated arrhythmias. Unfortunately, other antiarrhythmic drugs, including propranolol and lidocaine, have not proven reliably effective, and cardioversion, while necessary to terminte prolonged arrhythmias, does not prevent continued recurrences. For emergency control, an isoproterenol infusion has been recommended[101] which shortens the QT interval and suppresses ventricular irritability by the resultant sinus tachycardia.

The treatment of choice is overdrive atrial pacing.[21] Initially rates of up to 150 beats per minute may be necessary; subsequently, decremental reduction to slower rates is usually possible. Cardiac pacing can usually be discontinued after 24 to 48 h, by which time the underlying cause of delayed repolarization has often been corrected. Exceptions include patients with chronic AV block, who require permanent pacing, and patients with the long QT syndrome, who reportedly require regular propranolol therapy and/or partial sympathectomy for control.[111]

Pacemakers and Pacing Modes in the Treatment of Cardiac Arrhythmias (See Chaps. 90, 92, and 93)

A pacemaker is an electronic device that generates stimuli to be delivered to the endocardium or myocardium by electrodes (pacing leads). Pacemakers may be used on a temporary basis when reversible factors are present, or they may be permanently implanted. Transvenous pacing systems can be implanted under local anesthesia with minimal risks, and recent improvements—including the development of "tined" leads, enhancing fixation to the endocardium, and polyurethane leads—have favored a return to this approach. Direct placement of electrodes on the ventricles can also be achieved by transmediastinal exposure which does not enter the pleural cavities, although this approach carries a slightly higher risk than the transvenous alternative. The most common indication for permanent pacing is the presence of complete heart block.

Pacing systems have also been developed for the treatment of tachyarrhythmias. Radio-frequency pacemakers consisting of an implantable receiver and pacing leads and an external, patient-operated transmitter have proven useful in the treatment of supraventricular tachycardias and, to a lesser extent, ventricular tachycardias. However, concern over the possible induction of VF has limited this latter application. Fully implantable automatic pacemakers are also now available, with complex pacing and sensing capabilities.

Pacing Modes Available to Treat Arrhythmias

Cardiac Pacing (See Chaps. 92 and 93)

Until recently, all patients with complete heart block received a demand ventricular pacemaker, which senses spontaneous ventricular activity and generates a stimulus if this activity is not detected after a certain fixed interval. Units have now been developed that are capable of sensing and pacing both atria and ventricles, enabling each atrial contraction (spontaneous or paced) to be followed at a preselected PR interval by a ventricular contraction (spontaneous or paced). This type of unit, termed an *AV sequential pacemaker*, preserves the atrial contribution to ventricular filling and is likely to see increasing use, especially in younger patients. The development of external programming makes it now possible to noninvasively change many of the pulse generator parameters, such as rate or pulse width, although this capability is associated with a higher incidence of technical malfunctions.

Demand pacing of either the atria or the ventricles may also be used to suppress recurrent tachycardia. Here the underlying principle is that of overdrive suppression of ectopic beats due to either reentry or enhanced automaticity. Simple correction of bradycardia may alone prove sufficient, or faster pacing rates may be necessary.[112] Suppression of reentrant beats is achieved through direct effects upon conduction, refractoriness, and the temporal dispersion of recovery of excitability of cardiac cells. Enhanced atrial pacemakers are suppressed primarily by the release of acetylcholine, while latent Purkinje pacemakers appear to be suppressed both by an increase in extracellular potassium and by electrogenic extrusion of sodium.[113]

Overdrive and Underdrive Cardiac Pacing (See Chap. 90)

The principle common to both these modes of pacng is that penetration of a reentrant circuit by a paced beat will create refractoriness ahead of the circulating impulse, thereby terminating the tachycardia.[114] With underdrive pacing, a rate slower than the arrhythmia is chosen so that pacing stimuli fall randomly during tachycardia until, at a critical coupling interval, the reentrant circuit is invaded and reciprocation ended. Overdrive pacing employs a rate faster than the arrhythmia, so that rate-related shortening of refractoriness favors similar penetration of the reentrant circuit and extinction of tachycardia. The susceptibility of a reentrant tachycardia to termination is governed by the following factors: (1) the dimensions of the tachycardia circuit (with longer circuits the probability increases that paced beats will successfully interrupt reciprocation); (2) the distance separating the site of stimulation from the site of tachycardia (stimulation from the right ventricle may fail to terminate reentrant ventricular tachycardia rising from the left ventricle); (3) the heart rate during tachycardia (termination is difficult with very fast rates); (4) the electrophysiologic properties of the tissues between the site of stimulation and the tachycardia circuit (an intervening zone of depressed conduction may prevent paced beats from invading the reentrant circuit.[115] Occasionally overdrive pacing accelerates the rate of tachycardia, which may then require emergency cardioversion.

Other Pacing Modalities

Both paired depolarization of the heart and simultaneous atrial and ventricular stimulation have been used clinically. Paired stimulation may be achieved by driving the heart at a regular rate with two stimuli sufficiently close so that the second occurs early in the relative refractory period of the first complex and results only in electrical depolarization without mechanical contraction. A similar result may be achieved by coupling a single pacing stimulus to each atrial or ventricular complex. Although some success has been reported with this technique,[116] the risk of the second stimulus initiating VF limits its application to atrial arrhythmias. Simultaneous stimulation of the atrium and ventricle has been utilized in the treatment of patients with the permanent form of junctional tachycardia.[97] However in addition to the hemodynamic disadvantages of this pacing mode, very premature atrial beats falling within the refractory period of the atrial pacemaker may still sometimes initiate tachycardia.

Cardioversion

Direct-current cardioversion is a safe, reliable, and rapid treatment of reentrant arrhythmias in both elective and emergency situations. Conversely, although automatic rhythms may be briefly interrupted, resumption of tachycardia is to be expected as continued ectopic discharge resumes. The rationale underlying the method is the simultaneous depolarization of all cardiac tissue, with initial recovery of the dominant pacemaker, normally the sinus node.

Cardioversion has remained the definitive treatment of VF since its first successful use in 1947.[117] Because it is the current flow through the ventricles that actually defibrillates when pulse duration is held constant, a low-impedance pathway for defibrillation is very important.[118] Factors affecting impedance include the diameter of the paddle electrodes, the nature of the paddle/skin interface, the number of preceding direct-current shocks, and the time interval between any previous discharges.

Technique of Cardioversion

See Chap. 91.

Indications and Contraindications to Cardioversion

Cardioversion is indicated for any reentrant arrhythmia associated with circulatory collapse or severe symptoms. Elective cardioversion is commonly indicated to try and revert sustained AF to sinus rhythm, may be required for drug-resistant paroxysmal atrial tachycardia, and is often the preferred alternative to aggressive pharmacologic therapy for paroxysmal VT, especially when impaired ventricular function is present. Conversely, cardioversion should be avoided in situations where it is likely that the tachyarrhythmia will immediately recur or attempts at reversion may lead to more serious arrhythmias. These situations include long-standing AF (greater than 2 years), suspected digitalis toxicity, sick-sinus syndrome, active inflammatory conditions of the heart (e.g., pericarditis), and may occur following recent embolic episodes, when anticoagulation for 3 to 4 weeks is necessary prior to attempted cardioversion. Prior anticoagulation for any patient undergoing attempted reversion of chronic AF is also recommended.

Complications of Cardioversion

In the vast majority of cases, cardioversion may be carried out uneventfully if the precautions indicated above are observed. The complications of cardioversion relate chiefly to the induction of VF if the shock is not properly synchronized with the R wave, possible myocardial damage, and the appearance of postconversion arrhythmias.

At present the risk of myocardial damage with cardioversion employing conventional energies appears small. In anesthetized animals subjected to 10 consecutive dc shocks of 400 W·s, subepicardial foci of myocardial necrosis were observed by 4 days and were more severe in animals in whom smaller paddle sizes had been used.[119] In humans, MB-CPK elevations have been reported in 2 of 30 patients undergoing elective cardioversion who received a cumulative energy dose of greater than 425 W·s.[120] Increasing the size of the paddles used to deliver the charge both reduces the degree of myocardial damage and increases the effectiveness of defibrillation, although eventually, with very large paddle sizes, reduced current density decreases defibrillatory effectiveness.[118]

Postconversion arrhythmias may be partly due to myocardial injury, or partly related to the autonomic outflow associated with cardioversion. This autonomic outflow appears to include simultaneous cholinergic and adrenergic responses, the latter requiring an intact cardiac innervation, where cholinergic responses can still be elicited after surgical denervation of the heart.[121] Atrial arrhythmias are usually due to escape beats following transient overdrive suppression of the sinus node, increased atrial automaticity, or induction of atrial fibrillation. Cardiac standstill may occasionally occur in patients cardioverted from AF who are unrecognized to have an underlying sick-sinus syndrome. Ventricular arrhythmias are less common, though ventricular premature beats, VT, and even VF may occur. Postconversion arrhythmias are more likely to occur in digitalized patients, and the presence of digitalis toxicity is a contraindication to elective cardioversion.[122] VF following countershock in this situation has sometimes proved unresponsive to further shocks, possibly because the mechanism of fibrillation is now one of enhanced automaticity. Rarely, pulmonary edema or systemic embolism has followed the elective cardioversion of chronic AF to sinus rhythm.

References

1. Da Costa Andrade, E. N.: "Sir Isaac Newton," Doubleday and Company, Inc., Garden City, N.Y., 1958.
*2. Reynolds, E. W., and Vander Ark, C. R.: Quinidine Syncope and the Delayed Repolarization Syndromes, *Mod. Concepts Cardiovascular Dis.,* 45:117, 1976. (49 references)
3. Abildskov, J. A.: The Nervous System and Cardiac Arrhythmias, *Circulation,* 52(suppl. 3):116, 1975.
4. Engel, G. L.: Psychologic Factors in Instantaneous Sudden Death, *N. Engl. J. Med.,* 294:664, 1976 (editorial).
5. Isner, J. M., Sours, H. E., Paris, A. L., Ferrans, V. J., and Roberts, W. C.: Sudden Unexpected Death in Avid Dieters Using the Liquid-Protein–Modified-Fast Diet. Observations in 17 Patients and the Role of the Prolonged QT Interval, *Circulation,* 60:1401, 1979.
*6. Zipes, D. P., and Troup, P. J.: New Antiarrhythmic Agents. Amiodarone, Aprindine, Disopyramide, Ethmozin, Mexilitine, Tocainide, Verapamil, *Am. J. Cardiol.,* 41:1005, 1978. (234 references)
7. Gettes, L. S.: On the Classification of Antiarrhythmic Drugs, *Mod. Concepts Cardiovascular Dis.,* 48:13, 1979.
*8. Vaughan Williams, E. M.: Classification of Antidysrhythmic Drugs, *Pharm. Ther.,* 1:115, 1975. (140 references)
*9. Hauswirth, O., and Singh, B. N.: Ionic Mechanisms in Heart Muscle in Relation to Genesis and the Pharmacological Control of Arrhythmias, *Pharm. Rev.,* 30:5, 1978. (327 references)
10. Greenblatt, D. J., Pfeifer, H. J., Ochs, H. R., Franke, K., MacLaughlin, D. S., Smith, T. W., and J. Koch-Wester: Pharmacokinetics of Quinidine after Intravenous, Intramuscular, and Oral Administration, *J. Pharmacol. Exp. Ther.,* 202:365, 1977.
11. Kessler, K. M., Lowenthal, D. T., Warner, H., Gibson, T., Briggs, W., and Reidenberg, M. M.: Quinidine Elimination in Patients with Congestive Heart-Failure or Poor Renal Function, *N. Engl. J. Med.,* 290:706, 1974.
12. Prinzmetal, M., Ishikawa, K., Oishi, H., Ozkan, E., Wakayama, J., and Baines, J. M.: Effects of Quinidine on Electrical Behaviour in Cardiac Muscle, *J. Pharmacol. Exp. Ther.,* 157:659, 1967.
13. Johnson, E. A., and McKinnon, M. G.: Differential Effect of Quinidine and Pyrilamine on the Myocardial Action Potential at Various Rates of Stimulation, *J. Pharmacol. Exp. Ther.,* 120:460, 1957.
14. Wallace, A. G., Cline, R. E., Sealy, W. C., Young, W. G., and Troyer, W. G.: Electrophysiologic Effects of Quinidine. Studies Using Chronically Implanted Electrodes in Awake Dogs with and without Cardiac Denervation, *Circ. Res.,* 19:960, 1966.
15. Josephson, M. E., Seides, S. F., Batsford, W. P., Weisfogel, G. M., Akhtar, M., Caracta, A. R., Lau, S. H., and Damato, A. N.: The Electrophysiologic Effects of Intramuscular Quinidine on the Atrioventricular Conducting System in Man, *Am. Heart J.,* 87:55, 1974.
*16. Hoffman, B. F., Rosen, M. R., and Wit, A. L.: Electrophysiology and Pharmacology of Cardiac Arrhythmias. VII. Cardiac Effects of Quinidine and Procainamide. B. *Am. Heart. J.,* 90:117, 1975. (36 references)
17. Conrad, K. A., Molk, B. L., and Chidsey, C. A.: Pharmacokinetic Studies of Quinidine in Patients with Arrhythmias, *Circulation,* 55:1, 1977.
18. Ueda, C. T., Hirschfield, D. S., Scheinmann, M. M., Rowland, M., Williamson, B. J., and Dzindzio, B. S.: Disposition Kinetics of Quinidine, *Clin. Pharmacol. Ther.,* 19:30, 1976.
*19. Cohen, I. S., Hershel, J., and Cohen, S. I.: Adverse Reactions to Quinidine in Hospitalized Patients: Findings Based on Data from the Boston Collaborative Drug Surveillance Program, *Prog. Cardiovascular Dis.,* 20:151, 1977. (120 references)
20. Selzer, A., and Wray, H. W.: Quinidine Syncope, *Circulation,* 30:17, 1964.
*21. Smith, W. M., and Gallagher, J. J.: Les Torsades de Pointes, *Ann. Int. Med.,* 93:578, 1980. (98 references)
22. Hager, W. D., Fenster, P., Mayersohn, M., Perrier, D., Graves, P., Marcus, F. I., and Goldman, S.:

*This article is a review of the literature and contains additional references to the literature.

Digoxin-Quinidine Interaction Pharmacokinetic Evaluation, *N. Engl. J. Med.*, 300:1238, 1979.

23. Koch-Weser, J., and Klein, S. W.: Procainamide Dosage Schedules, Plasma Concentrations and Clinical Efffects, *J. Am. Med. Assoc.*, 215:1454, 1971.

*24. Woosley, R. L., and Shand, D. G.: Pharmacokinetics of Antiarrhythmic Drugs, *Am. J. Cardiol.*, 41:986, 1978. (53 references)

25. Rosen, M., Gelband, H., Merker, C., and Hoffman, B.: Effects of Procainamide on Electrophysiologic Properties of the Canine Ventricular Conducting System, *J. Pharmacol. Exp. Ther.*, 185:438, 1973.

26. Singer, D. H., Strauss, H. C., and Hoffman, B. F.: Biphasic Effects of Procainamide on Cardiac Conduction, *Bull. N.Y. Acad. Med.*, 43:1194, 1967.

27. Rosen, M. R., Gelband, H., and Hoffman, B. F.: Canine Electrocardiographic and Cardiac Electrophysiologic Changes Induced by Procainamide, *Circulation*, 46:528, 1972.

28. Josephson, M. E., Caracta, A. R., Ricauti, M. A., Lau, S. H., and Damato, A. N.: Electrophysiologic Properties of Procainamide in Man, *Am. J. Card.*, 33:596, 1974.

*29. Bigger, J. T., Jr., and Heissenbuttel, R. H.: The Use of Procainamide and Lidocaine in the Treatment of Cardiac Arrhythmias, *Prog. Cardiovasc. Dis.*, 11:515, 1969. (117 references)

*30. Kayden, H. J., Brodie, B. B., and Steele, J. M.: Procainamide—A Review, *Circulation*, 115:118, 1957. (78 references)

31. Stearns, N. S., Callahan, E. J., and Ellis, L. B.: Value and Hazards of Intravenous Procainamide ("Pronestyl") Therapy, *J. Am. Med. Assoc.*, 148:360, 1952.

32. Giardina, E. G. V., Heissenbuttel, R. H., and Bigger, J. T., Jr.: Intermittent Intravenous Procainamide to Treat Ventricular Arrhythmias, *Ann. Intern. Med.*, 78:183, 1973.

33. Branch, R. A., Shand, D. G., Wilkinson, G. R., and Nies, A. S.: The Reduction of Lidocaine Clearance by *dl*-Propranolol—An Example of a Hemo-dynamic Drug Interaction, *J. Pharmacol. Exp. Ther.*, 184:515, 1973.

34. Benowitz, N., Forsyth, R. P., Melmon, K. L., and Rowland, M.: Lidocaine Disposition Kinetics in Monkey and Man. I. Prediction by a Perfusion Model, *Clin. Pharmacol. Ther.*, 16:87, 1974.

35. Davis, L. D., and Temte, J. V.: Electrophysiological Actions of Lidocaine on Canine Ventricular Muscle and Purkinje Fibers, *Circ. Res.*, 24:639, 1969.

36. Singh, B. H., and Vaughan Williams, E. M.: Effect of Altering Potassium Concentration on the Action of Lidocaine and Diphenylhydantoin on Rabbit Atrial and Ventricular Muscle, *Circ. Res.*, 29:286, 1971.

37. Wittig, J., Harrison, L. A., and Wallace, A. G.: Electrophysiological Effects of Lidocaine on Distal Purkinje Fibers of the Canine Heart, *Am. Heart J.*, 86:69, 1973.

38. Weld, F. M., and Bigger, J. T., Jr.: The Effect of Lidocaine on Diastolic Transmembrane Currents Determining Pacemaker Depolarization in Cardiac Purkinje Fibers, *Circ. Res.*, 38:203, 1976.

39. Sugimoto, T., Schaal, S. F., Dunn, N. M., and Wallace, A. G.: Electrophysiologic Effects of Lidocaine in Awake Dogs, *J. Pharmacol. Exp. Ther.*, 166:146, 1969.

40. Rosen, K. M., Lau, S. H., Weiss, M. B., and Damato, A. N.: The Effect of Lidocaine on Atrioventricular and Intraventricular Conduction in Man, *Am. J. Cardiol.*, 25:1, 1970.

41. Marriott, H. J. L., and Bieza, C. F.: Alarming Ventricular Acceleration after Lidocaine Administration, *Chest*, 61:682, 1972.

42. Josephson, M. E., Caracta, A. R., Lau, S. H., Gallagher, J. J., and Damato, A. N.: Effects of Lidocaine on Refractory Periods in Man, *Am. Heart J.*, 84:778, 1972.

43. Roos, J. C., and Dunning, A. J.: Effects of Lidocaine on Impulse Formation and Conduction Defects in Man, *Am. Heart J.*, 89:686, 1975.

44. Gupta, P. K., Lichstein, E., and Dhadda, K. D.: Lidocaine Induced Heart-Block in Patients with Bundle-Branch Block, *Am. J. Cardiol.*, 33:487, 1974.

45. Cheng, T. O., and Wadhwa, K.: Sinus Standstill Following Intravenous Lidocaine Administration, *J. Am. Med. Assoc.*, 223:790, 1973.

46. Lippestad, C. T., and Forfang, K.: Production of Sinus Arrest by Lignocaine, *Br. Med. J.*, I:537, 1971.

47. Schumaker, R. R., Lieberson, A. D., Childress, R. H., and Williams, J. F., Jr.: Hemodynamic Effects of Lidocaine in Patients with Heart Disease, *Circulation*, 37:965, 1968.

48. Gianelly, R., Van der Groeben, J. D., Spivack, A. P., and Harrison, D. C.: Effect of Lidocaine on Ventricular Arrhythmias in Patients wth Coronary Heart Disease, *N. Engl. J. Med.*, 277:1215, 1967.

49. Le Lorier, J., Grenon, D., Caillé, Y., Dumont, G., Brosseau, A., and Sulignac, A.: Pharmacokinetics of Lidocaine after Prolonged Intravenous Infusions in Uncomplicated Myocardial Infarction, *Ann. Intern. Med.*, 87:700, 1977.

*50. Rosen, M. R., Hoffman, B. F., and Wit, A. L: Electrophysiology and Pharmacology of Cardiac Arrhythmias. V. Cardiac Antiarrhythmic Effects of Lidocaine, *Am. Heart J.*, 89:526, 1975. (61 references)

*51. Koch-Weser, J.: Pharmacokinetics of Antiarrhythmic Drugs, *Cardiol. Clin.*, 7:191, 1975. (56 references)

52. Strauss, H. C., Bigger, J. T., Jr., Bassett, A. L., and Hoffman, B. F.: Actions of Diphenylhydantoin on the Electrical Properties of Isolated Rabbit and Canine Atria, *Circ. Res.*, 23:463, 1968.

53. Bigger, J. T., Jr., Bassett, A. L., and Hoffman, B. F.: Electrophysiological Effects of Diphenylhydantoin on Canine Purkinje Fibers. *Circ. Res.*, 22:221, 1968.

54. Bigger, J. T., Jr., Weinberg, D. I., Kovalik, A. T. W., Harris, P. D., Cranefield, P. C., and Hoffman, B. F.: Effects of Diphenylhydantoin on Excitability and Automaticity in the Canine Heart, *Circ. Res.*, 26:1, 1970.

55. Rosati, R. A., Alexander, J. A., Schaal, S. F., and Wallace, A. G.: Influence of Diphenylhydantoin on Electrophysiological Properties of the Canine Heart, *Circ. Res.*, 21:757, 1967.

56. Caracta, A. R., Damato, A. N., Josephson, M. E., Ricciutti, M. A., Gallagher, J. J., and Lau, S. H.: Electrophysiologic Actions of Diphenylhydantoin, *Circulation*, 47:1234, 1973.

57. Lieberson, A. D., Schumaker, R. R., Childress, R. H., Boyd, D. L., and Williams, J. F.: Effect of Diphenylhydantoin on Left Ventricular Function in Patients with Heart Disease, *Circulation*, 36:692, 1967.

58. Hilmi, K. I., and Reagan, T. J.: Relative Effectiveness of Antiarrhythmic Drugs in Treatment of Digitalis-Induced Ventricular Tachycardia, *Am. Heart J.*, 76:365, 1968.

59. Rosen, M., Lisak, R., and Rubin, I. L.: Diphenylhydantoin in Cardiac Arrhythmias. *Am. J. Card.*, 20:674, 1967.

*60. Mercer, E. N., and Osborne, J. A.: Current Status of Diphenylhydantoin in Heart Disease, *Ann. Intern. Med.*, 67:1084, 1967. (121 references)

61. Bigger, J. T., Jr., Schmidt, D. H., and Kutt, H.: Relationship between the Plasma Level of Diphenylhydantoin Sodium and Its Cardiac Antiarrhythmic Effects, *Circulation*, 38:363, 1968.

62. Alquist, R. P.: A Study of the Adrenergic Receptors, *Am. J. Physiol.*, 153:586, 1948.

*63. Conolly, M. E., Kesting, F., and Dollery, C. T.: The Clinical Pharmacology of Beta-Adrenoreceptor-Blocking Drugs, *Prog. Cardiovasc. Dis.*, 19:203, 1976. (310 references)

64. Shand, D. G.: Individualization of Propranolol Therapy, *Med. Clin. North Am.*, 58:1063, 1974.

*65. Singh, B. N., and Jewitt, D. E.: β-Adrenergic Receptor Blocking Drugs in Cardiac Arrhythmias, *Drugs*, 7:426, 1974. (137 references)

*66. Wit, A. L., Hoffman, B. F., and Rosen, M. R.: Electrophysiology and Pharmacology of Cardiac Arrhythmias. IX. Cardiac Electrophysiologic Effects of Beta Adrenergic Receptor Stimulation and Blockade. Part C. *Am. Heart J.*, 90:795, 1975. (61 references)

67. Seides, S. F., Josephson, M. E., Batsford, W. P., Weisfogel, G. M., Lau, S. H., and Damato, A. N.: The Electrophysiology of Propranolol in Man, *Am. Heart J.*, 88:733, 1974.

68. Robin, E., Cowan, C., Puri, P., Ganguly, S., DeBoyne, E., Martinec, M., Stock, T., and Bing, R. J. A.: A Comparative Study of Nitroglycerine and Propranolol, *Circulation*, 36:175, 1967.

69. Stephen, S. A.: Propranolol in Acute Myocardial Infarction, A Multicenter trial, *Lancet*, 2:1435, 1966.

*70. Harrison, D. C., Meffin, P. J., and Winkle, R. A.: Clinical Pharmacokinetics of Antiarrhythmic Drugs, *Prog. Cardiovasc. Dis.*, 20:217, 1977. (158 references)

*71. Koch-Weser, J.: Drug therapy. Disopyramide, *N. Engl. J. Med.*, 300:957, 1979. (59 references)

72. Kus, T., and Sasyniuk, B. I.: Electrophysiological Actions of Disopyramide Phosphate on Canine Ventricular Muscle and Purkinje Fibers, *Circ. Res.*, 37:844, 1975.

73. Sasyniuk, B. I., and Kus, T: Cellular Electrophysiologic Changes Induced by Disopyramide Phosphate in Normal and Infarcted Hearts, *J. Intern. Med. Res.*, 4(I):20, 1976.

74. Josephson, M. E., Caracta, A. R., Lau, S. H., Gallagher, J. J., and Damato, A. N.: Electrophysiological Evaluation of Disopyramide in Man, *Am. Heart J.*, 86:721, 1973.

75. Mathur, P. P.: Cardiovascular Effects of a Newer Antiarrhythmic Agent, Disopyramide Phosphate, *Am. Heart J.*, 84:764, 1972.

76. Cathcart-Rake, W. F., Coker, J. E., Atkins, F. L., Huffman, D. H., Hassanein, K. M., Shen, D. D., and Azarnoff, D. L.: The Effect of Concurrent Oral Administration of Propranolol and Disopyramide on Cardiac Function in Healthy Man, *Circulation*, 61:938, 1980.

77. Wit, A. L., Steiner, C., and Damato, A. N.: Electrophysiological Effects of Bretylium Tosylate upon Single Fibers of the Canine Specialized Conducting System and Ventricle, *J. Pharmacol. Ther.*, 173:344, 1975.

78. Bacaner, M. B.: Quantitative Comparison of Bretylium and Other Antifibrillatory Drugs, *Am. J. Cardiol.*, 21:504, 1968.

79. Markis, J. E., and Koch-Weser, J.: Characteristics and Mechanism of Inotropic and Chronotropic Actions of Bretylium Tosylate, *J. Pharmacol. Exp. Ther.*, 178:94, 1971.

80. Bernstein, J. G., and Koch-Weser, J.: Effectiveness of Bretylium Tosylate against Refractory Ventricular Arrhythmias, *Circulation*, 45:1024, 1972.

81. Holder, D. A., Sniderman, A. D., Fraser, G., and Fallen, E. L.: Experience with Bretylium Tosylate by a Hospital Cardiac Arrest Team, *Circulation*, 55:541, 1977.

*82. Singh, B. N., Eilrodt, G., and Peter, C. T.: Verapamil: A Review of Its Pharmacological Properties and Therapeutic Use, *Drugs*, 15:169, 1978. (98 references)

83. Shigenobu, K., Scneider, J. A., and Sperelakis, N.: Verapamil Blockade of Slow Na^+ and Ca^{++} Responses in Myocardial Cells, *J. Pharmacol. Exp. Ther.*, 190:280, 1974.

84. Roy, P. R., Spurrell, R. A. J., and Sowton, G. E.: The Effect of Verapamil on the Conduction System in Man, *Postgrad. Med. J.*, 50:270, 1974.

85. Heng, M. K., Singh, B. N., Roche, A. H. G., Norris, R. M., and Mercer, C. J.: Effects of Intravenous Verapamil on Cardiac Arrhythmias and on the Electrocardiogram, *Am. Heart J.*, 90:487, 1975.

86. Krikler, D. M., and Spurrell, R. A. J.: Verapamil in the Treatment of Paroxysmal Supraventricular Tachycardia, *Postgrad. Med. J.*, 50:447, 1974.

87. Benaim, M. D.: Asystole after Verapamil, *Br. Med. J.*, 2:169, 1972.

88. Ferrier, M. I.: "The Sick Sinus Syndrome," Futura Publishing Company, Mount Kisco, N.Y., 1974.

89. Rosen, K. M., Loeb, H. S., Sinno, M. Z., Rahimtoola, S. H., and Gunnar, R. M.: Cardiac Conduction in Patients with Symptomatic Sinus Node Disease, *Circulation*, 43:1836, 1971.

90. Engel, T. R., and Schaal, S. F.: Digitalis in the Sick Sinus Syndrome. The Effects of Digitalis on Sinoatrial Automaticity and Atrioventricular Conduction, *Circulation*, 48:1201, 1973.

91. Damato, A. N., Varghese, P. J., Caracta, A. R., Akhtar, M., and Lau, S. H.: Functional 2:1 A-V Block within the His-Purkinje System. Simulation of Type II A-V Block, *Circulation*, 57:534, 1973.

92. Davies, M. J.: "Pathology of the Conducting Tissue of the Heart," Butterworth & Co. (Publishers), Ltd., London, 1971.

93. Lie, K. I., Wellens, H. J., and Schuilenburg, R. M.: Bundle Branch Block and Acute Myocardial Infarction, in H. J. Wellens, K. I. Lie, and M. J. Janse (eds.), "The Conduction System of the Heart," Lea & Febiger, Philadelphia , 1976.

94. Hagemeijer, F.: Verapamil in the Management of

Supraventricular Tachyarrhythmias Occurring after a Recent Myocardial Infarction, *Circulation,* 57:751, 1978.

95. Waldo, A. L., Maclean, W. A. H., Karp, R. B., Kouchoukos, N. T., and James, T. N.: Entrainment and Interruption of Atrial Flutter with Rapid Atrial Pacing. Studies in Man Following Open Heart Surgery, *Circulation,* 56:737, 1977.

*96. Batchelder, J. E., and Zipes, D. P.: Treatment of Tachyarrhythmias by Pacing, *Arch. Intern. Med.,* 135:1115, 1975. (59 references)

97. Coumel, P., Attuel, P., and Mugiea, J.: Junctional Reciprocating Tachycardia. The Permanent Form, in H. E. Kulbertus (ed.), "Reentrant Arrhythmias," University Park Press, Baltimore, 1976.

98. Lown, B., and Wolf, M.: Approaches to Sudden Death from Coronary Heart Disease, *Circulation,* 44:130, 1971.

99. Bigger, J. T., Jr., Wenger, T. L., and Heissenbuttel, R. H.: Limitations of the Lown Grading System for the Study of Human Ventricular Arrhythmias, *Am. Heart J.,* 93:727, 1977.

100. Winkle, R. A., Alderman, E. L., Fitzgerald, J. W., and Harrison, D. C.: Treatment of Recurrent Symptomatic Ventricular Tachycardia, *Ann. Intern. Med.,* 85:1, 1976.

101. Horowitz, L. N., Josephson, M. E., Farshidi, A., Spielman, S. R., Michelson, E. L., and Greenspan, A. M.: Recurrent Sustained Ventricular Tachycardia. 3. Role of the Electrophysiology Study in Selection of Antiarrhythmic Regimens, *Circulation,* 58:986, 1978.

102. Shapiro, W.: Correlative Studies of Serum Digitalis Levels and the Arrhythmias of Digitalis Intoxication, *Am. J. Cardiol.,* 41:852, 1978.

*103. Fisch, C., and Knoebel, S. B.: Recognition and Treatment of Digitalis Toxicity, *Prog. Cardiovasc. Dis.,* 12:71, 1970. (176 references)

*104. Mason, D. T., Zelis, R., Lee, G., Hughes, J. L., Spann, J. F., and Amsterdam, E. A.: Current Concepts and Treatment of Digitalis Toxicity, *Am. J. Cardiol.,* 27:546, 1971. (105 references)

105. Rabbino, M. D., Likoff, W., and Dreifus, L. S.: Complications and Limitations of Direct-Current Countershock, *J. Am. Med. Assoc.,* 190:417, 1964.

106. Smith, T. W., Haber, E., Yeatman, L., and Butler, V. P.: Reversal of Advanced Digoxin Toxication with Fab Fragments of Digoxin Specific Antibodies, *N. Engl. J. Med.,* 294:797, 1976.

107. Yeh, B. K., Chiang, B. N., and Sung, P. K.: Antiarrhythmic Activity of Potassium Canrenoate in Man, *Am. Heart J.,* 92:308, 1976.

*108. Gallagher, J. J., Pritchett, E. L. C., Sealy, W. C., Kasell, J., and Wallace, A. G.: The Pre-excitation Syndromes, *Prog. Cardiovasc. Dis.,* 20:285, 1978. (166 references)

109. Sellers, T. D., Bashore, T. M., and Gallagher, J. J.: Digitalis in the Preexcitation Syndrome: Analysis during Atrial Fibrillation, *Circulation,* 56:260, 1977.

110. Motté, G., Coumel, P., Abitol, G., Dessertenne, F., and Slama, R.: Le syndrome QT long et syncopes par "torsades de pointe," *Arch. Mal. Coeur.,* 63:831, 1970.

*111. Schwartz, P. J., Periti, M., and Malliani, A.: The Long Q-T Syndrome, *Am. Heart J.,* 89:378, 1975. (105 references)

112. Sowton, E., Leathem, A., and Carson, P.: The Suppression of Arrhythmias by Artificial Pacemaking, *Lancet,* 2:1098, 1964.

*113. Vassalle, M.: The Relationship among Cardiac Pacemakers, *Circ. Res.,* 41:269, 1977. (60 references)

*114. Wellens, H. J. J., Bar, F. W., Gorgels, A. P., and Muncharaz, J. F.: Electrical Management of Arrhythmias with Emphasis on the Tachycardias, *Am. J. Cardiol.,* 41:1025, 1978. (42 references)

115. Wellens, H. J. J.: "Electrical Stimulation of the Heart in the Study and Treatment of Tachycardias," University Park Press, Baltimore, 1971.

116. Braunwald, E., Ross, J., Jr., and Sonnenblick, E. H.: Clinical Observations on Paired Electrical Stimulation of the Heart, *Am. J. Med.,* 37:700, 1964.

117. Beck, C. S., Pritchard, W. H., and Feil, H.: Ventricular Fibrillation of Long Duration Abolished by Electric Shock, *J. Am. Med. Assoc.,* 135:985, 1947.

*118. Ewy, G. A.: Cardiac Arrest and Resuscitation: Defibrillators and Defibrillation, *Curr. Probl. Cardiol.,* II:8, 1978. (101 references)

119. Warnes, E. D., Dahl, C., and Ewy, G. A: Myocardial Injury from Transthoracic Defibrillator Countershock, *Arch. Pathol.,* 99:55, 1975.

120. Ehsani, A., Ewy, G. A., and Sobel, B. E.: Effects of Electrical Countershock on Serum Creatine Phosphokinase (CPK) Isoenzyme Activity, *Am. J. Cardiol.,* 37:12, 1976.

121. Cobb, F. R., Wallace, A. G., and Wagner, G. S.: Cardiac Inotropic and Coronary Vascular Responses to Countershock. Evidence for Excitation of Intracardiac Nerves, *Circ. Res.,* 23:731, 1968.

*122. Resnekov, L.: Present Status of Electroversion in the Management of Cardiac Dysrhythmias, *Circulation,* 47:1356, 1973. (46 references)

Section F Syncope

30

Syncope

Arnold M. Weissler, M.D.
Richard P. Lewis, M.D.
Harisios Boudoulas, M.D.
James V. Warren, M.D.

Syncope, or *fainting*, describes an episode characterized by a transient loss of consciousness. It is usually of cardiovascular origin. Clinically, it is to be separated from a large variety of "spells," meaning anything from transient and sudden weakness, a clouding or loss of consciousness, brief "fits" of cerebral origin, acute episodes of vertigo, and even sudden death.

Central to this larger cluster of disorders causing transient unconsciousness is the classic, common faint, probably best labeled *vasodepressor syncope*. Not only is it frequently seen, it is usually readily identifiable. It may appear in an incomplete or modified form in other types of episodes. Today, the physician, especially the cardiologist, sees an increasing number of patients who have sustained a transient loss of consciousness, the cause of which must be identified. This often requires a complex series of tests. The recognition of the vasodepressor syncope syndrome can save much unnecessary laboratory study. Knowledge of the clinical picture of the classic faint therefore becomes critical.

The Classic Faint—
Vasodepressor Syncope

Fainting can be a dramatic episode to all who view it. Probably no description is more vivid than that provided by Soma Weiss, one of the early clinical investigators of syncope:

> In the severe type with rapid onset the patient collapses instantly without warning. The body lies crumpled and motionless. The face and the body surface are ghastly pale. The pupils usually are dilated, and the conjunctival reflexes are absent. Respiration usually is either shallow and slow, or deep and sighing. The heart sounds are slow or normal in rate, barely audible. The radial pulse may be imperceptible or weak, but the carotid and femoral pulsations usually are easily palpable. There may be rather slow, clonic movements localized in the facial muscles or over the upper part of the body; in rare instances they may be generalized. There is no other condition including the deepest coma which so closely resembles death. No wonder that a simple benign syncope is often described as "an attack in which the patient almost died."[45]

The common faint is the most frequently encountered clinical form of syncope in the normal subject, although it may occur in the person with disease as well. It may occur as a response to sudden emotional stress or in a setting of real, threatened, or fantasied injury. The reaction is not infrequently brought on by venipuncture or the sight of blood, and it is also observed after sudden painful experience such as may occur during surgical manipulation or following severe tissue injury. It is particularly likely to occur in certain environmental settings, such as in a hot and crowded room, especially if the individual is fatigued, hungry, or ill or has experienced recent blood loss. The common faint is usually encountered when the patient is in the upright or sitting posture but may rarely occur while the patient is recumbent. Clinically, it is characterized by a fall in arterial pressure associated with impairment or loss of consciousness and accompanied by a marked degree of autonomic overactivity, as evidenced by pallor, sweating, nausea, mydriasis, hypotension, and bradycardia.

Less dramatic than the sudden collapse, but of equal importance in recognizing the clinical syndrome, are the premonitory symptoms of the fainting reaction. These more gradually occurring changes may appear minutes before the loss of consciousness and postural tone. One often observes first the occurrence of pallor accompanied by beads of perspiration. The subject soon experiences an epigastric discomfort which is frequently likened to nausea but often distinguished as a separate sensation. Associated yawning and sighing lead to frank hyperventilation. Close observation reveals the presence of pupillary dilation, and the individual reports the occurrence of visual blurring just prior to loss of consciousness. Although the sudden nature of the fainting episode, with precipitous fall in arterial pressure, is commonly emphasized, one observes in laboratory-induced syncope a relentless and more gradual fall in systolic and diastolic pressure prior to collapse. During this period, which we have referred to as *presyncope*, the patient has difficulty in concentration, gradually becomes unaware of the surroundings, and almost prefers the anticipated unconsciousness to the generalized distress in this presyncopal phase. Although bradycardia is regularly present at the time of unconsciousness, this premonitory phase of the fainting reaction is most often associated with a relatively rapid heart rate.[1] With continuing hypotension, progressive slowing of the pulse appears and may be marked at the moment that the individual loses consciousness. When the subject of a syncopal reaction is allowed to rest with the head down, consciousness is rapidly regained, while the relative bradycardia persists. Of additional importance in the overall clinical picture of vasodepressor syncope are the postsyncopal findings, characterized by a persistence of pallor, nausea, weakness, sweating, and oliguria and a tendency toward recurrence of the reaction if the individual is returning to the upright posture.

The hemodynamic mechanisms responsible for vasodepressor syncope have interested authors for over a century.[2] Although it was first felt that fainting might represent a severe depression of cardiac output, measurements have demonstrated little decline in cardiac output beyond that which occurs with assumption of the head-up posture.[3-5] The entire reaction may develop in the absence of diminished cardiac output. It is rather the marked and consistent fall in total peripheral vascular resistance that is the essential element responsible for the fall in arterial pressure and the diminished perfusion pressure to the brain in vasodepressor syncope. The peripheral hemodynamic factors responsible for the marked fall in arterial pressure were first suggested in observations by John Hunter in 1793, when he wrote,[6] "I bled a lady but she fainted and while she continued in the fit the colour of the blood that came from the vein was a fine scarlet." This description of arterialization of venous blood was the first observation reflecting on the greatly increased blood flow to the forearm during fainting, a finding which has been confirmed repeatedly in studies employing plethysmographic techniques.[7-9] From such studies

it is apparent that vascular resistance in the skeletal muscle bed is markedly reduced. Resistance is reduced, as well, in other major vascular areas, such as the mesenteric,[10] renal[11,12] and cerebral[13,14] beds. Of particular importance is the fact that the fall in total peripheral resistance is not compensated by a rise in cardiac output, as occurs in normal individuals in the presence of widespread vascular dilatation. Why the heart fails to respond to this stimulus is not entirely clear. Vagal inhibition may be a contributory factor. On the other hand, vasodepressor syncope may occur even when vagal activity is blocked by atropine.[5] This failure of the heart to respond appears to be related to postural shifts in blood volume in which the central venous volume is diminished.[15-18] The decrease in the central venous reservoir is sufficient to diminish the rate of ventricular filling. Recent evidence indicates that peripheral venodilatation, which could conceivably further impair ventricular filling during syncope, is not an important contributing factor. In fact, active venoconstriction appears to be the predominant response during vasodepressor syncope.[19] Thus, the failure of the cardiac output to increase in the face of a profound fall in peripheral resistance accounts for the marked decrease in arterial pressure and the diminished perfusion to the brain in vasodepressor syncope.

Although renin and aldosterone levels are known to increase in the upright posture, the renin-angiotensin system has been generally thought to function only in relation to long-term circulatory adjustments to the upright position. Studies have demonstrated a diminished rise in plasma renin activity among subjects who develop spontaneous vasodepressor syncope during upright tilt.[20] These observations suggest that the renin-angiotensin system may play a role in immediate postural circulatory adjustments and thus can influence the development of vasodepressor syncope.

The onset of unconsciousness in syncope is associated with the sudden appearance in the electroencephalogram of large-amplitude slow-wave activity.[1] This dramatic change in the electroencephalogram occurs only after severe diminution in mean arterial pressure (average pressure, 25 mmHg at heart level) and is accompanied by a fall in cerebral blood flow to 50 to 70 percent of normal.[1,6,14]

It is of interest to note that if one considers the average distance from the heart to the brain of 45 cm and the specific gravity of blood (1.058), an adequate pressure head of at least 31 mmHg at heart level is required to maintain cerebral perfusion in the upright posture. Considering the average decrease of 7 mmHg in venous pressure at the level of the brain when the upright posture is assumed, the arterial pressure at which fainting occurs in the upright tilt under laboratory conditions coincides well with that predicted on the basis of physical factors alone.

Accompanying the common faint there is usually

a moderate to severe degree of hyperventilation that is most probably the result of the associated anxiety as well as the cerebral hypoxia. Associated with the hyperventilation there is a fall in the arterial carbon dioxide content.[5] The recognized effect of hypocapnia in lowering cerebral blood flow may serve to accentuate the circulatory embarrassment in syncope.

A particularly intriguing aspect of the fainting reaction is the postsyncopal oliguria. It would appear that this antidiuresis is related to excessive secretion of antidiuretic hormone.[13] The possible role of the posterior pituitary substance in inducing some of the other alterations in syncope, viz., pallor and nausea, has been stressed by some investigators.

The underlying precipitating event in vasodepressor syncope has been the subject of considerable speculation. In the normal person vasodepressor syncope most frequently occurs in the upright posture and under circumstances that the person finds distasteful. Social behavior or other situational factors force the patient to stand his or her ground, and thus a state occurs in which the body reactions for fight or flight are in part mobilized, yet in part suppressed. Extensive peripheral arteriolar dilatation occurs, unaccompanied by a supporting cardiac response. The incomplete circulatory response results in a fall in arterial pressure and syncope. The emotional factors involved in the above interpretation were proposed initially by Darwin[21] and have been elaborated in later years by Engel and Romano.[22] A possible neurogenic network connecting the emotional and the cardiovascular changes in the syncopal responses was suggested by studies in animals, demonstrating a central vasomotor outflow pathway responsible for generalized arteriolar dilatation and a fall in arterial pressure.

Although vasodepressor syncope is most often observed in individuals with a normal circulation, the syncopal reaction is not at all uncommon in patients with cardiovascular disease. The mechanisms of the fainting reaction under these circumstances may be similar to that in the normal person, viz., fall in arterial pressure consequent upon a sudden decrease in peripheral vascular resistance, occurring in a setting in which the heart fails to compensate by an increase in output. The fall in peripheral resistance in these disease states may be induced by emotion or exercise. Syncope of this type may be observed in patients with aortic stenosis, in various forms of congenital heart disease, and in primary pulmonary hypertension.[23] Under these circumstances the cardiac lesion offers an additional impediment to cardiac responsiveness. Cardiac arrhythmias often contribute to the syncope in these conditions.

Syncope is often noted in patients with acute or chronic anemia and in individuals who have received surgical or pharmacologic sympathectomies.[6,24] Under these circumstances, the lowered blood volume or the diminished vascular responsiveness in the upright posture creates a hemodynamic setting predisposing to the fainting reaction. Occasionally, vasodepressor syncope occurs immediately following acute myocardial infarction or during a severe attack of angina pectoris. In addition to vasodepressor syncope, fainting due to cardiac arrhythmia must always be considered under these circumstances. Vasodepressor syncope of an unusual type may occur in the course of pregnancy. It is notable that this form of syncope may actually be precipitated by lying down and relieved by standing.[10,25] Syncope has also been noted to occur following strenuous exercise, after the intake of vasodilating drugs such as nitrites and nitroglycerin, in patients receiving various tranquilizing agents and L-dopa for Parkinson's disease. Fainting is particularly likely to occur in the course of acute febrile infections and following prolonged recumbency in chronic illness. Normal persons at bed rest for several days have a propensity for fainting, particularly when they arise abruptly from the recumbent position. A problem of importance in aviation and space medicine is the vasodepressor syncope occurring during acceleration, particularly when centrifugal force is applied in the head-to-foot position. Vasodepressor syncope is probably the most frequent cause of cardiovascular collapse during dental manipulations.

The therapy of vasodepressor syncope consists of placing the patient in a recumbent position with the head lower than the rest of the body. When profound bradycardia persists, intravenous atropine may be required. Rarely, vasodepressor therapy is needed to control prolonged hypotension associated with vasodepressor syncope.

Other Causes of Transient Unconsciousness

If the fainting episode is not classic vasodepressor syncope, it must be due to one of the many causes of acute cerebral dysfunction. Normally, effective cerebral blood flow is remarkably well maintained by the cardiovascular system of the human being. It can, however, become transiently disorganized from a variety of causes, including heart dysfunction, faulty arterial pressure control, local circulatory disease, or reflex and metabolic malfunctions. This may lead to fainting. The physician must then analyze the various components to determine the cause of a syncopal episode. They are considered here as outlined in Table 30-1.

Cardiac Syncope

Either severe obstruction to cardiac output or disturbances of cardiac rhythm can produce syncope. Obstructive lesions and arrhythmias frequently coexist, and indeed one abnormality may precipitate the other. The diagnosis of lesions producing ob-

TABLE 30-1   Types of Syncope

1. The classic faint—vasodepressor syncope
2. Cardiac syncope
    a. Obstruction to cardiac output
    b. Arrhythmia
3. Faulty arterial pressure control—orthostatic hypotension
4. Syncope in cerebrovascular disease
5. Reflex types of syncope
6. Carotid sinus syncope
7. Cough syncope
8. Postmicturition syncope
9. Glossopharyngeal neuralgia
10. Syncope in divers
11. Noncardiovascular syncope
    a. Hypoxia
    b. Hypoglycemia and hyperventilation
    c. Cerebral dysfunction
    d. Vertigo
    e. Hysteria
    f. Syncopal migraine

struction to flow can usually be made by physical examination. The recognition of arrhythmias is more difficult because of their transient nature.

Obstruction to Cardiac Output as a Cause of Syncope[26–30a]

Syncope, particularly with effort, is a major symptom of aortic stenosis. The mechanisms are unclear, but studies suggest an apparent reflex fall in peripheral vascular resistance as the usual cause. A failure of cardiac output to increase with exercise may also play a role. Finally, transient arrhythmias may also precipitate syncope. Syncope associated with effort is also observed in patients with idiopathic hypertrophic subaortic stenosis. It often occurs after exertion. Increased outflow obstruction due to a combination of increased contractility, a fall in peripheral resistance, and a decreased ventricular volume are probably explanations. Transient arrhythmias also play a role in some instances.

A left atrial myxoma may obstruct left ventricular filling, leading to low cardiac output and syncope. It may be related to body positions. Mitral stenosis, prosthetic valve malfunction, and cardiac tamponade may also produce syncope, particularly if tachycardia or other arrhythmias are present.

Primary pulmonary hypertension or pulmonary hypertension secondary to congenital heart disease may be complicated by syncope, particularly with effort. The right ventricle cannot increase the cardiac output on demand. Syncope has been reported as the initial or the predominant symptom of pulmonary embolism.

In the tetralogy of Fallot, the magnitude of the right-to-left shunt increases with effort because the right ventricular outflow obstruction is usually fixed while systemic resistance drops. The result is marked arterial hypoxia, which may result in syncope.

The history and physical examination usually suggest the diagnosis, but not always the severity, of the disease. The next step is to perform appropriate noninvasive tests. Dense calcifications of the aortic and/or mitral valves usually indicate a severe stenotic lesion. Fluoroscopy is the simplest method to define valvular calcification. It is also useful in the evaluation of prosthetic valve function and abnormalities in the pulmonary vasculature. The echocardiogram is the method of choice for the diagnosis of mitral stenosis; pericardial effusion, which may lead to tamponade; idiopathic hypertrophic subaortic stenosis; and left atrial myxoma. It is also useful for evaluation of prosthetic valve function and for the diagnosis of the tetralogy of Fallot and pulmonary hypertension. A prolonged left ventricular ejection time is consistent with significant aortic stenosis or idiopathic hypertrophic subaortic stenosis, and it is easily obtained from the systolic time intervals. The upstroke of the carotid pulse distinguishes between these two forms of aortic outflow obstruction. Radioisotopic techniques are useful for the diagnosis of pulmonary embolism. If the noninvasive tests are inconclusive, cardiac catheterization and angiography may be required.

Arrhythmias as a Cause of Syncope

Either extremes of ventricular rate can depress cardiac output to a point of critical hypotension and syncope. Arrhythmias are a common cause of syncope and must be considered in all cases without obvious cause. The most common arrhythmias producing syncope are summarized in Table 30-2. More than 50 percent of patients with rhythm disturbances leading to syncope or presyncope are not aware of their arrhythmias.

Syncope due to arrhythmias often depends on other factors. For example, patients with normal cardiac function can tolerate most of the arrhythmias listed in Table 30-2. This is not true if there is obstruction to flow or severe myocardial failure. Symptoms also may be related to the patient's position, blood pressure, or blood volume. Thus, the same arrhythmias may not always cause the same symptoms.

Methods used to study arrhythmias include the routine electrocardiogram, exercise testing, ambulatory monitoring, and electrophysiologic stud-

TABLE 30-2   Cardiac Causes of Syncope

Arrhythmias

Profound sinus bradycardia or sinoatrial exit block
Supraventricular tachycardia
High-grade atrioventricular block
Frequent premature ventricular beats (PVBs)
Repetitive pairs of PVBs
Ventricular tachycardia
Pacemaker malfunction
More than one arrhythmia

ies.[28,32–34] (See Chap. 4.) Due to the transient nature of most arrhythmias, the routine electrocardiogram is of limited value. The electrocardiogram is useful for identifying patients with Wolff-Parkinson-White syndrome and patients with prolonged QT interval, conditions known to be associated with arrhythmias. While identification of second- or third-degree atrioventricular block is very useful, the presence of bundle branch block has not proven to be a reliable predictor of syncope.

Exercise testing is a method for directly provoking arrhythmias, and many clinical and physiologic studies support this approach. The chance of detecting transient and random arrhythmias, however, is better achieved by prolonged monitoring. Although this can be done in the hospital, experience with monitor units has shown ambulatory monitoring to be superior. A 24-h period constitutes one complete diurnal wake-sleep cycle, but the optimal time for ambulatory monitoring is not clear. In some patients whose symptoms are intermittent, repetitive studies may be necessary until the abnormality is detected; otherwise the patient can be given a portable ECG transmission device.[31] Recent studies indicate that ambulatory monitoring is superior to exercise testing in detecting arrhythmia as a cause for syncope.[32]

In patients in whom ambulatory monitoring and exercise testing fail to reveal an arrhythmic basis of syncope, an electrophysiologic study may be indicated. Most of these patients are older and have diffuse conduction system disease. They usually fall into the "sick-sinus syndrome" category.[35]

Sinus node and atrial function is evaluated by measuring the sinoatrial recovery time, sinoatrial conduction time, and inter- and intraatrial conduction time. The conduction and automaticity of the atrioventricular junction can also be assessed. In patients with syncope due to tachycardia, both supraventricular or ventricular tachycardia can be reproduced by introduction of premature stimuli. This approach also allows definition of the mechanism of the tachycardia and evaluation of drug therapy.

Patients with an arrhythmic basis for syncope usually have two or more electrophysiologic abnormalities, while patients without syncope have either no electrophysiologic abnormalities or only one abnormality. The incidence of syncope increases as the number of abnormalities increases. Syncope is unlikely to be due to sinoatrial dysfunction or atrioventricular conduction defects if abnormalities are not detected by electrophysiologic stress testing.[33]

In our experience, in patients with no obvious cause of syncope or presyncope in whom arrhythmia is strongly suspected, the cause of symptoms is detected with ambulatory monitoring alone in approximately 50 percent of patients so treated, with electrophysiologic studies alone in 65 to 70 percent of patients so tested, and with exercise testing alone in approximately 10 percent of patients so tested. The combination of all methods will detect the cause of symptoms in 80 to 85 percent of patients (Fig. 30-1).

Faulty Arterial Pressure Control: Orthostatic Hypotension

When the normal individual assumes the upright posture, the attendant gravitational stresses on the circulation are compensated by several mechanisms, viz., reflex arteriolar and venous constriction, acceleration of heart rate, and mechanical factors including the venous valvular system, the mechanical pumping of the leg muscles, and decreased intrathoracic pressure. The increased autonomic activity during upright posture is reflected in an increase in plasma catecholamine levels. Chronic orthostatic hypotension is a disorder in which the autonomic factors compensating for the upright posture are inadequate or absent. Assumption of the upright posture in such patients is associated with a prompt fall in arterial pressure. Hypotension is progressive over a period of seconds to minutes, depending on the degree of loss in the adaptive responses, until perfusion pressure to the brain becomes inadequate to sustain consciousness. When the recumbent posture is resumed, there is rapid return toward normal in arterial pressure and consciousness is regained. The failure of reflex hemodynamic adaptation in the upright posture in chronic orthostatic hypotension is a reflection of an overall deficiency in autonomic function. Thus, during the presyncopal period in these patients there is little or no increase in heart rate, and there is absence of the autonomically induced pallor, sweating, and epigastric distress seen in vasodepressor syncope. Between episodes of fainting, the patients often demonstrate

FIGURE 30-1 Relative sensitivity of electrophysiologic studies (EP), ambulatory monitoring (AM), and exercise testing (ET) in detecting arrhythmias in patients with no obvious cause of syncope. Electrophysiologic studies are more sensitive than the ambulatory monitoring, and ambulatory monitoring is more sensitive than the exercise testing. However, each method could detect arrhythmias not detected by the other methods.

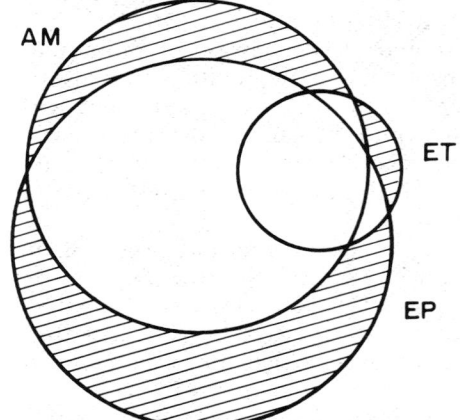

defects in autonomic function, including impotence, disturbances of bladder and bowel function, and absence of sweating. Urinary excretion of catecholamines may diminish, and plasma catecholamine levels fail to rise during head-up tilt.[36,37] Other manifestations of the autonomic imbalance include a decreased or absent arterial pressure overshoot in the Valsalva response, a fall in arterial pressure during supine exercise, an increased pressor and cardiac response to infused catecholamines,[38] and increased sensitivity to catecholamine-induced mobilization of free fatty acids from adipose tissue. When individuals with chronic orthostatic hypotension are observed under laboratory conditions, the role of mechanical factors in maintaining arterial pressure in the upright posture is reflected in transient elevations in arterial pressure induced by leg motion, deep inspiration, and infusions of blood volume expanders. There appears to be no impairment in the secretion of renin and aldosterone accompanying assumption of the upright posture in this syndrome.

Orthostatic hypotension with syncope is observed in a variety of clinical situations, including neurologic diseases involving the autonomic nervous system, such as tabes dorsalis, syringomyelia, diabetic neuropathy, and subacute combined sclerosis, and in peripheral neuritis, alcoholic neuropathy, Wernicke's syndrome, porphyria, amyloidosis, and spinal cord transsection. A similar but not identical picture is seen with prolonged recumbency during protracted illness, following surgical sympathectomy or pharmacologic blockade of the autonomic ganglions, and with pharmacologic suppression of sympathetic nerve activity. There is, in addition, an idiopathic form of chronic orthostatic hypotension in which no etiologic factor has yet been elucidated.[37] Current evidence indicates that the pathogenesis of this syndrome involves a defect in the biosynthesis of norepinephrine by sympathetic ganglia and neurons. Orthostatic hypotension also has been described in association with gradually progressive systemic neurologic abnormalities, including rigidity and tremor, ataxia, and upper and lower motor neuron abnormalities.[39] This association of autonomic with progressive neurologic abnormalities is usually sporadic but has been reported to have a familial association.

Orthostatic hypotension associated with prolonged bed rest can be lessened by early ambulation. When it is medically permissible, the chronically ill patient should spend some time in a chair each day. Orthostatic hypotension of the idiopathic variety or that associated with a known abnormality of the autonomic nervous system is difficult to manage. The treatment depends on the specific cause, when known, and is always tempered by the associated medical problems. Therapy ranges from the use of elastic stockings and pressure suits to high salt intake; use of corticosteroids, sympathomimetic amines and beta-adrenergic blocking agents; and expansion of the blood volume with volume ex-

panders or saline solution. Hypotensive agents such as ganglionic blocking agents, rauwolfia derivatives, monoamine oxidase inhibitors, diuretics, and potent tranquilizers should be avoided in such patients. In a recent report atrial pacing at a rate of 100 beats per minute has maintained effective symptomatic and hemodynamic improvement in a single patient with intractable orthostatic hypotension. This treatment modality will require additional clinical study.[40]

Syncope in Cerebrovascular Disease

With partial or complete occlusion of the major arteries of the neck, perfusion to the brain becomes a more direct function of the level of arterial pressure. The greater the degree of cerebral vascular involvement, the more likely it is that syncope will become a part of the clinical picture. The most common disorder involving the major arteries to the brain is atherosclerotic disease, frequently manifest in recurrent transient cerebral ischemic attacks. (See Chap. 64.) With extensive occlusive involvement of the origins of the brachiocephalic vessels such as occurs in patients with pulseless disease (aortic arch syndrome, Takayasu's arteritis), syncope occurs with a high degree of frequency. With lesser degrees of cerebral vascular inflow occlusion, transient lowering of arterial pressure, e.g., immediately following the assumption of the upright posture, may be followed by vague symptoms suggesting impaired or marginal cerebral blood flow. Such postural symptoms (i.e., lightheadedness, weakness, and visual disturbances) are common in elderly individuals in the absence of obvious carotid-vertebral disease and in patients with chronic hypertensive disease. Associated with such symptoms there may be signs of focal neurologic deficit, such as hemiparesis, unilateral sensory signs and symptoms, altered speech, and cranial nerve dysfunction. In patients with major occlusive disease of the carotid-vertebrobasilar arterial system, manual compression of either carotid artery may provoke syncope associated with focal neurologic signs. One must, therefore, be extremely cautious in using carotid sinus massage in patients with suspected occlusive cerebral vascular disease. Fainting induced in this manner may be erroneously interpreted as carotid sinus syncope. Transient losses or impairment of consciousness in patients with carotid-vertebral disease (transient ischemic attacks, TIA) that recurs frequently should be recognized as an ominous sign, often heralding a major cerebrovascular accident.

Impairment or loss of consciousness in relation to changing positions of the head, particularly hyperextension and lateral rotation, has been described in isolated occlusion of the vertebral arteries. Such symptoms have been observed in patients with disease of the upper cervical spine, such as the Klippel-Feil deformity, and in cervical osteoarthritis.

Impairment or loss of consciousness associated

with upper-extremity exercise has been described and characterized as the *subclavian steal syndrome.*[41,42] This syndrome is caused by major occlusive disease of the proximal subclavian artery. With the decrease in vascular resistance accompanying upper-extremity exercise, blood flow is shunted via the circle of Willis retrograde through the vertebral artery to the distal subclavian artery on the affected side. The consequent loss of blood flow to the cerebral circulation induces symptoms of cerebral ischemia. The propensity of a patient with proximal subclavian arterial occlusive disease to develop cerebral ischemic symptoms is related not only to the severity of occlusion but to such factors as existing carotid-vertebral vascular disease and the magnitude of exercise in the extremity. This syndrome is diagnosed by the findings of diminished brachial arterial pressure on the affected side, a bruit which is maximal over the supraclavicular area, and the precipitation of symptoms by exercise of the involved extremity.

Reflex Types of Syncope

Reflex suppression of atrial pacemaker activity and of atrioventricular conduction by the vagus plays an important role in several forms of syncope. Thus, in the course of vasodepressor syncope, sinus bradycardia and various levels of incomplete heart block are often noted. Although the vagal mechanism may not be the primary cause of fainting under these circumstances, the slowing of the heart rate to critically low levels is certainly a contributing factor. Vagal influences may also play an important role in the course of atrial arrhythmias when sudden slowing or acceleration in ventricular rate due to vagal-induced variation in atrioventricular block may occur. Similarly, alterations in vagal tone may account for episodes of syncope in patients with heart block, when changes from incomplete to complete block are responsible for the fainting reaction. The role of the vagus in the vasodepressor type of carotid sinus syncope will be discussed below. In the *cardioinhibitory* type of carotid sinus syncope, suppression of atrial pacemaker activity and of AV node conduction by the vagus is a primary cause of syncope.

In rare instances, syncope may occur in individuals without evidence of heart disease as a result of reflex cardiac asystole. The term *vagovagal syncope* is applied to such syncope, in which the entire reflex arc is located within the vagal system. Syncope associated with distension of an esophageal diverticulum and with pathologic lesions in the larynx and mediastinum has been explained on this basis. A similar mechanism for cardiac standstill arising from vagal reflex activity has been attributed to syncope following distension of the viscera, fainting associated with irritation of the pleura or peritoneum, the cardiac asystole associated with esophagoscopy or bronchoscopy, and the syncope associated with glossopharyngeal neuralgia and cardiospasm. Recurrent syncope of this type is often relieved or prevented by administration of anticholinergic agents, such as atropine sulfate, in adequate dosage.

Carotid Sinus Syncope[43–45a]

Massage or compression of the carotid sinus in normal persons is often attended by transient slowing of the heart rate and mild hypotension. In some patients with recurrent episodes of syncope such stimulation of the carotid sinus is followed by marked slowing in heart rate, a profound fall in arterial pressure, or a combination of these findings.[43] In these individuals the disorder is referred to as *carotid sinus syncope* or *hyperirritable carotid sinus syndrome.* This syndrome is observed most commonly in elderly patients, many of whom have diffuse atherosclerosis and organic heart disease (i.e., coronary arteriosclerosis with disease of the SA or AV node or aortic stenosis). Approximately 20 percent of men over age 65 with abnormal base-line electrocardiograms (i.e., left ventricular hypertrophy or old myocardial infarction in the absence of cardiac arrhythmia or heart block) have prolonged asystole or syncope with carotid sinus massage.[44] Such "carotid hypersensitivity" has not been observed in men of similar age without heart disease. These considerations have led to the impression that it is the associated cardiac disease and not age per se which predisposes to the problem of carotid sinus hypersensitivity and syncope in the aged. It is to be noted that not all patients with a hypersensitive response to carotid sinus massage experience recurrent syncope. The frequency of the syndrome and the potential for marked bradycardia and hypotension enjoin caution whenever carotid massage is attempted. Testing for carotid sinus hypersensitivity by digital massage should be done with gentle and very brief maneuvers at first and always when the patient is supine and while the heart is continuously monitored by auscultation or electrocardiography. The administration of digitalis appears to accentuate carotid sinus hypersensitivity. Carotid sinus syncope has been observed in patients with disease processes localized to the carotid sinus area, such as neoplasm and inflammatory masses in the neck. In patients with hypersensitive carotid sinus reflex, symptoms of lightheadedness and impaired consciousness may be initiated by relatively minor stimulation of the carotid sinus, and by head motion, shaving, or a tight collar.

Carotid sinus syncope of the vasodepressor type is that form of the syndrome in which fainting or impaired consciousness occurs in the absence of change in heart rate. Presyncopal signs such as nausea, sweating, and pallor are usually not observed under these circumstances, in which the fall in perfusion pressure to the brain is precipitous. Syncope due to a hypersensitive carotid sinus in other individuals is associated primarily with slowing of the heart rate because of marked sinus bradycardia, sinoatrial block, or high-degree atrioventricular block. In such circumstances syncope is related more to the prolonged asystole than to the marked fall in peripheral vascular resistance. Such episodes of carotid sinus syncope due to slowing of the heart rate are referred to as the *cardioinhibitory type of carotid sinus syncope*. The syncope may also occur as a result of combined cardioinhibitory and vasodepressor mechanisms; indeed, the vasodepressor component may not be evident until after atropine blockage, when carotid massage uncovers the hypotension without bradycardia.

In addition to carotid sinus syncope of the vasodepressor and cardioinhibitory types, Weiss[45a] has described a third form of syncope following carotid sinus massage in which loss of consciousness is unassociated with change in arterial pressure or pulse rate. In this type of carotid sinus syncope, symptoms may occur in any position, and the loss of consciousness may be preceded or accompanied by focal neurologic manifestations. It has been suggested that inhibition of the center for regulation of consciousness by a reflex mechanism or by secondary focal circulatory disturbances may account for these episodes. In view of reports of the occurrence of syncope during carotid sinus manipulation in patients with carotid-vertebroarterial insufficiency, some question has arisen as to whether some of these episodes are related primarily to cerebral ischemia. The possibility of *hysterical syncope* must also be raised in some instances in which a diagnosis of the *cerebral type of hypersensitive carotid sinus* is made. There are, however, a sufficient number of carefully observed episodes of syncope of this type to suggest that it is a clinical entity among the carotid sinus syndromes.

Tumors of the carotid sinus are rare. The common disorder associated with a hypersensitive carotid sinus reflex is coronary atherosclerosis, with impaired circulation to the SA and AV nodes. The use of atropine or its derivatives may be effective in preventing attacks. External stimulation of the carotid sinus, such as produced by turning the head, wearing a tight collar, or performing Valsalva's maneuver, should be avoided. The insertion of permanent-demand pacemakers has been reported as highly effective therapy in patients with an intractable cardioinhibitory type of carotid sinus syncope.

Cough Syncope

Although at one time fainting during paroxysms of cough was considered rare, coughing is now recognized as a relatively common cause of syncope. In cough syncope (also called *laryngeal vertigo* and *tussive syncope*), loss of consciousness occurs following a paroxysm of vigorous coughing. It is commonly observed in robust men and children, rarely in women. This syndrome is particularly frequent among individuals with chronic bronchitis and a "hacking cough." The impairment in cerebral blood flow is related to the marked increase in intrathoracic pressure during the coughing episode. Several factors may be implicated in the mechanism of cough syncope, including a sharp decrease in cardiac output, peripheral vasodilatation following cough, a marked increase in cerebrospinal fluid pressure with resultant compression of the intracranial capillary and venous beds, an increase in cerebral vascular resistance induced by the hypocapnia of coughing, and a "concussive" effect caused by the sudden rise in intracranial pressure transmitted from the thorax and abdomen via the cerebrospinal fluid.[46] The latter mechanism may explain those episodes of laboratory-induced cough syncope in which no change suggesting cerebral hypoxia has been observed in the electroencephalogram.

Omission of smoking is mandatory in the treatment of cough syncope. Therapy of associated bronchitis should be carried out. The patient should be informed of the deleterious effects of vigorous coughing.

Syncope related to more prolonged increases in intrathoracic pressure may be observed during a sustained Valsalva maneuver. With prolonged exhalation against a closed glottis, there is a progressive fall in arterial pressure and cardiac output, which may be of sufficient degree to impair cerebral circulation. The "fainting lark," a trick indulged in by schoolchildren and consisting of sudden manual compression of the chest of the victim made sensitive following a period of hyperventilation, is most probably caused by this mechanism. Syncope following a similar schoolchild prank in which the individual squats and hyperventilates and quickly stands and performs a Valsalva maneuver has a similar mechanism.

Postmicturition Syncope

Micturition syncope[47] or, more properly, postmicturition syncope is often seen in adult men with nocturia. During or immediately following voiding there is sudden loss of consciousness, often without premonitory symptoms. Many such persons give the history of drinking large quantities of an alcoholic beverage before retiring. A similar type of syncope may be observed following drainage of a distended bladder or after removal of large quantities of ascitic fluid. It has been suggested by some investigators that the loss of consciousness in these circumstances is related to a sudden reflex decrease in peripheral vascular resistance stimulated by the precipitous fall in intraabdominal volume. Others have thought the loss of consciousness in postmicturition syncope is related to typical vasodepressor syncope accentuated by such factors as the Valsalva maneuver and the widespread peripheral vasodilatation associated with a warm bed and recent alcohol consumption. A syndrome labeled *defecation syncope* has been observed in elderly patients and is thought to be of similar mechanism.

Glossopharyngeal Neuralgia and Syncope

This is a rare form of syncope associated with paroxysms of neuralgic pain in the throat and neck, accompanied by bradycardia, asystole, severe hypotension, and seizures.[48] The changes in cerebral function are felt generally to be secondary to the transient cerebral ischemia accompanying marked bradycardia and arterial hypotension. The cardiovascular changes in glossopharyngeal neuralgia can be reversed by parasympathetic blocking agents such as atropine. Diphenylhydantoin therapy, which has been found to be effective in relieving trigeminal neuralgia by raising the pain threshold, has been reported to be effective in relieving the pain, bradycardia, and syncope of glossopharyngeal neuralgia.

Syncope in Divers

Unusual and poorly understood forms of loss of consciousness and even sudden death may occur in underwater diving. Some may be forms of vasodepressor syncope. Hypoxia may be a factor, or the bradycardia of the "diving reflex" may be involved.

Noncardiovascular Syncope

The differential diagnosis of syncope often includes a group of disorders wherein altered consciousness is not primarily related to alterations in cardiac output, cardiac rhythm, or arterial pressure. These forms of syncope, which we refer to as *syncope of noncirculatory origin,* may be caused by primary disorders of cerebral function, profound alterations in cerebral metabolism, or psychologically induced behavioral mechanisms. The transient nature of the episodes creates sufficient suspicion of an underlying cardiovascular disorder to suggest syncope of circulatory origin. For this reason, the more common disorders of this nature are outlined in the following paragraphs, in which their differentiating features from syncope of circulatory origin are emphasized.

Hypoxia

Fainting due to hypoxia may be related primarily to the lack of oxygen or, as is often encountered, may be due to vasodepressor syncope initiated during a period of oxygen lack. The effect of hypoxia alone is best observed in persons studied in altitude chambers. Though there is considerable individual variation, the onset of the hypoxic symptoms under these circumstances depends primarily on the level of altitude and, in addition, on the rate of ascent. With exposure to altitudes of 10,000 ft or greater, the point in the oxyhemoglobin dissociation curve is reached at which an abrupt decrease in oxygen saturation occurs with further fall in oxygen tension. Oxygen saturation falls rapidly from approx-

imately 90 percent saturation at 10,000 ft (3048 m) to 80 percent at 15,000 ft (4572 m) and 60 percent at 20,000 ft (6096 m). At the latter altitudes there is an insidious progressive mental deterioration associated with visual disturbances, headache, and breathlessness. At the time of impairment of consciousness, one may note cyanosis; with severe oxygen deprivation, convulsive movements are seen. With cardiovascular disease, pulmonary insufficiency, and anemia, symptoms of hypoxia occur at lower levels of altitude. The impairment of consciousness due to hypoxia is accompanied by sinus tachycardia, but arterial pressure is preserved. The environmental setting in which impaired consciousness due to hypoxia occurs usually leaves little difficulty in differentiating it from other forms of syncope.

Hypoglycemia and Hyperventilation

Severe hypoglycemia is associated with weakness, sweating, and a sensation of hunger, confusion, and altered consciousness. The symptoms are unrelated to posture and usually respond promptly to food ingestion or intravenous glucose administration. Altered consciousness associated with overdosage of insulin, islet-cell adenomas of the pancreas, certain retroperitoneal tumors, and reactive hypoglycemia and in the presence of advanced adrenal, pituitary, or hepatic disease may be explained on this basis. Impaired consciousness associated with hypoglycemia is associated with a sinus rhythm and is rarely accompanied by hypotension; in contrast to syncope of circulatory origin, it is more gradual in onset.

In normal persons, anxiety is regularly accompanied by varying degrees of hyperventilation. In the hyperventilation syndrome, anxiety is associated with an inordinate degree of hyperventilation.[49] The symptoms of hypocapnia dominate the clinical picture under these circumstances and may actually replace the anxiety as the major discomfort. Early during the episode, the patient complains of smothering, a tightness in the chest, and a feeling of suffocation. Later, there appears confusion, a sense of unreality, bewilderment, and in time a feeling of panic. Symptoms of palpitation, precordial oppression, and dyspnea may suggest an acute cardiac or pulmonary catastrophe. Associated with the above, there are sensations of numbness or coldness of the extremities and the circumoral areas. The symptoms may last as long as 30 min, and in most severe episodes may occur in the sitting or recumbent posture; there is often slight hypotension, but not a profound drop in arterial pressure, and the heart rate is rapid. The episode is terminated usually after the patient is calmed and the hyperventilation ceases. One may aid the resolution of symptoms of hypocapnia by having the patient rebreathe in a paper or plastic bag. It is notable that although consciousness is impaired, actual loss of consciousness usually does not occur. Typical vasodepressor syncope may be superimposed in the hyperventilation attack, making identification of the syndrome more difficult.

The pathogenesis of the hyperventilation syndrome is incompletely understood. Though an underlying emotional disorder is almost invariably present, the factors leading to hyperventilation in these patients are not clearly defined. Much of the clinical findings in the hyperventilation syndrome, in particular the lowering of cerebral blood flow and the alkalosis, can be explained by the effects of hypocapnia. The reproduction of a typical episode by voluntary hyperventilation in patients with the syndrome is a helpful diagnostic maneuver and, in addition, aids in educating the patient regarding the prevention and control of attacks.

Cerebral Dysfunction
The differentiation of the various forms of syncope of circulatory origin from the transitory loss of consciousness during a generalized seizure is often made on the basis of history alone. One form of epilepsy, viz., the akinetic form of petit mal, does offer particular difficulty in differentiation. Epilepsy as a cause of sudden loss of consciousness is suggested in the dramatic nature of the onset of the attack, which is often preceded by an aura. Other observations which distinguish the loss of consciousness in epilepsy are the absence of hypotension and cardiac arrhythmia (other than sinus tachycardia) and the presence of tonic convulsive movements, upturning of the eyes, prolonged unconsciousness, urinary incontinence, and postictal drowsiness, headache, and confusion. Although any of the above findings may occur in individual episodes of syncope of circulatory origin, the frequent combination of these events in epilepsy allows differentiation of the cause of the event. The finding of an abnormal electroencephalographic picture suggesting cerebral arrhythmia between episodes of unconsciousness is most helpful in this differentiation.

Vertigo
Though recurrent episodes of vertigo may first be described by the patient as a loss or impairment of consciousness, careful direction of the history will often reveal the true nature of this symptom. In true vertigo there is a keen sense of movement, either of the environment or of the patient. Falling may be abrupt; it is due not to weakness of postural muscles but to loss of balance. Nausea, pallor, and cold perspiration may suggest vasodepressor syncope, but the lack of true loss or impairment of consciousness, the increased distress with head movement, and the associated nystagmoid movements of the eyes, together with the finding of a normal arterial pressure and pulse, will help differentiate the syndrome.

Hysterical Fainting
This is of particular importance because it may mimic altered consciousness of an organic origin.

Hysterical episodes occur most frequently in young adults, often with severe emotional illness. The episode usually occurs in the presence of an audience. The patient slumps gently and gracefully to the floor or in a convenient chair or sofa, typically without injury or awkwardness. The patient may be motionless at the time of the episode or may show symbolic and resistive movements. The episode is of varying duration and may last for as long as an hour or more. Although the patient is unresponsive to verbal stimulation, there is often evidence that consciousness is not lost, and there are no abnormalities in pulse, arterial pressure, or skin color. A distinctive characteristic in the hysterical faint is the calm emotional detachment with which the patient describes symptoms and the fact that there is no sharp reversal in their progress when the recumbent posture is assumed.

Syncopal Migraine
Symptoms suggesting syncope are rarely if ever encountered in ordinary types of migraine. In rare instances in which the basal arterial system is involved (as opposed to the more usually affected carotid system), the premonitory aura of migraine terminates in a period of unconsciousness lasting several minutes. When the patient awakens, there is severe headache, typically in the occipital area. This form of migraine usually afflicts adolescent girls. The period of unconsciousness is associated with no apparent circulatory change.[50]

Pursuit of the Diagnosis

Syncope, or presyncope, is among the most difficult symptoms to evaluate. While the vast majority of episodes are benign, the symptoms may be a harbinger of sudden death. A complete modern evaluation entails hospitalization and considerable expense. Clearly not all patients are candidates for this type of study.

The previous sections have described the various causes of syncope and various procedures employed to establish the diagnosis. Many causes of syncope require no more than a history, physical examination, chest x-ray, and electrocardiogram for diagnosis and appropriate therapy. These include classic vasodepressor syncope, orthostatic hypotension, reflex syncope, carotid sinus syncope, cough syncope, postmicturition syncope, and glossopharyngeal neuralgia syncope. Noncardiovascular syncope such as hypoglycemia, hyperventilation, hysteria, or epilepsy is usually suggested by history and relatively easily evaluated by neurologic or biochemical studies. Syncope due to obstructive cardiovascular disorders is also strongly suggested by physical examination, but often requires noninvasive cardiac evaluation and subsequent cardiac catheterization. Syncope due to cerebrovascular disease alone is uncommon. It is usually suspected on routine clinical examination. In such cases, cerebrovascular angiography and computer-assisted tomography or other studies may be required for a definitive diagnosis.

By far the most difficult class of patients to evaluate are those with syncope of suspected arrhythmic origin. Such patients often have evidence of underlying heart disease and/or cerebrovascular disease, but clear-cut evidence of an arrhythmic basis of the syncope is lacking after routine initial studies. Figure 30-2 provides a diagnostic schema for an approach to such patients. As noted earlier, a 24-h ambulatory monitoring study is the most useful initial approach. This will reveal approximately half of those arrhythmias that could cause the syncope. This is especially true for bradyarrhythmias. If the 24-h ambulatory monitoring study is negative, and no symptoms occur, a maximal treadmill test should be performed. This test will yield another 10 percent of arrhythmic causes of syncope—mostly ventricular arrhythmias. If these two tests are still inconclusive, an electrophysiologic study may be indicated. In addition to having the highest sensitivity for identifying arrhythmias, this test allows an opportunity to judge efficacy of pharmacologic or pacemaker therapy. Occasionally all three of these studies are negative, and a patient-activated monitoring device can be used if arrhythmia is still strongly suspected.

It should be emphasized that a given arrhythmia may not always produce symptoms, depending upon the state of the patient at the time of the occurrence (i.e., asleep, standing, dehydrated, etc.). Thus, it is not uncommon to be faced with a situation wherein a significant arrhythmia is documented but there is no clear relationship to syncope. In such instances, judgment is required in relation to the vigor with which one pursues therapy.

Finally, it should be emphasized that syncope due to arrhythmia is often precipitated by multiple factors; that is, the patient may have underlying cardiovascular disease with impaired hemodynamic response to arrhythmia or cerebrovascular disease, and/or may be taking medications that impair autonomic function. The occurrence of syncope may depend on what activity is being pursued at the time the arrhythmia occurs.

Therapy

Precise therapy will not be dealt with in this chapter since use of cardioactive drugs and pacemakers are described in Chaps. 29 and 92. A few general principles can, however, be stated. When surgically treatable obstructive heart disease is present, heart surgery is the primary treatment. When severe cerebrovascular disease is present, cerebrovascular surgery may be the primary approach. Syncope of noncirculatory origin has specific therapies. The various autonomic disorders (including vasodepressor syncope) are not ideally treated at present. Avoidance of precipitating factors is obviously important. In some instances a pacemaker is indicated (carotid sinus syncope), while other situations may require medical and surgical treatment of underlying disorders.

Syncope due to arrhythmias usually represents a very difficult therapeutic challenge. Often such patients are older and have diffuse conduction system disease and may have the tachycardia-bradycardia syndrome. In such patients, antiarrhythmic agents that suppress the tachyarrhythmia may aggravate the bradyarrhythmia. In this situation, the placement of a permanent transvenous pacemaker allows administration of appropriate antiarrhythmic agents. Finally, cardiac surgery may play a role in a limited

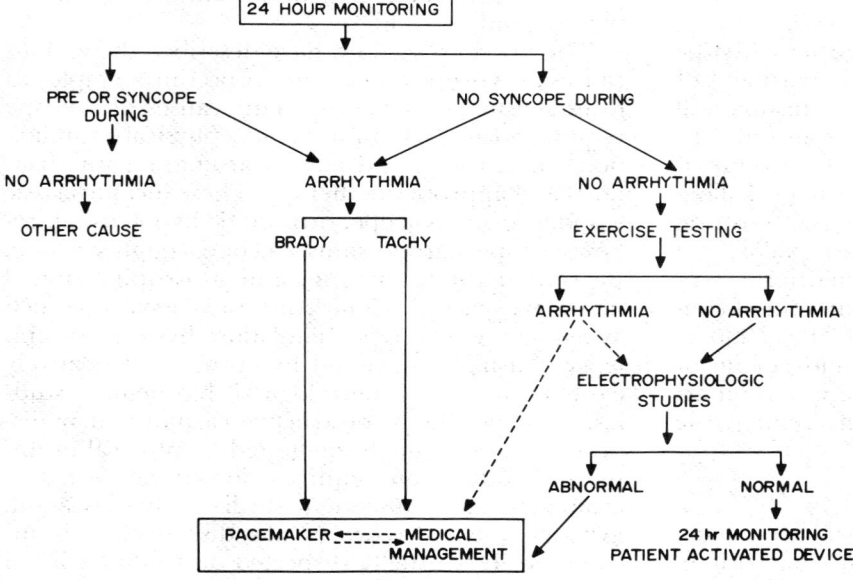

FIGURE 30-2 Diagnosis and management of syncope suspected secondary to arrhythmias.

number of patients, such as those with refractory Wolff-Parkinson-White syndrome and supraventricular tachyarrhythmias or those with ventricular tachycardia related to coronary artery disease and left ventricular aneurysm. (See Chap. 94.)

References

1. Karp, H. R., Weissler, A. M., and Heyman, A.: Vasodepressor Syncope: EEG and Circulatory Changes, *Arch. Neurol.*, 5:94, 1961.
2. Weissler, A. M., and Warren, J. V.: Vasodepressor Syncope, *Am. Heart J.*, 57:786, 1959.
3. Barcroft, H., Edholm, O. G., McMichael, J., and Sharpey-Schafer, E. P.: Posthemorrhagic Fainting: Study by Cardiac Output and Forearm Flow, *Lancet*, 1:489, 1944.
4. Warren, J. V., Brannon, E. S., Stead, E. A., Jr., and Merrill, A. J.: The Effect of Venesection and the Pooling of Blood in the Extremities on the Arterial Pressure and Cardiac Output in Normal Subjects: With Observations on Acute Circulatory Collapse in Three Instances, *J. Clin. Invest.*, 24:337, 1945.
5. Weissler, A. M., Warren, J. V., Estes, E. H., Jr., McIntosh, H. D., and Leonard, J. J.: Vasodepressor Syncope: Factors Influencing Cardiac Output, *Circulation*, 15:875, 1957.
6. Hunter, J.: "Words of John Hunter," J. F. Palmer, London, 1937, vol. 3.
7. Barcroft, H., and Edholm, O. G.: On the Vasodilatation in Human Skeletal Muscle during Posthemorrhagic Fainting, *J. Physiol.*, 104:161, 1945.
8. Anderson, D. P., Allen, W. J., Barcroft, H., Edholm, O. G., and Manning, G. W.: Circulatory Changes during Fainting and Coma Caused by Oxygen Lack, *J. Physiol.*, 104:426, 1946.
9. Bridgen, W., Howarth, S., and Sharpey-Shafer, E. P.: Postural Changes in the Peripheral Blood Flow of Normal Subjects: With Observations on Vasovagal Fainting Reactions as a Result of Tilting the Lordotic Posture, Pregnancy and Spinal Anaesthesia, *Clin. Sci.*, 9:79, 1950.
10. Bearn, A. G., Billing, B., Edholm, O. G., and Sherlock, S.: Hepatic Blood Flow and Carbohydrate Changes in Man during Fainting, *J. Physiol.*, 115:442, 1951.
11. DeWardener, H. E., and McSwiney, R. R.: Renal Haemodynamics in Vasovagal Fainting Due to Hemorrhage, *Clin. Sci.*, 10:209, 1951.
12. Brun, C., Knudsen, E. O. E., and Raaschou, F.: Kidney Function and Circulatory Collapse, Postsyncopal Oliguria, *J. Clin. Invest.*, 25:568, 1946.
13. Finnerty, F. A., Jr., Guillaudeu, R. L., and Fazekas, J. F.: Cardiac and Cerebral Hemodynamics in Drug-Induced Postural Collapse, *Circ. Res.*, 5:35, 1957.
14. McHenry, L. C., Fazekas, J. F., and Sullivan, J. F.: Cerebral Hemodynamics of Syncope, *Am. J. Med. Sci.*, 241:173, 1961.
15. Weissler, A. M., Leonard, J. J., and Warren, J. V.: Effect of Posture and Atropine on the Cardiac Output, *J. Clin. Invest.*, 36:1656, 1957.
16. Weissler, A. M., Leonard, J. J., and Warren, J. V.: The Hemodynamic Effects of Isoproterenol in Man: With Observations on the Role on the Central Blood Volume, *J. Lab. Clin. Med.*, 53:921, 1959.
17. Bevegard, S.: Studies on the Regulation of the Circulation in Man, *Acta Physiol. Scand.*, vol. 57, suppl. 200, 1962.
18. Weissler, A. M., Roehll, W. H., Jr., and Peeler, R. G.: Effect of Posture on the Cardiac Response to Increased Peripheral Demand, *J. Lab. Clin. Med.*, 59:1000, 1962.
19. Epstein, S. E., Stampfer, M., and Beiser, G. D.: Role of the Capacitance and Resistance Vessels in Vasovagal Syncope, *Circulation*, 37:524, 1968.
20. Oparil, S., Vassaux, C., Sanders, C. A., and Haber, E.: Role of Renin in Acute Postural Homeostasis, *Circulation*, 41:89, 1970.
21. Darwin, C.: "Expression of the Emotions," John Murray (Publishers), Ltd., London, 1972 (Philosophical Library, New York, 1955).
22. Engel, G. L., and Romano, J.: Studies of Syncope. IV. Biologic Interpretations of Vasodepressor Syncope, *Psychosom. Med.*, 9:288, 1947.
23. Dressler, W.: Effort Syncope as an Early Manifestation of Primary Pulmonary Hypertension, *Am. J. Med. Sci.*, 223:131, 1952.
24. Gambill, E. E., Hines, E. A., Jr., and Adson, A. W.: The Circulation in Man in Certain Postures before and after Extensive Sympathectomy for Essential Hypertension, *Am. Heart J.*, 27:360, 1944.
25. Howard, B. K., Goodson, J. H., and Mengert, W. F.: Supine Hypotensive Syndrome in Late Pregnancy, *Obstet. Gynecol.*, 1:371, 1953.
*26. Friedberg, C. F.: Syncope: Pathological Physiology: Differential Diagnosis and Treatment, *Mod. Concepts Cardiovasc. Dis.*, 10:55, 1971. (25 references)
27. Nobel, J. R.: The Patient with Syncope, *J. Am. Med. Assoc.*, 237:1372, 1977.
28. Hickler, R. B., and Howe, J. P., III: Syncope: Its Etiology, Pathophysiology, Management, *Primary Cardiology*, March 1979, pp. 46–51.
*29. Wright, K. E., Jr., and McIntosh, H. D.: Syncope: A Review of Pathophysiological Mechanisms, *Prog. Cardiovasc. Dis.*, 13:580, 1971. (56 references)
30. Schwartz, L. S., Goldfischer, J., Sprague, G. J., and Schwartz, S. P.: Syncope and Sudden Death in Aortic Stenosis, *Am. J. Cardiol.*, 23:647, 1969.
30a. Mark, A. L., Abboud, F. M., Schmid, P. G., and Heistad, D. D.: Vascular Responses to Left Ventricular Outflow Obstruction and Activation of Ventricular Baroreceptors in Dogs, *J. Clin. Invest.*, 52:1147, 1973.
31. Van Durme, J. P.: Tachyarrhythmias and Transient Cerebral Ischemic Attacks, *Am. Heart J.*, 89:538, 1975.
32. Boudoulas, H., Schaal, S. F., Lewis, R. P., and Robinson, J. L.: Superiority of 24-Hour Outpatient Monitoring over Multistage Exercise Testing for the Evaluation of Syncope, *J. Electrocardiol.*, 12:103, 1979.
33. Boudoulas, H., Schaal, S. F., and Lewis, R. P.: Electrophysiologic Risk Factors of Syncope, *J. Electrocardiol.*, 11:339, 1978.
34. Camm, J. A., Evans, K. E., Ward, D. E., Martin, A.: The Rhythm of the Heart in Active Elderly Subjects, *Am. Heart J.*, 99:598, 1980.
35. Scarpa, W. J.: The Sick Sinus Syndrome, *Am. Heart J.*, 92:648, 1976.

*This article is a review of the literature and contains additional references to the literature.

36. Kontos, H. A., Richardson, D. W., and Norvell, J. E.: Norepinephrine Depletion in Idiopathic Postural Hypotension, *Ann. Intern. Med.*, 82:336, 1975.

37. Benestad, A. M., and Boe, J.: Idiopathic Orthostatic Hypotension, *Acta Med. Scand.*, 150:1, 1954.

38. Hickler, R. B., Thompson, G. R., Fox, L. M., and Hamlin, J. T., III: Successful Treatment of Orthostatic Hypotension with 9-Alpha-Fluorohydrocortisone, *N. Engl. J. Med.*, 261:788, 1959.

39. Shy, G. M., and Drager, G. A.: A Neurological Syndrome Associated with Orthostatic Hypotension: A Clinical Pathologic Study, *Arch. Neurol.*, 2:511, 1960.

40. Moss, A. J., Glaser, W., and Topol, E.: Atrial Tachypacing in the Treatment of a Patient with Primary Orthostatic Hypotension, *N. Engl. J. Med.*, 302:1456, 1980.

41. Reivich, N., Holling, H. E., Roberts, B., and Toole, J. S.: Reversal of Blood Flow through the Vertebral Artery and Its Effect on Cerebral Circulation, *N. Engl. J. Med.*, 265:878, 1961.

42. Mannick, J. A., Suter, C. G., and Hume, D. G.: The "Subclavian Steal" Syndrome: A Further Documentation, *J. Am. Med. Assoc.*, 182:254, 1962.

43. Ferris, E. B., Capps, R. B., and Weiss, S.: Carotid Sinus Syncope and Its Bearing on the Mechanisms of the Unconscious State and Convulsions, *Medicine*, 14:377, 1935.

44. Smiddy, J., Lewis, H. D., Jr., and Dunn, M.: The Effect of Carotid Massage in Older Man, *J. Gerontol.*, 27:209, 1972.

45. Weiss, S.: Syncope and Related Syndromes, *Oxford Med.*, 2:250, 1935.

45a. Weiss, S., and Baker, J. P.: The Carotid Sinus Reflex in Health and Disease. Its Role in the Causation of Fainting and Convulsions, *Medicine*, 12:297, 1933.

46. McIntosh, H. D., Estes, E. H., and Warren, J. V.: The Mechanisms of Cough Syncope, *Am. Heart J.*, 52:70, 1956.

47. Lyle, C. B., Jr., Monroe, J. T., Jr., Flinn, D. E., and Lamb, L. E.: Micturition Syncope: Report of 24 Cases, *N. Engl. J. Med.*, 265:982, 1961.

48. Kong, Y., Heyman, A., Entman, M. L., and McIntosh, H. D.: Glossopharyngeal Neuralgia Associated with Bradycardia, Syncope, and Seizures, *Circulation*, 30:109, 1964.

49. Engel, G. L., Ferris, E. B., and Logan, M.: Hyperventilation Analysis of Clinical Symptomatology, *Ann. Intern. Med.*, 27:683, 1947.

50. Bickerstaff, E. R.: Impairment of Consciousness in Migraine, *Lancet*, 2:1057, 1961.

Section G Sudden Death

31

Pathology and Mechanisms of Sudden Death

Giorgio Baroldi, M.D., F.A.C.C.

The science of the precognition of sudden deaths is seen to be not merely useful but extremely necessary to physicians, since the Teacher of our Art [Hippocrates] clearly shows that man not only absolves himself from all blame, but acquires the name of and the admiration owed to a good physician, when he, unable to make everyone well, at least divines and foretells what is about to happen.

G. M. Lancisi, 1707[1]

For millennia, *mors subita,* as any unknown phenomenon, was interpreted in a mythical-religious sense. It took time to substitute a voodoo death concept with a more objective approach. From the sudden death of Phidippides the marathon runner in 490 B.C., one of the first examples mentioned in history, we waited until 1707 to have the first objective clinicopathologic report. In this year Lancisi[1] described an epidemic of sudden death which had occurred in Rome in 1705. The reader may recognize and translate in up-to-date medical language the close relationship that exists in many cases between cardiac disease and sudden death. Most were wealthy males living in a luxurious style. Common people were subsequently involved, but with less frequency. Females and people continent with respect to food, drink, and sexual life were preserved, a fact providing an early insight into risk factors and prevention. One of the more important contributions was to categorize different types of death. Among the three main categories of *natural, untimely,* and *violent,* the

death was defined as "slow" or "sudden" and in turn as "foreseen" and "forefelt" or "unforeseen, unperceptible, and unexpected."

Pathologic Definition of Sudden Cardiac Death

At present in defining this entity we are limited to (1) observation of the phenomenon, a fatal event which occurs in a short time without prodromes or with minor, unvalued ones and without notice or warning for the witnesses; (2) minimal clinical information, when fortunate conditions exist; and (3) the postmortem findings, the rationale being that these may explain the sudden death. However, two parameters have to be specified since the terms *unexpected* and *sudden* may have the same meaning colloquially. The first concerns *expectancy,* to distinguish a rapid death in apparently healthy subjects from that which may occur at any time (during the usual course, in the recovery phase, or in the inactive phase) in a manifest disease which may be responsible for the sudden demise. The second parameter concerns *timing.* According to different authors "sudden" ranges from 30 s to 1 h to 24 h from the onset of the fatal episode to death.[2-4] From the pathologic standpoint, both expectancy and survival time are essential to correctly evaluate the morphologic changes. Accordingly, as a working definition for proper selection of cases, *sudden cardiac death* can be defined as clinically unexplained, rapid death occurring in apparently healthy people, during their normal activity, without a history of pertinent disease and not receiving therapy of any type (*unwarned* or *unexpected*); or as an unusual, unexplained event in the course of an acute or chronic manifest disease (*warned* or *expected*). The pathologic findings are confined to the heart; the other organs are involved as a secondary phenomenon. In the present era of resuscitation, one point to be stressed

589

is that at postmortem examination the pathologic changes resulting from iatrogenic causes have to be distinguished from natural ones. Prospective studies in subjects dying without therapeutic interference of any type are required.

Pathologic Findings in Sudden Cardiac Death

Sudden death may occur in any type of cardiac disease. The aim should be to know the exact frequency of both warned and unwarned events in each type. Generally, in the literature, we deal more with impressions than with figures, the expectancy being variously interpreted. This chapter attempts to list the more frequent pathologic findings reported in sudden death, determining the frequency, when possible.

Coronary Arteries

Congenital Malformations

Sudden death is rarely observed in either minor (without abnormal connections) or major (with abnormal connections) coronary anomalies. Rare cases of persons with a single coronary artery or with severe hypoplasia of the right coronary artery dying suddenly after stressful exercise have been reported.[5] Only one variant of a minor abnormality, the dislocation of coronary ostia, shows a significantly higher frequency of sudden death. Among 51 subjects with this anomaly, both coronary arteries arose from the left sinus of Valsalva in 18, and from the anterior sinus of Valsalva in 33.[6] In the latter group, 8 (24.2 percent) subjects died suddenly and unexpectedly, while 1 died suddenly 4 months after a massive infarct. All subjects were young males (mean age 20.0 years, in contrast to 57.3 years in others dying from known causes), and death occurred during or after physical exercise. In contrast, there were no sudden deaths in the group where the coronary arteries originated from the left sinus of Valsalva. When the left coronary artery arises from the anterior sinus, it runs leftward, passing between the aorta and the pulmonary artery. In this anatomic disposition, the left ostium has a slitlike lumen due to its origin at an acute angle. It is postulated that increased physical activity with consequent aortic and pulmonary artery distension may induce a flaplike closure of the stretched anomalous artery, resulting in sudden, fatal ischemia.

Infectious-Immune and Thromboembolic Processes

In coronary arteritis, sudden death may ensue because of the rupture of an aneurysm (polyarteritis nodosa, benign mucocutaneous lymph node syn-

drome) or following secondary occlusive thrombosis.[7-10] Of 233 cases with luetic aortitis, 37 had mono- or bilateral obstruction of the coronary ostia and death was sudden in 17.[11] In 11 subjects with aortitis of various types (personally reviewed from the files of the Armed Forces Institute of Pathology), bilateral (sub)occlusion of the coronary ostia was associated with sudden and unexpected death in one instance.

Coronary embolism is frequently associated with sudden death. It has been reported in 60 percent of 74 cases. The underlying disorders were acute and subacute bacterial endocarditis (63.6 percent); thrombus of the heart chambers (10.9 percent); luetic aortitis (5.4 percent); ulcerated aortic plaque (4.1 percent); paradoxical emboli of various kinds (4.1 percent); aortic (2.7 percent) or proximal coronary thrombosis (2.7 percent); pulmonary thrombus, caseous tuberculous material, neoplastic tissue, fragment of calcific valve (1.3 percent); or of undetermined nature (1.3 percent). Frequent sites of embolization were the left main coronary trunk (32.4 percent), the left anterior descending branch (35.1 percent), the right coronary artery (12.2 percent), and the left circumflex (4.1 percent).[12]

Contradictory results have been reported regarding the frequency of platelet aggregates occluding the small intramural arterial vessels in sudden death. In one study[13] they were found with high frequency in sudden coronary deaths without acute coronary lesions; while in another study no difference was noted between sudden death cases and controls.[14]

Degenerative Processes

The atherosclerotic plaque is the most frequent postmortem finding in sudden death cases. This is the reason why, today, we speak of *sudden coronary death*. In a recent study of 208 selected cases (182 males, 26 females) of sudden and unexpected death (unrelated to physical effort), the maximal lumen/diameter reduction due to an atherosclerotic plaque was as follows: 28 (13.4 percent) cases with less than 50 percent, 23 cases (11.0 percent) between 50 and 69 percent, and 157 cases (75.4 percent) with more than 70 percent lumen reduction (29 cases between 70 and 79 percent, 53 between 80 and 84 percent, and 75 with more than 90 percent). In 53 cases only one main coronary vessel had a severe stenosis (≥70 percent); in 60 cases, two vessels had severe stenosis; and in 44 cases, three or more vessels were severely narrowed. Of 401 severe stenoses, 48 had a length of less than 2 mm, 139 were between 6 and 20 mm, and 214 were more than 20 mm long; most were concentric (345 concentric versus 56 semilunar). The structure of 216 plaques was mainly fibrous, while in 185 plaques atheromatous material prevailed. The right coronary artery, particularly its anterior segment, and the left anterior descending artery were the most compromised vessels. The left main trunk and the posterior descending branch only rarely showed severe stenosis (11 and 12 cases, respectively). In 32 cases (15.3 percent) an acute occlusive thrombus was located in an area of severe stenosis, generally longer than 20 mm and caused by a concentric atheromatous plaque. In 16 cases, the thrombus showed organization histologically, indicating that it antedated the sudden death by days. In 22 cases, a mural thrombus (thin, laminar, fibrin platelet deposition) was present, showing the same characteristics related to the plaque as the occlusive one.[15]

The rare primary dissecting aneurysm of coronary arteries is caused by an unknown "degenerative" process and leads to myocardial infarction and/or sudden death. The latter, if defined as unexpected, occurred in 18 (15 females, 3 males) of 24 cases reported in the literature.[16] Perhaps this is one of the few examples in which the frequency of sudden death is significantly higher in females than in males.

Heart Muscle and Cardiac Valves

Congenital Malformations

Among complications (heart failure, bacterial endocarditis, embolism, pulmonary hypertension, etc.) of congenital malformations of the heart,[17] sudden death seems to be a rare expected event. It is generally stated that it occurs more frequently in aortic stenosis, as well as in any condition producing obstruction of the left ventricular outflow tract. However, in a large series of children with congenital aortic stenosis, the frequency of sudden death was 1 percent (2 of 199 cases).[18]

Infectious-Immune Diseases

An inflammatory reaction in the myocardium during the course of an infectious or allergic disease may be the cause of sudden death.[19]

Of 45 human transplanted heart cases, 2 died suddenly and 2 had ventricular fibrillation which was successfully treated. In 72 percent there were atrial arrhythmias, and in 52 percent there were ventricular premature beats, frequently preceding episodes of acute rejection.[20]

On the other hand, foci of inflammatory reaction are frequently seen in the myocardium of people dying suddenly. In one of the first reports, sudden and unexpected death (three cases) was attributed to an "acute interstitial myocarditis." The latter consisted of rare microfoci of lymphocytes and occasional plasma cells, often associated with degenerative changes in myocardial cells.[21] Similar findings were observed in 81 percent of sudden death cases, in contrast to 33 and 31 percent of chronic coronary and noncoronary patients, respectively.[22] In our experience, microscopic foci of lymphocytes within "normal" myocardium were found in 66.8 percent of selected sudden death cases and in 53.6 percent of normal subjects. In the latter, however, the infiltrates were less numerous and extensive. Furthermore, lymphocytes and histiocytes were frequently associated with focal Zenker necrosis in a reparative stage.

Cardiomyopathies—Myocardial Necrosis

The *idiopathic* or *primary* cardiomyopathies, as well as the secondary cardiomyopathies, include a variety of conditions. Sudden death may occur in any of them. Among the four different morphofunctional categories (hypertrophic, congestive, obliterative, restrictive) into which they have been classified, hypertrophic cardiomyopathy shows the highest frequency of sudden death, even without prodromes. This idiopathic cardiomyopathy is characterized by massive hypertrophy, mainly of the interventricular septum, and by a pathognomonic, anomalous, widespread rearrangement of the myocardial fibers. In two series of 119 and 190 patients, followed for 10 to 15 years, the frequency of sudden death was 15.9 and 13.6 percent, respectively.[23] Of 26 other cases who died suddenly and unexpectedly, 19 were male and 7 female. There was no left ventricular outflow tract gradient in 6 of 12 catheterized patients, and all 19 had an abnormal electrocardiogram. A family history of sudden death was recorded in 9.[24]

With the present uncertainty as to the etiology and pathogenesis of many cardiomyopathies and the etiology and pathogenesis of the so-called ischemic myocardial lesions, it may be helpful to discriminate among the different types of irreversible myocardial degenerative processes found in these conditions, trying to determine when, how, and why each occurs. The term *myocardial necrosis* is used in a very broad sense, as a common end result of many causes. In medicine we try to understand disease and the mechanism of death; in this regard, the myocardial cell may die, not only for different reasons, but also in different ways. At present, at least three types of myocardial cell death may be recognized morphologically, each suggesting a different functional status of the cell. In the first type, the myocardial cell seems to lose its capability to contract and dies in irreversible relaxation (atonic death). Usually defined as a *coagulation necrosis*, it is the pathognomonic lesion of myocardial infarction on which the histologic diagnosis is made. In the second type, the myocardial cell dies in contraction, or more precisely in hypercontraction, losing its capability to relax (tetanic death). Observed in a variety of cardiomyopathies, it is a specific lesion in pheochromocytoma cardiomyopathy or following the experimental infusion of catecholamines. It has many synonyms (infarct-like necrosis, myofibrillar degeneration, contraction band necrosis, coagulative myocytolysis, etc.) but may be simply called *Zenker necrosis* because of its similarity to Zenker lesions in skeletal muscles. In the third type, the myocardial cell maintains its relaxation-contraction coupling, but its function progressively fails (failing death). This last type (colliquative myocytolysis or myocytolysis tout court) is found in cardiomyopathies with a low-output syndrome (e.g., alcoholic cardiomyopathy).[25]

In coronary atherosclerotic heart disease, all three types of necrosis can be seen, frequently together. Irrespective of the size of the coagulation necrosis, most infarcts show a more or less extensive associated Zenker necrosis in the surrounding normal myocardium. Also, in about 40 percent of cases, myocytolysis is observed in the noninfarcted subendocardial or perivascular myocardial layers. In sudden and unexpected coronary death cases, coagulation necrosis was found in 17 percent and Zenker necrosis in 86 percent, being the unique detectable acute lesion in 72 percent. In contrast, myocytolysis was seen in only 8 percent of the subjects. It was mainly associated with extensive myocardial fibrosis (Table 31-1). It may be pertinent to emphasize that there was no relation between both coagulation and Zenker necrosis and cardiac hypertrophy; the latter was in general unrelated to sudden death.

A general consideration is that one lesion may have several causes, but each cause produces one type of lesion. Accordingly, the clear-cut morphology of the histologic changes (Fig. 31-1) suggests that both the underlying biochemical disorder and the etiopathogenesis are specific for each type of myocardial cell death.

Heart Tumors

The frequency of both warned and unwarned sudden death according to clinical findings reported in a recent publication is summarized in Table 31-2.

In primary malignant tumors no sudden death was reported, but sudden death occurred in 2 of 39 patients with angiosarcoma and in 4 of 26 with rhabdomyosarcoma.[26] Sudden death may occur without any previous symptoms and signs, despite an extremely large tumor mass (Fig. 31-2).

Conduction System

Examination of the conduction system should be mandatory in any subject dying suddenly. A serial section study is required for the correct evaluation of this anatomic structure, and this requirement has

TABLE 31-1   Histologic Pattern in Different Types of Myocardial Necrosis in Coronary Heart Disease

Myocardium	Coagulation Necrosis	Coagulative Myocytolysis (Zenker Necrosis)	Colliquative Myocytolysis (Myocytolysis)
Functional status	Irreversible relaxation (atonic death) + stretching by intraventricular pressure	Irreversible contraction (tetanic death)	Progressive loss of function (failing death)
Muscle fiber	Early thinning	Normal or swollen	Increasing edema, vacuolization
Nucleus	Elongation, pyknosis, progressive fading	Normal	Normal
Myofibrils	Elongated sarcomeres in normal registered order, even in late stage	Rhexis, anomalous irregular cross-band formations (coagulation of hypercontracted sarcomeres)	Progressive disappearance
Vessels	Secondary wall degeneration and thrombosis	Normal	Normal
Infiltration	Massive polymorphonuclear exudation	No early infiltrates, possible late lymphocyte	No infiltrates
Extension-location	In general single massive focus of different size, internal to transmural	Multiple (mono- or pluri-cellular) disseminated or confluent foci of different size in any muscular layer	Focal subendocardial and perivascular, progressively spreading
Irreversible within	At least 20–60 min	Few minutes	?
Healing	Removal by macrophages; collagenization of empty sarcolemmal tubes	Removal by macrophages; collagenization of empty sarcolemmal tubes	Removal by macrophages; collagenization of empty sarcolemmal tubes
Frequency in coronary heart disease:			
Acute infarct	100%	100% external layer of infarct 77% in normal myocardium	43%
Sudden death	17% histologically demonstrated	72% only demonstrable lesion 86% including cases with coagulation necrosis	8%

Source: G. Baroldi, G. Falzi, and F. Mariani,[15] Sudden Coronary Death. Selected Cases Compared to 97 "Normal" Subjects, *Am. Heart J.,* 98:20, 1979. Reprinted with permission.

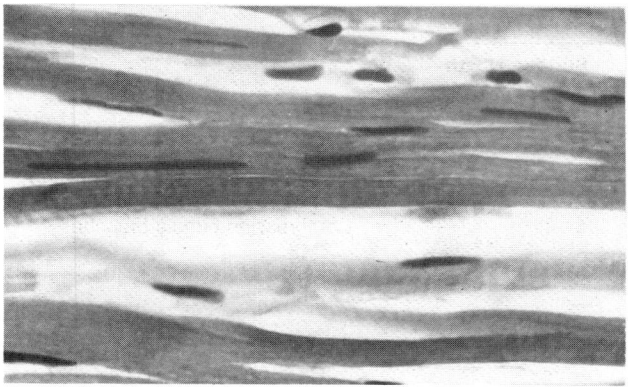

A

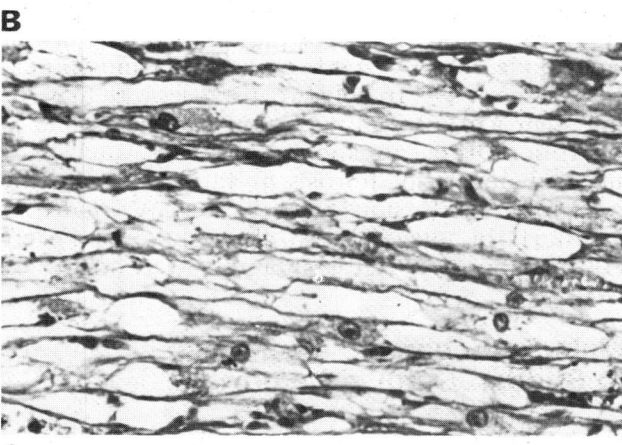

B

C

FIGURE 31-1 Early changes in different types of myocardial necrosis in coronary heart disease. *A*. Coagulation necrosis (atonic death). Thinning of the myocardial cells and elongation of the nuclei due to stretching by intraventricular pressure. The myofibrillar apparatus is undamaged. H&E; ×314. *B*. Zenker necrosis or coagulative myocytolysis (tetanic death). Hypercontraction with myofibrillar rhexis and anomalous cross-band formation. PTAH; ×431. *C*. Myocytolysis or colliquative myocytolysis (failing death). Disappearance of the myofibrils secondary to progressive vacuolization of the muscle fibers. H&E; ×216.

limited our source of information. A major contribution has been made in a series of 30 clinicopathologic reports ("De Subitaneis Mortibus") published in *Circulation* from August 1973 to June 1978.[27,28] The conduction system was examined by serial sections in a total of 77 sudden death cases (43 males and 34 females), excluding one instance of coronary embolism in a 20-week-old fetus (spontaneous abortion). In 60 cases the underlying diseases were asymmetric septal hypertrophy (22 cases), scleroderma (8 cases), long QT syndromes (8 cases), rupture of an infarcted interventricular septum (5 cases), pheochromocytoma (3 cases), type A Wolff-Parkinson-White syndrome (2 cases), persistent superior vena cava (2 cases), rheumatoid arthritis (2 cases), Pickwickian syndrome, homocystinuria, familial congenital heart block, Whipple's disease, ankylosing spondylitis, sarcoidosis, coarctation of aorta, and metastatic hypernephroma (1 case each). Most of the 60 cases presented with arrhythmias, while conduction disturbances (varying degrees of heart block, paroxysmal atrial fibrillation, premature ventricular beats, etc.) were the only signs in 7 cases. In 10 cases the history contributed nothing. In these cases, as well as in 17 cases with hypertrophic cardiomyopathy, the sudden death occurred without warning. The main pathologic findings within the conduction system were:

1. Benign tumor (fibroma compressing His bundle, polycystic tumor of the AV node, multifocal Purkinje cell tumor) was found in 4 cases.
2. Focal neuritis and neural degeneration occurred in the cases with long QT syndromes.
3. Structural anomalies (persistent fetal dispersion of AV node and His bundle in central fibrous body, loop or unusual connections, malformation of AV node and His bundle, venous lacunae, etc.) occurred in 25 cases.
4. Focal degeneration and/or fibrosis was found in more than half of the cases.
5. Focal or diffuse replacement by adipose tissue was found in 12 cases.
6. "Fibromuscular medial dysplasia" obstructing the sinus and AV node arterial vessels was an isolated finding in 6 patients and was frequently observed in cases with underlying diseases (7 with scleroderma, 13 with asymmetric hypertrophy, all 3 cases of pheochromocytoma, 3 cases with rupture of interventricular septum, 1 case with homocystinuria, rheumatoid arthritis, ankylosing spondylitis, sarcoidosis, coarctation of aorta, extensive acute myocarditis).
7. Other vascular lesions were panarteritis in the Whipple's disease case, disseminated intravascular coagulation in a pregnant woman with paroxysmal atrial fibrillation, platelet aggregates in the pheochromocytoma and homocystinuria cases, and occlusion of a normal sinus node artery by a fibromuscular polypoid mass. In only 10 of these 77 cases was there a severe obstruc-

TABLE 31-2 Sudden Death in Primary Benign Cardiac Tumors

| Type | Number of Cases | Sudden Death | | Annotations |
		Unwarned	Warned	
Myxoma	130	5	—	
Papillary fibroelastoma	42	3	—	13 aortic cusps (occl. cor. ostium)
Rhabdomyoma	36	?	—	
Fibroma, IV septum	10	6	—	Compression bundle branches
Fibroma, free wall	7	—	—	
Lipomatous hypertrophy, atrial septum	32	2	—	
Lipoma, heart/pericardium	5	—	1	
Hemangioma	15	—	—	
Mesothelioma, AV node	12	2	5	Symptoms lasted 5 months to 37 years
Teratoma	14	2	—	
Bronchogenic/pericardial cysts	89	—	—	

FIGURE 31-2 Fibroma of the left ventricle of the heart. Sudden and unwarned death following a swimming race in a 12-year-old girl. (*From D. Heath, Cardiac Fibroma, Br. Heart J., 31:656, 1969. Reproduced with permission.*)

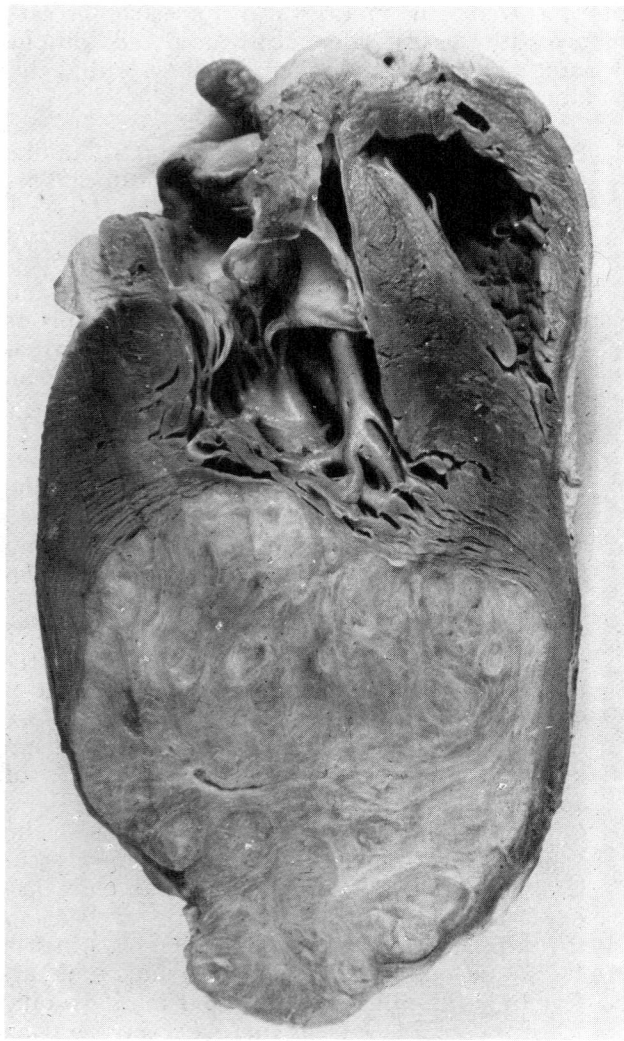

tion of the main subepicardial coronary arteries. In one instance it was located proximally to the origin of the AV node artery (case with Pickwickian syndrome), while in another (acute extensive myocarditis in a 19-year-old male with a history of atrial fibrillation) atresia of the left main trunk was observed.

In another serial section study[29] done on 49 cases of sudden death associated with severe coronary atherosclerosis with or without demonstrable myocardial infarction, no specific findings were noted in the conduction system. Intimal thickening with significant luminal narrowing was present in the sinus node or an AV node artery in 25 and 50 percent, respectively. In only two instances with massive interventricular septal infarction was the AV node necrotic. Other nonspecific findings, such as a marked degree of fibrosis or fatty replacement, were found in the sinus node (9 cases), AV node (21 cases), His bundle (22 cases), and right (4 cases), left (14 cases), or both (7 cases) bundle branches.

Main Pathogenetic Mechanisms in Sudden Cardiac Death

In about 90 percent of sudden death cases occurring out of a hospital, as well as in all but one of the reported patients who died suddenly while undergoing electrocardiographic monitoring, ventricular fibrillation (preceded by heart rate acceleration and ventricular ectopic activity) is the terminal cardiac disorder. Asystole, idioventricular rhythm, or electromechanical dissociation was observed in the remaining subjects (see Chap. 32). Despite this limited information confined to a selected group of sudden death patients with coronary atherosclerosis, ventricular fibrillation seems to be the leading cause of a cardiac arrest. The general belief is that the latter may be triggered by ischemia due to obstructive coronary vascular changes (absolute or co-ronarogenic ischemia) leading to electrical instability of the myocardium. Any other condition (anemia, hypertrophy of the heart, aortic stenosis, strenuous exercise, hypotension, hyperthyroidism, etc.) thought able to reduce either the oxygen supply or the coronary flow or to increase the metabolic demand may be responsible for inducing the fatal arrhythmias (relative or noncoronarogenic ischemia or relative coronary insufficiency).

From the pathologic standpoint, most people who died suddenly can be included in the ischemic group. In the small percentage of nonischemic cases, particularly those who died without warning, little is known as to the type of the terminal disorder. What they show are (1) extracardiac complications of a primary cardiac disease and/or dysfunction (cardiogenic embolism, pulmonary lesions, cerebral anoxia, etc.) causing sudden death by extracardiac damage or possibly by nervous reflexes affecting cardiac function; or (2) myocardial or conduction system changes (microfocal degenerative and/or inflammatory processes, structural abnormalities, neoplastic growth) associated or not associated with a specific disease. Both ischemic and nonischemic lesions may be present in combination in particular conditions, as in hypertrophic cardiomyopathy (compression of the intramural vessels, obstruction of the outflow tract, inflow resistance due to impaired relaxation, abnormal arrangement of the myocardial cells, deep clefts of the septum, vascular narrowing, fibrosis of the sinus node, cystic central fibrous body, etc.).

The basic question concerns the significance of the various lesions found in cases of sudden death in terms of their cause-effect relationship. Apart from situations in which the latter seems evident (e.g., cardiac tamponade following rupture of a necrotic cardiac wall, of a coronary aneurysm, or of the ascending aorta; of the 208 cases of sudden coronary death, wall rupture was observed in three with coagulation necrosis and in one with transmural Zenker necrosis), most, if not all, lesions are nonspecific and mainly reported in single case reports without a controlled study of their frequency in the general population, in which normal subjects and noncardiac patients have to be included. With but few exceptions and despite the need of more accurate prospective studies, it may be stated that, in general, these nonspecific lesions in the majority of cases are not associated with sudden death. Why then does sudden death occur?

Pathogenetic Significance of the Pathologic Findings in Sudden Cardiac Death

At present the true linkage between the pathologic findings and the fatal cardiac disorders is still unclear and often questionable; and sudden death remains for the majority of the cases an unanswered question. In an attempt to review this point we may distinguish primary vascular and myocardial lesions, both acute and chronic.

Vascular Lesions

Among *acute vascular lesions,* dissecting aneurysm and embolism of the main subepicardial coronary arteries appear as the lesions more frequently linked with sudden death. These rare events may be compared with an experimental acute occlusion of a normal coronary artery which is frequently followed by ventricular fibrillation. However, since the latter may be prevented by beta-adrenergic blocking drugs, the possibility arises that a mechanism other than ischemia could promote the cardiac disorders (see "Myocardial Lesions"). Subepicardial coronary thrombus is another acute event seen in a small percentage of sudden death cases associated with coronary atherosclerosis. Its significance in terms of blood flow reduction has been questioned, since the thrombus is always found at the site of a severe stenosis already bypassed by compensatory collateral flow (Fig. 31-3); this concept is supported by finding organizing occlusive thrombi without associated infarction and by the lack of any cardiac changes paralleled by a dramatic increase in collaterals after occlusion of an experimental stenosis which had lasted a few days. The thrombus can be interpreted as a secondary, ineffective multivariant phenomenon (with direct relation to degree and length of the stenosis, its concentric shape, atheroma extension, and infarct size) induced any time there is an increase in the peripheral resistance distal to stenosis (spasm, reduced inflow in infarcted area, etc.). The frequent occlusion of a stenosis surgically bypassed by a vein graft favors this view, the surgical bypass being the equivalent of natural collaterals at very high pressure and flow.[30-32]

Platelet aggregates formed in situ or embolized from major vessels into the intramural circulation are frequently reported as a cause of ischemic sudden death. In our experience, sudden death and control cases showed no difference in the frequency and number of vessels involved. Platelet aggregates appear to be linked with a protracted terminal type of blood stasis with separation of the blood elements. On the other hand, in 39 cases of thrombotic thrombocytopenic purpura (TTP) examined personally and in more than 200 cases reviewed from the literature, sudden death was a very rare event, as was ischemic heart disease in general, despite the demonstrable widespread platelet aggregation in small coronary vessels. Furthermore, this disease looks like an experimental pooling in human beings of several ischemic and hypoxic factors (extremely severe hemolytic anemia and obstructive microangiopathy, hemorrhagic diathesis, neurologic convulsive disorders, coma). If each factor was a true cause of absolute or relative ischemia, any TTP patient should be a "coronary" patient. In our cases,

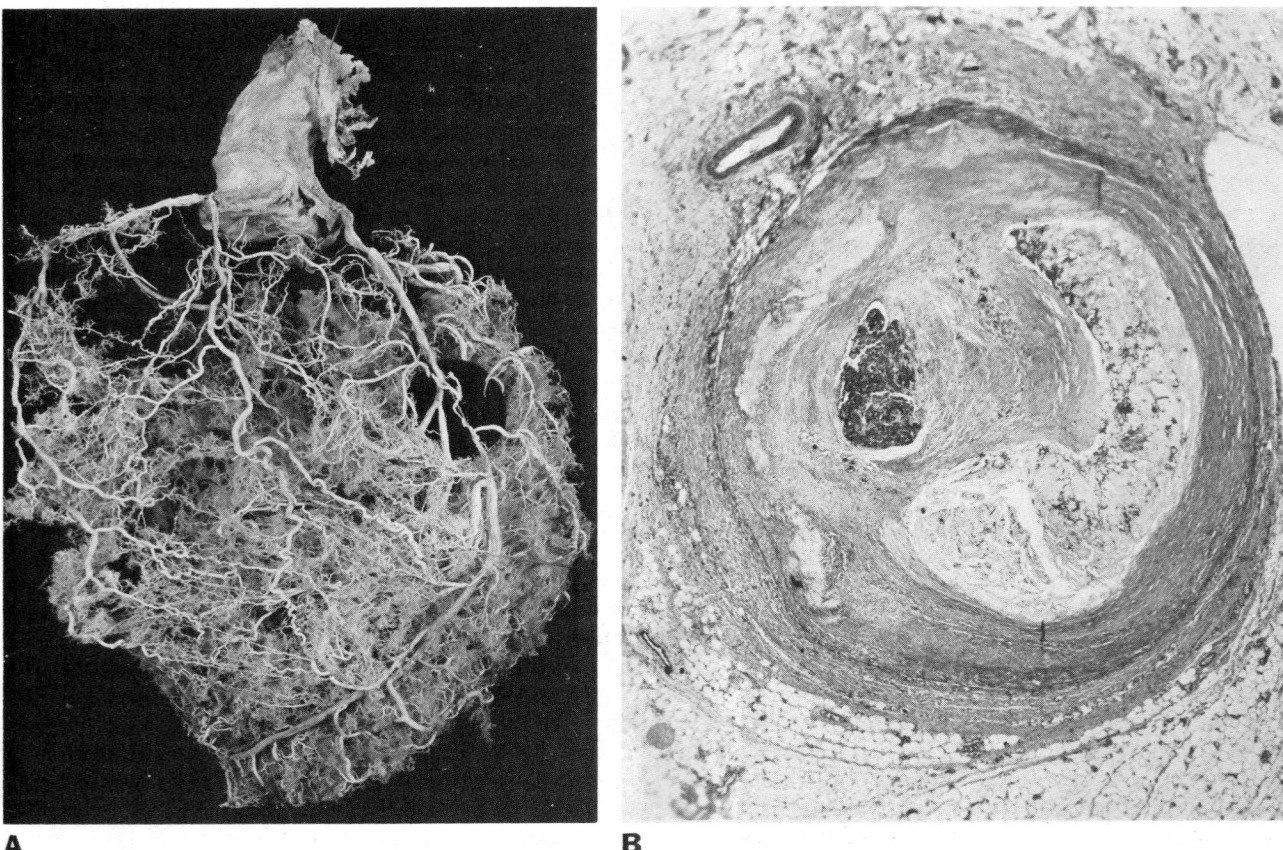

A **B**

FIGURE 31-3 Dramatic enlargement of the collaterals in presence of a severe stenosis. *A*. Tridimensional plastic cast view of a severe obstruction of the left anterior descending branch (within the black circle), with its distal segment filled by numerous collaterals. It seems unlikely that occlusion of an already bypassed stenosis can be effective in reducing the distal blood flow. *B*. Occlusive thrombus at the site of a severe stenosis. Movat; ×4. (*From G. Baroldi, F. Radice, G. Schmid, and A. Leone, Morphology of Acute Myocardial Infarction in Relation to Coronary Thrombosis, Am. Heart J., 87:65, 1974. Reproduced with permission.*)

no one had angina or infarction and only two died suddenly in the course of manifest disease. Finally, ischemic heart disease is a chronic pattern in which a continuous shower of platelet aggregates might be expected. Consequently, a TTP-like microangiopathy should also be expected in ischemic heart disease; but this is a finding never shown, as it was impossible to show any type of so-called small-vessel disease which could be considered responsible for sudden death.[14]

The previous example of TTP raises questions about many of the other proposed mechanisms of sudden death (anemia, disseminated intravascular coagulation, hypotension), as well as any other cause which implies an increased metabolic demand of the myocardium. Embolism of atheromatous material originating from a ruptured atherosclerotic plaque deserves a few words. This is a hypothesis often quoted but never demonstrated. Extensive examination of several hundred hearts (an average of 30 total wall samples per heart), both with acute infarction and from subjects dying suddenly, showed only one instance of chronic "cholesterol" embolus found in a septal branch surrounded by normal myocardium.

Among the *chronic vascular lesions,* the obstructive

atherosclerotic plaque is thought to be a major culprit in causing sudden death. However, three main facts question this point of view. First, there is a very high frequency of severe, multiple atherosclerotic obstructions found in normal subjects dying by accident and in atherosclerotic noncardiac patients dying in hospitals of diseases not involving the heart. Second, there is apparently no relationship between the degree of atherosclerotic damage and ischemic heart disease. In other words, one may have a first infarction or die suddenly without warning with no or minimal coronary stenosis or with one severe (lumen/diameter reduction greater than 70 percent) or three 90 percent stenoses, all or most of the main vessels being involved; there is apparently no critical degree of damage which causes ischemia. Third, severe atherosclerosis must be a very chronic process existing for a long time before the first clinical episode. This means that candidates for clinically overt disease are handling a normal, often stressful life-style despite severe coronary lesions. All these facts suggest that the increase in the number of enlarged collaterals (proportional to the number of stenoses, without relation to sex, age, and sudden death) demonstrated postmortem by tridimensional coronary casts is capable of maintaining an adequate compensatory flow to the myocardium. No proof exists that sudden death or infarction is due to an acute failure of this compensatory mechanism. The concept of spasm of the collaterals cannot be accepted since, in humans, the collaterals lack a muscular tunica. The same can be stated in the cases with bilateral occlusion of the coronary ostia where extracoronary collaterals are present, even in the presence of a greatly hypertrophied heart, but without signs of ischemia in most cases.[32]

The same criticism seems appropriate for the chronic obstructive lesions occasionally seen in the intramural vessels. We were unable to demonstrate any cause-effect relationship between these lesions (intimal or medial hyperplasia obliterans) and sudden death, their frequency being the same in sudden death, infarction, and control cases. Furthermore, it has been demonstrated in humans and experimentally that proliferative medial and intimal thickening is a phenomenon which occurs in the intramural arterial vessels surviving myocardial coagulation necrosis, or infarction. To find them around a scar means that they are a consequence and not the cause of the infarction.[32] In contrast, TTP is a good example, in this regard, to show that a severe microangiopathy does not induce ischemic heart disease.

Only a very small percentage of cases with aortic stenosis and/or cardiac hypertrophy die suddenly. The microfocal fibrosis seen in these conditions has been interpreted as ischemic. However, they may have a different nature (see "Myocardial Lesions"). In evaluating the possible ischemic effect of cardiac hypertrophy, there is an extreme example worthy of mention. In cor pulmonale, the right ventricle increases its muscular mass dramatically, approximating that of the left ventricle. In the hypertrophic right ventricle, even in the presence of severe obstruction of the right coronary artery, a primitive infarction has never been demonstrated in our material, and the patients died of congestive heart failure.

Myocardial Lesions

Scars of the myocardium found in sudden death cases are the anonymous end result of several degenerative processes and obviously have preceded the sudden death by a long time. Tumors of the heart may also exist for many years before being associated with sudden death. Their meaning in relation to the pathogenesis of the latter is still unclear, as are the microfocal lymphocytic infiltrates frequently found in sudden death cases but also present with a relatively high frequency in the normal controls. The nature of these infiltrates is totally unknown. One is reluctant to accept them as "foci of irritability" leading to ventricular fibrillation when found within a normal myocardium. On the other hand, lymphocytes and macrophages are often found as a secondary response to an acute lesion, namely Zenker necrosis found in the major-

ity of sudden death cases associated with coronary atherosclerosis.

This necrosis, however, is unrelated to the degree of the coronary damage, showing the same incidence in subjects with absent or minimal atherosclerosis. Therefore those studies which excluded subjects with less than 50 percent stenosis may not be representative of the so-called sudden coronary death. In discussing this lesion, four main facts seem pertinent: first, its identity with the necrosis induced by catecholamines; second, its constant presence around an infarct; third, its relation to ventricular fibrillation, both being prevented by beta blockers;[33] fourth, the increasing evidence that a sympathetic overactivity acts in sudden death as well as in acute infarct.[34,35] These facts suggest the following two pathogenic possibilities. The first is a sympathetic overstimulation of the normal myocardium to compensate for the loss of contraction of a large, overdistended, infarcted area, damage similar to that shown to produce cardiac hypertrophy in the early phase of experimental aortic stenosis. The second is a congenital or acquired sympathetic overactivity, since the same lesion, even extensive, can be seen in small infarcts which cannot mechanically affect the function of the pump. Coincidentally, the occurrence of Zenker necrosis may assume two possible meanings. It may be the hallmark (this necrosis is already visible in a few minutes) of a nondemonstrable large infarct (for unequivocal histologic demonstration of an infarct, 6 to 8 h of survival are needed, all other methods proposed for an earlier recognition being untenable), or it may be the histologic hallmark of a primitive metabolic disorder due to catecholamines or catecholamine-like agents. The cases of sudden death without myocardial infarction, in which different stages of organization of Zenker foci are shown, indicate that this may be the case,[36] a view further supported by the fact that 81 percent of subjects successfully resuscitated by defibrillation do not show evidence of an infarct, and 62 percent do not present lactic acid dehydrogenase isoenzymes (see Chap. 32). Keep in mind that enzymes may be released by Zenker necrosis and not necessarily by the coagulation necrosis of an infarct.

Myocardial Infarct in Relation to Sudden Death

From the previous data it seems possible to say that a patient with an infarct may die suddenly and that most of the sudden death subjects do not die because of an infarct. In the present terminological confusion in which terms such as *coronary thrombosis* (or *atherosclerosis, insufficiency, occlusion*), *cardiac infarct, sudden coronary death, myocardial necrosis*, etc., are all used without discrimination, it is time for a more precise definition according to the morphofunctional significance of the lesions found.

A cause-effect relationship means that any time

a cause acts the expected effect has to occur. Most, if not all, of the proposed causes of sudden death do not follow this basic law. The related pathologic findings or associated processes are too frequently present in controls. At the most they may be regarded as morphologic predisposing or risk factors. The case of the patient with an enormous tumor mass (shown in Fig. 31-2) who died suddenly without any prodromes or disease is a paradigmatic example of a long-standing impressive lesion which cannot be defined as a cause of the sudden death. One may speculate that in a heart with such a jeopardizing handicap—how could the person survive so long?—any stimulus increasing function may lead to a fatal arrhythmia, taking into consideration the different types of myocardial necrosis and their different possible meanings. In this context, myocardial infarction and sudden death can be considered two different aspects of a unique entity in which various pathogenic mechanisms appear to interact, leading to different types of death.

In this era of the coronary spasm, the pathologist also has to consider what he or she cannot see. Cineangiography has demonstrated that spasm is a fact, and that it occurs in angina and myocardial infarction. It still remains unknown if it is the cause of these events or if it is an associated, secondary phenomenon. Nevertheless, it is a provocative concept even for sudden death, both as an occlusive cause per se or as a cause of temporary occlusion. We know that reflow after a certain period of time induces contraction band necrosis and extensive interstitial hemorrhage, often associated with ventricular fibrillation. Contraction band necrosis, alias Zenker necrosis, is typical in sudden coronary death; however no interstitial hemorrhage is found.

References

1. Lancisi, G. M.: De Subitaneis Mortibus, Buegni, Roma, 1707. (Translated by P. D. White, and A. V. Boursey, St. John's University Press, New York, 1971).
2. Kuller, L., Perper, J., and Cooper, M.: Demographic Characteristics and Trends in Arteriosclerotic Heart Disease Mortality: Sudden Death and Myocardial Infarction, Circulation, 51/52(suppl. 3):1, 1975.
3. Fulton, M., Julian, D. G., and Oliver, M. F.: Sudden Death and Myocardial Infarction, Circulation, 40(suppl. 4):182, 1969.
4. Friedman, M., Manwaring, J. H., Rosenman, R. H., Donlon, G., Ortega, P., and Grube, S. M.: Instantaneous and Sudden Deaths. Clinical and Pathological Differentiation in Coronary Artery Disease, J. Am. Med. Assoc., 225:1319, 1973.
*5. Blake, H. A., Manion, W. C., Mattingly, T. W., and Baroldi, G.: Coronary Artery Anomalies, Circulation, 30:927, 1964. (70 references)
6. Cheitlin, M. D., De Castro, C. M., and McAllister, H. A.: Sudden Death as a Complication of Anomalous Left Coronary Origin from the Anterior Sinus of Valsalva. A Not-So-Minor Congenital Anomaly, Circulation, 50:780, 1974.
7. Sinclair, W., Jr., and Nitsch, E.: Polyarteritis Nodosa of the Coronary Arteries. Report of a Case with Rupture of an Aneurysm and Intrapericardial Hemorrhage, Am. Heart J., 38:898, 1949.
8. Kegel, S. M., Dorsey, T. J., Rowen, M., and Taylor, W. F.: Cardiac Death in Mucocutaneous Lymph Node Syndrome, Am. J. Cardiol., 40:282, 1977.
*9. Burns, C. J., and Manion, W. C.: Sudden Unexpected Death of a Two-Year-Old Child from Thrombosis of Both Coronary Arteries with Aneurysmal Dilatation of the Vessels, Med. Ann. D.C., 38:381, 1969. (48 references)
10. Ahronheim, J. H.: Isolated Coronary Periarteritis: Report of a Case of Unexpected Death in a Young Pregnant Woman, Am. J. Cardiol., 40:287, 1977.
11. Scharfman, W. B., Wallach, J. B., and Angrist, A.: Myocardial Infarction Due to Syphilitic Coronary Ostial Stenosis, Am. Heart J., 40:603, 1950.
*12. Wenger, N. K., and Bauer, S.: Coronary Embolism. Review of the Literature and Presentation of Fifteen Cases, Am. J. Med., 25:549, 1958. (102 references)
13. Haerem, J. W.: Platelet Aggregates in Intramyocardial Vessels of Patients Dying Suddenly and Unexpectedly of Coronary Artery Disease, Atherosclerosis, 15:199, 1972.
14. Baroldi, G., Falzi, G., Mariani, F., and Baroldi, L. A.: Morphology, Frequency and Significance of Intramural Arterial Lesions in Sudden Coronary Death, G. Ital. Cardiol., 10:644, 1980.
15. Baroldi, G., Falzi, G., and Mariani, F.: Sudden Coronary Death. A Post-mortem Study in 208 Selected Cases Compared to 97 "Control" Subjects, Am. Heart J., 98:20, 1979.
16. Claudon, D. G., Claudon, D. B., and Edwards, J. E.: Primary Dissecting Aneurysm of Coronary Artery. A Cause of Acute Myocardial Ischemia, Circulation, 45:259, 1972.
17. Edwards, J. E.: Congenital Malformations of the Heart and Great Vessels, in S. E. Gould (ed.), "Pathology of the Heart and Blood Vessels," 3d ed., Charles C Thomas, Publisher, Springfield, Ill., 1968, p. 262.
18. Glew, R. H., Varghese, J. P., Krovetz, J. L., Dorst, J. P., and Rowe, R. D.: Sudden Death in Congenital Aortic Stenosis. A Review of Eight Cases with an Evaluation of Premonitory Clinical Features, Am. Heart J., 78:615, 1969.
19. Gore, I., and Kline, I. K.: B. Myocarditis, in S. E. Gould (ed.), "Pathology of the Heart and Blood Vessels," 3d ed., Charles C Thomas, Publisher, Springfield, Ill., 1968, p. 731.
20. Schroeder, J. S., Berke, D. K., Graham, A. F., Rider, A. K., and Harrison, D. C.: Arrhythmias after Cardiac Transplantation, Am. J. Cardiol., 33:604, 1974.
21. Helwig, F. C., and Wilhelmy, E. W.: Sudden and Unexpected Death from Acute Interstitial Myocarditis: A Report of Three Cases, Am. Intern. Med., 13:107, 1939.
22. Haerem, J. W.: Myocardial Lesions in Sudden Unexpected Coronary Death, Am. Heart J., 90:562, 1975.
*23. Goodwin, J. F., and Krikler, D. M.: Sudden Death in Cardiomyopathy, in V. Manninen and P. I. Halonen (eds.), "Sudden Coronary Death," Adv. Cardiol., 25:98, 1978. (27 references)

*This article is a review of the literature and contains additional references to the literature.

*24. Maron, B. J., Roberts, W. C., Edward, J. E., Mc-
Allister, H. A., Jr., Foley, D. D., and Epstein, S. E.:
Sudden Death in Patients with Hypertrophic Cardiomyopathy: Characterization of 26 Patients without Functional Limitation, *Am. J. Cardiol.*, 41:803,
1978. (21 references)

*25. Baroldi, G.: Different Morphologic Types of My-
ocardial Cell Death in Man, in A. Fleckstein and
G. Rona (eds.), "Pathophysiology and Morphology
of Myocardial Cell Alteration," vol. 6: "Recent Advances in Studies on Cardiac Structure and Metabolism," University Park Press, Baltimore, 1975, p.
383. (77 references)

26. McAllister, H. A., and Fenoglio, J. J.: Tumors of the
Cardiovascular System, in W. H. Hartmann and
W. H. Cowan (eds.), "Atlas of Tumor Pathology,"
Armed Forces Institute of Pathology, Washington,
D.C., 1978.

27. James, T. N., Carson, D. J. L., and Marshall, T. K.:
De Subitaneis Mortibus. I. Fibroma Compressing
His Bundle, *Circulation*, 48:428, 1973.

28. James, T. N., Froggatt, P., Atkinsons, W. J., Jr., Lurie, P. R., McNamara, D. G., Miller, W. W., Schloss,
G. T., Carroll, J. F., and North, R. L.: De Subitaneis
Mortibus. XXX. Observations on the Pathophysiology of the Long QT Syndromes with Special Reference to the Neuropathology of the Heart, *Circulation*, 57:1221, 1978.

29. Lie, J. T.: Histopathology of the Conduction System
in Sudden Death from Coronary Heart Disease, *Circulation*, 51:446, 1975.

30. Baloldi, G.: Acute Coronary Occlusion as a Cause of
Myocardial Infarct and Sudden Coronary Heart
Death, *Am. J. Cardiol.*, 16:859, 1965.

31. Silver, M. D., Baroldi, G., and Mariani, F.: The Relationship between Acute Myocardial Infarction
Studied in 100 Consecutive Patients, *Circulation*,
61:219, 1980.

32. Baroldi, G., and Scomazzoni, G.: Coronary Circu-
lation in the Normal and Pathologic Heart, U.S.
Government Printing Office, American Registry of
Pathology, Armed Forces Institute of Pathology,
Washington, D.C., 1967.

33. Baroldi, G., Silver, M. D., Lixfield, W., and Mc-
Gregor, D. C.: Irreversible Myocardial Damage Resembling Catecholamine Necrosis Secondary to
Acute Coronary Occlusion in Dogs: Its Prevention
by Propranolol, *J. Mol. Cell. Cardiol.*, 9:687, 1977.

34. Raab, W.: Preventive Myocardiology, Fundamentals
and Targets, in N. I. Kugelmass (ed.), "Bannerstone
Division of American Lectures in Living Chemistry,"
Charles C Thomas, Publisher, Springfield, Ill., 1970.

*35. Lown, B.: Sudden Cardiac Death: The Major Chal-
lenge Confronting Contemporary Cardiology, *Am.
J. Cardiol.*, 43:313, 1979. (106 references)

36. Baroldi, G.: Different Types of Myocardial Necrosis
in Coronary Heart Disease: A Pathophysiological
Review of Their Functional Significance, *Am. Heart
J.*, 89:742, 1975.

32

Predictors and Prevention of Sudden Cardiac Death

Leonard A. Cobb, M.D.
Jeffrey A. Werner, M.D.

*In one sense, every CHD death in a population with
widespread atherosclerosis should be regarded as expected. But
some of these deaths are less expected than others.*
T. Gordon and W. B. Kannel, 1971[1]

For centuries there has been interest and speculation regarding death following unexpected collapse.
In many parts of the world it is now generally recognized that sudden, unexpected, and fatal collapse
is usually a primary cardiac event. Other nontraumatic causes of sudden or unexpected death are well
recognized; however, pulmonary, metabolic, neurologic, and vascular disorders in the aggregate represent only a small contribution to the numbers
of patients who develop cardiac arrest instanta-
neously or within minutes after onset of acute
symptoms.[2,3]

During the past two decades, several lines of investigation have led to a sharpened appreciation of
the magnitude and nature of a sudden cardiac death
(SCD) syndrome. Whereas prior knowledge had
largely been derived from selected cases coming to
autopsy, death certificates, or small series of reported cases, informative community studies[1,2] have
helped to clarify some of the epidemiologic aspects
of SCD. Moreover, the development of effective
prehospital emergency care systems in the past decade has resulted in increasing numbers of resuscitated patients who have "survived" sudden death
and have provided an opportunity for further study
and characterization of persons at risk for SCD. In
addition, advances in the understanding of factors
associated with myocardial electrical instability have
given support to the view that lethal ventricular arrhythmias may ultimately be controlled by pharmacologic or other interventions.[4–6]

Definition of Sudden Cardiac Death

Several definitions of SCD have been proposed. For
epidemiologic reasons and for practical purposes
SCD is commonly defined as *unexpected cardiac death*

occurring without symptoms or with symptoms of less than an hour's duration. When this or similar definitions are used, the majority of episodes occur outside of the hospital, usually without acute prodromal symptoms.[1,2,7,8]

Magnitude of the SCD Problem

In the United States, the incidence of SCD approximates 400,000 per year, the majority due to coronary atherosclerotic heart disease. The ultimate prevention of SCD obviously lies with the prevention, slowing, or reversal of the atherosclerotic process. However, until that can be attained, efforts to reduce mortality, once coronary atherosclerotic heart disease is present, rest largely with the prevention of SCD and to a lesser extent with the treatment of symptomatic complications, particularly myocardial infarction and congestive heart failure. Unfortunately, the difficulties in aborting an episode of SCD are compounded by the inherent nature of this disorder—first by the location of the incident, which is most often removed from a usual site of medical care, and second, by the lack of warning symptoms in 70 percent or more of cases.[7] Furthermore, the problem of SCD may not be resolved for a patient even after successful resuscitation from out-of-hospital cardiac arrest (see "Recurrence of the Sudden Cardiac Death Syndrome," below). Most victims of SCD are males whose average age is approximately 60 years.[4,8] SCD most often occurs during the routine activities of daily life.[9,10] However, in patients with recognized heart disease there appears to be an additional "risk" for SCD during physical exertion.[11,12] The magnitude of this additional hazard is unknown, but is probably not great.

Arrhythmias Responsible for Sudden Cardiac Death

Experiences in the hospital with patients who had acute myocardial infarction suggested that the primary mechanism for out-of-hospital sudden cardiac arrest was likely to be ventricular fibrillation. Furthermore, in animal experiments, ventricular fibrillation regularly follows both acute coronary artery occlusion and subsequent reperfusion of the ischemic myocardium.[13] Hence it has become generally accepted that the majority of sudden cardiac deaths outside the hospital are precipitated by ventricular fibrillation. Indeed, observations in patients seen shortly after collapse have confirmed this.[9,12,14] Although the electrical events immediately prior to SCD have been fortuitously recorded and reported in only a small number of patients, ventricular fibrillation has been confirmed with but one exception.[5] On the other hand, asystole, complete heart block, and electromechanical dissociation are common in the setting of cardiovascular collapse in

which there has been substantial delay in initiating emergency care or in situations where collapse has terminated a complicated systemic illness.[9,15]

Persons at Risk for Sudden Cardiac Death

More than three-fourths of sudden cardiac deaths are due to coronary atherosclerotic heart disease, usually with major obstruction of two or three coronary arteries.[2,3] However, many other cardiac lesions occasionally result in SCD.[16] In the absence of structural heart disease or evident conduction abnormalities, SCD due to arrhythmia is unusual.

Significance of Coronary "Risk Factors"

In view of the very high proportion of sudden deaths due to coronary atherosclerotic heart disease, it is to be expected that established coronary risk factors would be prevalent in patients at risk for SCD. Indeed, hypertension, cigarette smoking, and hypercholesterolemia have been commonly found in SCD victims.[1,17] An important emphasis in the Framingham report was an association with cigarette smoking: every one of the men who died before age 65 of coronary atherosclerotic heart disease, but without prior cardiovascular stigmata, was a cigarette smoker.[1]

Arterial Hypertension

Hypertension warrants special comment because it is often the sole recognized manifestation of cardiovascular disease prior to SCD. In the Framingham cohort, high blood pressure was the only recognized cardiovascular abnormality in nearly one-fourth of sudden deaths due to coronary atherosclerotic heart disease in men aged 65 and younger. Furthermore, left ventricular hypertrophy on the ECG was present (in the absence of symptomatic heart disease) in an additional 19 percent.[1]

Manifest Cardiovascular Disease

As shown in Fig. 32-1, patients successfully resuscitated from out-of-hopsital ventricular fibrillation usually have had one or more manifestations of cardiovascular disease prior to cardiac arrest. Histories of remote heart attack, angina, congestive heart failure, or hypertension were present in 78 percent of patients who had experienced an aborted episode of SCD due to coronary atherosclerotic heart disease. In the remaining 22 percent, out-of-hospital cardiac arrest was the first indication of cardiovascular disease. Comparable data were reported in the Framingham study: of 59 men who died suddenly, SCD was the first manifestation of cardiovascular disease in 20 percent of men younger than 65 years.[1]

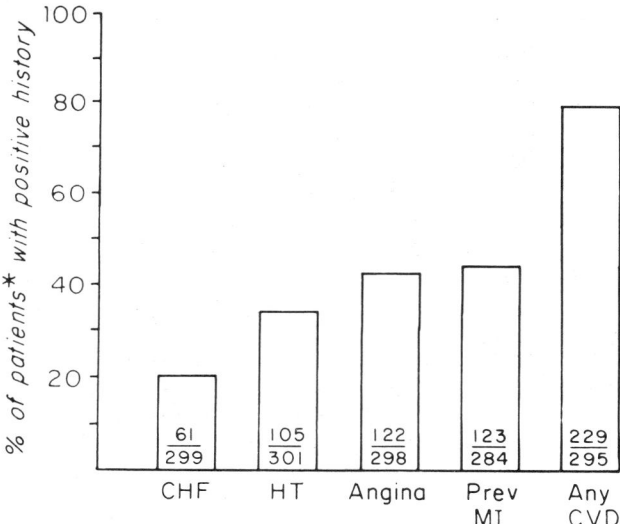

FIGURE 32-1   Manifestations of cardiovascular disease prior to out-of-hospital cardiac arrest from ventricular fibrillation (VF) in 305 patients with coronary artherosclerotic heart disease (ASHD). CHF = congestive heart failure; HT = hypertension; Prev MI = history of previous myocardial infarction; * = 305 patients with ASHD.

Recognition of High-Risk Patients

In patients with clinically evident coronary athero-sclerotic heart disease and/or hypertension, four major characteristics have been associated with en-hanced risk for SCD: (1) ventricular electrical insta-bility, (2) extensive coronary arterial narrowing, (3) abnormal left ventricular function, and (4) electro-cardiographic conduction and repolarization abnor-malities. The data in support of these predictors are limited by the populations studied and the necessity to use special clinical indications for study, e.g., eval-uation of selected patients undergoing coronary ar-teriography,[18,19] follow-up of patients after acute myocardial infarction,[20,21] and assessment of predic-tors for recurrences of the SCD syndrome in sur-vivors of out-of-hospital ventricular fibrillation.[6] In spite of differences in patient populations, a re-markable thread of consistency has emerged. Al-though these predictors appear to have unques-tioned statistical significance in identifying patients at risk for SCD, they are less than ideal in both sen-sitivity and specificity. This is further compounded by the seemingly erratic manner in which SCD com-monly occurs.

Ventricular Electrical Instability   Since SCD is pre-dominantly due to ventricular fibrillation, substan-tial attention has been directed to manifestations of myocardial electrical instability as harbingers of SCD. Several studies have shown that ventricular ectopic activity in patients with coronary athero-sclerotic heart disease is a predictor of SCD.[20–23] In a prospective study of patients who had sustained an acute myocardial infarction weeks to months pre-viously, Ruberman and colleagues[21] reported that complex ventricular premature depolarizations

(VPDs), i.e., multiform beats, repetitive forms, bi-geminy, or early (R on T) VPDs, were statistical pre-dictors of patients at high risk for SCD; sporadic, uniform VPDs during the single hour of monitoring were not predictive of subsequent SCD (Fig. 32-2). When large numbers of patients with coronary ath-erosclerotic heart disease have been examined, VPDs have commonly been found in ambulatory patients likely to develop SCD, even when evaluated with a single resting 12-lead ECG.[22,23] An additional group in whom ventricular ectopic activity has been shown to be a harbinger of SCD are patients in the recovery phase of acute myocardial infarction. Davis and colleagues reported that one or more VPDs noted on a predischarge, 6-h monitoring carried a significant risk for cardiac death during 1 to 5 years of follow-up.[20]

Clearly, complex VPDs are predictors of SCD *in patients with known coronary artherosclerotic heart dis-ease.* In persons without demonstrable heart disease, ventricular ectopic activity by itself appears to have little, if any, prognostic import.[5] At one time it was hoped that VPDs detected by ambulatory ECG mon-itoring or during exercise might prove to be sensi-tive and specific markers of patients at risk for SCD. However, VPDs in patients with recognized coro-nary atherosclerotic heart disease are ubiquitous, and even high grades of VPDs fall short in their

FIGURE 32-2   Mortality related to ventricular premature beats (VPB) identified in 1 h of ambulatory monitoring in patients with prior myocardial infarction. The abbreviation for premature ventric-ular depolarization (VDP) is used in the text instead of ventricular premature beats. Premature beats were considered complex if they were multiform or repetitive, or if bigeminy or R on T was present. (*From Ruberman et al.*[21] *Reproduced with permission of author and publisher.*)

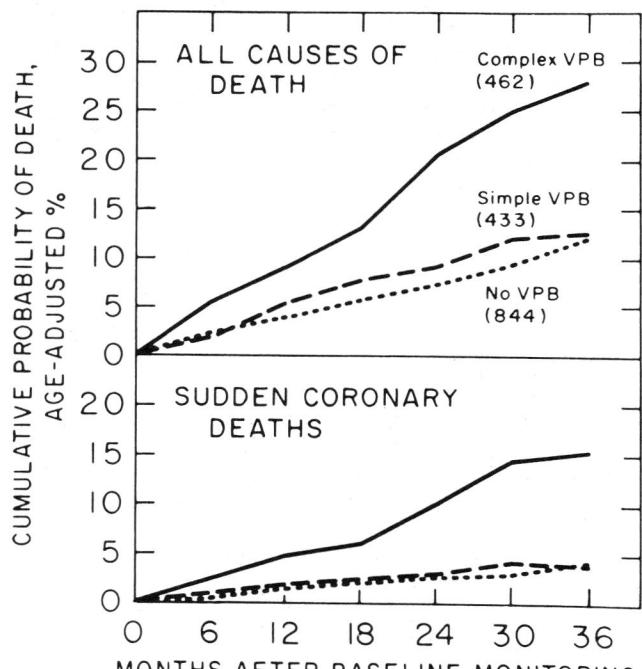

predictive value to discriminate among patient subgroups. For example, in a study by Ruberman et al.,[21] 41 percent of sudden cardiac deaths occurred in patients who *did not* have complex VPDs during 1 h of monitoring. Furthermore, only 10 to 15 percent of those with complex VPDs developed SCD during an average follow-up of 24 months.

Coronary Arterial Narrowing   Patients who develop SCD on the basis of coronary atherosclerotic heart disease usually have severe obstruction (70 percent or greater diameter narrowing) in two or three coronary arteries.[2,3,24,25] Although there is some evidence that SCD victims may have more involvement in the left anterior descending coronary artery than in other vessels,[26] other reports have shown that all three of the major coronary arterial systems appear to be equally affected.[24,25] Although disease involving the left main coronary artery is reported to have an ominous prognosis, severe obstruction of this vessel, in our experience, is infrequently encountered in both survivors and nonsurvivors of out-of-hospital cardiac arrest.[24,25]

In patients with angina pectoris, cardiac mortality has been shown to be related to the extent of coronary arterial narrowing.[18,19] In one report, the 5-year cardiac mortality was 15 percent in patients with single-vessel narrowing, 38 percent if two vessels were narrowed (by 50 percent or more), and 54 percent for three-vessel involvement.[19] In ambulatory patients who had been resuscitated from an episode of out-of-hospital ventricular fibrillation, recurrences of the SCD syndrome were reported in nearly 50 percent of patients (9 of 19) with triple-vessel narrowing, compared with only 10 percent of patients (2 of 20) with single-vessel narrowing.[24]

Abnormal Ventricular Function   It is well recognized that there is an association between left ventricular aneurysms and malignant ventricular arrhythmias, and surgical resection has been proposed as therapy in that situation.[27,28] In patients resuscitated from ventricular fibrillation, Weaver et al. reported a relatively high incidence of severe left ventricular wall motion abnormalities, particularly in patients who later developed recurrences of the SCD syndrome.[25] Of 14 patients who developed recurrent ventricular fibrillation or SCD, 10 had abnormal contraction patterns in over one-half of the left ventricular wall segments. Such extensive wall motion abnormalities were observed in only 9 of 45 patients who did not develop recurrences. Furthermore, half of the patients who developed recurrent ventricular fibrillation or SCD had one or more dyskinetic segments. Another example of the association between impaired ventricular function and SCD is the posthospital phase of acute myocardial infarction, where there is a relatively high mortality, mostly in SCD, during the first year after infarction.[20,29]

Because of the association between ventricular

ectopic activity and abnormal ventricular function, it is uncertain whether complex VPDs are *independent* predictors of SCD or whether they are merely reflective of myocardial dysfunction. In the report of Ruberman and colleagues, the predictive value of complex VPDs in identifying patients who later developed SCD appeared independent of clinical manifestations of heart failure.[21] In a study by Schulze et al., 81 patients were followed an average of 7 months after acute myocardial infarction; each of the 8 patients who developed SCD had both an impaired left ventricular ejection fraction (less than 40 per cent) and complex VPDs.[29] Although there is clearly an association between VPDs and ventricular dysfunction, their ability to predict SCD appears additive.

Because of considerations of cost, discomfort, and potential complications, extensive invasive cardiac procedures seem unsuitable for the primary purpose of establishing prognosis. On the other hand, noninvasive procedures, particularly two-dimensional echocardiography, may prove practical and useful for this purpose.

Electrocardiographic Abnormalities of Conduction and Repolarization   Resting ECG markers of patients with coronary atherosclerotic heart disease who are at greater-than-average risk for SCD include abnormalities of conduction, prolongation of the QT interval, and ST-T changes.[17,22,23] In a report by Haynes and coworkers,[23] abnormalities of repolarization, including prolongation of the QT interval were significantly more prevalent in ambulatory patients who had been resuscitated from an episode of out-of-hospital ventricular fibrillation than in a group of patients with prior myocardial infarction who had not developed the SCD syndrome. Although repolarization and conduction abnormalities are more prevalent in patients at high risk for SCD, it has yet to be shown that they are independent markers which provide additional prognostic information beyond that obtained by other assessments.

Lessons Learned from Survivors of the Sudden Cardiac Death Syndrome

To date the only *proven* means of preventing SCD is through the deployment of emergency medical services. If patients with ventricular fibrillation are treated with early initiation of cardiopulmonary resuscitation (CPR) and are promptly defibrillated, a substantial proportion can be resuscitated and ultimately discharged home after hospitalization.[12,14,30]

Experience Treating Ventricular Fibrillation

Experience in the management of out-of-hospital ventricular fibrillation in Seattle is shown in Fig. 32-3. The Seattle emergency care system operates with

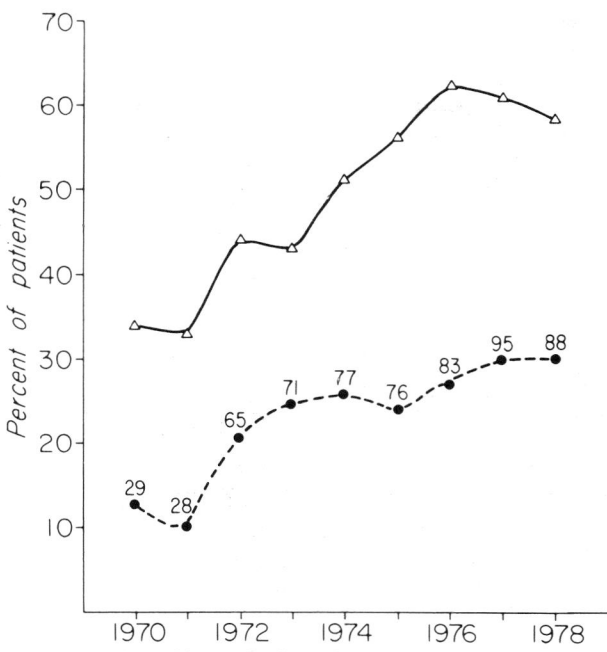

FIGURE 32-3 Outcomes in patients treated for out-of-hospital ventricular fibrillation during 9 years (1970–1978). All patients were in cardiac arrest at the time of arrival of paramedical personnel. Solid line shows percent of successful resuscitations; broken line shows percent discharged home. (*From Cobb, Werner, and Trobaugh.*[30] *Reproduced with permission of the author and publisher.*)

a tiered response, providing both basic and advanced life support. The major goal of this service is to deliver care comparable to that which a well-trained physician would provide on the scene. Paramedics are trained in such skills as tracheal intubation, use of common emergency drugs, arrhythmia recognition, and defibrillation. In Seattle the response time from dispatch until arrival of the first fire department unit averages 2.9 min. The advanced life-support (medic) units arrive on the scene approximately 4 min later. Except for cardiac arrest and hypovolemic shock, all therapy is carried out in conjunction with a physician who is in communication by radio or telephone with the paramedics.[30]

Each year the fire department paramedics treat approximately 300 patients who are in cardiac arrest with ventricular fibrillation when first seen—about 6 cases per 10,000 population per year. (An additional 40 to 50 patients typically develop ventricular fibrillation after arrival of the mobile units.) Over several years there has been a substantial increase in the rate of successful resuscitation and in the proportion of patients ultimately discharged home. In the initial years of the Seattle experience, 10 to 12 percent of patients found in ventricular fibrillation were ultimately discharged home; more recently, this figure has risen to approximately 30 percent. The proportion of patients resuscitated on the scene has increased from about 30 percent to 60 percent (Fig. 32-3).

Bystander-Initiated Cardiopulmonary Resuscitation

An important adjunct to the Seattle emergency care system is the involvement of the general public in the initiation of cardiopulmonary resuscitation.[31] By 1980, approximately 280,000 persons of high school age and older had requested and received CPR training by the fire department. Over one-third of resuscitations are initiated by bystanders prior to arrival of the fire department, and survival in those patients has been twice that of patients for whom initiation of CPR was delayed until arrival of fire department personnel.[31] Similar experiences have been reported in suburban King County, Washington, and in Oslo, Norway.[32,33]

Acute Myocardial Infarction versus Sudden Cardiac Death

Follow-up of patients resuscitated from out-of-hospital ventricular fibrillation has provided an opportunity to view the SCD syndrome from a somewhat different perspective than was heretofore possible. Although coronary atherosclerotic heart disease is responsible for most episodes of out-of-hospital ventricular fibrillation, only a minority of resuscitated patients appear to have developed ventricular fibrillation as a consequence of *acute* myocardial infarction. In the days following resuscitation, new Q waves of transmural myocardial infarction developed in only 19 percent of patients (Fig. 32-4). The majority of patients had either ST-segment (and/or T-wave) changes or no appreciable electrocardiographic changes during the postresuscitation hospitalization. Lactate dehydrogenase isoenzyme pat-

FIGURE 32-4 ECG changes during the days following resuscitation from out-of-hospital ventricular fibrillation. Acute transmural myocardial infarction (ATMI) was identified by the development of new Q waves in 19 percent of 305 patients with coronary atherosclerotic heart disease. NO CH = no change; UNK = unknown. (*From Cobb, Werner, and Trobaugh.*[30] *Reproduced with permission of author and publisher.*)

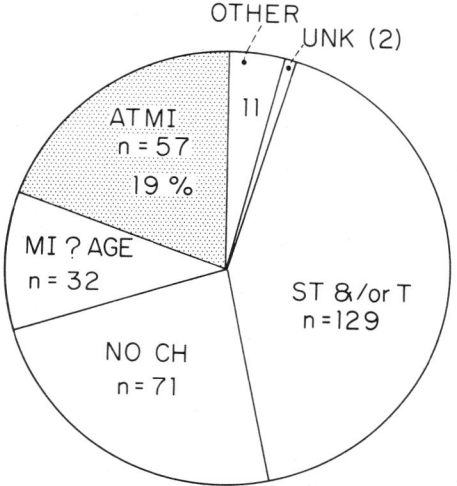

terns of myocardial necrosis were found in 38 percent of patients. The disparity between the incidence of electrocardiographically determined acute transmural infarction and the occurrence of isoenzyme evidence for necrosis may be explained by either acute nontransmural infarction or, perhaps more likely, by enzyme elevation secondary to cardiac arrest and resuscitation. In either case, the majority of patients appear to have developed ventricular fibrillation without acute transmural myocardial infarction as a precipitating event.[34,35] This relatively low incidence of acute infarction is in accord with the observation that most victims of SCD do not have antecedent chest pain,[7] and also with previously reported autopsy series.[2,3,25]

Recurrence of the SCD Syndrome

During the first year following hospitalization, there has been approximately a 30 percent mortality rate, with three-fourths of the deaths due to recurrence of the SCD syndrome.[34] When cardiac rhythms were recorded during the recurrent episodes, ventricular fibrillation was usually present if patients were monitored shortly after collapse.[9]

Predictors of Recurrent SCD Syndrome

Using easily obtained information from survivors of out-of-hospital ventricular fibrillation, multivariate risk profiles have been developed and validated (Table 32-1). Recurrences of the SCD syndrome were predominantly in patients whose initial episode of ventricular fibrillation was *not* associated with acute transmural myocardial infarction (Fig. 32-5). Historical factors associated with recurrences included remote myocardial infarction and congestive heart failure prior to the episode of ventricular fibrillation. Other predictors of recurrence were gender (males), abnormal left ventricular function, extensive coronary artery narrowing, and complex VPDs.[6,24]

Vulnerability to Ventricular Fibrillation

The contrasting rates of SCD recurrence in patients stratified according to the presence of acute transmural myocardial infarction are striking and war-

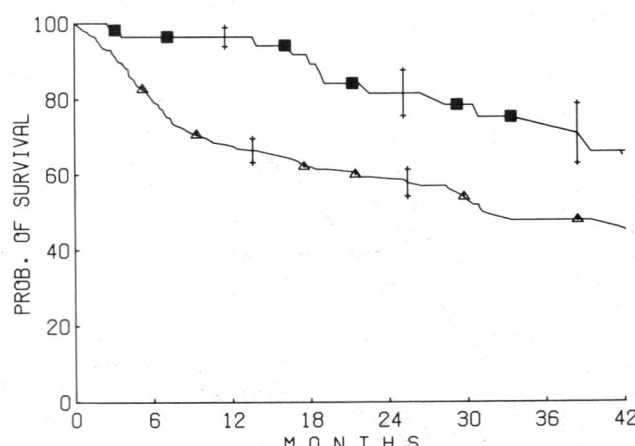

FIGURE 32-5 Survival following successful out-of-hospital resuscitation in 302 patients with coronary atherosclerotic heart disease. Patients who had ventricular fibrillation (VF) associated with acute transmural myocardial infarction (ATMI, ■) showed a markedly greater survival compared with those whose ECGs did not show ATMI during the postresuscitation hospitalization (▲). For those with ATMI, *N* = 57; there were 12 deaths. For those with other ECGs, *N* = 245; there were 101 deaths. *p* = 0.0008.

rant comment. First, this easily obtained information provides a simple, important prognostic indicator for an individual patient. Second, this comparison emphasizes the concept of continuing myocardial propensity to develop ventricular fibrillation. In patients with acute myocardial necrosis, there is a transient likelihood of developing ventricular fibrillation during the initial hours or days. In several studies, long-term survival following successful reversion of ventricular fibrillation complicating acute myocardial infarction was comparable to that of patients who did not experience ventricular fibrillation.[36,37] In patients whose ventricular fibrillation was not precipitated by an acute infarction, there appears to be a residual state of electrical instability which predisposes to recurrences of ventricular fibrillation. Whether this propensity is related to scarring from previous infarction, to chronic ischemia, or to intermittent acute ischemia is difficult to determine in most instances.[38] Other factors which may modulate myocardial vulnerability include physical and psychological stress, arousal of the autonomic nervous system[39] and such metabolic derangements as potassium depletion.[40]

Prevention of Sudden Cardiac Death

Because ventricular fibrillation is usually the immediate cause of SCD, attempts to prevent this disorder should be directed to the treatment of ventricular fibrillation as well as its prevention.

The Treatment of Ventricular Fibrillation

In the majority of victims, SCD appears to represent a primary arrhythmic event, which is potentially re-

TABLE 32-1 One-Year Risk of Recurrent SCD Syndrome in 425 VF Survivors with Coronary Atherosclerotic Heart Disease

Type of Survivor	Recurrence, %
ATMI	2% (2 of 85 patients)
No ATMI	22% (75 of 340 patients)
History of remote MI	30%
No history of remote MI	14%
With CHF	30%
Without CHF	11%

Notes: VF = ventricular fibrillation; ATMI = acute transmural myocardial infarction associated with VF; MI = myocardial infarction; CHF = history of congestive heart failure.

sponsive to electrical defibrillation. As described above (see "Experience Treating Ventricular Fibrillation"), the development of systems to provide advanced-level prehospital emergency care has resulted in the resuscitation of many persons who otherwise would clearly have died.

One criticism of emergency medical systems relates to their applicability in sprawling metropolitan areas where distances are great and where the surveillance and operation of such programs are made difficult by the juxtaposition of governmental and other agencies. Similarly, isolated urban areas will not likely benefit from systems which require a rapid response. Therefore, other means of providing rapid defibrillation have been proposed. Simple, portable defibrillators placed, under medical supervision, in the homes of high-risk patients or in public places has been considered.[41] Additionally, Mirowski and colleagues[42] have developed a prototype implantable defibrillator which provides electronic sensing of ventricular fibrillation and appropriate delivery of a defibrillatory current through implanted electrodes. While the feasibility and efficacy of these approaches are currently speculative, the major requirement for successful treatment of the SCD syndrome could be satisfied by their utilization: reversion of ventricular fibrillation moments after its onset. In spite of logistic and technical drawbacks, the evaluation and employment of these devices warrant consideration.

Prevention of Ventricular Fibrillation

Ventricular fibrillation can be prevented in animals with experimentally created myocardial ischemia or infarction.[13,39] The propensity to develop ventricular fibrillation may be modified by measures such as psychological adaptations, beta-adrenergic blocking agents, and antiarrhythmic drugs. Furthermore, clinical studies in coronary care units have suggested that pretreatment of patients at high risk for potentially fatal arrhythmias may prevent their emergence. In a randomized trial of patients with acute myocardial infarction Lie and associates[43] demonstrated that prophylactic administration of lidocaine reduced the incidence of ventricular arrhythmias and ventricular fibrillation when patients were treated within 6 h of the clinical onset of infarction.

In view of the association between complex ventricular ectopic activity and sudden cardiac death (see "Recognition of High-Risk Patients," above), attention has been directed to the possibility of preventing SCD through the reduction of VPDs. Although there is evidence that rigorous efforts to suppress complex VPDs may prevent ventricular fibrillation, this issue remains unsettled. The paradox of an acute lethal event occurring in the setting of long-standing ventricular dysfunction and chronic ventricular ectopy has stimulated a search for precipitating factors. Current knowledge suggests that the events leading to ventricular fibrillation may be electrical or mechanical, both of which are likely mediated at the cellular level and modulated by neural traffic. Recent studies have attempted to address the problem of detecting myocardial electrical instability by utilizing programmed ventricular stimulation techniques.[44,45] This approach, first proposed by Lown and coworkers,[46] is noteworthy in that it defines a state of electrical instability which may be related to the susceptibility to development of ventricular fibrillation. Such techniques also have potential therapeutic implications since the provoked responses may be modified by pharmacologic interventions.[45]

Clinical Trials to Prevent SCD

Clinical trials aimed at reduction of mortality from SCD have typically been carried out in ambulatory patients who had recently sustained an acute myocardial infarction.[47–50] Such studies have an important bearing on the problem of SCD. However, characteristics of patients in the early postinfarction period may not be representative of other patients with coronary atherosclerotic heart disease who are at risk for SCD. In patients resuscitated from out-of-hospital ventricular fibrillation, only 15 percent had sustained a recognized acute myocardial infarction in the year preceding the episode of ventricular fibrillation (Fig. 32-6). Although it is clear that postmyocardial infarction patients are at relatively high risk for SCD in the weeks to months following infarction, one should be somewhat circumspect in extrapolation of intervention data in this group to the broader clinical spectrum of patients with coronary atherosclerotic heart disease.

Beta-Adrenergic Blocking Agents Important studies carried out in Western Europe in the 1970s indicated that two beta-blocking drugs were probably efficacious in preventing SCD during the 2 years following myocardial infarction. Wilhelmsson et al.[48] treated 106 patients with the nonselective beta-blocking drug alprenolol and a comparable number with placebo in a prospective, randomized, postinfarction trial. When stratified for relative risk, the alprenolol-treated group had significantly fewer sudden deaths in the 2 years following infarction than the control group. Ahlmark and colleagues carried out a comparable study with alprenolol, with a similar outcome.[49] Practolol, a cardioselective beta-blocking drug, was evaluated in a large double-blind trial of over 3000 patients recently recovered from acute myocardial infarction. Although that study was prematurely terminated because of adverse side effects attributed to practolol, SCD was significantly lower in the group treated with practolol than in the placebo group.[47] Because of a relatively large number of dropouts in this study, there is some concern regarding the interpretation of these results. Nevertheless, these observations are in accord with the Swedish alprenolol studies. Interestingly, protection in the practolol study was limited to patients who

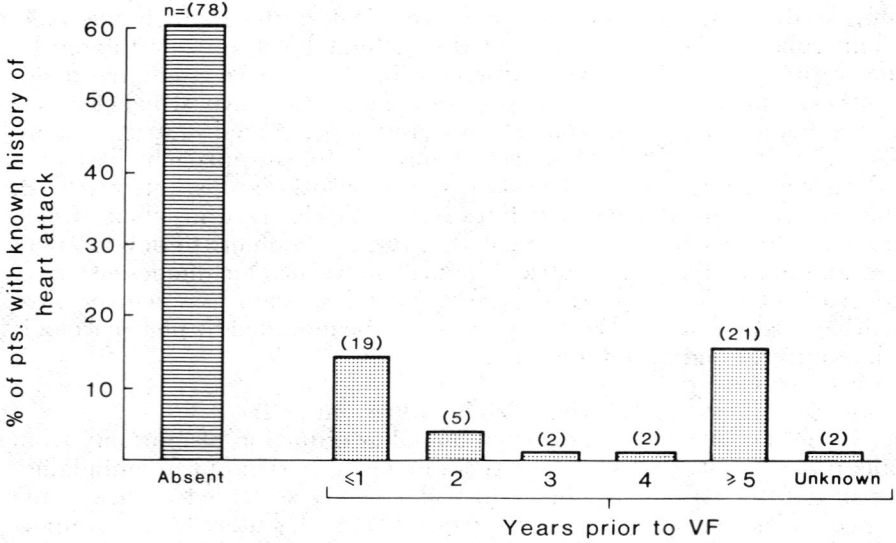

FIGURE 32-6 Proportion of 129 patients with coronary atherosclerotic heart disease who had a history consistent with remote myocardial infarction prior to out-of-hospital ventricular fibrillation (VF). Only 15 percent had a recognized heart attack in the 12 months prior to cardiac arrest. Such a history was entirely absent in more than 60 percent.

had previously sustained an anterior myocardial infarction. In spite of some uncertainties, the foregoing studies provide hope that one or more beta-blocking agents may diminish the incidence of cardiac mortality in the 1 or 2 years following acute myocardial infarction.

Antiarrhythmic Therapy It is of interest that ventricular ectopic activity was not used as a specific endpoint in the trials of beta-blocking drugs cited above. This contrasts to the approaches of others who have vigorously investigated and treated patients with advanced grades of ventricular ectopy, including previous VF patients who were considered to be at increased risk for SCD. In Lown's work,[4] the virtual abolition of high grades of ventricular arrhythmias was attempted through the use of acute drug testing and multidrug regimens—and was accomplished in 46 of 62 patients who had malignant ventricular arrhythmias. In these "controlled" patients the annual incidence of SCD was 3.9 percent. In contrast, 38 percent of the 16 patients who could not be controlled died suddenly. Although these results appear promising, they should be interpreted cautiously in view of the lack of a concomitant control population and the heterogeneous nature of the patient population studied. Other investigators have focused interest on suppression of recurrent, symptomatic ventricular tachycardia.[51,52] However it remains to be shown that observations in these patients can be extended to the very large numbers of patients at risk for SCD.

Myerburg and colleagues[53] have also advocated the use of antiarrhythmic agents in patients at high risk for SCD. These authors studied the long-term use of quinidine or procainamide in patients who had survived at least one episode of prehospital cardiac arrest. Of 16 patients treated intensively with doses adjusted by drug plasma levels, as well as by

the results of ambulatory ECG monitoring, 8 patients survived beyond 12 months, and 8 had a recurrence of the SCD syndrome. While the mean number of ventricular ectopic beats was not significantly different, all 8 who survived had stable drug plasma levels, which were in the so-called therapeutic range. In contrast, those who developed (recurrent) SCD had unstable plasma levels, often out of the therapeutic range. These observations suggested that attainment of adequate plasma levels of antiarrhythmic drugs, rather than suppression of VPDs per se, may be of primary importance in preventing the emergence of ventricular fibrillation.

Hence, the use of antiarrhythmic agents to reduce the incidence of SCD is hampered not only by unacceptable (and at times dangerous) side effects, but perhaps more importantly by the uncertainty of the appropriate therapeutic guidelines.

Other Drug Therapy An example of the use of alternate drugs to modify the likelihood of SCD following myocardial infarction is the large, randomized, double-blind trial comparing the effects of the antiplatelet drug, sulfinpyrazone, with a placebo.[50] In that multicenter trial involving over 1500 patients, there was an apparent reduction in SCD in the sulfinpyrazone-treated patients compared with the placebo group. This effect was evident at 7 months and persisted up to 24 months. While that report initially appeared encouraging, particularly because of the virtual absence of side effects, clarification of the mechanism through which such an effect might occur and the substantiation of these initial findings must be awaited. Similar studies comparing aspirin with placebo have also shown small but consistent trends favoring patients treated with that antiplatelet agent.[54]

Although a reduction in SCD by improvement of ventricular function has not been clearly shown, there is some evidence that VPD frequency may be reduced through measures which improve ventricular function with vasodilator drugs.[55,56]

Heart Surgery Since the overwhelming majority of patients experiencing SCD have atherosclerotic coronary artery obstruction, it might follow that improvement in coronary blood flow would enhance the survival of patients with atherosclerotic coronary heart disease, particularly by preventing or forestalling sudden death. Since coronary bypass surgery is performed on about 100,000 patients each year in the United States, it is proper to ask if this operation will prevent sudden cardiac death. Unfortunately, the answer is not yet available. Randomized, prospective trials of coronary artery bypass grafting have been carried out in patients with stable angina pectoris.[57–59] In spite of appreciable symptomatic relief from angina, the effects on overall long-term mortality have not consistently favored the surgically treated groups except for patients with left main coronary artery obstruction. In the European Coronary Surgery Study Group trial,[58] a subgroup of the surgically treated patients with triple-vessel disease showed improved survival, with reduction in total deaths and sudden cardiac deaths. However, this was not the case in the other prospective trials cited. Although uncertainties remain, evidence to date suggests that sudden death may be forestalled or prevented in subgroups of symptomatic patients with significant left main and triple-vessel coronary artery obstruction.[60,61] Available evidence suggests that ventricular ectopy is not affected by coronary artery bypass grafting.[62]

Coronary bypass surgery is rarely employed in patients without a history of, or symptoms of, coronary artery disease. Therefore asymptomatic patients who have sudden cardiac death have not had coronary bypass surgery, so its status is unknown in preventing sudden cardiac deaths in this large group of patients. Although there are encouraging preliminary reports concerning the efficacy of myocardial surgery for patients with recurrent, drug-resistant ventricular arrhythmias,[27,28] the numbers of patients who have undergone these operations are relatively small. It seems clear that if such surgical interventions are considered, electrophysiologic identification of abnormal foci should be done before and during surgery. The concept of "blind" aneurysm resection has been unrewarding, is probably an oversimplification, and may actually worsen the condition of some patients.

SCD in Patients with Cardiac Disease Other than Coronary Atherosclerotic Heart Disease

Although the vast majority (80 percent) of SCD victims have underlying coronary atherosclerotic heart disease, this should not minimize the importance of SCD in the remaining 20 percent who have other cardiac diagnoses. Uncommon causes of SCD, such as congenital anomalies of the coronary arteries and the Marfan syndrome, are discussed in Chaps. 36 and 47. For the purposes of this section, three major classifications are considered: (1) cardiomyopathic syndromes, (2) valvular lesions, and (3) primary electrical disturbances.

Cardiomyopathic Syndromes (See also Chap. 56)

Virtually any cardiomyopathy may on occasion result in SCD. However, SCD plays a particularly prominent role in the natural history of hypertrophic cardiomyopathy, including so-called idiopathic hypertrophic subaortic stenosis. Indeed SCD, probably due to ventricular fibrillation, is the most common mode of death in patients with that diagnosis. Most sudden deaths in hypertrophic cardiomyopathies occur during the early years (ages 10 to 35) and usually with minimal or no symptoms prior to the episode. Certain common characteristics of fatal cases have been noted: (1) family history of SCD, (2) markedly increased septal or left ventricular mass, (3) distinctly abnormal ECGs, and (4) advanced grades of VPDs. SCD occurs in patients with and without outflow pressure gradients.[63,64] It is not clear if treatment, particularly with beta blockade, has an effect on either the arrhythmias or SCD seen in these disorders.[65]

Valvular Lesions

Aortic valvular stenosis and mitral valve prolapse syndromes have been indicted specifically as causes of SCD.

Aortic Stenosis (See also Chaps. 36 and 38)
Approximately 30 percent of deaths from aortic valve stenosis occur suddenly. It is uncertain whether aortic valve replacement prevents SCD in patients with severe aortic stenosis. Intuitively, the answer is affirmative, but the precise documentation is not available. Fortunately, it is only a minority of patients with advanced aortic valve stenosis who develop SCD in the absence of symptoms. Hence, there is only an infrequent need to consider surgery solely for the purpose of preventing SCD.

Mitral Valve Prolapse (See Chap. 39)
Mitral valve prolapse is seemingly responsible for, or associated with, a host of maladies, including psychological disturbances, thromboembolic phenomena, and SCD. While the clinical implications of the auscultatory and echocardiographic findings of mitral valve prolapse are commonly overestimated, life-threatening arrhythmias do on occasion occur.[66] Sudden death solely due to mitral valve prolapse is uncommon; however the true incidence is not known. In patients referred to centers because of malignant ventricular tachycardia or ventricular fi-

brillation, mitral valve prolapse is occasionally found as the only recognized basis for these arrhythmias.[67] The mechanism for ventricular arrhythmias in such patients is not known, but speculation has centered on papillary muscle ischemia due to abnormal mechanical tension of chordae tendineae as well as on the coexistence of nonischemic wall motion abnormalities. Werner recently reported that echocardiograms performed in 124 consecutive survivors of the SCD syndrome indicated mitral valve prolapse as the major echocardiographic abnormality in four patients. However, two of the four patients had associated coronary artery disease, and another had important mitral regurgitation.[68]

Primary Electrical Disturbances (See Chaps. 28 and 29)

Of the primary electrical syndromes responsible for SCD, sinoatrial disorders, ventricular preexcitation, and prolonged QT syndromes are most commonly described. While such syndromes are frequently associated with other cardiac or metabolic abnormalities, the congenitally prolonged QT syndromes are worthy of note. Schwartz and colleagues reported a series of 203 patients with prolonged QT syndromes. There was an exceedingly high mortality (73 percent) in patients who received no treatment. This contrasted to a 6 percent mortality in patients treated with beta-blocking drugs or with ablation of the left stellate ganglion.[69]

Summary

Most deaths from coronary atherosclerotic heart disease are sudden, unexpected events which occur outside the hosital. In 80 percent of instances, there have been prior manifestations of heart disease, arterial hypertension, or both. In patients at risk for SCD, cessation of cigarette smoking and treatment of high blood pressure are prudent, albeit unproven, measures. In patients with some recognized cardiovascular diseases, complex VPDs have a statistical relationship to SCD. However, it is not clear that these markers are independent of the severity of myocardial dysfunction, which is also a predictor of SCD.

Following acute myocardial infarction, beta-blocking drugs, specifically practolol, alprenolol, and timolol,[70] have been shown to decrease SCD in the initial 2 years. The use of other antiarrhythmic drugs to prevent SCD is under intense study. This latter approach has its advocates, but at this time is unsettled. The essential purpose of drug therapy for control of SCD is to prevent the emergence of ventricular fibrillation with or without alteration of VPD frequency, i.e., antifibrillatory therapy.

The application of emergency medical services represents the major advance to date in preventing sudden cardiac death. Further steps to facilitate prompt initiation of cardiopulmonary resuscitation and rapid defibrillation will likely continue the trend of steadily improved rates of resuscitation and survival.

While coronary atherosclerosis is the underlying abnormality in most victims of SCD, coronary artery bypass grafting has not been shown convincingly to afford protection from either ventricular arrhythmias or SCD (see earlier discussion).

It should be clear that further interventions to alter the unacceptable burden from SCD must demonstrate first that there has been a decreased mortality in a specified group of patients whose risk is measurable, and second that there are neither excessive side effects nor unwarranted risks. Armed with the knowledge of the problem and a determination to reject the inevitability of SCD, these objectives seem attainable.

References

1. Gordon, T., and Kannel, W. B.: Premature Mortality from Coronary Heart Disease, *J. Am. Med. Assoc.*, 215:1617, 1971.
*2. Kuller, L. H.: Sudden Death—Definition and Epidemiologic Considerations, *Prog. Cardiovasc. Dis.*, 23:1, 1980. (41 references)
3. Spain, D. M., Bradess, V. A., and Mohr, C.: Coronary Atherosclerosis as a Cause of Unexpected and Unexplained Death, *J. Am. Med. Assoc.*, 174:384, 1960.
*4. Lown, B.: Sudden Cardiac Death: The Major Challenge Confronting Contemporary Cardiology, *Am. J. Cardiol.*, 43:313, 1979. (106 references)
*5. Moss, A. J.: Clinical Significance of Ventricular Arrhythmias in Patients with and without Coronary Artery Disease, *Prog. Cardiovasc. Dis.*, 23:33, 1980. (140 references)
6. Cobb, L. A., Werner, J. A., and Trobaugh, G. B.: Sudden Cardiac Death. II. Outcome of Resuscitation; Management, and Future Directions, *Mod. Concepts Cardiovasc. Dis.*, 49:37, 1980.
7. Gillum, R. F., Reinleid, M., Margolis, J. R., Fabsitz, R. R., and Brasch, R. C.: Delay in the Prehospital Phase of Acute Myocardial Infarction, *Arch. Intern. Med.*, 136:649, 1976.
8. Baum, R. S., Alvarez, H., and Cobb, L. A.: Survival after Resuscitation from Out-of-Hospital Ventricular Fibrillation, *Circulation*, 50:1231, 1974.
9. Schaffer, W. A., and Cobb, L. A.: Recurrent Ventricular Fibrillation and Modes of Death in Survivors of Out-of-Hospital Ventricular Fibrillation, *N. Engl. J. Med.*, 293:260, 1975.
10. Wikland, B.: Medically Unattended Fatal Cases of Ischemic Heart Disease in a Defined Population, *Acta Med. Scand.*, suppl. 524, 1971.
11. Burchell, H. B.: Patients with Coronary Artery Disease Should Avoid Strenuous Physical Exertion, in E. Rapaport (ed.), "Current Controversies in Cardiovascular Disease," W. B. Saunders Company, Philadelphia, 1980, p. 129.

*This article is a review of the literature and contains additional references to the literature.

12. Mead, W. F., Pyfer, H. R., Trombold, J. C., and Frederick, R. C.: Successful Resuscitation of Two Near Simultaneous Cases of Cardiac Arrest with a Review of Fifteen Cases Occurring during Supervised Exercise, *Circulation,* 53:187, 1976.

13. Lown, B., and Wolf, M.: Approaches to Sudden Death from Coronary Heart Disease, *Circulation,* 44:130, 1971.

14. Eisenberg, M. S., Copass, M. K., Hallstrom, A. P., Blake, B., Bergner, L., Short, F. A., and Cobb, L. A.: Treatment of Out-of-Hospital Cardiac Arrests with Rapid Defibrillation by Emergency Medical Technicians, *N. Engl. J. Med.,* 302:1379, 1980.

15. Iseri, L. T., Humphrey, S. B., and Sinner, E. J.: Prehospital Bradyasystolic Cardiac Arrest, *Ann. Intern. Med.,* 88:741, 1978.

16. Goldstein, S.: "Sudden Death and Coronary Heart Disease," Futura Publishing Company, Inc., Mt. Kisco, N.Y., 1974, p. 22.

17. Friedman, G. D., Klatsky, A. L., and Siegelaub, A. B.: Predictors of Sudden Cardiac Death, *Circulation,* 51, 52(suppl. 3):164, 1975.

18. Oberman, A., Ray, M., Turner, M. E., Barnes, G., and Grooms, C.: Sudden Death in Patients Evaluated for Ischemic Heart Disease, *Circulation,* 51, 52(suppl. 3):170, 1975.

19. Bruschke, A. U. G., Prudfit, W. L., and Sones, F. M.: Progress Study of 590 Consecutive Nonsurgical Cases of Coronary Disease Followed 5–9 Years. Angiographic Correlations, *Circulation,* 47:1147, 1973.

20. Davis, H. T., DeCamilla, J., Bayer, L. W., and Moss, A. J.: Survivorship Patterns in the Late Posthospital Phase of Myocardial Infarction, *Circulation,* 60:1259, 1979.

21. Ruberman, W., Weinblatt, E., Goldberg, J. D., Frank, C. W., and Shapiro, S.: Ventricular Premature Beats and Mortality after Myocardial Infarction, *N. Engl. J. Med.,* 297:750, 1977.

22. The Coronary Drug Project Research Group: Prognostic Importance of Premature Beats Following Myocardial Infarction, *J. Am. Med. Assoc.,* 223:1116, 1973.

23. Haynes, R. E., Hallstrom, A. P., and Cobb, L. A.: Repolarization Abnormalities in Survivors of Out-of-Hospital Ventricular Fibrillation, *Circulation,* 57:652, 1978.

24. Weaver, W. D., Lorch, G. S., Alvarez, H. A., and Cobb, L. A.: Angiographic Findings and Prognostic Indicators in Patients Resuscitated from Sudden Cardiac Death, *Circulation,* 54:895, 1976.

25. Reichenbach, D. D., Moss, N. S., Meyer, E.: Pathology of the Heart in Sudden Cardiac Death, *Am. J. Cardiol.,* 39:865, 1977.

26. Liberthson, R. R., Nagel, E. L., Hirschman, J. C., Nussenfeld, J. D., Blackbourne, B. D., and Davis, J. D.: Pathophysiologic Observations in Prehospital Ventricular Fibrillation and Sudden Cardiac Death, *Circulation,* 49:790, 1974.

*27. Gallagher, J. J.: Surgical Treatment of Arrhythmias: Current Status and Future Directions, *Am. J. Cardiol.,* 41:1035, 1978. (98 references)

28. Horowitz, L. N., Harken, A. H., Kastor, J. A., and Josephson, M. E.: Ventricular Resection Guided by Epicardial and Endocardial Mapping for Treatment of Recurrent Ventricular Tachycardia, *N. Engl. J. Med.,* 302:589, 1980.

29. Schultze, R. A., Strauss, H. W., and Pitt, B.: Sudden Death in the Year Following Myocardial Infarction, *Am. J. Med.,* 62:192, 1977.

*30. Cobb, L. A., Werner, J. A., and Trobaugh, G. B.: Sudden Cardiac Death. I. A Decade's Experience with Out-of-Hospital Resuscitation, *Mod. Concepts Cardiovasc. Dis.,* 19:31, 1980. (67 references)

31. Thompson, R. G., Hallstrom, A. P., and Cobb, L. A.: Bystander-Initiated Cardiopulmonary Resuscitation in the Management of Ventricular Fibrillation, *Ann. Intern. Med.,* 90:737, 1979.

32. Eisenberg, M., Bergner, L., and Hallstrom, A.: Paramedic Programs and Out-of-Hospital Cardiac Arrest. I. Factors Associated with Successful Resuscitation, *Am. J. Public Health,* 69:30, 1979.

33. Lund, I., and Skulberg, A.: Cardiopulmonary Resuscitation by Lay People, *Lancet,* 2:702, 1976.

34. Cobb, L. A., Baum, R. S., Alvarez, H., and Schaffer, W. A.: Resuscitation from Out-of-Hospital Ventricular Fibrillation: 4 Year Follow-Up, *Circulation,* 51, 52(suppl. 3):223, 1975.

35. Liberthson, R. R., Nagel, E. L., Hirschman, J. C., and Nussenfeld, S. R.: Prehospital Ventricular Fibrillation: Prognosis and Follow-Up Course, *N. Engl. J. Med.,* 291:317, 1974.

36. Stannard, M., and Sloman, G.: Ventricular Fibrillation in Acute Myocardial Infarction: Prognosis Following Successful Resuscitation, *Am. Heart J.,* 77:573, 1969.

37. Geddes, J. S., Adgey, A. H. J., and Pantridge, J. F.: Prognosis after Recovery from Ventricular Fibrillation Complicating Ischemic Heart Disease, *Lancet,* 2:273, 1967.

38. Trobaugh, G. B., Ritchie, J. L., Hallstrom, A. P., Hamilton, G. W., Werner, J. A., and Cobb, L. A.: Thallium-201 Myocardial Imaging in Survivors of Out-of-Hospital Ventricular Fibrillation, Part II, *Circulation,* 60:II-231, 1979. (Abstract.)

39. Lown, B., Verrier, R. L., and Rabinowitz, S. H.: Neural and Psychological Mechanisms and the Problems of Sudden Cardiac Death, *Am. J. Cardiol.,* 39:890, 1977.

40. Duke, M.: Thiazide Induced Hypokalemia: Association with Acute Myocardial Infarction and Ventricular Fibrillation, *J. Am. Med. Assoc.,* 239:43, 1978.

41. Freidberg, C. K.: Symposium—Myocardial Infarction 1972, Part 1, *Circulation,* 45:179, 1972.

42. Mirowski, M., Reid, P. R., Mower, M. M., et al.: Termination of Malignant Ventricular Arrhythmias with an Implantable Ventricular Defibrillator in Human Beings, *N. Engl. J. Med.,* 303:322, 1980.

43. Lie, K. I., Wellens, H. J, Van Capelle, F. J., and Durrer, D.: Lidocaine in the Prevention of Primary Ventricular Fibrillation. A Double-Blind Randomized Study of 212 Consecutive Patients, *N. Engl. J. Med.,* 291:1324, 1974.

44. Greene, H. L., Reid, P. R., and Schaeffer, A. H.: The Repetitive Ventricular Response in Man: A Predictor of Sudden Death, *N. Engl. J. Med.,* 399:729, 1978.

45. Mason, J. W., and Winkle, R. A.: Electrode-Catheter Arrhythmia Induction in the Selection and Assessment of Antiarrhythmic Drug Therapy for Recurrent Ventricular Tachycardia, *Circulation,* 58:971, 1978.

46. Lown, B., and Cannon, R.: Electrical Stimulation to Estimate the Degree of Digitalization. II. Experimental Studies, *Am. J. Cardiol.,* 22:251, 1968.

47. Multicentre International Study: Reduction in Mortality after Myocardial Infarction with Long-Term Beta-Adrenoceptor Blockade—Supplemental Report, *Br. Med. J.*, 2:419, 1977.

48. Wilhelmsson, C., Vedlin, J. A., Wilhelmsen, L., Tibblin, G., and Worko, L.: Reduction of Sudden Death after Myocardial Infarction by Treatment with Alprenolol, *Lancet*, 2:1157, 1974.

49. Ahlmark, G., and Saertre, H.: Long-Term Treatment with Beta Blockers after Myocardial Infarction, *Eur. J. Clin. Pharmacol.*, 10:77, 1976.

50. The Anturane Reinfarction Trial Research Group: Sulfinpyrazone in the Prevention of Sudden Death after Myocardial Infarction, *N. Engl. J. Med.*, 302:250, 1980.

51. Horowitz, L. N., Josephson, N. E., Farshidi, A., Spielman, S. R., Michelson, E. L., and Greenspan, A. M.: Recurrent Sustained Ventricular Tachycardia. 3. Role of Electrophysiologic Study in Selection of Antiarrhythmic Regimens, *Circulation*, 58:986, 1978.

52. Schaeffer, A. H., Greene, H. L., and Reid, P. R.: Suppression of the Repetitive Ventricular Response: An Index of Long-Term Antiarrhythmic Effectiveness of Aprindine for Ventricular Tachycardia in Man, *Am. J. Cardiol.*, 42:1007, 1978.

53. Myerburg, R. J., Conte, C., Sheps, D. S., Apel, R. A., Kiem, I., Sung, R. J., and Castellanos, A.: Antiarrhythmic Drug Therapy in Survivors of Prehospital Cardiac Arrest: Comparison of Effects of Chronic Ventricular Arrhythmias and Recurrent Cardiac Arrest, *Circulation*, 59:866, 1979.

54. Aspirin after Myocardial Infarction, *Lancet*, 1:1172, 1978 (editorial).

55. Salerno, D., Werner, J. A., Trobaugh, G. B., Hallstrom, A. P., and Cobb, L. A.: Reduced Ventricular Ectopy by Hydralazine in Survivors of Ventricular Fibrillation, *Clin. Res.*, 28:539, 1980. (Abstract.)

56. Kumpuris, A. G., Miller, R. R., Quinones, A. G., Hoffman, D. A., and Pratt, C. M.: Salutory Effect of Cardiac Unloading on Ventricular Ectopy, *Am. J. Cardiol.*, 43:360, 1979. (Abstract.)

57. Murphy, M. L., Hultgren, H. N., Detre, K., Thomsen, J., and Takaro, T.: Treatment of Chronic Stable Angina—A Preliminary Report of Survival Data of the Randomized Veterans Administration Cooperative Study, *N. Engl. J. Med.*, 297:621, 1977.

58. European Coronary Surgery Study Group: Prospective Randomised Study of Coronary Artery Bypass Surgery in Stable Angina Pectoris, *Lancet*, 2:491, 1980.

59. Kloster, F. E., Kremkau, E. L., Ritzman, L. W., Rahimtoola, S. H., Rosch, J., and Kanarek, P. H.: Coronary Bypass for Stable Angina: A Prospective Randomized Study. *N. Engl. J. Med.*, 300:149, 1979.

60. Takaro, T., Hultgren, H. N., Upton, M. J., and Detre, K. M.: VA Cooperative Randomized Study of Surgery for Coronary Arterial Occlusive Disease. II. Subgroup with Significant Left Main Lesion, *Circulation*, 54(suppl. 3):107, 1976.

61. Vismara, L. A., Miller, R. R., Price, J. E., Karem, R., De Maria, A. N., and Mason, D. T.: Improved Longevity Due to Reduction of Sudden Death by Aortocoronary Bypass in Coronary Atherosclerosis, *Am. J. Cardiol.*, 39:919, 1977.

62. Tilkian, A. G., Pfeifer, J. F., Barry, W. J., Lipton, M. J., and Hultgren, H. N.: The Effect of Coronary Bypass Surgery on Exercise-Induced Ventricular Arrhythmias, *Am. Heart J.*, 92:707, 1976.

63. Maron, B. J., Roberts, W. C., Edwards, J. E., McAllister, H. A., Foley, D. D., and Epstein, S. E.: Sudden Death in Patients with Hypertrophic Cardiomyopathy: Characterization of 26 Patients without Functional Limitation, *Am. J. Cardiol.*, 41:803, 1978.

64. Maron, B. J., Roberts, W. C., McAllister, H. A., Rosing, D. R., and Epstein, S. E.: Sudden Death in Young Athletes, *Circulation*, 62:218, 1980.

65. McKeena, W. J., Chetty, S., Oakley, C. M., and Goodwin, J. F.: Arrhythmia in Hypertrophic Cardiomyopathy: Exercise and 48 Hour Ambulatory Electrocardiographic Assessment with and without Beta Adrenergic Blocking Therapy, *Am. J. Cardiol.*, 45:1, 1980.

*66. Swartz, M. H., Teichholz, L. E., and Donoso, E.: Mitral Valve Prolapse—A Review of Associated Arrhythmias, *Am. J. Med.*, 62:377, 1977. (69 references)

67. Wei, J., Bulkley, B. H., Schaeffer, A. H., Greene, H. L., and Reid, P. R.: Mitral Valve Prolapse Syndrome and Recurrent Ventricular Tachyarrhythmias: A Malignant Variant Refractory to Conventional Drug Therapy, *Ann. Intern. Med.*, 89:6, 1978.

68. Werner, J. A., Salerno, D. M., Cobb, L. A., Trobaugh, G. B., Janko, C. L., and Hedgecock, M.: Echocardiographic Detection of Patients at High Risk for Recurrent Ventricular Fibrillation, *Am. J. Cardiol.*, 45:444, 1980. (Abstract.)

69. Schwartz, P. J., Periti, M., and Malliani, A.: The Long Q-T Syndrome, *Am. Heart J.*, 89:378, 1975.

70. The Norwegian Multicenter Study Group: Timolol-Induced Reduction in Mortality and Reinfarction in Patients Surviving Acute Myocardial Infarction, *N. Engl. J. Med.*, 304:801, 1981.

33

Cardiopulmonary Resuscitation and the Subsequent Management of the Patient

Myron L. Weisfeldt, M.D.
Nisha Chandra, M.D.

Then he went up and lay upon the child, putting his mouth upon his mouth, his eyes upon his eyes, and his hands upon his hands and he stretched himself upon him; the flesh of the child became warm.

2 Kings 4:34[1]

Since biblical times, humans have attempted to restore life to the dead or nearly dead individual. In the eighteenth century, it was a common practice in Europe to throw unconscious persons over the back of trotting horses or roll them over barrels in an attempt to move air in and out of their chests. Bellows were also used to inflate the lungs. One technique that gained broad use in this century was the Schafer prone pressure method of artificial respiration, in which the lower back was pressed cyclically, thus forcing air from the lungs.[2]

Although at the time all these methods were viewed as providing a means for lung ventilation, recent research suggests that circulation of blood might also have occurred. For example, pressure on the chest with the airway at least partially obstructed in the prone position would be an ideal way to increase intrathoracic pressure and thereby circulate blood (see below).

In 1954 Elam and his colleagues[3] showed that mouth-to-mouth or mouth-to-nose resuscitation was superior to the Schafer method in terms of efficacy of ventilation. The importance of circulation of blood was recognized and direct or internal cardiac massage became an accepted technique in 1916. Despite proven efficacy,[4] internal massage is fraught with complications and should only be employed by trained personnel. It was not until 1960 that Kouwenhoven, Jude, and Knickerbocker developed the present technique of external compression in the supine position and coupled this with artificial respiration.[5]

These investigators proposed that by using external sternal compression, the heart was squeezed or massaged between the sternum and vertebral column, thus expelling blood from the ventricles into the great vessels. This forward flow of blood was further facilitated by physiological functioning of the heart valves. This technique was shown to be effective,[6] although it now appears that the mechanism of blood flow during external sternal compression is usually related to the generalized rise in intrathoracic pressure, rather than cardiac compression.

In 1974 and 1980 (revised) the American Heart Association published "Standards for Cardiopulmonary Resuscitation and Emergency Cardiac Care."[7] They advised (1) 60 sternal compressions per minute, (2) 50 percent of each compression-relaxation cycle to be compression, and (3) 1 ventilation for every 5 compressions.

Diagnosis and Identification of Cardiac Arrest

Cardiac arrest is defined as the sudden cessation of effective cardiac pumping function as a result of either ventricular asystole (electrical or mechanical) or ventricular fibrillation. Rapid diagnosis is essential because (1) more than a few minutes of total cardiac arrest results in permanent cerebral anoxic damage and (2) the success of resuscitative measures is related to the rapidity with which they are instituted following arrest.[8]

Cardiac arrest should be considered in the differential diagnosis of sudden collapse in any patient. It can be clinically confirmed by pulseless major vessels and absent heart sounds. Although respirations may continue for a minute or two, the patient with cardiac arrest becomes rapidly cyanotic and unconscious.

If available, an electrocardiogram can confirm the diagnosis and identify asystole, ventricular fibrillation, or electromechanical dissociation as the mechanism of arrest. Cardiopulmonary resuscitation (CPR), however, should be initiated immediately once the clinical diagnosis is made without delaying to obtain this information. If a defibrillator but not an electrocardiogram is immediately available, a 200-joule (J) countershock should be administered without delay.

Respiratory Arrest

Respiratory arrest is the cessation of effective respiratory effort. It can result from airway obstruction (due to a foreign body or other causes), drug overdose, head trauma, cerebrovascular accident, or suffocation. When respiratory arrest occurs suddenly (as with foreign-body obstruction), the patient rapidly becomes cyanotic though a palpable pulse with blood pressure, consciousness, and ineffective respiratory efforts may be maintained for several minutes. Opening the airway and/or rescue breathing may be all that is necessary to resuscitate such a patient.

Three manual maneuvers are recommended for relieving foreign-body airway obstruction:

1. *Manual removal.* Open the victim's mouth and manually attempt to dislodge any obvious foreign body with a finger.
2. *Back blows.* Deliver four sharp blows with the heel of the hand high on the spine between the shoulder blades.
3. *Heimlich maneuver.* Deliver a series of sharp thrusts to the upper abdomen with a closed fist while standing behind the victim.[9] Abdominal thrusts can also be used directly in the unconscious supine patient to help mechanically dislodge a foreign body. If incorrectly administered, this maneuver can lead to visceral damage.[10]

Ventilation during Cardiopulmonary Resuscitation

Clearing the airway is of the utmost importance. Foreign bodies, loose dentures or any other oral obstruction should be removed. Next, the head tilt–chin lift technique, which results in moving the tongue anteriorly, is used to open the airway. The chin is lifted forward with the fingers of one hand supporting the jaw and the head tilted back by the other hand on the forehead of the patient.[11,12] The head tilt–neck lift method of opening the airway is also commonly employed and is an acceptable technique. Here the head is tilted back with one hand on the forehead; the other hand is placed behind the neck, lifting it upward to open the airway. If no spontaneous respirations are present, mouth-to-mouth ventilation is immediately initiated,[13] with adequacy being judged by the rise and fall of the patient's chest with each breath.

Equipped rescuers will use a bag-mask technique of ventilation together with a small plastic oral "airway" which moves the tongue anteriorly. Adequate ventilation is difficult with this method, and gastric distension and aspiration are common. An esophageal obturator with balloon obstruction of the esophagus and ventilation through proximal ports in the mouth avoids aspiration and appears to provide some but not optimal ventilation.[14] Skill is needed in placing and using this device properly. After successful resuscitation, balloon deflation frequently results in regurgitation of gastric contents.

In skilled hands endotracheal intubation is the ideal procedure, but much valuable time can be wasted by repeated unskilled attempts at intubation. If this technique is used, cardiopulmonary resuscitation should be discontinued for no more than 20 s while the tube is being passed into the airway. If more than 20 s elapse without successful intubation, the laryngoscope should be withdrawn and cardiopulmonary resuscitation reinstituted. Whenever possible a nasogastric tube should be inserted to drain the stomach and thus decrease the chances of aspiration.

Definitive Therapy

During cardiac arrest the electrocardiogram will usually show rapid ventricular tachycardia or fibrillation, asystole, or heart block, or it may be near normal.

Ventricular Tachycardia or Fibrillation

With ventricular fibrillation an attempt at electrical defibrillation should be made as quickly as possible. Direct-current defibrillation is employed with one electrode paddle placed at the right upper sternal edge and the other placed left of the cardiac apex. The paddles, coated with low-resistance gel, should be applied firmly to the chest and then discharged with 200 J and then 300 J if the first shock is unsuccessful. Prospective studies by Adgey, Pantridge, and Gascho[15–17] have shown 85 to 90 percent successful defibrillation using only 200 J in patients weighing up to 90 kg. Some advocate higher-energy defibrillation,[18] but few currently use more than 400 J.

When the electrocardiogram shows "fine" fibrillation waves, such defibrillation efforts are often unsuccessful. The administration of epinephrine (5 to 10 ml of 1:10,000) intravenously (IV) results in a more vigorous and coarse fibrillation which is more responsive to defibrillation. If defibrillation fails, it is likely that marked acidosis or hypoxemia is present. Emphasis should be on optimal ventilation with supplemental oxygen to correct both hypoxemia and acidosis.[19] Sodium bicarbonate should then be administered (1 meq/kg) to aid in the management of acidosis, and defibrillation should be repeated with 400 J.

For recurrent ventricular fibrillation, the administration of 75 to 100 mg of lidocaine IV followed by repeat defibrillation may increase the likelihood of returning to a stable rhythm. Bretylium tosylate, a quaternary ammonium compound, is the only available drug that may terminate ventricular fibrillation without electric shock. It should be employed when ventricular tachycardia or fibrillation has been unresponsive to lidocaine, procainamide, and repeated electrical shock. Initially, 5 mg/kg of bretylium is given IV followed by electrical defibrillation. The dose can be increased to 10 mg/kg and repeated at 15- to 30-min intervals until a maximum dose of 30 mg/kg has been given. For recurrent ventricular fibrillation, propranolol is another effective drug. It seems particularly helpful in the setting of primary ventricular fibrillation complicating acute myocardial infarction. The use of a permanent internal defibrillator is now being investigated for patients who had recurrent ventricular fibrillation.[19a]

Hyperkalemia is a readily treated condition that

can cause AV block and impaired intraatrial and intraventricular conduction and leads to ventricular fibrillation or, less commonly, asystole. It can be recognized by the development of tall, peaked T waves with a normal QT interval and sine wave–like ventricular tachycardia. Life-threatening hyperkalemia responds most readily to calcium infusion; 10 to 30 ml of 10% calcium gluconate is infused intravenously over 1 to 5 min under constant electrocardiographic monitoring. Calcium counteracts the adverse effects of potassium on the neuromuscular membranes, but does not alter plasma potassium. Its effect, though immediate, is transient. Hyperkalemia should subsequently be treated by either glucose-insulin infusion, sodium bicarbonate, or ion-exchange resins as outlined in Chap. 75.

With ventricular tachycardia, cough[20] and/or chest blows may revert the arrhythmia without defibrillation, and repeated cough will maintain the conscious state as a result of the rise in intrathoracic pressure.[21]

Asystole or Heart Block

Asystole due to vagal stimulation is the commonest cause of cardiac arrest associated with anesthesia induction and surgical procedures. Asystole also occurs as a result of heart block or sinus node disease (see Chaps. 27 and 28). Atropine (0.5 mg) given IV and repeated in 5 min can be used acutely to prevent or reverse severe bradycardia in many of these settings.

If asystole is diagnosed, vigorous blows to the precordium may sometimes be sufficient to restart the heart. Rhythmic chest blows may be continued if needed while palpating the femoral or carotid pulse until other treatment is available. If the chest blow fails, cardiopulmonary resuscitation should be initiated and intravenous epinephrine (5 to 10 ml of 1:10,000)—and if that fails, intracardiac epinephrine—should be administered. Efforts should be made to correct acidosis and hypoxemia by ventilation and sodium bicarbonate administration. Resuscitation measures may result in a slow ventricular rhythm returning, which can subsequently be supported with atropine (1 to 2 mg IV) or isoproterenol until a temporary pacemaker is placed. Attempts at external pacing are rarely helpful.

Electromechanical Dissociation

In electromechanical dissociation there is evidence of organized electrical activity on the electrocardiogram at a reasonable rate but failure of effective perfusion (no pulse or blood pressure). The most treatable causes of this condition are (1) hypovolemia due to severe hemorrhage, (2) pericardial tamponade, and (3) tension pneumothorax. Signs of these problems should be sought and definitive therapy undertaken with fluids and/or blood replacement, pericardiocentesis, or placement of a pleural needle or tube. These conditions should also be strongly considered if cardiopulmonary resuscitation results in no palpable pulse or evidence of perfusion. Unfortunately, many patients with electromechanical dissociation have primary myocardial failure. Epinephrine and calcium (5 to 7 mg/kg calcium chloride repeated every 10 min if necessary), after optimizing ventilation, may be helpful but are often not effective. In acute myocardial infarction sudden electromechanical dissociation is a sign of myocardial rupture. Only rarely do pericardiocentesis and surgical repair result in survival.

Establishment of an Intravenous Route

While external chest compression and artificial ventilation are continued, a plastic catheter should be inserted into a large peripheral vein. If a peripheral vein cannot be cannulated, a cutdown should be attempted or a central venous line placed by a percutaneous route. If cardiopulmonary resuscitation is properly performed, drugs administered through a peripheral line will reach the arterial circulation within 15 to 30 s.[19] Intracardiac injections are not necessary except when there is failure to obtain a peripheral line or in asystole after failure of peripherally administered epinephrine. If an intravenous route is not available, epinephrine (doses, 1 to 2 mg in 10 ml of sterile distilled water) and lidocaine (dose, 50 to 100 mg in 10 ml of sterile distilled water) can be administered via the endotracheal tube into the bronchial tree.

Termination of Cardiopulmonary Resuscitation

Despite resuscitative efforts, the patient in cardiac arrest may not regain spontaneous circulation. The decision to end cardiopulmonary resuscitation should be based on a physician's assessment of the cerebral, cardiovascular, and general status of the patient. Failure is likely if there is absence of organized ventricular electrocardiographic activity and/or perfusion after 10 to 15 min of adequate cardiopulmonary resuscitation and appropriate therapy. Persistent deep unconsciousness and absence of respiration, reflex response, or pupillary reaction suggest cerebral death, and resuscitative efforts are usually unproductive. These guidelines, however, should be altered in patients with hypothermia, barbiturate overdose, and perhaps following electrocution, where recovery has been seen even after hours of resuscitation.[22]

Postarrest Care

A patient who has been successfully resuscitated usually requires monitoring in an intensive care setting. That individual is prone to cardiac arrhythmias, hemodynamic and ventilatory instability, and ischemia encephalopathy. Ventilatory support with a respirator may well be necessary initially. Serial arterial blood gas determinations should be made to identify hypoxemia and assess the rapidly changing acid-base status.

The treatment of post-cardiac-arrest encephalopathies involves the prevention of further anoxia and hypotension. For cerebral edema after cardiac arrest methylprednisolone (60 to 100 mg) or dexamethasone sodium phosphate (12 to 20 mg intravenously every 6 h) has been recommended, but there is no conclusive evidence that these agents are beneficial. High-dose barbiturates, in animal studies, have also been shown to reduce postarrest brain injury;[23] the value of this therapy in human beings is uncertain. The prognosis of the patient with anoxic encephalopathy is related to the depth and continued duration of cerebral dysfunction.

Other potential life-threatening problems in the postarrest period include acute renal failure, bowel infarction, infection, and sepsis. Patients regaining consciousness may have a postarrest amnesia or may develop psychotic behavior.

Major Drugs Used during Cardiopulmonary Resuscitation

Drugs which are used for the treatment of various arrhythmias are mentioned above.

Catecholamines are used in cardiac arrest to (1) increase arterial and coronary perfusion during and following cardiopulmonary resuscitation, (2) stimulate spontaneous contraction during asystole, (3) make fine ventricular fibrillation more responsive to defibrillation, and (4) act as an inotropic agent.

Epinephrine is effective in achieving all these goals for catecholamine use. It is the most important drug for routine use during cardiac resuscitation. The recommended dose is 0.5 to 1.0 mg given IV. This dose should be repeated at approximately 5-min intervals.

Norepinephrine is a potent vasoconstrictor and generally produces a rise in blood pressure; it is also an inotropic agent. Its disadvantage is renal and mesenteric vasoconstriction, and it should not be used in the initial phase of resuscitation. This agent is most useful where severe hypotension is present but where the chronotropic effects of epinephrine are not desirable (such as in acute myocardial infarction or severe ischemia).

Similarly, *dopamine* (a chemical precursor of norepinephrine) and *dobutamine* (a synthetic catecholamine) are preferred for use as inotropic agents because of their less chronotropic effect. Both these drugs, however, have little use in the initial phases of resuscitation. Isoproterenol (a synthetic catecholamine) is a pure beta-adrenergic agonist and is useful for treatment of bradycardia due to heart block or asystole until a temporary pacemaker is placed.

Recent studies have shown that much less *sodium bicarbonate* is needed than had previously been thought necessary for adequate acid-base control during cardiac arrest. As with other types of metabolic acidosis, if adequate alveolar ventilation is achieved, metabolic acidosis is partially corrected through CO_2 excretion. Ideally, sodium bicarbonate should be given according to the results of measurement of arterial blood pH, P_{CO_2} determination, and calculation of the base deficit. Routinely, 1 meq/kg of sodium bicarbonate is administered after cardiopulmonary resuscitation is initiated and no more than half this dose repeated every 15 min. Excessive use of sodium bicarbonate can result in metabolic alkalosis, hypernatremia, and hyperosmolality.

Calcium chloride (5 to 7 mg/kg) enhances the contractile state of the heart and is indicated in treating severe hypotension and electromechanical dissociation refractory to catecholamines.

Mechanisms of Movement of Blood during Chest Compression

Since the advent of external chest compression as a means for creating artificial circulation in patients following cardiac arrest,[5] it was considered that the mechanism for movement of blood to the brain was well understood. The arrested heart was thought to function as a rubber ball filled with fluid with one-way valves at its entrance and exit. With the heart anatomically situated between the sternum and the vertebral column, it was suggested that direct cardiac compression resulted from compressing the heart between the sternum and the vertebral column. Such compression, like internal cardiac massage, resulted in movement of blood from the left ventricle into the aorta as the aortic valve opened under pressure from the external chest compression. Retrograde flow was prevented by mitral valve closure. Following the period of compression the left ventricle filled with blood as a result of opening of the mitral valve.

This widely held concept did not appear consistent with a number of observations in animal models[24] and humans,[25] but neither the investigators who made the observations in animal models nor the scientific readership of these papers suggested alternative mechanisms for the movement of blood.

Only recently did it become clear that other mechanisms besides cardiac compression operate during chest compression.[26] Our interest in this area was stimulated by a number of anecdotal observations in humans pointing to important features of maximally effective sternal compression. In general, it appeared that there was a correlation between a rise in intrathoracic pressure during sternal compression and the apparent magnitude of carotid flow and pressure.

Of considerable stimulus also were the observations of Criley and associates[21] dealing with "cough CPR." Criley was able to demonstrate that by continuous and early initiation of coughing, patients in ventricular fibrillation could maintain the conscious state as long as cough was continued. One ingredient of the cough is clearly a rise in intrathoracic pressure. If this is the active factor in moving blood during cough, then clearly a rise in intrathoracic pressure is a potent mechanism for the movement of blood to the brain in humans.

Experimental Observations

In large (20 to 40 kg) dogs[26] following cardiac arrest, chest compression resulted in an essentially equal rise in central venous, right atrial, pulmonary artery, and aortic pressures. Diastolic pressures were also similar, but were slightly higher in the aorta than the right atrium. These pressures in intrathoracic vascular structures were also nearly equal to general intrathoracic pressure as indexed by esophageal pressure.

In any fluid-filled system with an appreciable resistance to flow (such as is present in the peripheral vascular bed), there must be a pressure gradient across the resistance to allow the fluid to flow through it. If a pump is responsible for the generation of this pressure gradient across the resistance, there must be a pressure gradient across the pump itself. The lack of such a pressure gradient across the heart during chest compression eliminated compression of the heart as being the pump. Thus, the mechanism for the generation of the peripheral arteriovenous pressure gradient which *must* be present across the resistance bed, if there is a forward flow of blood, is unclear. But, as shown in Fig. 33-1, forward flow results from the fact that intrathoracic arterial pressure in the aorta is transmitted relatively completely into the extrathoracic arterial bed, whereas the intrathoracic venous pressure is not transmitted into the extrathoracic bed. This differential extrathoracic transmission of intrathoracic vascular pressures results in the generation of an extrathoracic arteriovenous pressure gradient required for forward blood flow.

At least three general mechanisms are now thought to contribute to the generation of the extrathoracic arteriovenous pressure gradient observed during conventional cardiopulmonary resuscitation in the dog. These factors are (1) the operation of various valving mechanisms, (2) the greater peripheral venous capacitance compared with arterial capacitance, and (3) the greater arterial resistance to collapse compared with venous resistance.

Thus, as shown in Fig. 33-1, a rise in intrathoracic pressure in the presence of venous valving mechanisms, unequal arterial and venous capacitance and collapsibility lead to the generation of an extrathoracic arteriovenous pressure gradient. The establishment of this pressure gradient is responsible for the generation of forward flow of blood through the peripheral resistance bed. From the point of view

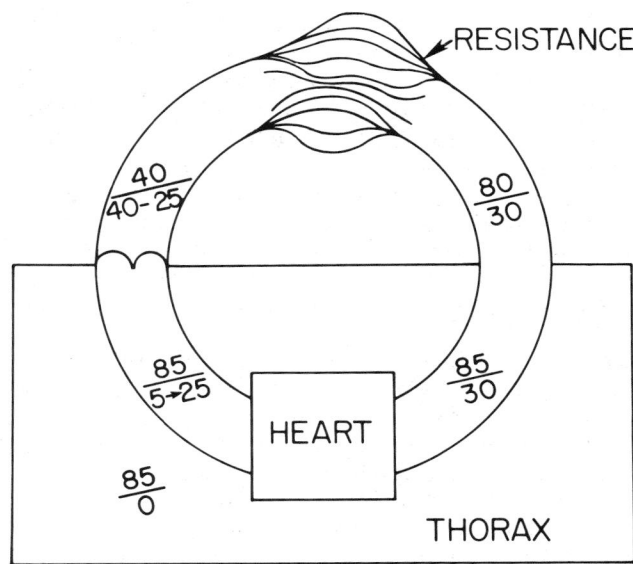

ALL PRESSURES IN mmHg

FIGURE 33-1 Representative pressures recorded during conventional cardiopulmonary resuscitation with forward carotid flow. Pressures are those recorded during compression. Intrathoracic pressures were indexed from esophageal pressures. There is no significant pressure gradient across the heart. The extrathoracic arterial pressure is similar to the intrathoracic aortic pressure. The extrathoracic venous pressure is markedly lower than the intrathoracic venous (right atrial) pressure. There is an extrathoracic arteriovenous pressure gradient which results in forward flow.

of these concepts, it would not be incorrect to say that the lower pressure in the extrathoracic venous bed is the major driving force for the forward flow of blood.

In several of over 200 dogs studied, a marked intrathoracic arteriovenous pressure gradient existed in which aortic pressure was markedly higher than right atrial pressure with chest compression. Thus, compression of the heart by sternal compression of animals with a chest structure such as the dog can result in direct cardiac compression, which can be identified hemodynamically by a net intrathoracic arteriovenous pressure gradient. In the absence of an intrathoracic arteriovenous pressure gradient, *even if the heart is physically compressed,* cardiac compression is not responsible for the peripheral or systemic blood flow since there is peripheral resistance to flow. If cardiac compression and a rise in intrathoracic pressure both occur, the effects will likely be additive.

Observations in Humans

Unfortunately, at this point in humans we can draw no final conclusion as to the frequency or importance of the use of the two mechanisms (chest compression or generalized increase in intrathoracic pressure) with conventional cardiopulmonary resuscitation. Clearly we can conclude that conventional cardiopulmonary resuscitation is remarkably effective in some patients in maintaining cerebral perfusion for long periods of time at a satisfactory level for long-term recovery.

In a number of patients we have easily been able to demonstrate[26] the presence of a pressure gradient at the thoracic inlet upon withdrawing intravascular catheters from the superior vena cava to the extrathoracic internal jugular vein. A pressure gradient at this site is the critical ingredient, as discussed above, for the forward flow of blood through manipulation of intrathoracic pressure. On the other hand, there are some patients (about 30 percent) who have readily measurable high arterial pressures with conventional cardiopulmonary resuscitation. These pressures are higher than those usually generated in humans during conventional cardiopulmonary resuscitation. In a few of these humans with higher blood pressures during conventional cardiopulmonary resuscitation, we have monitored simultaneous central venous pressures which have been lower than radial arterial pressures. Clearly, cardiac compression is occurring in these patients. In some patients, however, the higher arterial pressures may reflect higher generalized intrathoracic pressure during chest compression as a result of functional airway obstruction due to pulmonary congestion and/or bronchospasm. However, in the majority of the patients in whom we have measured radial artery pressures during cardiopulmonary resuscitation, the arterial pressure has been relatively low and similar to those seen in the dog during conventional cardiopulmonary resuscitation.

In human beings it is not essential to think about these mechanisms in an exclusive fashion. We can consider direct cardiac compression as useful when possible. Where this mechanism is not potent enough to maintain cerebral perfusion, it would not be surprising to see that manipulation of intrathoracic pressures would have a favorable additive effect on carotid blood flow.[27]

Potential Means for Improvement of Cardiopulmonary Resuscitation

We have explored two basic strategies for improvement of peripheral perfusion during cardiopulmonary resuscitation by utilizing the general principles of the mechanism of movement of blood through a rise in intrathoracic pressure. The first is to increase intrathoracic pressure per se. The second approach to augmenting blood flow during cardiopulmonary resuscitation relates to abdominal binding. Some years ago, abdominal binding had been shown to be useful in improving the hemodynamics of cardiopulmonary resuscitation.[28] One large study reported significant benefits in survival and hemodynamic improvement without resulting in any significant incidence of untoward complications. In contrast, another study seemed to show a high incidence of liver rupture resulting from abdominal binding.[29]

In the dog, carotid blood flow is increased through abdominal binding.[26] Abdominal binding is likely to be beneficial in improving carotid blood flow for a number of reasons. The first is that, with conventional cardiopulmonary resuscitation, abdominal binding alone increases esophageal pressure and vascular pressures during chest compression. Very likely this reflects a greater rise in intrathoracic pressure. Secondly, abdominal binding results in a diminished blood flow to organs below the diaphragm, thus directing flow to vital vascular beds. Thirdly, abdominal binding results in an increase in circulating blood volume.[26]

To this point we have applied abdominal binding[30] and ventilation at high airway pressures synchronous with chest compression[31] individually to small numbers of patients for only brief periods of time. Although the results are encouraging, factors such as adequacy of ventilation and the benefits of these procedures over a long period of time have yet to be studied. Ultimately the clinical benefits of these procedures in increasing survival and/or decreasing neurological or other complications must be explored. Thus, although the directional changes and the quantitative magnitude of the changes in humans are encouraging, at this point they should only provide the stimulus for performing further research.

References

1. The Holy Bible, King James Version, 2 Kings 4:34.
*2. Comroe, J. H.: Retrospectroscope, *Am. Rev. Respir. Dis.*, 119:803, 1972 (22 references).
3. Elam, J. O., Brown, E. S., and Elder, J. D.: Artificial Respiration by Mouth-to-Mask Method, *N. Engl. J. Med.*, 250:749, 1954.
*4. Turell, D. J., and Husni, E. A.: Cardiac Resuscitation after Documented Myocardial Infarction, *Am. J. Card.*, 7:736, 1961 (33 references).
5. Kouwenhoven, W. B., Jude, J. R., and Knickerbocker, G. G.: Closed Chest Cardiac Massage, *J. Am. Med. Assoc.*, 173:1064, 1960.
6. Jude, J. R., Kouwenhoven, W. B., and Knickerbocker, G. G.: Cardiac Arrest: Report of Application of External Cardiac Massage on 118 Patients, *J. Am. Med. Assoc.*, 178:1063, 1961.
7. American Heart Association: Standards for Cardiopulmonary Resuscitation and Emergency Cardiac Care, *J. Am. Med. Assoc.*, 227:833, 1974.
8. Chazen, J. A., Stevson, R., and Kurland, G. S.: The Acidosis of Cardiac Arrest, *N. Engl. J. Med.*, 278:360, 1968.
9. Heimlich, H. J.: A Life Saving Maneuver to Prevent from Choking, *J. Am. Med. Assoc.*, 234:398, 1975.
10. Visintine, R. E., and Baick, C. H.: Ruptured Stomach after Heimlich Maneuver, *J. Am. Med. Assoc.*, 234:415, 1975.
11. Elam, J. O., Greene, D. G., Schneider, M. A., Ruben, H. M., Gordon, A. S., Hustead, R. F., and Berson,

*This article is a review of the literature and contains additional references to the literature.

D. W.: Head Tilt Method of Oral Resuscitation, *J. Am. Med. Assoc.*, 172:812, 1960.

12. Greene, D. G., Elam, J. O., Dobkin, A. B., and Studley, C. L.: Cinefluorographic Study of Hypertension of the Neck and Upper Airway Patency, *J. Am. Med. Assoc.*, 176:570, 1961.

13. Safar, P., Escarraga, L. A., and Elam, J. O.: A Comparison of the Mouth to Mouth and Mouth to Airway Methods of Artificial Respiration with the Chest Pressures Arm Lift Methods, *N. Engl. J. Med.*, 258:671, 1958.

14. Bryson, T. K., Kenvmof, J. F., and Ward, C. F.: The Esophageal Obturator Airway. A Clinical Comparison to Ventilation with a Mask and Oropharnygeal Airway, *Chest*, 74:537, 1978.

15. Adgey, A. A. J., Patton, N. J., Campbell, N. P. S., and Webb, S. W.: Ventricular Defibrillation: Appropriate Energy Levels, *Circulation*, 60:219, 1979.

16. Pantridge, J. F., Adgey, A. A. J., Webb, S. W., and Anderson, J.: Electrical Requirements for Ventricular Defibrillation, *Br. Med. J.*, 2:313, 1975.

17. Gascho, J. A., Crampton, R. S., Cherwek, M. L., Siper, J. N., Cohen, F. P., and Obren, W. M.: Determinants of Ventricular Defibrillation in Adults, *Circulation*, 60:231, 1979.

18. Tacker, W. A., and Ewy, G. A.: Emergency Defibrillation Dose, Recommendation and Rationale, *Circulation*, 60:223, 1979.

19. Bishop, R. L., and Weisfeldt, M. L.: Sodium Bicarbonate Administration during Cardiac Arrest. Effect of arterial pH, PCO_2 and osmolality, *J. Am. Med. Assoc.*, 235:506, 1976.

19a. Mirowski, M., Reid, P. R., Mower, M. M., et al.: Termination of Malignant Ventricular Arrhythmias with an Implanted Automatic Defibrillator in Human Beings, *N. Engl. J. Med.*, 303(6):322, 1980.

20. Wei, J. Y., Greene, H. L., and Weisfeldt, M. L.: Cough Facilitated Reversion of Ventricular Tachycardia. The Cough Version, *Am. J. Cardiol.*, 45:174, 1980.

21. Criley, J. M., Blaufuss, A. N., and Kissel, G. L.: Cough-Induced Cardiac Compression, *J. Am. Med. Assoc.*, 236:1246, 1976.

22. Ravitch, M. M., Lane, R., Safar, P., Steichen, M. M., and Knowles, P.: Lightning Stroke. Report of a Case with Recovery after Cardiac Massage and Prolonged Artificial Respiration, *N. Engl. J. Med.*, 264:36, 1961.

23. Bleyaert, A. L., Nemoto, E. M., Safar, P., Stezoski, S. W., Michell, J. J., Moosy, J., and Rao, G. R.: Thiopental Amelioration of Brain Damage after Global Ischemia in Monkeys, *Acta Neurol. Scand.*, 56(suppl. 64):144, 1977, and *Anesthesiology*, 49:390, 1978.

24. Weale, F. E., and Rothwell-Jackson, R. L.: The Efficiency of Cardiac Massage, *Lancet*, 1:990, 1962.

25. MacKenzie, G. J., Taylor, S. H., McDonald, A. H., and Donald, K. W.: Hemodynamic Effects of External Cardiac Compression, *Lancet*, 1:1342, 1964.

26. Rudikoff, M. T., Maughan, W. L., Effron, M., Freund, P., and Weisfeldt, M. L.: Mechanisms of Blood Flow during Cardiopulmonary Resuscitation, *Circulation*, 61:345, 1980.

27. Chandra, N., Snyder, L., Tsitlik, J., and Weisfeldt, M. L.: Non-invasive Assisted Circulation by Synchronized Cyclical High Intrathoracic Pressure Support, *Clin. Res.*, 28:161A, 1980.

28. Redding, J. S.: Abdominal Compression in Cardiopulmonary Resuscitation, *Anesth. Analg.*, 50:668, 1971.

29. Harris, L. C., Kirimli, B., and Safar, P.: Augmentation of Artificial Circulation during Cardiopulmonary Resuscitation, *Anesthesiology*, 28:730, 1967.

30. Chandra, M. D., Snyder, L. D., Weisfeldt, M. L.: Abdominal Binding during CPR in Man, *J. Am. Med. Assoc.*, 1981, in press.

31. Chandra, N., Rudikoff, M., and Weisfeldt, M. L.: Simultaneous Chest Compression and Ventilation at High Airway Pressure during Cardiopulmonary Resuscitation, *Lancet*, 1:175, 1980.

PART IV Diseases of the Heart and Blood Vessels

The purpose of Part IV—"Diseases of the Heart and Blood Vessels"— is to present a discussion of the *disease processes* that can affect the heart and blood vessels. The reader should read the preface to Part III in order to understand the distinction we have made between a *disease process* and a *disorder*. Briefly, we define a *disease process* as a basic abnormality that exists in the tissue. The cause of the abnormality may be known or unknown. The pathologist can usually identify an abnormal disease process at autopsy when he or she examines the heart and blood vessels. A *disorder* is defined as a consequence of a disease process. A disorder is the derangement of function due to the disease process. A disorder is the final common pathway by which many different diseases make the patient ill. The pathologist may not be able to state that a patient had a disorder such as chest pain, ventricular dysfunction, a hyperdynamic circulation, arrhythmia, or syncope by examining the heart and blood vessels.

Whenever a physician identifies a disorder of the cardiovascular system, he or she must ask the question, "What cardiovascular disease caused this set of abnormalities?"

Whenever a physician identifies a disease process in a patient, he or she must ask the question, "Are any of the known consequences (disorders) of the disease present in my patient?"

34

Incidence, Prevalence, and Mortality of Cardiovascular Disease

William B. Kannel, M.D., M.P.H.

When meditating over a disease I never think of finding a remedy for it but instead a means of preventing it.

Louis Pasteur

Life expectancy has never been higher in the United States than at present, largely as a result of an improved standard of living and quality of life. The death rate is now declining at a rate of 2 percent per year, indicating that today's leading causes of death, cardiovascular diseases, are amenable to preventive and therapeutic management.

Cardiovascular Disease as a Major Health Hazard

General Mortality

Despite recent improvements, cardiovascular disease continues to be the most serious threat to life and health. One in every three males in the United States can expect to develop some major cardiovascular disease before reaching age 60; the odds for women are 1 in 10.[1] Coronary disease is the major cause of death after the age of 40 in men and after the age of 50 in women.

The cardiovascular diseases accounted for more than half of the deaths in the United States in 1979. Over 20 percent of these deaths occurred before age 65. Of all the deaths attributed to cardiovascular disease, 75 percent were caused by heart disease and 17 percent by stroke. An estimated 40 million persons in the United States (almost 20 percent) have one or more cardiovascular diseases, and at least 40 percent of these 40 million are limited in activity, even when persons in nursing homes and institutions are excluded from consideration (Fig. 34-1).

There were an estimated 4.8 million hospital admissions in 1978 attributed to cardiovascular disease.[2] Health expenditures and dollar value lost in productivity due to cardiovascular illness and death were estimated in 1980 to amount to $41 billion (Fig. 34-2).

Arteriosclerosis is the basis for 85 percent of deaths from heart and vascular disease. Hypertension afflicts 16 percent of the United States population, substantially increasing the risk of stroke, coronary heart disease, and cardiac failure. Cere-brovascular disease partially or completely disables more than half of the nearly 2 million persons who have survived a stroke. Coronary heart disease attacks 1.5 million persons in the United States each year. Congenital heart disease afflicts 8 of every 1000 children born each year, and 10 to 15 percent of them do not survive the first year of life. Acute rheumatic fever and subsequent rheumatic heart disease produce 7500 deaths and require 114,000 hospitalizations annually. Deep-vein thrombosis causes more than 90 percent of pulmonary emboli, which, in turn, are responsible for 50,000 deaths each year.[1-4]

The World Health Organization found that, internationally, the principal cause of mortality is heart and vascular disease, producing more than 40 percent of all deaths.[5-7]

General Prevalence

Accurate prevalence data based on actual examinations and acceptable criteria from representative general population samples are sparse. From health interviews it appears that some 66 million Americans are afflicted with cardiac or circulatory conditions. Heart conditions and hypertensive disease are the most commonly reported. The overall reported rate for heart conditions is 63 per 1000, rising from 25 per 1000 under age 45 to 215 per 1000 at ages 65 and over. Except for congenital anomalies, the prevalence increases markedly with age.

Estimates from the American Heart Association suggest that there are 40.8 million persons with cardiovascular disorders: 34 million with hypertensive disease, 4.2 million with coronary heart disease, 1.85 million with rheumatic heart disease, and 1.82 million with stroke (Fig. 34-1).

FIGURE 34-1 Estimated prevalence of the major cardiovascular diseases, United States, 1977. (*From American Heart Association.*)

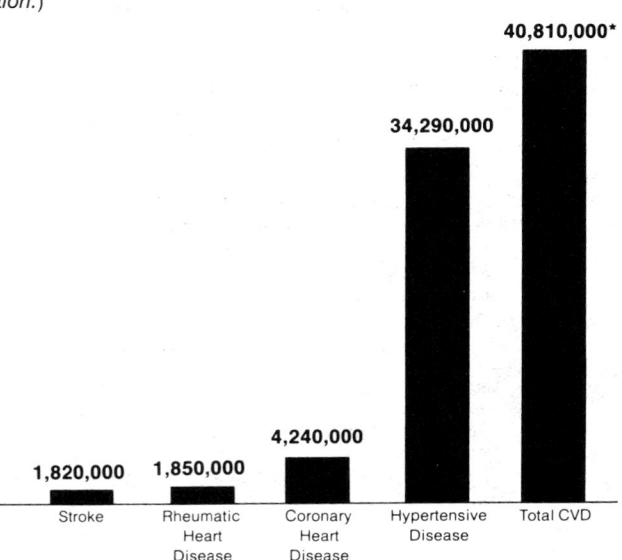

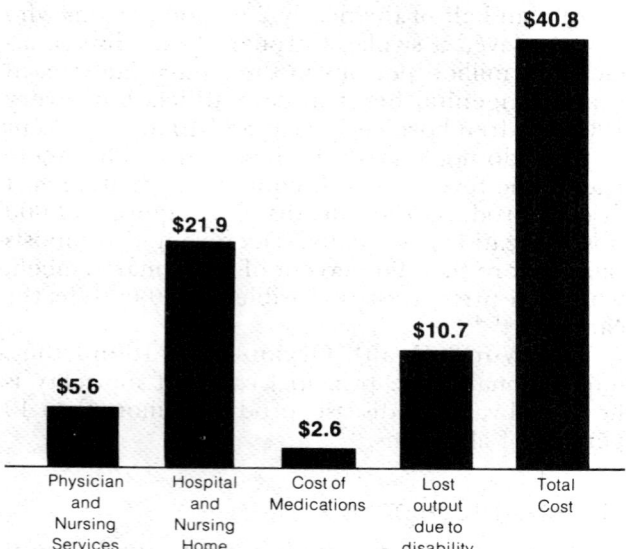

FIGURE 34-2 Estimated economic costs in billions of dollars of cardiovascular diseases by type of expenditure, United States, 1980. (*From American Heart Association.*)

General Incidence

Reliable incidence data for even the major cardiovascular diseases are also scarce. Data from the Framingham Study provide reliable estimates for 20 years of follow-up of a defined population sample of 5209 men and women, aged 45 to 74. Rates for men for combined atherosclerotic and hypertensive cardiovascular diseases rise from 12.8 per 1000 at ages 45 to 54 to 30.3 per 1000 at ages 65 to 74 (Table 34-1). For women, comparable rates are achieved 10 years later in life, with the gap closing with advancing age. This 10-year lag in incidence applies for coronary disease, occlusive peripheral arterial disease, and possibly for cardiac failure, but not for stroke. At all ages, the incidence of myocardial infarction exceeds that of brain infarction in men, while in women the infarction rates are similar.

Secular Trends

The long-term trend in deaths from cardiovascular disease since 1900 until recently has been upward because of an increasing proportion of older persons; control of infectious, parasitic, and nutritional deficiency diseases; and an epidemic increase in fatal coronary attacks. After adjustment for aging of the population, it became apparent that cerebrovascular and hypertensive cardiovascular disease mortality had been declining since 1928, antedating effective antihypertensive treatment (Fig. 34-3).

The long-term decline in cardiovascular mortality became more precipitous in the 1970s, falling 2.7 percent per year compared to just under a 1 percent decline between the 1950s and 1960s. More than 40 percent of the decline between 1950 and 1977 occurred in the 5 years following 1972. For stroke, the rate of decline since 1972 has exceeded 5 percent per annum.

A striking feature of this declining cardiovascular mortality has been its universal nature in all races, both sexes, all age groups, and all geographic areas in the United States. The greatest improvements have been noted in females, blacks, young adults, and higher socioeconomic subgroups. The largest decline was noted for hypertensive and cerebrovascular disease. However, except for cancer and chronic obstructive pulmonary disease, mortality from other natural causes has also been declining. Cardiovascular diseases account for half of all deaths, and, largely as a result of the decline in cardiovascular mortality, life expectancy in the United States is now the longest in history (73.2 years).

The decline in coronary heart disease (CHD) mortality reverses an earlier epidemic rise persisting into the 1960s; it coincides with improvements in the major cardiovascular risk factors, more vigorous and effective treatment of the acute episode, and greater efforts at secondary prevention. The United States decline in coronary heart disease mortality appears to exceed that elsewhere in the world, where some countries are still experiencing a rising mortality[8–10] (Fig. 34-3).

Unfortunately, except for stroke, there are no

TABLE 34-1 Incidence of Major Hypertensive and Atherosclerotic Cardiovascular Events: Framingham Study, 20-Year Follow-Up*

Age	Atherosclerotic and Hypertensive Cardiovascular Disease		Cardiovascular Disease (All Types)		Coronary Heart Disease		Occlusive Peripheral Arterial Disease		Cardiac Failure	
	Men	Women	Men	Women	Men	Women	Men	Women	Men	Women
45–54	128	46	20	9	99	31	18	6	18	8
55–64	262	136	32	29	208	95	51	19	43	27
65–74	303	234	84	86	204	145	63	38	82	68
45–74	199	107	34	29	153	72	37	16	37	25

*Average annual incidence rate per 10,000.

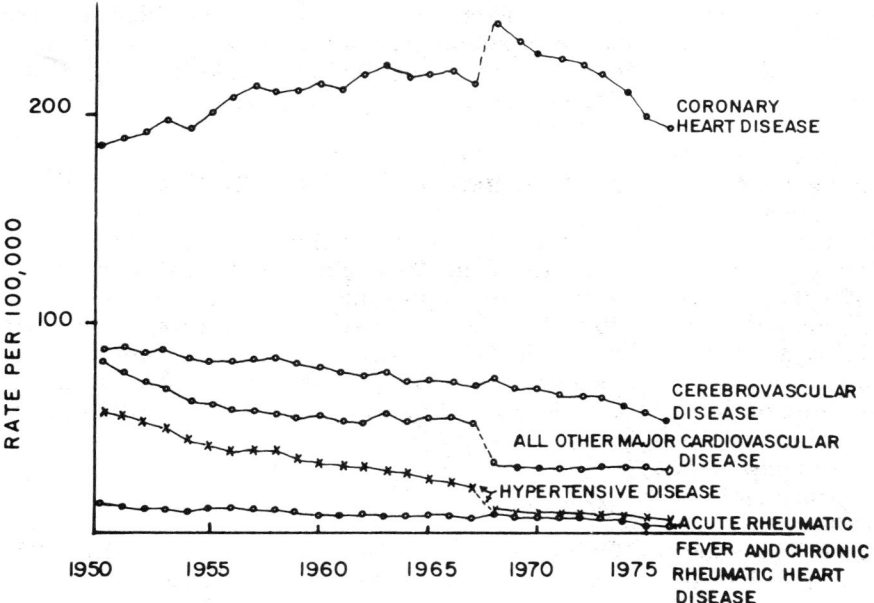

FIGURE 34-3   Age-adjusted death rates for components of major cardiovascular diseases. United States, 1950 to 1976. (*From National Center for Health Statistics, August 1978.*)

comparable data for trends in morbidity. This is important, since a reduction in mortality without a decline in attack rate indicates better medical care was responsible, while a reduction in both suggests environmental influences.

Coronary Heart Disease (See Chap. 45)

Coronary heart disease kills and disables people in their most productive years and accounts for most of the $10 billion spent annually for cardiovascular services. It is the most frequent cause for short-stay hospitalizations, and the per admission hospital costs for coronary heart disease are the highest. Coronary heart disease is the most prominent cause of premature disability in the American labor force, accounting for 22 percent of disability allowances granted by the Social Security Administration.

Prevalence

Health interviews indicate that about 2 percent of Americans (4 million) have coronary heart disease, over half below age 65. The prevalence rises from 1.3 per 1000 under age 45 to 41.6 per 1000 at ages 45 to 64 and to 84.8 per 1000 at 65 and over.

Incidence

Coronary disease causes as many as 500,000 heart attacks each year. The chances of an American male developing this disease before age 60 are one in five. Incidence in women lags by 10 years, and by 20 years for more serious clinical manifestations such

as myocardial infarction and sudden death (Table 34-2). Male predominance is least striking for uncomplicated angina pectoris.

The presenting complaint for women is more likely to be angina, whereas in men it is more likely to be manifest as myocardial infarction or sudden death. More angina in men occurs after infarction than afresh. Only 20 percent of coronary attacks are preceded by long-standing angina, less if the infarction is silent or unrecognized. Serious manifestations of coronary heart disease such as infarction or sudden death are rare in the premenopausal female. The incidence and severity of coronary heart disease increase precipitously after the menopause, with coronary heart disease rates in postmenopausal women 2 to 3 times that of those the same age remaining premenopausal. This applies whether the menopause is natural or surgical; and, in the latter, whether the ovaries are removed or not and whether or not estrogen replacement therapy is pre-

TABLE 34-2   Incidence of Specified Clinical Manifestations of Coronary Heart Disease: Framingham Study—20-Year Follow-Up*

Age	Angina Pectoris†		Myocardial Infarction		Sudden Death	
	Men	Women	Men	Women	Men	Women
45–54	28	17	48	9	11	3
55–64	75	56	91	19	27	4
65–74	46	68	111	51	26	12
Total	47	39	72	19	19	5

*Average annual incidence rate per 10,000.
†Uncomplicated by myocardial infarction.

scribed.[11] The gap in incidence between the sexes closes progressively with advancing age.

Mortality

Coronary heart disease is the leading cause of death in American adults, accounting for one-third of deaths in persons over age 35. It is estimated that a 30-year-old American male would survive to age 80 rather than 71 if coronary heart disease and stroke could be eliminated. In 1979 there were 545,000 coronary deaths; over 80 percent of the cardiac deaths in the age range 35 to 64 are attributed to this cause. While coronary heart disease mortality increases with age, it is the dominant cause of death in young adults at the peak of their productive lives.

Two of three coronary deaths are unexpected, occurring outside the hospital. Most are sudden deaths, which occur too rapidly to allow arrival at the hospital while the patient is still alive. These sudden deaths, which account for more than half of coronary fatalities, appear less likely to be sudden in women than men and in the elderly than the young.

A substantial part of coronary heart disease mortality progresses from inapparent disease to death rather swiftly. Much of the premature mortality from coronary heart disease comes on with little warning in a population prone to coronary heart disease.

Unrecognized myocardial infarctions are common, numbering at least one in five. Half are silent, and the rest are atypical so that neither the patient nor the physician entertains the possibility. More than half of these subjects eventually develop some overt clinical manifestation of coronary heart disease and hence come under medical care. Angina is less frequent in such subjects than in those with recognized symptomatic myocardial infarction, but the subsequent mortality is little different.

About 80 percent of coronary mortality in persons under age 65 occurs during the initial coronary attack. Thus, despite a higher risk of death with a prior coronary attack, most coronary deaths arise from the population still free of symptomatic coronary heart disease. Hence, primary prevention appears to offer more than secondary prevention. The first year following an attack is especially dangerous, with 20 percent of men and 45 percent of women with myocardial infarctions succumbing. Women have a higher recurrence rate than men once they sustain an infarction. Although the proportion of coronary deaths which are sudden is no greater after myocardial infarction, sudden deaths occur at four times the rate for the general population.

Epidemiologic studies indicate that the development of coronary heart disease is controlled by living habits and environment. It seems plausible that appropriate modifications could substantially reduce the premature mortality from this disease and lower overall mortality. Short of such an effort, it seems unlikely that there can be any major decrease in the appalling premature mortality. There is some evidence that this decline is taking place in the United States.

Hypertension (See Chaps. 49 and 50)

Hypertension is one of the most powerful contributors to cardiovascular morbidity and mortality. It is the most important factor contributing to the 500,000 cases of stroke which occur each year, resulting in 175,000 deaths. It is a major contributing factor in the 1,250,000 coronary events annually. It doubles overall mortality and triples cardiovascular mortality.

Mortality

Only 1.6 percent of cardiovascular deaths in 1978 were attributed to hypertensive disease, a gross underestimate of its impact on mortality. Hypertensive mortality is largely due to atherosclerotic sequelae such as coronary disease, stroke, and cardiac failure. Renal failure due to necrotizing arteriolar disease is uncommon, and malignant hypertension is vanishing as a cause of death. In 1970 only 6 percent of deaths directly attributed to hypertension were ascribed to malignant hypertension. The marked downward trend in hypertensive heart disease and stroke over the past decade strongly suggests that mortality from hypertension is on the decline and that the rate of decline has accelerated since the 1960s with more vigorous antihypertensive treatment and earlier detection of hypertensive subjects.

Prevalence

Data from the National Health and Nutrition Examination Survey for 1971 to 1972 indicated a prevalence of hypertension of 26 percent for persons 18 to 75 years of age in the United States;[12] hypertension was defined as blood pressures equal to or greater than 140/90 mmHg. Using a criterion of diastolic pressures of 95 mmHg or greater and/or use of antihypertensive medication, the Hypertension Detection and Follow-Up Program found 23.1 percent of subjects aged 30 to 69 hypertensive.[13]

Estimates are that 60 million Americans now have elevated blood pressures (above 140/90), and that 35 million of these, 15 percent of the population, have definite hypertension and face serious excess risks of cardiovascular sequelae. Since most of this excess risk is attributable to mild hypertension (90 to 104 mmHg diastolic pressure), there is a need for intervention through hygienic if not drug treatment. Risks of cardiovascular sequelae are proportional to the blood pressure level at any age, in either sex, whether the elevation is systolic or diastolic, labile or fixed.

Blacks and the elderly have a distinctly higher

prevalence of hypertension. Isolated systolic hypertension, particularly common in the elderly, is also a distinct hazard. The proportion of the population of hypertensive persons who are aware of their problem and are controlling it has doubled in recent years. However, the proportion aware but remaining untreated or uncontrolled has stayed constant.

Because of the higher prevalence of milder hypertension, almost 60 percent of the excess mortality attributable to hypertension comes from this blood pressure range. Epidemiologic evidence suggests that the increased cardiovascular risk in this subgroup is concentrated in those with other cardiovascular risk factors. The prevalence of hypertension is considerably lower than formerly over most of the nation.

In almost all populations, there is a rise in blood pressure with age in both sexes. This does not mean that blood pressures must inevitably rise with age or that those that do rise reflect a normal aging process. There is about a 20 mmHg systolic and 10 mmHg diastolic rise from age 30 to age 64. Systolic pressures continue to rise into the eighties in women and into the seventies in men. Diastolic pressures level off earlier and, in men, decline precipitously beyond age 55. The pressures start lower in women and rise more steeply so that they equal those of men in the fifties and then progressively exceed those of men in later life; this crossover is observed for both systolic and diastolic pressure. In some populations, blood pressure does not rise with age.

Incidence

Longitudinal observation of blood pressures as people age reveals a different pattern than cross-sectional data. Diastolic pressures are essentially parallel in the sexes, with women's pressure consistently below those of men. Systolic pressures, initially lower than those of men, rise more steeply in women to converge at age 60 with those of men, but never to exceed them. A progressive and disproportionate rise in systolic pressure with advancing age is presumed to result from loss of arterial elasticity.

Blacks have higher blood pressures than whites in most Western cultures. The crossover in blood pressures in the sexes appears to occur 10 years earlier in blacks than whites.

Determinants

While genetic susceptibility plays a large role, this may be only permissive, requiring one or more environmental cofactors such as salt intake, alcohol, or weight gain to bring on hypertension. New underlying causes of hypertension are discovered every decade, but the causes of the vast majority of cases remain undetermined. Of the identifiable causes, chronic renal disease, renovascular disease, and oral contraceptive–induced hypertension head the list.

Routine search for underlying causes not suggested by signs or symptoms is usually unrewarding and often counterproductive.

Stroke (See Chap. 64)

Mortality

In 1979 cerebrovascular disease was responsible for about 9 percent of the total mortality. Although formerly accounting for 250,000 deaths annually, 1979 estimates indicated that 167,000 deaths (47 per 100,000 population) would be attributed to stroke. Mortality from strokes accelerates with age, doubling with each 5-year increase in age. Although 85 percent of stroke deaths occur in persons over age 65, premature deaths are not uncommon. This is particularly true among blacks, who between ages 25 to 64 have 2.5 times the stroke mortality of whites, due largely to their high prevalence and increased severity of hypertension.[4] Stroke remains the third leading cause of death, behind heart disease and cancer.

Prevalence

There are about 8 stroke patients per 1000 population in the United States; the prevalence rises from 1 per 1000 under age 45, to 12 per 1000 at ages 45 to 64, to 45 per 1000 over age 65. The most common variety of stroke is atherothrombotic brain infarction, which accounts for 59 percent of all strokes. Next most common are cerebral embolus (14 percent), subarachnoid hemorrhage (10 percent), and intracerebral hemorrhage (5 percent). Intracerebral hemorrhage has apparently declined most in recent decades.

Incidence

The chances of having a stroke before age 70 in the United States are 1 in 20 for either sex. However, incidence rates vary depending on the age of the sample, whether derived from the general population or some select subgroup such as hospitalizations, and whether recurrent strokes are included. In 1972 the Joint Committee for Stroke Facilities estimated that stroke incidence increased from 1 per 1000 at ages 45 to 54 to 9 per 1000 at ages 65 to 74. These figures are similar to those in the Framingham Study. Although strokes occur most frequently late in life, 20 percent occur under age 65. The incidence reaches significant proportions only after age 55.

Until very recently, about 500,000 new strokes occurred each year in the United States. In the Framingham Study, brain infarctions occurred in men at one-third the rate of myocardial infarctions in the age range 45 to 74. For women, the incidence of brain and myocardial infarction is similar at all ages.

Unlike other hypertension- and atherosclerosis-related disease, there is no clear male predominance for stroke, except under age 55.

Disability

Strokes rank high on the list of crippling diseases. Many of the 250,000 Americans who survive strokes each year remain disabled by paralysis, speech disorders, and incontinence. Cerebrovascular disease accounts for half the patients hospitalized for neurological disease. Almost 10 percent of nursing home admissions for persons under age 65 are because of stroke. Residual disability is often substantial. In the Framingham Study, 31 percent of stroke survivors needed assistance in self-care, 20 percent required help in ambulation, and 71 percent had an impaired vocational capacity when examined an average of 7 years after their stroke.[14] Of the 1.6 million persons afflicted by stroke in the United States, 40 percent require special services and 10 percent total care.

Cerebrovascular disease need not be a result of aging. Modifiable contributing factors offer the possibility of prevention by identifying stroke candidates for corrective measures. Stroke prevention requires early treatment of persons with hypertension, cardiac disorders, and transient cerebral ischemic attacks.

Cardiac Failure (See Chap. 23)

Heart failure is the end stage of cardiac disease after the myocardium has used all its reserve and compensatory mechanisms. Once overt signs appear, half of the patients will be dead within 5 years despite modern medical management.[15] Cardiac failure is a tragic consequence of a variety of heart diseases, particularly hypertensive cardiovascular disease, coronary heart disease, rheumatic heart disease, and congenital heart disease. The dominant cause is hypertension, which precedes failure in 75 percent of cases. Coronary heart disease is responsible in 39 percent of cases, but in 30 percent of these it is accompanied by hypertension.[16] Precursive rheumatic heart disease, noted in 21 percent of cases of cardiac failure, was also accompanied by hypertension in 11 percent.

At least 1.5 million Americans have chronic heart failure and approximately 250,000 new cases occur each year, requiring 300,000 to 600,000 hospital admissions annually.

Reports of the incidence of cardiac failure in the United States vary from 0.05 to 2 per 1000 per annum.[17] From physician surveys, Gibson et al. estimated the occurrence at 3.8 to 5.0 per 1000 per annum.[18] The Framingham Study estimated the rate at 2.3 per 1000 per annum for men and 1.4 per 1000 per annum for women aged 30 to 79.[15]

Incidence increased with age, so that by the sixth decade the rate among men was five times that of the fourth decade. With an increasing geriatric population cardiac failure is a formidable problem. If preventive programs are to be developed, identification of factors that predispose and influence the course of the disease is essential.

Despite earlier recognition and more sophisticated treatment of cardiac failure, its clinical course and prognosis remain grim for the chief causes, hypertension and coronary heart disease; the outlook is not much better than for cancer. Greater emphasis must be given to preventive measures instituted before the heart has exhausted its reserve and compensatory mechanisms. Since hypertension is such an important predisposing factor, early and sustained treatment would seem a key to the prevention of most cardiac failure.

Rheumatic Fever and Rheumatic Heart Disease (See Chaps. 37 to 40)

Despite effective preventive measures for several decades and a known etiology and epidemiology, rheumatic fever and rheumatic heart disease have not been eradicated in the United States. There has been a dramatic decline in the occurrence of acute rheumatic fever in the United States since the 1930s, but the incidence in the 1960s was still 25 to 50 per 100,000 children aged 5 to 14 years. These diseases remain a substantial public health problem in developing countries. There is a need to better define the incidence and prevalence of rheumatic fever and rheumatic heart disease and the infective endocarditis which follows, as well as to better define those at risk.

Mortality

As late as the 1940s, rheumatic heart disease was the leading cause of death in school children aged 5 to 19 years. Mortality from rheumatic heart disease has since declined sharply, presumably as a result of antibiotic treatment of streptococcal infection. However, the decline antedated the widespread use of antibiotics and continued despite inadequate detection and prophylaxis. Acute rheumatic fever and rheumatic heart disease still cause 7500 deaths a year in the United States. About 1 percent of these deaths occur in people under age 20. The rate appears to be declining about 3 percent per year.

Prevalence

Rheumatic fever is the chief cause of serious valvular heart disease. Acute rheumatic fever and subsequent rheumatic heart disease remain one of the important cardiovascular problems throughout the world.[19] In contrast to the affluent Western world, rheumatic heart disease is often the most common form of heart disease in the tropical and subtropical developing countries. It occurs with a severity observed in the United States and Europe a century ago.[20] Rheumatic heart disease prevalence rates as high as 22 to 33 per 1000 have been reported in urban slum school children of some developing countries. Although theoretically preventable, this tragic toll occurs because of overcrowding, the deceptive self-limited nature of streptococcal pharyngitis, and the mild and often clinically inapparent nature of streptococcal infections.

With the decline in rheumatic fever in the United States, its clinical manifestations have also moderated so that carditis is detected in less than 20 percent of acute rheumatic fever patients.[21] Rheumatic fever in the United States tends to run in families and is more common in blacks, Puerto Ricans, Mexican Americans, and American Indians. Overcrowding, which facilitates spread of streptococcal infections, is the chief reason. Also, prophylaxis of first attacks in these groups is hampered by the huge size of the populations at risk and by imperfect and inconvenient methods for diagnosis of inapparent or self-limited streptococcal infections.

The prevalence of active rheumatic fever and chronic rheumatic heart disease has been roughly estimated at 5 percent for all ages, rising from 3.6 percent under age 45 to 9.7 percent at 45 to 64, and remaining at 7.3 percent at 65 and over. It is estimated that 24 percent of those afflicted must limit their activity. Of the estimated 114,000 hospitalizations in 1978, 6000 were for active rheumatic fever and 108,000 for chronic rheumatic heart disease.

Incidence

Despite the decrease in both incidence and severity of acute rheumatic fever in the United States and other developed areas, 100,000 new cases per year are still reported, concentrated largely in lower socioeconomic groups. The incidence of rheumatic valvular disease in adults has not declined to the same extent as has rheumatic fever in children.

Beginning in 1920, rheumatic fever has declined in more affluent countries. This has lately engendered an unfortunate complacency in the United States, considering that rheumatic fever and its cardiac sequelae are the most preventable of the serious cardiovascular disorders. Adequate treatment can reduce attacks by 90 percent.

Rheumatic fever is rare before age 3, occurring most frequently between 5 and 15 years of age, when streptococcal infections are most frequent. The geographic distribution, incidence, and severity of rheumatic fever coincide well with the frequency and severity of streptococcal infections. During epidemics of streptococcal pharyngitis, the rheumatic fever attack rate is 3 percent, whereas in endemic situations when infections are milder it is only 0.3

percent. However, once patients are afflicted with prior attacks, rheumatic fever attack rates accelerate to 10 to 50 percent with subsequent streptococcal infections.[21]

The availability of penicillin to treat streptococcal infection and living conditions that are less crowding than formerly have made rheumatic fever uncommon in the United States, although incidence rates remain high in disadvantaged subgroups. Rheumatic fever remains a major problem in many areas of South America, Africa, the Middle East, and Asia.[19]

Other Valvular Disease (See Chaps. 38 to 40)

In the two decades since mitral valve prolapse was described, the syndrome has changed from a curiosity to the most frequently diagnosed valvular deformity. The exact prevalence is not clear. It appears to occur in 6 to 10 percent of presumably normal young women[22] and is reported with similar frequency in healthy young men.[23] Although the condition may become manifest at any age, it is reported most frequently in young women aged 14 to 30, where it may reach a prevalence exceeding 10 percent. Echocardiographic studies indicate that it may be even more common, with 10 to 15 percent of the population possibly afflicted; however, many diagnosed by echocardiography exhibit neither clinical nor angiographic evidence of the syndrome. The fact that 6 to 10 percent of asymptomatic young women have this syndrome is prima facie evidence that it is generally a benign condition. The natural history is not well established. Limited follow-up suggests that few cases progress to a severe form, and initial reports of sudden death risk appear to have been overstated. The major importance may be the threat of endocarditis, which must be rare, and arrhythmias, which may be common.

Congenital Heart Disease (See Chap. 36)

The prevalence of congenital heart disease at birth as determined during the infant's brief stay in the hospital is likely to be underestimated, and recognition of specific lesions may be inaccurate. Most data are deficient for congenital heart disease diagnosed after the first week of life. Prevalence data based on autopsy findings are unreliable because they reflect a fraction of the deaths and relate only to fatal lesions. Most information comes from retrospective studies based extensively on referral practices.

Structural abnormalities of the heart or intrathoracic great vessels seem to affect 8 to 10 of every 1000 infants born alive in the United States. About 1 newborn per 1000 live births has a cardiac birth defect which cannot be managed medically or surgically. Many infants who previously would have died now survive to adult life because of improved treatment, but 5 to 6 per 1000 live births require frequent medical or surgical attention.

Except for the recent unexplained two-fold increase in ventricular septal defects and the threefold increase in patent ductus arteriosus, the incidence of most congenital heart diseases has remained stable. Rubella vaccine has reduced rubella-caused congenital heart disease, and congenital heart defects associated with Down's syndrome are less common because older women are having fewer babies. Preventive strategies are impeded by lack of knowledge of the cause of most congenital heart disease, although we have learned that alcohol, trimethadione, and lithium can cause cardiac defects. The majority of congenital heart disease may involve complex genetic-environmental interactions which remain to be elucidated.

About 72 of each 1000 live births in the United States are premature, with the infants weighing less than 2500 g. Almost half of premature infants weighing less than 1750 g will maintain patency of their ductus arteriosus, possibly because their immature lungs do not properly metabolize prostaglandins which cause the ductus to remain open.[24] The growing number of teratogens identified appear to account for only 5 percent of all human malformations. However, single mutant genes are said to be responsible for only 3 percent of cases.[25]

The overall congenital heart disease incidence rate is fairly uniform at 0.8 to 1 per 100 live births and has been fairly constant over time.[24,25] This often excludes bicuspid aortic valves which are found in 2 percent of the population and hence may be twice as frequent as all other congenital defects combined; this is usually identified in adult life.

In all evaluations of mortality from congenital heart disease, death in infancy predominates at 1.3 to 2.8 per 1000 live births. Later mortality is more speculative, about 0.4 per 1000 live births over the subsequent 3 years. About 25 percent of infants with congenital heart disease have a malformation incompatible with life beyond the first year; possibly half of these can be treated surgically to improve the quality of life if not to produce a cure. About 2.5 per 1000 live-born infants require specialized services for diagnosis and treatment of congenital heart disease shortly after birth, and another 2.5 per 1000 will need these resources later in childhood.[25]

Chagas' Disease (See Chap. 55)

Although cardiovascular disease is a worldwide problem, there are marked regional differences in its impact. In Latin America, Chagas' disease constitutes a serious cardiac public health problem. About 35 million Latin Americans are exposed to it and 7 million are infected, mostly in childhood.[7] Rates of infection with *Trypanosoma cruzi* approach 40 to 50 percent in the populations exposed; chronic-phase infection is around 15 percent.[26] Chronic Chagas' disease is the most common heart disease in some areas of South America, estimated to affect 7 million persons.[6] Since there is no known therapy to prevent the often overlooked acute stage from progressing to the chronic phase, prevention involving vector control is the only means to control the disease; the preponderance of cases occur in the third and fourth decade of life and in rural areas. Although encountered in the Southwestern United States, the disease is not a major problem in this country.

Venous Thromboembolism (See Chap. 52)

Estimates of mortality from pulmonary embolism vary widely, depending on the source and accuracy of data. It is probably directly responsible for 50,000 deaths annually in the United States and contributes to an equal number of deaths. It is the most common lethal pulmonary disease. If untreated, recurrent episodes are frequent and more than 25 percent will be fatal. Mortality is probably underreported, since more than half of cases found at autopsy were overlooked before death. More than 60 percent of fatalities occur within 1 h of onset; hence, pulmonary embolism is likely to be confused with sudden coronary death.

The incidence of pulmonary embolism is even more uncertain than the mortality. Only 10 percent of cases occur in normal persons without predisposing factors such as chronic cardiopulmonary and malignant disease, estrogen therapy, orthopedic trauma, immobilization, operative procedures, obesity, pregnancy, or blood dyscrasias. The elderly are more vulnerable.

Postoperative pulmonary emboli alone produce 4000 to 8000 deaths annually. It is a major cause of death postpartum and in patients hospitalized for orthopedic conditions. Evidence from Britain suggests that the annual mortality from pulmonary embolism has been increasing for several decades despite anticoagulant drugs. More than 5 million persons over age 40 undergo major surgery each year in the United States; 1 or 2 of each 1000 will die postoperatively from pulmonary embolism. The recent advent of low-dose heparin prophylaxis may substantially reduce this risk.[27]

Preventive Implications

Examination of the incidence, prevalence, mortality, and natural history of cardiovascular disease suggests the need for a preventive approach. It is not likely that any recent innovations in diagnosis and therapy for cardiovascular disease, impressive as they have been, nor any advances in the foreseeable future, can have a major impact on the continuing epidemic of cardiovascular disease. Only a preventive approach involving correction of predisposing factors in advance of the overt clinical expression of the disease can be expected to make a sizable impact. When the heart or brain is infarcted, no therapy can be expected to restore full function.

Coronary heart disease often strikes without warning; one in five coronary attacks presents as sudden death, and two-thirds of the deaths occur in the community too precipitously to be brought under medical attention.

While some strokes may give warning by transient ischemic attacks, most do not. Even when they do, intervention at that stage may not necessarily greatly delay a permanently damaging stroke or prolong life.

Heart valves damaged by rheumatic heart disease and infective endocarditis can be surgically repaired or replaced by prosthetic appliances; this approach often requires anticoagulants to prevent emboli, and valve failure and hemolysis are distressingly common. Although such patients live longer, more comfortable lives than formerly, their survival does not approach that of patients with rheumatic fever kept from progressing to severe valve damage by antibiotic prophylaxis against recurrent disease.

Hypertension which progresses to target organ involvement is less manageable than if vigorously treated prior to such manifestations. The first sign of target organ involvement is too often a stroke, myocardial infarction, or sudden death. Half such cardiovascular catastrophes occur before evidence of organ involvement can be discovered on biennial examinations.

Awaiting overt signs and symptoms of cardiovascular disease is no longer justified. In some respects, the occurrence of symptoms may be more properly regarded as a medical failure rather than as the initial indication for treatment.

The practice of preventive medicine, coupled with public health measures to alter the ecology to one more favorable to cardiovascular health and health education to inform people of what they must do to protect their cardiovascular health, should have major impact on cardiovascular morbidity and mortality. Reliance on therapeutic measures alone is not enough.

References

*1. Gordon, T., and Kannel, W. B.: Premature Mortal-

---

*This article is a review of the literature and contains additional references to the literature.

ity from Coronary Heart Disease: The Framingham Study, *J. Am. Med. Assoc.*, 215:1617, 1971. (21 references)

2. National Center for Health Statistics: "Vital Statistics of the U.S.," 1977.

3. Moriyama I., Krueger, E., and Stamler, J.: "Cardiovascular Diseases in the U.S.A.," Harvard University Press, Cambridge, 1971.

4. "Healthy People," the Surgeon General's Report on Health Promotion and Disease Prevention, DHEW Publication 79-55071, 1979.

5. World Health Organization: Cardiovascular Diseases—Care and Prevention, *Chronicle*, 28:55, 1974.

6. World Health Organization: Services for Cardiovascular Emergencies, *World Health Organization Technical Report Series*, report of a World Health Organization Expert Committee, 1975, p. 7.

7. World Health Organization: Cardiovascular Diseases—Care and Prevention, *Chronicle*, 28:62, 1974.

*8. Kannel, W. B., and Thom, T. J.: Implications of the Recent Decline in Cardiovascular Mortality, *Cardiovasc. Med.*, 4:983, 1979. (23 references)

9. National Center for Health Statistics: "Chartbook for the Conference on the Decline in Coronary Heart Disease," August 1978.

10. World Health Organization: "World Health Statistics—Annual I," 1971–1977.

11. Gordon, T., Kannel, W. B., Hjortland, M. C., and McNamara, P. M.: Menopause and Coronary Heart Disease, *Ann. Int. Med.*, 89:157, 1978.

12. U.S. Department of Health, Education, and Welfare: Blood Pressure of Persons 18–74 Years, U.S., 1971–1972, "National Health Survey," National Center for Health Statistics, series II, no. 150, 1975.

13. Hypertension Detection and Follow-Up Program Cooperative Group: Race, Education and Prevalence of Hypertension, *Am. J. Epidemiol.*, 106:351, 1977.

14. Gresham, G. E., Fitzpatrick, T. E., Wolf, P. A., McNamara, P. M., Kannel, W. B., and Dawber, T. R.: Residual Disability in Survivors of Stroke—The Framingham Study, *N. Engl. J. Med.*, 293:954, 1975.

*15. McKee, P. A., Castelli, W. P., McNamara, P. M., and Kannel, W. B.: The Natural History of Congestive Heart Failure: The Framingham Study. *N. Engl. J. Med.*, 285:1441, 1971. (26 references)

16. Kannel, W. B., Castelli, W. P., McNamara, P. M., McKee, P. A., and Feinleib, M.: Role of Blood Pressure in the Development of Congestive Heart Failure: The Framingham Study, *New Engl. J. Med.*, 287:781, 1972.

17. Klainer, L. M., Gibson, T. C., and White, K. L.: The Epidemiology of Cardiac Failure, *J. Chronic Dis.*, 18:797, 1965.

18. Gibson, T. C., White, K. L., Klainer, L. M.: The Prevalence of Congestive Heart Failure in Two Rural Communities, *J. Chronic Dis.*, 19:141, 1966.

*19. Bisno, A. L.: World Wide Control of Rheumatic Fever, *Ann. Int. Med.*, 91:918, 1979 (editorial). (10 references)

20. Elkholy A., Rotta, J., Wannamaker, L. W., et al.: Recent Advances in Rheumatic Fever Control and Future Prospects: A World Health Organization Memorandum, *Bull. WHO*, 56:887, 1978.

21. Persellin, R. H.: Acute Rheumatic Fever: Changing

Manifestations. *Ann. Int. Med.,* 89:1002, 1978 (editorial).

*22. Procacci, P. M., Savran, S. V., Schreiter, S. L., Bryson, A. L.: Prevalence of Clinical Mitral Valve Prolapse in 1169 Young Women, *N. Engl. J. Med.,* 294:1086, 1976. (18 references)

*23. Darsee, J. R., Mikolich, J. R., Nicoloff, N. B., and Lesser, L. E.: Prevalence of Mitral Valve Prolapse in Presumably Healthy Young Men, *Circulation,* 59:619, 1979. (18 references)

24. Proceedings of the Second Conference on the Epidemiology of Aging. DHEW Publication 80-969, pp. 65–89, July 1980.

25. Michaelsson, M.: Report on a Study of Congenital Cardiovacular Malformations—Etiology, Incidence, Natural History and Organization of Diagnostic and Therapeutic Services, World Health Organization, Regional Office for Europe, May 1979.

26. Puigbo, J. J., Rhode, J. R. N., Barrios, H. G., Suarez, J. A., and Yepez, C. G.: Clinical and Epidemiological Study of Chronic Heart Involvement in Chagas' Disease, *Bull. WHO,* 34:655, 1966.

27. Council on Thrombosis of the American Heart Association: Prevention of Venous Thromboembolism in Surgical Patients with Low Dose Heparin, *Circulation,* 55:423A, 1977.

35

Genetics and the Cardiovascular System

W. Jape Taylor, M.D.

If two plants which differ constantly in one or several characters be crossed, numerous experiments have demonstrated that the common characters are transmitted unchanged to the hybrids and their progeny.

G. Mendel, 1865[1]

Knowledge of the molecular mechanisms by which like begets like accrues at an ever-accelerating pace. DNA can now be synthesized,[2] and manufactured genes can induce bacteria to produce human insulin and other polypeptides. Interspecific cell hybrids are contributing to the rapid construction of a map which localizes our genes on the various chromosomes.

New techniques of cell biology have led to the recognition of new diseases and to increased understanding of old diseases. Over 50 entities can be diagnosed early in pregnancy, and as the biochemical bases of more heritable disorders are established, the list will grow. The prospects for the prevention of disease or for its amelioration with specific replacement therapy are bright.

In this chapter, emphasis is placed on entities in which genetic determinants have a prominent role, particularly those for which fundamental mechanisms are known.

Congenital Heart Disease

Evaluation of a possible genetic role in the etiology of congenital heart disease has been hampered by many factors. Deaths in early life have interrupted sequences in pedigree study, often at ages when the cardiac defect either was not recognized or was improperly diagnosed. Hospital records often contain inadequate family histories, and the stigma that some parents feel is associated with a congenital anomaly may make it difficult to obtain information. Finally, many investigators have grouped all congenital heart disease as one; lesions with a major genetic contribution may be masked by those in which environmental teratogens are more important.

Despite the objection to considering all congenital heart disease as a single group, it permits compiling data from a large number of patients. Numerous studies have demonstrated that the incidence of congenital cardiac lesions in the siblings of patients approximates 2 percent, which is significantly higher than the expected rate.[3] In studies of individual lesions the findings have been comparable; when multiple cases of congenital heart disease are found in one family, they are generally identical or similar defects. A slightly higher incidence has been found in the children of patients with congenital heart disease, giving an increased risk of 20- to 40-fold.[4]

In most large studies monozygotic twins were frequently not concordant with congenital heart disease in that one member of these single-egg twins would have a cardiac anomaly and the other would not. Concordance for congenital heart disease in monozygotic twins is clearly higher than in nonidentical twins but is far from complete, indicating an interaction between genetic and environmental factors.[5]

Environment influences the degree to which certain genetic disorders become manifest after birth, and the interaction between genes and their milieu undoubtedly begins in utero. This interplay between genetic and environmental forces is often referred to as multifactorial; however, in a given patient the causation may be fundamentally either genetic or environmental.

Recessive Inheritance of Congenital Heart Disease

The increased incidence of congenital heart disease in siblings of affected patients without a striking increase in more distant kin is suggestive of a recessive genetic effect, but the proof that a trait is due to a recessive gene may be difficult. In an autosomal recessive disorder, an affected offspring receives the gene from each heterozygous parent, who bears no overt evidence of the trait. The occurrence of multiple affected members of a single generation with normal preceding and following generations suggests recessive inheritance. If large groups are analyzed, the mathematical ratio of one homozygous recessive person demonstrating the trait to three phenotypical normal individuals is found. However, in relatively small families, now the rule in the United States and Europe, the number of isolated cases will outnumber those with a familial incidence.

Common ancestry can increase the likelihood that recessive genes may be present in both marriage partners, and evaluation of consanguinity has been widely applied to the study of recessive inheritance. Utilizing the Amish people of Lancaster County, Pennsylvania, McKusick et al. detected more individuals with the Ellis–van Creveld syndrome than had been reported in the entire earlier literature.[6] From the cardiovascular viewpoint, the recessive gene—which is responsible for the dwarfism, syndactyly, and chondroectodermal dysplasia which characterize this syndrome—also produces a single atrium or other congenital cardiac defect.

Only the heart disease of Ellis–van Creveld syndrome and that of complete transposition of the viscera seem established as congenital cardiac disorders which are related primarily to the effects of a single mutant recessive gene. However, data suggest a strong influence of other recessive genes on the occurrence of congenital heart disease.

Dominant Inheritance of Congenital Heart Disease

Because reproductive capacities of patients with the more severe cardiac anomalies were limited before the era of surgery, it seems unlikely that a dominant gene could be responsible for many such lesions. On the other hand, a defect well tolerated through early adult life, such as the secundum atrial septal defect, could have this mode of inheritance. Several kinships involving marriages between individuals with this defect and normal mates have produced atrial septal defects in approximately half of the children. Involved offspring have had at least one parent with an atrial septal defect, except in a few instances in which incomplete expression of the gene may be present (possibly a patent foramen ovale). These findings do not indicate the proportion of atrial septal defects which are the result of genetic influence, but indicate that a gene transmitted in classic auto-somal dominant fashion produces this defect. In such a family the odds are virtually 50:50 that further children from affected members will be involved, rather than the less precise figure derived from studying groups of all types of congenital anomalies.[7]

The dominant inheritance of supravalvular aortic stenosis was reviewed by Kahler et al.[8] In contrast with sporadic cases of supravalvular aortic stenosis, mental retardation and a readily identifiable facial appearance are not seen in the familial disorder.

The billowing, or prolapsing, mitral valve is a common lesion which is often congenital and in which a dominant genetic transmission is frequent, although many cases are sporadic.[9] The billowing valve is also seen in other disorders of genetic origin, such as Marfan's and Ehler-Danlos syndromes and osteogenesis imperfecta.

Chromosomal Aberrations

Cytogenetic techniques have shown clearly that a number of diseases are due to abnormalities of chromosome distribution. Triplication of chromosome 21 is the cause of Down's syndrome, the most common of the autosomal disorders. Congenital heart disease is present in approximately 50 percent of affected children, with about one-half of defects being some type of endocardial cushion defect; transposition of the great vessels, hypoplastic aorta, and coarctation are rare.[10]

Nondisjunction of a chromosome during meiosis is the genesis of the extra chromosome in Down's syndrome. More frequent occurrence of nondisjunction in the ovarian tissues of aging mothers is responsible for the increased incidence of Down's syndrome in babies born to older mothers. Trisomies of various other autosomes besides 21 have also been described. Multiple defects of many systems are present, including complicated congenital heart disease. The major autosomal defects often have characteristic external abnormalities and are lethal early in life.[11]

In contrast to the widespread somatic disturbances due to major autosomal abnormalities, disordered sex chromosomes are generally not associated with such disastrous effects. In gonadal dysgenesis (Turner's syndrome) only one sex chromosome—an X—is present, giving a total complement of 45. The individual develops as a female without ovarian function and with variable webbing of the neck, hypertelorism, minor skeletal defects, and congenital heart disease. Coarctation of the aorta is a frequent cardiac association in this entity, but by no means the only one.[12] Patients with Turner's syndrome in older age develop a high incidence of hypertension and atherosclerosis.[13] Most males with the Turner phenotype have normal karyograms, although chromosomal aberrations have been described and congenital heart disease is common.

Families in which Down's syndrome was present in several members of three or more generations could not be explained by nondisjunction. Subsequent observations indicated that one parent of some affected children has a translocation of chromosome 21 onto either 15 or another small chromosome.[14] Accordingly, this parent is monosomic for chromosomes 15 and 21 and has an abnormal translocation chromosome, for a total count of 45; however, the total genetic composition is normal, as is the phenotype of the carrier. Half of the children will have the equivalent of trisomy 21 and will have Down's syndrome when a gamete containing the abnormal chromosome is fertilized. The incidence of congenital heart disease is approximately the same in the translocation and trisomy types of Down's syndrome, but the type of heart disease associated with chromosomal aberrations in many cases is uncertain.

In addition to translocations and trisomies, chromosomal aberrations such as deletions and abnormal forms have been reported; in a number of these, congenital heart defects are cardinal features. Although routine surveys for chromosome defects in a random population of patients with congenital heart disease are not rewarding, defects of multiple organ systems should prompt chromosome analysis. Cytogenetic studies may be indicated for prenatal diagnosis and for identification of carrier states.

Noncardiac Abnormalities in Congenital Heart Disease

Patients with congenital heart disease have a greatly increased incidence of noncardiovascular defects. Approximately 20 percent of patients have other anomalies, although some entities, such as transposition of the great vessels and tricuspid atresia, are rarely associated with another defect.[15] The dominant inheritance of atrial septal defect and bony abnormalities of the upper extremities is frequently called the Holt-Oram syndrome. The skeletal aberration, although variable, usually consists of loss of apposition of the thumb and is distinctive. Subsequently, numerous families have been described in which cardiac abnormalities and upper limb as well as other skeletal defects coexist.

Cardiomyopathies

Hypertrophic Obstructive Cardiomyopathy

Angina, syncope, and sudden death are the dominant symptoms of obstructive cardiomyopathy. (See Chap. 56.)

The genetics of this disorder make it immediately suspected in any patient with apparent aortic stenosis and a dominant history of cardiac disease. Within the same family some members may present with a nonobstructive cardiomyopathy, while others have the typical obstructive findings. In many early

series isolated cases were common, leading to the designation of idiopathic hypertrophic subaortic stenosis. Echocardiography provided conclusive evidence of autosomal dominance; first-degree relatives of previously identified patients had asymmetric septal hypertrophy, although many had no clinical disease.[16]

The relationship between hypertension and acquired obstructive cardiomyopathy has been a recurrent theme; Darsee et al. used HLA (human histocompatibility leukocyte antigen) typing to evaluate the genetic relationship between hypertensive and nonhypertensive patients with obstructive cardiomyopathy.[17] Hypertensive individuals had no HLA linkage, while nonhypertensive patients had an increased incidence of HLA-B12. The authors concluded that a heritable form of obstructive cardiomyopathy is linked to the histocompatibility complex of chromosome 6, while a nongenetic form may be induced by hypertension.

The ultrastructural architecture of the outflow tract has extreme muscle cell and myofibrillar disorganization so that some myofibrils are perpendicular to the long axes of cells or may insert into the Z bands of contiguous myofibrils.[18] This arrangement suggests that the genetic defect involves an autosomal dominant gene which regulates the organization of embryonic heart cells.

Neuromuscular Syndromes

Most inherited peripheral muscle disorders are associated with cardiac disease. Specific ultrastructural and biochemical defects are delineated with increasing frequency. Although both myocardial failure and major conduction defects are seen in the various muscular dystrophies, one or the other seems to predominate. This relative segregation of effects is due to different biochemical mechanisms and may provide clues that will elucidate both the neuromuscular and cardiac pathophysiology.

Neuromuscular Diseases with Heart Failure as the Major Cardiac Manifestation

X-Linked Muscular Dystrophies The Duchenne type of muscular dystrophy is the most common of this group; it is characterized by early age of onset, rapid progression, pseudohypertrophy, elevated levels of serum creatine kinase (CK), and late occurrence of heart failure. It is a sex-linked recessive trait, and is transmitted to males by apparently healthy mothers. The phenotypically normal female carries the abnormal gene on one X chromosome but does not manifest the disease because of the normal gene on the other X chromosome. One-half of her male progeny receive the X chromosome bearing the mutant gene and develop the disorder, since their only other sex chromosome is a Y; the remaining male offspring are normal genetically and phenotypically (Fig. 35-1). Half of the daughters of heterozygous females are also carriers and many can be detected by mild elevations in serum CK levels. (See Chap. 56.)

Milder sex-linked recessive types of muscular dystrophy of a later age of onset and slower progression are sometimes referred to as the Becker type of dystrophy. Linkage data indicate that the Becker gene is near the glucose-6-phosphate dehydrogenase: deutan color-blindness cluster, while the Duchenne gene is not, indicating that the two genes are not alleles and the diseases are separate.[19] More than one type of benign X-linked dystrophy exists, but the cardiac findings, usually subclinical, have not been clearly defined; rarely, severe heart failure is seen relatively early.

Myotonia Dystrophica This is an autosomal dominant disorder with appearance in both sexes and transmission through consecutive generations, since the onset of symptoms is relatively late. Cataracts, testicular atrophy, baldness, and varying degrees of mental retardation combine with involvement of skeletal and cardiac muscle as symptoms of this disease. Variation in age of onset suggests considerable genetic heterogenicity, but no biochemical markers or linked traits permit clear distinction of subgroups, and cardiac involvement has been common in all types.[20] Rarely, patients with myotonia dystrophica die of heart failure, but electrocardiographic abnormalities are more usual, with a high incidence of atrioventricular and bundle branch conduction delays.

Friedreich's Ataxia Cardiac involvement is virtually a sine qua non for the diagnosis of this disease. Since the striking clinical abnormalities are neurological rather than dystrophic, the genesis of the cardiomyopathy has been puzzling. Biochemical studies have delineated a subset of patients with Friedreich's ataxia who have a decrease in lipoamide dehydrogenase activity in cultured fibroblasts or in platelet-enriched blood.[21] Although heterogeneity of the clinical picture still exists, in these patients the disease is inherited as an autosomal recessive trait and carriers have an intermediate degree of enzyme deficiency. Lipoamide dehydrogenase is involved in the last step of pyruvate oxidation and occupies a critical role in several metabolic pathways. Although the enzyme has not been assayed in the heart of patients with Friedreich's ataxia, a deficiency in the heart may be responsible for the cardiomyopathy. It is not clear how commonly cardiac disease is found in other hereditary ataxias.

Rare Neuromuscular Disorders *Refsum's Disease.* Heredopathia atactica polyneuritiformis is a recessive disorder characterized by retinitis pigmentosa, polyneuropathy, and cerebellar ataxia at an early age. Symptoms of heart failure are unusual, but sudden death is seen; cardiac hypertrophy and fibrosis are in keeping with the electrocardiographic findings of left ventricular hypertrophy and conduction delays. An enzymatic defect in degradation

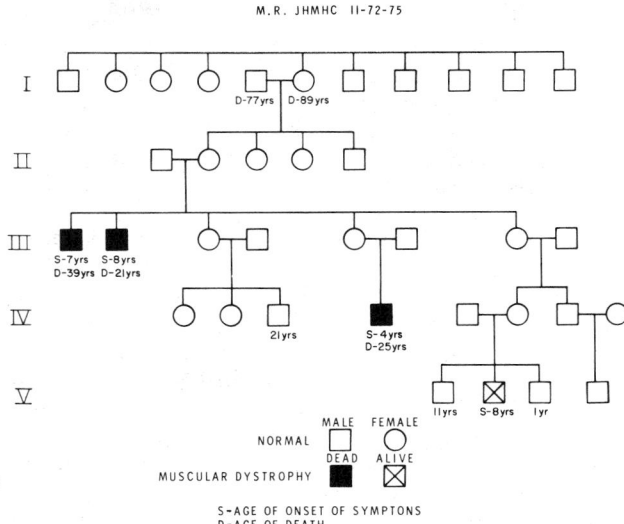

FIGURE 35-1 This pedigree demonstrates the transmission of the disease to males from healthy females, which is characteristic of a sex-linked recessive disorder, and the care which must be taken to uncover the genetic basis in many diseases. In view of the large number of normal males in generation I, the mutant gene may have arisen in the mother of generation I or II.

of phytanic acid of dietary origin is responsible for its accumulation in various tissues, and a restricted diet is of clinical benefit.[22]

Carnitine Deficiency. The syndromes of carnitine deficiency demonstrate that a marked deficiency in mitochondrial fatty acid can produce serious cardiac effects despite the fact that the heart can use glucose, lactate, and other substrates as well. Carnitine facilitates transport of fatty acids across the inner mitochondrial membrane. At least two syndromes of carnitine deficiency exist, with one (systemic carnitine deficiency) characterized by low serum and tissue levels and the other (muscle carnitine deficiency) by normal serum concentrations but low muscle values, presumably reflecting defects in synthesis and tissue uptake, respectively. A peripheral myopathy with an early age of onset characterizes both disorders and cardiac involvement has been demonstrated.[23]

The Glycogenoses

Pathological effects are produced by accumulation of excessive amounts of glycogen as well as by energy deprivation. In type II glycogen storage disease (Pompe's disease), heart failure is a common cause of death in infancy, although myopathic symptoms usually precede cardiac ones. The cardiomyopathy is hypertrophic with an occasional obstructive hemodynamic picture.[24] Deficiency of acid α-1,4-glucosidase (acid maltase) is responsible for this lethal disease of early life. Pompe's disease is inherited as an autosomal recessive trait and partial enzyme deficiency can be demonstrated in heterozygotes. Less severe varieties of acid maltase deficiency become symptomatic later in life and may be due to ineffective enzyme variants or a mutation affecting the rate of production or degradation of the enzyme.

Deficiency of amylo-1,6-glucosidase (debrancher enzyme) is the defect in type III glycogenosis. Childhood symptoms are due to liver involvement, which subsides, while peripheral myopathy becomes manifest in adult life.[25] Cardiac involvement in the late stages may be more common than suspected.

Muscle phosphorylase deficiency (McArdle's disease, type IV glycogenosis) involves primarily skeletal muscle and produces severe fatigue and pain with exertion because of an inability to utilize glycogen. Equivocal electrocardiographic abnormalities have been reported, but clinical evidence of heart disease is not seen. Muscle phosphorylase deficiency is usually inherited as an autosomal recessive disease, but appears to be genetically and biochemically heterogeneous.[25] Recently a fatal infantile form of myophosphorylase deficiency was described; electrophoresis revealed that two of the usual three cardiac enzymes were missing.[26]

Mitochondrial Myopathies Many myopathies with abnormal mitochondrial structure and function have been described. Most have clustered in siblings and consanguinity has been frequent, indicating autosomal recessive inheritance, but a sex-linked recessive pattern has also been noted. The myopathic symptoms vary, but all have mitochondria which are increased in number, enlarged, or bizarre in structure. On light microscopy the modified trichrome stain gives a "ragged-red" appearance due to the increased numbers of mitochondria and lipid deposits. The heart is usually hypertrophied, sometimes with obstructive physiology, which appears to be the response to excess metabolic demand. Abnormal mitochondria are striking in cardiac tissue, as in skeletal muscle.[27,28]

Neuromuscular Diseases with Major Conduction Abnormalities

Skeletal myopathies with major arrhythmias (complete heart block or the rare atrial standstill) are discussed separately, as the electrophysiological manifestations may provide a clue to the underlying biochemical defect. Cardiac dilatation, hypertrophy, and failure may or may not accompany the arrhythmias.

External Ophthalmoplegia with Heart Block Ptosis, paralysis of eye movements, retinal pigmentation, and heart block constitute an unusual syndrome; none of the early cases were familial, and debate has ensued about the entity because individuals with the major determinants may also have varying degrees of hearing loss, pharyngeal paralysis, or mental retardation. Recently familial cases have been described, but the genetics remain unclear.[29] Mitochondrial abnormalities have been found in some patients. The reason for the common vulnerability of ophthalmic muscles and the cardiac conduction system is unknown.

X-Linked Recessive Disorder In one X-linked recessive neuromuscular disorder, proximal upper extremity and distal leg involvement dominate the skeletal muscle symptoms, while arrhythmias, including arrest and sudden death, characterize the cardiac presentation.[30] In both peripheral muscle and heart, electrophysiological studies demonstrated a defect in electromechanical coupling. This may lead to persistent atrial standstill, sometimes preceded by atrial fibrillation or atrioventricular (AV) conduction delays.

Autosomal Disorders The peroneal muscular atrophies have a variable inheritance and clinical picture, but arrhythmias, including atrial standstill and third-degree AV block, are common. In the Kugelberg-Welander syndrome (juvenile progressive muscular atrophy), some cases are probably autosomal recessive disorders.[31]

Systemic Diseases

Hemochromatosis

Hemochromatosis, or iron storage disease, is a genetically determined disorder of variable expression in which myocardial iron deposits lead to cardiomegaly and congestive failure. Serum iron levels and liver biopsies can detect asymptomatic individuals with increased iron stores. Transmission of abnormal iron metabolism through multiple generations has been studied in conjunction with specific HLA linkage to indicate recessive inheritance with partial expression in heterozygotes.[32]

Amyloidosis

In one type of systemic amyloidosis cardiovascular manifestations are a dominant feature, sometimes mimicking constrictive pericarditis.[33] This type of amyloidosis is transmitted as an autosomal recessive trait and has widespread amyloid deposits in the vascular structures of many organs. Neurological or renal disease is the major feature of the more common autosomal dominant familial amyloidoses, but infiltration of the heart is usually present.

Tuberous Sclerosis Malformations of the brain which result in mental deficiency and epilepsy characterize this illness. It is associated with rhabdomyomas of the myocardium. Adenoma sebaceum of the skin leads to its recognition early in life. The gene for tuberous sclerosis may have a relatively high mutation rate since the reproductive capacity of affected patients is reduced, which, in the absence of new mutations, should lead to its extinction.

Isolated Idiopathic Cardiomyopathies

Endocardial Fibroelastosis Transmission of this disease from generation to generation has not been reported, but multiple occurrences in siblings and concordance in monozygotic twins is evidence for a recessive inheritance in some families. The disorder is more than 700 times as common in the siblings of affected patients as in the public at large.[34] Fibroelastosis, usually combined with complete heart block, has been reported in the children of mothers with systemic lupus erythematosus and may be familial.[35] This is a clear warning that *familial* and *genetic* are not synonymous terms.

Nonspecific Cardiomyopathies From time to time familial clusters of isolated myocardial disorders with heart failure, arrhythmias, or sudden death, but without a characteristic hemodynamic or pathological derangement, appear to be inherited as autosomal dominant traits.

Arrhythmias

The presence of conduction disturbances in multiple members of certain families indicates a genetic basis. Usually autosomal dominant transmission is present, although the age of onset of complete heart block varies from intrauterine to midadult life.[36] Advanced AV block is often preceded by sinus bradycardia and varying degrees of fascicular block. Familial congenital heart block is not as benign as isolated congenital heart block. In a few families conspicuous freckling has been noted as an associated hallmark.

Multiple siblings with heart block in infancy have been reported in a pattern which suggests an autosomal recessive inheritance. However, in some cases the mother had systemic lupus erythematosus; a variety of tissue antibodies can cross the placenta and damage the fetal conduction system as well as produce other cardiac anomalies.[35]

Familial tachycardias have been noted less frequently, but Gould reported a five-generation pedigree with 22 members in whom atrial fibrillation without other evidence of heart disease was well tolerated.[37] A similar suggestion of dominant inheritance of nodal rhythm has been made.[38] The preexcitation (Wolff-Parkinson-White) syndrome may occur in multiple family members in both single and subsequent generations, sometimes in association with obstructive cardiomyopathy.[39] Supraventricular tachycardias are a component of the billowing valve syndrome, sometimes inherited in an autosomal dominant fashion.

Prolongation of the QT interval of the electrocardiogram was described by Jervell and Lange-Neilsen as a part of a syndrome with recessive inheritance.[40] Congenital deafness and sudden death are other features; other investigators have reported dominant inheritance of QT interval prolongation without deafness.[41] The same ominous clinical implications are present in both syndromes.

Familial sudden death with minimal physical or psychic stimulation was described in apparently healthy teenaged siblings; unexpected death, often heralded by fainting episodes, appeared due to an autosomal dominant gene. Defects in the AV node and bundle were present, but no electrocardiographic or other clinical evidences of cardiac diseases were noted.[42]

Vascular Disorders

Atherosclerosis

Data remain inadequate about the genetic contribution to the etiology of atherosclerosis. The most persuasive evidence is derived from relatives of index patients with coronary artery disease. The incidence of coronary atherosclerosis in first-degree relatives of women who died of the disease before age 65 is seven times that of the population at large.[43] The male relatives of men who died of coronary disease under the age of 55 have a fivefold higher risk, and female relatives have an increased risk of over twofold. Twin studies have demonstrated a significant role for heredity; interestingly, heritable factors appear of more significance in women than men.

The Arterial Wall
Many factors which contribute to the development of atherosclerosis are subject to genetic variability. Increased susceptibility of the arterial wall is one factor which has been difficult to study and is considered significant only in rare disorders such as pseudoxanthoma elasticum, an autosomal dominant disease, and Werner's syndrome;[44] premature atherosclerosis and valve calcification with balding, cataracts, and atrophy of the skin produce a picture of precocious senility in this latter recessive disorder.

Some data suggest that atherosclerotic plaques have a monoclonal origin.[45] Electrophoretic variants of glucose-6-phosphate dehydrogenase (G6PD) are common in blacks, and random inactivation of either X chromosome in a given cell (Lyon hypothesis) produces black women who are mosaics for this enzyme. Plaques from women heterozygous for G6PD were reported to contain only one enzyme type, suggesting that mutational events produced these monoclonal lesions. This concept has been challenged by workers who demonstrated that a higher number of samples from aortic plaques reveals increasingly more with both G6PD variants.[46] Monotypism for G6PD in some plaques was considered due to differences in growth potential.

Hyperlipidemia
Familial hyperlipidemias are discussed in Chap. 42.

Familial hypercholesterolemia (type II hyperlipoproteinemia) is a group of closely related dominant disorders which in the usual heterozygous individual produce a serum cholesterol level of 350 to 450 mg/dl, normal triglyceride levels, corneal arcus, tuberous and tendinous xanthoma, and accelerated atherosclerosis. Homozygotic children, often produced by consanguineous parents, exhibit extreme hypercholesterolemia (600 to 1000 mg/dl), and death from vascular involvement is common in the first and second decades of life.

High-affinity receptors which bind low-density lipoproteins (LDL) at specific cell surface sites are absent in these extremely hypercholesterolemic individuals. Without LDL receptors, transfer of LDL cholesterol into the cells is deficient, leading to a lack of suppression of 3-hydroxy-3-methylglutaryl coenzyme A reductase (HMG-CoA reductase), the rate-limiting enzyme in cholesterol biosynthesis, and an impairment in LDL degradation and cellular cholesterol esterification.

Familial hypercholesterolemia is not the homogeneous entity which it had appeared to be. Individuals with a less marked deficiency of LDL binding, somewhat more responsive to dietary management, have been identified, as well as an intriguing variant in which LDL binding is normal but transfer of LDL cholesterol into the cell is impaired. The genes for LDL binding and internalization are alleles, suggesting that the LDL receptor is a bifunctional molecule with at least two active sites.[47] In an additional type of familial hypercholesterolemia, LDL from a hypercholesterolemic father and daughter did not suppress HMG-CoA reductase activity in either their own or normal leukocytes.[48] However, this apparent defect in LDL per se has not been confirmed in other laboratories or families. The LDL receptor pathway is a finely modulated mechanism which balances the transport and cellular needs for cholesterol. It can be overwhelmed by high levels of LDL, resulting in a nonspecific phagocytic uptake and accumulation of cholesteryl esters which Goldstein and Brown propose as a mechanism for susceptibility to atherosclerosis.[48a]

Other familial lipid abnormalities are more frequent than hypercholesterolemias, which have a heterozygote frequency of 0.1 to 0.2 percent. In relatives of survivors of myocardial infarction, the most common familial hyperlipidemia was an entity in which serum cholesterol and triglycerides were elevated individually or together;[49] this was termed combined hyperlipidemia, and is considered to be the result of a single dominant gene effect. The lipoprotein phenotypes in this disorder can be either IIa, IIb, or IV, and precise characterization of a lipid disorder requires family studies.

Familial hypertriglyceridemia is an autosomal dominant trait with a frequency between that of familial hypercholesterolemia and combined hyperlipidemia.[49] By electrophoretic classification, most of these individuals would be classified as type IV hyperlipoproteinemia.

In the rare type III hyperlipoproteinemia, an autosomal dominant variant, serum lipids are unusually sensitive to dietary manipulations; planar xanthoma and premature atherosclerosis are characteristic clinical manifestations.[50]

Type V hyperlipoproteinemia is another genetically heterogeneous group from which some families with an autosomal dominant inheritance can be dissected.[51] There is marked elevation of serum triglyceride levels; abnormal glucose tolerance is common. Clinical manifestations are pancreatitis, lipemia retinalis, and vascular disease.

Many individuals with elevation of serum lipid concentrations cannot be fitted into one of the single-gene disorders of lipid metabolism. In general population studies, a marked resemblance of cholesterol values within family groups is found, particularly for siblings below 16 or above 40 years of age.[52]

High levels of high-density lipoproteins (HDL) and the HDL:LDL ratio are negatively related to atherosclerosis. The HDL contain two major apoproteins (AI, AII), which have a major role in lipid transport.[53] Serum concentrations of HDL are to a degree regulated by genetic factors with an increased level segregating in an autosomal dominant fashion in some families. Higher HDL levels are found in American blacks than whites and may contribute to the lesser susceptibility of blacks to atherosclerosis despite a high incidence of hypertension.[54]

Antigenic polymorphisms have evolved among the lipoproteins, and two separate systems, the Ag and Lp, have been described in human beings. Increased vascular disease with specific alleles in each system has been reported.[55]

Other rare abnormalities of lipid metabolism associated with an atherogenic diathesis include familial lecithin: cholesterol acetyltransferase deficiency, cerebrotendinous xanthomatosis, β-sitosterolemia and xanthomatosis, Wolman's disease, and cholesterol ester storage disease.

Studies of a family from Tangier Island in Chesapeake Bay, in which two children had marked hypocholesterolemia and deposition of lipids in reticuloendothelial tissues, led to the definition of familial α-lipoprotein deficiency;[53] atherosclerosis is a component of this syndrome. Familial abetalipoproteinemia, an autosomal recessive disease, produces acanthocytes, neurological degeneration, and steatorrhea, with myocardial fibrosis, cardiac failure, and arrhythmias.[56] Hypobetalipoproteinemia is not the heterozygous state of the previous entity but a separate genetic disorder in which the serum cholesterol is low but precise clinical abnormalities are uncertain; a degenerative neurological defect may be associated.

Diabetes Mellitus

Although a familial predisposition to diabetes mellitus was noted early, a melding of classical genetic approaches and new immunochemistry has been required for more precise interpretations of the genetics of the disease.[57,58]

Twin studies have confirmed genetic heterogeneity in diabetes; virtually all identical-twin pairs are concordant for adult-onset insulin-insensitive diabetes, whereas only half of the juvenile insulin-dependent twins are both diabetics. The mode of inheritance of insulin-insensitive diabetes is not established, but in some patients a dominant inheritance is suggested by family pedigrees.[59] Population studies in ethnic groups with a high incidence of insulin-insensitive diabetes suggest single-gene inheritance, which cannot be clearly fitted into either a dominant or a recessive mode.

HLA antigens have provided a powerful tool for the study of genetic segregation in diabetes. No linkage is present between HLA-type and non-insulin-dependent diabetes, but juvenile insulin-dependent diabetes is related to specific HLA phenotypes.[57] The current consensus is that a gene (or genes) closely associated with the HLA-DRw3 and -DRw4 genes conveys increased susceptibility to viruses which, directly or through autoimmune responses, destroy the β cells of the pancreatic islets and produce insulin-dependent diabetes.[58] Debate continues as to whether more than one gene locus is involved and, assuming a single gene site, if it transmits diabetes in a dominant or recessive manner. An examination of the incidence of diabetes in American blacks, a racial outcross between Africans with no insulin-dependent diabetes and Caucasians, in which the disease is prevalent, reveals that the incidence of diabetes is comparable to the degree of genetic admixture, indicating a dominant inheritance.[60] About 20 percent of the American black gene pool (including the HLA diabetes-associated genes) is of Caucasian origin, and if a single recessive gene were responsible for diabetes, the frequency in American blacks should be approximately one-twenty-fifth $(\frac{1}{5})^2$, of the white incidence. An alternative proposal is that two susceptibility alleles interact with a normal gene in a codominant fashion.[61]

Systemic Hypertension

Most surveys of blood pressure in population groups demonstrate a unimodal distribution of blood pressure, suggesting a multifactorial genesis. However, evidence is accumulating that only a few genes are involved and that in any one individual or family group a single gene may be of major importance.

A familial clustering of blood pressure is found in population surveys, and identical twins have a high concordance rate for hypertension. Ethnic differences in frequency and severity of hypertension have been recognized for many years. Comparisons of the renal responsiveness to sodium loading and of plasma renin levels of black and white subjects demonstrate more sodium retention in blacks, which may relate to their increased incidence of hypertension.[62] The ethnic susceptibility, the familial clustering of blood pressure, and the twin studies all support a significant influence of genetic factors in the production of hypertension.

In uncommon forms of hypertension, single-gene influences have been recognized. Pheochromocytoma may occur in association with neurofibromatosis, a disorder with well-known genetic transmission. As an isolated lesion it has been described in multiple members of several kinships, although the exact mode of inheritance is unclear.[63] Hypertension is also present in the rarest of adrenogenital syndromes, an enzymatic defect in 11-hydroxylation of the steroid molecule, seemingly inherited as an autosomal recessive characteristic.[64]

Pulmonary Hypertension

Generally, hypertension in the lesser circulation is secondary to elevations of pulmonary venous pressure, left-to-right shunts, or alterations in the vascular bed due to intrinsic lung disease. However, the rise in pulmonary vascular resistance which causes this pulmonary hypertension is not uniform from individual to individual in response to apparently identical stimuli. A genetic basis for primary pulmonary hypertension, which develops without a known stimulus, suggests that the response to an abnormal load may be governed, in part, by inheritance. This infrequent illness is familial in about one-third of cases; autosomal dominant inheritance is suggested.[65]

Pulmonary hypertension is seen in a variety of inherited diseases[66] including cystic fibrosis, α_1-antitrypsin deficiency, Gaucher's disease, and tuberous sclerosis (Fig. 35-2). With the exception of the latter dominant illness, these are all autosomal recessive diseases.

Fabry's Disease

Angiokeratoma corporis diffusum (Fabry's disease) is a rare sex-linked recessive disorder in which deficiency of α-galactosidase leads to deposition of glycolipids in blood vessels, heart muscle, and other viscera.[67] Cardiac failure, hypertension, and angina are seen.

Systemic Diseases with Diffuse Cardiovascular Involvement

Mucopolysaccharidoses

The mucopolysaccharidoses constitute a large and diverse group of disorders relative to inheritance, age of symptomatic onset, and severity, but are unified by their underlying pathogenesis and sites of organ involvement.[68] Since they are due to deficiencies in the degradative lysosomal enzymes which catalyze dermatan sulfate and heparin sulfate (keratan sulfate in type IV), mucopolysacchariduria and widespread involvement of connective tissue cells and the musculoskeletal, cardiovascular, and central nervous systems are predictable.

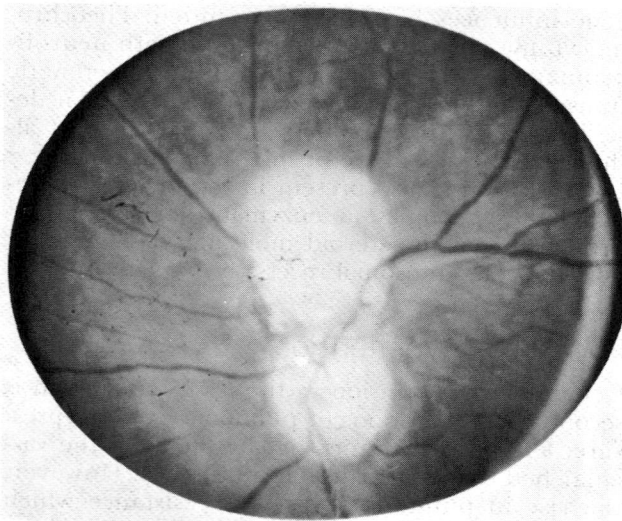

A

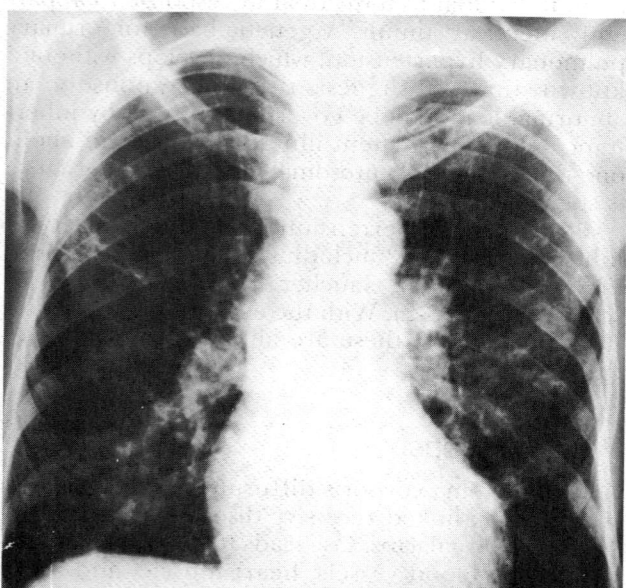

B

FIGURE 35-2 The phacoma with typical mulberry excrescences in the retinal fundus (A) led to the recognition of tuberous sclerosis as the cause of the marked pulmonary fibrosis in this patient (B).

Valvular and myocardial disease are characteristic in patients with Hurler's syndrome (Fig. 35-3). Increased consanguinity and involvement of multiple siblings of both sexes from normal parents provide the typical features of autosomal recessive inheritance, now proved by biochemical studies on the obligatory heterozygous carriers. This disorder is due to α-L-iduronidase deficiency, which is also defective in the much less severe Scheie's syndrome, in which intelligence is normal and life span is preserved. In both syndromes the same diffusible factor corrects the abnormal accumulation of mucopolysaccharides in cultured fibroblasts, indicating

that Hurler's and Scheie's syndromes are due to mutations at the same gene locus.

The severity of the cardiovascular manifestations parallels that of the generalized disease. Mucopolysaccharide accumulation may produce cardiac failure early in Hurler's syndrome, while more indolent valvular disease, most commonly aortic, is found in the less severe syndromes.

The use of cell cultures has permitted identification of enzyme defects in at least 12 distinct entities, most of which are autosomal recessive defects; two, including the classical Hurler's syndrome, are X-linked mutants.[68] Although effective enzyme replacement therapy is not available, intrauterine diagnosis with cultured amniotic fluid cells is now routine. Heterozygote detection is feasible with the use of enzyme detection in various tissues, including hair roots.[69]

The related autosomal recessive mucolipidoses not due to enzyme deficiencies are classified with the mucopolysaccharidoses.[68] Their clinical presentations are similar, but mucopolysacchariduria is not present. In the more severe form, mucolipidosis II, formerly called I-cell disease because of inclusions

FIGURE 35-3 The dwarfism, facial features, and bodily configuration of this child are characteristic of Hurler's syndrome, a heritable disease of mucopolysaccharide metabolism. (Courtesy of Dr. L. J. Krovetz.)

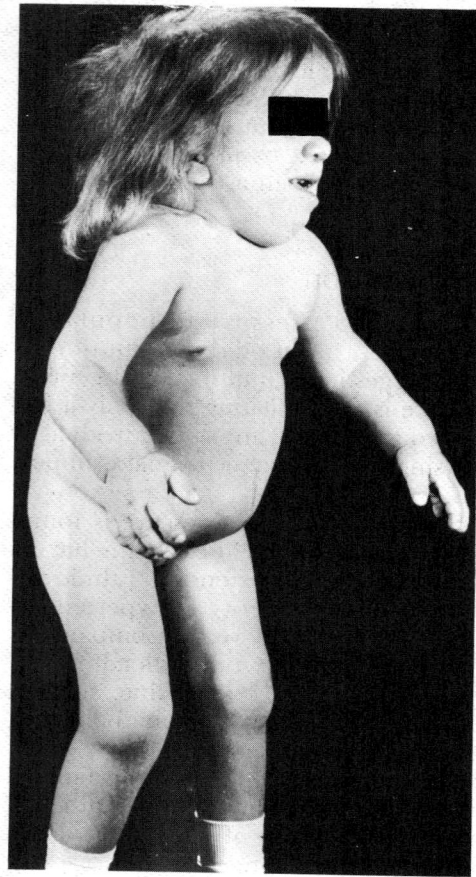

in cultured fibroblasts, heart failure is a common early manifestation. Only a modest deficiency of lysosomal hydrolases is found in cultured fibroblasts, while these enzymes are greatly increased in body fluids. It has been suggested that the defect is in packaging of the enzymes into lysosomes, perhaps because of a defect in a recognition site on the hydrolase.[70]

Connective Tissue Disorders

Research into the biochemical structure of connective tissue has confirmed the heterogeneity of Ehlers-Danlos syndrome, Marfan's syndrome, and osteogenesis imperfecta. Ehlers-Danlos syndrome has at least seven variants, with differing skin fragility, joint hypermobility, and visceral involvement. Specific enzyme deficiencies have been demonstrated in three variants, while type III collagen is deficient in the threatening Sack variety, which leads to rupture of major arteries.[71] The latter is usually inherited as a dominant disease, while sex-linked or autosomal recesssive modes are found in other variants.

Aortic dilatation and dissecting aneurysm are dominant cardiac features of Marfan's syndrome (Fig. 35-4). Although the severity of expression varies, a pattern of dominant inheritance is usual.

The cardiovascular manifestations in osteogenesis imperfecta include a billowing mitral valve and aortic dilatation; this is also a heterogeneous group.[72]

Immune-Mediated Disease

No clear-cut genetic marker for rheumatic fever has been identified. In systemic lupus erythematosus both vertical and horizontal grouping within families have been reported and concordance is high in identical twins.[73] Some heritable defects in the complement system are also associated with lupus erythematosus, additionally suggesting a strong genetic contribution. Impaired suppressor-cell function occurs in first-degree relatives of individuals with lupus erythematosus as well as the patients themselves.[74] An association of specific HLA type with lupus erythematosus has been noted, as well as a perplexing increase in antinuclear antibodies in both relatives and household contacts of individuals with this disease.[75] The development of active lupus erythematosus appears to require an environmental agent acting on a genetically prepared host.

Mulibrey Nanism

Myocardial fibrosis, pericardial constriction accompanied by calcification, in the context of multiple organ pathology is inherited in an autosomal fashion.[76] Mulibrey nanism was the name devised to indicate involvement of *mu*scle, *li*ver, *br*ain, and *ey*e.

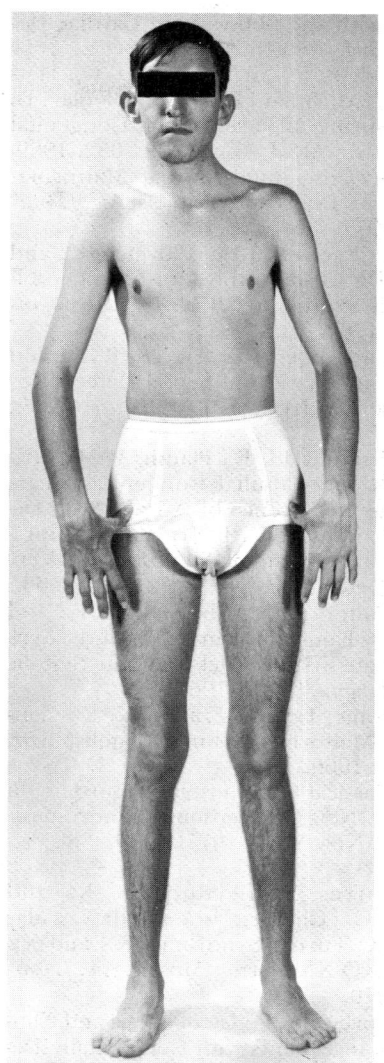

FIGURE 35-4 Absence of subcutaneous tissue, frail musculature, and scoliosis in this young man with aortic insufficiency and a cleft palate are hallmarks of Marfan's syndrome.

Gaucher's Disease

Gaucher's disease was the first disorder in which an attempt was made to administer the deficient enzyme.[77] Constrictive pericarditis and severe pulmonary hypertension may accompany the recessively inherited deficiency of glucocerebrosidase.

References

1. Mendel, G.: Experiment in Plant Hybridization, *Proceedings of the Natural History Society of Brünn,* 1865 (English translation).
2. Riggs, A. D., and Itakura, K.: Synthetic DNA and Medicine, *Am. J. Hum. Genet.,* 31:531, 1979.
3. Anderson, R. C.: Fetal and Infant Death, Twinning and Cardiac Malformations in Families of

2,000 Children with and 500 without Cardiac Defects, *Am. J. Cardiol.*, 38:218, 1976.

4. Nora, J. J., Dodd, P. F., McNamara, D. G., Hattwick, M. A. W., Leachman, R. D., and Cooley, D. A.: Risk to Offspring of Parents with Congenital Heart Defects, *J. Am. Med. Assoc.*, 209:2052, 1969.

5. Anderson, R. S.: Congenital Cardiac Malformations in 109 Sets of Twins and Triplets, *Am. J. Cardiol.*, 39:1045, 1977.

6. McKusick, V. A., Egeland, J. A., Eldridge, R., and Krusen, D. E.: Dwarfism in the Amish. I. The Ellis–van Creveld Syndrome, *Bull. Johns Hopkins Hosp.*, 115:306, 1964.

7. Lynch, H. T., Bachenberg, K., Harris, R. E., and Becker, W.: Hereditary Atrial Septal Defect. Update of a Large Kindred, *Am. J. Disease Child.*, 132:600, 1978.

8. Kahler, R. L., Braunwald, E., Plauth, W. H., Jr., and Morrow, A. G.: Familial Congenital Heart Disease: Familial Occurrence of Atrial Septal Defect with A-V Conduction Abnormalities; Supravalvular Aortic and Pulmonic Stenosis; and Ventricular Septal Defect, *Am. J. Med.*, 40:384, 1966.

9. Shell, W. E., Walton, J. A., Clifford, M. E., and Willis, P. W.: The Familial Occurrences of the Syndrome of Mid-Late Systolic Click and Late Systolic Murmur, *Circulation*, 39:327, 1969.

10. Berg, J. M., Crome, L., and France, N. E.: Congenital Cardiac Malformations in Mongolism, *Br. Heart J.*, 22:331, 1960.

*11. Gorlin, R. J.: Classical Chromosome Disorders, in J. J. Yunis (ed.), "New Chromosomal Syndromes," Academic Press, New York, 1977, p. 59. (380 references)

12. Nora, J. J., Torres, F. G., Sinha, A. K., and McNamara, D. G.: Characteristic Cardiovascular Anomalies of XO Turner Syndrome, XX and XY Phenotype and XO/XX Turner Mosaic, *Am. J. Cardiol.*, 25:639, 1970.

13. Engel, E., and Forbes, A. P.: Cytogenetic and Clinical Findings in 48 Patients with Congenitally Defective or Absent Ovaries, *Medicine*, 44:135, 1965.

14. Carter, C. O., Hamerton, J. L., Polani, P. E., Gunalp, A., and Weller, S. D. W.: Chromosome Translocation as a Cause of Familial Mongolism, *Lancet*, 2:679, 1970.

15. Boesen, I., Melchoir, J. C., Terslev, E., and Vendel, S.: Extracardiac Congenital Malformations in Children with Congenital Heart Diseases, *Acta Paediatr. (Suppl.)*, 146:28, 1963.

16. Clark, C. E., Henry, W. L., and Epstein, S. E.: Familial Prevalence and Genetic Transmission of Idiopathic Hypertrophic Subaortic Stenosis, *N. Engl. J. Med.*, 289:709, 1973.

17. Darsee, J. R., Heymsfield, S. B., and Nutter, D. O.: Hypertrophic Cardiomyopathy and Human Leukocyte Antigen Linkage. Differentiation of Two Forms of Hypertrophic Cardiomyopathy, *N. Engl. J. Med.*, 300:877, 1979.

18. Ferrans, V. J., Morrow, A. G., and Roberts, W. C.: Myocardial Ultrastructure in Idiopathic Hypertrophic Subaortic Stenosis. A Study of Operatively Excised Left Ventricular Outflow Tract Muscle in 14 Patients, *Circulation*, 45:769, 1972.

19. Zatz, M., Itskan, S. B., Sanger, R., Frota-Pessoa, O., and Saldanha, P. H.: New Linkage Data for the X-Linked Types of Muscular Dystrophy and G6PD Variants, Colour Blindness, and Xg Blood Groups, *J. Med. Genet.*, 11:321, 1974.

20. Bundery, S., and Carter, C. D.: Genetic Heterogeneity for Dystrophia Myotonica, *J. Med. Genet.*, 9:311, 1972.

21. Kark, R. A. P., Rodriguez-Budelli, M., Perlman, S., Gulley, W. F., and Toron, K.: Preclinical Diagnosis and Carrier Detection in Ataxia Associated with Abnormalities of Lipoamide Dehydrogenase, *Neurology (Minneap.)*, 30:502, 1980.

*22. Steinberg, D.: Elucidation of the Metabolic Error in Refsum's Disease: Strategy and Tactics, in R. A. P. Kark, R. N. Rosenberg, and L. J. Schut (eds.), "Advances in Neurology," Raven Press, New York, 1978, vol. 21, p. 113. (40 references)

23. Hart, Z. H., Chang, C-H., DiMauro, S., Farooki, Q., and Ayyar, R.: Muscle Carnitine Deficiency and Fatal Cardiomyopathy, *Neurology (Minneap.)*, 28:147, 1978.

24. Hohn, A. R., Lowe, C. V., Sokal, J. E., and Lambert, E. C.: Cardiac Problems in the Glycogenoses with Specific Reference to Pompe's Disease, *Pediatrics*, 35:313, 1965.

*25. Bosch, E. P., and Munsat, T. L.: Metabolic Myopathies, *Med. Clin. of N. Am.*, 63:759, 1979. (101 references)

26. Miranda, A. F., Nette, E. G., Hartlage, P. L., and DiMauro, S.: Phosphorylase Isoenzymes in Normal and Myophosphorylase-Deficient Human Heart, *Neurology (Minneap.)*, 29:1538, 1979.

*27. Stumpf, D. A.: Mitochondrial Multisystem Disorders: Clinical, Biochemical, and Morphologic Features, in H. R. Tyler and D. M. Dawson (eds.), "Current Neurology," Houghton Mifflin Professional Publishers, Medical Division, Boston, 1979, vol. 2, p. 117. (272 references)

28. Mackay, E. H., Brown, R. S., and Pickering, D.: Cardiac Biopsy in Skeletal Myopathy: Report of a Case with Myocardial Mitochondrial Abnormalities, *J. Pathol.*, 120:35, 1976.

29. Schnitzler, E. R., and Robertson, W. C., Jr.: Familial Kearns-Sayre Syndrome, *Neurology (Minneap.)*, 29:1172, 1979.

30. Waters, D. D., Nutter, D. O., Hopkins, L. C., and Dorney, E. R.: Cardiac Features of an Unusual X-Linked Humeroperoneal Neuromuscular Disease, *N. Engl. J. Med.*, 293:1017, 1975.

31. Tanaka, H., Vemura, N., Toyama, Y., Kudo, A., Okkatsu, Y., and Kanehisa, T.: Cardiac Involvement in the Kugelberg-Welander Syndrome, *Am. J. Cardiol.*, 38:528, 1976.

32. Kravitz, K., Skolnick, M., Cannings, C., Carmelli, D., Baty, B., Amos, B., Johnson, A., Mendell, N., Edwards, C., and Cartwright, G.: Genetic Linkage between Hereditary Hemochromatosis and HLA, *Am. J. Hum. Genet.*, 31:601, 1979.

33. Frederiksen, T., Gotzche, H., Harloe, N., Kiser, W., and Mellemgaard, K.: Familial Primary Amyloidosis with Severe Amyloid Heart Disease, *Am. J. Med.*, 33:328, 1962.

*This article is a review of the literature and contains additional references to the literature.

*34. Singh, A., Doyle, E. F., Danilowicz, D. A., and Finegold, J.: Familial Nonobstructive Cardiomyopathy with Endocardial Fibroelastosis Beyond Infancy, *Pediatrics*, 61:410, 1978. (27 references)

35. McCue, C. M., Mantakas, M. E., Tingelstad, J. B., and Ruddy, S.: Congenital Heart Block in Newborns of Mothers with Connective Tissue Disease, *Circulation*, 56:82, 1977.

*36. Sarchek, N. S., and Leonard, J. J.: Familial Heart Block and Sinus Bradycardia: Classification and Natural History, *Am. J. Cardiol.*, 29:451, 1972. (34 references)

37. Gould, W. L.: Auricular Fibrillation: Report on a Study of a Familial Tendency, 1920–1956, *A.M.A. Arch. Intern. Med.*, 100:916, 1957.

38. Bacos, J. M., Eagar, J. T., and Orgain, E. S.: Congenital Familial Nodal Rhythm, *Circulation*, 22:887, 1960.

39. Morooka, S., Kato, A., Murao, S., Ohsuzu, H.: A 17-Year Follow-Up Study of a Family with Idiopathic Hypertrophic Cardiomyopathy and WPW Syndrome, *Jap. Heart J.*, 19:332, 1978.

40. Jervell, A., and Lange-Neilsen, F.: Congenital Deaf-Mutism, Functional Heart Disease with Prolongation of the Q-T Interval and Sudden Death, *Am. Heart J.*, 54:59, 1957.

41. Garza, L. A., Vick, R. L., Nora, J. J., and McNamara, D. G.; Heritable Q-T Prolongation without Deafness, *Circulation*, 41:39, 1970.

42. Green, J. R., Jr., Krovetz, L. J., Shanklin, D. R., DeVito, J. J., and Taylor, W. J.: Sudden Unexpected Death in Three Generations, *A.M.A. Arch. Intern. Med.*, 124:359, 1969.

43. Slack, J., and Evans, K. A.: The Increased Risk of Death from Ischaemic Heart Disease in First Degree Relatives of 121 Men and 96 Women with Ischaemic Heart Disease, *J. Med. Genet.*, 3:239, 1966.

*44. Epstein, C. J., Martin, G. M., Schultz, A. L., and Motulsky, A. G.: Werner's Syndrome, *Medicine*, 45:177, 1966. (145 references)

45. Benditt, E. P., and Benditt, J. M.: Evidence for a Monoclonal Origin of Human Atherosclerotic Plaques, *Proc. Natl. Acad. Sci., USA*, 70:1753, 1973.

46. Thomas, W. A., Reiner, J. M., Jonakidevi, K., Florentin, R. A., and Lee, K. T.: Population Dynamics of Arterial Cells during Atherogenesis. X. Study of Monotypism in Atherosclerotic Lesions of Black Women Heterozygous for Glucose-6-Phosphate Dehydrogenase (G-6-PD), *Exp. Mol. Pathol.*, 31:367, 1979.

47. Goldstein, J. L., Brown, M. S., and Stone, N. J.: Genetics of the LDL Receptor: Evidence That the Mutations Affecting Binding and Internalization Are Allelic, *Cell*, 12:629, 1977.

48. Myant, N. B., Reichl, D., Thompson, G. R., Higgins, M. J. P., and Galton, D. J.: The Metabolism *in Vivo* and *in Vitro* of Plasma Low-Density Lipoprotein from a Subject with Inherited Hypercholesterolemia, *Clin. Sci. Mol. Med.*, 51:463, 1976.

*48a. Goldstein, J. L., and Brown, M. S.: The Low-Density Lipoprotein Pathway and Its Relation to Atherosclerosis, *Ann. Rev. Biochem.*, 46:897, 1977. (125 references)

49. Goldstein, J. L., Schrott, H. G., Hazzard, W. R., Bierman, E. L., and Motulsky, A. G.: Hyperlipi-demia in Coronary Heart Disease. II. Genetic Analysis of Lipid Levels in 176 Families and Delineation of a New Inherited Disorder, Combined Hyperlipidemia, *J. Clin. Invest.*, 52:1544, 1973.

50. Morganroth, J., Levy, R. I., and Fredrickson, D. S.: The Biochemical, Clinical, and Genetic Features of Type III Hyperlipoproteinemia, *Ann. Int. Med.*, 82:158, 1975.

51. Kwiterovich, P. D., Farah, J. R., Brown, W. V., Bachorik, P. S., Baylin, S. B., and Neill, C. A.: The Clinical, Biochemical and Familial Preservation of Type V Hyperlipoproteinemia in Childhood, *Pediatrics*, 59:513, 1977.

52. Deutscher, S., Epstein, F. H., Kjelsberg, M. D.: Familial Aggregation of Factors Associated with Coronary Heart Disease, *Circulation*, 33:911, 1966.

*53. Herbert, P. N., Gotto, A. M., and Fredrickson, D. S.: Familial Lipoprotein Deficiency (Abetalipoproteinemia, Hypobetalipoproteinemia, and Tangier Disease), in J. B. Stanbury, J. B. Wyngaarden, and D. S. Fredrickson (eds.), "The Metabolic Basis of Inherited Disease," 4th ed., McGraw-Hill Book Company, New York, 1978, p. 544. (374 references)

54. Srinivasan, S. R., Frerichs, R. R., Webber, L. S., and Berenson, G. S.: Serum Lipoprotein Profile in Children from a Biracial Community. The Bogalusa Heart Study, *Circulation*, 54:309, 1976.

*55. Rapacz, J.: Lipoprotein Immunogenetics and Atherosclerosis, *Am. J. Med. Genet.*, 1:377, 1978. (114 references)

56. Dische, M. R., and Porro, R. S.: The Cardiac Lesions of Bassen-Kornzweig Syndrome. Report of a Case with Autopsy Findings, *Am. J. Med.*, 49:568, 1970.

*57. Cudworth, A. G.: Type I Diabetes Mellitus, *Diabetologia*, 14:281, 1978. (74 references)

*58. Craighead, J. E.: Current Views on the Etiology of Insulin-Dependent Diabetes Mellitus, *N. Engl. J. Med.*, 299:1439, 1978. (68 references)

59. Tattersall, R. B., and Fajans, S. S.: A Difference between the Inheritance of Classical Juvenile-Onset and Maturity-Onset Type Diabetes of Young People, *Diabetes*, 24:44, 1975.

60. MacDonald, M. J.: The Frequencies of Juvenile Diabetes in American Blacks and Caucasians Are Consistent with Dominant Inheritance, *Diabetes*, 29:110, 1980.

61. Rotter, J. I., and Hodge, S. E.: Racial Differences in Juvenile-Type Diabetes Are Consistent with More than One Mode of Inheritance, *Diabetes*, 29:115, 1980.

62. Luft, F. C., Grim, C. E., Higgins, J. T., Jr., and Weinberger, M. H.,: Differences in Response to Sodium Administration in Normotensive White and Black Subjects, *J. Lab. Clin. Med.*, 90:555, 1977.

63. Carma, C. T., and Brasher, R. E.: Pheochromocytoma as an Inherited Abnormality, *N. Engl. J. Med.*, 263:419, 1960.

64. Wilkins, L.: Adrenal Disorders. II. Congenital Virilizing Adrenal Hyperplasia, *Arch. Dis. Child.*, 37:231, 1962.

65. Melmon, K. L., and Braunwald, E.: Familial Pulmonary Hypertension, *N. Engl. J. Med.*, 269:770, 1963.

66. Hodgson, C. H., Curchell, H. B., Good, C. A., II,

and Claggett, O. T.: Hereditary Hemorrhagic Telangiectasia and Pulmonary Arteriovenous Fistula: Survey of a Large Family, *N. Engl. J. Med.,* 261:625, 1959.

67. Ferrans, V. J., Hibbs, R. C., and Burda, C. D.: The Heart in Fabry's Disease: A Histochemical and Electronmicroscopic Study, *Am. J. Cardiol.,* 24:95, 1969.

*68. McKusick, V. A., Neufeld, E. F., and Kelly, T. E.: The Mucopolysaccharide Storage Diseases, in J. B. Stanbury, J. B. Wyngaarden, and D. S. Fredrickson (eds.), "The Metabolic Basis of Inherited Disease," 4th ed., McGraw-Hill Book Company, New York, 1978, p. 1282. (182 references)

69. Nwokoro, N., and Neufeld, E. F.: Detection of Hunter Heterozygotes by Enzymatic Analysis of Hair Roots, *Am. J. Hum. Genet.,* 31:42, 1979.

70. Hickman, S., and Neufeld, E. F.: A Hypothesis for I-Cell Disease: Defective Hydrolases That Do Not Enter Lysosomes, *Biochem, Biophys. Res. Comm.,* 49:992, 1972.

*71. Pinnell, S. R.: Disorders of Collagen, in J. B. Stanbury, J. B. Wyngaarden, D. S. Fredrickson (eds.), "The Metabolic Basis of Inherited Disease," 4th ed., McGraw-Hill Book Company, New York, 1978, p. 1366. (511 references)

72. Sillence, D. O., Senn, A., and Danks, D. M.: Genetic Heterogeneity in Osteogenesis Imperfecta, *J. Med. Genet.,* 16:101, 1979.

73. Arnett, F. C., and Shulman, L. E.: Studies in Familial Systemic Lupus Erythematosus, *Medicine,* 55:313, 1976.

74. Miller, K. B., and Schwartz, R. S.: Familial Abnormalities of Suppressor-Cell Function in Systemic Lupus Erythematosus, *N. Engl. J. Med.,* 301:803, 1979.

75. Cleland, L. G., Bell, D. A., Williams, M., and Saurino, B. C.: Familial Lupus. Family Studies of HLA and Serologic Findings, *Arthritis Rheum.,* 21:183, 1978.

76. Perheentupa, J., Aurio, S., Leisti, S., Raitta, C., and Tuuteri, L.: Mulibrey Nanism, Autosomal Recessive Syndrome with Pericardial Constriction, *Lancet,* 2;351, 1973.

*77. Brady, R. O.: Glucosyl Ceramide Lipidosis: Gaucher's Disease, in J. B. Stanbury, J. B. Wyngaarden, D. S. Fredrickson (eds.), "The Metabolic Basis of Inherited Disease," 4th Edition, McGraw-Hill Book Company, New York, 1978, p. 731. (98 references)

Section A Congenital Heart Disease

36

The Pathology, Abnormal Physiology, Clinical Recognition, and Medical and Surgical Treatment of Congenital Heart Disease

William H. Plauth, Jr., M.D.
Elizabeth W. Nugent, M.D.
Robert C. Schlant, M.D.
Jesse E. Edwards, M.D.
Willis H. Williams, M.D.
John W. Kirklin, M.D.

Incidence and Etiology

The incidence of congenital heart disease in the United States is approximately 8 per 1000 live births. The incidence among stillbirths is higher, but cardiac malformations are not accorded a significant role in fetal death.[1,2] Most of the infants born alive with cardiac defects will have anomalies that do not represent a threat to life, at least during infancy. Almost one-third, or 2.6 per 1000 live births, however, will have *critical disease*, defined as a malformation severe enough to result in cardiac catheterization, cardiac surgery, or death within the first year of life.[3] Two decades ago, the majority of these infants died within the first year of life with almost two-thirds of the deaths occurring within the first 4 weeks.[4] Today, with early detection, prompt referral, emergency cardiac catheterization, and remark-

able advances in operative and perioperative management, 60 percent of infants with critical disease can be expected to survive the first year of life.[3] Most of these survivors have malformations that have been or can be corrected by currently available surgical techniques. Therefore, the outlook for most children with congenital heart disease is quite good, even for those who are symptomatic within the first weeks of life.

Estimates of the incidence of specific lesions vary depending upon whether the data are drawn from infants or older children and upon whether the diagnosis is based on clinical, catheterization, surgical, or postmortem studies (Table 36-1). Hoffman has reviewed the problems of assessing incidence and natural history of congenital heart disease.[5] In a collaborative prospective study[1] of 56,109 total births at 12 medical centers in the United States, the diagnosis was verified by autopsy, surgery, or cardiac catheterization in 56 percent. In another prospective study[2] of 19,502 births among members of a health plan in the United States, the diagnosis was made by these methods in 48 percent with cumulative incidence increasing from 3.3 per 1000 at birth to 7.8 per 1000 at 1 year of age to 9.1 per 1000 at 5 years of age. The New England study[3] was also prospective, but it included only symptomatic infants to 1 year of age. Diagnosis was established by catheterization, surgery, or postmortem examination in all except 0.7 percent who died before any intervention and did not have autopsies performed. In the large series of 10,624 reported by Nadas,[4] 76 percent were diagnosed by catheterization, surgery, or postmorten examination. Incidence in other countries is remarkably similar to that reported for the United States.[6]

Despite these differences in case material, it is apparent that except for bicuspid aortic valve when older patients are included, ventricular septal defect is the most common malformation, occurring in about 30 percent of all patients with congenital heart disease (Table 36-1). Pulmonary stenosis, pat-

DISEASES OF THE HEART AND BLOOD VESSELS

TABLE 36-1   Incidence of Specific Lesions of Congenital Heart Disease

Lesion	Keith[6]	Nadas[4]	Collaborative Study[1]	Hoffman[2]	New England Study[3]
VSD	28.3	19.4	29.5	31.3	16.6
PS	9.9	7.5	8.6	13.5	3.5
PDA	9.8	15.5	8.3	5.5	6.5
ASD, secundum	7.0	4.5	7.4	6.1	3.1
VSD with PS*	9.7	10.5	6.4	3.7	9.4
AS	7.1	5.7	3.8	3.7	2.0
AO atresia	1.5	NL	3.1	0.6	7.9
AVC†	3.4	2.7	3.6	3.7	5.3
Coarctation AO	5.1	8.1	2.6	5.5	8.0
Peripheral PS	NL	1.0	3.6	NL	NL
EFE	0.9	NL	2.4	NL	NL
TGA	4.9	4.0	2.6	3.7	10.5
Truncus arteriosus	0.7	0.8	1.7	2.5	1.5
TAPVC	1.4	1.3	NL	0.6	2.8
Tricuspid atresia	1.2	1.0	1.2	NL	2.7
DORV	0.5	0.2	1.0	0.6	1.6
Pulmonary atresia without VSD	0.7	0.3	0.01	0.6	3.3
Number of patients	15,104	10,624	56,109	19,502	2,251

*Includes tetralogy of Fallot.
†Includes partial and complete.
Notes: NL = not listed; VSD = ventricular septal defect; PS = pulmonary stenosis; PDA = patent ductus arteriosus; ASD = atrial septal defect; AS = aortic stenosis; AVC = atrioventricular canal; AO = aorta; EFE = endocardial fibroelastosis; TGA = transposition of great arteries; TAPVC = total anomalous pulmonary venous connection; DORV = double-outlet right ventricle.

ent ductus arteriosus, atrial septal defect, tetralogy of Fallot, aortic stenosis, coarctation of the aorta, and transposition of the great arteries are also relatively common. These eight defects, including ventricular septal defect, constitute approximately 75 percent of all congenital heart disease in infants and children.

Of 2251 infants with critical congenital heart disease in the New England study,[3] 53.7 percent were male. Certain defects, however, are considerably more common in one sex than the other. The incidence among blacks does not differ significantly from that among white patients.[1] A seasonal influence on the incidence of certain defects has been demonstrated.[7]

The most popular concept regarding etiology is that cardiac defects are due to a combination of genetic and environmental interactions. This multifactorial etiology requires a genetic predisposition, probably polygenic, and an environmental teratogen to which the susceptible fetus is exposed in a critical or vulnerable period.[8,9] The incidence among siblings of those with congenital heart disease has been reported as 17 per 1000 compared to an incidence in the general population in the same series of only 7.6 per 1000 live births.[10] Genetic and environmental counseling for families with congenital heart disease is now a reality[9,11] (see Chap. 35).

Some examples of congenital heart disease can occur on a primarily genetic basis. Major chromosomal abnormalities such as trisomy, deletion, and mosaicism have an increased incidence of associated cardiac defects. Down's syndrome is a well-known example. Mendelian inheritance can be demonstrated in a few families with repeated occurrences of specific cardiac abnormalities, such as atrial septal defect or congenital atrioventricular block, which may be associated with other noncardiac anomalies.

Environmental factors can cause certain defects. Congenital heart disease, predominantly patent ductus arteriosus and peripheral pulmonary stenosis, in association with noncardiac abnormalities, can occur as a consequence of intrauterine rubella.[6] On the other hand, the aggressive management of very small premature infants, with a resultant increase in survival, has led to new and serious problems with patent ductus arteriosus, particularly when associated with respiratory distress.

Fetal Circulation and the Transition to the Neonatal and Adult Circulation[12–23]

Prior to birth, the fetus obtains all of its nutritional requirements, including oxygen, by the placental circulation. Consequently, there is a need for a high blood flow to the placenta, but there is no need to pass most of the blood through the uninflated fetal lungs. The fetal circulation accomplishes its special function with the aid of the following three vascular channels, all of which normally disappear after birth: (1) the *foramen ovale* in the atrial septum allows blood to pass from the right atrium to the left atrium in utero; (2) the *ductus arteriosus*, which develops from the dorsal part of the sixth left branchial arch, connects the relatively large pulmonary artery to the aorta about 5 to 10 mm distal to the origin of the left subclavian artery and enables most of the blood reaching the pulmonary artery to bypass the uninflated lungs; and (3) the *ductus venosus* shunts blood returning from the placenta in the umbilical cord by the liver to the inferior vena cava.

In the developed fetus, the total return of blood to the heart in the inferior vena cava is equal to 65 to 70 percent of the combined ventricular output (CVO); of this volume an amount equal to 25 to 28 percent of CVO passes through the foramen ovale to the left atrium, where it is joined by 5 to 10 percent of CVO returning from the lungs. The left ventricle thus receives and ejects only 33 percent of the CVO of the fetal heart. The preferential shunting of inferior vena cava blood to the left atrium is guided by the *crista dividens*, which is the lower rim of the septum secundum and which projects over the upper margin of the inferior vena cava. The remaining 38 to 42 percent of CVO returning in the inferior vena cava mixes with most of the 22 to 25 percent of CVO that returns in the superior vena cava and goes into the right ventricle, which thus receives and ejects about 66 percent of the CVO of the fetal heart prior to delivery. About 85 to 90 percent of the blood ejected by the right ventricle, or about 60 percent of the CVO, is diverted from the lungs through the ductus arteriosus to the aorta. Only 3 to 4 percent of the CVO passes through the pulmonary circulation from 0.4 to 0.7 gestation, but this increases progressively to 8 to 10 percent at term.[18] Prior to birth about 40 to 50 percent of the CVO goes to the placenta for the exchange of carbon dioxide, oxygen, and other metabolites. The CVO of the fetal lamb near term is about 5000 ml/kg/min; after birth the CVO decreases about 25 percent.[13]

Umbilical venous blood has a P_{O_2} of about 30 to 35 mmHg and an O_2 saturation of about 80 percent. As the result of the various mechanisms described above, fetal arterial blood in the ascending aorta has a P_{O_2} of about 26 to 28 mmHg and an O_2 saturation of 55 to 60 percent.

During delivery of the fetus, the umbilical cord is usually somewhat compressed, and the placenta may begin to separate. Simultaneously, the newborn baby is suddenly exposed to a cold, strange environment. Both the asphyxia and the cold environment are strong respiratory stimuli and the baby usually begins to breathe soon after birth. Within seconds after expansion of the lungs with air, the tremendous increase in blood flow to the lungs takes over the function of gas exchange from the placental circulation. Clamping or tying of the umbilical cord or, in natural childbirth, vasoconstriction of the umbilical arteries soon removes the placental circulation,

which had received about 40 to 50 percent of the combined ventricular output in utero. The acute decrease in placental blood flow markedly increases arterial resistance and decreases blood return from the inferior vena cava with a subsequent decrease in right atrial pressure.

The calculated fetal pulmonary vascular resistance is very high, about 6 mmHg/min/ml at 0.4 gestation, but falls progressively to 0.3 to 0.35 mmHg/min/ml at term. The marked decrease in resistance during gestation is probably due mainly to the growth of new pulmonary blood vessels.

The initial fall in pulmonary vascular resistance after birth is produced by two mechanisms. The first of these is a mechanical reduction in vascular resistance due to the physical expansion of lungs with air with a resultant decrease in the kinking and compression of the pulmonary vessels. The second and main mechanism is a marked diminution in the pulmonary arterial vasoconstriction related to the increased alveolar and interstitial P_{O_2}. It is not known whether oxygen exerts its vasodilator effect directly by causing relaxation of the smooth muscle in the pulmonary vasculature or whether it stimulates the release of a chemical mediator. Bradykinin may be involved as a supplementary mechanism in the immediate pulmonary vasodilatation after birth, but not thereafter since kinin blood concentration falls rapidly within the first hour after ventilation of fetal lambs. Distension of the lungs of adult animals results in the release of prostaglandins; the lungs produce predominantly prostaglandins of the E series. There is suggestive evidence that prostacycline (PGI_2) is involved in the fall in pulmonary vascular resistance associated with ventilation and distension of the newborn lungs.[15] In addition, the fetal pulmonary circulation is influenced by the autonomic nervous system, and it is possible that reflex autonomic effects contribute to the changes in pulmonary vascular resistance.

After birth, the pulmonary vascular resistance initially falls very rapidly and reaches adult levels by about 6 to 8 weeks after birth. During this time, there is a rapid regression of the medial muscle layer of the pulmonary arteries and arterioles. Infants who are born at high altitude with a decreased partial pressure of oxygen may fail to have the normal decrease in pulmonary vascular resistance or regression of pulmonary arterial smooth muscle after birth. On the other hand, premature infants, in whom the pulmonary vascular smooth muscle is less well developed, may have a much more rapid fall in pulmonary vascular resistance after birth than the full-term infant. In the presence of a patent ductus arteriosus or ventricular septal defect, this may permit the early onset of a large left-to-right shunt and heart failure. In infants with persistent pulmonary hypertension (persistent fetal circulation), prostacycline (PGI_2) may be used to lower pulmonary vascular resistance.[21] There is a further decrease in total pulmonary vascular resistance associated with growth of the lungs for several years.

Prior to birth the foramen ovale is held open by the large flow of blood from the inferior vena cava to the left atrium. After birth, the left atrial pressure increases due to the increase in pulmonary flow and the increase in systemic arterial resistance while the right atrial pressure decreases. These changes in left and right atrial pressure produce functional closure of the foramen ovale by the apposition of the valve of the foramen ovale, the septum primum, against the edge of the crista dividens. The septum primum usually becomes adherent with permanent closure in several months. In 15 to 20 percent of normal adults, however, a small opening or potential opening may persist. Rarely, this can allow a significant acquired left-to-right shunt if there is marked bulging and stretching of the septum associated with left atrial enlargement.

Prior to delivery, patency of the ductus arteriosus is probably an active condition produced by a prostaglandin formed intramurally. PGE_2, which is mainly degraded in the lungs, is a likely candidate for this role; its action may be complemented by that of PGI_2.

The ductus arteriosus usually is functionally closed 10 to 15 h after birth in a normal full-term infant, with complete closure within 10 to 21 days. The trigger for closure of the ductus arteriosus after birth is the postnatal rise in arterial P_{O_2} or oxygen tension. It is not clear, however, whether the effect of oxygen is exerted directly on the smooth-muscle cells of the ductus or whether other vasoactive agents are involved. Prostaglandins are probably involved, although the exact mechanism is not known. Several possible mechanisms have been suggested.[22] Patency of the ductus for several days after birth is relatively easy to detect by auscultation in calves, sheep, or foals. Patency in human infants is more difficult to detect, although occasional, intermittent patency can be demonstrated by special techniques. After birth, most of the flow through a ductus is probably from aorta to pulmonary artery; it may be bidirectional or even reversed, particularly if there is respiratory distress or crying.

Prior to birth, the pulmonary and systemic circuits are in communication by the relatively large ductus arteriosus. Consequently, the systolic pressures in both the ventricles, the aorta, and the pulmonary artery are almost identical. The pressures in the pulmonary artery and aorta increase progressively during gestation. The pressures are approximately 30 mmHg above amniotic cavity pressure at 0.4 gestation and increase to about 50 mmHg at term.[23] In association with the abrupt fall in pulmonary vascular resistance shortly after birth and the closure of the ductus arteriosus, the pulmonary artery pressure decreases, at first rather abruptly, to a mean pressure of about 20 to 30 mmHg; thereafter it decreases more slowly until it reaches normal childhood values in a few weeks.[13]

Although the right and the left ventricles are about the same thickness at birth, the markedly increased load on the left ventricle after birth causes it rapidly to increase in thickness and weight during the first few weeks after birth. The increase in left ventricular mass at this age is predominantly due to hyperplasia with an increase in the number of cells rather than to hypertrophy of individual cells. Since the right ventricular mass remains stable during this period, the ratio of left to right ventricular weights increases rapidly for 1 to 2 weeks and then increases more slowly. Interestingly, the electrocardiographic evidence of right ventricular predominance frequently persists for several months or even years after the development of anatomic left ventricular predominance.

Persistence of Fetal Circulation

Persistent fetal circulation,[24] or persistent pulmonary hypertension, in the newborn results in right-to-left shunting through the patent foramen ovale and/or patent ductus arteriosus. It most commonly occurs in full-term infants. The severe hypoxia is usually manifested in the first few hours of life with tachypnea, acidosis, and a chest roentgenogram that shows diminished vascular flow but no evidence of pulmonary parenchymal disease. Physical examination may reveal a parasternal heave, a loud second heart sound, and a systolic murmur.

Polycythemia, transient myocardial ischemia from hypoglycemia, and cyanotic congenital cardiac defects must be excluded. An oxygen level greater in the right radial artery than in the umbilical artery confirms right-to-left shunting through the ductus. Contrast echocardiography from a vein draining the upper segment of the body will demonstrate the right-to-left shunt at atrial level.

Initial treatment includes an increase in the inspired oxygen level and correction of acidosis with sodium bicarbonate. Frequently artificial ventilation is required. Hyperventilation[25] to diminish the partial pressure of carbon dioxide is often successful in lowering the pulmonary pressure and diminishing the right-to-left shunt. This may be monitored by an indwelling pulmonary arterial catheter in very critically ill newborns. Intravenous infusion of tolazoline[26] into the upper segment of the body to enhance flow to the lungs or directly into the pulmonary artery may be beneficial in those patients refractory to the other measures. Hypotension can be avoided to some extent by volume expansion as necessary. Gastrointestinal bleeding is a frequent complication of tolazoline.

Untreated, a majority of these infants will die of problems related to the hypoxia; survival is greatly improved by medical treatment.

Similar hemodynamic alterations may also be seen in premature infants with respiratory distress syndrome and other newborns with parenchymal lung disease. They require treatment specifically aimed at the underlying lung disease as well as the above measures.

Complications of Congenital Heart Disease

Congestive Heart Failure

Congestive heart failure is a common and serious complication of congenital heart disease, occurring in one patient in five at one time or another, usually within the first year of life.[27] In infants with congenital heart disease severe enough to produce death or require cardiac catheterization or surgery within the first year, over 80 percent have congestive failure as a major component of their illness.[28]

In general the onset of congestive failure is a phenomenon of the first year of life, the first 6 months in particular. Although heart failure may persist for many months or even years, its onset after 1 year of age is rare without a serious intercurrent problem such as infective endocarditis, pneumonia, anemia, arrhythmia, carditis, or cardiomyopathy. It is very important that failure be recognized in its earliest stages since it is frequently progressive in the infant, sometimes very rapidly so.

The time of onset of heart failure may provide a clue both to the type of lesion responsible and the degree of urgency for evaluation and treatment. Heart failure within the first 12 to 18 h of life is usually due to malformations that involve volume overload independent of pulmonary flow, such as severe tricuspid, pulmonary, aortic, or mitral regurgitation. Rarely, endocardial fibroelastosis or myocarditis may produce heart failure from the time of birth as may congenital complete heart block or supraventricular tachycardia. To be distinguished from primary cardiac disease at this time is the volume overload from a systemic arteriovenous fistula or severe polycythemia and depressed myocardial contractility from neonatal asphyxia, hypocalcemia, hypoglycemia, anemia, or sepsis.

The majority of infants presenting with severe heart failure during the remainder of the first week have critical obstruction to systemic arterial flow which, in many cases, is unmasked by narrowing or closure of the ductus arteriosus. Examples are aortic atresia, coarctation of the aorta, interruption of the aortic arch, and critical aortic stenosis. During the second week of life aortic coarctation and aortic atresia remain the most common causes of heart failure, but ventricular septal defect, transposition of the great arteries with a ventricular septal defect, and truncus arteriosus, malformations which require a pulmonary vascular bed with a reduced vascular resistance for full expression of their severity, make their appearance. During the third week and thereafter, ventricular septal defect is the primary cause of congestive failure followed by transposition, coarctation, complete atrioventricular canal,

and patent ductus arteriosus.[3] Less common malformations such as aortopulmonary window, double outlet right ventricle, single ventricle and total anomalous pulmonary venous return with mild pulmonary venous obstruction can be expected to follow a course similar to that of a large ventricular septal defect or complete atrioventricular canal.

Congestive failure in the infant may be fulminant and often is associated with respiratory tract infections. The most common symptom is difficulty in breathing. Rapid, grunting, or gasping breathing may be described in addition to breathlessness with breast or bottle feeding. Poor weight gain is the rule. Observation of the undisturbed infant will reveal tachypnea and dyspnea, recognized by nasal flaring and sub- or intercostal retractions, except in those rare instances of isolated right ventricular failure. A respiratory rate consistently above 60 is abnormal and rates in the range of 90 to 100 are not uncommon when failure is present. Wheezing may be observed. Neck vein distension is difficult to see in infants, but jugular venous pulsations can be seen above the clavicle in a few of the more slender infants if they are propped or held upright while sleeping. Edema, if present, usually is found in the periorbital area and on the dorsum of the feet and hands. Cool, moist skin, a subdued, rapid arterial pulse, and a liver edge 2 or more centimeters below the right costal margin are common signs of congestive failure in infancy. A gallop rhythm, pulmonary rales, and expiratory wheezes may be present. It may be difficult to distinguish the pulmonary findings of heart failure from those of pneumonia or bronchiolitis, and, indeed, many infants have both heart failure and concurrent pulmonary infection. Cardiac enlargement will be confirmed by chest roentgenogram. Infants with malformations such as total anomalous pulmonary venous connection, anomalous left coronary artery arising from the main pulmonary artery, or endocardial fibroelastosis, which are abnormalities usually not characterized by an impressive murmur, sometimes are referred only after weeks of tachypnea and failure to thrive or when a chest roentgenogram, taken to explore the possibility of lung disease, has revealed cardiac enlargement.

Hospitalization is recommended for the initial management of all infants in congestive failure with the possible exception of older infants with very mild failure associated with a typical ventricular septal defect or ductus arteriosus without evidence of pulmonary arterial hypertension. Breathing is made easier by elevation of the head and chest to an angle of approximately 30°. Administration of humidified oxygen by techniques that do not disturb the infant will help relieve dyspnea and cyanosis. Arterialized capillary or arterial P_{O_2} levels should be monitored in the newborn, particularly the premature, to avoid the risk of retrolental fibroplasia. Rest, aided by sedation with morphine 0.05 to 0.1 mg/kg intramuscularly, or chloral hydrate 50 mg/kg orally or rec-

DISEASES OF THE HEART AND BLOOD VESSELS

tally, is beneficial. With severe heart failure fluid intake should be restricted to 65 ml/kg/day for at least the first 24 h. With dyspnea or vomiting, oral feedings should be temporarily suspended and fluid requirements administered intravenously. When feedings are resumed, a formula low in sodium should be used (Table 36-2).[29] Abnormalities such as anemia, acidosis, hypoglycemia, or hypocalcemia should be sought and corrected. Serum sodium, potassium, BUN, and creatinine concentrations should also be determined. Because of the difficulty of recognizing the presence of infection in these very sick infants, a low threshold for the administration of antibiotics is appropriate.

Digitalis remains the most important medication for the management of congestive failure in infants and children. Digoxin is the form of digitalis used most commonly because of its excellent absorption when given orally, rapid onset of action, relatively rapid excretion, and convenience of administration. The recommended doses for daily oral maintenance therapy in milligrams per kilogram per day are given in Table 36-3. The daily dose is divided into two equal parts given as close to 12 h apart as is convenient for the family's schedule. The total oral digitalizing dose is three times the daily oral maintenance dose. Half of the digitalizing dose may be given initially, followed by the remaining two-quarters at 6-, 8-, or 12-h intervals depending upon the desired speed of total digitalization. Maintenance therapy may then be started 8 to 12 h after the last digitalizing dose. In less urgent situations, usually in an outpatient setting, full digitalization may be accomplished over an 8-day period by giving daily maintenance doses without an initial loading dose. In the severely ill infant, with depressed perfusion and unpredictable absorption, digitalization by the intravenous route is recommended. The parenteral dose of digoxin is approximately 75 percent of the oral dose for both full digitalization and maintenance therapy. The doses recommended in Table 36-3 are intended for patients with severe congestive heart failure but with normal renal function.

TABLE 36-2   Sodium and Potassium Concentrations in Milk and Infant Formulas

	Sodium, meq/liter	Potassium, meq/liter
Human milk	7	14
SMA-20	7	14
Similac PM 60/40	7	15
Similac-20	10	18
Enfamil-20	12	18
Isomil	13	18
Nutramigen	14	17
Cow's milk	25	35
Pedialyte	30	20

Source: "Composition of Foods," Agriculture Handbook No. 8, U.S. Department of Agriculture, 1963.

TABLE 36-3   Recommended Doses for Digoxin

Age	Daily Oral* Maintenance Dose†, mg/kg/day‡	Total Oral Digitalizing Dose, mg/kg
Premature:		
<1250 g	0.006	0.018
>1250 g	0.010	0.030
Newborn:	0.015	0.045
2 days–2 years	0.020	0.060
2–5 years	0.020–0.015	0.060–0.045
5–10 years	0.015–0.010	0.045–0.030
10–15 years	0.010–0.005	0.030–0.015
Adult	0.004–0.005	0.012–0.015

*Parenteral dose is 75 percent of the oral dose.
†Digitalizing dose is three times daily maintenance.
‡It is recommended that the daily dose be divided into two equal doses given every 12 h in the hospital and twice daily at home with approximately 12 h between doses, depending upon the family schedule.

Impaired renal function will lead to digoxin accumulation and toxicity, so the initial and maintenance doses should be adjusted accordingly.[30] Toxicity usually occurs within the first week of therapy. Its presence is considered likely with the appearance of anorexia, nausea, or vomiting or electrocardiographic evidence of premature ventricular contractions, ventricular tachycardia, atrioventricular dissociation, supraventricular tachycardia with atrioventricular block, or second-degree atrioventricular block. When any one of these occurs, digoxin is stopped and the serum digoxin level determined. Toxicity is probable if the level exceeds 3.0 ng/ml in the infant below 6 months of age or 2.0 ng/ml in the infant or child 6 months of age or older. Toxicity is considered confirmed if the symptoms or arrhythmia disappear after digoxin is withheld. We try to keep serum digoxin levels near but below 2.5 ng/ml in infants under 6 months of age and near but below 2.0 ng/ml in older infants and children.[31] Instructions for digoxin therapy at home should be written out in detail for the parents by the physician so that there is no confusion about the dose, schedule, or signs of toxicity. Warning should be given to prevent accidental ingestion by the patient or other children. If the need for digoxin continues, the dose is adjusted gradually as the patient grows and gains weight.

The diuretics furosemide (Lasix) or ethacrynic acid (Edecrin), used intravenously in doses of 1.0 mg/kg or orally in doses of 2.0 mg/kg, are very effective in the acute management of congestive failure. With severe congestive failure the dose of either drug may be increased by 1.0 mg/kg increments intravenously if no urinary response has been achieved after 45 min. For long-term oral diuretic therapy 2.0 mg/kg once daily, or if necessary, twice daily, is recommended. Since hypokalemia and hypochloremia can be induced with these potent diuretics, potassium supplementation is recommended, particularly in the presence of concomitant digitalis therapy. A total daily oral supplement of potassium chloride in the range of 1.0 to 1.5 meq/kg is recommended with adjustment depending upon the serum level. The serum potassium should not be allowed to fall below 3.5 meq/liter. Chlorothiazide (Diuril), a slightly less potent diuretic but with a longer duration of action, may be given orally in a dose of 20 to 40 mg/kg/day. If used alone, potassium supplements should be given. Spironolactone (Aldactone), an aldosterone antagonist, has proved useful in supplementing the diuresis and preventing the hypokalemia induced by the diuretics described above.[32] It may be given orally in a single daily dose of 2 to 3 mg/kg in combination with chlorothiazide, furosemide, or ethacrynic acid. A regimen of spironolactone, 2 mg/kg given every day, and chlorothiazide, 20 mg/kg given on alternate days, has been our preference for long-term diuretic therapy in most infants. This regimen is adequate for all but the most severe degrees of heart failure and does not require potassium supplementation. With more severe heart failure chlorothiazide may be given daily, the dose of both diuretics increased, or furosemide may be added. Under these circumstances potassium supplementation usually is necessary.

In emergency situations it may be necessary to provide an immediate inotropic stimulus to the heart. This may be accomplished by the intravenous administration of sympathomimetic amines in the form of isoproterenol, epinephrine, or dopamine by constant infusion pump. Isoproterenol (Isuprel), in a dose of 0.1 μg/kg/min, exerts a powerful inotropic effect, but its usefulness generally is limited by the induced tachycardia and peripheral vasodilatation, sometimes to the detriment of renal perfusion. Epinephrine in a dose of 0.1 to 1.0 μg/kg/min or dopamine in a dose of 5 to 15 μg/kg/min generally has been more helpful, with dopamine usually providing more adequate renal flow.[33] Systemic arterial blood pressure, urinary output, and the electrocardiogram should be monitored continuously. Vasodilator therapy in the form of intravenous sodium nitroprusside (Nipride) may be of considerable help in selected patients with severe congestive failure (see also Chaps. 22 and 23). The infusion rate at the start should be no greater than 0.5 μg/kg/min but may be increased gradually to 4.0 μg/kg/min to achieve the desired effect. Systemic arterial pressure should be monitored continuously to detect serious hypotension. Experience with the oral vasodilators hydralazine or prazosin in infants and children is limited to date, but preliminary reports suggest that vasodilator therapy may prove as beneficial in the pediatric age range as it has in adults with severe heart failure.[34]

Infants with potentially exhausting respiratory effort or with hypoxia or hypercapnia secondary to pulmonary edema or respiratory failure will benefit from endotracheal intubation and ventilation on a volume-controlled, positive pressure respirator, usually with the addition of positive end-expiratory pressure. These measures may permit additional therapy, cardiac catheterization, and surgical intervention with a much greater margin of safety. In patients with coarctation of the aorta or interruption of the aortic arch, in whom deterioration may be related to ductal closure, infusion of prostaglandin E₁ in a dose of 0.1 μg/kg/min usually will provide at least temporary relief sufficient to permit diagnosis and surgical treatment.

The response of heart failure to therapy should be documented by serial recordings of heart and respiratory rate, arterial pressure, urinary output, and body weight, and less objective criteria such as skin color and temperature, vigor and appetite. Note should be made of the regression of such initial abnormalities as cyanosis, gallop rhythm, pulmonary rales, liver and cardiac enlargement, and pulmonary venous congestion. Frequent review of the electrocardiogram and serum sodium and potassium, and periodic reappraisal of the blood glucose, calcium, hemoglobin, and blood gases also are indicated. A clear record of the patient's medications and the route and frequency of their administration is essential to avoid either under- or overtreatment or toxicity. A flow sheet for recording the above observations is recommended.

Finally, there will be infants and children in whom medical therapy is clearly inadequate or only temporarily successful. These patients will require surgical intervention for control or relief of their heart failure. There are exceptions, but, as a rule, the earlier the onset of congestive failure the more likely will be the need for surgery. At the very outset, consideration should be given to the logistics involved with surgical therapy as well as the prerequisite diagnostic studies, such as cardiac catheterization, so that these procedures may be carried out just as soon as optimal improvement or stability has been achieved.

Cyanosis

Cyanosis is one of the more frequent initial signs of congenital heart disease in the infant, but it may also be an early sign of pulmonary, central nervous system, or metabolic disease or of methemoglobinemia. The advent of nonsurgical palliation with prostaglandin,[35] as well as the rapid development of surgical techniques particularly for infants, makes prompt distinction between cardiac and noncardiac cyanosis even more important.

Respiratory distress syndrome of the newborn occurs most frequently in the premature infant, the infant of a diabetic mother, or the infant delivered by cesarean section. The cyanosis is almost invariably preceded by tachypnea and retraction of the chest wall, frequently with grunting respirations. The infant with cyanosis due to congenital heart disease may be tachypneic but otherwise appears comfortable unless the cyanosis is severe and prolonged with development of acidosis. In the infant with respiratory distress syndrome, there may be a striking parasternal lift, hepatomegaly, rales, a systolic murmur, and cardiomegaly later. Chest roentgenograms may show the characteristic reticulogranular appearance of the lungs and "air bronchograms" due to hypoaeration. Right-to-left shunting can occur through the foramen ovale and ductus arteriosus as well as in the lungs. With improvement in the lung disease, there is better oxygenation and a reduction in pulmonary vascular resistance. The right-to-left shunt diminishes in response.

The infant with cyanosis secondary to disease of the central nervous system will have other neurological manifestations. Periodic breathing and peripheral vasomotor instability found in the normal newborn may be accentuated. In methemoglobinemia, blood exposed to air will retain a brownish color instead of becoming a normal bright red. The syndrome of persistent fetal circulation is very important since it may be the most difficult to distinguish from cyanotic forms of congenital heart disease. Two-dimensional echocardiography is very helpful in distinguishing cyanotic heart disease[36] from other causes of cyanosis.

Cyanosis in congenital heart disease may be due to heart failure with pulmonary edema rather than intracardiac right-to-left shunting. Measurement of the partial pressure of oxygen with the infant breathing 100% oxygen can help since the hypoxia due to heart failure or lung disease with intrapulmonary shunting[37] will usually respond dramatically to oxygen administration, whereas that due to cyanotic defects will not. Low cardiac output and peripheral vasoconstriction can cause a grayish discoloration due to the underlying pallor, rather than typical cyanosis.

The "5 Ts" and "2 ATs" may be used to remember the most common cardiac defects causing cyanosis. These are *t*ransposition of the great arteries, *t*etralogy of Fallot, *t*ricuspid atresia, *t*otal anomalous pulmonary venous connection, *t*runcus arteriosus, aortic *at*resia, and pulmonary *at*resia.

The normal term newborn infant has a hemoglobin concentration of 17 to 21 g/dl. This normally drops to 10.4 to 12.2 g/dl by 3 months of age and then slowly rises to 12 to 13 g/dl by 2 years.[38] Systemic arterial desaturation will result in polycythemia with a higher hemoglobin level after the newborn period.

Cyanosis will lead to clubbing, which appears after the age of 3 months, initially as fullness at the base of the thumbnail with obliteration of the normal concavity. Tachypnea and dyspnea may be due to desaturation and are exaggerated with exercise. Squatting may also occur. Paroxysms of increased cyanosis, as seen in tetralogy of Fallot, can occur with an increase in the rate and depth of respiration without obstruction to airflow. Failure to gain weight is usually an indication of heart failure and not of cyanosis alone unless the hypoxia is extreme.[39]

The complications of cyanosis, to a large extent, result from polycythemia and paradoxical embolism. In those with prolonged polycythemia, the resultant hyperuricemia can precipitate a secondary form of gout.[40] Most frequently the central nervous system is the target organ, with cerebrovascular accidents and brain abscess occurring[6] due to the effects of polycythemia and paradoxical embolism, especially in the setting of dehydration or excessive temperatures. Paradoxical embolism is a potential complication whenever a right-to-left shunt exists. An infected venous thrombus or unfiltered blood during a bacteremia can cause a cerebral abscess. Brain abscess is rare under 2 years of age and occurs most frequently in patients with tetralogy of Fallot and transposition of the great arteries. The incidence and mortality are directly related to the degree of hypoxia.[41] Thrombosis, embolism, and hemorrhage can cause cerebrovascular accidents. Venous thrombosis is a common finding at autopsy, particularly in tetralogy of Fallot or transposition of the great arteries. A majority of instances occur in infants up to 1 year of age with relatively few after 4 or 5 years of age. The younger patients very frequently have relative iron deficiency anemia, whereas the older patients have polycythemia.[42,43] Recent rheological studies have demonstrated impaired deformability of microcytic erythrocytes.[44]

Disturbances in hemostasis also occur with polycythemia.[6] Coagulation factors are commonly abnormal in patients with hematocrits in excess of 60 percent.[45,46] Actual platelet counts may be normal, but they can be increased initially in some with subsequent decreases related to persistent and worsening desaturation.[47] There is evidence of shortened platelet survival time in patients with cyanotic heart disease.[48] Laboratory evaluation of coagulation status requires that correction be made for the diminished volume of plasma and the volume of anticoagulant used in the blood samples to avoid false results.

The major consequences of cyanosis can be avoided in many instances with advances in management. Prevention of iron deficiency by dietary supplementation in infants and of excessive polycythemia by surgical intervention in children should decrease the number of cerebrovascular accidents. Surgical correction under 2 years of age for defects amenable to early correction can help prevent the occurrence of brain abscess.

Pulmonary Arterial Hypertension and Pulmonary Vascular Obstructive Disease

Pulmonary arterial hypertension (PAH) and pulmonary vascular obstructive disease (PVOD) are very serious and feared complications of congenital heart disease. PAH usually is the result of direct transmission of systemic arterial pressure to the right ventricle or pulmonary artery via a large communication. Less frequently, it is due to severe obstruction to blood flow through the left side of the heart at the pulmonary venous level or beyond. PVOD refers to a process involving structural changes in the smaller muscular arteries and arterioles of the lung that gradually diminishes and eventually destroys the ability of the pulmonary vascular bed to transmit blood from the larger pulmonary arteries to the pulmonary veins without an abnormal elevation of the proximal pulmonary arterial pressure.

The muscular medial layer of the small pulmonary arteries of the fetus is very thick in relation to overall external vessel diameter and enables the fetus to maintain a high level of pulmonary vascular resistance. At birth the normal increase in alveolar and interstitial P_{O_2} and, to a much lesser extent, the physical expansion of the lung itself with air, produces dilatation of these muscular arteries and a sharp diminution in pulmonary resistance.[13] Pulmonary blood flow increases dramatically in response to this fall in resistance, but pulmonary arterial pressure tends to remain elevated, at least until closure of the ductus arteriosus. With spontaneous closure of the ductus, usually within 10 to 15 h after birth, the pulmonary arterial pressure can vary independently of the systemic arterial pressure and declines rapidly in the face of a diminishing pulmonary resistance, reaching normal adult levels of 15 to 30 mmHg systolic, 5 to 10 mmHg diastolic, and 10 to 20 mmHg mean by about 7 days of age.[49] Pulmonary resistance may be as high as 8 to 10 units/m² immediately after birth but falls rapidly throughout the first week and by 6 to 8 weeks usually has reached the normal adult levels of 1 to 3 units/m².[4] These changes are accompanied by a gradual regression or maturation of the medial layer of the muscular pulmonary arteries,[13] growth of existing arteries, and the development of new arteries and arterioles; the latter process contributes over 90 percent of the smaller or intraacinar pulmonary arterial vessels present in the older child and adult.[50] The presence of congenital heart disease may seriously alter these normal changes in pressure and resistance by creating a setting in which normal pulmonary vascular maturation and growth are retarded and in which, over a period of time, direct injury may be inflicted upon the pulmonary vascular bed.

Unlike the adult, in whom a threefold increase in pulmonary blood flow can be accommodated without a significant rise in pulmonary arterial pressure, the neonate responds to a significant increase in pulmonary blood flow with an increase in pulmonary arterial pressure, a reflection of the limited compliance of the thick-walled muscular pulmonary arteries. The resulting hypertension increases arterial wall stress which, in turn, stimulates persistence of or further development and extension of medial muscular hypertrophy. Thus, increased pulmonary arterial pressure, whether it be a consequence of *increased pulmonary blood flow* or of *pulmonary venous obstruction* or *direct transmission of systemic arterial pressure* via a large systemic-pulmonary communication, has an adverse effect on the normal maturation of the pulmonary vascular bed. Finally, medial hypertrophy renders the pulmonary vascular bed of the neonate more responsive than that of the older child or adult to the vasoconstrictive effects of *hypoxia* or *acidemia,* abnormalities characteristically present in infants with right-to-left shunts, pulmonary venous congestion, chronic respiratory obstruction, or among those infants living at high altitude. Under these adverse conditions, the pulmonary vascular resistance tends to fall at a much slower rate and may never attain the very low level reached by the normal child or adult. It should be pointed out that there is considerable individual variation in the pulmonary arterial pressures and resistances observed among patients with similar degrees of increased pulmonary arterial blood flow, pulmonary venous hypertension, or systemic arterial oxygen desaturation associated with congenital heart disease, or among individuals living at the same high altitude or with similar degrees of chronic lung disease. While the direction of the response is predictable and conforms to the pattern described above, the degree of response of the pulmonary vascular bed to any given stimulus varies significantly from one individual to another.[51]

Operating singly or in combination, the abnormal conditions described above are present in many infants and children with congenital heart disease. Increased flow is provided by such malformations as ventricular septal defect, patent ductus arteriosus, complete atrioventricular canal—examples of a direct communication between the pulmonary and systemic circuits. If the opening between the two circuits is large, the pulmonary arterial pressure cannot vary independently of systemic pressure and little if any fall in pulmonary pressure will occur in response to the sharp decline of pulmonary vascular resistance (R_p) at birth. Instead, pulmonary flow will increase as pulmonary vascular resistance falls. The diminution in pulmonary muscle mass and pulmonary resistance is less rapid and of less magnitude under these circumstances than in the normal infant in these early weeks of life. Usually, however, it is sufficient to permit a large pulmonary blood flow and, as a result, congestive failure. Pulmonary arterial pressure usually remains at or near systemic levels throughout by virtue of the large interventricular or systemic–pulmonary arterial communication. In the premature infant in whom the medial muscle mass is less than in the full-term infant, the fall in pulmonary vascular resistance may be much more rapid, and, in the face of a large systemic–pulmonary communication, congestive failure may become severe within a matter of days. The stimulus of hypoxia, either from alveolar hy-

DISEASES OF THE HEART AND BLOOD VESSELS

poventilation or altitude, added to that of increased pressure and flow, permits even less involution of the muscular medial layer and less fall in the R_p. Clinically, this is expressed in the lower incidence of congestive failure observed among infants with a large ventricular septal defect born and living at high altitude and by the increase in pulmonary blood flow and the appearance of congestive failure in such infants if transported from high altitude to sea level.[52] Examples of pulmonary venous hypertension exerting a retarding effect upon the maturation of the pulmonary vascular bed are found among infants with pulmonary vein stenosis, mitral stenosis, cor triatriatum, severe coarctation of the aorta, or aortic stenosis. Rarely an infant will maintain a very high pulmonary vascular resistance in the face of an anatomically large systemic–pulmonary communication, without evidence of significant hypoxia or acidemia, and remain free of the signs and symptoms of congestive failure. It is unclear why pulmonary vascular resistance falls to levels low enough to permit a large pulmonary blood flow and severe congestive failure in one infant, while it falls considerably less and is associated with little or no failure in another infant. This variation in response to the stimuli of pressure, flow, and hypoxia, mentioned earlier, is felt to present the spectrum of pulmonary vascular reactivity, with infants with low resistance and severe failure occupying one end of the spectrum and infants with a more reactive pulmonary vascular bed, perhaps "hyperreactors," occupying the other.[51]

Infants with an isolated atrial septal defect characteristically do not follow the course described above. Although pulmonary blood flow is considerably increased in the older infant and child, it usually does not reach these high levels during the neonatal period. Maturation of the pulmonary vascular bed appears to proceed on a schedule similar to that of the normal infant, and, with the exception of a relatively small number of young women in whom PVOD may develop quite rapidly, responds to the chronically increased pulmonary blood flow only after several decades with an increase in pulmonary vascular resistance and pulmonary arterial pressure.

Chronic PAH or increased flow or both produce a characteristic series of histological changes within the pulmonary vascular bed. These changes, described by Heath and Edwards,[53] consist of the following:

Grade I—Increased medial thickness of the small pulmonary arteries and proximal pulmonary arterioles, with extension of smooth muscle into smaller and more peripheral arteries than normal for age. The latter appears related to increased flow rather than pressure[50] (Fig. 36-1). These changes, noted as early as 4 to 6 weeks of age among infants with a ventricular septal defect,[54,55] probably are completely reversible.

Grade II—Concentric or eccentric cellular intimal proliferation and thickening within the smaller pul-

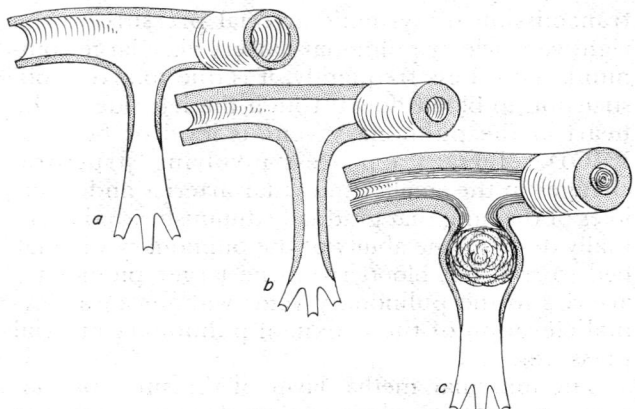

FIGURE 36-1 Pulmonary vascular obstructive disease. *a.* Normal mature muscular pulmonary artery and arteriole. *b.* Hypertrophy and abnormal distal extension of medial smooth muscle (grade I). *c.* Intimal thickening, initially the result of cellular proliferation (grade II) but progressing to intimal fibrosis (grade III), with occlusion of the arteriolar lumen, formation of the plexiform lesion, and distal arteriolar dilatation (grade IV).

monary arteries and arterioles, which are capable, in the extreme, of producing vascular occlusion. Increased shearing stresses, induced by increased velocity of blood flow within the narrowed muscular arteries, are considered to play a role in the production of these intimal lesions. Whether or not these changes are completely reversible is uncertain; but if the changes are mild, it seems unlikely that significant residual obstruction will result even if complete regression does not occur.

Among patients with isolated atrial septal defect, the earliest evidence of PVOD is such cellular intimal proliferation. Little if any medial hypertrophy is present since PAH usually is not a feature of the natural history of patients with atrial septal defect until the onset of PVOD. Once proliferation has begun and progressed, however, pulmonary arterial pressure rises and medial hypertrophy appears.

Grade III—Relatively acellular intimal fibrosis with the accumulation of concentric or eccentric masses of fibrous tissue leading to widespread occlusion of the smaller pulmonary arteries and arterioles superimposed upon marked hypertrophy and widespread cellular intimal proliferation of grades I and II. Isolated examples of dilatation in smaller arteries and arterioles with thinning of their medial wall distal and proximal to foci of occlusion warn of the generalized, progressive arterial dilatation characteristic of grades IV and V (Fig. 36-1). Grade III changes may be seen as early as 2 months of age in patients with transposition of the great arteries with either a large ventricular septal defect or ductus arteriosus. Similar changes are seen in infants with complete atrioventricular canal as early as 10 or 12 months of age but are seldom seen before 1 year of age in the infant with an isolated ventricular septal defect.[54,55] It is unlikely that grade III changes are reversible to any significant degree.

Grade IV—Progressive, generalized dilatation of the muscular arteries and the appearance of plexiform lesions, complex vascular structures comprised of a network or plexus of proliferating endothelial tissue, frequently accompanied by thrombus, within a dilated thin-wall sac. Whether these are the result of aneurysms of the media, vasculitis, or thrombosis is unclear, but their appearance signifies very severe PVOD. Grade IV changes may be seen as early as 2 to 4 months in infants with transposition with ventricular septal defect and 10 to 12 months among infants with complete atrioventricular canal. They are rare before 2 years of age among infants with isolated ventricular septal defect. Grade IV changes are considered irreversible.[54,55]

Grade V—Thinning and fibrosis of the media superimposed upon the formation of numerous complex dilatation lesions.

Grade VI—Necrotizing arteritis within the media with necrosis of muscle accompanied by surrounding areas of inflammatory reaction and granulation tissue. This form of PVOD is extremely rare among patients with congenital heart disease and is found more commonly among patients with primary pulmonary hypertension.

Techniques appropriate for open lung biopsy and designed to permit quantitation of changes such as wall thickness and vessel size and number indicate that the development of new arteries and growth of existing arteries are significantly retarded by PAH. This retardation, recognized as early as 5 months of age in some instances, is evident in most, if not all, infants beyond 2 years of age with significant PAH.[50]

Estimation of pulmonary vascular resistance from data obtained at cardiac catheterization remains the most widely used means of assessing the state of the pulmonary vascular bed. Hypoxia from oversedation, atelectasis, or pneumonia at the time of study should be scrupulously avoided. If pulmonary vascular resistance is elevated, its responsiveness to vasodilatation induced by the inhalation of 100% oxygen or the intravenous administration of tolazoline, or both, should be tested.

Pulmonary vascular resistance values of 3 units/m^2 or less are considered normal, although in infants with a large ventricular septal defect and high pulmonary blood flow, a resistance of 2 units undoubtedly reflects an elevation since the normal pulmonary vascular bed responds to such a high flow with a reduction of resistance to levels of 0.5 units or less. The level of pulmonary vascular resistance may also be expressed as a ratio of pulmonary vascular resistance to systemic vascular resistance (R_p/R_s) since oxygen consumption is often estimated rather than measured. Severe elevations of systemic vascular resistance can, however, yield a deceptively low R_p/R_s ratio. Pulmonary to systemic resistance ratios of less than 0.2 are considered normal, with 0.2 to 0.49 a moderate elevation and 0.5 to 0.69 a severe elevation.

As pulmonary vascular resistance increases, pulmonary blood flow generally decreases. Therefore a point is reached where surgical closure of the defect will produce only a small diminution of blood flow, a proportionately small decrease in pulmonary arterial pressure, and no significant change in the factors contributing to the progression of the vascular disease. Patients in this category are considered prohibitive risks for surgery because of the increased mortality associated with the procedure and the early postoperative period. A pulmonary to systemic vascular resistance ratio of 0.7 or greater, or a pulmonary vascular resistance of 11 units/m^2 or more with a pulmonary to systemic blood flow ratio of less than 1.5 are the criteria generally used to define this situation. Unoperated, these patients survive as examples of Eisenmenger syndrome where pulmonary vascular resistance is equal to or greater than systemic vascular resistance and in whom at least some right-to-left shunting occurs at rest or with exercise. These patients may survive for several decades, leading a productive life with relatively mild symptoms or limitation until death. The reader is referred to reviews of the Eisenmenger syndrome by Graham[56] and Hallidie-Smith.[57]

The decision regarding surgery for patients with less severe PVOD is a clinical one. Experience indicates that the higher the resistance at any given age, or the older the patient with any given level of elevated resistance, the less likely the outcome will be satisfactory. If one defines a satisfactory outcome from surgery as surviving operation and having a mean pulmonary arterial pressure of less than 25 mmHg 5 years or more later, the data compiled by Blackstone and colleagues would indicate that the chances of a 2-year-old infant having such an outcome are 90 percent if the pulmonary vascular resistance is 4 units, 75 percent if the resistance is 8 units, and only 55 percent if the resistance is 12 units, provided the pulmonary to systemic blood flow ratio is greater than 1.3. By the same token the chance of having a satisfactory outcome with a pulmonary vascular resistance of 8 units would be in the range of 75 percent for the 2-year-old, 65 percent for the 3-year-old, and about 50 percent for the 4-year-old child.[58] Open lung biopsy[50] or magnification pulmonary wedge angiography[59] may prove to be of value in this group of patients.

The prevention of PVOD is of far greater service to the patient than an accurate estimate of the degree of its severity. For prevention one needs first to identify those patients at risk, namely all patients with a systemic-pulmonary communication and a pulmonary arterial systolic pressure greater than half the systemic arterial systolic pressure. Also included would be all patients with transposition, regardless of pressure or flow, with the possible exception of those with severe pulmonary stenosis or pulmonary arterial banding with documented pulmonary arterial pressures in the normal range. Ideally all patients at risk should undergo correction or pulmonary arterial banding unless there is proof that the pulmonary arterial systolic pressure has fallen to or is less than half the systemic systolic pressure before the end of the first year of life. Among patients with transposition with a large ventricular septal defect, action must be taken within the first 6 months of life, whereas among those with normally related great arteries and ventricular septal defect, correction or banding at the end of the first year usually is acceptable. Today there is little or no excuse for the discovery of unsuspected, severe PVOD among infants and children.

Infective Endocarditis[60,61]

Infective endocarditis is discussed more fully in Chap. 54. This section will deal with certain aspects that relate to the pediatric age group and those with congenital heart disease.

A retrospective review in patients under 25 years of age[62] demonstrated some changes that have ensued over a 40-year period. The survival increased from almost 0 percent in the initial preantibiotic decade to 81 percent from 1963 through 1972. The mean age increased to 12.7 years in the last decade of the study period. There was an increase in absolute number of episodes and number relative to total hospital admissions. The absolute number with rheumatic heart disease or no significant underlying heart disease was stable, but the number with congenital heart disease increased, accounting for 91 percent of the total episodes from 1963 through 1972. Risk appears to be higher for certain forms of congenital heart disease such as tetralogy of Fallot, ventricular septal defect, and aortic stenosis.

Although infective endocarditis is rare under 2 years of age, a clinical and pathological study suggests that congenital heart disease also predisposes to endocarditis in infancy. A review of the records of 847 infants who died with bacterial sepsis found that 10 percent of 61 infants dying with bacterial sepsis associated with congenital heart disease acquired endocarditis, whereas only 0.8 percent of 786 infants without heart disease did so.[63]

M-mode and cross-sectional echocardiography can identify vegetations in many patients with infective endocarditis. This may help clarify the diagnosis in some and is particularly helpful in pediatrics with the high frequency of febrile illnesses. It may also provide a means of identifying patients who will require early operative intervention. Information available suggests that the two methods of echocardiography are of equal value since neither detects small vegetations[64] (see Chaps. 54 and 95).

Antibiotics have favorably altered the natural history of infective endocarditis. The addition of early surgical intervention in selected patients can further improve survival. One review of 182 patients recommended early valve replacement of all cases of staphylococcal endocarditis and native or prosthetic valve endocarditis with moderate or severe heart failure. Major embolism and fungal endocarditis are also indications for early surgery.[65]

Certain procedures, such as dental extraction, clearly produce bacteremia[66] that can cause infective endocarditis in patients at risk. Guidelines for prevention have been published,[67] including appropriate dosages for pediatric patients. All forms of congenital heart disease are considered at risk with the exception of uncomplicated secundum atrial septal defect. The only two exceptions after cardiac surgery are suture repair of secundum atrial septal defect and ligation of patent ductus arteriosus more than 6 months after surgery.

Retardation of Growth and Development

Growth failure among infants and children with congenital heart disease is common and is of serious concern to both the physician and the parents. To the extent that normal or maximal attainable growth is a by-product of successful management, attention must be directed at the removal or diminution of those factors which produce growth failure.

Physical growth can be assessed by plotting the measurements of height and weight at each examination on a standard growth chart where the normal range of values for age is expressed in terms of percentiles, the 16th percentile line representing one standard deviation and the 3d percentile line two standard deviations below the mean. In general, children growing normally track along a given percentile for their height or weight. Children with mild congenital abnormalities of the heart tend to grow normally, but a significant proportion of those with more severe malformations have evidence of serious growth abnormality, namely height and weight measurements near or below the 3d percentile or weight measurements 20 percentile points or more below those for height.[68]

Interference with growth is most severe among those children with overtly cyanotic lesions and those with large left-to-right shunts caused by ventricular septal defect, patent ductus arteriosus, or atrioventricular canal defect.[69] Patients with cyanotic lesions tend to have a rather parallel retardation of both height and weight, while those with large left-to-right shunts tend to have a greater retardation of weight than height. This discrepancy is accentuated by the presence of congestive heart failure (Fig. 36-2). Skeletal retardation, reflected by bone age, usually occurs along with height and weight retardation and, among children with cyanotic heart disease, can be correlated with the severity of hypoxia.[39] In general girls are more resistant than boys to factors producing growth retardation.

In addition to hypoxia and overt congestive failure, a number of factors probably play a role in the growth retardation in many of these infants, namely insufficient caloric intake caused by anorexia, dyspnea, frequent infections or psychological disturb-

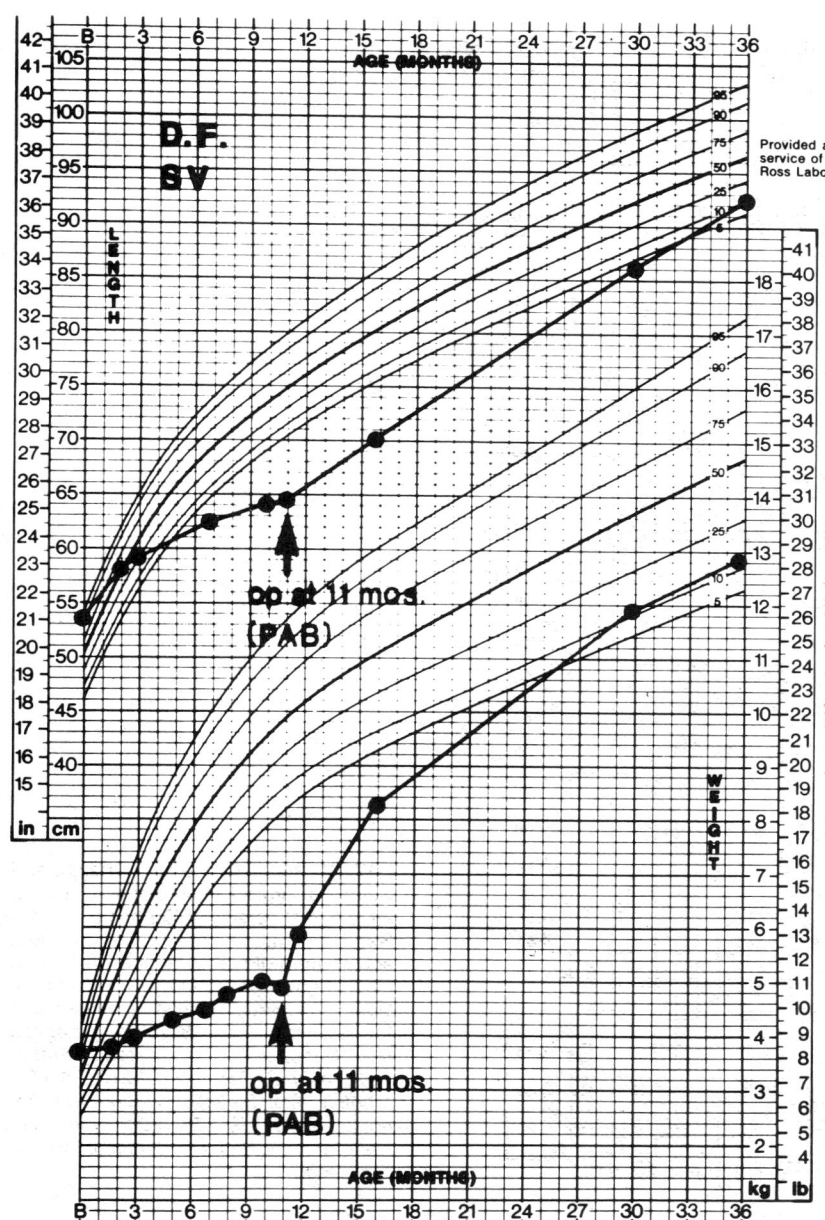

FIGURE 36-2 Response of height and weight to surgical pulmonary arterial banding (PAB) in an infant with a single ventricle (SV) and congestive heart failure due to severe pulmonary overcirculation. Chart shows physical growth [National Center for Health Statistics percentiles) for boys from birth to 18 months. [*Adapted from National Center for Health Statistics, NCHS Growth Charts, 1976, Monthly Vital Statistics Report, vol. 25, no. 3, suppl. (HRA) 76-1120, June 1976. Data from the Fels Research Institute, Yellow Springs, Ohio. Copyright 1976 by Ross Laboratories.*]

ances, malabsorption, hypermetabolism, and, particularly among those with severe congenital heart disease recognized within the first year of life, a significantly increased incidence of subnormal birth weight, intrauterine growth retardation (6.1 percent), and major extracardiac anomalies (19.9 percent).[70] Finally, a relatively small number of children will have associated syndromes known to be characterized by growth retardation, such as rubella, Noonan's, Turner's, or Down's syndrome.

If growth retardation is related primarily to the congenital heart disease, surgical correction or palliation of the malformation usually is followed by an impressive acceleration of growth with a return to or toward normal measurements (Fig. 36-3). As might be expected, acceleration of height and

weight gain tends to be greatest in children operated on in the first year or two of life, with weight gain showing a more abrupt change than height. Girls tend to experience a more complete return to normal than boys. While the above is a general trend, in some children the acceleration of weight gain and linear growth is small, and in these patients such factors as additional unrecognized heart disease or inadequate repair or palliation must be considered. Those children in whom small size is largely or in part the result of hereditary, genetic, or intrauterine influences will have only a modest response.

While cardiac surgery seldom is recommended on the basis of growth failure alone, this undesirable trend should be recognized as early as possible and, until proved otherwise, considered as an index of

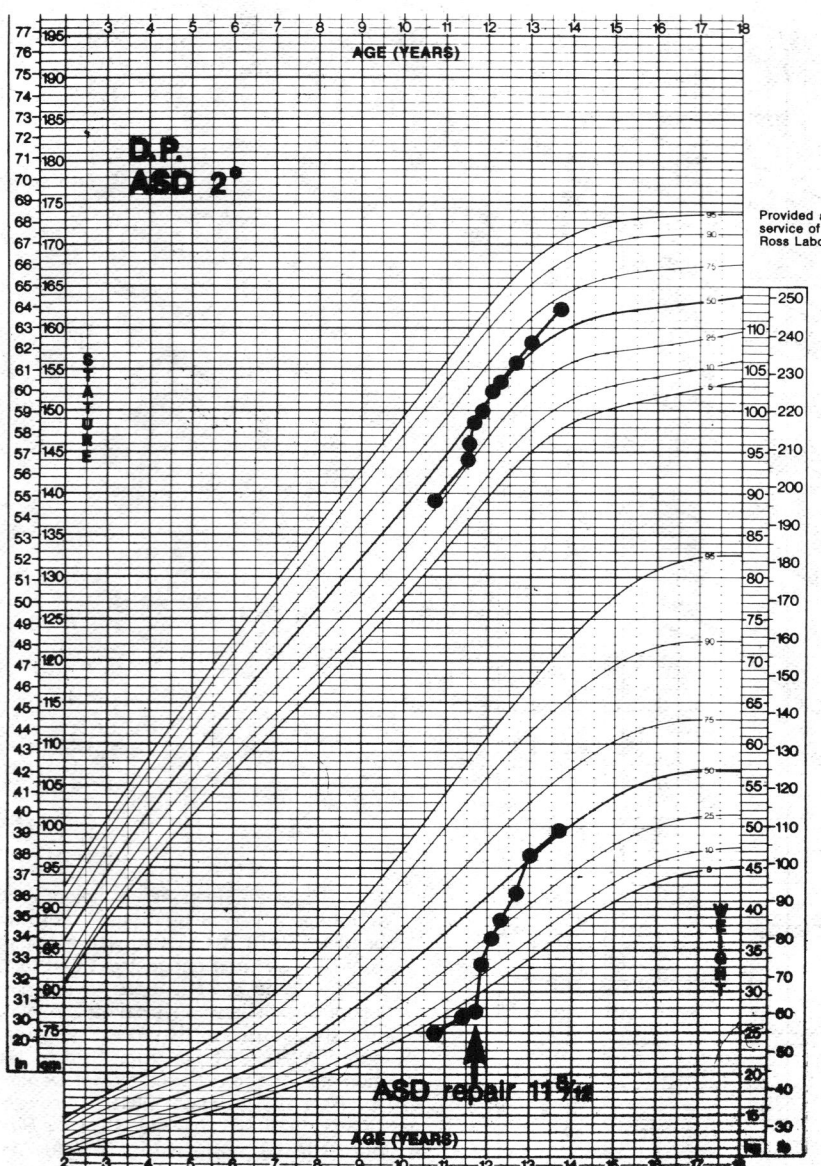

FIGURE 36-3 Response of height and weight to surgical closure of a secundum atrial septal defect (ASD 2°) in a preadolescent girl with a large left-to-right shunt and normal pulmonary arterial pressures. Chart shows physical growth (National Center for Health Statistics percentiles) for girls from 2 to 18 years. [*Adapted from National Center for Health Statistics, NCHS Growth Charts, 1976, Monthly Vital Statistics Report, vol. 25, no. 3, suppl. (HRA) 76-1120, June 1976. Data from the National Center for Health Statistics.*]

the severity of the heart disease. In general the earlier and the more successful the surgery, the less will be the retardation of growth and development with its sequelae of physical, psychological, and intellectual problems.[68]

Exertional Intolerance and Restrictions

Certain infants and children with congenital heart disease may manifest exertional intolerance that is clinically overt. The infant with heart failure uncontrolled by medical management frequently demonstrates intolerance with feeding since this is a major form of exercise for the infant. Feeding is slow due to the increased respiratory rate and is interrupted frequently for periods of rest because of fatigue. The total volume consumed each feeding is usually small so intervals between feedings are shortened as hunger recurs rapidly. Infants with heart failure usually must be fed on a schedule based on individual need. Even so, caloric intake may be inadequate and failure to gain weight appropriately can result. The child with a significant degree of cyanosis may squat or breathe more deeply and rapidly during play. Increased need for sleep or rest can parallel changes in the degree of motor activity seen with increasing age. In general, infants and children with such overt manifestations of intolerance to exercise will restrict their own activities based on their physical capacity so that there is usually no need for parental or other external restrictions.

For the less severely restricted or asymptomatic child, the questions of parents usually revolve around the potential harm of exercise. How much a child can do and how the heart responds to exercise should be used as guides when making recommendations concerning the need for and the degree of external restrictions of activity. Exercise testing with measurement of work capacity, electrocardiographic, and cardiorespiratory responses is useful in evaluating these children.

Data on the response to exercise of normal children, measured using bicycle and treadmill protocols,[71-73] and that of children with specific defects are available.[6,71,72] In general terms, exertional endurance is commonly affected in those children with heart disease,[74,75,76] but usually it is adequate for participation in childhood activities. Only children with cyanosis or other severe disease have consistently reduced exercise capacity. Individual variability is expected. Radionuclide angiography can be combined with exercise to assess reserve more definitively in selected patients.[77]

Restrictions other than those due to limited physical capacity exist for young people with congenital heart disease. Problems with insurability and employability[78] are recognized and efforts to minimize these are ongoing.

The Examination of the Individual Suspected of Having Congenital Heart Disease

In most instances questions concerning symptoms will, of necessity, be directed to the parents. It may be helpful for the interviewer to think in terms of three broad categories of congenital heart disease, to pick a malformation that is representative of each category, and to ask questions designed to uncover the symptoms of that particular malformation. *Obstructive lesions* would be exemplified by aortic stenosis, and questions would include those related to easy fatigue, light-headedness, syncope, shortness of breath with exercise, and angina. *Left-to-right shunts* would be represented by ventricular septal defect, and questions would be directed toward the presence of rapid or labored breathing, shortness of breath with effort, excessive sweating, and frequent or prolonged respiratory infections. *Cyanotic lesions* would be best represented by tetralogy of Fallot and the interviewer would ask about cyanosis at rest or with exercise, unprovoked episodes of breathlessness or cyanosis, and squatting. It is unlikely that symptoms would be undetected after this brief and easily remembered series of questions.

The apprehensive infant or child represents a challenge for the examiner. Infants or children through the ages of 3 or even 4 years usually are best examined in their mother's or father's lap, first sitting and then supine. Youngsters in this age range do not seem to mind being handled by a stranger nearly as much as they mind being looked at, at close quarters, by a stranger. For this reason the examiner usually will find it advantageous not to make eye contact with the subject even to the point of shielding one's eyes and face with a hand, low-

ering one's head so that the infant sees only the top, or looking directly away. If the child becomes so restless that it is difficult to obtain an adequate examination, one should have no hesitancy in using sedation. Chloral hydrate, 50 mg/kg orally or rectally, is recommended with the expectation that the child would be drowsy and cooperative or fully asleep within about 15 min.

Time should be taken to inspect before approaching or touching the subject. A mental note should be taken of at least five items, easily remembered by the letters ABCDE if necessary, and these are *a*ctivity, *b*reathing, *c*olor, *d*evelopment, and *e*xternal signs of cardiac abnormality. *Activity* would include observations such as asleep or awake, quiet, apprehensive, or unmanageable. *Breathing* refers to the rate, counted for at least 15 s, and a judgment as to whether or not air hunger or dyspnea exists. Attention would be directed to inter- or subcostal retractions, nasal flaring, or grunting. *Color* refers to the presence or absence of pallor, jaundice, cyanosis, or rubor. Inspection for cyanosis will lead one to look for the earliest degrees of clubbing, usually found in the thumbs and first fingers or toes, and to examine for differential cyanosis. *Development* refers broadly to the overall body build, state of nutrition, and any unusual facial features or hand or limb abnormalities that might be present. *External signs* include abnormal jugular venous or precordial pulsations, deformity of the chest, and edema. With the patient sitting, an easily reproducible position, visible venous *a* or *v* waves in the neck are abnormal. Prominence of the left hemithorax usually suggests cardiac enlargement of some duration.

Palpation should include attention to the pulses, precordium, and abdomen. Femoral, brachial, and, in the infant, temporal pulses should be surveyed to be certain that they are present, with particular attention paid to the femoral pulses where a diminution in volume compared to the brachial or delay compared to the radial pulse would suggest the presence of coarctation. An assessment should be made of the rate, volume, speed of upstroke, and any irregularity that might suggest the presence of an arrhythmia, pulsus paradoxus, or pulsus alternans, the latter two phenomena being best documented with a blood pressure cuff and auscultation. The precordium should be felt for the presence of thrills and abnormal ventricular systolic or presystolic pulsations. A reasonable estimate of heart size can be gained by a combination of palpation and percussion, particularly in the child, but the final decision on heart size should await review of the chest roentgenogram. The position of the liver and, when possible, the spleen should be noted, with the liver size estimated by the measured distance between its lower edge and the respective costal margin or xiphoid.

At some point in the examination—the timing depending upon the cooperation of the subject—the blood pressure should be obtained and recorded. This should be taken in the supine infant and seated child in whichever arm is more convenient, provided there is no inequality of pulses, in which event pressures should be taken in both arms and in one leg. The blood pressure should be measured in all individuals at least at the time of their initial cardiovascular examination, whether they be newborn, older infant, or child.

Techniques of auscultation vary widely, but the one recommended would include attention to, first, the heart sounds in order, e.g., S_1, S_2, S_3, S_4, clicks, opening snaps, and rubs, and then, if present, systolic, diastolic, or continuous murmurs.

From the chest roentgenogram the viewer should make a judgment on at least the following five items: (1) overall heart size (normal, mild, moderate, or marked enlargement); (2) pulmonary arterial blood flow (normal or a definite increase or decrease); (3) pulmonary arterial segment (prominence, diminution, or absence); (4) left atrium (normal or enlarged by displacement of the barium-filled esophagus); and (5) aortic arch (position and abnormalities causing esophageal indentation).

The electrocardiogram, an indispensable tool for evaluation of congenital heart disease, may reveal abnormalities of QRS orientation. These abnormalities may be characteristic of certain malformations, such as the superior orientation with atrioventricular canal malformations, or they may suggest more or less dominance of the right ventricle than is normal for age, such as the right axis deviation associated with tetralogy of Fallot or the normal axis in the newborn with pulmonary atresia and intact ventricular septum. One should also be particularly interested in abnormally small or large voltages of either P waves or QRS complexes, which would suggest absence, hypoplasia, enlargement, or hypertrophy of one or more of the four cardiac chambers. Abnormalities are judged by comparison of the observed axis and voltages with those of normal children of the same age.[79] Observed values that fall beyond the 5th or 95th percentile are likely to be abnormal.

If the examiner establishes a set of observations to be obtained for every infant or child examined, and then correlates these observations with the information supplied by echocardiography, cardiac catheterization, surgery, or postmortem examination, it will not be long before he or she will become quite skillful in detecting even rather subtle congenital abnormalities of the heart.

Intracardiac Communications between the Systemic and Pulmonary Circulations Usually without Cyanosis

When a communication occurs between the two circulations, the lesion usually takes the form of a septal defect or a communication between the aorta, on one hand, and the pulmonary arterial system, on the other. Less commonly, a vessel of the systemic circulation, such as the aorta or a coronary artery, communicates with a right-sided cardiac chamber.

In the uncomplicated state, such communications are responsible for left-to-right shunts, and cyanosis is absent. When occlusive pulmonary vascular disease appears, the resulting increase in pulmonary vascular resistance may be of sufficient magnitude to cause a right-to-left shunt. Under the latter conditions cyanosis may appear as a late phenomenon.

Conditions which allow shunts to occur may be divided into those in which the shunt is *intracardiac* and those in which it is *extracardiac*. The intracardiac shunts result from defects in either the atrial septum or the ventricular septum. In some cases the lesion is an isolated one; in others it is part of a complex anomaly as in common atrioventricular canal, or the so-called endocardial cushion defect. Because a partial anomalous pulmonary venous connection may resemble an atrial septal defect functionally and clinically, the former condition will also be considered in this section. Conditions in which a shunt begins in an extracardiac structure and leads to the right atrium or to the ventricle or pulmonary vascular system are considered under "Extracardiac Shunts."

The major individual factors that determine the magnitude and direction of intracardiac or extracardiac shunts are (1) the size (diameter and length) of the communication between the involved chambers and vessels, (2) the pressure differences between the involved chambers and vessels, (3) the diastolic compliance of the chambers and vessels, (4) the afterload or outflow resistances of the chambers and vessels, including the systemic and pulmonary vascular resistances, and (5) the systolic functioning or emptying of the respective ventricles.

The diagnosis of intracardiac or extracardiac shunting of blood is often based on changes in oxygen content or saturation of blood samples obtained during catheterization of the right side of the heart and pulmonary artery. Since there is normally more oxygen in blood returning to the heart in the inferior vena cava than in superior vena cava blood and since there is incomplete mixing of blood in the right atrium and in the right ventricle, it is important to know the range of variation in oxygen content or saturation that may be encountered in the chamber of normal subjects without a shunt. Table 36-4 gives these values as reported by two groups of investigators.[80,81] It should also be noted that there may be streaming of the shunted blood, causing it to be detected first in the downstream chamber. In addition, valvular regurgitation may occasionally cause shunted blood to be detected in the chamber upstream to the shunt. Special diagnostic techniques, such as hydrogen or radioactive gas inhalation indicator-dilution curves and angiography, may enable one to establish the presence of left-to-right shunts that are too small to detect by measurements of oxygen content.

TABLE 36-4 Normal Variations in Venous Oxygen Content and Saturation

| Site | Maximum Variation in Oxygen Content of Successive Samples, vol %* | | Oxygen Saturation† | |
	Within Chambers	Between Chambers‡	Mean	Range (95% band)
Pulmonary artery:				
Right and/or left	0.4			
Main		+0.5	78	73–83
Right ventricle:				
Below pulmonary valve	0.8			
Midventricle	1.0	+0.9	79	71–87
Right atrium:§				
Lower	1.5			
Mid	2.3		80	74–86
Upper		+1.9 (superior) −1.5 (inferior)		
Vena cava:				
Superior	0.6		77	67–87
Inferior	0.8		83	77–89

*From Dexter, Haynes, Burwell, Eppinger, Sagerson, and Evans.[80]

†From Barrett-Boyes and Wood.[81]

‡+ = maximum increase over the more proximal chamber; − = maximal decrease over the more proximal chamber.

§Occasionally, sampling near the coronary sinus will give an abnormally low oxygen content out of line with other atrial samples.

Atrial Septal Defect

Definition
An atrial septal defect is a through-and-through communication between the atria at the septal level. The condition is to be distinguished from the valvular-competent foramen ovale, a condition that is a potential opening. The latter is common in the population (approximately 35 percent) in adults.[82]

Pathology
Atrial septal defects are usually sufficiently large to allow free communication between the atria. They may be subdivided according to anatomic location (Fig. 36-4).[83] These will be considered first, followed by features that are common to all anatomic types. These are given in order of decreasing frequency in the following coverage.

Anatomic Types *Defect at the Fossa Ovalis (Ostium Secundum).* The isolated atrial septal defect (so-called ostium secundum defect) classically involves the region of the fossa ovalis and is the most common type (Fig. 36-4*A* and *C*, and Fig. 36-5). Its posterior border may be so deficient that the posterior atrial wall forms a boundary for the defect. Separating the inferior edge of the defect from the atrioventricular

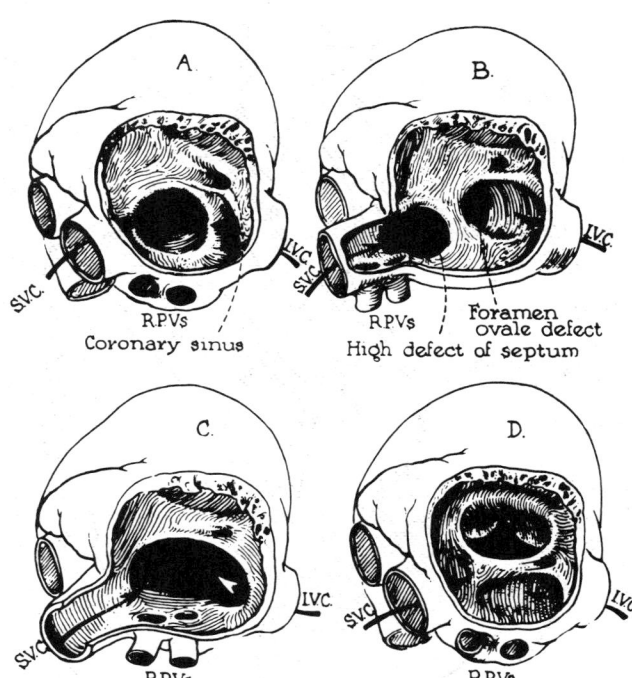

FIGURE 36-4 Types of interatrial communications. *A.* Large ostium secundum type of atrial septal defect. *B.* So-called sinus venosus type of defect—one high in the atrial septum associated with anomalous connection of the right superior pulmonary vein to the junctional area of the superior vena cava and right atrium. *C.* Very large ostium secundum type of atrial septal defect with absence of the posterior rim. *D.* Partial form of common atrioventricular canal with cleft mitral valve. S.V.C. = superior vena cava; R.P.Vs = right pulmonary veins; I.V.C. = inferior vena cava. (*From F. J. Lewis, P. Winchell, and F. A. Bashour, Open Repair of Atrial Septal Defects: Results in Sixty-Three Patients, J. Am. Med. Assoc., 165:922, 1957.*[83] *Reproduced with permission.*)

valves is atrial septal tissue. By virtue of its position, the defect has its posteroinferior zone in close proximity to the right atrial orifice of the inferior vena cava and its valve.

Various causes of left atrial enlargement, such as patent ductus arteriosus, ventricular septal defect, mitral valvular disease, or right atrial enlargement as in primary pulmonary hypertension, may cause tensions or disproportions at the site of an initially valvular-competent foramen ovale so as to yield a septal defect.[84] Removal of the underlying condition may result in spontaneous closure of the defect.[85] When present, the defect may be indistinguishable from a congenital defect. The association of mitral stenosis and atrial septal defect is commonly called *Lutembacher's syndrome.*[86] The floppy mitral valve has been found in association with atrial septal defect.[87] Here, too, the defect may be an ultimate effect of the mitral insufficiency of the floppy valve.

The Holt-Oram syndrome may be associated with the fossa ovalis type of atrial septal defect.[88]

Defect Inferior to the Fossa Ovalis. Defects of the atrial septum which lie inferior to the fossa ovalis usually are part of a complex malformation known as common atrioventricular canal defect (Fig. 36-

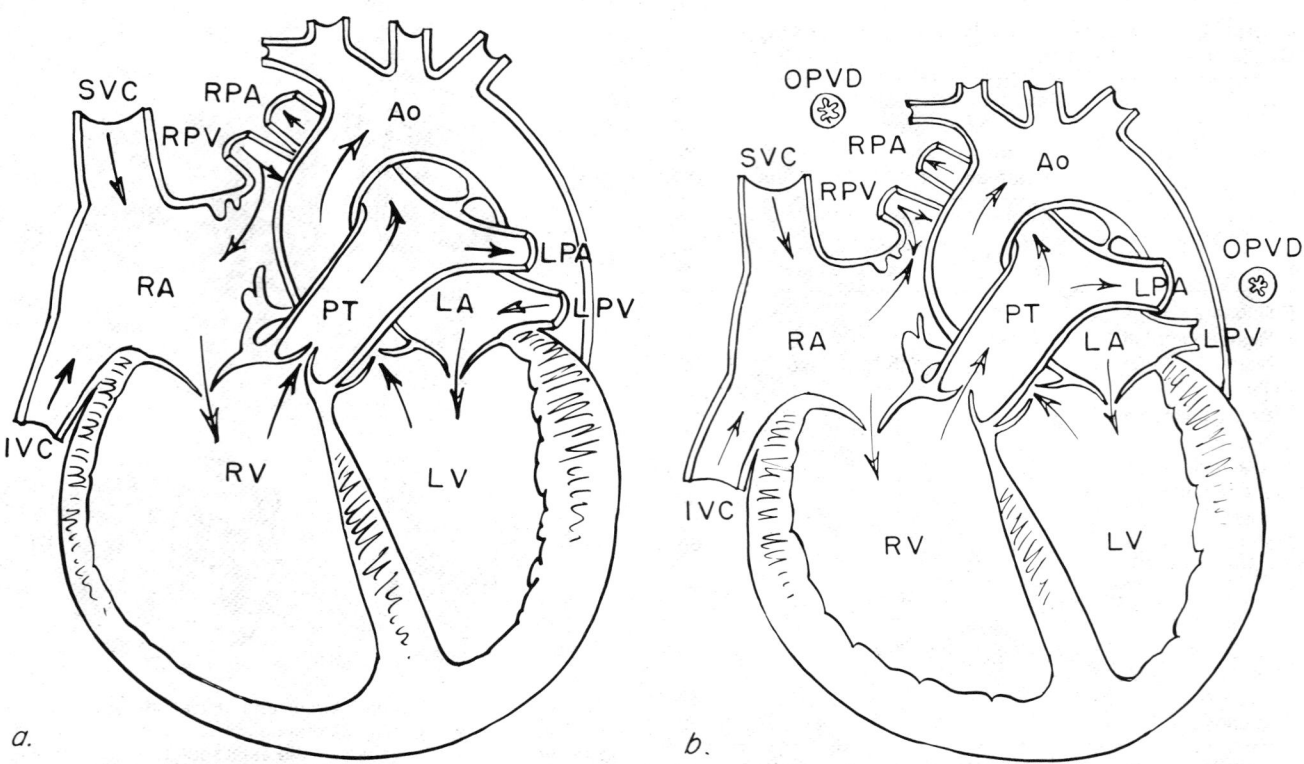

FIGURE 36-5   Atrial septal defect at fossa ovalis. *a.* With left-to-right shunt. *b.* With right-to-left shunt. The latter situation depends on complicating pulmonary hypertension with right ventricular hypertrophy. OPVD = obstructive pulmonary vascular disease; SVC = superior vena cava; IVC = inferior vena cava; RA = right atrium; RV = right ventricle; PT = main pulmonary arterial trunk; RPA = right pulmonary artery; LPA = left pulmonary artery; RPV = right pulmonary vein; LPV = left pulmonary vein; LA = left atrium; LV = left ventricle; Ao = aorta. [*From J. E. Edwards, Classification of Congenital Heart Disease in the Adult, in W.C. Roberts (ed.), "Congenital Heart Disease in Adults," Cardiovasc. Clin. Series 10/1, F. A. Davis Company, Philadelphia, 1979, pp. 1–26. Reproduced with permission.*]

4D). This type of defect will be considered later in this section under "Common Atrioventricular Canal Defects."

Defect Superior to the Fossa Ovalis (Sinus Venosus Type). Some atrial septal defects lie superior to the fossa ovalis in close relation to the right atrial ostium of the superior vena cava (Fig. 36-4B and Fig. 36-6). Commonly called sinus venosus in type, such defects are but one of two parts of an entity in which the second element involves anomalous termination of right-sided pulmonary veins, either into the superior vena cava near its right atrial junction or into the right atrium near the superior vena caval junction.[89] Most often the anomalous connection is made by one vein or several veins from the upper lobe of the right lung, while the veins of the remaining part of the right lung and of the entire left lung join the left atrium normally. Less commonly, the venous system of the entire right lung is involved in the anomalous connection. It is to be emphasized that there are other instances in which anomalous venous connection from the right lung to the superior vena cava or to the right atrium is not associated with an atrial septal defect, or if an interatrial communication is present, it takes the form of a patent foramen ovale.

Defect Posteroinferior to the Fossa Ovalis. An uncommon type of atrial septal defect is located in the posteroinferior angle of the atrial septum in the position normally occupied by the right atrial ostium of the coronary sinus (Fig. 36-7). From the left atrial aspect, the defect is centered above the posteromedial commissure of the mitral valve. This defect is part of a developmental complex described by Raghib and associates.[90] Associated with this type of atrial septal defect are the two other parts of the complex, that is, (1) absence of the coronary sinus and (2) entry of the left superior vena cava into the left atrium. The latter feature is responsible for a right-to-left shunt into the left atrium, while a left-to-right shunt occurs through the atrial septal defect. In some instances, this type of atrial septal defect is associated with persistent common atrioventricular canal. Under this circumstance the atrial septal defects of the two associated entities are continuous, resulting in a large defect involving the lower part of the atrial septum. This phenomenon commonly occurs in the syndrome of asplenia with congenital cardiac disease, but it may be seen in cases in which the spleen is present.

Conditions Common to All Anatomic Types   *The Cardiac Chambers.* In uncomplicated atrial septal defect with left-to-right shunt, the two atria and the right

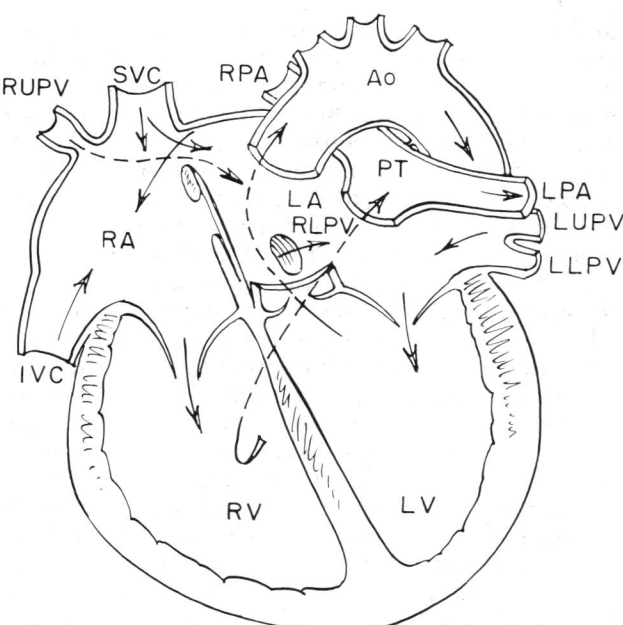

FIGURE 36-6 Sinus venosus type of atrial septal defect. The classic association of anomalous termination of right pulmonary veins to the right atrium or to the superior vena cava is shown. RUPV = right upper pulmonary vein; RLPV = right lower pulmonary vein; LUPV = left upper pulmonary vein; LLPV = left lower pulmonary vein. [*From J. E. Edwards, Classification of Congenital Heart Disease in the Adult, in W. C. Roberts (ed.), "Congenital Heart Disease in Adults," Cardiovasc. Clin. Series 10/1, F. A. Davis Company, Philadelphia, 1979, pp. 1–26. Reproduced with permission.*]

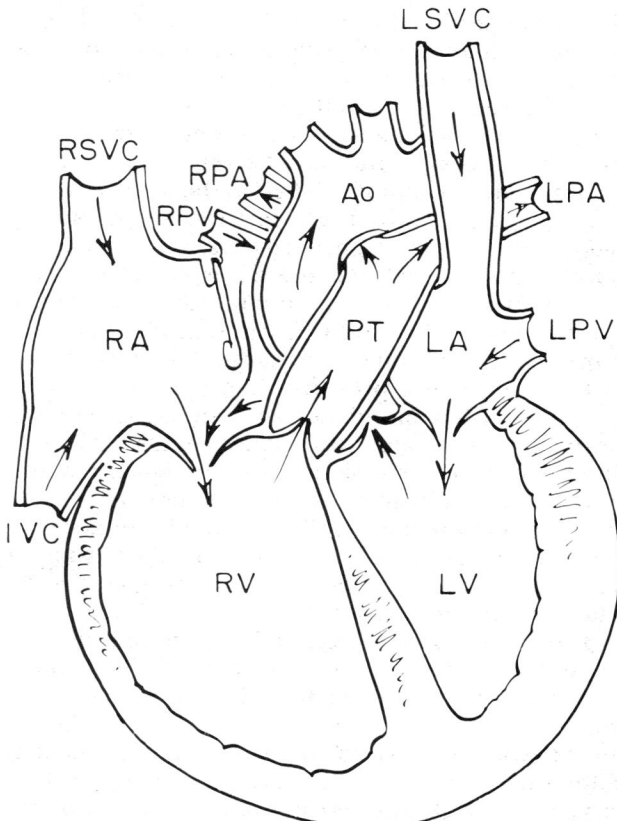

FIGURE 36-7 Termination of the left superior vena cava (LSVC) into the left atrium associated with absence of the coronary sinus. RSVC = right superior vena cava; RA = right atrium; IVC = inferior vena cava; RV = right ventricle; PT = main pulmonary arterial trunk; RPA = right pulmonary artery; LPA = left pulmonary artery; RPV = right pulmonary vein; LPV = left pulmonary vein; LA = left atrium; LV = left ventricle; Ao = aorta. [*From J. E. Edwards, Classification of Congenital Heart Disease in the Adult, in W. C. Roberts, (ed.), "Congenital Heart Disease in Adults," Cardiovasc. Clin. Series 10/1, F. A. Davis Company, Philadelphia, 1979, pp. 1–26. Reproduced with permission.*]

ventricle participate in carrying the shunt. The left ventricle does not participate and remains normal. The right atrial and ventricular chambers become grossly enlarged, but their walls are not hypertrophied. The left atrium has a tendency not to become enlarged. This is explained on the basis of the assumption that as the shunted blood enters the left atrium, it is not retained in this chamber but, instead, flows immediately into the right atrium. When atrial septal defect becomes complicated by pulmonary hypertension, the right ventricular wall becomes hypertrophied, but the signs of the previously occurring large left-to-right shunt remain in the form of enlargement of the right atrial and ventricular chambers.

Pulmonary Vasculature. In uncomplicated atrial septal defect, the major pulmonary arteries are dilated and the pulmonary trunk is considerably wider than the aorta. The absolute caliber of the latter vessel may be less than normal. As the pulmonary trunk dilates, the individual cusps of the pulmonary valve are stretched.

When pulmonary hypertension enters as a complication, atherosclerosis occurs in the major pulmonary arteries. Saccular aneurysm and thrombosis of the major pulmonary arteries may occur. Dissecting aneurysm or rupture of the pulmonary trunk are among the rare complications.

Among patients with atrial septal defect and left-to-right shunt, pulmonary hypertension may develop but usually not before the third decade. In such cases, occlusive pulmonary vascular lesions are apparent. The earliest lesion appears to be characterized by cellular fibrous intimal thickening in the proximal segments of arterioles. Following the development of this process, the pulmonary arterial pressure rises; then follow the development of medial hypertrophy of muscular arteries and the appearance of plexiform lesions. In the final state, the pulmonary vascular bed may be difficult to distinguish from that in ventricular septal defect with occlusive pulmonary vascular disease.[53]

Abnormal Physiology

In secundum atrial septal defect the mean left atrial pressure may be slightly higher, usually less than 3 mmHg, than that in the right atrium if the cross-sectional area of the defect is not over 2 cm². If the total cross-sectional area of the defect(s) is larger, however, there is essentially no resistance to blood flow across the defect and hence no significant pressure difference between the two atria, which may be considered functionally to be a common atrial chamber.[84,91–96] Most of the blood from the functional common atrial chamber will go to the right ventricle (Fig. 36-5A), producing a left-to-right shunt of blood since (1) the right atrial system is more distensible than the left, (2) the tricuspid valve is normally more capacious than the mitral valve, and (3) the thinner-walled right ventricular chamber will more readily accommodate a larger volume of blood at the same filling pressure than the left ventricle (i.e., after a few months of age, the right ventricle normally has greater compliance or distensibility). In about 70 percent of cases, a very small amount of blood passes from right atrium to left atrium, but this is so slight that it usually does not lower systemic arterial saturation below normal. This right-to-left shunt often may be detected only by special indicator-dilution techniques.

It has usually been assumed that there is little or no left-to-right shunt in atrial septal defects immediately after birth and before the rapid increase in left ventricular mass decreases the compliance of the left ventricle relative to that of the right ventricle. Subsequent studies,[97] however, have shown that large left-to-right shunts can sometimes occur in this period and during infancy, perhaps related to a greater right ventricular emptying with lower right ventricular end-systolic volume and pressure. In most instances of secundum atrial septal defect the right ventricle accommodates the large, "torrential" left-to-right shunt with moderate dilatation but with no elevation of end-diastolic pressure and only slight elevation of systolic pressure. The preferential shunting of the blood returning to the left atrium from the right pulmonary veins is due to their proximity to the atrial septal defect. The massive flow across the tricuspid valve often is associated with a diastolic flow murmur, which at times may be misinterpreted as being produced by mitral stenosis. The large flow across the normal pulmonary valve not only produces a midsystolic murmur, but it also may produce a systolic gradient across the pulmonary valve because of a "relative" or "functional" stenosis. The peak systolic pressure difference across the pulmonary valve in patients with secundum atrial septal defect is usually less than 10 mmHG, although occasionally it may be 10 to 20 mmHg; very rarely, it has been reported to be 50 to 60 mmHg in the absence of pulmonary stenosis.

In patients with secundum atrial septal defect the pulmonary arterial system undergoes regression after birth, following which most patients tolerate the tremendous volume load on the right ventricle and pulmonary circuit quite well for many years. In a minority of patients, however, pulmonary vascular disease develops and alters the situation considerably. The pulmonary vascular disease and associated increased vascular resistance develop as a consequence of both the tremendous volume of pulmonary blood flow and the slight increase in pulmonary artery pressure. Severe pulmonary vascular disease rarely occurs before the age of 20, and it has been suggested that the rare cases in which severe pulmonary vascular disease occurs earlier are instances of coincidental primary pulmonary hypertension.[93,95,96] In those patients who do develop pulmonary vascular disease with high vascular resistance and pulmonary artery hypertension, the left-to-right shunt decreases, largely because of the increased thickness and decreased compliance or distensibility of the right ventricle. In some patients the process continues until there is no significant left-to-right shunting of blood, and eventually the shunt may be from right-to-left (Fig. 36-5B). If there is a significant right-to-left shunt, arterial desaturation and cyanosis will develop, clinical characteristics of the so-called Eisenmenger syndrome.[98,99]

In patients with a secundum atrial septal defect, left ventricular failure (as from systemic hypertension) is associated with a decrease in left ventricular diastolic compliance and a decrease in left ventricular emptying, and with increases in left ventricular end-systolic pressure and volume. These changes tend to increase the left-to-right shunt and the pulmonary congestion. In such patients the pressure in the common atrial chamber appears to be related predominantly to the diastolic compliance or function of the left ventricle.[95]

The key role played by the pulmonary vasculature in the physiology of atrial septal defect should be emphasized. In most patients with atrial septal defect who have a large pulmonary blood flow and a normal or only slightly elevated pulmonary artery pressure, there is actually a decrease in calculated pulmonary vascular resistance. This is thought to be due both to utilization of all pulmonary vascular channels, many of which are thought to be only partially or intermittently utilized in normal individuals, and to dilatation of the pulmonary vasculature. It is not known why some patients with atrial septal defect have a progressive course and develop pulmonary vascular disease while other patients with the same apparent hemodynamics do not suffer the same fate. It is probable that the genetic characteristics of their pulmonary blood vessels are significantly different.

Atrial Septal Defect Associated with Mitral Stenosis Atrial septal defect associated with mitral stenosis, referred to as Lutembacher's syndrome, has varying hemodynamic patterns, depending mainly on the size of the atrial septal defect and the severity of the pulmonary vascular disease. If the mitral stenosis is severe, there must be an elevation of left atrial pressure to provide an adequate gradient across the mitral valve to force enough blood into the left ventricle to sustain life. If the atrial septal defect is large and there is equal pressure in both atria, there will be a large flow into the right ventricle and pulmonary artery. In such patients the jugular venous pressure provides a simple estimate of pressure in the two atria and a useful estimate of the severity of mitral obstruction. Rarely, patients with acquired or congenital mitral valve disease may stretch the interatrial septum and develop a left-to-right shunt through the foramen ovale.

Clinical Manifestations

Atrial septal defect is a relatively common cardiac malformation. It is found in approximately 10 percent of children surviving beyond the first year of life with congenital heart disease,[4] and if one excludes the congenitally bicuspid aortic valve, it is the most common form of congenital heart disease among adults.[6] Somewhere between 20 to 25 percent of interatrial communications are of the ostium primum type. These represent the partial form of the atrioventricular canal malformation and are discussed below. The remainder, about 75 to 80 percent of atrial septal defects, are considered clinically to be of the secundum type. When these defects are identified surgically, approximately 70 percent prove to be limited to the central portion of the atrial septum (Fig. 36-4*A* and *C* and Fig. 36-5), 20 percent extend to the posterior septal wall and inferior vena cava, and about 6 percent are found to be sinus venosus type defects adjacent to the superior vena cava (Fig. 36-4*B* and Fig. 36-6).[100] The remaining 3 or 4 percent are identified as multiple defects or other rare forms of interatrial communication such as the coronary sinus defect.[101]

Atrial septal defects are more common among females with the female/male ratio being approximately 2:1. Although the mode of transmission is best explained in most instances on a multifactorial basis where the risk would be approximately 2.5 percent for first-degree relatives of a single affected family member, examples of autosomal dominant transmission are recognized either as an isolated entity,[102] associated with severe atrioventricular conduction disturbances,[103] or with upper extremity malformations as in the Holt-Oram syndrome.[104] Examples of Mendelian autosomal recessive transmission are found in the Ellis–van Creveld and thrombocytopenia–absent radius syndromes.[105]

History The majority of children are considered asymptomatic by themselves and by their parents. Probably most have some mild diminution of stamina, however, since it is not unusual for the patient or the parents to comment on the increased endurance and strength that follows surgical correction. Symptoms of mild fatigue and dyspnea tend to be recognized in the late teens and early twenties with unrepaired defects, and approximately three-quarters of individuals will be definitely symptomatic as adults.[91] Congestive heart failure is rare in childhood, but a few infants, perhaps 5 percent, will have congestive heart failure in the first year of life.[106]

Failure becomes more common again in the fourth and fifth decades, usually associated with the onset of arrhythmias. Approximately 40 percent of adults develop severe symptoms such as easy fatigue, dyspnea, orthopnea, chest pain, and syncope.[107]

Physical Examination Many children tend to have a slender habitus, but normal growth and development are not unusual. Color, breathing, and the jugular venous pulse are normal in the absence of congestive failure or severe pulmonary arterial hypertension. Prominence of the left anterior chest is common, and a hyperdynamic right ventricular, systolic lift can usually be felt along the entire left sternal border. The first heart sound may be slightly accentuated at the lower left sternal border, and the two components of the second heart sound are characteristically widely split with the interval of splitting relatively fixed despite expiration or the Valsalva maneuver. The pulmonary component of the second heart sound may be slightly to moderately accentuated even in the absence of pulmonary arterial hypertension. With increasing pulmonary arterial pressure and resistance, the interval between the aortic and pulmonary components of the second heart sound narrows and the pulmonary component becomes louder, but the lack of respiratory influence on the interval between the two components persists. A midsystolic, spindle-shaped murmur of grade 2 to 3 intensity at the left upper sternal border, reflecting increased right ventricular stroke volume, is to be expected. A low- to medium-pitched, early diastolic murmur over the lower left sternal border, denoting increased diastolic flow across the tricuspid valve, is present in most individuals with large shunts. A soft, early systolic ejection click may be heard during expiration in the same area, but a prominent systolic ejection click or a loud midsystolic murmur with a thrill favors associated valvular pulmonary stenosis. Occasionally, a midsystolic click and, less frequently, a holosystolic murmur at the apex will suggest concomitant mitral valve prolapse and mitral regurgitation. Patients with biatrial hypertension, almost always adults, on the basis of associated left ventricular, aortic, or mitral disease, may have pulmonary rales, jugular venous distension, and hepatomegaly. The presence of an accentuated first heart sound at the apex, an opening snap of the mitral valve, or an apical diastolic rumble in this setting would suggest the presence of concomitant mitral stenosis, an association referred to as Lutembacher's syndrome.[86] Cyanosis and clubbing reflect right-to-left shunting, which is usually the result of severe pulmonary vascular disease and altered right ventricular compliance. In this setting the murmurs of tricuspid and pulmonary regurgitation are not uncommon.

Chest Roentgenogram Mild to moderate cardiac enlargement and prominence of the main and branch pulmonary arteries are characteristic of this lesion.

DISEASES OF THE HEART AND BLOOD VESSELS

The ascending aorta is inconspicuous. The absence of left atrial displacement of the barium-filled esophagus in the lateral view helps to distinguish atrial septal defect from other large left-to-right shunts such as ventricular septal defect and patent ductus arteriosus (Fig. 36-8). With advanced pulmonary vascular disease the proximal pulmonary arterial segment may become markedly dilated or aneurysmal, while in contrast, the peripheral pulmonary vascular markings become attenuated.

Electrocardiogram An rsR′ QRS pattern over the right precordium indicating mild right ventricular conduction delay or mild right ventricular hypertrophy is characteristic. The PQ interval is slightly prolonged in approximately 20 percent of patients. The mean QRS axis in the frontal plane is 90° or greater in 60 percent of patients, while a few, a little over 2 percent, will have superior QRS axis lying between −10 and −160°. About half of these will have apparently uncomplicated secundum defects, while the remainder will be found to have a variety of unusual features such as mitral valve prolapse, hypertrophic cardiomyopathy, Noonan's syndrome, or single coronary artery.[108] Serious arrhythmias are usually, though not invariably, limited to adults; atrial fibrillation and atrial flutter are the most common.

Echocardiogram M-mode studies reflect the right ventricular diastolic volume overload by an increase in right ventricular end-diastolic dimensions. Abnormal anterior systolic motion of the interventricular septum is usually, though not invariably, present as well (Fig. 36-9). Two-dimensional, cross-sectional echocardiography can provide direct imaging of the atrial septum from the subxiphoid approach in infants and, somewhat less reliably, from the apex in older children and adults.[109] With the use of intravenously injected echo-producing solutions, both left-to-right and right-to-left shunting of blood at the atrial level can be identified.[110,111] Coexistent mitral valve prolapse, present in anywhere from 30 to 95 percent of patients, may also be demonstrated.[112]

Cardiac Catheterization There will be a significant increase in oxygen saturation in the blood samples drawn from the right atrium compared with those from the superior or inferior venae cavae. Saturations similar to those in the right atrium will be found in the right ventricle and pulmonary arteries. Pulmonary arterial and right ventricular systolic pressures usually are normal or only slightly elevated. A systolic pressure gradient of up to 20 mmHg across the right ventricular outflow tract is accepted as secondary to flow rather than to organic obstruction. The right and left atrial mean and phasic pressures will be virtually identical with little if any elevation above normal. A mean pressure gradient of 3 mmHg or more between the two atria should alert the operator to the possibility that the oxygen step-up at atrial level is due to a left ventricular–right atrial communication, to partial anomalous pulmonary venous connection with an intact atrial septum, or that the interatrial opening is a stretched foramen ovale associated with left atrial hypertension. The cardiac catheter, if passed from the inferior vena cava, usually crosses a central interatrial opening easily. In the presence of a sinus venosus defect, passage across the defect may be difficult or impossible from this route. The site of connection of pulmonary veins can often be established by selective injections of contrast material in

FIGURE 36-8 Frontal and lateral chest roentgenograms of a 4-year-old child with a secundum atrial septal defect, a large left-to-right shunt, and normal pulmonary arterial pressures. Right ventricular enlargement, seen in the lateral view, accompanies prominence of the main pulmonary arterial segment and increased blood flow. No left atrial dilatation is present.

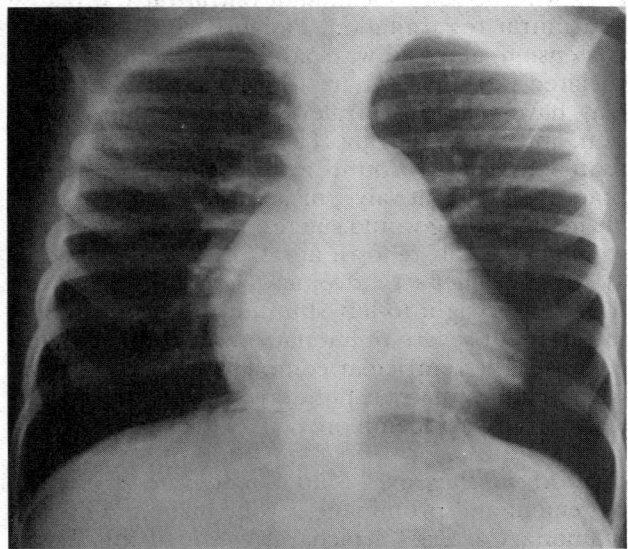

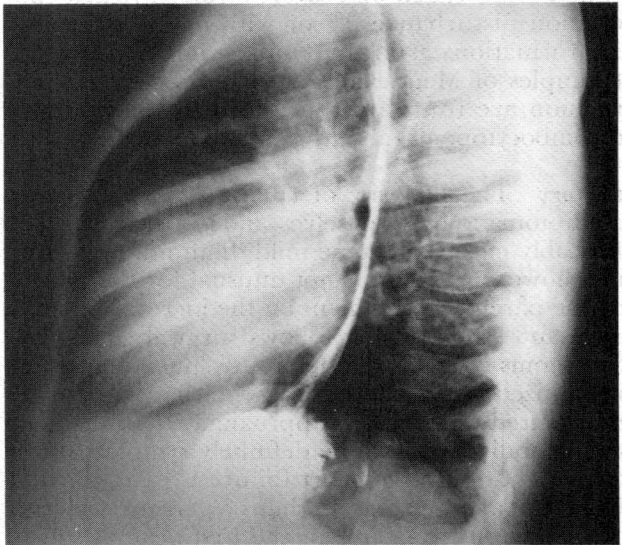

A

B

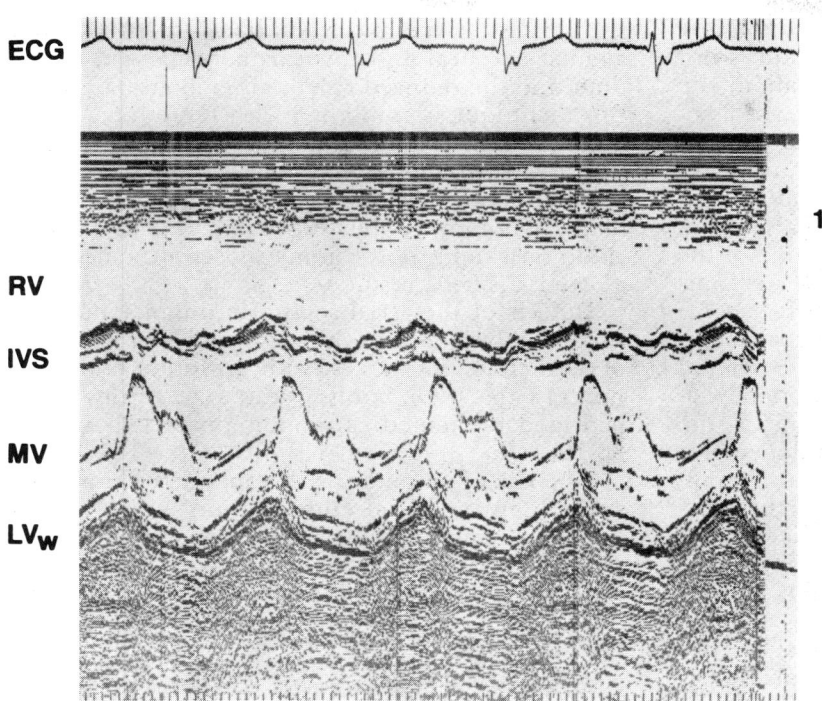

ECG

1 cm

RV

IVS

MV

LV$_W$

FIGURE 36-9 M-mode echocardiogram from a child with a secundum atrial septal defect demonstrating the increased right ventricular cavity dimension (2.4 cm end-diastolic diameter) and anterior systolic motion of the interventricular septum (IVS) characteristic of right ventricular diastolic overload. ECG = electrocardiogram; RV = right ventricle; MV = mitral valve; LVW = posterior left ventricular wall; cm = centimeter.

the individual veins or by dye-dilution studies. Selective left ventricular angiography is indicated if mitral valve disease is suspected or if a superior QRS axis is present on the electrocardiogram.

Natural History and Prognosis

Atrial septal defects of the secundum type usually go undetected in the first year or two of life because of the lack of symptoms and unimpressive auscultatory findings. A soft systolic murmur, perhaps considered innocent initially, is the usual reason for referral. Aside from the small number of infants in the first year with congestive heart failure, most children and adolescents lead a relatively normal life. In the late teens and twenties, symptoms become more common and by age 40, the majority, but not all, of individuals are symptomatic, some severely so.[107] Though rare in childhood, pulmonary vascular disease with serious pulmonary hypertension begins to make its appearance in the early twenties. It affects approximately 15 percent of young adults, particularly women, and may be rapidly progressive, especially with pregnancy. The incidence of atrial fibrillation or flutter also increases with each decade and is closely linked to the onset of congestive failure. Cleft anterior or posterior leaflets, rheumatic heart disease, and a variety of other lesions may occur in patients with atrial septal defect. Mitral valve prolapse is implicated in some, though usually a minority. The influence of prolapse, detected either clinically, angiographically, or echocardiographically, on the natural history of a patient with operated or unoperated atrial septal defect is still unclear.[113,114] However, echocardiographic evidence of disappearance or dimunition of prolapse

following surgery suggests that a reversible distortion of the left ventricular cavity may be responsible for this abnormality rather than an intrinsic anatomic deformity of the mitral valve itself.[115] Spontaneous closure of secundum defects is thought to be rare beyond the first year of life, but below that age such closure may be relatively frequent, perhaps even approaching 50 percent.[85] Although longevity is possible in the absence of closure, it is quite clear that the passage of time, certainly after adolescence, is associated with a steady increase in the frequency and the severity of symptoms, a higher prevalence of pulmonary arterial hypertension and pulmonary vascular disease, a greater number of individuals with important right ventricular dilatation and hypertrophy, a greater frequency of arrhythmias and congestive failure, and a higher mortality and morbidity with and following corrective surgery.[107] Congestive failure is the most common cause of death among patients with unoperated atrial septal defects. Other causes of death include pulmonary embolism or thrombosis, paradoxical emboli, brain abscess, and infection. The average age of death among patients with severe pulmonary vascular disease is 36 years, with the mode of exitus being sudden collapse, heart failure, or hemoptysis.[98] Congestive failure is an indication for prompt cardiac catheterization and surgical correction.

Medical Management

Asymptomatic infants and children are usually followed at yearly intervals and surgery is recommended just prior to their entry into school or shortly thereafter. Restrictions on activity or exercise are usually unnecessary in childhood. If the physical and laboratory findings are completely characteristic, preoperative catheterization is not necessary; but if there is any suspicion about the accuracy of the diagnosis or the possibility of associated defects, other than partial anomalous pulmonary venous connection, catheterization is indicated. Surgery is recommended if the pulmonary to systemic blood flow ratio is 1.7:1 or greater, provided no serious malfunction of the left side of the heart is present. Surgical closure is also recommended for those patients with ratios between 1.5 and 1.7:1 if right ventricular volume overload is evident on clinical examination or pulmonary arterial hypertension is documented by catheterization. Closure would seem prudent prior to pregnancy or the use of contraceptives in view of the tendency of a few individuals to develop rapidly progressive pulmonary vascular obstructive disease under these circumstances. Postoperative follow-up is recommended to determine the completeness of surgical repair, to document the extent of return to normal of the clinical and laboratory abnormalities, to manage arrhythmias dating from either before or after the time of surgery, and to be certain no previously undetected heart disease, particularly of the mitral valve, is present. As an alternative to open heart surgery, transvenous closure of atrial septal defects using an umbrella-like patch placed with a cardiac catheter is under investigation.[116] Genetic counseling is in order. In the absence of a syndrome transmitted dominantly or recessively in a Mendelian pattern and if the patient is the only first-degree relative affected, the risk of the next sibling having congenital heart disease is in the order of 2.5 percent. The risk to offspring of the patient is the same.[117] Since existing siblings and parents of the patient are also first-degree relatives and since the signs and symptoms of atrial septal defect may be subtle, careful examination of these family members is indicated. Infective endocarditis is rare, but antibiotic coverage at the times of possible bacteremia is recommended if there is associated mitral valve disease.

Surgical Management

Defects of the interatrial septum are closed by direct suture or placement of a pericardial or Dacron patch, depending upon the location of the defect, its size, and the firmness of its margins. Several ingenious operative techniques have been devised for closure of interatrial communications. Gross[118] developed the atrial well technique for blind closure of atrial septal defects through the blood-filled right atrium of the beating heart. Many defects have been closed using moderate hypothermia and circulatory arrest without cardiopulmonary bypass.[119] Gibbon's closure of an atrial septal defect was the first operation ever performed using extracorporeal circulatory support.[120] Cardiopulmonary bypass with total-body perfusion and moderate hypothermia (30 to 32°C) is now used routinely for closure of atrial sep-

tal defects. Excellent visualization, protection against cerebral and myocardial ischemia, ample time, and the reduced risk of air embolization when this technique is combined with temporary aortic occlusion and cardioplegia have virtually eliminated operative mortality.

Operation is usually performed through a median sternotomy. A bilateral submammary skin incision or a right thoracotomy is used in females for a better cosmetic result.

Defects of the atrial septum in infants and very small children can be closed during a brief period of total circulatory arrest with profound hypothermia (18 to 20°C), cooling and rewarming being provided by limited cardiopulmonary bypass (Fig. 36-10).

The risk of air entering the open left atrium with subsequent cerebral embolization is avoided by cross-clamping the aorta prior to opening the right atrium. Cardiac standstill is produced by the injection of cardioplegic solution into the ascending

FIGURE 36-10 *A.* Large atrial septal defect in the secundum position. *B.* Same defect, now closed by a knitted Dacron patch. (*Courtesy of S. Bert Litwin, M.D.*)

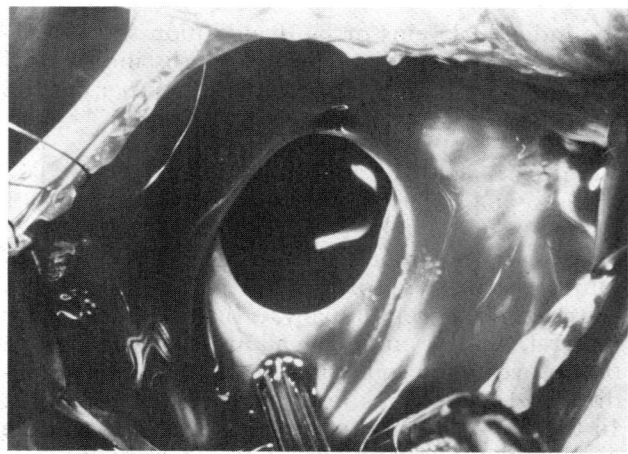

A

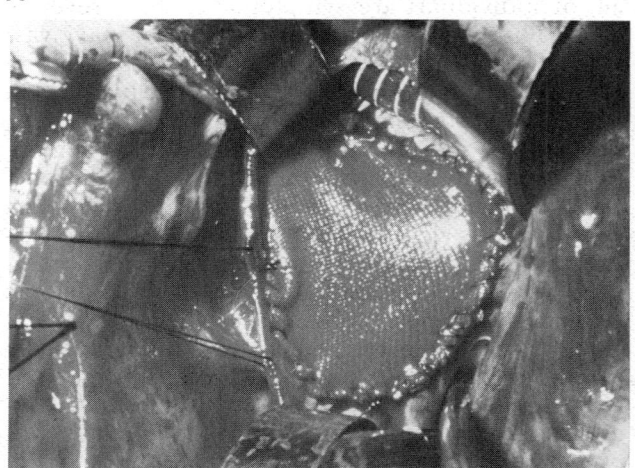

B

aorta and coronary arteries. Blood remains within the left ventricle and left atrium during closure of the defect. After removal of the cross-clamp, blood and air bubbles are aspirated continuously from the ascending aorta using a perforated plastic needle connected to suction from the heart-lung machine.

Foramen ovale defects are closed by simple suture during intracardiac repair of complex defects such as tetralogy of Fallot. Ostium secundum defects can be closed by direct suture if the margins are firm. If the entire membranous septum has multiple fenestrations and tenuous margins, closure will require placement of a patch of pericardium or Dacron.

High atrial septal defects of the sinus venosus type are usually associated with anomalous drainage of the right superior pulmonary vein into the lower lateral portion of the superior vena cava. These defects are corrected by placement of a pericardial or tubular Dacron patch from above the abnormally draining vein down to and around the atrial septal defect (Fig. 36-11). Pulmonary venous blood is thus diverted through the defect into the left atrium.[121] The superior vena cava is cannulated as high as possible to allow space for the patch. Pericardial gusset enlargement of the superior vena cava at the caval-atrial junction may be required to avoid obstruction.[122]

Closure of ostium primum atrial septal defects is described in the discussion of partial atrioventricular canal.

Hospital death following closure of simple atrial defects in children and young adults is extremely rare.[122,123] Postoperative atrial dysrhythmias are relatively common but usually transient. Mortality in patients over 40 years of age is about 5 percent.[124] Long-term results in patients undergoing closure of an uncomplicated atrial septal defect are excellent.

Consequences of an atrial septal defect in older patients include right atrial dilatation and hypertrophy, supraventricular arrhythmias, chronic congestive heart failure, tricuspid and mitral valvular incompetence secondary to ventricular and annular dilatation, and mild to moderate pulmonary vascular obstructive disease.[124] Although clinical improvement can be anticipated following closure of atrial septal defects in adults with these complications, mortality is higher and the degree of improvement uncertain. The frequency of these complications in adults and the low risk of surgical closure in the young child mandates operation in the preschool or preadolescent years.[125] The possibility that even earlier operation at about 2 years of age would avoid late right ventricular dysfunction encourages closure of an atrial septal defect when the child is quite young.

Single Atrium

Definition

Single atrium (cor triloculare biventriculare) refers to the condition in which either no atrial septal tissue is present or the atrial septum is so rudimentary as to yield a common chamber involving both atria.

Pathology

In its simple form, single atrium is observed in adolescents or adults. Its secondary effects are essentially like those in atrial septal defect. Except in

FIGURE 36-11   *A.* Sinus venosus type of atrial septal defect, with its constantly accompanying anomalous pulmonary venous connection of superior pulmonary vein (SPV) to superior vena cava (SVC). *B.* Repair is effected with a pericardial patch, so placed as to divert pulmonary venous blood across the defect into the left atrium and to divert superior vena caval blood to the right atrium.

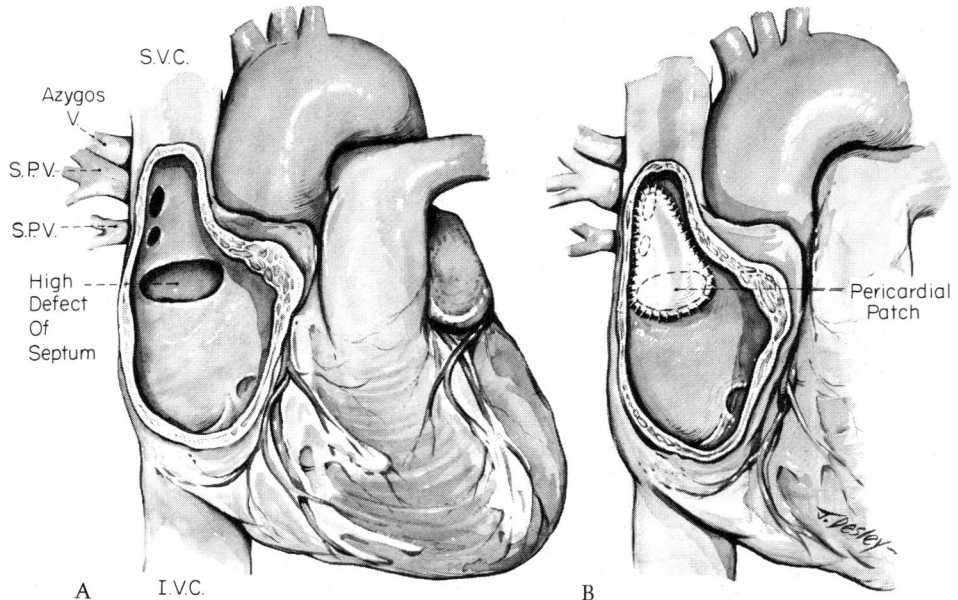

asplenia, the great vessels are usually normally related. There is a strong tendency for the atrioventricular valves to be anomalous, characteristic of the common atrioventricular canal defects.[126] In this way a ventricular septal defect may be present or absent. In adults an interventricular communication is usually absent.

A special form of single atrium is present in the syndrome of asplenia and is commonly associated with other malformations, including pulmonary stenosis and malposed great vessels.

Clinical Manifestations

The clinical features of this malformation are those of a very large atrial septal defect of the atrioventricular canal variety.[127] Though rare, it is the characteristic malformation described among patients with the autosomal recessive Ellis–Van Creveld syndrome.

History Symptoms of shortness of breath and easy fatigue usually appear within the first year of life. Mild cyanosis is commonly observed with crying. Weight gain tends to be slow and lower respiratory tract infections are frequent.

Physical Examination Mild tachypnea, mild cyanosis, and clubbing of the fingers and toes are characteristic. Prominence of the left precordium, a hyperdynamic right ventricular lift, and fixed splitting of the second heart sound reflect the right ventricular volume overload and the unobstructed interatrial opening. A holosystolic, regurgitant murmur at the apex would indicate mitral regurgitation, a common feature of this malformation.[128]

Laboratory Mild to moderate polycythemia reflects the mild systemic arterial oxygen desaturation usually found with this lesion.

Chest Roentgenogram Cardiac enlargement is usual with prominence of the main and branch pulmonary arteries and an impressive increase in pulmonary blood flow, but little, if any, left atrial enlargement. Dextrocardia, mesocardia, or levocardia with situs ambiguus also may be present.

Electrocardiogram The mean QRS axis is superior, as with other varieties of atrioventricular canal defect. Mild first-degree atrioventricular block, a mild to moderate right ventricular conduction delay, and right ventricular hypertrophy complete the picture. Ectopic atrial rhythms and junctional escape rhythms are frequent.

Echocardiogram Both M-mode and two-dimensional studies show the characteristic feature of an atrioventricular canal defect.

Cardiac Catheterization Complete or nearly complete mixing of systemic venous and pulmonary venous blood is found at the atrial level, and mild

systemic arterial oxygen desaturation is the rule. Pulmonary arterial hypertension is common, with a mild to moderate increase in the pulmonary vascular resistance in some cases. Selective angiography with injections in both systemic and pulmonary veins is recommended to define abnormalities of venous return. Left ventricular angiography will assess the presence and degree of mitral regurgitation and the presence of an associated ventricular septal defect, establish the relationship of the great arteries, and demonstrate the "gooseneck" deformity characteristic of atrioventricular canal defects.

Natural History, Prognosis, and Medical Management

The natural history, management, and indications for surgery are the same as those for the ostium primum type of atrioventricular canal defects. Abnormalities of pulmonary and systemic venous return may add considerably to the complexity of the surgery, however.

Surgical Management

Through a median sternotomy the common atrial chamber is partitioned with a pericardial or Dacron patch sutured under conditions of total cardiopulmonary bypass, whole-body perfusion, moderate hypothermia (25 to 28°C), and cardioplegia. Total circulatory arrest with profound hypothermia is used in infants. Suture lines and patch are placed so that pulmonary venous blood is diverted to the mitral orifice and left ventricle. Superior and inferior caval flow is directed to the tricuspid orifice and right ventricle. Hepatic veins may enter the atrium directly and should be placed on the right side of the atrial partition. The coronary sinus may be placed in either the pulmonary or the systemic venous atrium. Since single atrium is a type of atrioventricular canal defect, anomalies of the atrioventricular valves and coexisting ventricular septal defects should be repaired at the same operation.

Care is required to avoid injury to the atrioventricular node near the coronary sinus. Conduction disturbances and supraventricular arrhythmias are common preoperatively in patients with single atrium, but postoperative complete heart block can usually be avoided by meticulous surgical technique and an understanding of the anatomy of the conduction system.

Long-term results depend upon the severity of associated anomalies but are generally quite good when single atrium is the only defect.

Partial Anomalous Pulmonary Venous Connection

Definition

In partial anomalous pulmonary venous connection one or more, but not all, of the pulmonary veins enter the right atrium or its venous tributaries.

Pathology
The atrial septum may be intact, but an atrial septal defect is usually present. There are many patterns of anomalous pulmonary venous connection, but the four most common, in order of decreasing frequency, are (1) the right upper and/or middle lobe pulmonary veins to the superior vena cava, usually with a sinus venosus atrial septal defect; (2) all the right pulmonary veins to the right atrium, usually in the polysplenia syndrome; (3) all the right pulmonary veins or the right middle and lower lobe veins to the inferior vena cava entering the systemic vein just above or below the diaphragm; and (4) the left upper or both left pulmonary veins to an anomalous vertical vein draining to the left brachiocephalic vein (Fig. 36-12).

When right pulmonary veins connect to the inferior vena cava, the atrial septum may be intact or patent. This venous anomaly may be isolated or part of the *scimitar syndrome*. The latter includes hypoplasia of the right lung, bronchial abnormalities, and anomalous systemic pulmonary arterial supply to the right lung from branches of the descending and/or the abdominal aorta, and dextroposition of the heart.[129] The right pulmonary artery, as well as the left, is present.

Abnormal Physiology
Partial anomalous pulmonary venous connection with or without associated atrial septal defect is hemodynamically similar to an uncomplicated atrial

FIGURE 36-12   Partial anomalous pulmonary venous connection of left upper pulmonary vein (LUPV) to left innominate (brachiocephalic) vein (LI).

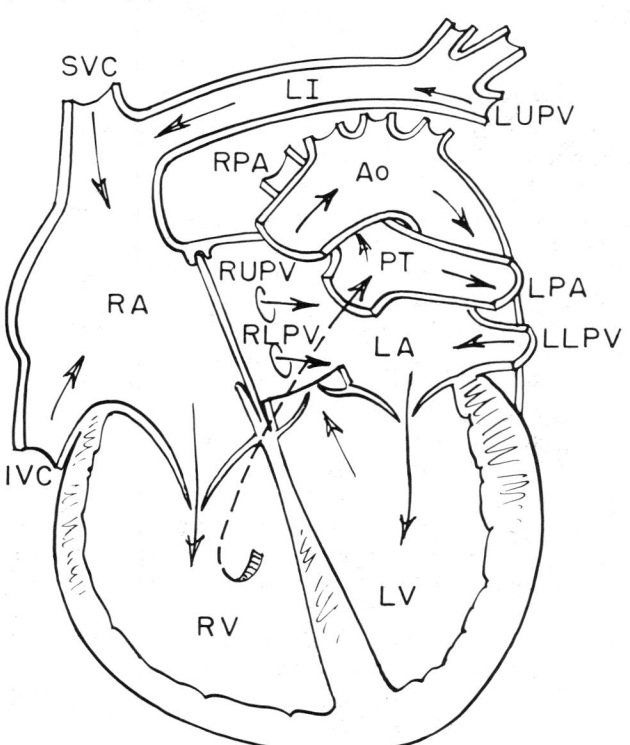

septal defect; however, the magnitude of pulmonary blood flow rarely reaches the very high values found in atrial septal defect. Arterial unsaturation and cyanosis are rare unless there is an associated atrial septal defect with the development of pulmonary hypertension.

Clinical Manifestations
This malformation occurs in approximately 1 in every 160 individuals, or 0.6 percent of the population.[130] There is no sex predilection. Most examples are found in association with atrial septal defects where the drainage is, with few exceptions, from part or all of the right lung to the right atrium or superior vena cava. Approximately 15 percent of all atrial septal defects have this coexisting anomaly; but in the case of the sinus venosus type defect, the association is in the range of 85 percent.[131] Anomalous connection of a single pulmonary vein also may be discovered, usually accidentally at the time of catheterization, in combination with more complex cardiac malformations such as tetralogy of Fallot, truncus arteriosus, single ventricle, or ventricular septal defect. The remaining examples are found as an isolated abnormality with an intact atrial septum. In the latter situation abnormal connections from the right lung continue to outnumber those from the left but only in a ratio of approximately 3:1.

History   When partial anomalous pulmonary venous connection coexists with an atrial septal defect, the symptoms, as well as the electrocardiographic and, usually, the roentgenologic findings, are indistinguishable from those of an isolated atrial septal defect. Isolated, uncomplicated anomalous connection of a single pulmonary vein usually goes undetected clinically since in this circumstance only about 20 percent of the pulmonary venous flow returns to the right atrium or its tributaries. When two pulmonary veins or the entire venous return from one lung are connected anomalously, approximately 65 percent of the pulmonary venous flow returns to the right side of the heart and symptoms are similar to those of an atrial septal defect with a comparable increase in pulmonary blood flow. Easy fatigue, dyspnea, and occasionally heart failure, particularly during early infancy, may be present.[131] Respiratory symptoms in individuals with the scimitar syndrome may, at least in part, be due to hypoplasia of the right lung.

Physical Examination   The findings are the same as those in patients with an atrial septal defect. The volumes of left-to-right shunting are comparable, with the notable exception that the two components of the second heart sound, though usually widely split, move normally with respiration if the atrial septum is intact. Hypoplasia of the right hemithorax and rightward shift of the heart within the chest would suggest the possibility of scimitar syndrome.

DISEASES OF THE HEART AND BLOOD VESSELS

Chest Roentgenogram Right ventricular enlargement, pulmonary arterial dilatation, and increased pulmonary blood flow in the lung fields are characteristic when more than one pulmonary vein connects anomalously. Only occasionally can one detect dilatation of the superior vena cava, azygous vein, or a left vertical vein, which would suggest anomalous pulmonary venous connection to that vessel. An exception, however, is found with anomalous connection of the right pulmonary veins to the inferior vena cava, where the pulmonary venous pattern assumes a crescent-shaped or scimitar curve in the right lower lung field along the right lower heart border. This syndrome usually is associated with varying degrees of hypoplasia of the right lung and right hemithorax with displacement of the heart toward the midline or into the right chest (Fig. 36-13).

Electrocardiogram The electrocardiographic findings are either normal, in instances of anomalous connection of a single pulmonary vein, or reflect volume overload of the right side of the heart, which is indistinguishable from that of an atrial septal defect.

Echocardiogram If more than one pulmonary vein drains anomalously, the volume usually is sufficient to produce the characteristic pattern of right ventricular diastolic overload, which is indistinguishable from that of an atrial septal defect. Failure to visualize an atrial septal opening with two-dimensional imaging or the characteristic displacement of echoes within the right atrium with intravenous contrast studies should arouse suspicion of an intact atrial septum.

FIGURE 36-13 Frontal view of the chest roentgenogram of an 8-year-old boy with scimitar syndrome. The crescent-shaped curve of the right common pulmonary vein (arrows) lies behind the heart, which is rotated into the right hemithorax due to hypoplasia of the right lung.

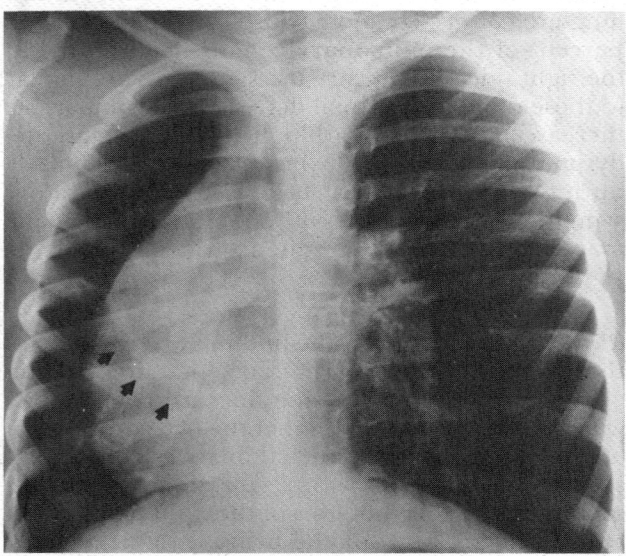

Cardiac Catheterization Anomalously connected pulmonary veins may be entered directly with the cardiac catheter from the right atrium, superior or inferior venae cavae, or their tributaries. Selective biplane angiograms in these vessels will document their site of connection. While indicator-dilution curves with injection in the individual veins and systemic arterial sampling usually will provide similar information, the particular value of this technique lies in its ability to distinguish partial anomalous pulmonary venous connection with an atrial septal defect from partial anomalous pulmonary venous connection with an intact atrial septum. A large step-up in oxygen saturation at the atrial level favors the presence of an atrial septal defect since left-to-right shunting with partial anomalous pulmonary venous connection and an intact atrial septum is usually small or moderate. The presence of anomalous connection of a single, isolated pulmonary vein and its site of entry may go undetected by oximetry techniques unless multiple blood samples are drawn and a localized increase in oxygen saturation can be demonstrated. Even with drainage of the entire right lung to the inferior vena cava, as in the case of scimitar syndrome, the increase in oxygen saturation within the right atrium may be unimpressive because of hypoplasia and diminished volume of the right pulmonary vascular bed and the normal relatively high saturation of the inferior vena cava samples due to blood contributed by the renal veins. In these situations selective indicator-dilution curves in the right and left pulmonary arteries with systemic arterial sampling can detect the lung with the anomalous pulmonary venous connection, and selective biplane angiograms in the pulmonary artery branches will visualize these connections.

Natural History and Prognosis

Patients with partial anomalous pulmonary venous connection with atrial septal defect appear to follow a course similar, if not identical, to that of those with an isolated atrial septal defect. When the atrial septum is intact, the course depends primarily upon the volume of pulmonary venous blood returning to the right atrium or its tributaries. A large flow leads eventually to disability, pulmonary arterial hypertension, and pulmonary vascular disease. Rarely, pulmonary vascular obstructive disease may be found even in the presence of a single anomalously connected pulmonary vein and an intact atrial septum.[132] Finally, increasing left atrial pressure, due either to mitral valve disease or diminishing left ventricular compliance, will, in the course of time, encourage a greater redistribution of pulmonary arterial blood flow to that portion of the lung drained by the more compliant right atrium. Thus, patients, initially asymptomatic and with a very modest volume of anomalous pulmonary venous return in youth, may become symptomatic and even develop congestive failure in adult life.

Medical Management

Medical management does not differ significantly from that of the patient with atrial septal defect. Asymptomatic patients with small shunts require no treatment, while those with symptoms, larger pulmonary blood flows, congestive failure, or pulmonary arterial hypertension require surgical correction. Preoperative identification of partial anomalous venous connection in the presence of an atrial septal defect is not essential since, with extracorporeal circulation, the pulmonary venous drainage can be identified and, if necessary, corrected at the time of surgery. With an intact atrial septum, however, precise preoperative identification of the site of the anomalous venous connection is essential. Long-term follow-up in unoperated patients is indicated to ensure the detection of increasing flow or the appearance of pulmonary arterial hypertension. A relatively low threshold for postoperative cardiac catheterization is appropriate in view of the subtle, but important, effects of either persistent pulmonary venous hypertension or pulmonary arterial volume overload on the pulmonary vascular bed.[133]

Surgical Management

Anomalous connection of the *right superior* pulmonary vein to the superior vena cava is usually asso-

ciated with an atrial septal defect of the sinus venosus type. Operative management of this anomaly is described in the discussion of atrial septal defect (Fig. 36-11).

Anomalous connection of the *right inferior* pulmonary vein to the right atrium or to the inferior vena cava above or below the diaphragm is corrected by placement of an intracardiac patch diverting the orifice of the anomalous vein into the left atrium through a surgically created atrial septal defect.[134] Cardiopulmonary bypass is used, sometimes with a period of hypothermic circulatory arrest to facilitate exposure within the inferior vena cava (Fig. 36-14).

When the *right inferior* pulmonary vein passes *anterior* to the pulmonary hilum to enter the supradiaphragmatic inferior vena cava, the vein may be transplanted directly into the left atrium posterior to the interatrial groove without cardiopulmonary bypass.

Individual *left* pulmonary veins draining into the brachiocephalic venous system usually have sufficient length for transplantation to the left atrial appendage without cardiopulmonary bypass.[135]

Rare cases of bilateral partial anomalous pulmonary venous connection require individualized and combined operations. Mortality from operation ap-

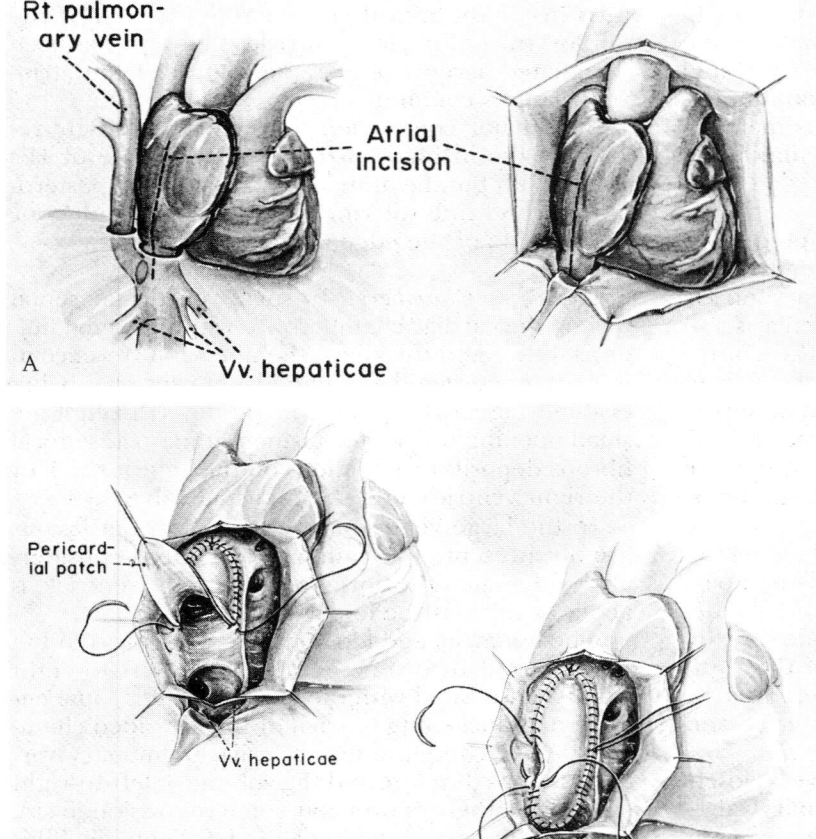

FIGURE 36-14 The anomalous vein draining the entire right lung pierces the diaphragm to join the inferior vena cava near the right hepatic vein. *Right.* The pericardium has been opened. The proposed right atrial incision is carried onto the intrapericardial portion of the inferior vena cava. *B.* Placement of pericardial patch so as to divert blood from anomalously connected right pulmonary vein to left atrium. (*From Murphy, Kerr, and Kirklin.*[134] *Reproduced with permission.*)

proaches zero. Morbidity is low. Long-term results are excellent.

Ventricular Septal Defect

Definition

Ventricular septal defect represents an opening between that part of the ventricular septum that separates the two ventricles. (Left ventricular–right atrial communication is a special type of ventricular septal defect and is ordinarily not included under the category of ventricular septal defect.)

Pathology

A defect of the ventricular septum represents the most common alteration among malformed hearts. In some this is the only condition. In others a defect of the ventricular septum is part of a complex malformation in which additional structures participate. In still other subjects, a ventricular septal defect is isolated but may be associated with an additional malformation that is not a recognized complex.

Usually, ventricular septal defect is a solitary opening varying in diameter from a few millimeters, but often early equaling the diameter of the aortic orifice. When more than one defect is present, it is either a coincidence of two anatomic types being present or a multiplicity of muscular defects appearing as a recognized form. Defects may be divided into two functional types: the small, when there is an obstructive element to the defect, and the large, when there is unobstructive communication between the two ventricles.[136] Defects may also be classified according to right ventricular landmarks.[137]

Anatomic Types The most common type of ventricular septal defect is the paramembranous type. It lies in the outflow portion of the right ventricle immediately below the crista supraventricularis and posterior to the papillary muscle of the conus. Three-fourths of all ventricular septal defects lie in this region.[138] Less common are the conal or supracristal defects (8 percent), defects lying posteriorly and beneath the septal leaflet of the tricuspid valve in the region of atrioventricular canal defects (4 percent), and, finally, defects toward the apex of the right ventricle in the muscular septum (Fig. 36-15).

About one-third of defects lie toward the apex. Multiplicity of such defects is characteristic, the defects being represented by tortuous channels within the septum. Defects lying in the wall of the right ventricular outflow tract are, from the left ventricular aspect, closely related to the aortic valve and may be overhung by it.

In the supracristal defect the aortic valve is closely allied through the defect with the pulmonary valve.

A special form of defect of the paramembranous type tends to run at right angles to the long axis of the right ventricular infundibulum and cuts into the

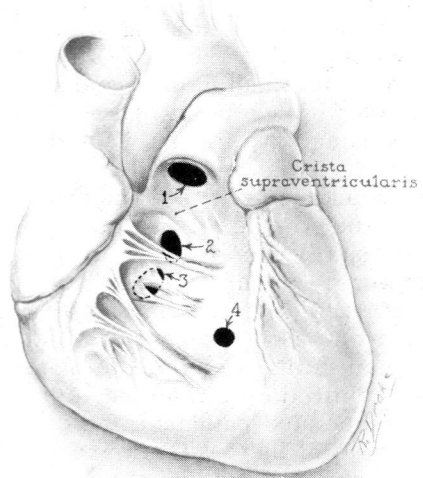

FIGURE 36-15 Diagrammatic representation of types of ventricular septal defects. *1.* A high defect immediately under the pulmonary valve. *2.* The typical high ventricular septal defect. *3.* The atrioventricular canal type of ventricular septal defect. *4.* A defect in the muscular portion of the septum. (*From J. W. Kirklin, H. G. Harshbarger, D. E. Donald, and J. E. Edwards, Surgical Correction of Ventricular Septal Defect: Anatomic and Technical Considerations, J. Thorac. Surg., 33:45, 1957. Reproduced with permission.*)

septal band. When viewed from the left side, the defect runs obliquely from the posteromedial commissure of the mitral valve across the wall of the outflow tract of the left ventricle. This type has been designated a ventricular septal defect of the atrioventricularis communis type.[139]

The major conduction tissue is most closely related to the infracristal defect. The bundle of His and the left bundle branches lie close to the posteroinferior and inferior rim of the defect[140] and favor the left side of the edge of the defect.

The Cardiac Chambers In small ventricular septal defect, the cardiac chambers are within normal limits as to size and thickness, the normal difference in thickness between the left and right ventricles being evident (Fig. 36-16). As the blood flows through the small opening in a jetlike fashion, it may cause focal fibrous deposits or jet lesions on the anterior wall of the right ventricle and the tricuspid valve.

In the large ventricular septal defect, jet lesions are not present. The pulmonary trunk is considerably wider than the aorta, and the right ventricle is about as thick as the left (Fig. 36-16).

The left atrial and left ventricular cavities tend to be enlarged in instances with large left-to-right shunts. Associated with the enlargement is some endocardial thickening of each of the left-sided chambers. After complicating occlusive pulmonary vascular lesions develop, and the volume of left-to-right shunt falls, there is probably some regression in size of the chambers, notably of the left ventricle. This chamber may assume a normal size but continues to exhibit endocardial thickening.

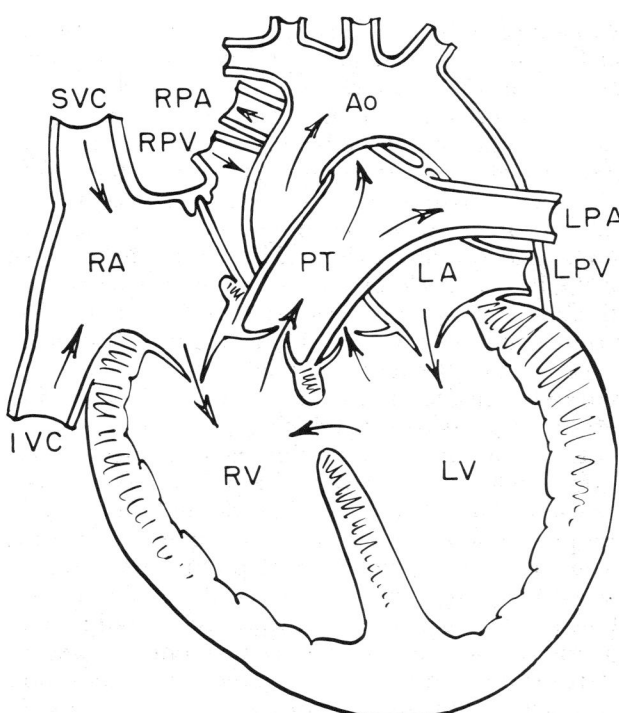

FIGURE 36-16 Ventricular septal defect with left-to-right shunt. Large defect. SVC = superior vena cava; IVC = inferior vena cava; RA = right atrium; RV = right ventricle; PT = main pulmonary arterial trunk; RPA = right pulmonary artery; LPA = left pulmonary artery; RPV = right pulmonary vein; LPV = left pulmonary vein; LA = left atrium; LV = left ventricle; Ao = aorta. [*From J. E. Edwards, Classification of Congenital Heart Disease in the Adult, in W. C. Roberts (ed.), Congenital Heart Disease in Adults, Cardiovasc. Clin. Series 10/1, F. A. Davis Company, Philadelphia, 1979, pp. 1–26. Reproduced with permission.*]

Associated Conditions Ventricular septal defect is frequently associated as an additional anomaly with which it does not form a recognized complex. The most common conditions which were found to be associated with ventricular septal defect as coincidental malformations among 46 specimens studied by Girod and associates[141] were, in order of decreasing frequency, as follows: (1) obstructive anomalies of the aorta (13 of 46 cases), of which coarctation was the most common; (2) additional shunts, most commonly atrial septal defect of the fossa ovalis type and patent ductus arteriosus; (3) intracardiac obstructions such as subaortic stenosis, mitral stenosis, and anomalous muscle bundle of the right ventricle; and (4) incompetent valves.

An intriguing condition that may be associated with ventricular septal defect is the so-called straddling tricuspid valve or double inlet left ventricle. The mitral valve leads into the left ventricle, while the tricuspid valve straddles the ventricular septum so as to open into each ventricle. The tensor apparatus of the tricuspid valve is anchored partly in each ventricle.[142,143]

Complications In small ventricular septal defect, the main potential complication is infectious endo-

carditis. This may begin at the edges of the defect or at the site of a right ventricular jet lesion; aortic valvular endocarditis may occur uncommonly. Except for the accompanying infections, small ventricular septal defects are well tolerated and may be found occasionally as incidental findings in the adult. The pulmonary vascular bed is normal.[136]

In large ventricular septal defect, the effects of the large left-to-right shunt may be evident in infancy and characterized by left ventricular failure. This is associated with congestive changes in the lungs. Secondary pneumonia may occur. The dominant effects are upon the lungs.[144]

Aortic regurgitation may develop in childhood or adolescence as a consequence of lack of support of the aortic root and is seen typically in supracristal defects and in some infracristal defects (Fig. 36-17).[145]

Abnormal Physiology[144,146–149]
The physiology of ventricular septal defect is largely dependent upon the area of the defect and the reaction of the pulmonary vasculature. Generally, patients with isolated ventricular septal defect may be divided into three groups, depending on the size of the defect. In the first group of patients, the defect is less than 0.5 cm^2 per square meter of body surface area, and consequently the defect itself offers a large resistance to flow from the left ventricle to the right ventricle. The magnitude of the shunt is determined mainly by size of the defect. In such patients there is usually no elevation of right ventricular or pulmonary artery pressures. The left-to-right shunt may be so small that it is not detected

FIGURE 36-17 Necropsy specimen (viewed from left ventricular aspect) from a patient with ventricular septal defect and aortic valve incompetence. Note prolapse and deformity of right aortic cusp. (*From F. H. Ellis, Jr., P. A. Ongley, and J. W. Kirklin, Ventricular Septal Defect with Aortic Incompetence: Surgical Considerations, Circulation, 27:789, 1963. Reproduced with permission of the American Heart Association.*)

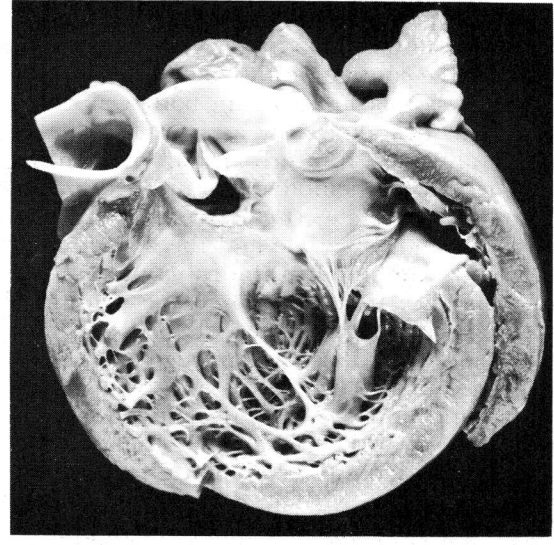

DISEASES OF THE HEART AND BLOOD VESSELS

by oxygen analysis or blood samples from the right side of the heart and pulmonary artery, but the shunt can be detected only by special indicator (hydrogen, krypton, nitrous oxide, dye) techniques. Usually, this type of defect imposes little burden on the heart except for the danger of infective endocarditis; however, it is possible that it is a contributing factor to congestive failure in patients with other forms of heart disease, such as coronary heart disease or systemic hypertension.

In the second group of patients, the ventricular septal defect is 0.5 to 1.0 cm^2 per square meter of body surface area in effective cross-sectional area. In this situation there are three main areas of resistance to the left-to-right shunting of blood: (1) the orifice of the defect itself, which offers some resistance to the passage of blood from left to right ventricle; (2) the right ventricle, which slightly increases in mass during the first 2 weeks so that its diastolic compliance is less than normal; (3) the pulmonary vasculature, which in this situation with moderate increase in flow (about 1.5 to 3.0 times systemic) and with moderate increase in systolic pressure in the right ventricle and pulmonary artery, does not regress normally but rather develops some degree of increased pulmonary vascular resistance and, eventually, some degree of pulmonary vascular disease. The pulmonary hypertension may stay mild or moderate and not change for many years or may, for unknown reasons, become progressive with a marked elevation of pulmonary vascular resistance. As the pulmonary vascular resistance becomes elevated, the right ventricle will usually become thicker and less distensible and its systolic pressure rises. Consequently, the pressure difference across the defect may be less, and the left-to-right shunt actually decreases or may even reverse.

In the third group of patients with ventricular septal defect, the effective area of the defect is approximately equal to or greater than the aortic valve orifice, or at least 1.0 cm^2 per square meter. As a result of this large defect, which offers virtually no resistance to the flow of blood, the two ventricles are essentially in free communication at all times. Consequently, the systolic pressure in both ventricles, the aorta, and the pulmonary artery is essentially the same at all times, in utero and after birth. In this situation, which is hemodynamically very similar to a common ventricle, there are two outlets, namely, the pulmonary valve and the aortic valve, through which the blood in the functional single pumping chamber may pass when the ventricles contract. The relative proportion of blood going to the two circulations is directly governed by the relative resistance of the two valves and two circulations. Any condition or drug affecting either of these resistances will therefore affect the distribution of blood flow from the common pressure ventricles.

At birth, the pulmonary vasculature in infants with a large (over 1.0 cm^2 per square meter of body surface area) ventricular septal defect has high resistance and there may be little if any left-to-right shunt. After birth, the normal decrease in pulmonary vascular resistance begins and results in an increasing left-to-right shunt over the first few weeks of life. This produces a progressively greater amount of blood flow through both ventricles, the lungs, and the left atrium. The high-volume work of the left ventricle produces an increase in its end-diastolic volume and pressure, which increases the stroke volume by the Frank-Starling mechanism. In some infants, the left ventricle "fails" and develops markedly elevated left ventricular end-diastolic and left atrial pressures, producing pulmonary edema. At the same time, if the pulmonary arteries and arterioles regress excessively, the pulmonary capillaries will be "unprotected" from the high pressure in the pulmonary arteries. The consequences of these events may be an elevation of pulmonary capillary pressure, pulmonary edema, and possible death. This syndrome is in part produced by pulmonary arteriolar "failure," i.e., failure to maintain a degree of resistance adequate to protect the pulmonary capillaries from high pulmonary artery pressure and failure to protect the left ventricle by limiting the volume of the shunt.

Some of the other factors that may determine whether or not the ventricle fails include the degree of prematurity, the degree of maturation of the myocardial contractile mechanism, the sympathetic innervation of the myocardium, the time available to increase ventricular mass by hyperplasia and hypertrophy, anemia, and the presence of additional stress due to fever or infection. In addition, left ventricular function may be impaired by a decrease in left ventricular coronary blood flow secondary to elevation of left ventricular diastolic pressure or to tachycardia.[150] Occasionally, the increased left atrial pressure can stretch the atrial septum and produce an opening of the foramen ovale with a considerable left-to-right shunt at the atrial level, which perhaps may be of benefit to the overloaded left ventricle.

As a result of the above changes, clinical pulmonary congestion may occur at about 8 to 12 weeks in mature infants born at sea level with a large ventricular septal defect. In premature infants in whom the poorly developed pulmonary vasculature regresses more rapidly, failure is frequently noted at 2 to 4 weeks. On the other hand, in infants born at high altitude with a large ventricular septal defect, the lower partial pressure of inspired oxygen significantly delays and lessens the normal decrease in pulmonary vasculature resistance. As a result, heart failure is less common, less severe, and of later onset.

In most mature infants born at sea level with a large ventricular septal defect, the pulmonary vasculature eventually responds to the combined high-pressure and high-flow stimulus with the apparent "redevelopment" of high pulmonary vascular resistance, which results in a decreased pulmonary blood flow, a lessened left-to-right shunt across the interventricular septum, and decreased volume load on both ventricles. Indeed, for the survival of patients with a large ventricular septal defect, it is *necessary* to have an increased resistance to outflow from the right ventricle. Initially the high pulmonary vascular resistance is caused both by hypertrophy and by increased vasomotor tone and vasoconstriction of the pulmonary arteries and arterioles. In some unfortunate patients, however, progressive pulmonary vascular disease develops during subsequent years, and eventually the pulmonary vascular resistance may equal or exceed systemic resistance. When the pulmonary vascular disease is very severe, there may be little or no vasoconstrictive element to the pulmonary vascular resistance which is then relatively "fixed" and is associated with severe intimal changes. When the two resistances are equal in such patients, the pulmonary and systemic net flows are also virtually equal, with either no shunting of blood or bidirectional shunting of an equal, small amount of blood in each direction. When the pulmonary resistance is higher than the systemic resistance, the right-to-left shunt predominates and may be sufficient to produce detectable cyanosis—*Eisenmenger's complex.* The expressions *Eisenmenger syndrome* and *Eisenmenger physiology* have been rather loosely applied to *any* condition with a left-to-right shunt that subsequently develops severe pulmonary vascular disease and a predominant right-to-left shunt.

At times, patients with medium- or large-sized ventricular septal defect develop right ventricular hypertrophic infundibular muscular stenosis.[151] This obstruction, not present at birth, may also serve to protect the pulmonary vasculature from the high pressure and flow to which it otherwise would be exposed.

Clinical Manifestations

Ventricular septal defect is the most commonly recognized form of congenital heart disease except for a bicuspid aortic valve. It occurs as an isolated defect in approximately 23 percent of infants and children so affected and in combination with other important malformations, such as complete atrioventricular canal, coarctation of the aorta, pulmonary stenosis, and transposition of the great arteries, in an additional 26 percent.[6] Its incidence is 2 per 1000 live births, while its prevalence among school-age children has been estimated as 1 per 1000.[152] Ventricular septal defects constitute about 10 percent of the congenital cardiac malformations found among adults.[153] Males and females are affected equally. The mode of transmission usually is best explained on a multifactorial basis. It is the most common defect found among infants with chromosomal abnormalities, with the notable exceptions being trisomy 21 (Down's syndrome) and Turner's syndrome (XO syndrome), in which it ranks second to complete

atrioventricular canal and coarctation of the aorta, respectively.[154]

History Infants or children with a small isolated defect are asymptomatic. The murmur is usually detected at the first routine pediatric office examination following discharge from the hospital, traditionally at 4 weeks of age. The murmur may actually be present within the first 24 to 36 h of life since a small defect permits the normal rapid fall in pulmonary arterial pressure and pulmonary vascular resistance. The rate of weight gain and breathing usually are normal. Larger defects permit greater exposure of the right ventricle, pulmonary artery, and pulmonary vascular bed to the left ventricular systolic pressure, resulting in continued right ventricular and pulmonary arterial hypertension and an ever-increasing left-to-right shunt as pulmonary vascular resistance gradually falls. Characteristically, these infants present with congestive failure, frequently with associated lower respiratory tract infections, between 2 to 10 weeks of age. Parents frequently describe tachypnea, grunting respirations, and fatigue, particularly with feedings. Excessive sweating is common and weight gain is slow.

Physical Examination With a small defect, the child is quite comfortable. A soft systolic thrill at the lower left sternal border is common, although with very small defects this may not be present. The second heart sound splits normally without accentuation of the pulmonary component. Toward the end of the second year, a few children will develop an early systolic sound at the lower left sternal border, reflecting the presence of an aneurysm of the membranous septum. The systolic murmur, usually grade 2 to 4 in intensity along the lower left sternal border, is characteristically holosystolic, but may be decrescendo and limited to early or midsystole. These latter features would suggest a defect in the muscular rather than the membranous ventricular septum. A middiastolic, low-pitched, flow murmur at the apex usually indicates a pulmonary to systemic blood flow ratio (Q_P/Q_S) of 2:1 or greater and is seldom heard with small defects.

In contrast, children with large defects, large flows, and pulmonary arterial hypertension tend to be restless, irritable, and underweight. Linear growth is usually fairly well preserved, but weight is seldom above the 3d percentile. Moderate respiratory distress, even to the point of flaring of the nostrils and intercostal retractions, may be present, and respiratory rates of 80 to 100 are not unusual in those infants under 3 or 4 months of age. Both the right and left ventricular systolic impulses are impressively hyperdynamic, frequently tumultuous, to palpation. A thrill at the lower left sternal border is the rule. The first heart sound is loud at the lower left sternal border, and the second heart sound is narrowly split with a loud, frequently palpable, pulmonary component. Third heart sound gallops at the apex are common. Characteristically, the systolic murmur is holosystolic at the lower left sternal border and accompanied by a middiastolic rumble of grade 2 to 3 intensity at the apex. Hepatic enlargement, a helpful guide to the severity of congestive heart failure, can be identified below the right costal margin. Pulmonary rales are relatively common with severe failure, but overt peripheral edema is seldom observed. Impressive diminution of the arterial pulses is not a characteristic of ventricular septal defect, and this finding would suggest the presence of aortic stenosis. Selective diminution or absence of the femoral pulses would suggest an associated coarctation. Similarly, cyanosis and clubbing are not features of uncomplicated ventricular septal defect and would indicate the presence of associated abnormalities.

With the passage of time, the left-to-right shunt may diminish in size, and one can expect an improved rate of weight gain, less dyspnea, a diminution of the precordial hyperactivity, and disappearance of the apical diastolic flow rumble. This clinical improvement may be the result of the defect becoming smaller, the development of subvalvular pulmonary stenosis with little or no appreciable change in the size of the defect, or, most worrisome, the development of pulmonary vascular obstructive disease with continued severe pulmonary arterial hypertension. As the defect narrows, the lower sternal systolic murmur usually becomes more localized and softer and occasionally shortens in duration. The second heart sound splits easily with respiration and the pulmonary component returns to normal intensity. With developing subpulmonary stenosis, the systolic murmur radiates more and more impressively to the upper left sternal border and the second heart sound becomes more widely split, with a progressive diminution in the intensity of the pulmonary component. Decreased flow due to pulmonary vascular disease is characterized by a gradual reduction in the intensity and duration of the systolic murmur, more narrow splitting of the second heart sound, and marked accentuation of the pulmonary component. The clinical picture of advanced pulmonary vascular disease, or Eisenmenger syndrome, is that of a relatively comfortable older child, adolescent, or young adult with mild cyanosis and clubbing in whom one finds a prominent *a* wave in the jugular venous pulse. Prominence of the left anterior precordium may suggest cardiac enlargement during early childhood. Palpation usually reveals a mild left parasternal right ventricular lift, a second heart sound which is narrowly split or virtually single with a very loud, usually palpable, pulmonary component. An early pulmonary systolic ejection sound, reflecting dilatation of the main pulmonary artery, may be heard, and the systolic murmur is usually confined to early systole, or, with dominant right-to-left shunting, there may be no systolic murmur at all. In older adolescents and adults, the early, high-pitched diastolic murmur of

pulmonary regurgitation (Graham Steell murmur) or a holosystolic murmur of tricuspid regurgitation may appear.[98]

Chest Roentgenogram In the presence of a small defect the heart size and shape are barely altered. Slight dilatation of the left atrium may be appreciated in the lateral view by indentation of the barium-filled esophagus. The pulmonary blood flow may appear to be at the upper limits of normal. With large defects there will be moderate to marked enlargement of the heart with prominence of the main pulmonary arterial segment and impressive overcirculation in the peripheral lung fields. Interstitial edema is not uncommon when congestive failure is severe. The left atrium is impressively dilated in the absence of an associated atrial septal defect, and partial or complete atelectasis of the left lower lobe of the lung from bronchial compression is not unusual. With increasing pulmonary vascular disease, there is diminution in heart size toward normal while the central pulmonary arteries remain dilated. The peripheral pulmonary arterial markings become attenuated and a "pruned" effect is produced in the outer third of the lung fields (Fig. 36-18).

Electrocardiogram In the infant with a small defect, one can expect the normal progression of the mean QRS axis from right to left and the normal gradual diminution of the prominent right ventricular voltages characteristic of the newborn. The left ventricular forces will either remain within normal

FIGURE 36-18 Frontal view of the chest roentgenogram of a 12-year-old child with a large ventricular septal defect and Eisenmenger syndrome. The main and central pulmonary arteries are markedly dilated while the peripheral segmental branches appear attenuated.

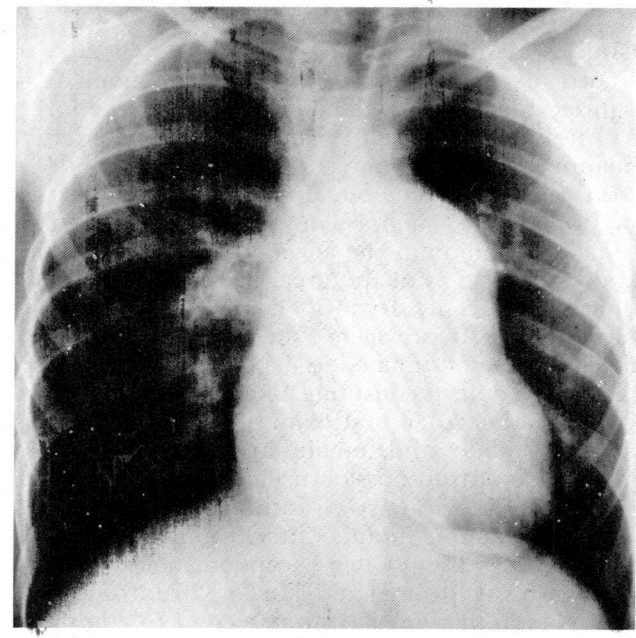

limits or become slightly augmented as a reflection of the mild left ventricular volume overload. With large defects, the mean QRS axis tends to remain oriented to the right, and there is little or no regression in right ventricular voltage. The left ventricular forces gradually increase resulting in a pattern of biventricular hypertrophy within the first few weeks of life. Left atrial hypertrophy is usually present and frequently right atrial hypertrophy as well. With the development of pulmonary vascular disease or significant pulmonary stenosis, the mean QRS axis remains and progresses even further to the right, while the evidence of left ventricular hypertrophy and left atrial hypertrophy lessens or even disappears. Pure right ventricular hypertrophy remains and usually right atrial hypertrophy as well. A superior QRS is not characterisitic of an isolated defect and would suggest the presence of an atrioventricular canal–type malformation.

Echocardiogram M-mode imaging can provide valuable information concerning the position and orientation of the ventricular septum and can distinguish the uncomplicated ventricular septal defect from more complex malformations such as single ventricle, truncus arteriosus, double outlet right ventricle, and tetralogy of Fallot. The ratio of the left atrial diameter to that of the ascending aorta (LA/Ao ratio) can identify the majority of infants and older children with significant left-to-right shunts in the absence of an associated atrial septal defect.[155] A combination of echo- and vectorcardiographic findings, namely a ratio of right ventricular preejection period to right ventricular ejection time (RPEP/RVET) of greater than 0.3 determined by echocardiography and a counterclockwise or anterior figure-of-eight QRS loop in the horizontal plane determined vectorcardiographically, appears promising as a technique for predicting those infants beyond 2 months of age in whom the ventricular septal defect is nonrestrictive (right ventricular systolic pressure at least 75 percent of the systemic systolic pressure).[156] Two-dimensional echocardiography is capable of imaging the defect directly by using the left parasternal long axis, the apical four-chamber, or the subxiphoid four-chamber view.[157]

Cardiac Catheterization An increase in oxygen saturation at the right ventricular level reflects the left-to-right shunt via the ventricular septal defect. With small defects, the right ventricular and pulmonary arterial systolic pressures are normal or only very slightly elevated. With large defects, these pressures are at or near systemic levels and the mean left atrial pressure may be elevated to the 10 to 15 mmHg range. In the absence of a true atrial septal defect left-to-right shunting also may be present at the atrial level due to a stretched foramen ovale when pulmonary blood flow is very large and the left atrium is hypertensive and dilated.

In these particular infants, in whom the catheterization findings are so important, it is wise to obtain the following in addition to the routine right-sided heart pressures and blood samples: (1) simultaneous pulmonary and systemic arterial pressures and oxygen saturations, followed immediately by pressures and a blood sample from either the superior vena cava or right atrium, whichever is felt to best represent the mixed systemic venous blood; (2) left atrial or pulmonary arterial wedge pressures or both; (3) left atrial or pulmonary arterial wedge pressures and left ventricular end-diastolic pressures in a manner that permits assessment of possible mitral valve obstruction; (4) selective left ventricular angiography in the anteroposterior, lateral, and oblique views to note the spatial relationship of the great arteries to each other and to the ventricles and to determine the exact site, size, and number of septal defects (Fig. 36-19); and (5) aortography to eliminate the possibility of an associated ductus arteriosus or unsuspected coarctation of the aorta.

Natural History and Prognosis

Fortunately, the majority of ventricular septal defects are small and do not present a serious clinical problem. In approximately 24 percent of these small defects, spontaneous closure can be expected by 18 months, 50 percent by 4 years, and 75 percent by 10 years.[158] Even large defects tend to become smaller and many eventually close. Blackstone and associates estimate that approximately 75 percent of defects judged to be large at 6 months of age will either close or become small enough that one would expect them to eventually close by 10 years of age.[58]

FIGURE 36-19 Left anterior oblique view of the left ventricular angiogram from a 5-year-old child with a small, membranous ventricular septal defect (arrow). RV = right ventricle; LV = left ventricle; Aa = ascending aorta; PA = pulmonary artery.

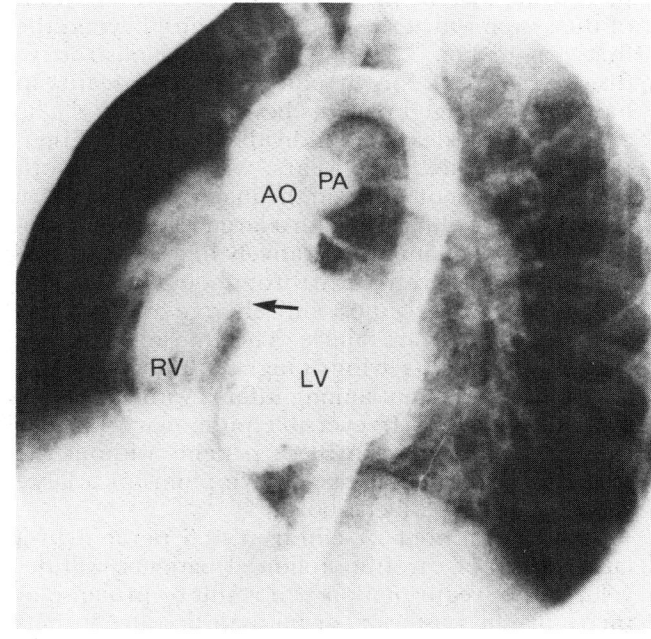

As with small defects, the tendency to close or diminish significantly in size is greatest in the first year or two of life.

Congestive failure is a threatening and almost inevitable complication of large ventricular septal defects. It becomes evident toward the end of the first month of life in full-term infants, but it may appear much earlier, particularly among premature infants, who are less well equipped to maintain pulmonary vascular resistance at a protective level. Approximately 35 percent of infants with a large defect will be symptomatic enough to warrant hospitalization by 4 weeks of age, and almost 80 percent will have required similar management by the age of 4 months.[3] The onset of failure beyond the age of 8 months is unusual and suggests additional complications, such as infective endocarditis, anemia, pneumonia, or myocardial disease. The risk of death with congestive failure is in the range of 11 percent, with slightly more than half of the deaths being among those infants with major noncardiac malformations and very low birth weights (under 2000 g).[3] Spontaneous improvement in the failure, the result of diminishing left ventricular volume overload, may be the result of narrowing of the defect, the development of subvalvular pulmonary stenosis, or the appearance of pulmonary vascular obstructive disease. Significant subvalvular pulmonary stenosis develops in approximately 3 percent of these infants and children and may progress even to the point of cyanosis, squatting, and hypoxic spells characteristic of severe tetralogy of Fallot. Pulmonary vascular obstructive disease is seldom severe and rarely irreversible in the first 12 months of life but becomes progressively more common and less likely to regress, even with surgical closure of the septal defect, after the first year.[58] At risk of this complication are those infants and children with a pulmonary systolic pressure in excess of 50 percent of the systemic arterial systolic pressure beyond the first year of life.[159] Pulmonary vascular obstructive disease accounts for virtually all of the deaths in medically managed patients beyond infancy.[159] The average age of death for individuals with the Eisenmenger complex is 33 years, with sudden death being the mode of exitus in the majority.[98,159] A very small number of infants with a large ventricular septal defect will maintain a relatively high level of pulmonary vascular resistance throughout the first year of life and remain almost entirely free of symptoms and congestive heart failure. This unusual course is seen among infants living at high altitude and is also surprisingly frequent among infants with associated Down's syndrome. Irreversible pulmonary vascular disease may develop in these patients without the usual and expected signs and symptoms of a large septal defect described above.[160]

A small number of children, 0.6 percent in a large group of carefully followed patients, will develop aortic regurgitation as a result of prolapse of the right, the posterior, or both aortic valve leaflets into the defect.[159] This complication is more prevalent among males in a ratio of 2:1 and seems particularly likely to occur with defects in the supracristal or conal septum region. Shunt size appears unrelated to the development of this complication. The characteristic aortic diastolic murmur may appear anywhere between the age of 18 months and 20 years and is not infrequently mistaken for the murmur of an associated ductus arteriosus. Regurgitation is usually progressive, sometimes rapidly so, and appears to predispose these individuals to infective endocarditis. The risk of infective endocarditis in patients with an uncomplicated ventricular septal defect managed medically is approximately 10 percent for the first 30 years of life, with the risk being some six times greater for the interval between 20 and 30 years than that from birth to 20 years.[159]

Medical Management

It is important to identify as early as possible those patients in whom the defect is of sufficient size to permit a large left-to-right shunt and the transmission of systemic systolic pressure directly from the left ventricle to the right ventricle or pulmonary vascular bed since these are the patients at special risk of developing congestive failure, pulmonary vascular disease, or serious pulmonary stenosis. The newborn suspected of having a sizable defect should be reexamined at 1- and then 2-week intervals for the first 4 to 6 weeks in order to detect early signs of increasing cardiac volume overload, namely slow weight gain, tachypnea, dyspnea, easy fatigue, cardiac hyperactivity and enlargement, a diastolic rumble or gallop, and an enlarged liver. The electrocardiogram, repeated frequently in the early weeks, is particularly helpful in identifying those infants in whom the right ventricular systolic pressure is remaining at or near systemic levels. Heart failure is treated with digitalis and, if necessary, oral diuretics. Anemia is prevented or corrected and respiratory infections are treated promptly. The success of medical management depends so heavily upon the accuracy of the diagnosis and a knowledge of the pulmonary arterial pressure that it is appropriate to adopt a relatively low threshold for the recommendation of cardiac catheterization and angiography in these infants. Greater experience with echocardiography and other techniques may bring a change in criteria, but at present we recommend cardiac catheterization for those infants who develop overt congestive heart failure or who retain impressive right ventricular or biventricular voltage in the electrocardiogram or both. If the pulmonary arterial systolic pressure is found to be greater than half the systemic systolic pressure and congestive failure is difficult to manage medically, the defect should be closed surgically. Exceptions would be those infants with multiple septal defects or large defects in the muscular septum for whom pulmonary arterial banding is recommended. If congestive failure is not severe, medical management is continued with the hope that spontaneous narrowing of the defect will occur. This trial of medical management is limited to no longer than 6 months, and at that point, with or without clinical improvement, the patient undergoes repeat cardiac catheterization. If the pulmonary arterial systolic pressure is still greater than half of the systemic systolic pressure, the defect should be closed without delay. If the pulmonary pressure has fallen to less than half the systemic pressure, the infant may be managed medically into the second year of life with the expectation that the size of the defect will continue to diminish and the pulmonary arterial pressure will continue its fall to normal levels.[159] This course must be supported by diminishing right ventricular potentials in the electrocardiogram and continued clinical improvement. If by the second birthday the pulmonary arterial pressure has not returned to normal (a mean pulmonary arterial pressure of less than 20 mmHg) as judged by persistent right or biventricular hypertrophy or direct measurement at catheterization, the defect should be closed. A few children will remain symptomatic or continue to have cardiac enlargement beyond the second year of life due to a large left-to-right shunt despite a normal pulmonary arterial pressure. At present, surgical closure is recommended before the child enters school if the pulmonary to systemic blood flow ratio (Q_P/Q_S) is above 1.8 or if symptoms or cardiac enlargement persists and the Q_P/Q_S is above 1.4. Finally, closure of a defect in an adult is usually recommended if the flow ratio is above 1.4 and if severe pulmonary vascular disease is not present.

Unfortunately, not all patients with a large defect are encountered during the first or even the second year of life, when reduction of a seriously elevated pulmonary arterial pressure and flow, either by banding of the pulmonary artery or direct closure of the defect, will prevent permanent injury to the pulmonary vascular bed. If significant pulmonary arterial hypertension (pulmonary arterial systolic pressure greater than half the systemic arterial systolic pressure) is allowed to persist, one can expect the development of mild, moderate, and then severe and irreversible pulmonary obstructive disease. Although the speed of this reaction varies from individual to individual, it is clearly related to age and the pulmonary arterial pressure. For this reason prompt surgical closure of defects is recommended in all individuals beyond the age of 2 years if the pulmonary arterial systolic pressure is greater than half the systemic arterial systolic pressure, the mean pulmonary pressure exceeds 20 mmHg, or the pulmonary to systemic vascular resistance ratio exceeds 0.2. With severe pulmonary vascular obstructive disease a point is reached eventually where the risks of death at operation or in the months or years immediately following operation due to progressive vascular disease more than offset the possible benefits from surgical closure. At present, surgery is rec-

ommended if the calculated pulmonary vascular resistance is less than 11 units/m^2 or if the ratio of the pulmonary to systemic vascular resistance is less than 0.7 provided the Q_P/Q_S is still 1.5 or greater. In adults, the upper limit of pulmonary vascular resistance for surgery is approximately 800 dyn·s/cm^5.

Those patients in whom the defect is judged clinically to be small or modest by 2 or 3 months of age may be reexamined at 1- or 2-month intervals through the age of 6 months to be certain that the initial impression is supported by a normal weight gain, lack of symptoms, and a normal regression of the right ventricular forces in the electrocardiogram. Periodic examinations after that, at 1- or 2-year intervals, are advisable to reassure the patient and family, to reemphasize the importance of antibiotic protection against infective endocarditis, to document the further narrowing or closure of the defect, and, in a very small number of patients, to detect the first signs of aortic valve prolapse.

If the murmur of an otherwise uncomplicated ventricular septal defect evolves into a crescendo, harsh, holosystolic murmur at the upper left sternal border, the physician should be alerted to the possibility of a conal or supracristal defect, a predisposing factor for aortic valve prolapse. Selective left ventricular angiography will identify these supracristal lesions, with or without mild regurgitation, for which surgical closure is recommended. With existing moderate regurgitation, aortic valve leaflet plication and septal defect closure may or may not correct or prevent further regurgitation. Severe regurgitation usually requires valve replacement. Particular emphasis on prevention of infective endocarditis is advisable for these patients.[161]

Those individuals with a large ventricular septal defect and severe pulmonary arterial hypertension and in whom the pulmonary vascular resistance approaches, is equal to, or exceeds systemic vascular resistance are referred to as having *Eisenmenger's complex*.[98] Stamina is limited by systemic arterial hypoxia and, in some, right-sided heart failure. Complications to be anticipated include syncope, hemoptysis, brain abscess, hyperuricemia, and congestive failure. Pregnancy, with a mortality of 27 percent, and oral contraceptives are contraindicated. Transient symptomatic relief from symptomatic extreme polycythemia may be achieved by careful erythrophoresis. Travel to or living at high altitude is poorly tolerated, and supplemental oxygen should be provided and used in commercial airlines if the cabin altitude is permitted to rise above sea level.[56]

Patients who have undergone surgical banding of the pulmonary artery and who continue to do well usually undergo repeat cardiac catheterization 2 or 3 years after the procedure in anticipation of total correction at 3 or 4 years of age. Those who undergo surgical closure as a primary procedure or at the time of band removal receive diuretics and usually digitalis in the immediate postoperative period, particularly if pulmonary hypertension has been present preoperatively. Diuretics may be discontinued after the first few weeks if progress is satisfactory. Digitalis is usually continued until the heart returns to normal or near normal size. The development of complete heart block at surgery is managed by pacing with the temporary epicardial electrodes placed at the time of surgery. If sinus rhythm, as judged by a brief discontinuation of pacing under direct surveillance, has not returned by 14 to 21 days after surgery, permanent transthoracic epicardial electrodes are placed and permanent pacing is instituted. Individuals with preoperative pulmonary arterial hypertension or elevated pulmonary vascular resistance should be restudied by cardiac catheterization 1 or 2 years following surgery. Earlier restudy is indicated if there is a persistent loud murmur, unexplained cardiac enlargement, or congestive failure. Following the surgery, precautions against infective endocarditis are continued for at least 1 year in all patients and indefinitely in patients with any residual murmur. Symptoms suggesting an arrhythmia, particularly in a setting of postoperative right bundle branch block and left anterior hemiblock, should be evaluated by 24-h ambulatory monitoring of the electrocardiogram.

Genetic counseling should establish the risk of congenital heart disease for a subsequent sibling of a single affected child to be in the order of 3 to 4 percent.[154] Pregnancy in the presence of a small defect and normal pulmonary vascular resistance does not appear to carry an increased risk to the patient or infant, although precautions against infective endocarditis should be observed. The risk to the offspring of having congenital heart disease with a single parent with ventricular septal defect is estimated at 4 percent.[154]

Finally, when a patient with a residual defect or one who has undergone corrective surgery leaves the pediatric age group, arrangements should be made with an adult cardiologist for future care.

Surgical Management

Although reduction of pulmonary blood flow by pulmonary arterial banding played an important role in the management of ventricular septal defect prior to predictably successful infant open heart surgery, banding is now used only for complex and uncorrectable defects.[162,163] Complications of pulmonary arterial banding include marked deformity of the pulmonary arteries, unpredictable palliation, progressive right ventricular hypertrophy, and acquired subaortic left ventricular outflow tract obstruction. Subsequent removal of the band, repair of the pulmonary artery, and closure of the ventricular septal defect are more difficult than primary repair. Early closure of ventricular septal defects is preferred in centers offering precise angiographic diagnosis and skillful infant cardiac surgery.[164–166]

Ventricular septal defects are closed through a median sternotomy on total cardiopulmonary bypass with cardioplegia, moderate hypothermia (25 to 28°C), and whole-body perfusion in children over 1 year old and weighing more than 10 kg. In younger and smaller infants we prefer to use total circulatory arrest with profound hypothermia (18 to 20°C) and cardioplegia.[167] Limited cardiopulmonary bypass employing a single right atrial cannula for venous drainage is used for cooling and rewarming. Whole-body hypothermia induced by surface cooling (ice bags, water bath, or hypothermia chamber) is no longer used in our institutions. Cardiopulmonary bypass is convenient, safe, and faster, although adequate time must be allowed during the cooling phase to achieve uniform total-body hypothermia. Moderate hemodilution (hematocrit 15 to 20 percent) is used in conjunction with hypothermia to reduce the volume of blood in the heart-lung machine prime, lower blood viscosity, and minimize hemolysis.

Closure of the ventricular septal defect is usually accomplished through the right atrium and the tricuspid valve orifice (Fig. 36-20).[168] This approach is particularly useful in patients with elevated pulmonary resistance where it is desirable to avoid injury to the right ventricle. Appropriately placed traction sutures, magnifying glasses, the surgical headlight, miniature instruments, and the ideal operating conditions of circulatory arrest allow excellent visualization of the defect. Occasionally the septal leaflet of the tricuspid valve is incised near the annulus to facilitate exposure. The outflow tract of the right ventricle may be incised transversely or longitudinally for adequate exposure of high defects (see Fig. 36-101). A right ventriculotomy is used routinely for closure of supracristal (type I) defects where a prolapsing aortic valve leaflet may be encountered.[169]

Care is required to avoid injury to the atrioven-

FIGURE 36-20 Exposure of the usual high ventricular septal defect through the atrial approach. Cardiopulmonary bypass has been established. The right atrium is opened. The aorta has been cross-clamped. The ventricular septal defect is adequately exposed through the intact tricuspid valve. (*From Cartmill, DuShane, McGoon, and Kirklin.*[168] *Reproduced with permission.*)

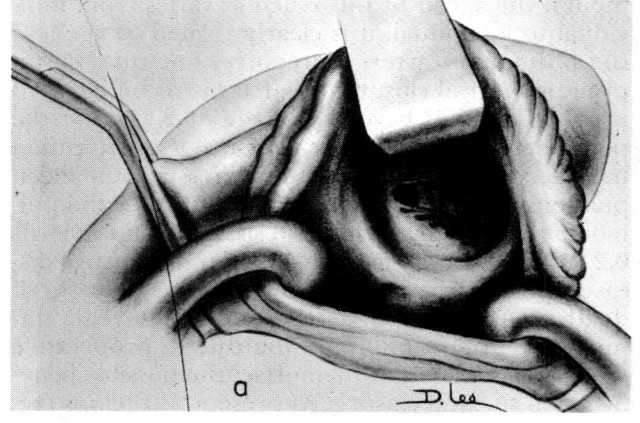

tricular node near the ostium of the coronary sinus and to the bundle of His as it courses inferiorly near the tricuspid annulus, passing to the left side of the ventricular septum near the posterocaudal margin of the septal defect.[170] A Dacron patch is secured over the right side of the septal defect using a series of fine interrupted mattress sutures buttressed with Teflon felt pledgets. Sutures are placed in fibrous tissue, well away from the inferior rim on the right side of the septum, and parallel to the axis of the conduction system to avoid complete heart block.[171] The portion of the patch adjacent to the tricuspid valve is anchored to the fibrous tricuspid annulus. Small septal defects with firm fibrous margins may be closed by direct suture. Posterior type III defects of the atrioventricular canal type are always closed with a Dacron patch.

Defects in the muscular septum (type IV) are frequently multiple—the so-called Swiss cheese septum. They are usually small and can be closed by direct suture, but they may be difficult to locate through either the tricuspid orifice or a right ventriculotomy.[172] Exposure of muscular defects through an apical or posterior left ventriculotomy facilitates closure; care is required to avoid trauma to coronary arteries and mitral papillary muscles.[173] Left ventricular function and immediate postoperative cardiac output are probably compromised somewhat by the left ventriculotomy, but we have found this approach quite satisfactory.

The results achieved by primary closure of ventricular septal defects are generally excellent. Operative risk is 1 to 2 percent in older children with normal pulmonary vascular resistance. When growth retardation has existed preoperatively in a young child, an acceleration of growth and marked improvement in symptoms can be anticipated postoperatively. The pulmonary vasculature responds quite favorably when the left-to-right shunt is eliminated prior to the age of 2 years.

Poor postoperative results are largely due to preexisting pulmonary vascular obstructive disease, an occasional technical error producing complete heart block, a rare significant residual shunt, or the presence of anatomically complex or multiple ventricular septal defects. Patients having undergone previous pulmonary arterial banding may obtain inadequate relief of right ventricular outflow tract obstruction at the time of ventricular septal defect closure and may develop acquired subaortic left ventricular outflow tract obstruction.

Rein and colleagues at the Boston Childrens' Hospital Medical Center[164] reviewed their experience with primary closure of ventricular septal defects during the first year of life for control of intractable congestive heart failure and failure to thrive. There were three hospital deaths (6 percent), all in the second month of life. There were no late deaths. Only 1 of the 24 children subjected to repeat cardiac catheterization had a significant residual shunt. These good results in a relatively high risk

group of infants with ventricular septal defect indicate the excellent prognosis to be expected in less critically ill older children, provided their pulmonary vascular resistance remains normal.

Common Atrioventricular Canal Defects

Definition

The condition variously called atrioventricular (AV) canal, persistent common AV canal, and endocardial cushion defect is characterized by an atrial septal defect in the lowermost part of the atrial septum, a cleft condition of the mitral valve, either alone or in combination with that of the tricuspid valve, and deficiency of ventricular septal tissue.

The condition appears to result from incomplete growth of the AV endocardial cushions.[174] Fusion of the two cushions not only divides the canal into tricuspid and mitral orifices but also gives origin to the anterior mitral and septal tricuspid leaflets. Incomplete growth of the cushions underlies cleft states of the AV valves. In fusing with the developing atrial septum and the ventricular septum, the cushions provide anchors for these structures. Deficiency in cushion growth fails to provide such anchors and allows for an atrial septal defect to form and for the ventricular septum to be deficient.

Pathology

Common to the condition is an atrial septal defect of the *ostium primum type* and deficiency of the ventricular septum. The atrial septal defect is characterized by having a crescent-shaped upper border and no septal tissue forming its lower border. The lower aspect of the defect is bounded by the atrial surfaces of the AV valves and in the complete type (see below) in part by the upper edge of the ventricular septum. The center of the anteroposterior extent of the defect lies about midway between the anterolateral and posteromedial papillary muscles of the mitral valve. A small amount of septal tissue separates the defect from the posterior atrial wall.

The deficiency of the ventricular septum is at the basal aspect and particularly prominent beneath the aortic valve. The deficiency may, however, involve the complete anteroposterior extent of the basal aspect.

Anatomic Types Variations occur with respect to the nature of the AV valves. The terms *partial* and *complete* were first introduced to describe these types.[175] Later, a transitional or intermediate type was recognized.[176]

Partial Type. The partial type of common AV canal, the so-called ostium primum atrial septal defect with cleft mitral valve, constitutes about one-fourth of all atrial septal defects. It is characterized by a cleft in the anterior mitral leaflet and an ostium primum atrial septal defect (Figs. 36-4D and 36-21). The tricuspid valve is either not cleft or shows minor

DISEASES OF THE HEART AND BLOOD VESSELS

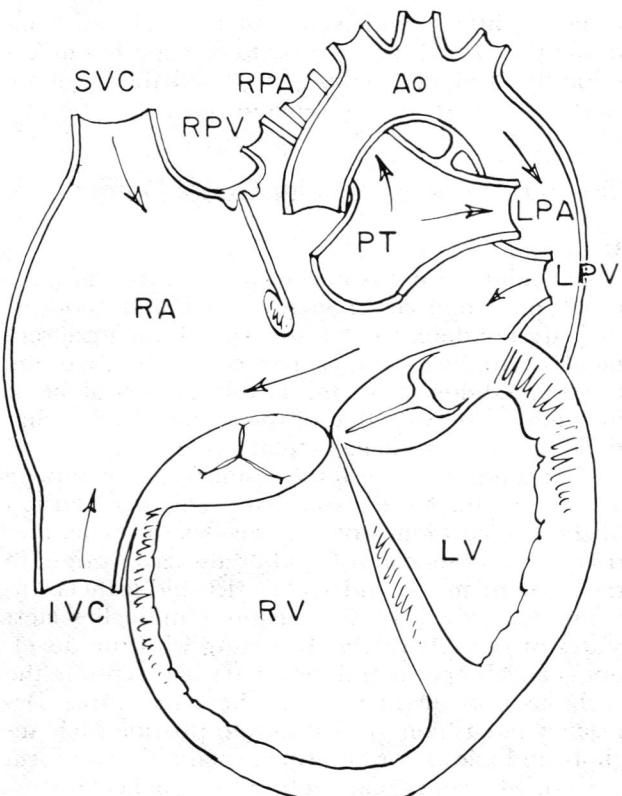

FIGURE 36-21 Common AV canal of the partial type. The mitral valve shows a cleft in its anterior leaflet, while the tricuspid valve is undisturbed. SVC = superior vena cava; IVC = inferior vena cava; RA = right atrium; RV = right ventricle; PT = main pulmonary arterial trunk; RPA = right pulmonary artery; LPA = left pulmonary artery; RPV = right pulmonary vein; LPV = left pulmonary vein; LV = left ventricle; AO = aorta. [*From J. E. Edwards, Classification of Congenital Heart Disease in the Adult, in W. C. Roberts. (ed.), Congenital Heart Disease in Adults, Cardiovasc. Clin. Series 10/1, F. A. Davis Company, Philadelphia, 1979, pp. 1–26. Reproduced with permission.*]

central deficiency. The ventricular aspects of the anterior mitral valve elements are usually fused to the upper edge of the deficient ventricular septum, precluding an interventricular communication.

Of the several anatomic types, the partial may allow survival to adult life. The characteristics of the chambers are like those in classical atrial septal defect.

Complete Type. The complete type of common AV canal is characterized by failure of partitioning of the primitive canal into separate AV orifices. The orifice between the atria and ventricles is guarded by a common valve, of which the anterior leaflet is derived from the ventral AV endocardial cushion and represents the anterior halves of the anterior mitral and septal tricuspid leaflets. The posterior leaflet is derived from the dorsal AV endocardial cushion and represents the posterior halves of the anterior mitral and septal tricuspid leaflets.

Usually, considerable space exists between the anterior and posterior leaflets, above, and the ven-

tricular septum, below, in that in most cases of the complete type there is free communication between the ventricles and the various anatomic characteristics of large ventricular septal defect pertain. Included in these are congestive pulmonary changes which account for a high incidence of infant death in contrast to the partial type.

Rastelli and associates[177] subdivided the complete variety into three subgroups as follows:

Type A: The anterior common leaflet is subdivided into mitral and tricuspid halves, with chordae from the edges inserting into appropriate ventricles. Spaces between chordae allow free communication between the ventricles.

Type B: As in type A, the anterior leaflet is subdivided. Chordae from the mitral side insert into the right ventricular wall.

Type C: There is no subdivision of the anterior common leaflet and no chordae run from this leaflet to the ventricular septum. The anterior common leaflet may be said to be "free-floating."

With regard to the posterior common leaflet, there is variation among the three foregoing types as to presence or absence of subdivision and as to whether the posterior leaflet is attached to the ventricular septum by chordae or an imperforate membrane. The transitional type of common AV canal defect shows clefts in both the anterior mitral and septal tricuspid leaflets. A bridge of tissue joins the anterior and posterior elements of the cleft leaflets so that true mitral and tricuspid orifices are present. In this type there is variation as to whether or not one interventricular communication is present and, if present, its extent.

Variations from the foregoing classic types of common AV canal defects are recognized, of which the most common is the AV canal type of isolated ventricular septal defect. Other variations include isolated ostium primum atrial septal defect without malformed AV valves, and isolated cleft of the anterior mitral or septal tricuspid valve.

Associated Conditions Among children with Down's syndrome, 45 percent have some form of congenital heart disease. Malformations of the AV canal types, usually of the complete variety, comprise 25 to 36 percent of these abnormalities.[178,179] In the asplenic syndrome the complete variety is almost universal and occurs in about one-quarter of cases with polysplenia.

An atrial septal defect of the fossa ovalis type is present in about half of the cases.[180] Double orifice of the mitral valve was observed by Wakai and Edwards[180] in 5 instances among 28 cases.

The tetralogy of Fallot may be associated with the complete type. This association tends to allow survival longer than occurs in cases with only the features of the complete type.[181–183] The longer survival appears to depend upon the features of the tetralogy applying a "band" to control the potential effects of the wide interventricular communication. The association of double-outlet right ventricle with common AV canal defects is usually also attended by pulmonary stenosis.[184]

Complications   The complications of the partial variety are essentially like those in atrial septal defect, and survival to adult life is not uncommon.[185]

In the complete variety fatal pulmonary complications of left ventricular failure, as in isolated large ventricular septal defect, are common.

Among survivors of infancy it has been claimed that obstructive pulmonary vascular disease occurs earlier on the average in those with Down's syndrome than in subjects with the complete type but without Down's syndrome. Plett and associates have not been able to confirm this.[186] Infective endocarditis is a rare complication and, when present, tends to occur in adults.[180]

Abnormal Physiology

If the communication is mainly at the ventricular level, the right ventricular and pulmonary artery pressures will be elevated and the pulmonary flow will be increased unless the pulmonary vascular resistance is severely elevated. Hemodynamically, these patients are often similar to patients with large ventricular septal defects.[187] Patients with the main communication at the atrial level have normal pressures in the right side of the heart and a large pulmonary blood flow, as in the secundum type of atrial septal defect. Defects in the tricuspid or mitral valve, or both, may result in severe regurgitation or direct shunting of blood from the left ventricle to the right atrium.

Clinical Manifestations

Approximately 3 percent of infants and children with congenital heart disease have AV canal (endocardial cushion) defects. Fortunately, the majority, some 60 to 70 percent, have the partial or incomplete form, consisting of a primum type atrial septal defect, a cleft in the anterior leaflet of the mitral valve, and variable degrees of tricuspid valve leaflet deficiency.[4] The female to male ratio is approximately 1.3:1. A little over half of the patients with the complete form will have associated Down's syndrome.[3]

History   Only if the mitral valve is incompetent do the symptoms of patients with partial AV canal differ from those associated with a secundum type atrial septal defect. Mild mitral regurgitation may be tolerated quite well, but moderate or severe regurgitation is associated with poor weight gain, easy fatigue, dyspnea, repeated respiratory infections, and congestive heart failure. Those infants and children with complete AV canal are almost invariably very sick. Heart failure appears early and is severe. Almost 40 percent of infants with this malformation will require hospitalization within the first month of

life, and if management is limited to medical therapy only, death will occur in approximately 60 percent within the first year of life. Dyspnea, sweating, difficulty feeding, and extremely poor weight gain are the rule. A small number of infants will maintain an elevated pulmonary vascular resistance throughout the first months of life, will gain weight acceptably, and will have surprisingly few symptoms.

Physical Examination   The findings on inspection, palpation, and auscultation among patients with the partial defect are those of an atrial septal defect unless the cleft anterior mitral leaflet is incompetent. In this event the murmur of mitral regurgitation will be heard, and if regurgitation is severe, this murmur will be accompanied by a diastolic filling sound and a middiastolic flow rumble at the apex. A hyperdynamic apical impulse will be felt in addition to the expected right ventricular parasternal lift.

The physical findings with the complete canal are those of a very large ventricular septal defect usually with full-blown congestive failure. The murmur of mitral regurgitation may not be heard or recognized as such, but fixed splitting of the second heart sound would suggest the presence of an associated atrial septal defect and hence the possibility of complete canal. With the development of pulmonary vascular obstructive disease the examination is virtually indistinguishable from that of a patient with a large ventricular septal defect and a similar elevation of the pulmonary vascular resistance, with the exception of the second heart sound which remains split and fixed. In some patients the murmur of tricuspid regurgitation may also be present.

Chest Roentgenogram   Overall cardiac enlargement, out of proportion to the degree of pulmonary plethora, or a cardiac silhouette suggesting combined ventricular dilatation may serve to distinguish the uncomplicated secundum atrial septal defect from the primum defect with significant mitral regurgitation. Marked cardiac enlargement with severe pulmonary overcirculation are features of the complete canal. Absence of impressive left atrial dilatation with the clinical and radiological features of a very large left-to-right shunt and congestive failure would suggest the presence of an associated atrial septal defect and also lead to the suspicion of complete AV canal. With the development of pulmonary vascular obstructive disease cardiac enlargement usually diminishes while central pulmonary arterial dilatation persists in contrast to progressive attenuation of the distal pulmonary vascular markings.

Electrocardiogram   Certainly the most helpful diagnostic feature in distinguishing individuals with AV canal defects from those with isolated atrial or ventricular septal defects is the characteristic superior orientation of the mean QRS axis in the frontal plane (Fig. 36-22). Between 92 and 95 percent of both types of canal will have a QRS axis lying between 0 and −150°. The axis also is of value within the canal family since 70 percent of patients with a partial canal will have an axis between 0 and −90° and only 22 percent between −91 and −150°. On the other hand 70 percent of patients with complete canal will have an axis between −91 and −150° and only 23 percent between 0 and −90°. About 3 percent of both forms will have right axis deviation, i.e., +91 to +180°.[127] The PQ interval is slightly prolonged in the majority of both partial and complete defects. Mild right ventricular hypertrophy is characteristic of partial canal and is indistinguishable from the pattern associated with an uncomplicated atrial septal defect of the secundum type. The presence of associated left ventricular hypertrophy reflects moderate or severe mitral regulitation. With complete AV canal, biatrial and biventricular hypertrophy is characteristic (Fig. 36-22). In the presence of severe pulmonary vascular obstructive disease or important pulmonary stenosis, the pattern is one of right atrial and right ventricular hypertrophy. Accompanying left ventricular hypertrophy would reflect mitral regurgitation.

Echocardiogram M-mode study of the partial defect will demonstrate the increased right ventricular dimensions and anterior systolic movement of the ventricular septum consistent with the diastolic volume overload of an atrial septal defect. Features characteristic of AV defects include prolonged diastolic aposition of the anterior mitral valve leaflet to the interventricular septum, multiple anterior leaflet systolic echoes, narrowing of the left ventricular outflow tract, and the appearance of the tricuspid valve opening from within the ventricular septal echoes (Fig. 36-23). A feature favoring the presence of a complete canal would be apparent diastolic

movement of the anterior mitral valve leaflet echoes through the ventricular septum with an associated absence of ventricular septal echoes in the region of this passage (Fig. 36-24). While this continuity of the mitral and tricuspid valve echoes is a virtually constant finding in complete AV canal, it can also be demonstrated in approximately half of patients with a partial defect, although usually without absence of ventricular septal echoes. Inability to demonstrate this mitral-tricuspid diastolic continuity would favor an incomplete defect. Ventricular septal motion usually is normal in the presence of a complete canal, and hence systolic anterior movement of the ventricular septum would favor an incomplete defect. Measurement of the right and left ventricular end-diastolic dimensions and their ratio appears promising as a technique for distinguishing those patients with serious and perhaps surgically prohibitive hypoplasia of either ventricle.[188] Two-dimensional sector scanning is capable of visualizing the atrial septal defect and mitral valve attachment to the ventricular septum in partial canal, the atrial and ventricular components of the complete canal, and the cleft anterior mitral valve leaflet with or without an associated atrial or ventricular septal defect (Figs. 36-25 and 36-26). The anatomic features of the anterior AV leaflet and its connections may be visualized with sufficient clarity to permit subdivision of complete AV canal defects into types A, B, or C (Fig. 36-27). Straddling AV valves, right- or left-sided inflow obstruction, and right or left ventricular outflow obstruction can also be documented with this technique.[189]

Cardiac Catheterization A significant increase in oxygen saturation between the superior vena cava and the right atrium is present in both the uncomplicated incomplete and complete forms of AV canal. Serious right ventricular and pulmonary arterial systolic hypertension are unusual with a partial defect, and a right ventricular or pulmonary arterial systolic pressure in excess of 60 percent of the systemic systolic pressure favors the presence of a complete canal. With a large communication between the two ventricles below the AV valves, the right ventricular, pulmonary arterial, and systemic arterial pressures are identical. Passage of the venous catheter through a defect low in the atrial septum, direct catheter passage from the right atrium to the left ventricle, and unintentional passage of the catheter from the right ventricular outflow tract to the left atrium during attempts to enter the pulmonary artery help to distinguish complete AV canal from a large ventricular septal defect. Left ventricular angiography in the frontal view demonstrates the gooseneck deformity of the left ventricular outflow tract characteristic of AV canal malformations (Fig. 36-28) and allows a semiquantitative assessment of the degree of mitral regurgitation and left ventricular to right atrial shunting. The left anterior oblique view, with or without craniocaudal

FIGURE 36-22 Electrocardiogram from an infant with complete AV canal, a large left-to-right shunt, and severe pulmonary arterial hypertension. The superior mean QRS axis (−70°C) is accompanied by first-degree heart block, biatrial and biventricular hypertrophy.

| I | II | III | aVR | aVL | aVF |

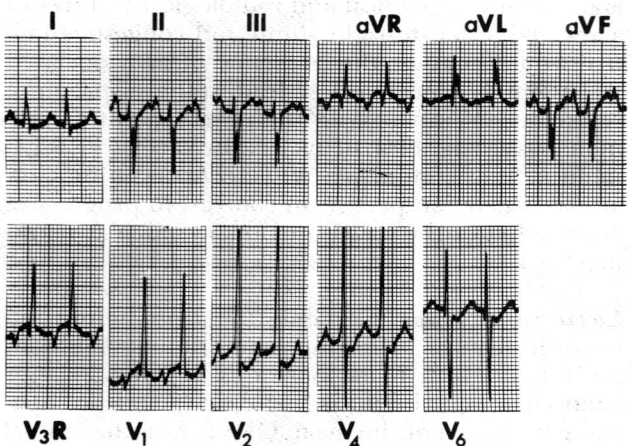

| V₃R | V₁ | V₂ | V₄ | V₆ |

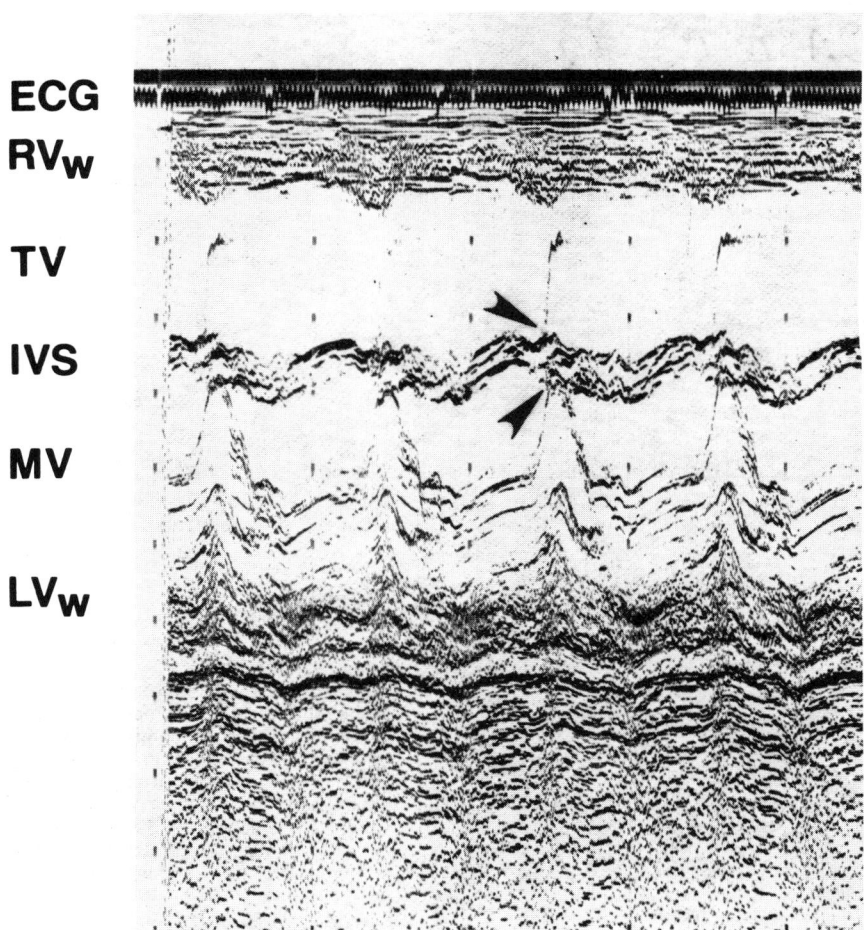

ECG
RV_W

TV

IVS

MV

LV_W

FIGURE 36-23 M-mode echocardiogram from a child with a primum atrial septal defect. The increased right ventricular cavity dimension and anterior systolic motion of the interventricular septum (IVS) are characteristic of diastolic overload of the right ventricle (RV), while diastolic aposition of the anterior mitral valve (MV) leaflet (lower arrowhead) to the IVS and near continuity of the anterior mitral and tricuspid valve (TV) echoes (lower and upper arrowheads) without absence of IVS echoes are characteristic of a partial AV canal defect. ECG = electrocardiogram; RV_W = anterior right ventricular wall; LV_W = posterior left ventricular wall.

angulation, is recommended for visualizing the interventricular defect and judging the extent of ventricular septal deficiency.[190,191] Aortography is essential in the presence of pulmonary arterial hypertension to eliminate the possibility of a patent ductus arteriosus.

Natural History and Prognosis

Partial defects without significant mitral regurgitation follow a course similar to that described for secundum-type atrial septal defects. An exception would be the greater likelihood of infective endocarditis because of the mitral valve deformity. Moderate or severe mitral regurgitation produces heart failure with the resulting symptoms and growth retardation. Infants with a complete AV canal without protective pulmonary stenosis develop and continue in congestive failure until the course is altered either by death, the development of severe, frequently irreversible, pulmonary vascular obstructive disease, or surgical intervention in the form of pulmonary arterial banding or complete repair. Spontaneous narrowing or closure of the atrial or ventricular portion of a complete AV canal defect does not seem to occur.

Medical Management

Children with partial defects are managed, if possible, in the same manner as children with uncomplicated atrial septal defect. Those who are symptomatic with or without mitral regurgitation should undergo surgical closure of their primum atrial septal defect and plication of the cleft of the anterior mitral valve leaflet. Those few patients with significant residual mitral regurgitation are managed medically until such time as mitral valve replacement can be accomplished.

The clinical approach to the infant with complete AV canal is the same as described for infants with a large ventricular septal defect but tempered by the knowledge that spontaneous improvement is very unlikely except at the expense of the pulmonary vascular bed. For very young infants, under 3 or 4 months of age, in severe congestive heart failure with a documented large interventricular defect and little or no mitral regurgitation, banding of the pulmonary artery is still recommended. In the older infant, or in the presence of moderate or severe mitral regurgitation, complete correction is recommended. For those infants in whom failure is more manageable and pulmonary arterial pressure some-

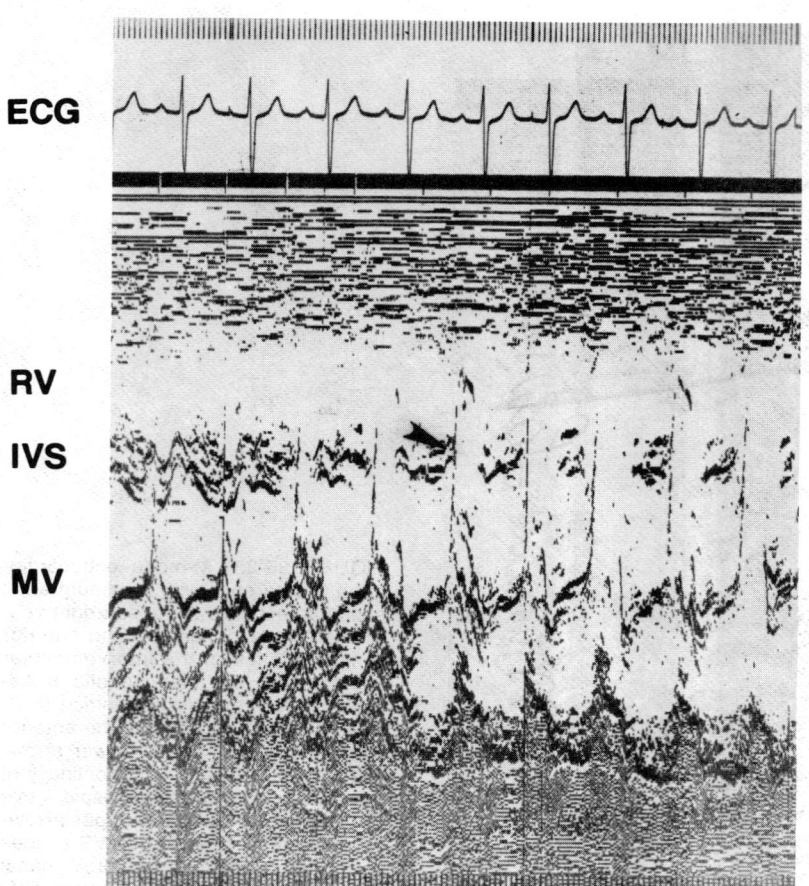

FIGURE 36-24 M-mode echocardiogram from a child with complete AV canal which demonstrates continuity (arrowhead) of the anterior mitral valve (MV) and tricuspid valve (TV) echoes across the interventricular septum (IVS) with absence of IVS echoes. IVS motion is normal. ECG = electrocardiogram; RV = right ventricle; TV = tricuspid valve.

what lower, perhaps due to a smaller interventricular communication, the indications for recatheterization and surgery are the same as those for a ventricular septal defect.

Complete heart block is an uncommon complication of surgical correction today, but it carries the same serious consequences whether it is induced during correction of the partial or complete form of AV canal or whether it develops in the months and years following surgery. Permanent ventricular pacing is indicated.

Antibiotic coverage at times of special risk of bacteremia is indicated indefinitely for all forms of AV canal, operated or unoperated, in view of the complexity of the lesion and the mitral valve deformity which must persist.

With regard to genetic counseling, the risk of a subsequent sibling having heart disease in the presence of a single affected family member is in the range of 2 percent and is probably the same for the offspring of an affected parent. Interestingly, there is evidence to suggest that the offspring of family members with a superiorly oriented QRS axis but without overt heart disease may also be at risk. Concordance for AV canal defects among affected siblings or offspring is much higher than with other forms of congenital heart disease and approaches 90 percent.[154]

Surgical Management

The excellent results achieved in several medical centers[192–195] following total correction of complete AV canal defects in infancy have encouraged early correction. Banding of the pulmonary artery is rarely practiced but still deserves consideration in the occasional very tiny or critically ill infant having a large left-to-right shunt rather than AV valvular regurgitation.[196] When associated right ventricular outflow tract obstruction is severe, a systemic arterial to pulmonary arterial shunt such as the Blalock-Taussig subclavian arterial to pulmonary arterial anastomosis will effectively reduce hypoxia and its complications, allowing subsequent anatomic correction.

Anatomic correction of complete AV canal is carried out through a median sternotomy. The patient is supported on total cardiopulmonary bypass with moderate hypothermia (22 to 28°C) and cardioplegia. In infants less than 1 year old weighing less than 10 kg, we prefer to operate under conditions of total circulatory arrest with profound hypothermia (18 to 20°C), limited cardiopulmonary bypass being used for cooling and rewarming.

The interior of the heart is exposed through a generous right atriotomy. Details of repair are dictated by the anatomy in each case (Fig. 36-27).[197] Fibrous attachments from the anterior and poste-

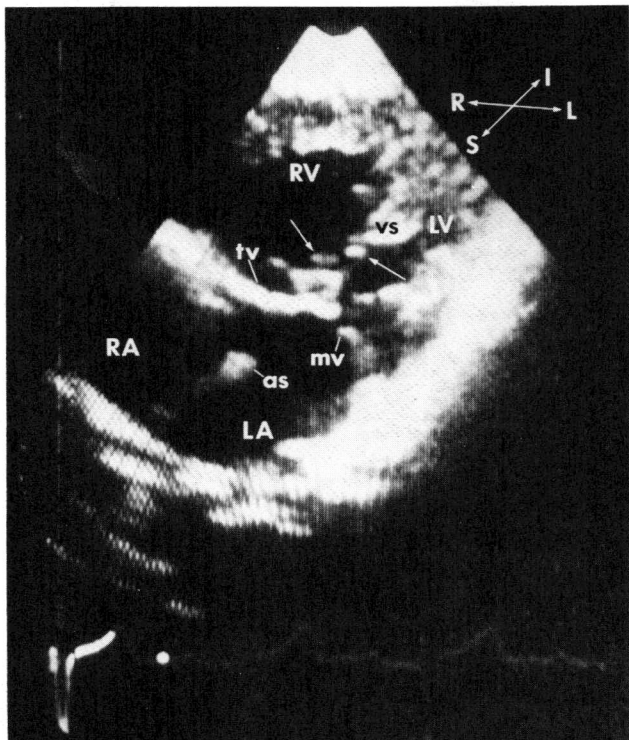

FIGURE 36-25 Two-dimensional echocardiogram in the apex view from a child with type A complete atrioventricular canal. The common anterior leaflet of the tricuspid (tv) and mitral (mv) valves appears to be attached to the crest of the ventricular septum (vs) by multiple chordae (arrows). The areas of the ostium primum atrial septal defect lies between the lowermost edge of the atrial septum (as) and the mitral valve (mv). R = right; S = superior; I = inferior; L = left; RV = right ventricle; LV = left ventricle; RA = right atrium; LA = left atrium. (*From Hagler, Tajik, Seward, Mair, and Ritter.*[189] *Reproduced with permission of the American Heart Association, Inc.*)

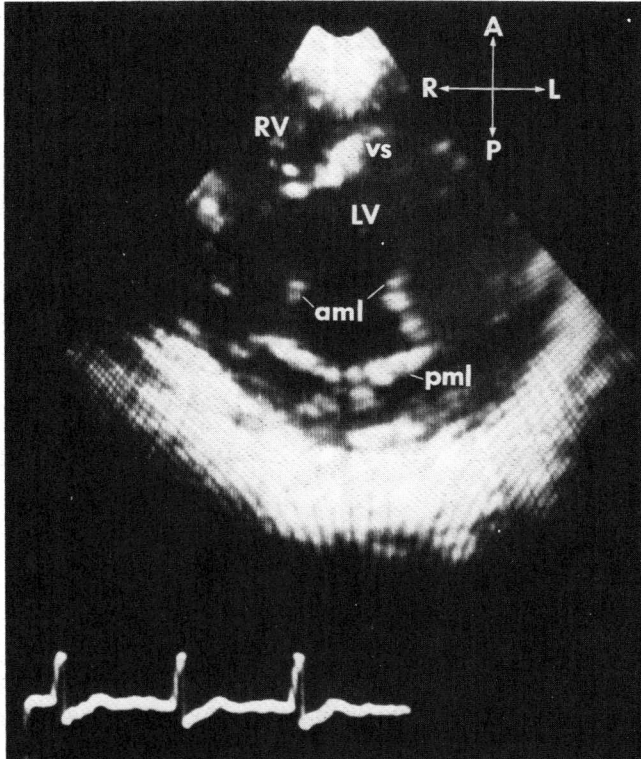

FIGURE 36-26 Two-dimensional echocardiogram in the parasternal short axis view of a child with an AV canal-type ventricular septal defect, intact atrial septum, and mitral valve cleft. The cleft in the anterior mitral valve leaflet (aml) is noted during diastole. R = right; A = anterior; P = posterior; L = left; RV = right ventricle; LV = left ventricle; VS = ventricular septum; pml = posterior mitral valve leaflet. (*From Hagler, Tajik, Seward, Mair, and Ritter.*[189] *Reproduced with permission of the American Heart Association, Inc.*)

rior common bridging leaflets to the rim of the ventricular septum are divided. One or both of the common bridging leaflets may require division to create separate mitral and tricuspid components (Fig. 36-29). Construction of an adequate mitral orifice and competent mitral valve is of foremost concern; tricuspid incompetence rarely poses a postoperative problem. A Dacron patch is attached to fibrous endocardium on the right side of the ventricular septum away from the rim of the septal defect to obliterate the interventricular communication while avoiding the areas of the bundle of His and the AV node. The anterior and posterior components of the anterior mitral valve leaflet are approximated with sutures; this newly formed leaflet is sutured to the Dacron septal patch at an appropriate level. The tricuspid valve is reconstructed in a similar manner. Mitral valve competence is assessed by gentle distension of the left ventricle with saline injected across the valve with an irrigating syringe. Severe residual mitral regurgitation may require subsequent mitral valve replacement,[198] but we have not had to insert

a prosthetic valve in any patient during the initial correction.

The interatrial communication is closed using the remaining portion of the septal patch or a separate piece of pericardium, the latter reducing the likelihood of life-threatening hemolysis if residual mitral regurgitation is present.[199] Associated right ventricular outflow tract obstruction is relieved by pulmonary commissurotomy and excision of hypertrophic infundibular myocardium. A previously placed pulmonary arterial band is incised and removed, the main pulmonary artery being enlarged with a gusset of pericardium. Previously constructed systemic arterial to pulmonary arterial shunts are closed as described elsewhere (see tetralogy of Fallot). To facilitate postoperative management, left and right atrial pressure monitoring catheters are inserted; atrial and ventricular pacing wires are attached.

Hospital mortality for total correction of AV canal in infancy is about 20 percent, the highest mortality being encountered during the first few months of life and in those infants with severe AV valve regurgitation or elevated pulmonary vascular

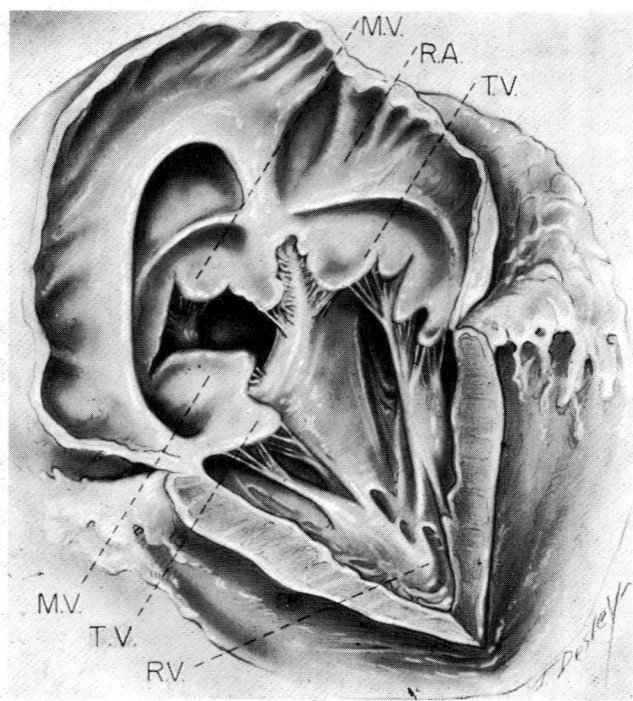

FIGURE 36-27 Complete form of common AV canal, type A. The common anterior leaflet has recognizable mitral component, MV, and tricuspid component, TV. In type B, not illustrated, those components are attached by chordae to a papillary muscle in the right ventricle. In type C, not illustrated, the common anterior leaflet is a single unit without any attachment to the underlying ventricular septum. Type A is most amenable to repair. (*From G. C. Rastelli, P. A. Ongley, J. W. Kirklin, and D. C. McGoon: Surgical Repair of the Complete Form of Persistent Common Atrioventricular Canal, J. Thorac. Cardiovasc. Surg., 55:299, 1968. Reproduced with permission.*)

FIGURE 36-28 Posteroanterior view of the left ventricular angiogram from a child with complete AV canal demonstrating the characteristic gooseneck deformity (arrows) of the outflow tract of the left ventricle (LV). Opacification of the right ventricular outflow tract (RVO) and main pulmonary artery (MPA) before or in the absence of atrial opacification reflects the presence of the interventricular communication. Ao = aorta.

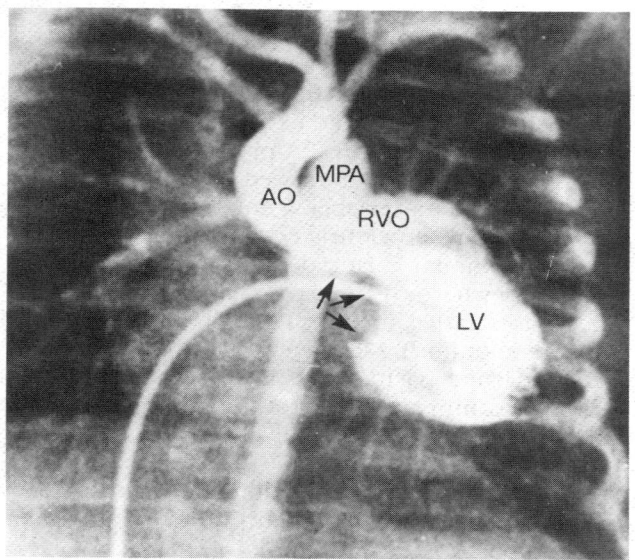

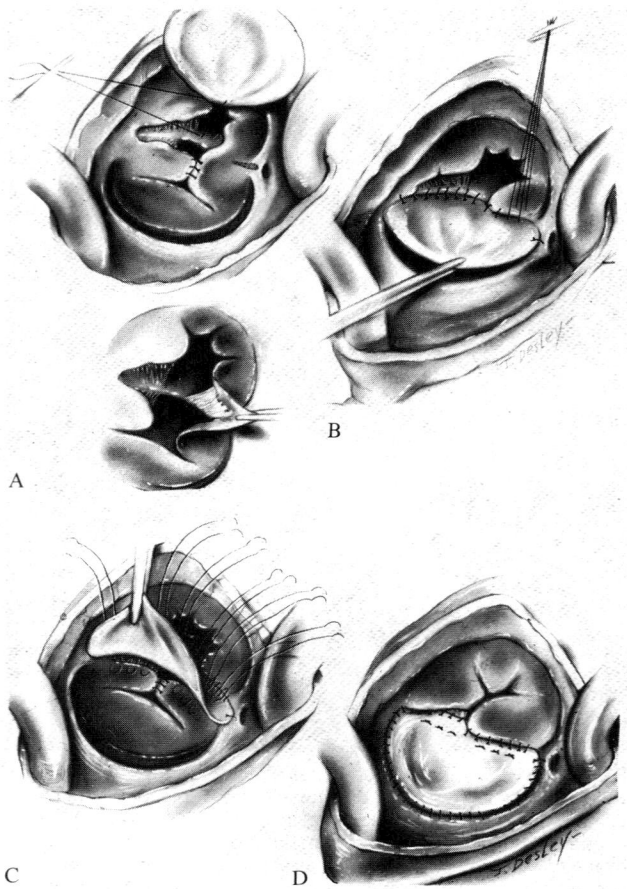

FIGURE 36-29 Steps in the repair of the complete form of common AV canal, type A. *A* and *B.* A pericardial patch is sutured to the ventricular septum. *C* and *D.* The anterior leaflet of the mitral valve is reconstructed and attached to the patch. *D.* A portion of the tricuspid leaflet is attached to the patch. (*From G. C. Rastelli, P. A. Ongley, J. W. Kirklin, and D. C. McGoon, Surgical Repair of the Complete Form of Persistent Common Atrioventricular Canal, J. Thorac. Cardiovasc. Surg., 55:299, 1968. Reproduced with permission.*)

resistance.[192,193] Survival to the age of 5 years without operation occurs in only 4 percent.[194] Berger and his associates at the University of Alabama Medical Center reported a 5-year survival of 91 percent for patients discharged from the hospital following total correction.[194] They found that the greatest likelihood for "surgical cure" (alive 5 years later with a mean pulmonary arterial pressure of 25 mmHg or less) was greatest (73 percent) if the operation was performed when the child was about 14 months old. Operation may be required before this age if symptoms dictate.

Danielson[197] reviewed 49 patients operated upon at the Mayo Clinic between 1963 and 1976. This series included several older patients, the oldest being 30 years. Operative mortality was 14 percent. Late results were excellent.

Successful correction of complete AV canal associated with common ventricle,[200] tetralogy of Fallot, or double-outlet right ventricle,[201] and other complex anomalies[202,203] has been reported.

Ostium primum atrial septal defect with or without mitral valve incompetence secondary to a cleft in the anterior (aortic) leaflet—partial AV canal—is repaired through a median sternotomy on cardiopulmonary bypass with moderate hypothermia (25 to 30°C) and cardioplegia (Fig. 36-10). The right atrium is opened by enlargement of the appendage cannulation site. When mitral regurgitation has been demonstrated by angiocardiography, a cleft in the anterior mitral leaflet is sought and closed with a few simple interrupted sutures. Only the edges of the leaflets free of chordae are approximated. The atrial septal defect is closed by placement of a pericardial patch. Dacron is avoided when possible because of the risk of hemolysis imposed by its use. Care is exercised to avoid injury to the bundle of His in the area of contiguous mitral and tricuspid valves by confining the sutures to fibrous tissue to the left of the annulus. The AV node is avoided near the ostium of the coronary sinus by placement of superficial interrupted sutures on the left atrial side of the atrial septum.

Severe mitral regurgitation is difficult to correct even by closure of the cleft between the anterior and posterior portions of the anterior mitral valve leaflet. Excessive or inaccurate closure of the cleft may produce mitral stenosis. The leaflet itself may be deficient or severely deformed. Mitral valve competence can be evaluated by gentle distension of the left ventricle with saline injected through a small rubber catheter passed across the valve; however, there is relatively poor correlation between auscultatory, angiographic, and intraoperative assessment of mitral regurgitation.[197]

McMullan and his colleagues at the Mayo Clinic[204] reviewed 232 patients between the ages of 3 months and 50 years operated upon between 1955 and 1972. Hospital mortality was 6 percent; risk of death was greater in patients having severe preoperative disability, those having a cardiothoracic ratio exceeding 0.60, and in infants under 1 year of age. Eight (3.8 percent) of 210 patients for whom follow-up data were available required mitral valve replacement 3 months to 14 years after the initial operation. Permanent complete heart block contributed substantially to early mortality and morbidity but is now extremely rare. A very low operative mortality and excellent late results can be anticipated from correction of partial AV canal in all but those few patients having severe mitral valvular incompetence. In some of these, valve replacement may be necessary.

Left Ventricular–Right Atrial Communication

Definition

A left ventricular–right atrial communication is a defect that allows direct communication of the two chambers named. The defect is usually small.

Pathology

In this uncommon condition one of several anatomic arrangements is observed, of which the most common is characterized by an infracristal ventricular septal defect associated with a cleft in the septal leaflet of the tricuspid valve (Fig. 36-30). The edges of the valvular cleft are attached to the edges of the defect, thereby committing the left ventricle to communicate with the right atrium. Less commonly there is a defect in that part of the membranous septum that normally separates the two chambers involved.[205–207]

The left ventricle may be somewhat enlarged, while right ventricular hypertrophy is absent (except in cases of associated transposition). The right atrium is enlarged.

Associated conditions that have been observed are complete transposition,[208] Ebstein's malformation of the tricuspid valve, and subaortic stenosis.

Clinical Manifestations

This uncommon but interesting malformation makes up somewhat less than 1 percent of all congenital cardiac defects. Females are slightly more commonly affected than males.[9]

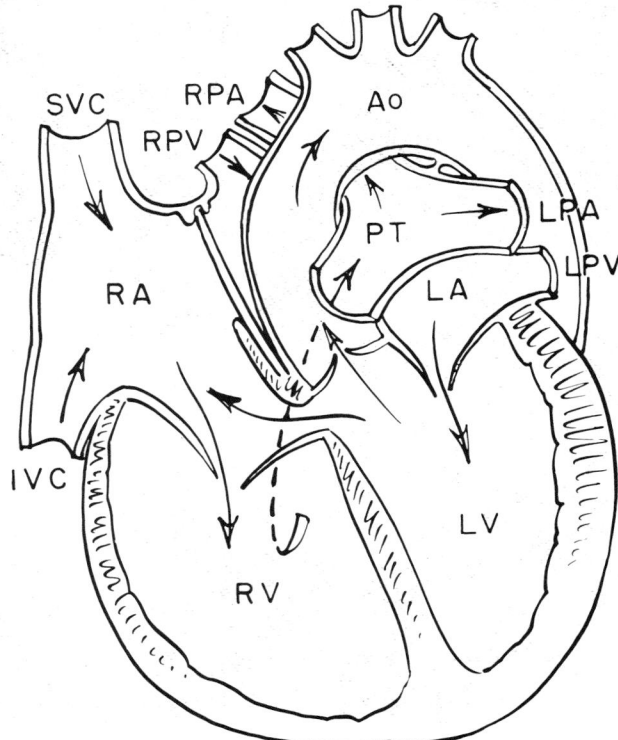

FIGURE 36-30 Left ventricular–right atrial communication. SVC = superior vena cava; IVC = inferior vena cava; RA = right atrium; RV = right ventricle; PT = main pulmonary arterial trunk; RPA = right pulmonary artery; LPA = left pulmonary artery; RPV = right pulmonary vein; LPV = left pulmonary vein; LA = left atrium; LV = left ventricle; Ao = aorta. [*From J. E. Edwards, Classification of Congenital Heart Disease in the Adult, in W. C. Roberts. (ed.), Congenital Heart Disease in Adults, Cardiovasc. Clin. Series 10/1, F. A. Davis Company, Philadelphia, 1979, pp. 1–26. Reproduced with permission.*]

DISEASES OF THE HEART AND BLOOD VESSELS

History The murmur frequently is detected within the first day of life since flow through the defect is not dependent upon a reduced pulmonary vascular resistance. Slow weight gain, tachypnea, repeated lower respiratory infections, and congestive failure appearing within the first few months of life are typical if the defect is large, but many individuals with small defects are entirely asymptomatic.

Physical Examination A holosystolic murmur typical of a ventricular septal defect is present at the lower left sternal border but may radiate unusually well to the right midsternal border area. A diastolic flow rumble at the apex is common with large shunts. A hyperdynamic left parasternal lift, with or without an early diastolic flow murmur at the lower left sternal border, reflects the right ventricular volume overload one might expect from an associated atrial septal defect, but normal movement of the aortic and pulmonary components of the second heart sound indicates an intact atrial septum.

Chest Roentgenogram The pulmonary vascular engorgement, cardiac enlargement, and left atrial dilatation support the diagnosis of ventricular septal defect. Impressive right atrial enlargement, best seen in the frontal view, an unexpected finding with typical ventricular septal defect, should suggest this variant malformation.

Electrocardiogram The QRS axis in the frontal plane may be superior if the septal defect is in the canal position, but in the majority of patients the QRS axis is normal. Left ventricular hypertrophy and usually right ventricular hypertrophy are present unless the shunt is small. Tall, peaked P waves are not uncommon in this setting and provide a valuable clue to the correct diagnosis.

Echocardiogram M-mode studies have demonstrated high-frequency systolic fluttering of the anterior tricuspid leaflet, coinciding in time with the holosystolic murmur, at least in those patients where the stream of left ventricular blood must traverse the tricuspid leaflets to reach the right atrium.[209]

Cardiac Catherization A step-up in oxygen saturation will be found at the right atrial level together with mean and phasic pressure differences between the left and right atria, which indicate an intact interatrial septum. The diagnosis may be made by selective left ventricular angiography in the frontal view where immediate opacification of the dilated right atrium will be seen (Fig. 36-31).

Natural History and Prognosis
The clinical course is similar to that described for ventricular septal defect.

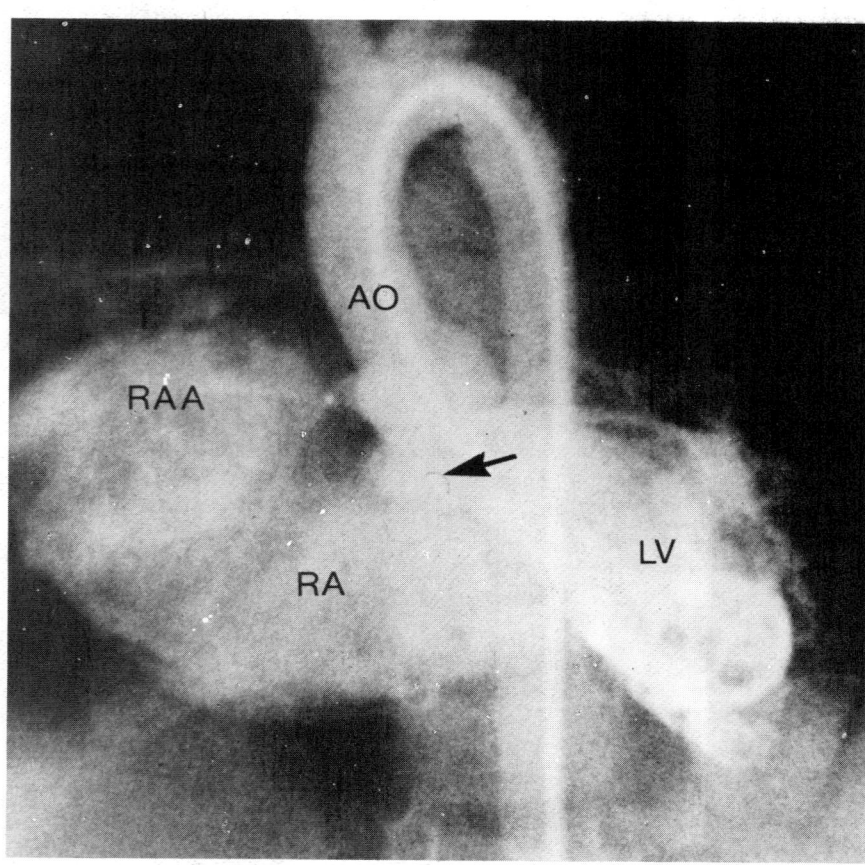

FIGURE 36-31 Posteroanterior view of the left ventricular angiogram from a child with a left ventricular–right atrial shunt demonstrating opacification of the dilated right atrium (RA) and right atrial appendage (RAA) through a high ventricular septal defect (arrow). LV = left ventricle; AO = aorta.

Medical Management

The management of congestive failure, the indications for operation, and the other features of management are as described for ventricular septal defect.

Surgical Management

Operation is performed through a median sternotomy on complete cardiopulmonary bypass with moderate hypothermia (28 to 30°C) and cardioplegia. Profound hypothermia (18 to 20°C) and circulatory arrest are used in infancy.[165] The left ventricular–right atrial communication is exposed through a right atriotomy. The defect is usually near or actually within the tricuspid annulus, lying just superior to the septal leaflet of the tricuspid valve. The edges of a cleft in the septal leaflet of the tricuspid valve may be fused to the edges of the defect. Closure is accomplished by direct suture of the fibrous margin or placement of a small Dacron patch after freeing the tricuspid leaflet edges,[171] sutures being carefully placed to avoid injury to the atrioventricular node and the bundle of His. If present, the small cleft in the septal leaflet of the tricuspid valve is closed with a few simple interrupted sutures. Hemodynamic results are excellent; morbidity and mortality are very low.[168]

Extracardiac Communications between the Systemic and Pulmonary Circulations Usually without Cyanosis

Patent Ductus Arteriosus

Definition

Patent ductus arteriosus, the most common type of extracardiac shunt, represents persistent patency of the vessel in the fetus that normally connects the pulmonary arterial system and the aorta (Fig. 36-32).

Etiology

Delayed closure of the ductus is observed in premature infants.[210] It has been recognized that patent ductus arteriosus may follow maternal rubella during the first 2 months of gestation, and it may be associated with certain extracardiac abnormalities, including mental retardation and various ophthalmic changes.[211] Cardiovascular abnormalities other than patent ductus following maternal rubella include atrial septal defects, ventricular septal defects, tetralogy of Fallot, coarctation of the aorta, aortic stenosis, transposition of the great arteries, and tricuspid atresia. In older children, pulmonary stenosis associated with mental retardation has been described.[212]

Pathology

The ductus arteriosus usually closes within 2 or 3 weeks after birth and becomes the ligamentum ar-

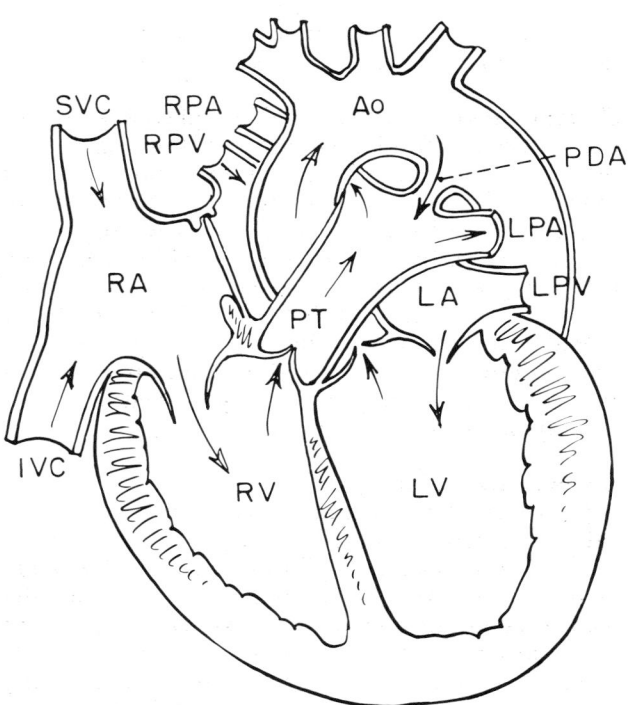

FIGURE 36-32 Patent ductus arteriosus (PDA), classic type. In this type of patent ductus arteriosus the abnormal channel offers sufficient resistance to flow as to prevent equalization of aortic and pulmonary arterial pressures. The wide ductus allows free communication between the great arteries with equalization of pressures between them. SVC = superior vena cava; IVC = inferior vena cava; RA = right atrium; RV = right ventricle; PT = main pulmonary arterial trunk; RPA = right pulmonary artery; LPA = left pulmonary artery; RPV = right pulmonary vein; LPV = left pulmonary vein; LA = left atrium; LV = left ventricle; Ao = aorta. [*From J. E. Edwards, Classification of Congenital Heart Disease in the Adult, in W. C. Roberts (ed.), Congenital Heart Disease in Adults, Cardiovasc. Clin. Series 10/1, F. A. Davis Company, Philadelphia, 1979, pp. 1–26. Reproduced with permission.*]

teriosum,[213] but it may remain patent as long as 8 weeks postnatally.[214] It runs from the origin of the left pulmonary artery, below, to the lower aspect of the aortic arch just beyond the level of origin of the left subclavian artery, above. The recurrent branch of the left vagus nerve hooks around its lateral and inferior aspects.

The hearts of subjects with patent ductus arteriosus show varying degrees of enlargement of the left atrium and ventricle. The character of the right ventricle depends upon the state of the ductus, whether narrow (obstructive) or wide (so-called hypertensive ductus). In the former the right ventricle is normal; in the latter its wall is hypertrophied.

Associated Conditions Many cardiovascular anomalies may be associated with a patent ductus, the most common being coarctation of the aorta and ventricular septal defect. Patent ductus arteriosus is an integral part of interruption of the aortic arch. In certain anomalies, such as pulmonary atresia with intact ventricular septum (so-called ductus-depend-

DISEASES OF THE HEART AND BLOOD VESSELS

ent conditions), persistent patency of the ductus is desirable, but this tends to close at a normal rate.

Complications The potential complications of patent ductus are fundamentally like those in ventricular septal defect. Infective endocarditis in patent ductus involves the pulmonary artery at the site of impact of the shunt coming from the aorta. Pulmonary arterial aneurysm resulting either from pulmonary hypertension or infection occurs. In subjects surviving into adult life, calcification of the ductal wall is common. Ductal aneurysm may occur and potentially be confused with an aneurysm of the aortic arch if the pulmonary end is either closed or only narrowly patent.[215]

Abnormal Physiology[216–220]
Patients with patent ductus arteriosus may be divided into groups according to those in whom the vascular resistance through the ductus itself is small, moderate, or large. Since the resistance of the ductus is related not only to its cross-sectional area but also to its length, it is difficult to define the anatomic size of the ductus in each group. In patients with a ductus of small internal diameter and high resistance, the flow across the ductus will be relatively small. The extra volume of work on the left ventricle is tolerated well and the pulmonary pressure and resistance are not elevated. Patients with only moderate resistance in the ductus have some increase in pulmonary artery pressure with a moderately greater volume of shunting across the ductus.

In patients with a large patent ductus which offers minimal resistance to blood flow, the aorta and pulmonary artery are essentially in free communication; the systolic pressure in the pulmonary artery will be nearly equal to that in the aorta. In patent ductus, the volume load is on the left ventricle, which may "fail." Pulmonary congestion results from left ventricle failure with increased pressure in the left atrium and pulmonary capillaries and the failure of the pulmonary vasculature to "protect" the pulmonary capillaries from the high pulmonary artery pressure and flow. With time, the left ventricle compensates with dilatation and hypertrophy to carry the volume load, and the pulmonary vasculature responds to the high pressure by developing and maintaining adequate vasomotor tone and resistance to protect the pulmonary capillaries. It is likely that the high pressure in the pulmonary circuit induces a "reactive" type of muscular hypertrophy, probably giving the arteries and arterioles greater ability to have and to maintain greater vasoconstriction. When hypertrophy decreases the cross-sectional area of a vascular vessel, any additional narrowing produced by vasomotion will be proportionately even more effective in increasing the resistance of the vessel. The role of reflexes in the development and maintenance of "functional" pulmonary vasoconstriction is uncertain.

In patients with a moderate or large ductus, the right ventricle is burdened mainly by a pressure load in the pulmonary circuit caused largely by pulmonary vasoconstriction.

In patients with extreme degrees of pulmonary vascular disease, the structural changes in the vessels themselves account for most of the vascular resistance, which can no longer be decreased with pulmonary vasodilators such as oxygen administration or acetylcholine infusion. When this stage is reached, the pulmonary resistance may equal or exceed the resistance of systemic circulation and there may be shunting of unsaturated blood from pulmonary artery to aorta. This often causes the arterial saturation to be higher in the arms, especially the right arm, than in the legs.

Clinical Manifestations

History The history of the mother's pregnancy and of perinatal events may provide helpful clues that are associated with a high incidence of patent ductus arteriosus.[6] Exposure to rubella in the first trimester by a nonimmunized mother is an example. Patent ductus is also more common in the premature infant, especially those with birth asphyxia or respiratory distress syndrome.[217,221–223] There is a much higher incidence in females, except in rubella syndrome, where the sexes are affected equally.[224] Extensive review of the literature[6] and series of large numbers of patients[224] can be referred to for more detail.

Symptoms are usually restricted to those with large shunts that produce heart failure or with other complicating problems such as respiratory distress in the premature infant. The symptoms related to heart failure were discussed earlier. Heart failure is most likely to develop in the first few weeks or months of life. If it does not appear during infancy, it is unlikely to occur before the third decade. The clinical presentation in the premature infant is usually very different from the full-term infant. This is particularly true in those with a birth weight under 1.5 kg, who are more likely to have moderate to severe respiratory distress requiring continuous positive airway pressure or assisted ventilation with oxygen administration. In these infants, the clinical features of respiratory distress often blend over the course of several days into those of heart failure. Increasing ventilatory or oxygen requirements with carbon dioxide retention or episodic apnea and bradycardia are often the first signs that a patent ductus may be complicating the picture. Growth problems can occur in the symptomatic or otherwise asymptomatic patient with patent ductus,[225] but is clearly due to, and not just associated with, the ductus only in those with large shunts and failure.

Physical Examination In the full-term infant or child with patent ductus arteriosus, there is frequently a systolic thrill over the pulmonary artery and in the suprasternal notch. The peripheral pulses are generally brisk and bounding, especially with the larger shunts. Blood pressure measurement in older patients with significant shunts will frequently demonstrate a pulse pressure of 45 mmHg or more.[224] Diffuse cyanosis may be present if there is pulmonary edema. The patient with elevated pulmonary vascular resistance and shunt reversal will have cyanosis and clubbing of the toes and occasionally the fingers on the left side. The apex impulse may be increased or displaced in those with large shunts. The right ventricular impulse is increased in the premature infant with respiratory distress or in infants and children with significant pulmonary hypertension. Auscultatory findings will vary with age, size of the shunt, and the pulmonary vascular status. The typical murmur is a continuous or machinery murmur that is best heard at the left upper sternal border and below the left clavicle. It is usually a rough or crackling murmur with eddy sounds that are helpful in making the diagnosis. This murmur peaks at or near the second heart sound. The murmur may have a more abbreviated diastolic component, especially in newborns and those with very small shunts or pulmonary hypertension. A nonspecific systolic murmur is present in a small percentage of patients, more commonly the premature or very young infant. Uncommonly, the murmur may vary widely[226] or be absent.[227] In infants and children with at least a moderate shunt, there is a middiastolic rumble occasionally associated with an opening snap at the apex. The second heart sound may be difficult to hear due to the continuous murmur, but it is usually normal. The pulmonary component of the second heart sound will be accentuated in those with pulmonary hypertension. Careful auscultation is particularly important in the diagnosis of patent ductus. Other causes of continuous murmurs, such as aorticopulmonary septal defect and ruptured aneurysm of the sinus of Valsalva, are extemely uncommon. They are discussed later in this chapter and have been reviewed elsewhere.[228]

Chest Roentgenogram Findings on chest roentgenogram are also dependent on the magnitude of the shunt. In those with a small shunt, it is normal or may suggest that the aorta and pulmonary artery are dilated by the contour produced. With larger shunts, the heart size is increased. In addition to the enlarged aorta and pulmonary artery, the left atrium is enlarged with posterior indentation on a barium-filled esophagus or elevation of the left mainstem bronchus. With large shunts, the left ventricle is also enlarged. Increases in pulmonary arterial flow also parallel the magnitude of the shunt. In the presence of heart failure, there are signs of pulmonary edema. In older patients who have developed Eisenmenger's physiology, the only abnormality may be marked prominence of the central pulmonary arteries with rapid tapering to the periphery of the lung fields with a normal heart size.

Electrocardiogram In patent ductus with a small shunt, the electrocardiogram may be normal. The QRS axis is usually normal, but it may be deviated to the left in some patients. Left atrial hypertrophy is probably the most common abnormality found, but left ventricular hypertrophy of the volume overload type with deep Q waves and increased R-wave voltage in the left precordial leads is also common. Right ventricular hypertrophy is unusual, but is seen in premature infants with respiratory distress syndrome and in others with pulmonary hypertension.

Echocardiogram M-mode echocardiography is a noninvasive method for detection of left atrial enlargement, although not specific for patent ductus (Fig. 36-33). The ratio of left atrial to aortic diameters[229] offers an internal correction for body size and has been used for assessment of the shunt in premature infants with a patent ductus.[230] The ratio of left atrial to aortic diameters was 1.28 ± 0.23 in those with a ductus and 0.86 ± 0.10 in the control group. Rapid changes to normal after surgical ligation and the value of serial measurements were also discussed. Others have found that the left atrial dimension corrected for body surface area is more accurate than the ratio.[231] The left ventricular end-diastolic dimension is increased in symptomatic premature infants with patent ductus.[232] The mean velocity of circumferential fiber shortening is significantly increased in infants with large shunts in addition to the increased ratio.[233] A simpler measure of left ventricular performance, the percent shortening of the internal diameter of the left ventricle, is increased in ill premature infants with patent ductus and left cardiac enlargement until myocardial performance deteriorates, and it then decreases.[234]

Cardiac Catheterization In those with a typical, uncomplicated patent ductus, cardiac catheterization is not a necessity for diagnosis. When catheterization is performed, the catheter usually passes quite easily from the pulmonary artery to the descending aorta, except when the ductus is too small. The saturation will be increased in the pulmonary artery to a degree relative to the size of the shunt. In infants with a very large ductus, the saturation may be increased in the right atrium due to shunting across a patent foramen ovale. The systemic arterial saturation is normal in the absence of pulmonary edema. The pulmonary arterial and right ventricular pressures are usually normal, but they are elevated in those with a large ductus. The pulmonary vascular resistance is almost always normal in infants and young children. It will be elevated in older patients who have developed irreversible changes in the pulmonary vascular bed. These patients will also have diminished saturation in the descending aorta once the pulmonary resistance reaches a level that will reverse the shunt. Aortography will opacify the ductus and pulmonary arteries.

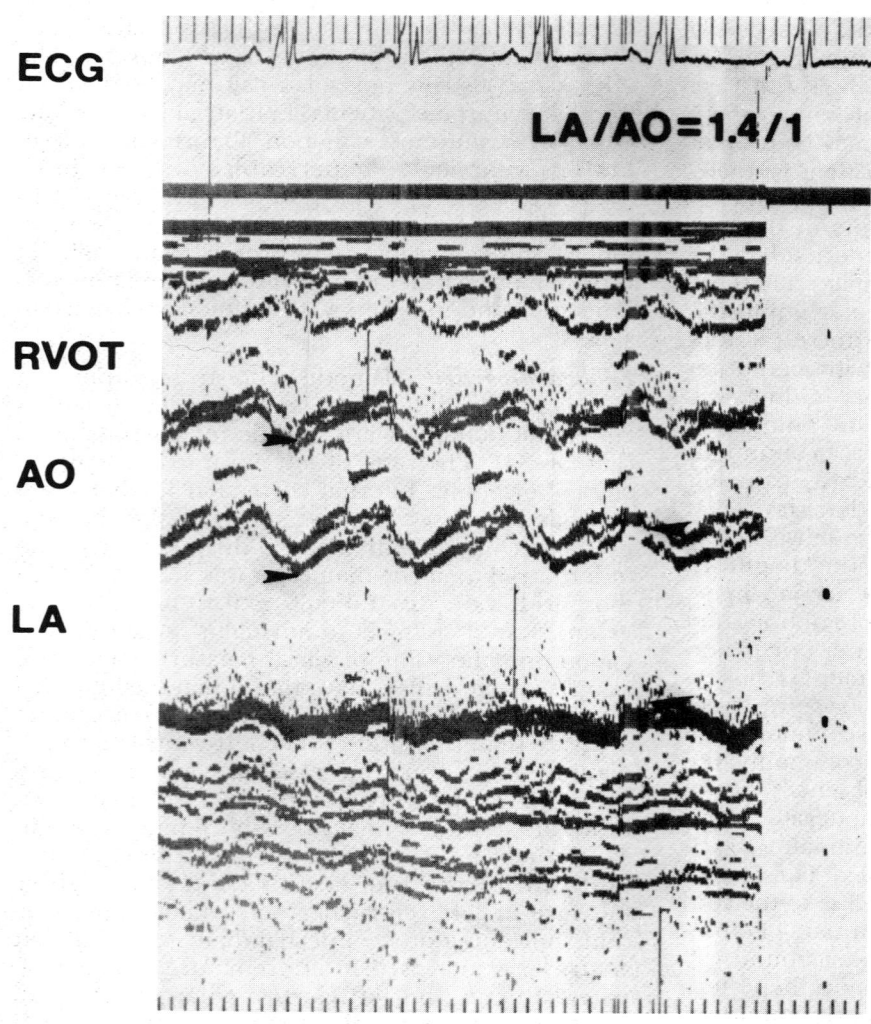

ECG

LA/AO=1.4/1

RVOT

AO

LA

FIGURE 36-33 M-mode echocardiogram of a premature infant with a large patent ductus arteriosus. Aortic and left atrial dimensions (arrows) yield increased ratio due to left atrial enlargement. ECG = electrocardiogram; RVOT = right ventricular outflow tract; AO = aortic root; LA = left atrium.

Natural History and Prognosis[6,216]

The complications related to patent ductus include infective endarteritis, heart failure, and pulmonary hypertension with vascular damage. Infection of the ductus is a risk regardless of its size. The risk increases with length of survival. This can lead to development of a mycotic aneurysm with the potential to compress the recurrent laryngeal nerve, embolize septic material to the lungs, or rupture.

In those with large shunts, heart failure can cause significant morbidity and mortality, particularly in the premature and young infant, and sudden death can occur. Progressive damage to the pulmonary vascular bed can occur in some, but it is rarely to an irreversible degree in the first year or two of life. Once irreversible damage occurs, premature death in late adolescence or early adulthood can be anticipated. Although there is disagreement in the literature, present evidence strongly suggests that untreated patent ductus leads to premature death, but studies with unbiased patient selection and comparison among groups with differing hemodynamic status are not available and will not become available in view of current management.

Medical Management

Primary prevention will require obstetrical measures to decrease the incidence of prematurity. Primary prevention by widespread immunization of children has already been largely successful in reducing the number of those born with rubella syndrome. For women in the child-bearing years who have not been immunized and who have not had the documented disease, serologic study will further elucidate their immunologic status. For those who are immunologically unprotected and exposed during the first trimester of pregnancy, abortion offers a controversial form of prevention.

Medical management centers around the symptomatic patients and the prevention of infection of the ductus. For prevention and treatment of infection, refer to the preceding section on infective endocarditis and to Chap. 54. Prevention is important regardless of the size of the ductus and can be accomplished most effectively in the older infant and child by surgical ligation.

For symptomatic patients, usually premature and young infants, standard medical measures for treatment of heart failure are initiated. Management will be more successful if anemia is also prevented. In the premature infant, attempts to improve oxygenation, with increasing concentration of inspired oxygen and ventilatory assistance as necessary with monitoring of arterial oxygen levels, can promote spontaneous ductal closure. The use of prolonged continuous positive airway pressure has been described.[235] A relationship of volume of fluid administration to the incidence of ductus in premature infants has been demonstrated.[236] Difficulties related to achieving a balance between the need for supplying adequate calories to very small infants and excessive fluid administration may explain some of the differences in incidence of the clinically significant ductus on an iatrogenic basis. Other ways that the problem might be iatrogenic have been suggested.[237]

For those who do not respond to this type of management, alternatives to surgery have been sought, particularly for the higher-risk patients. Methods of transfemoral catheter closure using an Ivalon plug[238] and a foam-covered prosthesis with hooks[239] have been used successfully in selected patients. Such techniques continue to be done on an investigational basis, but they have not been accepted for widespread clinical use at the present time. Successful pharmacologic closure of the ductus in premature infants using inhibitors of prostaglandin synthesis, aspirin and indomethacin, was first reported in 1976.[219,220] These reports were followed by an editorial urging caution in this area.[240] Subsequent reports include further assessment of responses[241,242] as well as significant side effects, such as changes in renal function[243] and other complications.[244] In addition, since anatomic closure is delayed beyond functional closure, the ductus may be a recurrent problem in these infants. Currently, prostaglandin inhibitors should only be used in major centers under a strict clinical research protocol until further data on effectiveness and toxicity are accumulated. Until then, surgical ligation and/or division is the safest alternative for others, since accumulated experience here is great.[245–248]

The current indications for surgery include uncontrollable heart failure in the newborn and young infant, failure to grow properly in association with signs of a significant shunt in the infant, and continued patency with any size shunt beyond the first year or so of life. Recommended age for elective surgical ligation is usually 1 to 2 years of age. The tendency in the premature has been toward earlier intervention in attempts to decrease development of chronic pulmonary disease. The presence of irreversible pulmonary vascular disease is a contraindication to surgery.

Intraoperative and postoperative management require special care with a team approach in the ill newborn. Most patients demonstrate increases in the systemic systolic and diastolic pressures in the immediate postoperative period. In a few patients, this rise can produce significant hypertension that is sustained[6] and may require medical treatment.

Surgical Management

The patent ductus arteriosus is exposed through a posterolateral left thoracotomy in the fourth intercostal space. The ductus is mobilized by careful dissection, avoiding injury to the recurrent laryngeal nerve as it passes around the inferior margins. Details of the operation are described by Jones.[249]

Interruption of the ductus is accomplished by division or multiple ligation. A short, broad, or thin-walled ductus is usually divided between vascular clamps and the ends closed with fine continuous suture (Fig. 36-34). A long, narrow, thick-walled ductus can be divided as just described or ligated with two or three sutures spaced a few millimeters apart. The suture ligatures at each end are passed through the adventitia and media to avoid migration and to assure multiple points of obliteration. This technique is preferred by some surgeons who believe it to be safer and faster.

The fragile, thin-walled patent ductus of the premature infant is obliterated by ligation with a relatively thick suture to minimize accidental disruption. We have found the placement of two metallic surgical Hemoclips to be an effective method for obliterating the patent ductus in an infant.

Closure of a patent ductus arteriosus in an adult requires particular caution because of possible calcification and diminished pliability of the ductus wall. Placement of a Dacron patch over the aortic orifice of the ductus from within the aorta may be advisable, the aorta being occluded briefly by vascular clamps placed above and below the origin of the ductus. Proximal hypertension is controlled by intravenous infusion of sodium nitroprusside while the clamps are in place. In some cases of calcified patent ductus arteriosus, operation may be facilitated by the use of femoral vein to femoral arterial bypass using the heart-lung machine, left atrial to femoral arterial bypass using a roller pump, or the use of a Gott shunt to transfer blood from the aorta above to the aorta below the ductus.

We usually infiltrate the intercostal spaces subpleurally with Marcaine 0.25%, a long-acting local anesthetic, to reduce postoperative discomfort and improve spontaneous ventilation. A small plastic tube is placed through the incision to evacuate air from the chest; the tube is removed as the muscles of the chest wall are approximated. Subcuticular skin closure provides an excellent cosmetic result.

Mortality for elective closure of uncomplicated patent ductus arteriosus by experienced surgeons is now virtually zero. Hemodynamics improve immediately; stroke volume and heart rate fall to nearly normal. In children showing growth retardation,

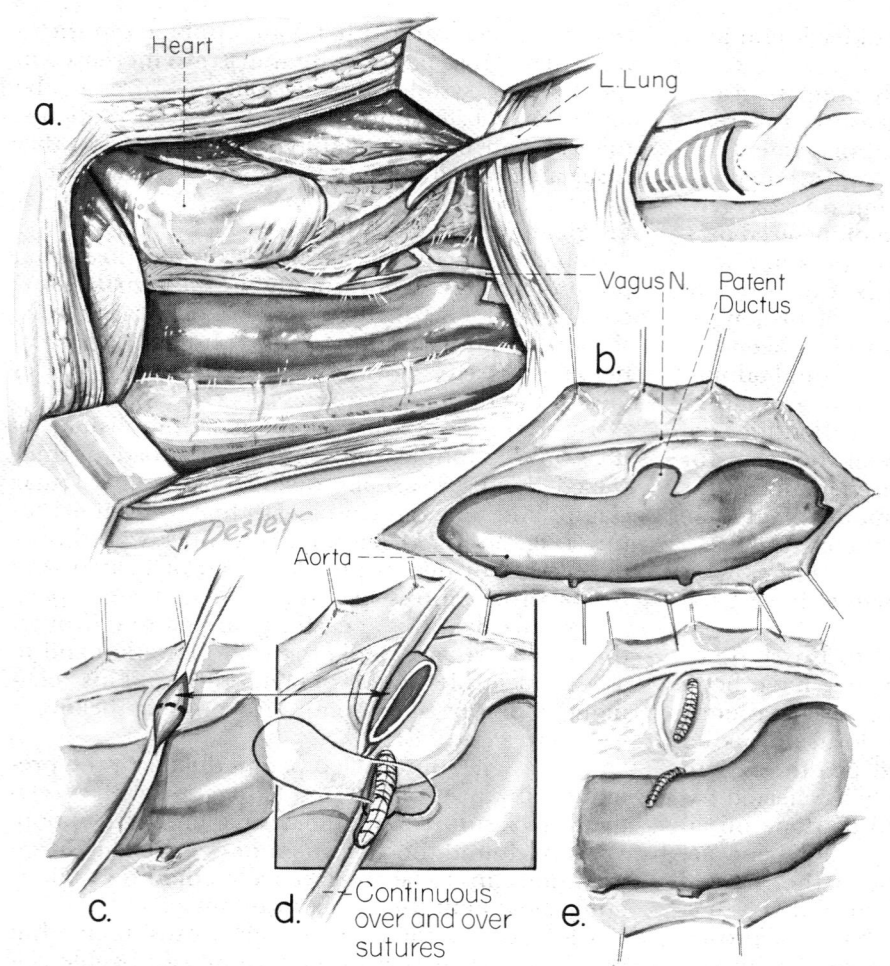

FIGURE 36-34 Division of patent ductus arteriosus. *a.* Mediastinal pleura is opened over the upper part of the descending thoracic aorta, and pleural flaps are retracted with fine silk sutures. *b.* Ductus arteriosus is nicely exposed as the vagus and recurrent laryngeal nerves are reflected medially. *c* and *d.* Ductus is appropriately clamped. *e.* Aortic and pulmonary ends are oversewn with two rows of continuous No. 5-0 silk sutures.

acceleration can be anticipated following ductus obliteration. Long-term results are excellent with very few late complications. In a multi-institutional review of nearly 4000 patent ductus arteriosus obliterations published 25 years ago, even before recent advances in pediatric anesthesia and intensive care, operative mortality was about 2 percent for children and about 4.5 percent for adults.[250] The risks of ductus closure remain somewhat higher in adults and in those patients with elevated pulmonary vascular resistance. In fact, the risk of operation in patients with severe elevation of pulmonary vascular resistance is prohibitive; death even after closure is likely within 1 or 2 years.[251] Those patients with moderately elevated pulmonary vascular resistance will be benefited but not cured by operation.

In a review of 21 published reports of patent ductus ligation in 361 premature infants supposedly having idiopathic respiratory distress syndrome, Edmunds[252] found only 6 deaths attributable to the surgical procedure. Although this low mortality certainly does not include those infants dying of other complications of prematurity and seems overly optimistic, ductus ligation can be carried out safely with marked clinical improvement in infants

weighing as little as 600 g. A carefully controlled multi-institutional study of the relative safety and effectiveness of indomethacin (a prostaglandin synthetase inhibitor) versus operation for closure of a patent ductus arteriosus in the premature infant is now under way.

Aorticopulmonary Septal Defect (Window)

Definition
An aorticopulmonary septal defect, also called aorticopulmonary window, is a communication between the ascending aorta and pulmonary trunk.

Pathology
The condition is usually represented by a solitary opening between the left side of the ascending aorta and the right side of the pulmonary trunk (Fig. 36-35). On the pulmonary side the opening lies close to the origin of the right pulmonary artery. Classically, the defect is wide and unobstructive.[253] Uncommonly, it is narrow.

The condition results from focal deficiency in the septum that divides the primitive truncus arteriosus.

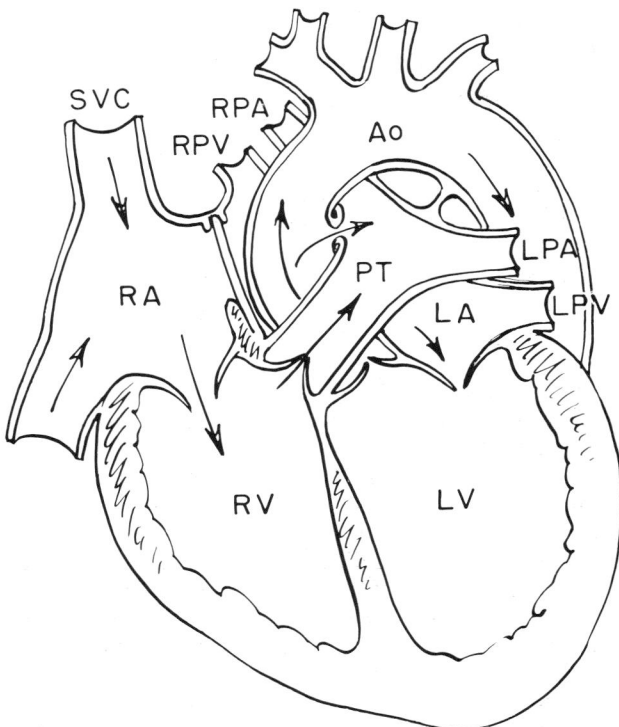

FIGURE 36-35 Aorticopulmonary window. The communication is between the ascending aorta and the pulmonary trunk. In the latter vessel the opening lies near the origin of the right pulmonary artery. SVC = superior vena cava; RA = right atrium; RV = right ventricle; PT = main pulmonary arterial trunk; RPA = right pulmonary artery; LPA = left pulmonary artery; RPV = right pulmonary vein; LPV = left pulmonary vein; LA = left atrium; LV = left ventricle; Ao = aorta. [*From J. E. Edwards, Classification of Congenital Heart Disease in the Adult, in W. C. Roberts (ed.), Congenital Heart Disease in Adults, Cardiovasc. Clin. Series 10/1, F. A. Davis Company, 1979, pp. 1–26. Reproduced with permission.*]

Secondary cardiac effects are like those in widely patent ductus arteriosus.

Associated conditions are relatively uncommon and include patent ductus arteriosus, ventricular septal defect,[254] the tetralogy of Fallot,[255] and subaortic stenosis.[256]

Abnormal Physiology[257]

The hemodynamic pattern in patients with aorticopulmonary septal defect is basically the same as that of patients with a large patent ductus arteriosus.

Clinical Manifestations

History The history in patients with aorticopulmonary septal defect is dependent on the size of the communication. Infrequently, it may be small, with a small shunt and no pulmonary hypertension. In this case, the patient is usually asymptomatic. In most patients, the defect is large, with the clinical picture being similar to a large patent ductus with heart failure and pulmonary hypertension. The presence of associated defects may be confusing.[254]

Physical Examination When the defect is small, the findings are similar to a small patent ductus, although a systolic ejection click at the left sternal border may be heard.[257] In large defects, the murmur is usually systolic, harsh, and heard lower at the left sternal border. Other findings are similar to a large patent ductus with pulmonary hypertension.

Chest Roentgenogram The findings on chest roentgenogram are similar to a large patent ductus, although the aortic knob is not enlarged. A right aortic arch is occasionally associated.[254]

Electrocardiogram With a small defect, the electrocardiogram may be normal. In larger ones, there is usually biventricular hypertrophy similar to the larger ventricular septal defects. Isolated right ventricular hypertrophy occurs in very young infants and older patients with severe pulmonary vascular disease.[257]

Cardiac Catheterization Findings at catheterization are similar to a large patent ductus with pulmonary hypertension. The venous catheter may cross the defect and enter the ascending aorta. Aortography will elucidate the diagnosis and demonstrate associated defects such as patent ductus arteriosus and abnormalities of the coronary arteries.[257]

Natural History and Prognosis

Unfortunately, the diagnosis of aorticopulmonary septal defect may not be suspected until the time of surgery or at autopsy, since it mimics the clinical picture of patent ductus so closely and is uncommon in comparison. Performance of catheterization and aortography is recommended in patients suspected of having a patent ductus with any atypical findings or evidence of pulmonary hypertension, and in all patients with ventricular septal defect.

Since most defects are large, the complications of heart failure and pulmonary vascular disease are very common.[257] Death occurs frequently in those with failure managed medically. Most others will succumb in childhood with complications resulting from pulmonary vascular disease. There is also a risk of infective endarteritis.

Medical Management

Medical management is similar to that for a large patent ductus. Although reported surgical risk is high,[257] repair should be recommended because of the poor prognosis otherwise. Irreversible pulmonary vascular disease is a contraindication to surgery.

Surgical Management

Although it is occasionally possible to close an aorticopulmonary window by ligation or division between vascular clamps without the use of cardiopulmonary bypass, these techniques are generally unsatisfactory and ill advised. Ligation often resulted in recurrence, incomplete closure, or intraoperative hemorrhage.[258] Division of the aorticopulmonary communication on cardiopulmonary bypass with suture closure of the resulting defects in both the aorta and the pulmonary artery is tedious and likely to produce distortion of one or both great vessels.

We prefer to obliterate the aortic orifice of the aorticopulmonary window from within the aorta using a Dacron patch placed during a brief period of cardiopulmonary bypass or, in infants, circulatory arrest with profound hypothermia (18 to 20°C).[255,256,259,260] The great vessels are exposed through a median sternotomy incision. The aorta is cross-clamped cephalad to the communication; an aortotomy is made in a position appropriate for exposure and closure of the orifice of the aorticopulmonary window (Fig. 36-36). No dissection is required outside the aorta. The leaflets of the aortic valve and the coronary arterial ostia are identified and protected. The aortotomy is closed by continuous suture.

Most reported series are small and include patients operated upon by techniques no longer used; results in the literature are thus not as good as might be expected with present methods and early operation before the development of increased pulmonary vascular resistance. Survival of about 90 percent should be anticipated following closure of an uncomplicated aorticopulmonary window.[161,261] Long-term results are excellent—equivalent to those expected following division of a patent ductus arteriosus—in patients having normal pulmonary vascular resistance and no other defects.

FIGURE 36-36 Technique for repair of aorticopulmonary window. *A.* Position of aortotomy may be as shown. We more commonly make a transverse incision. *B.* Closure by a patch is illustrated. In infants we usually repair the window by direct suture. Note the proximity of the orifice of the left coronary artery. (*From Deverall, Aberdeen, Bonham-Carter, and Waterston.*[260] *Reproduced with permission.*)

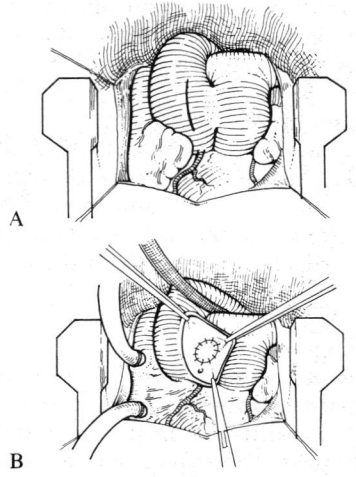

One Pulmonary Artery from the Ascending Aorta

Pathology[263]
The origin of one pulmonary artery from the ascending aorta and one from the right ventricle, sometimes called *hemitruncus,* is a rare anomaly. The anomalous pulmonary artery is usually on the side opposite the aortic arch. The more commonly associated defects are patent ductus in approximately 75 percent, tetralogy of Fallot in 12 percent, and ventricular septal defect in 8 percent.

Clinical Manifestations
The origin of one pulmonary artery from the ascending aorta and one from the right ventricle presents in a similar clinical manner to that of a large patent ductus. Keane and coworkers have reported 6 new cases and reviewed the literature on 44 others.[263] Heart failure occurs in most reported cases within the first weeks or months of life. Cyanosis is associated in over half of the patients. The pulses are usually increased. Auscultation commonly reveals a nonspecific systolic murmur and an accentuated pulmonary closure sound caused by pulmonary hypertension. The clinical picture may be further confused by the presence of associated defects.

The electrocardiogram shows right ventricular hypertrophy in most and combined ventricular hypertrophy in some. Chest roentgenogram demonstrates cardiomegaly, and unilaterally increased pulmonary flow is frequent on the side of the anomalous pulmonary artery and opposite to the side of the aortic arch. Pulmonary flow can be increased bilaterally, particularly in the presence of a patent ductus. Lung scans show uptake on the side supplied by the normally arising pulmonary artery, usually the left if there is no right-to-left intracardiac shunt. Cardiac catheterization reveals pulmonary hypertension on both sides with diagnosis confirmed by angiograms in the aorta and right ventricle.

Natural History and Prognosis
Deaths frequently occur in early infancy and appear to be because of heart failure or complications thereof, although associated defects may contribute. Histological examination of the lungs at autopsy[263] has not revealed significant obstructive changes in most of the infants dying at less than 6 months of age. Of 10 patients over 6 months of age, 6 did have significant vascular changes more predominant in the lung supplied by the anomalous artery. Thus, the natural history is a rapidly progressive one with death occurring in infancy or young childhood for most of those untreated or managed medically.

Medical Management
Medical treatment of heart failure after prompt diagnosis may temporarily improve the status of the

patient. This should be followed by surgical correction as soon as possible, except in patients with severe pulmonary vascular disease.

Surgical Management

Correction requires excision of the origin of the anomalous pulmonary artery from the ascending aorta and establishment of continuity between the main pulmonary artery and the anomalous pulmonary artery. Operation is performed through a median sternotomy. Cardiopulmonary bypass is usually not required but should be available in case the patient does not tolerate the placement of a partial occlusion clamp on the main pulmonary artery. The clamp is necessary for anastomosis of the anomalous pulmonary artery to the main pulmonary artery. The loss of pulmonary blood flow through the anomalous artery and the simultaneous reduction in blood flow through the main pulmonary artery to the other lung may produce severe hypoxia and acute cardiac failure, requiring cardiopulmonary bypass. A prosthetic vascular graft may be needed to extend the anomalous pulmonary artery when it is too short for a tension-free and undistorted anastomosis. Ductus-like tissue, if present near the origin of the vessel, should be excised before the anastomosis is constructed.

Richardson and associates[262] in a 1979 review of the literature found that 60 patients with this anomaly have been reported, 18 of whom had successful correction by the methods described above. Other palliative procedures, including banding of the aberrant pulmonary artery, ligation of a patent ductus arteriosus and the anomalous pulmonary artery, and ligation of a patent ductus alone, have failed.[263] Operation should be carried out as early as possible to minimize the development of pulmonary vascular obstructive disease, a contraindication to correction. Changes in pulmonary vessels occur bilaterally but are more severe on the side receiving pulmonary blood flow directly from the aorta.[264]

Aortic Sinus Aneurysm

Definition

An aneurysm of the aorta at its very origin that is not caused by acquired disease is considered to be of congenital origin.

Pathology

The condition is uncommon. Based on assumed intrinsic weakness at the union of the aorta with the heart, the aortic media may separate from the aortic annulus and retract upward. The structure that lies between becomes aneurysmal and may rupture.[265] The usual sites are the posterior (noncoronary) and right sinuses.[266,267] Posterior sinus aneurysms rupture through the atrial septal wall into the right atrium (Fig. 36-37A). Those of the right sinus rupture into the right ventricular infundibulum (Fig. 36-37B). The aneurysm is represented by a gray pouch with multiple perforations in the wall. The principal associated condition is that of supracristal ventricular septal defect in cases with aneurysms of the right sinus (about 50 percent).

Congenital aneurysm of the left aortic sinus is rare. As it presents toward the epicardium, it may compress the left coronary artery.[268] Shunts do not occur. Though not described, rupture of a left aortic sinus aneurysm would be expected to lead to hemopericardium.

Clinical Manifestations

Ruptured aortic sinus of Valsalva aneurysms are most common in adults. When the rupture is secondary to bacterial endocarditis,[269] evidence of preceding infection is found, whereas this is not so with spontaneous rupture. If the rupture occurs slowly, a small fistulous tract into the right atrium or ventricle will develop. These patients will present with recent onset findings of a small left-to-right shunt. With sudden rupture, there is usually a tearing pain in the midchest associated with dramatically rapid development of pulmonary congestion due to the sudden onset of a large shunt. Characteristically the murmur is loud and continuous but heard lower on the chest than the murmur of a patent ductus. A to-and-fro murmur rather than a continuous one may be heard at times. The apex impulse is hyperdynamic and the pulse pressure is widened. Aneurysms of the right sinus have been frequently associated with a ventricular septal defect, so this may complicate the clinical picture. The chest roentgenograms are similar to those of patent ductus and are dependent on the magnitude of the shunt. The electrocardiogram may show biventricular diastolic overload patterns. In addition, first- and second-degree heart block can occur due to compression of the atrioventricular node.[270]

In general, patients with unruptured aneurysms discovered incidentally are asymptomatic. A few cases, however, have been reported to cause tricuspid regurgitation if the noncoronary sinus is involved, or pulmonary stenosis if the right sinus is involved.[271]

Cardiac catheterization will confirm the level of the shunt. Aortography is necessary for a definite confirmation of the diagnosis. A pressure difference across the right ventricular outflow tract may be present if the right sinus is involved. Tricuspid regurgitation is a difficult diagnosis to establish by catheterization alone, but right ventricular angiography is helpful. At times, it may be reliably diagnosed if the right ventricle is adequately visualized by aortography.

Natural History and Prognosis

With slow rupture and a small shunt, the major risk is infective endocarditis or perhaps extension of the rupture with an increasing shunt. With a large shunt, the heart failure is usually rapidly progres-

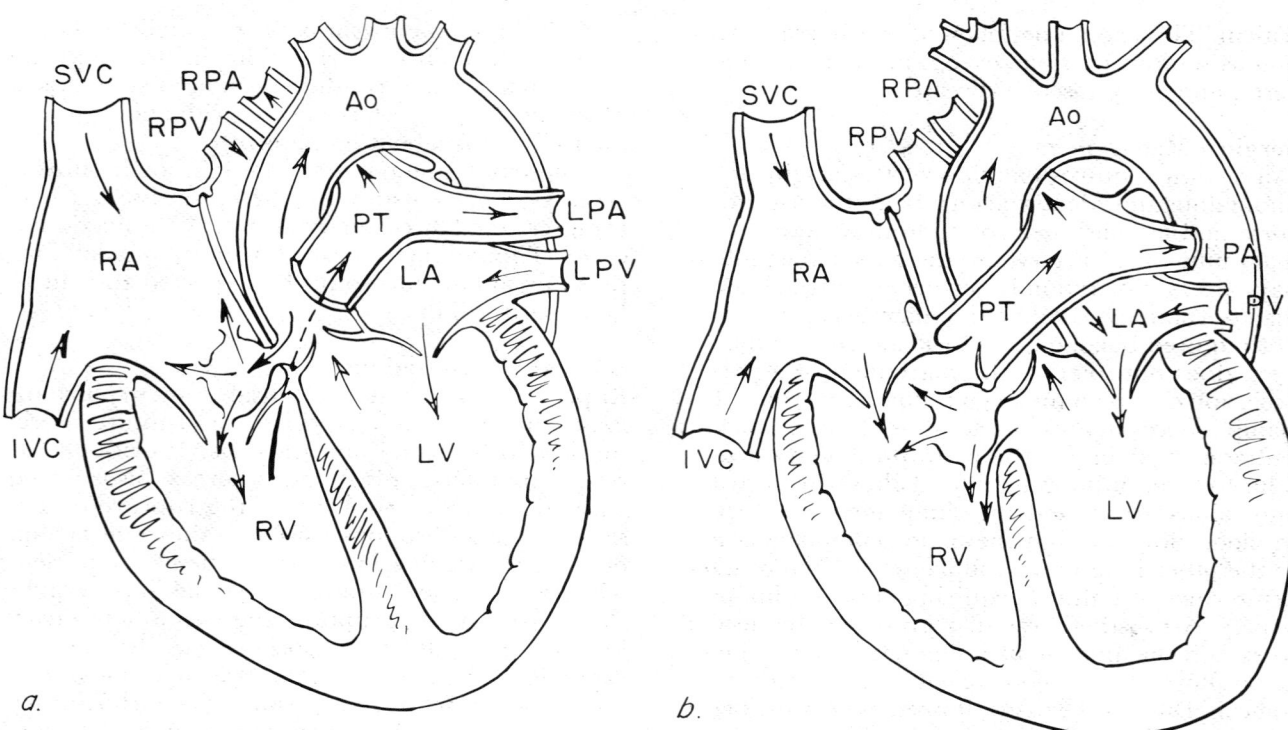

FIGURE 36-37   Ruptured aortic sinus aneurysms. *a.* Aneurysm involves the posterior aortic sinus and ruptures into the right atrium. *b.* Aneurysm involves right aortic sinus and ruptures into the right ventricle. A ventricular septal defect is commonly associated, as illustrated. SVC = superior vena cava; IVC = inferior vena cava; RA = right atrium; RV = right ventricle; PT = main pulmonary arterial trunk; RPA = right pulmonary artery; LPA = left pulmonary artery; RPV = right pulmonary vein; LPV = left pulmonary vein; LA = left atrium; LV = left ventricle; Ao = aorta. [*From J. E. Edwards, Classification of Congenital Heart Disease in the Adult, in W. C. Roberts (ed.), Congenital Heart Disease in Adults, Cardiovasc. Clin. Series 10/1, F. A. Davis Company, Philadelphia, 1979, pp. 1–26. Reproduced with permission.*]

sive and may result in death very quickly. A few patients seem to stabilize in this situation.[270] All five patients reported[271] with pulmonary stenosis and tricuspid insufficiency died suddenly, with the majority also having evidence of heart failure.

Medical Management

Appropriate cultures should be drawn and antibiotics begun if endocarditis is suspected. Treatment of heart failure should be instituted rapidly. Because of the natural history, all patients with rupture or significant tricuspid regurgitation or pulmonary stenosis should be corrected surgically.[272] Others should be followed for development of any of these problems and infective endocarditis should be prevented.

Surgical Management

Ruptured or unruptured aneurysms of the noncoronary or right coronary sinuses are repaired through a median sternotomy on total cardiopulmonary bypass with moderate hypothermia (25 to 28°C) and cardioplegia. We prefer to repair these aneurysms through an aortotomy which allows precise visualization of the aortic valve leaflets, the margins of the aneurysm, and the coronary arterial orifices. When the mouth of the aneurysm is small and

the margin is firm, the orifice can be obliterated by direct suture of the media distally to the aortic annulus proximally. Larger orifices are closed by the placement of a Dacron patch. A supracristal (type I) ventricular septal defect must be looked for and closed either through the aortic valve or the right ventricular outflow tract when an aneurysm of the right coronary sinus of Valsalva has ruptured into the right ventricle. If the ventricular septal defect extends to the tricuspid valve, approach should be through the right ventricle to avoid damage to the His bundle. Occasionally, associated right ventricular outflow tract obstruction requires resection of hypertrophic infundibular myocardium. Aortic valve replacement was required to correct aortic regurgitation in 24 of the 45 patients with aneurysm or fistula of the sinus of Valsalva reported by Meyer.[272]

Aneurysms of the noncoronary sinus may be approached and repaired through the right atrium; those arising from the right coronary sinus are accessible through the right ventricle. Care is required to avoid injury to the conduction bundle just proximal to the aortic annulus.[273]

In 1977, Nowicki and colleagues[274] reviewed 176 cases of aortic fistula to the heart published in the English literature between 1839 and 1972. Of these,

126 underwent operative repair, successful in 108 (86 percent). Current results in major centers are better than this earlier combined series. In a group of 21 patients operated upon at the Mayo Clinic and reviewed in 1971,[275] there were no hospital deaths, although 3 patients required reoperation to correct dehiscence of the repair. Congestive heart failure is effectively controlled by successful closure of the fistula.

Anomalous Systemic Arterial Supply to the Lung

Pathology[276,277]

Anomalous systemic arterial supply to the lung originates from the descending thoracic or abdominal aorta. Commonly, sequestration of a portion of the lung, usually one of the lower lobes, is associated. In this situation, there is no communication with the tracheobronchial tree and no supply from the pulmonary arterial system is present. Less commonly, the anomalous systemic arterial supply is to a portion of the lung in communication with the tracheobronchial tree. Rarely, the anomalous vessels are multiple, bilateral, or large.

Clinical Manifestations

Clinical manifestations vary with the anatomic spectrum of associated defects.[276] About one-half are diagnosed by 10 years of age.[278] If sequestration of a portion of the lung is associated, there may be no symptoms or, more frequently, there are pulmonary symptoms with recurrent infections.[277] If the anomalous systemic arterial supply is to a portion of the lung in communication with the tracheobronchial tree, there are usually no symptoms. Rarely, the arterial supply is large and high output can result in congestive heart failure in infancy.[278,279] This situation is emphasized in the following discussion.

The clinical picture may be similar to that of a large patent ductus, but there may be no precordial murmur or a nonspecific systolic murmur. The peripheral pulses are increased. This is distinguished from pulmonary arteriovenous fistula, since there is no cyanosis unless pulmonary edema is severe. The chest roentgenogram will show cardiomegaly and pulmonary edema if there is heart failure,[279] and a density in the right or left lower lobe if there is sequestration. The electrocardiogram may reveal left ventricular hypertrophy with a volume overload pattern if the shunt is large. Cardiac catheterization will exclude left-to-right shunts, which are usually expected, by the finding of normal saturations throughout the right side of the heart. Pulmonary hypertension is rare.[279] Aortography will demonstrate the anomalous vessel from the descending aorta with pulmonary venous return to the left atrium. We have encountered a rare case with bilateral vessels (Fig. 36-38). If sequestration is

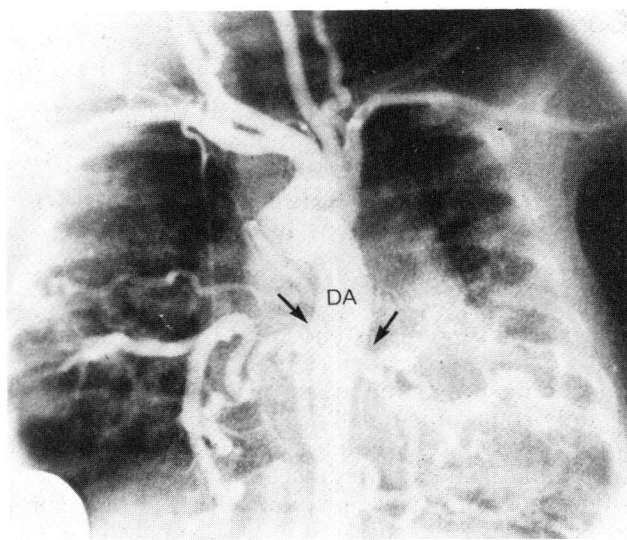

FIGURE 36-38   Aortogram in an infant with bilateral anomalous systemic arterial supply to the lungs originating (arrows) from the descending aorta (DA).

present, pulmonary arteriography will show no branch to the involved area of the lung.[277]

Natural History and Prognosis

The complications of recurrent infection and heart failure are recognized, but asymptomatic adults are reported.[278]

Medical Management

Medical management consists of vigorous treatment of infection and heart failure if they occur. Surgery is indicated for those who are symptomatic.

Surgical Management

Angiographic demonstration of the location and size of anomalous systemic arteries is required before operation. The descending thoracic aorta is exposed through a thoracotomy, usually on the left. The anomalous systemic arteries to the lung are thoroughly mobilized, ligated, and divided.[279] A vessel may pass upward through the diaphragm, originating from the abdominal aorta. These vessels are usually located in the inferior pulmonary ligament. When the anomalous arteries are associated with pulmonary sequestration, lobectomy or excision of the sequestered pulmonary tissue is carried out during the same operation.[276]

Although recent reports describe obliteration of anomalous arteries by embolization of a variety of materials, including silicone balloons or bucrylate tissue adhesive through intravascular catheters,[280,281] the low morbidity, minimal mortality, and the definitiveness of surgical interruption of the vessels remains appealing.[282] Dramatic clinical improvement has followed operation in our small series of patients with this abnormality.

Coronary Arteriovenous Fistula

See section on congenital abnormalities of the coronary arterial circulation, below.

Valvular and Vascular Malformations of the Left Side of the Heart with Right-to-Left, Bidirectional, or No Shunt

Aortic Arch Anomalies

Aortic arch anomalies encompass all of the variations of the aortic arch with regard to its position and branching. Some are sufficiently common and unimportant functionally as to be considered *variations*. A common origin for the innominate and left common carotid arteries is seen in about 10 percent of individuals. In a like proportion, the left vertebral artery arises from the arch just proximal to the left subclavian origin. Others cause compression of the esophagus and trachea with the potential for disturbance in function of these tubes. Such anomalies are often broadly grouped under the heading of *vascular rings*. Still others, although not functioning as vascular rings, may simply incite interest from their nature alone, or be responsible for peculiar circulatory derangements.

Between the primitive bilaterally symmetrical system of six aortic arches and the fully developed fetus are (1) numerous adjustments in shape, (2) interruption and loss of segments, and, importantly, (3) a shift of the subclavian artery of each side so as to arise cephalad to the sixth aortic arch.

Deviations from the normal lead to a variety of structural patterns of the aortic arch system. Some of these are of clinical significance. For details as to the variety of patterns and the developmental bases for these, the reader is referred to the literature.[283–285]

The following will identify the morphological highlights of the more common variations and significant anomalies of the aortic arch system.

Aberrant Subclavian Artery

Pathology In about 0.5 percent of persons with a left aortic arch, the right subclavian artery arises as the fourth branch of the aortic arch. From the aorta it runs behind the esophagus to reach the position normally occupied by the right subclavian artery.

Aberrant left subclavian artery may be associated with a right aortic arch. Further discussion of this subject will be given under the heading "Right Aortic Arch."

Clinical Manifestations Though occasionally implicated in instances of dysphagia, it would appear that an aberrant right subclavian artery with an otherwise normal left aortic arch seldom if ever produces symptoms. It may be found in association with the rare vascular ring created by a left aortic arch that crosses the midline and descends on the right of the spine. In this instance the aberrant right subclavian artery is connected by a persistent ductus or ligamentum arteriosum to the right pulmonary artery, but the symptoms and radiological features are due primarily to the retroesophageal position of the aorta itself.[286,287] An aberrant right subclavian artery arising below coarctation of the aorta or interruption of the aortic arch with its subdued or absent pulses may lead one to suspect aortic atresia or critical aortic stenosis in the newborn or may yield deceptively normotensive pressures in the older child with coarctation if the disparity in the pulses between the two arms goes undetected. An aberrant left subclavian artery arising from a right aortic arch almost invariably is part of a loose, but complete, vascular ring by virtue of its connection with the left pulmonary artery via a persistent left patent ductus arteriosus or ligamentum arteriosum. This is the most common of vascular rings but only rarely produces symptoms. Atresia or stenosis of the origin of a subclavian artery appears to be more common if its origin is aberrant. Finally, failure to recognize an aberrant left or right subclavian artery prior to attempted Blalock-Taussig anastomosis increases the difficulty of operation and jeopardizes its successful outcome.

On chest roentgenogram the aberrant right subclavian artery creates a shallow, oblique, posterior indentation of the barium-filled esophagus which slants upward from left to right. The aberrant left subclavian artery associated with right aortic arch and tetralogy of Fallot creates a similar shallow, oblique indentation slanting upward from right to left. In contrast, the aberrant left subclavian artery associated with no heart disease or with heart disease other than tetralogy of Fallot arises from the right arch via an aortic diverticulum of relatively large diameter, which creates a larger posterior esophageal indentation and assumes a more horizontal course from right to left. If an aberrant right subclavian artery arises below a significant coarctation, characteristic rib notching may be limited to the left hemithorax.

Medical Management Infants or children with persistent symptoms of respiratory obstruction and evidence of an aberrant subclavian artery should undergo bronchoscopy and, if external compression is demonstrated, aortography. Those who are asymptomatic may be followed medically. Individuals with either atresia or stenosis of an aberrant subclavian artery or with unrelieved or recurrent coarctation of the aorta above its origin are at risk of developing the subclavian steal syndrome.

Surgical Management Although this anomaly rarely produces symptoms and rarely requires operation,[288,289] we have operated upon one patient with a large aneurysm of an aberrant right subclavian artery producing both respiratory distress and dysphagia. When required because of dysphagia, operation consists of ligation and division of the anomalous artery through a left thoracotomy. The vessel is freed of its retroesophageal attachments, allowing it to retract into the right hemithorax. Development of the subclavian steal syndrome following interruption of anterograde arterial flow is a possible consequence of subclavian artery division.

Right Aortic Arch

Pathology Right aortic arch is characterized by the aortic arch passing over the right, rather than the left, bronchus. Two types are recognized: that with a retroesophageal aortic segment and that without[290] (Fig. 36-39). In the absence of a retroesophageal segment, the cases of right aortic arch are usually associated with congenital heart disease, of which the tetralogy is the most common type. There is variation of branching. The most common pattern is that of mirror-image branching, a left innominate artery being the first branch (Fig. 36-39A). The ductus arteriosus may be absent, right-sided, or left-sided. If left-sided, the ductus runs between the origin of the left subclavian artery, above, and the left pulmonary artery, below.

Less common than mirror-image branching is that in which the left subclavian artery is aberrant and, in effect, represents a mirror image of the common aberrant right subclavian artery. The aberrant left subclavian artery indents the posterior aspect of the esophagus, and this is accentuated if a left ductus is present, as this structure runs between the origins of the left subclavian and the left pulmonary arteries.

Isolation of the left subclavian artery forms the third and least common pattern of branching in right aortic arch without retroesophageal segment.

In right aortic arch *with retroesophageal segment*, congenital heart disease is usually not present, and the condition is observed at all ages.[291] If other anomalies are associated, there does not appear to be a particular type in association.

In this pattern of aortic malformation, the aortic arch, after passing over the right bronchus, turns to the left behind the esophagus (Fig. 36-39B). At the left aspect of the junction of the right arch with the descending thoracic aorta, a diverticulum is present. The left subclavian artery arises from the upper aspect of the diverticulum, and the aortic end of the ductus arteriosus or ligamentum arteriosum inserts into the lower aspect of the diverticulum. Compression of the trachea and eosphagus results from a complexity of vascular structures oriented around these tubes. The vascular structures are, anteriorly, the bifurcation of the pulmonary trunk; on the right, the right aortic arch; posteriorly, the retroesophageal segment of the aorta; and on the left, the ductus arteriosus or ligamentum arteriosum.[291–293]

FIGURE 36-39 Two types of right aortic arch. *a.* Without retroesophageal segment. This type usually is associated with congenital heart disease, principally tetralogy of Fallot. Variations in branching occur. This illustration shows the most common type, which is that of mirror-image branching, in which frequently a left ductus arteriosus (L. Ductus) runs from the base of the left subclavian artery (L.S.) to the left pulmonary artery (L.P.A.). *b.* Right aortic arch with retroesophageal segment. The left subclavian artery (L.S.) arises as a fourth branch of the aorta from a diverticulum which lies at the junction of the right aortic arch and the descending aorta. A left ductus arteriosus, or ligamentum arteriosum, runs from the left pulmonary artery (L.P.) to the diverticulum. The bifurcation of the pulmonary trunk (P.T.) is held against the bifurcation of the trachea by the ductus arteriosus, if short. A. = ascending aorta; R.S. = right subclavian artery; R.C. = right carotid artery; L.C. = left carotid artery; L.S. = left subclavian artery. (*From J. E. Edwards, Anomalies of the Aortic Arch System, Birth Defects: Original Article Series, 13:47, 1977. Reproduced with permission of the National Foundation—March of Dimes.*)

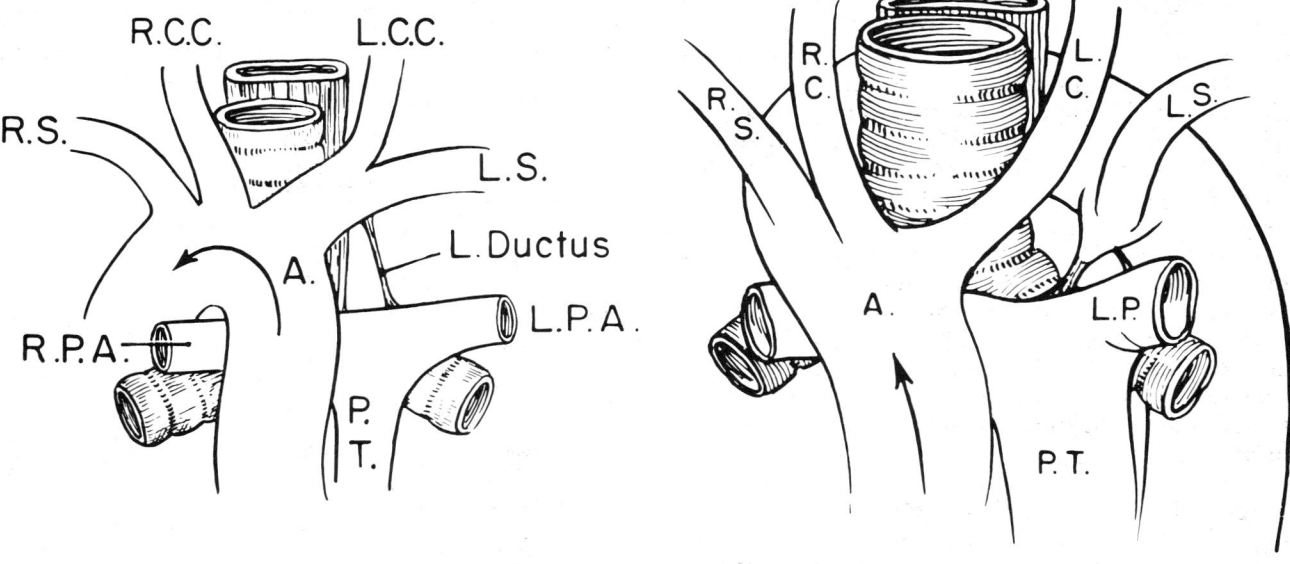

a.   *b.*

Clinical Manifestations   This anomaly occurs in approximately 0.1 to 0.14 percent of the population.[294] Its importance lies in its use as a predictor of the presence or absence of congenital disease in general and its association with several important cardiac malformations in particular. In addition, its connection with a left patent ductus or ligamentum arteriosus creates the possibility of a complete and symptomatic vascular ring. When there is mirror-image branching, the incidence of congenital heart disease is 98 percent, with the majority of patients having tetralogy of Fallot. In the presence of an aberrant left subclavian artery the incidence of cardiac anomalies is estimated at only 10 percent.[295] A right aortic arch is found in approximately 53 percent of patients with pulmonary atresia and ventricular septal defect,[296] 31 percent of patients with tetralogy, 31 percent of patients with truncus arteriosus, 20 percent of patients with double-outlet right ventricle, and 5 percent among patients with tricuspid atresia.[6] The incidence may also be slightly higher among individuals with transposition of the great arteries associated with a ventricular septal defect and pulmonary stenosis. With mirror-image branching, the usual site of origin of the ductus arteriosus is the left subclavian artery arising from the innominate artery, and no vascular ring is created (Fig. 36-39A). Persistence of a right ductus is uncommon, and no ring is formed in this situation either. A complete vascular ring is created when the ductus or ligamentum arteriosum connects the left pulmonary artery to an aberrant left subclavian artery or directly to the descending aorta, with or without mirror-image branching. Symptoms are related to the associated heart disease, to the presence of a restrictive vascular ring, or to a combination of both. In the absence of heart disease or with a nonrestrictive vascular ring, individuals with a right aortic arch are asymptomatic.

On the chest roentgenogram the right aortic arch is seen as a prominent vascular shadow to the right of the esophagus and trachea in the frontal view. The lateral margin of the descending aorta is usually seen to the right of the thoracic spine as well. There is no vascular shadow on the left to suggest a left aortic arch or left descending aorta. When these structures are obscured by the thymus, one may still see a slight deviation of the air-filled trachea to the left, leaving little or no room for a normal left aortic arch within the mediastinal shadow. Similarly, the barium-filled esophagus will show the aortic indentation on the right and reveal the presence or absence of a retroesophageal vascular structure in the form of an aberrant left subclavian artery, ductus or ligamentum arteriosum, or the aorta itself.

Surgical Management   The presence of a right aortic arch assumes surgical significance when associated lesions cause tracheal and esophageal compression[289] or when creation of a systemic arterial to pulmonary arterial shunt is required for palliation of patients with congenital heart defects causing reduced pulmonary blood flow.

In symptomatic patients having a right aortic arch with a retroesophageal left subclavian artery and a left ligamentum arteriosum, the ligamentum arteriosum is divided through a left thoracotomy, relieving tracheoesophageal compression. It is unnecessary and inadvisable to divide the left subclavian artery.

The vascular ring created by a right aortic arch with mirror-image origin of the bracheocephalic vessels and a left ligamentum arteriosum is also released by division of the ligamentum through a left thoracotomy. Fibrous adhesions between the aorta, trachea, and esophagus are divided. Some surgeons suspend the right aortic arch from the posterior aspect of the sternum, pulling it away from the trachea;[297] we have not found this necessary in situations other than anomalous origin of the innominate or carotid arteries.

Double Aortic Arch

Pathology   Double aortic arch is characterized by persistence of two aortic arches. Arising from the ascending aorta and after passing over the respective bronchi, the left and right arches join at a level posterior to the esophagus to form the descending thoracic aorta. Each common carotid and subclavian artery arises independently from its respective aortic arch (Fig. 36-40). Usually, the right aortic arch is wider than the left.[292]

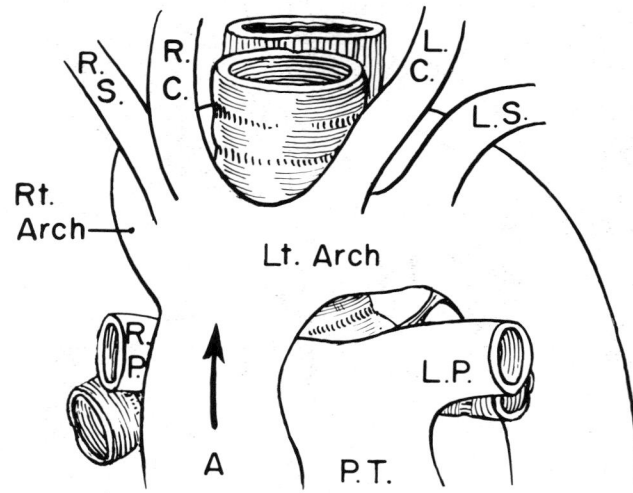

FIGURE 36-40   Double aortic arch. The classic picture is that in which the right arch (Rt. Arch) passes behind the esophagus to join the left arch (Lt. Arch). There are independent origins of the common carotid (R.C. and L.C.) and subclavian (R.S. and L.S.) arteries from the homolateral arch. A. = ascending aorta; P.T. = main pulmonary arterial trunk; R.P. = right pulmonary artery; L.P. = left pulmonary artery. (*From J. E. Edwards, Anomalies of the Aortic Arch System, Birth Defects: Original Article Series, 13:47, 1977. Reproduced with permission of the National Foundation–March of Dimes.*)

The relatively narrow state of the left arch compared to the right varies from minor differences to atresia of a segment of the left arch.

The ductus arteriosus or ligamentum is left-sided, running between the distal part of the left arch and the left pulmonary artery.

Clinical Manifestations Double aortic arch is the most common type of symptomatic vascular ring.[285] Approximately one-fifth of patients will have associated congenital heart disease, with ventricular septal defect and tetralogy of Fallot being the most frequent malformations.[6] About 75 percent of affected individuals are symptomatic with symptoms ranging from mild to life-threatening respiratory obstruction and apnea. A few individuals remain asymptomatic and are detected accidentally as older children and young adults. Inspiratory stridor, dyspnea, and wheezing, which are accentuated with feeding, crying, or respiratory infections, are characteristic. Fluids are usually better tolerated with feeding than solids. A brassy cough may be described.

Suprasternal and intercostal retractions, bilateral rhonchi, and even cyanosis may be found with severe obstruction. The head and neck may be held in hyperextension and ill-advised flexion by the examiner may completely obstruct the airway and precipitate a respiratory crisis. A heart murmur and other features of associated heart disease may be present.

Since the right arch is the larger of the two arches in somewhere between 75 and 85 percent of patients, the usual picture on the chest roentgenogram is that of a vascular shadow to the right of the esophagus and trachea simulating an isolated right aortic arch. A barium swallow or esophagram will reveal, in the frontal view, bilateral compression of the esophagus with the larger and more superior indentation indicating the dominant arch. In the lateral view, a large posterior esophageal indentation will be seen as the dominant arch crosses the midline. Emphysema, atelectasis, or pneumonia may also be present. Aortography is recommended to evaluate the relative size and the patency of the two arches and to identify the brachiocephalic arterial branches. Approximately 16 percent will have atresia of the left arch, usually just distal to the origin of the left subclavian artery.[6] In the presence of suspected, associated heart disease, complete cardiac catheterization is always indicated.

Natural History, Prognosis, and Medical Management A few patients remain asymptomatic and require no therapy. The majority present within the first month or two of life with symptoms that may have been present since birth. Once present, symptoms persist and usually progress.

For symptomatic patients, a brief period of stabilization for treatment of pneumonia and diagnostic studies is justified, but surgical relief of the constricting ring is recommended as soon as possible. Preoperative bronchoscopy adds little in these particular patients. Despite the immediate and dramatic diminution in symptoms, mild degrees of respiratory obstruction may persist for weeks and even months before disappearing completely.

Surgical Management All vascular rings, including double aortic arch and the anomalies associated with a right aortic arch described previously, are exposed through a left thoracotomy. Thorough dissection is required before division of any vessel. The recurrent laryngeal nerve must be protected as it passes around the ligamentum arteriosum or ductus arteriosus. The left or anterior component of the double aortic arch is usually the smaller of the two, and hence it is the one most often divided to break the compressing ring.[289] An atretic or stenotic area in the smaller arch may limit the possible sites for division. The surgeon should verify the presence of carotid or temporal arterial pulses prior to division of the arch while a clamp occludes the arch at the point of anticipated division. The arch is incised between vascular clamps at the appropriate point and the ends are sutured (Fig. 36-41). Adhesions between vessels, trachea, and esophagus are freed to assure the relief of tracheal compression. Suspension of the remaining arch is rarely required but has been useful in the infant with secondary tracheomalacia,[297] particularly when the left or anterior arch is larger and remains intact after division of the smaller posterior arch.

Isolation of Subclavian Artery

Pathology Isolation of a subclavian artery, a designation first introduced by Stewart and associates,[283] is an uncommon condition, usually observed in subjects with other cardiovascular anomalies, the most common being the tetralogy of Fallot and interruption of the aortic arch. The condition is characterized by the involved subclavian artery not having connection with the aorta. Instead, it arises from the homolateral pulmonary artery by way of the ductus arteriosus or ligamentum arteriosum of that side.

Cases with normally arising arteries but with atresia of origin of a subclavian or the innominate artery have also been included under the designation of isolation.[298] From a developmental viewpoint, such cases are different from the term *isolation* as defined above.

The isolated subclavian artery is always on the side opposite the aortic arch. Isolation of the left subclavian artery is about four times more common than isolation of the right artery. The periphery of the isolated artery is fed by systemic collaterals, including the vertebral arteries that arise from the contralateral subclavian artery.[284]

Clinical Manifestations This malformation does not cause symptoms and is usually detected at the

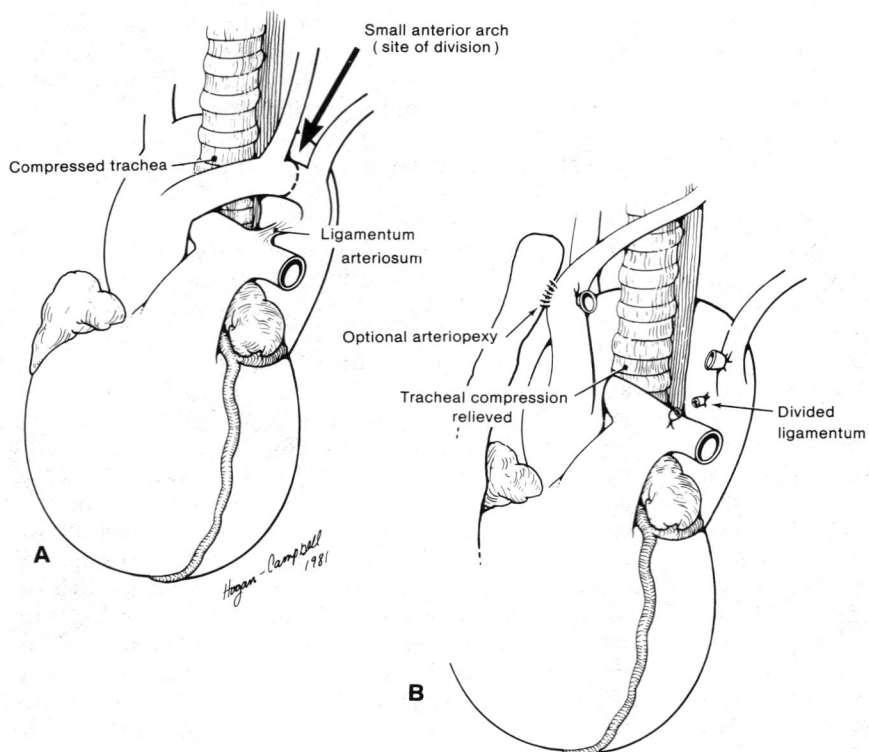

FIGURE 36-41 Relief of tracheal compression caused by double aortic arch (vascular ring). The great vessels are exposed through a left thoracotomy. The anatomy must be assessed carefully prior to division of vessels. In this case, the smaller anterior arch is divided between the left carotid and the left subclavian arteries. The ligamentum arteriosum is divided. The anterior arch may be sutured to the posterior sternal periosteum to pull the vessels away from the trachea. Fibrous attachments between vessels and trachea are not divided.

time of aortography and catheterization for intracardiac malformations, particularly tetralogy of Fallot. Since the blood supply of the isolated subclavian artery may derive from the pulmonary artery via a patent ductus or from systemic arterial collaterals, subdued and delayed pulses and diminution of blood pressure readings in the affected arm would be expected. These findings generally go unrecognized, however, prior to catheterization or surgery.

The chest roentgenogram usually reveals the aortic arch on the side opposite the arm with the delayed, diminished, or absent pulses, and the esophagram will not demonstrate the posterior indentation characteristic of an aberrant subclavian artery to that arm.

Aortography will fail to opacify the subclavian artery arising from either the innominate artery or as the fourth branch of the aortic arch. Later frames usually will reveal opacification of the isolated subclavian artery by collateral circulation or retrograde flow in the ipsilateral vertebral artery. Rarely, the subclavian artery may be entered with a catheter from the main pulmonary artery via a patent ductus.[299]

Natural History, Prognosis, and Medical Management This malformation should be given specific consideration in all individuals with cyanotic heart disease in whom the Blalock-Taussig anastomosis is contemplated. The arterial pulses in both arms should be compared and preferably blood pressures taken and recorded. Careful identification of all the great arteries arising from the aortic arch is essential at the time of preoperative review of aortograms if this anomaly is not to be missed. Over the course of time, individuals with this malformation are candidates for the subclavian steal syndrome.

Surgical Management The subclavian artery arising from the main pulmonary artery or its proximal branches can be ligated through a thoracotomy on the side of the anomaly—usually the left. If the artery is of sufficient diameter and length, it should be anastomosed to the aorta at a convenient point. An excellent outcome should be anticipated. Obviously the association of this anomaly with other cardiac defects producing cyanosis due to diminished pulmonary blood flow would preclude the use of this vessel in the construction of a Blalock-Taussig shunt, where it would already be serving as a source of collateral pulmonary blood flow.

Origin of Left Pulmonary Artery from Right Pulmonary Artery (Pulmonary Arterial Sling)

Pathology In this condition, after the usual site of origin of the ductus arteriosus, the pulmonary trunk continues simply as the right pulmonary artery. The left pulmonary artery arises to the right of the midline from the right pulmonary artery just proximal to the normal branching of the latter. The left pulmonary artery then arches over the origin of the right main bronchus and proceeds leftward behind the trachea and anterior to the esophagus to reach the left lung. The anterior aspect of the esophagus is indented.[300–302] If a bronchus sinus (independent origin of the right upper bronchus from the trachea) is present, as is commonly associated, the left pulmonary artery arches over the origin of the intermediate bronchus (Fig. 36-42).[303]

As the left pulmonary artery passes over the right main bronchus or the intermediate bronchus, the pertinent structure is indented by the artery.

Pulmonary arterial sling may be an independent gross malformation or may be associated with congenital heart disease, as tetralogy of Fallot, ventricular septal defect, persistent truncus arteriosus, or interruption of the aortic arch.

Tracheomalacia[304] and complete cartilaginous encirclement of the trachea[305] have been described.

Clinical Manifestations Somewhere between 60 to 80 percent of patients with this rare cause of respiratory distress have associated cardiovascular disease and almost 50 percent have associated tracheobronchial abnormalities as well. The male-to-female ratio is equal.[302] The majority present with symptoms of respiratory obstruction and distress either at birth or within the first 6 months of life. Symptoms tend to be progressive and consist of expiratory wheezing, stridor, apneic episodes, and cyanosis. Signs of unequal aeration and mediastinal shift are characteristic. A few individuals are asymptomatic.

Unilateral obstructive emphysema characteristically is present on the chest roentgenogram, and although either lung may be involved, hyperaera-

FIGURE 36-42 Vascular sling associated with *bronchus suis.* In the latter situation, as illustrated, the eparterial bronchus (E.B.) arises from the trachea (Tr.). The vascular sling consists of the anomalous left pulmonary artery (A. Left Pul. A.) arising from the right pulmonary artery (Right Pul. A.). This arches over the right bronchus in a situation of normal tracheal bifurcation. When bronchus suis is present as shown, the left pulmonary artery arches over the origin of the hyparterial bronchus (H.B.) from the trachea (T) and causes compression of the origin of that airway. P.T. = main pulmonary arterial trunk; D.A. = ductus arteriosus; L.B. = left bronchus. (*From Jue and Associates.*[303] *Reproduced with permission.*)

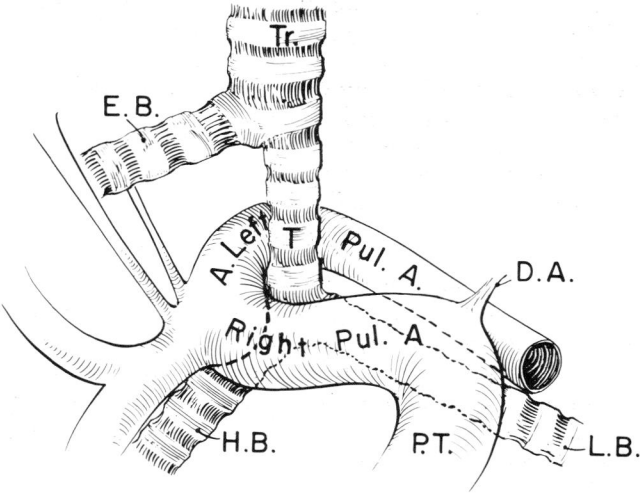

tion of the right lung with mediastinal shift to the left is the more common pattern. The left hilar shadow is displaced inferiorly, and the esophagram usually, although not invariably, will demonstrate an anterior indentation of the esophagus at the level of the carina.

Bronchoscopy will demonstrate posterior compression of the distal trachea by a pulsatile mass and, in addition, identify complicating bronchotracheal abnormalities. Selective pulmonary angiography in the frontal view with the patient propped to a sitting position of 60° from the horizontal will demonstrate the vascular deformity and is the definitive diagnostic procedure. If there is any suggestion of associated congenital disease, complete cardiac catheterization is warranted, since palliative corrective surgical procedures may be possible at the time of the surgical approach to the aberrant left pulmonary artery.

Natural History and Prognosis Death from airway obstruction is the fate of untreated patients with severe symptoms. Symptoms of respiratory obstruction may persist for weeks and months before finally clearing, and those symptoms due to associated anomalies of the trachea or bronchi, such as major segments of hypoplasia or stenosis, will not be relieved by the vascular surgery. Hemoptysis, the result of extensive compensatory collateral circulation to the left lung with a thrombosed pulmonary artery, may be a later complication.

Medical Management Prompt diagnosis and surgical therapy are indicated for symptomatic infants. At present surgical reimplantation of the left pulmonary artery to the proximal portion of the main pulmonary artery is the treatment of choice. Postoperative cardiac catheterization for measurement of pulmonary arterial pressures and pulmonary arteriography is recommended.

Surgical Management In 1954 Potts[306] described dramatic improvement in a 5-month-old infant with recurring attacks of dyspnea and cyanosis following ligation and reimplantation of the anomalous left pulmonary artery into the main pulmonary artery. Since that description, this has been the most commonly performed operation for relief of symptomatic pulmonary arterial sling. Other procedures have included division and repositioning of the trachea, left mainstem bronchus division, and division of a patent ductus arteriosus. Results of operation have been disappointing, with surgical mortality approaching 50 percent. Left pulmonary arterial patency has rarely persisted following anastomosis to the main pulmonary artery.[301]

Management of pulmonary arterial sling is often complicated by associated cardiovascular abnormalities which occur in half of these patients. Severe deformity of the right mainstem bronchus and the lower trachea is frequently present prior to surgical intervention and is not relieved by reimplantation of the left pulmonary artery; symptoms of airway obstruction commonly persist following operation.[307]

In symptomatic patients with pulmonary arterial sling, we prefer to detach the left pulmonary artery from the right pulmonary artery and to anastomose the tangentially bevelled end of the left pulmonary artery to the main pulmonary artery through a median sternotomy incision. A right thoracotomy offers inadequate exposure; a left thoracotomy compromises postoperative respiratory function of the unobstructed lung.

The mere presence of this anatomic abnormality does not justify operation. Symptoms of respiratory obstruction, bronchoscopic evidence of right mainstem bronchial and lower tracheal compression, and arteriographic confirmation of the anomaly should encourage operation, even though long-term patency of the left pulmonary artery cannot be ensured. When evaluated 24 years following operation, the patient operated upon by Potts and associates in 1954 had normal exercise tolerance with only minimal perfusion to the left lung.[301]

Cervical Aortic Arch

Pathology   In cervical aortic arch the right or left aortic arch lies at a higher level than normal and is evident in the supraclavicular area. The branches are usual for the type of arch. No significant pathological processes result from this condition. While the condition has been considered to result from persistence of the right second or third aortic arches of the embryo, we would agree with Massumi and associates[308] that the condition represents an arrest in downward migration of the usual structures that form the right aortic arch.

Clinical Manifestations   This anomaly is usually recognized during childhood when attention is drawn to a pulsating mass in either the right or left supraclavicular area, usually the right. Most patients are asymptomatic. A few will have symptoms of stridor or dysphagia, suggesting the presence of a vascular ring. A murmur and thrill usually are present over the mass but not over precordium. Occasionally a delay in arterial pulse transmission can be appreciated by simultaneous palpation of the radial and femoral arterial pulses. Digital compression of the mass may produce a discernible diminution in femoral arterial pulses.

The chest roentgenogram will reveal widening of the upper mediastinum, reflecting the vascular shadow of the aortic arch on the side of the supraclavicular mass. The trachea may be displaced to the opposite side. Posterior indentation of the barium-filled esophagus at the level of a normal aortic arch will be seen if the descending aorta crosses the midline.

Aortography will demonstrate the cervical aortic arch, establish the pattern of branching of the great vessels to the head, neck, and arms, and eliminate other possible alternative diagnoses such as carotid arterial aneurysm or arteriovenous fistula.

Natural History, Prognosis, and Medical Management   This developmental anomaly is considered benign and is very infrequently associated with cardiac malformations. In the absence of signs or symptoms of vascular ring, medical or surgical intervention is unnecessary.[309]

Tracheal Compression by the Innominate Artery or Left Carotid Artery

Pathology   Either of these two great arteries can, in rare instances, produce anterior compression of the trachea and severe symptoms of respiratory obstruction. No diagnostic deformity of the esophagus is present. In the case of innominate artery compression of the trachea, the more common of the two situations, the innominate artery appears to arise in a position more posterior or "later" than usual from the normal aortic arch. On its course back to the right, the innominate artery compresses the trachea anteriorly. The left carotid artery, arising either more to the right than usual from the aortic arch or arising as a third branch of the innominate artery, crosses the trachea from right to left and may have a similar compressing effect.

Clinical Manifestations   The symptoms of stridor, wheezing, and apneic episodes may be no different than those seen with complete vascular rings or double aortic arch, and usually begin within the first month or two or life. A series of lateral chest roentgenograms will show a constant anterior indentation of the tracheal air shadow just below the thoracic inlet. A similar indentation is present in normal infants but will be seen to vary in depth from film to film, depending on the phase of breathing.

Aortography is of limited help since the variation in the vascular pattern of the symptomatic patient usually falls within the wide range of normal seen among asymptomatic individuals. Bronchoscopy will reveal significant pulsatile anterior compression of the trachea in symptomatic infants.

Natural History, Prognosis, and Medical Management   The majority of infants with mild symptoms can be managed conservatively with the expectation of gradual improvement as tracheal rigidity increases with age. Those infants with severe symptoms will benefit dramatically from surgery.[6]

Surgical Management   The ascending aorta and the innominate artery are exposed through a right anterior submammary incision. The thymus is excised up to the level of the innominate vein. The pericardium is opened longitudinally well anterior to the phrenic nerve. A series of Teflon felt pledget–reinforced mattress sutures are placed in the adventitia and media of the ascending aorta and innominate artery; these sutures are then passed through the posterior periosteum of the manubrium and the sternum. The arteries are *not* dissected free from the trachea. As the sutures are tied, pulling the vessels anteriorly toward the sternum, the remaining fibrous attachments to the trachea tend to open the tracheal lumen.[297] Pressure is relieved; symptomatic improvement is dramatic.

We have encountered no significant complications from operation in our patients with this anomaly. No patient has required further treatment for airway obstruction, even though some had sustained preoperative cardiac arrest. The most crucial diagnostic consideration justifying operation is the bronchoscopic visualization of severe pulsatile anterior or right anterolateral tracheal compression in the symptomatic child.

Abnormalities of left carotid arterial origin that produce tracheal compression are treated as described above by suspension of the vessels from the posterior aspect of the sternum, usually through a left thoracotomy. Detachment of the carotid artery and anastomosis in a different location has been advised, but we have not found this necessary.

Coarctation of the Aorta

Definition

Coarctation of the aorta is a discrete narrowing of the distal segment of the aortic arch.

Pathology

The characteristic lesion is a deformity of the media of the aorta. The deformity, involving the anterior, superior, and posterior walls, is represented by a curtain-like infolding of the wall which causes the lumen to be narrowed and eccentric[310] (Figs. 36-43 and 36-44).

The lesion most commonly lies just distal to the entrance of the ductus arteriosus or ligamentum into the aorta. In symptomatic infants the lesion lies either opposite the ductus or in a preductal location. In adolescents and adults it is usually distal to the ligamentum arteriosum. In uncommon cases the lesion lies proximal to the origin of the left common carotid artery. In such a pattern the left subclavian artery "lags," occupying a primitive position caudal to the aortic entrance of the ductus.[311]

The principal cardiac abnormality is left ventricular hypertrophy. In some infants left ventricular endocardial fibroelastosis may be associated. Proximal to the obstruction, the aorta may show moderate degrees of cystic medial necrosis. Beyond the coarctation the lining may show a localized jet lesion.[311]

Prominent collaterals are evident anatomically, especially in the adolescent and adult (Fig. 36-45). The collaterals may be divided into anterior and posterior systems, the source for each being the subclavian arteries.[312] The anterior system originates with the internal mammary arteries and makes use of the epigastric arteries in the abdominal wall to

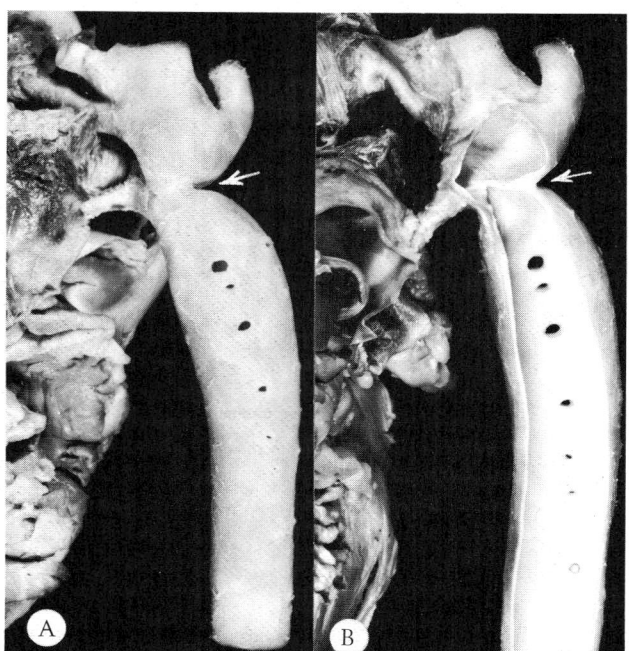

FIGURE 36-43 Coarctation of aorta. *A.* Exterior of thoracic aorta from in front. At point of arrow is an indentation in the superior wall of the aorta corresponding to the narrowed zone within the lumen. Dilated intercostal arterial ostia. *B.* Interior of the aorta. Corresponding to the indentation in the external aspect of the aorta is a diaphragmatic membrane which protrudes across the lumen of the aorta to cause major narrowing of this channel.

FIGURE 36-44 Model of coarctation of aorta demonstrating that the lumen through the coarctate area is always smaller than would be suspected from the external appearance. (*From J. E. Edwards, T. J. Dry, R. L. Parker, H. B. Burchell, E. H. Wood, and A. H. Bulbulian, "An Atlas of Congenital Anomalies of the Heart and Great Vessels," Charles C Thomas, Publisher, Springfield, Ill., 1954. Reproduced with permission.*)

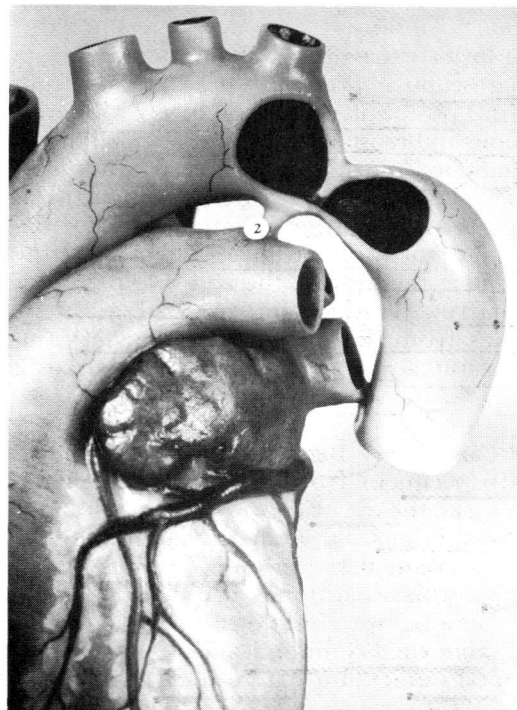

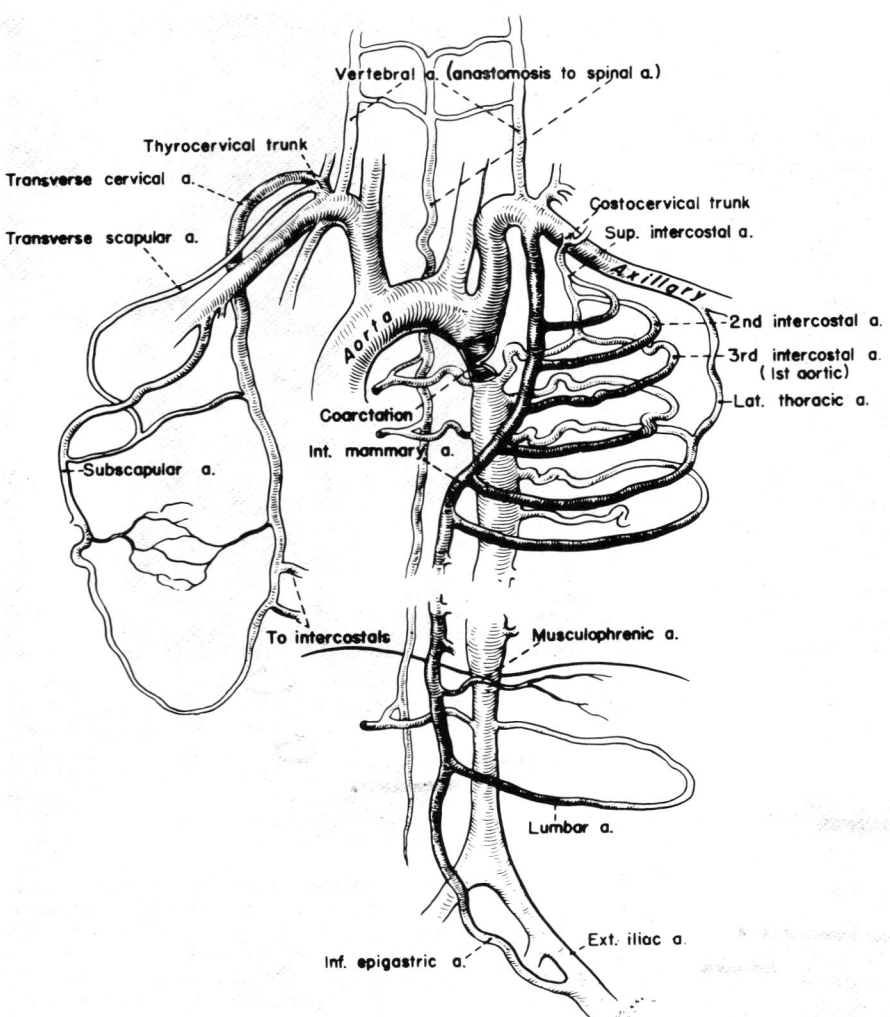

FIGURE 36-45 Diagrammatic portrayal of collateral circulation in coarctation of the aorta. (*From Edwards and Associates.*[312] *Reproduced with permission.*)

supply the lower extremities. The posterior system involves parascapular arteries. These, in turn, connect with the posterior intercostal arteries (the dilated tortuous intercostal arteries cause notching of ribs that may not be evident until early adult life), which carry blood to the distal aortic compartment principally for supply of the abdominal viscera. Anatomic support for this concept is that beyond the origins of the renal arteries, the abdominal aorta is unusually narrow. The anterior spinal artery receiving branches from the proximal and distal compartments of the aorta is dilated and tortuous, as it also participates in collateral function.

Associated Conditions Becker and associates[313] reviewed 100 specimens from patients with coarctation of the aorta, the majority of whom were infants. Associated conditions with the coarctation, in order of decreasing frequency, were *tubular hypoplasia of the aortic arch* (this condition is characterized by a narrow segment but with histologically normal characteristics); abnormal communications, mainly ventricular septal defect and patent ductus; left ven-

tricular outflow obstruction, mainly subaortic stenosis; left ventricular inflow obstruction; and a variety of transpositions of the great vessels. A bicuspid aortic valve was present in 46 percent of the cases. Aberrant right subclavian artery may be associated. In about one-half of such cases the vessel arises proximal to the coarctation and is distal to the coarctation in the other half. A ductus arteriosus, while patent, may mask the presence of aortic obstruction when the coarctation lies opposite the ductus.[314]

Rosenquist[315] studied the mitral valves in 53 specimens from subjects with aortic coarctation. In 31 of these some abnormality of the mitral valve was considered to be present. The abnormalities were (1) fused or closely related chordae, (2) underdevelopment in the space between the papillary muscles and ventricular wall, and (3) parachute mitral valve (one case).

Complications The major complications[316] in coarctation of the aorta include congestive cardiac failure; dissecting aneurysm of the aorta, usually proximal and uncommonly distal to the coarctation; infective endocarditis of the bicuspid aortic valve; uncommonly bacterial endaortitis at the site of the jet lesion in the distal compartment; aortic valvular insufficiency,[317] and rupture of an aneurysm of the circle of Willis. Rupture of the aorta without dissection, rupture of an aneurysm of an intercostal artery, and thrombosis of anterior spinal artery are among the rare complications. Development of calcific aortic stenosis is a complication of long-term survival.

Abnormal Physiology[318,319]

By obstructing the flow of blood in the aorta, coarctation of the aorta increases the resistance to aortic flow. In most blood vessels the resistance to flow is increased relatively little until the cross-sectional area is decreased by about 60 to 70 percent; however, the resistance increases strikingly if the cross-sectional area is further decreased. In most coarctations that produce hemodynamic alterations, there is a significant narrowing of the aortic lumen, which is often only 1 to 2 mm in diameter. The degree of aortic obstruction produced by coarctation often appears to be progressive after birth. In addition to the increased resistance to left ventricular output, the coarctation produces other important hemodynamic changes. In most instances both the systolic and the diastolic arterial pressures above the coarctation are elevated above normal levels, whereas the pressure pulse in the femoral artery below the coarctation has a systolic pressure that is lower than that in the upper extremities, and a diastolic pressure that is usually above the normal range (Fig. 36-46). As a result of the damping effect on the transmission of the pulse wave, the onset of the femoral pulse wave is delayed about 0.03 s beyond that of the radial pulse wave, and the femoral pulse wave has a prolongation of the buildup time; i.e., the systolic upstroke time, or the time from the onset to the peak of the pulse wave, is prolonged.

The mechanism of the hypertension in the upper limbs has been the subject of numerous investiga-

FIGURE 36-46 Characteristic tracings above and below a coarctation of the aorta. The arterial pressure pulse below the coarctation is damped by the coarctation and is characterized by a slow rate of rise of pressure and a delayed peak pressure.

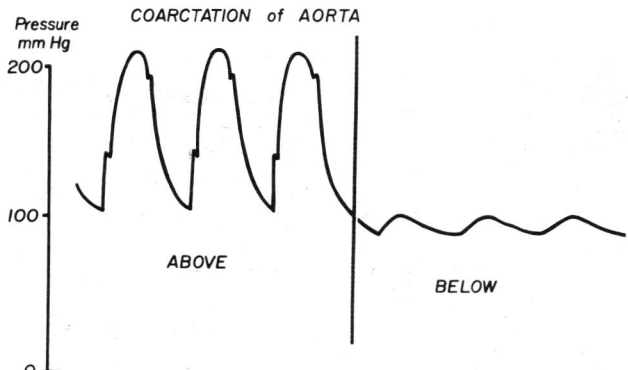

tions. It appears to involve mechanical factors (the increased resistance to aortic flow produced by the coarctation and the decreased capacity and distensibility of the vessels into which the left ventricle ejects its contents during systole) and possibly humoral factors. Plasma renin activity does not appear to be increased. Once the pressure is increased by other mechanisms, it is also probable that the hypertension is maintained, in part, by an increased capability of the blood vessels to respond to increased intraluminal pressure secondary to increased tone and muscular hypertrophy. At present there is little good evidence of a significant neurogenic mechanism in the production of the hypertension above the coarctation. As a result of the upper body hypertension and the development of extensive collateral channels, some patients are surprisingly symptom-free even with moderately severe coarctation of the aorta. In most cases surgical removal of the coarctation results in marked improvement of the circulatory dynamics with long-lasting correction of the hypertension. There is some evidence that patients who have had surgical correction of a coarctation have an increased risk of developing hypertension in subsequent years. A bicuspid aortic valve has been reported to occur in up to 80 percent of patients with coarctation of the aorta. The major importance of the bicuspid valve lies in its susceptibility to the later development of calcific aortic stenosis and to infective endocarditis, although on occasion it may produce significant obstruction to left ventricular outflow, or, less commonly, significant regurgitation.

Clinical Manifestations

This malformation accounts for approximately 8 percent of congenital heart disease in infants and children, ranking only behind ventricular septal defect and patent ductus arteriosus in frequency.[4] Of all individuals born with coarctation, approximately half will present within the first months of life with varying degrees of heart failure, usually severe. Of these infants, 60 percent will require hospitalization by the end of 2 weeks and the majority of the rest will require similar management in the next few weeks.[5] About 22 percent of infants so admitted will have uncomplicated coarctation, and a similar proportion a patent ductus. Almost half will have an associated ventricular septal defect.[5] The timing of ductal tissue constriction, both in terms of ductal closure and, perhaps, aortic constriction as well, appears to play a decisive role in the onset or worsening of symptoms in some of these patients.[320] The male-to-female ratio is approximately 3:1 with isolated coarctation, but only 1.1:1 with complicated coarctation. Approximately 45 percent of children with Turner's syndrome will have coarctation. Familial occurrence has been described.[321]

History The clinical picture in the symptomatic infant is one of dyspnea, difficulty feeding, and poor

DISEASES OF THE HEART AND BLOOD VESSELS

weight gain. Beyond the age of infancy patients are for the most part asymptomatic, although a few will complain of mild fatigue or dyspnea or symptoms of claudication in their legs when running. Symptoms again appear in the unoperated patient in the twenties, with congestive heart failure being a major complication after the age of 40.

Physical Examination   In the infant, tachypnea and labored breathing are characteristic. Rales are frequent, and impressive enlargement of the liver reflects the degree of heart failure. Right and left ventricular impulses are hyperdynamic. A gallop rhythm is common and a murmur of ventricular septal defect, mitral regurgitation, patent ductus, or, posteriorly in the interscapular area, from the coarctation itself, may be heard. Frequently, these murmurs are either inaudible or nondescript on admission and become characteristic when congestive failure is brought under control. In the older, usually asymptomatic child, disproportionate development of the arms, chest, and shoulder girdle compared to that of the legs may be noted. Prominent arterial pulses may be visible in the suprasternal notch and carotid arteries. The left ventricular impulse usually is forceful and the first heart sound at the apex accentuated. The aortic component of the second heart sound frequently is accentuated. An early systolic ejection click at the apex suggests the presence of a bicuspid aortic valve. The murmur from the coarctation itself, which is presumably the result of turbulent flow across the narrowed aortic segment, is medium-pitched, systolic, and blowing in quality. It is best heard posteriorly in the interscapular area, usually with some degree of radiation to the left axilla, apex, and anterior precordium. Low-pitched, continuous murmurs of collateral circulation may be heard over the chest wall, particularly posteriorly, but seldom before adolescence. Murmurs consistent with mitral regurgitation, mitral stenosis, or aortic regurgitation or stenosis, may be heard in a few patients. A short, middiastolic rumble at the apex without clinical evidence of mitral disease is relatively common.

The characteristic clinical feature of coarctation, namely a significant systolic blood pressure difference between the upper and lower extremities, may be difficult to appreciate or measure in infants with severe congestive failure or with a large ventricular septal defect or ductus. Usually all pulses are subdued with severe failure, but with improved compensation those in the upper extremities become readily palpable. The femoral pulses remain weak, delayed, or absent. In these very young infants, it is important that the pulses in both brachial arteries and in both carotids or temporals be assessed, since weak or absent pulses in all sites are characteristic of critical aortic stenosis or aortic atresia, while normal pulses in one or both carotids would raise the possibility of coarctation or interruption of the aortic arch, with one or both subclavian arteries or even

one carotid artery arising below the coarctation or interruption.

In older children and adults, the radial arterial pulses typically are strong while those in the femoral arteries are either diminished, delayed, or absent. A measured systolic pressure difference between the upper and lower extremities is diagnostic, whereas the diastolic pressure will be either the same or only slightly greater in the arms than in the legs. The pulse pressure in the leg is reduced, and in some patients no pressure can be measured by cuff. Approximately one-third of children have little or no hypertension. Two-thirds have mild or severe hypertension with the latter being defined here as a systolic pressure above 150 mmHg or a diastolic pressure above 100 mmHg, or both. A systolic pressure difference between the two arms suggests the origin of one subclavian artery at or below the obstruction. It is useful to measure the blood pressure difference between the arms and legs before and after exercise in order to evaluate patients with only mild pressure differences at rest.

Chest Roentgenogram   For the symptomatic infant the pattern will be one of impressive cardiac enlargement, venous congestion, and, in the presence of ventricular septal defect or patent ductus, pulmonary arterial overperfusion. In the older and asymptomatic child, the heart size is generally at the upper limits of normal with a left ventricular prominence. A figure-three configuration of the left margin of the aorta at the level of the coarctation may be seen in overpenetrated films, with the upper curve formed by the slightly dilated aorta just above the coarctation, the central indentation by the coarctation itself, and the lower curve by the poststenotic dilatation below the coarctation. The mirror image of this, or *E sign*, may be outlined by the barium-filled esophagus along the right margin of the aorta. Notching of the inferior margin of the ribs by tortuous intercostal arteries acting as collaterals is seldom present before 7 or 8 years of age. Notching signifies clinically important coarctation and localizes the obstruction to the thoracic aorta. Prominent enlargement of the left ventricle and dilatation of the left atrium are not uncommon in older individuals with unoperated coarctation.

Electrocardiogram   The electrocardiogram of the symptomatic infant will show right-axis deviation, right atrial hypertrophy, and right or biventricular hypertrophy during the first 3 months of life. Isolated left ventricular hypertrophy is rare. T-wave inversion in the left precordial leads is common (Fig. 36-47). Among older children, the electrocardiogram is usually normal or may indicate mild left ventricular and left atrial hypertrophy. Among older individuals there is a higher incidence than normal of conduction abnormalities, including left anterior hemiblock and ventricular bigeminy.

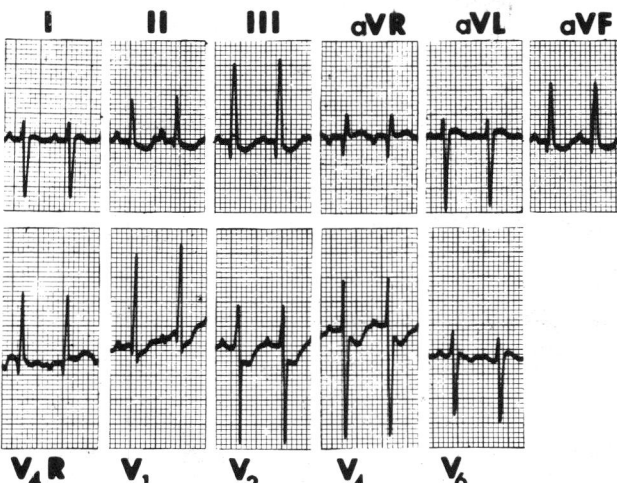

FIGURE 36-47   Electrocardiogram from an 8-year-old infant with symptomatic coarctation of the aorta. The mean QRS axis is normal for age (+120°) but the qR pattern in leads V$_4$R and V$_1$ indicates severe right ventricular hypertrophy. The abnormal T waves and ST segments reflect serious left ventricular ischemia.

Echocardiogram   M-mode echocardiography may be useful to follow left ventricular function in infants managed medically.[322] Two-dimensional echocardiographic imaging of the aortic arch from the suprasternal notch permits visualization of the coarctation, and prediction of anatomic variations such as isthmic hypoplasia.[323] The precordial and subxiphoid views are of great value in assessing the presence and severity of associated defects.

Cardiac Catheterization   Study of symptomatic infants, usually after 24 h of vigorous medical management, characteristically reveals left atrial and left ventricular hypertension and a significant systolic pressure difference between the left ventricle and femoral artery, particularly if the coarctation is isolated. In the presence of a large ventricular septal defect or patent ductus, the left ventricular hypertension and the systolic pressure difference between the left ventricle and femoral artery are much less impressive and may not exist at all. In these patients with combined defects, the diagnosis depends upon high-quality angiographic studies. Every attempt should be made to define the nature and severity of associated defects. Aortography is necessary to demonstrate the exact site and length of the coarctation as well as unusual features of the collateral circulation that may be of importance to the surgeon (Fig. 36-48).

Natural History and Prognosis

Approximately one-fifth of those infants admitted with heart failure within the first weeks of life will have coarctation without significant associated defects. The majority, though not all, of these infants will respond well to medical management and, usually, reach a stage at 2 or 3 years of age where they are indistinguishable from the asymptomatic children whose coarctation is first detected at that age because of a soft heart murmur, modest upper-extremity hypertension, or absence or diminution of the femoral pulses on a routine physical examination. Upper-extremity hypertension usually increases during the first several months of life and then tends to diminish again, presumably as collateral circulation improves. Cardiac enlargement, tachypnea, and other signs of failure diminish at the same time and digitalis can usually be discontinued during the second year of life. For those infants with failure and serious associated defects such as a large patent ductus, ventricular septal defect, or transposition of the great arteries, chances of survival are extremely slim despite the most vigorous medical management. These patients, and those few with isolated coarctation in whom the response to medical management has been marginal, require prompt surgical relief of the coarctation and simultaneous correction or palliation of associated defects. These patients generally do extremely well, although most will require correction of residual significant associated defects at some point in the future. Recoarctation in these very young infants undergoing end-to-end anastomosis of the aorta in the first year of life is in the order of 33 percent over the course of the next several years.[324] In a small number of patients this generally optimistic postoperative course will be complicated by rapidly recurrent coarctation or the development of moderate or severe mitral stenosis or regurgitation.

Unoperated older children in the 3 to 10 age range on the whole do well, but the consequences of persistent hypertension appear in the second and third decades in the form of aortic rupture or intracranial hemorrhage from an aneurysm of the circle of Willis, or in the fourth decade in the form of

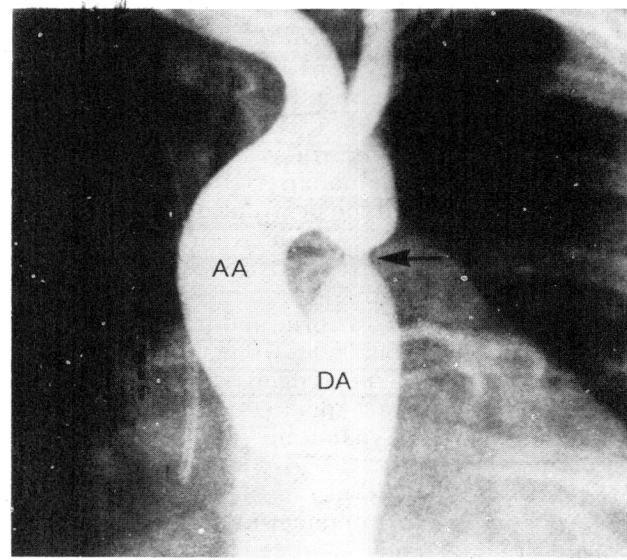

FIGURE 36-48   Posteroanterior view of an aortogram demonstrating discrete coarctation of the aorta. AA = ascending aorta; DA = descending aorta.

congestive heart failure often complicated by mitral or aortic valve disease or atherosclerosis. Dissecting aneurysm of the aorta may occur. The risk of endocarditis on the aortic or mitral valves or endarteritis at the site of coarctation appears spread relatively evenly over the course of years. The median age of death of patients surviving infancy with unoperated coarctation is 31 years.[325]

Surgical correction of coarctation has proved extremely effective in removing the serious obstruction to left ventricular output and in providing relief for the upper portion of the body from the deleterious effects of prolonged hypertension. For infants with severe failure, particularly those with associated defects, surgery provides virtually the only chance of survival. Among older adults with congestive failure, the results of surgery, though less dramatic, are decidedly beneficial in most instances. Normal blood pressures are achieved in at least 80 percent of patients if surgery is performed during childhood and if those individuals with recurrent coarctation are excluded.[325,326] The prevalence of recoarctation, which may be defined as a systolic pressure gradient between the upper and lower extremities of greater than 10 mmHg at rest, diminishes sharply from the 33 percent quoted above for patients undergoing correction during infancy, to approximately 10 percent or less for those undergoing correction as older children. Recently, significant pressure gradients have been documented by exercise testing among patients formerly judged to be free of significant residual obstruction. This observation will undoubtedly lead to a reassessment of all postoperative patients, particularly those in whom the blood pressure has not returned to normal following surgery.[327]

Residual or recurrent hypertension among patients without demonstrable recurrent coarctation, renal disease, or significant aortic regurgitation appears related to the duration of hypertension prior to surgery. This complication seems rare among individuals operated before the age of 6 years but becomes progressively more common as surgery is delayed and may be present in anywhere from 20 percent to 50 percent of individuals operated at 20 years of age or beyond.[325,328] Similarly, the risk of premature death from cardiovascular disease in the form of aortic or cerebral arterial rupture, congestive heart failure, or myocardial infarction is increased if surgical correction is delayed into the third decade.[328] Finally, survivors of surgery may carry with them residual congenital heart disease primarily in the form of aortic and mitral valve malformations. While some 60 to 70 percent of patients fall in this category and remain at risk of infective endocarditis, in only a small proportion will these lesions prove hemodynamically significant.

Medical Management

Vigorous medical treatment with digitalis, intravenous diuretics, oxygen, and sedation are indicated for those infants with severe failure. Cardiac catheterization, usually after 24 h of medical management is recommended to detect and assess the severity of associated lesions. An occasional infant will require intravenous infusion of prostaglandin E_1 to reopen the closing ductus, thereby controlling pulmonary edema and providing a sufficiently stable patient to permit catheterization and operation.[329] Surgical correction of the coarctation is recommended for those infants in whom there is one or more associated defects and for infants with isolated coarctation as well, unless the response to medical management has been dramatic and sustained. A patent ductus is ligated at the same operation. If a large ventricular septal defect is present, the pulmonary arterial systolic pressure is measured at the end of the procedure. If it still is at systemic levels, a pulmonary arterial band is applied. These patients are recatheterized toward the end of the first year of life, and if the septal defect is found to be small, the pulmonary arterial band is removed. If the defect is still large, the band is removed, and the septal defect closed directly. In any event, operated infants should be followed closely to detect the occasional patient with rapid redevelopment of coarctation or with continuing or progressive symptoms related to severe aortic or mitral stenosis or insufficiency. Infants not requiring surgery generally improve steadily despite impressive hypertension in the first months of life. The persistence of failure or its appearance for the first time beyond the age of 6 months suggests a complication or an associated lesion.

Elective correction of coarctation is now recommended between the ages of 4 and 6 years in order to avoid the relatively high rate of recoarctation found among patients corrected under 1 year of age and the complication of residual persistent or recurrent hypertension without demonstrable recoarctation among those individuals operated beyond 6 years of age. Increasing fatigue or dyspnea, progression of hypertension with or without symptoms suggesting impending encephalopathy or cerebral vascular accident, significant cardiac enlargement, or severe left ventricular hypertrophy in the electrocardiogram, also would indicate a need for earlier correction. Restriction from strenuous sports or exercise is recommended prior to correction.

Older children and adults should undergo correction without delay and even older adults who are symptomatic with hypertension and associated lesions usually benefit significantly from repair.

A serious postoperative syndrome may occur in patients of any age between the second and tenth postoperative day. The syndrome is characterized by persistent or recurrent severe hypertension, abdominal distension, abdominal pain, and leukocytosis. This has been attributed to mesenteric arteritis which, untreated, may lead to necrosis of the bowel and death. Symptoms subside quickly if the blood pressure, particularly the diastolic pressure, is brought within normal limits and maintained at normal levels by parenteral antihypertensive therapy. Usually this hypertensive reaction subsides spontaneously within 8 to 12 days and therapy may be tapered and discontinued (see Chap. 50).

With or without surgical correction, patients with coarctation should be followed indefinitely. For those individuals with significant recoarctation expressed as a systolic pressure gradient of 30 mmHg or more at rest between the upper and lower extremities, angiography and, if feasible, reoperation, is recommended. Postoperative patients, with or without resting hypertension, with insignificant or small resting gradients, but who manifest abnormal upper-extremity hypertension and significant gradients with exercise probably should undergo reoperation as well. Patients with persistent hypertension without gradients either at rest or exercise and those patients described above in whom reoperation seems unjustified or unduly hazardous, will probably benefit from restricted activity and antihypertensive medication. Pregnancy carries a mortality rate of approximately 10 percent and a complication rate of 90 percent among women with uncorrected coarctation. With correction the mortality rate does not differ significantly from the normal, while complications are on the order of 15 percent.[330] The risk of congenital heart disease in the offspring of a single affected parent or in a sibling of a single affected family member is estimated at 2 percent with about a 50 percent chance of the defect being coarctation.[154]

Surgical Management

Coarctation of the aorta should be corrected surgically in all symptomatic infants and in asymptomatic children prior to the age of 5 or 6 years.[331,332] In fact, elective repair by the subclavian flap technique in the first year of life may offer the best chance for long-term cure.

The coarctation is exposed and thoroughly mobilized through a left thoracotomy. It is usually possible to resect the narrow area of aorta and restore continuity by direct end-to-end anastomosis[333,334] (Fig. 36-49). Occasionally a tubular Dacron prosthesis or similar graft is required to bridge the gap between the two ends of the aorta when the coarctation is unusually long, the aortic isthmus is hypoplastic, or there is an associated aneurysm.[335] In adults with a relatively nonelastic or partially calcified aorta, a tubular vascular prosthesis may be used to bypass the unresected coarctation, the conduit being anastomosed to the side of the left subclavian artery above and to the side of the descending thoracic aorta below the point of narrowing.[336,337]

The infant and small child with coarctation pose

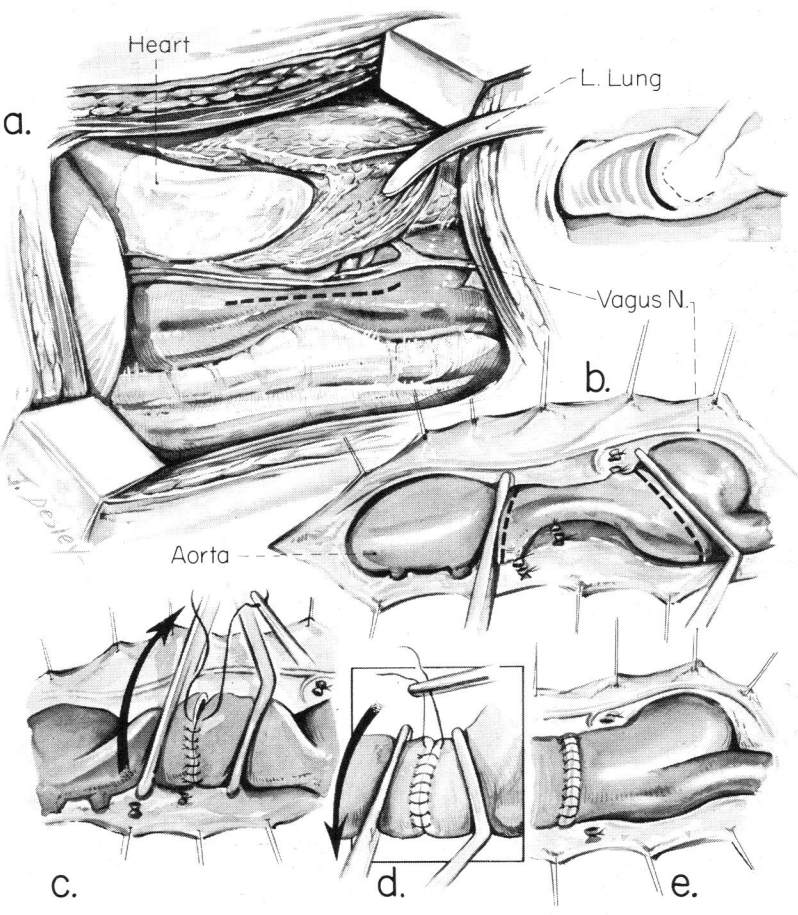

FIGURE 36-49 Steps in operative repair of coarctation of aorta. *a.* Mediastinal pleura is opened over the upper part of the descending thoracic aorta. *b.* After appropriate mobilization of the coarctate area and division of ligamentum arteriosum, appropriate clamps are placed above and below the stricture. At times the distal clamp must be placed more downstream than in the illustration, and then the intercostal arteries are temporarily controlled with bulldog clamps. *c, d,* and *e.* End-to-end anastomosis is made with interrupted simple sutures of No. 5-0 silk.

a unique problem. Growth of a circular suture line at the site of an end-to-end anastomosis will probably not be adequate; recurrent stenosis as the child grows is likely.[324] This problem may be reduced somewhat when the end of the distal aorta is sutured to the opened underside of the transverse aortic arch.[338] Techniques offering promise of reducing the incidence of recurrent coarctation include the Dacron patch angioplasty[339-341] and the subclavian arterial flap angioplasty[342] described by Waldhausen (Fig. 36-50). We have been pleased with our own experience using the Waldhausen technique and the still attached but open subclavian artery as a flap of viable tissue to widen the narrow portion of the aorta in infants. The patent ductus arteriosus is ligated at the time of coarctation repair.

When a significant ventricular septal defect is present, distal pulmonary arterial pressure is reduced to about one-third of the systemic arterial pressure by placement of a pulmonary arterial band. The ventricular septal defect is closed if required and the band removed at a later operation, usually during the second 6 months of life. If the ventricular septal defect is of an anatomically complex form and adequate palliation has been achieved, repair is deferred until the child is about 2 years old. Tiraboschi[343] has reported excellent results, however, with *simultaneous* repair of coarctation and closure of the ventricular septal defect in a few older infants, an aggressive approach deserving further consideration.

Adequacy of collateral circulation is important to the successful repair of coarctation. Collaterals should be assessed clinically and angiographically. In the operating room the aorta is cross-clamped prior to resection of the coarctation. A rise in proximal systemic arterial pressure of more than 20 mmHg suggests marginal collateral blood supply to the descending aorta. In such situations we begin an intravenous infusion of sodium nitroprusside and administer additional intravascular volume. The pressure in the descending aorta may be monitored to ensure adequate perfusion of the spinal cord and kidneys during the period of aortic interruption. Left side of the heart cardiopulmonary bypass techniques have been used as an adjunct to resection of coarctation in patients with underdeveloped collateral circulation, but we have not found this approach necessary with the use of volume expansion and vasodilators. Others have used moderate hypothermia to 33°C to further protect the spinal cord from ischemia.[334]

Postoperative paradoxical hypertension is common[344] and may contribute to the postcoarctation syndrome in which ileus, abdominal pain, mesenteric vasculitis, and even visceral infarction may occur. We have not encountered this syndrome in patients in whom we have maintained the postoperative diastolic blood pressure within normal range for age with sodium nitroprusside, propranolol, or reserpine, and in whom nasogastric tube decompression

FIGURE 36-50 *A.* Coarctation repair using Dacron patch angioplasty. A longitudinal incision extends from the normal aorta below the coarctation to a point well above the coarctation on the subclavian artery. A relatively large patch is cut from a Dacron tube graft and sutured across the coarctation after excision of any intraluminal membrane. Circular suture lines are thus avoided. The patch is large, allowing for growth. *B.* Subclavian arterial flap angioplasty repair of coarctation of the aorta. The subclavian artery is divided in the apex of the left pleural cavity. The lateral wall of the artery is incised downward, the incision continuing across the coarctation onto normal aorta below. The flap thus created is sutured across the coarctation, after excision of intraluminal membrane, using fine continuous monofilament suture. Circular suture lines are avoided. The viable flap should grow as the child and aorta grow, minimizing recurrent coarctation. (*From V. M. Herrmann, H. Laks, L. Fagan, D. Terschluse, and V. L. William, Repair of Aortic Coarctation in the First Year of Life, Ann. Thorac. Surg., 25:57, 1978. Reproduced with permission.*)

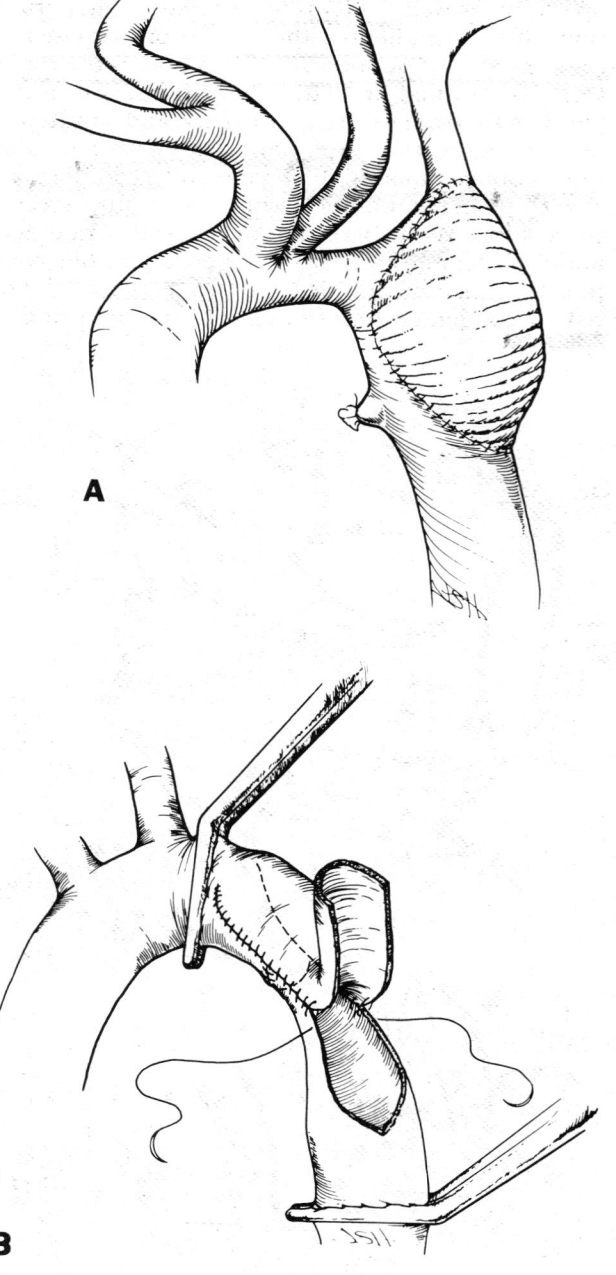

A

B

of the gastrointestinal tract has been maintained postoperatively for 48 h.

Williams[345] reviewed 191 infants less than 1 year old who underwent repair of coarctation of the aorta during a recent 14-year period. Operative mortality was 4 percent for infants with isolated coarctation, but 25 percent when other cardiovascular defects were present. There were no subsequent deaths in hospital survivors with isolated coarctation but the 5-year mortality for those having coarctation with other defects was 25 percent. Recurrent coarctation evidenced by a gradient between arm and leg blood pressures at rest occurred in 54 percent of survivors within 7 years. Hypertension was present in 27 percent of children followed more than 5 years after repair.

Maron[318] reported data from 248 older patients (over 2 years) followed 11 to 25 years after correction of coarctation. Twelve percent of these patients have died. Seventy-eight percent had persistent evidence of cardiovascular disease. Premature death was believed to correlate with the duration of hypertension present preoperatively.

Sehested[331] reviewed 182 patients undergoing repair of coarctation between the ages of 3 weeks and 60 years. Four operative deaths occurred in children less than 14 months old, all having other cardiac defects. Two patients sustained lower limb paralysis. There were no operative or late deaths in patients with uncomplicated coarctation, but about one-third of the patients remained hypertensive on follow-up.

Earlier diagnosis and correction of coarctation in infancy is suggested[332] by the dismal prognosis of untreated coarctation, the excellent hemodynamic results achieved by aortoplasty, and the relatively low mortality now expected when this technique is used by experienced surgical groups.[342]

Interruption of the Aortic Arch

Definition
Interruption of the aortic arch is characterized by lack of a channel between the aortic arch and the descending aorta. In almost all cases there is no connection between the two segments of the aorta. Unusually an atretic strand connects the two segments, so-called atresia of the aortic arch.

Pathology
The descending aorta is connected with the pulmonary arterial system by the ductus arteriosus. Classically, the ductus is left-sided, as is the descending aorta. Rarely, the ductus and the descending aorta are right-sided.[346]

Variations occur in the origin of branches of the arch.[347] In over half of the cases (53 percent) the left subclavian artery arises from the descending aorta. In about 42 percent all of the branches of the arch arise proximal to the interruption (Fig. 36-51).

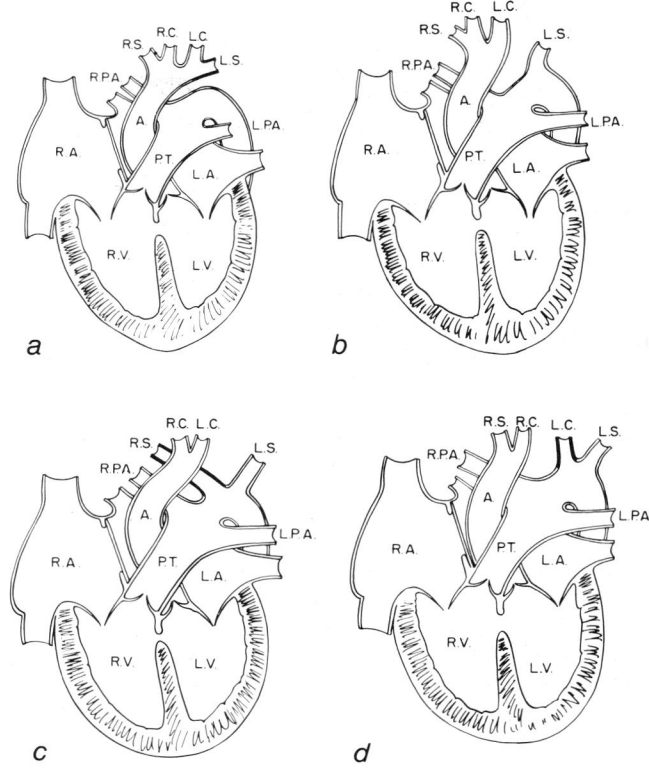

FIGURE 36-51 Variations in manner of origin of branches of the aortic arch in association with interruption of the aortic arch and ventricular septal defect. *a.* Each of the standard branches of the aortic arch arises from the arch. *b.* The left subclavian artery (L.S.) arises from the descending aorta; the other branches arise from the aortic arch. *c.* The left subclavian and right subclavian (R.S.) arteries each arise from the descending aorta. *d.* The left common carotid (L.C.) and left subclavian arteries arise from the descending aorta. Although this pattern has been described, it may represent a misinterpretation of the condition shown in *c.* R.A. = right atrium; R.V. = right ventricle; P.T. = main pulmonary arterial trunk; R.P.A. = right pulmonary artery; L.P.A. = left pulmonary artery; L.A. = left atrium; L.V. = left ventricle; A. = aorta; R.C. = right carotid artery. (*From Moller and Edwards.[347] Reproduced with permission.*)

Less common patterns are (1) origin of both subclavian arteries from the descending aorta, (2) origin of the right subclavian artery from the descending aorta, (3) isolation of the subclavian artery on the side opposite the descending aorta, and (4) very rarely, origin of the left common carotid and left subclavian arteries from the distal compartment.

In some cases enlargement of the intercostal arteries may be noted.

Associated Conditions Only rarely is the heart normal. The most common abnormality is ventricular septal defect, either alone or, more commonly, associated with a subaortic spur of muscle that causes subaortic stenosis downstream from the ventricular septal defect.[348] Less commonly associated anomalies are complete transposition, persistent truncus arteriosus, and origin of both great vessels from the right ventricle.

Complications Only rarely does the natural history show survival beyond infancy, the most common complication being pulmonary in nature. In the rare cases of right ductus and right descending aorta there may be right bronchial compression by the right ductus.[346]

Clinical Manifestations

This very rare malformation accounts for about 4 percent of the deaths among infants with congenital heart disease in the first month of life.[349] The median age of death among unoperated patients is 4 days.[350] There is no sex predilection. The clinical picture is the same as that of the newborn with severe complicated coarctation, except that in approximately half of these infants the left subclavian arterial pulse is weak or absent. If both subclavian arteries arise below the interruption, pulses in all extremities will be weak or absent. Preservation of a right carotid pulse will distinguish these patients from those with aortic atresia or critical aortic stenosis. Similarly, M-mode and two-dimensional studies will distinguish infants with interruption or coarctation from those with aortic atresia.

The pressure and oxygen saturation data at catheterization will be similar to those of infants with severe coarctation, ventricular septal defect, and patent ductus arteriosus, but high-quality biplane angiography will reveal the absence of an aortic isthmus (Fig. 36-52).

Natural History and Prognosis

Survival is uncommon even with the most vigorous medical or surgical management. Rarely an individual with this malformation may survive to adulthood. In these instances the ductus and the intracardiac or supracardiac communication remained patent, and a marked elevation of the pulmonary vascular resistance prevented overwhelming flooding of the pulmonary vascular bed, or ductal closure was delayed long enough to permit compensatory collateral circulation to develop between the two segments of the aorta.[351] Only the latter individuals are candidates for correction.

Medical Management

Despite intensive therapy to control congestive failure, the course is usually one of rapid and relentless deterioration. Intravenous infusion of prostaglandin E_1 is beneficial and usually will permit cardiac catheterization and surgery under somewhat less critical conditions.[329] Only very limited success has been achieved with either palliative or corrective surgery.

Surgical Management

Gradual spontaneous closure of the patent ductus arteriosus and development of collateral vascularization to the distal aorta occasionally allows survival to childhood. Repair is then accomplished by the interposition of a prosthetic vascular graft between the ascending aorta and the descending aorta. It is unusual to find a ventricular septal defect requiring closure in these older patients.

Palliation has been accomplished by creation of a "permanent" patent ductus arteriosus using a prosthetic vascular graft between the main pulmonary artery and the descending aorta.[352] The main pulmonary artery is banded distal to the origin of the vascular graft. Results have been poor.

The left subclavian artery or the left common carotid artery has been used to bridge the gap between the ascending aorta and descending aorta.[353] Severe obstruction owing to the small size of the vessels usually persists or evolves as the child grows. In infancy the aorta is usually too small to allow the safe placement of a partially occluding vascular clamp without producing cerebral ischemia during anastomosis of a graft to the side of the ascending aorta. The experience with palliation has been reviewed by Copeland.[353]

Although the risk of total correction in these critically ill infants is high, this approach probably offers the greatest likelihood for long-term survival. Several case reports have recently appeared describing the successful one-stage repair of interrupted aortic arch in infancy.[354–356] Barratt-Boyes[357] placed a prosthetic graft between the ascending aorta and the descending aorta, closed a ventricular septal defect, and repaired anomalous pulmonary venous drainage. Murphy[358] used an allograft vein as a conduit and closed a ventricular septal defect. Bowman[359] described the successful management of three patients using a technique originally demonstrated by Trusler[360]—mobilization of the descending aorta through a median sternotomy incision, ex-

FIGURE 36-52 Posteroanterior view of an arteriogram in the ascending aorta demonstrating interruption of the aortic arch between the left carotid artery (LC) and left subclavian artery (type b). AA = ascending aorta; I = innominate artery.

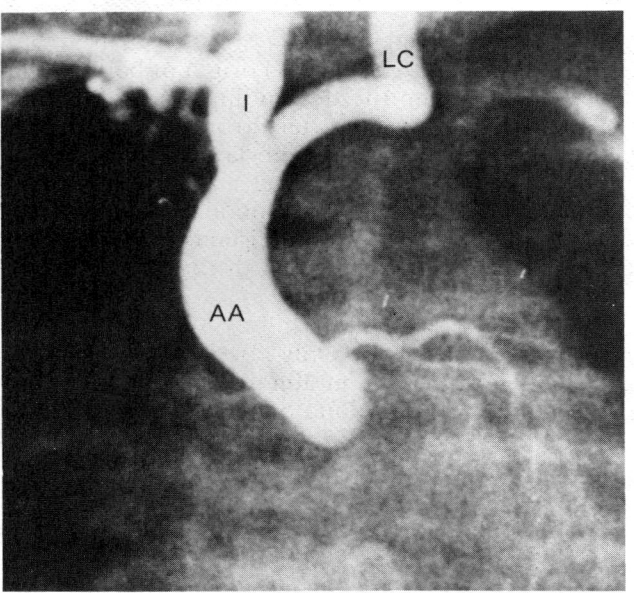

cision of ductus tissue, anastomosis of the end of the descending aorta to the side of the ascending aorta, and closure of associated ventricular or atrial septal defects. Operation is carried out during a period of circulatory arrest, with profound hypothermia provided by surface cooling or the pump oxygenator, the latter being used for rewarming and resuscitation. Survival will most likely be influenced by the adequacy of left ventricular function, usually compromised in this anomaly. Subsequent stenosis of the circular vascular suture line requiring revision would be anticipated.

Valvular Aortic Stenosis

Definition
As used here, aortic stenosis is defined as obstruction in the channel of left ventricular outflow. The channel of left ventricular outflow is always patent, the obstruction exhibiting varying degrees of severity. In order of decreasing frequency, the sites of obstruction are (1) valvular, (2) subvalvular, and (3) supravalvular (Fig. 36-53).[361]

Pathology
In congenital valvular stenosis there is only one commissure, the valvular tissue being a modified dome, the so-called unicommissural, unicuspid aortic valve.[362,363] Two shallow raphes lie opposite and equidistant from the commissure. The orifice is often slitlike in shape, at first glance suggesting a bicuspid valve. Uncommonly a true dome is present, resembling the valve of congenital isolated pulmonary stenosis. The orifice varies in caliber. When survival to adult life occurs, varying degrees of calcification may appear in the valvular tissue, leading to major rigidity of the valve. In the majority of cases manifesting cardiac dysfunction in infancy, the left ventricular wall is hypertrophied, but the chamber is small and significant degrees of endocardial fibroelastosis occur. Hearts so altered are included under the broad condition of *"hypoplastic left heart."* In such cases the left atrium is stretched and the

valve of the foramen ovale is herniated into the right atrium. In an occasional case of this type a connection of a pulmonary vein with a systemic vein is associated.

Among those cases of valvular stenosis in which the left ventricular cavity is of normal dimension, some patients reach adult life. Others become complicated by mitral insufficiency as a consequence of infarction of the left ventricular wall, including papillary muscles.[364]

In all cases, poststenotic dilatation of the ascending aorta occurs to some degree.

Coarctation of the aorta is the most common associated anomaly.

Abnormal Physiology[85,365–368]
The hemodynamics of *congenital valvular aortic stenosis* are similar to that of acquired aortic stenosis (see Chap. 38) except that a persistent ductus arteriosus in the immediate postnatal period may shunt blood away from the lungs and may lessen the severity of pulmonary edema by decreasing left atrial pressure.

Occasionally, in an infant with severe aortic stenosis and with a markedly increased left atrial pressure, the left atrial septum is stretched enough to open the foramen ovale, producing a large left-to-right shunt with pulmonary arterial hypertension. The normal aortic valve in infancy and childhood is about 2 cm^2/m^2, and normally the valve increases in size appropriately for body growth. Serial studies in infants and children with congenital aortic stenosis suggest that the valve frequently fails to increase in size and area proportionately to body size and cardiac output needs.[369,370]

Clinical Manifestations
About 7 percent of infants and children with clinically identified congenital heart disease will have aortic stenosis in one of its several forms. Approximately 80 percent of these patients will have valvular aortic stenosis, while the remainder will have discrete fibrous, fibromuscular, or muscular subvalvular aortic stenosis, or supravalvular aortic steno-

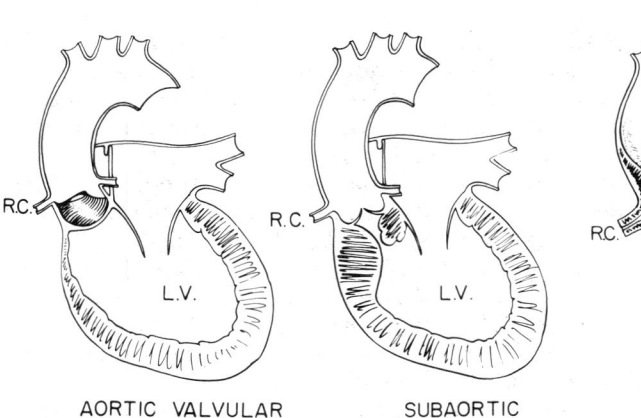

AORTIC VALVULAR
STENOSIS

SUBAORTIC
STENOSIS

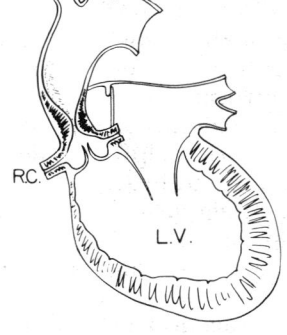

SUPRAVALVULAR
AORTIC STENOSIS

FIGURE 36-53 Types of left ventricular outflow obstruction in order of decreasng frequency moving from left to right. R.C. = right coronary artery; L.V. = left ventricle. (*From J. E. Edwards, Pathology of Left Ventricular Outflow Tract Obstruction, Circulation, 31:586, 1965. Reproduced with permission.*)

sis.[6] Valvular aortic stenosis is much more common among males than females in a ratio of 4:1. Associated intracardiac anomalies are infrequent. Severity usually is judged by the peak systolic pressure gradient across the aortic valve and the calculated aortic valve area. In the presence of a normal cardiac output, a gradient of 80 mmHg or more or an aortic valve area of less than 0.5 cm^2/m^2 is considered severe; a gradient between 50 to 79 mmHg or a valve area between 0.5 to 0.8 cm^2/m^2 moderate; and a gradient of less than 50 mmHg or a valve area greater than 0.8 cm^2/m^2 is considered mild.[9,371]

History The detection of a systolic murmur leads to the discovery of this malformation in most patients. Although it may be heard within the first 24 to 48 h of life, the murmur is detected within the first year in slightly less than half of the patients. Growth and development usually are normal and the vast majority of children are asymptomatic. Easy fatigue or dyspnea suggests severe obstruction, although severe obstruction may exist in the absence of any symptoms. Similarly, angina or syncope warns of severe disease. Sudden death may occur from this malformation but in most cases death is preceded by symptoms or electrocardiographic changes.[371] A few infants with critical stenosis from birth will present with congestive failure within the first week or two of life, and these patients represent true medical emergencies. A similar small number of patients with less critical but still very severe obstruction is detected over the course of the next 4 to 6 months. Dyspnea, easy fatigue with feedings, and slow weight gain usually have been noticed.

Physical Examination The arterial blood pressure and the quality of the peripheral arterial pulses of the older infant and child usually are normal, and a measured pulse pressure of less than 20 mmHg suggests severe stenosis. Visible prominence of the left precordium is seldom seen, and the heart is usually not detectably enlarged to palpation or percussion. The cardiac impulse, maximal at the apex, may be heaving and sustained. A systolic thrill along the right upper sternal border and over the carotid arteries is present in about 90 percent of patients, and the absence of such a thrill at the right upper sternal border suggests a systolic pressure gradient of 30 mmHg or less. Paradoxical splitting of the second heart sound is rare and is associated either with very severe obstruction or with coexisting myocardial disease. Intermittent third or fourth heart sounds are fairly frequent, and, while not particularly helpful among young children, a fourth heart sound heard in patients between 12 and 40 years of age usually signifies severe obstruction. (See Chap. 38.) An early systolic ejection click at the apex is characteristic and serves to distinguish valvular aortic stenosis from other forms of left ventricular outflow tract obstruction. The classic auscultatory finding is a grade 3 to 6 harsh systolic murmur, loudest at the right upper

sternal border with radiation into the carotid arteries and down the left sternal border to the apex. The configuration of this murmur may be of some help in diagnosis, in that peaking in the latter half of systole frequently is associated with severe degrees of obstruction. A soft, early diastolic blowing murmur of aortic regurgitation may be heard in perhaps 30 percent of patients with mild to moderate aortic stenosis and in about 8 percent of those with severe stenosis.[372] Among infants with critical obstruction there may be no palpable peripheral pulses with a return of weak pulses only after decongestive therapy and the administration of digitalis. Marked respiratory distress usually is evident with pulmonary rales and, not uncommonly, cyanosis. A gallop rhythm is characteristic. There may be no murmur heard initially or a soft, nondescript murmur may be present along the left sternal border. The murmur of aortic stenosis, characteristic in its location and quality, will emerge as congestive failure is controlled. A systolic ejection click may also appear with improved compensation. Occasionally, the murmur of mitral regurgitation may be present or appear, as well.

Chest Roentgenogram The overall heart size usually is normal, but the left ventricle may appear prominent. Cardiac enlargement indicates severe disease in most instances. Poststenotic dilatation of the ascending aorta is characteristic. Calcification of the aorta is not seen during childhood but appears with increasing frequency after adolescence. Infants with failure will have generalized cardiac enlargement, left atrial dilatation, and varying degrees of pulmonary edema.

Electrocardiogram The QRS axis usually is normal regardless of severity. Left ventricular hypertrophy, as indicated by voltage criteria in the left precordial leads, seldom is helpful in distinguishing those patients with severe obstruction from those with mild to moderate obstruction. However, diminished anterior forces in the right precordial leads and a deep SV_1 of 30 mV or more suggests severe stenosis, as does absence of the Q wave in V_6. The T wave in V_6 may be helpful in diagnosis in that virtually all patients with pressure gradients of less than 50 mmHg will have a normal, upright T wave in V_6, while 20 percent of patients with moderate and 50 percent of patients with severe obstruction will have a flat, biphasic, or inverted T wave in V_6. It should be noted, however, that the other 50 percent of patients with severe stenosis will have a perfectly normal, upright T wave in V_6. A superior T-wave vector in the frontal plane between 270 and 359° also favors severe obstruction (Fig. 36-54). Severe and even critical obstruction may be present with none of the electrocardiographic abnormalities mentioned above.[372] Symptomatic infants may show right, left, or biventricular hypertrophy, frequently with T-wave inversion over the left precordium.

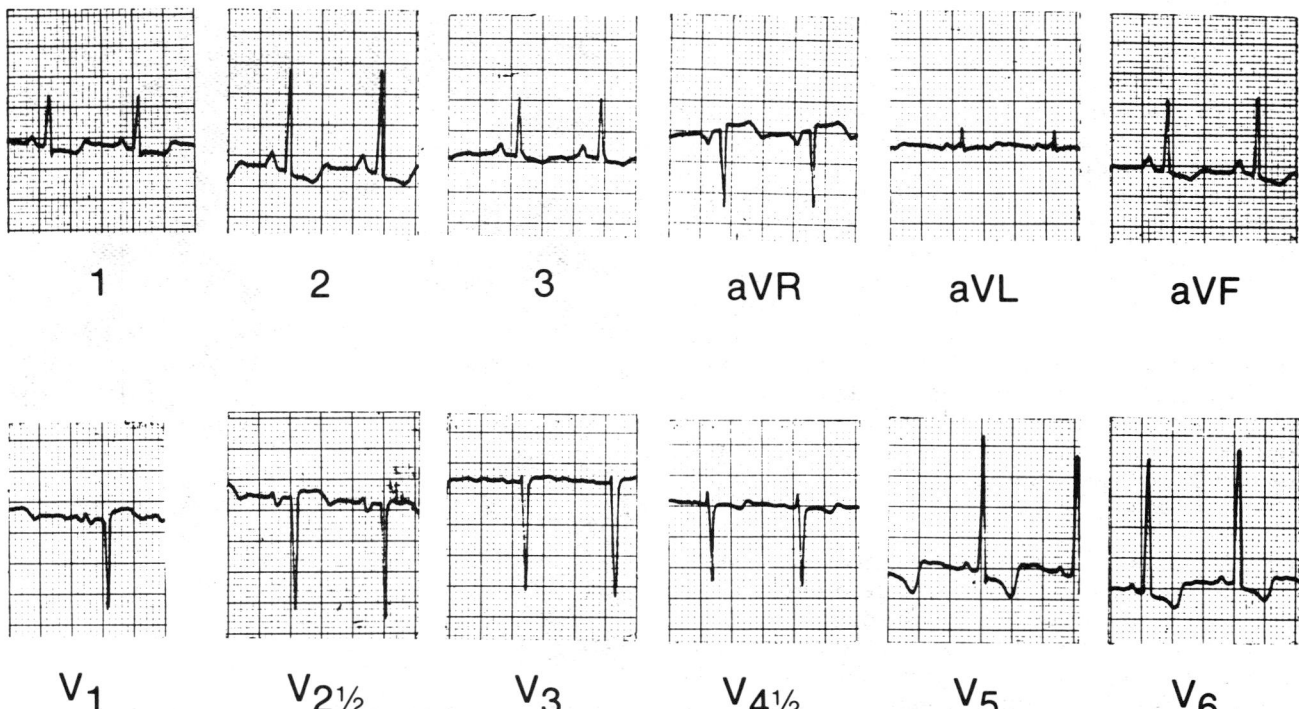

FIGURE 36-54   Electrocardiogram from an 8-year-old boy with valvular aortic stenosis and a 94 mmHg peak systolic pressure gradient. The small anterior QRS forces (rV_1, rV_2, and rV_3), abnormally large posterior QRS forces (SV_2), absent Q waves in leads V_5 and V_6, and abnormal T waves and ST segments reflect severe left ventricular systolic pressure overload with ischemia.

Monitoring of the ST segment in leads V_5 through V_7 during exercise appears to be a reliable method of detecting those children in whom a significant pressure gradient (greater than 50 mmHg) has developed and in whom that gradient might represent a threat of sudden death if the obstruction were not relieved.[373]

Echocardiogram   M-mode technique may show an abnormally eccentric closure of the aortic cusps and multiple diastolic echoes characteristic of a bicuspid valve. Multiple nonmoving echoes may fill the aortic root in those infants with critical aortic stenosis and a unicuspid valve, but with this exception, diminished valve movement, as visualized by the M-mode echocardiogram, is not a distinctive feature of valvular aortic stenosis in children. The diminished left ventricular end-diastolic volume resulting from concentric ventricular hypertrophy is reflected in the shortening fraction (SF) and can be used in children without evidence of congestive failure or myocardial ischemia as a semiquantitative guide to the systolic pressure gradient. [SF = LVIDd − (LVIDs/LVIDd), where LVIDd = left ventricular end-diastolic internal dimension and LVIDs = left ventricular end-systolic internal dimension.] Those patients with gradients in excess of 45 mmHg usually have SF values of 0.41 or greater, while those with gradients of less than 45 mmHg usually have SF values less than 0.41. A decreasing SF in the face of long-standing unrelieved obstruction suggests deterioration of left ventricular function. These ob-

servations appear to be unaffected by at least mild aortic regurgitation and may be of value in the postoperative patient as well.[157] Since the magnitude of left ventricular hypertrophy appears dependent upon left ventricular wall stress, and this in turn is dependent upon left ventricular systolic pressure and cavity dimensions [wall stress = pressure × (cavity diameter/wall thickness)], an estimate can be made of the left ventricular peak systolic pressure if the wall stress and the cavity dimensions remain relatively constant. The most commonly used formulas for this estimation in children with normal ventricular function are as follows:

1. LVP = 225 × Ws/Ds

   where LVP = left ventricular peak systolic pressure in mmHg

         Ws = left ventricular posterior wall end-systolic thickness

         Ds = left ventricular end-systolic cavity dimension

2. LVP = 312.12 × $h/4$ ± 28.01 h/r (SEE)

   where h = the mean value of the septal and left ventricular posterior wall end-diastolic thickness

         r = ½ of the left ventricular end-diastolic cavity dimension

      SEE = standard error of the estimate[374,375]

An estimate of the left ventricular peak systolic pressure gradient may be obtained by subtracting

DISEASES OF THE HEART AND BLOOD VESSELS

the arterial systolic pressure obtained by cuff at the time of the echocardiographic recording from the estimated left ventricular peak systolic pressure. Unfortunately, these estimates are not valid in the postoperative patient.[375] Two-dimensional echocardiography can distinguish valvular from supravalvular or subvalvular obstruction. In addition the measurement of maximal aortic cusp separation correlates well with the calculated aortic valve area for any given patient and, expressed as a percent of simultaneously recorded and measured aortic root diameter, provides a semiquantitative guide to the peak systolic pressure gradient.[376] Both M-mode and two-dimensional techniques are capable of identifying those critically ill infants in whom the left ventricular cavity dimensions and aortic root diameter are hypoplastic to a degree that would preclude survival in the first week or so of life.[377]

Cardiac Catheterization In infants symptomatic with severe aortic obstruction there often is a left-to-right shunt at the atrial level through a stretched foramen ovale. Pulmonary arterial and right ventricular hypertension are the rule, and there may be also a right-to-left shunt through a patent ductus arteriosus which temporarily provides adequate systemic arterial perfusion and relieves some of the burden on the already congested pulmonary venous bed. A marked increase in left ventricular end-diastolic pressure usually is present. The systolic pressure gradient between the left ventricle and central aorta or femoral artery should be documented whenever possible. If left ventricular output is markedly diminished, this gradient may be relatively small, even in the presence of severe obstruction. Left ventricular angiography will confirm the site of obstruction and outline the size of the left ventricular cavity (Fig. 36-55). Mitral stenosis, mitral regurgitation, and fibroelastosis are common complicating features. In older infants and children pressures on the right side of the heart usually are normal, although the pulmonary arterial wedge or left atrial pressures may be elevated. Simultaneous recording of central aortic and left ventricular pressures or a pressure tracing upon catheter withdrawal from the left ventricle to the aorta, coupled with an accurate estimate of cardiac output, is necessary for reliable assessment of severity. Left ventricular angiography will document the site of obstruction. The aortic leaflets typically will be thickened and domed, with a central or eccentric jet of contrast material entering the ascending aorta. Poststenotic dilatation is characteristic. Supravalvular aortography is recommended to assess the presence and severity of the aortic regurgitation and, again, the degree of the aortic valve deformity.

Natural History and Prognosis
About half of the infants born with severe valvular aortic stenosis are symptomatic enough to require hospitalization within the first week of life.[9] The re-

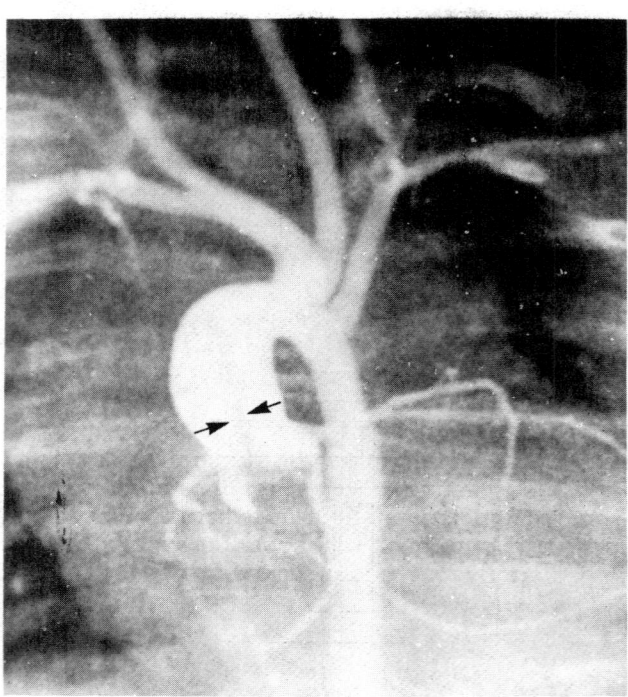

FIGURE 36-55 Posteroanterior view of the aortogram from an infant with critical valvular aortic stenosis. Note the extremely narrow jet of unopacified blood (between arrows) entering the ascending aorta from the left ventricle. Moderate poststenotic dilatation of the ascending aorta is present.

mainder develop congestive failure over the course of the next 6 months. Not uncommonly, the murmur is mistaken for that of a ventricular septal defect. Failure beyond infancy and before adolescence is usually not seen without the presence of complicating factors such as endocarditis, aortic regurgitation, or cardiomyopathy. Symptomatic infants require prompt surgery, but the mortality approaches 30 percent under the best of circumstances.[377] Endocardial fibroelastosis, papillary muscle necrosis, associated intracardiac and extracardiac deformities, and a small left ventricular cavity contribute to this mortality. Anywhere from 30 to 90 percent of survivors will have significant aortic regurgitation, but the majority can be managed medically until such time as valve replacement is feasible.

Among the infants and children with milder degrees of aortic valvular stenosis, gradual progression in severity of the systolic pressure gradient during childhood can be expected in about a third, and the appearance of symptoms and signs such as fatigue, dyspnea, angina or syncope, cardiac enlargement, or the development of a left ventricular strain pattern in the electrocardiogram in about 40 percent of children followed over a 4 to 8 year period, including some with mild gradients at the outset.[371] Sudden unexpected death is a very uncommon but definite threat to those with at least a moderate gradient. Of 67 patients with systolic pressure gradients greater than 50 mmHg followed medically within the framework of the Joint Study on the Natural

History of Congenital Heart Defects, 4 died suddenly, without warning; 2 had a left ventricular strain pattern in the electrocardiogram and were shown by cardiac catheterization to have gradients of 55 and 46 mmHg 5 and 6 years prior to death, respectively. The other 2 patients, with no strain pattern, died 1½ years after gradients of 82 and 68 mmHg were documented. Conceivably, with the noninvasive techniques available today, warning might have been obtained either of progressive stenosis or of ischemia related to exercise that would have averted death.[371] Infective endocarditis on the aortic valve poses an extremely serious threat in the form of systemic arterial emboli; the production of serious, chronic aortic regurgitation; or the appearance of sudden catastrophic regurgitation with congestive failure, shock, and death. Surgical mortality, except for those infants in the first 2 months of life, is relatively low, being in the range of 2 percent among the 179 patients operated on in the joint study. Six percent of survivors developed serious aortic regurgitation. In that study, only one-third of the survivors had systolic pressure gradients of less than 25 mmHg, while another third had residual gradients ranging between 25 and 50 mmHg. The final third were found to have either recurrent or residual gradients above 50 mmHg, and half of these were in the severe range. Of the 26 patients undergoing two postoperative catheterizations, 6, or about 20 percent, could be documented to be developing significant restenosis.[371] Surgery, then, while reducing the risk of sudden death and relieving symptoms, is palliative in most if not all instances. Despite evidence of improved myocardial perfusion, persistent elevation of left ventricular end-diastolic pressures by catheterization and left ventricular hypertrophy by echocardiogram indicate that the heart seldom returns to a completely normal state.[375,378]

Medical Management
Infants with the characteristic murmur detected in the first weeks of life should be observed very carefully to be certain that the obstruction is not severe. Those who develop failure should be operated on without delay. Beyond infancy yearly reexaminations usually are adequate. Careful questioning regarding symptoms, a thorough cardiac examination including recording of blood pressure, yearly electrocardiograms, periodic echocardiograms and exercise electrocardiograms, and less frequent chest roentgenograms should prevent progression from going unrecognized. Indications for cardiac catheterization include the appearance or presence of any symptoms such as fatigue, dyspnea, syncope or angina, a pulse pressure of less than 20 mmHg on physical examination, cardiac enlargement by chest roentgenogram, small anterior forces with an SV_1 of 33 mV or more, flattening or inversion of the T wave in V_6, abnormality of the ST-T segments on exercise testing, or an estimated peak systolic pressure gradient of 50 mmHg or greater by echocardiogram. At present we recommend surgical relief of valvular aortic stenosis with a peak systolic pressure gradient of 75 mmHg or more or if the calculated aortic valve area is 0.5 cm^2/m^2 or less. We would recommend surgery for a systolic pressure gradient as low as 40 mmHg if the patient were clearly symptomatic, the heart enlarged, or the electrocardiogram showed ST-T wave changes. Children with more than mild aortic stenosis are restricted from strenuous organized athletics, isometric exercises, and activities that require a good deal of stamina and produce shortness of breath. Since stenosis is usually progressive and since at least some degree of left ventricular obstruction persists in most children into adult life, even following surgery, it would seem reasonable to counsel the parents of a young child with moderate and perhaps even mild aortic stenosis to channel the youngster's energies into activities and sports that do not require strenuous exercise or stamina and that will not need to be forbidden later. For genetic counseling, the risk of congenital heart disease is estimated at 2 percent for siblings and 4 percent for offspring of affected patients. Aortic stenosis, alone or in conjunction with such defects as ventricular septal defect, patent ductus, or coarctation, is found in about half of affected siblings or offspring.[54]

Surgical Management
Operation is carried out through a median sternotomy incision on total cardiopulmonary bypass with moderate hypothermia and cardioplegia. In infants the aortic valve may be exposed during a brief period of circulatory arrest with hypothermia, cooling and rewarming being provided by a limited period of cardiopulmonary bypass. A transverse oblique aortotomy is made just distal to the aortic valve. Appropriate retractors and traction sutures allow visualization and careful inspection of the entire aortic valve prior to incision of the fused commissures. Care is required to discriminate between true commissures and abortive raphes, incision of the latter producing intolerable aortic valvular regurgitation. Relief of aortic valvular stenosis is accomplished by a carefully placed incision in the middle of each fused but well-supported true commissure (Fig. 36-56).

A conservative attitude is important when treating aortic stenosis in the infant or small child; some degree of residual stenosis is preferred over intolerable aortic regurgitation in infants where aortic valve replacement is virtually impossible.

A second valvotomy can occasionally be performed, but eventual aortic valve replacement due to calcification and restenosis should be anticipated in all children requiring surgical relief of aortic stenosis.[379] We prefer to salvage the child's own valve for as long as possible because the ideal valve substitute for pediatric use does not exist.[380,381] (See

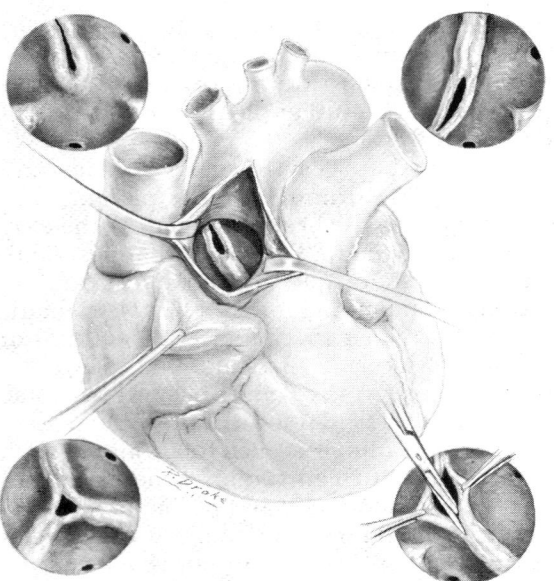

FIGURE 36-56 Types of valvular deformities in patients with congenital valvular aortic stenosis. (*From F. H. Ellis, Jr., and J. W. Kirklin, Congenital Valvular Aortic Stenosis: Anatomic Findings and Surgical Technique, J. Thorac. Surg., 43:199, 1962. Reproduced with permission.*)

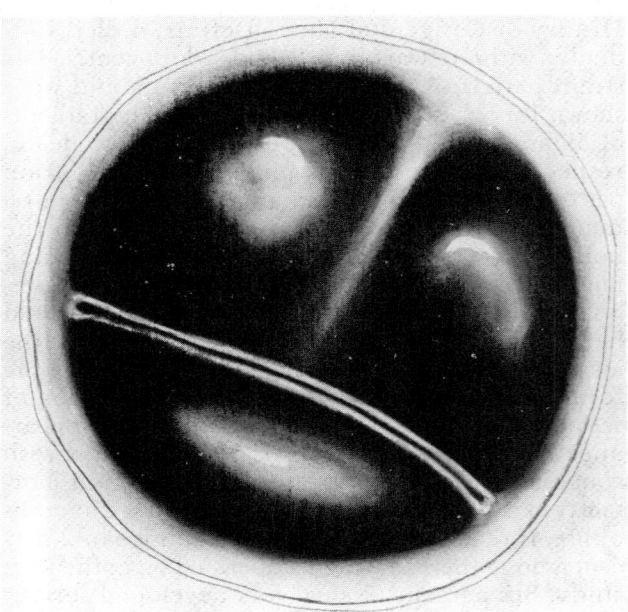

FIGURE 36-57 Congenital bicuspid aortic valve. The conjoined cusp shows a raphe or ridge that runs from the aortic wall onto the cusp and blends with the structure of the latter.

"Congenital Aortic Regurgitation" for further discussion of aortic valve replacement.)

The risks associated with aortic valvotomy in the older child are low; results are excellent.[368,382] Risk of operation is much higher in the critically ill infant[383] in whom the natural history of aortic stenosis is also dismal.[367] Late deaths are usually secondary to a small left ventricle, endocardial fibroelastosis, or arrhythmias.[377,384]

Survival and eventual outcome depend upon the degree to which stenosis can be relieved without the development of intolerable aortic regurgitation. When the aortic valve is tricuspid in configuration a good result can be anticipated.[379] Satisfactory results with some reduction in left ventricular pressure are usually obtained when the valve is bicuspid, but moderate aortic insufficiency is often present postoperatively. A unicommissural valve cannot be opened surgically without the production of severe valvular incompetence.

A small aortic annulus limits severely the degree of relief of left ventricular hypertension which can be achieved without resorting to radical operations in which the annulus is divided and an artificial valve inserted[385] or a conduit placed from the apex of the left ventricle to the descending aorta.[386]

Subvalvular Aortic Stenosis

Pathology

Subvalvular stenosis (Fig. 36-57) may result from one of several anatomic situations. Three classic varieties involve the left ventricular outflow tract primarily: the membranous, the tunnel, and the muscular.[361] The membranous type is characterized by a localized fibrous encirclement of the left ventricular outflow tract a short distance below the aortic valve. The anterior leaflet of the mitral valve is involved in receiving attachment to this membrane. The tunnel type shows hypoplasia of the aortic annulus and a fibrous-lined channel in the subjacent left ventricular outflow tract.[387]

The muscular type is variously known as *asymmetric septal hypertrophy* (ASH), *hypertrophic obstructive cardiomyopathy* (HOCM), or *hypertrophic obstructive subaortic stenosis.* There is major hypertrophy of the left ventricle with accentuation of the hypertrophy in the basal part of the ventricular septum. Overlying the prominence, the mural endocardium may be thickened as a reaction to friction upon this area by the anterior mitral leaflet.[361]

Histologically, the site of asymmetric hypertrophy shows varying abnormalities of the myocardial fibers and their arrangement, commonly called disarray. Similar fibers may be distributed in other ventricular locations, particularly in cases without left ventricular outflow obstruction.[388]

Other forms of subvalvular stenosis result from abnormalities of the mitral valve, including accessory tissue and abnormal adhesions to the ventricular septum of either the anterior mitral leaflet or ectopic chordae emanating from it. Abnormal adhesions may be observed in certain instances of the atrioventricular canal malformation.[389]

Infective endocarditis of the aortic valve is a complication associated particularly with the membranous type of subvalvular stenosis.

Abnormal Physiology

With subvalvular aortic stenosis the systolic pressure immediately below the aortic valve is the same as that in the ascending aorta, while the systolic pressure in the body and apex of the left ventricle is significantly higher by virtue of the fibrous or muscular obstruction.

Clinical Manifestations

Discrete subvalvular aortic stenosis is present in about 9 percent of children with left ventricular outflow tract obstruction.[6] It is more frequent among males, with a male-to-female ratio of approximately 2.5:1.[387]

History The majority of patients are referred because of the detection of a murmur which, not uncommonly, is mistaken initially for that of a ventricular septal defect. Symptoms of fatigue, dyspnea, angina, and syncope have the same implications as they do for valvular aortic stenosis.

Physical Examination The findings are similar to those of valvular aortic stenosis with the exceptions that an early systolic ejection click is not heard at the apex and an early diastolic murmur of aortic regurgitation is present in approximately one-half of these patients. In a few, particularly those with mild obstruction, the murmur may be best heard at the mid left sternal border and may have musical overtones.

Chest Roentgenogram Among patients with uncomplicated subvalvular obstruction, the features will be similar to those of valvular aortic stenosis with the exception that poststenotic dilatation of the ascending aorta will not be seen. The high frequency of associated lesions such as ventricular septal defect, patent ductus, coarctation, and aortic regurgitation may alter this typical pattern significantly in terms of heart size and pulmonary vascularity.

Electrocardiogram The findings are similar to those of valvular aortic stenosis.

Echocardiogram M-mode studies document what appears to be a characteristic narrowing of the left ventricular outflow tract. Systolic fluttering of the aortic valve leaflets and early systolic partial closure of the aortic leaflets are seen in most patients, but the membrane itself is very infrequently demonstrated. Evidence of associated muscular obstruction may be present in the form of asymmetric septal hypertrophy and anterior systolic mitral valve motion.[390] Two-dimensional studies (Fig. 36-58), particularly from the subxiphoid approach, permit excellent visualization of the obstructing membrane or fibromuscular ridge.[391] Estimation of the left ventricular peak systolic pressure and left ventricular–aortic systolic pressure gradient from

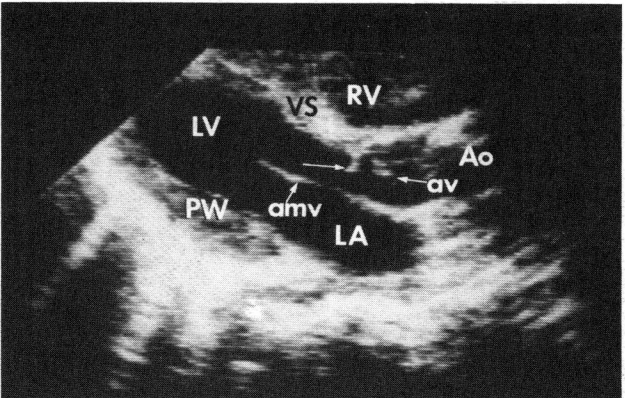

FIGURE 36-58 Two-dimensional echocardiogram in the parasternal, long-axis view from a patient with discrete, fibrous subvalvular aortic stenosis. A thin, discrete membrane (unlabeled arrow) is seen attached to the interventricular septum (VS) in the left ventricular (LV) outflow tract immediately below the aortic valve (av). RV = right ventricle; Ao = ascending aorta; PW = posterior left ventricular wall; amv = anterior leaflet of the mitral valve; LA = left atrium.

M-mode echocardiographic measurements, as described for valvular aortic stenosis, appear valid.[375]

Cardiac Catheterization As with valvular aortic stenosis, a careful pullback pressure tracing across the left ventricular outflow tract is important to document the severity of the gradient and to establish the site of the obstruction. Left ventricular biplane angiography, usually in angled as well as conventional views, will visualize the subvalvular ridge or membrane, its extent, and the presence or absence of associated diffuse outflow tract, annular, or supravalvular narrowing (Fig. 36-59). Since over half of the patients with subvalvular obstruction will have associated intra- or extracardiac malformations, it is important that a careful and complete right-sided and left-sided heart catheterization be performed with appropriate angiography. Supravalvular aortography is recommended to evaluate the degree of aortic regurgitation and eliminate the possibility of associated supravalvular stenosis or patent ductus.

Natural History and Prognosis

Unlike valvular aortic stenosis, severe congestive failure in infancy is unusual with subvalvular aortic stenosis and, if present, is almost invariably associated with complicating defects such as patent ductus, ventricular septal defect, or coarctation. Cardiac catheterization and corrective surgery for the associated lesions may be carried out prior to the discovery of subvalvular aortic obstruction.[371] Obstruction is progressive in most instances, sometimes rapidly so. The associated aortic regurgitation also tends to be progressive and appears to result, at least in part, from prolonged turbulence with secondary thickening and deformity of the valve leaflets. Sudden unexpected death has been described but, fortunately, is rare.[387] Results of surgery depend on

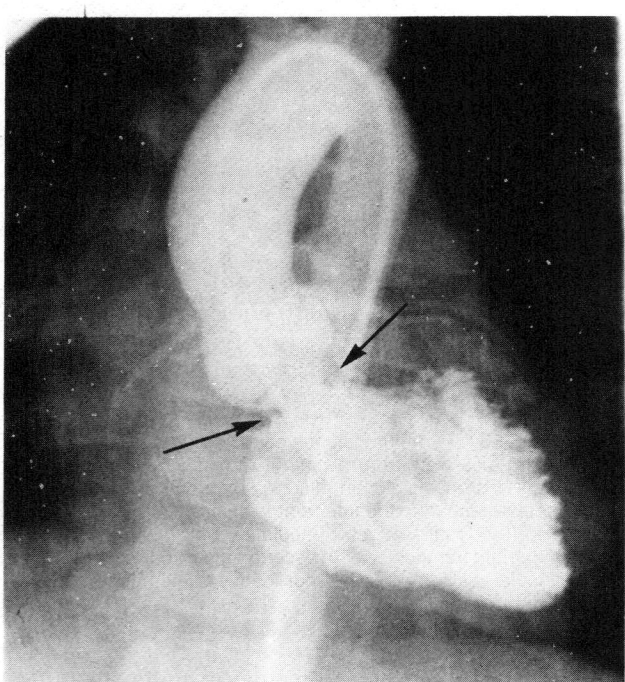

FIGURE 36-59   Posteroanterior view of the left ventricular angiogram from an 8-year-old boy with discrete subvalvular aortic stenosis (arrows) producing a 55 mmHg peak systolic pressure gradient.

the extent of involvement of the entire left ventricular outflow tract, with the best results being obtained in those patients with a thin, discrete subvalvular membrane. Usually good but sometimes disappointing results are obtained among those patients with a more diffuse fibromuscular ridge extending onto and involving the anterior leaflet of the mitral valve.[387] The least satisfactory results in terms of residual gradient or recurring obstruction occur in those patients with tunnel obstruction,[392] or asymmetrical septal hypertrophy.[393]

Medical Management

The medical treatment and indications for surgery are similar to those for patients with valvular aortic stenosis. Surgery usually is recommended for a considerably lower pressure gradient, however, because of the possibility of rapid progression of obstruction, the likelihood of progressive aortic valvular deformity and increasing aortic regurgitation with time, and the likelihood of complete and lasting relief if the membrane can be removed entirely. At present surgery is recommended for those patients with discrete subvalvular obstruction with systolic pressure gradients of 30 mmHg or more. For those patients with severe tunnel subaortic obstruction, either a plastic reconstruction of the outflow tract with seating of a prosthetic valve in the subannular position[394] or venting of the left ventricle via a valved conduit from the left ventricular apex to the descending aorta[386] appear to be the only options.

Continued follow-up for the assessment of reobstruction, progression of aortic regurgitation, and a reemphasis of the precautions against infective endocarditis are essential in all patients.

Surgical Management

Left ventricular outflow tract obstruction below the level of the aortic valve is approached through the aortic root in a manner similar to that described for the aortic valve itself (Fig. 36-60). The use of a nasal speculum and special retractors to protect the aortic valve leaflets allows exposure of the subaortic fibromuscular tissue which is attached to the ventricular septum and the anterior leaflet of the mitral valve. Traction sutures or tiny nerve hooks are placed in the obstructing tissue to pull it clearly into view. The abnormal tissue is then excised from the ventricular septum and the anterior leaflet of the mitral valve, care being taken to avoid trauma in the area of the bundle of His and to the mitral valve leaflet.[395] The aortic valve leaflets must be carefully protected to avoid accidental fenestration of the base of a cusp. Extensive excision is possible only beneath the contingent right and left coronary arterial leaflets.

Diffuse tunnel obstruction in the left ventricular outflow tract poses a very difficult therapeutic problem,[396] perhaps best treated by insertion of a valve-containing conduit from the apex of the left ventricle to the descending or abdominal aorta.[386]

The recognition that subaortic stenosis can occur in association with a ventricular septal defect is important and demands special intraoperative consideration.[397]

Even though immediate and early operative results are quite good, residual, recurrent, and progressive fibromuscular subaortic obstruction is well documented, demanding continued reevaluation.[398]

Treatment of idiopathic hypertrophic subaortic stenosis (IHSS) or asymmetric septal hypertrophy

FIGURE 36-60   Localized subvalvular aortic stenosis. Obstruction is immediately upstream from the aortic valve. (*From J. W. Kirklin and F. H. Ellis, Jr., Surgical Relief of Diffuse Subvalvular Aortic Stenosis, Circulation, 24:739, 1961. Reproduced with permission.*)

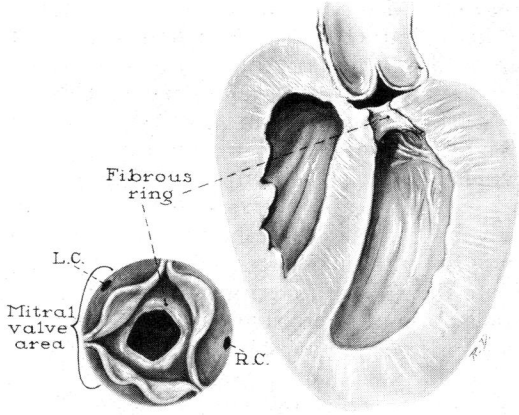

by transaortic septal myotomy and myectomy[399] is discussed elsewhere.

Supravalvular Aortic Stenosis

Pathology

In supravalvular stenosis the obstruction is in the ascending aorta downstream from the coronary ostia (Fig. 36-53). The three types are (1) hourglass, (2) hypoplastic, and (3) membranous.[400] The process may be viewed as more widespread than the valvular or subvalvular types, as it tends to be associated with obstruction in the pulmonary trunk,[401] peripheral pulmonary arteries, and branches of the aortic arch; valvular abnormalities, including myxomatous mitral valve; deformities of the mandible;[402,403] and mental retardation.[401–403]

The hourglass type may be associated with coronary arterial stenosis[400] or atresia of the left coronary artery.[404]

Among the complications specific to this type of aortic stenosis are hypertrophy of the coronary arterial walls and premature coronary atherosclerosis.

Abnormal Physiology

With supravalvular aortic stenosis, the systolic pressure in the chamber immediately above the aortic valve is the same as that in the left ventricle but significantly higher than that in the aorta above the obstruction. The diastolic pressure in the chamber is essentially the same as in the aorta. The arterial systolic pressure in the subclavian artery which originates from the brachiocephalic artery is higher than in the other subclavian artery; i.e., the right subclavian and brachial artery systolic pressures are higher than the left unless there is dextrocardia.[405,406]

Clinical Manifestations

Supravalvular stenosis may be familial,[407] associated with characteristic facies and mental retardation,[408] sporadic,[409] or, rarely, the result of congenital rubella.[410] All forms may, and usually are, associated with varying degrees of peripheral or branch pulmonary arterial stenosis. The familial form is transmitted as an autosomal dominant trait with variable expression. Mental retardation is not present and there are no characteristic facial features. Supravalvular aortic stenosis associated with mental retardation, frequently called Williams' syndrome, is sporadic and associated with a high, prominent forehead, epicanthal folds, underdevelopment of the bridge of the nose and mandible, and a broad, overhanging upper lip (Fig. 36-61). It has been linked with idiopathic hypercalcemia of infancy, but in the majority of patients recognized beyond infancy hypercalcemia is not present.[408]

History In general the symptoms are similar to those of valvular and subvalvular aortic stenosis, although critical obstruction with congestive failure in

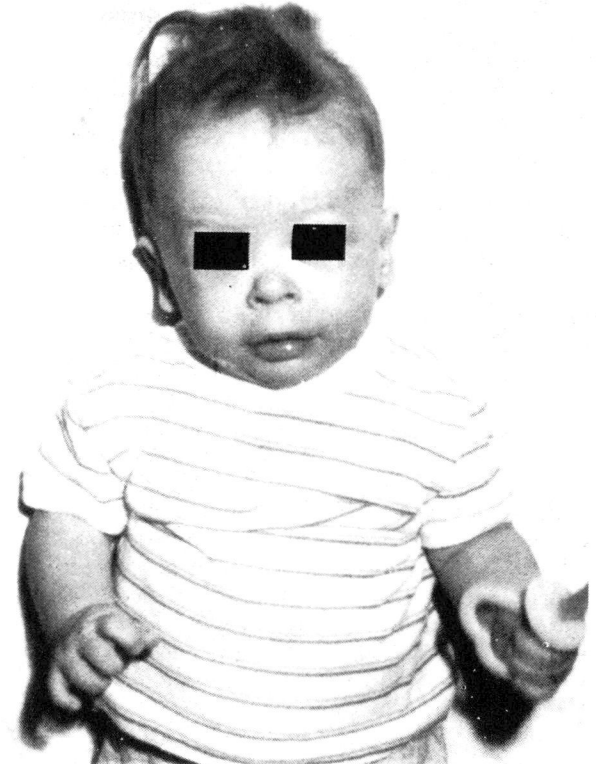

FIGURE 36-61 Photograph of a 14-month-old male infant with severe supravalvular aortic stenosis, mild supravalvular pulmonary stenosis, mental retardation, and the characteristic facies of Williams' syndrome.

the neonatal period is exceedingly rare.[3] Those with characteristic facies and mental retardation usually have a history of irritability, vomiting, and hypotonia in early life, an observation lending support to the hypothesis of hypercalcemia in these infants. Those with the familial form usually have a distinctive family history, but one which seldom emerges in its entirety on initial questioning.

Physical Examination A systolic thrill, frequently very prominent, can be felt over the carotid arteries, in the suprasternal notch, and, to a lesser degree, at the right upper sternal border area. The midsystolic murmur is maximal in the same areas and somewhat less well heard along the right upper sternal border. The murmur of mitral regurgitation may also be present. Usually no systolic ejection click is heard. A systolic blood pressure difference may be recorded between the two arms and, on occasion, between the arms and legs as well, since coarctation is occasionally present in these patients. The characteristic facies are described above.

Chest Roentgenogram No dilatation of the ascending aorta will be seen. Considerable cardiac enlargement and left atrial dilatation may be present with significant mitral regurgitation.

Electrocardiogram The findings are similar to those of other forms of aortic stenosis with the exception that right ventricular hypertrophy may be present if associated pulmonary arterial stenosis is severe.

Echocardiogram M-mode technique may demonstrate the narrowed diameter of the aortic lumen just distal to the aortic valve, but two-dimensional technique visualizes this much more clearly and permits an estimation of the degree of severity both in terms of narrowing of the aortic lumen and the extent of ascending aortic involvement.[411]

Cardiac Catheterization A systolic pressure gradient can be demonstrated just above the aortic valve by careful pullback pressure tracings from the left ventricular cavity to the aortic arch. Supravalvular aortography or left ventricular angiography will visualize the supravalvular narrowing (Fig. 36-62). Pressure recordings in the branch pulmonary arteries should be obtained and right ventricular or pulmonary arterial angiography performed in the presence of any significant right ventricular systolic pressure elevation to rule out associated stenoses of the pulmonary arteries.

Natural History and Prognosis

The sequence of progressive obstruction, the appearance of symptoms and electrocardiographic changes, and the possibility of sudden death appears to apply for this malformation as well as for valvular aortic stenosis. Infective endocarditis rep-

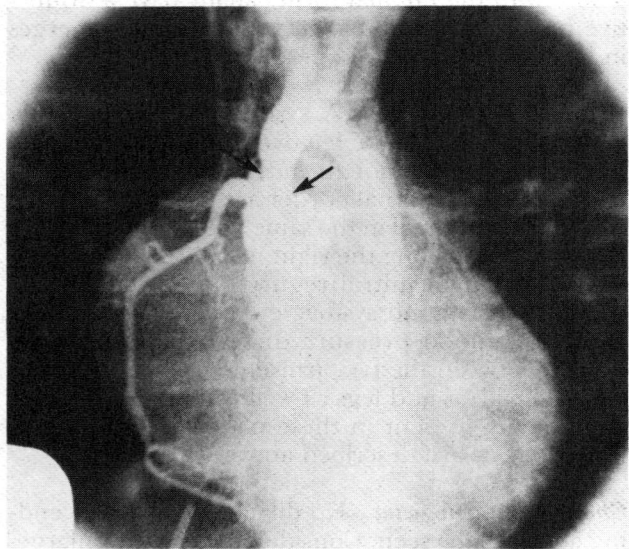

FIGURE 36-62 Posteroanterior view of the aortogram from an infant with severe supravalvular aortic stenosis (arrows) and hypoplasia of the ascending aorta. Contrast material in the left ventricle is the result of catheter-induced aortic regurgitation.

resents a threat to these patients throughout life. Surgical relief of the obstruction may be complicated by marked hypoplasia and diffuse thickening of a considerable length of the ascending aorta. In these circumstances plastic revision or replacement of the entire hypoplastic segment of aorta is necessary. In addition a few patients will have severe pulmonary arterial stenoses which may or may not be amenable to repair and the presence of which may increase the risk of aortic surgery considerably.

Medical Management

The indications for cardiac catheterization and surgery are the same as for valvular aortic stenosis. The patient and the parents of the patient with the familial variety of supravalvular aortic stenosis will need genetic counseling. The parents of the child with mental retardation also will benefit from genetic counseling, from referral to resources which aid in the care and training of these children, and, eventually, from advice regarding contraception for the retarded adolescent female.

Surgical Management

Discrete supravalvular aortic stenosis is relieved by placement of a longitudinal incision across the narrow portion of the ascending aorta, the incision being carried well down into the noncoronary sinus of Valsalva (Fig. 36-63). Ridges of obstructing fibrous tissue are excised and the aorta is enlarged by the insertion of a gusset of prosthetic vascular graft material to increase the circumference at the point of aortic constriction.[412,413] Rigidity of the aortic wall at the site of constriction and fibrous thickening may prevent the aorta from opening up adequately even after insertion of the usual oval gusset. An extended aortoplasty in which the fibrous ring is incised at two points, the aorta being further enlarged with a tailored tubular Dacron prosthesis, has been successfully applied in several patients with this problem.[414] A good result can be expected postoperatively in most cases of *discrete* supravalvular aortic stenosis.

Diffuse tubular hypoplasia of the ascending aorta is a technically challenging problem associated with a high mortality and poor postoperative hemodynamic results.[415,416] Use of a conduit from the apex of the left ventricle to the descending or abdominal aorta is appealing,[386] although most attempts at repair have used an extensive prosthetic enlargement of the ascending aorta.

Aortic valvular regurgitation and/or stenosis may coexist with supravalvular stenosis. Fusion of commissures should be relieved at the time of aortoplasty, but treatment of valvular insufficiency should await postoperative reassessment. Intimal obstruction of the coronary arterial ostia may require debridement, dilatation, or even saphenous vein bypass grafting.[416]

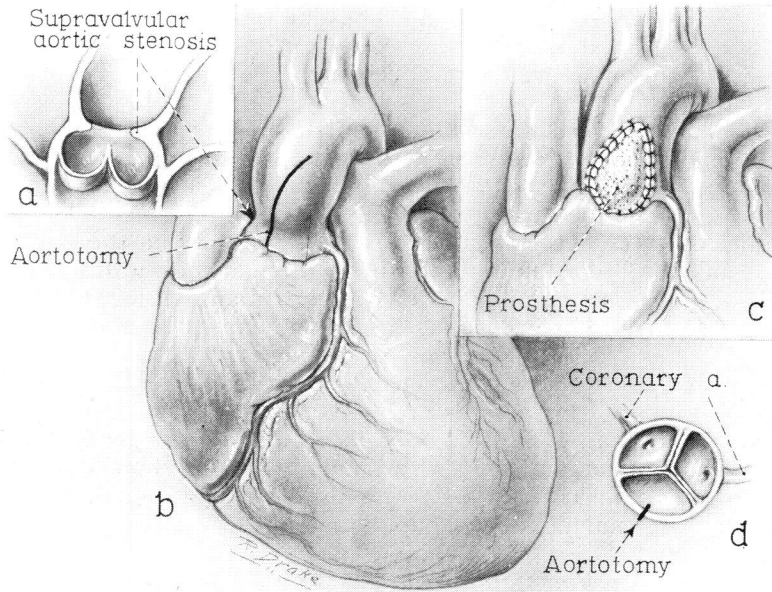

FIGURE 36-63 *a* to *d*. Supravalvular aortic stenosis and its repair. Obstruction is almost diaphragmatic in nature (*a*) and is not easily recognized externally (*b*). *c*. The complete repair. (*From D. C. Mc-Goon, H. T. Mankin, P. Vlad, and J. W. Kirklin, The Surgical Treatment of Supra-valvular Aortic Stenosis, J. Thorac. Cardiovasc. Surg., 41:125, 1961. Reproduced with permission.*)

Bicuspid Aortic Valve

Definition
In congenital bicuspid aortic valve two cusps represent the aortic valve.

Pathology
Classically, the cusps are oriented anteriorly and posteriorly, the anterior or conjoined cusp being the larger, and from its sinus the two coronary arteries arise. A raphe, or ridge, is present along the aortic aspect of the larger cusp. The ridge runs from the aortic wall toward or to the free edge of the cusp (Fig. 36-57). In some cases the ridge may be tall and even bifid, resembling the ridge of an acquired bicuspid valve.[417]

Associated Conditions It has been estimated that the congenital bicuspid valve occurs in up to 2 percent of the population, and in most of these no significant associated malformation is present.[370] The most common associated conditions of significance are coarctation of the aorta and interruption of the aortic arch. Origin of the posterior descending coronary artery from the left circumflex artery has been observed in about 30 percent of cases with biscuspid aortic valves, in contrast to an incidence of such arterial origin in about 10 percent of subjects with tricuspid aortic valves.[418]

Complications Some individuals with bicuspid valves reach the age of three score and ten or older without significant complications. These are in the minority.[370] The most common complication is calcification of the valve with resulting stenosis. In about 85 percent of cases of calcific aortic stenosis the fundamental valve is congenitally bicuspid. Aortic regurgitation from prolapse of the larger cusp is

a less common complication and usually is not evident until adolescence or adult life. Infectious endocarditis is a significant potential complication and may occur at any age. Dissecting aneurysm of the aorta may complicate the bicuspid aortic valve, whether or not it is associated with calcific stenosis and/or coarctation of the aorta.[419]

Abnormal Physiology[370]
Although it may occasionally produce significant aortic stenosis or regurgitation in infancy or childhood, it is statistically more important in middle and later periods of life when it is the most common underlying cause of isolated calcific aortic stenosis.

Clinical Manifestations
The incidence of this malformation approaches 2 percent and makes it the most common congenital abnormality of the heart or great vessels. Its importance lies in its frequent association with other forms of congenital heart disease, its predisposition to become stenotic as a result of fibrosis and deposition of calcium over the course of years, its tendency to become regurgitant, and, finally, in its susceptibility to infective endocarditis. A bicuspid aortic valve is found, then, among patients with coarctation of the aorta, primary endocardial fibroelastosis, isolated ventricular septal defect, and atrioventricular canal malformations.[6] It is also found among patients with valvular aortic stenosis, where bicuspid aortic valve is the underlying malformation in some 60 percent of patients between the ages of 15 and 65 years,[420] patients with isolated or dominant aortic regurgitation, patients with infective endocarditis with or without a history of predisposing heart disease, and, probably most frequently, among otherwise normal individuals who come to the physician's attention because of unrelated illnesses. The incidence among

DISEASES OF THE HEART AND BLOOD VESSELS

males is approximately 2.5 times that among females.

History Patients with uncomplicated bicuspid aortic valve are asymptomatic, while those with aortic stenosis, aortic regurgitation, or infective endocarditis have symptoms related to these complications.

Physical Examination The characteristic feature is auscultatory and consists of an early systolic, loud, high-pitched ejection sound or click that is best heard at the apex and does not vary with respiration. This sound follows the first heart sound by 43 to 91 ms and can be demonstrated to coincide with the halting of the opening movement of the aortic valve cusps. The aortic component of the second heart sound is usually accentuated at the apex unless the leaflets are fibrotic or calcified. A soft, early, or midsystolic murmur of no greater than grade 3 intensity frequently is present at the right upper sternal border. Less commonly, a soft murmur of aortic regurgitation may be heard. In patients with a demonstrated pressure difference between the left ventricle and aorta, the aortic ejection sound occurs slightly earlier, about 30 to 65 ms after the first heart sound.[421]

Chest Roentgenogram No abnormality will be noted with uncomplicated bicuspid aortic valve, but the presence of aortic stenosis or aortic regurgitation will usually produce dilatation of the ascending aorta and, if significant, a left ventricular contour to the overall cardiac silhouette. Among older patients calcification of the aortic valve may be seen. (See Chap. 38.)

Electrocardiogram The only abnormalities would be those reflecting complications of aortic stenosis or regurgitation. (See Chap. 38.)

Echocardiogram Eccentric closure of the aortic valve leaflets within the aortic lumen is characteristic of bicuspid aortic valve and this can be demonstrated using the M-mode technique (Fig. 36-64). The eccentricity index (EI), measured at the onset of diastole as the ratio of one-half the width of the aortic lumen divided by the minimum distance from the aortic cusp echoes to the nearest aortic margin, is 1.3 or greater in approximately 75 percent of individuals with a bicuspid aortic valve. The EI among individuals with a tricuspid aortic valve does not exceed 1.25. The only exceptions to this are found among patients with a high ventricular septal defect, particularly those with prolapse of an aortic valve leaflet.[422] (See Chap. 38.)

Cardiac Catheterization In most instances, the distinction between a tricuspid and bicuspid aortic valve can be made by high-quality selective aortography.[422]

Natural History and Prognosis

It is generally accepted that the majority, if not all, of congenitally bicuspid aortic valves are nonobstructive at birth, but with the passage of time a few of these valves will become fibrotic, stiffer, and more obstructive, and eventually be the site of calcium deposition. Uncommonly, this process of fibrosis, deformity, and stenosis may be rapid enough to produce severe obstruction during childhood; but it is primarily among individuals between the ages of 15

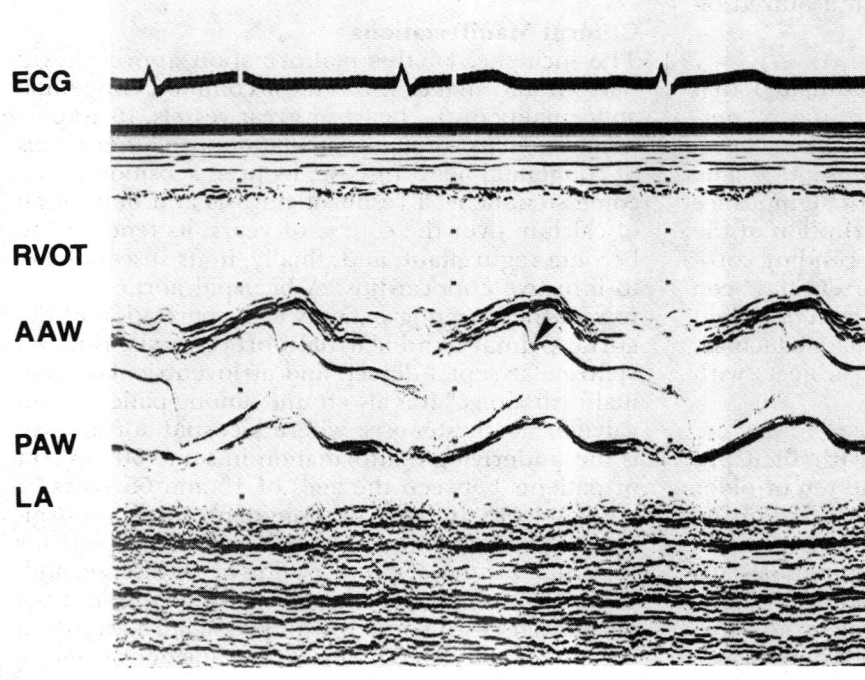

FIGURE 36-64 Echocardiogram from a patient with a bicuspid aortic valve. Eccentric aortic valve closure is present (arrow) with an eccentricity index of 1.6 (see text). ECG = electrocardiogram; RVOT = right ventricular outflow tract; AAW = anterior aoritc wall; PAW = posterior aortic wall; LA = left atrium.

and 65 that one finds the bicuspid valve as the most common cause of serious aortic valvular obstruction. Important calcium deposition is unusual before the age of 30, whereas large, grossly visible deposits of calcium are present in the valves of virtually all patients with severe stenosis beyond that age. A much smaller number of individuals born with a bicuspid aortic valve will develop isolated aortic regurgitation. In approximately one-third, this will be the result of fibrosis and retraction of the leaflets, and in the remainder regurgitation will be the result of infective endocarditis on an apparently functionally normal bicuspid valve. Why one individual with a bicuspid valve will develop stenosis, another regurgitation, and still others live a functionally normal life is not known. It is estimated that among these individuals with an aortic ejection sound but no evidence of aortic stenosis or regurgitation, the passage of a decade will find about 12 percent to have developed aortic stenosis. The majority of these will be beyond the age of 45 at that point and will have evidence of calcium deposition. Mild aortic regurgitation will have been developed by 6 percent, 8 percent will have experienced infective endocarditis, 8 percent will have died of unrelated causes, and a little over 60 percent will have remained without complications.[423] (See Chap. 38.)

Medical Management

Patients suspected of having a bicuspid aortic valve should be followed expectantly, without restrictions but with particular attention paid to the prevention of infective endocarditis.

Surgical Management

Operation is required only when significant aortic stenosis or regurgitation is present. (See "Valvular Aortic Stenosis" and "Congenital Aortic Regurgitation.")

Congenital Aortic Regurgitation

Definition

Under this heading is included the condition in which aortic regurgitation results from a primary anomaly of the aortic valve. Aortic regurgitation resulting from complications of congenital disease is not included, as, for example, aortic regurgitation following infectious endocarditis of a bicuspid valve. Such conditions as shunts from the aorta or major arteries that may simulate aortic regurgitation are also not included.

Pathology

Two principal anomalies underlie the uncommon condition of aortic regurgitation as defined. These are congenital bicuspid aortic valve and cystic medial necrosis of the aorta, as in Marfan's syndrome.

In the first condition, prolapse of the larger of the two cusps is the cause.[424] In extensive cystic me-

dial necrosis of the aorta incompetence of the valve results from dilatation of the aorta or associated flappy aortic valve or the two together.

Associated Conditions In bicuspid aortic valve with primary regurgitation some, but not all, cases are associated with coarctation of the aorta. In extensive cystic medial necrosis some cases show the body features of Marfan's syndrome. Features of associated mitral valve prolapse may be present.

Complications The complications of congenital aortic regurgitation are no different from acquired types of aortic regurgitation. (See Chap. 38.)

Clinical Manifestations

True aortic valvular regurgitation as an isolated entity is unusual among children and particularly unusual among infants. In most instances isolated regurgitation is related to a congenital bicuspid aortic valve as described above.[420] Aortic regurgitation also is recognized in association with valvular, subvalvular, or supravalvular aortic stenosis; coarctation of the aorta; ventricular septal defect with prolapse of one or more aortic valve cusps; fibroelastosis; or during or after an episode of infective endocarditis. It may also develop as a consequence of connective tissue disorders such as cystic medial necrosis with or without the stigmata of Marfan's syndrome, osteogenesis imperfecta, Ehlers-Danlos syndrome, relapsing polychondritis, and ankylosing spondylitis. Occasionally, the diastolic murmur of pulmonary regurgitation, particularly in the presence of pulmonary arterial hypertension, may be confused with that of aortic regurgitation, and the diastolic murmurs heard with a coronary arterial fistula or even patent ductus arteriosus may simulate aortic regurgitation in individual patients. In the newborn, the diastolic murmurs of aortic–left ventricular tunnel and truncal valve insufficiency with truncus arteriosus may simulate that of isolated aortic regurgitation. The history, physical, and laboratory findings are characteristic of valvular aortic regurgitation in adults. (See Chap. 38.)

Natural History, Prognosis, and Medical Management

Mild and even moderate isolated aortic valvular regurgitation usually is well tolerated during childhood with slow or barely detectable progression in most patients. Catastrophic acceleration of this course may be associated with complicating infective endocarditis.[425] Careful assessment of the possible etiologies of aortic regurgitation is recommended because of the differing natural history and approach to therapy with each associated disease or malformation. Medical management of isolated valvular aortic regurgitation may include, as necessary, restriction of activity, digitalis, diuretics, and vasodilators, but valve replacement is recommended for patients with more than moderate regurgitation.

Surgical Management

Surgical correction of congenital aortic regurgitation almost always requires aortic valve replacement, a difficult procedure at best in small children. A possible exception is the suspension valvuloplasty advocated for the management of aortic regurgitation associated with supracristal (type I) ventricular septal defects.[426,427] Small prosthetic valves are intrinsically obstructive. The need for a larger valve and an annulus-enlarging procedure must be anticipated if the child survives and grows following initial valve replacement.

Porcine heterografts have proved unsatisfactory as a valve substitute in children.[428] We prefer the Bjork-Shiley tilting disk prosthesis for use in children, even though mechanical prosthetic valves require the administration of anticoagulants to avoid thromboembolic complications.[429]

When aortic valve replacement has been required in a child, we have been pleased with the results of enlarging the aortic annulus by incision across the annulus in the noncoronary sinus of Valsalva into the anterior leaflet of the mitral valve.[430] A gusset of low-porosity prosthetic vascular graft material is placed in the defect thus created; a considerably larger valve may then be inserted.

We have also enlarged the aortic annulus by creation of a ventricular septal defect, extending the aortotomy incision into the outflow tract of the right ventricle between the right and left coronary arteries.[431] Again, a prosthetic gusset is inserted to increase the circumference of the annulus. This is a technically more difficult operation and the likelihood of postoperative complete heart block is greater, but the annular circumference gained is quite a bit more than with the simpler operation described above.

Aortic regurgitation secondary to cystic medial necrosis may require composite replacement of the aortic valve and the ascending aorta, the coronary arteries usually being reimplanted into the aortic graft.[432]

In older children and adults, aortic valve replacement provides quite satisfactory treatment of congenital aortic regurgitation.

Aortic–Left Ventricular Tunnel

Definition

Aortic–left ventricular tunnel is a channel beginning in the ascending aorta, proceeding into the epicardium, and then penetrating the ventricular septum to empty into the subaortic region of the left ventricle.

Pathology

The aortic aspect of the anomalous channel lies in the anterior wall of the aorta, slightly above the levels of the origins of the coronary arteries. At its beginning, and while in the epicardium, the channel has an arterial structure. While in the ventricular septum, it exhibits a sinusoidal structure. While in the ventricular septum, the tunnel lies in the posterior wall of the right ventricular infundibulum and may distort the structure of the latter. In the same position it lies close to the aortic valve.[433]

The left ventricle shows eccentric hypertrophy and there is major dilatation of the ascending aorta.

Associated Conditions A fibrotic, sometimes bicuspid, aortic valve may be associated.

Complications In its epicardial segment the tunnel may develop a saccular aneurysm.[433] The principal complications are those associated with excessive diastolic volume of the left ventricle and are comparable to those of classic aortic regurgitation. Incompetence of the aortic valve may also occur.[434]

Clinical Manifestations

This very rare malformation, which characteristically presents in very early infancy, is amenable to correction and is seldom associated with other defects.

History The majority of infants are only mildly symptomatic in the first week or two after birth, presumably due to compensatory myocardial hypertrophy developed in utero. A few develop congestive heart failure within the first day or two of life, and the majority develop symptoms of dyspnea, easy fatigue with activity, and growth failure as the weeks and months go by.

Physical Examination Physical findings are those of gross aortic regurgitation. Bounding arterial pulses, sometimes visible, a wide pulse pressure, and a hyperdynamic left ventricular lift are characteristic. The murmur usually is to-and-fro, but the diastolic component is almost invariably louder than the systolic. It is inclined to be harsh and is frequently associated with a thrill at the left sternal border.

Chest Roentgenogram The heart is enlarged with a left ventricular configuration and the ascending aorta is impressively dilated. Pulmonary venous congestion may be present in very symptomatic patients.

Electrocardiogram Left ventricular hypertrophy is present from birth in the majority of patients. ST- and T-wave changes of myocardial ischemia are present at the outset or may develop with time.

Cardiac Catheterization The characteristic abnormality is visualized best with selective aortography in the ascending aorta. A paravalvular tunnel, seen best in the lateral view, creates a mass anterior and superior to the aortic valve and slightly to the left of the aortic root in the frontal projection. Marked ascending aortic dilatation and left ventricular dilatation are characteristic (Fig. 36-65).

Natural History and Prognosis

In most instances, the characteristic loud diastolic murmur is heard within the first 3 months of life, frequently within the first few days. Although the hemodynamic burden is tolerated reasonably well in most patients initially, the course appears to be one of progressive paravalvular regurgitation and progressive dilatation of the aortic root and left ventricle. Sudden onset of congestive failure and sudden death have been described. There is reason to believe that turbulence within the aortic root and progressive aortic root dilatation lead to secondary aortic valvular regurgitation with the passage of time.[435]

Medical Management

Prompt cardiac catheterization and early repair of this defect are recommended before the deformity of the ascending aorta, aortic ring, and the aortic valves themselves produce permanent aortic valvular regurgitation.[435,436] The natural history of the intracardiac portion of the tunnel following surgical closure of the aortic opening is unclear, but in the majority of patients it appears to persist without complications. Long-term follow-up of these patients is indicated to monitor any residual aortic regurgitation or stenosis and enforce the precautions against infective endocarditis.

Surgical Management

This rare anomaly should be repaired as soon as the diagnosis is established to avoid progressive dilatation of the tunnel, deformity of the aortic valve with aortic valvular regurgitation or left ventricular outflow tract obstruction, and elevation of the posterior wall of the right ventricle with right ventricular outflow tract obstruction.[437]

Operation is carried out through a median sternotomy incision. The patient is supported on cardiopulmonary bypass with hypothermia and cardioplegia. The aorta is opened cephalad to the aortic end of the tunnel. The orifice is identified within the aorta and distinguished from the nearby orifice of the right coronary artery. The aortic end of the tunnel is closed by direct suture or the placement of a small patch, care being taken to avoid injury to the right coronary arterial orifice and the right coronary cusp of the aortic valve. The use of a patch is believed to reduce the likelihood of aortic regurgitation being produced by deformity and separation of the leaflet edges.[436] In most reported cases the ventricular end of the tunnel has not been closed due to inaccessibility and the fear of injury to the conduction system. In a few cases the tunnel has been obliterated by sutures placed a short distance away from the point of entry into the ventricle.[438] Results have been satisfactory in the few reported cases, although recurrence of the tunnel has required a second operation. The tissue in which sutures must be placed for obliteration of the tunnel may be quite thin and friable.

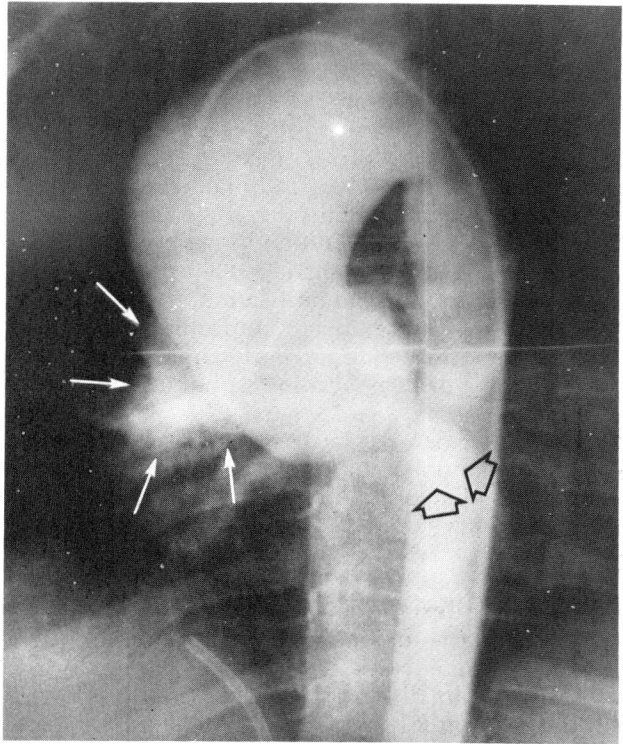

A

B

FIGURE 36-65 Posteroanterior (A) and lateral (B) view of the aortogram from a newborn infant with aortic–left ventricular tunnel. The tortuous channel (solid arrows) lies superior to the origin of the right coronary artery (RCA), and anterior and to the right of the aortic root. Contrast material in the left ventricular outflow tract (open arrows) appears after opacification of the tunnel. (*The Department of Cardiology, Children's Hospital Medical Center, Boston, Massachusetts. Reproduced with permission.*)

Aortic Atresia

Definition
In aortic atresia the region of the aortic valve shows no patency.

Pathology
Usually, the ventricular septum is intact and the aorta is normally related to the pulmonary trunk and the left ventricle. The atretic segment lies proximal to the coronary arterial origins. The left ventricle shows major hypertrophy of its wall, but the cavity is tiny and the mitral valve, although formed, is hypoplastic, as is the left ventricular cavity (Fig. 36-66). The right-sided heart chambers are enlarged and the ventricle hypertrophied.[439,440] The usual route of escape of blood from the left side of the heart is at the foramen ovale, of which the valve is herniated into the right atrium. Rarely, when the foramen ovale is sealed or narrow, alternate routes for the flow of blood are present. Among these are (1) connection between a pulmonary vein and a systemic vein, and (2) prominent sinusoids in the left ventricular wall which connects the left ventricular cavity with coronary arteries. The ductus arteriosus is wide and the ascending aorta is hypoplastic.

Associated Conditions In exceptional cases a ventricular septal defect is present.[440–442] Under this condition the left ventricular cavity and the mitral valve are near normal in size.

Aortic atresia may be associated with mitral atresia.[440] This combination occurs in about 15 percent of cases of aortic atresia and, when present, has a male-to-female ratio of 3:1 in contrast to a male-to-female ratio of about 10:1 in isolated aortic atresia.

When atresia of the mitral valve is associated, the left ventricle is a tiny blind endocardial-lined cavity in the wall of the right ventricle that usually requires microscopic study for identification.[443]

Coarctation of the aorta manifesting varying degrees of stenosis is common both when aortic atresia appears alone or in association with mitral atresia.[444]

Complications Aortic atresia uncommonly allows survival beyond 1 week of age. The principal complication is that of pulmonary venous obstruction with secondary congestive and edematous states of the lungs.

Clinical Manifestations
Aortic atresia is an uncommon cardiac malformation, but it is the leading cause of death among children with heart disease in the first 2 weeks of life.[3] Although familial occurrence has been reported, the transmission of this defect usually appears to be on a multifactorial basis. The recurrence risk in siblings for this specific defect is approximately 0.5 percent and for all types of congenital heart disease is 2.2 percent.[154] Males are more commonly affected than females in a ratio of 1.8:1.

History The clinical situation usually is that of a 2- or 3-day-old infant, considered entirely well until then, who develops the sudden onset of severe respiratory distress and slate gray cyanosis.

Physical Examination Signs are those of systemic arterial hypoperfusion and congestive failure. Pulses are weak or absent in all areas including the carotids, but may wax and wane initially as the ductus opens and closes. The disparity between the forceful heart action felt on palpation and the weak arterial pulses is striking. The second heart sound is single and loud and a gallop rhythm is frequent. Murmurs, if present at all, usually are soft and nondistinctive. Moist rales and severe hepatomegaly complete the clinical picture.

Chest Roentgenogram Moderate to marked cardiac enlargement is seen with a combination of pulmonary arterial and pulmonary venous engorgement.

Electrocardiogram Right axis deviation and marked right ventricular hypertrophy, frequently with a qR pattern in the right precordial leads, are characteristic. Very rarely, a pattern compatible with left ventricular hypertrophy may be present.

Echocardiogram Both M-mode and two-dimensional studies usually are diagnostic. In both, the

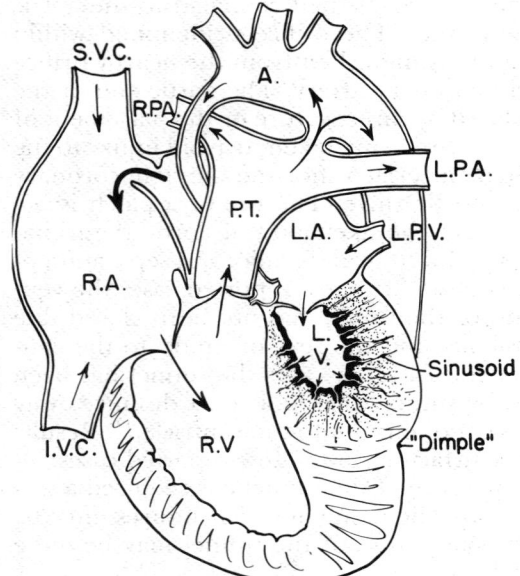

FIGURE 36-66 Diagrammatic portrayal of the central circulation in aortic atresia. The mitral valve is hypoplastic, as is the left ventricle (L.V.). The aortic channel (A.) is supplied from the right ventricle (R.V.) through the ductus arteriosus. Blood flows in a retrograde fashion in the ascending aorta. The only outlet for blood from the left side of the heart is a communication between the left atrium (L.A.) and right atrium (R.A.) at the level of the fossa ovalis (bold arrow). S.V.C. = superior vena cava; I.V.C. = inferior vena cava; P.T. = main pulmonary arterial trunk; R.P.A. = right pulmonary artery; L.P.A. = left pulmonray artery; L.P.V. = left pulmonary vein.

aortic root echoes are small or absent and the mitral valve echoes are small, distorted, or absent. The posterior ventricle is small or nondemonstrable, while the anterior ventricular chamber is large (Fig. 36-67).[445] Easily identifiable anterior tricuspid valve echoes can be seen. Rarely, in the presence of a sizable ventricular septal defect, the left ventricular chamber size and mitral valve echoes may be normal or near normal.[157]

Cardiac Catheterization This invasive study usually is not necessary, but if performed, a large right-to-left shunt will be found at the atrial level with virtually complete mixing of systemic and pulmonary venous blood within the right atrium. Right ventricular and pulmonary arterial systolic pressures will be equal to or, in the case of a closing ductus, greater than those in the systemic circuit. Pulmonary arterial or aortic angiography will demonstrate a greatly dilated main pulmonary artery with a patent ductus supplying the descending aorta and, in a retrograde fashion, the brachiocephalic vessels and the extremely hypoplastic ascending aorta.

Natural History and Prognosis
This malformation is almost invariably fatal, with 80 percent of affected infants dying within the first week and only 6 percent surviving beyond the first month. The mean age of death, related directly to ductal closure and deprivation of flow to the systemic arterial circulation, is 5 days.[440]

Medical Management
Treatment is symptomatic and directed toward the control of congestive failure and the comfort of the patient. Emotional support and genetic counseling for the parents are of utmost importance in this devastating situation. Palliative surgery is not recommended. Rarely, in perhaps 4 percent of infants with aortic atresia, a ventricular septal defect permits normal or near normal development of the left ventricular cavity and mitral valve. In this unusual circumstance, it is conceivable that palliative surgery may be of some benefit.[446]

Surgical Management
Aortic atresia has not been corrected successfully, but possible approaches and morphological features pertinent to surgical consideration have been reviewed.[446] Palliation in management of the hypoplastic left side of the heart syndrome has been reported by Doty[447] and Norwood;[448] these methods are possibly applicable to management of aortic atresia, although one must question the advisability of intervening surgically in this basically lethal defect.

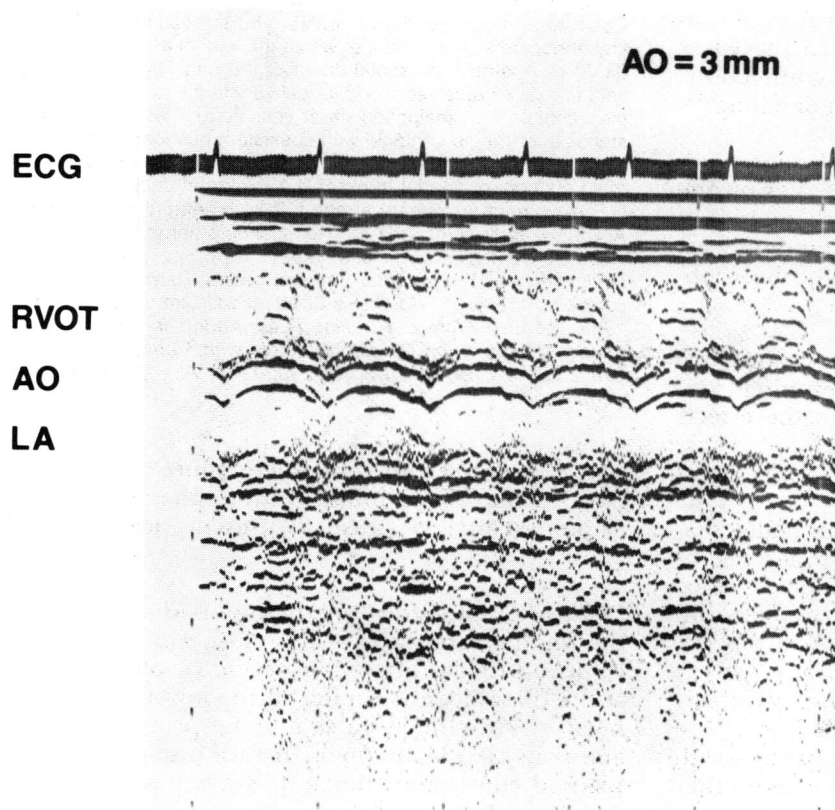

FIGURE 36-67 M-mode echocardiogram from a 2-day-old infant with aortic atresia. An extremely small aortic root diameter (3 mm) and normal left atrial dimension are demonstrated. No aortic valve leaflets could be recorded. ECG = electrocardiogram; RVOT = right ventricular outflow tract; AO = aorta; LA = left atrium.

Mitral Atresia

Definition

Mitral atresia is characterized by the lack of an opening between the left atrium and the ventricular portion of the heart.

Pathology

In most instances, there is a depression at the anticipated location of the mitral valve, but no opening or valvular tissue is present.[449] Uncommonly, valvular tissue without an orifice exists (so-called membranous mitral atresia). In about half the cases, mitral atresia coexists with aortic atresia (Fig. 36-68A), a condition that has been discussed under "Aortic Atresia," above.

The balance of this discussion relates to those cases of mitral atresia with a patent aortic valve (Fig. 36-68B through D).

In about one-half of the cases in which only the mitral valve is atretic, the great vessels are normally related and two ventricles are present, of which the left is relatively hypoplastic, as is the ascending aorta. The ventricular septum shows one or, usually, multiple defects. When the great vessels are malposed, the ventricular portion of the heart exhibits features of a single ventricle either with or without an inverted infundibulum.[449]

The usual route for exit of blood from the left atrium is through the foramen ovale, of which the valve is herniated into the right atrium. When the foramen ovale is sealed or narrow, alternate routes exist, like a vein from the left atrium to a systemic vein (levoatrial cardinal vein) or a vein from a pulmonary vein to a systemic vein.[450,451] In the latter state anomalous pulmonary venous connections may occur between lungs and/or within one lung.[452]

Associated Conditions Coarctation of the aorta and double outlet right ventricle, either together or one alone, is fairly common. In cases with malposed great vessels, pulmonary atresia is uncommonly associated.[453] Straddling tricuspid valve has been observed.[454]

Complications The principal complications are either pulmonary congestive changes resulting from pulmonary venous obstruction or from the effects of a large left-to-right shunt.

Clinical Manifestations

The clinical features of this uncommon malformation are determined by the presence or absence of significant pulmonary stenosis and the presence or absence of adequate left atrial decompression. There is no sex predilection.

History The majority of patients with mitral atresia are detected within the first 2 weeks of life. Those without significant pulmonary stenosis present with respiratory distress that is usually severe, and other

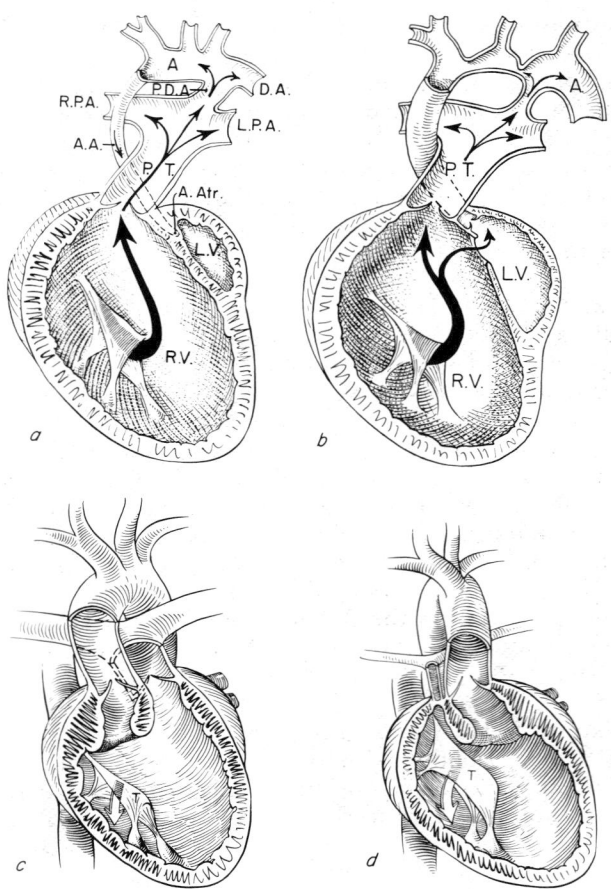

FIGURE 36-68 Variations in intracardiac detail among cases exhibiting mitral atresia. *a* and *b*. Normally related great vessels. *a*. Coexistent mitral and aortic atresia. The left ventricle (L.V.) is a tiny endocardial-lined channel within the wall of the right ventricle (R.V.) *b*. A ventricular septal defect is the route by which the left ventricle (L.V.) received blood for delivery to the aorta (A.). *c*. Single ventricle with malposed great vessels and without pulmonic stenosis. *d*. Single ventricle with coexistent pulmonary atresia, as well as malposed great vessels. A.A. = ascending aorta; P.T. = main pulmonary arterial trunk; P.D.A = patent ductus arteriosus; R.P.A. = right pulmonary artery; L.P.A. = left pulmonary artery; A. Atr. = aortic atresia; D.A. = descending aorta; T. = tricuspid valve. (*a from Eliot and Associates.*[449] *b from E. Chesler, J. H. Moller, and J. E. Edwards, The Congenital Cardiovascular Anomalies Underlying "Reversed Coarctation," Am. Heart J., 75:34, 1968. c and d From L. P. Elliot, R. C. Anderson, and J. E. Edwards, The Common Cardiac Ventricle with Transposition of the Great Vessels, Br. Heart J., 26:289, 1964. All reproduced with permission.*)

symptoms of severe congestive failure and pulmonary edema. Those infants with pulmonary stenosis or pulmonary atresia usually present with severe cyanosis.

Physical Examination Without pulmonary stenosis, the findings are those of dyspnea, a hyperdynamic right ventricular lift, a nonspecific systolic murmur, and a diastolic flow rumble at the lower left sternal border. Pulmonary rales may be present and cyanosis usually is minimal. In rare instances, a low-pitched continuous murmur may be heard at the left sternal border due to flow from the left to the right atrium through an incompetent and restrictive foramen ovale. With pulmonary stenosis, the findings are similar to those of patients with tetralogy of Fallot. With pulmonary atresia, there is usually no murmur and cyanosis is intense.

Chest Roentgenogram Cardiac enlargement, the degree of pulmonary arterial overperfusion, and the severity of pulmonary venous congestion will reflect the presence or absence of pulmonary stenosis and the size of the interatrial opening. Left atrial dilatation rarely is present.

Electrocardiogram Right axis deviation and right atrial and right ventricular hypertrophy are the rule. Left atrial hypertrophy may or may not be present.

Echocardiogram M-mode and two-dimensional techniques will demonstrate absence of mitral valve echoes and will permit estimation of the size of the aortic root and the left ventricular cavity.[455,157]

Cardiac Catheterization There will be a step up in oxygen saturation at the right atrial level, with complete mixing of systemic venous and pulmonary venous blood at that site and beyond. This finding alone should alert the physician to the possibility of mitral atresia. Varying degrees of left atrial and pulmonary arterial wedge hypertension will be present, depending upon the adequacy of left atrial decompression and the volume of pulmonary arterial blood flow. Left atrial angiography is diagnostic. Balloon atrial septostomy should be attempted in all patients under 1 month of age.

Natural History and Prognosis
Rapid deterioration and death within the first few weeks of life either from pulmonary edema or hypoxia is characteristic unless a fortuitous balance of pulmonary stenosis and adequate left atrial decompression exists. Such a natural balance is rare, but if pulmonary blood flow can be adjusted to a near normal level and adequate left atrial runoff ensured by balloon septostomy or surgical atrial septectomy, survival beyond infancy is possible.[456]

Medical Management
Early recognition combined with prompt left atrial decompression and adjustment of pulmonary arterial blood flow either by banding of the pulmonary artery, ligation of a ductus arteriosus, or the creation of a systemic to pulmonary arterial anastomosis are essential. Among survivors there will be a continuing need to maintain pulmonary arterial blood flow at an optimal level and to reassess the adequacy of the interatrial opening, either by repeat cardiac catheterization or two-dimensional echocardiography.

Surgical Management
No operation exists for the total correction of mitral atresia. The usefulness of palliative operations depends upon the adequacy of the interatrial communication, the size of the ventricular septal defect, and the relative degree of right ventricular outflow tract obstruction. Excision of the interatrial septum reduces left atrial hypertension and pulmonary congestion. Pulmonary arterial banding is required when pulmonary blood flow is excessive. The creation of a systemic arterial to pulmonary arterial shunt is helpful when right ventricular outflow tract obstruction is severe. Ductus ligation and coarctation repair may be required. The operative details of these palliative operations are dictated by the specific pathophysiology in each patient.

In a recent review of 40 patients with left atrioventricular valve atresia,[456] 23 patients (56 percent) required palliation. Of these operated patients, 15 died—a mortality of 65 percent. Prognosis was best in patients with mild to moderate pulmonary stenosis and poorest in those with pulmonary atresia. Surgical palliation definitely improved the quality of life and was thus believed to be worthwhile.

Mitral Stenosis

Definition
Mitral stenosis represents an effective barrier between the left atrium and left ventricle during the period of ventricular diastole.

Pathology
The stenotic lesion may be at the inlet to the valve, called the *supravalvular ring,* or at the valve.

The supravalvular ring is a fibrous encirclement at the inlet to the mitral valve, the lesion lying downstream from the left atrial appendage. Varying degrees of this condition may exist, the degree determining whether or not effective stenosis is present.[457,458]

Stenotic lesions at the valve are of two principal types, the *parachute mitral valve* and the *dysplastic mitral valve.*

In the parachute mitral valve only one papillary muscle is present in the left ventricle, and the chordae of the two leaflets converge to insert into this single muscle (Fig. 36-69).[459] Blood must flow in the interchordal spaces to reach the left ventricle, and when these spaces are narrow, mitral stenosis occurs.

In the dysplastic valve the leaflets are nodular and the chordae are poorly developed and unusually short, causing the papillary muscles to be held close to the valvular orifice. Valvular commissures are poorly developed.[460] The condition previously designated as *anomalous mitral arcade* is probably better classified as dysplasia of the valve.

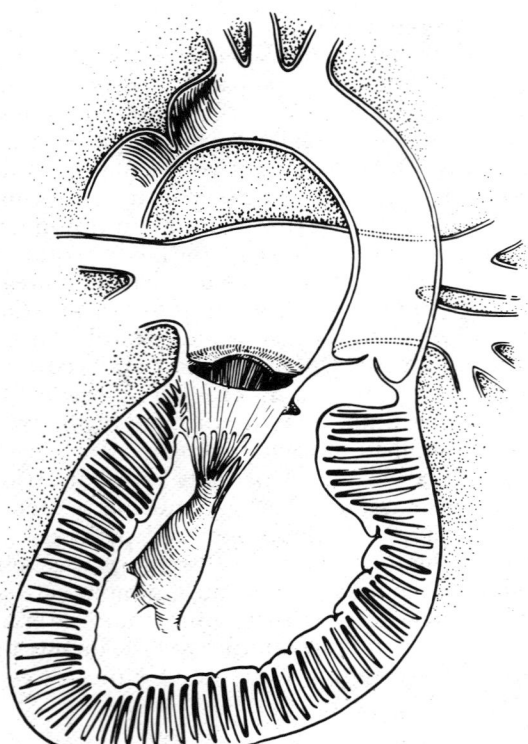

FIGURE 36-69 Diagrammatic portrayal of the four obstructive anomalies in the complex described by Shone and associates. These are (1) stenosing ring of left atrium, (2) parachute deformity of mitral valve, (3) subaortic stenosis, and (4) coarctation of aorta. (*Shone et al.*[459] *Reproduced with permission.*)

Associated Conditions The supravalvular ring may either appear as an isolated condition, or it may be associated with the parachute mitral valve and the other two conditions associated with the parachute valve, namely coarctation of the aorta and subaortic stenosis.[459] A bicuspid aortic valve is commonly present; a ventricular septal defect is uncommon.

The dysplastic mitral valve may be associated with dysplasia of all or any of the other valves and with supravalvular aortic and pulmonary arterial stenosis.

Complications The principal complications are those of pulmonary venous hypertension, the principal effect being either respiratory or right ventricular failure.

Clinical Manifestations

This is a rare malformation found in only 0.42 percent of children with congenital heart disease. Approximately 75 percent of patients so affected have important associated cardiac malformations, and in these situations it is not uncommon for mitral stenosis to be detected for the first time at cardiac catheterization, operation, or postmortem examination. The male-to-female ratio is estimated at 2.2:1.[461]

History Although symptoms may appear during the neonatal period, they are, on the average, most commonly detected in the second year of life. Symptoms consist of exertional dyspnea, cyanosis, episodes of respiratory distress suggesting pulmonary edema, repeated and persistent lower respiratory tract infections, and poor weight gain.

Physical Examinations A prominent right ventricular lift and a loud pulmonary component of the second heart sound reflect right ventricular and pulmonary arterial hypertension. The first heart sound usually is loud at the apex, and an opening snap can be detected in a few patients. The characteristic murmur is a relatively harsh, well-localized, low-pitched diastolic murmur at the apex with presystolic accentuation. The presystolic component helps to distinguish this murmur from that of increased diastolic flow across the mitral valve, which is associated with ventricular septal defect or patent ductus. A thrill to palpation is relatively common. On initial examination, this harsh, abrupt, apical diastolic murmur with a thrill frequently is mistaken for a systolic murmur, particularly if no systolic murmur is present to aid with timing. Soft murmurs of mitral, pulmonary, or tricuspid regurgitation may be heard. In some patients, particularly those with diminished pulmonary blood flow as with tetralogy of Fallot, no murmur is audible.

Chest Roentgenogram Mild to moderate cardiac enlargement is not unusual and generally reflects right ventricular dilatation. Pulmonary venous engorgement, Kerley B lines, and prominence of the left atrium and left atrial appendage are characteristics of important obstruction.

Electrocardiogram Varying degrees of normal or right axis deviation are present with left atrial, right ventricular, and right atrial hypertrophy.

Echocardiogram M-mode study can detect the signs of left ventricular inflow obstruction, namely anterior motion of the posterior valve leaflet during diastole, and a markedly decreased E-to-F slope, diminished excursion, and a reduced rate of diastolic closure of the anterior leaflet, but M-mode study is of limited value in defining the precise structural malformation or providing an estimate of severity.[461,462] Two-dimensional echocardiography appears capable of distinguishing the parachute mitral valve deformity with a single papillary muscle from valvular mitral stenosis and supravalvular stenosis in the form of an obstructing membrane. The distinction between a supravalvular membrane or ring and the membrane of cor triatriatum is less secure.[463]

Cardiac Catheterization A diastolic pressure gradient between the left ventricle and the left atrium is diagnostic. Left atrial or pulmonary arterial wedge hypertension is present in most patients, but in circumstances of reduced pulmonary blood flow or a sizable interatrial opening, this hypertension and the mitral diastolic pressure gradient may only be relative and their significance may go unrecognized. Pulmonary arterial hypertension and elevation of the pulmonary vascular resistance also are characteristic. Left atrial angiography in the right anterior oblique view will show left atrial size and may demonstrate a supravalvular chamber created by a supravalvular ring, restriction of mitral leaflet motion, or a subvalvular funnel converging on a single papillary muscle, which is characteristic of parachute mitral valve. Left ventricular angiography will permit identification of the papillary muscles, evaluation of mitral valve leaflet motion, and an estimate of the breadth and width of the column of unopacified blood entering the ventricle from the left atrium.

Natural History and Prognosis

In general, the outlook for symptomatic infants and young children is poor, since the congenitally malformed mitral apparatus usually does not lend itself to successful palliative or corrective surgery. Exceptions are found among patients with a supravalvular ring, where removal of the ring, usually with additional valvulotomy, may produce excellent and permanent relief of obstruction. Those children able to survive to an age and size when mitral valve replacement is feasible also can expect relief of symptoms and the return of the pulmonary arterial pressure and vascular resistance to normal or near normal levels. Without surgery the course is one of progressive stenosis with increasing pulmonary venous congestion. Dyspnea becomes more pronounced, orthopnea appears, lower respiratory tract infections are more frequent and protracted, and weight gain is slow. There will also be clinical and laboratory evidence of increasing pulmonary arterial hypertension, pulmonary vascular obstructive disease, and right-sided heart failure.

Medical Management

The physician must be alert to the possibility of mitral obstruction in any patient with an apical diastolic murmur or a disproportionate elevation of left atrial pressure as judged either by unusual dyspnea, radiological evidence of pulmonary venous congestion, or by direct measurement at catheterization. This is particularly true among patients with coarctation of the aorta and valvular or subvalvular aortic stenosis, but it also is true for those patients in whom the mitral orifice has not yet been subjected to normal or increased flow. Examples would be patients with tetralogy of Fallot or atrial septal defect in whom corrective or palliative surgery is contemplated. Early study is recommended to identify those patients in whom palliative or corrective surgery would be feasible, as well as those in whom correction of a complicating lesion such as coarcta-

tion of the aorta, ventricular septal defect, patent ductus, or aortic stenosis might permit more successful management. Medical therapy includes the use of digitalis, diuretics, restriction of activity, prompt treatment of respiratory infections, and protection against infective endocarditis. With the exception of those patients with a supravalvular mitral ring, who comprise about 20 percent of individuals with congenital mitral obstruction and in whom palliative or even corrective surgery might be possible, management consists of supportive measures to permit survival until valve replacement is feasible or necessary. In the interim, serial noninvasive or invasive studies are indicated to assess left atrial and pulmonary arterial hypertension and pulmonary vascular resistance.

Surgical Management

The variety of pathological conditions producing mitral valvular stenosis—hypoplastic annulus, commissure fusion, the "hammock valve," the parachute valve, and the funnel-shaped valve—require individualized surgical approaches.[461,464] The mitral orifice is exposed through a median sternotomy incision on cardiopulmonary bypass with moderate hypothermia and cardioplegia. The left atrium is entered posterior to the interatrial groove on the right or through the right atrium and atrial septum. Circulatory arrest with profound hypothermia is used in infants and small children. Depending upon the specific anatomy encountered, fused commissures are incised, thickened chordae are excised, and obstructing subvalvular tissue is fenestrated or excised when possible. The results achieved by these difficult reconstructive valvuloplasty procedures are variable and unpredictable. Overall surgical mortality in children having congenital mitral stenosis in association with other defects is about 50 percent; mortality for operation on the mitral valve alone is about 25 percent.[461]

Mitral valve replacement may be required to achieve adequate relief of obstruction while avoiding intolerable mitral regurgitation. There were 6 early deaths and 2 late deaths following mitral valve replacement in 26 children reported by Berry and his associates at the Mayo Clinic.[465] The small child requiring mitral valve replacement will undoubtedly require the insertion of a larger prosthetic valve as growth occurs. Sequential mitral valve replacement with the necessary enlargement of the mitral annulus has been successfully performed in growing children.[466]

Mitral Regurgitation

Definition

Mitral regurgitation represents incomplete closure of the mitral valve during ventricular systole (Fig. 36-70).

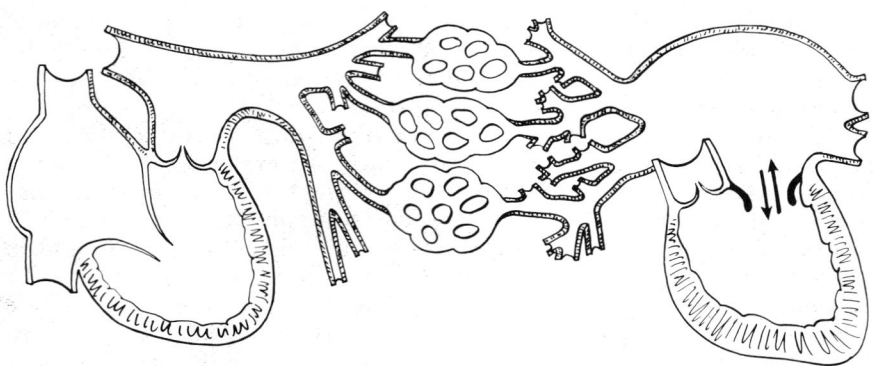

FIGURE 36-70   Central circulation laid flat in diagrammatic form showing incompetence of the mitral valve.

Pathology

Mitral insufficiency resulting from congenital disease may be a consequence of a primary anomaly of the valve or it may be secondary, either a systemic condition or primary anomaly in a nonvalvular structure. The most common cause is the mitral deformity that is part of the common atrioventricular canal defect. (See preceding discussion.) Further consideration of the pathology of mitral regurgitation will not consider the features of that malformation. Davachi and associates[467] found that among 55 infants with mitral valvular disease, there were 29 in which the mitral valve was the site of primary malformation, in 26 of which it was affected secondarily through myocardial infarction. Among these 26 cases, infarction of the papillary muscles was associated with endocardial fibroelastosis in 10 cases, aortic stenosis in 15, coarctation of the aorta in 6, and anomalous origin of the left coronary artery from the pulmonary trunk in 5.

Systemic diseases associated with mitral regurgitation include mucopolysaccharidosis[468] and Marfan's syndrome.

Associated Conditions   The principal associated conditions relate to the processes of which mitral regurgitation is a secondary effect. In cases of mitral regurgitation resulting from primary anomalies of the valve, few associated conditions are present, with the exception of corrected transposition (see later section). In that condition, inversion of the ventricles and atrioventricular valves places the tricuspid valve on the left side of the heart, functioning as a "mitral" valve. In corrected transposition, the inverted tricuspid valve has a strong tendency to be associated with an Ebstein-like malformation, and incompetence of the valve may occur. Mitral regurgitation may be part of the syndrome of congenital polyvalvular disease.[469]

Complications   Left ventricular failure is the usual result of mitral regurgitation. When the regurgitation is secondary, the complications are contributed to, in part, by the effects of the underlying conditions.

Clinical Manifestations

Isolated mitral regurgitation is uncommon during childhood. In addition to those mentioned above, a variety of rare primary malformations have been implicated, including isolated clefts of the anterior or posterior leaflets, absence of leaflet tissue, fenestration, duplication of the mitral orifice, as well as malformations and ectopic insertions of the papillary muscles and chordae tendineae.[6]

History   Easy fatigue, dyspnea with exertion, excessive sweating, numerous episodes of lower respiratory tract infection, and slow weight gain are symptoms of significant mitral regurgitation.

Physical Examination   The patient is usually a slender, dyspneic infant or child, frequently with cool and clammy skin and a prominent left precordial bulge. The left ventricular lift is hyperdynamic to palpation, with a diffuse and sustained impulse. The second heart sound is widely split but varies normally with respiration. The pulmonary component is accentuated in the presence of pulmonary arterial hypertension. A third heart sound at the apex is common. The characteristic holosystolic blowing murmur is loudest at the apex with radiation to the axilla. In the presence of leaflet fenestration, the murmur may radiate to the base of the heart and simulate aortic stenosis. A middiastolic rumble at the apex accompanies significant regurgitation.

Chest Roentgenogram   Both left ventricular and left atrial enlargement are present. The left mainstem bronchus may be displaced upward and left lower lobe atelectasis is not uncommon.

Electrocardiogram   Left ventricular and left atrial hypertrophy with deep Q waves in leads aV_L, V_5, and V_6 are characteristic. Flattening and inversion of the T waves over the left precordium usually reflect severe regurgitation.

Echocardiogram   M-mode technique will demonstrate slightly hyperkinetic motion of the interventricular septum and posterior ventricular wall, as well as enlargement of both the left ventricle and atrium, but these findings are nonspecific. Regurgitation associated with left atrium myxoma, prolapse, or flail mitral valve leaflet can be distinguished. Two-dimensional echocardiography may, in addition, be able to identify an isolated cleft of the mitral leaflet, displacement of the left atrioventricular valve associated with corrected transposition of the great arteries, and the single papillary muscle associated with parachute mitral valve deformity.[470,471]

Cardiac Catheterization With severe mitral regurgitation, there will be elevation of the left ventricular end-diastolic, left atrial, and pulmonary arterial wedge pressures. Tall V waves in the left atrial or wedge pressure tracings are characteristic. Pulmonary arterial hypertension usually reflects the severity of regurgitation. Left ventricular angiography documents the regurgitation, the degree of left ventricular and left atrial dilatation, and it provides a semiquantitative as well as a quantitative estimate of severity. A measured regurgitant volume of 50 percent or more of the left ventricular stroke volume is considered indicative of severe mitral regurgitation in children.

Natural History and Prognosis

While mild and even moderate isolated mitral regurgitation may be tolerated well for many years, the clinical course among patients with severe regurgitation usually is one of increasing dyspnea, frequent respiratory infections, recurrent left lower lobe atelectasis, and marked retardation of growth. There will be clinical and laboratory evidence of increasing left ventricular and left atrial dilatation, as well as pulmonary congestion and pulmonary arterial hypertension. Arrhythmias may appear in late childhood but are uncommon in infancy. The response to successful surgical valve annuloplasty or valve replacement in children usually is dramatic. Symptoms are relieved, cardiac enlargement is markedly reduced, and, perhaps most striking, growth and weight gain resume at a normal or even accelerated pace.

Medical Management

Decongestive measures in the form of digitalis, diuretics, vasodilator agents, and restriction of activity are indicated with severe regurgitation. Prompt and vigorous therapy of respiratory infections, including postural drainage, is important to avoid pulmonary complications. Protection against infective endocarditis is emphasized. Every attempt should be made to remove or relieve complicating associated cardiac lesions such as patent ductus, ventricular septal defect, coarctation of the aorta, and aortic stenosis. Fortunately, medical therapy is sufficient in most instances to permit the infant or young child to reach a size sufficient to allow mitral valve replacement if necessary. Among severely symptomatic infants and children with growth failure, increasing

heart size, and pulmonary arterial hypertension, surgical plication of the mitral annulus may be offered. Finally, it should be emphasized that rheumatic fever is still a very important cause of isolated mitral regurgitation during childhood. Unless it can be established that the regurgitation is congenital or the result of some well-documented disorder or disease, antibiotic prophylaxis against streptococcal infections and recurrent rheumatic fever is indicated.

Surgical Management

Incompetence of the mitral valve may result from annular dilatation, clefts in the leaflets, agenesis of a portion of the leaflet tissue, or fenestration of otherwise normal leaflets. In addition, subvalvular abnormalities, including agenesis or retraction of chordae, elongation of the chordae, and a variety of abnormalities of the papillary muscle apparatus, produce mitral regurgitation.[467] These abnormalities demand individualized surgical treatment.[464]

The left atrium is entered anterior to the right pulmonary veins while the patient is supported on complete cardiopulmonary bypass with moderate hypothermia. Circulatory arrest under conditions of profound hypothermia may be used in infants and small children. Simple clefts are closed by direct suture. The dilated annulus may be constricted by suture plication, suture annuloplasty, or prosthetic ring annuloplasty.[472] Partial valvular agenesis may be corrected by annular plication. Small fenestrations are closed by direct suture. Abnormalities of the chordae tendineae and papillary muscles have been managed by a variety of unpredictable plastic procedures which are not generally successful.

Clinically significant mitral regurgitation not correctable by reconstructive procedures requires mitral valve replacement, subsequent insertion of another larger valve being anticipated as the child grows toward maturity. Porcine heterograft valves have calcified, become stenotic, and deteriorated when used in children.[428] Mechanical prosthetic valves require anticoagulation therapy to avoid thromboembolic complications.[429] Injury to the bundle of His with subsequent complete heart block is more likely to occur in mitral valve replacement for congenital abnormalities than for rheumatic disease. The mitral annulus is likely to be smaller than normal when the mitral valve is congenitally abnormal, further complicating the insertion of an adequate-sized prosthetic valve. No good operation exists for enlargement of the mitral annulus.

Cor Triatriatum

Definition

Cor triatriatum is characterized by the presence in the left atrium of a perforated muscular membrane which separates the atrium into upper and lower chambers.

Pathology

The dividing membrane lies horizontally above the level of the atrial appendage (Fig. 36-71).[473,474] Its structure is that of cardiac muscle covered on its superior and inferior aspects by endocardial tissue. In adolescents and adults the edges of the perforation may show fibroelastosis. The pulmonary veins enter the upper chamber, and blood must pass through the opening in the membrane to reach the lower aspect of the left atrium. The caliber of the perforation in the membrane determines the degree of obstruction to pulmonary venous flow. In cases with severe degrees of obstruction, all the secondary signs comparable to those seen in mitral stenosis are present, including right ventricular hypertrophy and pulmonary venous hypertensive vascular changes.

Although the mitral valve is intrinsically normal, jet lesions may appear on the atrial aspect of the leaflets and on the mural endocardium of the lower atrial compartment.

Associated Conditions   A defect in the atrial septum is uncommonly present and may allow communication between the upper left atrial compartment and the right atrium.

In an occasional case, a pulmonary vein may connect anomalously with a systemic vein.[475] Tetralogy[474] and pulmonary stenosis have been observed uncommonly.[476]

Complications   The usual complication is comparable to that of mitral stenosis.

Clinical Manifestations

This malformation is one of the rarest congenital cardiac deformities. In most instances it lends itself to complete surgical correction, but the absence of a heart murmur, certainly a distinctive murmur, frequently leads to an initial diagnosis of primary pulmonary vascular or parenchymal disease.

History   Almost invariably patients are considered normal at birth and in the immediate neonatal period. Symptoms are those of pulmonary venous congestion and include dyspnea, orthopnea, difficulty with feeding, poor weight gain, and frequent lower respiratory tract infections. Episodes of pulmonary edema, particularly associated with exertion, may occur.

Physical Examination   Signs of pulmonary arterial and right ventricular hypertension are present, with a prominent *a* wave in the jugular venous pulse, forceful right ventricular lift, accentuated pulmonary second sound, and, occasionally, a soft early diastolic murmur of pulmonary regurgitation. Dyspnea, orthopnea, and basal lung rales reflect the pulmonary venous congestion. Right-sided heart failure with jugular venous distension, hepatomegaly, and peripheral edema occurs in the extreme. Murmurs described with this malformation usually are soft and nondescript. An apical diastolic murmur is extremely rare. Occasionally, a soft, continuous murmur is present and is most likely due to continuous flow across the small aperture in the obstructing membrane.[6]

Chest Roentgenogram   At least mild cardiac enlargement is the rule, with prominence of the pulmonary arterial segment and evidence of pulmonary venous congestion. The latter may include Kerley B lines and the "ground-glass" pattern of acute pulmonary edema in the hilar areas. Left atrial dilatation rarely is present.

Electrocardiogram   The characteristic pattern is one of right axis deviation and right atrial and right ventricular hypertrophy, the latter frequently associated with a deeply negative T wave in the right chest leads reflecting right ventricular ischemia.

Echocardiogram   Although the M-mode technique may demonstrate abnormal echoes posterior to the anterior mitral valve leaflet which presumably are reflected from the fibromuscular membrane itself,[477] two-dimensional echocardiography offers

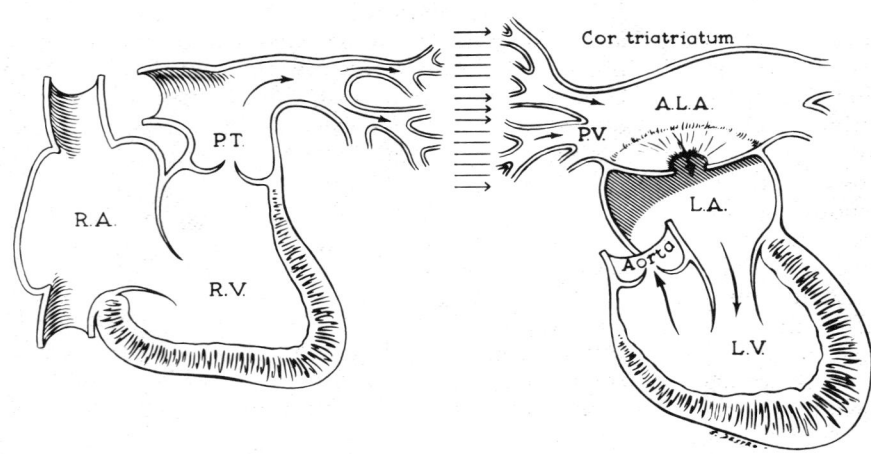

FIGURE 36-71   Central circulation laid flat in diagrammatic form showing cor triatriatum. The accessory left atrium (A.L.A.) lies above a perforated membrane between that chamber and the true left atrium (L.A.) below. R.A. = right atrium; R.V. = right ventricle; P.T. = main pulmonary arterial trunk; P.V. = pulmonary vein; L.V. = left ventricle.

a more definitive view of this intraatrial membrane.[157]

Cardiac Catheterization Severe elevation of the pulmonary arterial wedge pressure is characteristic and usually is associated with severe pulmonary arterial and right ventricular hypertension as well. A normal left ventricular diastolic pressure places the obstruction at the mitral, left atrial, or pulmonary venous level. Occasionally it is possible to enter the distal, low-pressure, left atrial chamber via a patent foramen ovale. Pulmonary arterial angiography usually will permit visualization of the obstructed dorsal chamber with its delayed emptying and lack of contraction, as well as the diminutive ventral chamber with its characteristic crescent shape and left atrial appendage. In the frontal view, the membrane may be seen as a thin, oblique, radiolucent line slanted from an inferior medial to a superior lateral position. Since a little over 10 percent of patients with cor triatriatum will have partial anomalous venous return, angiography also will be helpful in distinguishing this variant from total anomalous pulmonary venous return with pulmonary venous obstruction.

Natural History and Prognosis

The course is one of progressive pulmonary venous hypertension and congestion with pulmonary edema and right-sided heart failure. The majority of patients are recognized during childhood, while a few become symptomatic in early infancy. A rare patient may develop symptoms for the first time as a young adult. Surgical removal of the membrane results in relief of symptoms and, usually, a return of the pulmonary arterial pressure and vascular resistance to normal.

Medical Management

Prompt diagnostic studies are indicated to identify this curable cause of serious pulmonary venous and pulmonary arterial hypertension. Surgical removal of the obstructing membrane should be carried out with dispatch. Digitalis and diuretics may be indicated in the circumscribed preoperative management and in the immediate postoperative period until the right ventricular and pulmonary arterial pressures and the pulmonary vascular resistance return to normal.

Surgical Management

The heart is exposed through a median sternotomy incision. In older children cardiopulmonary bypass is used with moderate hypothermia and cardioplegia. A brief period of circulatory arrest during hypothermic cardiopulmonary bypass provides optimal exposure in infants and small children. The left atrium is entered posterior to the interatrial groove on the right, just anterior to the right pulmonary veins. The obstructing fibrous membrane is widely excised, allowing all of the pulmonary veins unre-

stricted access to the mitral valve orifice. An associated atrial septal defect is closed.[478] Clinical improvement is dramatic; mortality and morbidity are low if operative correction is carried out before the development of severe pulmonary vascular obstructive disease and right ventricular failure.

Stenosis of Pulmonary Veins and Venules

Definition

Obstruction in major pulmonary veins is usually designated as *stenosis of individual pulmonary veins,* while obstruction in the venules and small veins is designated as *pulmonary venoocclusive disease.*

Pathology

Stenosis of individual pulmonary veins may be characterized either by hypoplasia of involved veins or, more commonly, by a fibrous intimal lesion at the junction of a vein with the left atrium.[479] All or only some of the veins may be involved in a given case.

In pulmonary venoocclusive disease, venules and small veins are obstructed by connective tissue that at many sites shows vascular spaces (Fig. 36-72). This picture suggests an acquired process, namely organized thrombosis.[480] Pulmonary hemosiderosis and other features of pulmonary venous hypertension are present and particularly prominent in the occasional adult with this condition.

Associated Conditions Stenosis of individual pulmonary veins may be an isolated condition, but in the few reported cases atrial septal defect was common.[479,481] Other anomalies may be associated, such as corrective transposition,[482] but there does not appear to be a particular association.

Pulmonary venoocclusive disease characteristically is not associated with cardiovascular anomalies.

Complications Complications of stenosis of individual pulmonary veins depend on the extend of the disease. In significant obstruction of all or most of the veins, the complications resemble those of mitral stenosis, as they do in pulmonary venoocclusive disease.

Clinical Manifestations

Stenosis of the individual pulmonary veins and pulmonary venoocclusive disease are both very rare conditions and both, particularly the latter, carry an extremely poor outlook for survival.

History Symptoms are those of dyspnea, easy fatigue, frequent lower respiratory tract infections, and poor weight gain. Venous stenosis tends to occur somewhat earlier in life, frequently within the first year, while venoocclusive disease has a somewhat wider age distribution. Hemoptysis may occur in both, but syncope, cough, and chest pain are more typical venoocclusive disease.

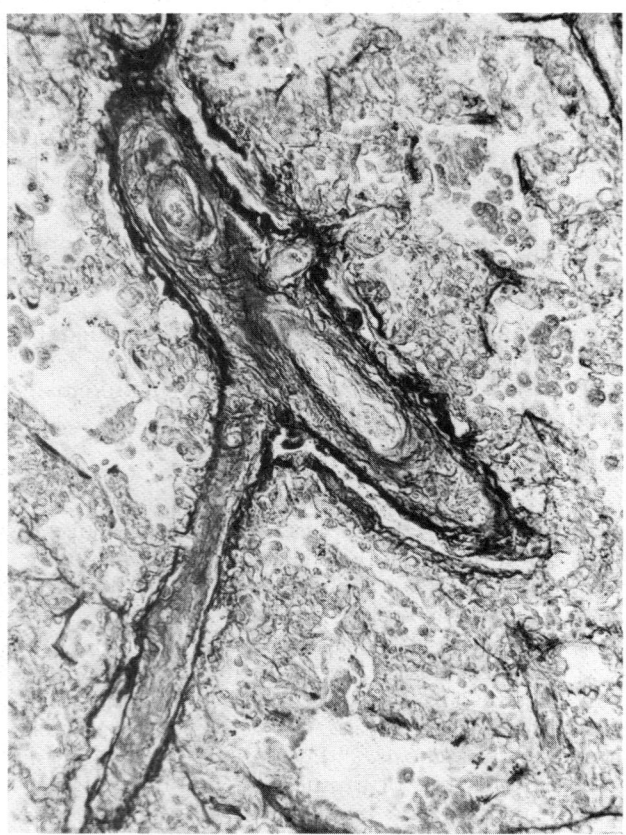

A

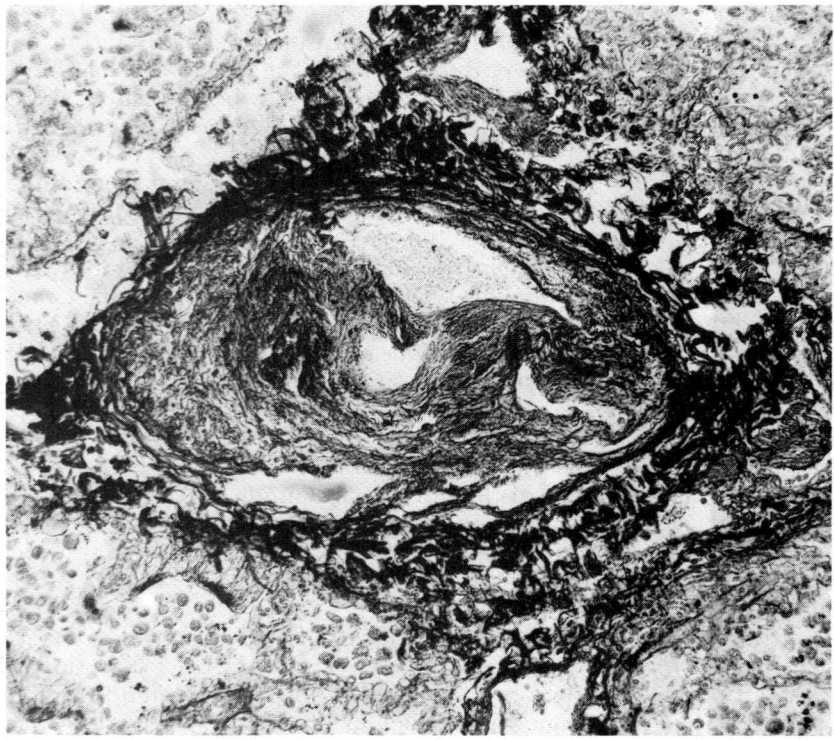

B

FIGURE 36-72 Pulmonary venoocclusive disease. *A.* A vein and its tributaries show narrowing of the lumen by fibrous tissue. *B.* An intrapulmonary vein shows its lumen to be filled by vascular connective tissue suggesting an organized thrombus. Each elastic tissue stain × 100. [*From J. E. Edwards, Pulmonary Vascular Disease, in K. M. Moser (ed.), "Congenital Pulmonary Vascular Disorders," Marcel Dekker, Inc., New York, 1979, pp. 527–571. Reproduced with permission.*]

Physical Examination   Both tend to show evidence of central cyanosis, and in both the physical findings are those of severe pulmonary arterial hypertension and pulmonary venous congestion. A forceful right ventricular lift and a loud pulmonary second sound are characteristic. Moist rales may be heard over the lung fields. There are no distinctive murmurs.

Chest Roentgenogram   A diffuse pattern of pulmonary venous congestion with Kerley B lines and effusions in the major and minor interlobar fissures may be seen. A ground-glass pattern in the hilar areas is not unusual. The central pulmonary arteries will be enlarged and usually there is mild cardiac enlargement due to right ventricular dilatation. No left atrial enlargement is present.

Echocardiogram   M-mode and two-dimensional studies are helpful in documenting the absence of mitral stenosis or cor triatriatum.

Cardiac Catheterization   Both conditions are characterized by severe pulmonary arterial hypertension and varying degrees of systemic arterial oxygen desaturation. With stenosis of the individual pulmonary veins, the corresponding pulmonary arterial wedge pressures are elevated, whereas in pulmonary venoocclusive disease, the pulmonary arterial wedge pressures usually are normal. Left atrial pressures are normal. Stenosis of the individual pulmonary veins may be visualized by high-quality pulmonary arterial angiography, but selective pulmonary venous angiography is preferable.

Natural History and Prognosis

The prognosis is grave in both conditions. In the case of stenosis of the individual pulmonary veins, the course is usually relatively short, ending in death within a year or two. The average age of death is estimated to be 4 years, with a range from 5 months to 10 years.[130] Among children with pulmonary venoocclusive disease, the course also is one of rapid deterioration, with an average survival of 20 months from the onset of symptoms.[483]

Medical Management

At least temporary control of right-sided heart failure and relief of pulmonary edema can be achieved with digitalis, diuretics, and restricted activity. Oxygen therapy in the acute situation is helpful. Among patients with stenosis of individual pulmonary veins, surgical relief of obstruction has met with little or no success unless the obstruction has been discrete and limited to one or two relatively large veins.[484] As yet, there is no specific therapy for pulmonary venoocclusive disease and only supportive measures can be offered.

Surgical Management

Stenoses of individual pulmonary veins have seldom been relieved by operation. The appropriate procedure depends upon the form of the obstruction and its location. Stenosis of the orifice or of a length of extraparenchymal vein is best repaired by pericardial patch angioplasty. Atretic segments or very severe stenoses at or near the atrial orifice can be resected, the dilated proximal vein being anastomosed directly to the left atrium. Rarely, a membranous diaphragm can be excised.[485] Unfortunately, there is no surgical treatment for the most common form of this disease, which is diffuse pulmonary venoocclusive disease or hypoplastic pulmonary veins.

When attempts to relieve obstruction have failed or where there appears little hope of providing adequate venous drainage to a relatively small area of lung, the affected pulmonary tissue should be resected to prevent intrapulmonary hemorrhage and pneumonitis.

Endocardial Fibroelastosis

Definition

Endocardial fibroelastosis is characterized by a proliferation of elastic and collagenous fibers within the endocardium.

Pathology

Grossly, the endocardium is abnormally thickened and has a smooth, glistening, milky white or "porcelain" appearance. The left ventricle is involved either exclusively or, less commonly, along with the right ventricle.[486] In the left ventricle two types are recognized, the dilated, which is more common, and the contracted.

In the dilated type, the left ventricular cavity is enlarged and the wall thick. The condition may be said to be primary or secondary (Fig. 36-73). Even the primary type may be secondary to prenatal myocardial failure, either idiopathic or through infection. The secondary type is associated with a variety of conditions, principally aortic valvular stenosis, coarctation of the aorta, and anomalous origin of the left coronary artery from the pulmonary trunk, and lesser degrees may be observed in states with left-to-right shunts, such as ventricular septal defect and patent ductus arteriosus. It may follow primary myocardial disease.[487]

The contracted type is characterized by the presence of a smaller than normal left ventricular cavity. The most severe forms of left ventricular hypoplasia are seen in association with aortic atresia, and to a lesser degree in those cases of aortic stenosis with a hypoplastic left ventricle.

An unusual variety of the contracted type appears as an isolated condition. While the left ventricle is smaller than normal, the left atrium is enlarged and the right ventricle hypertrophied.[488]

Complications   In the dilated type, mitral insufficiency is a common complication. When underlying

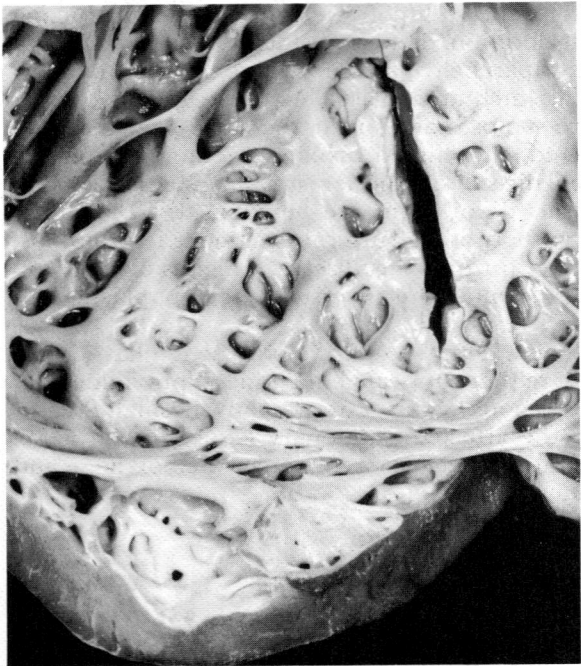

FIGURE 36-73 Endocardial fibroelastosis. Interior of left ventricle shows hypertrophy of wall, enlargement of chamber, and marked endocardial fibrous thickening.

conditions are present, the complications are principally those of the particular underlying condition.

Clinical Manifestations

Primary fibroelastosis is a disease chiefly of infants, with approximately 80 percent of affected patients being symptomatic by 10 months of age.[9] When related to a total clinical population of infants and children affected with congenital heart disease, its incidence is slightly less than 1 percent. It would appear that this incidence is distinctly less today than in years past.[6] The female-to-male ratio lies between 1.3 and 1.6:1.[9] Familial occurrence is uncommon but well described. The risk of fibroelastosis for a sibling of an affected infant is estimated at 4 percent by Nora,[154] although the risk to later-born siblings may be higher.[489]

History Patients are almost always in heart failure when first seen, but generally have normal growth and development until that time. Approximately 1 in 10 patients is symptomatic from birth. The onset is rapid, with dyspnea, grunting respirations, cough, irritability, weakness, and pallor being the most common observations. In over half the infants, the onset of congestive failure is linked with an immediately preceding respiratory infection.

Physical Examination Respiratory distress is evident with flaring of the nostrils and intercostal retractions. Fine, moist rales are frequent in the lung fields, the heart is enlarged, and a gallop rhythm is almost invariably present. A soft systolic murmur of mitral regurgitation may be heard, but characteris-

tically no significant murmur is present early in the illness.

Chest Roentgenogram The heart is massively enlarged, usually with left atrial dilatation. Left lower lobe atelectasis due to bronchial compression is present in almost one-fifth of these patients.

Electrocardiogram The electrocardiogram indicates isolated left ventricular hypertrophy in almost all instances with tall R waves in leads V_5 and V_6 and a small rS ratio and deep S wave in V_1. Flat or inverted T waves over the left precordium are characteristic. Left or biatrial hypertrophy usually is present as well (Fig. 36-74). Rarely, one finds a low-voltage pattern more typical of myocarditis. With the contracted type of fibroelastosis, right ventricular hypertrophy is present with normal or small left precordial voltages.

Echocardiogram M-mode study will demonstrate a markedly dilated left ventricle, a thin free wall, and very diminished contractility. Posterior displacement of the mitral apparatus due to marked ventricular dilatation is characteristic.[455]

Cardiac Catheterization A wide systemic arteriovenous oxygen content difference, a diminished cardiac output, and elevated left ventricular end-diastolic, left atrial, and pulmonary arterial wedge pressures are the usual findings. Left ventricular angiography reveals a markedly dilated chamber with prolonged opacification and little change in chamber size from systole to diastole. Left ventricular end-diastolic and end-systolic volumes are increased, and the ejection fraction diminished.

Natural History and Prognosis

This disease formerly was considered almost invariably fatal, but there is now reason to believe that

FIGURE 36-74 Electrocardiogram of a 4-month-old infant with endocardial fibroelastosis (verified pathologically) shows a normal mean QRS axis, an abnormal T vector, and left ventricular hypertrophy. The P wave is hidden in the terminal portion of the preceding T wave.

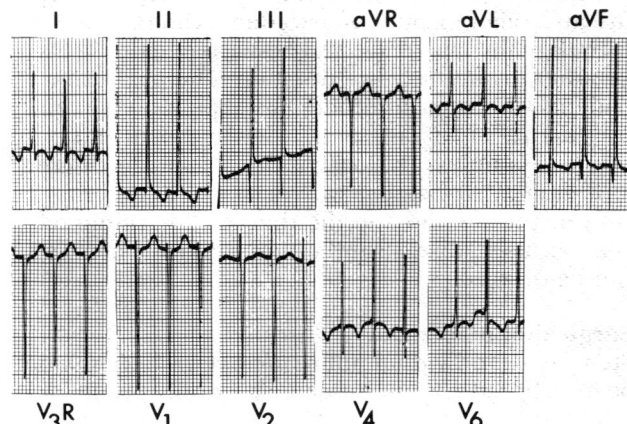

early recognition and prompt, diligent, and prolonged therapy may salvage as many as 60 percent of affected infants and children. Death, if it is to occur, takes place in the first year of life in about 80 percent of patients. The course in these infants usually is one of recurrent episodes of congestive failure with persistent cardiac enlargement and electrocardiographic abnormalities. Death is from congestive heart failure or tachyarrhythmias in most instances. Systemic or pulmonary emboli from mural thrombi occur in approximately 10 percent of patients. Early recognition, a prompt response to decongestive measures, a rapid return of heart size to normal, disappearance of abnormal T waves, and a gradual resolution of left ventricular hypertrophy are favorable signs. Survival to the fifth birthday suggests continued survival with little or no handicap. Unfortunately, deaths have been described in a few children several years after an excellent initial clinical response, albeit usually with some residual electrocardiographic or roentgenologic abnormality. The diagnosis of fibroelastosis is documented by postmortem examination in those who succumb. Whether the same disease process existed and then resolved or became tolerable in the survivors is open to question.

Medical Management

Prompt, vigorous, and sustained treatment of heart failure with adequate amounts of digitalis and diuretics is essential. Rest, with sedation if necessary, and restriction of activity are advised. Anemia should be corrected promptly and recurrence prevented. Complicating congenital cardiac lesions should be corrected or relieved if possible. The value of steroids in patients with fibroelastosis is unproved, but since a few patients with inflammatory myocarditis appear to benefit from its use early in the course of the illness, a trial of therapy should be considered. Full medical support, including digitalis and diuretics, should be continued at least until the electrocardiogram and chest roentgenogram have returned to normal and probably considerably longer. The aim of such therapy is to control congestive failure, reduce heart size, and extend life with the hope that the disease will resolve and permit long-term survival. In selected patients, mitral valve replacement for mitral regurgitation may be indicated.[6,9]

Valvular and Vascular Malformations of the Right Side of the Heart with Right-to-Left, Bidirectional, or No Shunt

Valvular Pulmonary Stenosis with Intact Ventricular Septum

Pathology

Valvular pulmonary stenosis with intact ventricular septum is usually characterized by the so-called dome-shaped stenosis of the pulmonary valve and

only uncommonly by dysplasia of the valve (Fig. 36-75). In dome-shaped stenosis, the valvular tissue is represented by a cone or dome-shaped structure perforated at its distal end with the opening representing the effective orifice of the pulmonary valve (Fig. 36-76).[490,491] Great disproportion may occur between the diameter of the pulmonary trunk and the effective orifice at the stenotic valve; the pulmonary trunk exhibits poststenotic dilatation. In adult patients, including those reaching the fifth decade, calcification of the valve may appear.[492]

In pulmonary valvular dysplasia, the annulus of the valve may be abnormally narrow, but the most dramatic changes are related to the cusps, of which three are identifiable. The cusps are exceedingly thickened by mucoid and dense connective tissue. This process may extend into the sinuses of the pulmonary valve.[493]

Concentric hypertrophy of the right ventricle is present, its degree reflecting the degree of obstruction at valve level. The right ventricular thickness may exceed that of the left ventricle. The hypertrophy, as it affects the infundibular musculature, may cause secondary muscular infundibular stenosis.[494]

FIGURE 36-75 Congenital pulmonary valvular stenosis with intact ventricular septum. Major hypertrophy of the right ventricular wall resulting from dome-shaped stenosis of the pulmonary valve is present. SVC = superior vena cava; IVC = inferior vena cava; RA = right atrium; RV = right ventricle; PT = main pulmonary arterial trunk; RPA = right pulmonary artery; LPA = left pulmonary artery; RPV = right pulmonary vein; LPV = left pulmonary vein; LA = left atrium; LV = left ventricle; Ao = aorta. [*From J. E. Edwards, Classification of Congenital Heart Disease in the Adult, in W. C. Roberts (ed.), "Congenital Heart Disease in Adults," Cardiovasc. Clin. Series 10/1, F. A. Davis Company, Philadelphia, 1979, pp. 1–26. Reproduced with permission.*]

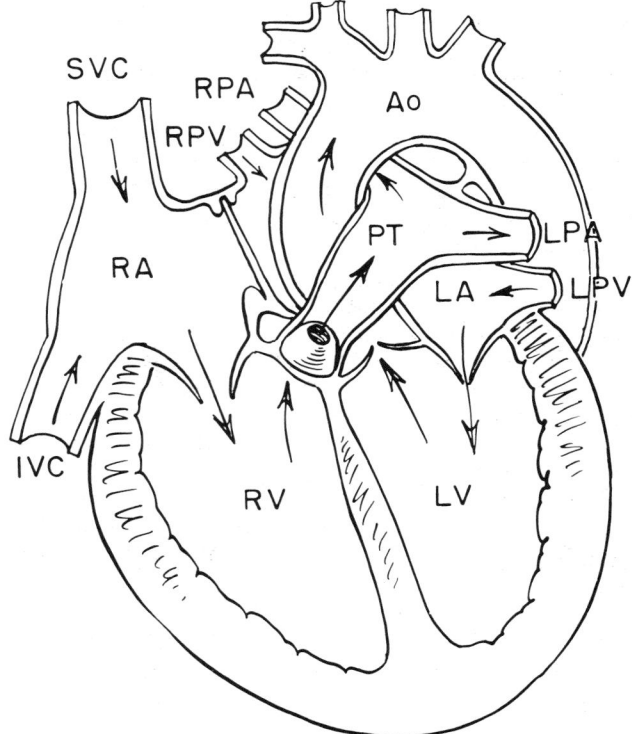

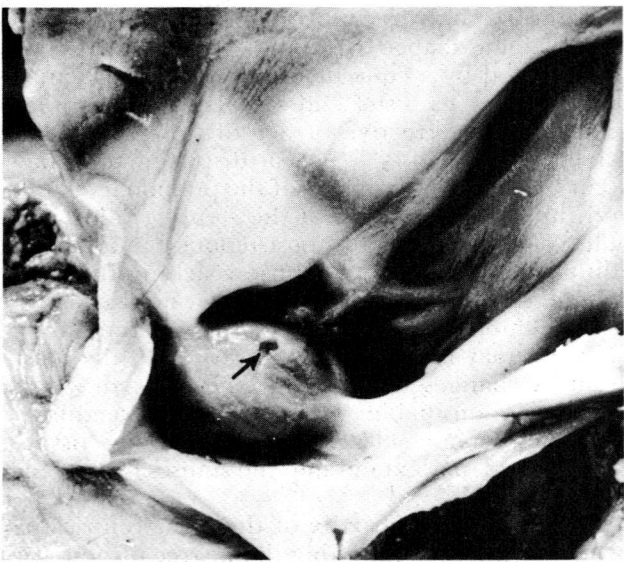

FIGURE 36-76 Pulmonary valvular stenosis with intact ventricular septum. Pulmonary valve viewed from above. Valve is a dome-shaped structure with a narrow central opening (arrow). (*From J. E. Edwards, L. S. Carey, H. N. Neufeld, and R. G. Lester, "Congenital Heart Disease: Correlation of Pathologic Anatomy and Angiocardiography," W. B. Saunders Company, Philadelphia, 1965, vol. II, p. 601. Reproduced with permission.*)

The tricuspid valve may show fibrous thickening with secondary contracture of leaflets and chordae. The atrial septum varies.[495] In some instances, the foramen ovale is anatomically sealed, in others patent. In cases of dome-shaped stenosis with patent foramen ovale the term *trilogy of Fallot* is applied by some.

Associated Conditions Among conditions associated with the dome-shaped valve are anomalous muscle bundle of the right ventricle[496] and focal stenosis of the pulmonary arteries. In pulmonary valvular dysplasia, familial dome-shaped valvular pulmonary stenosis has been observed. In affected subjects there is a tendency for peculiar facies in which a wide forehead and a narrow chin are present.[493]

Complications Although right ventricular failure may occur, it is not common in the young and the condition is classically free of major complications until adult life. Significant complications in the young are usually those of systemic hypoxia, seen in cases with severe degrees of stenosis and a patent foramen ovale.

Among the complications of pulmonary stenosis is tricuspid insufficiency. Infective endocarditis, usually seen in adults, may occur upon the dome-shaped valve, upon the pulmonary trunk, or upon the edges of secondary infundibular stenosis.

Cerebral abscess, also classic in the adult, is confined to those individuals with a patent foramen ovale.[491]

Abnormal Physiology[497–500]

As a result of valvular pulmonary stenosis with intact interventricular septum, there is a pressure difference during systole between the main right ventricular cavity and the pulmonary artery. The area of the pulmonary valve orifice is normally 2 cm²/m² or about 0.5 cm at birth and increases in size with body growth. In general, the effective valve area must be decreased by about 60 percent before there is hemodynamically significant obstruction to flow.

In patients with severe valvular stenosis, the pulmonary artery pressure is usually lower than normal and has a pulse wave which is less distinct than normal. Just distal to the stenotic valve, there may be negative systolic waves, referred to as *Venturi waves*. As the catheter is withdrawn to the right ventricle, there is an abrupt change to a high ventricular pressure (Fig. 36-77). The right ventricular pressure pulse typically has a rapid rate of increase in pressure to a delayed but sharp peak pressure and then a rapid fall in pressure. In pulmonary stenosis the peak systolic pressure difference may reach 150 to 240 mmHg; rarely, it may be higher. A proper appreciation of the degree of obstruction requires knowledge not only of the mean systolic pressure gradient but also of the amount of flow across the valve, since a relatively mild degree of stenosis may have a significant pressure difference if the pulmonary flow is very high. Conversely, severe stenosis may be associated with a relatively small pressure difference if the flow is very low as a result of right ventricular failure. If pulmonary flow is normal, most patients with peak pressure differences at rest less than 50 mmHg have mild stenosis, and patients with a pressure difference over 100 mmHg have severe stenosis.

When the pulmonary stenosis is severe, the right ventricle may fail and the cardiac output may be decreased, even at rest, associated with elevation of both the right ventricular end-diastolic pressure and the right atrial mean pressure. The elevated right atrial pressure may produce signs of systemic venous congestion. At times, it may cause the foramen ovale to open and allow some shunting of blood from the right atrium to the left atrium. Arterial unsaturation and cyanosis result from this shunt. In addition, peripheral cyanosis can also result from a decreased cardiac output, with "peripheral" or "stagnant" cyanosis resulting from the low flow to the peripheral tissues in severe pulmonary stenosis without a patent foramen ovale. In the latter situation, the arterial saturation is normal. At times, significant fibrosis of the right ventricular endocardium occurs in adults and contributes to the right ventricular failure and elevated diastolic pressure.

In most adolescent or adult patients with significant pulmonary stenosis, the resting cardiac output is within normal limits, although it does not usually increase normally during exercise. In contrast, children may be able to increase their cardiac output during exercise.[370] Since a doubling of flow across

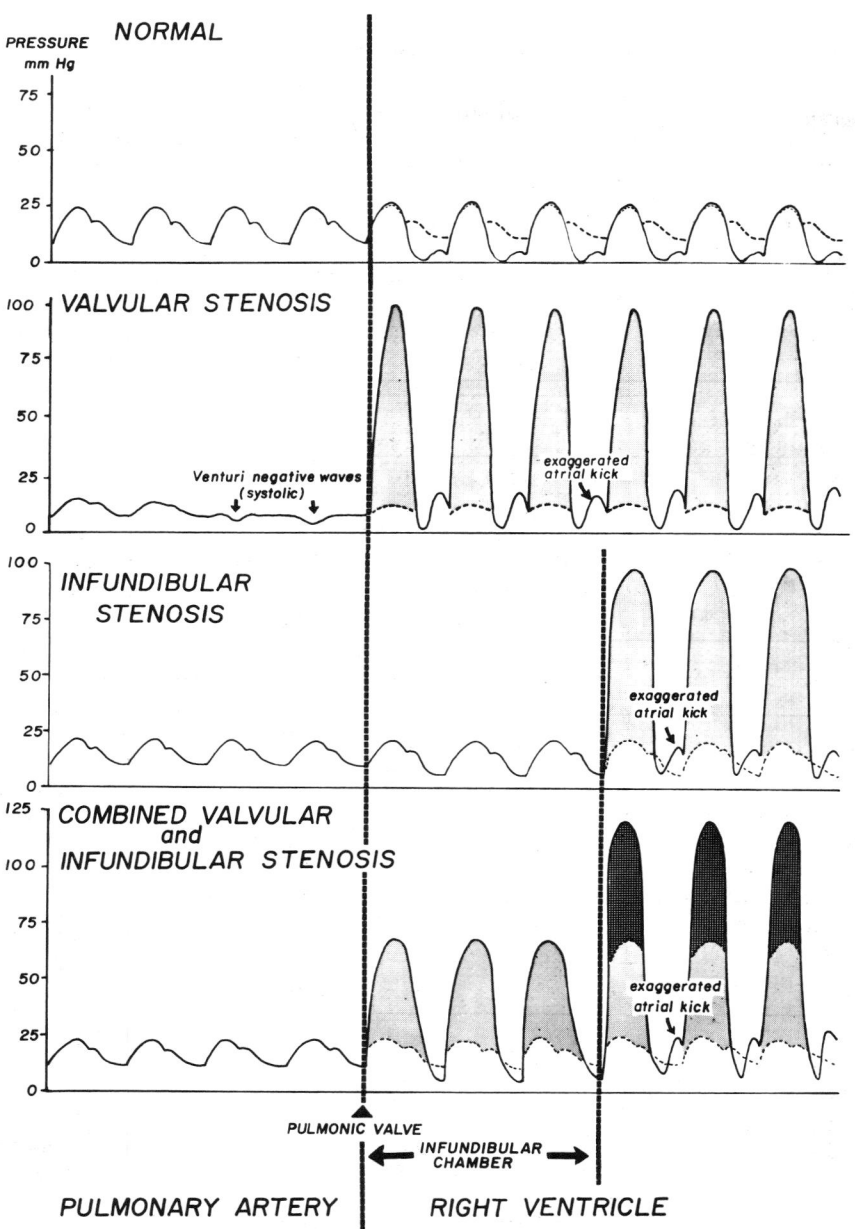

FIGURE 36-77 Characteristic pressure tracings during withdrawal of catheter from pulmonary artery to right ventricle. *Upper tracing.* Normal pressure tracings with no significant pressure difference between right ventricle and pulmonary artery during systole. *Second tracing.* The characteristic findings in pure valvular pulmonary stenosis—a systolic pressure difference between right ventricle and pulmonary artery indicated by the shaded areas, a sharp rise of pressure in the right ventricle, an exaggerated atrial kick in the right ventricular tracings, a prolonged systolic ejection period of the right ventricle, negative systolic ejection period of the right ventricle, negative systolic waves (Venturi waves) in the pulmonary artery just above the pulmonary valve, and damped, low-amplitude pressure pulses in the pulmonary arterial system. *Third tracing.* The findings in infundibular pulmonary stenosis, characterized by an "infundibular chamber," which has a systolic pressure lower than in the main right ventricular cavity but equal to the systolic pressure in the pulmonary artery. During diastole the pressure in the infundibular chamber is equal to that in the main right ventricular chamber. The right ventricular pressure tracing has an exaggerated atrial kick, and the rate of increase in pressure in the main right ventricular cavity during systole is less than in valvular stenosis. The systolic pressure difference between the main right ventricular chamber and the infundibular chamber is indicated by the shaded areas. *Lower tracing.* The findings in combined valvular and infundibular stenosis. The systolic pressure difference between the main right ventricular chamber and the infundibular chamber is indicated by cross-hatching; the pressure difference between the infundibular chamber and the pulmonary artery is indicated by the shaded areas.

a stenotic valve requires a *fourfold* increase of pressure, and since the peak pressure in either ventricle rarely exceeds 320 mmHg, flow through a severely stenotic valve is limited. In patients with severe pulmonary stenosis, right ventricular function, especially during exercise, may also be hindered by poor coronary blood flow.

In some infants, the pressure difference increases significantly with body growth, suggesting either that the valve fails to change in orifice size proportionately with body size, or that infundibular hypertrophy is producing secondary obstruction. On the other hand, some patients with mild or moderate degrees of stenosis may have no change in right ventricular systolic pressure with significant growth over many years, suggesting that the valve orifice can enlarge.

Trilogy of Fallot[492] Atrial septal defect associated with pulmonary stenosis, referred to as the trilogy (triad) of Fallot, presents a wide spectrum of hemodynamic alterations, mainly depending on the severity of the pulmonary stenosis. If the stenosis is mild, the shunt may be predominantly left-to-right, although it seldom has the "torrential" volume found in uncomplicated atrial septal defect. If the stenosis is more severe or the right ventricle "fails," the shunting of blood at the atrial level may be predominantly right-to-left with arterial unsaturation and cyanosis.

Clinical Manifestations

Pulmonary stenosis is one of the most common congenital heart defects, accounting for about 10 percent in most large study populations (see Table 36-1). The stenosis is at the level of the pulmonary valve in most instances, but it can occur within the right ventricle or in the pulmonary arteries. Distinguishing clinical features will be discussed separately, although combinations occur in some patients. Approximately one-quarter of patients with stenosis of the pulmonary valve also have an atrial shunt,[501] but this frequency is probably dependent on the age group studied.

History Most infants and children are asymptomatic, but a small percentage with very severe obstruction will manifest symptoms. The most common symptoms are mild fatigue or shortness of breath with exertion. Young infants with critical obstruction present with symptoms related to heart failure and may have cyanosis if there is a patent foramen ovale or atrial septal defect.[502] Squatting and syncope are rare in childhood. Growth and development are normal. There is no sex preference, and familial transmission is reported,[503] especially when the valve is dysplastic and associated with certain dysmorphisms described by Noonan.[493,504]

Physical Examination Only those with a dysplastic valve have consistent noncardiac abnormalities. These patients frequently have short stature, hypertelorism, ptosis, low-set ears, and mental retardation.[504] Cyanosis is uncommon, except with severe obstruction and an atrial communication.[496] Tachypnea, hepatomegaly, and the murmur of tricuspid regurgitation may be present in these infants. In those with at least moderate obstruction, a prominent *a* wave is seen on examination of the jugular venous pulse. A systolic thrill in the suprasternal notch and at the left upper sternal border is present. The right ventricular parasternal impulse becomes increasingly forceful with more severe obstruction. On auscultation an early systolic click accentuated with expiration is heard at the left upper sternal border unless the obstruction is severe or the valve is dysplastic. As obstruction increases in severity, the pulmonary component of the second heart sound becomes progressively softer and more delayed. As the right ventricular pressure reaches systemic levels or greater, it becomes inaudible. A fourth heart sound is heard if obstruction is severe. The characteristic systolic murmur is harsh, crescendo-decrescendo in shape, and best heard at the left upper sternal border with radiation toward the left clavicle. The duration of the murmur and timing of peak intensity correlate well with the severity of obstruction. With mild to moderate stenosis, the murmur peaks in midsystole and ends at or before the aortic component of the second heart sound. In patients with severe stenosis, the murmur peaks late in systole and extends beyond the aortic component (A_2) of the second heart sound.[505]

There is an entity called *idiopathic dilatation of the pulmonary artery,* which may be a mild valvular abnormality with little obstruction or an arterial wall abnormality. It mimics very mild stenosis, except that the murmur of pulmonary regurgitation is more frequently heard.[6]

Chest Roentgenogram Most patients have a normal or only slightly increased heart size. Significant enlargement is seen with critical obstruction and is an ominous sign. Characteristically, the main and proximal left pulmonary arteries are prominent due to poststenotic dilatation (Fig. 36-78). This finding may be absent with very severe obstruction, a dysplastic valve, or in very young infants. The pulmonary vascular pattern is normal in most, but diminished in those with a right-to-left shunt at atrial level.

Electrocardiogram Right ventricular forces in the anterior precordial leads correlate reasonably well with the degree of obstruction.[506] They will be normal or demonstrate mild hypertrophy with an rsR′ pattern if there is mild obstruction. With severe stenosis, there is right axis deviation, right atrial hypertrophy, and very tall R waves in the anterior precordial leads. The presence of a qR pattern in these leads is almost always a sign of very severe obstruction. Infants with critical pulmonary stenosis and severe cyanosis may have a leftward QRS axis between +30 and +120° with diminished right ventricular forces indistinguishable from the electrocardiogram of pulmonary atresia with intact ventricular septum.[496] Those with a dysplastic valve frequently have a superior QRS axis.[493]

Vectorcardiogram The Frank vectorcardiogram provides an estimate of peak right ventricular systolic pressure, using the right maximum spatial volt-

FIGURE 36-78 Chest roentgenogram in a 10-year-old girl with a dilated main pulmonary artery due to mild valvular pulmonary stenosis.

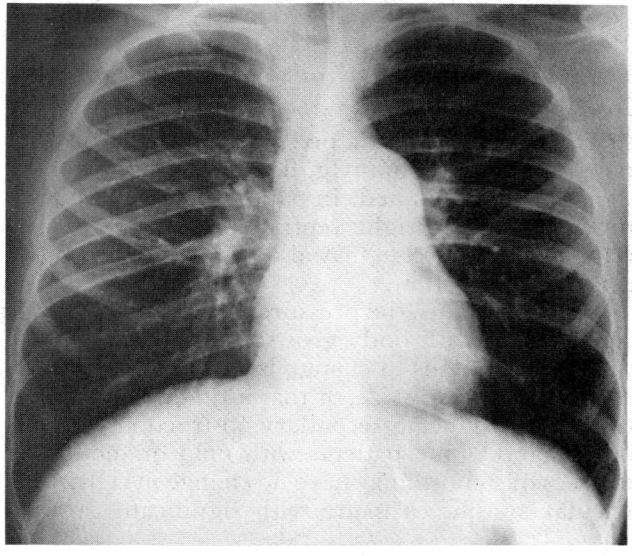

age (RMSV) in the following regression equation: $41.5(RMSV) + 24.1$ mmHg.[507] Accuracy of estimation from physical and electrocardiographic data has been shown to be nearly equal to this.[506,508]

Echocardiogram   With moderate or severe pulmonary valvular stenosis, there is exaggeration of the maximal *a* wave depth of the pulmonary valve recorded with inspiration, and when anterior and posterior leaflets are recorded, presystolic opening of the valve occurs. The latter finding is probably the most specific.[509] Absence of these findings does not exclude the diagnosis, particularly if the stenosis is mild.

Cardiac Catheterization   There is elevated right ventricular systolic pressure with a distinct systolic pressure difference across the valve on slow withdrawal of the catheter from the pulmonary artery to the right ventricle. If critical obstruction is suspected, it may be wise not to attempt to advance the catheter to the pulmonary artery due to the risk of compromising an already marginal opening. Simultaneous measurement of systemic arterial and right ventricular pressures with measurement of flow are necessary to assess severity accurately. The right ventricular end-diastolic pressure and right atrial *a* wave may be elevated. Systemic saturation will be diminished only in those with more severe obstruction and a patent foramen ovale or, less commonly, a true septal defect. A left-to-right shunt at atrial level is detected in some patients with mild to moderate obstruction.[501] Right ventricular angiography will demonstrate thickened and doming valve leaflets and a jet of contrast material entering the dilated pulmonary artery (Fig. 36-79). Doming is not

characteristic of the dysplastic valve (Fig. 36-80).[493] Secondary infundibular subvalvular narrowing due to muscular hypertrophy may be seen.[510] The degree varies and is of importance in choosing the surgical approach. Studies of ventricular volume characteristics have demonstrated depressed ventricular function in those with right-to-left shunts.[500]

Natural History and Prognosis

The clinical course is favorable in most patients with mild to moderate obstruction. In a national cooperative study,[508] 86 percent of patients had no significant increase in their pressure gradients over a 4- to 8-year interval. Those with a significant increase were less than 4 years of age and had at least moderate stenosis initially. Progression during the period of growth seems the most likely explanation for most of the increases, but a few developed subvalvular muscular hypertrophy, which increased the obstruction. Even mild obstruction may progress significantly in some infants during the first year of life.[499] The prognosis of those with severe obstruction is poor, especially for infants with critical obstruction. With severe obstruction, right ventricular damage and dysfunction can ensue over the years and heart failure or arrhythmias can cause premature death in adults.[499] Brain abscess can occur if a right-to-left shunt is present.

Medical Management

Management will obviously depend on the severity of obstruction. For those with mild to moderate stenosis, periodic reexamination with electrocardiogram is indicated to detect any evidence of progression, with more frequent evaluation for those less than 1 year of age. Measures to treat heart fail-

FIGURE 36-79   Lateral view of a right ventricular (RV) angiogram demonstrating the typical features of valvular pulmonary stenosis with doming of the pulmonary valve (arrow) and a narrow jet of contrast entering the dilated main pulmonary artery (MPA).

FIGURE 36-80   Lateral view of a right ventricular (RV) angiogram with very thickened dysplastic pulmonary valve (arrow) and mild poststenotic dilatation of the main pulmonary artery (MPA).

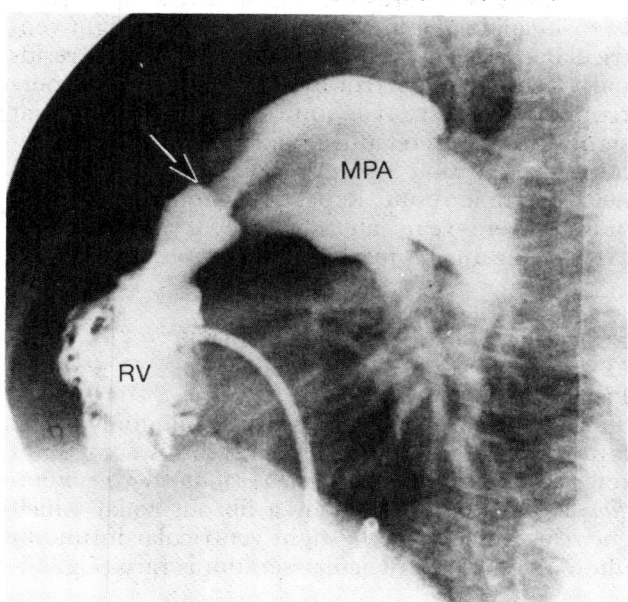

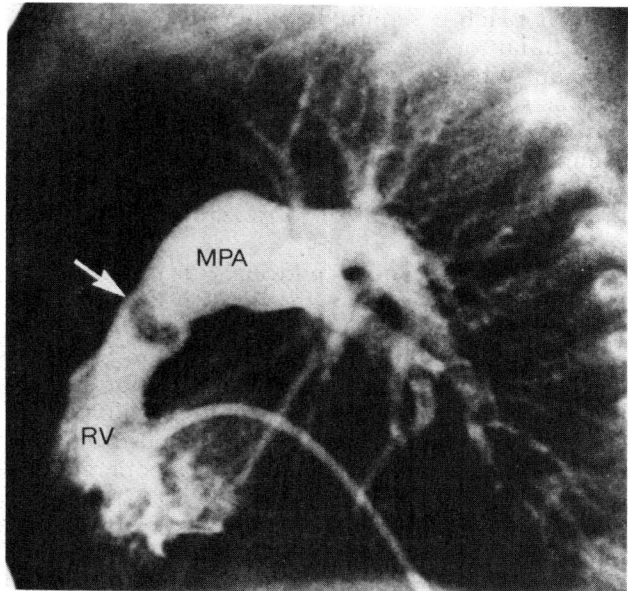

ure should be instituted in the infant with critical stenosis, but prompt surgical intervention is mandatory. Cyanosis or a right ventricular systolic pressure well above systemic levels also are indications for prompt surgery. In asymptomatic older infants and children, elective surgery is usually recommended when the right ventricular systolic pressure is near 70 mmHg or the gradient is near 50 mmHg or more. For those beyond infancy, there is some suggestion that surgery gives better overall results, even in the group with pressures somewhat less than this.[508] Exercise studies[497] during catheterization have demonstrated that altered cardiac function observed in some children is reversible by surgery. This does not appear to be true for adults, so the best results are likely if surgery is done relatively early in childhood. Prophylaxis against infective endocarditis is recommended for all patients whether or not surgery is done.

Surgical Management

Valvular pulmonary stenosis is relieved surgically through a median sternotomy on cardiopulmonary bypass with mild to moderate hypothermia and total-body perfusion. The valve is exposed through a short longitudinal or transverse incision in the main pulmonary artery. Fused commissures are incised to the annulus. Each leaflet is detached slightly from the annulus adjacent to the commissures to improve mobility. Minor valvular regurgitation thus produced is well tolerated.

The dysplastic pulmonary valve requires total excision—valvectomy; the thick, mucocartilaginous, deformed, and immobile leaflet tissue otherwise remains as an obstruction in the right ventricular outflow tract.[511,512] When a patch is required because an obviously small annulus is present, the size of the reconstructed outflow tract is determined by data describing the normal annular diameter in individuals of equivalent body surface area.

The right ventricle is not incised unless a transannular patch is required or there is coexisting infundibular or subvalvular obstruction requiring excision. When the annulus is adequate, the hypertrophic subvalvular muscle can be excised through the valve and pulmonary artery. Fused valvular commissures can be incised through a right ventriculotomy when extensive subvalvular muscle resection or the placement of a transannular gusset is required.

In infants and small children with life-threatening valvular pulmonary stenosis,[513] valvotomy can be accomplished during about 90 s of venous inflow occlusion and circulatory arrest (Fig. 36-81). The empty heart continues to beat; resuscitation usually requires only the restoration of cardiac filling by release of caval clamps.[514] For longer exposure or the placement of a transannular patch, the operation is conducted during circulatory arrest with profound hypothermia. Cooling and rewarming are provided by limited cardiopulmonary bypass. Cardiopulmo-

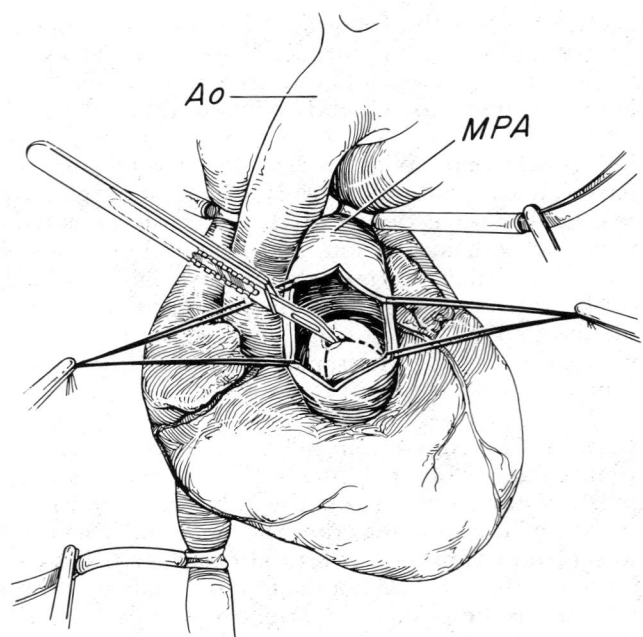

FIGURE 36-81 Pulmonary valvotomy in the infant using brief circulatory arrest with inflow occlusion. Tourniquets around the inferior and superior venae cavae interrupt blood flow into the heart, allowing exposure and excision or incision of the obstructing valve or membrane in the right ventricular outflow tract. Operation can be accomplished in 60 to 90 s of circulatory arrest. Resuscitation usually requires no more than release of the tourniquets to restore blood flow through the heart. Air is aspirated from the ascending aorta as forward flow is resumed. MPA = main pulmonary artery; Ao = aorta.

nary bypass with or without circulatory arrest and hypothermia allows closure of a stretched foramen ovale or atrial septal defect, eliminating the possibility of a postoperative right-to-left shunt and consequent hypoxia.

Beyond the first few months of life mortality is virtually nil; morbidity is low. Nearly normal right ventricular pressures can eventually be expected. Occasionally the immediate postoperative right ventricular pressure will remain elevated due to residual muscular hypertrophy, but will fall as hypertrophy regresses. It is important, however, that significant discrete subvalvular obstruction be relieved at the time of operation to assure a good hemodynamic result. Repeat valvotomy may be required several years later if the initial valvotomy was carried out during infancy.

Subvalvular Pulmonary Stenosis

Pathology

Subvalvular pulmonary stenosis is commonly at the infundibular level. Infundibular stenosis, sometimes referred to as *stenosis of the lower ostium of the infundibulum,* is characterized by a fibrous collar which encircles the inlet to the right ventricular infundibulum. An intact ventricular septum is rare (Fig. 36-

82). When the ventricular septum is defective, the cases resemble the tetralogy of Fallot. In all cases the right ventricular hypertrophy is limited to that part of the right ventricle proximal to the obstructing ring.

In some cases of hypertrophic obstructive cardiomyopathy the asymmetrical hypertrophy of the ventricular septum may cause infundibular stenosis.

Abnormal Physiology

The continuous recording of pressure while withdrawing a cardiac catheter from the pulmonary artery will frequently reveal whether stenosis is valvular, infundibular, or both (Fig. 36-77). Pressure tracings will not usually distinguish between muscular infundibular obstruction, infundibular obstruction produced by a fibrous band, or obstruction produced by both. If the evidence of infundibular obstruction on the pressure tracings becomes apparent or more marked during the administration of an inotropic drug such as isoproterenol or norepinephrine, it is likely that there is a muscular element in the infundibular obstruction.

If the stenosis is of the "pure" infundibular type, it may be possible to identify an "infundibular chamber" from pressure tracings at cardiac catheterization, although the catheter tip frequently flips through the area. Typically, as the catheter is withdrawn from the pulmonary artery across the pulmonary valve into the infundibular chamber, systolic pressure stays the same, but the diastolic pressure decreases to right ventricular level (Fig. 36-77). When the catheter is further withdrawn to the main right ventricular cavity, the systolic pressure is significantly higher than in the infundibular chamber or pulmonary artery. If both infundibular and valvular stenosis are present, the pressure tracings will be similar, except that the systolic pressure in the infundibular chamber will be at a level between that in the main right ventricle and that in the pulmonary artery.

Clinical Manifestations

Isolated subvalvular pulmonary stenosis in the infundibular area or from an anomalous muscle bundle is uncommon.[515] The clinical picture varies with the associated defects, most commonly ventricular septal defect, valvular pulmonary stenosis, and tetralogy of Fallot. The reader is referred to sections of this chapter on these specific defects.

Patients have a clinical picture similar to that of valvular pulmonary stenosis, but a thrill in the suprasternal notch is usually not present and the systolic murmur is best heard lower along the left sternal border. There is no ejection click. The electrocardiogram is similar to valvular stenosis, but chest roentgenogram shows no poststenotic dilatation of the pulmonary artery. Echocardiogram usually shows fluttering of the pulmonary valve leaflets,[509] but this is not specific for this defect. It is helpful as a distinction from valvular obstruction.

Cardiac catheterization will show a pressure difference as the catheter is slowly withdrawn from the right ventricular outflow tract to the inflow portion. If the obstruction is due to a muscle bundle rather than at the infundibular area, the pressure difference will be lower in the ventricle and careful positioning near the apex will sometimes be helpful in demonstrating the higher pressure area. Right ventricular angiography will further define the nature of the obstruction (Fig. 36-83). Associated ventricular septal defect is common, and some feel that it almost always occurs with subvalvular obstruction, but it may be small or close spontaneously.[6] Thus, even a small defect should be excluded by sensitive methods such as hydrogen electrode study, reverse dye curves, or selective left ventricular angiography.

The muscular hypertrophy and severity of obstruction frequently increase with time. Otherwise, the clinical course, medical management, and indications for surgery are the same as those described for valvular stenosis.

Surgical Management

Subvalvular pulmonary stenosis is relieved surgically through a median sternotomy on complete cardiopulmonary bypass with moderate hypothermia (28 to 30°C). Circulatory arrest with profound hypothermia (18 to 20°C) is used for infants and small children, cooling and rewarming being provided by

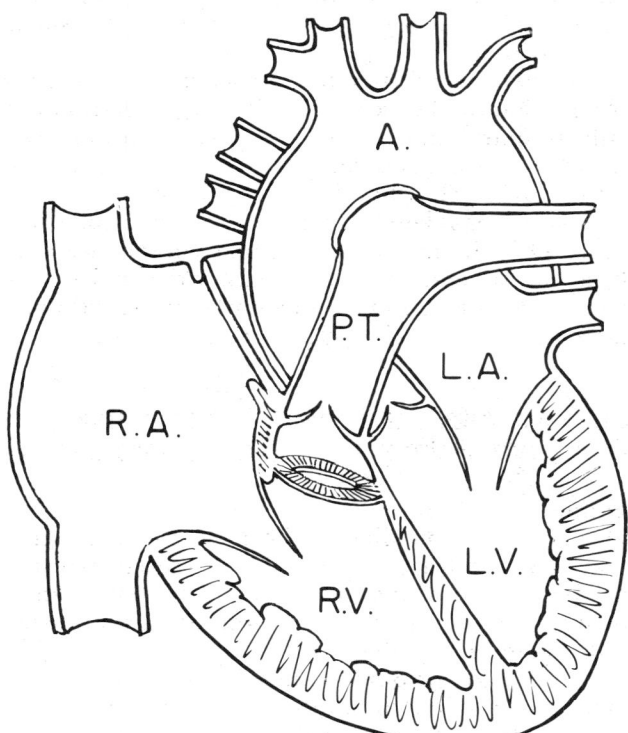

FIGURE 36-82 Localized membranous infundibular stenosis of the right ventricle (R.V.) with intact ventricular septum. R. A. = right atrium; P.T. = main pulmonary arterial trunk; L.A. = left atrium; L.V. = left ventricle; A. = aorta.

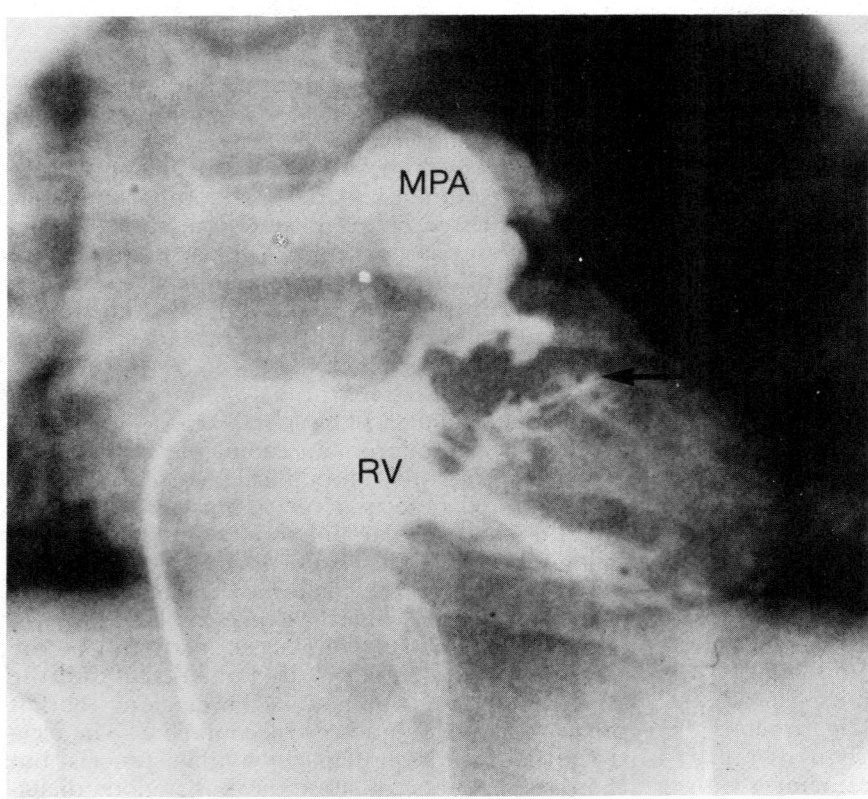

FIGURE 36-83   Posteroanterior view of a right ventricular (RV) angiogram demonstrating large anomalous muscle bundles (arrow) creating obstruction between the inflow and outflow areas of the ventricle. MPA = main pulmonary artery.

limited cardiopulmonary bypass. Cardioplegia facilitates myocardial preservation and exposure for longer procedures.

A small right ventriculotomy is made in the infundibulum parallel to the axis of the right ventricular outflow tract (Fig. 36-92). Large coronary arteries are avoided. Hypertrophic parietal and septal muscle bands constituting the fibrous orifice of the os infundibulum are excised; the ventriculotomy is extended through the anterior rim of the infundibular orifice (Fig. 36-100). The crista supraventricularis forming the posterior wall of the infundibulum can be thinned somewhat, but such excision is limited by the aortic valve lying directly beneath this muscle. Obstructing moderator bands or muscle bundles within the body of the right ventricle are incised, caution and good visualization being required to avoid injury to tricuspid papillary muscles and chordae tendineae. A frequently associated ventricular septal defect is sought and closed if present. (See discussions of ventricular septal defect and tetralogy of Fallot.) Associated valvular pulmonary stenosis is relieved by incision of the valve commissures back to the annulus; exposure is quite adequate through the ventriculotomy. (See discussion of valvular pulmonary stenosis.) Direct suture closure of the right ventriculotomy is usually satisfactory, but a small oval pericardial or Dacron gusset can be used if necessary to avoid narrowing the infundibulum as the myocardium is reapproximated. Right ventricular function is only minimally com-

promised by the placement of a small patch proximal to the annulus; a greater degree of functional compromise must be anticipated if a large patch is extended across the annulus. A patent foramen ovale is routinely sought and closed through a small right atriotomy.

Excellent relief of right ventricular outflow tract obstruction can be expected following operation for subvalvular pulmonary stenosis. Postoperative death is unusual and complications are rare. Operation during childhood reduces the likelihood of complications related to severe right ventricular hypertrophy, diminished ventricular compliance and function, subendocardial ischemia, tricuspid valvular regurgitation, and supraventricular arrhythmias associated with marked right atrial hypertrophy.

Supravalvular Pulmonary Stenosis and Peripheral Pulmonary Arterial Coarctations

Pathology

Obstructive anomalies of the pulmonary arteries may take the form of stenosis or atresia. Atresias will be covered in another section. The stenosis may be localized to any segment of the pulmonary arterial system (Fig. 36-84).

From angiographic studies, D'Cruz and associates[516] classified the anomalies into four types, namely (1) localized stenosis with poststenotic dilatation, (2) segmental stenosis, (3) diffuse hypoplasia,

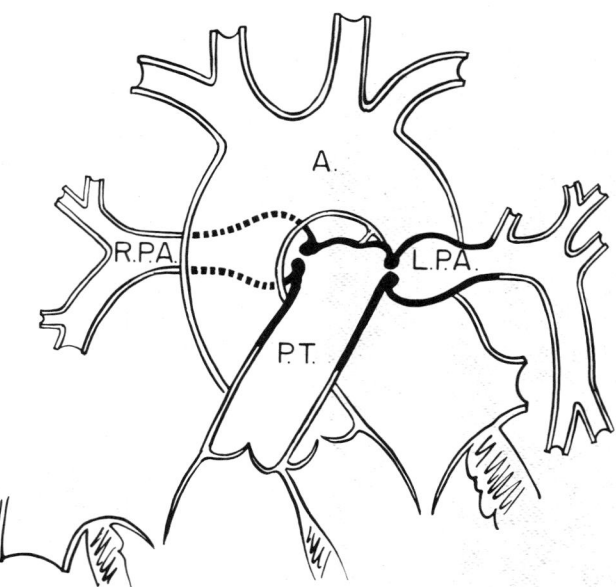

FIGURE 36-84 Stenosis, so-called coarctation, of each pulmonary artery as it arises from the pulmonary trunk (P.T.) R.P.A. = right pulmonary artery; L.P.A. = left pulmonary artery; A. = aorta. [From J. E. Edwards, Pulmonary Vascular Disease, in K. M. Moser (ed.), "Congenital Pulmonary Vascular Disorders," Marcel Dekker, Inc., New York, 1979, pp. 527–571. Reproduced with permission.]

and (4) multiple peripheral stenoses. They found that the process was unilateral in about one-third of the cases and bilateral in two-thirds. Pulmonary arterial stenosis is commonly (about 75 percent), though not universally, associated with other cardiovascular anomalies, among which are ventricular septal defect and pulmonary stenosis, supravalvular aortic stenosis, coarctation of the aorta, and the tetralogy of Fallot. Pulmonary arterial stenosis has been identified in some as one of the sequelae of maternal rubella.[517]

Abnormal Physiology[518]

Coarctation in the pulmonary arterial system is established by demonstrating a systolic pressure difference while withdrawing a cardiac catheter from a free position in a small peripheral pulmonary artery into the main pulmonary artery. The hemodynamic consequences are basically similar to those of valvular pulmonary stenosis.

Clinical Manifestations

There are many clinically associated abnormalities that give some clues to etiology.[6] It can occur as part of the syndrome described by Noonan, which was discussed under valvular stenosis, and it is a frequent abnormality in rubella syndrome with cataracts, sensorineural deafness, microcephaly, and other cardiac anomalies, most commonly patent ductus. It may be found in patients with Williams' syndrome or idiopathic hypercalcemia in association with characteristic facies, dental anomalies, mental retardation, and supravalvular aortic stenosis. There is also a familial occurrence associated with

supravalvular aortic stenosis, but not with the other characteristics of Williams' syndrome.

Manifestations are similar to valvular stenosis. The stigmata of the above-mentioned syndromes should be looked for on examination and careful histories of the pregnancy, neonatal period, and familial abnormalities obtained. The second heart sound is usually normal and there is no ejection click. A spindle-shaped midsystolic murmur is heard at the left upper sternal border, but it is equally or even better heard in the axillae and back. It may be heard unilaterally if only one side has significant obstruction. A similar murmur may be heard during the first weeks of life in premature infants, but this will disappear.[519] Occasionally, a continuous murmur is heard in those with severe stenosis in whom a diastolic gradient is demonstrable.[6] The electrocardiogram is similar to valvular obstruction. There is usually no poststenotic dilatation on chest roentgenogram. Cardiac catheterization will reveal a systolic pressure difference or differences with careful exploration of the entire pulmonary arterial tree. A widened pulse pressure in the proximal main pulmonary artery with a low dicrotic notch and low diastolic pressure reflecting distal pressure are typical of the more severe obstructions when they are bilateral.[9] Pulmonary arterial or right ventricular angiography will demonstrate the sites of obstruction in the main pulmonary artery and branches (Fig. 36-85). Study of the left side of the heart should also be done because of the frequency of associated supravalvular aortic stenosis or abnormalities of the left ventricular morphology and function.

Natural History and Prognosis

Although natural history[6] is not well defined, available information suggests that there is little change in severity with time. Those with severe obstructions may thrombose or rupture the thin-walled distal vessels with hemoptysis resulting.

Medical Management

Medical management is the same as with valvular stenosis, but should include special attention to the noncardiac handicaps in many of these patients. Surgical relief is possible for those with severe stenosis in whom the stenoses are proximal and relatively discrete.

Surgical Management

Isolated or multiple coarctations of main and branch pulmonary arteries are correctable by pericardial patch angioplasty if poststenotic dilatation is present. Proximal coarctations in the larger portion of the pulmonary arterial tree are more readily corrected than those located in smaller distal branches. Results are poor when stenoses are located at or beyond the bifurcation of either the right or left pulmonary artery. Stenosis of the main pulmonary artery or hypoplasia of the bifurcation of the main pulmonary artery is corrected by the placement of

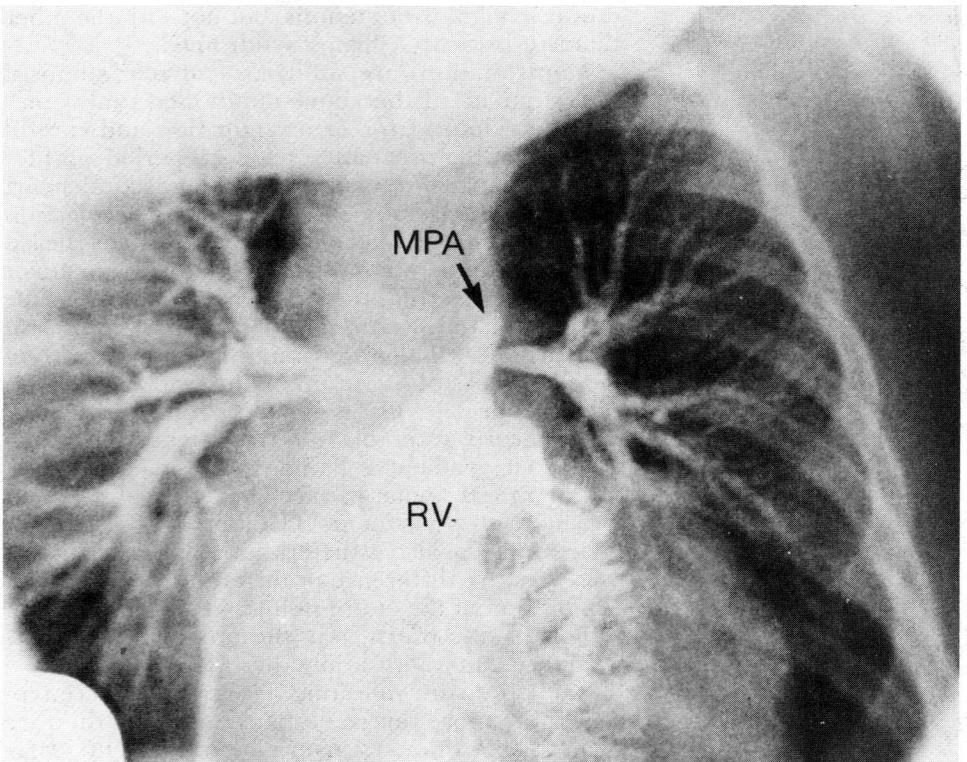

FIGURE 36-85 Posteroanterior view of a right ventricular (RV) angiogram showing diffuse hypoplasia of the main pulmonary artery (MPA) and proximal branches.

an oval or stellate pericardial gusset across the narrow point while the patient is supported on cardiopulmonary bypass. Discrete stenoses of the right or left pulmonary arteries can be widened with a similar pericardial patch angioplasty; cardiopulmonary bypass, although not absolutely necessary, allows more proximal placement of a clamp across the main pulmonary artery bifurcation for better exposure and a longer arteriotomy. Prosthetic graft materials such as Dacron or Gore-Tex can be substituted for pericardium if necessary, but these are probably more subject to thrombosis. Tubular conduits can be placed to "bypass" obstructions but are usually not necessary. Such conduits and the associated circular suture lines do not grow and hence are subject to restenosis as the child grows. The same potential for restenosis exists when discrete pulmonary arterial coarctations are excised and arterial continuity established by direct end-to-end anastomosis.

Pulmonary Atresia with Intact Ventricular Septum

Definition
Pulmonary atresia with intact ventricular septum is characterized by the pulmonary valve being an atretic membrane.

Pathology
The valve may be either a horizontal fibrous plate or a dome-shaped structure without an opening.[520,521] Three equidistant raphes of varying length are present along the arterial aspect of the valve. Cases tend to fall into two groups, depending on the size of the right ventricular chamber.[522] In one the chamber is smaller than normal, in some instances even diminutive (Fig. 36-86A). In the other, the chamber of the right ventricle is either of normal size or grossly enlarged. The difference in size of the chamber among patients with this valvular anomaly appears to depend on the state of the tricuspid valve. Patients with a functionally competent (although hypoplastic) tricuspid valve tend to have a smaller than normal right ventricular cavity. In contrast, when the tricuspid valve is incompetent, the right ventricular cavity develops to a normal size or is even enlarged (Fig. 36-86B). When the right ventricular cavity is small, the wall is grossly hypertrophied. In the subvalvular area the hypertrophy causes an accentuation of the proximity of right ventricular myocardium with the inferior aspect of the pulmonary valvular tissue.[523] Also, in cases with the small right ventricle, large sinusoids are present in the wall of the ventricle. These communicate with the coronary arteries.[524] Vital channels for the flow of blood are the foramen ovale and the ductus arteriosus.

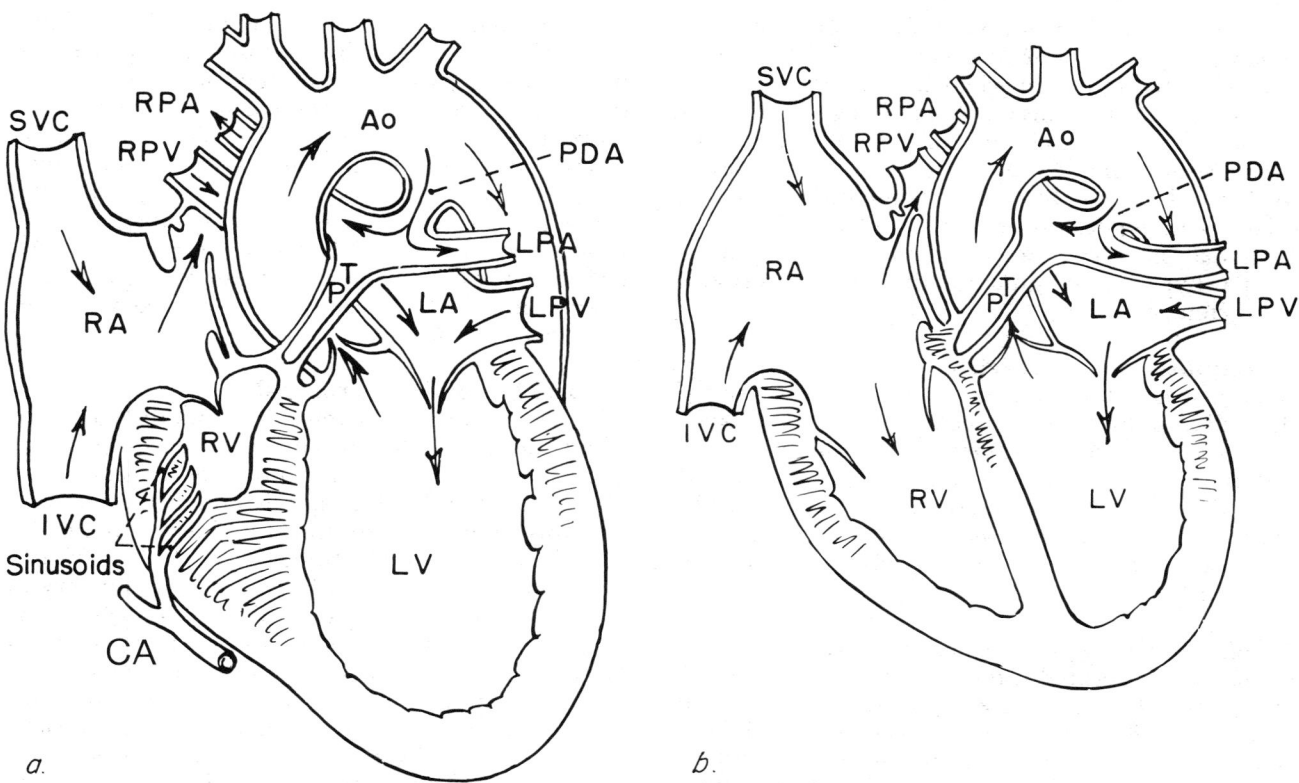

FIGURE 36-86 Pulmonary valvular atresia with intact ventricular septum. *a.* With small right ventricular (RV). As a consequence of the high pressure built up in the right ventricle, sinusoids may carry blood from the right ventricular cavity to coronary arterial branches (CA) in the epicardium. The essential route for the flow of blood from the right atrium (RA) is through a patent foramen ovale into the left side of the heart. Pulmonary circulation depends on flow from the aorta (Ao) through a patent ductus arteriosus (PDA). *b.* With large right ventricle. As a consequence of coexistent tricuspid insufficiency (often as a result of associated Ebstein's malformation of the tricuspid valve), the right ventricle may enlarge in the presence of pulmonary valvular atresia with intact ventricular septum. Except for the tricuspid insufficiency, the route for the flow of blood is like that in *a.* SVC = superior vena cava; IVC = inferior vena cava; PT = main pulmonary arterial trunk; RPA = right pulmonary artery; LPA = left pulmonary artery; RPV = right pulmonary vein; LPV = left pulmonary vein; LA = left atrium; LV = left ventricle.

Associated Conditions In a rare case, the tricuspid valve is also atretic. In such cases, the right ventricular cavity is a blind, tiny structure. Ebstein's deformity of the tricuspid valve is common both in cases with small and large right ventricles.[525]

Complications The principal complication is closure of the ductus arteriosus. Uncommonly, this is brought about by ductal thrombosis. Usually, closure is through the usual processes of anatomic ductal closure. In cases with massive enlargement of the right ventricle, failure of that chamber may be a complication.

Clinical Manifestations

History Although pulmonary atresia with intact ventricular septum is uncommon, it is one of the most frequent causes of cyanosis and death in the neonatal period.[3] Cyanosis and tachypnea appear soon after birth. Since these infants are dependent on an atrial communication and patency of the ductus, progressive cyanosis or hypoxic attacks occur as the ductus undergoes spontaneous closure. Acidosis and death will ensue if there is no intervention.

Physical Examination These infants are usually extremely cyanotic; tachypnea is associated. The precordium is quiet. The second heart sound is single. There may be no murmur, but the continuous or abbreviated murmur of a ductus may be heard intermittently. In some infants a blowing holosystolic murmur of tricuspid regurgitation resembling that of a ventricular septal defect is heard at the lower sternal border.[9] Progressive hepatomegaly and a prominent *a* wave in the jugular venous pulse may appear later.

Chest Roentgenogram Diminished pulmonary flow is invariably seen on the chest roentgenogram. The heart size may be near normal to grossly enlarged. The latter is primarily due to right atrial enlargement, particularly if there is tricuspid regurgitation.

Electrocardiogram The findings on electrocardiogram vary to a large extent, depending on the size of the right ventricle, although this is not completely reliable as an indicator of cavity size. In those with a hypoplastic right ventricle, which is the most common type, the QRS axis is normal to slightly leftward for age and there is absence of the usual right ventricular dominance for age (Fig. 36-87). Right atrial hypertrophy is common. Less commonly there is a dilated and hypertrophied right ventricle. These infants may have right axis deviation and right ventricular hypertrophy similar to those with severe valvular stenosis.[9]

Echocardiogram The echocardiographic findings will also depend on cavity size. Commonly, there are delayed and diminished tricuspid excursion, diminished right ventricular dimension, no demonstrable pulmonary valve, and normal to slightly increased left heart diameter.[526] Less commonly, the right ventricular size is increased and the pulmonary valve can be recorded with only presystolic motion or *a* dip.[527]

Cardiac Catheterization Immediate cardiac catheterization is indicated if the diagnosis of pulmonary atresia is suspected, since rapid deterioration can occur. The right atrial pressure is elevated and there is a right-to-left shunt at atrial level. Right ventricular pressure is markedly elevated, frequently above left ventricular level. Occasionally, only a dampened diphasic pressure can be recorded if the right ventricle is extremely diminutive. Arterial oxygen saturations are usually very low and acidosis may be present. Right ventricular angiography will dem-

onstrate cavity size, shape of the infundibulum, and any pinpoint opening in the pulmonary valve that might exist (Fig. 36-88). Enlarged sinusoids are frequent and may opacify the coronary arteries and aortic root. The degree of tricuspid regurgitation can be estimated. Volume studies may be performed for prognostic implications.[528,529] Aortography with simultaneous right ventricular injection can help to define the length of the atretic segment more accurately.[530] Left ventricular or aortic angiogram is needed to assess the size of the pulmonary arteries filled via the ductus.

Natural History and Prognosis

The natural history generally follows the course of events outlined. Most infants will die as the ductus closes in the first month of life. An occasional survivor to a slightly older age is noted if the ductus remains open long enough for development of a collateral circulation. Unoperated, death inevitably ensues in the first year, but even with surgery in competent centers, only one of four infants will survive to 1 year of age.[3] The postoperative course is largely dependent on right ventricular size. Growth of the cavity has been reported and eventual outcome is better for those with a large right ventricle, usually associated with a regurgitant tricuspid valve, who have had continuity established between the right ventricle and pulmonary arteries.[529]

Medical Management

Medical management includes supportive measures. Once the diagnosis is established, prostaglandin in-

FIGURE 36-87 Twelve-lead electrocardiogram of a young infant with pulmonary atresia with intact ventricular septum and hypoplastic right ventricle with a mean QRS axis of +80° and diminished right ventricular forces for age. There is also biatrial hypertrophy.

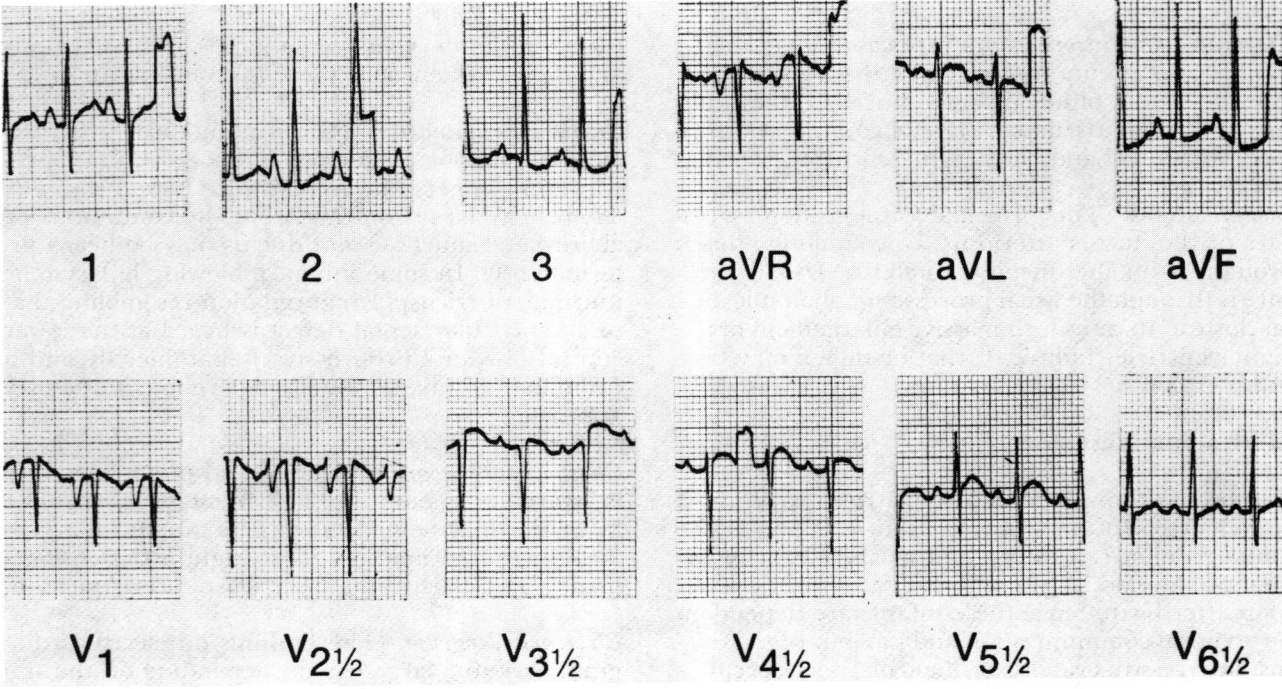

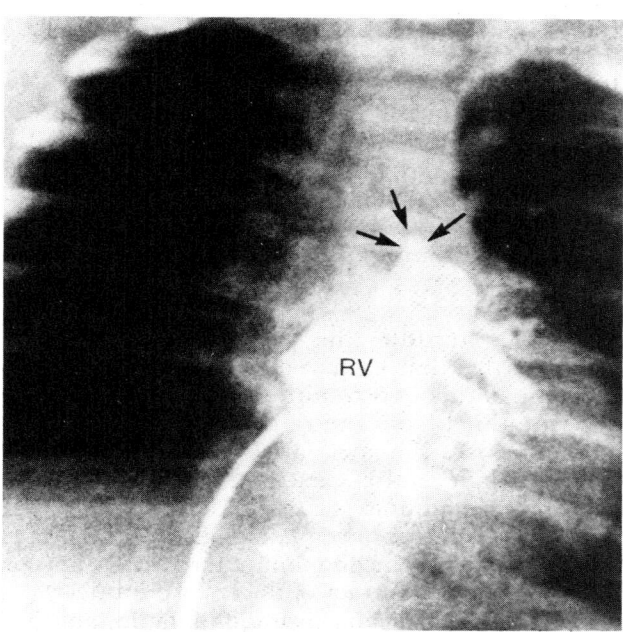

FIGURE 36-88 Posteroanterior view of right ventricular (RV) angiogram in an infant with pulmonary atresia (arrows) with intact ventricular septum and hypoplasia of the right ventricle.

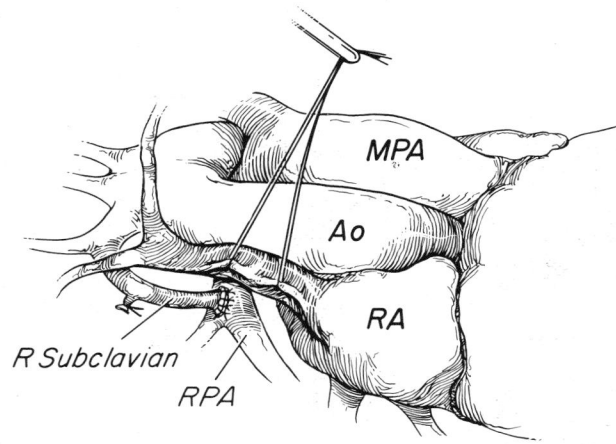

FIGURE 36-89 The Blalock-Taussig shunt. The divided end of the subclavian artery, usually on the side opposite the aortic arch, is anastomosed to the cephalad side of the ipsilateral pulmonary artery. This was the first, and still preferred, method for increasing pulmonary blood flow. Complications are rare, and closure at the time of subsequent total correction of the intracardiac defect is relatively simple.

fusion will usually result in ductal dilatation so that oxygenation is improved and acidosis can be corrected.[531] This should be continued until surgery can be done, to keep the infant in optimal condition and, it is hoped, to diminish surgical risks. Surgery is recommended for all. The operation may be creation of a systemic to pulmonary arterial anastomosis and/or reconstruction of the right ventricular outflow tract. The type of surgery is largely dependent on the anatomic variations[520] of right ventricular and tricuspid size, length of atresia, and size of the pulmonary arteries.

Surgical Management

Survival and quality of life for children with pulmonary atresia and intact ventricular septum are largely dependent upon the size, growth, and function of the right ventricle. Infants with a tiny right ventricle require the construction of a systemic to pulmonary arterial shunt to maintain adequate pulmonary blood flow after the ductus closes. We prefer the Blalock-Taussig subclavian to pulmonary arterial anastomosis, but other shunts, including the Waterston ascending aorta to right pulmonary artery shunt, ascending aorta to main pulmonary arterial "window," or the Gore-Tex central shunt can be used (Figs. 36-89, 36-90, and 36-91). (See discussion of tetralogy of Fallot.) Infants having a larger right ventricle will benefit from excision of the obstructing diaphragm by open or closed techniques at the same or a subsequent operation. The small noncompliant right ventricle rarely provides adequate pulmonary blood flow even when the obstruction is relieved by a transannular patch, but the es-

tablishment of forward flow through the right ventricle appears essential for subsequent ventricular growth. Decompression by relief of the outflow tract obstruction probably reduces the severity of arrhythmias associated with subendocardial ischemia. Tricuspid regurgitation and a right-to-left shunt at atrial level through a stretched foramen ovale cause hypoxia and low pulmonary blood flow, often resulting in death following operation. A pros-

FIGURE 36-90 Waterston shunt. The right pulmonary artery is anastomosed side-to-side to the posterior aspect of the ascending aorta, care being exercised to restrict the size of the orifice to 4 mm in infants and 5 mm in older children. Continuous monofilament suture is used to restrict growth. The anastomosis must lie directly posterior, not to the right, to avoid excessive flow to the right lung. Kinking and distortion of the right pulmonary artery have limited the usefulness of this shunt.

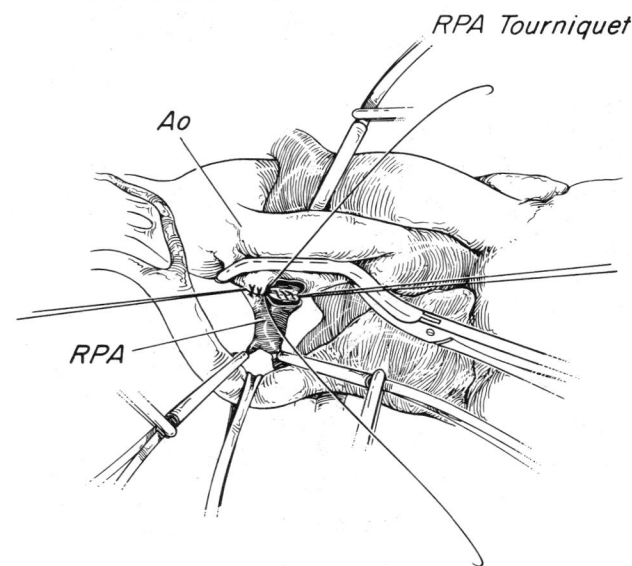

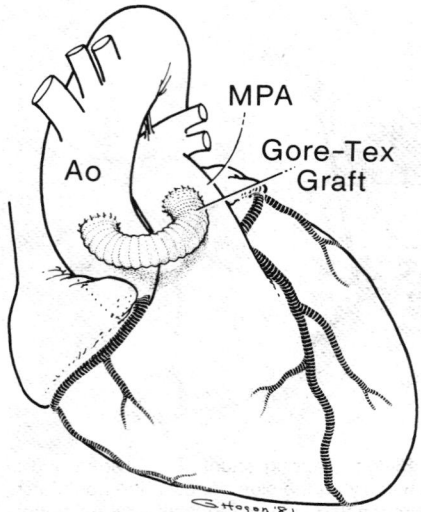

FIGURE 36-91   Central Gore-Tex shunt. A conduit of tubular Gore-Tex graft material is sutured to the ascending aorta and the main pulmonary artery through a median sternotomy incision. Graft sizes range from 4 mm in infants to 6 mm in older children.

taglandin infusion will temporarily maintain adequate pulmonary blood flow via the ductus arteriosus until a shunt can be constructed, if relief of right ventricular outflow tract obstruction fails to raise the systemic oxygen saturation.

Because of the relatively dismal long-term outlook for these children with small right ventricles, a definitive operation—placement of a transannular patch and closure of the atrial septal defect during circulatory arrest with profound hypothermia—may prove to be the appropriate initial procedure in spite of the anticipated high early mortality (Fig. 36-92).[532] Most surgeons still prefer palliation with both a shunt and a valvotomy.[533,534]

Tetralogy of Fallot

Definition
The tetralogy of Fallot is characterized by biventricular origin of the aorta above a large ventricular septal defect, right ventricular hypertrophy, and obstruction to pulmonary flow. When the obstruction is complete (pulmonary atresia) the term *pseudotruncus arteriosus* is applied.

Pathology
The aorta straddles the ventricular septum and arises partly from each ventricle with varying degree, usually about two-thirds from the left ventricle and one-third from the right (Fig. 36-93). In uncommon cases the aorta arises almost exclusively from the right ventricle (extreme dextroposition).[535] Yet fibrous continuity of the aortic origin and the anterior mitral valve are maintained, as in all cases of the tetralogy. Uncommonly there is also fibrous continuity of the aorta and the tricuspid valve.[536]

The right ventricular infundibulum lies anterior to the position of the ventricular septal defect and is bounded by the anterior and septal walls anteriorly and medially, while the posterior wall is said to be a vertical crista supraventricularis or displaced conus septum.[537] The right ventricular infundibulum is a distinctive channel that has been termed a third ventricle. The caliber of the channel varies. Uncommonly it is only mildly obstructive. Usually it exhibits a significant degree of stenosis and is the dominant site of the obstruction to pulmonary flow characteristic of the tetralogy. In the young, the lining of the infundibulum is normal, but in adolescents and adults it shows varying degrees of endocardial fibroelastosis, especially at its inlet.

The pulmonary valve is often malformed, usually being either bicuspid or unicuspid. The valve may contribute to pulmonary stenosis, but only uncom-

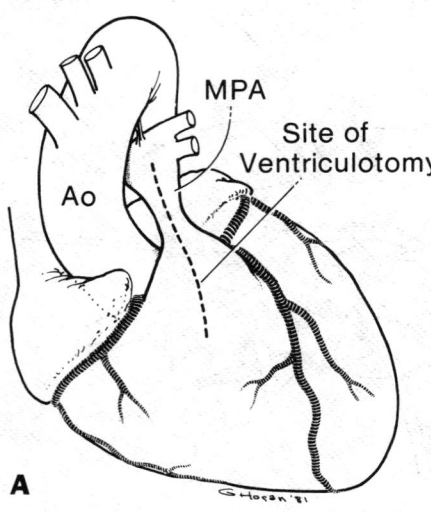

A

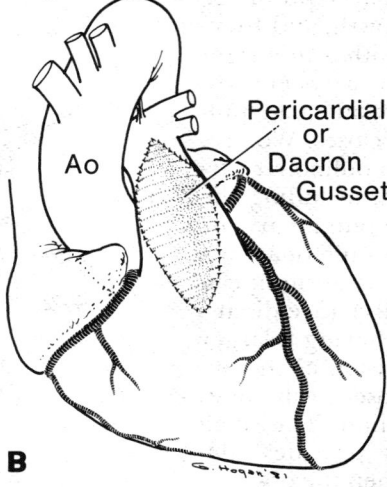

B

FIGURE 36-92   *A.* Site of incision for enlargement of the right ventricular outflow tract. Major coronary arteries are avoided. The incision is carried well out onto the main pulmonary artery to the bifurcation when the annulus and main pulmonary are small. The ventricular septal defect in tetralogy of Fallot is exposed through the caudal right ventricular portion of this incision. *B.* Pericardial or Dacron gusset used to widen the restrictive right ventricular outflow tract. Pericardial patches have become aneurysmal when elevated pulmonary vascular resistance or distal obstruction has resulted in persistent elevation of right ventricular pressures postoperatively.

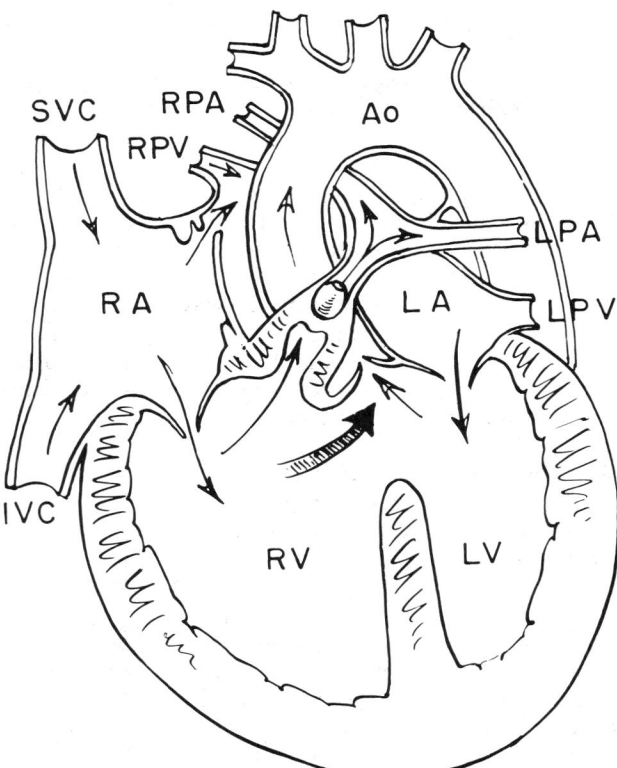

FIGURE 36-93   Classical tetralogy of Fallot. There is infundibular and pulmonary valvular stenosis. The major shunt is right-to-left at the ventricular level. A patent foramen ovale is also frequently present. SVC = superior vena cava; IVC = inferior vena cava; RA = right atrium; RV = right ventricle; RPA = right pulmonary artery; LPA = left pulmonary artery; RPV = right pulmonary vein; LPV = left pulmonary vein; LA = left atrium; LV = left ventricle; Ao = aorta. [*From J. E. Edwards, Classification of Congenital Heart Disease in the Adult, in W. C. Roberts (ed.), "Congenital Heart Disease in Adults," Cardiovasc. Clin.. Series 10/1, F. A. Davis Company, Philadelphia, 1979, pp. 1–26. Reproduced with permission.*]

monly will it be the only site of significant obstruction to pulmonary flow.[538] Characteristically, the pulmonary trunk is thin-walled and its lumen is more narrow than normal, but usually it is wider than either the right ventricular infundibulum or the orifice of the pulmonary valve. The aorta is wider than normal, its caliber roughly inverse to that of the pulmonary trunk. The foramen ovale is usually patent in patients of all ages.

In the pseudotruncus form of the tetralogy, the atretic segment usually lies either at the valve level or in the uppermost aspect of the infundibulum. Only uncommonly is the atretic site in the pulmonary trunk. In all cases of the tetralogy with significant pulmonary obstruction, collateral branches to the lungs arise from the aorta.

Associated Conditions   The most commonly associated condition with the tetralogy of Fallot is right aortic arch (about 30 percent).[538] It is usually of the

type that does not have a retroesophageal segment (see "Aortic Arch Anomalies"). A double aortic arch occurs uncommonly. A persistent left superior vena cava has been described in 10.6 percent of cases. The ductus arteriosus may be absent, present unilaterally on either the right or left side, or bilateral. Common atrioventricular canal malformations as well as isolated anomalies of the tricuspid or mitral valves may be associated. A particular type of tricuspid anomaly is that of an accessory flap on the septal leaflet. This flap may serve to obstruct the ventricular septal defect.[539] Coronary arterial anomalies characterized by a major artery crossing the infundibulum are seen in a few cases.

Complications   Among the complications of tetralogy of Fallot are (1) hypoxic fainting spells, (2) cerebral abscess, and (3) infective endocarditis. In cases with shunts the infection may be related to the site of the shunt, usually at the pulmonary end.

In cases of the tetralogy with mild pulmonary stenosis, hypertensive pulmonary vascular disease may appear, and rarely such changes may occur in severe pulmonary stenosis or even pulmonary atresia, the changes evidently being responsive to the effects of major flow through well-established collaterals. In patients treated by shunt procedures, hypertensive pulmonary vascular disease occurs uncommonly. The tendency for this complication is most often seen in cases with wide shunts, such as the Pott's or Waterston types.[540] In untreated cases with significant pulmonary stenosis, thrombi in varying stages are seen in small arteries of the lung. The distribution, however, is usually not wide enough to be responsible for significant obstruction to flow through the pulmonary vascular bed. The incidence of thrombotic lesions has a direct relationship to the degree of pulmonary stenosis and the occurrence of thrombosis may be abetted by the associated polycythemia.[541]

Abnormal Physiology[542–546]
It is probable that the altered relation of the aortic root to the ventricular septal defect plays a minor role in the altered hemodynamics of this condition. Since the ventricular septal defect is usually large, with an area about as large as the aortic valve, both ventricles and the aorta have essentially the same systolic pressures. The basic hemodynamic factor that determines how well these patients tolerate their disease is the ratio between the resistance to flow into the aorta and the resistance to flow across the stenotic right ventricular infundibular and/or stenotic pulmonary valve. If the resistances to right ventricular outflow are not large, the pulmonary flow may be twice the systemic flow and the arterial saturation may be normal (so-called acyanotic tetralogy of Fallot). On the other hand, the resistance to the pulmonary flow may be markedly increased with a right-to-left shunt, arterial unsaturation, and

cyanosis, even at rest. When the pulmonary stenosis is very severe, much or most of the pulmonary blood flow may be by way of collateral blood flow in large, tortuous bronchial arteries, particularly after childhood. The infundibular obstruction, which is very dynamic, is increased by drugs, maneuvers, or activities that increase myocardial contractility or heart rate or that decrease right ventricular volume. In addition, the infundibular hypertrophy may gradually increase over many years.[547] Since the systolic pressure in the right ventricle cannot exceed that in the left ventricle because of the large ventricular septal defect, the right ventricle is "protected" from excessive pressure-work, although exercise tolerance may be very limited. This may also explain why cardiac failure is so rare during childhood.

The pressure tracing in the right ventricle resembles that in the left ventricle, with a rapid upstroke, a relatively flat top, and a sharp descent, in contrast to the triangular pulse characteristic of isolated valvular stenosis.

The precise mechanism by which squatting relieves breathlessness and faintness after exercise in patients with tetralogy of Fallot is unknown. It is known that the arterial saturation returns to its resting value more rapidly if the patient squats after exercise. In normal subjects, it is probable that squatting also produces an increase in systemic arterial blood pressure, an increase in venous return to the heart, and in systemic cardiac output. Presumably squatting produces these same changes in patients with tetralogy. It is possible that in these patients the increase in arterial saturation produced by squatting is also related to an increase in peripheral resistance by compression and kinking of the femoral arteries. Squatting does not obstruct the return of markedly unsaturated blood from the legs. Actually, it usually increases venous return to the heart with an increase in right ventricular stroke volume, pressure, and pulmonary blood flow.

Hypercyanotic episodes in patients with tetralogy are of uncertain origin. It is possible that some episodes are caused by periods of unusual hyperactivity of muscular fibers in the right ventricular outflow tract producing, or exaggerating, the infundibular stenosis. Some spells may be caused by a decrease in peripheral resistance and systemic arterial pressure, which cause the right ventricular pressure and pulmonary blood flow to decrease. Cyanosis is also often much worse during crying, presumably due to decreased pulmonary blood flow from a combination of performing a Valsalva maneuver, breath holding, and sympathetic excitation.

As a result of arterial unsaturation, patients with tetralogy develop marked polycythemia. This may be severe enough to increase the viscosity of blood and impede blood flow, particularly in small vessels. Polycythemia may increase the tendency to thrombosis, particularly in the cerebral and pulmonary vessels.

Combined tetralogy of Fallot and atrial septal defect is referred to as *pentalogy (pentad) of Fallot*. The presence of the additional defect at the atrial level does not significantly modify the basic hemodynamics.

Clinical Manifestations

Tetralogy of Fallot is one of the most common congenital cardiac defects causing cyanosis. Of cyanotic patients over age 2 years and not requiring surgery, approximately three-fourths have tetralogy of Fallot.[6] An associated atrial septal defect, or pentalogy of Fallot, is not distinguishable clinically. The reader is referred to the section on cyanosis and its complications earlier in this chapter.

History The majority of patients are first seen by 6 months of age because of cyanosis. If the right ventricular outflow obstruction is very severe, marked cyanosis is present at birth or as soon as the ductus closes. Other patients slowly develop progressively more severe obstruction and cyanosis; such patients will present later in infancy, childhood, or even in adulthood. Some patients with a large ventricular septal defect and left-to-right shunt in early infancy may acquire infundibular pulmonary stenosis and become clinically indistinguishable from the usual patient with tetralogy of Fallot. Dyspnea with exertion occurs commonly. Attacks of suddenly increasing cyanosis associated with hyperpnea, or hypoxic spells,[548,549] are common between the ages of 2 months and 2 years. There are many precipitating events, including infection, exertion, and summer heat. They occur most often in the morning and the infant is usually irritable. Frequency and duration vary widely, but prolonged episodes can lead to syncope, seizures, and death. During these spells, the systolic murmur, which may have been quite loud before the attack, decreases or even disappears due to the reduced flow across the obstruction. Cyanosis increases dramatically because of the increased right-to-left shunting. Squatting with exercise is common from $1\frac{1}{2}$ to 10 years of age and is almost pathognomonic of this diagnosis.

Physical Examination Growth is usually normal unless cyanosis is extreme.[39] Clubbing occurs after 3 months of age and is proportional to the level of cyanosis. Signs of congestive heart failure do not appear in tetralogy of Fallot during childhood unless there is a superimposed illness such as anemia, acute glomerulonephritis, or infective endocarditis. There is increased right ventricular activity. A systolic thrill is frequently palpable at the left midsternal border, with a harsh midsystolic murmur in this location. Softer murmurs signal more severe obstruction and are common when presentation is in the newborn period or during hypoxic spells. The murmur ends before the second heart sound, which is characteristically single. A continuous murmur is heard if a patent ductus or large bronchial collateral vessels are present. An early systolic ejection sound at the left sternal border and apex is common.

Chest Roentgenogram (Fig. 36-94) The total heart size is usually normal on chest roentgenogram, but right ventricular enlargement is present in the lateral projection. The aorta arches to the right in 25 percent or more of cases.[290] Pulmonary flow is diminished. The pulmonary segment is concave and the apex elevated, giving the coeur en sabot contour. The very young infant may have only diminished pulmonary flow.

Electrocardiogram The mean QRS axis of the electrocardiogram is usually to the right, between $+90$ and $+210°$. If the axis is superior, endocardial cushion defects, single ventricle, or double outlet right ventricle with pulmonary stenosis should be suspected. There is right ventricular hypertrophy with a tall R wave in the right precordial leads and a deep S wave in the left. A small percent have right atrial hypertrophy.

Echocardiogram M-mode echocardiography[550] will show abrupt ending of the septal echoes just below the overriding aorta (Fig. 36-95). Frequently right ventricular enlargement and hypertrophy, narrowing of the outflow tract, and aortic dilatation also occur. The pulmonary valve may be difficult to record, and if unsuccessful, truncus arteriosus and ventricular septal defect with pulmonary atresia are not excluded. The left atrium is usually small in tetralogy and normal to enlarged in truncus arteriosus. Continuity of the anterior mitral leaflet and posterior aortic wall excludes double outlet of the right ventricle with pulmonary stenosis.[551] Associated en-

docardial cushion defect can be excluded. False overriding of the aorta can be created by a transducer position that is too high along the sternal border. Cross-sectional echocardiography[36,552] is extremely helpful in delineating the anatomy and is more specific for definitive diagnosis (Figs. 36-96, 36-97, and 36-98).

Hematologic and Other Laboratory Studies (Refer to section on cyanosis, earlier in this chapter.) Measurement of hemoglobin and hematocrit should be done in all patients at initial evaluation, and periodically both for determination of the degree of polycythemia and the early detection of anemia relative to the degree of cyanosis. The latter is common, especially in those under 2 years of age, and in those in this age group with cerebrovascular accidents. Platelet counts and clotting studies may be advisable in patients with marked polycythemia, particularly if a surgical procedure is planned. Serum uric acid levels should be measured periodically in older children and adults with severe polycythemia.

Cardiac Catheterization The right ventricular systolic pressure is equal to that in the left ventricle and aorta, except in the rare case with a small ventricular septal defect when the right ventricular pressure will be above systemic. The right atrial pressure is almost always normal. If the pulmonary artery can be entered, the pressure will be normal or low. The level(s) of obstruction can be evaluated by careful pullback to the right ventricle. An infundibular chamber can usually be demonstrated. Caution should be observed if the pulmonary artery is entered, as the catheter may critically reduce the pulmonary flow and cause a hypoxic episode. Time with the catheter across the obstruction should be kept to a minimum. It is unnecessary to attempt to enter the pulmonary artery in those with very severe cyanosis or with a history of severe hypoxic spells, since the diagnosis can be made without this maneuver, which has a high risk. Systemic arterial saturation is low because of right-to-left shunting from the right ventricle. If a patent foramen ovale or atrial septal defect (pentalogy of Fallot) is present, there will be an additional right-to-left or bidirectional shunt at the atrial level, confirmed by dye curves or by normal pulmonary venous but diminished left atrial oxygen saturations. Selective biplane right ventricular angiography (Fig. 36-99) is extremely valuable to demonstrate the levels of obstruction, size of the pulmonary arteries, size and position of the ventricular defect, and opacification of the left ventricular outflow tract and aorta, which will frequently demonstrate the aortic-mitral relationship. Left ventricular angiography may be necessary at times to aid in exclusion of double outlet of the right ventricle. Aortography should be done on all patients preoperatively to demonstrate the

FIGURE 36-94 Chest roentgenogram in a 3-year-old boy with tetralogy of Fallot demonstrating a "boot-shaped" heart with a right aortic arch and mildly diminished pulmonary flow.

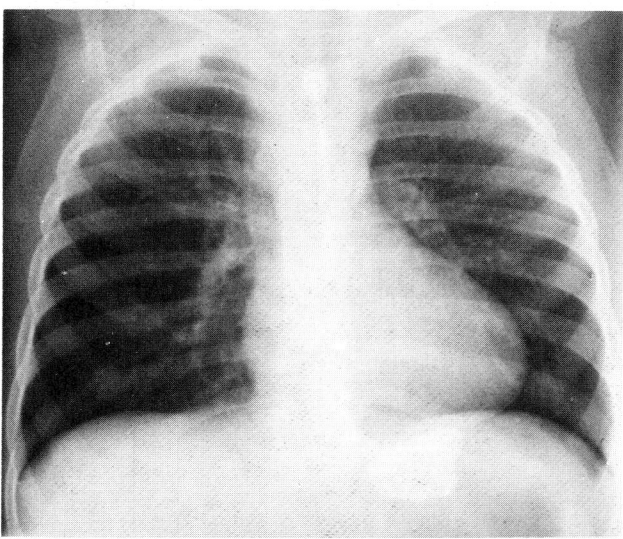

DISEASES OF THE HEART AND BLOOD VESSELS

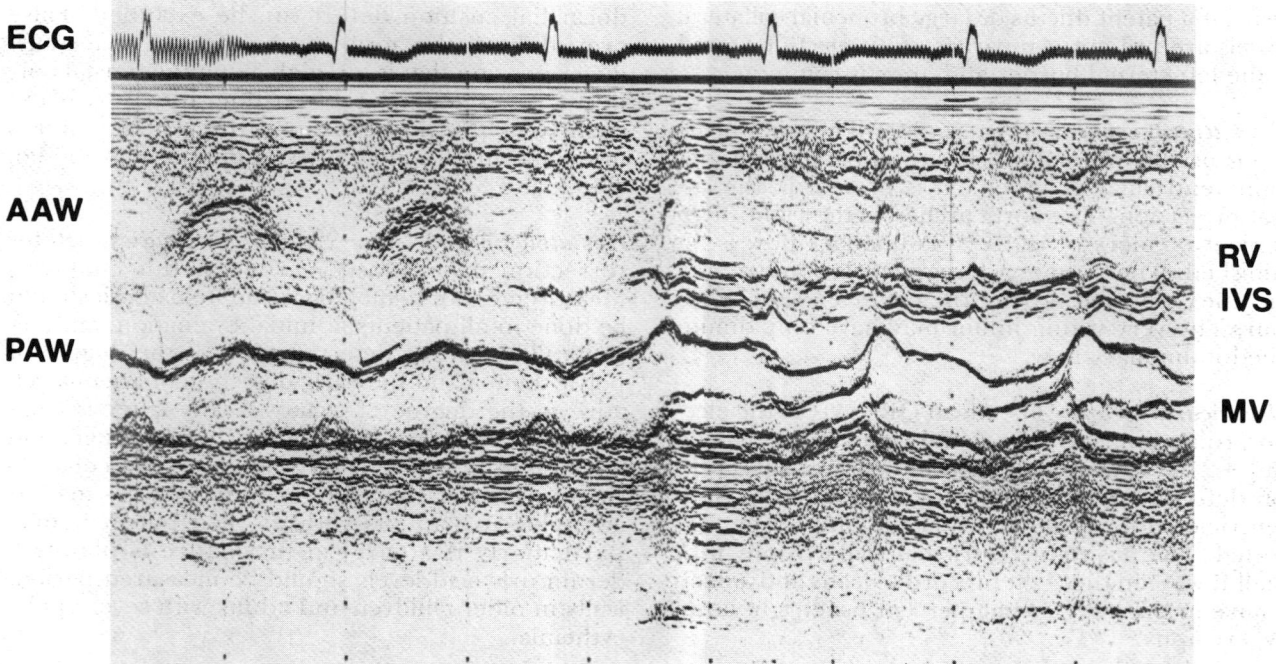

ECG

AAW

PAW

RV

IVS

MV

FIGURE 36-95   M-mode echocardiogram in a child with tetralogy of Fallot demonstrating aortic override of the interventricular septum (IVS), aortic-mitral (MV) continuity, and a small left atrium. ECG = electrocardiogram; AAW = anterior aortic wall; PAW = posterior aortic wall; RV = right ventricle.

coronary arterial pattern.[553] Selective coronary angiography can be done if necessary for better delineation.[554,555]

Natural History and Prognosis

Prognosis is poorest in very young infants who present with severe cyanosis due to the severity of obstruction and size of the pulmonary arteries, which are usually very small.[544] Hypoxic spells offer a poor prognosis if they are allowed to continue untreated. Obstruction to pulmonary flow tends to progress even to atresia[547] with increasing cyanosis

FIGURE 36-96   Two-dimensional echocardiogram in a patient with tetralogy of Fallot. The view is short-axis from the parasternal area. There is a dilated aortic root (AO), hypoplastic right ventricular outflow, and small pulmonary valve (PV). (*From Hagler et al.*[552] *Reproduced with permission*)

FIGURE 36-97   Two-dimensional echocardiogram in a patient with ventricular septal defect and pulmonary atresia. The view is the same as Fig. 36-96, for comparison. There is a dilated aortic root (AO) and the right ventricular outflow tract appears to end blindly. LA = left atrium. (*From Hagler et al.*[552] *Reproduced with permission.*)

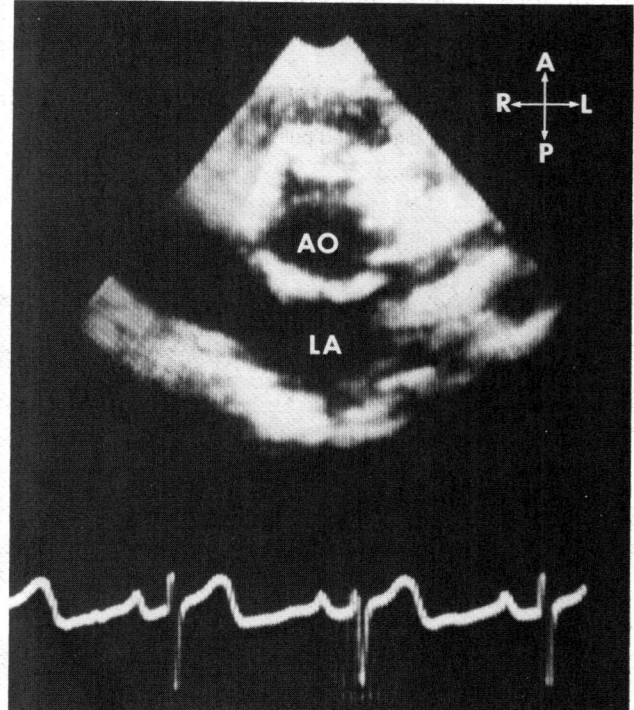

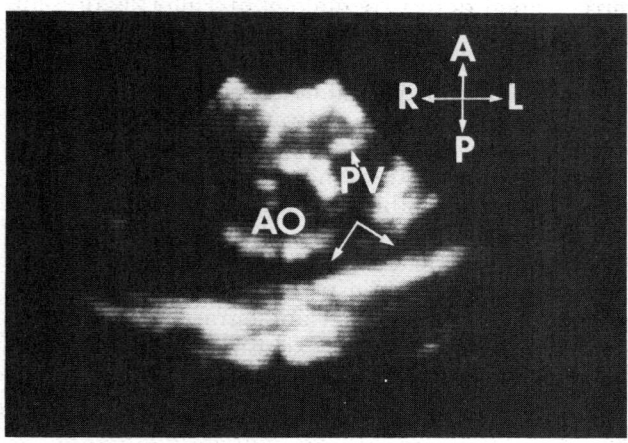

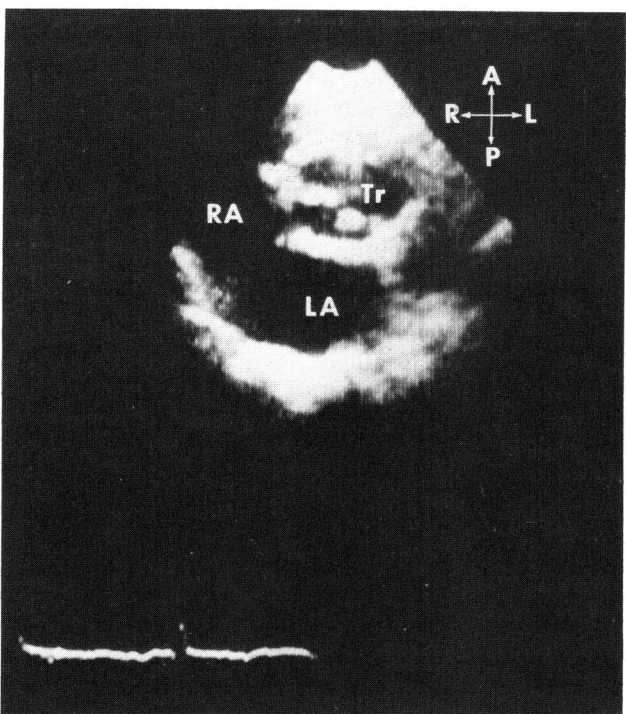

FIGURE 36-98   Two-dimensional echocardiogram in a patient with truncus arteriosus. The view is the same as Fig. 36-96 and 36-97, for comparison. There is a dilated truncal (Tr) root, but no evidence of a right ventricular outflow tract. LA = left atrium; RA = right atrium. (*From Hagler et al.*[552] *Reproduced with permission.*)

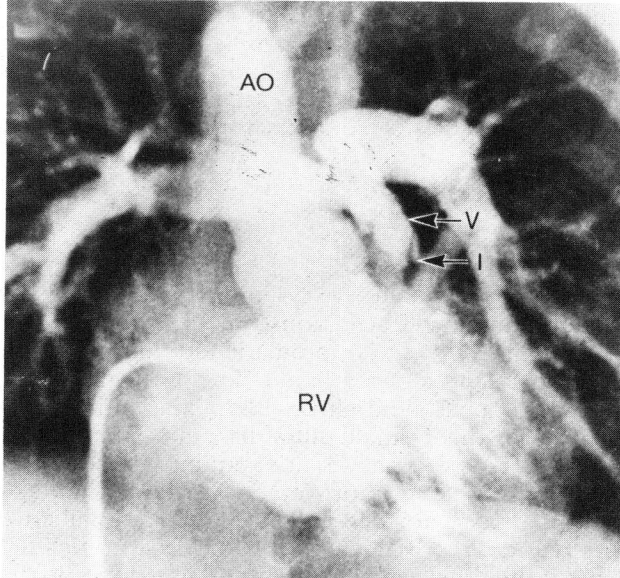

FIGURE 36-99   Posteroanterior view of a right ventricular (RV) angiogram in a child with tetralogy of Fallot with severe infundibular (I) and valvular (V) narrowing creating an outflow chamber (between arrows), and with right-to-left shunting into the aorta (AO), which arches to the right.

and polycythemia. The complications of polycythemia, including cerebrovascular accident and brain abscess, are discussed above. With polycythemia and decreased flow, multiple thrombi in small pulmonary vessels can occur.[556] The risk of infective endocarditis is high. Without surgery, approximately one-third die by age 1 year, one-half by age 3 years, three-quarters by age 10 years, with less than 5 percent surviving beyond age 30 years.[557]

Medical Management

The medical management in tetralogy of Fallot is directed primarily toward prevention and treatment of complications. Iron deficiency anemia should be promptly treated with iron supplementation. Fever or other common pediatric illness that would lead to dehydration and possible thrombotic complications should also be treated promptly. Hypoxic spells in infants should be treated initially by placing the infant in the knee-chest position. Parental education will help in prevention or management of all three of these problems. Further treatment of hypoxic spells includes administration of a high concentration of oxygen and morphine sulfate. If acidosis is present and does not correct spontaneously and promptly, intravenous sodium bicarbonate should be given. Propranolol is useful in the acute treatment and prevention of prolonged hypoxic spells.[558,559] Propranolol, a beta-adrenergic blocker,

should be given intravenously only for severe hypoxic spells, and orally for prevention. If for some reason the hematocrit should reach a level of 70 to 75 percent, erythrophoresis is recommended, using fresh frozen plasma or a colloid equivalent. This will temporarily diminish viscosity, but more definitive surgical treatment is indicated. Early and vigorous treatment should be given for intercurrent infections. Prophylactic antibiotics are recommended for prevention of infective endocarditis.

For the severely cyanotic newborn, prostaglandin administration may be of benefit, as with pulmonary atresia,[35,531] to open the ductus until surgery can be done. Prompt surgical intervention is indicated. Surgical correction is recommended in children for progressive symptoms or polycythemia with hematocrit approaching 65 percent. Elective surgical correction should be done in early childhood, since further delay offers no advantage and the continuing risks of complications of cyanosis are significant.

The infant who is symptomatic may be treated in three ways: palliation with propranolol and delayed correction, palliation with a systemic to pulmonary arterial shunt and delayed correction, or early correction. There is currently much debate on this issue. Clearly, certain anatomic variables, such as tiny pulmonary arteries or a coronary arterial abnormality, make early correction less attractive. Otherwise, early correction seems desirable if risk is no more than the total risk of other choices and outcome is equally as favorable. There are centers where this is possible in selected patients. One group has reported a method of looking at results in a statistical manner.[560] They found that propranolol and delayed correction was the best choice at their center, but that early correction is probably best at centers where early operative mortality is 10 percent or less. This type of analysis seems warranted. Additional variables, such as anatomic characteristics, should also be included to offer a firmer basis for recommendation of mode of treatment in the symptomatic infant.

Surgical Management

For many years palliative systemic to pulmonary arterial shunts have been constructed in infants and small children with symptomatic tetralogy of Fallot to increase pulmonary blood flow, prevent hypercyanotic "spells" and chronic hypoxia, and to promote growth of small pulmonary arteries.[561] Cardiopulmonary bypass is not required, recovery is usually rapid, and improvement is dramatic.

The first-performed and still preferred palliative operation is the Blalock-Taussig shunt, in which the end of the subclavian artery on the side opposite the aortic arch is anastomosed to the side of the ipsilateral pulmonary artery (Fig. 36-89). A modification described by Laks and Castaneda[562] utilizes a small arterioplasty across the orifice of the origin of the subclavian artery on the side of the aortic arch, making possible the construction of a shunt on this side without kinking the subclavian artery at its origin. In the first month of life, another useful option is the placement of a Gore-Tex graft between an undissected subclavian artery and the pulmonary artery. The Blalock-Taussig anastomosis almost always provides adequate but not excessive pulmonary blood flow, since the subclavian artery is usually of appropriate size. Deformity of the pulmonary artery at the site of the anastomosis is minimal. The development of pulmonary hypertension is rare. Excellent palliation is provided by this shunt until the child is considered a candidate for total correction. Closure of the shunt at the time of intracardiac repair is accomplished simply by ligation of the subclavian artery. Microvascular surgical technique, improved monofilament sutures, use of the operating headlight and magnifying glasses, and intraoperative systemic heparinization maintained for 2 to 3 days postoperatively by constant infusion have made possible the construction of an adequate classical or modified Blalock-Taussig shunt in newborns and small children.[563]

The Waterston anastomosis (Fig. 36-90) was for several years a popular and rapidly constructable systemic to pulmonary arterial shunt, but it has fallen into disfavor because of the deformity of the right pulmonary artery frequently produced at the anastomosis. This communication between the posterior aspect of the ascending aorta and the side of the right pulmonary artery is closed at the time of total repair by direct suture from within the ascending aorta or placement of a tiny Dacron patch over the orifice. Care is required to avoid creation of an excessively large shunt. Constriction, kinking, and even total obstruction of the right pulmonary artery by this anastomosis have caused technical difficulties at the time of total repair.[564]

Although the choice between a two-stage repair versus routine primary repair of tetralogy of Fallot remains controversial, improvements in perioperative support, a large experience with intracardiac correction under conditions of circulatory arrest and profound hypothermia, and the interim mortality and complications experienced in children having undergone palliative operations have altered our approach over the past decade.[565] We now prefer complete anatomic correction of all infants and children with symptomatic tetralogy of Fallot having pulmonary arteries and annulus of adequate size as determined by angiographic criteria. A small subgroup of infants with small pulmonary arteries and annulus are still managed by the initial construction of a Blalock-Taussig anastomosis.[561]

Total repair of tetralogy of Fallot is accomplished through a median sternotomy incision. Infants less than 1 year of age and weighing less than 10 kg are operated upon under conditions of circulatory arrest with profound hypothermia (18 to 20°C), cooling and rewarming being provided by cardiopulmonary bypass. Larger children are corrected on total cardiopulmonary bypass with moderate hypothermia and cardioplegia.

Details of the intracardiac operation are dictated by the level and severity of the right ventricular outflow tract obstruction. A small longitudinal incision (Fig. 36-92) is made in the infundibulum of the right ventricle through which hypertrophic parietal and septal muscle bands are excised (Fig. 36-100). Pulmonary valvular stenosis is relieved by valvotomy. The ventricular septal defect is closed through the right ventriculotomy by placement of a woven Dacron patch (see discussion of ventricular septal defect) (Fig. 36-101). When the pulmonary annulus and main pulmonary artery are of adequate caliber, the right ventriculotomy is closed by direct suture. Commonly the right ventricular outflow tract requires enlargement with a pericardial or synthetic fabric gusset which may cross a small annulus onto the main pulmonary artery (Fig. 36-92). Pulmonary valvular incompetence produced by a transannular gusset is generally well tolerated. When we elect not to insert a transannular patch, right ventricular pressure is measured after the child has been weaned from cardiopulmonary bypass. If right ventricular pressure exceeds 75 percent of the systemic arterial pressure, a patch is inserted during a subsequent period of cardiopulmonary bypass. A patent foramen ovale is routinely sought and closed by direct suture through a small right atriotomy.

The coronary arterial anatomy must be known before undertaking intracardiac total repair of tetralogy of Fallot.[566] When the left anterior descending coronary artery arises from a large conus branch of the right coronary artery traversing the right ventricular outflow tract, initial palliation by a Blalock-

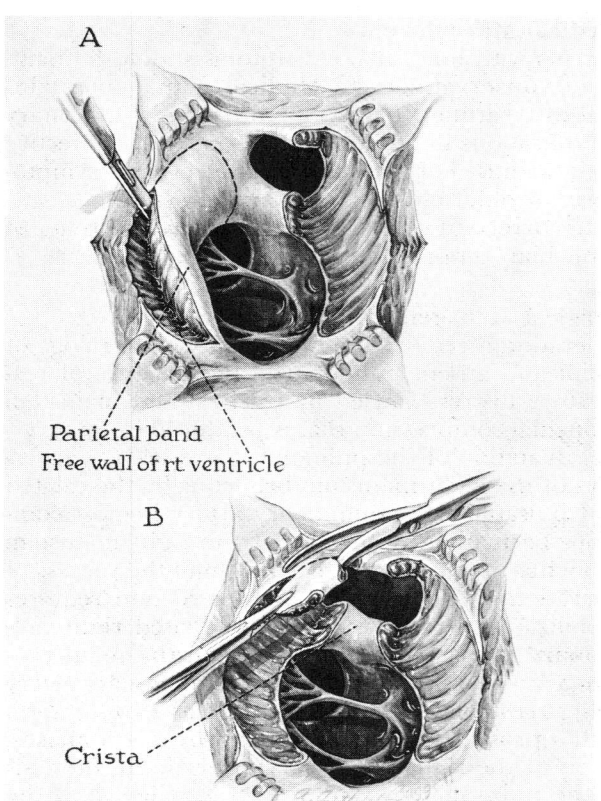

FIGURE 36-100 Relief of infundibular stenosis in a patient with tetralogy of Fallot. *A.* The septal band has been resected, and the parietal band is being mobilized. *B.* The parietal band has been excised and the free wall of the right ventricle is being mobilized. (*From Kirklin and Karp.*[542] *Reproduced with permission.*)

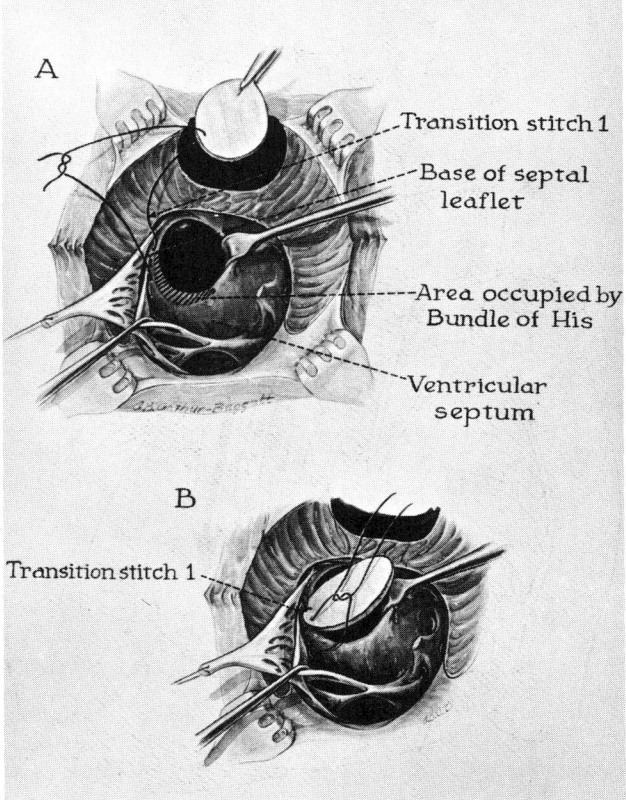

FIGURE 36-101 The repair of the ventricular septal defect in a patient with tetralogy of Fallot is being made. A patch of knitted Dacron is sewn into place with continuous sutures, placing the stitches so as to avoid the area occupied by the bundle of His. (*From Kirklin and Karp.*[542] *Reproduced with permission.*)

Taussig anastomosis is preferred. Eventual total correction may require the insertion of a conduit from the right ventricle over the anomalous coronary artery to the main pulmonary artery.

Absent Pulmonary Valve

Definition
Total or effective absence of the pulmonary valve is designated by the term *absent pulmonary valve.*

Pathology
All vestiges of the pulmonary valve may be absent or only remnants of tissue at valve level are identified.[567] The right ventricular infundibulum is wider than normal. The pulmonary trunk is distinctly enlarged, and bronchial compression may result. The basic features of the tetralogy are usually present (Fig. 36-102). In only a rare case are there no intracardiac anomalies.

Clinical Manifestations
Although absent or hypoplastic pulmonary valve is an uncommon defect, it can cause significant problems in infancy[567] with cyanosis and heart failure.

In the newborn, pulmonary hypertension, which is normally present, can lead to marked pulmonary regurgitation since valve tissue is very deficient. Commonly, the pulmonary valve ring is small and causes obstruction to pulmonary flow and there is an associated ventricular septal defect. Thus, some compare this entity to tetralogy of Fallot, but there are notable distinctions in the hemodynamics and clinical picture. Aneurysmal dilatation of the central pulmonary arteries occurs and causes bronchial compression with obstructive emphysema and resulting atelectasis.[568] Respiratory symptoms[569] frequently dominate the clinical picture and can lead to impressive respiratory distress in infants. Superimposed infection causes recurrent and episodic increases in the respiratory systems. Congestive heart failure can occur if the pulmonary regurgitation is great, especially in the newborn or if the annulus is not very restrictive so that significant left-to-right shunting through an associated ventricular septal defect occurs. Cyanosis can occur with heart failure but is more frequently due to some right-to-left or bidirectional shunting across the ventricular defect with a restrictive pulmonary valve annulus.

A hyperdynamic left parasternal impulse and harsh systolic and diastolic murmurs with a to-and-

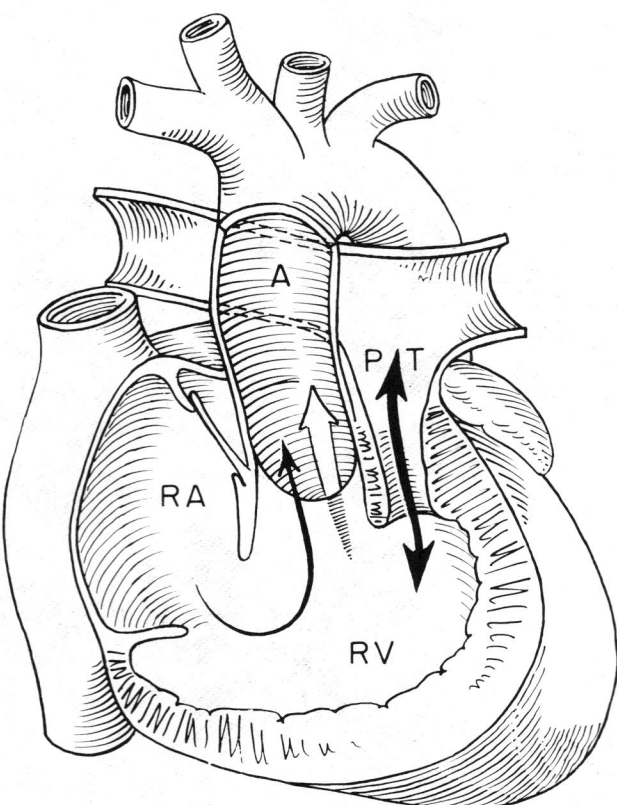

FIGURE 36-102 Tetralogy of Fallot with absent pulmonary valve. Significant dilatation of major pulmonary arteries occurs. RA = right atrium; RV = right ventricle; PT = main pulmonary arterial trunk; A = aorta.

fro quality are found. The second heart sound may be inaudible or single. The electrocardiogram usually shows right axis deviation and right ventricular hypertrophy. The chest roentgenogram shows cardiomegaly and aneurysmal dilatation of the central pulmonary arteries. There are frequently signs of hyperinflation, atelectasis, or pneumothorax and shift of the mediastinum that may make interpretation difficult.

Cardiac catheterization will reveal associated shunts. Difficulty may be encountered entering the pulmonary arteries, but assessment of the annular pressure difference is important. Angiography (Fig. 36-103) demonstrates the massive size of the pulmonary arteries and pulmonary valve anatomy, particularly the annular size, as little leaflet tissue is usually present.

Natural History and Prognosis

The natural history is not well defined due to small numbers of patients.[567] The newborn with heart failure may respond to medical management as the pulmonary vascular resistance decreases. Infants can succumb to severe hypoxia, rarely, or pulmonary complications, more commonly.

Medical Management

Infants with mild or no symptoms should be managed conservatively.[567] Medical management includes treatment of heart failure and pulmonary complications in addition to prevention of infective endocarditis. For infants who are severely symptomatic or older children with milder symptoms, surgical correction of intracardiac defects and relief of bronchial compression should be attempted.[570]

Surgical Management

Operation is required in the infant with tetralogy of Fallot and absent pulmonary valve because of respiratory distress caused by tracheal and mainstem bronchial compression that is produced by aneurysmal dilatation of the pulmonary arteries. Compression of the right mainstem bronchus by the dilated and pulsatile right pulmonary artery is most common. Permanent deformity of the right mainstem bronchus and lower trachea may limit the success of operation.[569] Relief of airway obstruction requires mobilization and division of the dilated right pulmonary artery, continuity between the main pulmonary artery and the distal right pulmonary artery being reestablished anterior to the ascending aorta with a prosthetic vascular graft or by direct anastomosis of the right pulmonary artery itself. Stenosis at the pulmonary annular level is relieved by the placement of a transannular patch. The ventricular septal defect is closed as described in the discussion of tetralogy of Fallot. Operation in the infant is conducted through a median sternotomy incision during a period of circulatory arrest with profound hypothermia (18 to 20°C).

In the older child with absent pulmonary valve, operation consists of plication or partial excision

FIGURE 36-103 Right anterior oblique view of right ventricular (RV) angiogram in a child with absent pulmonary valve with narrowing of the pulmonary annulus (arrows) and aneurysmal dilatation of the main (MPA) and proximal right (RPA) pulmonary arteries.

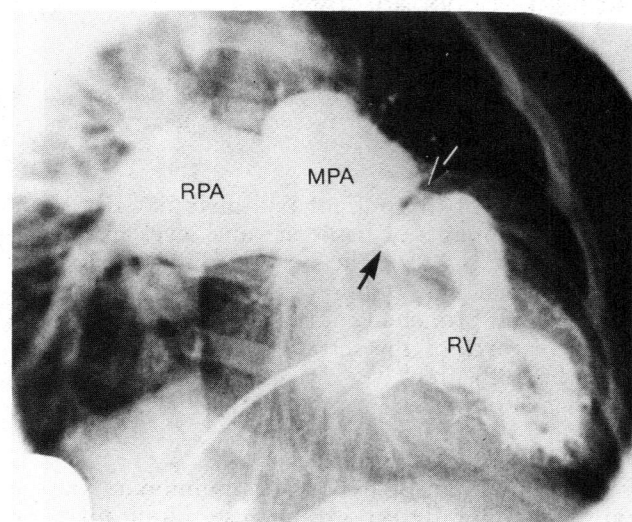

and repair of the dilated branch pulmonary arteries and possibly replacement of the pulmonary valve. Stenosis at the annular level is relieved by the placement of a large pericardial gusset over the portion of the prosthetic valve which cannot be anchored to the patient's natural annulus. The need for a prosthetic valve in the right ventricular outflow tract is controversial.[569] Reduction in the size of the branch pulmonary arteries, relief of the right ventricular outflow tract obstruction, and closure of the ventricular septal defect would probably constitute adequate correction. The presence of associated pulmonary vascular disease or tricuspid valvular insufficiency would encourage the use of a substitute pulmonary valve. Right ventricular function, especially during exercise, would probably be better when a valve is used, although one must weigh this advantage against the risk of deterioration and restenosis of a biprosthesis.

Results of operation in critically ill infants with airway obstruction are poor.[569] The operative mortality in older children is somewhat higher than that expected from the repair of tetralogy of Fallot, but late results in survivors are equal to those achieved in patients having tetralogy with a pulmonary valve.[571]

Absence of Anatomic Origin of Pulmonary Arterial System from Heart: With and without Confluence of Right and Left Pulmonary Arteries

Classification
Among some patients there is a common phenomenon of a ventricular septal defect and no direct connection of the pulmonary arterial supply with the heart. From the surgical point of view, one of the crucial points is whether the arterial supply to one lung is connected with that to the other (confluence), or whether each supply is independent of the other (nonconfluence). With this pivotal point in mind, the following classification is modified from that of Edwards and McGoon.[572]

1. Confluent origin of pulmonary arteries.
   a. With remnant of pulmonary trunk (pseudotruncus).
      (1) Proximal atresia and distal patency (pseudotruncus with patent pulmonary trunk) (Fig. 36-104).
      (2) Uniform cordlike atresia (psuedotruncus with atretic pulmonary trunk) (Fig. 36-105A).
   b. Without remnant of pulmonary trunk (isolated confluent pulmonary arteries) (Fig. 36-105B).
   c. From persistent truncus arteriosus, types I and II (Fig. 36-106).
2. Nonconfluent origin of pulmonary arterial supply.

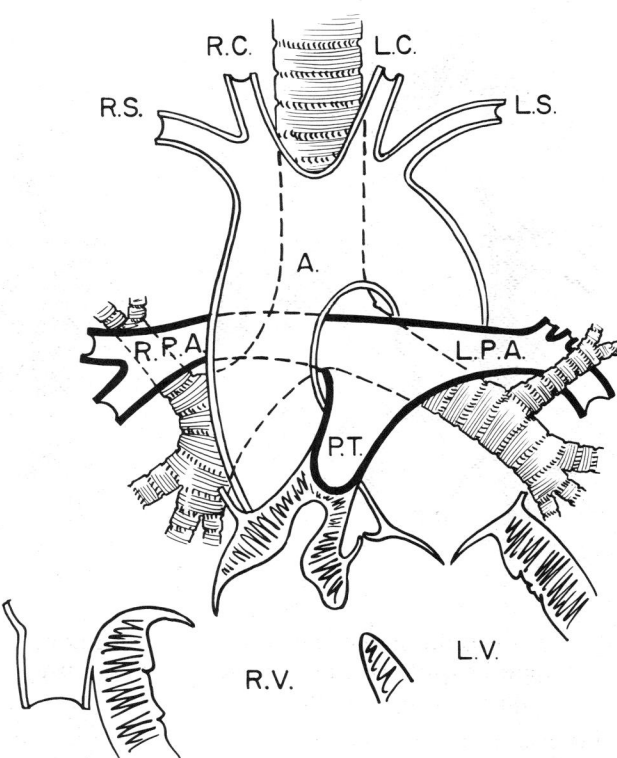

FIGURE 36-104   Tetralogy of Fallot with pulmonary atresia at the valve level. Condition is sometimes referred to as pseudotruncus arteriosus. There is confluence of the two pulmonary arteries. R.V. = right ventricle; L.V. = left ventricle; P.T. = main pulmonary arterial trunk; R.P.A. = right pulmonary artery; L.P.A. = left pulmonary artery; A. = aorta; R.S. = right carotid artery; L.C. = left carotid artery; L.S. = left subclavian artery. (*From Edwards and McGoon.[572] Reproduced with permission.*)

   a. True pulmonary arteries present and arising from:
      (1) Persistent truncus arteriosus, type III (Fig. 36-107).
      (2) Ductus arteriosus.
      (3) Bronchial arteries.

FIGURE 36-105   Pseudotruncus arteriosus with confluent pulmonary arteries. *A.* The pulmonary trunk is identified but atretic. *B.* The pulmonary trunk is not identifiable. R.V. = right ventricle; R.P.A. = right pulmonary artery; L.P.A. = left pulmonary artery; A. = aorta; R.S. = right subclavian artery; L.S. = left subclavian artery; L.V. = left ventricle. (*From Edwards and McGoon.[572] Reproduced with permission.*)

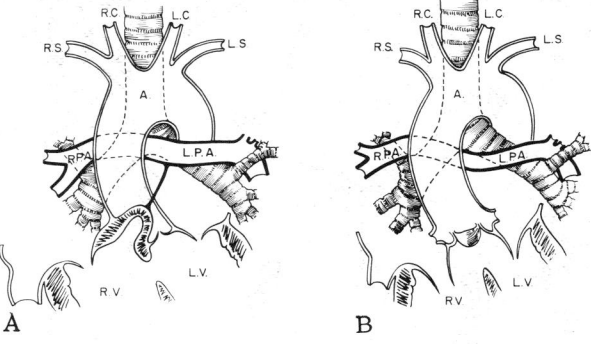

A   B

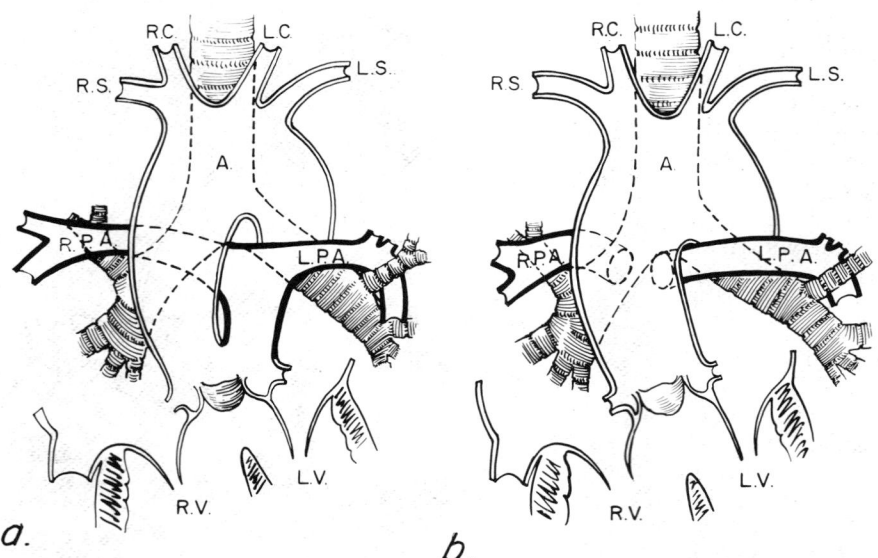

FIGURE 36-106 Persistent truncus arteriosus, type I (*a*) and type II (*b*). R.V. = right ventricle; R.P.A. = right pulmonary artery; L.P.A. = left pulmonary artery; A. = aorta; R.S. = right subclavian artery; R.C. = right carotid artery; L.C. = left carotid artery; L.S. = left subclavian artery; L.V. = left ventricle. (*From Edwards and McGoon.*[572] *Reproduced with permission.*)

b. True pulmonary arteries absent. Pulmonary blood supply from bronchial arteries (truncus type IV) (Fig. 36-108).

This classification will be rearranged into three clinical groups for ease of discussion concerning the clinical manifestations, natural history, and management.

Pathology

In all cases under this heading there is a ventricular septal defect. Usually the ventricles are not inverted, and the aorta or truncus arteriosus shows biventricular origin and fibrous continuity with the mitral valve. Uncommonly, the aorta or truncus arteriosus arises entirely from the right ventricle, as in double outlet right ventricle.

Rarely, the ventricles are inverted, with the aorta (and theoretically the truncus arteriosus) arising

FIGURE 36-107 Persistent truncus arteriosus, type III. R.V. = right ventricle; R.P.A. = right pulmonary artery; L.P.A. = left pulmonary artery; A. = aorta; R.S. = right subclavian artery; R.C. = right carotid artery; L.C. = left carotid artery; L.S. = left subclavian artery; L.V. = left ventricle. (*From Edwards and McGoon.*[572] *Reproduced with permission.*)

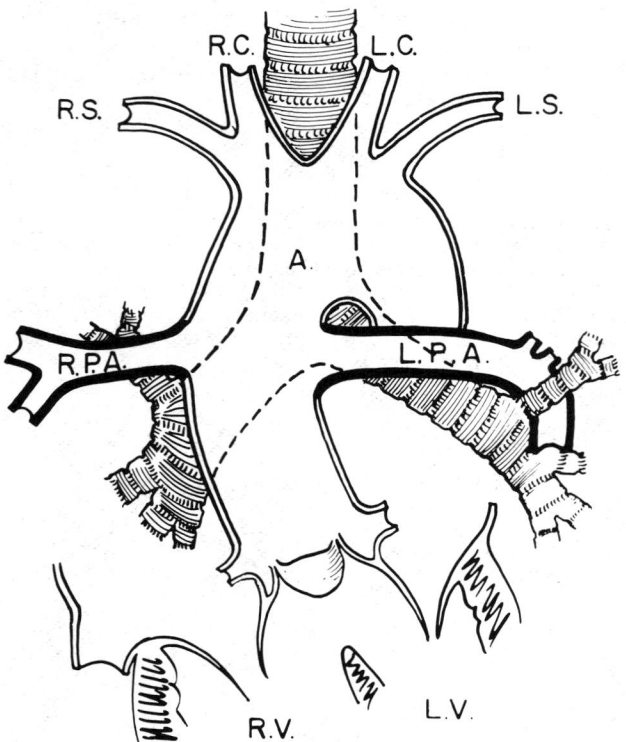

FIGURE 36-108 Persistent truncus, type IV. R.V. = right ventricle; A. = aorta; R.S. = right subclavian artery; R.C. = right carotid artery; L.C. = left carotid artery; L.S. = left subclavian artery; R.B.A. = right bronchial artery; L.B.A. = left bronchial artery; L.V. = left ventricle. (*From Edwards and McGoon.*[572] *Reproduced with permission.*)

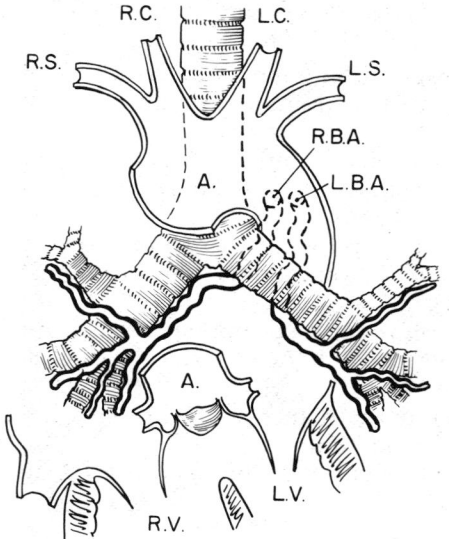

from the inverted right ventricle. Such cases may be viewed as variants of corrected transposition.

Confluence and Origin of Pulmonary Arteries When confluence of pulmonary arterial supply is present, several variations are possible.

With Remnant of Pulmonary Trunk. When there is a remnant of a pulmonary trunk identifiable, its origin is from the right ventricle. The atresia may involve simply the valve level and a short segment of the pulmonary trunk, while the more distal part of the pulmonary trunk is patent and of varying width. In other cases the pulmonary trunk is represented by a cordlike structure leading to confluence of the right and left pulmonary arteries. The ductus arteriosus may be present or absent. If present, it may be patent. Cases with a remnant of a pulmonary trunk are usually considered variants of the tetralogy of Fallot and may be so termed along with the qualification of "with pulmonary atresia" or simply as "pseudotruncus arteriosus."

Without Remnant of Pulmonary Trunk. This type of condition may be referred to as *isolated confluent pulmonary arteries.* The patent aspects of the pulmonary arterial system are like those in pseudotruncus arteriosus with atretic pulmonary trunk except for the absence of any vestige of a pulmonary trunk. As with the foregoing condition, a patent ductus may lead to the pulmonary arterial confluence, although not necessarily.

Persistent Truncus Arteriosus, Types I and II. The condition referred to as *persistent truncus arteriosus* is characterized by one arterial vessel leaving the heart above a ventricular septal defect. From this vessel the coronary and pulmonary arteries, as well as the aorta, arise. There are several subdivisions of this condition according to the classification of Collett and Edwards.[573] Apropos of the condition discussed in this section are the types referred to as *persistent truncus arteriosus types I and II.* Type I is characterized by partial septation of the truncus so that a pulmonary trunk of varying length, usually very short, arises from the truncus and, in turn, the pulmonary arteries arise from the vestigial pulmonary trunk. There is no pulmonary stenosis. In persistent truncus arteriosus type II, the two pulmonary arteries arise separately from the posterior wall of the truncus. In truncus arteriosus type I, the site of pulmonary arterial origin is usually from the left side of the truncus, only rarely from the right.

Associated conditions of all types of truncus arteriosus are fairly numerous.[574,575] A right aortic arch is present in about 20 percent of the cases. Single coronary artery is fairly common (about 5 percent), and unusually high origin of the coronary arteries is about twice as common. The most significant feature is that branches of the right coronary artery have a tendency to cross the anterior wall of the right ventricle.[576] Interruption of the aortic arch is present in about 10 percent of cases. So-called absence of a pulmonary artery occurs in about 2 percent, more commonly on the side of the aortic arch than contralateral to it.

In these, as in other types of persistent truncus arteriosus, the truncal semilunar valve may show a variety of alterations characterized by thickening of the cusps with mucoid connective tissue.[577] This process, if severe, may be responsible either for stenosis or insufficiency.[578]

Hypertensive pulmonary vascular disease is common and reflects the early death in untreated patients. Unusually long survival may be complicated by obstructive pulmonary arterial lesions like those in large ventricular septal defect.[579]

Nonconfluent Origin of Pulmonary Arteries When nonconfluence of pulmonary arterial supply is present, a number of variations are possible, the simplest being persistent truncus arteriosus, type III.

Origin from Persistent Truncus Arteriosus (Truncus Type III). In rare instances of persistent truncus arteriosus, each pulmonary artery arises independently from the lateral aspect of the truncus, the latter form being type III.

Origin from Ductus Arteriosus. When there is ductal pulmonary arterial origin, two basic patterns exist, namely, (1) bilateral origin of the pulmonary arteries from ductus arteriosi, and (2) origin of a pulmonary artery from the homolateral ductus, while the other pulmonary artery has a normal site of origin, but there is atresia of the pulmonary trunk and/or the normally arising pulmonary artery.[580]

Origin from the Descending Aorta through Bronchial Arteries. Hypothetically, a situation may occur in which true pulmonary arteries may arise from the descending thoracic aorta, the stems of origin for the vessels being bronchial arteries.

Pulmonary Arterial Supply from Bronchial Arteries (Truncus Type IV); Pulmonary Arteries Absent. As the description implies, this condition is characterized by no true pulmonary arterial system being present, while the arterial supply to the lung is by way of bronchial arteries. A synonym for this condition, *persistent truncus type IV,* was contributed by Collett and Edwards.[573]

While such a condition may exist, some cases considered to be examples of truncus type IV are, in fact, examples either of confluent or nonconfluent origin of the pulmonary arteries associated with atresia of these vessels in the mediastinum. Dissection of the pulmonary hili in cases thought to be examples of truncus type IV usually reveals patent pulmonary arteries of varying caliber at the hili.[580]

Pulmonary Atresia with Ventricular Septal Defect with and without Pulmonary Arterial Confluence

The anatomic types[572] of the preceding classification included here are those with:

1. Confluence of pulmonary arteries originating from the pulmonary trunk with patency of some

portion of the pulmonary trunk (pseudotruncus) or isolated confluence without remnant of pulmonary trunk.

2. Nonconfluence of pulmonary arteries with origin of true pulmonary arteries through bilateral ductus arteriosi or bronchial arteries.

Clinical Manifestations[296]   These defects create a clinical picture with many similarities to severe tetralogy of Fallot. The size of the pulmonary arteries and ductus and/or bronchial collateral vessels determine the clinical manifestations. In the large majority, they are small so that pulmonary blood flow is diminished. Marked cyanosis is then present from birth or shortly thereafter. Most are dependent on ductal patency for their pulmonary flow so that rapid deterioration can occur as the ductus frequently undergoes spontaneous closure. For those in whom the ductus remains patent or who have adequate bronchial supply, the course in the newborn period is more stable. With growth of the infant and increasing physical activity, the cyanosis progresses gradually. In only a few patients, usually those with numerous large collateral vessels, the cyanosis will be mild and heart failure may ensue from increased pulmonary flow.

On auscultation, the second heart sound is single and there may be no murmur. Soft, continuous murmurs from the ductus or collateral vessels may be heard. The electrocardiogram and chest roentgenogram are indistinguishable from tetralogy of Fallot. Approximately 50 percent will have a right aortic arch.[296] The M-mode echocardiogram is similar to tetralogy of Fallot, which can be distinguished only if the pulmonary valve can be recorded. Two-dimensional echocardiography (Fig. 36-97) is very helpful. In the small number of patients with large collateral flow, the continuous murmur will be most prominent, biatrial and biventricular hypertrophy may be present on the electrocardiogram, and the chest roentgenogram will show cardiomegaly and increased pulmonary flow.

Findings at cardiac catheterization are similar to tetralogy of Fallot, except the pulmonary artery cannot be entered from the right ventricle (Fig. 36-109). The combination of aortography and selective arteriography in collateral vessels (Fig. 36-110) will usually demonstrate the origin of pulmonary flow, the size of the pulmonary arteries, and the presence or absence of confluence between the right and left pulmonary arteries.[581] Pulmonary venous angiography may be necessary for this in some.[582,583]

Natural History and Prognosis[296]   Outlook is, in general, much worse than for tetralogy of Fallot. Without intervention, only those with large collateral vessels are likely to survive beyond infancy. The complications of cyanosis and endocarditis were discussed earlier in this chapter.

Medical Management   This is the same as that for severe tetralogy of Fallot except that propranolol is

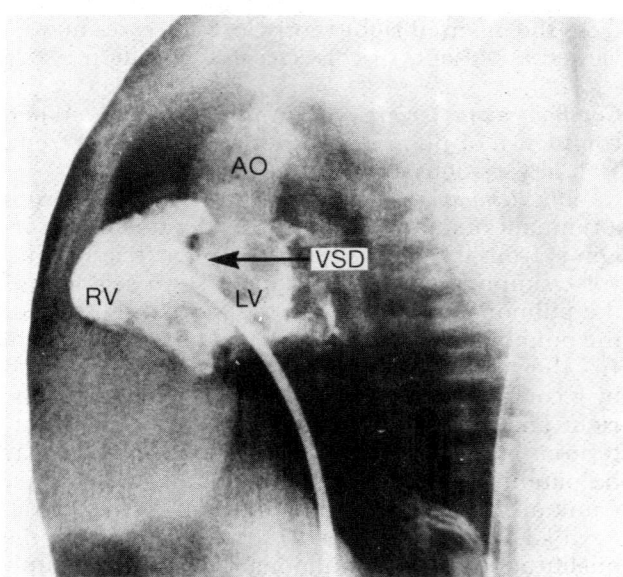

FIGURE 36-109   Lateral view of a right ventricular (RV) angiogram in an infant with pulmonary atresia and ventricular septal defect (VSD) with the RV outflow tract ending bluntly and a right-to-left shunt opacifying the left ventricle (LV) and aorta (AO).

not useful. Prostaglandin infusion has been extremely helpful in newborns with critical cyanosis and acidosis.[35,531] If there are pulmonary arteries of adequate size, surgery can be done.[584] This usually consists of palliation with correction deferred until a larger body size is obtained.

Surgical Management   Infusion of prostaglandin has enhanced the success of urgent surgical palliation. A systemic arterial to pulmonary arterial shunt is constructed. We prefer the Blalock-Taussig subclavian artery to pulmonary artery anastomosis us-

FIGURE 36-110   Posteroanterior view of selective arteriogram in a large bronchial collateral (B) from the descending aorta in a patient with pulmonary atresia and ventricular septal defect. There is opacification of tiny right (RPA) and left (LPA) pulmonary arteries with confluence.

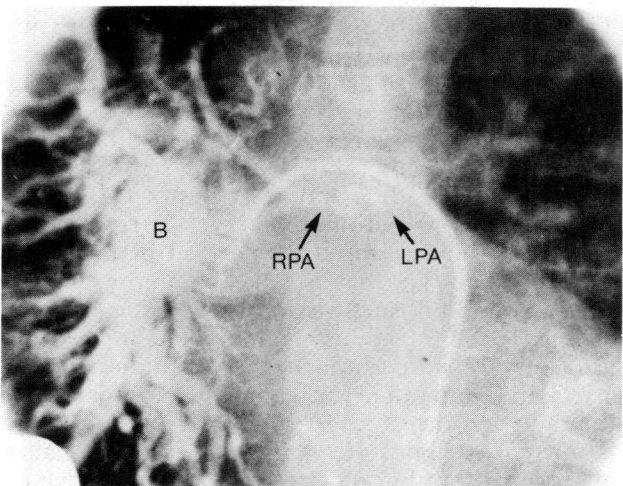

ing magnification, fine monofilament suture, coronary arterial surgical technique, and systemic heparinization. Alternatively, a Waterston side-to-side ascending aortic to pulmonary arterial anastomosis can be constructed or a segment of synthetic Gore-Tex graft can be interposed between aorta and pulmonary artery. When confluence of right and left pulmonary arteries is absent, bilateral shunts are required if growth of the pulmonary arteries is to be achieved.

Satisfactory palliation has been obtained in a few patients having pulmonary atresia with ventricular septal defect, confluence of small pulmonary arteries, and a patent pulmonary trunk by placement of a pericardial patch across the right ventricular outflow tract to establish continuity between the right ventricle and the pulmonary trunk. The ventricular septal defect is left open. Cyanosis is reduced and the pulmonary arteries grow. The ventricular septal defect is closed at a subsequent operation before the development of congestive heart failure and pulmonary vascular obstructive disease.

Infants with confluent pulmonary arteries judged adequate to carry the required systemic cardiac output have been corrected primarily in some centers. A valve-containing extracardiac conduit is placed between the right ventricle and the pulmonary arteries; the ventricular septal defect is closed (Fig. 36-111).[585] The small conduit used in the infant will require eventual replacement with a larger conduit as the child grows.

Infants having numerous aorticopulmonary communications—collateral sources of pulmonary blood flow—may survive for several years without operative intervention. These children then require ventricular septal defect closure and establishment of right ventricular to pulmonary arterial continuity with a conduit placed through a median sternotomy incision. The aorticopulmonary communications must then be interrupted, usually through a separate left thoracotomy (Fig. 36-112).[584]

Experience with correction in infancy is limited. Survival following palliation is about 75 percent. Children first operated upon between the ages of 5 and 10 years have experienced excellent late hemodynamic results with a hospital mortality of 5 to 10 percent.[584–586]

Truncus Arteriosus Types I, II, and III

Clinical Manifestations These defects are grouped together whether there is (types I and II) or is not (type III) pulmonary arterial confluence, since clinical distinction is impossible. A rare form of truncus has been described in which there is no ventricular septal defect.[587] The reader is referred to the preceding section on aorticopulmonary septal defect, which is a clinically indistinguishable condition.

FIGURE 36-112 Repair of pseudotruncus arteriosus. Through a lateral thoracotomy incision the collateral or bronchial arteries are ligated after cardiopulmonary bypass is established. (*From Doty, Kouchoukos, Kirklin, Barcia, and Bargeron.*[584] *Reproduced with permission.*)

FIGURE 36-111 Repair of pseudotruncus arteriosus. *A.* The valved conduit is anastomosed to the confluent left and right pulmonary arteries. *B.* The ventricular septal defect is repaired. *C.* The completion of the operation. (*From Doty, Kouchoukos, Kirklin, Barcia, and Bargeron.*[584] *Reproduced with permission.*)

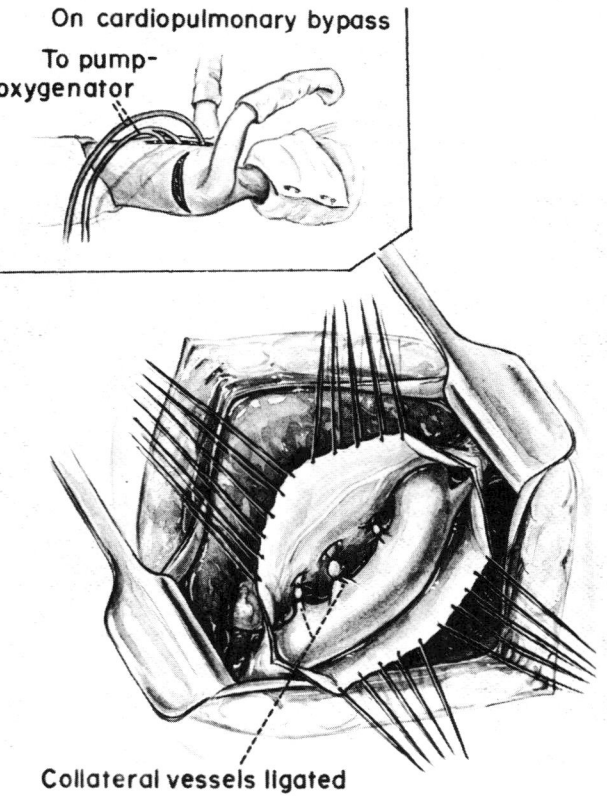

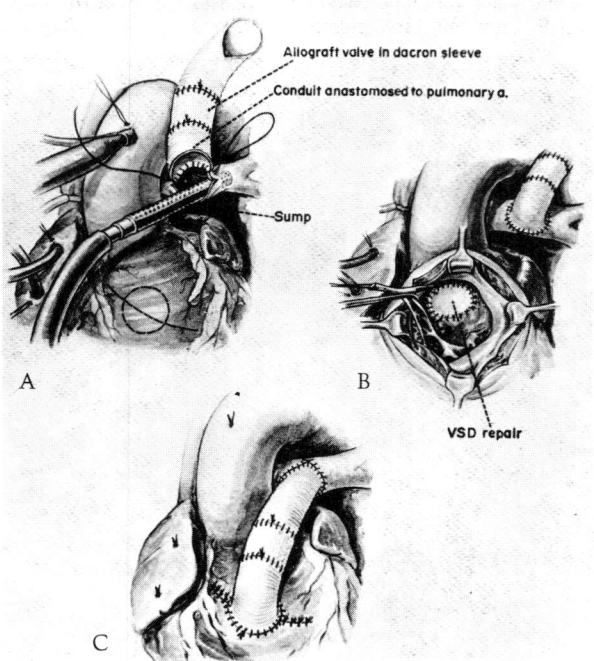

Clinical manifestations depend on the size of the pulmonary arteries and thus the amount of pulmonary flow. Most patients with truncus arteriosus have increased pulmonary flow and mild cyanosis with heart failure. Severe congestive failure and poor growth are observed in the first few weeks of life. If the pulmonary arteries are small, cyanosis will predominate and heart failure will be absent or mild. A prominent left parasternal lift and apical impulse are palpated. A loud, constant systolic click and a single second heart sound are common, but splitting may be thought present because of loud multiple sounds occurring near the second sound. Elevated jugular venous pulsations, hepatomegaly, tachypnea, and rales are frequent. After the first month of life, 70 percent will have a systolic murmur, occasionally accompanied by a thrill, in the third and fourth left intercostal spaces.[4,6] A continuous murmur may be heard over the lung fields if pulmonary resistance is low. Approximately one-third of these patients[578] will have a decrescendo diastolic murmur of truncal valvular regurgitation at the left sternal border and apex. If this is severe, a more rapid downhill course with heart failure occurs. There are bounding pulses and a wide pulse pressure.

The electrocardiographic findings are nonspecific with a mean QRS axis within normal range and biventricular hypertrophy. The chest roentgenogram (Fig. 36-113) will show moderate to severe cardiomegaly with increased pulmonary flow. The "aorta" may be enlarged, and a right arch is frequently present. The latter finding is a helpful clue in distinguishing this from other large left-to-right shunts. In the rare patient with small pulmonary arteries, the heart size is less impressive and pulmonary flow is normal to diminished. The M-mode echocardiographic findings are similar to tetralogy of Fallot except two semilunar valves can never be recorded and the left atrium is more commonly enlarged. Two-dimensional echocardiography (Fig. 36-98) is very helpful. (See section on tetralogy of Fallot earlier in this chapter.)

Cardiac catheterization will demonstrate bidirectional shunting with more severe systemic arterial desaturation in those with small pulmonary arteries or pulmonary vascular disease. Initially, the diagnosis may not be apparent since the catheter may advance easily from the right ventricle into the pulmonary trunk with a near normal appearance of the catheter course. There is usually pulmonary hypertension at or near systemic levels. Attempts to enter both right and left pulmonary arteries should be made to evaluate the pulmonary vascular resistance completely, especially in those beyond the newborn period. Right ventricular angiography will demonstrate the ventricular septal defect, but angiography in the proximal truncus (Fig. 36-114) will show the severity of any truncal regurgitation and usually is necessary to visualize the origin of the pulmonary arteries. Biplane angiography is particularly useful in this defect.

Natural History and Prognosis[4,6,588] The majority die before 1 year of age from congestive heart failure and its complications. Severe pulmonary vascular disease occurs early in these patients. It is usually present to some degree by 6 months of age and

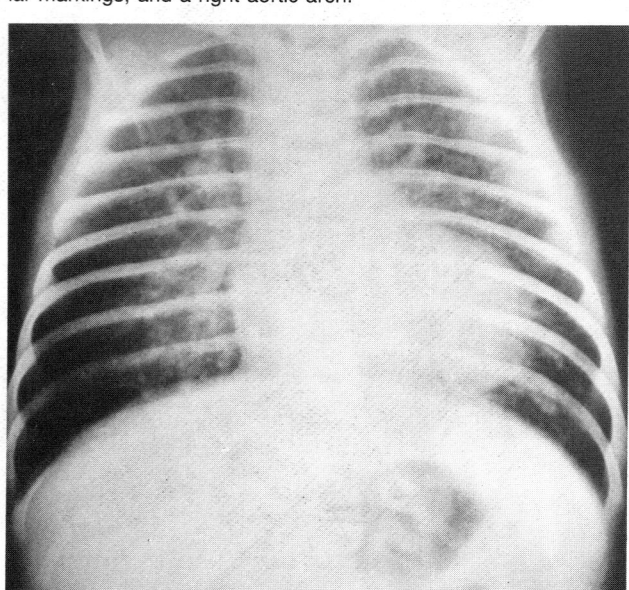

FIGURE 36-113 Chest roentgenogram in a newborn with truncus arteriosus shows mild cardiomegaly, increased pulmonary vascular markings, and a right aortic arch.

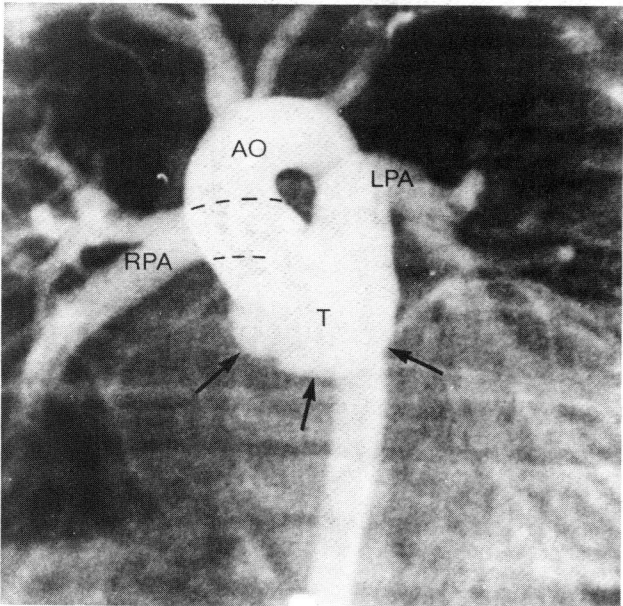

FIGURE 36-114 Posteroanterior view of an angiogram in truncus arteriosus showing the common truncus (T) with a broad distorted semilunar valve (arrows) which gives rise to the aorta (AO) and right (RPA) and left (LPA) pulmonary arteries.

progresses thereafter. The majority of children surviving to age 5 years have severe pulmonary vascular disease, although a teenager with only mild to moderate disease may be rarely seen. Those who have small pulmonary arteries that restrict pulmonary flow survive somewhat longer, although survival to early adulthood is extremely rare. The complications of cyanosis discussed earlier in this chapter can occur, but polycythemia is usually not as marked as in those with obstruction to pulmonary flow until pulmonary vascular disease becomes severe. Infective endocarditis also occurs.

Medical Management Medical management is primarily directed toward treatment of heart failure and prevention of the complications of cyanosis and endocarditis. Numerous anatomic features delineated by angiography are important when considering surgery.[574,589] Infants with severe heart failure should have surgical intervention in the first few months of life. This may be banding of the pulmonary arteries or early primary correction with anticipated replacement of the outflow tract conduit at a later age. The latter is done in small infants with reasonable mortality and comparable outcome at very few centers. In most centers, banding is performed in early infancy and correction must be delayed until several years of age because of differences in risk and outcome.[590–592] In those patients with restrictive flow and very small pulmonary arteries, systemic to pulmonary arterial anastomosis may be necessary prior to correction at a later age if the pulmonary arteries grow. Severe pulmonary vascular disease is a contraindication to surgery. Patients with severe truncal valve regurgitation may require valve replacement in the aortic position early or late after initial correction. This is associated with all of the problems attendant to valve replacement in children and should not be done unless the degree of regurgitation allows no medical alternative.

Surgical Management The excellent results achieved from total correction in infancy of truncus arteriosus types I, II, and III by Ebert and associates,[593] extending concepts applied earlier in older children by McGoon, Rastelli, and Ongley,[594] have changed the approach to these complex anomalies. Repair is now carried out in the first few months of life, hopefully before the child has suffered irreversibly from congestive heart failure and the development of pulmonary vascular obstructive disease.

Operation is conducted through a median sternotomy during circulatory arrest with profound hypothermia (18 to 20°C). Cooling and rewarming is accomplished while the child is supported on partial cardiopulmonary bypass. Total cardiopulmonary bypass with moderate hypothermia (25 to 28°C) and cardioplegia is used for older children and those

who have previously undergone bilateral pulmonary arterial banding for control of congestive heart failure.

The ventricular septal defect is closed with a patch placed through a right ventriculotomy, the truncal valve being placed entirely on the left side of the patch (Fig. 36-115). The pulmonary arteries and a portion of adjacent aortic wall are excised from the ascending aorta; the defect thus created in the aortic wall is repaired directly or with a patch (Fig. 36-116). Right ventricular–pulmonary arterial continuity is established with a valve-containing conduit (Fig. 36-111). We prefer a Dacron conduit with a bioprosthetic porcine valve, although the early experience with correction of truncus arteriosus was accumulated using homograft aortas with their retained valves. Conduits inserted during infancy will require replacement with a larger one before the child reaches adolescence; this has been accomplished with less difficulty and better results than one might anticipate.

A major complicating factor in truncus arteriosus—truncal valvular regurgitation—reduces the likelihood of a good operative result. Replacement of the truncal valve with a prosthetic valve may be required.

Hospital survival of 80 percent has been achieved following total correction in infancy; 90 percent of

FIGURE 36-115 Steps in the repair of truncus arteriosus. The ventricular septal defect is repaired with a patch. An aortic homograft with its valve is used to connect the right ventricle to the previously disconnected pulmonary arteries. (*From D. C. McGoon, Technics of Open-Heart Surgery for Congenital Heart Disease, Curr. Probl. Surg., April, 1968. Reproduced with permission.*)

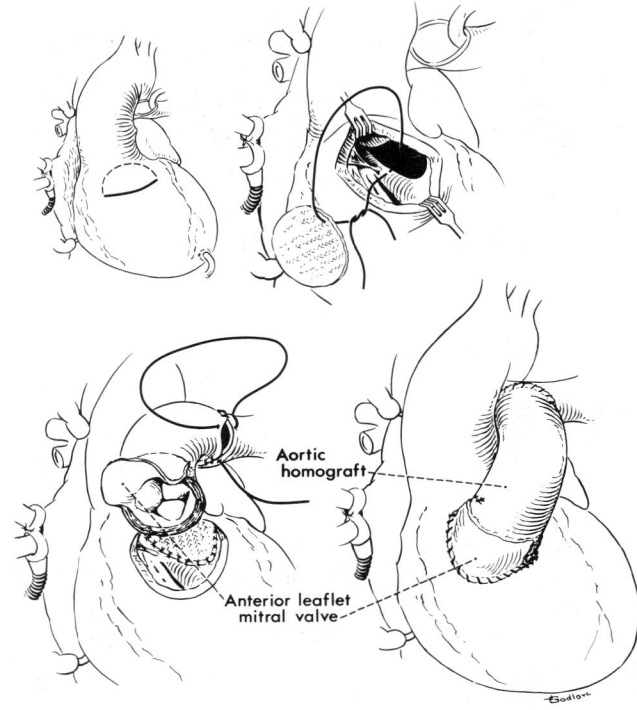

Aortic homograft

Anterior leaflet mitral valve

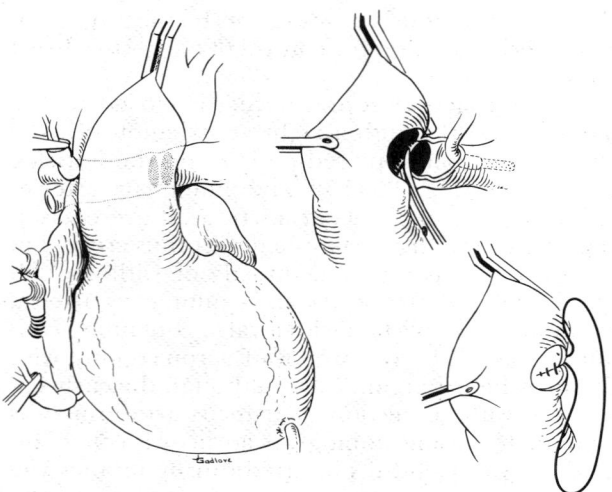

FIGURE 36-116 Steps in the repair of truncus arteriosus. After cardiopulmonary bypass has been established and the aorta cross-clamped, the pulmonary arteries are disconnected from the common arterial trunk. The defect in the trunk is repaired. (*From D. C. McGoon, Technics of Open-Heart Surgery for Congenital Heart Disease, Curr. Probl. Surg., April, 1968. Reproduced with permission.*)

older children, appropriately selected, should survive.[595] These results certainly support a policy of early total correction, since most infants with truncus arteriosus will die without operation. Results of palliation by bilateral pulmonary arterial banding have been discouraging.

Truncus Arteriosus Type IV

Fortunately this is a rare defect, but the clinical picture is similar to that described above for ventricular septal defect and pulmonary atresia with pulmonary arteries. The distinction is made only with selective angiography, which demonstrates no true pulmonary arteries and only bronchial collateral circulation to the lungs. These patients are usually severely hypoxic and die early in life. Occasionally with larger collateral flow, survival to older age is possible. Since there are no true pulmonary arteries, there is no effective surgical treatment.

Tricuspid Atresia

Definition

In tricuspid atresia, there is no channel of communication of the right atrium with the ventricular portion of the heart.

Pathology

Classically, there is neither a tricuspid orifice nor valvular tissue. A dimple lies in the floor of the right atrium at the anticipated location of the tricuspid orifice.

The great arteries may be normally related or,

less commonly, malpositioned[596] (Fig. 36-117). In a study of 45 specimens, Tandon and Edwards[597] found that in 25 the great vessels were normally related (one had pulmonary atresia as well). Malposition of the great vessels was found in the remaining 19 cases. In 16 of these there was a single (subaortic) conus; the malposition was dextro-type in 12 of these, levo-type in 4, and 3 cases had double (subaortic and subpulmonary) coni. Persistent truncus arteriosus was present in one case.

Pulmonary valvular atresia or stenosis may occur with either of the major configurations of the great vessels. When the great vessels are normally related, there is a greater tendency for pulmonary stenosis than when malposition occurs, the basis for the stenosis being the narrow state of the ventricular septal defect. In this type in particular the ventricular septal defect may, over time, narrow or close.[598] In cases with malposition the ventricular configuration is like that in single or common ventricle, the aorta arising from the infundibulum of that chamber. An interatrial communication, usually a patent foramen ovale, of varying caliber is present in all cases.

A fairly commonly associated condition of cases with malposition of the great vessels is juxtaposition of the *atrial appendages.*[599] This condition is characterized by both atrial appendages lying to one side, more commonly the left side, of the great vessels. While this condition is rare in normal hearts and uncommon in classic ventricular septal defect, it is usually seen in conditions such as complete transposition and most commonly in the condition under discussion.

Coarctation of the aorta and patent ductus arteriosus have been described as occurring in about 25 percent of cases with tricuspid atresia and dextromalposition.[13]

Abnormal Physiology[600,601]

The only outlet for blood returning to the right atrium is through an interatrial communication, which is usually a patent foramen ovale. In the left atrium, the systemic venous blood mixes with oxygenated blood returning from the pulmonary veins. Consequently, there is always arterial unsaturation, the extent of which is inversely proportional to pulmonary blood flow. In most cases there is an associated ventricular septal defect through which blood passes to the right ventricle and the lungs. If the ventricular septum is intact, the ductus arteriosus and the bronchial arteries must provide the entire pulmonary circulation. In most cases of tricuspid atresia, the right ventricle is diminutive. Cardiac catheterization demonstrates an elevation of right atrial pressure, often with a prominent or giant *a* wave, particularly if the interatrial communication is not large. The catheter cannot be passed into the right ventricle but rather passes into the left atrium, which may have a slightly lower pressure than the right atrium. The arterial saturation is low.

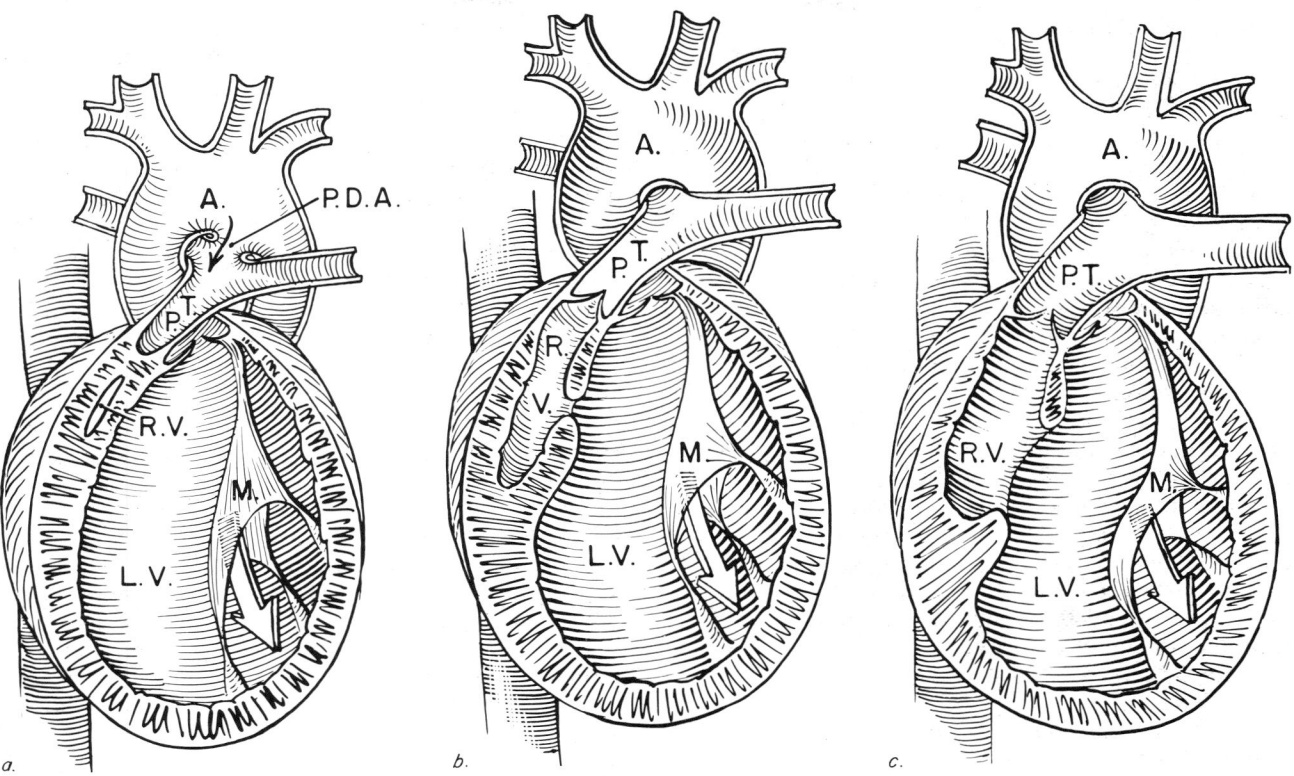

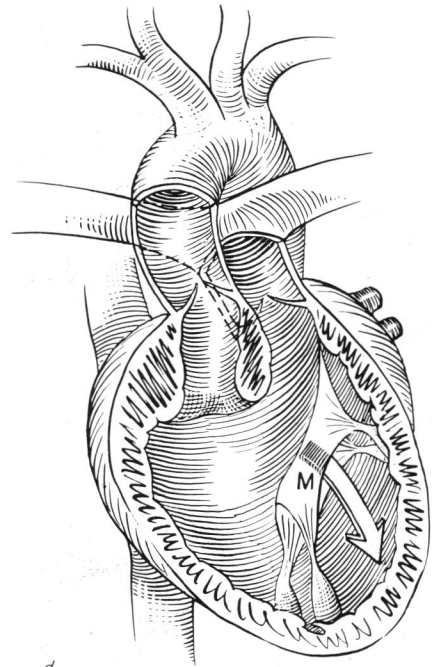

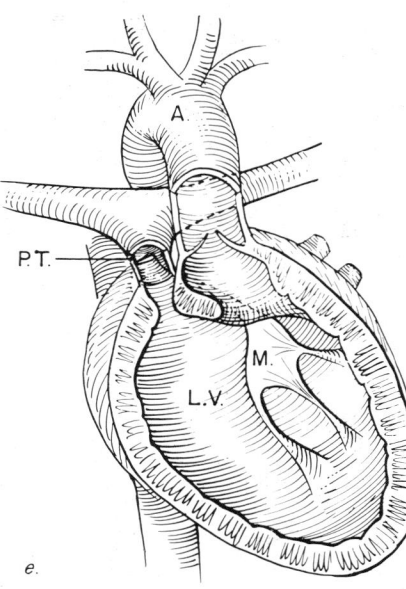

FIGURE 36-117   Tricuspid atresia. *a, b,* and *c.* With normally related great vessels. *d* and *e.* With malposition of great vessels. *a.* Type Ia. Pulmonary atresia is associated. *b.* Type Ib. Subpulmonary stenosis by virtue of small ventricular septal defect. *c.* Type Ic. No pulmonary stenosis resulting from a large ventricular septal defect. *d.* Type IIa. Associated with dextro malposition of the great vessels. *e.* Type IIb. Associated with levo malposition of the great vessels. Pulmonary stenosis is also present. R.V. = right ventricle; L.V. = left ventricle; M. = mitral valve; P.T. = main pulmonary arterial trunk; A. = aorta; P.D.A. = patent ductus arteriosus. (*From Tandon and Edwards.*[597] *Reproduced with permission.*)

Clinical Manifestations[6,600]

History The clinical picture varies with associated defects. The most common combination occurring with tricuspid atresia is normally related great arteries, a small ventricular septal defect and right ventricle, and pulmonary stenosis. The predominant problem in these infants is cyanosis, usually presenting quite early in the newborn period. When the ventricular septal defect and right ventricle are large and there is no pulmonary stenosis or, more commonly, when there is transposition of the great arteries without pulmonary stenosis, the pulmonary flow is increased and clinical manifestations are due to congestive heart failure with only very mild cyanosis. These patients may present at a few weeks to months of age. Those patients with pulmonary atresia with or without transposition are ductal dependent and frequently will present with severe cyanosis immediately after birth. Growth failure may occur, particularly in those with large pulmonary flow. Paroxysmal hypoxic spells similar to those in tetralogy of Fallot can occur. Squatting occurs at a later age.

Physical Examination In those with predominant cyanosis, tachypnea and even hypoxic episodes may be seen. Clubbing is not seen until later in infancy. A prominent *a* wave is noted in the jugular venous pulse and the liver may be moderately enlarged. The apex impulse is prominent. The second heart sound is single. Murmurs will depend on associated defects. If a ductus is present, a soft systolic or continuous murmur may be heard. If the pulmonary stenosis is not extremely severe, there may be a midsystolic murmur at the left sternal border. With pulmonary atresia or severe stenosis, there may be no murmur. In those with increased pulmonary flow, the parasternal and apical impulses are hyperdynamic and the second heart sound is usually split. There is a systolic thrill with a long systolic murmur at the lower left sternal border similar to that of a ventricular septal defect. A middiastolic rumble may be audible at the apex. Signs of heart failure are also found. A pulse discrepancy should be looked for since coarctation or aortic interruption has been reported to be common in those with transposition.[602]

Chest Roentgenogram Total heart size by chest roentgenogram is usually normal, but it may be at least moderately increased in those with increased flow. A straight border of the right side of the heart is considered characteristic. Commonly, the pulmonary segment and flow are markedly diminished. The opposite is true in the minority described above with increased flow.

Electrocardiogram[603] The electrocardiographic manifestations (Fig. 36-118) generally show diminished right ventricular forces for age and left ventricular hypertrophy. Right atrial hypertrophy is

FIGURE 36-118 Twelve-lead electrocardiogram in a 2-month-old infant with tricuspid atresia, ventricular septal defect, and pulmonary stenosis with hypoplasia of the right ventricle. The mean QRS axis of −45° is deviated to the left, and there is left ventricular hypertrophy with diminished right ventricular forces for age.

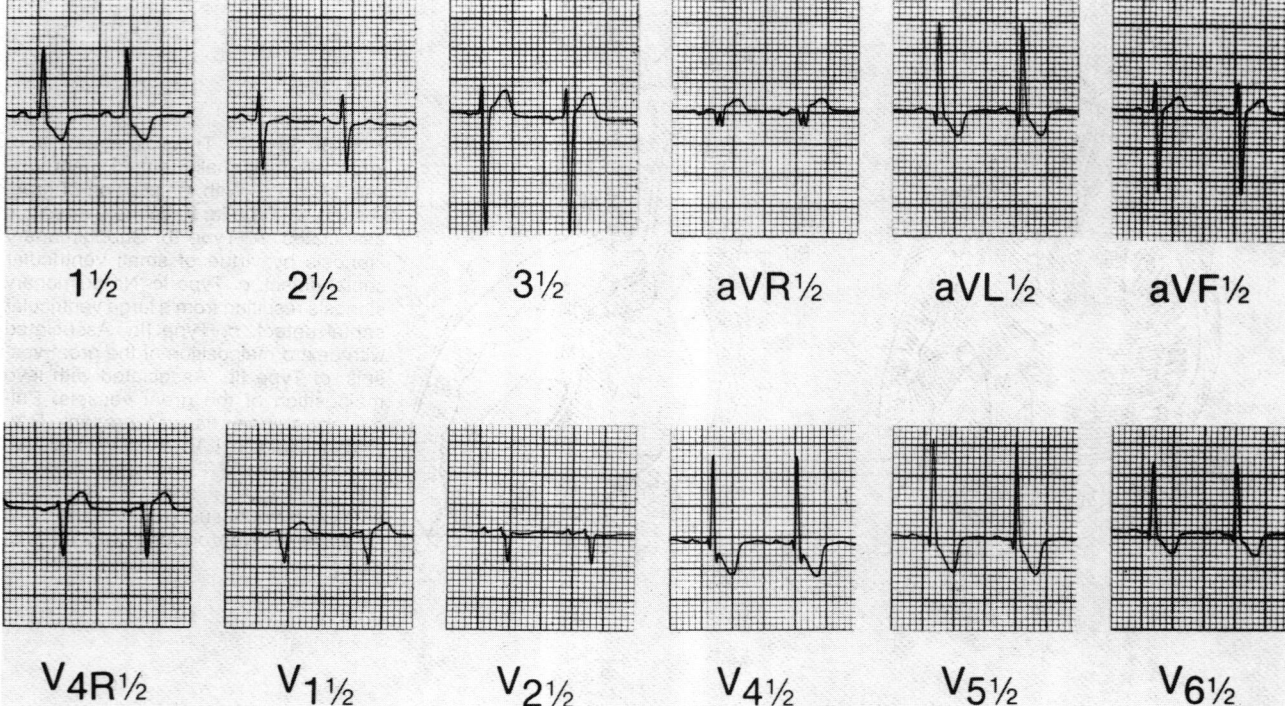

frequently present. In those without transposition, the mean QRS axis is between 0 and −90° in three-fourths of the cases. It is usually between 0 and +90° in those with transposition.[600]

Echocardiogram The common findings on M-mode echocardiography[526] are those of a hypoplastic right side of the heart in most (Fig. 36-119). There is failure to record the tricuspid valve, but in those with pulmonary stenosis, the pulmonary valve also may not be recorded. In this case, the diagnosis is not distinguishable from that of pulmonary atresia with intact ventricular septum. Cross-sectional echocardiography[36] offers clearer distinction and better evaluation of associated abnormalities such as transposition.

Cardiac Catheterization There is usually a mean pressure difference between the atria with the right atrium being the higher because at least two-thirds of cases have a patent foramen ovale rather than an atrial septal defect.[6] The mean gradient and height of the *a* wave in the right atrium correspond to the size of the atrial communication. There is always desaturation throughout the left side of the heart, but the degree is dependent on the pulmonary flow. With the help of flow-directed catheters, the right ventricle and great vessels can be entered from the left ventricle. Measurement of pulmonary pressure in this manner is most important in those with increased pulmonary flow. Right atrial angiography

will demonstrate the flow pattern with a triangular, nonopacified area in the usual region of the inflow portion of the right ventricle. Pulmonary atresia with intact ventricular septum and very diminutive right ventricle can occasionally mimic this pattern. Left ventricular biplane angiography will demonstrate the relationship of ventricular sizes, the ventricular septal defect, and the great vessels (Fig. 36-120). Studies of left ventricular function may be of prognostic significance.[604]

Natural History and Prognosis
Over 50 percent of patients present with cyanosis on the first day of life.[600] Cyanosis is usually progressively severe due to ductal closure, increasing pulmonary stenosis, or spontaneous diminution or closure of the ventricular defect.[598]

The overall prognosis[6] is poor with an average life expectancy of less than 3 months in those with pulmonary atresia. Overall, one-half die by 6 months of age, two-thirds by 1 year, and 90 percent by 10 years. The best-tolerated combination with an average life expectancy of over 7 years is that of transposition with pulmonary stenosis. Hypoxia is the most common cause of death, but death can result from congestive heart failure or pulmonary vascular disease.

Medical Management
Medical management of cyanosis and heart failure have been previously discussed. Prostaglandin is of

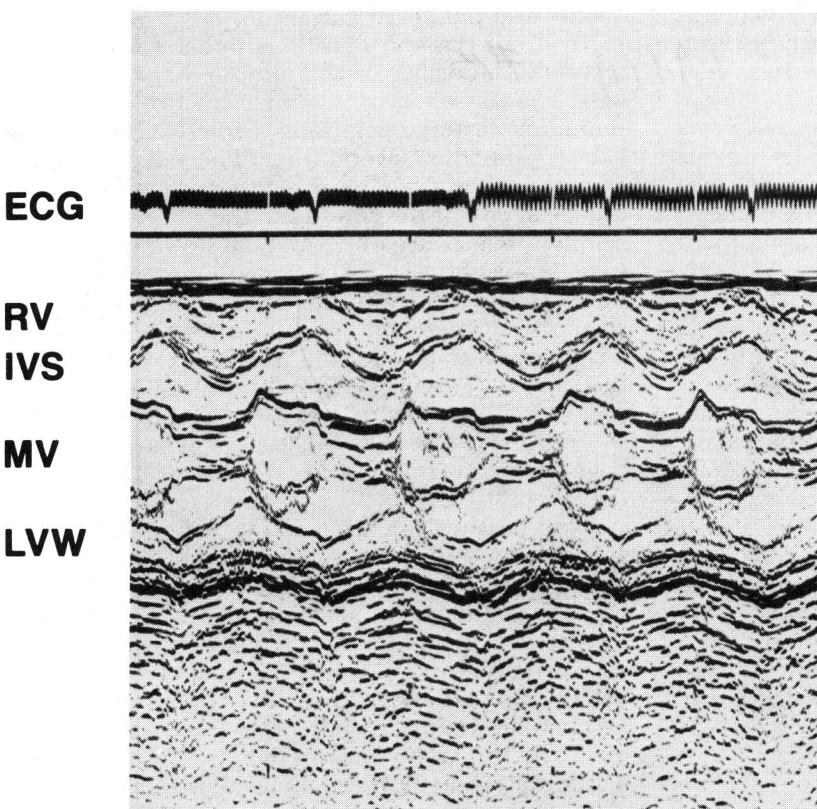

FIGURE 36-119 M-mode echocardiogram from the patient in Fig. 36-118 demonstrates the tiny right ventricular size in comparison to the left ventricle. ECG = electrocardiogram; RV = right ventricle; IVS = interventricular septum; MV = mitral valve; LVW = posterior left ventricular wall.

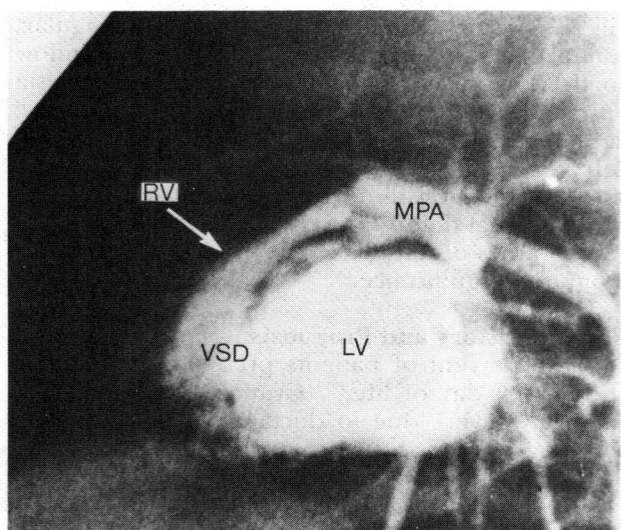

FIGURE 36-120 Lateral view of the left ventricular (LV) angiogram from the same patient in Fig. 36-118 demonstrates the ventricular septal defect (VSD), small right ventricle (RV), and narrowed outflow tract with a slightly thickened pulmonary valve filling a larger main pulmonary artery (MPA).

temporary help in the critically cyanotic newborn.[35] Hypoxic spells should be treated as discussed with tetralogy of Fallot.[605] Prompt and vigorous treatment of intercurrent infections and prophylaxis against endocarditis is recommended.

Occasionally there is evidence for an inadequate opening between the two atria with extremely tall P waves on electrocardiogram, progressively enlarging liver, and a large pressure difference between the atria measured at catheterization. In a very young infant, balloon atrial septostomy may help. Commonly, the atrial septum is thickened in this situation and is normally too thick in older infants for this procedure to be performed safely. Surgical creation of an atrial defect should then be done.

For infants and children with severe hypoxia, prompt surgical intervention with creation of a systemic to pulmonary arterial shunt is indicated. For those who have uncontrollable heart failure and poor growth, the pulmonary artery should be banded. This should be done only after an adequate trial of medical therapy since some of these patients will have a progressive decrease in their pulmonary flow over a few months such that the failure may spontaneously resolve and surgery can be avoided. Such patients should be recatheterized by 3 to 6 months of age to evaluate pulmonary pressure and resistance. Overall, surgery definitely increases life expectancy.[600] Newer surgical approaches, such as right atrial–pulmonary arterial anastomosis,[606,607] are being tried on selected older patients in certain centers and may offer more prolonged survival for those with normally related great arteries.

Surgical Management

Only within the past decade has physiological correction of tricuspid atresia become a realistic consid-

eration. Initial palliation should now be planned with eventual correction in mind. Factors determining the need for palliation include the amount of pulmonary blood flow and the adequacy of the interatrial communication. Palliation may include (1) a systemic arterial to pulmonary arterial shunt, (2) a systemic venous to pulmonary arterial shunt, (3) pulmonary arterial banding, (4) balloon atrial septostomy, and (5) surgical atrial septectomy.

Insufficient pulmonary blood flow with consequent systemic hypoxia—the most common indication for palliation—requires creation of a systemic to pulmonary arterial shunt. We prefer the Blalock-Taussig subclavian to pulmonary arterial anastomosis even in the newborn, although some surgeons prefer a Potts or Waterston shunt (see discussion of tetralogy of Fallot).

In the presence of excessive pulmonary blood flow, pulmonary arterial banding provides acceptable palliation. Gradual spontaneous closure of the ventricular septal defect may lead to progressive cyanosis requiring a systemic arterial to pulmonary arterial shunt.

Low cardiac output and elevated systemic venous pressure with peripheral edema, ascites, hepatic engorgement, and distended, pulsatile neck veins suggest the presence of an inadequate interatrial communication. A balloon atrioseptostomy can be performed in newborns; in older children the atrial septum should be surgically excised.

Fontan first accomplished physiological correction of tricuspid atresia in 1968 by joining the right atrium and pulmonary artery using a valve-containing conduit (Fig. 36-121).[606] Another valve was inserted in the orifice of the inferior vena cava. This basic concept of using the right atrium to provide pulmonary arterial perfusion through a conduit has been modified in several ways. The valve in the inferior vena cava has been omitted. Anastomosis of the distal end of the conduit to the right ventricular remnant makes use of the patient's own pulmonary valve and right ventricular contribution to pressure development.[608] A valveless conduit may be used in such cases. Combined use of Glenn's operation and a right atrial to pulmonary arterial conduit reduces the work required of the right atrium. Valves and prosthetic conduits may be omitted entirely from the right-sided circulation, the right atrial appendage and pericardium being used as a valveless conduit (Fig. 36-122).[758]

Prerequisites for application of Fontan's operation are low pulmonary vascular resistance, normal sinus rhythm, pulmonary arteries of adequate caliber, and adequate left ventricular function. Morbidity includes arrhythmias, systemic venous hypertension with visceral and hepatic manifestations, deterioration of allograft valves in the conduits, and low cardiac output, especially when supraventricular arrhythmias occur secondary to surgical trauma or right atrial hypertension and hypertrophy.

In appropriately selected patients early survival following physiological correction has been satisfac-

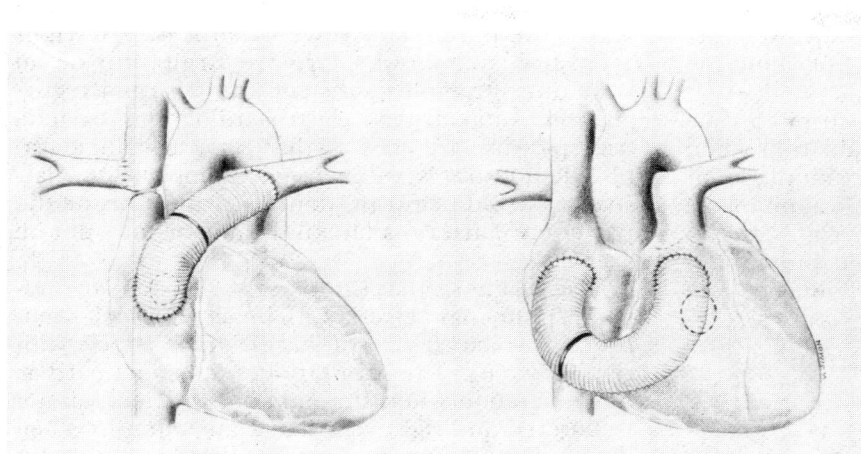

FIGURE 36-121 Fontan repairs of tricuspid atresia. On the left, a porcine valve–containing conduit is used to divert right atrial blood to the pulmonary artery in a patient having a previously constructed superior vena caval to right pulmonary arterial anastomosis (Glenn shunt). The dotted line indicates the atrial septal defect, closed with a patch. On the right, a porcine-valved conduit is used to divert right atrial blood to the right ventricular outflow tract. The dotted line indicates the small ventricular septal defect which was closed with a patch. (*From H. Laks, W. G. Williams, M. D. Hellenbrand, R. M. Freedom, N. S. Talner, R. D. Rowe, and G. A. Trusler, Results of Right Atrial to Right Ventricular and Right Atrial to Pulmonary Artery Conduits for Complex Congenital Heart Disease, Ann. Surg., 192:382, 1980. Reproduced with permission of author and publisher.*)

tory. Fontan described operation in 15 consecutive patients without a death. Bowman and associates reported nine patients in whom a modified Fontan operation resulted in only one operative death.[608] The eight survivors were described as clinically well as long as 42 months following operation. Behrendt and Rosenthal[609] reported six survivors of nine patients undergoing operation. Five of their surviving patients have been carefully evaluated postoperatively. Two are in NYHA functional class 1; three are in functional class 2. This series includes some patients with serious arrhythmias including complete heart block which appeared to be tolerated without serious ill effects.

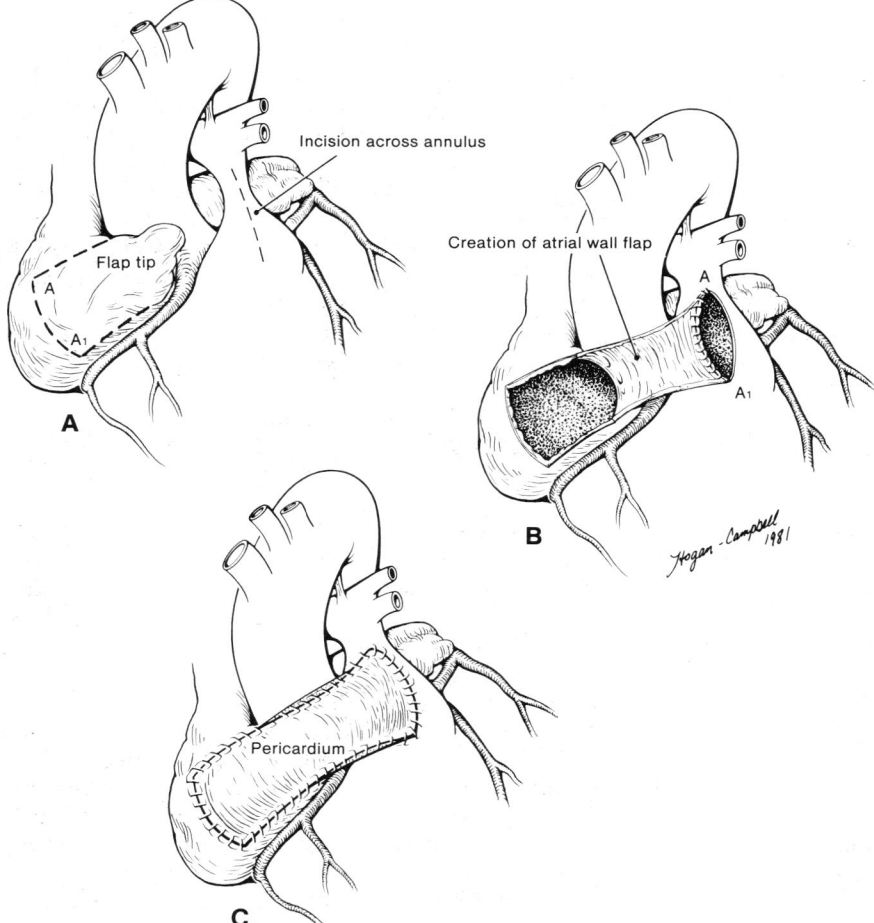

FIGURE 36-122 Bjork modification of the Fontan right atrial to pulmonary arterial shunt. A large flap of right atrial anterolateral wall is created, sutured to the right side of an incision in the right ventricular outflow tract and main pulmonary artery, and covered anteriorly with a large piece of pericardium to create a valveless conduit of entirely autologous material. Interatrial communications are closed with a patch. When applied in cases of single ventricle, the tricuspid orifice is closed with a patch.

Trusler and Williams[610] recently reviewed the late results of shunt procedures for palliation of tricuspid atresia. They found that 84 percent of children surviving a first shunt procedure were alive 10 years later; 72 percent were alive 15 years following the first operation.

Management of the infant with tricuspid atresia should include carefully planned palliation when symptoms demand, followed by consideration of physiological correction using a modification of the Fontan operation between the ages of 5 and 8 years, prior to the development of elevated pulmonary vascular resistance or left ventricular failure.

Tricuspid Regurgitation

Pathology

Tricuspid regurgitation based upon intrinsic anomalies of the valve is uncommon as an isolated entity. It may be part of Ebstein's anomaly, either alone or associated with pulmonary atresia and intact ventricular septum. It may be observed in cases of multiple dysplasia of valves.[469] Although uncommon, the usual basis for regurgitation based on an anomalous condition involving the tricuspid valve other than Ebstein's anomaly is dysplasia of the valve. This is characterized by poor differentiation of the leaflets and the chordae.[611] A rare case with no valvular tissue guarding the tricuspid orifice in association with pulmonary atresia has been reported.[612] A patent foramen ovale is usually present regardless of the basis for the tricuspid regurgitation.

Clinical Manifestations

Clinical manifestations vary somewhat depending on the etiology of the tricuspid regurgitation since there are primary and secondary forms. Endocardial cushion defects and Ebstein's anomaly are discussed in separate sections of this chapter. In general, many of those with tricuspid regurgitation present at, or shortly after, birth with profound cyanosis and congestive heart failure.

In reports on a small number of cases[613,614] that distinguish those with isolated tricuspid valvular dysplasia, most presented with cyanosis at less than 1 day of age and all within the first week. Failure occurred in most. Prenatal history and delivery were uncomplicated. There is tachypnea, hepatomegaly, a prominent left parasternal impulse with a thrill, and loud holosystolic murmur in this area. Occasionally, a middiastolic murmur at the lower left sternal border or a ductal murmur is also heard. Chest roentgenograms show extreme cardiomegaly, and pulmonary flow, when visible, is diminished or normal. The electrocardiogram shows right axis deviation, right atrial enlargement and right bundle branch block or right ventricular hypertrophy. The right ventricle is dilated by echocardiogram. Cardiac catheterization demonstrates a right-to-left shunt at atrial level and right ventricular pressures that are normal to moderately elevated, but less than systemic level in all. The pulmonary artery is occasionally not entered, but there is no pressure difference across the pulmonary valve when it is. The right atrial pressure shows a large regurgitant (r or cv) wave during systole consistent with tricuspid regurgitation. Intracavitary electrocardiograms exclude tricuspid displacement. Right ventricular angiography demonstrates an enlarged chamber with massive tricuspid regurgitation. Opacification of the pulmonary artery is late and faint or may not be visible.

The diagnosis that can present very similar findings is pulmonary atresia with intact ventricular septum, in which there is a large right ventricle with severe tricuspid regurgitation.[613,615] Even cardiac catheterization when the pulmonary artery cannot be entered and right ventricular angiography when the pulmonary artery is not visualized may not distinguish between the atretic valve and the normal valve that does not open. In both diagnoses, the pulmonary flow is by way of a ductus, and distinction is critical to management since infants with isolated tricuspid regurgitation should not have unnecessary surgery, but surgery is imperative if there is pulmonary atresia. Recently, aortography has been reported to be valuable since those with primary tricuspid abnormality have associated pulmonary regurgitation.[616]

The clinical manifestations of those with secondary forms of tricuspid regurgitation vary from this in some patients so that clinical distinction may be possible. There are numerous causes of persistently elevated pulmonary resistance in newborns that may cause this murmur. The entity of persistent fetal circulation discussed earlier in this chapter can create a similar clinical picture. Upper airway obstruction with birth defects such as choanal atresia should be suspected on the basis of the respiratory pattern. Chest roentgenogram will distinguish those with pulmonary parenchymal disease. In a number of infants, transient tricuspid regurgitation has been found to be due to myocardial dysfunction.[617] These infants have a birth history of asphyxia, and preceding hypoglycemia has occurred in many. The electrocardiographic abnormalities include ST depression in the midprecordial leads with T-wave inversion in the left precordial leads. Thus this etiology can be strongly suspected on clinical grounds alone. Diseases, such as myocarditis, are clinically distinguishable due to additional findings related to the left-sided involvement.

Natural History and Prognosis

The course of those with an isolated tricuspid valvular abnormality seems to be widely divergent. They may die of hypoxia and related problems in the first week of life,[613] or if they survive this critical period,[614] the cardiovascular abnormalities improve drastically although they continue to have a soft murmur of tricuspid regurgitation with or without mild cardiomegaly and right ventricular hypertrophy. This natural history is also true of those with tricuspid regurgitation related to persistent fetal circulation or myocardial dysfunction related to asphyxia. Survivors in these groups usually have complete resolution including disappearance of the murmur.[617]

Medical Management
Medical management of those with primary tricuspid abnormalities includes administration of oxygen, assisted ventilation when necessary, and treatment of congestive heart failure. Potentially additive problems such as hypoglycemia must be prevented. Surgery for the mistaken diagnosis of pulmonary atresia should be avoided whenever possible.[613] There is no surgical management for this in the newborn.

Surgical Management
Surgical management of tricuspid regurgitation associated with endocardial cushion defects and Ebstein's anomaly has been described in the discussions of these anomalies.

Most infants with tricuspid regurgitation secondary to dysplasia of the valve are too small, hypoxic, and acidotic to allow successful operative intervention. In the rare child who survives with unresolved tricuspid regurgitation, suture annuloplasty, prosthetic ring annuloplasty, commissural plication, or tricuspid valve replacement should be considered. An atrial septal defect or patent foramen ovale, if present, should be closed at the same operation.

Ebstein's Anomaly

Definition
Ebstein's anomaly is characterized by malinsertion of part of the tricuspid apparatus so that part of the inflow portion of the right ventricle is common with the right atrium.

Pathology
The anterior leaflet of the tricuspid valve is attached normally to the annulus, while varying portions of the posterior and the septal leaflets are displaced downward, being attached to the ventricular wall below the annulus. The proximal part of the right ventricle is thin-walled and continuous with the right atrium. The functional right ventricle is small and made up of the apical and infundibular portions of the right ventricle[618] (Fig. 36-123). An additionally common finding is that the papillary muscles and chordae are highly malformed so that great variation occurs in the manner of attachment of the two involved leaflets to the right ventricular wall. Commonly, multiple direct attachments of valvular tissue to the right ventricular mural endocardium occur.[611]

An interatrial communication is present in most cases, usually taking the form of a patent foramen

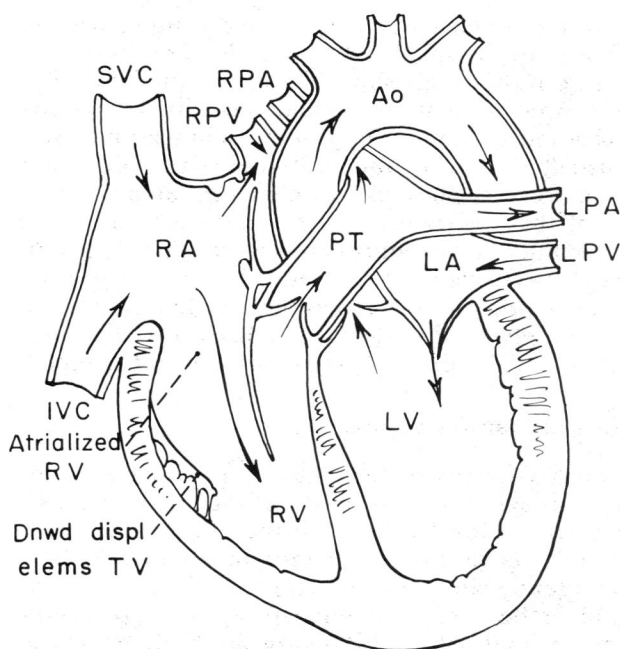

FIGURE 36-123 Ebstein's malformation of the tricuspid valve. Low attachment of elements of the tricuspid valve (TV) functions in such a way that part of the right ventricle (RV) is common with the right atrium (RA). The effective right ventricular cavity is reduced in size. SVC = superior vena cava; IVC = inferior vena cava; PT = main pulmonary arterial trunk; RPA = right pulmonary artery; LPA = left pulmonary artery; RPV = right pulmonary vein; LPV = left pulmonary vein; LA = left atrium; LV = left ventricle; Ao = aorta. [*From J. E. Edwards, Classification of Congenital Heart Disease in the Adult, in W. C. Roberts (ed.), Congenital Heart Disease in Adults, Cardiovasc. Clin. Series 10/1, F. A. Davis Company, Philadelphia, 1979, pp. 1–26. Reproduced with permission.*]

ovale. Continuity of right atrial and right ventricular myocardial tissues, in addition to the usual connections by way of the main conduction pathways, has been observed. Atrophy of right ventricular myocardium is common, principally in that part proximal to the tricuspid valve.

Associated Conditions In subjects reaching adult life, significantly associated conditions are uncommon. In symptomatic infants, pulmonary atresia is commonly associated. Pulmonary stenosis or ventricular septal defect is observed in isolated cases.

Complications Among the complications of Ebstein's anomaly without associated pulmonary atresia are congestive heart failure and abscess of the brain, the latter being a complication that is usually not observed until late childhood or even adult life.

Abnormal Physiology[619,620]
Ebstein's anomaly results in obstruction to right ventricular filling because of a decrease in size of the right ventricle, part of which is incorporated into the huge right atrium. The deformed tricuspid valve also frequently allows tricuspid regurgitation.

As a consequence of the decreased compliance and capacity of the small right ventricle, there is usually a large right-to-left shunt through either the foramen ovale or an atrial septal defect with arterial hypoxia and cyanosis. The right atrial mean pressure is usually normal or moderately elevated. The right atrial pressure pulse usually has a prominent *a* wave, and if there is tricuspid regurgitation, it may have a prominent *v* or regurgitant *r* wave. The right ventricular systolic pressure tends to be low, and the diastolic pressure resembles that of the right atrium with an elevated end-diastolic pressure. The pulmonary artery pressure is usually low and damped.

Clinical Manifestations

History Approximately one-half of reported cases develop symptoms in early infancy with cyanosis and right-sided heart failure. The remainder present because of a murmur or abnormal chest roentgenogram with no symptoms in early childhood or because of gradual progression of symptoms through late childhood or adult life.[621] Those with associated defects may be more symptomatic. The most common symptom is dyspnea on exertion at all ages.[621] Growth and development are usually normal.[622] Palpitations due to supraventricular tachyarrhythmias occur.[619] Occasionally, syncope occurs due to arrhythmia or low cardiac output if the atrial septum is intact.

Physical Examination The newborn with elevated pulmonary vascular resistance has severe cyanosis. In most other newborns, cyanosis and clubbing are mild. Only a small percentage do not have an atrial septal defect or patent foramen ovale and thus are not cyanotic. The precordium is generally quiet even in those with striking cardiomegaly. The liver is frequently enlarged, and the jugular venous pulse may be elevated. The murmur of tricuspid regurgitation is heard at the lower left sternal border and may be accompanied by a "scratchy" diastolic murmur of tricuspid stenosis. The first heart sound is split and loud, and the second heart sound is widely and persistently split. Loud third and fourth heart sounds are usual in older patients.

Chest Roentgenogram Heart size by chest roentgenogram varies, but it is ordinarily very large, predominantly due to a very dilated right atrium (Fig. 36-124). In those with cyanosis, pulmonary blood flow will be diminished correspondingly.

Electrocardiogram Giant peaked P waves are common with a prolonged PQ interval and right ventricular conduction delay or complete right bundle branch block. Electrophysiological correlates of these abnormalities have been reported.[623] In approximately 10 percent, the pattern of Wolff-Parkinson-White syndrome is seen with a short PQ interval and delayed conduction of initial QRS forces, or a delta wave.[621]

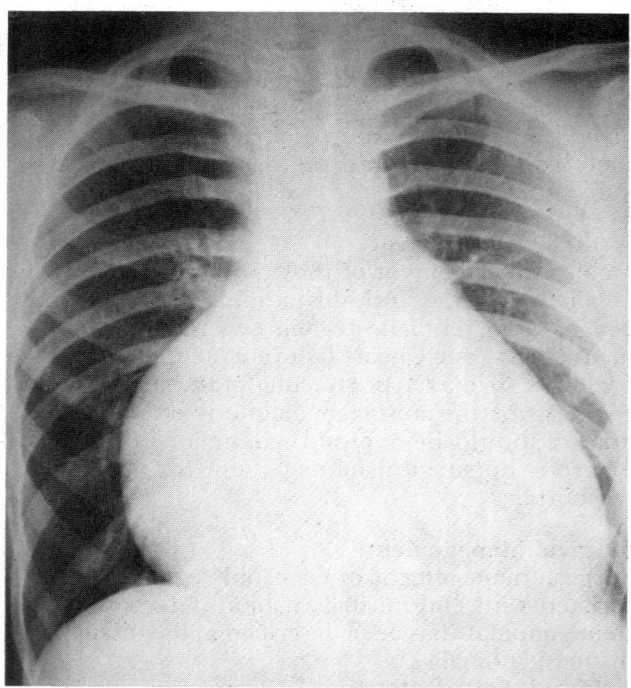

FIGURE 36-124 Chest roentgenogram in a 12-year-old boy with Ebstein's anomaly with marked cardiomegaly and diminished pulmonary flow.

Echocardiogram A large tricuspid valve is recorded widely by echocardiogram, but the most specific finding is that of delayed closure compared to the mitral valve.[624,625] Two-dimensional echocardiography is very helpful.[622]

Cardiac Catheterization There is higher risk than usual associated with cardiac catheterization because of the frequency of rhythm disturbances. Proper precautions and prompt use of cardioversion when necessary will minimize this risk. There is usually right-to-left shunting at atrial level and right atrial hypertension. The characteristic right ventricular pressure recording is not obtained until the catheter is advanced to the apex or outflow tract. Intracardiac electrocardiogram[626] will demonstrate an area on pullback from the right ventricle where the electrocardiogram is ventricular but the pressure is atrial in contour. This method is not infallible, but it is good evidence of tricuspid displacement with an "atrialized" portion of the right ventricle. The pulmonary artery may be difficult to enter, but it is very important in the cyanotic newborn to exclude pulmonary atresia, which can occur with Ebstein's anomaly. (See section on tricuspid regurgitation for further discussion of methods.) Right ventricular angiography will demonstrate tricuspid regurgitation and the right ventricular morphology. Definitive diagnosis of mild forms is difficult. Frequent abnormalities of the left ventricle and mitral valve are reported,[619,627] so left ventricular angiography should be considered.

Natural History and Prognosis

Natural history varies greatly with the severity of the abnormality. Fifty percent of those diagnosed in infancy die early, whereas late survival is reported into the ninth decade.[622] Significant associated cardiac defects will lead to a worse prognosis with almost one-half of an autopsy series in this group.[618]

Symptomatically, most patients tend to progress. In one study,[622] mortality was highly correlated to one or more of these factors: severe symptoms, cardiothoracic ratio greater than 0.65 by chest roentgenogram, cyanosis, and diagnosis in infancy. Premature death can result from heart failure, complications of cyanosis, arrhythmias, and low cardiac output if the atrial septum is intact.

Medical Management

Medical management involves treatment of heart failure and arrhythmias and prevention and treatment of complications of cyanosis and endocarditis. Treatment of infants is medical alone. Surgical success has varied, so a conservative approach toward surgery is recommended. Surgical results may offer lower morbidity and mortality for older patients with severe disease.[622]

Surgical Management

Historically, the Glenn shunt (superior vena cava to right pulmonary artery) was used for palliation of cyanotic patients with Ebstein's anomaly. Systemic arterial to pulmonary arterial shunts were poorly tolerated. The atrial septal defect was closed as an isolated procedure in some patients with adequate right ventricular function and minimal tricuspid regurgitation. More recently a modification of Fontan's operation using a valve-containing conduit from the right atrium to the right ventricular outflow tract has been applied in the management of Ebstein's anomaly, the tricuspid orifice being closed surgically.[628]

When symptoms justify operation for Ebstein's anomaly, the atrial septal defect is closed and the aneurysmal atrialized portion of the right ventricle is obliterated by plication of the spiral line of attachment of the posterior and septal tricuspid valve leaflets to the annulus fibrosis (Fig. 36-125).[629] Tricuspid valvular incompetence is corrected by an annuloplasty, if possible, or by replacement with a low-profile prosthesis. Results of this approach have been encouraging, 10 of the 11 patients operated upon by Shigenobu[630] and associates having survived operation. They have been followed for 4 to 13 years. Seven of these patients are working full-time without difficulty. All patients improved at least one class in the NYHA functional classification. Barbero-Marcial[631] and colleagues have described 20 patients with Ebstein's anomaly operated upon between 1965 and 1978. All but 1 of the 13 long-term survivors are in functional class 1.

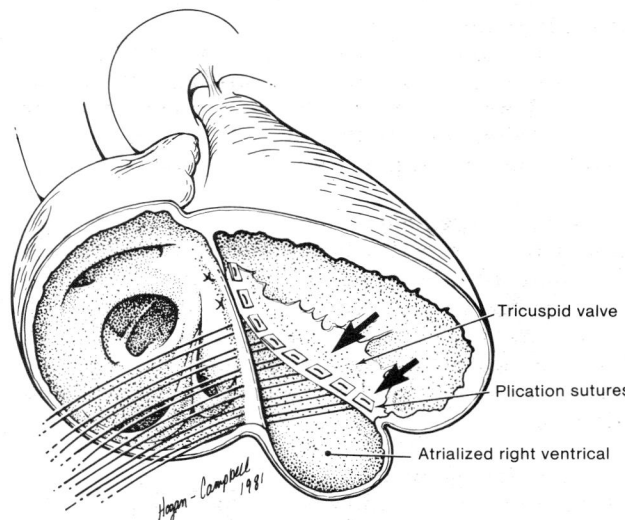

FIGURE 36-125 Plication for Ebstein's malformation. The atrialized aneurysmal portion of right ventricle is obliterated by the placement of Teflon-felt reinforced mattress sutures between the spiral line of attachment of the inferiorly displaced tricuspid valve and the true annulus fibrosus. Tricuspid valve replacement may be required. Associated atrial septal defects are closed.

Uhl's Malformation

This rare malformation, also called *parchment heart*, is characterized by the tricuspid valve being normal, while the right ventricular wall is atrophic and the chamber is noticeably dilated. Histologically, much of the right ventricular wall is fibrotic with irregular distribution of islands of myocardial tissue.[632]

Clinical Manifestations

This rare anomaly was first described in 1952.[633] A total of 18 cases[634] have been reviewed recently. In many ways, it is similar to Ebstein's anomaly. The age of presentation is 1 day to 57 years of age with progressive cyanosis, dyspnea, and fatigue with exercise. Chest pain and syncope related to exertion are common. Growth and development are normal.

Physical examination shows a quiet precordium, cyanosis, prominent *a* wave in the jugular venous pulse, widely split and soft second heart sound, and a nonspecific systolic murmur. Chest roentgenogram usually shows significant cardiomegaly. The electrocardiogram shows diminished right ventricular forces, some with a Qr pattern in mid precordial leads, and very tall, peaked P waves. Echocardiogram[635] demonstrates right ventricular dilatation, delayed tricuspid closure, and diastolic opening of the pulmonary valve. Cardiac catheterization reveals an atrial pressure wave with predominant *a* wave throughout the right side of the heart since the atrium is the driving force. A right-to-left shunt through a patent foramen ovale or atrial septal defect is usually found. Intracardiac electrocardiography and angiography exclude Ebstein's anomaly and demonstrate the large, noncontractile right ventricle.

Natural History and Prognosis

Of the 18 cases reviewed,[634] only one 14-year-old was alive. Cause of death was heart failure in a majority and otherwise similar to those discussed under Ebstein's anomaly. Right ventricular thrombi have been found on postmortem examination.

Medical Management

Supportive therapy for heart failure and treatment of cyanotic complications and arrhythmias are necessary. Surgery is not generally recommended. Surgical intervention with systemic to pulmonary shunts is uniformly unsuccessful. Closure of the atrial septal defect has been tried with one reported survivor.[634]

Surgical Management

Although not to our knowledge reported, patch closure of the tricuspid valve orifice, establishment of right atrial to pulmonary arterial continuity with a valve-containing conduit (Fontan's operation), and closure of the atrial septal defect might offer relief of congestive heart failure and cyanosis in patients with Uhl's malformation.

Pulmonary Arteriovenous Fistula

Definition

A direct connection between a pulmonary arterial branch and a pulmonary vein has variously been termed pulmonary arteriovenous fistula, pulmonary arteriovenous aneurysm, and cavernous hemangioma of the lung.

Pathology

The process, which tends to involve the subpleural part of the lung, may occur in any segment of either lung, but the right middle and both lower lobes seem most commonly involved. Classically, the site of communication is represented by a thin-walled, aneurysm-like structure into which is fed one or more arterial branches and from which one or several veins leave. A rare variation is direct connection of a pulmonary artery with the left atrium at the site of anticipated entrance of a pulmonary vein.[636] Among 63 cases of classic pulmonary arteriovenous fistula studied by Dines and associates,[637] there were single lesions in 41 cases and multiple lesions in 22 cases. Among the latter, bilateral involvement was present in five cases.

A familial tendency has been observed, and either involved individuals or relatives may show telangiectasis of various organs as part of the Rendu-Osler-Weber syndrome.[637,638] Dines and associates[637] found that when the Rendu-Osler-Weber syndrome was identified, there was an increased incidence of multiplicity of pulmonary arteriovenous fistulas.

The most severe complication is either cerebral abscess or infarction from paradoxical embolism.[639]

Bacterial infection of the fistula is uncommon, and rupture of the fistula is rare.

Clinical Manifestations

Clinical manifestations depend on the size of the connecting vessels between the pulmonary artery and the pulmonary vein. This is usually manifested with cyanosis and heart failure, with large defects presenting in early infancy.[640] Smaller ones may go undetected into the adult years. Those with pulmonary arteriovenous fistula due to hereditary hemorrhagic telangiectasia[641] have angioma of the skin and mucous membranes and a positive family history. These are usually multiple small defects that increase in number with age and do not have frank cyanosis or failure in childhood. There are commonly no precordial murmurs, but a continuous murmur may be heard over the area of the fistula. Chest roentgenogram will show a mass or multiple ones in the lung fields in the larger fistulas. The heart is frequently enlarged, and the mediastinum may be shifted due to the space-occupying mass. Pulmonary arteriography will establish the diagnosis except in the very small defects.

Medical Management

Medical management is aimed at treatment of heart failure. Prompt diagnosis can be followed by surgery[640] to prevent complications of cyanosis if the lesion is single or multiple lesions are confined to one area. Continued support with particular attention to respiratory care is important postoperatively.

Surgical Management

Conservative resection of involved lung tissue should be carried out when the diagnosis of a pulmonary arteriovenous fistula is established.[637] Occasionally the thin-walled subpleural saccular aneurysms can be dissected free of adjacent pulmonary parenchyma and excised after ligation of the artery and vein. More often segmental resection, wedge resection, or lobectomy is required. Resection should be limited to the smallest possible volume of lung tissue permitting excision of the aneurysmal sac and vessels. Resection is safe; morbidity is low; improvement is dramatic. The potential for life-threatening complications in the natural history of pulmonary arteriovenous fistulas justifies early excision even when presenting symptoms are minimal.

Abnormalities of the Pulmonary Venous Connections

Pulmonary veins terminating anomalously may involve either some of the pulmonary veins (partial anomalous connection; see earlier section of this chapter) or all of the veins.

Total Anomalous Pulmonary Venous Connection

Definition

When all pulmonary veins fail to join the left atrium but instead terminate in a systemic vein or the right atrium, the term *total anomalous pulmonary venous connection* is applied (Fig. 36-126). Synonyms include *anomalous pulmonary venous drainage* or *anomalous pulmonary venous return.*

Pathology

When all of the pulmonary venous supply terminates in a systemic vein or the portal venous system, the usual veins leave the lung and then join a chamber-like confluence. The latter lies superior to the left atrium and inferior to the tracheal bifurcation. From the confluence of veins, one vessel leads to the anomalous termination into a systemic vein or an element of the portal venous system. The sites of anomalous connection may be either supradiaphragmatic or subdiaphragmatic.

Sites of supradiaphragmatic termination in order of decreasing frequency are the left innominate vein, the coronary sinus, the right atrium, the superior vena cava and the azygous vein.[642,643]

Usually supradiaphragmatic termination is not associated with pulmonary venous obstruction, but exceptions occur. The most common of these relates to total anomalous pulmonary venous connection to the left brachiocephalic (innominate) vein. More commonly, the vein that ascends from the confluence of pulmonary veins to the brachiocephalic vein runs anteriorly to the left pulmonary hilus. Less commonly, the ascending vein runs between the left pulmonary artery, anteriorly, and the left main bronchus, posteriorly. In this position the ascending anomalous vein is compressed by what has been called a *hemodynamic vise,*[644] and pulmonary venous obstruction occurs. In addition, such a vein may be narrow and contain foci of intrinsic stenosis to compound the obstructive process. A process of hemodynamic vise may also occur in anomalous connection to the superior vena cava when the vein ascending from the pulmonary venous confluence to its anomalous termination runs between the right pulmonary artery, anteriorly, and the right main bronchus, posteriorly.

When there is total anomalous connection of pulmonary veins to the coronary sinus, the latter is markedly dilated and may be confused with an accessory atrial chamber lying posteriorly to the left atrium.

When there is total anomalous pulmonary venous connection to the portal venous system, the anomalous vein leaving the confluence of pulmonary veins descends into the abdomen alongside the esophagus, accompanying this structure through

FIGURE 36-126   Three common types of total anomalous pulmonary venous connection. In each instance blood from the lungs is ultimately delivered to the right atrium (R.A.), whence it traverses an interatrial communication for delivery to the left atrium (L.A.). *a.* Total anomalous pulmonary venous connection to the left brachiocephalic (innominate) vein (L.I.). *b.* Total anomalous pulmonary venous connection to the coronary sinus (C.S.). *c.* Total anomalous pulmonary venous connection of the infradiaphragmatic type. In the details shown, the anomalous pulmonary vein inserts into the ductus venosus (D.V.). In other instances, such an anomalous pulmonary vein may connect with the portal vein or with the left gastric vein. R.V. = right ventricle; L.V. = left ventricle.

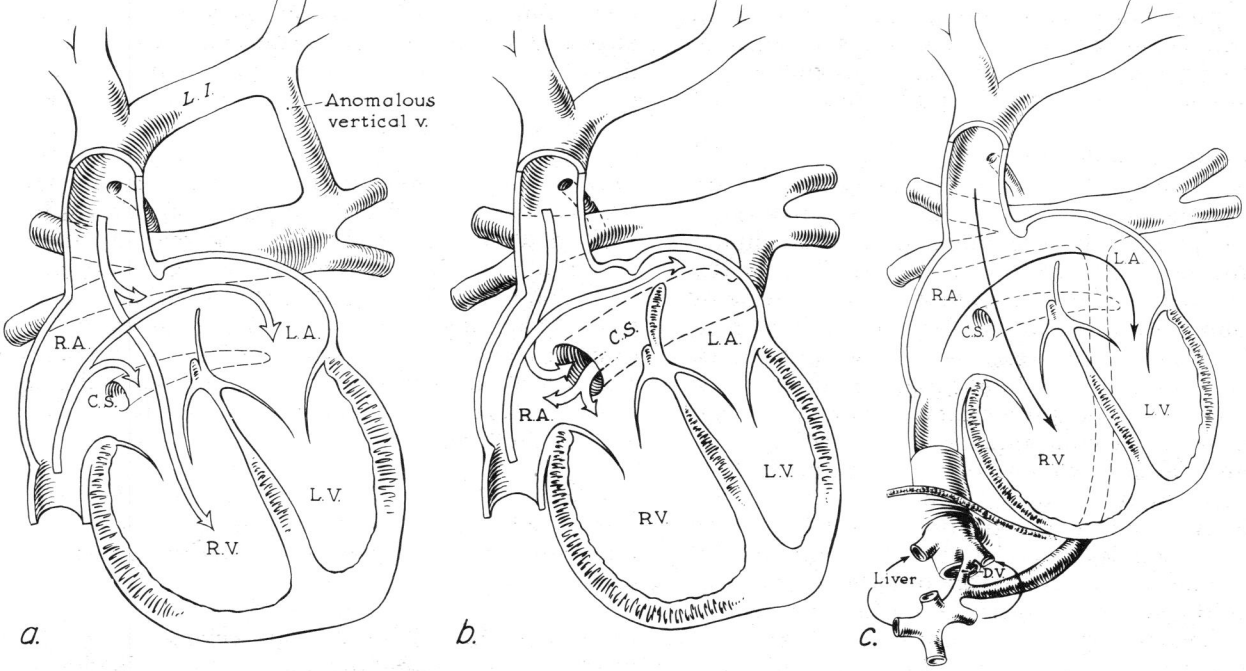

esophageal hiatus of the diaphragm. Having reached the abdominal cavity, the vein then deviates toward the right to terminate in the portal venous system. In this position, veins that receive the anomalous vein include one of the following: the ductus venosus, the portal vein, or the left gastric vein. Pulmonary venous obstruction characteristically is manifested in all cases of infradiaphragmatic connection with the portal venous system.[645]

A particular type of total anomalous pulmonary venous connection has been termed *atresia of the common pulmonary vein*. In this condition, as in classic examples of total anomalous pulmonary venous connection, there is a chamber-like confluence of the pulmonary veins leaving the lungs. In contrast, there is no gross channel of exit from the confluence of veins.[646] Small veins running from the confluence enter the esophageal wall.

In all cases of total anomalous pulmonary venous connection to a vein, there is a patent foramen ovale. The atrium and ventricle of the left side are small compared to the right-sided chambers but within normal limits as to absolute size.

Total anomalous pulmonary venous connection to the right atrium may be part of the polysplenia syndrome. In the absence of asplenia or polysplenia, associated anomalies are not common among cases of total pulmonary venous connection to systemic veins or the portal venous system. When present, there is usually asplenia or polysplenia and the various cardiovascular anomalies of that syndrome (refer to later discussion).

Complications of total anomalous pulmonary venous connection depend in part upon whether or not pulmonary venous obstruction exists. When present, survival beyond infancy is not common. Among instances of supradiaphragmatic termination of pulmonary veins there are adult subjects. In these the right-sided cardiac chambers are dilated, resembling those of partial anomalous pulmonary venous connection or atrial septal defect.[647]

Abnormal Physiology[536,647–649]

In this anomaly all the blood from both pulmonary and systemic circulations returns to the right atrium. It is compatible with life only if there is a communication between the right and left sides of the heart, which usually is a patent foramen ovale or less commonly an atrial septal defect. In most situations the pulmonary resistance is low, and a large volume of blood from the right atrium flows to the right ventricle and pulmonary circuit, somewhat analogous to a secundum atrial septal defect. Consequently, a large volume of fully saturated blood returns to the right atrium, where it mixes with a smaller volume of unsaturated blood returning from the systemic circulation. Since systemic arterial blood comes from this mixture of blood in the right atrium, the systemic arterial saturation may remain high. The systemic arterial saturation will be low if pulmonary blood flow is decreased because of either increased pulmonary vascular resistance or obstruction to pulmonary venous flow or if the oxygen content of blood returning from the systemic circulation is decreased by exercise.

Clinical Manifestations[648]

History   Male predominance, particularly of the subdiaphragmatic type of total anomalous pulmonary venous connection, has been noted in some reports and familial instances are very unusual. Almost all patients are cyanotic with over one-half presenting with cyanosis in the first month of life. Most also have congestive heart failure, including all of those with and two-thirds of those without pulmonary hypertension. The symptoms of congestive heart failure occur in almost two-thirds before 3 months of age. All patients who present in the first year of life are thin and most gain little weight after birth. In the few who gain weight, there is no pulmonary hypertension. Association with complex defects, particularly common in the asplenia syndrome, will not be discussed here.

Physical Examination   These infants are dusky, tachypneic, and diaphoretic. The jugular venous pulse is elevated and hepatomegaly appears early. There is a diffuse and hyperdynamic right ventricular impulse. The second heart sound is split and relatively fixed. The pulmonary component is increased. There is usually a grade 2 to 3 midsystolic murmur at the left sternal border. At the lower sternal border, there is a middiastolic rumble and prominent third and fourth heart sounds. Rales may be heard over the lung fields and periorbital edema. A continuous murmur may be heard over the common venous channel. If there is significant obstruction to pulmonary venous flow, most common in the subdiaphragmatic type, the cyanosis is more marked. The heart is not as hyperkinetic, and auscultation may reveal little or no murmur with a very loud second heart sound.

Chest Roentgenogram   With the unobstructed types, the heart is enlarged and the pulmonary flow is increased. Pulmonary edema may be seen. In those with return to the left innominate vein, there may be a characteristic bulging of the superior mediastinum bilaterally, producing a "snowman" or figure-of-eight contour.[6] With obstructed types, the heart size is near normal and there is very marked pulmonary edema, which may give a granular appearance to the lungs.

Electrocardiogram   There is right axis deviation, right atrial and right ventricular hypertrophy. Commonly, there is a qR pattern in the right precordial leads.

Echocardiogram   The M-mode echocardiogram[650] usually shows volume overload of the right side of the heart in the unobstructed types. The only abnormality in obstructed types may be abnormal right ventricular systolic time intervals due to pulmonary hypertension. Occasionally, an echo-free space, thought to be the common pulmonary venous channel, is seen behind the left atrium. Cross-sectional echocardiography is more specific and may outline the site of drainage.[651]

Cardiac Catheterization There will be an increase in saturation at the level of the abnormal connection, with similar saturations in the remainder of the chambers on the right and left sides of the heart. Right atrial, right ventricular, and pulmonary arterial pressures are elevated to a variable degree. Pulmonary pressures above systemic can occur if there is marked pulmonary venous or pulmonary vascular obstruction. Pulmonary capillary wedge pressures are elevated in proportion to the degree of venous obstruction. The atrial communication can rarely be obstructive,[648,652] with a mean gradient of 3 mmHg or more from right to left atrium suggesting this. Pulmonary arteriography will usually show the anomalous venous connection (Figs. 36-127 and 36-128). Angiography directly in the common venous channel, if entered, will outline its course and any sites of obstruction optimally.[653] Left ventricular angiography will demonstrate its volume[654] as well as exclude an associated ventricular septal defect or, more commonly, a patent ductus. Balloon atrial septostomy may be helpful in the uncommon case

FIGURE 36-127 Venous phase in posteroanterior projection of an arteriogram in the main pulmonary artery (MPA) in an infant with total anomalous pulmonary venous connection. The left upper (LU) pulmonary vein drains to the left vertical vein (LVV) and innominate vein (IV). The right upper (RU), right lower (RL), and left lower (LL) pulmonary veins drain into the coronary sinus (CS) and subsequently the right atrium (RA).

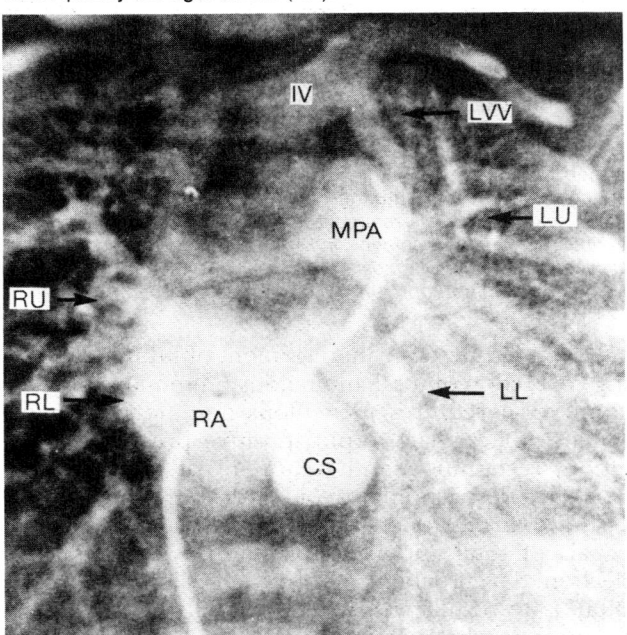

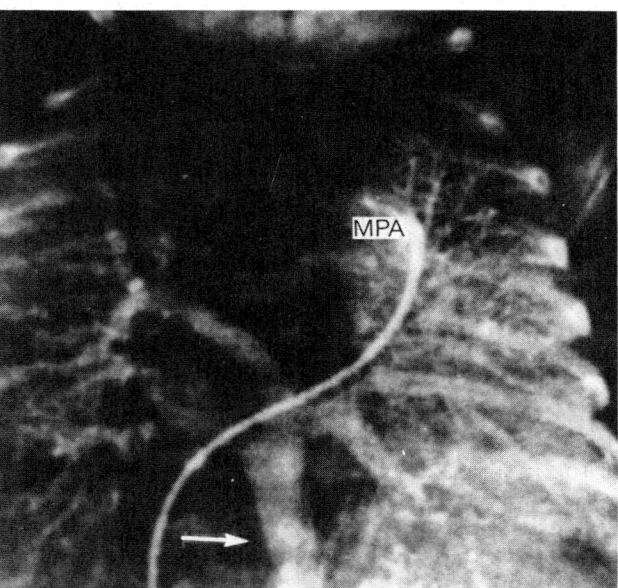

FIGURE 36-128 Venous phase in the posteroanterior projection of an arteriogram in the main pulmonary artery (MPA) in an infant with total anomalous pulmonary venous connection to a common trunk (arrow) draining subdiaphragmatically.

where there is significant obstruction demonstrated at this level.[652,655]

Natural History and Prognosis

The clinical course is usually that of progressive congestive heart failure with death in the first year of life.[648,649] There are significant differences among those with varying degrees of pulmonary hypertension. The majority of those with severe pulmonary hypertension and pulmonary vascular obstruction die by the age of 3 months, whereas those with significant pulmonary hypertension alone may survive to 1 year of age. The best clinical course is seen in those with pulmonary pressures less than one-half systemic. The majority of these patients survive to 1 year and some do not develop congestive heart failure. Severe growth failure occurs in all but a few of this latter group. At postmortem examination, structural changes in the pulmonary vascular bed are present to some degree at all ages, but changes are more severe in those with obstruction.[656,657]

Medical Management

Medical management involves vigorous treatment of congestive heart failure and intercurrent respiratory infections and prevention of endocarditis.

Initial surgical success in the 1960s was followed by numerous reports outlining the high risk involved. Surgical mortality for the early 1970s was still high, varying from 20 to 40 percent,[655,658,659] so a conservative attitude toward surgical correction except in the very ill infant continued. Some of the factors contributing to this high risk, particularly in the subdiaphragmatic type,[660] have been examined.

More recent reports indicate that a lower risk, 13 percent, can be achieved now[661] with improvements in surgical technique and intensive postoperative care. In this series, age did not appear to be a major factor in survival. Because of this success and the poor outlook with medical management alone, surgery is being recommended at even younger ages. Any newborn or young infant with severe obstruction or pulmonary edema should have prompt surgical correction. Surgery may be delayed for a few months in those without critical obstruction. Failure to grow usually occurs in those with pulmonary hypertension and surgery should be done at a few months of age. For infants with less than one-half systemic pressure in the pulmonary artery who grow, surgery may be deferred until the latter half of the first year.

Surgical Management

Correction of total anomalous pulmonary venous connection requires (1) creation of a large communication between the left atrium and the pulmonary venous system, (2) obliteration of the anomalous pulmonary venous connection, and (3) closure of the associated atrial septal defect (Fig. 36-129). Operation is carried out through a median sternotomy incision during total circulatory arrest with profound hypothermia (18 to 20°C). Cooling and rewarming is accomplished with limited cardiopulmonary bypass. Total cardiopulmonary bypass with moderate hypothermia may be used for repair of the rare child who survives beyond infancy before requiring operation. Details of the operation depend upon the precise anatomy of the anomalous connection.[478]

Supracardiac anomalous connection to the left brachiocephalic vein and infracardiac connections to the portal venous system or the inferior vena cava are corrected by the creation of a wide anastomosis between the posterior aspect of the left atrium and the common pulmonary venous sinus. The stretched foramen ovale or associated atrial septal defect is closed. The ascending or descending anomalous pulmonary venous connection is ligated.

Anomalous pulmonary venous connection to the coronary sinus is repaired by creation of a large fenestration in the common wall between the coronary sinus and the left atrium (Fig. 36-130). The coronary sinus orifice is diverted into the left atrium by placement of an intracardiac patch. The atrial septal defect is closed by the same patch.

Total anomalous pulmonary venous connection to the right atrium is repaired by excision of the atrial septum followed by placement of a patch diverting the opening of the anomalous pulmonary venous connection across into the left atrium.

Mixed forms of total anomalous pulmonary venous connection pose particular technical difficulties and require a combination of operations, some of which have been described in the discussion of partial anomalous venous connection.

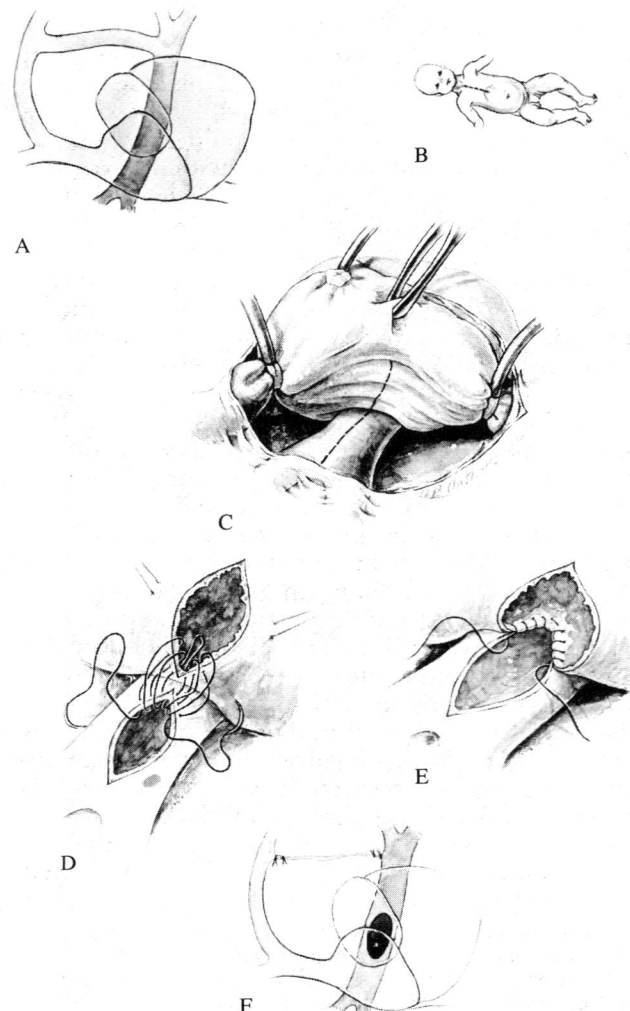

FIGURE 36-129 Correction of total anomalous venous connection draining to a left vertical vein. *A.* Schematic representation of anatomy, as seen from surgeon's side, of total anomalous pulmonary venous connection to left brachiocephalic vein. *B.* Median sternotomy incision. *C.* Appearance after cutting posterior pericardial attachments. Retraction forcep is on right atrium. Proposed incisions in posterior wall of left atrium and in anterior wall of common pulmonary venous sinus are shown. *D.* The two incisions are made, and the first few stitches of a double-armed monofilament suture are placed. *E.* These have been snugged up and the suturing continued. *F.* Final result. [*From J. W. Kirklin, Surgical Treatment for Total Anomalous Pulmonary Venous Connection in Infancy, in B. G. Barratt-Boyes (ed.), "Heart Disease in Infancy: Diagnosis and Surgical Treatment," Churchill Livingstone, Edinburgh, 1973. Reproduced with permission.*]

The postoperative management of infants following correction of total anomalous pulmonary venous connection requires meticulous attention to maintenance of cardiac output, positive pressure ventilation, recognition and treatment of arrhythmias, and fluid restriction to avoid overhydration.

Katz, Kirklin, and Pacifico[662] reviewed 51 cases of repair of total anomalous pulmonary venous connection. Seven patients (14 percent) died in the hospital. Late results were excellent. Patients surviving to operation later in life are obviously less critically

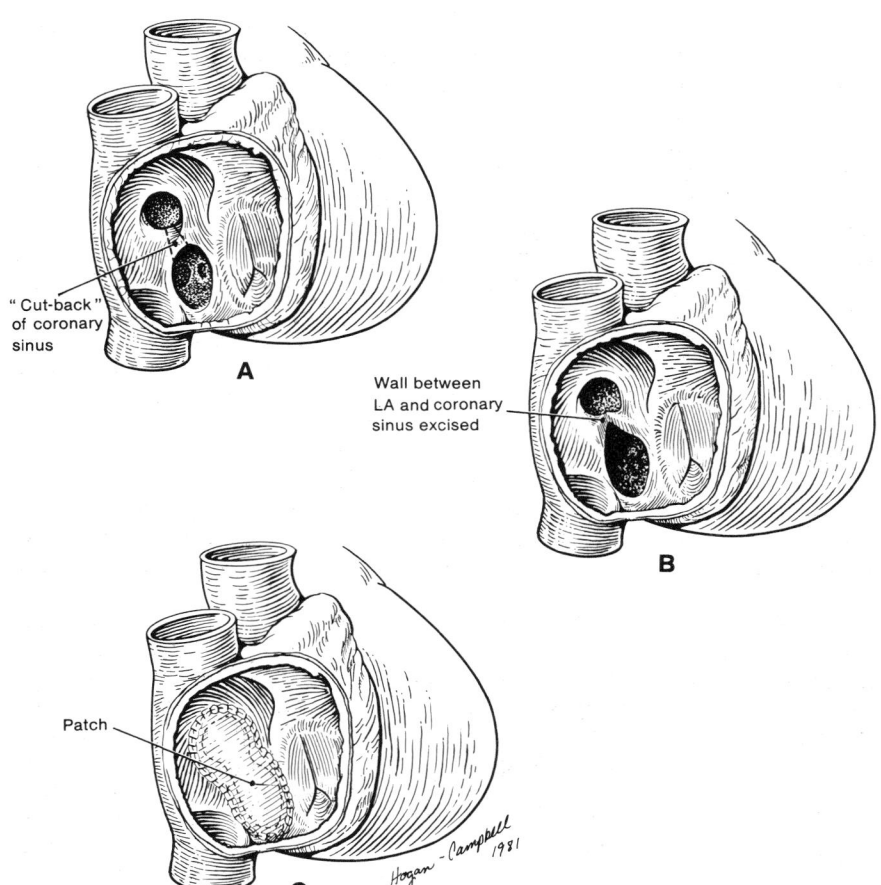

"Cut-back" of coronary sinus

A

Wall between LA and coronary sinus excised

B

Patch

C

Hogan-Campbell 1981

FIGURE 36-130 Correction of total anomalous pulmonary venous drainage to the coronary sinus. The tissue between the coronary sinus and the interior of the left atrium is excised, "cutting back" the coronary sinus orifice well away from the area of the atrioventricular node. A Dacron patch is then sutured over the orifice of the coronary sinus and the associated atrial septal defect, pulmonary venous and coronary venous blood being diverted to the left atrium. The patch must be anchored in areas remote from the atrioventricular node to avoid conduction disturbances.

ill; a lower operative mortality—about 7 percent for patients older than 1 year—would be expected.[663] Operation is indicated in all symptomatic infants and in asymptomatic infants by the age of 6 to 12 months. Determinants of survival are primarily the degree of pulmonary venous obstruction, depression of left ventricular function, and the specific type of anatomic defect.[661]

Abnormalities of Systemic Venous Connections

Union of Superior or Inferior Vena Cava with Left Atrium

When a vena cava joins the left atrium, it is rare that the inferior cava is involved. More commonly, the situation is one in which a left superior vena cava is present. The union of the left superior cava with the left atrium lies just posterior to the base of the atrial appendage. In this condition, the coronary sinus is not formed. Union of a left superior vena cava with the left atrium is usually observed in association with one of three phenomena: (1) asplenia, (2) polysplenia, or (3) presence of an atrial septal defect in the posteroinferior angle of the atrial septum. The latter condition has been discussed under

the subject of atrial septal defect (Fig. 36-7). In asplenia there is commonly a single atrium, for practical purposes, in that only a narrow strand of tissue representing the atrial septum runs between the posterior and anterior walls of the common atrium. The right superior vena cava joins the right side of the common atrium in the normal manner. In polysplenia, union of the left superior vena cava with the left atrium is less common than in asplenia. There is usually an atrial septum, but defective. Union of the inferior vena cava with the left atrium is rare.[664]

The frequently associated defects of asplenia and polysplenia syndromes and atrial septal defect are discussed in other sections of this chapter. In the rare isolated case, cyanosis is usually detected. Cardiac catheterization and venous angiography will establish that the superior vena cava or more rarely the inferior vena cava or both return to the left atrium. If both do so, there is hypoplasia of the right side of the heart. Medical treatment is directed toward the prevention and management of the complications of cyanosis. Surgical treatment is recommended to prevent these complications.[665]

An interatrial pericardial or Dacron patch baffle is placed to divert the desaturated systemic venous blood from the left atrial orifices of the anomalous cavae to the right atrium. Care is required to avoid injury to the atrioventricular node near the orifice of the coronary sinus when present. A portion of the atrial septum is excised if necessary for proper baffle placement. Pulmonary venous obstruction by the ballooning baffle is avoided by careful tailoring and proper placement of suture lines. Occasionally the hepatic veins enter the inferior aspect of the atrium directly rather than the inferior vena cava; this, too, is corrected by individualized baffle placement. Cannulation of the venae cavae for cardiopulmonary bypass may be more difficult than usual; we prefer hypothermic circulatory arrest (18 to 20°C) for correction of these rare anomalies of systemic venous return. Reports of repair are limited to individual cases; results in general are good.

Persistent Left Superior Vena Cava

Usually, malformations of the systemic intrathoracic veins are of incidental significance. Persistent left superior vena cava, the most common of these malformations, may occur either as an isolated condition or in association with other cardiovascular malformations. The right brachiocephalic vein descends in the position of the superior vena cava and, after receiving the azygous vein, enters the right atrium, as the superior vena cava does normally. On the left side, the left brachiocephalic vein is formed by its usual tributaries and descends as the left superior vena cava. It passes ventrally to the aortic arch and root of the left lung to become continuous with the coronary sinus. The latter, because of carrying the additional blood it receives through the anomalous connection, is wider than normal. The coronary sinus terminates in the right atrium. Therefore, the blood from the left arm and left side of the head and neck, despite its abnormal path, finally reaches the right atrium. Among some, but not all, cases of *atresia of the right atrial ostium of the coronary sinus*[666] a persistent left superior vena cava is present.

Winter,[667] who presented an extensive review on the subject of persistent left superior vena cava, found that in about 60 percent of cases studied a bridge connected the two brachiocephalic veins. Usually, the *hemiazygous vein* joins the left superior vena cava after arching over the left main bronchus to form a mirror image of the normal arrangement of the azygous vein and superior vena cava on the right.

In rare cases the venous system in the neck is essentially a mirror image of the normal. The right brachiocephalic vein crosses to the left and joins the left brachiocephalic vein to form a left superior vena cava; the latter then follows the usual course of a left superior vena cava and terminates in the coronary sinus. In a review of 29 cases of nonfunctional right superior vena cava, Kanegis and associates[668] found that in 26 instances there was no anatomic remnant of the right superior vena cava. In four cases such a remnant was present.

The presence of a persistent left superior vena cava is hemodynamically insignificant. Chest roentgenogram may show fullness of the left superior mediastinum. Technical difficulties may be encountered if cardiac catheterization is done from the left arm. Identification by catheter course to the left brachiocephalic vein through the coronary sinus or angiography is usual if cardiac catheterization is performed from the leg since the coronary sinus ostium is very large and easily entered. Recognition is of importance only if open heart surgery is anticipated since special bypass techniques are required.[669]

We look for a persistent left superior vena cava at the time of operation in all patients undergoing procedures requiring total cardiopulmonary bypass. When a left superior vena cava persists, the right superior vena cava is usually smaller than normal. The left superior vena cava poses no problems during operations carried out under circulatory arrest, but the operative field is obscured by blood during total cardiopulmonary bypass unless the left superior vena cava draining to the coronary sinus is either occluded or cannulated. Since an adequate communication between right and left venae cavae exists in only about 40 percent of patients, we prefer to drain the extracardiac left superior vena cava posterior to the left atrial appendage using a right-angled cannula to assure a bloodless operative field and adequate decompression of the cephalic venous system. When adequate communication between left and right venae cavae has been demonstrated at catheterization, the persistent left superior vena cava may be occluded with a clamp or tourniquet during operations carried out on total cardiopulmonary bypass. Although not routine, monitoring of the central venous pressure in the left jugular or brachial vein assures adequate venous decompression during occlusion of a persistent left superior vena cava. An increase in the pressure measured above a clamp placed temporarily on the left superior vena cava indicates the need for drainage of the left-sided venous system.

Continuity of Inferior Vena Cava with Azygous Venous System

In this condition, at times called *absence of inferior vena cava,* the hepatic portion of the inferior vena cava is absent. Under this circumstance, the inferior vena cava remains a posterior structure and joins either the azygous or hemiazygous vein. In this way the inferior vena caval blood is carried into either the right superior vena cava or a persistent left superior vena cava. The hepatic veins converge to form a relatively narrow trunk which joins the right atrium at the usual location of the inferior vena caval junction with this cardiac chamber. This venous pattern has also been termed the *candy cane* deformity or *absence of hepatic segment of inferior vena cava.* Polysplenia is usually associated.[670]

This abnormality is of clinical significance in those with congenital heart disease only by the technical problems it poses during cardiac catheterization. On chest roentgenogram, there may be fullness of the right or left superior mediastinum, depending on whether the drainage is via the azygous or hemiazygous system. On the lateral view, absence of the inferior vena caval shadow below the atrium posteriorly may also be a clue to the diagnosis. Superior orientation of the mean P axis on the electrocardiogram is frequently associated. Venous angiography from the leg will demonstrate the anomaly. In small infants, it may be safer and easier to approach cardiac catheterization from the arm if this is strongly suspected clinically.[671]

Transpositions and Malpositions of the Great Arteries

Definition and Terminology

The subject of transpositions and malpositions tends to create apprehension and at times confusion. In approaching this subject it is important for the one doing the analysis of a given case to realize consciously that the purpose of the circulation is to carry systemic venous blood to the lungs and to carry blood that has passed through the lungs to the systemic arterial system. With this in mind there are but two basic types of circulation, that which fulfills the purpose of the circulation and that which does not. Therefore, if normality is achieved, it does not, in reality, matter what specific connections of the chambers and vessels are, nor where the various chambers lie. These features will be brought out in the next section dealing with the segmental approach to the diagnosis of congenital heart disease. In order for that section to be understood, certain definition of terms is essential.

The following definitions are offered:

Inversion: When a structure exhibits a mirror image position from the "normal" with regard to left and right, it is said to exhibit inversion.
Situs solitus: Distribution of all the organs according to what is generally recognized as normal, as for example a left-sided stomach and spleen, a trilobed right lung, a bilobed left lung, and union of the left gonadal vein with the left renal vein.
Situs inversus (totalis): The organs show a perfect mirror image, as regarding left and right, to that of situs solitus. Anteroposterior relations are not disturbed.
Situs ambiguus: When, because of the nature of the atria and the position of abdominal organs, either situs solitus or situs inversus cannot be identified, situs ambiguus is said to be present. This usually applies in cases of asplenia or polysplenia.
Cardiac chambers: While each cardiac chamber usually shows particular connections, these may vary. Regardless of these, each chamber exhibits features from which it may be identified, regardless

of whether or not that chamber lies on the usual side of the heart.

Before defining the specific characteristics of the chamber, it is important to indicate certain principles that pertain when splenic anomalies are absent. With the rarest of exceptions the atria follow the body situs (morphological right atrium on the right in situs solitus and on the left in situs inversus). The ventricles do not necessarily follow the body situs so that the morphological right ventricle may be on either side in either situs solitus or situs inversus. Each atrioventricular valve is part of the specific ventricle into which it leads. Of the two great arteries the anterior one usually joins the anatomic right ventricle.

The *morphological right atrium* is characterized by the foramen ovale lying in its septal wall.

The *morphological left atrium* shows interatrial ostium II in its septal wall.

In a segmental designation of the heart, situs solitus position of the atria is designated as S and the situs inversus position (left-sided right atrium and right-sided left atrium) is designated as I.

The *morphological right ventricle* is characterized by possessing a *conus,* the latter being a cardiac tube interposed between tricuspid and semilunar valves.

The *anatomic* left ventricle is characterized by fibrous continuity between the semilunar and mitral valves and so does not exhibit a conus.

d-loop and l-loop:[672] When the morphological right ventricle lies to the right of the morphological ventricle, the ventricular portion of the heart is said to exhibit a d-loop. When the ventricular relationships are reversed, an l-loop is said to be present. In a segmental definition of the heart, a d-loop is designated as D and an l-loop as L.
Cardiac apex: If the cardiac apex points to the left, *levocardia* is designated; if to the right, *dextrocardia;* and toward the midline, *mesocardia.*
Great arteries: The great arteries may deviate from the usual both with respect to their anteroposterior and lateral (left to right) relationships.[673]
Normal: In situs solitus the aortic origin lies to the right of and posterior to the position of the pulmonary valve. In situs inversus the anteroposterior relationships are not disturbed by laterality is, the aortic origin lying to the left of the pulmonary arterial origin. In the former, it may be said that the great vessels are *normally related:* in the latter, inversion of a normal relationship.
Malposition and transposition: Abnormal relationship between the great arteries or inappropriate ventriculoarterial connection may be termed malposition. Transposition may be considered a particular variety of malposition.

In *transposition* (of the great arteries), the aorta arises from the anatomic right ventricle and the pulmonary artery from the anatomic left ventricle. Usually, the aortic origin is more anterior than that of the pulmonary artery.

When the transposed aortic origin is to the right of the pulmonary origin, the transposition is called dextro transposition (d-transposition; see discussion of complete transposition of great arteries below). When the reverse is the case, levo transposition (l-transposition) is present (see the section on corrected transposition, below). When the transposed aorta lies directly anterior to the pulmonary artery, it is a-transposition.

Malposition (of the great arteries) may also be termed d-malposition or l-malposition, depending on the laterality in relationships between the origins of the two great arteries. When malposition does not involve specific types as complete or corrected transposition, the term malposition is used. Two specific types of malposition have been described. The first is characterized by one artery arising from the appropriate ventricle, while the other artery also arises from the same (or inappropriate) ventricle, yielding a situation either of *double-outlet* right ventricle (DORV) or double-outlet left ventricle (DOLV).

The second type of malposition has been termed *anatomically corrected malposition*.[674] This is characterized by the great arteries having the same laterality as the ventricles from which they arise.

The reader should not confuse the rare condition of anatomically corrected malposition with the condition commonly called *classical corrected transposition* or simply *corrected transposition*. In that condition the course for the flow of blood is normal. In anatomically corrected malposition the route for the flow of blood may be normal or abnormal, depending upon the atrioventricular connections.

The terms *concordance and discordance* refer to the connections of the atria with the ventricles and connections of the ventricles with the great arteries and may be applied regardless of body situs. Thus, whether in situs solitus or situs inversus, the connection of the morphological right atrium with the morphological right ventricle and connection of the morphological left atrium with the morphological left ventricle represents *atrioventricular concordance*. When the right atrium connects with the left ventricle and the left atrium with the right ventricle, *atrioventricular discordance* is present.

When the anatomic right ventricle connects with the pulmonary artery and the anatomic left ventricle with the aorta, *ventriculoarterial concordance* exists. *Ventriculoarterial discordance* is present when the morphological right ventricle connects with the aorta and the left ventricle with the pulmonary trunk. The connections between the chambers and great vessels are more important in determining whether or not the circulation is normal than their positions. A workable rule regarding the concept of concordance and discordance is that "one wrong (discordance) is bad, while two wrongs make a right." Obviously, two rights make for right also.

Various additional terms are used. *Mirror-image dextrocardia* is synonymous with situs inversus. *Iso-lated dextrocardia* or *levocardia* refers to the location of the cardiac apex inappropriate with the body situs. *Isolated ventricular inversion* is said to be present when in situs solitus the ventricles are inverted and the great vessels are in normal relationship. *Isolated ventricular noninversion* is present when, in situs inversus, the ventricles are noninverted (d-loop), while the great vessels are normally interrelated. When, as is common in asplenia or polysplenia, the orientation of some or all of the abdominal organs do not conform either to situs solitus or inversus, the term *abdominal heterotaxia* is used.

The Segmental Approach to Diagnosis of Transpositions and Malpositions of the Great Arteries

The segmental or step-by-step approach is a valuable tool for arriving at the correct diagnosis in patients with complex congenital heart disease. This approach is independent of cardiac position and as such can be applied equally well to hearts in the normal position or to those with dextrocardia, mesocardia, or levocardia. In order, one determines (1) the location of the right and left atria, (2) the location of the right and left ventricles and the nature of their atrioventricular connections, and (3) the position of the great arteries and their relationship to the ventricle, ventricles, or outlet chamber. In addition, one must search for associated malformations between and within each of these segments.[675,676]

Determining atrial situs can be accomplished in most instances by taking advantage of the high degree of abdominal visceroatrial concordance. With abdominal situs solitus (S) the liver is on the right and the right atrium will almost invariably be on the right as well, while with abdominal situs inversus (I) the liver is on the left and the right atrium will almost invariably be on the left. With abdominal situs ambiguus (A) the liver may be almost symmetrically placed across the midline or predominantly to the right or to the left and the atria may be normally located, inverted, or both atria may have morphological characteristics of either the right or the left atrium. When both atria have the characteristics of a right atrium (i.e., bilateral superior venae cavae and no pulmonary venous connections), dextroisomerism of "bilateral right-sidedness" is said to be present. This situation usually, though not invariably, is accompanied by asplenia. When both atria have characteristics of a left atrium (i.e., pulmonary venous drainage from the ipsilateral lung) levoisomerism or "bilateral left-sidedness" is said to exist. This usually, but again not invariably, is accompanied by polysplenia. It is in the recognition of, or rather the failure in recognition of, abdominal situs ambiguus, and hence atrial situs ambiguus, that the greatest number of errors occurs since a symmetrical liver, a good predictor if present, is present in only a little over one-third of patients with situs ambiguus. Lateralization of the liver, evident in the remainder, may simulate either situs solitus or situs inversus.

Bronchial situs, determined by overpenetrated chest roentgenogram or bronchial tomography, has proved to be a more accurate predictor of atrial situs than abdominal situs. The longer of the two main bronchial lengths, measured from the carina to the proximal wall of the upper lobe bronchus, is divided by the shorter. A ratio of 2.0 or greater indicates lateralization of the bronchi, and hence the atria, with the longer being the left bronchus. A ratio of 1.5 or less indicates bronchial situs ambiguus with either dextro- or levoisomerism. Tomography may be necessary at this point to permit distinction, on the basis of bronchial morphology, between bilateral left or bilateral right bronchi. Among those patients with ratios between 1.5 and 2.0, tomography will also permit accurate bronchial length measurements corrected for magnification, which can be used to identify each main bronchus by comparison with measurements from normal controls of the same age.[676]

Of all the techniques for determining atrial situs, the most accurate appears to be identification of the hepatic portion of the inferior vena cava, which almost always enters the morphologically right atrium.[676] The location of the hepatic portion of the inferior vena cava as it enters the right atrium can be determined either by catheter position, angiography, or two-dimensional echocardiography.[677]

Additional clues to atrial situs may be provided by a superiorly oriented P-wave vector in the electrocardiogram and absence of the suprarenal and infrahepatic portion of the inferior vena cava with azygous extension to the superior vena cava—characteristics of levoisomerism and polysplenia—or the presence of Howell-Jolly bodies in the peripheral blood smear—a characteristic of dextroisomerism and asplenia. Selective atrial angiography at the time of catheterization may permit visualization of the triangular right atrium with its broad, pyramidal atrial appendage or the elliptical left atrium with its narrow, "crooked-finger" appendage.

The second step is to determine the atrioventricular and ventricular relationships. High-quality, selective biplane ventricular angiography is essential for visualization of the distinctive right and left ventricular morphology. The right ventricle, with its globular shape, blunt apex, coarse trabeculations, and, usually, semilunar-atrioventricular valve discontinuity, may be distinguished from the left ventricle, with its footlike shape in diastole and tail shape in systole, its fine trabeculations, and two papillary muscles. Two-dimensional echocardiography appears capable of permitting recognition of these morphological features and perhaps other, more distinctive features as well.[678] Normally, the straight cardiac tube of the embryo, either as a result of folding or looping to the right or of internal organization or both, becomes oriented in such a fashion

that the proximal bulbus cordis or future right ventricle comes to occupy a position to the right of the ventricle portion of the bulboventricular loop, or future left ventricle. Thus, in the usual or normal situation the sinus or inflow portion of the right ventricle lies to the right of the left ventricle, with the sequence of internal organization of the U-shaped right ventricular being from right to left. That is, the tricuspid valve is on the right, followed by the sinus or inflow portion somewhat more to the left, the septal and moderator bands still further to the left, and, finally, the outflow tract or infundibulum also to the left and superior. Occasionally, the embryonic straight cardiac tube folds to the left or develops in such a way that the right ventricle lies to the left of the left ventricle with the sequence of internal organization of the right ventricle being from left to right. If the right ventricular inflow tract or sinus lies to the right of the left ventricle and the organization of the right ventricle is from right to left, angiographically or echocardiographically, the patient is said to have a d-loop. If the patient's right ventricular inflow tract or sinus lies to the left of the left ventricle and the right ventricular organization is oriented from left to right, the patient is said to have an l-loop. If the type of loop cannot be determined, it is designed as X. The sequence of right ventricular internal organization takes on particular importance in situations of crisscross atrioventricular connections and superoinferior ventricles where the major portion of the right ventricular cavity lies directly above or even somewhat to the left of the left ventricle but the ventricular loop is still identifiable as a D-loop by virtue of the internal sequence.[679] When the morphologically right atrium connects with the morphologically right ventricle and the morphologically left atrium to the morphologically left ventricle, the atrioventricular connection is said to be *concordant*. When the right atrium connects with the left ventricle and the left atrium to the right ventricle, the connection is described as *discordant*. When atrial situs cannot be determined, the connection is said to be *ambiguus*.

Finally, the ventriculoarterial relationships or connections and the type of conus must be established, again either angiographically or echocardiographically. If the great arteries are normally related and their ventricular connections normal, they are designated as solitus (S) or normally inverted (I). With transposition of the great arteries (TGA), where the aorta arises from the right ventricle and the pulmonary artery from the left ventricle, and among examples of malposition of the great arteries (MGA), double-outlet right ventricle (DORV), double-outlet left ventricle (DOLV), and anatomically corrected malposition (ACM), the symbol D is used to indicate that the aorta arises to the right of the pulmonary artery and the symbol L to designate that the aorta arises to the left of the pulmonary artery. The symbol A may be used when the aorta arises directly anterior to the pulmonary artery.

The symbols used to designate the combination or sequence of segments are arranged in order as follows: (1) the viscero- or bronchoatrial situs, (2) the ventricular loop, and (3) the relationship of the great arteries. These are included within parentheses and preceded by words or abbreviations which indicate the ventriculoarterial interconnection, for example, TGA, DORV, or single ventricle (SV). Associated malformations such as ventricular septal defect, pulmonary stenosis, and straddling tricuspid valve are listed after the parentheses. Thus, the typical or usual transposition of the great arteries with situs solitus, D-ventricular loop, aorta arising from the right ventricle and to the right of the pulmonary artery, with an intact ventricular septum (IVS) would be designated TGA (SDD) IVS. The designation for typical corrected transposition with situs solitus, L-ventricular loop, aorta arising from the morphologically right ventricle and lying to the left of the pulmonary artery, with ventricular septal defect and pulmonary stenosis would be TGA (SLL), VSD, PS. These designations apply to these particular transpositions with situs solitus, whether the heart lies in the right or the left chest (dextrocardia or levocardia, respectively). It should be noted that the description of the position of the heart within the chest would offer no additional information referable to the intracardiac anatomy or great-vessel connections.

Transposition of the Great Arteries

Definition
In this condition, wherein there is atrioventricular concordance, there is ventriculoarterial discordance (SDD or ILL).

Pathology
In the majority of cases the atria are in a situs solitus (S), and there is atrioventricular concordance, the right ventricle lying to the right of the left ventricle (d-loop, D). The aorta arises from the right ventricle and the pulmonary trunk from the left, the pulmonary and mitral valves showing fibrous continuity (Fig. 36-131). The aorta lies to the right of the pulmonary arterial origin (d-transposition, D), and usually the aorta is somewhat more anterior. Less commonly the aorta is distinctly anterior to the pulmonary trunk, and rarely the pulmonary artery is more anterior. Of the communications between the two sides of the circulation, a narrow patent foramen is common. Patent ductus is common in young infants. The ventricular septum may be intact (Fig. 36-131A). A ventricular septal defect of significant size and varying location occurs in somewhat over one-third of cases (Fig. 36-131B).[680]

The incidence of associated pulmonary stenosis varies with the state of the ventricular septum. Liebman and associates[680] found pulmonary stenosis in 4 percent of cases with intact ventricular septum and in 28 percent of those with ventricular septal defect

(Fig. 36-131C). Anatomic causes of pulmonary stenosis include (1) the presence of bilateral coni with a narrow state of the subpulmonary conus, (2) a membranous collar encircling the left ventricular outflow tract, (3) anomalous adhesion of the anterior mitral leaflet to the ventricular septum, and (4) stenotic deformity of the pulmonary valve.[681]

The coronary arteries usually arise from the left and posterior sinuses, the right artery arising from the latter location. A fairly frequent variation is origin of the left circumflex artery from the right coronary artery,[682] while that vessel arising from the left sinus is the anterior descending artery.

Associated Conditions Associated conditions are relatively uncommon. Among these are right aortic arch and juxtaposition of the atrial appendages.

Malformations of the cardiac valves may be associated with complete transposition. Among 88 specimens studied by Layman and Edwards,[683] 23 specimens collectively exhibited 31 valvular malformations. Among the significant valvular malformations observed were aortic valvular stenosis, cleft of the tricuspid valve associated with left ventricular–right atrial communication, cleft of the mitral valve, and adhesion of anomalous chordae of the mitral valve to the ventricular septum causing left ventricular outflow obstruction.

Total situs inversus may occur rarely (ILL).

Complications Peripheral desaturation and acidosis constitute the principal cause of death. In cases with valvular abnormalities these may contribute to congestive cardiac failure.

Hypertensive pulmonary vascular disease may occur at an inordinately early age and may even occur with intact ventricular septum.[684]

Miscellaneous Transpositions. An uncommon type of transposition was described by Elliott and associates.[685] This was characterized by normal orientation of the cardiac chambers, while the aorta arose from the right ventricle and the pulmonary trunk arose above a ventricular septal defect from both ventricles. There was fibrous continuity between the pulmonary valve and mitral valve. The fundamental arrangement was that of a transitional state between classic complete transposition of the great vessels, on one hand, and double right ventricle of the Taussig-Bing type, on the other.

A somewhat related condition was described by Van Praagh and associates.[673] In four cases, also with normally positioned cardiac chambers, the great vessels lay side by side and the aorta arose from the right ventricle, while the pulmonary trunk arose from the left ventricle. There was fibrous continuity between the aortic and the tricuspid valves in three of the four cases, while in the fourth case there was continuous fibrous continuity between the left aortic leaflet and the anterior leaflet of the mitral valve through an associated subaortic ventricular septal defect.

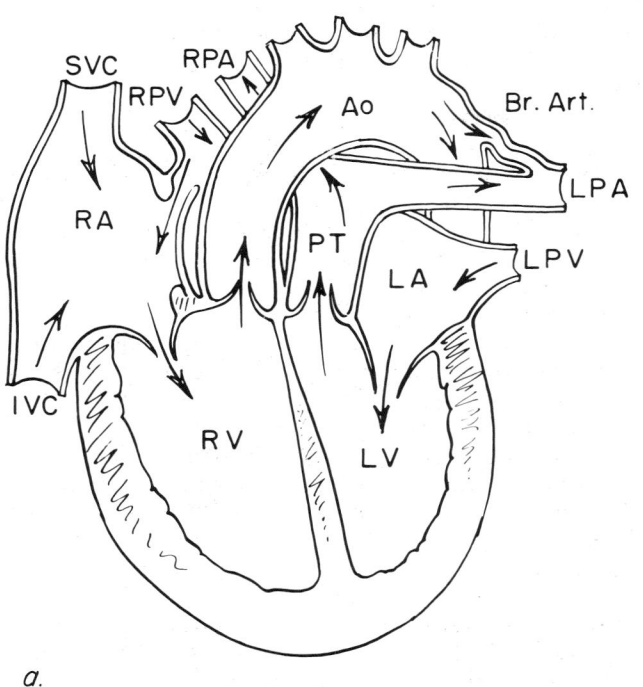

a.

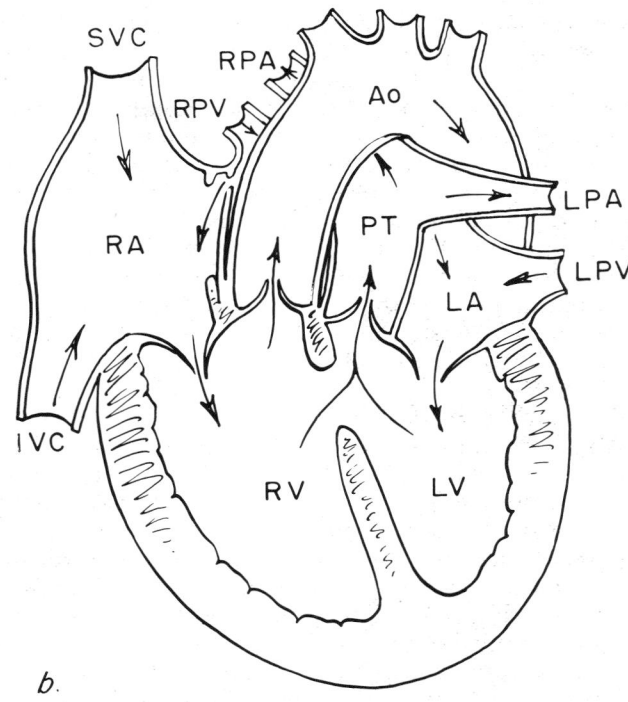

b.

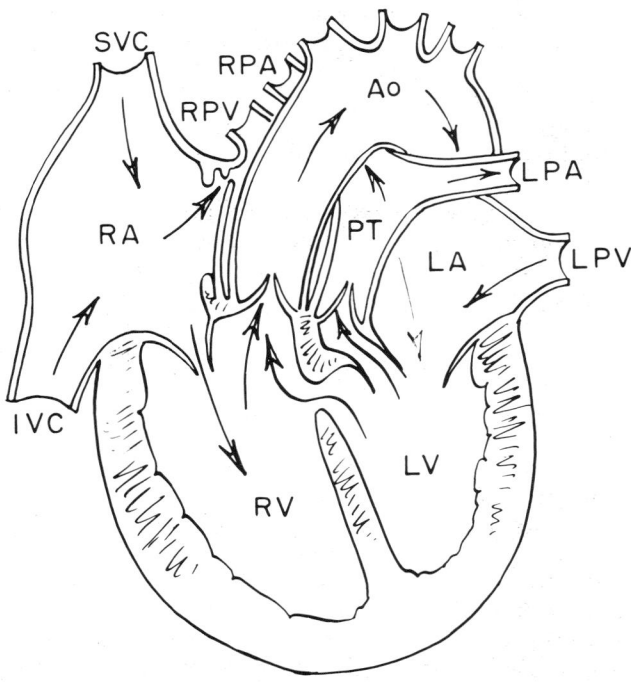

c.

FIGURE 36-131 Complete transposition. *a.* With intact ventricular septum. A patent foramen ovale and enlarged bronchial arteries (Br. Art.) are present. *b.* With ventricular septal defect and without pulmonary stenosis. *c.* With ventricular septal defect and subpulmonary stenosis. SVC = superior vena cava; IVC = inferior vena cava; RA = right atrium; RV = right ventricle; Ao = aorta; LA = left atrium; LV = left ventricle; PT = main pulmonary arterial trunk; RPA = right pulmonary artery; LPA = left pulmonary artery; RPV = right pulmonary vein; LPV = left pulmonary vein.

Yet another condition is to be considered among the miscellaneous types of transposition. This is characterized by the presence of normally related great vessels while there is isolated ventricular inversion. In this state, the anatomic left ventricle lies on the right side and joins the aorta, while the anatomic right ventricle lies on the left side and joins the pulmonary trunk.[686,687] Thus, while the great vessels are not transposed, the anatomic arrangements allow venous blood to be delivered to the aorta, yielding a functional state identical with that in classic complete transposition of the great vessels.

Abnormal Physiology[688–691]

In complete transposition (d-transposition) of the great arteries with situs solitus, the systemic and pulmonary circulations are arranged so that the systemic venous return is conducted back to the systemic arterial system and the pulmonary venous returns back to the pulmonary arterial system with no obligatory mixing or interchange. For survival there must be communication between the two circulations in the form of either an atrial septal defect, patent ductus arteriosus, or ventricular septal defect. The hemodynamics are dependent on the combination of defects present and particularly on the amount of mixing between the systemic and pulmonary circulations. The characteristic finding at cardiac catheterization is a smaller oxygen content in blood from the aorta, which originates from the right ventricle, than in blood from the pulmonary artery, which originates from the left ventricle. The right ventricular systolic pressure will be essentially the same as systemic arterial pressure. There is evidence of shunts at various levels. Usually the atrial shunt is from left to right if a patent ductus arteriosus is present, but bidirectional if the interatrial opening is the only site of systemic-pulmonary mixing. The shunt via a patent ductus usually is from aorta to pulmonary artery. Ventricular shunting is commonly bidirectional, although the magnitude of the shunt and the pressure in the left ventricle and pulmonary artery depend upon the size of the ventricular defect and the relative resistances in the pulmonary and systemic circulations, as in uncomplicated ventricular septal defects.

Clinical Manifestations

Approximately 9 percent of children with recognized congenital heart disease will have transposition of the great arteries,[6] an extremely serious malformation with a mortality rate, untreated, of 30 percent within the first week and 50 percent within the first month.[9] Transposition, usually with an intact ventricular septum, is the most common diagnosis among infants admitted to the hospital with heart disease within the first week of life and ranks second only to ventricular septal defect in frequency among infants with heart disease serious enough to produce death or to require cardiac catheterization or cardiac surgery within the first year of life. Males are more commonly afflicted than females in a ratio of between 2 and 3:1. Three-quarters or more of those patients with d-transposition, situs solitus, and d-loop [TGA (SDD)], either have no significant associated cardiac defects or relatively simple malformations in the form of ventricular septal defect, atrial septal defect, patent ductus arteriosus, or pulmonary stenosis. The remainder generally will have more complicated lesions such as tricuspid or mitral atresia, single ventricle, atrioventricular canal defects, or aortic atresia.[3] The more common and relatively uncomplicated form of transposition is the subject of this section.

History Approximately half of infants with transposition will have an intact ventricular septum, and very early, severe, and progressive cyanosis is the presenting symptom or sign in this group. Approximately 60 percent of these infants require transfer to a cardiac center within the first 2 days of life and 75 percent within the first week. In a very few, a patent ductus in combination with an incompetent foramen ovale or a small ventricular septal defect will permit survival for several weeks, but narrowing or closure of any of the three will produce critical hypoxia. Those infants with a sizable ventricular septal defect present with severe congestive failure and only mild or barely detectable cyanosis toward the middle or latter part of the first month of life. Tachypnea, dyspnea, and failure to thrive are characteristic. Those infants or children with a large ventricular septal defect and significant pulmonary stenosis may present within the first days of life with

cyanosis if stenosis is severe, but with more moderate stenosis they may present with cyanosis and little if any congestive failure somewhat later within the first year.

Physical Examination Among infants with an intact ventricular septum, the most prominent feature is intense cyanosis. Tachypnea and mild dyspnea are present. Arterial pulses are easily felt. The right ventricular lift is forceful, and the first sound is usually loud at the lower left sternal border. In most patients the second heart sound may be heard to be split narrowly, confirming the presence of two semilunar valves. Murmurs are seldom impressive or distinctive. Signs of congestive failure such as gallop rhythm, hepatomegaly, or pulmonary rales are uncommon unless the infant is beyond the first week of life and a large ductus is present. Among infants with a large ventricular septal defect, slenderness and mild cyanosis or a grayish pallor are apparent. Breathing is labored, usually with nasal flaring, and both right and left ventricular impulses are hyperactive. A thrill is uncommon. A systolic murmur at the lower left sternal border usually is present, but it is seldom very loud or completely holosystolic. A gallop rhythm and a diastolic flow rumble at the apex are typical. Infants and children with ventricular septal defect and significant pulmonary stenosis generally are severly cyanotic. A forceful or hyperdynamic right ventricular lift, an audible sound of pulmonary closure, or a stenotic murmur of greater intensity and duration than one might expect in tetralogy of Fallot, with a similar degree of cyanosis, would suggest the possibility of transposition.

Chest Roentgenogram With an intact ventricular septum, the heart size and pulmonary vascularity appear normal or at the upper limits of normal during the first week. A narrow base due to the displaced pulmonary artery may give rise to the characteristic "egg-on-side" contour. Impressive cardiomegaly, pulmonary plethora, and this characteristic contour are more common during the second week and beyond. With a large ventricular septal defect, marked cardiac enlargement involving all chambers, impressive pulmonary plethora, and the egg-on-side contour are present. With significant pulmonary stenosis, the heart resembles that of tetralogy of Fallot, but it is usually slightly larger and the pulmonary vascularity less diminished than one would expect for the degree of clinical cyanosis. A right aortic arch is present in about 4 percent of patients with an intact ventricular septum, 11 percent with a ventricular septal defect, and 16 percent of those with a ventricular septal defect and pulmonary stenosis.[692]

Electrocardiogram With an intact ventricular septum, the electrocardiogram may reveal tall or peaked P waves by the second or third day of life, but clearly abnormal right ventricular forces are not usually apparent until the latter part of the first week. The persistence of an upright T wave in leads V_1 and V_3R beyond 4 days of age would provide an early clue that the right ventricular systolic pressure is at systemic levels. The older infant will have abnormal right axis deviation and marked right ventricular hypertrophy. A large ventricular septal defect and a large pulmonary blood flow usually will produce biatrial and biventricular hypertrophy. If pulmonary blood flow is reduced toward normal, either by significant pulmonary stenosis, by pulmonary arterial banding, or by severe pulmonary vascular obstructive disease, the pattern becomes one of right ventricular and right atrial hypertrophy. Diminutive right ventricular forces or isolated left ventricular hypertrophy suggests right ventricular hypoplasia, frequently associated with overriding of the tricuspid valve.

Echocardiogram With the M-mode technique the anterior great artery can be identified as the aorta and the posterior great artery as the pulmonary artery by the reversal of the normal ratios of the left to right ventricular systolic ejection times (normal being 0.80) and the left to right ventricular preejection periods (the normal being 1.25). The anterior great artery or aorta usually, though not invariably, is displaced medially and lies to the right of the posterior great artery of pulmonary artery.[455] Two-dimensional study, either from the subxiphoid or precordial approach, can document the pulmonary artery arising from the left ventricle and the aorta from the right ventricle and provides information regarding associated anomalies (Fig. 36-132).[693] The success of balloon septostomy or surgical septectomy can be judged by visualizing the atrial septal opening directly using the subxiphoid approach.[109] The

FIGURE 36-132 Two-dimensional echocardiogram in the parasternal, long-axis view from a patient with transposition of the great arteries and intact ventricular septum. Both great arteries are visualized with the pulmonary artery (PA) identified as posterior to the aorta (AO) by the sharp posterior angulation of the PA around the superior aspect of the left atrium (LA). MV = mitral valve; A = anterior; I = inferior; S = superior; P = posterior. (*From Hagler, Tajik, Seward, Mair, and Ritter.*[552] *Reproduced with permission.*)

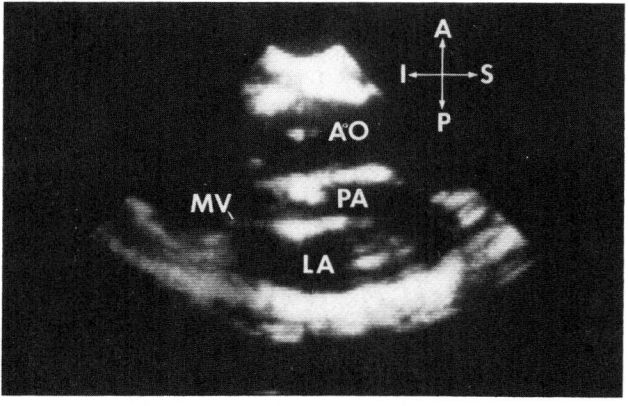

ratio of left ventricular preejection period to left ventricular ejection time, determined by the M-mode technique, can be used to estimate pulmonary arterial pressure in the weeks and months beyond the newborn period. In the absence of bundle branch block, atrioventricular dissociation, or arrhythmias, values of less than 0.26 almost invariably predict a pulmonary arterial diastolic pressure of less than 20 mmHg and a pulmonary arterial mean pressure less than 30 percent of the systemic arterial mean pressure. A ratio greater than 0.30 strongly suggests a pulmonary arterial diastolic pressure greater than 20 mmHg and a mean pulmonary arterial pressure greater than 50 percent of the systemic arterial mean pressure.[694] Valvular and subvalvular pulmonary stenosis can be visualized by two-dimensional echocardiography, and such visualization may permit semiquantitative assessment of the degree of obstruction and its progression.

Cardiac Catheterization Systemic arterial oxygen desaturation will be present in all patients, with saturation values ranging from 18 to 70 percent among those with an intact ventricular septum and from 70 to 90 percent in those with a large ventricular septal defect without pulmonary stenosis. The pulmonary arterial oxygen saturation invariably is higher than the systemic arterial saturation. The right ventricular systolic pressure will be at systemic levels, and the left ventricular pressure will be also if a large ventricular septal defect, ductus arteriosus, or significant pulmonary stenosis is present. A wide pressure difference between the two ventricles or between the two atria indicates an intact or virtually intact ventricular or atrial septum, respectively, but the lack of such a gradient certainly does not guarantee the presence of an adequate opening at either level. Selective ventricular angiography will document the anteriorly located aorta arising from the right ventricle with the aortic valve displaced superiorly and anteriorly by the subaortic conus. The pulmonary artery will arise from the left ventricle posteriorly and to the left (Fig. 36-133). The presence and size of a ventricular septal defect should be noted as well as the morphology and size of both ventricular chambers. The presence or absence of a patent ductus should be established by aortography if possible. The pulmonary artery can and should be entered, usually with the use of a balloon-guided catheter, in all patients with transposition with the possible exception of very small infants with critical hypoxia and those with extremely severe pulmonary stenosis. All newborns with transposition will benefit from balloon atrial septostomy by virtue of the increased mixing of the pulmonary and systemic venous circulations and the decompression of the left atrium that will result. This procedure is usually lifesaving in infants with an intact ventricular septum, in whom it should be performed at the time of the initial catheterization.

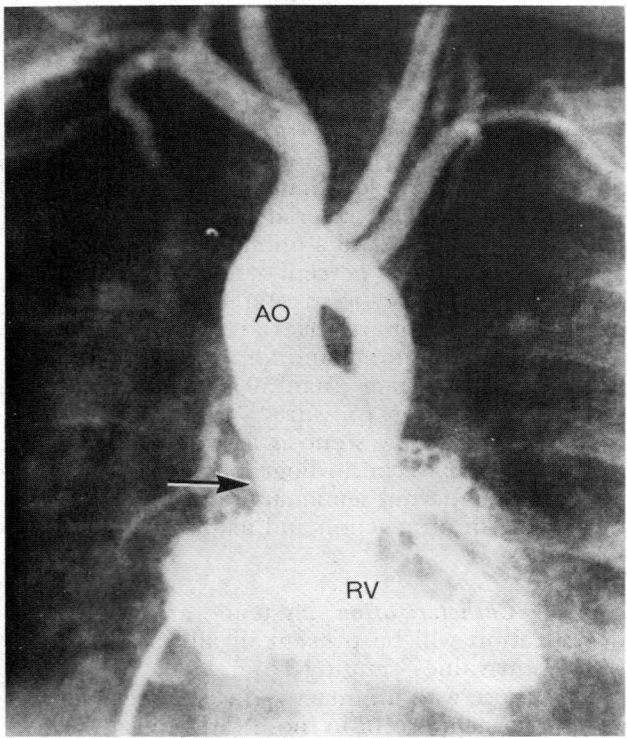
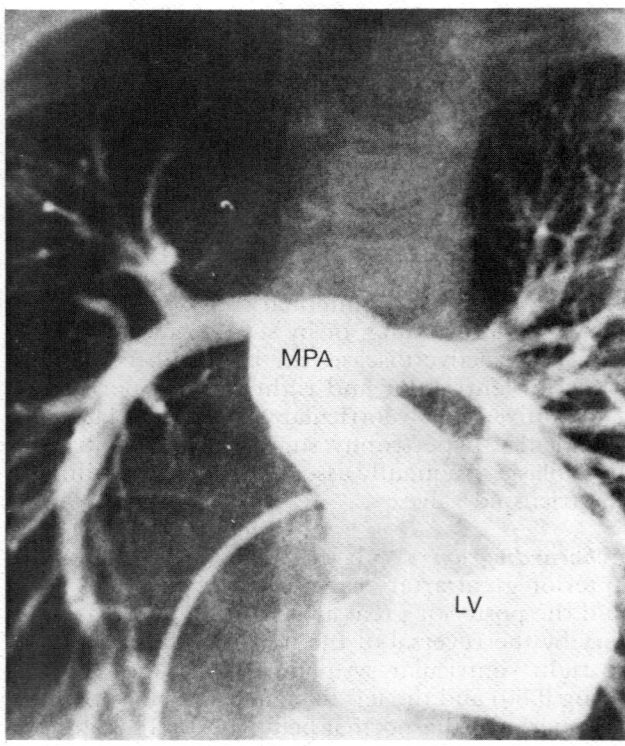

A   **B**

FIGURE 36-133   Posteroanterior views of (*A*) the right ventricular and (*B*) the left ventricular angiograms from a patient with D-transposition of the great arteries and intact ventricular septum. The aorta (AO) arises from the heavily trabeculated right ventricle (RV) above a subaortic conus (arrow). The main pulmonary artery (MPA) arises from the smooth-walled left ventricle (LV).

Natural History and Prognosis

Without balloon septostomy or surgical intervention, 50 percent of infants with transposition will die within the first month and 90 percent within the first year of life. Those with an intact ventricular septum die very early from hypoxia. Those with a large ventricular septal defect usually live somewhat longer, but the majority die in the first months with congestive failure, while the few survivors will have severe pulmonary vascular obstructive disease. Those with a large ventricular septal defect and pulmonary stenosis have the best outlook, but the average life expectancy is barely 5 years even with this combination of defects. With an adequate interatrial opening, whether it be natural, balloon-induced, or surgically created, infants with an intact ventricular septum do relatively well during the first year. Easy fatigue and slow weight gain are common, and mild to moderate cyanosis is present, but congestive failure is seldom troublesome. Continuing significant failure following atrial septal defect creation in patients with documented absence of a ventricular septal defect indicates a complicating lesion, most commonly a persistent ductus. Documented spontaneous closure of small ventricular septal defects occurs in perhaps 10 percent of patients; and subvalvular pulmonary stenosis, usually though not invariably mild, develops in approximately one out of seven patients. Increasing cyanosis during the first year in these patients may be due to a gradual diminution of the size of the atrial septal opening, narrowing or closure of a persistent patent ductus or small ventricular septal defect, the gradual development of subvalvular pulmonary stenosis, or the development of pulmonary vascular obstructive disease. Cerebrovascular accidents are a hazard to these hypoxic infants and occur, almost invariably, in a setting of relative anemia rather than extreme polycythemia below the age of 2 years. The appearance of pulmonary vascular obstructive disease is unusual within the first 12 months of life but is described and becomes more frequent, approaching 10 percent in the second year of life and thereafter.[695] Infants with a large ventricular septal defect and no significant pulmonary stenosis will develop pulmonary vascular obstructive disease and become prohibitive risks for corrective surgery by the end of the first year of life unless the defect has been closed or the pulmonary artery banded. After a banding procedure, these infants usually do well and await total repair as older children. Those with a ventricular septal defect and severe pulmonary stenosis usually become progressively more cyanotic and require systemic to pulmonary artery shunting procedures.

Corrective surgery, whether by the intraatrial techniques of Senning or Mustard or by a variety of other ingenious surgical interventions, has enabled a relatively large group of patients to survive beyond infancy and early childhood. Among some of these survivors will be found residual abnormalities such as pulmonary stenosis or pulmonary vascular obstructive disease as well as complications that are the result of surgery or a consequence of the greater longevity. A small number of patients will develop serious pulmonary venous obstruction following intraatrial repair as a result either of direct encroachment upon the pulmonary veins by the intraatrial baffle or of a pulmonary venous atrium of inadequate size. This complication may be fatal if unrecognized and requires either prompt replacement of the baffle or enlargement of the pulmonary venous atrium. A small number of patients will develop serious systemic venous obstruction by the same mechanisms and will require appropriate corrective surgery. Whether the result of injury to the sinus node or its artery or to interruption of internodal pathways, postoperative arrhythmias, consisting of tachyarrhythmias, sinus node dysfunction with slow junctional escape rhythms, or atrioventricular conduction abnormalities, occur at one time or another in perhaps 40 percent of patients. While the majority of these arrhythmias are not clinically troublesome, late sudden death has been described in about 3 percent of survivors and is very possibly the result of these or related arrhythmias. Finally, right ventricular dysfunction with or without tricuspid regurgitation has been documented in many of the somewhat older survivors and raises the question of whether the right ventricle can function adequately as the systemic arterial ventricle beyond adolescence and early adult life.

Medical Management
Among patients with an intact ventricular septum, the first step is to establish an adequate interatrial opening. Balloon septostomy should be performed without delay. The adequacy of this opening can be determined by a sustained increase in the systemic arterial oxygen saturation above 60 percent or P_{O_2} above 30 torr, or by direct visualization with two-dimensional echocardiography. If the relief of hypoxia is unsatisfactory and the interatrial opening is judged by echocardiography to be small, we recommend surgical atrial septectomy without delay. Another alternative would be to proceed directly with corrective surgery, although the risk of the Mustard or Senning procedure appears to be significantly greater under the age of 4 months than beyond that age.[3] If the response to balloon septostomy is unsatisfactory, but the size of the interatrial opening is judged by echocardiography to be adequate, a trial of intravenous prostaglandin E_1 is recommended.[696] If the response is still not adequate, the alternatives would be to create a systemic to pulmonary arterial shunt or to proceed with total correction. In the circumstances of a large, persistent ductus arteriosus, an adequate interatrial opening, judged by echocardiography, should be created and the ductus closed with indomethacin or operation prior to discharge.

Once an adequate atrial septal defect has been created, infants with transposition may be followed during the first year of life with the expectation of corrective surgery at approximately 12 months. Care is taken to prevent anemia or infective endocarditis. Echocardiographic assessment of pulmonary arterial pressure at intervals is recommended. Increasing hypoxia or a suspicion of increasing pulmonary arterial pressure is indicated for prompt recatheterization. Even if the course is uncomplicated, our preference has been to recatheterize these infants electively at 10 or 11 months of age and to proceed with elective surgical repair using the Mustard technique at about 12 months of age. Ambulatory electrocardiographic monitoring is performed preoperatively and at intervals postoperatively in order to detect arrhythmias. Careful observation for development of pulmonary venous or systemic venous obstruction in the weeks and months following corrective surgery is important as are the continued precautions against infective endocarditis. Whether or not digitalis should be continued indefinitely in view of the possibility of existing or potential right ventricular dysfunction is unknown, but we have a low threshold for its use. Postoperative catheterization a year or two following corrective surgery is appropriate to assess pressure gradients, residual intracardiac shunting, pulmonary vascular resistence, and ventricular function.

Infants with transposition, a large ventricular septal defect, and pulmonary arterial hypertension should either be repaired or undergo banding of the pulmonary artery within the first 4 to 6 months of life if severe pulmonary vascular obstructive disease is to be prevented. Our preference has been pulmonary arterial banding because of the high mortality associated to date with correction of this group during infancy. Those patients with ventricular septal defects and severe pulmonary stenosis do well with shunting procedures. Children with banding or shunting procedures will require correction at an older age but may benefit from the increased medical and surgical experience that will be available at that time. Finally, the severe hypoxia present in those children with a large ventricular septal defect and severe pulmonary vascular obstructive disease may be reduced, in selected patients, by the Mustard procedure performed as a palliative procedure with no attempt at closure of the ventricular septal defect.

Surgical Management
Infants with transposition of the great arteries are managed during initial cardiac catheterization by balloon atrioseptostomy[697] to improve interatrial mixing of systemic venous and pulmonary venous blood. Improvement in systemic oxygen saturation is immediate and dramatic but often temporary. In-

fants failing to maintain a systemic P_{O_2} of greater than 30 mmHg in room air undergo surgical excision of the interatrial septum by the technique of Blalock and Hanlon[698] or during a brief period of inflow occlusion[699] Persistence of severe hypoxia in the presence of an adequate interatrial communication is usually due to left ventricular outflow tract obstruction or elevated pulmonary vascular resistance and may demand the creation of a small systemic arterial to pulmonary arterial shunt.[700] We prefer a Blalock-Taussig subclavian arterial to pulmonary arterial anastomosis, but the Waterston ascending aortic to right pulmonary arterial window or a central shunt using a Gore-Tex graft from the ascending aorta to the main pulmonary artery is used occasionally.

A significant patent ductus arteriosus is ligated to control congestive heart failure and minimize the development of pulmonary vascular obstructive disease, provided an adequate interatrial communication exists. Severe congestive heart failure in an infant with transposition of the great arteries and a ventricular septal defect may require palliative reduction in pulmonary blood flow by banding the main pulmonary artery or by early correction.[700]

Attrition and morbidity between palliation and planned correction, complications of correction induced by palliation, and improvements in corrective cardiac surgery during the first year of life have prompted some centers to advocate primary correction rather than surgical palliation in most cases of transposition, regardless of age.[701]

Correction of transposition of the great arteries requires transposition of systemic venous and pulmonary venous return at the atrial level utilizing methods proposed by Albert,[702] first performed successfully by Senning,[703] and modified by Mustard,[704] Brom,[705] and others.[706,707] Anatomic correction—translocation of the aorta and pulmonary artery with reimplantation of the coronary arteries—was performed successfully by Jatene[708] and is being evaluated by a few centers in selected patients. The current high mortality for this otherwise physiologically appealing operation discourages its widespread application.

The commonly used Mustard and Senning operations are usually performed when the child is 6 to 12 months old or earlier if the clinical course dictates. Both procedures divert systemic venous blood to the mitral valve, left ventricle, and pulmonary artery, while pulmonary venous blood is directed to the tricuspid valve, right ventricle, and aorta (Figs. 36-134 and 36-135). Operation is carried out through a median sternotomy during total circulatory arrest with profound hypothermia (18 to 20°C) in infants. Total cardiopulmonary bypass with venous drainage directly from each vena cava using special right-angle cannulas facilitates operation in larger children and when more operating time is required for the correction of associated defects, including left ventricular outflow tract obstruction or a ventricular septal defect.

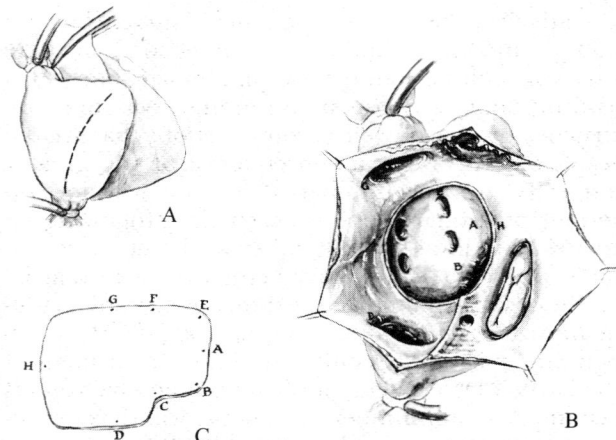

FIGURE 36-134   Interatrial transposition of venous return. *A.* The incision in right atrium is made so as to minimize damage to internuncial bundles. *B.* The atrial septum is excised. *C.* A patch of knitted Dacron is trimmed. [*From J. W. Kirklin, Surgery for Transposition of the Great Arteries and Other Types of Malpositions of the Great Arteries, in B. G. Barratt-Boyes (ed.), "Heart Disease in Infancy: Diagnosis and Surgical Treatment," Churchill Livingstone, Edinburgh, 1973. Reproduced with permission.*]

FIGURE 36-135   *A, B,* and *C.* The patch is sutured into place so as to divert systemic venous return to the mitral valve. Pulmonary and coronary venous blood pass to the tricuspid valve. [*From J. W. Kirklin, Surgery for Transposition of the Great Arteries and Other Types of Malpositions of the Great Arteries, in B. G. Barratt-Boyes (ed.), "Heart Disease in Infancy: Diagnosis and Surgical Treatment," Churchill Livingstone, Edinburgh, 1973. Reproduced with permission.*]

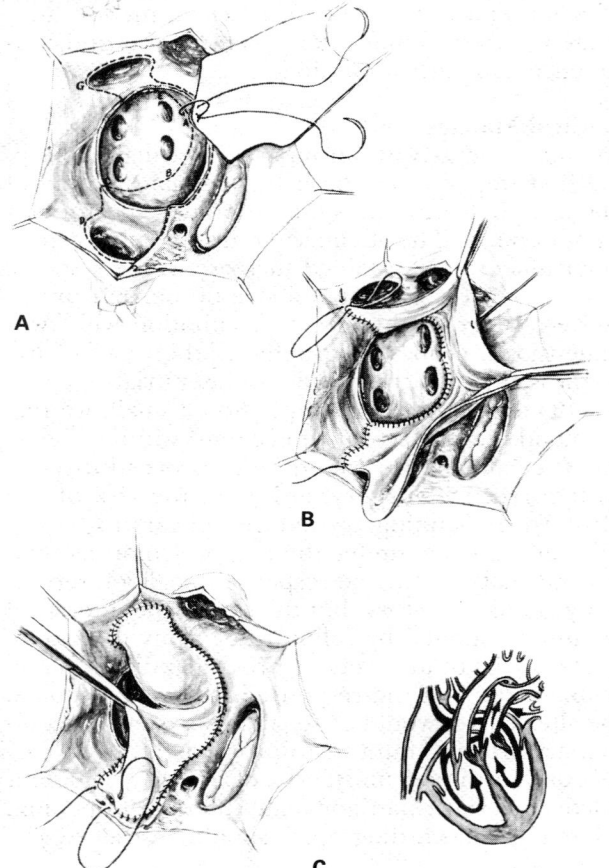

Mustard's operation employs a trouser-shaped baffle of pericardium, Dacron, or Teflon. Complications of systemic venous and pulmonary venous obstruction,[709,710] usually occurring several months after operation, and the relatively high incidence of atrial dysrhythmias and conduction disturbance following Mustard's procedure[711,712] have renewed enthusiasm for a modification of Senning's original intraatrial transposition operation, which uses little or no prosthetic material and preserves atrial tissue (Fig. 36-136).[713] The atrial septum and the lateral right atrial wall are used in the construction of the intraatrial baffle. Available data suggest little difference in the early results of these two operations; long-term comparative assessment is needed. Other late complications—right ventricular failure[714] and tricuspid regurgitation[715]—occur occasionally after both the Mustard and the Senning operations.

Transposition of the great arteries complicated by the presence of a ventricular septal defect requires early surgical intervention to control congestive heart failure and to prevent the rapid progression of pulmonary vascular obstructive disease.[700] These infants are usually treated by transatrial closure of the ventricular septal defect and simultaneous intraatrial venous transposition by either the Mustard or Senning technique.[716,717] Alternatively, palliative pulmonary arterial banding may be followed by correction as proposed by Rastelli and associates[718] for transposition, ventricular septal de-

fect, and pulmonary stenosis. In this complex lesion the ventricular septal defect is closed with a patch which diverts the left ventricular blood through the ventricular septal defect to the aorta; the pulmonary artery is ligated just above the valve and right ventricular blood is diverted to the distal pulmonary artery through an extracardiac conduit. The ventricular septal defect must occasionally be enlarged surgically along its anterior and cephalad margins to allow unobstructed egress of left ventricular blood.

Lindesmith[719] demonstrated that intraatrial transposition of venous return *without* closure of the ventricular septal defect (the so-called palliative Mustard procedure) often offered remarkable benefit to patients with transposition of the great arteries and ventricular septal defect who had developed otherwise inoperable pulmonary vascular obstructive disease.

Simple valvular, fibrous, or membranous obstruction of the left ventricular outflow tract can usually be relieved by excision through the main pulmonary artery at the time of interatrial transposition of venous return.[700] Severe fibromuscular tunnel obstruction or obstruction related to accessory mitral valve tissue poses technically difficult problems. The likelihood of progression of acquired left ventricular outflow tract obstruction is believed to be reduced by early corrective transposition of venous return.

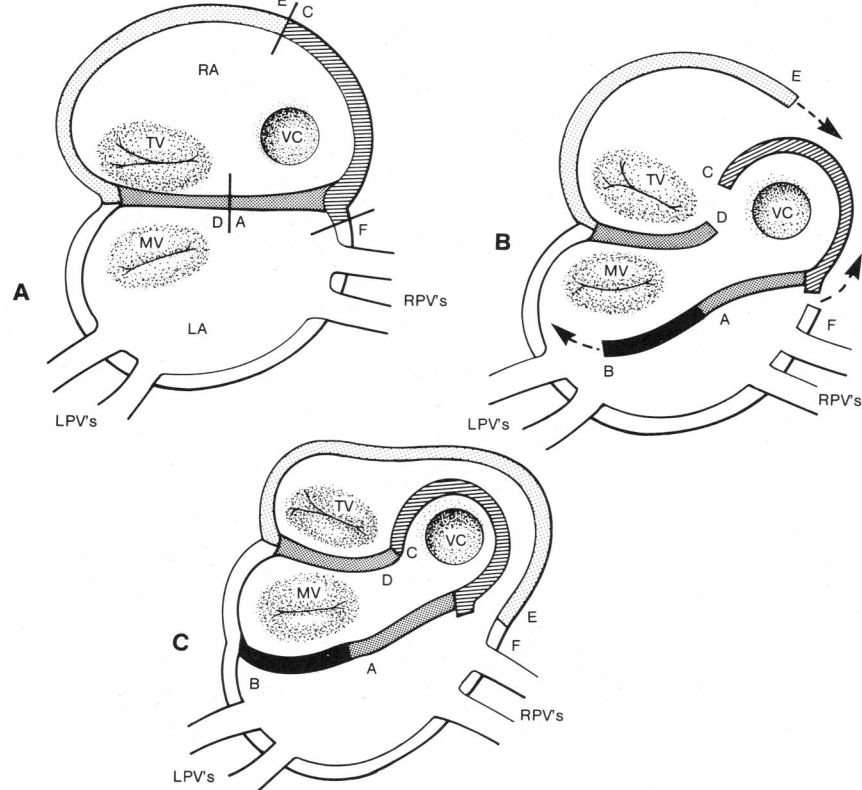

FIGURE 36-136 Senning operation for interatrial transposition of venous return to correct transposition of the great arteries. Incisions in the right atrium (E/C) and left atrium just anterior to the right pulmonary veins (F) combined with detachment of the atrial septum (D/A) allow the creation of an interatrial baffle directing systemic venous blood from the vena cavae (VC) through the mitral valve (MV) while pulmonary venous blood is directed through the tricuspid orifice (TV). The atrial septum is sutured anteriorly and to the left of the left pulmonary veins (B). When deficient, the atrial septum is augmented with a small prosthetic patch (solid dark line). The posterior edge of the right atrial wall is attached to the atrial septum between the mitral and tricuspid orifices (D). Right and left atria are approximated just anterior to the right pulmonary veins (E/F) to create the pulmonary venous atrium. Enlargement of this chamber with a small pericardial patch is occasionally required. In many cases the use of prosthetic material can be avoided entirely, a possible advantage of the Senning operation over the Mustard procedure.

DISEASES OF THE HEART AND BLOOD VESSELS

Double-Outlet Right Ventricle

Definition
Double-outlet right ventricle is characterized by origin of both great arteries from the morphological right ventricle.

Pathology
Situs solitus (S) is usual. In most cases the ventricles display a d-loop (D), and the pulmonary arterial origin is normally positioned, arising from a conus of the right ventricle, while the aorta also arises from the right ventricle above a second conus. The two semilunar valves are at about the same level and there is no fibrous continuity between either the semilunar valve, on one hand, and the mitral valve, on the other (Fig. 36-137).

In most cases the aortic origin is to the right (d-malposition) of the pulmonary arterial origin, the two vessels usually displaying a side-by-side relationship. Unusually, the aortic origin is distinctly anterior to the pulmonary origin. Uncommonly the aorta arises to the left (l-malposition) of the pulmonary artery.[720]

With the exception of unusual cases in which the ventricular septum is intact, there is a ventricular septal defect. The condition may be further subdivided on the basis of the position of the ventricular septal defect with regard to the arterial origins. Among 31 cases with ventricular septal defect, Zamora and associates[721] found the following distribution in position of the defect: (1) subaortic, 15 cases; (2) subpulmonary (synonym, Taussig-Bing

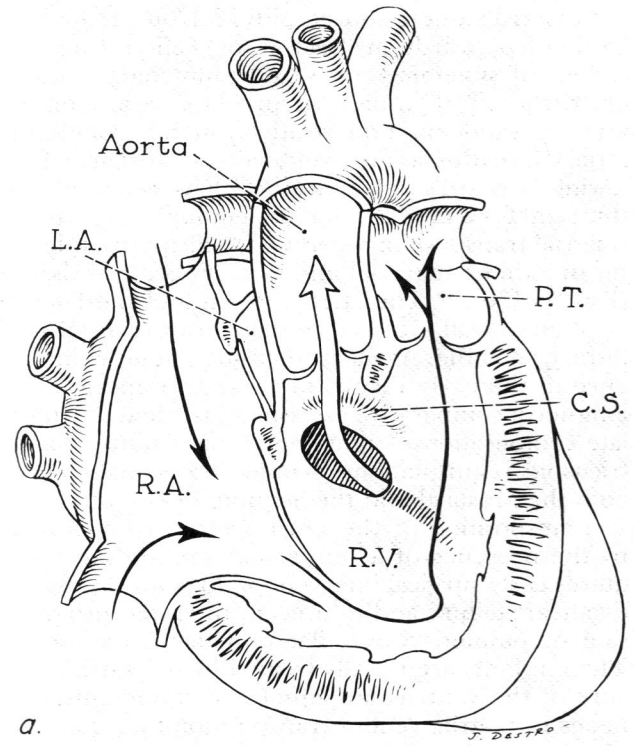

a.

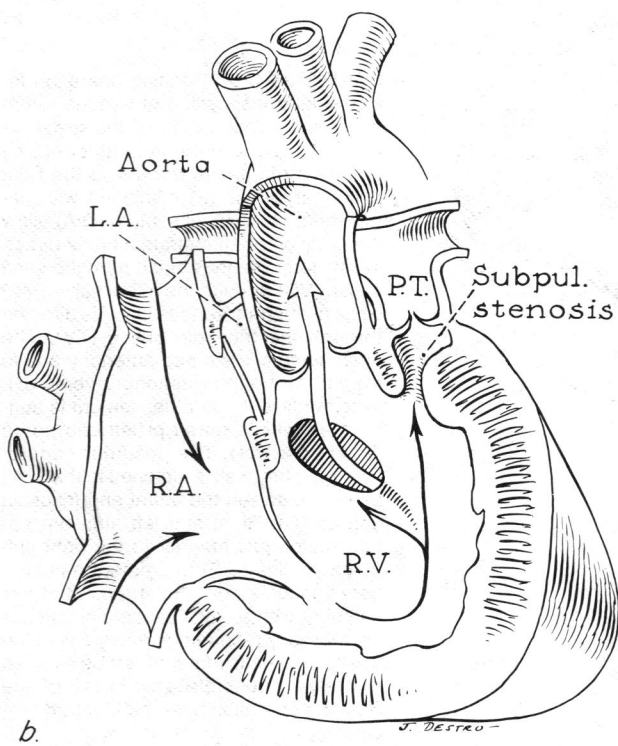

b.

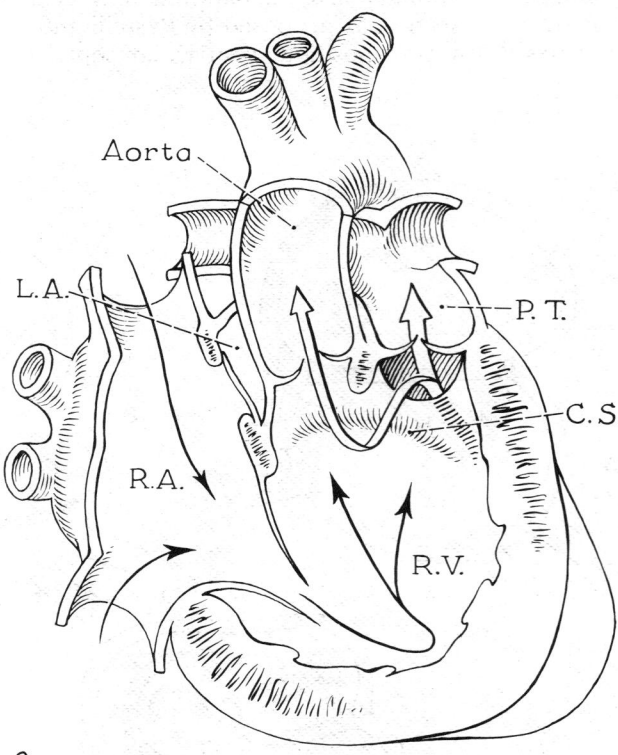

c.

FIGURE 36-137 Double-outlet right ventricle. *a.* Subaortic ventricular septal defect without pulmonary stenosis. *b.* With subaortic ventricular septal defect and subpulmonary stenosis (Subpul. stenosis). *c.* With subpulmonary ventricular septal defect, the so-called Taussig-Bing complex. R.A. = right atrium; R.V. = right ventricle; C.S. = crista suraventricularis; L.A. = left atrium; P.T. = main pulmonary arterial trunk.

heart), 9 cases; (3) subaortic and subpulmonary ("doubly committed" of Lev and associates[722], 4 cases; and (4) remote ("uncommitted" of Lev and associates[722]), 3 cases.

When in situs solitus there is ventricular inversion (atrioventricular discordance) and double-outlet right ventricle, both great vessels arise from the left-sided anatomic right ventricle. From a purely anatomic viewpoint such cases should not be confused with the condition considered in the next section, namely double-outlet left ventricle.

Also, it is to be recognized that double-outlet right ventricle may occur in situs inversus with atrioventricular concordance.

Associated Conditions Pulmonary stenosis occurs in about 20 percent of cases, the condition usually resulting from a narrow subpulmonary conus. Obstruction to systemic flow, either at the subaortic conus or by coarctation of the aorta, may occur in half of the cases. The type with subpulmonary defect has a particular tendency to be associated with coarctation. Obstruction at the mitral valve, including supravalvular ring, parachute mitral valve, and mitral atresia, may be observed in about one-fifth of cases of double-outlet right ventricle.[721] Common atrioventricular canal may be associated.[184]

A rare association is that the mitral valve straddles the ventricular septal defect, leading to a state of "double-inlet–double-outlet right ventricle."[723]

Clinical Manifestations

Double-outlet right ventricle or origin of both great arteries from the right ventricle is a relatively rare malformation, found in only 0.5 percent of patients with congenital heart disease,[6] but is of considerable importance because its clinical and laboratory features frequently resemble those of more common and more easily correctable malformations. The incidence among males and females is equal except in the presence of pulmonary stenosis where two-thirds are male.[3] An association with trisomy 18 has been described. The clinical picture depends almost entirely upon the presence or absence of pulmonary stenosis and the relationship of the ventricular septal defect to the aortic and pulmonary valves. Survival prior to surgical correction depends almost always upon the continued patency of the ventricular septal defect.

History and Physical Examination Patients with a subaortic ventricular septal defect without pulmonary stenosis (Fig. 36-137A) have the findings of patients with a large isolated ventricular septal defect. Congestive failure with tachypnea, dyspnea, and slow weight gain appears within a few weeks of birth. Cyanosis is seldom described. Those with a subaortic ventricular septal defect and pulmonary stenosis (Fig. 36-137B) usually present after the newborn period and follow a course not unlike that of tetralogy of Fallot. Patients with a subpulmonary

defect without pulmonary stenosis (Fig. 36-137C), the Taussig-Bing malformation, resemble patients with transposition of the great arteries and a large ventricular septal defect without pulmonary stenosis. The findings are those of a large ventricular septal defect, severe congestive failure, and impressive cyanosis.

Chest Roentgenogram Cardiomegaly with pulmonary overperfusion are characteristic of all types without pulmonary stenosis. The similarity of double-outlet right ventricle with subaortic ventricular septal defect and pulmonary stenosis to tetralogy of Fallot extends to a 30 percent incidence of right aortic arch, but the cardiac contour is seldom boot-shaped and heart size tends to be somewhat larger than in patients with classic tetralogy of Fallot. With subpulmonary ventricular septal defect without pulmonary stenosis, the pulmonary artery usually lies beside rather than posterior to the aorta and this clearly visible dilated main pulmonary artery may permit distinction from transposition, which this malformation mimics so closely.

Electrocardiogram Right axis deviation and right atrial and right ventricular hypertrophy are characteristic of double-outlet right ventricle. Among patients with subaortic ventricular septal defect without pulmonary stenosis a superior QRS axis is relatively common. Patients with pulmonary stenosis usually have more marked right ventricular and right atrial hypertrophy than do patients with classic tetralogy of Fallot.

Echocardiogram M-mode echocardiography may distinguish double-outlet right ventricle from uncomplicated ventricular septal defect and tetralogy of Fallot[455] by demonstrating a lack of continuity between echoes from the anterior mitral leaflet and those of the posterior margin of the aortic annulus as well as an abrupt anterior displacement of the posterior margin of the aorta. Two-dimensional echocardiography is capable of demonstrating the commitment of both great arteries to the right ventricle as well as mitral-semilunar discontinuity (Fig. 36-138).[552]

Cardiac Catheterization There will be an increase in oxygen saturation at the right ventricular level. The pulmonary arterial saturation usually is slightly lower than that of the aorta in patients with a subaortic ventricular septal defect and invariably higher than the aortic in those with a subpulmonary septal defect. Aortic and right ventricular and left ventricular systolic pressures usually are equal, but the left ventricular systolic pressure may be higher than the right if the ventricular septal defect is small and restrictive.[724] Simultaneous left ventricular and systemic arterial pressures should be recorded to evaluate this possibility. The possibility of mitral valve atresia, stenosis, or straddling of the ventricular sep-

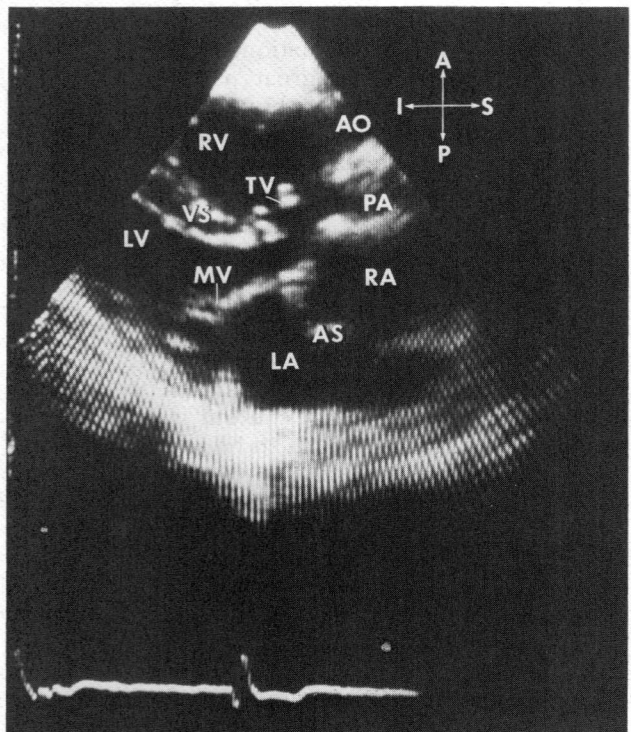

FIGURE 36-138 Two-dimensional echocardiogram in the parasternal, long-axis view from a patient with double-outlet ventricle and ventricular septal defect. The aorta (AO) and pulmonary artery (PA) both arise from the right ventricle (RV) in a parallel orientation anterior to the ventricular septum (VS). There is no continuity between the posterior aortic wall and the mitral valve (MV). A = anterior; I = inferior; S = superior; P = posterior; TV = tricuspid valve; LV = left ventricle; RA = right atrium; LA = left atrium; AS = atrial septum. (*From D. J. Hagler, A. J. Tajik, J. B. Seward, D. D. Mair, and D. C. Ritter, Double-Outlet Right Ventricle: Wide-Angle Two-Dimensional Echocardiographic Observations, Circulation, 63:419, 1981. Reproduced with permission of author and publisher.*)

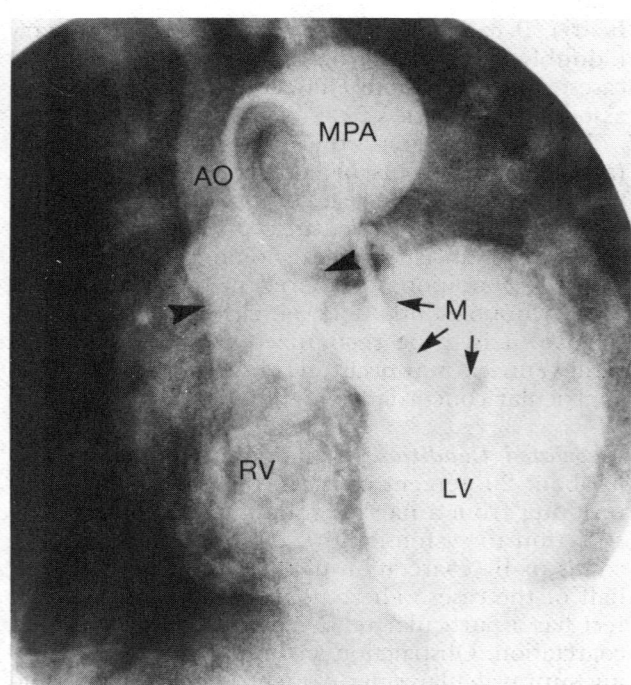

FIGURE 36-139 Left anterior oblique view of left ventricular angiogram from a child with double-outlet right ventricle and ventricular septal defect. The ascending aorta (AO), right ventricle (RV), and main pulmonary artery (MPA) fill from the left ventricle (LV) via a large, high ventricular septal defect. The aortic valve (dark arrowheads) is displaced superiorly and anteriorly with a resulting lack of continuity between the aortic valve and the mitral valve (M). Arrows = mitral valve annulus.

tum should be investigated and the presence or absence of pulmonary or aortic stenosis determined. Selective right and left ventricular biplane angiography is recommended to determine the size of the ventricular septal defect and its relationship to the great arteries. In most instances angiography will demonstrate the presence of conal tissue beneath both semilunar valves with displacement of the aortic valve anteriorly and superiorly to the level of the pulmonary valve. In the most common situation both great arteries lie side by side, as seen from the lateral view, with the aorta to the right of the pulmonary artery. Less frequently the aorta will be slightly anterior and either to the right (d-malposition) or to the left (l-malposition) of the pulmonary artery. Lack of mitral aortic continuity can be seen in the lateral view (Fig. 36-139). An aortogram is recommended to exclude anomalies of the coronary arterial distribution that might interfere with the surgical approach to the subvalvular pulmonary stenosis.

Natural History and Prognosis

The clinical course of each variety of double-outlet right ventricle is determined by the associated defects. Without surgical intervention, those with an unguarded pulmonary artery either die in infancy with congestive failure or develop pulmonary vascular obstructive disease. Amelioration of signs and symptoms due to spontaneous narrowing of a large ventricular septal defect is not an option open to these patients, unfortunately, and is one of several reasons why early recognition and distinction of this malformation from uncomplicated ventricular septal defect is essential. Spontaneous narrowing or closure of the ventricular septal defect may indeed occur and is life-threatening. Increasing dyspnea, increasing intensity of the systolic murmur, and progressive left ventricular hypertrophy in the electrocardiogram suggest this complication. Patients with pulmonary stenosis tend to have progressive obstruction and cyanosis.

Medical Management

The majority of patients with double-outlet right ventricle are correctable surgically. Until recently it has been our recommendation to band the pulmonary artery of all infants with double-outlet right ventricle with increased pulmonary blood flow and significant pulmonary arterial hypertension. Selected infants with these findings and a subaortic ventricular septal defect are probably best managed today by total correction between the age of 3 and 12 months. For those infants with Taussig-Bing malformation or subpulmonary ventricular septal defect we still prefer a combination of pulmonary arterial banding, atrial septal defect creation, and a Blalock-Taussig shunt. Corrective surgery for this group is postponed until the age of 5 or 6 years. Systemic to pulmonary arterial shunts are performed in those patients with cyanosis and diminished pulmonary blood flow, with correction postponed until the patient is large enough to accept, if necessary, an external valved conduit. All patients, corrected or uncorrected, in whom the left ventricular output must pass through the ventricular septal defect should be observed continuously for the possibility of spontaneous narrowing and obstruction at that site.

Surgical Management

Although many variations exist in the anatomic spectrum of which double-outlet right ventricle is a part, the surgeon is confronted with four basic problems: (1) closure of the ventricular septal defect (in most cases), (2) relief of pulmonary stenosis (in about 20 percent), (3) routing of pulmonary venous blood to the aorta, and (4) diversion of vena caval blood to the pulmonary artery.[725]

The relative challenges posed by these four problems depend primarily upon the anatomic relationships to each other of the aorta, the pulmonary artery, and the ventricular septal defect. When the ventricular septal defect is near and below the aortic valve, a Dacron semiconduit or tunnel-shaped patch can be placed to obliterate the interventricular communication while diverting the left ventricular blood through the ventricular septal defect to the aorta.

In cases where the ventricular septal defect is committed to the pulmonary artery, consideration should still be given to the establishment of correct intracardiac ventriculoatrial continuity using an intracardiac tunnel in order to preserve the systemic work potential of the left ventricle (Fig. 36-140). When this is not possible, it is necessary to place a patch diverting left ventricular blood through the ventricular septal defect into the pulmonary artery. The "transposition" thus created is then corrected by intraatrial transposition of venous return by the Mustard or Senning technique (see discussion of transposition of the great arteries).

When double-outlet right ventricle occurs in the presence of ventricular inversion (atrioventricular discordance), a modification of the techniques of Rastelli and associates is preferred.[726] The ventricular septal defect is closed with a patch placed to the right of both the aortic and pulmonary valves; the pulmonary artery is divided just above the valve; systemic venous blood is diverted to the distal pulmonary artery through an extracardiac conduit from the right-sided ventricle. Earlier attempts at totally intracardiac repair of double-outlet right ventricle with atrioventricular discordance resulted in a moderate mortality, frequent heart block, and inadequate relief of pulmonary stenosis.[727]

Pulmonary stenosis associated with double-outlet right ventricle is corrected by a valvotomy and placement of the usual transannular patch, if required. When demanded by the position of the pulmonary outflow tract or the presence of an abnormal coronary artery, an extracardiac conduit is placed between the systemic venous ventricle and the pulmonary artery.[728]

Because of the relative complexity of intracardiac repair of some forms of double-outlet right ventricle, palliation in infancy plays a greater role than for simple ventricular septal defect or tetralogy of Fallot. Congestive heart failure and the develop-

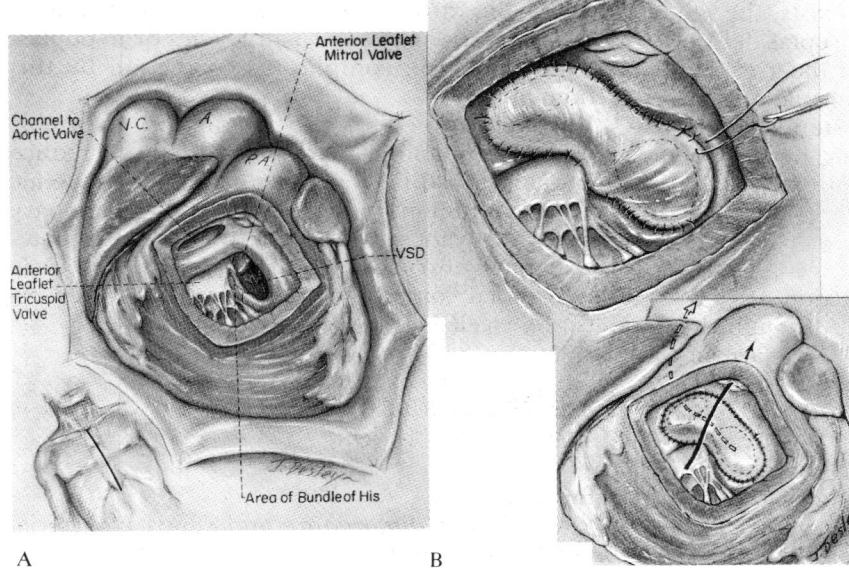

FIGURE 36-140 *A.* The anatomy of double-outlet right ventricle with subaortic ventricular septal defect as viewed through the right ventriculotomy incision. Note that there is no continuity between atrioventricular valves and semilunar valves and that the ventricular septal defect is more in relation to the aortic valve than to the pulmonary valve. *B.* The patch has been sutured into place so as to close the interventricular communication and to conduct blood from the ventricular septal defect to the aorta. (*From J. W. Kirklin, R. A. Karp, and D. C. McGoon, Surgical Treatment of Origin of Both Vessels from Right Ventricle, Including Cases with Pulmonary Stenosis, J. Thorac. Cardiovasc. Surg., 48:1026, 1964. Reproduced with permission.*)

A   B

ment of pulmonary vascular obstructive disease can be controlled by pulmonary arterial banding. Hypoxia and its complications are managed by the creation of a systemic arterial to pulmonary arterial anastomosis when possible.

Recent results of total correction for patients with relatively uncomplicated double-outlet right ventricle are very encouraging,[729,730] but mortality remains high for those requiring a transannular patch to relieve pulmonary stenosis, those having an uncommitted ventricular septal defect, and those with Taussig-Bing anomaly. Mortality is high, of course, in patients having significant pulmonary vascular obstructive disease, a complication which might now be avoided by earlier total correction.

Double-Outlet Left Ventricle

Pathology

When both great vessels arise from the left-sided ventricle, the usual situations are either situs inversus with double-outlet right ventricle or situs solitus with isolated ventricular inversion.

Rarely in instances with atrioventricular concordance the two arteries arise from the morphological left ventricle (Fig. 36-141). The aorta may lie either to the left or the right of the pulmonary artery.

Among the few cases reported, a ventricular septal defect and pulmonary stenosis are usually associated.[731] In the case of Paul and associates[732] the ventricular septum was intact.

Clinical Manifestations

The clinical manifestations of this extremely rare anomaly are similar to those of tricuspid atresia, tetralogy of Fallot, or transposition of the great arteries with ventricular septal defect. Most patients, then, are cyanotic.[783] The diagnosis in each case depends upon high-quality selective biplane angiography with special attention paid to the location of the ventricular septal defect, if such exists, the relationship of the great arteries to the septal defect, and the interrelationship and origin of the great arteries themselves. Tricuspid valve abnormalities, including Ebstein's anomaly, atresia, stenosis, and straddling, are common as are varying degrees of right ventricular hypoplasia.[9] This malformation is correctable in some patients.[733]

Surgical Management

Reported experience with total correction of double-outlet left ventricle is small.[733–735] Although the first successful repair of this anomaly was accomplished by Sakakibara[736] in 1964 using an intraventricular baffle to direct right ventricular blood through the ventricular septal defect to the pulmonary artery, this approach has limited anatomic applicability.[733,734] A more generally useful and simpler approach includes (1) closure of the ventricular septal defect through a right ventriculotomy, leav-

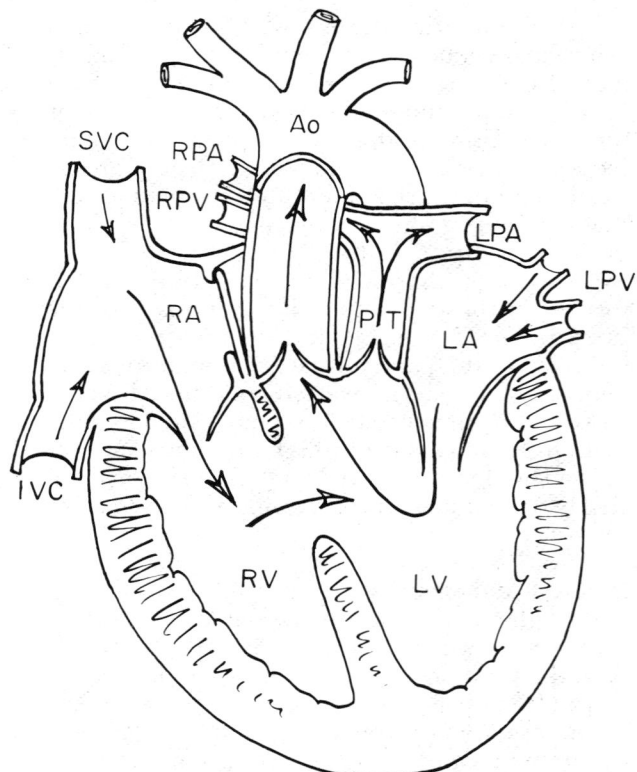

FIGURE 36-141 Double-outlet left ventricle. A ventricular septal defect is associated. SVC = superior vena cava; IVC = inferior vena cava; RA = right atrium; RV = right ventricle; Ao = aorta; PT = main pulmonary arterial trunk; RPA = right pulmonary artery; LPA = left pulmonary artery; RPV = right pulmonary vein; LPV = left pulmonary vein; LA = left atrium; LV = left ventricle.

ing orifices of both great vessels on the left side of the patch, (2) closure of the pulmonary valve orifice or ligation of the proximal main pulmonary artery, and (3) establishment of pulmonary blood flow from right ventricle to distal main pulmonary artery through an extracardiac conduit.[734] The presence of associated tricuspid valve anomalies or hypoplastic right ventricle complicates correction by this technique.

When required in the infant, palliation is achieved by pulmonary arterial banding to reduce pulmonary blood flow or the creation of a systemic arterial to pulmonary arterial shunt if pulmonary stenosis and cyanosis are severe. When an adequate-sized right ventricle and pulmonary arteries are present, total correction is preferred; reported results are excellent.

Corrected Transposition of the Great Arteries

Definition

Atrioventricular discordance and ventriculoarterial discordance form the characteristics of corrected transposition (it should not be confused with anatomically corrected malposition).

Pathology

Usually situs solitus is present (S), while the ventricles are inverted showing an l-loop (L). The great vessels are transposed and in the l-position so that the pulmonary artery arises from the right-sided morphological left ventricle and the anteriorly l-transposed aorta arises from the left-sided right ventricle yielding an SLL pattern (Fig. 36-142). Along with the ventricular inversion there is atrioventricular valve inversion. The mitral valve is on the right and shows fibrous continuity with the pulmonary valve, while the tricuspid valve is on the left.[737]

The aortic arch is left-sided. The anterior of the three aortic sinuses is the noncoronary one, while the two coronary arteries arise from the right and left (posteriorly positioned) sinuses. The courses of the arteries are inverted so that the right-sided artery gives rise to the anterior descending and circumflex arteries. The left-sided coronary artery courses in the left atrioventricular sulcus and ter-

FIGURE 36-142 Corrected transposition with ventricular septal defect. "RV" and "LV" represent the right-sided and left-sided ventricles, respectively. Anatomically, "RV" is the morphological left ventricle, and "LV" is the morphological right ventricle. SVC = superior vena cava; IVC = inferior vena cava; RA = right atrium; PT = main pulmonary arterial trunk; RPA = right pulmonary artery; LPA = left pulmonary artery; RPV = right pulmonary vein; LPV = left pulmonary vein; LA = left atrium; Ao = aorta.

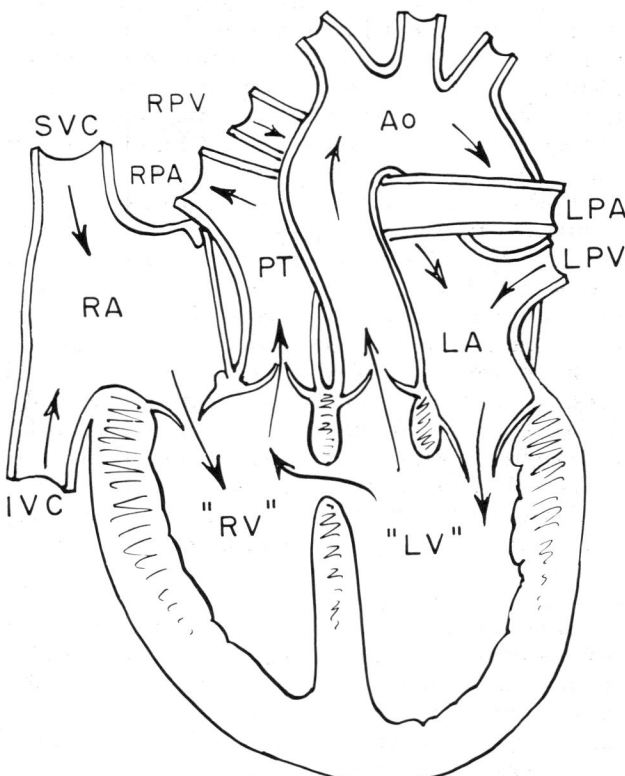

minates as the posterior descending artery. The cardiac apex points to the right in about 25 percent of cases and in some is not committed to either side.

Associated Conditions In a rare case no associated conditions are present and the circulation is normal. In the majority of cases (over 60 percent) a ventricular septal defect is present. Two types of ventricular septal defect have been described,[738] one that lies beneath both semilunar valves and the other lying beneath the pulmonary valve but remote from the aortic valve, the latter being essentially in an inverted position from the common paramembranous isolated ventricular septal defect.

In about half the cases, whether or not a septal defect is present, the inverted left-sided tricuspid valve shows some degree of an Ebstein-like malformation and may be incompetent.[739]

Pulmonary atresia or stenosis, the latter at times with an intact ventricular septum, is seen in about 10 percent of cases. The obstruction is usually subvalvular, being a mirror image of membranous subaortic stenosis or resulting from accessory tissue of the anterior mitral leaflet that projects into and obstructs the outlet of the right-sided anatomic left ventricle.[740]

Uncommonly, situs inversus is present giving a segmental pattern of IDD.

Abnormal Physiology[741]

In an individual with uncomplicated corrected transposition of the great arteries, the circulation could be considered normal since the pulmonary and systemic circulation are in series. On the other hand, more than 95 percent of these patients do have associated abnormalities, including large ventricular septal defect or single ventricle, pulmonary stenosis, left atrioventricular valve regurgitation, paroxysmal atrial tachycardia, and varying degrees of atrioventricular heart block. In 85 to 90 percent of cases, there is either a ventricular septal defect or a single ventricle with a left-to-right shunt, which is reflected by a large step-up in oxygen content as soon as the catheter enters the venous ventricle. The saturation of systemic arterial blood, however, is higher than or at least equal to the saturation of blood from the pulmonary artery. The pressures in the venous ventricle and the pulmonary artery are usually elevated to systemic levels. If either valvular or subvalvular pulmonary stenosis is present, however, the pressure in the pulmonary artery will be low. If there is left atrioventricular regurgitation, the pulmonary capillary wedge pressure or the left atrial pressure may be elevated with a large regurgitant R wave. Angiography demonstrates the position of the great arteries, the heart valves, the basket-weave pattern of the anatomic right ventricle, and the smooth surface of the anatomic left ventricle.

Clinical Manifestations

This is an uncommon malformation occurring in slightly less than 1 percent of children with congenital heart disease. Males are slightly more commonly affected than females in a ratio of 1.4:1.[6] The importance of this anomaly lies in its frequent association with serious atrioventricular conduction disturbances and intracardiac malformations, and the medical and surgical implications of the ventricular inversion. The clinical picture is determined primarily by the associated anomalies. About 15 percent will have either second-degree or third-degree atrioventricular block, and almost one-quarter of patients will have clinically detectable left-sided atrioventricular valve regurgitation. Fully 80 percent of patients will have a ventricular septal defect, and of these almost half will have associated pulmonary stenosis.[741] The clinical manifestations described below will pertain to those patients with left atrioventricular valve regurgitation or atrioventricular block, ventricular septal defect without pulmonary stenosis, and ventricular septal defect with significant pulmonary stenosis.

History A slow, irregular heart rate, often detected in utero, may lead to the diagnosis of second- or third-degree atrioventricular block, and about 10 percent of patients with congenital complete block will prove to have corrected transposition. Those patients with a large ventricular septal defect without pulmonary stenosis usually present within the first month or so of life with symptoms of dyspnea, difficulty feeding, frequent and severe lower respiratory tract infections, and slow weight gain, which is a course indistinguishable from that of infants with a large septal defect without ventricular inversion. Patients with ventricular septal defect and pulmonary stenosis generally present with symptoms of cyanosis and resemble patients with tetralogy of Fallot.

Physical Examination The murmur of left atrioventricular valve regurgitation may be best heard either at the apex or lower left sternal border and is described as not radiating as well to the axilla as the murmur of rheumatic mitral regurgitation. Occasionally an inordinately accentuated second heart sound at the upper left sternal border will suggest the presence of pulmonary arterial hypertension, although in reality it represents the sound of aortic valve closure augmented to auscultation by the anterior and superior displacement of the aorta. The second heart sound frequently is very soft or inaudible along the right sternal border. Dyspnea, a hyperdynamic precordium, a pansystolic ventricular septal defect murmur, and an apical middiastolic rumble are characteristic of the patient with a large ventricular septal defect. Those with a ventricular septal defect and associated pulmonary stenosis have the physical findings of tetralogy of Fallot, although an accentuated second heart sound at the

upper left sternal border would be an unexpected finding with tetralogy. In a few patients the murmur of pulmonary stenosis may be louder to the right of the sternum than to the left.

Chest Roentgenogram The usual, slightly convex shadow of the ascending aorta along the upper right border of the heart will be absent. The right pulmonary artery, angled upward slightly and emerging at the same level as the left pulmonary artery, may create a "water fall" appearance as it curves inferiorly. The main pulmonary artery will not be a part of the left cardiac contour and may, if enlarged, indent the left margin of the esophagus in its more centrally located position. Similarly, among those patients with increased pulmonary blood flow, pulmonary arterial hypertension, or both, in whom dilatation of the main and left pulmonary arteries would be expected, the absence of this characteristic enlargement as the usual location should suggest the possibility of a displaced main pulmonary artery. A straight or gently curved convex upper left heart border, representing the contour of the transposed ascending aorta, is characteristic and is seen most frequently in those patients with a ventricular septal defect and pulmonary stenosis, in whom there is a mild dilatation of the ascending aorta.

Electrocardiogram Varying degrees of atrioventricular conduction delay are present in almost a third of patients, with half of these having second- or third-degree block. The initial forces of ventricular depolarization are oriented anteriorly and to the left rather than anteriorly and to the right as in the normal patient with noninversion of the ventricles. This is well demonstrated in the horizontal plane loop of the vectorcardiogram but is reflected in the scalar electrocardiogram by Q waves being present in the right precordial leads and absent in leads I, V_5, and V_6. In the presence of volume overloading of the arterial ventricle, with either left atrioventricular valve regurgitation or a large ventricular septal defect, absence of left precordial Q waves should raise the suspicion of corrected transposition. Absence of left precordial Q waves is not invariable among patients with corrected transposition, however.[741] With normal or near normal pressure in the systemic venous or morphologically left ventricle, a QS pattern in the right and an RS pattern in the left precordial leads is usual. Similarly upright T waves in the right precordial leads and somewhat flattened T waves in the left are a frequent pattern among patients with corrected transposition.

Echocardiogram With the M-mode technique, it may be difficult or impossible to record ventricular septal echoes since the long axis of the septum lies nearly perpendicular to the anterior chest wall and parallel to the transducer beam. The left superior and anterior semilunar valve and the right posterior semilunar valve can be identified as the aortic and pulmonary valves, respectively, by analysis of the systolic time intervals. Absence of continuity between the left atrioventricular valve and a semilunar valve with continuity between the right atrioventricular valve and the posterior semilunar valve is characteristic of ventricular inversion.[455] Two-dimensional echocardiography permits demonstration of the characteristic morphology of the right and left ventricles, and identification of the aorta and pulmonary artery. The most helpful feature in identifying the right ventricle is the more caudal attachment of the tricuspid valve than that of the mitral valve to the interventricular septum.[677]

Cardiac Catheterization From the right atrium the morphologically left ventricle is entered, and, in the presence of a ventricular septal defect, the catheter may cross the defect, traverse the morphologically right ventricle, and enter the ascending aorta in the position normally occupied by the pulmonary artery in patients with normally related great arteries. Entry into the medially placed pulmonary artery may be much more difficult, but the use of flow-guided catheters will permit successful entry and measurement of the pulmonary arterial and pulmonary arterial wedge pressures in most instances. Selective angiography in the right-sided morphologically left ventricle will reveal the characteristic "sock" shape and smooth walls as well as the medially placed main pulmonary artery with its almost symmetrical right and left branches. Angiography in the left-sided morphologically right ventricle, best accomplished by the retrograde approach, permits assessment of

chamber size and competency of the left atrioventricular valve. The ventricular septum usually lies in a plane almost perpendicular to the frontal plane, and the presence, size, and location of a ventricular septal defect may be seen best in the frontal view (Fig. 36-143). Gentle manipulation of the catheter within the heart is indicated since the production of varying degrees of transient atrioventricular block is not uncommon. In a rare instance, block induced at catheterization may prove permanent in patients with this malformation.

Natural History and Prognosis

The clinical course is determined primarily by the severity of the associated defects. It is estimated that only about 1 percent of individuals with corrected transposition have an otherwise normal heart. Even with complicating anomalies survival to adulthood is possible, with one-quarter of the patients in a large clinical series being over 16 years of age.[741] Congestive heart failure associated with a large ventricular septal defect has been the most common cause of death, with most fatalities occurring within the first year of life. Atrioventricular conduction abnormalities tend to be progressive and complete atrioventricular block may appear for the first time in the older child, adolescent, or adult. Similarly left atrioventricular valve regurgitation may present at any age, but in the majority this is detected in infancy and early childhood. Even without associated malformations, or following correction of these abnormalities, the question remains as to whether the morphologically right ventricle is capable of sustaining adequate cardiac output over a normal life span.

FIGURE 36-143   Posteroanterior view of (*A*) the left ventricular (LV) and (*B*) the right ventricular (RV) angiograms in a child with corrected transposition of the great arteries. The main pulmonary artery (MPA) arises from the smooth-walled LV, which receives the systemic venous blood. The ascending aorta (AO) arises to the left of the pulmonary artery from the more heavily trabeculated RV, which receives the pulmonary venous blood. The ventricular septum, seen here perpendicular to the frontal plane, is intact.

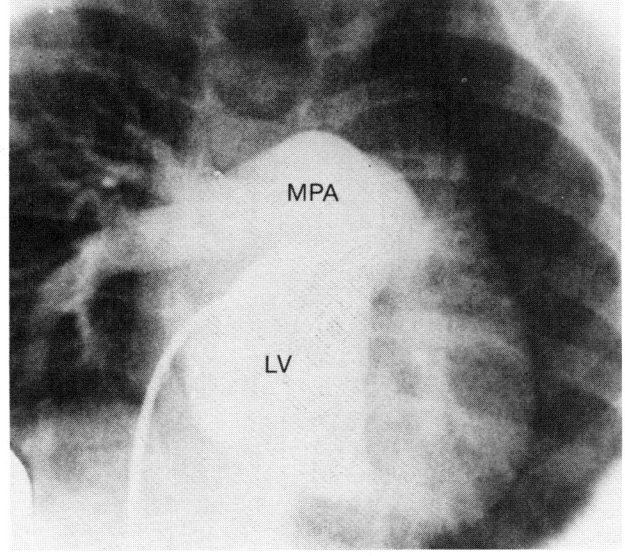

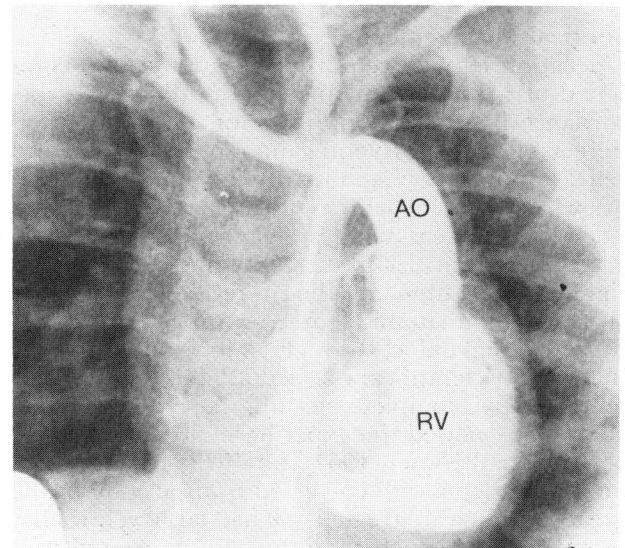

A   **B**

Medical Management

This includes the treatment of congestive failure and the prevention of infective endocarditis. Patients with large ventricular septal defects and severe pulmonary hypertension or congestive heart failure should undergo early banding of the pulmonary artery or repair of the defect. Similarly those patients with a ventricular septal defect, severe pulmonary stenosis, and cyanosis will benefit from systemic to pulmonary artery shunting procedures or total correction. The vulnerability of the ventricular conduction system, and the difficulty in visualization of the septal defect and the subpulmonary region of the morphologically left ventricle, have influenced us to recommend the palliative approach in both groups of patients, especially during infancy. The incidence of complete atrioventricular block has been reduced substantially, although not eliminated, with intraoperative mapping of the conduction system which arises from an anterior atrial node, crosses anterior to the pulmonary artery, and descends along the anterior and superior aspect of the ventricular septal defect in patients with situs solitus. Surgical correction of somewhat older children can now be accomplished with a mortality of somewhere between 10 and 15 percent in centers with a particular interest and experience with this malformation.[676] Patients with complete atrioventricular block induced surgically should be managed, without exception, by the insertion of a permanent pacemaker. Those with congenital block may require pacemaker therapy if symptomatic. Patients symptomatic with left atrioventricular valve regurgitation will require valve replacement. Regularly scheduled follow-up examinations are recommended for all patients with corrected transposition of the great arteries, with or without associated anomalies, in order to detect progressive atrioventricular conduction disorders and the late appearance of left ventricular valve incompetence.

Surgical Management

Operation may be required in patients with combined atrioventricular and ventriculoarterial discordance for correction of one or more associated defects. Closure of ventricular septal defects and relief of pulmonary stenosis are the operations most often required in patients with corrected transposition of the great arteries. The conduction system is particularly at risk in these patients because of its right-sided location and the surgeon's lack of familiarity with its anatomic course. Approach to the ventricular septal defect through an incision in the left-sided ventricle appears to reduce the incidence of postoperative complete heart block.[742]

Fox[743] reviewed the experience at the University of Alabama between 1967 and 1975, during which time 17 patients with corrected transposition of the great arteries were treated. All had large ventricular septal defects of which eight had associated pulmonary stenosis. Three had tricuspid valve incompetence requiring tricuspid valve replacement. All underwent closure of ventricular septal defects. Seven required relief of pulmonary stenosis, insertion of a valve-containing extracardiac conduit being required in four. There were four hospital deaths (23.5 percent), two late deaths (11.8 percent), six instances of atrioventricular dissociation (37.5 percent), and six cases of postoperative tricuspid valvular incompetence.

Single Ventricle

Definition

As used here single ventricle, also called common ventricle, is characterized by the entire flow from the two atria being carried directly through the mitral and tricuspid valves into a single ventricular chamber. As used here cases of either mitral or tricuspid atresia are excluded, as are cases of straddling tricuspid or mitral valves.

Pathology

The most common type is that in which the base of the large ventricular chamber communicates through an opening, the bulboventricular foramen, with an infundibulum, the latter probably representing a rudiment of the right ventricle (Fig. 36-144). The large chamber usually (78 percent) shows characteristics of a left ventricle, the so-called type A of Van Praagh and associates.[744] It is claimed that in 5 percent of cases the large ventricle shows the features of a right ventricle (type B) and that in 7 percent the ventricle shows equal amounts of right and left ventricular sinus features but without a ru-

FIGURE 36-144 Common ventricle with dextro malposition and without pulmonary stenosis. T = tricuspid valve; M = mitral valve.

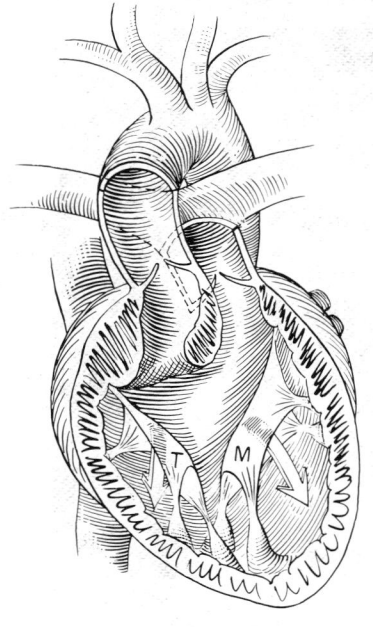

diment of a ventricular septum (type C). In 10 percent neither ventricular sinus could be identified (type I), the so-called primitive ventricle. Attempts at distinction between the latter three types by most examiners are not readily made.[745]

In some instances a clear-cut infundibulum is not easily identified, and uncommonly there are two coni. In about 80 percent of cases of single ventricle the great vessels are malposed (about equally levo and dextro in position), the aorta arising from the infundibulum when one is present. The position of the infundibulum corresponds to the position of the aorta.

Single ventricle with normally related great vessels is uncommon (so-called Holmes heart). Marin-Garcia and associates[745] found 7 examples (22 percent) among 32 cases of single ventricle. Subpulmonary stenosis is usual. Continuity of the aortic and mitral valves exists.[746]

Associated Conditions In single ventricle with malposition of the great vessels, pulmonary stenosis or atresia may be observed in about 25 percent of cases when not associated with asplenia. If the latter condition is present, obstruction to pulmonary flow occurs in most cases.

Subaortic stenosis may result from a narrow bulboventricular foramen.

The main tendency for associated cardiovascular abnormalities is observed when asplenia is present. Under this circumstance many cardiovascular and positional anomalies characteristic of the asplenic syndrome are present.[747]

Complications The complications depend in part on whether pulmonary stenosis is present or not. In cases with pulmonary stenosis the complications simulate those of the tetralogy of Fallot. When pulmonary stenosis is absent, the complications simulate those of large ventricular septal defect, including obstructive pulmonary vascular disease in patients reaching adolescence or adulthood.

Cerebral abscess is a potential complication, particularly in subjects with pulmonary stenosis.

Clinical Manifestations

This complex and challenging malformation is relatively rare and is found in only 1.5 percent of individuals with congenital heart disease.[6] Males are slightly more commonly afflicted than females in a ratio of 1.6 to 1.[3] Interestingly 70 percent of patients reported with single ventricle of the left ventricular type, pulmonary stenosis, and normally related great arteries have been female.[748] The clinical picture is determined largely by the associated defects, of which pulmonary stenosis, present in a little over half of the patients, is the most important.

History All patients will have some degree of systemic arterial oxygen desaturation, although cyanosis, appreciated clinically, may range from barely detectable to severe. Infants without significant pulmonary stenosis will present with little or no cyanosis but with tachypnea, dyspnea, poor weight gain (Fig. 36-2), and other features of congestive failure. Those with severe pulmonary stenosis or atresia will be hypoxic and resemble patients with tetralogy of Fallot. Approximately 60 percent of all patients with single ventricle will require hospitalization with the first month of life because of congestive failure, severe hypoxia, or both.[3]

Physical Examination The findings on palpation and auscultation are not distinctive of single ventricle but mimic those of patients with a large ventricular septal defect, tetralogy of Fallot, or transposition. The presence of a left-sided or symmetrical liver should arouse suspicion of a more complicated lesion than ventricular septal defect, tetralogy of Fallot, or the usual uncomplicated transposition.

Chest Roentgenogram Almost all patients with single ventricle have at least some degree of cardiac enlargement. Those with little or no pulmonary stenosis generally have very large hearts with marked pulmonary plethora. Only those patients with atresia or very severe pulmonary stenosis show a near-normal heart size and diminished pulmonary arterial blood flow. Those patients with normally related great arteries, a minority of some 15 percent, will have a clearly visible or prominent pulmonary arterial segment. The remainder will have either the narrow cardiac base characteristic of d-transposition or the mildly convex left upper cardiac border reflecting the left-sided ascending aorta of l-transposition.

Electrocardiogram Among those patients with single ventricle of the left ventricular type and d-loop (ventricular noninversion) the pattern usually is one of left ventricular hypertrophy with an rS pattern in the right and an Rs pattern in the left precordial leads. Q waves usually are absent in all precordial leads. The QRS axis characteristically lies between 0 and +90°. A superior QRS axis would suggest the presence of an associated atrioventricular canal malformation, but this is also noted among those few patients with this ventricular morphology, pulmonary stenosis, normally related great arteries but without atrioventricular canal. Patients with single ventricle of the left ventricular type but with an l-loop (ventricular inversion) generally have a pattern of right or biventricular hypertrophy with Q waves in the right precordial leads as well as in leads III and aV_F. These patients may also show evidence of significant atrioventricular block. The characteristic pattern of single ventricle of the right ventricular type is less well defined although right ventricular hypertrophy appears to be the rule. A few patients with single ventricle will have an rS pattern across the entire precordium.[9]

Echocardiography   M-mode echocardiography may establish the diagnosis by simultaneous recording of two atrioventricular valves without interposing septal echoes and by confirming the absence of septal echoes on a base-to-apex scan. An anterior outflow chamber, if present, usually can be identified anterior to both atrioventricular valves.[749] Two-dimensional echocardiography will confirm the absence of the ventricular septum and identify the number and position of the atrioventricular valves.[750]

Cardiac Catheterization   An increase in oxygen saturation will be found at the ventricular level and frequently at the atrial level as well. A degree of systemic arterial oxygen desaturation will be present in all patients. While a mild degree of preferential streaming of pulmonary venous blood to either the aorta or pulmonary artery may occur from patient to patient, the level of systemic arterial saturation appears to be related more to the volume of pulmonary blood flow than to the orientation of the great arteries or the type of single ventricle. Careful recording of intracardiac and arterial pressures is essential in order to detect significant or potentially significant obstruction to blood flow across either atrioventricular valve, across the atrial septum, or between the single ventricle and the aorta or pulmonary artery. The mode of atrioventricular connection is of particular importance. The presence of two atrioventricular valves, with or without straddling of one, or the presence of a single atrioventricular valve in the form of a common orifice or as the result of atresia of one or two atrioventricular valves can be confirmed by a combination of selective catheter passage, visualization of the common or separate orifices as negative-contrast areas following ventricular angiography, or by the technique of contrast echocardiography with atrial or caval injections.[751,752] The presence or absence of an outflow chamber or trabecular pouch, the morphological features of the main ventricular chamber, and the relationship of the aorta and pulmonary artery to the ventricle and atrioventricular valves can be established by high-quality selective ventricular angiography using specially angled views to supplement conventional views (Fig. 36-145).[751]

Natural History and Prognosis

Patients with single ventricle usually present within the first month or two of life with cyanosis, congestive failure, or a combination of both. Almost half of these patients expire before the age of 1 year as a result of these complications or attempted surgical palliation.[3] Those in whom the pulmonary arterial pressure and blood flow are not already reduced by significant natural pulmonary stenosis require surgical banding of the pulmonary artery to avoid death from congestive heart failure or the development of severe and progressive pulmonary vascular obstructive disease. Those patients with severe pulmonary stenosis and serious hypoxia will require

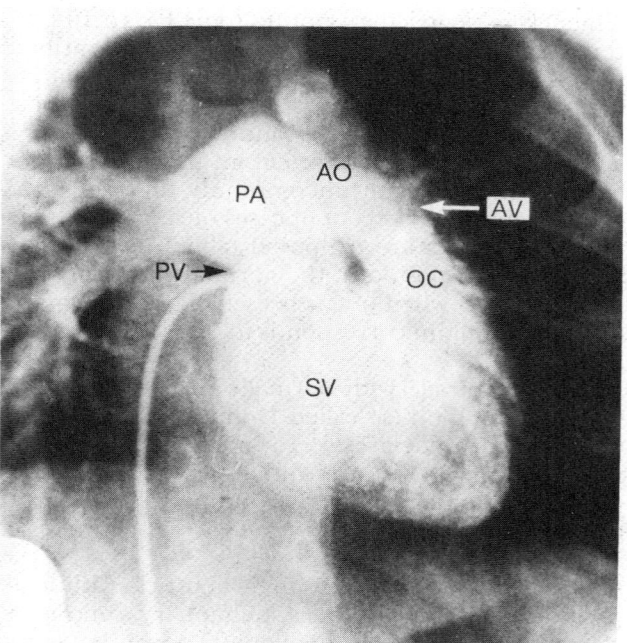

FIGURE 36-145   Posteroanterior view of the ventricular angiogram in an infant with single ventricle (SV), subaortic outflow chamber (OC), and levo transposition of the great arteries. The OC and left-sided aorta (AO) fill via the bulboventricular foramen, while the medially placed pulmonary artery (PA) fills directly from the single ventricle. The plane of the pulmonary valve (PV) is slightly below that of the aortic valve (AV).

systemic to pulmonary arterial shunting procedures. Among patients with single ventricle there is a propensity for the development of subaortic obstruction, usually in the form of progressive narrowing of the bulboventricular foramen between the single ventricle and the outflow chamber. In addition survivors are subject to the threats of infective endocarditis, brain abscess, the complications of progressive pulmonary vascular obstructive disease or Eisenmenger syndrome, and, finally, ill-advised surgical procedures when single ventricle is mistaken for a more common and more easily correctable malformation. Longevity, nevertheless, is possible with this condition. Of 18 patients who survived systemic to pulmonary arterial anastomoses during the early year of experience with that procedure, 11 were alive at the end of 15 years and 8 alive at the end of 20 years.[753] In all, some 33 patients are described as having survived beyond the age of 15 years, the eldest being 56 years old.[754]

Medical Management

Early recognition and identification of these patients are important if successful palliative surgical procedures are to be carried out for the relief of congestive failure or cyanosis. Corrective surgery is not recommended during infancy and usually is delayed until the age of 7 to 10 years, or even later if the child is doing well. In the interim, digitalis and diuretics may be necessary for those patients with continuing heart failure. Care is taken that anemia or severe polycythemia does not develop and that these patients are adequately protected against infective endocarditis. If surgical correction in the future is to be considered, the pulmonary vascular bed must be preserved, in a condition as near to normal as possible, by natural pulmonary stenosis or by surgical banding of the pulmonary artery. The adequacy of this preservation should be confirmed by cardiac catheterization and direct pressure measurements if possible, even in the face of an acceptable clinical course. Corrective surgery in the form of septation of the univentricular heart, although producing some remarkable examples of success, has been characterized by a high initial mortality and a high incidence of complete heart block despite intraoperative mapping of the conduction system. In view of this, increasing attention has been directed toward right atrium to pulmonary artery diversion via a valved or nonvalved conduit with surgical closure of the right atrioventricular valve. Progressive postoperative narrowing of the bulboventricular foramen, right atrial failure, and arrhythmias represent threats to patients undergoing this latter procedure.[755] The long-term outlook for the survivors of either surgical approach has yet to be determined. At present it would seem wise to postpone definitive surgical procedures as long as patients with single ventricle are doing reasonably well with medical management or as the result of earlier palliative procedures.

Surgical Management

Palliation of patients with univentricular heart without pulmonary stenosis is accomplished by banding of the main pulmonary artery to reduce pulmonary blood flow, control congestive heart failure, and prevent the development of pulmonary vascular obstructive disease. Hypoxia occurring as a consequence of univentricular heart with associated pulmonary stenosis is treated by the creation of a systemic arterial to pulmonary arterial shunt, usually the Blalock-Taussig subclavian arterial to pulmonary arterial anastomosis.

Two operations—septation[756] and atriopulmonary anastomosis[757]—are currently employed for correction of the univentricular heart. Historically the first of these operations used successfully was septation of the single ventricle, functional "right" and "left" ventricles being created by the placement of a fabric patch within the chamber (Fig. 36-146). When pulmonary stenosis is present, pulmonary blood flow is usually directed through an extracardiac conduit from the new "right ventricle" to the pulmonary artery. The septation patch in these cases is sutured to the right of both semilunar valves; the pulmonary artery is divided just distal to the stenotic valve. Direct resection or reconstruction

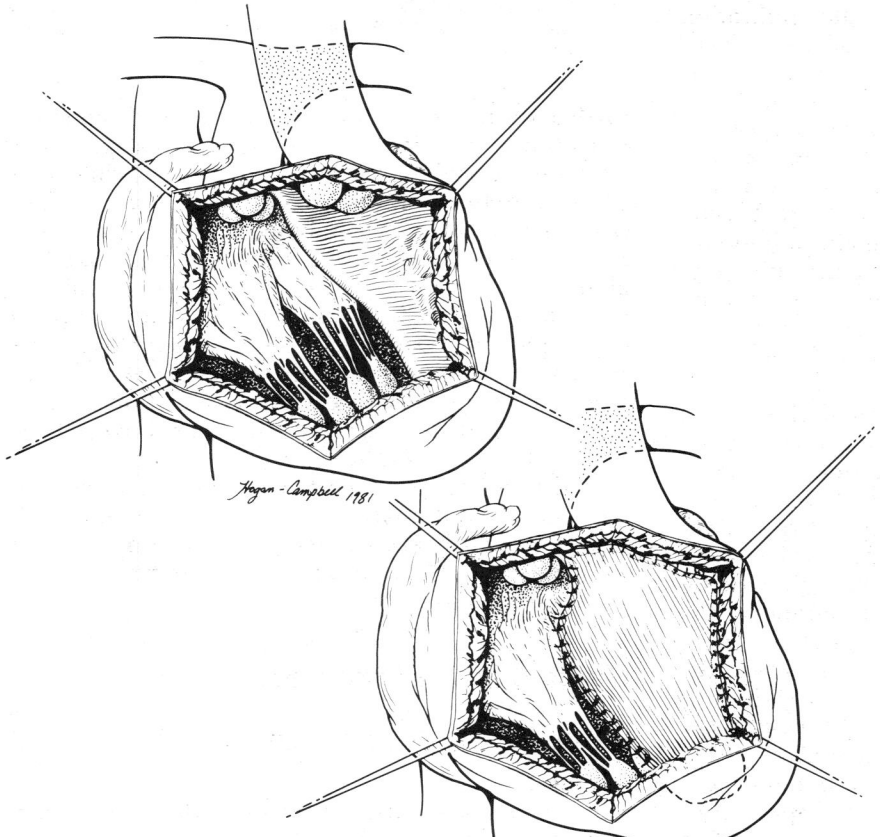

FIGURE 36-146 Septation of the univentricular heart. A large Dacron or Teflon patch is placed in the ventricle so that systemic venous blood from the tricuspid orifice is directed to the pulmonary artery while pulmonary venous blood from the mitral orifice is directed to the aorta. Knowledge of the course of the conduction system, facilitated by intracardiac electrophysiological mapping during operation, is required to avoid heart block. The bulboventricular foramen must usually be enlarged surgically in cases having a subaortic outflow chamber. Injury to major coronary arteries must be avoided.

of the obstructed pulmonary outflow tract is avoided because of its relatively inaccessible posterior position and the proximity of the conduction bundle and a major coronary artery.

Postoperative low cardiac output, complete heart block, and residual left-to-right shunting across the prosthetic septum are relatively common, but the incidence of each of these complications has lessened with increased surgical experience. Certain anatomic types of univentricular heart—notably A-III, in which the aorta arises anterior, to the left, and from a left-sided outlet chamber, and those with pulmonary stenosis—appear more favorable for repair.

McGoon and associates at the Mayo Clinic[756] reviewed their series of 35 corrections of univentricular heart by septation in 1977. There were 14 hospital deaths, most due to inadequate postoperative cardiac output. Two late deaths occurred. Fewer than half of the patients undergoing septation were judged to have obtained a satisfactory result. Neither the age of the patient, the pulmonary vascular resistance (if less than 10 units/m^2), the preoperative cardiothoracic ratio, nor the presence of a previous Blalock-Taussig shunt appeared to alter the outcome in this group of patients. Preexisting atrioventricular valve abnormalities were nearly always associated with a poor result.

The encouraging results achieved in the treatment of tricuspid atresia by establishment of right atrial to pulmonary arterial continuity as advocated by Fontan and Baudet[606] stimulated the application of this concept to the management of the univentricular heart and other complex congenital cardiac defects. Operation requires (1) closure of any atrial septal defect, (2) prosthetic patch closure of the right atrioventricular valve orifice, (3) division and closure of the proximal main pulmonary artery, and (4) diversion of all systemic venous blood directly from the right atrium to the distal main pulmonary artery through any of several possible conduits (Fig. 36-147). The right atrial appendage can often be anastomosed directly to the pulmonary artery, the anterior wall of this natural conduit being enlarged with a pericardial patch.[758]

Although early reports[759] advocated the use of bioprosthetic valves in both the inferior vena caval orifice and the atriopulmonary conduit, recent experience[757] indicates that neither of these valves is necessary for the achievement of a good result. Indeed, deterioration and stenosis of such valves used in this situation suggests that they should be avoided. The presence of normal pulmonary vascular resistance is essential if the right atrium is to function as a right ventricle; atriopulmonary anastomosis is contraindicated in any patient with even modest elevation of pulmonary vascular resistance.

Gale and his colleagues at the Mayo Clinic[757] reported 14 patients with univentricular heart corrected by a modification of Fontan's operation. There were four hospital deaths, three due to low

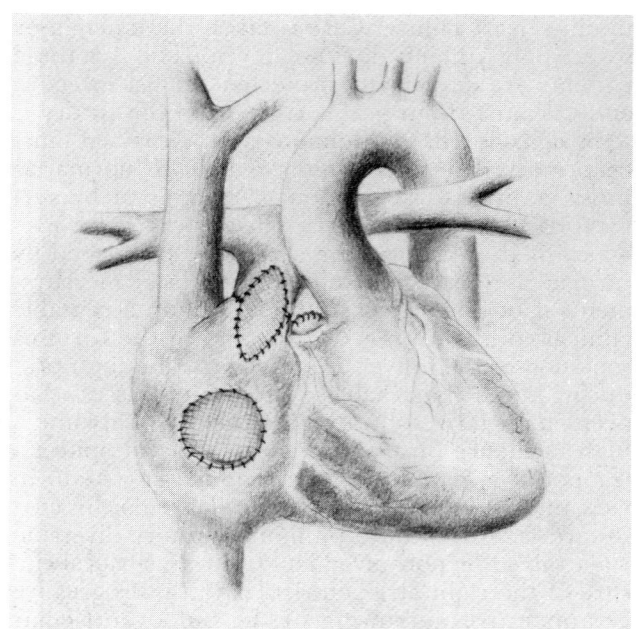

FIGURE 36-147   Establishment of direct right atrial to pulmonary arterial continuity by anastomosis of the appendage to the pulmonary artery, lying to the right of the aorta in the transposed position. This illustration depicts the repair of tricuspid atresia, but identical methods are applicable in correction of the univentricular heart. The tricuspid orifice and the atrial septal defect are closed with patches. The atrioarterial anastomosis is widened with a pericardial gusset. (*From H. Laks, W. G. Williams, W. E. Hellenbrand, R. M. Freedom, N. S. Talner, R. D. Rowe, and G. A. Trusler, Results of Right Atrial to Right Ventricular and Right Atrial to Pulmonary Artery Conduits for Complex Congenital Heart Disease, Ann. Surg., 192: 382, 1980. Reproduced with permission of author and publisher.*)

cardiac output even in the presence of systemic venous filling pressures exceeding 25 mmHg. It was necessary to maintain right atrial pressures in excess of 16 mmHg in all patients and all required inotropic support, often combined with nitroprusside. Bilateral pleural effusions and ascites occurred in all patients and transient renal failure was common. Complete heart block occurred in about one-third of the patients. Dehiscence of the patch closing the tricuspid valve occurred in three patients, all of whom underwent successful reoperation. There were no late deaths. Eight of the ten survivors have obtained a good result.

Only continued surgical experience in a few centers and careful analysis of surviving patients with univentricular heart will determine the operation of choice for this defect and the optimum time for surgical intervention.

Malpositions of the Heart

Levocardia, Dextrocardia, and Mesocardia

Pathology

The cardiac apex usually forms a dominant characteristic of the heart. The position of the apex, therefore, usually indicates a condition of levocardia, dextrocardia, or mesocardia. While a left-sided apex (levocardia) represents the common situation, this may be "abnormal" for certain situations. Most attention is directed to a right-sided apex (dextrocardia). As the left ventricle has a strong tendency to form the cardiac apex, dextrocardia may mean that the anatomic left ventricle lies toward the right side. This, however, is not always the case, as the heart may be shifted to the right because of other intrathoracic abnormalities. The latter condition may be termed *dextroposition*. There are rare cases in which the anatomic left ventricle lies on the left side, yet the shape of the ventricular portion is so distorted from the normal as to yield a right-sided apex. This might be termed *dextrocardia with normal orientation of the cardiac chambers or dextroversion.*

When the anatomic left ventricle lies on the right side of the heart, the ventricles may be said to be inverted, or the heart showing an l-loop. In one situation, this is part of the total inversion of all the organs, namely situs inversus, in which the heart may be normal fundamentally except for total inversion in keeping with the status of the other organs. Dextrocardia of this type has been referred to as *mirror-image dextrocardia*. Under other circumstances, the various organs of the body are normally oriented, yet the anatomic left ventricle lies on the right. This is usually seen in corrected transposition. Since the right-sided left ventricle is discordant with the other organs, this type of dextrocardia may be termed *isolated dextrocardia*. It usually means that there is corrected transposition, although not always.

As stated, *levocardia* is the anticipated normal, but in certain instances of total situs inversus wherein the apex is anticipated to be on the right side, it does, in fact, lie on the left side. In this situation, termed *isolated levocardia*, one may anticipate that the ventricles are inverted from the total inversion of situs inversus, as in corrected transposition of the great vessels associated with situs inversus.

Mesocardia is a term reserved for a midline apex. This tends to be observed in cases of polysplenia.

Cardiac malformations associated with isolated dextrocardia or levocardia or mesocardia usually, though not invariably, are severe and complex.[760] The most common anomalies are corrected transposition, double-outlet right ventricle and single ventricle.

Clinical Manifestations

Because they do not provide any significant information beyond what is already known, the trend today is to discard the terms *dextroposition, dextroversion, mirror-image dextrocardia*, and *isolated dextrocardia* and to use the broad term *dextrocardia* for all right-sided hearts followed by a description of the visceroatrial situs. In the case of those patients in whom the heart appears to have been pulled or pushed into the right chest by massive atelectasis,

hypoplasia of the right lung, diaphragmatic hernia, eventration of the diaphragm, pleural effusion, obstructive emphysema, or pneumothorax, an appropriate descriptive phrase should be added. The term *isolated levocardia* is applied to all left-sided hearts with situs inversus or situs ambiguus and a description of the visceroatrial situs should follow.

Dextrocardia with complete situs inversus occurs in approximately 2 per 10,000 live births.[9] The incidence of congenital heart disease is relatively low among these individuals and is estimated to be about 3 percent. Dextrocardia with situs solitus or situs ambiguus is considerably less common and occurs in perhaps 1 per 20,000 live births. The incidence of congenital heart disease is extremely high in this situation, however, and is probably in the range of 90 percent or greater.[6] From these figures one could project that approximately 16 percent of individuals found to have dextrocardia and congenital heart disease would have complete situs inversus. This estimate compares favorably with the figure of 18 percent observed in large autopsy series.[9] About half the patients with dextrocardia and heart disease have situs solitus and the remainder are about equally divided, depending upon the series, between situs inversus and situs ambiguus.[9,761] An l-ventricular loop is found in the majority of all patients with dextrocardia regardless of situs but is most common, as one might expect, among those patients with situs inversus, where it approaches 80 percent. Cardiac malformations usually, although not invariably, are severe and complex. The most common lesions and their approximate frequency are as follows: transposition of the great arteries, 50 to 75 percent; double-outlet right ventricle, 10 to 18 percent; ventricular septal defect, 60 to 80 percent; single ventricle, 15 to 40 percent; and pulmonary stenosis or atresia, 70 to 80 percent.[6,9,761,762] Approximately three-quarters of the transposed great arteries will have the segmental arrangement of corrected transposition. Tetralogy of Fallot is distinctly uncommon. One or the other of the associated noncardiac anomalies of polysplenia and asplenia are found in about one-quarter of patients with dextrocardia and almost invariably with situs ambiguus. Kartagener's syndrome, which is the triad of situs inversus, sinusitis, and bronchiectasis, is present in approximately 20 percent of patients with dextrocardia and situs inversus totalis.[763] The incidence of *isolated levocardia* is estimated at approximately 0.6 per 10,000 live births. Although less is known about this entity, it is estimated that over 90 percent of affected individuals will have associated heart disease.[9] Situs inversus is present in approximately 20 percent while the remainder have situs ambiguus, with the ratio of asplenia to polysplenia or accessory spleens being anywhere from 2.5 or 1.5:1. Regardless of situs, the ventricular loop is almost exclusively of the D type. Transposition of the great arteries, almost always of the corrected transposition configuration, and double-outlet right ventricle are present in the majority and are of about equal frequency. The associated defects are comparable in complexity and severity to those associated with dextrocardia. *Mesocardia* may exist either as a variant position of the normal heart or as a variant position of dextrocardia or isolated levocardia.

Medical Management

Medical management of patients with cardiac malpositions is similar to that of patients with normally located hearts, with the exceptions of continuous daily antibiotic coverage and pneumococcal vaccine for patients with asplenia and the particular attention to detail that is necessary to establish the correct diagnosis in those individuals with unusual and complex malformations. Surgical management differs in the technical considerations imposed by the malposition of the heart itself, the frequency of the l-ventricular loop, and the variability of the intracardiac conduction system.

Crisscross Heart

Definition

Crisscross heart is characterized by an atrioventricular spatial relationship that places or appears to place each ventricle in a contralateral position relative to its associated atrium.

Pathology

Among individuals with situs solitus and atrioventricular concordance (d-loop), the major portion of the right ventricular chamber occupies a left, superior position, while the left ventricle lies in a right, inferior position.[764] This relationship also has been called the "upstairs downstairs" heart or the superoinferior heart.[765] This situation, with a virtually horizontal ventricular septum, appears to result from underdevelopment of the inflow or sinus portion of the right ventricule, which, in turn, permits a greater than normal clockwise ventricular rotation among patients with a d-ventricular loop and counterclockwise rotation among those with an l-ventricular loop along the longitudinal axis of the heart as seen from below. In the case of situs solitus and d-ventricular loop (atrioventricular concordance), a normally located right atrium is connected to and supplies, via a superiorly and anteriorly displaced tricuspid valve, a right ventricle whose major portion, namely the infundibulum, is positioned anteriorly, superiorly, and to the left in relation to the left ventricle. The normally positioned left atrium supplies a left ventricle, which, by virtue of the clockwise rotation and diminutive right ventricular sinus, now occupies the posterior and inferior portion of the heart, at times extending almost to the right side of the heart border. With situs solitus and an l-ventricular loop (atrioventricular discordance), a normally located right atrium is connected to and

supplies a left ventricle which lies posteriorly, inferiorly, and to the left. The normally located left atrium supplies a right ventricle whose dominant infundibular portion is located anteriorly, superiorly, and to the right by virtue of counterclockwise rotation. Atrioventricular discordance has been present in almost one-third of recorded cases to date.[766] The connections of the ventricles with the great arteries are almost invariably abnormal. A very few patients have ventriculoarterial concordance, in which case the basic circulation may be normal. The majority have ventriculoarterial discordance, in which case the circulation has been that of d-transposition, l-transposition, or double-outlet right ventricle. A ventricular septal defect, usually large, is present in the majority and pulmonary stenosis, either valvular or subvalvular, is found in about half of the patients with this anomaly. Straddling of either of the atrioventricular valves, particularly the right-sided mitral valve in the presence of l-loop, is common. The tricuspid valve displays varying degrees of hypoplasia, reflecting the right ventricular inflow underdevelopment, and may override the ventricular septum as well. With l-ventricular loop the tricuspid valve is almost invariably abnormal with resultant tricuspid regurgitation, stenosis, or both.

Clinical Manifestations

Only 40 patients with superoinferior ventricles or crisscross atrioventricular relations have been reported to date.[766] The history and physical examination appear to be indistinguishable from those of patients with d-transposition, corrected transposition, or double-outlet right ventricle with a large ventricular septal defect with or without significant pulmonary stenosis. The presentation, then, is dominated by cyanosis or heart failure or both.

Cardiac Catheterization Selective right atrial angiography at cardiac catheterization will create the illusion of a right atrium connected to and filling a contralateral left-sided right ventricular chamber, and hence the term "crisscross atrioventricular connection." However, the inflow portion of the right ventricle, diminutive and less obvious than the enlarged infundibular portion, can still be seen to arise on the right and still demonstrate the right-to-left sequence which identifies it as a right ventricle that is part of a d-ventricular loop, i.e., the right-to-left sequence of tricuspid valve, right ventricular inflow or sinus region, septal and moderator bands, and then the infundibulum. This sequence is always from right-to-left in the presence of a d-loop and from left-to-right in the presence of an l-loop, as explained in the preceding section, "Segmental Approach to the Diagnosis of Congenital Heart Disease." High-quality selective biplane angiography in both ventricles is essential to define the precise ventriculoarterial relationships and connections. The coronary arterial distribution should be established by aortography in those patients being considered for corrective surgery.[767,768]

Natural History, Prognosis, and Medical Management
Palliative rather than corrective surgical procedures are recommended in infants unless associated complicating malformations can be excluded with reasonable certainty and the corrective surgery performed in a center with particular interest and experience with this malformation. Among older children the principal limiting factors would appear to be the size of the right ventricular chamber and the presence of atrioventricular valve overriding.

Asplenia and Polysplenia Syndromes

The association of congenital heart disease, usually severe, with thoracic or abdominal visceral heterotaxia has been recognized for many years. Abdominal visceral heterotaxia (Greek, *heteros* = "other," *taxis* = "arrangement") is characterized by varying degrees of malposition of the liver and stomach, varying degrees of malrotation of the gastrointestinal tract, and, usually, abnormalities of the spleen. The latter includes absence (asplenia) and the presence of multiple small masses of splenic tissue (polysplenia). In the case of the bronchopulmonary viscera, heterotaxia usually takes the form of isomerism with the presence of either (1) bilateral right or eparterial bronchi (above the pulmonary artery) and trilobed lungs, or (2) bilateral left or hyparterial bronchi (below the pulmonary artery) and bilobed lungs. These abdominal and thoracic anomalies appear to represent an abnormal persistence of the embryonal pattern of symmetry which gives way to lateralization somewhere between the thirtieth and thirty-sixth day of fetal life. This state of heterotaxia, lying between situs solitus and its mirror image situs inversus, has been termed *situs ambiguus* by Van Mierop and is the situs found in approximately one-third of patients with dextrocardia and over 80 percent of those with isolated levocardia.[769] From this picture of visceral heterotaxia or situs ambiguus has emerged at least two rather distinct syndromes, namely the asplenia syndrome and the polysplenia syndrome.

The *asplenia syndrome* is characterized by duplication or persistence of right-sided structures and absence or displacement of left-sided structures. This situation has been termed dextroisomerism or "bilateral right-sidedness," a mnemonic which, although unsound from an embryological viewpoint, provides a helpful reminder of the features of the asplenia syndrome. These include an abnormally symmetrical liver placed across both sides of the upper abdomen, a stomach displaced to the right side in approximately half of patients, and bilateral trilobed lungs and eparterial bronchi. The inferior

vena cava may lie to the right or left of the spine. Both atria frequently have the morphological characteristics of a right atrium with bilateral superior venae cavae, absence of the coronary sinus, and total anomalous pulmonary venous return. The characteristic cardiovascular malformations are presented in Table 36-5.[770] Note should be taken of the high incidence of dextrocardia, transposition of the great arteries, pulmonary atresia or stenosis, total anomalous pulmonary venous connection, complete atrioventricular canal, and single ventricle. Males are more commonly affected than females in a ratio of 1.7:1.

The usual clinical picture is that of a very young male infant with severe cyanosis and a symmetrical liver. The P-wave axis in the electrocardiogram is

TABLE 36-5 Cardiovascular Abnormalities in Asplenia and Polysplenia Syndromes

	Asplenia, %	Polysplenia, %
Cardiac position:		
Dextrocardia	41	42
Levocardia	59	58
Great arteries:		
Normally related	19	84
Transposition	72	8
Double-outlet RV	9	8
Pulmonary valve:		
Normal	22	58
Pulmonary stenosis	34	33
Pulmonary atresia	44	9
Great veins:		
Normal	16	50
TAPVC	72	0
PAPVC	6	42
Absent infrahepatic/suprarenal IVC	0	84
Bilateral SVC	53	33
Atrial septum:		
Intact	0	16
Primum ASD	100	42
Secundum ASD	66	26
Single atrium	0	16
Atrioventricular valves:		
Two	13	50
Single or common	87	16
Ventricular septum:		
Intact	6	25
Single ventricle	44	8
Atrioventricular canal	50	33
Other VSD	3	33
Coronary arteries:		
Single	19	0
Coronary sinus:		
Absence	85	42

Note: RV = right ventricle; TAPVC = total anomalous pulmonary venous connection; PAPVC = partial anomalous pulmonary venous connection; IVC = inferior vena cava; SVC = superior vena cava; ASD = atrial septal defect; VSD = ventricular septal defect.
Source: Modified from Rose, Izukawa, and Moes.[770]

normal, while the QRS axis is superior in most instances, reflecting the presence of an atrioventricular canal. The pulmonary blood flow is usually diminished on chest roentgenogram and an abnormal position of the stomach may be recognized. An overpenetrated chest roentgenogram may permit identification of bilateral eparterial bronchi. Howell-Jolly and Heinz bodies may be seen on the stained smear of peripheral blood,[771] and no splenic tissue will be demonstrated by radioisotope scanning.[772] Approximately one-third of these infants will die within the first week of life, and only a very small number, perhaps 15 to 20 percent, will survive to the end of the first year. Shunting procedures to increase pulmonary blood flow are necessary for survival in most instances. Renal and gastrointestinal malformations are present in some 10 to 15 percent of patients. Sudden, overwhelming bacterial sepsis is a constant hazard for these patients with asplenia. The most common offending organisms for survivors below 6 months of age are *Klebsiella* and *E. coli* and for those beyond 6 months of age are pneumococcus and *H. influenzae*. Continuous daily oral antibiotic coverage is recommended for all individuals with this syndrome, with the antibiotic of choice being amoxicillin for children under the age of 10 years and penicillin for those older than 10 years.[773]

Polysplenia, defined as two or more splenic masses and usually consisting of two somewhat larger spleens accompanied by a number of smaller splenules, tends to be characterized by levoisomerism or "bilateral left-sidedness." The liver is abnormally symmetrical in about one-quarter of patients, and the stomach is on the right in about two-thirds of patients. Isomerism of the lungs is not nearly as constant as with asplenia, but bilateral hyparterial bronchi and bilobed lungs are found in perhaps two-thirds of these patients. Partial, rather than total, anomalous pulmonary venous connection is frequent, with the most frequent pattern being that of pulmonary venous drainage of each lung to the corresponding atrium on that side. The other characteristic cardiovascular malformations are listed in Table 36-5. Despite the relatively high incidence of cardiac malposition, it can be seen that the anomalies, in general, are less severe than those associated with asplenia. More patients have normally related great arteries and fewer have transposition, pulmonary atresia, complete atrioventricular canal, or single ventricle. Somewhere between 50 and 85 percent of patients have absence of the infrahepatic to suprarenal portion of the inferior vena cava with azygos or hemiazygos vein continuation of the suprarenal inferior vena cava to the ipsilateral superior vena cava. A superior and leftward P-wave vector in the frontal plane, falling between −30 and −90°, is extremely common among these patients and would warn of difficulties that might be encountered with catheter passage from the femoral vein to the right atrium at the time of cardiac cath-

eterization. A superior QRS axis is present in one-third of patients. Chest roentgenogram tends to show increased pulmonary blood flow. Splenic tissue may be demonstrated in the dorsal mesogastrium on both sides of the abdomen using radioisotopic scanning techniques.[772] Renal and gastrointestinal anomalies are present in approximately 15 percent of patients. Survival of patients with polysplenia is considerably better than that of patients with asplenia with almost 40 percent living into and beyond the second year of life.

It should come as no surprise, however, that exceptions to and overlap between these two syndromes have been identified. Bilateral eparterial bronchi, trilobed lungs, situs ambiguus, and cardiac malformations characteristic of asplenia have been described in the presence of a normal spleen. Bilateral eparterial bronchi with bilobed lungs and bilateral hyparterial bronchi with trilobed lungs have also been described.[676] Asplenia with bilateral bilobed lungs does occur rarely, but, to our knowledge, asplenia with bilateral hyparterial bronchi has not been reported. At present it appears that bronchial situs and the location of the hepatic portion of the inferior vena cava are the most accurate predictors of dextro- or levoisomerism, with their characteristic cardiac malformations, and of atrial situs, respectively.[676] The state of the spleen is a less accurate predictor but remains of importance in terms of the possibility of lethal sepsis and as a colorful reminder of the different patterns of cardiovascular and visceral abnormalities.

Ectopia Cordis

Pathology

Ectopia cordis is the rare condition in which the heart lies in some location outside of the thorax.[774]

Abdominal heart is a very rare condition in which the heart lies within the abdominal cavity. The vascular connections pass a defect in the diaphragm. A diverticulum of the left ventricle walled by cardiac muscle may extend through a diaphragmatic defect as, in effect, a forme fruste of abdominal heart. Intracardiac abnormalities are common, the most consistent one being ventricular septal defect.[775]

Clinical Manifestations

This is an extremely rare malformation but one easily recognized, particularly in its thoracic form. The heart, almost invariably lacking any covering, lies on the anterior chest wall with its apex pointing cephalad and, at times, touching the infant's chin. The great arteries and veins exit and enter the heart through a cleft in the sternum of variable size. The thoracic cavity has no provision for the heart and thus a return of the heart to its usual position is precluded. Ravitch, in 1977, collected and described 20 examples of true thoracic ectopia cordis in whom a surgical attempt had been made to position the heart within the chest or to provide a protective covering of skin. There was only one survivor. Death was due either to kinking of the great arteries or veins, to tamponade of the heart itself as a result of repositioning, or to associated intracardiac defects. The latter consisted of ventricular septal defect in nine, single ventricle in three, transposition in one, and coarctation in two. In two patients only a patent ductus was noted and in three the internal structure of the heart was not known. Among those patients with a ventricular septal defect, three had pulmonary atresia and four severe pulmonary stenosis. There are, then, a few patients with intracardiac anomalies that would permit survival if the malposition of the heart could be managed successfully. True abdominal ectopia cordis appears to be rarer still, with only 1 or 2 reported instances of the heart lying completely within the abdomen.[776]

Patients with thoracic ectopia cordis are to be distinguished from those with an isolated cleft of the sternum, either of the superior portion or of the entire sternum except for the xiphoid. In this situation the heart can be seen to pulsate beneath a covering of skin or cutaneous tissue which has the appearance of scar tissue. The heart may protrude anteriorly and superiorly with crying, but true ectopia or displacement of the heart from the thorax does not exist. There does not appear to be a propensity for intracardiac malformations with this condition, and the sternal defect lends itself to surgical repair.[776]

Finally, both thoracic and abdominal ectopia cordis are to be distinguished from the syndrome of five associated defects described by Cantrell, Haller, and Ravitch and referred to as Cantrell's pentalogy. In its complete form this syndrome consists of (1) a midline supraumbilical abdominal wall defect, (2) a defect of the lower sternum, (3) a deficiency of the anterior diaphragm, (4) a defect of the diaphragmatic pericardium, and (5) a congenital intracardiac malformation, usually a ventricular septal defect.[777] The ventral abdominal defect may take the extreme form of an omphalocele, covered by a translucent membrane and containing liver, bowel, and the cardiac apex, or of merely an area of wrinkled, hyperpigmented skin overlying a wide supraumbilical diastasis. Similarly, the sternal defect may be either quite striking or inconspicuous. Mesocardia usually is present with the heart appearing to have undergone a counterclockwise rotation as seen from below, but the heart is not totally displaced from the thoracic cavity. Approximately 80 percent of patients with this syndrome will have a ventricular septal defect, particularly in the form of tetralogy of Fallot, but isolated instances of tricuspid atresia, total anomalous pulmonary venous return, and common atrium have been described.[776] In addition, almost two-thirds will have a muscular diverticulum of the apical portion of the left ventricle, which may present along with an omphalocele or as a small, pulsating, frequently tubular, midline mass in the epigastrium. The diverticulum may be enclosed by pericardium or extend through a defect in the pericardium. A murmur and rarely a thrill may be observed. The electrocardiogram may be normal or show a mild intraventricular conduction delay. Left ventricular angiography, performed with care to avoid injection into the diverticulum itself, will reveal this abnormal structure.[778] Spontaneous rupture of the diverticulum with death has been reported in over half of the patients with this anomaly. Amputation of the diverticulum with suture closure of its base is the treatment of choice, and this may be done at the time of operative repair of the intracardiac defect or at the time of repair of the abdominal, sternal, and diaphragmatic defects.

Congenital Abnormalities of the Coronary Arterial Circulation

Coronary Arteriovenous Fistulas

Definition
A coronary arteriovenous fistula is represented by a gross communication between a coronary artery, on one hand, and a cardiac chamber, the coronary sinus, or the pulmonary trunk, on the other (Fig. 36-148).

Pathology
The site of origin may involve any of the epicardial coronary arteries, and the anomalous termination may be into any of the sites mentioned in the definition. The right coronary artery is the site of origin in somewhat over half of the cases, and the two most common sites into which the fistula feeds is a cardiac vein (usually the coronary sinus) and the right ventricle. Although solitary communication is the rule, rare cases may show multiple sites of termination into the involved site of reception.[779]

A fistula into the pulmonary trunk is usually characterized by one or more vessels opening into the pulmonary trunk and making connection with branches of each of the two main coronary arteries. The artery or arteries feeding the fistula are grossly enlarged and tortuous. Saccular aneurysms may develop in segments of dilated vessels; such aneurysms are usually observed in the adult and frequently show calcification of the wall.[780] A part of the large flow through the fistulas is contributed from various noncoronary mediastinal arteries.

Clinical Manifestations[781,782]
Many patients with a coronary arteriovenous fistula are asymptomatic. In some, the magnitude of the shunt into the right side of the heart is great enough to cause congestive heart failure, with a tendency for this to occur in early infancy or after 40 years of age. The classic finding is that of a continuous murmur with an unusual location since it is loudest over the fistula. It may have a louder diastolic com-

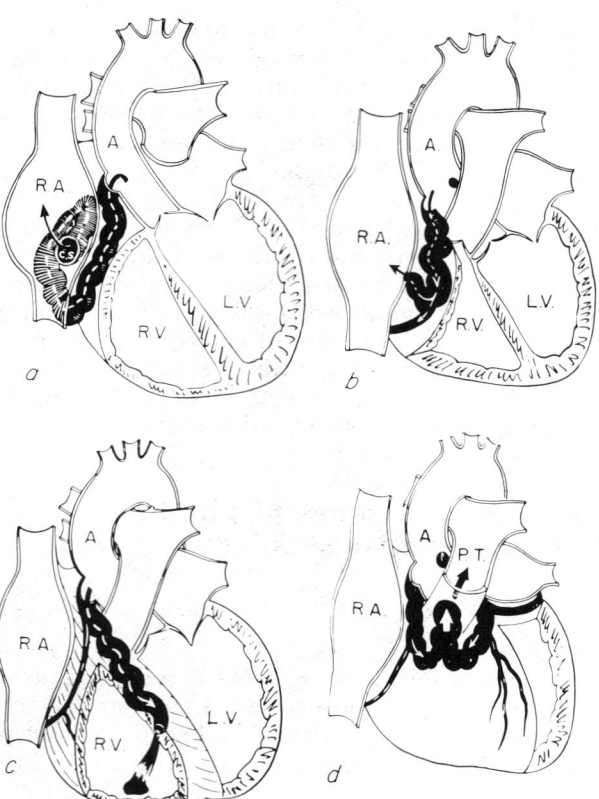

FIGURE 36-148 Anomalous communications of coronary arteries. *a.* Right coronary artery communicates with coronary sinus. *b.* Right coronary artery communicates with right atrium (R.A.). *c.* Anomalous communication of right coronary artery with right ventricle (R.V.). *d.* Two coronary arteries arise from the aorta (A.) and make collateral communication with accessory coronary artery arising from pulmonary trunk (P.T.). L.V. = left ventricle.

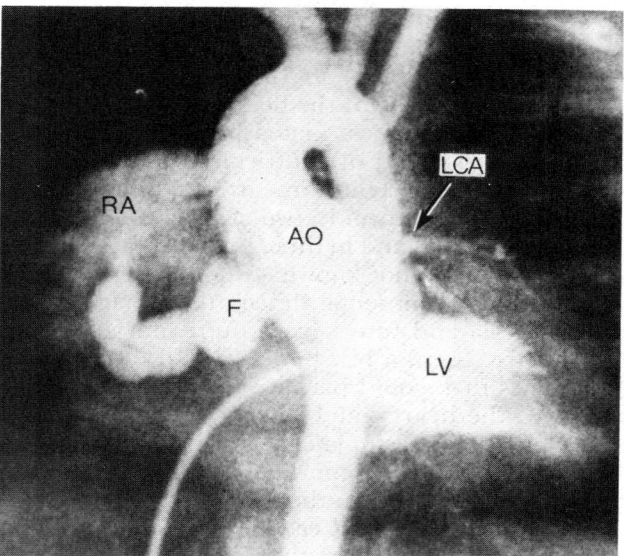

FIGURE 36-149 Posteroanterior view of left ventricular (LV) angiogram in a child with a coronary arteriovenous fistula (F) from the left coronary artery (LCA) to the right atrium (RA).

ponent, especially if communication is with the right ventricle. In those with large shunts, there may be cardiomegaly and increased pulmonary flow by chest roentgenogram and left ventricular hypertrophy on electrocardiogram. At cardiac catheterization, an increase in oxygen saturation may be encountered, usually in the right atrium or right ventricle, if the shunt is large enough. Pressures are normal. Aortography or selective coronary arteriography (Fig. 36-149) will demonstrate the involved coronary artery and site of entry of the fistula.[554,783] The most common complication is infective endocarditis, but thrombosis, myocardial ischemia, and rupture may occur.

Medical Management
Medical management involves treatment and prevention of the complications. Surgical closure is recommended.[784]

Surgical Management
Closure of coronary arteriovenous fistulas requires obliteration of the fistula at its point of entry into the atrium, ventricle, coronary sinus, or pulmonary trunk, *and* preservation of the continuity of the coronary artery. In some cases this can be accomplished without the use of cardiopulmonary bypass by lateral arteriorrhaphy—the placement of a series of obliterating mattress sutures across the fistula beneath the coronary artery as it passes over the surface of the heart.[785] Cardiopulmonary bypass is preferred for safe exposure of large or multiple fistulas such as those entering the right atrium near the superior vena caval–right atrial junction and arising from the artery to the sinus node. The orifice of the fistula is obliterated from within the heart by direct suture or placement of a Dacron patch. Associated aneurysms, common when the artery to the sinus node arises from a branch of the left coronary artery, are mobilized and resected or obliterated with multiple sutures. Fistulas have been closed from within the opened coronary artery, the artery then being repaired by direct suture or venous patch angioplasty.

Only four deaths occurred in 116 reported cases of coronary arteriovenous fistulas which were surgically closed.[784] Operation is safe, simple, and effective.

Origin of the Left Coronary Artery from the Pulmonary Artery

The right coronary artery arises from the aorta, while the left coronary artery arises from the left anterior pulmonary arterial sinus (Fig. 36-150). This is also known as the Bland-White-Garland syndrome. The course and branching of the vessel is normal. In the young, the coronary arteries are of normal size, but if survival occurs beyond infancy, there is noticeable dilatation of these vessels. In the uncommon case reaching adult life, both coronary

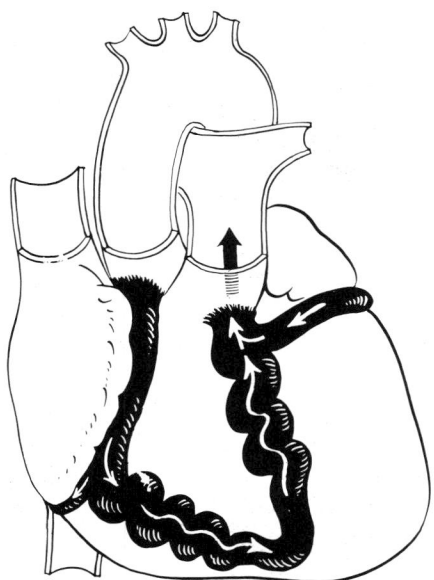

FIGURE 36-150 Diagrammatic portrayal of anomalous origin of the left coronary artery from the pulmonary trunk. With time, wide collaterals develop between the two coronary systems, so that right coronary arterial blood is shunted into the left coronary system and thence into the pulmonary trunk.

arterial systems are huge and tortuous. In cases of infant death from this condition, the left ventricle is dilated and may show sites of infarction with calcification of infected myocardium. In subjects surviving infancy, there is often scarring of the left ventricular papillary muscles and of the left ventricular wall, particularly in the distribution of the left coronary artery. The left ventricular cavity is dilated and the chamber shows endocardial fibroelastosis. The mitral valve may become incompetent.[786,787]

Uncommon variations are those in which only one of the two branches of the left coronary artery arises from the pulmonary artery, while the other branch arises from the aorta. Associated conditions are uncommon, a ventricular septal defect[788] and the tetralogy of Fallot[789] having been reported.

An extensive literature review helped elucidate the clinical spectrum and mode of presentation in patients with this abnormality.[790] The majority of patients present in the first few months of life. Acute episodes of irritability, profuse cold sweating, pallor, and respiratory distress occur with evidence of heart failure. Less often the patients present at any age with mitral regurgitation and heart failure. A few reach adolescence or adulthood with relatively few symptoms, other than occasional exertional angina or palpitations. Sudden death may be the first and only sign of this diagnosis.

On physical examination, the heart is enlarged with an abnormal left ventricular apex impulse. Other signs of failure are usually present. Pallor and "clammy" skin are common. In some, a soft continuous murmur is heard at the upper left sternal border. This murmur is more prominent in the older patients, presumably due to development of a more extensive collateral circulation. The murmur of mitral regurgitation may be heard at the apex radiating to the axilla, but in young infants with heart failure there can be a surprising degree of regurgitation without a distinctive murmur.

The chest roentgenogram typically shows marked enlargement of the heart with posterior displacement of the esophagus by a large left atrium. There is pulmonary edema, and there may be atelectasis of the left lower lobe due to bronchial compression.

The electrocardiogram demonstrates the pattern of anterolateral infarction (Fig. 36-151) with a deep Q wave in leads I and aV_L and abnormal R-wave progression across the precordium. Arrhythmias are frequent. The horizontal loop of the vectorcardiogram is clockwise and posteriorly oriented. Echocardiogram shows marked enlargement of the left atrium and ventricle with little or no left ventricular wall motion. Thallium 201 myocardial perfusion imaging can help distinguish this from congestive cardiomyopathy.[791]

At cardiac catheterization, there may be an increase in saturation in the pulmonary artery if there is enough retrograde flow. There is usually some pulmonary hypertension with very elevated pulmonary wedge pressure. Left ventricular angiography will delineate the left ventricular volume and function as well as the degree of mitral regurgitation. Aortography or selective right coronary arteriography[554,783] will demonstrate the collateral circulation filling the left coronary artery retrogradely with at least faint opacification of the main pulmonary artery (Fig. 36-152).

Natural history and prognosis is indicated by the modes of presentation. Most will die in infancy. Medical management is aimed at control of congestive heart failure and arrhythmias. Surgical anastomosis to the aorta should be attempted to improve myocardial blood flow and prevent further myocardial damage.[792]

Several operations have been proposed.[793] Ligation of the anomalous left coronary artery near its pulmonary arterial orifice reduces the "run-off" of coronary arterial blood into the low-resistance pulmonary vascular bed. Late results are good.[794]

Establishment of anterograde left coronary arterial flow has been accomplished by interposition of autologous venous grafts and synthetic grafts between the aorta and the anomalous left coronary artery followed by ligation of the artery near its pulmonary arterial orifice.[795] The end of the left subclavian artery has been anastomosed to the side of the left coronary artery after ligation of the anomalous vessel. These operations can be performed without the use of cardiopulmonary bypass, but late prognosis probably depends upon long-term graft patency, as yet unpredictable.

In most cases the orifice of the anomalous left coronary artery can be excised through the open

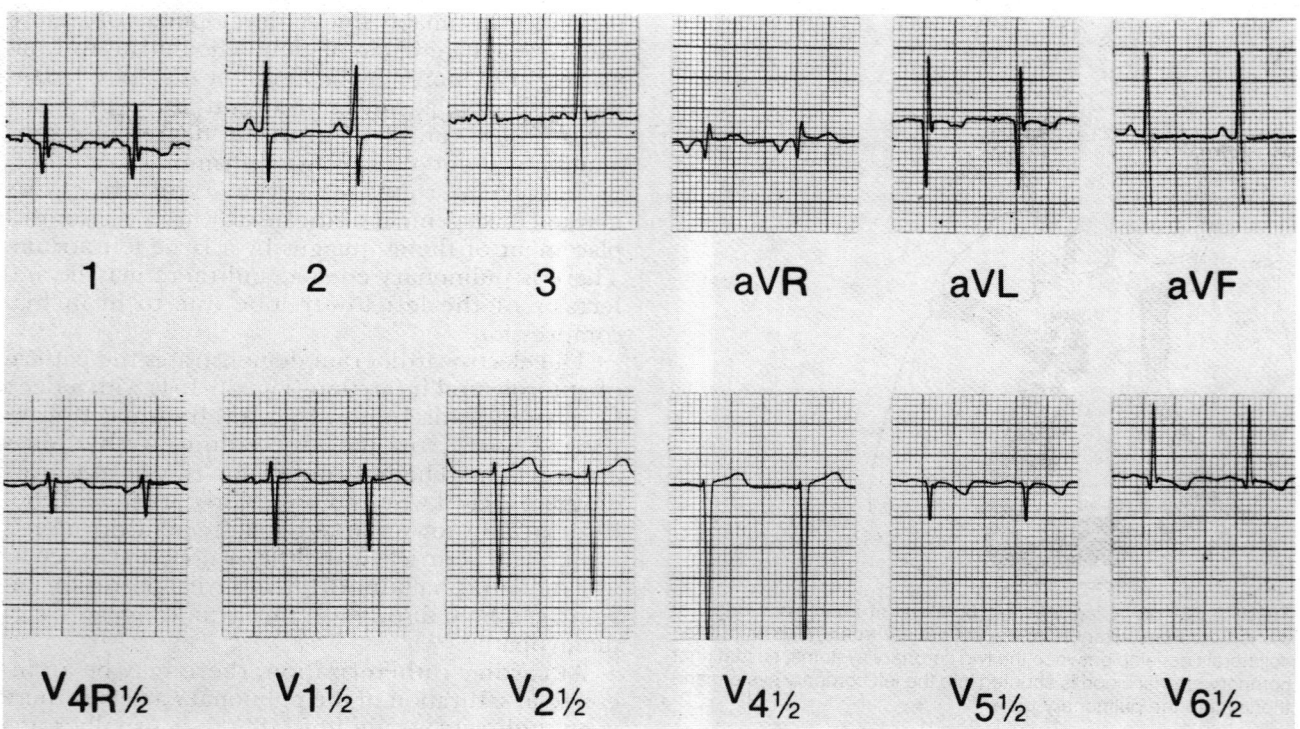

1   **2**   **3**   **aVR**   **aVL**   **aVF**

V4R½   **V1½**   **V2½**   **V4½**   **V5½**   **V6½**

FIGURE 36-151 Twelve-lead electrocardiogram in an infant with origin of the left coronary artery from the pulmonary artery, demonstrating the pattern of anterolateral infarction. Chest leads are recorded at one-half standard.

pulmonary artery with a cuff of surrounding pulmonary arterial wall. The left main coronary artery is carefully mobilized over a length sufficient to allow direct anastomosis (Fig. 36-153)[262] with care to

FIGURE 36-152 Posteroanterior view of a left ventricular (LV) angiogram in an infant with an anomalous left coronary artery demonstrating origin of the right coronary artery (RCA) from the aorta (AO) with collaterals filling the left coronary artery (LCA) and subsequently the pulmonary artery (PA).

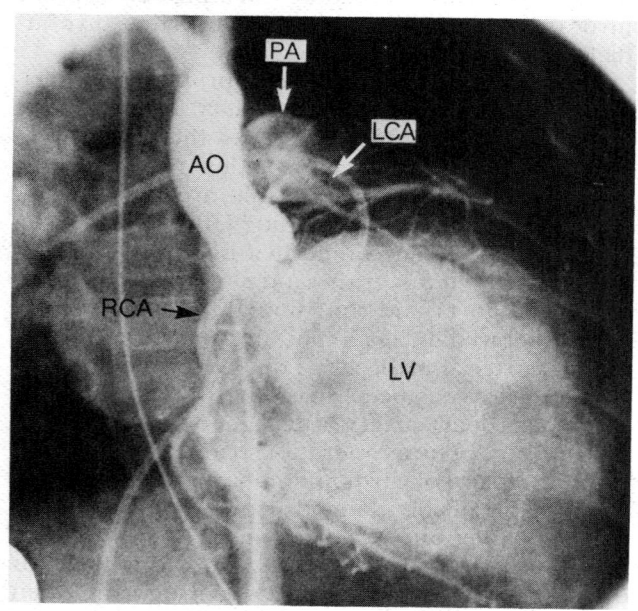

avoid injury to the circumflex branch. Tension on the artery must be avoided if long-term patency is to be achieved. When insufficient length prevents direct anastomosis, a segment of vein or prosthetic graft can be interposed between the aorta and the end of the excised left coronary artery, or the end of the left subclavian artery can be sutured to the end of the coronary artery.[796]

Operations requiring removal of the coronary artery from the pulmonary artery are best performed on cardiopulmonary bypass or during a period of circulatory arrest with profound hypothermia (18 to 20°C). Some form of circulatory support is required when the pulmonary artery is opened.

Assuming the usual measures of intraoperative myocardial protection, postoperative mortality is largely attributable to preexisting left ventricular infarction and failure, ventricular arrhythmias, and mitral regurgitation secondary to papillary muscle dysfunction and annular dilatation. These problems are most prevalent in critically ill infants requiring urgent operation. Improvement in ventricular function following operation has been reported.[797] Low mortality and good hemodynamic result should be anticipated in older patients.

Origin of the Right or Both Coronary Arteries from the Pulmonary Artery

Origin of the right coronary artery from the pulmonary artery while the left arises from the aorta is highly uncommon. Some infants and, more com-

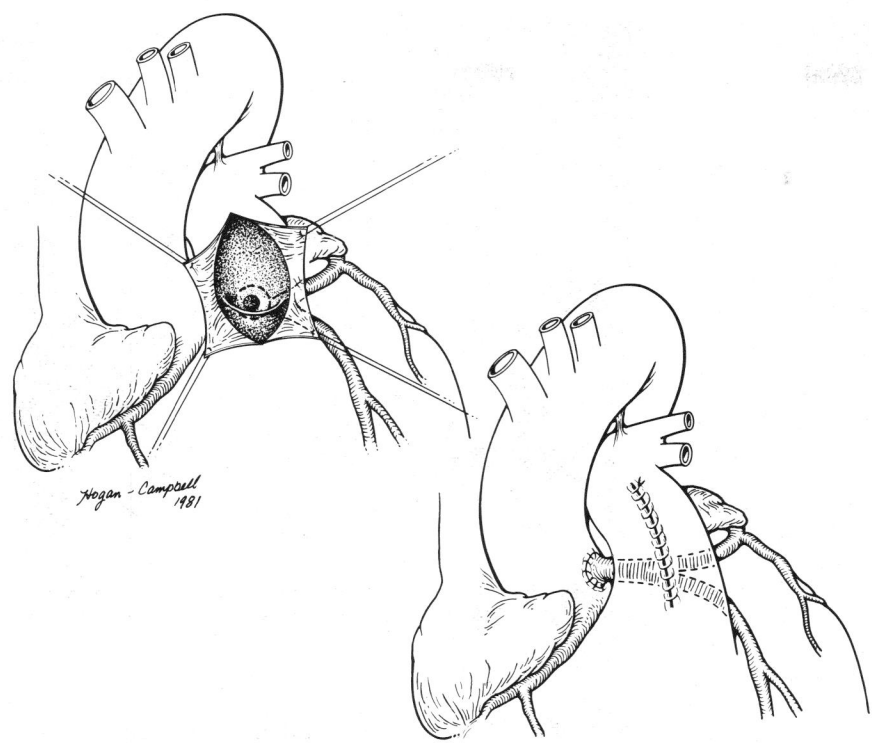

FIGURE 36-153 Transposition of anomalous left coronary artery from the pulmonary artery to the aorta. The orifice of the left coronary artery is excised from within the opened pulmonary artery (on cardiopulmonary bypass). The proximal segment of left coronary artery and its branches, the circumflex and the left anterior descending branches, are mobilized to provide sufficient length for a tension-free anastomosis of the orifice and surrounding cuff of pulmonary arterial wall to the left posterolateral wall of the aorta.

monly, adults manifest evidence of inadequate perfusion of the myocardium.[798] Origin of both coronary arteries from the pulmonary trunk is rare,[799] as is usually the case when there is a single coronary artery and this vessel arises from the pulmonary trunk.[800,801]

Anomalous origin of the right coronary artery from the pulmonary artery usually has a good prognosis, but sudden death has been described.[802] If both coronary arteries arise from the pulmonary artery, early death almost always occurs.[801]

Since anomalous origin of the right coronary artery from the pulmonary artery has been associated with sudden death, operative correction is justified even in the asymptomatic patient. Normal coronary arterial circulation is established by excision of the right coronary artery from the pulmonary artery followed by direct implantation of the coronary artery with a cuff of surrounding pulmonary artery into the ascending aorta. Cardiopulmonary bypass should be available but is not necessary in most cases. In adults, the anomalous coronary artery can be ligated near its point of entry into the pulmonary artery, anterograde coronary blood flow being established with a saphenous vein graft from the ascending aorta to the distal right coronary artery. Direct implantation of the right coronary artery is safe, simple, and probably the procedure of choice for long-term patency.[803]

Origin of both coronary arteries from the pulmonary artery has not been corrected surgically, no patient having survived to operation.

Origin of the Left Coronary Artery from the Right Aortic Sinus

In this condition both coronary arteries arise from the right aortic sinus, the left arising anterior to the origin of the right. After penetrating the epicardium, the left coronary artery takes a sharp turn to the left and, after passing behind the pulmonary artery, courses and branches in a normal manner.[804]

Sudden death during exercise has been reported when the left coronary artery coursed behind the right ventricular outflow tract in these cases.[804,805] If symptomatic and demonstrated angiographically, surgery should be considered.

Origin of the left coronary artery from the right sinus with a course anterior to the right ventricular outflow tract or similar origin of the left anterior descending branch alone is not clinically significant. In patients such as those with tetralogy of Fallot,[553] preoperative diagnosis is important to avoid incision at the time of surgery (see the section in this chapter discussing tetralogy of Fallot).

Origin of the Circumflex Coronary Artery from the Right Aortic Sinus or Right Coronary Artery

In less than 0.5 percent of individuals, the left circumflex coronary artery arises either from the proximal segment of the right coronary artery or from the right aortic sinus just posterior to the origin of the right artery. From either site of origin the vessel courses along the posterior aspect of the aorta to reach the proximal part of the left atrioventricular sulcus. The anterior descending artery arises from the usual position of origin of the left coronary artery.

In the absence of coronary atherosclerosis, this anomaly probably has no clinical significance.

Atresia of the Left Coronary Ostium

Atresia of the origin of the left coronary artery is an unusual basis for ischemic heart disease in the young. Each coronary artery has a normal site of origin. The atresia usually affects the entire length of the main left coronary artery, and various degrees and lengths of stenosis may involve the proximal segments of the anterior descending and left circumflex arteries.[404] There is an association with a forme fruste of supravalvular aortic stenosis, wherein this vessel may histologically show a mosaic pattern to its media. The mitral valve may show features of prolapse.

This rare abnormality has been recently reviewed with the addition of another case.[806] The clinical picture is identical to anomalous left coronary artery from the pulmonary artery. The diagnosis can be suspected by angiography[783] if it is noted that there is no filling of the pulmonary artery once the main left coronary fills via collaterals. Successful coronary bypass grafting has been reported in a 14-year-old boy.[807]

Aneurysm of Coronary Artery

Localized congenital aneurysms are uncommon and tend to favor the male and to be located in the right coronary artery. The basis is probably a dysplastic condition of the arterial media. The potential danger is thrombosis with either occlusion of the parent artery or embolism downstream. In cases with coronary arterial fistula, saccular aneurysms may be of acquired nature. Multiple aneurysms have been reported in the young. While some of these may be of congenital origin, some are probably secondary to the mucocutaneous lymph node syndrome.[808]

In general, the diagnosis of aneurysm of the coronary arteries[809] has been made at postmortem examination. Some patients are apparently asymptomatic, but rupture may occur. The clinical picture is one of angina and myocardial infarction. It may be suspected clinically if these findings occur in a very young person. The history should exclude mucocutaneous lymph node syndrome. A systolic or systolic and diastolic murmurs may be heard. The chest roentgenogram will show cardiomegaly with an unusual round shadow at the cardiac margin, particularly common along the distribution of the right coronary artery. Patterns of ischemia or infarction will be evident on the electrocardiogram. The diagnosis is made by coronary arteriography (Fig. 36-154).[810] Coronary artery bypass grafting[811]

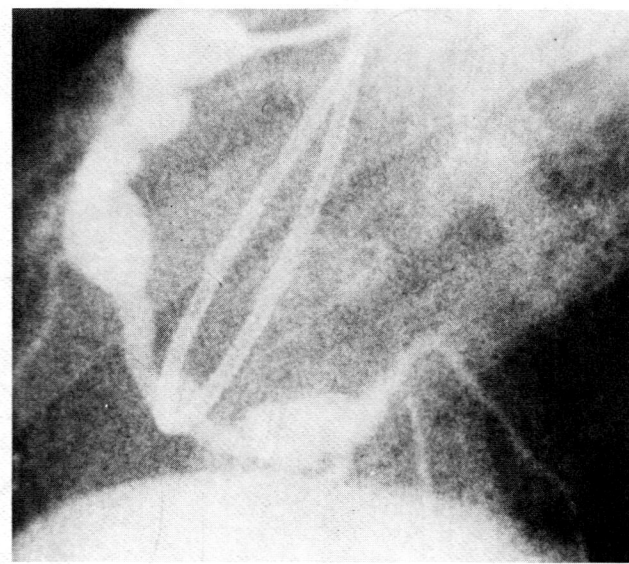

FIGURE 36-154   Right anterior oblique view of a selective right coronary arteriogram in a patient with multiple saccular aneurysms. (*From McMartin et al.*[810] *Reproduced with permission.*)

and, if possible, resection of the aneurysm are recommended.

Congenital Abnormalities of the Coronary Venous Circulation

Coronary Sinus Malformations

A comprehensive review of anomalies involving the coronary sinus was presented by Mantini and associates.[812] These relate to enlargement of the sinus, absence of the sinus, atresia of its right ostium and hypoplasia.

Enlargement of the coronary sinus results from delivery of blood foreign to the coronary sinus into this channel. The most common situation is that in which no left-to-right shunt is associated. Persistent left superior vena cava joining the coronary sinus is the most common cause. Less common is that in which the inferior vena cava is continuous with the left superior vena cava by way of the hemiazygous vein. This, in turn, causes inferior vena caval blood ultimately to reach the right atrium through the coronary sinus. When a left-to-right shunt into the coronary sinus occurs, it may be of either the high-pressure or low-pressure type. The high-pressure types are the result of a communication between a coronary artery and the coronary sinus, such as a congenital fistula. A low-pressure left-to-right shunt into the coronary sinus results from unusual circumstances in which there is a communication between the coronary sinus and the left atrium, or from the more common circumstance in which the pulmonary veins join the sinus.

Absence of the coronary sinus occurs when there is

direct communication of the left superior vena cava with the left atrium or with the left side of a common atrium.

Atresia of the right atrial ostium of the coronary sinus may occur as an independent abnormality or may be associated with other conditions. Cardiac venous blood may leave the coronary sinus through a persistent left superior vena cava and through the bridging left brachiocephalic vein into the right superior vena cava. More commonly, the left superior vena cava is absent, and multiple connections between the coronary sinus and the atria provide a route for exit of blood from the coronary sinus.[666]

The clinical importance of coronary sinus malformations is mainly limited to the technical aspects of cardiac catheterization and cardiac surgery in those who have associated defects. Abnormalities resulting in enlargement of the coronary sinus were discussed in preceding sections of this chapter.

In the absence of the coronary sinus[813] or atresia of the ostium, there may be minimal desaturation of systemic arterial blood if the coronary venous blood returns to the left side of the heart. The magnitude of flow is usually not sufficient to cause cyanosis which is clinically apparent.

Congenital Abnormalities of the Pericardium

Deficiency

Moore[814] classified pericardial defects into three groups as follows: (1) heart and left lung in a common cavity, 60 percent; (2) foramen between the pericardial and left pleural sacs, 21 percent; and (3) pericardium absent or rudimentary, 19 percent.

Nasser and associates[815] reported six cases of pericardial defect, two with partial absence and two with complete absence, each condition involving the left side of the pericardium.

Defects are three times more common in males than females. Commonly associated conditions involve the heart, lungs, pleural cavities, peritoneum, or kidneys. Two of Nasser's six patients had atrial septal defect. Other associated defects reported by Hipona and associates[816] were patent ductus arteriosus in four patients, bifid heart in two, tetralogy of Fallot in two, tricuspid insufficiency in one, bicuspid aortic valve in one, bronchogenic cysts in six, and aberrant pulmonary lobe in one. Bronchial cysts and enterogenous thoracic cysts have been reported as associated defects. Diaphragmatic pericardial defects may be combined into a pentalogy with abdominal wall defects, lower sternal defects, deficiency of the anterior diaphragm, and congenital intracardiac defects.[817]

Cysts and Diverticula

A true diverticulum communicates with the pericardial cavity; a cyst does not. These abnormalities were classified by Loehr[820] into the following three varieties:

1. Congenital true cysts: coelomic (mesodermal), lymphangiomatous, bronchial, or teratomatous
2. Acquired secondary to hematoma, neoplasm, or parasitic disease
3. Pseudocysts, pericardial diverticula encapsulating pericardial exudate

Pericardial cysts and diverticula are not rare. The cysts may be congenital pericardial coelomic cysts, which are usually not connected with the pericardium except by loose connective tissue. Lymphangiomatous cysts may arise from the pericardium and are usually multilocular. When the fibrous structure of the pericardium is weak, the serosa may herniate to form a diverticulum. When the diverticulum loses its connection with the pericardial sac, a pericardial cyst is formed.

Giant left atrial appendage has the potential of being confused with a pericardial cyst or diverticulum.[821]

Congenital pericardial deficiency[5,814,815,818] may not produce symptoms. Associated cardiac defects and defects of the thoracoabdominal wall can occur and dominate the clinical picture. A partial defect on the right can produce symptoms of obstruction of the superior vena cava due to herniation of the lung into the pericardium. The chest radiograph is diagnostic.

Partial defects on the left are rare causes of chest pain. The pain may be related to position. The left atrial appendage and ventricle can herniate and strangulate. Sudden death has been reported with left ventricular strangulation. There is also an increased risk of infection due to the communication of the pleural and pericardial cavities.

On physical examination with defects on the left, the apex impulse is displaced to the left and even posteriorly in some. The chest roentgenogram will demonstrate this leftward displacement and prominence of the pulmonary arterial segment. An unusual convexity on the left is seen with herniation of the left atrial appendage. Fluoroscopy is helpful. In those with defects on the left, the electrocardiogram may show right axis deviation and, less commonly, right ventricular hypertrophy. Echocardiographic study in patients with large defects on the left may mimic the findings of volume overload of the right ventricle.[819]

Surgery is usually recommended to remove any constrictive, or potentially constrictive, portions of the pericardium in symptomatic patients and in those with partial defects on the left in whom left ventricular strangulation is a risk.

A pericardial cyst or diverticulum[820] does not usually cause symptoms but is commonly discovered when a chest roentgenogram is obtained for an unrelated reason. A mass is then noted, usually in the right anterior cardiophrenic angle. Surgical exploration is required to exclude other diagnoses, such as tumors or a Morgagni hernia.

References

1. Mitchell, S. C., Korones, S. B., and Berendes, H. W.: Congenital Heart Disease in 56,109 Births: Incidence and Natural History, *Circulation,* 43:323, 1971.

2. Hoffman, J. I. E., and Christianson, R.: Congenital Heart Disease in a Cohort of 19,502 Births with Long-Term Follow-Up, *Am. J. Cardiol.,* 42:641, 1978.

3. Fyler, D. C.: Report of the New England Regional Infant Cardiac Program, *Pediatrics,* 65(suppl.):375, 1980.

4. Nadas, A. S., and Fyler, D. C.: "Pediatric Cardiology," 3d ed., W. B. Saunders Company, Philadelphia, 1972.

5. Hoffman, J. I. E.: Natural History of Congenital Heart Disease: Problems in Its Assessment with Special Reference to Ventricular Septal Defects, *Circulation,* 37:97, 1968.

6. Keith, J. D., Rowe, R. D., and Vlad, P.: "Heart Disease in Infancy and Childhood," 3d ed., The Macmillan Company, New York, 1978.

7. Miettinen, O. S., Reiner, M. L., and Nadas, A. S.: Seasonal Incidence of Coarctation of the Aorta, *Br. Heart J.,* 32:103, 1970.

8. Jaffee, O. C. (ed.): "Cardiac Development with Special Reference to Congenital Heart Disease" (proceedings, international symposium), University of Dayton Press, Dayton, Ohio, 1968.

9. Moss, A. J., Adams, F. H., and Emmanouilides, G. C.: "Heart Disease in Infants, Children, and Adolescents," 2d ed., The Williams & Wilkins Company, Baltimore, 1977.

10. Anderson, R. C.: Fetal and Infant Death, Twinning and Cardiac Malformations in Families of 2,000 Children with and 500 without Cardiac Defects, *Am. J. Cardiol.,* 38:218, 1976.

11. Nora, J. J., and Nora, A. H.: The Evolution of Specific Genetic and Environmental Counseling in Congenital Heart Diseases, *Circulation,* 57:205, 1978.

12. Comline, K. S., Cross, K. W., Dawes, G. S., and Nathanielze, P. W. (eds.): "Fetal and Neonatal Physiology" (proceedings, Sir Joseph Barcroft Centenary Symposium), Cambridge University Press, Cambridge, 1973.

13. Rudolph, A. M.: "Congenital Diseases of the Heart. Clinical-Physiologic Considerations in Diagnosis and Management," Year Book Medical Publishers, Inc., Chicago, 1974.

14. Rudolph, A. M., and Heymann, M. A.: Neonatal Circulation and Pathophysiology of Shunts, in H. J. Levine (ed.), "Clinical Cardiovascular Physiology," Grune & Stratton, Inc., New York, 1976, p. 597.

15. Young, M.: The Fetal and Neonatal Circulation, in W. F. Hamilton and P. Dow (eds.), "Handbook of Physiology," sec. 2, "Circulation," vol. 2, American Physiological Society, Washington, D.C., 1963, p. 1619.

16. Dawes, G. S.: "Foetal and Neonatal Physiology," Year Book Medical Publishers, Inc., Chicago, 1968.

17. Rudolph, A. M., and Heymann, M. A.: The Fetal Circulation, *Ann. Rev. Med.,* 19:195, 1968.

18. Rudolph, A. M.: The Changes in the Circulation after Birth: Their Importance in Congenital Heart Disease, *Circulation,* 41:343, 1970.

19. Heymann, M. A., and Rudolph, A. M.: Effects of Congenital Heart Diseases on Fetal and Neonatal Circulation, *Prog. Cardiovasc. Dis.,* 15:115, 1972.

20. Melmon, K. L., Cline, M. J., Hughes, T., and Nies, A. S.: Kinins: Possible Mediators of Neonatal Circulatory Changes in Man, *J. Clin. Invest.,* 47:1295, 1968.

21. Olley, P. M., and Coceani, F.: Use of Prostaglandins in Cardiopulmonary Diseases of the Newborn, in M. A. Heymann (ed.), "Prostaglandins in the Perinatal Period," Grune & Stratton, Inc., New York, 1980, p. 135.

22. Coceani, F., and Olley, P. M.: Role of Prostaglandins, Prostacyclin, and Thromboxanes in the Control of Prenatal Patency and Postnatal Closure of the Ductus Arteriosus, in M. A. Heymann (ed.), "Prostaglandins in the Perinatal Period," Grune & Stratton, Inc., New York, 1980, p. 109.

23. Rudolph, A. M.: Fetal and Neonatal Pulmonary Circulation, *Ann. Rev. Physiol.,* 41:383, 1979.

24. Levin, D. L., Heymann, M. A., Kitterman, J. A., Gregory, G. A., Phibbs, R. H., and Rudolph, A. M.: Persistent Pulmonary Hypertension of the Newborn Infant, *J. Pediatr.,* 89:626, 1976.

25. Peckham, G. J., and Fox, W. W.: Physiologic Factors Affecting Pulmonary Artery Pressure in Infants with Persistent Pulmonary Hypertension, *J. Pediatr.,* 93:1005, 1978.

26. Goetzman, B. W., Sunshine, P., Johnson, J. D., Wennberg, R. P., Hackel, A., Merten, D. F., Bartoletti, A. L., and Silverman, N. H.: Neonatal Hypoxia and Pulmonary Vasospasm: Response to Tolazoline, *J. Pediatr.,* 89:617, 1976.

27. Keith, J. D.: Congestive Heart Failure, in J. D. Keith, R. D. Rowe, and P. Vlad (eds.), "Heart Disease in Infancy and Childhood," 3d ed., The Macmillan Company, New York, 1978.

*28. Talner, N. S.: Heart Failure, in A. J. Moss, F. H. Adams, and G. C. Emmanouilides (eds.), "Heart Disease in Infants, Children, and Adolescents," 2d ed., The Williams & Wilkins Company, Baltimore, 1977. (60 references)

29. "Composition of Foods," Agriculture Handbook No. 8, USDA, 1963.

30. Jelliffe, R. W., and Brooker, G.: A Nomogram for Digoxin Therapy, *Am. J. Med.,* 57:64, 1974.

31. Halkin, H., Radomsky, M., Blieden, L., Frand, M., Millman, P., and Boichis, H.: Steady State Serum Digoxin Concentrations in Relation to Digitalis Toxicity in Neonates and Infants, *Pediatrics,* 61:184, 1978.

32. Baylen, B. G., Johnson, G., Tsang, R., Srivastava, L., and Kaplan, S.: The Occurrence of Hyperaldosteronism in Infants with Congestive Heart Failure, *Am. J. Cardiol.,* 45:305, 1980.

33. Lang, P., Williams, R. G., Norwood, W. I., and Castaneda, A. R.: The Hemodynamic Effects of

*This article is a review of the literature and contains additional references to the literature.

Dopamine in Infants after Corrective Cardiac Surgery," *J. Pediatr.*, 96:630, 1980.

34. Dillon, T. R., Janos, G. G., Meyer, R. A., and Kaplan, S.: Vasodilator Therapy for Congestive Heart Failure, *J. Pediatr.*, 96:623, 1980.

35. Olley, P. M.: Nonsurgical Palliation of Congenital Heart Malformations, *N. Engl. J. Med.*, 292:1292, 1975.

36. Houston, A. B., Gregory, N. L., and Coleman, E. N.: Two-Dimensional Sector Scanner Echocardiography in Cyanotic Congenital Heart Disease, *Br. Heart J.*, 39:1076, 1977.

37. Shannon, D. C., Lusser, M., Goldblatt, A., and Bunnell, J. B.: The Cyanotic Infant—Heart Disease or Lung Disease, *N. Engl. J. Med.*, 287:951, 1972.

38. Avery, G. B.: "Neonatology. Pathophysiology and Management of the Newborn," J. B. Lippincott Company, Philadelphia, 1975.

39. Danilowicz, D. A.: Delay in Bone Age in Children with Cyanotic Congenital Heart Disease, *Radiology*, 108:655, 1973.

40. Somerville, J.: Gout in Cyanotic Congenital Heart Disease, *Br. Heart J.*, 23:31, 1961.

41. Fischbein, C. A., Rosenthal, A., Fisher, E. G., Nadas, A. S., and Welch, K.: Risk Factors for Brain Abscess in Patients with Congenital Heart Disease, *Am. J. Cardiol.*, 34:97, 1974.

42. Cottrill, C. M., and Kaplan, S.: Cerebral Vascular Accidents in Cyanotic Congenital Heart Disease, *Am. J. Dis. Child.*, 125:484, 1973.

43. Phornphutkul, C., Rosenthal, A., Nadas, A. S., and Berenberg, W.: Cerebrovascular Accidents in Infants and Children with Cyanotic Congenital Heart Disease, *Am. J. Cardiol.*, 32:329, 1973.

44. Linderkamp, O., Klose, H. J., Betke, K., Brodherr-Heberlein, S., Buhlmeyer, K., Kelson, S., and Sengespeik, C.: Increased Blood Viscosity in Patients with Cyanotic Congenital Heart Disease and Iron Deficiency, *J. Pediatr.*, 95:567, 1979.

45. Wedemeyer, A. L., Edson, J. R., and Krivit, W.: Coagulation in Cyanotic Congenital Heart Disease, *Am. J. Dis. Child.*, 124:656, 1972.

46. Henriksson, P., Varendh, G., and Lundstrom, N.: Hemostatic Defects in Cyanotic Congenital Heart Disease, *Br. Heart J.*, 41:23, 1979.

47. Gross, S., Keefer, V., and Liebman, J.: The Platelets in Cyanotic Congenital Heart Disease, *Pediatrics*, 42:651, 1968.

48. Waldman, J. D., Czapek, E. E., Paul, M. H., Schwartz, A. D., Levin, D. L., and Schindler, S.: Shortened Platelet Survival in Cyanotic Heart Disease, *J. Pediatr.*, 87:77, 1975.

49. Krovetz, L. J., and Goldbloom, S.: Normal Standards for Cardiovascular Data. II. Pressures and Vascular Resistances, *Johns Hopkins Med. J.*, 130:187, 1972.

50. Rabinovitch, M., Haworth, S. G., Castenada, A. R., Nadas, A. S., and Reid, L. M.: Lung Biopsy in Congenital Heart Disease: A Morphometric Approach to Pulmonary Vascular Disease," *Circulation*, 58:1107, 1978.

*51. Vogel, J. H. K.: Pulmonary Hypertension, in A. J. Moss, F. H. Adams, and G. C. Emmanouilides (eds.), "Heart Disease in Infants, Children, and Adolescents," 2d ed., The Williams & Wilkins Company, Baltimore, 1977. (99 references)

52. Blount, S. G., Jr.: Comparison of Patients with Ventricular Septal Defect at High Altitude and Sea Level, in A. S. Nadas (ed.), Report from the Joint Study on the Natural History of Congenital Heart Defects, *Circulation*, 56(suppl. 1):1, 1977.

53. Heath, D., and Edwards, J. E.: The Pathology of Hypertensive Pulmonary Vascular Disease. A Description of Six Grades of Structural Changes in the Pulmonary Arteries with Special Reference to Congenital Cardiac Septal Defects, *Circulation*, 18:533, 1958.

54. Newfeld, E. A., Paul, M. H., Muster, A. J., and Idriss, F. S.: Pulmonary Vascular Disease in Complete Transposition of the Great Arteries: A Study of 200 Patients. *Am. J. Cardiol.*, 34:75, 1974.

55. Newfeld, E. A., Sher, M., Paul, M. H., and Nikaidoh, H.: Pulmonary Vascular Disease in Complete Atrioventricular Canal Defect, *Am. J. Cardiol.*, 39:721, 1977.

56. Graham, T. P., Jr.: The Eisenmenger Reaction and Its Management, in W. C. Roberts (ed.), "Congenital Heart Disease in Adults," F. A. Davis Company, Philadelphia, 1979.

57. Hallidie-Smith, K. A., and Goodwin, J. F.: The Eisenmenger Syndrome, in "Progress in Cardiology," Lea & Febiger, Philadelphia, 1974, vol. 3.

58. Blackstone, E. H., Kirklin, J. W., Bradley, E. L., DuShane, J. W., and Applebaum, A.: Optimal Age and Results in Repair of Large Ventricular Septal Defects, *J. Thorac. Cardiovasc. Surg.*, 72:661, 1976.

59. Nihill, M. R., and McNamara, D. G.: Magnification Pulmonary Wedge Angiography in the Evaluation of Children with Congenital Heart Disease and Pulmonary Hypertension, *Circulation*, 58:1094, 1978.

60: Kaplan, E. L., and Taranta, A. V. (eds.): "Infective Endocarditis: An American Heart Association Symposium" (Monograph No. 52), The American Heart Association, Inc., 1977.

61. Kaplan, E. L., Rich, H., Gersony, W., and Manning, J.: A Collaborative Study of Infective Endocarditis in the 1970s: Emphasis on Infections in Patients Who Have Undergone Cardiovascular Surgery, *Circulation*, 59:327, 1979.

62. Johnson, D. H., Rosenthal, A., and Nadas, A. S.: A Forty-Year Review of Bacterial Endocarditis in Infancy and Childhood, *Circulation*, 51:581, 1975.

63. Johnson, D. H., Rosenthal, A., and Nadas, A. S.: Bacterial Endocarditis in Children under 2 Years of Age, *Am. J. Dis. Child.*, 129:183, 1975.

64. Wann, L. S., Hallam, C. C., Dillon, J. C., Weyman, A. E., and Feigenbaum, H.: Comparison of M-Mode and Cross-Sectional Echocardiography in Infective Endocarditis, *Circulation*, 60:728, 1979.

65. Richardson, J. V., Karp, R. B., Kirklin, J. W., and Dismukes, W. E.: Treatment of Infective Endocarditis: A 10-Year Comparative Analysis, *Circulation*, 58:589, 1978.

66. Peterson, L. J., and Peacock, R.: The Incidence of Bacteremia in Pediatric Patients Following Tooth Extraction, *Circulation*, 53:676, 1976.

67. Committee on Rheumatic Fever and Bacterial Endocarditis of the Council on Cardiovascular Disease in the Young of the American Heart Association: Prevention of Bacterial Endocarditis, *Circulation*, 56:139A, 1977.

*68. Rosenthal, A., and Castaneda, A. R.: Growth and

Development after Cardiovascular Surgery in Infants and Children, *Prog. Cardiovasc. Dis.*, 18:27, 1975. (58 references)

69. Mehrizi, A., and Drash, A.: Growth Disturbance in Congenital Heart Disease, *J. Pediatr.*, 61:418, 1962.

70. Levy, R. J., Rosenthal, A., Fyler, D. C., and Nadas, A. S.: Birthweight of Infants with Congenital Heart Disease, *Am. J. Dis. Child.*, 132:249, 1978.

71. Godrey, S.: "Exercise Testing in Children: Applications in Health and Disease," W. B. Saunders Company, London, 1974.

72. James, F. W., Kaplan, S., Glueck, C. J., Tsay, J., Knight, M. J. S., and Sarwar, C. J.: Responses of Normal Children and Young Adults to Controlled Bicycle Exercise, *Circulation*, 61:902, 1980.

73. Riopel, D. A., Taylor, A. B., and Hohn, A. R.: Blood Pressure, Heart Rate, Pressure-Rate Product and Electrocardiographic Changes in Healthy Children during Treadmill Exercise, *Am. J. Cardiol.*, 44:697, 1979.

74. Cumming, G. R.: Maximal Exercise Capacity of Children with Heart Defects, *Am. J. Cardiol.*, 42:613, 1978.

75. Goldberg, S. J., Weiss, R., and Adams, F. H.: A Comparison of the Maximal Endurance of Normal Children and Patients with Congenital Cardiac Disease, *J. Pediatr.*, 69:46, 1966.

76. Goldberg, S. J., Weiss, R., Kaplan, E., and Adams, F. H.: Comparison of Work Required by Normal Children and Those with Congenital Heart Disease to Participate in Childhood Activities, *J. Pediatr.*, 69:56, 1966.

77. Reduto, L. A., Berger, H. J., Johnstone, D. E., Hellenbrand, W., Wackers, F. J. T., Whittemore, R., Cohen, L. S., Gottschalk, A., and Zaret, B. L.: Radionuclide Assessment of Right and Left Ventricular Exercise Reserve after Total Correction of Tetralogy of Fallot, *Am. J. Cardiol.*, 45:1013, 1980.

78. Manning, J. A.: Insurability and Employability of Young Cardiac Patients, *Pediatrics*, 60:126, 1977.

79. Liebman, J., and Plonsey, R.: Electrocardiography, in A. J. Moss, F. H. Adams, and G. C. Emmanouilides (eds.), "Heart Disease in Infants, Children, and Adolescents," 2d ed., The Williams & Wilkins Company, Baltimore, 1977.

80. Dexter, L., Haynes, F. W., Burwell, C. S., Eppinger, E. C., Sagerson, R. P., and Evans, J. M.: Studies of Congenital Heart Disease. II. The Pressure and Oxygen Content of Blood in the Right Auricle, Right Ventricle, and Pulmonary Artery in Control Patients, with Observations on the Oxygen Saturation and Source of Pulmonary "Capillary" Blood, *J. Clin. Invest.*, 26:554, 1947.

81. Barratt-Boyes, B. G., and Wood, E. H.: The Oxygen Saturation of Blood in the Vessels of Healthy Subjects, *J. Lab. Clin. Med.*, 50:93, 1957.

82. Schroeckenstein, R. F., Wasenda, G. J., and Edwards, J. E.: Valvular Competent Patent Foramen Ovale in Adults, *Minnesota Med.*, 55:11, 1972.

83. Edwards, J. E.: The Pathology of Atrial Septal Defect, *Semin. Roentgenol.*, 1:24, 1966.

84. Tandon, R., and Edwards J. E.: Atrial Septal Defect in Infancy, Common Association with Other Anomalies, *Circulation*, 49:1005, 1974.

85. Mody, M. R.: Serial Hemodynamic Observations in Secundum Atrial Septal Defect with Special Ref-

erence to Spontaneous Closure, *Am. J. Cardiol.*, 32:978, 1973.

86. Steinbrunn, W., Cohn, K. E., and Selzer, A.: Atrial Septal Defect Associated with Mitral Stenosis: The Lutembacher Syndrome Revisited, *Am. J. Med.*, 48:295, 1970.

87. Betriu, A., Wigle, E. D., Felderhof, C. H., and McLoughlin, M. J.: Prolapse of the Posterior Leaflet of the Mitral Valve Associated with Secundum Atrial Septal Defect, *Am. J. Cardiol.*, 35:363, 1975.

88. Holt, M., and Oram, S.: Familial Heart Disease with Skeletal Malformations, *Br. Heart J.*, 22:236, 1960.

*89. Bedford, D. E., Sellors, T. H., Somerville, W., Belcher, J. R., and Besterman, E. M. M.: Atrial Septal Defect and Its Surgical Treatment, *Lancet*, 1:1255, 1957. (37 references)

90. Raghib, G., Ruttenberg, H. D., Anderson, R. C., Amplatz, K., Adams, P., Jr., and Edwards, J. E.: Termination of Left Superior Vena Cava in Left Atrium, Atrial Septal Defect, and Absence of Coronary Sinus: A Developmental Complex, *Circulation*, 31:906, 1965.

91. Craig, R. J., and Selzer, A.: Natural History and Prognosis of Atrial Septal Defect, *Circulation*, 37:805, 1968.

92. Andersen, M., Lyngborg, K., Moller, I., and Wennevold, A.: Natural History of Small Atrial Septal Defects—Long-Term Follow-Up with Serial Heart Catheterizations, *Am. Heart J.*, 92:302, 1976.

93. Dave, K. S., Parkrashi, B. C., Wooler, G. H., and Ionescu, M. I.: Atrial Septal Defects in Adults. Clinical and Hemodynamic Results of Surgery, *Am. J. Cardiol.*, 31:7, 1973.

94. Hynes, K. M., Frye, R. L., Brandenburg, R. O., McGoon, D. C., Titus, J. L., and Guiliani, E. R.: Atrial Septal Defect (Secundum) Associated with Mitral Regurgitation, *Am. J. Cardiol.*, 34:333, 1974.

95. Popio, K. A., Gorlin, R., Teichholz, L. E., Cohn, P. F., Bechtel, D., and Herman, M. V.: Abnormalities of Left Ventricular Function and Geometry in Adults with an Atrial Septal Defect: Ventriculographic, Hemodynamic, and Echocardiographic Studies, *Am. J. Cardiol.*, 36:302, 1975.

96. Nasrallah, A. T., Hall, R. J., Garcia, E., Leachman, R. D., and Cooley, D. A.: Surgical Repair of Atrial Septal Defect in Patients over 60 Years of Age, Long-Term Results, *Circulation*, 53:329, 1976.

97. Hoffman, J. I. E., Rudolph A. M., and Danilowicz, D.: Left to Right Atrial Shunts in Infants, *Am. J. Cardiol.*, 30:868, 1972.

98. Wood. P.: The Eisenmenger Syndrome, *Br. Med. J.*, 2:701 and 755, 1958.

99. Brammell, H. L., Vogel, J. H. K., Pryon, R., and Blount, S. G., Jr.: The Eisenmenger Syndrome. A Clinical and Physiologic Reappraisal, *Am. J. Cardiol.*, 28:679, 1971.

100. Bedford, D. E.: The Anatomical Types of Atrial Septal Defect: Their Incidence and Clinical Diagnosis, *Am. J. Cardiol.*, 6:568, 1960.

101. Lee, M. E., and Sade, R. M.: Coronary Sinus Septal Defect: Surgical Considerations, *J. Thorac. Cardiovasc. Surg.*, 78:563, 1979.

102. Lynch, H. T., Bachenberg, K., Harris, R. E., and Becker, W.: Hereditary Atrial Septal Defect, *Am. J. Dis. Child.* 132:600, 1978.

103. Maron, B. J., Borer, J. S., Lau, S. H., Damato,

A. N., Scott, L. P., and Epstein, S. E.: Association of Secundum Atrial Septal Defect and Atrioventricular Nodal Dysfunction. A Generally Transmitted Syndrome, *Br. Heart J.*, 40:1293, 1978.

104. Kaufman, R. L., Rimoin, D. L., McAlister, W. H., and Hartmann, A. F.: Variable Expression of the Holt-Oram Syndrome, *Am. J. Dis. Child.*, 127:21, 1974.

*105. Noonan, J. A.: Association of Congenital Heart Disease with Syndromes or Other Defects, in "The Pediatric Clinics of North America," W. B. Saunders Company, Philadelphia, 1978, vol. 25, p. 797. (80 references).

106. Hunt, C. E., and Lucas, R. V., Jr.: Symptomatic Atrial Septal Defect in Infancy, *Circulation*, 47:1042, 1973.

107. Hamilton, W. T., Haffajee, C. I., Dalen, J. E., Dexter, L., and Nadas, A. S.: Atrial Septal Defect Secundum: Clinical Profile with Physiologic Correlates in Children and Adults, in W. C. Roberts and A. N. Brest (eds.), "Congenital Heart Disease in Adults," F. A. Davis Company, Philadelphia, 1979.

108. Tan King-Twok, T., Hashimoto, A., and Sato, T.: Electrocardiogram of Secundum Type Atrial Septal Defect Simulating Endocardial Cushion Defects, *Br. Heart J.*, 37:209, 1975.

109. Bierman, F. Z., and Williams, R. G.: Subxiphoid Two-Dimensional Imaging of the Interatrial Septum in Infants and Neonates with Congenital Heart Disease, *Circulation*, 60:80, 1979.

110. Weyman, A. E., Wann, L. S., Caldwell, R. L., Hurwitz, R. A., Dillon, J. C., and Feigenbaum, H.: Negative Contrast Echocardiography: A New Method for Detecting Left-to-Right Shunts, *Circulation*, 59:498, 1979.

111. Kronik, G., Slany, J., and Moesslacher, H.: Contrast M-Mode Echocardiography in Diagnosis of Atrial Septal Defect in Acyanotic Patients, *Circulation*, 59:372, 1979.

112. Lieppe, W., Scallion, R., Behar, V. S., and Kisslo, J. A.: Two Dimensional Echocardiographic Findings in Atrial Septal Defect, *Circulation*, 56:447, 1977.

113. Somerville, J., Katu, S., and Saravalli, O.: Prolapsed Mitral Cusps in Atrial Septal Defect: Erroneous Radiologic Interpretation, *Br. Heart J.*, 40:58, 1978.

114. Boucher, C. A., Liberthson, R. R., and Buckley, M. J.: Secundum Atrial Septal Defect and Significant Mitral Regurgitation, *Chest*, 75:6, 1979.

115. Schreiber, T. L., Feigenbaum, H., and Weyman, A. E.: Effect of Atrial Septal Defect Repair on Left Ventricular Geometry and Degree of Mitral Valve Prolapse, *Circulation*, 61:888, 1980.

116. Rashkind, W. J.: Experimental Transvenous Closure of Atrial and Ventricular Septal Defects, *Circulation*, 51/52(suppl. 2):8, 1975.

117. Nora, J. J., and Fraser, F. C.: "Medical Genetics: Principles and Practice," Lea & Febiger, Philadelphia, 1974.

118. Gross, R. E., Pomeranz, A. A., Watkins, E. Jr., and Goldsmith, E. I.: Surgical Closure of Defects of the Interauricular System by Use of an Atrial Well, *N. Engl. J. Med.*, 247:455, 1952.

119. Lewis, F. J., and Taufic, M.: Closure of Atrial Septal Defect with Aid of Hypothermia, *Surgery*, 33:1, 1953.

120. Gibbon, J. H.: Application of a Mechanical Heart and Lung Apparatus to Cardiac Surgery, *Minnesota Med.*, 37:171, 1954.

121. Kirklin, J. W., Ellis, F. H., Jr., and Wood, E. H.: Treatment of Anomalous Pulmonary Venous Connections in Association with Interatrial Communications, *Surgery*, 39:389, 1956.

122. Kyger, E. R., III, Frazier, O. H., Cooley, D. A., Gillette, P. C., Reul, G. J., Jr., Sandiford, F. M., and Wukasch, D. C.: Sinus Venous Atrial Septal Defect: Early and Late Results Following Closure in 109 Patients, *Ann. Thorac. Surg.*, 25:44, 1978.

123. Rahimtoola, S. H., Kirklin, J. W., and Burchell, H. B.: Atrial Septal Defect, *Circulation*, 37/38(suppl. 5):2, 1968.

124. Daicoff, G. R., Brandenburg, R. O., and Kirklin, J. W.: Results of Operation for Atrial Septal Defect in Patients Forty-Five Years of Age and Older, *Circulation*, 35/36(suppl. 1):143, 1967.

125. Kolbjorn, F., Simonsen, S., Andersen, A., and Efskind, L.: Atrial Septal Defect of Secundum Type in the Middle-Aged: Clinical Results of Surgery and Correlations between Symptoms and Hemodynamics, *Am. Heart J.*, 94:44, 1977.

126. McGoon, D. C., DuShane, J. W., and Kirklin, J. W.: The Surgical Treatment of Endocardial Cushion Defects, *Surgery*, 46:185, 1959.

127. Feldt, R. H.: "Atrioventricular Canal Defects," W. B. Saunders Company, Philadelphia, 1976.

128. Feldt, R. H., and Weidman, W. H.: Defects of the Atrial Septum and Endocardial Cushion, in A. J. Moss, F. H. Adams, and G. C. Emmanouilides (eds.), "Heart Disease in Infants, Children, and Adolescents," 2d ed., The Williams & Wilkins Company, Baltimore, 1977.

*129. Kiely, B., Filler, J., Stone, S., and Doyle, E. F.: Syndrome of Anomalous Venous Drainage of the Right Lung to the Inferior Vena Cava. A Review of 67 Reported Cases and Three New Cases in Children, *Am. J. Cardiol.*, 20:102, 1967. (67 references)

*130. Lucas, R. V., Jr., and Schmidt, R. E.: Anomalous Venous Connections, Pulmonary and Systemic, in A. J. Moss, F. H. Adams, and G. C. Emmanouilides (eds.), "Heart Disease in Infants, Children, and Adolescents," 2d ed., The Williams & Wilkins Company, Baltimore, 1977. (114 references)

131. Rowe, R. D.: Anomalies of Venous Return, in J. D. Keith, R. D. Rowe, and P. Vlad (eds.), "Heart Disease in Infancy and Childhood," The Macmillan Company, New York, 1978.

132. Saalouke, M. G., Shapiro, S. R., Perry, L. W., and Scott, L. P.: Isolated Partial Anomalous Pulmonary Venous Drainage Associated with Pulmonary Vascular Obstructive Disease, *Am. J. Cardiol.*, 39:439, 1977.

133. Friedli, B., Guerin, R., Davignon, A., Fouron, F. C., and Stanley, P.: Surgical Treatment of Partial Anomalous Pulmonary Venous Drainage: A Long-Term Follow-Up Study, *Circulation*, 45:159, 1972.

134. Murphy, J. W., Kerr, A. R., and Kirklin, J. W.: Intracardiac Repair for Anomalous Pulmonary Venous Connection of Right Lung to Inferior Vena Cava, *Ann. Thorac. Surg.*, 11:38, 1971.

135. Geraci, J. E., and Kirklin, J. W.: Transplantation of Left Anomalous Pulmonary Vein to Left

Atrium: Report of a Case, *Proc. Staff Meet. Mayo Clin.*, 28:472, 1953.

136. Edwards, J. E.: The Lewis A. Conner Memorial Lecture. Functional Pathology of the Pulmonary Vascular Tree in Congenital Cardiac Disease, *Circulation*, 15:164, 1957.

137. Becu, L. M., Swan, H. J. C., DuShane, J. W., and Edwards, J. E.: Ebstein Malformation of the Left Atrioventricular Valve in Corrected Transposition of the Great Vessels with Ventricular Septal Defect, *Proc. Mayo Clin.*, 30:483, 1955.

138. Goor, D. A., Edwards, J. E., and Lillehei, C. W.: The Development of the Interventricular Septum of the Human Heart. Correlative Morphogenetic Study, *Chest*, 58:453, 1970.

139. Neufeld, H. N., Titus, J. L., DuShane, J. W., Burchell, H. B., and Edwards, J. E.: Isolated Ventricular Septal Defect of the Persistent Common Atrioventricular Canal Type, *Circulation*, 23:685, 1961.

140. Titus, J. L., Daugherty, G. W., Kirklin, J. W., and Edwards, J. E.: Lesions of the Atrioventricular Conduction System after Repair of Ventricular Septal Defect. Relation to Heart Block, *Circulation*, 28:82, 1963.

141. Girod, D. A., Raghib, G., Adams, P., Jr., Anderson, R. C., Wang, Y., and Edwards, J. E.: Cardiac Malformations Associated with Ventricular Septal Defect, *Am. J. Cardiol.*, 17:73, 1966.

142. Liberthson, R. R., Paul, M. H., Muster, A. J., Arcilla, R. A., Eckner, F. A. O., and Lev, M.: Straddling and Displaced Atrioventricular Orifices and Valves with Primitive Ventricles, *Circulation*, 43:213, 1971.

143. Bharati, S., McAllister, H. A., Jr., and Lev, M.: Straddling and Displaced Atrioventricular Orifices and Valves, *Circulation*, 60:673, 1979.

144. Edwards, J. E.: Ventricular Septal Defect, Unresolved Problems, *Am. J. Cardiol.*, 19:832, 1967.

*145. Tatsuno, K., Konno, S., and Sakakibara, S.: Ventricular Septal Defect with Aortic Insufficiency, *Am. Heart J.*, 85:13, 1973. (14 references)

146. Campbell, M.: Natural History of Ventricular Septal Defect, *Br. Heart J.*, 33:246, 1971.

147. Jarmakani, J. M., Graham, T. P., Jr., and Canent, R. V., Jr.: Left Ventricular Contractile State in Children with Successfully Corrected Ventricular Septal Defect, *Circulation*, 45(suppl. 1): 102, 1972.

148. Collins, G., Calder, L., Rose, V., Kidd, L., and Keith, J.: Ventricular Septal Defect: Clinical and Hemodynamic Changes in the First Five Years of Life, *Am. Heart J.*, 84:695, 1972.

149. Allen, H. D., Anderson, R. A., Noren, G. R., and Moller, J. H.: Postoperative Follow-Up of Patients with Ventricular Septal Defect, *Circulation*, 50:465, 1974.

150. Buckberg, G. B., Fixler, D. E., Archie, J. P., and Hoffman, J. I. E.: Experimental Subendocardial Ischemia in Dogs with Normal Coronary Arteries, *Circ. Res.*, 30:67, 1972.

151. Shepherd, R. L., Glancy, D. L., Jaffe, R. B., Perloff, J. K., and Epstein, S. F.: Acquired Subvalvular Right Ventricular Outflow Obstruction in Patients with Ventricular Septal Defect, *Am. J. Med.*, 53:446, 1972.

152. Hoffman, J. I. E., and Rudolph, A. M.: The Natural History of Isolated Ventricular Septal Defect, *Adv. Pediatr.*, 17:57, 1970.

*153. Engle, M. A., and Kline, S. A.: Ventricular Septal Defect in the Adult, in W. C. Roberts (ed.), "Congenital Heart Disease in Adults," F. A. Davis Company, Philadelphia, 1979. (100 references)

154. Nora, J. J., and Nora, A. H.: "Genetics and Counseling in Cardiovascular Diseases," Charles C Thomas, Springfield, Ill., 1978.

155. Ahmad, M., and Hallidie-Smith, K. A.: Assessment of Left-to-Right Shunt and Left Ventricular Function in Isolated Ventricular Septal Defect, *Br. Heart J.*, 41:147, 1979.

156. Riggs, T., Mehta, S., Hirschfeld, S., Borkat, G., and Liebman, J.: Ventricular Septal Defect in Infancy: A Combined Vectorgraphic and Echocardiographic Study, *Circulation*, 59:385, 1979.

157. Breitweser, J. A., and Meyer, R. A.: Use of Echocardiography to Evaluate Structure and Function in Congenital Heart Disease, *Prog. Cardiol.*, 8:97, 1979.

158. Alpert, B. S., Cook, D. H., Varghese, P. J., and Rowe, R. D.: Spontaneous Closure of Small Ventricular Septal Defects: 10 Year Follow-Up, *Pediatrics*, 63:204, 1979.

159. Weidman, W. H., Blount, S. G., Jr. Du Shane, J. W., Gersony, W. M., Hayes, C. J., and Nadad, A. S.: Clinical Course in Ventricular Septal Defect, *Circulation*, 56(suppl. 1):1, 1977.

160. Blount, S. G., Jr.: Clinical Course in Adults with Ventricular Septal Defect at High Altitude and Sea Level, *Circulation*, 56(suppl. 1):1, 1977.

161. Keane, J. F., Plauth, W. H., Jr., and Nadas, A. S.: Ventricular Septal Defect with Aortic Regurgitation, *Circulation*, 56(suppl. 1): 1, 1977.

162. Muller, W. H., Jr., and Dammann, J. F., Jr.: The Treatment of Certain Congenital Malformations of the Heart by the Creation of Pulmonic Stenosis to Reduce Pulmonary Blood Flow: A Preliminary Report, *Surg. Gynecol. Obstet.*, 95:213, 1952.

163. Hallman, G. L., Cooley, D. A., and Bloodwell, R. D.: Two-Stage Surgical Treatment of Ventricular Septal Defect: Results of Pulmonary Artery Banding in Infants and Subsequent Open-Heart Repair, *J. Thorac. Cardiovasc. Surg.*, 52:476, 1966.

164. Rein, J., Freed, M. D., Norwood, W. I., and Castaneda, A. R.: Early and Late Results of Closure of Ventricular Septal Defect in Infancy, *Ann. Thorac. Surg.*, 24:19, 1977.

165. Barratt-Boyes, B. G., Neutze, J. M., Clarkson, P. M., Shardey, G. C., and Brandt, P. W. T.: Repair of Ventricular Septal Defect in the First Two Years of Life Using Profound Hypothermia—Circulatory Arrest Techniques, *Ann. Surg.*, 184:376, 1976.

166. Kirklin, J. W., and DuShane, J. W.: Repair of Ventricular Septal Defect in Infancy, *Pediatrics*, 27:961, 1961.

167. Barratt-Boyes, B. G., Simpson, M., and Neutze, J. M.: Intracardiac Surgery in Neonates and Infants Using Deep Hypothermia with Surface Cooling and Limited Cardiopulmonary Bypass, *Circulation*, 43/44(suppl. 1):25, 1971.

168. Cartmill, T. B., DuShane, J. W., McGoon, D. C., and Kirklin, J. W.: Results of Repair of Ventricular Septal Defect, *J. Thorac. Cardiovasc. Surg.*, 52:486, 1966.

169. Trusler, G. A., Moes, C. A. F., and Kidd, B. S. L.: Repair of Ventricular Septal Defect with Aortic Insufficiency, *J. Thorac. Cardiovasc. Surg.*, 66:394, 1973.

170. Milo, S., Ho, S. Y., Wilkinson, J. C., and Anderson, R. H.: Surgical Anatomy and Atrioventricular Conduction Tissues of Hearts with Isolated Ventricular Septal Defects, *J. Thorac. Cardiovasc. Surg.*, 79:244, 1980.

171. Malm, J. R.: Ventricular Septal Defects—Single Ventricle, in M. M. Ravitch, K. J. Welch, C. D. Benson, E. Aberdeen, and J. G. Randolph (eds.), "Pediatric Surgery," Year Book Medical Publishers, Inc., Chicago, 1979, p. 731.

172. Breckenridge, I. M., Stark, J., Waterston, D. J., and Bonham-Carter, R. E.: Multiple Ventricular Septal Defects, *Ann. Thorac. Surg.*, 13:128, 1972.

173. Aaron, B. L., and Lower, R. R.: Muscular Ventricular Septal Defect Repair Made Easy, *Ann. Thorac. Surg.*, 19:568, 1975.

174. Van Mierop, L. H. S., Alley, R. D., Kausel, H. W., and Stranahan, A.: The Anatomy and Embryology of Endocardial Cushion Defects, *J. Thorac. Cardiovasc. Surg.*, 43:71, 1962.

*175. Rogers, H. M., and Edwards, J. E.: Incomplete Division of the Atrioventricular Canal with Patent Interatrial Foramen Primum (Persistent Common Cardioventricular Ostium). Report of Five Cases and Review of the Literature, *Am. Heart J.*, 36:28, 1948. (54 references)

176. Wakai, C. S., and Edwards, J. E.: Developmental and Pathologic Considerations in Persistent Common Atrioventricular Canal, *Proc. Mayo Clin.*, 31:487, 1956.

177. Rastelli, G. C., Kirklin, J. W., and Titus, J. L.: Anatomic Observations on Complete Form of Persistent Common Atrioventricular Canal with Special Reference to Atrioventricular Valves, *Proc. Mayo, Clin.*, 41:296, 1968.

178. Cullum, L., and Liebman, J.: The Association of Congenital Heart Disease with Down's Syndrome (Mongolism), *Am. J. Cardiol.*, 24:354, 1969.

179. Laursen, H. B.: Congenital Heart Disease in Down's Syndrome, *Br. Heart J.*, 38:32, 1975.

*180. Wakai, C. S., and Edwards, J. E.: Pathologic Study of Persistent Common Atrioventricular Canal, *Am. Heart J.*, 66:779, 1958. (32 references)

181. Lev, M., Agustsson, M. H., and Arcilla, R.: The Pathologic Anatomy of Common Atrioventricular Orifice Associated with Tetralogy of Fallot, *Am. J. Clin. Pathol.*, 36:408, 1961.

182. Tandon, R., Moller, J. H., and Edwards, J. E.: Tetralogy of Fallot Associated with Persistent Common Atrioventricular Canal (Endocardial Cushion Defect), *Br. Heart J.*, 36:197, 1974.

183. Fisher, R. D., Bone, D. K., Rowe, R. D., and Gott, V. L.: Complete Atrioventricular Canal Associated with Tetralogy of Fallot. Clinical Experience and Operative Methods, *J. Thorac. Cardiovasc. Surg.*, 70:265, 1975.

184. Sridaromont, S., Feldt, R. H., Ritter, D. G., Davis, D. C., McGoon, D. C., and Edwards, J. E.: Double-Outlet Right Ventricle Associated with Persistent Common Atrioventricular Canal, *Circulation*, 52:933, 1975.

185. Tandon, R., Moller, J. H., and Edwards, J. E.: Unusual Longevity in Persistent Common Atrioventricular Canal, *Circulation*, 50:619, 1974.

186. Plett, J. A., Tandon, R., Moller, J. H., and Edwards, J. E.: Hypertensive Pulmonary Vascular Disease, *Arch. Path.*, 97:187, 1974.

187. Somerville, J.: Atrioventricular Defects, *Mod. Concepts Cardiovasc. Dis.*, 40:33, 1971.

188. Mehta, S., Hirschfeld, S., Riggs, T., and Liebman, J.: Echocardiographic Estimation of Ventricular Hypoplasia in Complete Atrioventricular Canal, *Circulation*, 59:888, 1979.

189. Hagler, D. J., Tajik, A. J., Seward, J. B., Mair, D. D., and Ritter, D. G.: Real-Time Wide-Angle Sector Echocardiography: Atrioventricular Canal Defects, *Circulation*, 59:140, 1979.

190. Bargeron, L. M., Jr., Elliott, L. P., Soto, B., Bream, P. R., and Curry, G. C.: Axial Cineangiography in Congenital Heart Disease. Sec. 1. Concept, Technical and Anatomical Considerations, *Circulation*, 56:1075, 1977.

191. Macartney, F. J., Rees, P. G., Daly, K., Piccoli, G. P., Taylor, J. F. N., DeLeval, M. R., Stark, J., and Anderson, R. H.: Angiographic Appearances of Atrioventricular Defects with Particular Reference to Distinction of Ostium Primum Atrial Septal Defect from Common Atrioventricular Orifice, *Br. Heart J.*, 42:640, 1979.

192. Culpepper, W., Kolff, J., Lin, C. Y., Vitullo, D., Lamberti, J., Arcilla, R. A., and Replogle, R.: Complete Common Atrioventricular Canal in Infancy—Surgical Repair and Postoperative Hemodynamics, *Circulation*, 58:550, 1978.

193. Berger, T. J., Kirklin, J. W., Blackstone, E. H., Pacifico, A. D., and Kouchokos, N. T.: Primary Repair of Complete Atrioventricular Canal in Patients Less than 2 Years Old, *Am. J. Cardiol.*, 41:906, 1978.

194. Berger, T. J., Blackstone, E. H., Kirklin, J. W., Bargeron, L. M., Jr., Hazelrig, J. B., and Turner, M. E., Jr.: Survival and Probability of Cure without and with Operation in Complete Atrioventricular Canal, *Ann. Thorac. Surg.*, 27:104, 1979.

195. Kirklin, J. W., and Blackstone, E. H.: Management of the Infant with Complete Atrioventricular Canal, *J. Thorac. Cardiovasc. Surg.*, 78:32, 1979.

196. Epstein, M. L., Moller, J. H., Amplatz, K., and Nicoloff, D. M.: Pulmonary Artery Banding in Infants with Complete Atrioventricular Canal, *J. Thorac. Cardiovasc. Surg.*, 78:28, 1979.

197. Danielson, G. K.: Endocardial Cushion Defects, in M. M. Ravitch, K. J. Welch, C. D. Benson, E. Aberdeen, and J. G. Randolph (eds.), "Pediatric Surgery," Year Book Medical Publishers, Inc., Chicago, 1979, p. 720.

198. Castaneda, A. R., Nicoloff, D. M., Moller, J. H., and Lucas, R. V., Jr.: Surgical Correction of Complete Atrioventricular Canal Utilizing Ball-Valve Replacement of the Mitral Valve: Technical Considerations and Results, *J. Thorac. Cardiovasc. Surg.*, 62:926, 1971.

199. Hines, G. L., Finnerty, T. T., Doyle, E., and Isom, O. W.: Near Fatal Hemolysis Following Repair of Ostium Primum Atrial Septal Defect, *J. Cardiovasc. Surg.*, 19:7, 1978.

200. Danielson, G. K., Guiliani, E. R., and Ritter, D. G.: Successful Repair of Common Ventricle Associated with Complete Atrioventricular Canal, *J. Thorac. Cardiovasc. Surg.*, 67:152, 1974.

201. Pacifico, A. D., Kirklin, J. W., and Bargeron, L. M., Jr.: Repair of Complete Atrioventricular Canal Associated with Tetralogy of Fallot or Double-Outlet Right Ventricle: Report of 10 Patients, *Ann. Thorac. Surg.*, 29:351, 1980.

202. Danielson, G. K., Tabry, I. F., Ritter, D. G., and Maloney, J. D.: Successful Repair of Double-Outlet Right Ventricle, Complete Atrioventricular Canal, and Atrioventricular Discordance Associated with Dextrocardia and Pulmonary Stenosis, *J. Thorac. Cardiovasc. Surg.*, 76:710, 1978.

203. Danielson, G. K., McMullan, M. H., Kinsley, R. H., and DuShane, J. W.: Successful Repair of Complete Atrioventricular Canal Associated with Dextroversion, Common Atrium, and Total Anomalous Systemic Venous Return, *J. Thorac. Cardiovasc. Surg.*, 66:817, 1973.

204. McMullan, M. H., McGoon, D. C., Wallace, R. B., Danielson, G. K., and Weidman, W. H.: Surgical Treatment of Partial Atrioventricular Canal, *Arch. Surg.*, 197:705, 1973.

205. Perry, E. L., Burchell, H. B., and Edwards, J. E.: Congenital Communication between the Left Ventricle and the Right Atrium. Coexisting Ventricular Septal Defect and Double Tricuspid Orifice, *Proc. Mayo Clin.*, 24:198, 1949.

206. Berbode, F., Hultgren, H., Melrose, D., and Osborn, J.: Syndrome of Left Ventricular–Right Atrial Shunt, *Ann. Surg.*, 148:433, 1958.

207. Lynch, D. L., Alexander, J. K., Hershberger, R. L., Mise, J., Dennis, E. W., and Cooley, D. A.: Congenital Ventriculo-Atrial Communication with Anomalous Tricuspid Valve, *Am. J. Cardiol.*, 1:404, 1958.

208. Elliott, L. P., Carey, L. S., Adams, P., Jr., and Edwards, J. E.: Left Ventricular–Right Atrial Communication in Complete Transposition of the Great Vessels, *Am. Heart J.*, 66:29, 1963.

209. Mills, P., McLaurin, L., Smith, C., Murray, G., and Craige, E.: Echocardiographic Findings in Left Ventricular to Right Atrial Shunts, *Br. Heart J.*, 39:594, 1977.

210. Jones, R. W. A., and Pickering, D.: Persistent Ductus Arteriosus Complicating Respiratory Distress Syndrome, *Arch. Dis. Child.*, 52:274, 1977.

211. Swan, C., Tostevin, A. L., Moore, B., Mayo, H., and Black, G. H. B.: Congenital Defects in Infants Following Infectious Diseases during Pregnancy, with Special Reference to the Relationship between German Measles and Cataract, Deaf-Mutism, Heart Disease and Microcephaly, and to the Period of Pregnancy in Which the Occurrence of Rubella is Followed by Congenital Anomalies, *Med. J. Aust.*, 2:201, 1943.

212. Hastreiter, A. R., Joarabchi, B., Pujatti, G., van de Horst, R. L., Patacsil, G., Sever, J. L.: Cardiovascular Lesions Associated with Congenital Rubella, *J. Pediatr.*, 71:59, 1967.

213. Wells, H. G., Persistent Patency of the Ductus Arteriosus, *Am. J. Med. Sci.*, 136:381, 1908.

214. Christie, A.: Normal Closing Time of the Foramen Ovale and the Ductus Arteriosus, *Am. J. Dis. Child.*, 40:323, 1930.

*215. Falcone, M. W., Perloff, J. K., and Roberts, W. C.: Aneurysm of the Nonpatent Ductus Arteriosus, *Am. J. Cardiol.*, 29:422, 1972.

216. Campbell, M.: Natural History of Persistent Ductus Arteriosus, *Br. Heart J.*, 30:4, 1968.

217. Kitterman, J. A., Edmonds, H., Jr., Gregory, G. A., Heymann, M. A., Tooley, W. H., and Rudolph, A. M.: Patent Ductus Arteriosus in Premature Infants, Incidence, Relation to Pulmonary Disease and Management, *N. Engl. J. Med.*, 287:473, 1972.

218. Heymann, M. A., and Rudolph, A. M.: Control of the Ductus Arteriosus, *Physiol. Rev.*, 55:62, 1975.

219. Friedman, W. F., Hirschklau, M. J., Printz, M. F., Pitlick, P. T., and Kirkpatrick, S. E.: Pharmacologic Closure of Patent Ductus Arteriosus in the Premature Infant, *N. Engl. J. Med.*, 295:526, 1976.

220. Heymann, M. A., Rudolph, A. M., and Silverman, N. H.: Closure of the Ductus Arteriosus by Prostaglandin Inhibition, *N. Engl. J. Med.*, 295:530, 1976.

221. Neal, W. A., Bessinger, F. B., Jr., Hunt, C. E., and Lucas, R. V., Jr.: Patent Ductus Arteriosus Complicating Respiratory Distress Syndrome, *J. Pediatr.*, 86:127, 1975.

222. Thibeault, D. W., Emmanouilides, G. C., Nelson, R. J., Lachman, R. S., Rosengart, R. M., and Oh, W.: Patent Ductus Arteriosus Complicating the Respiratory Distress Syndrome in Preterm Infants, *J. Pediatr.*, 86:120, 1975.

223. Siassi, B., Blanco, C., Cabal, L. A., and Coran, A. G.: Incidence and Clinical Features of Patent Ductus Arteriosus in Low-Birthweight Infants: A Prospective Analysis of 150 Consecutively Born Infants, *Pediatrics*, 57:347, 1976.

224. Krovetz, L. J., and Warden, H. E.: Patent Ductus Arteriosus: An Analysis of 515 Surgically Proven Cases, *Dis. Chest*, 42:46, 1962.

225. Krovetz, L. J.: Weight Gain in Children with Patent Ductus Arteriosus, *Dis. Chest*, 44:274, 1963.

226. Thapar, M. K., Rao, P. S., Rogers, J. H., Jr., Moore, H. V., and Strong, W. B.: Changing Murmur of Patent Ductus Arteriosus, *J. Pediatr.*, 92:939, 1978.

227. McGrath, R. L., McGuinness, G. A., Way, G. L., Wolfe, R. R., Nora, J. J., and Simmons, M. A.: The Silent Ductus Arteriosus, *J. Pediatr.*, 93:110, 1978.

228. Zuberbuhler, J. R., Lenox, C. C., Park, S. C., and Neches, W. H.: Continuous Murmurs in the Newborn, in D. J. Leon and J. A. Shaver (eds.), "Physiologic Principles of Heart Sounds and Murmurs," (American Heart Association Monograph no. 46), American Heart Association, New York, 1975, p. 209.

229. Brown, O. R., Harrison, D. C., and Popp, R. L.: An Improved Method for Echocardiographic Detection of Left Atrial Enlargement, *Circulation*, 50:58, 1974.

230. Silverman, N. H., Lewis, A. B., Heymann, M. A., and Rudolph, A. M.: Echocardiographic Assessment of Ductus Arteriosus Shunt in Premature Infants, *Circulation*, 50:821, 1974.

231. Bloom, K. R., Rodrigues, L., and Swan, E. M.: Echocardiographic Evaluation of Left-to-Right Shunt in Ventricular Septal Defect and Persistent Ductus Arteriosus, *Br. Heart J.*, 39:260, 1977.

232. Baylen, B. G., Meyer, R. A., Kaplan, S., Ringenburg, W. E., and Korfhagen, J.: The Critically Ill Premature Infant with Patent Ductus Arteriosus and Pulmonary Disease—An Echocardiographic Assessment, *J. Pediatr.*, 86:423, 1975.

233. Sahn, D. J., Vaucher, Y., Williams, D. E., Allen, H. D., Goldberg, S. J., and Friedman, W. F.: Echocardiographic Detection of Large Left to Right Shunts and Cardiomyopathies in Infants and Children, *Am. J. Cardiol.*, 38:73, 1976.

234. Baylen, B., Meyer, R. A., Korfhagen, J., Benzing, G., III, Bubb, M. E., and Kaplan, S.: Left Ventricular Performance in the Critically Ill Premature Infant with Patent Ductus Arteriosus and Pulmonary Disease, *Circulation*, 55:182, 1977.

235. Roberton, N. R. C.: Prolonged Continuous Positive Airways Pressure for Pulmonary Oedema Due to Persistent Ductus Arteriosus in the Newborn, *Arch. Dis. Child.*, 49:585, 1974.

236. Stevenson, J. G.: Fluid Administration in the Association of Patent Ductus Arteriosus Complicating Respiratory Distress Syndrome, *J. Pediatr.*, 90:257, 1977.

237. Krovetz, L. J., and Rowe, R. D.: Patent Ductus, Prematurity and Pulmonary Disease, *N. Engl. J. Med.*, 287:513, 1972.

238. Porstmann, W., Wierny, L., Warnke, H., Gerstberger, G., Romaniuk, P. A.: Catheter Closure of Patent Ductus Arteriosus: 62 Cases Treated without Thoracotomy, *Radiol. Clin. N. Am.*, 9:203, 1971.

239. Rashkind, W. J., and Cuaso, C. C.: Transcatheter Closure of Patent Ductus Arteriosus: Successful Use in a 3.5 Kilogram Infant, *Pediatr. Cardiol.*, 1:3, 1979.

240. Nadas, A. S.: Patent Ductus Revisited, *N. Engl. J. Med.*, 295:563, 1976.

241. Alpert, B. S., Lewins, M. J., Rowland, D. W., Grant, M. J. A., Olley, P. M., Soldin, S. J., Swyer, P. R., and Rowe, R. D.: Plasma Indomethacin Levels in Preterm Newborn Infants with Symptomatic Patent Ductus Arteriosus—Clinical and Echocardiographic Assessments of Response, *J. Pediatr.*, 95:578, 1979.

242. Merritt, T. A., White, C. L., Jacob, J., Kurlinski, J., Martin, J., DiSessa, T. G., Edwards, D., Friedman, W. F., and Gluck, L.: Patent Ductus Arteriosus Treated with Ligation or Indomethacin: A Follow-Up Study, *J. Pediatr.*, 95:588, 1979.

243. Cifuenks, R. F., Olley, P. M., Balfe, J. W., Radde, I. C., and Soldin, S. J.: Indomethacin and Renal Function in Premature Infants with Persistent Patent Ductus Arteriosus, *J. Pediatr.*, 95:583, 1979.

244. Halliday, H. L., Hirata, T., and Brady, J. P.: Indomethacin Therapy for Large Patent Ductus Arteriosus in the Very Low Birth Weight Infant: Results and Complications, *Pediatrics*, 64:154, 1979.

245. Edmunds, L. H., Jr., Gregory, G. A., Heymann, M. A., Kitterman, J. A., Rudolph, A. M., and Tooley, W. H.: Surgical Closure of the Ductus Arteriosus in Premature Infants, *Circulation*, 48:856, 1973.

246. Gay, J. H., Daily, W. J. R., Meyer, B. H. P., Trump, D. S., Cloud, D. T., and Moltham, M. E.: Ligation of the Patent Ductus Arteriosus in Premature Infants: Report of 45 Cases, *J. Pediatr. Surg.*, 8:677, 1973.

247. Lewis, C. E., Jr., Coen, R. W., Talbot, W., and Edwards, W. S.: Early Surgical Intervention in Premature Infants with Respiratory Distress and Patent Ductus Arteriosus, *Am. J. Surg.*, 128:829, 1974.

248. Murphy, D. A., Outerbridge, E., Stern, L., Karn, G. M., Jegier, W., and Rosales, J.: Management of Premature Infants with Patent Ductus Arteriosus, *J. Thorac. Cardiovasc. Surg.*, 67:221, 1974.

249. Jones, J. C.: Twenty-Five Years' Experience with Surgery of Patent Ductus Arteriosus, *J. Thorac. Cardiovasc. Surg.*, 50:149, 1965

250. Waterman, D. H., Samson, P. C., and Bailey, C. P.: The Surgery of Patent Ductus Arteriosus. A Report of the Section on Cardiovascular Surgery, *Dis. Chest*, 29:102, 1956.

251. Ellis, F. H., Jr., Kirklin, J. W., Callahan, J. A., and Wood, E. H.: Patent Ductus Arteriosus and Pulmonary Hypertension: Analysis of Patients Treated Surgically, *J. Thorac. Cardiovasc. Surg.*, 31:268, 1956.

252. Edmunds, L. H., Jr.: Operation or Indomethacin for the Premature Ductus, *Ann. Thorac. Surg.*, 26:586, 1978.

253. Neufeld, H. N., Lester, R. G., Adams, P., Jr., Anderson, R. C., Lillehei, C. W., and Edwards, J. E.: Aorticopulmonary Septal Defect, *Am. J. Cardiol.*, 9:12, 1962.

254. Tandon, R., daSilva, C. L., Moller, J. H., and Edwards, J. E.: Aorticopulmonary Septal Defect Coexisting with Ventricular Septal Defect, *Circulation*, 50:188, 1974.

255. Cooley, D. A., McNamara, D. G., and Latson, J. R.: Aorticopulmonary Septal Defect: Diagnosis and Surgical Treatment, *Surgery*, 42:101, 1957.

256. Morrow, A. G., Greenfield, L. J., and Braunwald, E.: Congenital Aortopulmonary Septal Defect. Clinical and Hemodynamic Findings, Surgical Technic, and Results of Operative Correction, *Circulation*, 25:463, 1962.

257. Blieden, L. C., and Moller, J. H.: Aorticopulmonary Septal Defect. An Experience with 17 Patients, *Br. Heart J.*, 36:630, 1974.

258. Putnam, T. C., and Gross, R. E.: Surgical Management of Aortopulmonary Fenestration, *Surg.*, 59:727, 1966.

259. Clarke, C. P., and Richardson, J. P.: The Management of Aortopulmonary Window. Advantages of Transaortic Closure with a Dacron Patch, *J. Thorac. Cardiovasc. Surg.*, 72:48, 1976.

260. Deverall, P. B., Aberdeen, E., Bonham-Carter, R. E., and Waterston, D. J.: Aortopulmonary Window, *J. Thorac. Cardiovasc. Surg.*, 57:479, 1969.

261. Aberdeen, E.: Aortic-Pulmonary Septal Defect, in M. M. Ravitch, K. J. Welch, C. D. Benson, E. Aberdeen, and J. G. Randolph (eds.), "Pediatric Surgery," Year Book Medical Publishers, Inc., Chicago, 1979, p. 720.

262. Richardson, J. V., Doty, D. B., Rossi, N. P., and Ehrenhaft, J. C.: The Spectrum of Anomalies of Aortopulmonary Septation, *J. Thorac. Cardiovasc. Surg.*, 78:21, 1979.

*263. Keane, J. F., Maltz, D., Bernhard, W. F., Corwin, R. D., and Nadas, A. S.: Anomalous Origin of One Pulmonary Artery from the Ascending Aorta: Diagnostic, Physiologic, and Surgical Considerations, *Circulation*, 50:588, 1974. (24 references)

264. Matsuda, H., Zavanella, C., Lee, P., and Subramanian, S.: Aortic Origin of the Right Pulmonary Artery, *Ann. Thorac. Surg.*, 24:374, 1977.

265. Edwards, J. E., Burchell, H. B., and Christensen, N. A.: Specimen Exhibiting the Essential Lesion in Aneurysm of the Aortic Sinus, *Proc. Mayo Clin.*, 31:407, 1956.

266. Edwards, J. E., and Burchell, H. B.: Pathologic Anatomy of Deficiencies between the Aortic Root

and the Heart Including Aortic Sinus Aneurysms, *Thorax*, 12:125, 1957.

*267. Sakakibara, S., and Konno, S.: Congenital Aneurysm of the Sinus of Valsalva. Anatomy and Classification, *Am. Heart J.*, 63:405, 1962. (109 references)

268. Eliot, R. S., Wolbrink, A., and Edwards, J. E.: Congenital Aneurysm of the Left Aortic Sinus. A Rare Lesion and a Rare Cause of Coronary Insufficiency, *Circulation*, 28:951, 1963.

269. Shumaker, H. B., Jr.: Aneurysms of the Aortic Sinuses of Valsalva Due to Bacterial Endocarditis with Special Reference to Their Operative Management, *J. Thorac. Cardiovasc. Surg.*, 63:896, 1972.

270. Kakos, G. S., Kilman, J. W., Williams, T. E., and Hosier, D. M.: Diagnosis and Management of Sinus of Valsalva Aneurysm in Children, *Ann. Thorac. Surg.*, 17:474, 1974.

271. Bulkley, B. H., Hutchins, G. M., and Ross, R. S.: Aortic Sinus of Valsalva Aneurysms Simulating Primary Right-Sided Valvular Heart Disease, *Circulation*, 52:696, 1975.

272. Meyer, J., Wukasch, D. C., Hallman, G. L., and Cooley, D. A.: Aneurysm and Fistula of the Sinus of Valsalva: Clinical Considerations and Surgical Treatment in 45 Patients, *Ann. Thorac. Surg.*, 19:170, 1975.

273. Shumacker, H. B., Jr., and Judson, W. E.: Rupture of Aneurysm of Sinus of Valsalva into Left Ventricle and Its Operative Repair, *J. Thorac. Cardiovasc. Surg.*, 45:650, 1963.

274. Nowicki, E. R., Aberdeen, E., Friedman, S., and Rashkind, W. J.: Congenital Left Aortic Sinus—Left Ventricle Fistula and Review of Aortocardiac Fistulas, *Ann. Thorac. Surg.*, 23:378, 1977.

275. Bonfils-Roberts, E. A., DuShane, J. W., McGoon, D. C., and Danielson, G.: Aortic Sinus Fistula—Surgical Considerations and Results of Operation, *Ann. Thorac. Surg.*, 12:492, 1971.

*276. Sade, R. M., Clouse, M., and Ellis, R. H., Jr.: The Spectrum of Pulmonary Sequestration, *Ann. Thorac. Surg.*, 18:644, 1974. (79 references).

*277. Telander, R. L., Lenox, C. C., and Sieber, W.: Sequestration of the Lung in Children, *Proc. Mayo Clin.*, 51:578, 1976. (36 references)

278. Ransom, J. M., Norton, J. B., and Williams, G. D.: Pulmonary Sequestration Presenting as Congestive Heart Failure, *J. Thorac. Cardiovasc. Surg.*, 76:378, 1978.

279. Litwin, S. B., Plauth, W. H., Jr., and Nadas, A. S.: Anomalous Systemic Arterial Supply to the Lung Causing Pulmonary-Artery Hypertension, *N. Engl. J. Med.*, 283:1098, 1970.

280. White, R. I., Jr., Kaufman, S. L., Barth, K. H., DeCaprio, V., and Strandberg, I. D.: Embolotherapy with Detachable Silicone Balloons: Technique and Clinical Results, *Radiology*, 131:619, 1979.

281. Zuberbuhler, J. R., Dankner, E., Zoltun, R., Burkholder, J., and Bahnson, H. T.: Tissue Adhesive Closure of Aortopulmonary Communications, *Am. Heart J.*, 88:41, 1974.

282. Thurer, R. J.: Communication between the Pulmonary and Systemic Circulation, *Ann. Thorac. Surg.*, 21:114, 1976.

283. Stewart, J. R., Kincaid, O. W., and Edwards, J. E.: "An Atlas of Vascular Rings and Related Malformations of the Aortic Arch System," Charles C Thomas, Publisher, Springfield, Ill., 1965.

*284. Edwards, J. E.: Congenital Cardiovascular Causes of Tracheobronchial and/or Esophageal Obstruction, in B. L. Tucker and G. G. Lindesmith (eds.), "Congenital Heart Disease," Grune & Stratton, Inc., New York, 1979, p. 49. (39 references)

285. Shuford, W. H., and Sybers, R. G.: "The Aortic Arch and its Malformations: With Emphasis on the Angiographic Features," Charles C Thomas, Inc., Springfield, 1973, p. 264.

286. Park, S. C., Siewers, R. D., Neches, W. H., Lenox, C. C., and Zuberbuhler, J. R.: Left Aortic Arch with Right Descending Aorta and Right Ligamentum Arteriosum, A Rare Form of Vascular Ring, *J. Thorac. Cardiovasc. Surg.*, 71:779, 1976.

287. Velasquez, G., Nath, P. H., Castaneda-Zuniga, W. R., Amplatz, K., and Formanek, A.: Aberrant Left Subclavian Artery in Tetralogy of Fallot, *Am. J. Cardiol.*, 45:811, 1980.

288. Gross, R. E.: Surgical Treatment for Dysphagia Lusoria, *Ann. Surg.*, 124:532, 1946.

289. Arciniegas, E.: Vascular Anomalies Compressing the Trachea and Esophagus, in M. M. Ravitch, K. J. Welch, C. D. Benson, E. Aberdeen, and J. G. Randolph (eds.), "Pediatric Surgery," Year Book Medical Publishers, Inc., Chicago, 1979, p. 649.

290. Knight, L., and Edwards, J. E.: Right Aortic Arch. Types and Associated Cardiac Anomalies, *Circulation*, 50:1047, 1974.

291. Rogers, H. M., Wilcox, A. Y., Jr., Reilly, L. E., and Edwards, J. E.: Congenital Vascular Ring: Report of a Case with Survival to 62 Years, *Am. Heart J.*, 60:281, 1960.

292. Edwards, J. E.: Pathology of Anomalies of the Thoracic Aorta, *Am. J. Clin. Pathol.*, 23:1240, 1953.

293. Klinkhamer, A. C.: Esophagography, in "Anomalies of the Aortic Arch System," Excerpta Medica Foundation, Amsterdam, 1969.

294. Hastreiter, A. R., D'Cruz, I. A., and Cantez, T.: Right-Sided Aorta. 1. Occurrence of Right Aortic Arch in Various Types of Congenital Heart Disease, *Br. Heart J.*, 28:722, 1966.

295. Stewart, J. R., Kincaid, O. W., and Titus, J. L.: Right Aortic Arch: Plain Film Diagnosis and Significance, *Am. J. Roentgenol.*, 97:377, 1966.

296. Miller, W. W., Nadas, A. S., Bernhard, W. F., and Gross, R. E.: Congenital Pulmonary Atresia with Ventricular Septal Defect, *Am. J. Cardiol.*, 21:673, 1968.

297. Gross, R. E.: Vascular Anomalies of the Thorax Producing Compression of the Trachea and Esophagus, in "The Surgery of Infancy and Childhood," W. B. Saunders Company, Philadelphia, 1953, p. 913.

298. Victorica, B. E., Van Mierop, L. H. S., and Elliott, L. P.: Right Aortic Arch Associated with Contralateral Congenital Subclavian Steal Syndrome, *Am. J. Roentgenol.*, 108:582, 1970.

299. Rodriguez, L., Iwkawa, T., Moes, C. A. F., Trusler, G. A., and Williams, W. G.: Surgical Implications of Right Aortic Arch with Isolation of Left Subclavian Artery, *Br. Heart J.*, 37:931, 1975.

300. Quist-Hanssen, S. V.: Mutual Compression of the Right Main Bronchus and an Abnormal Left Pulmonary Artery as Causes of the Death of a 7-Week Old Child, *Acta Paediatr. Scand.*, 37:87, 1949.

*301. Campbell, C. D., Wernly, J. A., Koltip, P. C., Vitullo, D., and Replogle, R. L.: Aberrant Left Pulmonary Artery (Pulmonary Artery Sling): Successful Repair and 24 Year Follow-Up Report, *Am. J. Cardiol.*, 45:316, 1980. (17 references)

*302. Gumbiner, C. H., Mullins, C. E., and McNamara, D. G.: Pulmonary Artery Sling, *Am. J. Cardiol.*, 45:311, 1980. (40 references)

303. Jue, K. L., Raghib, G., Amplatz, K., Adams, P., and Edwards, J. E.: Anomalous Origin of the Left Pulmonary Artery from the Right Pulmonary Artery, *Am. J. Roentgenol.*, 95:598, 1965.

304. Koopot, R., Nikaidoh, H., and Idriss, F. S.: Surgical Management of Anomalous Left Pulmonary Artery Causing Tracheobronchial Obstruction. Pulmonary Artery Sling, *J. Thorac. Cardiovasc. Surg.*, 69:239, 1975.

305. Cohen, S., and Landing, B.: Tracheostenosis and Bronchial Abnormalities Associated with Pulmonary Artery Sling, *Ann. Otol. Rhinol. Laryngol.*, 85:582, 1976.

306. Potts, W. C., Holinger, P. H., and Rosenblum, A. H.: Anomalous Left Pulmonary Artery Causing Obstruction to the Right Mainstem Bronchus, *J. Am. Med. Assoc.*, 155:1409, 1954.

307. Sade, R. M., Rosenthal, A., Fellows, K., and Castaneda, A. R.: Pulmonary Artery Sling, *J. Thorac. Cardiovasc. Surg.*, 69:333, 1975.

308. Massumi, R., Wiener, L., and Charif, P.: The Syndrome of Cervical Aorta: Report of a Case and Review of the Previous Cases, *Am. J. Cardiol.*, 11:678, 1963.

*309. McCue, C. M., Mauck, H. P., Jr., Tingelstad, J. B., and Kellett, G. N., Jr.: Cervical Aortic Arch, *Am. J. Dis. Child.*, 125:738, 1973. (19 references)

310. Edwards, J. E., Christensen, N. A., Clagett, O. T., and McDonald, J. R.: Pathologic Considerations in Coarctation of the Aorta, *Proc. Mayo Clin.*, 23:324, 1948.

311. Clagett, O. T., Kirklin, J. W., and Edwards, J. E.: Anatomic Variations and Pathologic Changes in 124 Cases of Coarctation of the Aorta, *Surg. Gynecol. Obstet.*, 98:103, 1954.

312. Edwards, J. E., Clagett, O. T., Drake, R. L., and Christensen, N. A.: The Collateral Circulation in Coarctation of the Aorta, *Proc. Mayo Clin.*, 23:333, 1948.

313. Becker, A. E., Becker, M. J., and Edwards, J. E.: Anomalies Associated with Coarctation of Aorta. Particular Reference to Infancy, *Circulation*, 41:1067, 1970.

314. Talner, N. S., and Berman, M. A.: Postnatal Development of Obstruction in Coarctation of the Aorta: Role of the Ductus Arteriosus, *Pediatrics*, 56:562, 1975.

315. Rosenquist, G. C.: Congenital Mitral Valve Disease Associated with Coarctation of the Aorta. A Spectrum That Includes Parachute Deformity of the Mitral Valve, *Circulation*, 49:985, 1974.

316. Reifenstein, G. H., Levine, S. A., and Gross, R. E.: Coarctation of the Aorta: A Review of 104 Autopsied Cases of the "Adult Type," 2 Years of Age or Older, *Am. Heart J.*, 33:146, 1947.

317. Drouin, B., Graisely, B., and Bouvrain, Y.: Insuffisance aortique et coarctation. À propos de deux observations, *Coeur Med. Intern.*, 15:109, 1976.

318. Maron, B. J., Humphries, J. O., Rowe, R. D., and Mellits, E. D.: Prognosis of Surgically Corrected Coarctation of the Aorta: A 20-Year Postoperative Appraisal, *Circulation*, 47:119, 1973.

319. Nanton, M. A., and Olley, P. M.: Residual Hypertension after Coarctectomy in Children, *Am. J. Cardiol.*, 37:769, 1976.

320. Ho, S. Y., and Anderson, R. H.: Coarctation, Tubular Hypoplasia, and the Ductus Arteriosus. Histological Study of 35 Specimens, *Br. Heart J.*, 41:268, 1979.

321. Simon, A. B., Zloto, A. E., Perry, B. L., and Sigmann, J. M.: Familial Aspects of Coarctation of the Aorta, *Chest*, 66:687, 1974.

322. Wing, J. P., Findlay, W. A., Sahn, D. J., McDonald, G., Allen, H. D., and Goldberg, S. J.: Serial Echocardiographic Profiles in Infants and Children with Coarctation of the Aorta, *Am. J. Cardiol.*, 41:1270, 1978.

323. Sahn, D. J., Allen, H. D., McDonald, G., and Goldberg, S. J.: Real Time Cross-Sectional Echocardiographic Diagnosis of Coarctation of the Aorta. A Prospective Study of Echocardiographic Angiographic Correlations, *Circulation*, 56:762, 1977.

324. Connors, J. P., Hartmann, A. F., and Weldon, C. S.: Considerations in the Surgical Management of Infantile Coarctation of Aorta, *Am. J. Cardiol.*, 36:489, 1975.

*325. Liberthson, R. R., Pennington, D. G., Jacobs, M. L., and Daggett, W. M.: Coarctation of the Aorta: Review of 234 Patients with Clarification of Management Problems, *Am. J. Cardiol.*, 43:835, 1979. (54 references)

*326. Hubbell, M. M., Jr., O'Brien, R. G., Krovetz, L. J., Mauck, H. P., and Tompkins, D. G.: Status of Patients 5 or More Years after Correction of Coarctation of the Aorta over Age 1 Year, *Circulation*, 60:74, 1979. (18 references)

*327. Freed, M. D., Rocchini, A., Rosenthal, A., Nadas, A. S., and Castaneda, A. R.: Exercise Induced Hypertension after Surgical Repair of Coarctation of the Aorta, *Am. J. Cardiol.*, 43:253, 1979. (16 references)

*328. Maron, B. J.: Coarctation of the Aorta in the Adult, in W. C. Roberts (ed.), "Congenital Heart Disease in Adults," F. A. Davis Company, Philadelphia, 1979. (21 references)

329. Heymann, M. A., Berman, W., Rudolph, A. M., and Whitman, V.: Dilatation of the Ductus Arteriosus by Prostaglandin E-1 in Aortic Arch Abnormalities, *Circulation*, 59:169, 1979.

330. Barash, P. G., Hobbins, J. C., Hook, R., Stansel, H. C., Jr., Whittemore, R., and Hehre, F.: Management of Coarctation of the Aorta during Pregnancy, *J. Thorac. Cardiovasc. Surg.*, 69:781, 1975.

331. Sehested, J.: Evaluation of Optimum Time for Surgical Repair of Coarctation of the Aorta, *Surg. Gynecol. Obstet.*, 146:593, 1978.

332. Kirklin, J. W., and Nadas, A. S.: Editorial Comments in W. P. Harvey, W. M. Kirkendall, J. W. Kirklin, A. S. Nadas, O. Paul, and E. H. Sonnenblick (eds.), "The Year Book of Cardiology—1979," Year Book Medical Publishers, Inc., Chicago, 1979, p. 286.

333. Craaford, C., and Nylin, G.: Congenital Coarctation of the Aorta and Its Surgical Treatment, *J. Thorac. Surg.*, 14:347, 1945.

334. Gross, R. E., and Hufnagel, C. A.: Coarctation of

the Aorta: Experimental Studies Regarding Its Surgical Correction, *N. Engl. J. Med.*, 233:287, 1945.

335. Gross, R. E.: Treatment of Certain Aortic Coarctations by Homologous Grafts: Report of 19 Cases, *Ann. Surg.*, 134:753, 1951.

336. Morris, G. C., Cooley, D. A., DeBakey, M. E., and Crawford, E. S.: Coarctation of the Aorta with Particular Emphasis upon Improved Techniques of Surgical Repair, *J. Thorac. Cardiovasc. Surg.*, 40:705, 1960.

337. Edie, R. N., Janani, J. Attai, L. A., Malm, J. R., and Robinson, G.: Bypass Grafts for Recurrent or Complex Coarctations of the Aorta, *Ann. Thorac. Surg.*, 20:558, 1975.

338. Amato, J. J., Rheinlander, H. F., and Cleveland, R. J.: Method of Enlarging the Distal Transverse Arch in Infants with Hypoplasia and Coarctation of the Aorta, *Ann. Thorac. Surg.*, 23:261, 1977.

339. Venturini, A., Perna, A. M., and Bianchi, G.: Repair of Coarctation of Thoracic Aorta without Resection: Patch Graft Aortoplasty: Follow-Up Study of 46 Cases, *J. Cardiovasc. Surg.* (Torino), 19:49, 1978.

340. Vosschulte, K.: Surgical Correction of Coarctation of the Aorta by an "Isthmusplastic" Operation, *Thorax*, 16:338, 1961.

341. Reul, G. J., Jr., Kabbani, S. S., Sandiford, F. M., Wukasch, D. C., and Cooley, D. A.: Repair of Coarctation of the Thoracic Aorta by Patch Graft Angioplasty, *J. Thorac. Cardiovasc. Surg.*, 68:696, 1974.

342. Pierce, W. S., Waldhausen, J. A., Berman, W., Jr., and Whitman, V.: Late Results of the Subclavian Flap Procedure in Infants with Coarctation of the Thoracic Aorta, *Circulation*, 58(suppl. 1):78, 1978.

343. Tiraboschi, R., Alfieri, O., Carpentier, A., and Parenzan, L.: One-Stage Correction of Coarctation of the Aorta Associated with Intracardiac Defects in Infancy, *J. Cardiovasc. Surg.* (Torino), 19:11, 1978.

344. Fox, S., Pierce, W. S., and Waldhausen, J. A.: Pathogenesis of Paradoxical Hypertension after Coarctation Repair, *Ann. Thorac. Surg.*, 29:135, 1980.

345. Williams, W. G., Shindo, G., Trusler, G. A., Dische, M. R., and Olley, P. M.: Results of Repair of Coarctation of the Aorta during Infancy, *J. Thorac. Cardiovasc. Surg.*, 69:603, 1980.

346. Pierpont, M. E. M., Zollikofer, C. L., Moller, J. H., and Edwards, J. E.: Interruption of the Aortic Arch with Right Descending Aorta. A Rare Condition and a Cause of Bronchial Compression, unpublished data.

347. Moller, J. H., and Edwards, J. E.: Interruption of Aortic Arch. Anatomic Patterns and Associated Cardiac Malformations, *Am. J. Roentgenol.*, 95:557, 1965.

348. Becu, L. M., Tauxe, W. N., DuShane, J. W., and Edwards, J. E.: A Complex of Congenital Cardiac Anomalies: Ventricular Septal Defect, Biventricular Origin of the Pulmonary Trunk, and Subaortic Stenosis, *Am. Heart J.*, 50:901, 1955.

349. Van Praagh, R., Bernhard, W. F., Rosenthal, A., Parisi, L. F., and Fyler, D. C.: Interrupted Aortic Arch: Surgical Treatment, *Am. J. Cardiol.*, 27:200, 1971.

*350. Collins-Nakai, R. L., Dick, M., Paresi-Buckley, L., Fyler, D. C., and Castaneda, A. R.: Interrupted Aortic Arch in Infancy, *J. Pediatr.*, 88:959, 1976. (30 references)

351. Dische, M. R., Tsai, M., and Baltaxe, H. A.: Solitary Interruption of the Arch of the Aorta. Clinicopathologic Review of Eight Cases, *Amer. J. Cardiol.*, 35:271, 1975.

352. Jones, E. L., Plauth, W. H., and Hatcher, C. R., Jr.: A Palliative Operation for All Types of Aortic Arch Interruption in the Neonate, *J. Thorac. Cardiovasc. Surg.*, 69:579, 1975.

353. Copeland, J. G., Record, J. A., Salomon, N. W., Sahn, D. J., Allen, H. D., and Goldberg, S. J.: Successful Palliation Using Partial Cardiopulmonary Bypass in a Two-Day-Old Infant with Type B Interruption of the Aortic Arch, *J. Thorac. Cardiovasc. Surg.*, 76:495, 1980.

354. Monro, J. L., Brawn, W., and Conway, N.: Correction of Type B Interrupted Aortic Arch with Ventricular Septal Defect in Infancy, *J. Thorac. Cardiovasc. Surg.*, 74:618, 1977.

355. Muraoka, R., Yokota, M., Aoshima, M., Nomoto, S., Osaragi, M., Kyoku, I., Nakano, H., Ueda, K., and Saito, A.: Simplified Method for Total Correction of Interrupted Aortic Arch with Ventricular Septal Defect in Infancy, *J. Thorac. Cardiovasc. Surg.*, 78:744, 1979.

356. Ito, K., Kohguchi, N., Ohkawa, Y., Akasaka, T., Ohara, H., Takarada, M., Aoki, H., Ogata, M., Nishibatake, M., Fukatsu, O., and Matsushima, K.: Total One-Stage Repair of Interrupted Aortic Arch Associated with Aortic Septal Defect and Patent Ductus Arteriosus, *J. Thorac. Cardiovasc. Surg.*, 74:913, 1977.

357. Barratt-Boyes, B. G., Nicholls, T. T., Brandt, P. W. T., and Neutze, J. M.: Aortic Arch Interruption Associated with Patent Ductus Arteriosus, Ventricular Septal Defect, and Total Anomalous Pulmonary Venous Connection, *J. Thorac. Cardiovasc. Surg.*, 63:367, 1972.

358. Murphy, D. A., Lemire, G. G., Tessler, I., and Dunn, G. L.: Correction of Type B Aortic Arch Interruption with Ventricular and Atrial Septal Defects in a Three-Day-Old Infant, *J. Thorac. Cardiovasc. Surg.*, 65:882, 1973.

359. Bowman, F. O., in discussion of Fishman, N. H., Bronstein, M. H., Berman, W., Jr., Rol, B. B., Edmunds, L. H., Jr., Robinson, S. J., and Rudolph, A. M.: Surgical Management of Severe Aortic Coarctation and Interrupted Aortic Arch in Neonates, *J. Thorac. Cardiovasc. Surg.*, 71:35, 1976.

360. Trusler, G. A., and Izukawa, T.: Interrupted Aortic Arch and Ventricular Septal Defect. Direct Repair through a Median Sternotomy Incision in a 13-Day Old Infant, *J. Thorac. Cardiovasc. Surg.*, 69:126, 1975.

361. Roberts, W. C.: Valvular, Subvalvular, and Supravalvular Aortic Stenosis: Morphologic Features, *Cardiovasc. Clin. Series* 5/1, F. A. Davis Company, Philadelphia, 1973, p. 98.

362. Edwards, J. E.: Pathologic Aspects of Cardiac Valvular Insufficiency, *Arch. Surg.*, 77:634, 1958.

363. Roberts, W. C., and Morrow, A. G.: Congenital Aortic Stenosis Produced by a Unicommissural Valve, *Br. Heart J.*, 27:505, 1965.

364. Moller, J. H., Nakib, A., and Edwards, J. E.: Infarction of Papillary Muscles and Mitral Insufficiency Associated with Congenital Aortic Stenosis, *Circulation*, 34:87, 1966.

365. Vincent, W. R., Buckberg, G. D., and Hoffman, J. I. E.: Left Ventricular Subendocardial Ischemia in Severe Valvular and Supravalvular Aortic Stenosis: A Common Mechanism, *Circulation*, 49:326, 1974.

366. Lewis, A. B., Heymann, M. A., Stanger, P., Hoffman, J. I. E., and Rudolph, A. M.: Evaluation of Subendocardial Ischemia in Valvular Aortic Stenosis in Children, *Circulation*, 49:978, 1974.

367. Lakier, J. B., Lewis, A. B., Heymann, M. A., Stanger, P., Hoffman, J. I. E., and Rudolph, A. M.: Isolated Aortic Stenosis in the Neonate: Natural History and Hemodynamic Considerations, *Circulation*, 50:801, 1974.

368. Conkle, D. M., Jones, M., and Morrow, A. G.: Treatment of Congenital Aortic Stenosis: An Evaluation of the Late Results of Aortic Valvotomy, *Arch. Surg.*, 107:649, 1973.

369. Rudolph, A. M., Heymann, M. A., and Spitznas, U.: Hemodynamic Considerations in the Development of Narrowing of the Aorta, *Am. J. Cardiol.*, 30:514, 1972.

370. Roberts, W. C.: The Congenitally Bicuspid Aortic Valve. A Study of 85 Autopsy Cases, *Am. J. Cardiol.*, 26:72, 1970.

371. Wagner, H. R., Ellison, R. C., Keane, J. F., Humphries, J. O., and Nadas, A. S.: Clinical Course in Aortic Stenosis, in A. S. Nadas (ed.), "Pulmonary Stenosis, Aortic Stenosis, Ventricular Septal Defect: Clinical Course and Indirect Assessment" (report from the Joint Study on the Natural History of Congenital Heart Defects), *Circulation*, 55(suppl. 1):1, 1977.

372. Wagner, H. R., Weidman, W. H., Ellison, R. C., and Miettinen, O. S.: Indirect Assessment of Severity in Aortic Stenosis, in A. S. Nadas (ed.), "Pulmonary Stenosis, Aortic Stenosis Ventricular Septal Defect: Clinical Course and Indirect Assessment" (report from the Joint Study on the Natural History of Congenital Heart Defects), *Circulation*, 55(suppl. 1):1, 1977.

*373. Chandramouli, B., Ehmke, D. A., and Lauer, R. M.: Exercise-Induced Electrocardiogram Changes in Aortic Stenosis, *J. Pediatr.*, 87:725, 1974. (24 references)

374. Gewitz, M. H., Werner, J. C., Kleinman, C. S., Hellenbrand, W. E., and Talner, N. S.: Role of Echocardiography in Aortic Stenosis: Pre and Post Operative Studies, *Am. J. Cardiol.*, 43:67, 1979.

375. Berry, T. E., Aziz, K. U., and Paul, M. H.: Echocardiographic Assessment of Discrete Subaortic Stenosis in Childhood, *Am. J. Cardiol.*, 43:957, 1979.

376. Weyman, A. E., Feigenbaum, H., Hurwitz, R. A., Girod, D. A., and Dillon, J. C.: Cross Sectional Echographic Assessment of the Severity of Aortic Stenosis in Children, *Circulation*, 55:773, 1977.

377. Kugler, J. D., Campbell, E., Vargo, T. A., McNamara, D. G., Hallman, G. L., and Cooley, D. A.: Results of Aortic Valvulotomy in Infants with Isolated Aortic Valvular Stenosis, *J. Thorac. Cardiovasc. Surg.*, 78:553, 1979.

378. Orsmond, G. S., Bessinger, F. B., Jr., and Moller, J. H.: Rest and Exercise Hemodynamics in Children before and after Aortic Valvotomy, *Am. Heart J.*, 99:76, 1980.

379. Lawson, R. M., Bonchek, L. I., Menashe, V., and Starr, A.: Late Results of Surgery for Left Ventricular Outflow Tract Obstruction in Children, *J. Thorac. Cardiovasc. Surg.*, 71:334, 1976.

380. Smith, J. M., III, Cooley, D. A., Ott, D. A., Ferreira, W., and Reul, G. J., Jr.: Aortic Valve Replacement in Preteenage Children, *Ann. Thorac. Surg.*, 29:512, 1980.

381. Wada, J., Yokoyama, M., Hashimoto, A., Imai, Y., Kitamura, N., Takao, A., and Momma, K.: Long-Term Follow-Up of Artificial Valves in Patients under 15 Years Old, *Ann. Thorac. Surg.*, 29:519, 1980.

382. Jack, W. D., II, and Kelly, D. T.: Long-Term Follow-Up of Valvulotomy for Congenital Aortic Stenosis, *Am. J. Cardiol.*, 38:231, 1976.

383. Chiariello, L., Agosti, J., Vlad, P., and Subramanian, S.: Congenital Aortic Stenosis—Experience with 43 Patients, *J. Thorac. Cardiovasc. Surg.*, 72:182, 1976.

384. Keane, J. F., Bernhard, W. F., and Nadas, A. S.: Aortic Stenosis Surgery in Infancy, *Circulation*, 52:1138, 1975.

385. Rastan, H., and Koncz, J.: Aortoventriculoplasty, *J. Thorac. Cardiovasc. Surg.*, 71:920, 1976.

386. Norman, J. C., Cooley, D. A., Hallman, G. L., and Nihill, M. R.: Left Ventricular Apical–Abdominal Aortic Conduits for Left Ventricular Outflow Tract Obstructions, *Circulation*, 56:62, 1977.

387. Newfeld, E. A., Muster, A. J., Paul, M. H., Idriss, F. S., and Riker, W. L.: Discrete Subvalvular Aortic Stenosis in Childhood. Study of 51 Patients, *Am. J. Cardiol.*, 38:53, 1976.

388. Maron, B. J., Ferrans, V. J., Henry, W. L., Clark, C. E., Redwood, D. R., Roberts, W. C., Morrow, A. G., and Epstein, S. E.: Differences in Distribution of Myocardial Abnormalities in Patients with Obstructive and Nonobstructive Asymmetric Septal Hypertrophy (ASH). Light and Electron Microscopic Findings, *Circulation*, 50:436, 1974.

389. Sellers, R. D., Lillehei, C. W., and Edwards, J. E.: Subaortic Stenosis Caused by Anomalies of the Atrioventricular Valves, *J. Thorac. Cardiovasc. Surg.*, 48:289, 1964.

390. Krueger, S. K., French, J. W., Forker, A. D., Caudill, C. C., and Popp, R. L.: Echocardiography in Discrete Subaortic Stenosis, *Circulation*, 59:506, 1979.

391. Lange, L. W., Sahn, D. J., Allen, H. D., and Goldberg, S. J.: Subxiphoid Cross-Sectional Echocardiography in Infants and Children with Congenital Heart Disease, *Circulation*, 59:513, 1979.

392. Maron, B. J., Redwood, D. R., Roberts, W. C., Henry, W. L., Morrow, A. G., and Epstein, S. E.: Tunnel Subaortic Stenosis, *Circulation*, 54:404, 1976.

393. Sung, C. S., Price, E. C., and Cooley, D. A.: Discrete Subaortic Stenosis in Adults, *Am. J. Cardiol.*, 42:283, 1978.

394. Bjornstad, P. G., Rastan, H., Keutel, J., Buren, A. J., and Koncz, J.: Aortoventriculoplasty for Tunnel Aortic Stenosis and Other Obstructions of the Left Ventricular Outflow Tract. Clinical and Hemodynamic Results. *Circulation*, 60:59, 1979.

395. Bjork, V. D., Holtquist, G., and Lodin, H.: Subaortic Stenosis Produced by Abnormalcy Plated Anterior Mitral Leaflet, *J. Thorac. Cardiovasc. Surg.*, 41:659, 1961.

396. Reis, R. L., Peterson, L. M., Mason, D. T., Simon, A. L., and Morrow, A. G.: Congenital Fixed Sub-

valvular Aortic Stenosis: An Anatomical Classification and Correlations with Operative Results, *Circulation*, 43/44(suppl. 1):11, 1971.

397. Manouguian, S., Kirchoff, P., Koncz, J., Corovic, D., and Dahn, D.: Ventricular Septal Defect Associated with Fibrous Subvalvular Aortic Stenosis: Diagnostic Problems and Surgical Management, *Thoraxchirurgie*, 23:444, 1975.

398. Katz, N. M., Buckley, M. J., and Liberthson, R. R.: Discrete Membranous Subaortic Stenosis: Report of 31 Patients, Review of the Literature, and Delineation of Management, *Circulation*, 56:1034, 1977.

399. Morrow, A. G.: Hypertrophic Subaortic Stenosis: Operative Methods Used to Relieve Left Ventricular Outflow Obstruction, *J. Thorac. Cardiovasc. Surg.*, 76:423, 1978.

400. Peterson, T. A., Todd, D. B., and Edwards, J. E.: Supravalvular Aortic Stenosis, *J. Thor. Cardiovasc. Surg.*, 50:734, 1965.

401. Blieden, L. C., Lucas, R. V., Jr., Carter, J. B., Miller, K., and Edwards, J. E.: A Developmental Complex Including Supravalvular Stenosis of the Aorta and Pulmonary Trunk, *Circulation*, 49:585, 1974.

402. Beuren, A. J., Schulze, G., Eberle, P., Harmjanz, D., and Apitz, A.: The Syndrome of Supravalvular Aortic Stenosis, Peripheral Pulmonary Stenosis, Mental Retardation and Similar Facial Appearance, *Am. J. Cardiol.*, 13:471, 1964.

403. Char, F., and Rowe, R. D.: Infantile Hypercalcemia Syndrome with Mitral Regurgitation and Hypoplasia of Aorta, *Birth Defects: Original Article Series* (The National Foundation—March of Dimes), 8:258, 1972.

404. Chernausek, S. D., Swan, D. S., Moller, J. H., Vlodaver, Z., and Edwards, J. E.: Supravalvular Aortic Stenosis Forme Fruste, with Left Coronary Ostial Stenosis; Neonatal Acute Myocardial Infarction; Persistent Truncus Arteriosus, Type II; Right Aortic Arch with Aberrant Left Subclavian Artery; Atrial Septal Defect, Small, *Am. Heart J.*, 91:249, 1976.

405. French, J. W., and Guntheroth, W. G.: An Explanation of Asymmetric Upper Extremity Blood Pressures in Supravalvular Aortic Stenosis: The Coanda Effect, *Circulation*, 42:31, 1970.

406. Martin, E. C., and Moseley, I. F.: Supravalvular Aortic Stenosis, *Br. Heart J.*, 35:758, 1973.

*407. Johnson, L. W., Fishman, R. A., Schneider, B., Parker, F. B., Jr., Husson, G., and Webb, W. R.: Familial Supravalvular Aortic Stenosis, *Chest*, 70:494, 1976. (23 references)

*408. Folger, G. M., Jr.: Further Observations on the Syndrome of Idiopathic Infantile Hypercalcemia Associated with Supraventricular Aortic Stenosis, *Am. Heart J.*, 93:455, 1977. (32 references)

*409. Pansegrau, D. G., Kioshos, J. M., Durnin, R. E., and Kroetz, F. W.: Supravalvular Aortic Stenosis in Adults, *Am. J. Cardiol.*, 31:635, 1973. (71 references)

*410. Varghese, P. J., Izukawa, T., and Rose, R. D.: Supravalvular Aortic Stenosis as Part of Rubella Syndrome, with Discussion of Pathogenesis, *Br. Heart J.*, 31:59, 1969.

*411. Weyman, A. E., Caldwell, R. L., Hurwitz, R. A., Girod, D. A., Dillon, J. C., Feigenbaum, H., and Green, D.: Cross-Sectional Echocardiographic Characterization of Aortic Obstruction. I. Supravalvular Aortic Stenosis and Aortic Hypoplasia, *Circulation*, 57:491, 1978.

412. Rastelli, G. C., McGoon, D. C., Ongley, P. A., Mankin, H. T., and Kirklin, J. W.: Surgical Treatment of Supravalvular Aortic Stenosis: Report of 16 Cases and Review of Literature, *J. Thorac. Cardiovasc. Surg.*, 51:873, 1966.

413. Williams, J. C. P., Barratt-Boyes, B. G., and Lowe, J. B.: Supravalvular Aortic Stenosis, *Circulation*, 24:1311, 1961.

414. Doty, D. B., Polansky, D. B., and Jenson, C. B.: Supravalvular Aortic Stenosis: Repair by Extended Aortoplasty, *J. Thorac. Cardiovasc. Surg.*, 74:362, 1977.

415. Keane, J. F., Fellows, K. E., LaFarge, C. G., Nadas, A. S., and Bernhard, W. F.: Surgical Management of Discrete and Diffuse Supravalvular Aortic Stenosis, *Circulation*, 54:112, 1976.

416. Landes, R. G., Zavoral, J. H., Emery, R. W., Moller, J. H., Lindsay, W. G., and Nicoloff, D. M.: The Surgical Management of Vascular Abnormalities Associated with Supravalvular Aortic Stenosis, *J. Thorac. Cardiovasc. Surg.*, 75:80, 1978.

417. Waller, B. F., Carter, J. B., Williams, H. J., Jr., Wang, K., and Edwards, J. E.: Bicuspid Aortic Valve. Comparison of Congenital and Acquired Types, *Circulation*, 48:1140, 1973.

418. Scholz, D. G., Lynch, J. A., Willerscheidt, A. B., Sharma, R. K., and Edwards, J. E.: Coronary Arterial Dominance Associated with Congenital Bicuspid Aortic Valve, *Arch. Pathol. Lab. Med.*, 104:417, 1980.

419. Edwards, W. D., Leaf, D. S., and Edwards, J. E.: Dissecting Aortic Aneurysm Associated with Congenital Bicuspid Aortic Valve, *Circulation*, 57:1022, 1978.

420. Roberts, W. C. (ed.): "Congenital Heart Disease in Adults," *Cardiovasc. Clin.* 10/1, F. A. Davis, 1979.

421. Leech, G., Mills, P., and Leatham, A.: The Diagnosis of a Non-Stenotic Bicuspid Aortic Valve, *Br. Heart J.*, 40:941, 1978.

422. Radford, D. J., Bloom, K. R., Izukawa, T., Moes, C. A. F., and Rowe, R. D.: Echocardiographic Assessment of Bicuspid Aortic Valves: Angiographic and Pathological Correlates, *Circulation*, 53:80, 1976.

423. Mills, P., Leech, G., Davies, M., and Leatham, A.: The Natural History of Non-Stenotic Bicuspid Aortic Valve, *Br. Heart J.*, 40:951, 1978.

424. Edwards, J. E.: The Congenital Bicuspid Aortic Valve, *Circulation*, 23:485, 1961.

425. Morganroth, J., Perloff, J. K., Zeldis, S., and Dunkman, W. B.: Acute Severe Aortic Regurgitation, Pathophysiology, Clinical Recognition and Management, *Ann. Intern. Med.*, 87:223, 1977.

426. Spencer, F. C., Bahnson, H. T., and Neill, C. A.: The Treatment of Aortic Regurgitation Associated with a Ventricular Septal Defect, *J. Thorac. Cardiovasc. Surg.*, 43:222, 1962.

427. Murphy, D. A., and Poirier, N.: A Technique of Aortic Valvuloplasty for Aortic Insufficiency Associated with Ventricular Septal Defect, *J. Thorac. Cardiovasc. Surg.*, 64:800, 1972.

428. Geha, A. S., Laks, H., Stansel, H. C., Cornhill, J. F., Kilman, J. W., Buckley, M. J., and Roberts,

W. C.: Late Failure of Porcine Valve Heterografts in Children, *J. Thorac. Cardiovasc. Surg.*, 78:351, 1979.

429. Murphy, E. S., and Kloster, F. E.: Late Results of Valve Replacement Surgery. II. Complications of Prosthetic Heart Valves, *Mod. Concepts Cardiovasc. Dis.*, 48:59, 1979.

430. Blank, R. H., Pupello, D. F., Bessone, L. N., Harrison, E. E., and Sbar, S.: Method of Managing the Small Aortic Annulus during Valve Replacement, *Ann. Thorac. Surg.*, 22:356, 1976.

431. Konno, S., Imai, Y., Iida, Y., Nakajima, M., and Tatsuno, K.: New Method for Prosthetic Valve Replacement in Congenital Aortic Stenosis Associated with Hypoplasia of the Aortic Valve Ring, *J. Thorac. Cardiovasc. Surg.*, 70:909, 1975.

432. Mayer, J. E., Lindsay, W. G., Wang, Y., Jorgensen, C. R., and Nicoloff, D. M.: Composite Replacement of the Aortic Valve and Ascending Aorta, *J. Thorac. Cardiovasc. Surg.*, 76:816, 1978.

433. Levy, M. J., Lillehei, C. W., Anderson, R. C., Amplatz, K., and Edwards, J. E.: Aortico–Left Ventricular Tunnel, *Circulation*, 27:841, 1963.

434. Somerville, J., English, T., and Ross, D. N.: Aorto–Left Ventricular Tunnel: Clinical Features and Surgical Management, *Br. Heart J.*, 36:321, 1974.

435. Somerville, J., English, T., and Ross, D. N.: Aorto–Left Ventricular Tunnel. Clinical Features and Surgical Management, *Br. Heart J.*, 36:321, 1974.

436. Bjork, V. O., Eklof, O., Wallgren, G., and Zetterquist, P.: Successful Surgical Treatment of an Aortico–Left Ventricular Tunnel in a Four Month-Old Infant, *J. Thorac. Cardiovasc. Surg.*, 78:35, 1979.

437. Bernhard, W. F., Plauth, W., and Fyler, D.: Unusual Abnormalities of the Aortic Root or Valve Necessitating Surgical Correction in Early Childhood, *N. Engl. J. Med.*, 282:68, 1970.

438. Spooner, E. W., Dunn, J. W., and Behrendt, D. M.: Aortico–Left Ventricular Tunnel and Sinus of Valsalva Aneurysm, *J. Thorac. Cardiovasc. Surg.*, 75:232, 1978.

439. Lev, M.: Pathologic Anatomy and Interrelationships of Hypoplasia of the Aortic Tract Complexes, *Lab. Invest.*, 1:61, 1952.

440. Roberts, W. C., Perry, L. W., Chandra, R. S., Myers, G. E., Shapiro, S. R., and Scott, L. P.: Aortic Valve Atresia: A Study of 73 Necropsy Patients, *Am. J. Cardiol.*, 37:753, 1976.

441. Pellagrino, P. A., and Thiene, G.: Aortic Valve Atresia with a Normally Developed Left Ventricle, *Chest*, 69:121, 1976.

*442. Freedom, R. M., Williams, W. G., Dishe, M. R., and Rowe, R. D.: Anatomical Variants in Aortic Atresia: Potential Candidates for Ventriculoaortic Reconstruction, *Br. Heart J.*, 38:821, 1976. (18 references)

443. Kanjuh, V. I., Eliot, R. S., and Edwards, J. E.: Coexistent Mitral and Aortic Valvular Atresia. A Pathologic Study of 14 Cases, *Am. J. Cardiol.*, 15:611, 1965.

444. Von Rueden, T. J., Knight, L., Moller, J. H., and Edwards, J. E.: Coarctation of the Aorta Associated with Aortic Valvular Atresia, *Circulation*, 52:951, 1975.

445. Bass, J. L., Ben-Shaghar, G., and Edwards, J. E.:

Comparison of M-Mode Echocardiography and Pathologic Findings in the Hypoplastic Left Heart Syndrome, *Am. J. Cardiol.*, 45:79, 1980.

446. Thiene, G., Gallucci, V., Macartney, F. J., Torso, S. D., Pellegrino, P. A., and Anderson, R. H.: Anatomy of Aortic Atresia, Cases Presenting with a Ventricular Septal Defect, *Circulation*, 59:173, 1979.

447. Doty, D. B., Marvin, W. J., Jr., Schieken, R. M., and Lauer, R. M.: Hypoplastic Left Heart Syndrome. Successful Palliation with a new Operation, *J. Thorac. Cardiovasc. Surg.*, 80:148, 1980.

448. Norwood, W. I., Kirklin, J. K., and Sanders, S. P.: Hypoplastic Left Heart Syndrome: Experience with Palliative Surgery, *Am. J. Cardiol.*, 45:87, 1980.

449. Eliot, R. S., Shone, J. D., Kanjuh, V. I., Ruttenberg, H. D., Carey, L. S., and Edwards, J. E.: Mitral Atresia. A Study of 32 Cases, *Am. Heart J.*, 70:6, 1965.

450. Lucas, R. V., Jr., Lester, R. G., Lillehei, C. W., and Edwards, J. E.: Mitral Atresia with Levatriocardinal Vein. A Form of Congenital Pulmonary Venous Obstruction, *Am. J. Cardiol.*, 9:607, 1962.

451. Beckman, C. B., Moller, J. H., and Edwards, J. E.: Alternate Pathways to Pulmonary Venous Flow in Left-Sided Obstructive Anomalies, *Circulation*, 52:509, 1975.

452. Shone, J. D., and Edwards, J. E.: Mitral Atresia Associated with Pulmonary Venous Anomalies, *Br. Heart J.*, 26:241, 1964.

453. Watson, D. G., Rowe, R. D., Conen, P. E., and Duckworth, J. W.: Mitral Atresia with Normal Aortic Valve. Report of 11 Cases and Review of the Literature, *Pediatrics*, 25:450, 1960.

454. Rosenquist, G. C.: Over-Riding Right Atrioventricular Valve in Association with Mitral Atresia, *Am. Heart J.*, 87:26, 1974.

455. Meyer, R. D.: "Pediatric Echocardiography," Lea & Febiger, Philadelphia, 1977.

*456. Mickell, J. J., Mathews, R. A., Park, S. C., Lenox, C. C., and Fricker, F. J.: Left Atrioventricular Valve Atresia: Clinical Management, *Circulation*, 61:123, 1980. (13 references)

457. Rogers, H. M., Waldon, B. R., Murphey, D. F. H., and Edwards, J. E.: Supravalvular Stenosing Ring of the Left Atrium in Association with Endocardial Sclerosis (Endocardial Fibroelastosis) and Mitral Insufficiency, *Am. Heart J.*, 50:777, 1955.

458. Benrey, J., Leachman, R. D., Cooley, D. A., Klima, T., and Lufschanowski, R.: Supravalvular Mitral Stenosis Associated with Tetralogy of Fallot, *Am. J. Cardiol.*, 37:111, 1976.

459. Shone, J. D., Sellers, R. D., Anderson, R. C., Adams, P., Jr., Lillehei, C. W., and Edwards, J. E.: The Developmental Complex of "Parachute Mitral Valve," Supravalvular Ring of Left Atrium, Subaortic Stenosis, and Coarctation of Aorta, *Am. J. Cardiol.*, 11:714, 1963.

460. Daoud, G., Kaplan, S., Perrin, E. V., Dorst, J. P., and Edwards, F. K.: Congenital Mitral Stenosis, *Circulation*, 27:185, 1963.

*461. Collins-Nakai, R. L., Rosenthal, A., Castaneda, A. R., Bernhard, W. F., and Nadas, A. S.: Congenital Mitral Stenosis: A Review of 20 Years' Experience, *Circulation*, 56:1039, 1977. (28 references)

462. Driscoll, D. J., Gutgesell, H. P., and McNamara,

D. G.: Echocardiographic Features of Congenital Mitral Stenosis, *Am. J. Cardiol.*, 42:259, 1978.

463. Snider, A. R., Roge, C. L., Schiller, N. B., and Silverman, N. H.: Congenital Left Ventricular Inflow Obstruction Evaluated by Two-Dimensional Echocardiography, *Circulation*, 61:848, 1980.

464. Carpentier, A., Branchini, B., Cour, J. C., Asfaou, E., Villani, M., Deloche, A., Relland, J., D'Allaines, C., Blondeau, P., Piwnica, A., Parenzan, L., and Brom, G.: Congenital Malformations of the Mitral Valve in Children, *J. Thorac. Cardiovasc. Surg.*, 72:854, 1976.

465. Berry, B. E., Ritter, D. G., Wallace, R. B., McGoon, D. C., and Danielson, G. K.: Cardiac Valve Replacement in Children, *J. Thorac. Cardiovasc. Surg.*, 68:705, 1974.

466. Nudelman, I., Schachner, A., and Levy, M. J.: Repeated Mitral Valve Replacement in the Growing Child with Congenital Mitral Valve Disease, *J. Thorac. Cardiovasc. Surg.*, 79:765, 1980.

467. Davachi, F., Moller, J. H., and Edwards, J. E.: Diseases of the Mitral Valve in Infancy: An Anatomic Analysis of 55 Cases, *Circulation*, 43:565, 1971.

*468. Krovetz, L. J., Lorincz, A. E., and Schiebler, G. L.: Cardiovascular Manifestations of the Hurler Syndrome. Hemodynamic and Angiocardiographic Observations in 15 Patients, *Circulation*, 31:132, 1965. (56 references)

469. Bharati, S., and Lev, M.: Congenital Poly-Valvular Disease, *Circulation*, 47:575, 1973.

470. Felner, J. M., and Schlant, R. C.: "Echocardiography: A Teaching Atlas," Grune & Stratton, New York, 1976.

471. Mintz, G. S., Kotler, M. N., Segal, B. L., and Parry, W. R.: Two Dimensional Echocardiographic Evaluation of Patients with Mitral Insufficiency, *Am. J. Cardiol.*, 44:670, 1979.

472. Kahn, D. R., Stern, A. M., Sigmann, J. M., Kirsh, M. M., Lennox, S., and Sloan, H.: Long-Term Results of Valvuloplasty for Mitral Insufficiency in Children, *J. Thorac. Cardiovasc. Surg.*, 53:1, 1967.

473. Borst, M.: Ein Cor Triatriatum, *Verhandl. d. deutsch. path. Gesellsch.*, 9:178, 1905.

*474. Van Praagh, R., and Corsini, I.: Cor Triatriatum: Pathologic Anatomy and a Consideration of Morphogenesis Based on 13 Post-Mortem Cases and a Study of Normal Development of the Pulmonary Vein and Atrial Septum in 83 Human Embryos, *Am. Heart J.*, 78:379, 1969. (100 references)

475. Becu, L. M., Tauxe, W. N., DuShane, J. W., and Edwards, J. E.: Anomalous Connection of Pulmonary Veins with Normal Pulmonary Venous Drainage. Report of a Case with Pulmonary Venous Stenosis and Cor Triatriatum, *Arch. Pathol.*, 59:563, 1955.

476. From, A. H. L., Mazzitello, W. F., Judd, A. S., and Edwards, J. E.: Ebstein's Malformation of the Tricuspid Valve Associated with Valvular Stenosis and Cor Triatriatum, *Chest*, 64:248, 1973.

477. Moodie, D. S., Hagler, D. J., and Ritter, D. G.: Cor Triatriatum: Echocardiographic Findings, *Mayo Clin. Proc.*, 51:289, 1976.

478. Hallman, G. L., and Cooley, D. A.: "Surgical Treatment of Congenital Heart Disease," 2d. ed., Lea & Febiger, Philadelphia, 1975. p. 192.

479. Reye, R. D. K.: Congenital Stenosis of the Pulmonary Veins in Their Extrapulmonary Course, *Med. J. Aust.*, 1:801, 1951.

480. Wagenvoort, C. A.: Pulmonary Veno-Occlusive Disease. Entity or Syndrome? *Chest*, 69:82, 1976.

481. Moller, J. H., Noren, G. R., David, P. R., Amplatz, K., Kanjuh, V. I., and Edwards, J. E.: Congenital Stenosis of Individual Pulmonary Veins without Intracardiac Anomalies, *Am. Heart J.*, 72:530, 1966.

482. Becker, A. E., Becker, M. J., and Edwards, J. E.: Occlusion of Pulmonary Veins, "Mitral" Insufficiency, and Ventricular Septal Defect. Functional Resemblance to Ventricular Aneurysm, *Am. J. Dis. Child.*, 120:557, 1970.

*483. Rosenthal, A., Vawter, G., and Wagenvoort, C. A.: Intrapulmonary Veno-Occlusive Disease, *Am. J. Cardiol.*, 31:78, 1973. (18 references)

*484. Park, S. C., Neches, W. H., Lenox, C. C., Zuberbuhler, J. R., Siewers, R. D., and Bahnson, H. T.: Diagnosis and Surgical Treatment of Bilateral Pulmonary Vein Stenosis, *J. Thorac. Cardiovasc. Surg.*, 67:755, 1974. (17 references)

485. Sade, R. M., Freed, M. D., Matthews, E. C., and Castaneda, A. R.: Stenosis of Individual Pulmonary Veins, *J. Thorac. Cardiovasc. Surg.*, 67:953, 1974.

486. Dennis, J. L., Hansen, A. E., and Corpening, T. N.: Endocardial Fibroelastosis, *Pediatrics*, 12:130, 1953.

487. Hutchins, G. M., and Vie, S. A.: The Progression of Interstitial Myocarditis to Idiopathic Endocardial Fibroelastosis, *Am. J. Pathol.*, 66:483, 1972.

488. Moller, J. H., Fisch, R. O., From, A. H. L., and Edwards, J. E.: Endocardial Fibroelastosis Occurring in a Mother and Son, *Pediatrics*, 38:918, 1966.

489. Chen, S., Thompson, M. W., and Rose, V.: Endocardial Fibroelastosis: Family Studies with Special Reference to Counseling, *J. Pediatr.*, 79:385, 1971.

490. Currens, J. H., Kinney, T. D., and White, P. D.: Pulmonary Stenosis with Intact Interventricular Septum: Report of Eleven Cases, *Am. Heart J.*, 30:491, 1945.

491. Parker, R. L.: Pulmonary Stenosis: Tetralogy of Fallot, *Med. Clin. N. Am.*, 32:855, 1948.

*492. Hardy, W. E., Gnoj, J., Ayres, S. M., Giannelli, E., and Christianson, L. C.: Pulmonic Stenosis and Associated Atrial Septal Defects in Older Patients. Report of Three Cases, Including One with Calcific Pulmonic Stenosis, *Am. J. Cardiol.*, 24:130, 1969. (16 references)

493. Koretzky, E. D., Moller, J. H., Korns, M. E., Schwartz, C. J., and Edwards, J. E.: Congenital Pulmonary Stenosis Resulting from Dysplasia of Valve, *Circulation*, 40:43, 1969.

494. Kirklin, J. W., Connolly, D. C., Ellis, F. H., Jr., Burchell, H. B., Edwards, J. E., and Wood, E. H.: Problems in the Diagnosis and Surgical Treatment of Pulmonic Stenosis with Intact Ventricular Septum, *Circulation*, 13:849, 1953.

495. Wood, P.: Congenital Pulmonary Stenosis, with Left Ventricular Enlargement Associated with Atrial Septal Defect, *Br. Heart J.*, 4:11, 1942.

496. Lucas, R. V., Jr., Varco, R. L., Lillehei, C. W., Adams, P., Jr., Anderson, R. C., and Edwards, J. E.: Anomalous Muscle Bundle of the Right Ven-

tricle. Hemodynamic Consequences and Surgical Considerations, *Circulation*, 25:443, 1962.

497. Stone, F. M., Bessinger, F. B., Jr., Lucas, R. V., Jr., and Moller, J. H.: Pre- and Postoperative Rest and Exercise Hemodynamics in Children with Pulmonary Stenosis, *Circulation*, 49:1102, 1974.

498. Danilowicz, D., Hoffman, J. I. E., and Rudolph, A. M.: Serial Studies of Pulmonary Stenosis in Infancy and Childhood, *Br. Heart J.*, 37:808, 1975.

499. Mody, M. R.: The Natural History of Uncomplicated Valvular Pulmonic Stenosis, *Am. Heart J.*, 90:317, 1975.

500. Nakazawa, M., Marks, R. A., Isabel-Jones, J., and Jarmakam, J. M.: Right and Left Ventricular Volume Characteristics in Children with Pulmonary Stenosis and Intact Ventricular Septum, *Circulation*, 53:884, 1976.

501. Roberts, W. C., Shemin, R. J., and Kent, K. M.: Frequency and Direction of Interatrial Shunting in Valvular Pulmonic Stenosis with Intact Ventricular Septum and without Left Ventricular Inflow or Outflow Obstruction, *Am. Heart J.*, 99:142, 1980.

502. Freed, M. D., Rosenthal, A., Bernhard, W. F., Litwin, S. B., and Nadas, A. S.: Critical Pulmonary Stenosis with Diminutive Right Ventricle in Neonates, *Circulation*, 48:875, 1973.

503. Campbell, M.: Factors in the Aetiology of Pulmonary Stenosis, *Br. Heart J.*, 24:625, 1962.

504. Noonan, J. A.: Hypertelorism with Turner Phenotype: A New Syndrome with Associated Congenital Heart Disease, *Am. J. Dis. Child.*, 116:373, 1968.

505. Gamboa, R., Hugenholtz, P. G., and Nadas, A. S.: Accuracy of the Phonocardiogram in Assessing Severity of Aortic and Pulmonic Stenosis, *Circulation*, 30:35, 1964.

506. Cayler, G. C., Ongley, P., and Nadas, A. S.: Relation of Systolic Pressure in the Right Ventricle to the Electrocardiogram, *N. Engl. J. Med.*, 258:979, 1958.

507. Hugenholtz, P. G., and Gamboa, R.: Effect of Chronically Increased Ventricular Pressure on Electrical Forces of the Heart: A Correlation between Hemodynamic and Vectorcardiographic Data (Frank System) in 90 Patients with Aortic or Pulmonic Stenosis, *Circulation*, 30:511, 1964.

508. Nadas, A. S. (ed.): Pulmonary Stenosis, Aortic Stenosis, Ventricular Septal Defect: Clinical Course and Indirect Assessment (Report from the Joint Study on the Natural History of Congenital Heart Defects), *Circulation*, 56(suppl. 1):1, 1977.

509. Weyman, A. E., Dillon, J. C., Fiegenbaum, H., and Chang, S.: Echocardiographic Differentiation of Infundibular from Valvular Pulmonary Stenosis, *Am. J. Cardiol.*, 36:21, 1975.

510. Lester, R. G., Osteen, R. T., and Robinson, A. E.: Infundibular Obstruction Secondary to Pulmonary Valvular Stenosis, *Am. J. Roentgenol.*, 94:78, 1965.

511. Schieken, R. M., Friedman, S., and Pierce, W. S.: Severe Congenital Pulmonary Stenosis with Pulmonary Valvular Dysplasia Syndrome, *Ann. Thorac. Surg.*, 15:570, 1973.

512. Vancini, M., Roberts, K. D., Silove, E. D., and Singh, S. P.: Surgical Treatment of Congenital Pulmonary Stenosis Due to Dysplastic Leaflets and Small Valve Annulus, *J. Thorac. Cardiovasc. Surg.*, 79:464, 1980.

513. Litwin, S. B., Williams, W. H., Freed, M. D., and Bernhard, W. F.: Critical Pulmonary Stenosis in Infants: A Surgical Emergency, *Surgery*, 74:880, 1973.

514. Mistrot, J., Neal, W., Lyons, G., Moller, J., Lucas, R., Castaneda, A., Varco, R., and Nicoloff, D.: Pulmonary Valvulotomy under Inflow Stasis for Isolated Pulmonary Stenosis, *Ann. Thorac. Surg.*, 21:30, 1976.

515. Li, M. D., Coles, J. C., and McDonald, A. C.: Anomalous Muscle Bundle of the Right Ventricle: Its Recognition and Surgical Treatment, *Br. Heart J.*, 40:1040, 1978.

*516. D'Cruz, I. A., Agustsson, M. H., Bicoff, J. P., Weinberg, M., Jr., and Arcilla, R. A.: Stenotic Lesions of the Pulmonary Arteries. Clinical and Hemodynamic Findings in 84 Cases, *Am. J. Cardiol.*, 13:441, 1964. (34 references)

517. Rowe, R. D.: Cardiovascular Disease in the Rubella Syndrome, *Cardiovasc. Clin.*, 5:62, 1972.

518. Rios, J. C., Walsh, B. J., Massumi, R. A., Sims, A. J., and Ewy, G. A.: Congenital Pulmonary Artery Branch Stenosis, *Am. J. Cardiol.*, 24:318, 1969.

519. Dunkle, L. M., and Rowe, R. D.: Transient Murmur Simulating Pulmonary Artery Stenosis in Premature Infants, *Am. J. Dis. Child.*, 124:666, 1972.

520. Zuberbuhler, J. R., and Anderson, R. H.: Morphological Variations in Pulmonary Atresia with Intact Ventricular Septum, *Br. Heart J.*, 41:281, 1979.

*521. Celermajer, J. M., Bowdler, J. D., Gengos, D. C., Cohen, D. H., and Stuckey, D. S.: Pulmonary Valve Fusion with Intact Ventricular Septum, *Am. Heart J.*, 76:452, 1968. (17 references)

522. Davignon, A. L., Greenwold, W. E., DuShane, J. W., and Edwards, J. E.: Congenital Pulmonary Atresia with Intact Ventricular Septum: Clinicopathologic Correlation of Two Anatomic Types, *Am. Heart J.*, 62:591, 1961.

523. Arom, K. V., and Edwards, J. E.: Relationship between Right Ventricular Muscle Bundles and Pulmonary Valve. Significance in Pulmonary Atresia with Intact Ventricular Septum, *Circulation*, 54(suppl. 3):79, 1976.

*524. Freedom, R. M., and Harrington, D. P.: Contributions of Intramyocardial Sinusoids in Pulmonary Atresia and Intact Ventricular Septum to a Right-Sided Circular Shunt, *Br. Heart J.*, 36:1061, 1974. (20 references)

525. Elliott, L. P., Adams, P., Jr., and Edwards, J. E.: Pulmonary Atresia with Intact Ventricular Septum, *Br. Heart J.*, 25:489, 1963.

526. Solinger, R., Elbl, F., and Minhas, K.: Echocardiography: Its Role in the Severely Ill Infant, *Pediatrics*, 57:543, 1976.

527. Lewis, B. S., Amitai, N., Simcha, A., Merin, G., and Gotsman, M. S.: Echocardiographic Diagnosis of Pulmonary Atresia with Intact Ventricular Septum, *Am. Heart J.*, 97:92, 1979.

528. Graham, T. P., Jr., Bender, H. W., Atwood, G. F., Page, D. L., and Sell, C. G. R.: Increase in Right Ventricular Volume Following Valvulotomy for

Pulmonary Atresia or Stenosis with Intact Ventricular Septum, *Circulation*, 50(suppl. 2):69, 1974.

529. Patel, R. G., Freedom, R. M., Moes, C. A. F., Bloom, K. R., Olley, P. M., Williams, W. G., Trusler, G. A., and Rowe, R. D.: Right Ventricular Volume Determinations in 18 Patients with Pulmonary Atresia and Intact Ventricular Septum: Analysis of Factors Influencing Right Ventricular Growth, *Circulation*, 61:428, 1980.

530. Freedom, R. M., White, R. I., Jr., Ho., C. S., Gingell, R. L., Hawker, R. E., and Rowe, R. D.: Evaluation of Patients with Pulmonary Atresia and Intact Ventricular Septum by Double Catheter Technique, *Am. J. Cardiol.*, 33:892, 1974.

531. Heymann, M. A., and Rudolph, A. M.: Ductus Arteriosus Dilatation by Prostaglandin E_1 in Infants with Pulmonary Atresia, *Pediatrics*, 59:325, 1977.

532. Rigby, M. L., Silove, E. D., Astley, R., and Abrams, L. D.: Pulmonary Atresia with Intact Ventricular Septum: Open Heart Surgical Correction at 32 Hours, *Br. Heart J.*, 39:573, 1977.

533. Moulton, A. L., Bowman, F. O., Jr., Edie, R. N., Hayes, C. J., Ellis, K., Gersony, W. M., and Malm, J. R.: Pulmonary Atresia with Intact Ventricular Septum: Sixteen-Year Experience, *J. Thorac. Cardiovasc. Surg.*, 78:527, 1979.

534. Trusler, G. A., Yamamoto, N., Williams, W. G., Izukawa, T., Rowe, R. D., and Mustard, W. T.: Surgical Treatment of Pulmonary Atresia with Intact Ventricular Septum, *Br. Heart J.*, 38:957, 1976.

535. Lev, M., and Eckner, F. A. O.: The Pathologic Anatomy of Tetralogy of Fallot and Its Variations, *Dis. Chest*, 45:251, 1964.

536. Rosenquist, G. C., Sweeney, L. J., Stemple, D. R., Christianson, S. D., and Rowe, R. D.: Ventricular Septal Defect in Tetralogy of Fallot, *Am. J. Cardiol.*, 31:749, 1973.

*537. Becker, A. E., Connor, M., and Anderson, R. H.: Tetralogy of Fallot: A Morphometric and Geometric Study, *Am. J. Cardiol.*, 35:402, 1975. (27 references)

538. Rao, B. N. S., Anderson, R. C., and Edwards, J. E.: Anatomic Variations in the Tetralogy of Fallot, *Am. Heart J.*, 81:361, 1971.

539. Neufeld, H. N., McGoon, D. C., DuShane, J. W., and Edwards, J. E.: Tetralogy of Fallot with Anomalous Tricuspid Valve Simulating Pulmonary Stenosis with Intact Septum, *Circulation*, 22:1083, 1960.

540. Hofschire, P. J., Rosenquist, G. C., Ruckerman, R. N., Moller, J. H., and Edwards, J. E.: Pulmonary Vascular Disease Complicating the Blalock-Taussig Anastomosis, *Circulation*, 56:124, 1977.

541. Heath, D., DuShane, J. W., Wood, E. H., and Edwards, J. E.: The Aetiology of Pulmonary Thrombosis in Cyanotic Congenital Heart Disease with Pulmonary Stenosis, *Thorax*, 13:213, 1958.

542. Kirklin, J. W., and Karp, R. B.: "The Tetralogy of Fallot," W. B. Saunders Company, Philadelphia, 1970.

543. Higgins, C. B., and Mulder, D. G.: Tetralogy of Fallot in the Adult, *Am. J. Cardiol.*, 28:837, 1972.

544. Bonchek, L. I., Starr, A., Sunderland, C. O., and Menashe, V. D.: Natural History of Tetralogy of Fallot in Infancy: Clinical Classification and Therapeutic Implications, *Circulation*, 48:386, 1973.

545. Ruzyllo, W., Nihill, M. B., Mullins, C. E., and McNamara, D. G.: Hemodynamic Evaluation of 221 Patients after Intracardiac Repair of Tetralogy of Fallot, *Am. J. Cardiol.*, 34:565, 1974.

546. Taussig, H. B., Kallman, C. H., Nagel, D., Baumgardner, R., Momberger, N., and Kirk, H.: Long-Time Observations on the Blalock-Taussig Operation. VIII. 20- to 28-Year Follow-Up on Patients with a Tetralogy of Fallot, *Johns Hopkins Med. J.*, 137:13, 1975.

547. Roberts, W. C., Friesinger, G. C., Cohen, L. S., Mason, D. T., and Ross, R. S.: Acquired Pulmonary Atresia. Total Obstruction to Right Ventricular Outflow after Systemic to Pulmonary Arterial Anastomoses for Cyanotic Congenital Cardiac Disease, *Am. J. Cardiol.*, 24:335, 1969.

548. Morgan, B. C., Guntheroth, W. G., Bloom, R. S., and Fyler, D. C.: A Clinical Profile of Paroxysmal Hyperpnea in Cyanotic Congenital Heart Disease, *Circulation*, 31:66, 1965.

549. Guntheroth, W. G., Morgan, B. C., and Mullins, G. L.: Physiologic Studies of Paroxysmal Hyperpnea in Cyanotic Congenital Heart Disease, *Circulation*, 31:70, 1965.

550. Morris, D. C., Felner, J. M., Schlant, R. C., and Franch, R. H.: Echocardiographic Diagnosis of Tetralogy of Fallot, *Am. J. Cardiol.*, 36:908, 1975.

551. Story, W. E., Felner, J. M., and Schlant, R. C.: Echocardiographic Criteria for the Diagnosis of Mitral-Semilunar Valve Continuity, *Am. Heart J.*, 93:575, 1977.

552. Hagler, D. J., Tajik, A. J., Seward, J. B., Mair, D. D., and Ritter, D. G.: Wide-Angle Two-Dimensional Echocardiographic Profiles of Conotruncal Abnormalities, *Mayo Clin. Proc.*, 55:73, 1980.

553. Fellows, K. E., Freed, M. D., Keane, J. F., Van Praagh, R., Bernard, W. F., and Castaneda, A. C.: Results of Routine Preoperative Coronary Angiography in Tetralogy of Fallot, *Circulation*, 51:561, 1975.

554. Formanek, A., Nath, P. H., Zollikofer, C., and Moller, J. H.: Selective Coronary Arteriography in Children, *Circulation*, 61:84, 1980.

555. Dabizzi, R. P., Caprioli, G., Aiazzi, L., Castelli, C., Baldrighi, G., Parenzan, L., and Baldrighi, V.: Distribution and Anomalies of Coronary Arteries in Tetralogy of Fallot, *Circulation*, 61:95, 1980.

556. Ferencz, C.: The Pulmonary Vascular Bed in Tetralogy of Fallot. I. Changes Associated with Pulmonary Stenosis, *Bull. Johns Hopkins, Hosp.*, 106:81, 1960.

557. Bertranaou, E. G., Blackstone, E. H., Hazelrig, J. B., Turner, M. E., Jr., and Kirklin, J. W.: Life Expectancy without Surgery in Tetralogy of Fallot, *Am. J. Cardiol.*, 42:458, 1978.

558. Honey, M., Chamberlain, D. A., and Howard, J.: The Effect of Beta-Sympathetic Blockade on Arterial Oxygen Saturation in Fallot's Tetralogy, *Circulation*, 30:501, 1964.

559. Ponce, F. E., Williams, L. C., Webb, H. M., Riopel, D. A., and Hohn, A. R.: Propranolol Palliation of Tetralogy of Fallot: Experience with Long-Term Drug Treatment in Pediatric Patients, *Pediatrics*, 52:100, 1973.

560. Garson, A., Jr., Gorry, G. A., McNamara, D. G., and Cooley, D. A.: The Surgical Decision in Tetralogy of Fallot: Weighing Risks and Benefits with Decision Analysis, *Am. J. Cardiol.,* 45:108, 1980.

561. Kirklin, J. W., Bargeron, L. M., Jr., and Pacifico, A. D.: Enlargement of Small Pulmonary Arteries by Preliminary Palliative Operations, *Circulation,* 56:612, 1977.

562. Laks, H., and Castaneda, A. R.: Subclavian Arterioplasty for the Ipsilateral Blalock-Taussig Shunt, *Ann. Thorac. Surg.,* 19:319, 1975.

563. Marbarger, J. P., Jr., Sandza, J. G., Jr., Hartmann, A. F., Jr., and Weldon, C. S.: Blalock-Taussig Anastomosis: Preferred Shunt in Infants and Newborns, *Circulation,* 58(suppl. 1):73, 1978.

564. Somerville, J., Barbosa, R., Ross, D., and Olsen, E.: Problems with Radical Corrective Surgery after Ascending Aorta to Right Pulmonary Artery Shunt (Waterston's Anastomosis) for Cyanotic Congenital Heart Disease, *Br. Heart J.,* 37:1105, 1975.

565. Kirklin, J. W., Blackstone, E. H., Pacifico, A. D., Brown, R. N., and Bargeron, L. M., Jr.: Routine Primary Repair vs. Two-Stage Repair of Tetralogy of Fallot, *Circulation,* 60:373, 1979.

566. Meyer, J., Chiariello, L., Hallman, G. L., and Cooley, D. A.: Coronary Artery Anomalies in Patients with Tetralogy of Fallot, *J. Thorac. Cardiovasc. Surg.,* 69:373, 1975.

*567. Lakier, J. B., Stanger, P., Heymann, M. A., Hoffman, J. I. E., and Rudolph, A. M.: Tetralogy of Fallot with Absent Pulmonary Valve. Natural History and Hemodynamic Considerations, *Circulation,* 50:167, 1974. (43 references)

568. Borg, S. A., Young, L. V., and Roghair, G. D.: Congenital Avalvular Pulmonary Artery and Infantile Lobar Emphysema: A Diagnostic Correlation, *Am. J. Roentgenol. Radium Ther. Nucl. Med.,* 125:412, 1975.

569. Pinsky, W. W., Nihill, M. R., Mullins, C. E., Harrison, G., and McNamara, D. G.: The Absent Pulmonary Valve Syndrome: Considerations of Management, *Circulation,* 57:159, 1978.

570. Litwin, S. B., Rosenthal, A., and Fellows, K.: Surgical Management of Young Infants with Tetralogy of Fallot, Absence of the Pulmonary Valve, and Respiratory Distress, *Am. J. Thorac. Cardiovasc. Surg.,* 65:552, 1973.

571. Stafford, E. G., Mair, D. D., McGoon, D. C., and Danielson, G. K.: Tetralogy of Fallot with Absent Pulmonary Valve: Surgical Considerations and Results, *Cardiovasc. Surg.,* 47:24, 1973.

572. Edwards, J. E., and McGoon, D. C.: Absence of Anatomic Origin from Heart of Pulmonary Arterial Supply, *Circulation,* 47:393, 1973.

573. Collett, R. W., and Edwards, J. E.: Persistent Truncus Arteriosus: A Classification According to Anatomic Types, *Surg. Clin. N. Am.,* 29:(Mayo Clin. No.)1245, 1949.

*574. Bharati, S., McAllister, H. A., Jr., Rosenquist, G. C., Miller, R. A., Tatooles, C. J., and Lev, M.: The Surgical Anatomy of Truncus Arteriosus Communis, *J. Thorac. Cardiovasc. Surg.,* 67:501, 1974. (44 references)

*575. Calder, L., Van Praagh, R., Van Praagh, S., Sears, W. P., Corwin, R., Levy, A., Keith, J. D., and Paul, M. H.: Truncus Arteriosus Communis. Clinical, Angiocardiographic, and Pathologic Findings in 100 Patients, *Am. Heart J.,* 92:23, 1976. (48 references)

576. Anderson, K. R., McGoon, D. C., and Lie, J. T.: Surgical Significance of the Coronary Arterial Anatomy in Truncus Arteriosus Communis, *Am. J. Cardiol.,* 41:76, 1978.

577. Becker, A. E., Becker, M. J., and Edwards, J. E.: Pathology of the Semilunar Valves in Persistent Truncus Arteriosus, *J. Thorac. Cardiovasc. Surg.,* 62:16, 1961.

578. Gelband, H., Van Meter, S., and Gersony, W. M.: Truncal Valve Abnormalites in Infants with Persistent Truncus Arteriosus. A Clinicopathologic Study, *Circulation,* 45:397, 1972.

579. Carter, J. B., Blieden, L. C., and Edwards, J. E.: Persistent Truncus Arteriosus. Report of Survival to Age of 52 Years, *Minnesota Med.,* 56:280, 1973.

580. Sotomora, R. F., and Edwards, J. E.: Anatomic Identification of So-Called Absent Pulmonary Artery, *Circulation,* 57:624, 1978.

581. Jefferson, K., Simon, R., and Somerville, J.: Systemic Arterial Supply to the Lungs in Pulmonary Atresia and Its Relation to Pulmonary Artery Development, *Br. Heart J.,* 34:418, 1972.

582. Nihill, M. R., Mullins, C. E., and McNamara, D. G.: Visualization of the Pulmonary Arteries in Pseudotruncus by Pulmonary Vein Wedge Angiography, *Circulation,* 58:140, 1978.

583. Singh, S. P., Rigby, M. L., and Astley, R.: Demonstration of Pulmonary Arteries by Contrast Injection into Pulmonary Vein, *Br. Heart J.,* 40:55, 1978.

584. Doty, D. B., Kouchoukos, N. T., Kirklin, J. W., Barcia, A., and Bargeron, L. M., Jr.: Surgery for Pseudotruncus Arteriosus with Pulmonary Blood Flow Originating from Upper Descending Thoracic Aorta, *Circulation,* 45(suppl. 1):121, 1972.

585. Ross, D. N., and Somerville, J.: Correction of Pulmonary Atresia with a Homograft Aortic Valve, *Lancet,* 2:1446, 1966.

586. Kouchoukos, N. T., Barcia, A., Bargeron, L. M., Jr., and Kirklin, J. W.: Surgical Treatment of Congenital Pulmonary Atresia with Ventricular Septal Defect, *J. Thorac. Cardiovasc. Surg.,* 61:70, 1971.

587. Van Praagh, R., and Van Praagh, S.: The Anatomy of Common Aorticopulmonary Trunk (Truncus Arteriosus Communis) and Its Embryologic Implications: A Study of 57 Necropsy Cases, *Am. J. Cardiol.,* 16:406, 1965.

588. Marcelletti, C., McGoon, D. C., and Mair, D. D.: The Natural History of Truncus Arteriosus, *Circulation,* 54:108, 1976.

589. Mair, D. D., Ritter, D. G., Davis, G. D., Wallace, R. B., Danielson, G. K., and McGoon, D. C.: Selection of Patients with Truncus Arteriosus for Surgical Correction: Anatomic and Hemodynamic Considerations, *Circulation,* 49:144, 1974.

590. Parker, R. K., McGoon, D. C., Danielson, G. K., Wallace, R. B., and Mair, D. D.: Repair of Truncus Arteriosus in Patients with Prior Banding of the Pulmonary Artery, *Surgery,* 78:761, 1975.

591. Wallace, R. B., Rastelli, G. C., Ongley, P. A., Titus, J. L., and McGoon, D. C.: Complete Repair of

Truncus Arteriosus Defects, *J. Thorac. Cardiovasc. Surg.,* 57:95, 1969.

592. Appelbaum, A., Bargeron, L. M., Jr., Pacifico, A. D., and Kirklin, J. W.: Surgical Treatment of Truncus Arteriosus, with Emphasis on Infants and Small Children, *J. Thorac. Cardiovasc. Surg.,* 71:436, 1976.

593. Ebert, P. A., Robinson, S. J., Stanger, P., and Engle, M. A.: Pulmonary Artery Conduits in Infants Younger than Six Months of Age, *J. Thorac. Cardiovasc. Surg.,* 72:351, 1976.

594. McGoon, D. C., Rastelli, G. C., and Ongley, P. A.: An Operation for Correction of Truncus Arteriosus, *J. Am. Med. Assoc.,* 205:69, 1968.

595. Marcelletti, C., McGoon, D. C., Danielson, G. K., Wallace, R. B., and Mair, D. D.: Early and Late Results of Surgical Repair of Truncus Arteriosus, *Circulation,* 55:636, 1977.

596. Edwards, J. E., and Burchell, H. B.: Congenital Tricuspid Atresia: A Classification, *Med. Clin. N. Am.,* 33:(Mayo Clin. No.)1177, 1949.

597. Tandon, R., and Edwards, J. E.: Tricuspid Atresia. A Re-evaluation and Classification, *J. Thorac. Cardiovasc. Surg.,* 67:530, 1974.

*598. Rao, P. S.: Natural History of the Ventricular Septal Defect in Tricuspid Atresia and Its Surgical Implications, *Br. Heart J.,* 39:276, 1977. (50 references)

599. Charuzi, Y., Spanos, P. K., Amplatz, K., and Edwards, J. E.: Juxtaposition of the Atrial Appendages, *Circulation,* 47:620, 1973.

*600. Dick, M., Fyler, D. C., and Nadas, A. S.: Tricuspid Atresia: Clinical Course in 101 Patients, *Am. J. Cardiol.,* 36:327, 1975. (52 references)

601. Shariatzadeh, A. N., King, H., Girod, D., and Schumacher, H. B.: Tricuspid Atresia. Review of 68 Cases, *Chest,* 71:538, 1977.

602. Marcano, B. A., Riemenschneider, T. A., Ruttenberg, H. D., Goldberg, S. J., and Gyepes, M.: Tricuspid Atresia with Increased Pulmonary Blood Flow: An Analysis of 13 Cases, *Circulation,* 40:399, 1969.

603. Davachi, F., Lucas, R. V., Jr., and Moller, J. H.: The Electrocardiogram and Vectorcardiogram in Tricuspid Atresia: Correlation with Pathologic Anatomy, *Am. J. Cardiol.,* 25:18, 1970.

604. La Corte, M. A., Dick, M., Scheer, G., LaFarge, C. G., and Fyler, D. C.: Left Ventricular Function in Tricuspid Atresia: Angiographic Analysis in 28 Patients, *Circulation,* 52:996, 1975.

605. Van der Horst, R. L., Winship, W. S., and Gotsman, M. S.: Beta-Adrenergic Blockade in the Relief of Paroxysmal Cyanotic Spells in Tricuspid Atresia, *S. Afr. Med. J.,* 46:494, 1972.

606. Fontan, F., and Baudet, E.: Surgical Repair of Tricuspid Atresia, *Thorax,* 26:240, 1971.

607. Tatooles, C. J., Ardekani, R. G., Miller, R. A., and Serratto, M.: Operative Repair for Tricuspid Atresia, *Ann. Thorac. Surg.,* 21:499, 1976.

608. Bowman, F. O., Jr., Malm, J. R., Hayes, C. J., and Gersony, W. M.: Physiological Approach to Surgery for Tricuspid Atresia, *Circulation,* 58(suppl. 1):83, 1977.

609. Behrendt, D. M., and Rosenthal, A.: Cardiovascular Status after Repair by Fontan Procedure, *Ann. Thorac. Surg.,* 29:322, 1979.

610. Trusler, G. A., and Williams, W. G.: Long-Term Results of Shunt Procedures for Tricuspid Atresia, *Ann. Thorac. Surg.,* 29:312, 1978.

611. Becker, A. E., Becker, M. J., and Edwards, J. E.: Pathologic Spectrum of Dysplasia of the Tricuspid Valve. Features in Common with Ebstein's Malformations, *Arch. Path.,* 91:167, 1971.

612. Kanjuh, V. I., Stevenson, J. E., Amplatz, K., and Edwards, J. E.: Congenitally Unguarded Tricuspid Orifice with Coexistent Pulmonary Atresia, *Circulation,* 30:911, 1964.

*613. Barr, P. A., Celermajer, J. M., Bowdler, J. D., and Cartmill, T. B.: Severe Congenital Tricuspid Incompetence in the Neonate, *Circulation,* 49:962, 1974. (21 references)

614. Boucek, R. J., Graham, T. P., Jr., Morgan, J. R., Atwood, G. F., and Boerth, R. C.: Spontaneous Resolution of Massive Congenital Tricuspid Insufficiency, *Circulation,* 54:795, 1976.

615. Berman, W., Jr., Whitman, V., Stanger, P., and Rudolph, A. M.: Congenital Tricuspid Incompetence Simulating Pulmonary Atresia with Intact Ventricular Septum: A Report of Two Cases, *Am. Heart J.,* 96:655, 1978.

616. Freedom, R. M., Culham, G., Moes, F., Olley, P. M., and Rowe, R. D.: Differentiation of Functional and Structural Pulmonary Atresia: Role of Angiography, *Am. J. Cardiol.,* 41:914, 1978.

617. Bucciarelli, R. L., Nelson, R. M., Egan, E. A., II, Eitzman, D. V., and Gessner, I. H.: Transient Tricuspid Insufficiency of the Newborn: A Form of Myocardial Dysfunction in Distressed Newborns, *Pediatrics,* 59:330, 1977.

*618. Lev, M., Liberthson, R. R., Joseph, R. H., Seten, C. E., Kunske, R. D., Eckner, F. A. O., and Miller, R. A.: The Pathologic Anatomy of Ebstein's Disease, *Arch. Path.,* 90:334, 1970. (38 references)

619. Kumar, A. E., Fyler, D. C., Miettinen, O. S., and Nadas, A. S.: Ebstein's Anomaly. Clinical Profile and Natural History, *Am. J. Cardiol.,* 28:84, 1971.

620. Bialostozky, D., Horwitz, S., and Espino-Vela, J.: Ebstein's Malformation of the Tricuspid Valve. A Review of 65 Cases, *Am. J. Cardiol.,* 29:826, 1972.

621. Watson, H.: Natural History of Ebstein's Anomaly of the Tricuspid Valve in Childhood and Adolescence: An International Cooperative Study of 505 Cases, *Br. Heart J.,* 36:417, 1974.

*622. Giuliani, E. R., Fuster, V., Brandenburg, R. O., and Mair, D. D.: Ebstein's Anomaly: The Clinical Features and Natural History of Ebstein's Anomaly of the Tricuspid Valve, *Mayo Clin. Proc.,* 54:163, 1979. (31 references)

623. Kastor, J. A., Goldreyer, B. N., Josephson, M. E., Perloff, J. K., Scharf, D. L., Manchester, J. H., Shelburne, J. C., and Hirschfeld, J. W., Jr.: Electrophysiologic Characteristics of Ebstein's Anomaly of the Tricuspid Valve, *Circulation,* 52:987, 1975.

624. Kotler, M. N.: Tricuspid Valve in Ebstein's Anomaly, *Circulation,* 49:194, 1974.

625. Farooki, Z. Q., Henry, J. G., and Green, E. W.: Echocardiographic Spectrum of Ebstein's Anomaly of the Tricuspid Valve, *Circulation,* 53:63, 1976.

626. Hernandez, F. A., Rochkind, R., and Cooper, H. R.: The Intracavitary Electrocardiogram in the Diagnosis of Ebstein's Anomaly, *Am. J. Cardiol.,* 1:181, 1958.

627. Monibi, A. A., Neches, W. H., Lenox, C. C., Park,

S. C., Mathews, R. A., and Zuberbuhler, J. R.: Left Ventricular Anomalies Associated with Ebstein's Malformation of the Tricuspid Valve, *Circulation*, 57:303, 1978.

628. Marcelletti, C., Duren, D. R., Schuilenburg, R. M., and Becker, A. E.: Fontan's Operation for Ebstein's Anomaly, *J. Thorac. Cardiovasc. Surg.*, 76:63, 1980.

629. Hardy, K. L., and Roe, B. B.: Ebstein's Anomaly: Further Experience with Definitive Repair, *J. Thorac. Cardiovasc. Surg.*, 58:553, 1969.

630. Shigenobu, M., Mendez, M. A., Zubiate, P., and Kay, J. H.: Thirteen Years' Experience with the Kay-Shiley Disc Valve for Tricuspid Replacement in Ebstein's Anomaly, *Ann. Thorac. Surg.*, 29:423, 1980.

631. Barbero-Marcial, M., Verginelli, G., Awad, M., Ferreira, S., Ebaid, M., and Zerbini, E. J.: Surgical Treatment of Ebstein's Anomaly: Early and Late Results in Twenty Patients Subjected to Valve Replacement, *J. Thorac. Cardiovasc. Surg.*, 78:416, 1979.

632. Gasul, B. M., Lendrum, B. L., and Arcilla, R. A.: Congenital Aplasia or Marked Hypoplasia of the Myocardium of the Right Ventricle (Uhl's Anomaly), *Circulation*, 22:752, 1960.

633. Uhl, H. S. M.: Previously Undescribed Congenital Malformation of the Heart: Almost Total Absence of the Myocardium of the Right Ventricle, *Bull. Johns Hopkins Hosp.*, 91:197, 1952.

*634. Vecht, R. J., Carmichael, D. J. S., Gopal, R., and Philip, G.: Uhl's Anomaly, *Br. Heart J.*, 41:676, 1979. (21 references)

635. French, J. W., Baum, D., and Popp, R.: Echocardiographic Findings in Uhl's Anomaly. Demonstration of Diastolic Pulmonary Valve Opening, *Am. J. Cardiol.*, 36:349, 1975.

636. Lucas, R. V., Jr., Lund, G. W., and Edwards, J. E.: Direct Communication of a Pulmonary Artery with the Left Atrium. An Unusual Variant of Pulmonary Arteriovenous Fistula, *Circulation*, 29:1409, 1961.

637. Dines, D. E., Arms, R. A., Bernatz, P. E., and Gomes, M. R.: Pulmonary Arteriovenous Fistulas, *Proc. Mayo Clin.*, 49:460, 1975.

638. Goldman, A.: Arteriovenous Fistula of the Lung. Its Hereditary and Clinical Aspects, *Am. Rev. Tuberc.*, 57:266, 1948.

*639. Sisel, R. J., Parker, B. M., Bahl, O. P.: Cerebral Symptoms in Pulmonary Arteriovenous Fistula. A Result of Paradoxical Emboli (?), *Circulation*, 41:123, 1970. (28 references)

640. Crosby, I. K., Tompkins, D. G., and Carpenter, M. A.: Pulmonary Arteriovenous Fistula and Patent Ductus Arteriosus in the Newborn Infant, *J. Pediatr.*, 86:986, 1975.

641. Hodgson, C. H., Burchell, H. B., Good, C. A., and Clagett, O. T.: Hereditary Hemorrhagic Telangiectasia and Pulmonary Arteriovenous Fistula, *N. Engl. J. Med.*, 261:65, 1959.

642. Burroughs, J. T., and Edwards, J. E.: Total Anomalous Pulmonary Venous Connection, *Am. Heart J.*, 59:913, 1960.

643. Blake, H. A. R., Hall, J., and Manion, W. C.: Anomalous Pulmonary Venous Return, *Circulation*, 32:406, 1965.

644. Elliott, L. P., and Edwards, J. E.: The Problem of

Pulmonary Venous Obstruction in Total Anomalous Pulmonary Venous Connection to the Left Innominate Vein, *Circulation*, 25:913, 1962.

645. Lucas, R. V., Jr., Adams, P., Jr., Anderson, R. C., Varco, R. L., Edwards, J. E., and Lester, R. G.: Total Anomalous Pulmonary Venous Connection to the Portal Venous System: A Cause of Pulmonary Venous Obstruction, *Am. J. Roentgenol.*, 86:561, 1961.

646. Lucas, R. V., Jr., Woolfrey, B. F., Anderson, R. C., Lester, R. G., and Edwards, J. E.: Atresia of the Common Pulmonary Vein, *Pediatrics*, 29:729, 1962.

*647. Jensen, J. B., and Blount, S. G., Jr.: Total Anomalous Pulmonary Venous Return. A Review and Report of the Oldest Surviving Patient, *Am. Heart J.*, 82:387, 1971. (45 references)

648. Gathman, G. E., and Nadas, A. S.: Total Anomalous Pulmonary Venous Connection. Clinical and Physiologic Observations of 75 Pediatric Patients, *Circulation*, 42:143, 1970.

649. Delisle, G., Ando, M., Calder, A. L., Zuberbuhler, J. R., Rochenmacher, S., Alday, L. E., Mangini, O., Van Praagh, S., and Van Praagh, R.: Total Anomalous Pulmonary Venous Connection: Report of 93 Autopsied Cases with Emphasis on Diagnostic and Surgical Considerations, *Am. Heart J.*, 91:99, 1976.

650. Paquet, M., and Gutgesell, H.: Echocardiographic Features of Total Anomalous Pulmonary Venous Connection, *Circulation*, 51:599, 1975.

651. Sahn, D. J., Allen, H. D., Lange, L. W., and Goldberg, S. J.: Cross-sectional Echocardiographic Diagnosis of the Sites of Total Anomalous Pulmonary Venous Drainage, *Circulation*, 60:1317, 1979.

652. Mullins, C. E., El-Said, G. M., Neches, W. H., Williams, R. L., Vargo, T. A., Nihill, M. R., and McNamara, D. G.: Balloon Atrial Septostomy for Total Anomalous Pulmonary Venous Return, *Br. Heart J.*, 35:752, 1973.

653. Tynan, M., Behrendt, D., Urquhart, W., and Graham, G. R.: Portal Vein Catheterization and Selective Angiography in Diagnosis of Total Anomalous Pulmonary Venous Connection, *Br. Heart J.*, 36:1155, 1974.

654. Mathew, R., Thilenius, O. G., Replogle, R. L., and Arcilla, R. A.: Cardiac Function in Total Anomalous Pulmonary Venous Return before and after Surgery, *Circulation*, 55:361, 1977.

655. Galioto, F. M., Jr., Fyler, D. C., and Chameides, L.: Total Anomalous Pulmonary Venous Drainage (TAPVD): A 5 Year Review in New England, *Am. J. Cardiol.*, 35:138, 1975.

656. Haworth, S. G., and Reid, L.: Structural Study of Pulmonary Circulation and of Heart in Total Anomalous Pulmonary Venous Return in Early Infancy, *Br. Heart J.*, 39:80, 1977.

657. Newfeld, E. A., Wilson, A., Paul, M. H., and Reisch, J. S.: Pulmonary Vascular Disease in Total Anomalous Pulmonary Venous Drainage, *Circulation*, 61:103, 1980.

658. Wukasch, D. C., Deutsch, M., Reul, G. J., Hallman, G. L., and Cooley, D. A.: Total Anomalous Pulmonary Venous Return: Review of 125 Patients Treated Surgically, *Ann. Thorac. Surg.*, 19:622, 1975.

659. Clarke, D. R., Stark, J., DeLeval, M., Pincott, J. R., and Taylor, J. F. N.: Total Anomalous Pulmonary Venous Drainage in Infancy, *Br. Heart J.*, 39:436, 1977.

660. Duff, D. F., Nihill, M. R., and McNamara, D. G.: Infradiaphragmatic Total Anomalous Pulmonary Venous Return: Review of Clinical and Pathological Findings and Results of Operation in 28 Cases, *Br. Heart J.*, 39:619, 1977.

661. Turley, K., Tucker, W. Y., Ullyot, D. J., and Ebert, P. A.: Total Anomalous Pulmonary Venous Connection in Infancy: Influence of Age and Type of Lesion, *Am. J. Cardiol.*, 45:92, 1980.

662. Katz, N. M., Kirklin, J. W., and Pacifico, A. D.: Concepts and Practices in Surgery for Total Anomalous Pulmonary Venous Connection, *Ann. Thorac. Surg.*, 25:479, 1978.

663. Gomes, M. M. R., Feldt, R. H., McGoon, D. C., and Danielson, G. K.: Total Anomalous Pulmonary Venous Connection, *J. Thorac. Cardiovasc. Surg.*, 60:116, 1970.

664. Gardner, D. L., and Cole, L.: Long Survival with Inferior Vena Cava Draining into Left Atrium, *Br. Heart J.*, 17:93, 1955.

665. Roberts, K. D., Edwards, J. M., and Astley, R.: Surgical Correction of Total Anomalous Systemic Venous Drainage, *J. Thorac. Cardiovasc. Surg.*, 64:803, 1972.

666. Fieldstein, L. E., and Pick, J.: Drainage of the Coronary Sinus into the Left Auricle. Report of a Rare Congenital Cardiac Anomaly, *Am. J. Clin. Path.*, 12:66, 1942.

667. Winter, F. S.: Persistent Left Superior Vena Cava: Survey of World Literature and Report of Thirty Additional Cases, *Angiology*, 5:90, 1954.

668. Karnegis, J. N., Wang, Y., Winchell, P., and Edwards, J. E.: Persistent Left Superior Vena Cava, Fibrous Remnant of the Right Superior Vena Cava and Ventricular Septal Defect, *Am. J. Cardiol.*, 14:573, 1964.

669. Fraser, R. S., Dvorkin, J., Rossall, R. E., and Eidem, R.: Left Superior Vena Cava: A Review of Associated Congenital Heart Lesions, Catheterization Data, and Roentgenologic Findings, *Am. J. Med.*, 31:711, 1961.

670. Freedom, R. M., and Ellison, R. C.: Coronary Sinus Rhythm in the Polysplenia Syndrome, *Chest*, 63:952, 1973.

671. Merrill, W. H., Pieroni, D. R., Freedom, R. M., and Ho, C. S.: Diagnosis of Infrahepatic Interruption of the Inferior Vena Cava, *Johns Hopkins Med. J.*, 133:329, 1973.

672. Van Praagh, R.: The Segmental Approach to Diagnosis in Congenital Heart Disease, *Birth Defects: Original Article Series* (The National Foundation—March of Dimes), 8:4, 1972.

673. Van Praagh, R., Perez-Trevino, C., Lopez-Cuellar, M., Baker, F. W., Zuberbuhler, J. R., Quero, M., Perez, V. M., Moreno, F., and Van Praagh, S.: Transposition of the Great Arteries with Posterior Aorta, Anterior Pulmonary Artery, Subpulmonary Conus, and Fibrous Continuity between Aortic and Atrio-Ventricular Valves, *Am. J. Cardiol.*, 28:621, 1971.

674. Anderson, R. H., Becker, A. E., Losekott, T. G., and Gerlis, L. M.: Anatomically Corrected Mal-

position of Great Arteries, *Br. Heart J.*, 37:993, 1975.

675. Van Praagh, R., and Vlad, P.: Dextrocardia, Mesocardia, and Levocardia: The Segmental Approach to Diagnosis in Congenital Heart Disease, in J. D. Keith, R. D. Rowe, and P. Vlad (eds.), "Heart Disease in Infancy and Childhood," Macmillan Publishing Company, Inc., New York, 1978.

676. Anderson, R. H., and Shenebourne, E. A. (eds.): "Paediatric Cardiology 1977," Churchill Livingston, Edinburgh, 1978.

677. Foale, R. A., Stefanini, L., Richards, A. F., and Somerville, J.: Two-Dimensional Echocardiographic Features of Corrected Transposition, *Am. J. Cardiol.*, 45:466, 1980.

678. Hagler, D. J., Tajik, A. J., Seward, J. B., Mair, D. D., and Ritter, D. G.: Wide-Angle Two-Dimensional Echocardiographic Criteria for Ventricular Morphology, *Am. J. Cardiol.*, 45:466, 1980.

679. Van Praagh, R., Weinberg, P. M., and Van Praagh, S.: Malposition of the Heart, in A. J. Moss, F. H. Adams, and G. C. Emmanouilides (eds.), "Heart Disease in Infants, Children and Adolescents," 2d. ed., The Williams & Wilkins Company, Baltimore, 1977.

*680. Liebman, J., Cullum, L., and Belloc, N. B.: Natural History of Transposition of the Great Arteries. Anatomy and Birth and Death Characteristics, *Circulation*, 40:237, 1969. (42 references)

681. Shrivastava, S., Tadavarthy, S. M., Fukuda, T., and Edwards, J. E.: Anatomic Causes of Pulmonary Stenosis in Complete Transposition, *Circulation*, 54:154, 1976.

682. Shaher, R. M., and Puddu, G. C.: Coronary Arterial Anatomy in Complete Transposition of the Great Vessels, *Am. J. Cardiol.*, 17:355, 1966.

683. Layman, T. E., and Edwards, J. E.: Anomalies of the Cardiac Valves Associated with Complete Transposition of the Great Vessels, *Am. J. Cardiol.*, 19:247, 1967.

684. Edwards, W. D., and Edwards, J. E.: Hypertensive Pulmonary Vascular Disease in D-Transposition of the Great Arteries, *Am. J. Cardiol.*, 41:921, 1978.

685. Elliott, L. P., Adams, P., Jr., Levy, M. J., and Edwards, J. E.: Right Ventricular Aorta and Biventricular Pulmonary Trunk. An Uncommon Form of Transposition, *Am. Heart J.*, 66:478, 1963.

686. Van Praagh, R., and Van Praagh, S.: Isolated Ventricular Inversion: A Consideration of the Morphogenesis, Definition and Diagnosis of Nontransposed and Transposed Great Arteries. *Am. J. Cardiol.*, 17:395, 1966.

687. Stanger, P., Benassi, R. C., Korns, M. E., Jue, K. L., and Edwards, J. E.: Diagrammatic Portrayal of Variations in Cardiac Structure: Reference to Transposition, Dextrocardia and the Concept of Four Normal Hearts, *Circulation*, 37/38(suppl. 4):1, 1968.

688. Plauth, W. H., Jr., Nadas, A. S., Bernhard, W. F., and Fyler, D. C.: Changing Hemodynamics in Patients with Transposition of the Great Arteries, *Circulation*, 42:131, 1970.

689. Tynan, M.: Transposition of the Great Arteries. Changes in the Circulation after Birth, *Circulation*, 46:809, 1972.

690. Mair, D. D., and Ritter, D. G.: Factors Influencing

Systemic Arterial Oxygen Saturation in Complete Transposition of the Great Arteries, *Am. J. Cardiol.,* 31:742, 1973.

691. Newfeld, E. A., Paul, M. H., Muster, A. J., and Idriss, F. S.: Pulmonary Vascular Disease in Complete Transposition of the Great Arteries: A Study of 200 Patients, *Am. J. Cardiol.,* 34:75, 1974.

692. Mathew, R., Rosenthal, A., and Fellows, K.: The Significance of Right Aortic Arch in D-Transposition of the Great Arteries, *Am. Heart J.,* 87:314, 1974.

693. Bierman, F. Z., and Williams, R. G.: Prospective Diagnosis of D-Transposition of the Great Arteries in Neonates by Subxiphoid Two-Dimensional Echocardiography, *Circulation,* 60:1496, 1979.

694. Gutgesell, H. P.: Echocardiographic Estimation of Pulmonary Artery Pressure in Transposition of the Great Arteries, *Circulation,* 57:1151, 1978.

695. Newfeld, E. A., Paul, M. H., Muster, A. J., and Idriss, F. S.: Pulmonary Vascular Disease in Transposition of the Great Vessels and Intact Ventricular Septum, *Circulation,* 59:525, 1979.

696. Lang, P., Freed, M. D., Bierman, F. Z., Norwood, W. I., Jr., and Nadas, A. S.: Use of Prostaglandin E in Infants with D-Transposition of the Great Arteries and Intact Ventricular Septum, *Am. J. Cardiol.,* 44:76, 1979.

697. Rashkind, W. J., and Miller, W. W.: Creation of an Atrial Septal Defect without Thoracotomy: A Palliative Approach to Complete Transposition of the Great Arteries, *J. Am. Med. Assoc.,* 196:173, 1966.

698. Blalock, A., and Hanlon, C. R.: Surgical Treatment of Complete Transposition of the Aorta and Pulmonary Artery, *Surg. Gynec. Obstet.,* 90:1, 1950.

699. Litwin, S. B., Plauth, W. H., Jr., Jones, J. E., and Bernhard, W. F.: Appraisal of Surgical Atrial Septectomy for Transposition of the Great Arteries, *Circulation,* 43/44(suppl. 1):7, 1971.

700. Kirklin, J. W., Barcia, A., Deverall, P. B., Kouchoukos, N. T., and Bargeron, L. M., Jr.: Surgical Treatment of Complex Forms of Transposition, *Br. Heart J.,* 33(suppl.):73, 1971.

701. Zavanella, C., and Subramanian, S.: Review: Surgery for Transposition of the Great Arteries in the First Year of Life, *Ann. Surg.,* 187:143, 1978.

702. Albert, H. M.: Surgical Correction of Transposition of the Great Vessels, *Surg. Forum,* 5:74, 1954.

703. Senning, A.: Surgical Correction of Transposition of the Great Vessels, *Surgery,* 45:966, 1959.

704. Mustard, W. T.: Successful Two-Stage Correction of Transposition of the Great Vessels, *Surgery,* 55:469, 1964.

705. Quaegebeur, J. M., and Brom, G. A.: Trousers-Shaped Baffle for Use in the Mustard Operation, *Ann. Thorac. Surg.,* 25:240, 1978.

706. Aberdeen, E.: Correction of Uncomplicated Cases of Transposition of the Great Arteries, *Br. Heart J.,* 33(suppl.):66, 1971.

707. Stark, J.: Primary Definitive Cardiac Operations in Infants: Transposition of the Great Arteries, in J. W. Kirklin (ed.), "Advances in Cardiovascular Surgery," Grune & Stratton, Inc., New York, 1973, p. 101.

708. Jatene, A. D., Fontes, V. F., Paulista, P. P., Souza, L. C. B., Neger, F., Galantier, M., and Souza, J. E. M. R.: Anatomic Correction of Transposition

of the Great Vessels, *J. Thorac. Cardiovasc. Surg.,* 72:364, 1976.

709. Stark, J., Silove, E. D., Taylor, J. F. N., and Graham, G. R.: Obstruction to Systemic Venous Return Following the Mustard Operation for Transposition of the Great Arteries, *J. Thorac. Cardiovasc. Surg.,* 68:742, 1974.

710. Berman, M. A., Barash, P. S., Hellenbrand, W. E., Stansel, H. C., Jr., and Talner, N. S.: Late Development of Severe Pulmonary Venous Obstruction Following the Mustard Operation, *Circulation,* 56(suppl. 2):91, 1977.

711. Lewis, A. B., Lindesmith, G. G., Takahashi, M., Stanton, R. E., Tucker, B. L., Stiles, Q. R., and Meyer, B. W.: Cardiac Rhythm Following the Mustard Procedure for Transposition of the Great Vessels, *J. Thorac. Cardiovasc. Surg.,* 73:919, 1977.

712. El-Said, G., Rosenberg, H. S., Mullins, C. E., Hallman, G. L., Cooley, D. A., and McNamara, D. G.: Dysrhythmias after Mustard's Operation for Transposition of the Great Arteries, *Am. J. Cardiol.,* 30:526, 1972.

713. Quaegebeur, J. M., Rohmer, J., and Brom, A. G.: Revival of the Senning Operation in the Treatment of Transposition of the Great Arteries, *Thorax,* 32:517, 1977.

714. Graham, T. P., Jr., Atwood, G. F., Boucek, R. J., Jr., Boerth, R. C., and Bender, H. W., Jr.: Abnormalities of Right Ventricular Function Following Mustard's Operation for Transposition of the Great Arteries, *Circulation,* 52:678, 1975.

715. Tynan, M., Aberdeen, E., and Stark, J.: Tricuspid Incompetence after the Mustard Operation for Transposition of the Great Arteries, *Circulation,* 45/46(suppl. 1):111, 1972.

716. Castaneda, A. R., Metras, D., and Buckley, L. P.: Transposition of the Great Arteries with Ventricular Septal Defect: Surgical Experience with the Mustard Operation and Closure of the Ventricular Septal Defect, *Proc. 7th Eur. Congr. Cardiol.,* Amsterdam, 1976, p. 566.

717. Idriss, F. S., Aubert, J., Paul, M. H., Nikaidoh, H., Lev, M., and Newfeld, E. A.: Transposition of the Great Vessels with Ventricular Septal Defect, *J. Thorac. Cardiovasc. Surg.,* 68:732, 1974.

718. Rastelli, G. C., McGoon, D. C., and Wallace, R. B.: Anatomic Correction of Transposition of the Great Arteries with Ventricular Septal Defect and Subpulmonary Stenosis, *J. Thorac. Cardiovasc. Surg.,* 58:545, 1969.

719. Lindesmith, G. G., Stiles, Q. R., Tucker, B. L., Gallaher, M. E., Stanton, R. E., and Meyer, B. W.: The Mustard Operation as a Palliative Procedure, *J. Thorac. Cardiovasc. Surg.,* 63:75, 1972.

*720. Sridaromont, S., Feldt, R. H., Ritter, D. G., Davis, G. D., and Edwards, J. E.: Double Outlet Right Ventricle: Hemodynamic and Anatomic Correlations, *Am. J. Cardiol.,* 38:85, 1976. (26 references)

721. Zamora, R., Moller, J. H., and Edwards, J. E.: Double-Outlet Right Ventricle. Anatomic Types and Associated Anomalies, *Chest,* 68:672, 1975.

722. Lev, M., Bharati, S., Meng, L., Liberthson, R. R., Paul, M. H., and Idriss, F.: A Concept of Double-Outlet Right Ventricle, *J. Thor. Cardiovasc. Surg.,* 64:271, 1972.

723. Tandon, R., Moller, J. H., and Edwards, J. E.:

Communication of Mitral Valve with Both Ventricles Associated with Double Outlet Right Ventricle, *Circulation*, 48:904, 1973.

724. Sridaromont, S., Ritter, D. G., Feldt, R. H., Davis, G. D., and Edwards, J. E.: Double-Outlet Right Ventricle: Anatomic and Angiocardiographic Correlations, *Mayo Clin. Proc.*, 53:555, 1978.

725. Stewart, S.: Double-Outlet Right Ventricle: A Collective Review with Surgical Viewpoint, *J. Thorac. Cardiovasc. Surg.*, 71:355, 1976.

726. Tabry, I. F., McGoon, D. C., Danielson, G. K., Wallace, R. B., Davis, Z., and Maloney, J. D.: Surgical Management of Double-Outlet Right Ventricle Associated with Atrioventricular Discordance, *J. Thorac. Cardiovasc. Surg.*, 76:336, 1978.

727. Kiser, J. C., Ongley, P. A., Kirklin, J. W., Clarkson, P. M., and McGoon, D. C.: Surgical Treatment of Dextrocardia with Inversion of Ventricles and Double-Outlet Right Ventricle, *J. Thorac. Cardiovasc. Surg.*, 55:6, 1968.

728. Gomes, M. M. R., Weidman, W. H., McGoon, D. C., and Danielson, G. K.: Double-Outlet Right Ventricle with Pulmonary Stenosis, *Circulation*, 43:889, 1971.

729. Harvey, J. C., Soundheimer, H. M., Williams, W. G., Olley, P. M., and Trusler, G. A.: Repair of Double-Outlet Right Ventricle, *J. Thorac. Cardiovasc. Surg.*, 73:611, 1977.

730. Stewart, R. W., Kirklin, J. W., Pacifico, A. D., Blackstone, E. H., and Bargeron, L. M., Jr.: Repair of Double-Outlet Right Ventricle: An Analysis of 62 Cases, *J. Thorac. Cardiovasc. Surg.*, 78:502, 1979.

*731. Brandt, P. W. T., Calder, A. L., Barratt-Boyes, B. G., and Neutze, J. M.: Double Outlet Left Ventricle. Morphology, Cineangiocardiographic Diagnosis and Surgical Treatment, *Am. J. Cardiol.*, 38:897, 1976. (25 references)

732. Paul, M. H., Muster, A. J., Sinha, S. N., Cole, R. B., and Van Praagh, R.: Double-Outlet Left Ventricle with an Intact Ventricular Septum: Clinical and Autopsy Diagnosis and Developmental Implications, *Circulation*, 41:129, 1970.

733. Bharati, S., Lev, M., Stewart, R., McAllister, H. A., and Kirklin, J. W.: The Morphologic Spectrum of Double Outlet Left Ventricle and Its Surgical Significance, *Circulation*, 58:558, 1978.

734. Pacifico, A. D., Kirklin, J. W., Bargeron, L. M., Jr., and Soto, B.: Surgical Treatment of Double-Outlet Left Ventricle, *Circulation*, 47/48(suppl. 3):19, 1973.

735. Villani, M., Lipscombe, S., and Ross, D. N.: Double Outlet Left Ventricle: How Should We Repair It? *J. Cardiovasc. Surg.*, 20:413, 1979.

736. Sakakibara, S., Takao, A., Arai, T., Hashimoto, A., and Nogi, M.: Both Great Vessels Arising from the Left Ventricle, *Bull. Heart Inst. Jap.*, 66, 1967.

*737. Schiebler, G. L., Edwards, J. E., Burchell, H. B., DuShane, J. W., Ongley, P. A., and Wood, E. H.: Congenital Corrected Transposition of the Great Vessels: A Study of 33 Cases, *Pediatrics*, 27(part II):851, 1961. (98 references)

738. Okamura, K., and Konno, S.: Two Types of Ventricular Septal Defect in Corrected Transposition of the Great Arteries: Reference to Surgical Approaches, *Am. Heart J.*, 85:483, 1973.

739. Edwards, J. E.: Differential Diagnosis of Mitral

Stenosis: A Clinicopathologic Review of Simulating Conditions, *Lab. Invest.*, 3:89, 1954.

740. Levy, M. J., Lillehei, C. W., Elliott, L. P., Carey, L. S., Adams, P., Jr., and Edwards, J. E.: Accessory Valvular Tissue Causing Subpulmonary Stenosis in Corrected Transposition of Great Vessels, *Circulation*, 27:494, 1963.

741. Friedberg, D. Z., and Nadas, A. S.: Clinical Profile of Patients with Congenital Corrected Transposition of the Great Arteries. A Study of Sixty Cases, *N. Engl. J. Med.*, 282:1053, 1970.

742. Nagai, I., Kawashima, Y., Fujita, T., Mori, T., and Manabe, H.: Successful Closure of Ventricular Septal Defect through a Left-Sided Ventriculotomy in Corrected Transposition of the Great Arteries, *Ann. Thorac. Surg.*, 21:491, 1976.

743. Fox, L. S., Kirklin, J. W., Pacifico, A. D., Waldo, A. L., and Bargeron, L. M., Jr.: Intracardiac Repair of Cardiac Malformations with Atrioventricular Discordance, *Circulation*, 54:123, 1976.

744. Van Praagh, R., Ongley, P. A., and Swan, H. J. C.: Anatomic Types of Single or Common Ventricle in Man. Morphologic and Geometric Aspects of 60 Necropsied Cases, *Am. J. Cardiol.*, 13:367, 1964.

745. Marin-Garcia, J., Tandon, R., Moller, J. H., and Edwards, J. E.: Single Ventricle with Transposition, *Circulation*, 49:994, 1974.

746. Marin-Garcia, J., Tandon, R., Moller, J. H., and Edwards, J. E.: Common (Single) Ventricle with Normally Related Great Vessels, *Circulation*, 49:565, 1974.

747. Ruttenberg, H. D., Neufeld, H. N., Lucas, R. V., Jr., Carey, L. S., Adams, P., Jr., Anderson, R. C., and Edwards, J. E.: Syndrome of Congenital Cardiac Disease with Asplenia. Distinction from Other Forms of Congenital Cyanotic Cardiac Disease, *Am. J. Cardiol.*, 13:387, 1964.

748. Saalouke, M. G., Perry, L. W., Okoroma, E. O., Shapiro, S. R., and Scott, L. P.: Primitive Ventricle with Normally Related Great Vessels and Stenotic Subpulmonary Outlet Chamber. Angiographic Differentiation from Tetralogy of Fallot, *Br. Heart J.*, 40:49, 1978.

749. Seward, J. B., Tajik, A. J., Hagler, D. J., Guiliani, E. R., Gau, G. T., and Ritter, D. G.: Echocardiograms in Common (Single) Ventricle: Angiographic-Anatomic Correlation, *Am. J. Cardiol.*, 39:217, 1977.

750. Silverman, N. H., and Schiller, N. B.: Apex Echocardiography: A Two-Dimensional Technique for Evaluating Congenital Heart Disease, *Circulation*, 57:503, 1978.

751. Soto, B., Bertranou, E. G., Bream, P. R., Souza, A., Jr., and Bargeron, L. M., Jr.: Angiographic Study of Univentricular Heart of Right Ventricular Type, *Circulation*, 60:1325, 1979.

752. Seward, J. B., Tajik, A. J., Hagler, D. J., and Ritter, D. G.: Contrast Echocardiography in Single or Common Ventricle, *Circulation*, 55:513, 1977.

753. Taussig, H. B.: Long-Time Observations on the Blalock-Taussig Operation. IX. Single Ventricle (with Apex to the Left), *Johns Hopkins Med J.*, 139:69, 1976.

754. Graham, T. P., Jr., and Friesinger, G. C.: Complex Cyanotic Congenital Heart Disease in Adults, in W. C. Roberts (ed.), "Congenital Heart Disease in

Adults," F. A. Davis Company, Philadelphia, 1979.

755. Moreno-Cabral, R. J., Miller, D. C., Oyer, P. E., Stinson, E. B., Reitz, B. A., and Shumway, N. E.: A Surgical Approach for S.L.L. Single Ventricle Incorporating Total Right Atrium–Pulmonary Artery Diversion," *J. Thorac. Cardiovasc. Surg.*, 79:202, 1980.

756. McGoon, D. C., Danielson, G. K., Ritter, D. G., Wallace, R. B., Maloney, J. D., and Marcelletti, C.: Correction of the Univentricular Heart Having Two Atrioventricular Valves, *J. Thorac. Cardiovasc. Surg.*, 74:218, 1977.

757. Gale, A. W., Danielson, G. K., McGoon, D. C., and Mair, D. D.: Modified Fontan Operation for Univentricular Heart and Complicated Congenital Lesions, *J. Thorac. Cardiovasc. Surg.*, 78:831, 1979.

758. Bjork, V. O., Olin, C. L., Bjarke, B. B., and Thoren, C. A.: Right Atrial–Right Ventricular Anastomosis for Correction of Tricuspid Atresia, *J. Thorac. Cardiovasc. Surg.*, 77:452, 1979.

759. Yacoub, M. H., and Radley-Smith, R.: Use of a Valved Conduit from Right Atrium to Pulmonary Artery for "Correction" of Single Ventricle, *Circulation,* 54(suppl.3):63, 1976.

*760. Stanger, P., Rudolph, A. M., and Edwards, J. E.: Cardiac Malpositions. An Overview Based on Study of Sixty-Five Necropsy Specimens *Circulation*, 56:159, 1977. (48 references)

761. Calcaterra, G., Anderson, R. H., Lau, K. C., and Shinebourne, E. A.: Dextrocardia—Value of Segmental Analysis in Its Categorisation, *Br. Heart J.*, 42:497, 1979.

762. Squarcia, U., Ritter, D. G., and Kincaid, O. W.: Dextrocardia: Angiographic Study and Classification, *Am. J. Cardiol.*, 32:965, 1973.

763. Miller, R. D., and Divertie, M. B.: Kartagener's Syndrome, *Chest*, 62:130, 1972.

764. Anderson, R. H., Shinebourne, E. A., and Gerlis, L. M.: Criss-Cross Atrioventricular Relationships Producing Paradoxical Atrioventricular Concordance or Discordance: Their Significance to Nomenclature of Congenital Heart Disease, *Circulation*, 50:176, 1974.

*765. Van Praagh, S., La Corte, M., Fellows, K. E., Bossina, K., Busch, H. J., Keck, E. W., Weinberg, P. M., Van Praagh, R.: Superoinferior Ventricles: Anatomic and Angiographic Findings in Ten Post Mortem Cases, in R. Van Praagh and A. Takao (eds.), "Etiology and Morphogenesis of Congenital Heart Disease," Futura Publishing Company, Mount Kisco, New York, 1980. (11 references)

*766. Attie, F., Munoz-Castellanos, L., Ovseyevitz, J., Flores-Delgado, I., Testelli, M. R., Buendia, A., Kuri, J., and Molina, B.: Crossed Atrioventricular Connections, *Am. Heart J.*, 99:163, 1980. (28 references)

767. Sieg, K., Hagler, D. J., Ritter, D. G., McGoon, D. C., Maloney, J. D., Seward, J. B., and Davis, G. D.: Straddling Right Atrioventricular Valve in Criss-Cross Atrioventricular Relationship, *Mayo Clin. Proc.*, 52:561, 1977.

768. Freedom, R. M., Culham, G., and Rowe, R. D.: The Criss-Cross and Superoinferior Ventricular Heart: An Angiocardiographic Study, *Am. J. Cardiol.*, 42:620, 1978.

*769. Van Mierop, L. H. S., Gessner, I. H., and Schie-

bler, G. L.: Asplenia and Polysplenia Syndromes, *Birth Defects: Original Article Series* (National Foundation—March of Dimes), 8:36, 1972. (41 references)

770. Rose, V., Izukawa, T., and Moes, C. A. F.: Syndromes of Asplenia and Polysplenia. A Review of Cardiac and Non-Cardiac Malformations in 60 Cases with Special Reference to Diagnosis and Prognosis, *Br. Heart J.*, 37:840, 1975.

771. Padmanabhan, J., Risemberg, H. M., and Rowe, R. D.: Howell-Jolly Bodies in the Peripheral Blood of Full Term and Premature Neonates, *Johns Hopkins Med. J.,* 132:146, 1973.

772. Freedom, R. M., and Treves, S.: Splenic Scintigraphy and Radionuclide Venography in the Heterotaxy Syndrome, *Radiology,* 107:381, 1973.

773. Waldman, J. D., Rosenthal, A., Smith, A. L., Shurin, S., and Nadas, A. S.: Sepsis and Congenital Asplenia, *J. Pediatr.*, 90:555, 1977.

774. Byron, F.: Ectopia Cordis—Case with Attempted Operative Correction, *J. Thorac. Surg.*, 7:717, 1948.

775. Knight. L., Neal, W. A., Williams, H. J., Huseby, T. L., and Edwards, J. E.: Congenital Left Ventricular Diverticulum. Part of a Syndrome of Cardiac Anomalies and Midline Defects, *Minnesota Med.*, 59:372, 1976.

*776. Ravitch, M. M.: "Congenital Deformities of the Chest Wall and Their Operative Connection," W. B. Saunders Company, Philadelphia, 1977. (37 references)

777. Cantrell, J. R., Haller, J. A., and Ravitch, M. M.: A Syndrome of Congenital Defects Involving the Abdominal Wall, Sternum, Diaphragm, Pericardium, and Heart, *Surg. Gynec. Obst.*, 107:602, 1958.

778. Galioto, F. M., Jr., Reitman, M. J., Vargo, T. A., Gillette, P. C., and McNamara, D. G.: Congenital Diverticulum of the Left Ventricle, *Am. Heart J.*, 87:109, 1974.

779. McNamara, J. J., and Gross, R. E.: Congenital Coronary Artery Fistula, *Surgery*, 65:59, 1969.

780. Edwards, J. E., Gladding, T. C., and Weir, A. B., Jr.: Congenital Communication between the Right Coronary Artery and the Right Atrium, *J. Thor. Surg.*, 35:662, 1958.

*781. Liberthson, R. R., Sagar, K., Berkoben, J. P., Weintraub, R. M., and Levine, F. H.: Congenital Coronary Arteriovenous Fistula: Report of 13 Patients, Review of the Literature and Delineation of Management, *Circulation*, 59:849, 1979. (70 references)

782. Jaffee, R. B., Glancy, D. L., Epstein, S. E., Brown, B. G., and Morrow, A. G.: Coronary Arterial–Right Heart Fistula: Long-Term Observations in Seven Patients, *Circulation*, 47:133, 1973.

783. Levin, D. C., Fellows, K. E., and Abrams, H. L.: Hemodynamically Significant Primary Anomalies of the Coronary Arteries: Angiographic Aspects, *Circulation*, 58:25, 1978.

784. Oldham, H. N., Jr., Ebert, P. A., Young, W. G., and Sabiston, D. C., Jr.: Surgical Management of Congenital Coronary Artery Fistula, *Ann. Thorac. Surg.*, 12:503, 1971.

785. Liotta, D., Hallman, G. L., Hall, R. J., and Cooley, D. A.: Surgical Treatment of Congenital Coronary Artery Fistula, *Surgery*, 70:876, 1971.

786. Noren, G. H., Raghib, G., Moller, J. H., Amplatz,

K., Adams, P., Jr., and Edwards, J. E.: Anomalous Origin of the Left Coronary Artery from the Pulmonary Trunk with Special Reference to the Occurrence of Mitral Insufficiency, *Circulation,* 30:171, 1964.

787. Burchell, H. B., and Brown, A. L., Jr.: Anomalous Origin of Coronary Artery from Pulmonary Artery Masquerading as Mitral Insufficiency, *Am. Heart J.,* 63:388, 1962.

788. Rao, B. N. S., Lucas, R. V., Jr., and Edwards, J. E.: Anomalous Origin of the Left Coronary Artery from the Right Pulmonary Artery Associated with Ventricular Septal Defect, *Chest,* 59:616, 1970.

789. Masel, L.: Tetralogy of Fallot with Origin of the Left Coronary Artery from the Right Pulmonary Artery, *Med. J. Aust.,* 1:213, 1960.

*790. Wesselhoeft, H., Fawcett, J. S., and Johnson, A. L.: Anomalous Origin of the Left Coronary Artery from the Pulmonary Trunk: Its Clinical Spectrum, Pathology, and Pathophysiology Based on a Review of 140 Cases with 7 Further Cases, *Circulation,* 38:403, 1968. (71 references)

791. Gutgesell, H. P., Pinsky, W. W., and DePuey, E. G.: Thallium-201 Myocardial Perfusion Imaging in Infants and Children: Value in Distinguishing Anomalous Left Coronary Artery from Congestive Cardiomyopathy, *Circulation,* 61:596, 1980.

792. Wilson, C. L., Dlabal, P. W., and McGuire, S. A.: Surgical Treatment of Anomalous Left Coronary Artery from Pulmonary Artery: Follow-Up in Teenagers and Adults, *Am. Heart J.,* 98:440, 1979.

793. Cooley, D. A., Hallman, G. L., and Bloodwell, R. D.: Definitive Surgical Treatment of Anomalous Origin of Left Coronary Artery from Pulmonary Artery: Indications and Results, *J. Thorac. Cardiovasc. Surg.,* 52:798, 1966.

794. Shrivastava, S., Castaneda, A. R., and Moller, J. H.: Anomalous Left Coronary Artery from Pulmonary Trunk: Long-Term Follow-Up After Ligation, *J. Thorac. Cardiovasc. Surg.,* 76:130, 1978.

795. Chiariello, L., Meyer, J., Reul, G. J., Hallman, G. L., and Cooley, D. A.: Surgical Treatment for Anomalous Origin of Left Coronary Artery from Pulmonary Artery, *Ann. Thorac. Surg.,* 19:443, 1975.

796. Meyer, B. W., Stefanik, G., Stiles, Q. R., Lindesmith, G. G., and Jones, J. C.: A Method of Definitive Surgical Treatment of Anomalous Origin of Left Coronary Artery, *J. Thorac. Cardiovasc. Surg.,* 56:104, 1968.

797. Levitsky, S., van der Horst, R. L., Hastreiter, A. R., and Fisher, E. A.: Anomalous Left Coronary Artery in the Infant: Recovery of Ventricular Function Following Early Direct Aortic Implantation, *J. Thorac. Cardiovasc. Surg.,* 79:598, 1980.

798. Tingelstad, J. B., Lower, R. R., Eldredge, W. J.: Anomalous Origin of the Right Coronary Artery from the Main Pulmonary Artery, *Am. J. Cardiol.,* 30:670, 1972.

*799. Blake, H. A., Manion, W. C., Mattingly, R. W., and Baroldi, G.: Coronary Artery Anomalies, *Circulation,* 30:927, 1964. (70 references)

800. Ogden, J. A.: Origin of a Single Coronary Artery from the Pulmonary Artery, *Am. Heart J.,* 78:251, 1969.

801. Feldt, R. H., Ongley, P. A., and Titus, J. L.: Total Coronary Arterial Circulation from Pulmonary Artery with Survival to Age Seven: Report of a Case, *Proc. Mayo Clin.,* 40:539, 1965.

802. Neufeld, H. N., and Blieden, L. C.: Coronary Artery Disease in Children, *Prog. Cardiol.,* 4:119, 1975.

803. Lerberg, D. B., Ogden, J. A., Zuberbuhler, J. R., and Bahnson, H. T.: Anomalous Origin of the Right Coronary Artery from the Pulmonary Artery, *Ann. Thorac. Surg.,* 27:87, 1979.

*804. Cheitlin, M. D., De Castro, C. M., and McAllister, H. A.: Sudden Death as a Complication of Anomalous Left Coronary Origin from the Anterior Sinus of Valsalva. A Not-So-Minor Congenital Anomaly, *Circulation,* 50:780, 1974. (12 references)

805. Liberthson, R. R., Dinsmore, R. E., and Fallon, J. T.: Aberrant Coronary Artery Origin from the Aorta: Report of 18 Patients. Review of Literature and Delineation of Natural History and Management, *Circulation,* 59:748, 1979.

806. Byrum, C. J., Blackman, M. S., Schneider, B., Sondheimer, H. M., and Kavey, R. W.: Congenital Atresia of the Left Coronary Ostium and Hypoplasia of the Left Main Coronary Artery, *Am. Heart J.,* 99:354, 1980.

807. Mullins, C. E., El-Said, G., McNamara, D. G., Cooley, D. A., Treistman, B., and Garcia, E.: Atresia of the Left Coronary Ostium: Repair by Saphenous Vein Graft, *Circulation,* 46:989, 1972.

808. Radford, D. J., Sondheimer, H. M., Williams, G. J., and Fowler, R. S.: Mucocutaneous Lymph Node Syndrome with Coronary Artery Aneurysm, *Am. J. Dis. Child.,* 130:596, 1976.

809. Wilson, C. S., Weaver, W. F., Zeman, E. D., and Forker, A. D.: Bilateral Nonfistulous Congenital Coronary Arterial Aneurysms, *Am. J. Cardiol.,* 35:319, 1975.

810. McMartin, D. E., Stone, A. J., and Franch, R. H.: Multiple Coronary-Artery Aneurysms in a Child with Angina Pectoris, *N. Engl. J. Med.,* 290:669, 1974.

811. Mattern, A. L., Baker, W. P., McHale, J. J., and Lee, D. E.: Congenital Coronary Aneurysms with Angina Pectoris and Myocardial Infarction Treated with Saphenous Vein Bypass Graft, *Am. J. Cardiol.,* 30:906, 1972.

812. Mantini, E., Grondin, C. M., Lillehei, C. W., and Edwards, J. E.: Congenital Anomalies Involving the Coronary Sinus, *Circulation,* 33:317, 1966.

813. Foale, R. A., Baron, D. W., and Richards, A. F.: Isolated Congenital Absence of Coronary Sinus, *Br. Heart J.,* 42:355, 1979.

814. Moore, R. L.: Congenital Deficiencies of the Pericardium, *Arch. Surg.,* 11:765, 1925.

815. Nasser, W. K., Helmen, C., Tavel, M. E., Feigenbaum, H., and Fisch, C.: Congenital Absence of the Left Pericardium, *Circulation,* 41:469, 1970.

816. Hipona, F. A., and Crummy, A. J., Jr.: Congenital Pericardial Defect Associated with Tetralogy of Fallot, *Circulation,* 29:132, 1964.

817. Spitz, L., Bloom, F., Milner, S., and Levin, S. E.: Combined Anterior Abdominal Wall, Sternal, Diaphragmatic, Pericardial, and Intracardiac Defects: A Report of 5 Cases and Their Management, *J. Pediat. Surg.,* 10:481, 1975.

818. Ellis, K., Leeds, N. E., Himmelstein, A.: Congenital Deficiencies of the Parietal Pericardium, *Amer. J. Roentgenol. Radium Ther. Nucl. Med.,* 82:125, 1959.

819. Payvandi, M. N., and Kerber, R. E.: Echocardiography in Congenital and Acquired Absence of the Pericardium, *Circulation,* 53:86, 1976.

820. Loehr, W. M.: Pericardial Cysts, *Am. J. Roentgenol.,* 68:584, 1952.

821. Bramlet, D. A., and Edwards, J. E.: Congenital Aneurysm of the Left Atrial Appendage, *Br. Heart J.,* 45:97, 1981.

Section B Valvular Heart Disease

37

Acute Rheumatic Fever and Its Management

Gene H. Stollerman, M.D.

Definition

Rheumatic fever is a diffuse inflammatory disease which is a delayed nonsuppurative sequela of pharyngeal infection with group A streptococci. In its typical form, the disease is an acute febrile illness characterized by inflammation of the joints, heart, skin, and nervous system. The clinical manifestations usually include migratory polyarthritis, pancarditis, Sydenham's chorea, erythema marginatum, and subcutaneous nodules, in varying combinations. Although the name *acute rheumatic fever* (ARF) emphasizes involvement of the joints, the disease owes its major importance to the involvement of the heart. The disease can be fatal during the acute attack or can lead to rheumatic heart disease, a chronic condition characterized by scarring and deformity of the heart valves. Patients who have suffered an initial attack of rheumatic fever are at high risk of developing recurrences following group A streptococcal infections.

Etiology and Pathogenesis

Etiology

Several lines of evidence have established the etiologic relationship between group A streptococcal infection and rheumatic fever.[1] Outbreaks of ARF tend to accompany epidemics of streptococcal sore throat and scarlet fever. Approximately two-thirds of rheumatic fever patients recall having a recent sore throat, and virtually all ARF patients have immunologic evidence of recent streptococcal infection.[2] In long-term prospective follow-up studies, rheumatic fever recurs only as a result of intercurrent streptococcal infections. Both primary and secondary attacks of the disease can be prevented by prompt treatment or prevention of streptococcal infections by antimicrobial therapy.[1,3]

Pathogenesis

To initiate the rheumatic process, group A streptococci must infect the pharynx. Streptococcal infections of the skin or other extrapharyngeal sites will not cause the disease.[4,5] Furthermore, throat infections with some group A strains appear to produce rheumatic fever rarely or not at all.[6] A relatively small percentage of patients who sustain a streptococcal throat infection subsequently develop ARF. The organism cannot be found in the lesions when rheumatic fever appears after a latent period of several days or weeks after the acute streptococcal infection. No streptococcal product has been identified as a cause of the rheumatic lesions, and the latter have not been identified as due to a direct effect of a tissue toxin or an immunologic process. Gamma globulin has been demonstrated repeatedly in the sarcolemma of the myocardial fibers of patients who have died of rheumatic carditis and in the biopsied auricular appendages of patients operated upon for mitral stenosis. Purified proteins from streptococcal cell membranes have been shown to be immunologically cross-reactive with sarcolemmal tissue,[7] and patients with rheumatic fever (with or without carditis) often have circulating antibodies to heart tissue.[8] Experimentally, tissue cultures of embryonic guinea pig heart can be damaged by lymphocytes sensitized to group A streptococci.[9] These findings have suggested that the myocardial lesions of rheumatic fever are the result of autoimmunity induced by streptococcal antigens. This concept has not been proved, however, since the immunologic phenomena might be secondary to cardiac tissue damage rather than a cause of it.

A possible explanation for the disparity in the rheumatogenicity of pharyngeal and cutaneous streptococcal infections relates to differences in the bacterial strains responsible for each. Group A streptococci commonly isolated from pyoderma lesions belong to different serotypes from those classically associated with acute exudative tonsillopharyngeal infections. Although these "pyoderma" strains commonly colonize the pharynx, they tend to produce less virulent infections by both clinical and immunologic criteria.[10] A relatively limited number of streptococcal M-protein serotypes have been clearly associated with outbreaks of rheumatic fever,[6] and, in general, these so-called rheumatogenic strains have properties associated with high degrees of virulence, such as large hyaluronate capsules, large amounts of M protein, striking resistance to phagocytosis in human blood, and the capacity to evoke very strong immune responses, particularly to M-associated proteins.[11] Whether rheumatogenicity is, therefore, a reflection of the virulence and intensity of the streptococcal pharyngeal infection per se or a *qualitative* distinction of certain strains of group A streptococci is not yet clear.

Incidence and Epidemiology

ARF appears most frequently between the ages of 5 and 15 when streptococcal pharyngitis is most intense. It is extremely rare in infancy but may appear at any age. The geographic distribution, incidence, and severity of rheumatic fever are closely correlated with the frequency and severity of streptococcal disease in a given population. In epidemics of severe exudative streptococcal pharyngitis, the attack rate of rheumatic fever averages approximately 3 percent of untreated patients.[12] The attack rate, however, appears to be very much lower when streptococcal pharyngitis is sporadic and mild and due to strains of lesser rheumatic potential.[11] Two variables known to affect the attack rate of ARF are (1) the magnitude of the immune response to the antecedent streptococcal infection and (2) the duration of the throat infection prior to antibiotic therapy. Eradication of the infection by penicillin can reduce the attack rate when treatment is begun up to 10 days after the onset of pharyngitis. Treatment which fails to suppress the immune response and which fails to eradicate the bacteria from the throat also fails to prevent rheumatic fever.

Such factors as latitude, altitude, crowding, dampness, economic conditions, and age all affect the incidence of rheumatic fever because they are all related to the incidence and transmission of streptococcal pharyngitis.

Secondary rheumatic attack rates (those following streptococcal infections in patients who have had previous attacks of rheumatic fever) are increased to as high as 5 to 50 per 100 streptococcal infections and are also related to the virulence of reactivating infections.[13] Moreover, the frequency of secondary attacks of rheumatic fever is much greater in subjects with rheumatic heart disease than in those who had ARF but escaped rheumatic carditis during the prior rheumatic attack. With the passage of years, the tendency to suffer recurrences of rheumatic fever following streptococcal infections declines but remains higher than the attack rate in the general population even after more than a decade. Certain host variables, therefore, as well as probable qualitative and quantitative differences in the nature of streptococcal infection to which the rheumatic host may be exposed, appear to condition variations in the secondary rheumatic fever attack rate, and such variables have an important bearing upon strategies for rheumatic fever prevention (see below).

Whether these variables are genetic, acquired, or both has not been settled. A family history of rheumatic fever is commonly elicited and yet the concordance of the disease in identical twins is approximately 20 percent,[14] a figure which does not exceed that of poliomyelitis or tuberculosis, suggesting only a limited penetrance of genetic predisposition to rheumatic fever. Although vigorously investigated, the association of ARF with specific histocompatibility antigens has not yet been established.

The incidence of ARF, and certainly its mortality, like that of septic streptococcal sore throat and scarlet fever, has been decreasing for several years in countries where housing and economic conditions have been improving steadily. The rate of decrease has probably been accelerated by the wide use of antimicrobial therapy. The decrease may also be due to a change in the prevalence of rheumatogenic streptococcal strains. Despite its dramatic decline in relatively affluent countries, ARF is a major cause of death and disability from heart disease wherever in the world poor economic conditions, overcrowding, and substandard housing are most common. Thus, rheumatic fever and rheumatic heart disease retain an important place in the priorities for public health programs in the poorest countries and populations in the world, and particularly in such regions as India, the Middle East, China, Southeast Asia, Micronesia, and many parts of South America. It is noteworthy that even in countries with a good record of rheumatic fever control, pockets of the disease persist within these nations among economically depressed populations such as Australian aborigines, American Indians, inner-city-dwelling blacks and Hispanics, New Zealand Maoris, and the Arab population of Israel.[15]

Pathology

The pathology of rheumatic fever is characterized by diffuse proliferative and exudative inflammatory lesions in the connective tissues, particularly around small blood vessels.

Cardiovascular Lesions

The disease has a distinct personality pathologically because of its unique lesions of the heart and in its tendency to spare other organs from serious damage. All of the layers of the heart—endocardium, myocardium, and pericardium—may be involved, giving rise to the term *rheumatic pancarditis*. The most distinctive and specific pattern of rheumatic inflammation is found in the myocardial *Aschoff body*. This lesion, a submiliary granuloma, when present in its classic form, is considered to be pathognomonic of rheumatic fever. The earliest features of the lesion are swelling and fragmentation of collagen fibers and alteration in the staining properties of the ground substance of the connective tissues, a change described as *fibrinoid degeneration* of collagen. The chemical basis of this change is still not known. Around and between the altered collagen, lymphocytes accumulate and, in addition, large cells appear which have a ragged basophilic cytoplasm and one or more nuclei with a very characteristic arrangement of chromatin condensed into patterns like an "owl's eye" or "sawtooth" edges and surrounded by a very sharp and clear nuclear membrane. These Aschoff cells, or *Anitschkow myocytes*, have been the subject of controversy over whether they are myocytes or whether they are of interstitial origin.[16] Aschoff bodies with more productive and less exudative changes may persist for many years after clinical evidence of carditis has subsided and remain as the lingering traces of chronic rheumatic inflammation in patients with rheumatic heart disease, particularly those who go on to develop mitral stenosis.[17] Eventually the Aschoff body heals, taking the form of a spindle-shaped triangular scar lying between the muscle bundles and surrounding blood vessels.

Rheumatic endocarditis is characterized by a verrucous valvulitis which causes swelling, edema, and deformity of the valves and leads to the most serious permanent cardiac damage once the risk of heart failure from the "toxic," exudative phase of myocarditis is over. Healing of the valvulitis may occur with fibrous thickening and adhesion of the valve commissures and chordae tendineae, leading to variable degrees of valvular regurgitation and stenosis. Valvular deformity occurs most commonly in the mitral and aortic valves, less frequently in the tricuspid valves, and almost never in the pulmonary valves.

Rheumatic pericarditis consists of a serofibrinous effusion, causing "shaggy" elements of fibrin to be deposited on the heart's surface. Despite such heavy fibrinous and sometimes sanguineous effusions, pericardial constriction does not occur, although the pericardium may become calcified.

Extracardiac Lesions

The joints are affected by an exudative, nonspecific synovitis and not by proliferative changes, and healing occurs without significant scarring or deformity. During the acute phase of the disease subcutaneous nodules, which are composed of granulomas with localized areas of fibrinoid necrosis may appear. The nodules also contain perivascular collections of large cells with pale, prominent nuclei resembling somewhat the Aschoff lesions of the myocardium. Pulmonary and pleural lesions are less definite and less characteristic. Fibrinous pleurisy and rheumatic pneumonitis may occur with exudative and proliferative lesions which may be difficult to differentiate from lung lesions associated with severe heart failure, hypoxia, and pulmonary thrombosis. Because patients with pure Sydenham's chorea rarely die during the active stage of this condition, the pathological findings which have been reported in the central nervous system are not consistent and no characteristic lesion has been found which explains the choreiform activity. During active chorea the spinal fluid remains normal and is free of cells, it contains normal levels of protein, and no change in the relative concentrations of various proteins occurs. Perivascular changes described in the brains of patients dying with fulminating rheumatic carditis occur whether or not chorea is also present.

Clinical Features

The major clinical manifestations of rheumatic fever are polyarthritis, carditis, chorea, erythema marginatum, and subcutaneous nodules. These major manifestations may occur singly or in various combinations following a latent period of 1 to 5 weeks (mean of 18 days) after streptococcal infection (usually much later in the case of chorea, as discussed below). Surprisingly, as many as one-third of patients with ARF cannot recall the antecedent streptococcal sore throat.

Arthritis

The classic attack of rheumatic fever presents as an acute migratory polyarthritis associated with the usual signs and symptoms of an acute febrile illness and cannot be distinguished from many other forms of acute infectious polyarthritis when joint involvement is the only major manifestation of the disease. The large joints of the extremities are most frequently affected, but any joint may be involved; the arthritis may include the hands, feet, and spine as well. Joint effusions occur but are not persistent. As pain and swelling subside in one joint, others tend to become involved in "migratory" fashion, although such migration is not invariable and several large joints may become inflamed simultaneously. For polyarthritis to be acceptable as a criterion for the diagnosis of rheumatic fever, it should involve at least two joints; should be associated with at least two minor manifestations such as fever and elevation of erythrocyte sedimentation rate (ESR); and most important, should be associated with a high titer of one or more streptococcal antibodies.[18]

Acute Rheumatic Carditis

Carditis, if it is to occur, usually does so within the first 3 weeks of the attack.[19] It first manifests itself by the appearance of the heart murmurs of either mitral or aortic regurgitation or both (the former more frequently). When acute polyarthritis is the presenting symptom, attention of the physician is drawn to the heart, and carditis can usually be detected by the presence of the murmurs early in the attack. If isolated carditis is the initial manifestation, however, the onset may be insidious or even subclinical. In its most severe form, carditis causes death from acute myocardial failure. The fulminating form of rheumatic carditis has now become relatively rare, however. In contrast to the seriousness of its prognosis, rheumatic carditis most often causes no symptoms of its own and is often diagnosed only because arthritis or chorea directs the patient to a physician, unless isolated carditis is associated with the pain of pericarditis or is severe enough to cause symptoms of heart failure or fever and constitutional symptoms such as weakness, fatigue, and anorexia. For this reason, patients whose rheumatic fever is manifested only by carditis are frequently not diagnosed and in later life may be discovered to have rheumatic heart disease without a definite history of rheumatic fever.

Carditis occurs in 40 to 50 percent of first attacks of ARF, although the incidence of various rheumatic manifestations varies with age. Carditis is most frequent during an initial rheumatic attack in the youngest age groups and is relatively rare in adult cases. Moreover, there tends to be an inverse relationship between the severity of the arthritis and the severity of carditis.

The hallmarks of clinically active rheumatic carditis are (1) organic heart murmurs not previously present or a distinct change in the character of a preexisting heart murmur, (2) cardiac enlargement, (3) congestive heart failure, and (4) pericardial friction rubs or signs of effusion. In actuality, rheumatic carditis is almost always associated with one or more characteristic murmurs. The diagnosis must be suspect in the absence of such murmurs unless they are obscured by a loud pericardial friction rub or severe tachycardia. Among patients who develop carditis in their first rheumatic attack, the murmurs are present in 75 percent during the first week of the illness and in 85 percent by the third week.[19] Virtually all murmurs appear within 3 months except, perhaps, for those patients with slight degrees of aortic or mitral regurgitation, which may be heard for the first time some months later, after maximal exercise or effort is permitted. The three murmurs of rheumatic carditis are apical systolic, apical middiastolic, and basal diastolic.

The murmur of mitral regurgitation is high-pitched and blowing and occupies most of systole. It is best heard at the apex, radiates toward the axilla, and does not change significantly with position or respiration. It must be distinguished from functional murmurs so frequently heard in children and adolescents. These functional murmurs have a vibratory quality often described as moaning or groaning, are often louder along the left sternal border or at the pulmonary area than at the apex, and are accentuated in recumbency.

The apical middiastolic murmur, also known as the *Carey-Coombs murmur,* begins immediately following the third heart sound and ends prior to the first heart sound. It is low-pitched and does not radiate widely. The murmur can also be heard in other situations characterized by rapid flow across the mitral valve (e.g., established mitral regurgitation in chronic rheumatic heart disease, other forms of carditis with marked cardiac dilatation, thyrotoxicosis, anemia).

The basal diastolic murmur of aortic regurgitation begins immediately following the second heart sound. It is soft, high-pitched, and decrescendo; at times it is heard best in the third intercostal space at the left sternal border, and at times in the second intercostal space just to the right of the sternum. The aortic regurgitation murmur may be heard only intermittently. Occasionally one hears transiently a cooing or high-pitched crying ("sea gull") quality to the murmur during the active stage of rheumatic valvulitis of either mitral or aortic valves.

In addition to murmurs, cardiomegaly, frank congestive failure, and pericarditis, other manifestations of carditis in ARF include tachycardia, which persists during sleep, and gallop rhythms of S_3, S_4, or summation types. Abnormalities of atrioventricular conduction are quite common. The most common of these is first-degree heart block. Second-degree heart block, complete heart block, and atrioventricular dissociation may also be observed. Atrial fibrillation, on the other hand, is usually a feature of chronic rather than acute rheumatic heart disease. Prolongation of the PR interval and other changes in the ECG are very common but do not in themselves indicate acute carditis, and their presence or absence is unrelated to the subsequent development of chronic rheumatic heart disease.[20]

Chronic Rheumatic Carditis

The presenting picture in this syndrome is one of chronic heart failure in a patient with a markedly dilated heart and with physical, electrocardiographic, and x-ray findings compatible with mitral regurgitation. The differentiation from other forms of chronic myocarditis may be difficult, if not impossible, when the other associated extracardiac features of rheumatic fever are absent. Although rheumatic fever does not produce *isolated* myocarditis and is almost invariably a pancarditis, the pericardial inflammation may not be evident and the mitral valvulitis might not be distinguishable from mitral regurgitation due to dilatation of the mitral ring. In such cases one must search diligently for clues such as evanescent pericardial rubs, pericardial effusion, transient aortic regurgitation, subcutaneous nodules, erythema marginatum, and subtle signs of chorea.

Chronic rheumatic myocarditis may run a fatal course over a period of months or even several years. Often, however, the patient improves, sometimes rather suddenly, and may even recover cardiac reserve dramatically in association with the disappearance of systemic manifestations of the chronic inflammatory process. The heart may remain large or may decrease somewhat in size. In occasional instances it may even return to normal size, leaving varying degrees of valvular insufficiency. Such a course signals the termination of the toxic phase of the rheumatic process, and thereafter the course of rheumatic heart disease depends on the variables in healing cited below.

Chorea

This manifestation is a disorder of the central nervous system characterized by sudden, aimless, irregular movements and is often accompanied by emotional instability. Chorea may appear after a long latent period, as long as several months after the antecedent streptococcal infection, and at a time when all other manifestations of rheumatic fever have abated and antistreptococcal antibodies have returned to normal. When no previous rheumatic manifestations are present, the syndrome is called *pure chorea*. More often chorea begins 1 to 3 months after the antecedent streptococcal infection, but always later than polyarthritis.[21] When the former is absent, chorea may first call the physician's attention to the presence of active carditis and other manifestations of the acute rheumatic attack.

The clinical onset of chorea is often insidious. The patient may be unusually nervous, fidgety, emotionally labile, suffer behavioral disorders, and have difficulty in writing and handiwork. Stumbling, grimacing, falling, and dropping objects due to sudden weakness of muscle groups is characteristic. As symptoms become more severe, movements become grossly spasmodic and violent so that walking, talking, and even sitting up become impossible. The weakness may simulate paralysis, and when present unilaterally (hemichorea) may be particularly confusing. Symptoms are exaggerated by excitement or fatigue but subside completely during sleep. All degrees of speech disturbances are seen.

The duration of chorea in hospitalized patients is usually between 2 and 4 months, but this neurological manifestation of ARF may last for only a week or may persist for several years. Chorea is the only manifestation of ARF which shows a striking difference in sex incidence. Before puberty the incidence is the same in boys and girls, but as the male matures sexually, chorea becomes rare and is not found in the fully mature adult male. On the other hand, female hormones tend to aggravate chorea and the disease may be exacerbated by pregnancy.

Subcutaneous Nodules

These are usually small, painless, firm, discrete, and freely movable swellings ranging in size from a few millimeters to 2 cm, and found over bony prominences and along extensor tendons. They are frequently unnoticed by the patient and need to be sought for carefully on physical examination. They are often evanescent and easily overlooked. These nodules are most often observed in patients with protracted carditis and are seldom observed in mild rheumatic fever.

Erythema Marginatum

This nonpruritic, pink, erythematous rash occurs on the trunk and proximal extremities—never on the face or hands. It begins as pink or red macules which fade centrally and extend peripherally in the pattern of enlarging circles. The erythema blanches completely and may change before one's eyes. It is often accentuated by a hot bath and is difficult to discern in the dark-skinned races. Erythema marginatum appears to be a vasomotor phenomenon, and anatomical lesions are not found. Individual lesions may come and go in minutes or hours, but the process may go on intermittently for weeks or months. It may appear early in the attack but sometimes is seen only during convalescence, and its course seems to be uninfluenced by anti-inflammatory therapy nor is its persistence necessarily an adverse prognostic sign.

Minor Clinical Criteria

These clinical features occur quite regularly in rheumatic fever but are also common to many other inflammatory diseases and are, therefore, of minor diagnostic value except as they support the major manifestations as diagnostic criteria. They include fever, arthralgia, abdominal pain, tachycardia, and epistaxis.

Laboratory Findings

No laboratory test is pathognomonic for the diagnosis of rheumatic fever. The appraisal of rheumatic activity by laboratory findings is, however, of value, since various tests are useful to indicate the persistence of rheumatic inflammation when clinical manifestations subside.

Streptococcal Antibody Tests for Preceding Streptococcal Infection

Because of the latent period between streptococcal sore throat and the onset of the early manifestations of rheumatic fever, streptococcal antibodies should always be increased, except when rheumatic fever is not discovered until many months after the pharyngeal infection, such as may happen in the case of pure chorea or chronic rheumatic carditis.[21] The antibodies may already be declining, or low, if the interval between the acute streptococcal infection and the detection of rheumatic fever has been longer than 2 months. Except in these instances, one should be reluctant to make the diagnosis of ARF in the absence of serological evidence of a recent streptococcal infection. The most widely used and best standardized test is the antistreptolysin O titer (ASO). In general, single titers of at least 250 Todd units per milliliter in adults and at least 333 Todd units per milliliter in children over 5 years of age are considered to be increased. A varying percentage of the normal population may show titers of this magnitude depending upon the general prevalence and intensity of streptococcal infections. In the early stages of rheumatic fever, about 20 percent of patients may have a low or borderline ASO titer, and in such cases it is advisable to obtain another streptococcal antibody test such as the antideoxyribonucleotidase B (anti-DNase B) or antihyaluronidase titers. The antistreptozyme (ASTZ) test is a hemagglutination reaction to a concentrate of extracellular streptococcal antigens absorbed to red blood cells. It is a very sensitive indicator of streptococcal infection in that virtually all patients with ARF have titers in excess of 200 Todd units per milliliter.[22] The actual value of all streptococcal antibody tests is in ruling out rheumatic fever when no antibody rise can be detected, especially in the case of polyarthritis, which invariably occurs within 4 to 5 weeks of streptococcal infection at a time when streptococcal antibody responses are maximal.

However, increased streptococcal antibodies do not reflect rheumatic activity per se, and their rate of decline is independent of the course of the rheumatic attack.[2]

Isolation of Group A Streptococci

Throat cultures are less satisfactory than antibody tests as supporting evidence of recent streptococcal infection. Throat cultures usually fail to reveal group A streptococci when the rheumatic attack begins or when such organisms are present in very small numbers and difficult to find. In addition, a significant number of normal individuals, especially children, carry group A streptococci in their throats intermittently, and positive cultures may be difficult to interpret.

Acute Phase Reactants

The erythrocyte sedimentation rate (ESR) and the test for C-reactive protein (CRP) in serum are useful although nonspecific detectors of the presence of an inflammatory process. Unless the patient has received corticosteroids, salicylates, or other aspirin-like compounds, these reactions are almost invariably abnormal in patients presenting with arthritis or carditis, whereas they are often normal in patients with the delayed onset of chorea. Other laboratory tests reflecting the presence of active inflammation include leukocytosis, increased serum complement, mucoproteins, and immunoglobulins. Prolongation of the PR interval of the electrocardiogram is frequent in ARF (about 25 percent of all cases with and without carditis), and other ECG changes are common but nondiagnostic. Anemia is common due to the suppression of erythropoiesis found in many inflammatory diseases.

Course and Prognosis

The course of rheumatic fever cannot be predicted at the onset of the disease, but despite its variability in any given case, generalizations can be made on a statistical basis. Thus, 75 percent of acute rheumatic attacks abate within 6 weeks, 90 percent within 12 weeks, and less than 5 percent persist more than 6 months. The persistent forms of the disease are the stubborn, prolonged attacks of Sydenham's chorea. Once all evidence of rheumatic inflammation has abated, however, and more than 2 months has elapsed after withdrawal of all antirheumatic suppressive therapy with adrenal corticosteroids or aspirin-like compounds, rheumatic fever does not recur in the absence of new streptococcal infections. The frequency of recurrences is then dependent upon the frequency and severity of streptococcal infections, and further influenced by the presence or absence of rheumatic heart disease and the duration of freedom from the last attack.[13]

Rheumatic Carditis and the Course of Rheumatic Heart Disease

The long-term prognosis of ARF is correlated most closely with the severity of carditis during the acute attack. Approximately 95 percent of patients who escape rheumatic carditis during their initial attack and are kept free of recurrences by careful prophylactic therapy (see below) will have no stigmata of rheumatic heart disease when examined a decade later.[23] Patients who show evidence of mild acute carditis (i.e., apical systolic murmur of mild mitral regurgitation without heart failure or pericarditis) have a fairly good prognosis in that only 30 percent will have organic heart murmurs after 10 years of observation. Approximately 40 percent of subjects with basal or apical *diastolic* murmurs and 70 percent of those with heart failure and/or pericarditis during their acute attack will have residual heart disease, and prognosis is the worst for those who have rheumatic heart disease and suffer recurrent rheumatic attacks. Patients with "pure" chorea represent an exception to the rule that the absence of acute carditis in an initial attack insures a good prognosis. In a long-term follow-up study, 25 percent of such patients eventually developed rheumatic heart disease, particularly late-onset mitral stenosis.[24]

In the longest prospective study of ARF, two forms of mitral stenosis could be distinguished: (1) the early appearance of a severely deformed valve within 5 years of the acute attack, which occurred with equal distribution in both sexes and often carried a fatal prognosis due to the hemodynamics of severe valvular dysfunction, and (2) the insidious development of mitral stenosis, primarily in women and in those who had experienced mild mitral valvulitis and who had no recurrent attacks to explain the progression of the disease.[23]

Thus, the remarkable variability in the course of rheumatic heart disease stems from several factors: (1) the variability in the duration and severity of rheumatic inflammation, (2) the amount of scarring of the valves and myocardium following the abatement of the acute inflammation, (3) the location and severity of the hemodynamic lesion due to valvular insufficiency and stenosis, (4) the frequency of recurrent bouts of carditis, and (5) the progression of valvular sclerosis and calcification which occurs as a secondary phenomenon in a deformed or injured valve without recurrent or persistent rheumatic inflammation (as seen in congenital valvular disease or following healed bacterial endocarditis). These factors and probably others not yet appreciated produce striking variations in the clinical syndromes of rheumatic heart disease.

Differential Diagnosis

Diagnosis is most difficult when rheumatic fever presents as isolated polyarthritis. In this form it cannot be readily distinguished from a long list of bacteremic diseases. In the young adult population, gonococcal polyarthritis is a particularly common differential diagnosis that can only be excluded by the prompt response of early cases of disseminated gonococcal disease to a therapeutic trial of penicillin. If streptococcal antibodies are not increased, polyarthritis should be attributed to some cause other than rheumatic fever. In rheumatoid arthritis, joint involvement will persist and characteristic joint deformities appear. The latter are not seen in rheumatic fever nor is rheumatoid factor or other autoantibodies observed in ARF. Pericarditis and myocarditis do not occur as isolated findings in ARF; associated endocarditis and attendant murmurs are virtually always present in rheumatic carditis.

Unless ill-defined febrile syndromes are clearly associated with major rheumatic manifestations, the diagnosis of rheumatic fever should not be made. A common error is premature treatment of an ill-defined syndrome with corticosteroids or salicylates and suppression of the diagnostic features of the disease before they are unmistakable. In the absence of a curative agent of rheumatic inflammation, there should be no great urgency to suppress inflammation before the diagnosis is clear. The rapidity with which the arthritis of ARF is suppressed with salicylates is characteristic of this disease but by no means diagnostic because other forms of acute synovitis may respond just as well.

In order to help clarify the diagnosis of rheumatic fever and to avoid overdiagnosis, the American Heart Association has published a modification of the *Jones criteria* (Table 37-1). They are not meant to substitute for sound medical judgment but are recommended as a guide for the diagnosis of questionable cases. The finding of two major or of one major and two minor criteria indicates a high probability of the presence of rheumatic fever if supported by evidence of preceding streptococcal infection. The absence of the latter should always make the diagnosis suspect except when rheumatic manifestations are discovered long after the antecedent infection, as in chorea or low-grade carditis. Because the prognosis may vary greatly according to the major manifestations, for recording purposes the diagnosis of ARF should be followed by a list of the major manifestations present, e.g., rheumatic fever manifested by polyarthritis and carditis. An indication of the severity of carditis (cardiac enlargement, congestive heart failure) is also advisable for future reference.

Treatment

No measures are known which will cure rheumatic fever or change the course of the attack. Good supportive therapy, however, may reduce its morbidity and mortality.

TABLE 37-1   Jones Criteria (Revised)

Major Manifestations	Minor Manifestations
Carditis	Fever
Polyarthritis	Arthralgia
Chorea	Previous rheumatic fever or rheumatic heart disease
Erythema marginatum	
Subcutaneous nodules	Elevated ESR or positive CRP
	Prolonged PR interval

Plus, supporting evidence of preceding streptococcal infection: history of recent scarlet fever; positive throat culture for group A streptococcus; increased ASO titer or other streptococcal antibodies.

Source: G. H. Stollerman, M. Markowitz, A. Taranta, and L. W. Wannamaker, Jones Criteria (Revised) for Guidance in the Diagnosis of Rheumatic Fever, *Circulation,* 32:664, 1965. Reproduced with permission.

Antibiotic Therapy

As soon as ARF is diagnosed, a course of penicillin should be given to ensure the elimination of group A streptococci from the throat, even when throat cultures are negative. An effective course is either a single injection of 1.2 million units of benzathine penicillin G intramuscularly or 600,000 units of procaine penicillin intramuscularly daily for 10 days. Penicillin, even in large doses, will not reduce ultimate heart damage or influence the course of the attack, but once initiated it should be given continuously as prophylaxis against intercurrent streptococcal infection with one of the regimens described below.

Suppressive Therapy

Acute arthritis can be relieved with codeine or with salicylates or other nonsteroidal anti-inflammatory drugs. Although codeine will relieve pain but not inflammation, the rheumatic attack will be briefer with this drug than when agents are used to suppress inflammation. Nonetheless, the brilliance with which aspirin and aspirin-like compounds suppress the arthritis of ARF makes it difficult to deny patients the symptomatic benefits of these drugs. For patients without carditis, corticosteroids are unnecessary. When aspirin is used in the therapy of ARF, the dosage should be increased until the drug produces either a clinical effect or systemic toxicity characterized by tinnitus, headache, dizziness, blurred vision, or hyperpnea (salicylism). A starting daily dose of 100 to 150 mg/kg in children and 6 to 8 g in adults given in five to six divided doses is recommended as a full therapeutic test. Of the various salicylates or other nonsteroidal anti-inflammatory compounds having similar inhibiting effects upon prostaglandin synthesis, aspirin is cheapest and is not exceeded in efficacy. Gastric intolerance can be reduced by administering antacids or enteric-coated aspirin preparations that are well absorbed. For patients who are intolerant of aspirin despite these measures, indomethacin or other aspirin-like compounds effective in lower doses may be employed.

Despite the lack of a demonstrated advantage of adrenocorticosteroids in controlled clinical trials,[25] many physicians prefer these agents to aspirin for the treatment of carditis. Corticosteroids are more potent anti-inflammatory agents but are more likely to be followed by posttherapeutic "rebounds" of rheumatic activity and may thus prolong the rheumatic attack. Moreover, corticosteroids have the additional disadvantage of more frequent side effects such as acne, hirsutism, Cushingoid changes in facies and body habitus, and salt and water retention. It is preferable, therefore, to begin treatment of patients with carditis with salicylates or compounds with similar pharmacologic action. If these drugs fail to reduce fever and to relieve heart failure, cor-

ticosteroid therapy may be promptly substituted. Prednisone, the corticosteroid most commonly employed, is administered in initial doses of 60 to 120 mg or higher when necessary in four divided doses daily. After the signs and symptoms of rheumatic inflammation have been brought under control by anti-inflammatory agents, treatment should be continued until the ESR approaches near-normal values and the test for CRP is negative. Treatment should be maintained for several weeks thereafter before tapering the dose. Poststeroid rebounds can often be avoided by an overlapping course of salicylate therapy when steroids are slowly withdrawn over a 2-week period. Salicylates may then be continued for an additional 2 to 3 weeks. Mild rheumatic rebounds are best allowed to abate spontaneously without resuming anti-inflammatory treatment so as to avoid further prolongation of the attack. About 5 percent of rheumatic attacks persist for more than 6 months. These chronic attacks are most likely to occur in patients with severe carditis and in those who have had previous episodes. The healing process should be followed with weekly tests for CRP and ESR.

Treatment of Chorea

The manifestations of chorea do not respond well to antirheumatic therapy, and sedatives and tranquilizers are usually necessary along with complete physical and emotional rest. Because of the great variation in the course of chorea, it is difficult to evaluate and to compare various agents. It is well to remember that chorea is a self-limited disease and that good results are almost invariably attained by patient, attentive nursing care and conservative medical management. Various neuroleptic drugs such as the phenothiazines are useful in controlling violent involuntary movements.

Prevention of Recurrence

Recurrences are preventable by continuous chemoprophylaxis against recurrent streptococcal sore throat. The most efficient and effective regimen for this purpose is a monthly injection of 1.2 million units of benzathine penicillin G.[26] The discomfort and disadvantages of this regimen have to be weighed against the probability of recurrence in each case. Those with recent rheumatic fever, rheumatic heart disease, multiple previous attacks, and, particularly, exposure to an environment in which the risk of streptococcal pharyngitis is great deserve the most effective form of protection. A second choice is an oral regimen of either 1 g sulfadiazine daily in a single dose or 200,000 units of penicillin G given twice daily on an empty stomach. The duration for which chemoprophylaxis must be sustained depends upon several variables. A minimum period of 5 years or until age 18—whichever is longer—is recommended for patients who develop rheumatic fever without carditis. The decision to continue prophylaxis beyond this period should be conditioned by the following variables: the presence of rheumatic heart disease (which greatly increases the risk and seriousness of recurrences), previous bouts of carditis, exposure to epidemiologic settings with a high incidence of streptococcal disease, and, particularly, exposure to populations in which ARF is prevalent. Such variables should be carefully considered before prophylaxis is terminated.

Prevention of Initial Rheumatic Attacks

First attacks of rheumatic fever may be prevented if group A streptococcal pharyngitis is treated promptly and adequately.[3] In communities where group A streptococcal pharyngitis has been diagnosed early and treated well and where socioeconomic standards are high, the group A streptococci found in schoolchildren's throats may be of relatively low virulence and may cause rheumatic fever less frequently than do more virulent strains prevalent in epidemic settings.[27] It is always appropriate, however, to treat streptococcal pharyngitis with chemotherapeutic regimens that are effective in eradication of the organisms and in terminating their spread through the population.

Streptococcal pharyngitis is adequately treated by a single intramuscular injection of 600,000 units of benzathine penicillin G in very young children or 1.2 million units in patients age 10 or older. Alternative plans of parenteral therapy or combined parenteral and oral therapy should provide for consistent penicillinemia over a period of at least 10 days. If oral penicillin is employed, 200,000 units four times daily is recommended. Erythromycin in daily doses of 1 g for 10 days may be substituted in penicillin-sensitive individuals, although erythromycin resistance is a growing problem in some populations[28] where this antibiotic is used extensively for upper respiratory infections. Tetracycline is no longer recommended because of increasing worldwide frequency of strains of group A streptococci resistant to this antibiotic. So far, all group A streptococci have remained extremely sensitive to penicillin G.

References

*1. Stollerman, G. H.: "Rheumatic Fever and Streptococcal Infection," Grune & Stratton, New York, 1975. (Extensively referenced)
2. Stollerman, G. H., Lewis, A. J., Schultz, L., and Taranta, A.: Relationship of Immune Response to Group A Streptococci to the Course of Acute, Chronic and Recurrent Rheumatic Fever, *Am. J. Med.*, 20:163, 1956.
3. Denny, F. W., Wannamaker, L. W., Brink, W. R., Rammelkamp, C. H., Jr., and Custer, E. A.: Prevention of Rheumatic Fever: Treatment of the Preceding Streptococcal Infection, *J. Am. Med. Assoc.*, 143:151, 1950.
4. Wannamaker, L. W.: The Chain That Links the Heart to the Throat, *Circulation*, 48:9, 1973.
5. Stollerman, G. H.: Nephritogenic and Rheumatogenic Group A Streptococci, *J. Infect. Dis.*, 120:258, 1969.
6. Bisno, A. L.: The Concept of Rheumatogenic and Nonrheumatogenic Group A Streptococci, in S. E. Read and J. B. Zabriskie (eds.), "Streptococcal Diseases and the Immune Response," Academic Press, Inc., New York, 1980, p. 789.
7. Van de Rijn, I., Zabriskie, J. B., and McCarty, M.: Group A Streptococcal Antigens Cross-Reactive with Myocardium: Purification of Heart-Reactive Antibody and Isolation and Characterization of the Streptococcal Antigen, *J. Exp. Med.*, 146:579, 1977.
8. Kaplan, M. H., and Svec, K. H.: Immunologic Relation of Streptococcal and Tissue Antigens. III. Presence in Human Sera of Streptococcal Antibody Cross-Reactive with Heart Tissue. Association with Streptococcal Infection, Rheumatic Fever, and Glomerulonephritis, *J. Exp. Med.*, 119:651, 1964.
9. Yang, L. C., Soprey, P. R., Wittner, M. K., and Fox, E. N.: Streptococcal-Induced Cell-Mediated Immune Destruction of Cardiac Myofibers in Vitro, *J. Exp. Med.*, 146:344, 1977.
10. Bisno, A. L., Pearce, I. A., Wall, H. P., Moody, M. D., and Stollerman, G. H.: Contrasting Epidemiology of Acute Rheumatic Fever and Acute Glomerulonephritis: Nature of the Antecedent Streptococcal Infection, *N. Engl. J. Med.*, 283:561, 1970.
11. Stollerman, G. H.: The Relative Rheumatogenicity of Strains of Group A Streptococci, *Mod. Concepts Cardiovasc. Dis.*, 64:35, 1975.
12. Rammelkamp, C. H., Denny, F. W., and Wannamaker, L. W.: Studies on the Epidemiology of Rheumatic Fever in the Armed Services, in L. Thomas, "Rheumatic Fever," University of Minnesota Press, Minneapolis, 1952, pp. 72–89.
*13. Taranta, A., Kleinberg, E., Feinstein, A. R., Wood, H. F., Tursky, E., and Simpson, R.: Rheumatic Fever in Children and Adolescents: A Long-Term Epidemiologic Study of Subsequent Prophylaxis, Streptococcal Infections, and Clinical Sequelae. V. Relation of the Rheumatic Fever Recurrence Rate per Streptococcal Infection to Preexisting Clinical Features of the Patients, *Ann. Intern. Med.*, 60(suppl. 5):58, 1964. (23 references)
14. Taranta, A., Metrakos, J. D., and Uchida, I.: Rheumatic Fever in Monozygotic and Dizygotic Twins, *Circulation*, 20:778, 1959 (abstract).
15. Stollerman, G. H.: The Streptococcus, Rheumatic Fever and Rheumatic Heart Disease, in A. G. Shaper, M. S. R. Hutt, and Z. Fejfar (eds.), "Cardiovascular Disease in the Tropics," British Medical Association, London, 1974, pp. 7–21.
16. Becker, C. G., and Murphy, G. E.: On the Pathology of Rheumatic Heart Disease, in S. E. Read and J. B. Zabriskie (eds.), "Streptococcal Diseases and the Im-

*This article is a review of the literature and contains additional references to the literature.

mune Response," Academic Press, Inc., New York, 1980, p. 23.

17. Virmani, R., and Roberts, W. C.: Aschoff Bodies in Operatively Excised Atrial Appendages and in Papillary Muscles. Frequency and Clinical Significance, *Circulation*, 55:559, 1977.

18. Stollerman, G. H., Markowitz, M., Taranta, A., and Wannamaker, L. W.: Jones Critiera (Revised) for Guidance in the Diagnosis of Rheumatic Fever, *Circulation*, 32:664, 1965.

19. Massell, B. F., Fyler, D. C., and Roy, S. B.: The Clinical Picture of Rheumatic Fever. Diagnosis, Immediate Prognosis, Course and Therapeutic Implications, *Am. J. Cardiol.*, 1:436, 1958.

20. Feinstein, A. R., Wood, H. F., Spagnuolo, M., et al.: Rheumatic Fever in Children and Adolescents. VII. Cardiac Changes and Sequelae, *Ann. Intern. Med.*, 60(suppl. 5):87, 1964.

21. Taranta, A., and Stollerman, G. H.: The Relationship of Sydenham's Chorea to Infection with Group A Streptococci, *Am. J. Med.*, 20:170, 1956.

22. Bisno, A. L., and Ofek, I.: Serologic Diagnosis of Streptococcal Infection: Comparison of a Rapid Hemagglutination Technique with Conventional Antibody Tests, *Am. J. Dis. Child.*, 127:676, 1974.

*23. United Kingdom and United States Joint Report: The Natural History of Rheumatic Fever and Rheumatic Heart Disease: Ten-Year Report of a Coop-

erative Clinical Trial of ACTH, Cortisone and Aspirin, *Circulation*, 32:457, 1965. (2 references)

24. Bland, E. F.: Chorea as a Manifestation of Rheumatic Fever. A Long-Term Perspective, *Trans. Am. Clin. Climatol. Assoc.*, 73:209, 1961.

*25. Combined Rheumatic Fever Study Group: A Comparison of the Effect of Prednisone and Acetylsalicylic Acid on the Incidence of Residual Rheumatic Heart Disease, *N. Engl. J. Med.*, 262:895, 1960. (10 references)

26. Wood, H. F., Feinstein, A. R., Taranta, A., Epstein, J. A., and Simpson, R.: Rheumatic Fever in Children and Adolescents: A Long-Term Epidemiologic Study of Subsequent Prophylaxis, Streptococcal Infections, and Clinical Sequelae. III. Comparative Effectiveness of Three Prophylaxis Regimens in Preventing Streptococcal Infection and Rheumatic Recurrences, *Ann. Intern. Med.*, 60(suppl. 5):31, 1964.

27. Siegel, A. C., Johnson, E. E., and Stollerman, G. H.: Controlled Studies of Streptococcal Pharyngitis in a Pediatric Population. I. Factors Related to the Attack of Rheumatic Fever, *N. Engl. J. Med.*, 265:559, 1961.

28. Maruyama, S., Yoshioka, H., Fujita, K., Takimoto, M., and Satake, Y.: Sensitivity of Group A Streptococci to Antibiotics: Prevalence of Resistance to Erythromycin in Japan, *Am. J. Dis. Child.*, 133:1143, 1979.

38

Aortic Valve Disease

Charles E. Rackley, M.D.
Jesse E. Edwards, M.D.
Robert B. Karp, M.D.
John W. Kirklin, M.D.

Aortic Stenosis

Strong action of the left ventricle; extremely loud and musical murmur at the extent of the arterial tree; the heart's action generally regular.

William Stokes, 1854[1]

Etiology

The most frequent causes of aortic stenosis are congenital aortic stenosis with a unicuspid or bicuspid valve, rheumatic aortic stenosis, and calcific stenosis

of the elderly. The incidence and prevalence of the various etiologies of aortic stenosis have been influenced by the change in frequency of diseases, such as a significant decline in acute rheumatic fever, reinterpretation of pathological studies, and an increasing life span of the adult population. Pathological studies during this century first ascribed aortic stenosis to inflammation or valvular sclerosis, but a series in 1947 suggested rheumatic valvulitis as the major cause.[2,3] Subsequent studies suggested congenital valvular stenosis as the most common cause, and in recent years the bicuspid valve seems to have been established as a major cause of aortic stenosis.[4,5]

The age of the patient when the clinical findings of aortic stenosis are first recognized suggests an important characteristic of the mechanism of the disease. If the patient is under the age of 30 years, a congenitally stenotic aortic valve is most likely the mechanism.[6] From ages 30 to 70 years, rheumatic disease may play a role, and beyond 70 years calcification of the aortic valve is the usual cause.[7,8] Isolated aortic stenosis has a rheumatic basis in 6 to 24 percent of affected individuals, but if the aortic stenosis is combined with mitral valve disease the likelihood of a rheumatic basis is increased even higher.[9,10] In the younger age range males have a greater frequency of aortic stenosis, whereas in older individuals with calcific stenosis there may be an increased predominance in women.

Pathology

Acquired stenosis results primarily either from commissural fusion, yielding the fibrous type of stenosis, or from calcification of the cusps of the valve. While a rheumatic etiology may underlie each of these types, calcific stenosis is most commonly engrafted upon nonrheumatic valves, either congenitally bicuspid valves or, uncommonly, on a tricuspid valve.

The Fibrous Type
Recurrent rheumatic endocarditis causes fibrous contracture with shortening of cusps and a tendency for fusion of adjacent cusps at commissures.

When commissural adhesion occurs only at one aortic commissure, the valve becomes bicuspid (acquired bicuspid valve). In a valve so affected, the orifice is somewhat reduced, but usually not measurably. Such valves offer (as do congenital bicuspid valves) the tendency for acquired calcification of the cusps.

If there is fusion at two or three commissures the cusps are sufficiently restrained so as to cause obstruction at the valve level. The valve that is stenotic because of commissural fusion may show varying degrees (sometimes heavy) of calcification, but the primary basis for stenosis resides in adhesions of one cusp to another, yielding the fibrous type of aortic stenosis.[11] This is usually of rheumatic origin. Because of associated shortening of cusps, this type of aortic stenosis is usually accompanied by some degree of aortic insufficiency (Fig. 38-1). Also, it is common that some degree of rheumatic change be present in the mitral valve and, in some cases, the tricuspid valve also.

FIGURE 38-1 Fibrous (rheumatic) aortic stenosis. There is fusion of all three commissures. (*From J. E. Edwards, Pathology of Acquired Valvular Disease of the Heart, Seminars in Roentgenol., 14:96, 1979. Reproduced with permission.*)

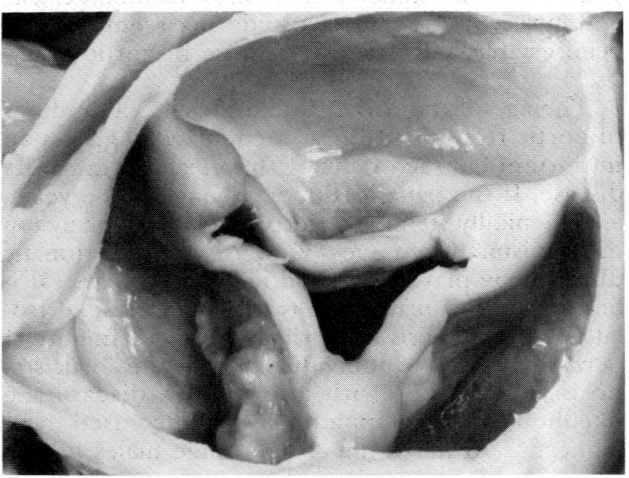

The Calcific Type
Aortic stenosis resulting primarily from rigidity of cuspid tissue incident to calcification usually occurs in a bicuspid valve, and relatively uncommonly in a tricuspid or unicuspid aortic valve.[7,12] There are two etiologies for the bicuspid state, either acquired through rheumatic disease (Fig. 38-2A) or congenital (Fig. 38-2B). In instances of the calcific type of aortic stenosis, the congenital bicuspid valve is more common than the acquired bicuspid valve by a ratio of about 4:1. Classically, the aortic valve is competent and, in instances of the congenital bicuspid valve, no other valve of the heart is diseased.

In the congenital bicuspid valve the large, conjoined cusp as a rule lies anteriorly, and the two coronary arteries arise from its sinus. In acquired bicuspid valve the conjoined cusp may occupy the same position or be oriented toward the right or left.

It is common for some degree of calcification to appear in the normal aortic valves of persons 70 years and older.[13] Usually, the calcification is inadequate to cause stenosis, although it may be responsible for a murmur. In exceptional cases, each of the three cusps is highly calcified, making the valve stenotic. This uncommon type of aortic stenosis may be called the senile type of calcific aortic valvular sclerosis (Fig. 38-2C).

Miscellaneous Types
Aortic stenosis observed from infancy to adolescence is usually of congenital origin, the valve displaying the unicommissural, unicuspid character. Occasionally, individuals with such valves may reach adulthood before they display significant signs of aortic stenosis. This phenomenon may result from calcification with secondary incompetence of a congenitally deformed but intrinsically mildly stenotic valve (Fig. 38-2D). The resultant effects of the incompetence may then serve to bring the element of stenosis into evidence.

Uncommonly, aortic stenosis may result from the presence of a congenital papillary mass or flap of endocardial tissue that obstructs an otherwise normal valve. Extensive thrombosis at the valve site has been a cause of aortic stenosis in lupus erythematosus.[14] The secondary effects of aortic stenosis include left ventricular hypertrophy and poststenotic dilatation of the ascending aorta.

Numbered among the common complications of aortic stenosis are sudden death and congestive cardiac failure. Other complications include embolism, including coronary embolism of valvular fragments in calcific aortic stenosis.[15] In aortic stenosis, as in aortic insufficiency, as the left ventricle enlarges downward there may be undue restraint upon the mitral chordae, and secondary mitral insufficiency may result.[16] Mitral insufficiency may also result from congenital aortic stenosis through fibrosis of papillary muscles and related left ventricular free wall.[17] Dissecting or saccular aneurysm of the aorta

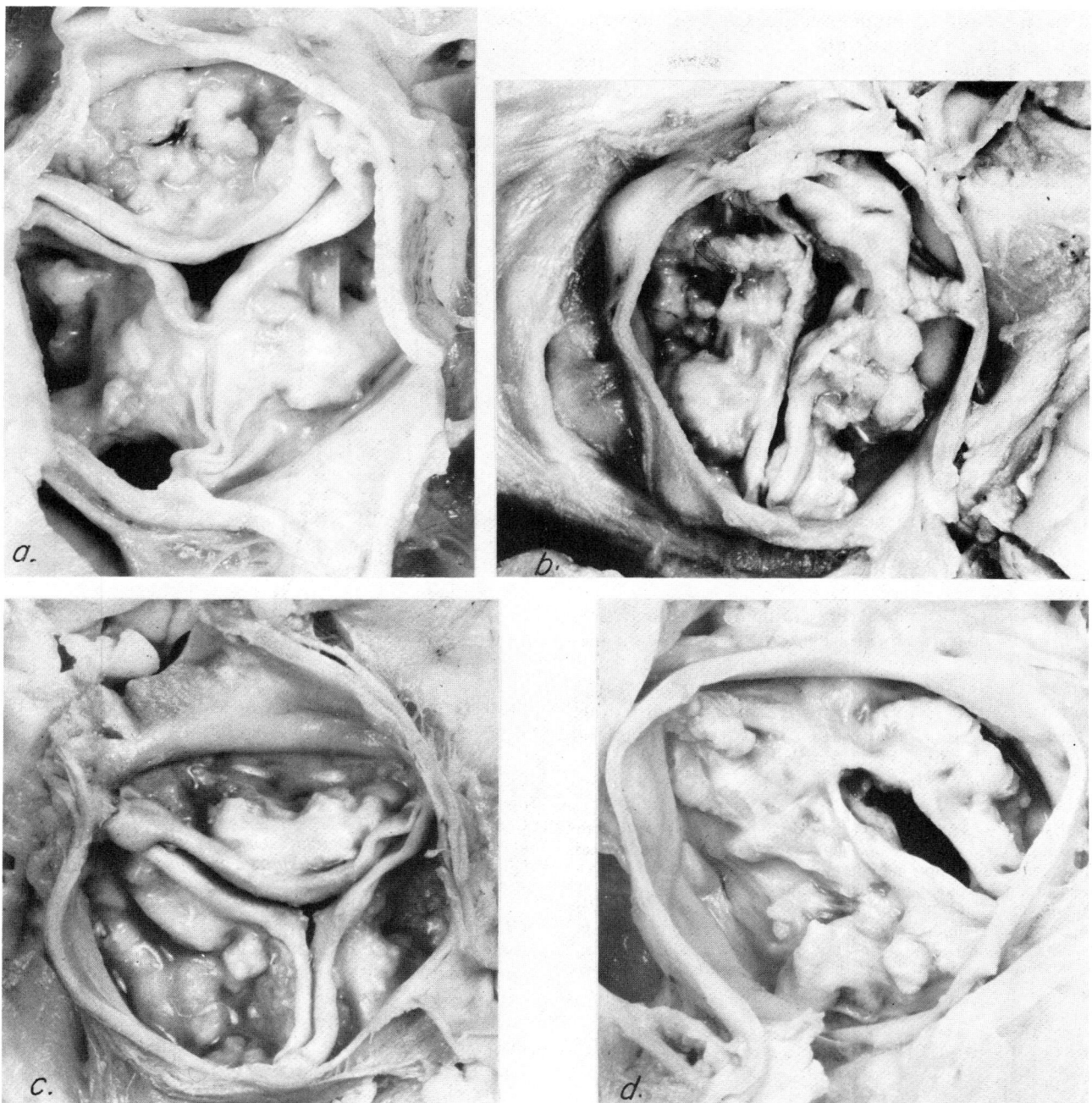

FIGURE 38-2   Four types of calcific aortic stenosis. In each, the unopened aortic valve is viewed from above. *a.* Acquired bicuspid aortic valve with secondary calcification. At the center of the conjoined cusp (lower center) are elements of two preexisting cusps, now fused. *b.* Congenital bicuspid valve. The characteristic raphe of the congenital bicuspid aortic valve appears at the lower portion of the illustration. *c.* Senile type. None of the commissures are fused, but there is major intrinsic calcification of the three cusps. *d.* Unicuspid unicommissural congenital aortic stenosis with secondary calcification. (*From J. E. Edwards, Pathology of Acquired Valvular Disease of the Heart. Seminars in Roentgenol., 14:96, 1979. Reproduced with permission.*)

may occur as a consequence of the cystic medial necrosis of the aorta that may accompany aortic stenosis.[18]

Although aortic stenosis has been claimed as protective against coronary atherosclerosis, studies indicate that the average degree of coronary atherosclerosis among patients with aortic stenosis is not materially different from that in persons with normal aortic valves.[19]

Abnormal Physiology

The physiological abnormality imposed on the left ventricle by stenosis of the aortic valve is resistance

DISEASES OF THE HEART AND BLOOD VESSELS

to ejection, and a systolic pressure gradient develops between the left ventricle and systemic arterial system. The gradual reduction in the orifice size of the aortic valve from the normal 2 to 3 cm² is accompanied by a progressive increase in the left ventricular pressure during systole. This increase in left ventricular systolic pressure creates a pressure overload on the left ventricle, which compensates by an increase in the thickness of the ventricular wall and left ventricular mass or hypertrophy of the myocardium (Figs. 38-3 and 38-4).[20] This concentric form of hypertrophy without chamber dilatation is developed to normalize the systolic force or stress in the ventricular wall and thus to preserve the mechanical function of the ventricle in terms of ejection fraction and cardiac output.[21] Compensatory hypertrophy to a pressure overload is not associated with dilatation of the left ventricular chamber until significant depression of the contractile state of the myocardium occurs. In this manner the increased systolic pressure in the left ventricular chamber is normalized by an increase in the cross-sectional area of the ventricular wall during diastole and systole so that wall stress remains within the normal range throughout the cardiac cycle.[22]

The increase in left ventricular mass and hypertrophy in aortic stenosis results in a significant elevation of the left ventricular end-diastolic pressure, which is further raised by atrial systole. In aortic stenosis, atrial systole has been shown to contribute significantly to the percent of the volume ejected during ventricular systole as compared to the normal ventricle.[23] However, the suggested mechanism

FIGURE 38-3 Left ventricular pressure-volume diagram in compensated aortic stenosis and left ventricular pressure overload. The significant abnormality is the abnormally elevated systolic pressure, but end-diastolic volume, end-systolic volume, and ejection fraction remain normal. [From C. E. Rackley, Value of Ventriculography in Cardiac Function and Diagnosis: Diagnostic Methods in Cardiology, in N. O. Fowler (ed.), "Cardiovascular Clinics," F. A. Davis Company, Philadelphia, 1975. Reproduced with permission.]

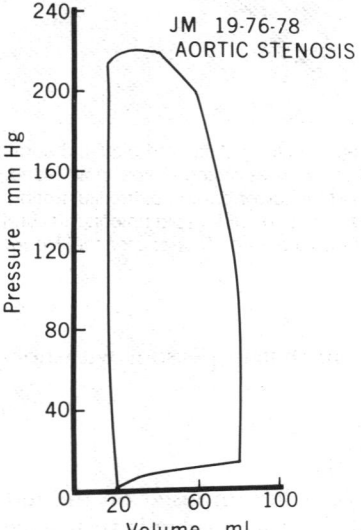

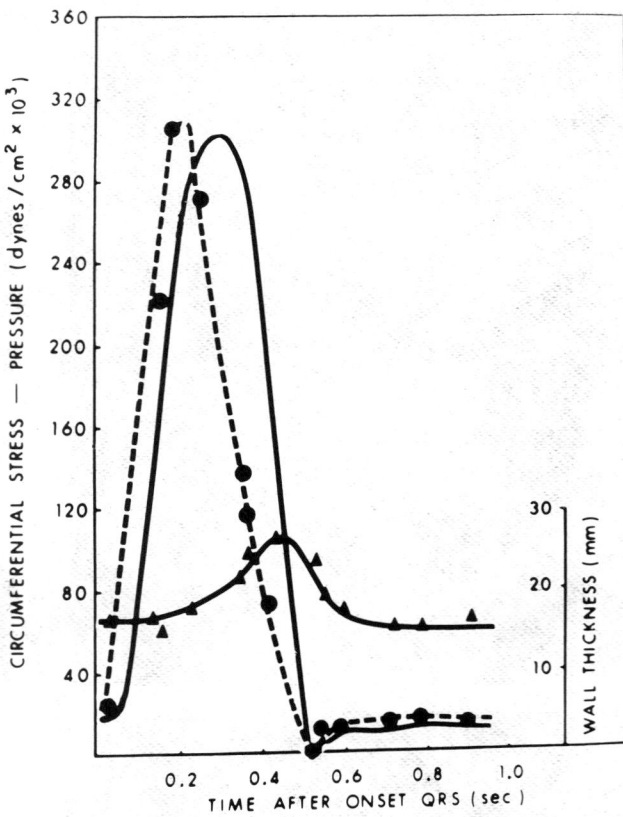

FIGURE 38-4 Left ventricular pressure, circumferential wall stress, and wall thickness in compensated aortic stenosis and pressure overload. Diastole wall thickness is abnormally increased, and further thickening occurs during systolic ejection which results in a rapid decline of circumferential wall stress. (–●–, stress; ——, pressure; ▲——▲, wall thickness.) [From C. E. Rackley and W. P. Hood, Jr., Aortic Valve Disease, in H. J. Levine (ed.), "Clinical Cardiovascular Physiology," Grune & Stratton, Inc., New York, 1976. Reproduced with permission.]

that atrial systole augments the Frank-Starling mechanism by elevation of left ventricular end-diastolic pressure is not supported by the finding of a normal end-diastolic wall stress in the hypertrophied left ventricle of aortic stenosis.[24] The increased left ventricular end-diastolic pressure produced by atrial systole in the hypertrophied ventricle of aortic stenosis probably reflects a decrease in the compliance of the hypertrophied myocardium. This elevation of left atrial systolic pressure will eventually cause enlargement of the left atrium.

In the course of severe chronic aortic stenosis the sustained pressure overload on the myocardium will lead to depression of the contractile state of the ventricular myocardium.[25] At this stage the ventricle dilates in order to maintain forward cardiac output. In the early stages of aortic stenosis the increased systolic pressure in the chamber produces hypertrophy of the myocardium which is able to normalize the systolic wall stress, but eventual depression of the contractile state will lead to dilatation of the chamber, decreased ejection fraction, reduction in cardiac output, and marked elevation of the left ventricular filling pressure with pulmonary hypertension.

Clinical Manifestations

The characteristic clinical manifestations of aortic stenosis are chest pain, syncope, and heart failure.[26] The patient's age at the onset of symptoms may be helpful in attributing the pathological lesion to a congenital, rheumatic, or calcific valve. On the other hand, symptoms of aortic stenosis tend to occur late in the course of the disease, when a critical reduction in valve size has developed. Furthermore, chest pain and symptoms of left ventricular failure may be difficult to extract from children. In adults the presentation of the usual manifestations of aortic stenosis may be complicated by other underlying cardiac lesions, such as coronary artery disease.

Angina pectoris is the most frequent symptom of aortic stenosis and occurs in 50 to 70 percent of affected individuals.[27,28] Life expectancy has been estimated at an average of 5 years after the development of chest pain. Special features have been ascribed to the chest discomfort of aortic stenosis in an attempt to differentiate this discomfort from the discomfort associated with underlying coronary artery disease. These features include the development of chest discomfort after the completion of physical exertion and a higher incidence of nitroglycerin-induced syncope.[29] However, coronary arteriography has demonstrated that anatomical coronary artery disease is frequent in adults with aortic stenosis whether chest pain has developed or is absent.[30] The mechanism of the chest pain has been attributed to a difference in myocardial oxygen demands and oxygen availability. Myocardial oxygen consumption in aortic stenosis is greater than normal due to the increase in left ventricular mass, and oxygen availability can be diminished at the subendocardial level whether there is patency of coronary vessels or coronary artery disease.[31] Systolic wall stress is a major determinant of myocardial oxygen consumption, and in the hypertrophied myocardium wall stress is highest at the subendocardium.[32] Calcific emboli have been incriminated as a rare mechanism for impaired blood flow in the coronary arteries.[33]

Effort syncope is another typical symptom of aortic stenosis, and as the term suggests this occurs with or immediately follows physical exertion.[27] Survival has been estimated to be 3 to 4 years in patients developing syncope from aortic stenosis.[26] One proposed mechanism of the syncope is left ventricular failure and an abrupt fall in cardiac output.[34] Arrhythmias may also play a role in the syncope of stenosis of the aortic valve, but some researchers have contended that the arrhythmia develops in the late stages of syncope.[35] Exercise-induced peripheral vasodilatation may aggravate the systolic pressure gradient and further reduce the perfusing

pressure of the myocardium. In older patients with calcific aortic stenosis, transient cerebral ischemia from cerebrovascular disease must also be considered.

Left ventricular failure is a third significant symptom of severe aortic stenosis, but dyspnea may be described quite differently by children and adults and is influenced by the amount of exercise in different age groups.[36] If the patient is quite active physically, the development of dyspnea may not necessarily be associated with other signs of pulmonary congestion such as orthopnea and paroxysmal noctural dyspnea. The symptoms of heart failure may portend a shorter average survival in older patients than in the younger age group. In adults with aortic stenosis average survival has been estimated at 2 years after symptoms of left ventricular failure develop.[26,36] Other symptoms attributable to significant aortic stenosis include palpitations, fatigue, and visual defects. Fatigue may be an early symptom in children. In elderly patients with calcific aortic stenosis, carotid and cerebrovascular disease may produce additional symptoms referable to the central nervous system. Finally, visual field defects can result from embolization from the aortic valve, but are rare symptoms.[33]

Physical Examination
Characteristic hemodynamic alterations in the vital signs in patients with aortic stenosis are reflected in the peripheral pulse and blood pressure. The pulse pressure is typically narrowed in significant aortic stenosis with a reduction in systolic pressure and maintenance of the diastolic level. A systemic systolic pressure above 200 mmHg is rarely encountered in severe aortic stenosis.[27] However, in elderly patients with calcific aortic stenosis and loss of arterial elasticity, pressures above 180 mmHg can be observed with significant pressure gradients across the aortic valve.[37]

In the case of valvular aortic stenosis, examination of the blood vessels in the neck does not reveal abnormal venous pulsations, and visible changes in the carotid arteries will not be detected. A conspicuous *a* wave in the jugular vein should suggest other conditions, such as idiopathic hypertrophic subaortic stenosis, which could cause decreased compliance of the right ventricle. The characteristic delay in upstroke and decline in slope of the pulse contour can be palpated in the carotid artery, but the examiner should be cautious in palpating the carotid arteries to recognize these waveform abnormalities, since in elderly patients carotid sinus sensitivity and cerebral ischemia can produce a sudden bradycardia and impairment of consciousness (Fig. 38-5). Occasionally faint vibrations can be detected as transmitted from the aortic valve. The brachial artery is a much more accessible artery to palpate and assess arterial waveform abnormalities in aortic stenosis. A single finger can occlude the brachial artery and upon gradual release of pressure an anacrotic

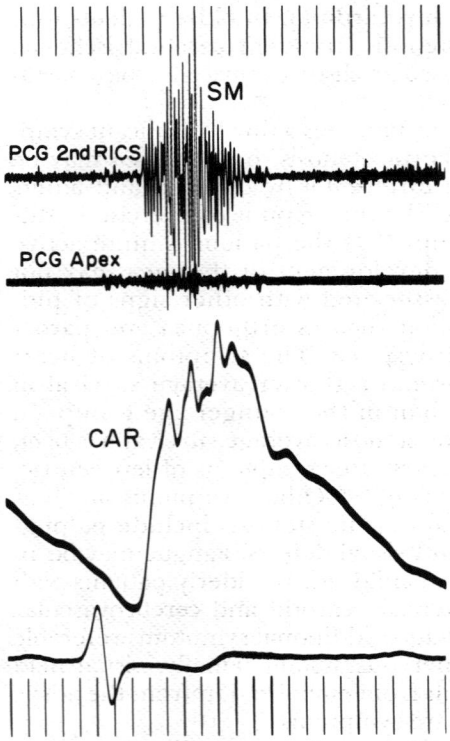

FIGURE 38-5 Phonocardiogram and carotid pulse recording in aortic stenosis. A loud crescendo-decrescendo, diamond-shaped systolic murmur is recorded in the aortic area and the carotid pulse shows the delayed upstroke with a jagged appearance corresponding with the vibrations of a thrill. PCG = phonocardiogram; RICS = right intercostal space; SM = systolic murmur; CAR = carotid artery. (*Courtesy of Dr. Ernest Craige.*)

notch can sometimes be recognized.[27] This notch is attributed to peak turbulence across the aortic valve, and the more severe the stenosis the more proximal to the initial upstroke the anacrotic notch appears. Associated aortic regurgitation may lengthen the duration from onset of the upstroke to the anacrotic notch. The delayed peak of the pulse, diminished amplitude, and gradual downslope are characteristically described by the term *pulsus parvus et tardus*. The lung fields remain clear to auscultation until the patient has developed heart failure, pulmonary venous hypertension, and characteristic rales.

Inspection of the precordium is often nonrevealing in aortic stenosis, and even with marked left ventricular hypertrophy the apical impulse may remain focal and within the midclavicular line. The apical impulse can be hyperactive to palpation. A systolic thrill should be sought, particularly over the aortic area and the right second interspace. This is best detected by using the palm of the hand over the area while the patient sits or leans forward in full expiration. If palpable vibrations during systolic ejection can be detected, the gradient across the aortic valve usually exceeds 40 mmHg. Rarely, systolic vibrations can accompany the systolic murmur of relative aortic stenosis in severe aortic regurgitation.

The auscultatory characteristics of aortic stenosis include an aortic ejection click, the characteristic diamond-shaped crescendo-decrescendo murmur, delayed closure of the aortic valve, and a detectable diastolic blow along the left sternal border. The ejection sound is high-pitched and may be audible at the apex or along the left sternal border shortly after the first heart sound.[38] This sound occurs with the systolic elevation of the central aortic pulse and probably originates from the aortic valve leaflets. The ejection click is related to the mobility of the valve and not the severity of the gradient. The intensity of the click often correlates with the prominence of the aortic second sound.

Characteristics of the systolic murmur include a harsh crescendo-decrescendo or diamond-shaped pattern to the systolic components. An interval between the first sound and onset of the murmur can be appreciated, and the murmur usually terminates before the second sound. However, if the aortic second sound is sufficiently diminished, the pulmonic closure sound may be identified as the aortic second sound, and the murmur interpreted as holosystolic.

The aortic second sound is characteristically delayed in significant aortic stenosis and may result in paradoxical splitting of the second sound. Rather than the normal inspiratory splitting of the first and second heart sounds, the delayed closure of the aortic valve coincides with the pulmonic delay during inspiration, and therefore the pulmonic sound moves toward the first heart sound during expiration, producing paradoxical splitting.[27] However, as the aortic valve loses mobility and becomes calcified, there may be a diminution and eventual loss of aortic second-sound vibrations.

In one-third to one-half of patients with isolated aortic valve stenosis, careful auscultation will detect a high-pitched diastolic blow of aortic regurgitation.[39] This murmur has been attributed to the fixed stenosis of the aortic valve, which remains slightly open during diastole.

Calcific aortic stenosis in the elderly may produce different auscultatory features.[40] These audible changes in the aortic stenotic murmur can be attributed to the nodular calcification at the bases of the aortic cusps and root, with preservation of leaflet mobility. Therefore, the ejection click often disappears and the murmur becomes musical and heard more prominently at the apex and along the left sternal border. The location of the murmur at the apex can raise the possibility of mitral annulus calcification and regurgitation across the mitral valve.

In addition to these auscultatory variations of calcific aortic stenosis, sclerosis and loss of compliance in peripheral arteries can obscure the characteristic pulse deformities. Thus noncompliant vessels in the elderly may normalize pulse contour abnormalities.

Chest Roentgenogram

Despite the severity of aortic stenosis and the pressure overload on the left ventricle, radiographic heart size initially remains within normal limits.[41]

The apical curvature may be prominent or bulging, which suggests concentric hypertrophy. Poststenotic dilatation of the ascending aorta is a common feature of aortic stenosis. The final radiographic abnormality in aortic stenosis is calcification of the valve, but this cannot be excluded unless fluoroscopy of the heart is performed. Calcification of the aortic valve is commonly encountered in significant stenosis in the patient over 40 years of age. Minimal enlargement of the left atrium may occur, but excessive left atrial dilatation should raise other possibilities, such as mitral valve stenosis and idiopathic hypertrophic subaortic stenosis.

Electrocardiogram

The most frequent abnormalities in the electrocardiogram in aortic stenosis are changes produced by left ventricular hypertrophy and reflected in the amplitude of the QRS complex and ST-T wave changes.[27,42] The systolic overload or left ventricular strain pattern or left ventricular hypertrophy consists of increased S waves in right precordial leads and elevated R waves in left precordial leads, coupled with depression of the ST segment and inversion of the T waves. Conduction defects are not rare, and first-degree heart block as well as left bundle branch block can be present. Complete heart block is infrequent but has been associated with aortic stenosis.

Special Laboratory Studies

Echocardiogram Echocardiography has proved useful in aortic stenosis, not only in delineating valve structure and mobility but also in the recognition of nonvalvular forms of aortic stenosis and the assessment of ventricular function.[43] Echocardiography can record characteristic changes of thickening, calcification, and reduced mobility of the aortic leaflet.[44] Left ventricular echocardiographic dimensions of septal wall thickness can demonstrate the extent of left ventricular hypertrophy as well as asymmetrical septal hypertrophy in idiopathic subaortic stenosis. Left ventricular chamber dimensions from echocardiography can estimate end-diastolic and end-systolic volumes and ejection fraction. Echocardiography has been used occasionally to recognize a bicuspid aortic valve, to detect asymmetry of the two leaflets, and to calculate an eccentricity index.[45]

Based on the assumption that the increase in wall thickness in aortic stenosis is a compensatory mechanism to normalize wall stress, left ventricular peak systolic pressure has been estimated from the relationship of systolic wall thickness to systolic internal diameter.[46] In this manner the aortic valve gradient can be extrapolated from the predicted left ventricular systolic pressure and the measured systemic systolic pressure.

Cardiac Catheterization Cardiac catheterization is clinically performed in aortic stenosis to determine the gradient across the valve and estimate the severity of the stenosis, to evaluate left ventricular function, and to delineate coronary artery anatomy (Fig. 38-6).

Normal aortic systolic valve area is 2 to 3 cm², and calculations indicate that reduction has to be 75 percent or more with orifice size less than 0.8 cm² before significant impairment to flow and forward cardiac output develops.[47] This degree of reduced orifice size is usually accompanied by a gradient exceeding 50 mmHg, but one must remember that a decline in cardiac output will reduce the gradient across the valve[48] (Fig. 38-7).

Quantitative angiography can provide measurements of end-diastolic and systolic volume, along with the ejection fraction and an estimate of left ventricular mass[49] (Fig. 38-8). Chamber dimensions, pressure, and wall thickness allow calculation of wall stress at end-diastole and during systolic valve opening, which indicate preload and afterload, respectively (Fig. 38-8).

Coronary arteriography in aortic stenosis has shown a high incidence of underlying coronary artery disease whether patients have a prior history of exertional chest pain or not[30] (Fig. 38-9). Therefore, physical findings suggestive of aortic stenosis war-

FIGURE 38-6 Left ventricular pressure and volume in compensated aortic stenosis. The end-diastolic volume is normal, the ejection fraction slightly higher than normal, and left ventricular mass significantly increased. These measurements indicate concentric hypertrophy of the ventricle in response to a pressure overload. End-diastolic volume (EDV) = 78; end-systolic volume (ESV) = 13; stroke volume (SV) = 65; ejection fraction (EF) = 65/78 = 0.83; left ventricular weight (LVwt) = 270; left ventricular end-diastolic pressure (LVedp) = 13). [*From C. E. Rackley and W. P. Hood, Jr., Measurements of Ventricular Volume, Mass and Ejection Fraction, in W. Grossman (ed.), "Cardiac Catheterization and Angiography," Lea & Febiger, Philadelphia. Reproduced with permission.*]

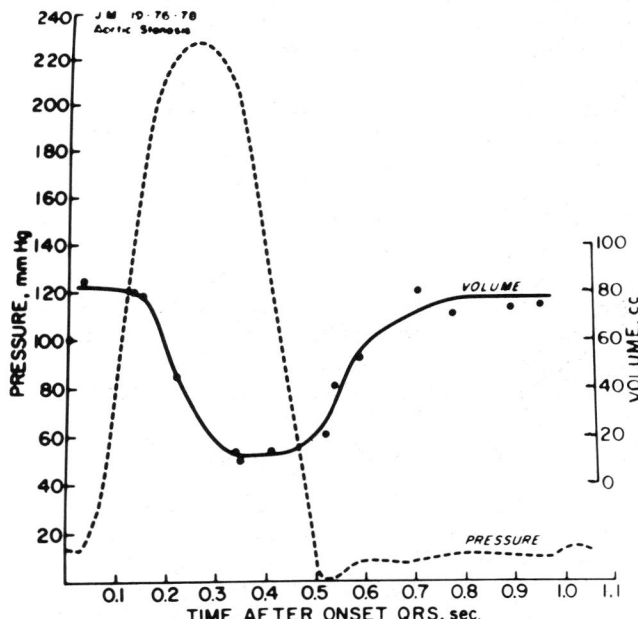

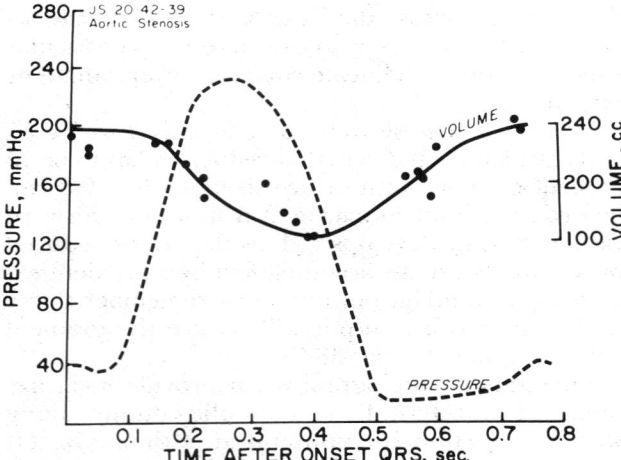

FIGURE 38-7 Left ventricular pressure and volume in decompensated aortic stenosis. The stroke volume has remained normal, but end-diastolic and end-systolic volumes are significantly increased with a reduced ejection fraction. End-diastolic pressure is elevated, and there is a marked increase in left ventricular mass. EDV = 238; ESV = 163; SV = 75; EF = 75/238 = 0.31; LVwt = 557; LVedp = 34. [*From C. E. Rackley and W. P. Hood, Jr., Aortic Valve Disease, in H. J. Levine (ed.), "Clinical Cardiovascular Physiology," Grune & Stratton, Inc., New York, 1976. Reproduced with permission.*]

rant coronary arteriography for both diagnostic and therapeutic reasons. Coronary artery surgery should be performed at the time of replacement of the aortic valve.

Radionuclide Studies Radionuclide techniques can be utilized to assess ventricular function and myocardial perfusion in aortic stenosis.[50] Left ventricular ejection fraction at rest and during exertion may demonstrate deterioration of left ventricular function before clinical symptoms have developed. Impaired myocardial radionuclide perfusion may raise the possibility of underlying coronary disease in addition to aortic valve stenosis. These radionuclide studies on left ventricular function and myocardial perfusion can be repeated in the serial evaluation of patients with aortic stenosis before and following valve surgery.

Exercise Studies In patients with symptomatic aortic stenosis, particularly those with a history of syncope, exercise testing should be performed with extreme caution or with very minimal effort. Under carefully monitored conditions, the exercise test can be combined with radionuclide studies to assess ventricular function as well as the clinical response.[50]

Natural History and Prognosis

The incidence of bicuspid aortic valve has been estimated at 4 out of 1000 live births with a predominance of males to females at 4:1.[4] Leaflets may thicken by age 40 and almost invariably by age 50, with calcium deposits rarely observed before 40

years of age. Although symptoms occur late in the course of aortic stenosis, 3 to 5 percent of patients may be subject to sudden death during the asymptomatic period, probably caused by an arrhythmia.[26,51] Any of the triad of symptoms of angina pectoris, syncope, or heart failure heralds a significantly shortened life expectancy. In one large series, the average age at clinical presentation was 48 years, whereas the average age at death was 63 years.[52] However, once patients develop symptoms, average survival is usually less than 5 years, and the incidence of sudden death in symptomatic patients increases to 15 to 20 percent.[53] The development of exertional chest pain is associated with an average life expectancy of about 5 years, and less than 5 percent of patients survive 10 to 20 years.[27] The prognosis after the development of syncope is usually 3 to 4 years, and the average survival after symptoms of left ventricular failure is 2 years.[26,36] Thus, development of symptoms in patients with aortic stenosis carries a much worse long-term prognosis than any other valve lesion affecting either the aortic or mitral valve.

Management

Medical
The medical management of aortic stenosis prior to the development of symptoms is prophylactic to prevent bacterial endocarditis with elective dental

FIGURE 38-8 Left ventricular pressure-volume diagram is decompensated aortic stenosis. The systolic pressure remains abnormally elevated, but left ventricular stroke volume is maintained by abnormal increases in end-diastolic and end-systolic volume. The left ventricular end-diastolic pressure is also abnormally elevated. [*From C. E. Rackley and W. P. Hood, Jr., Aortic Valve Disease, in H. J. Levine (ed.), "Clinical Cardiovascular Physiology," Grune & Stratton, Inc., New York, 1976. Reproduced with permission.*]

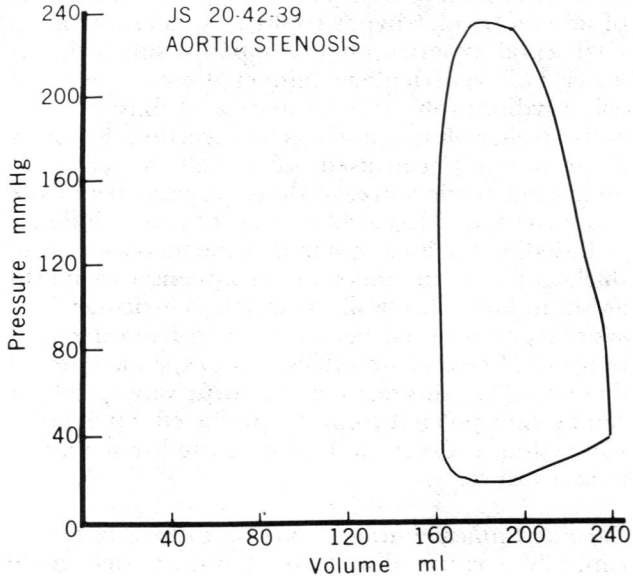

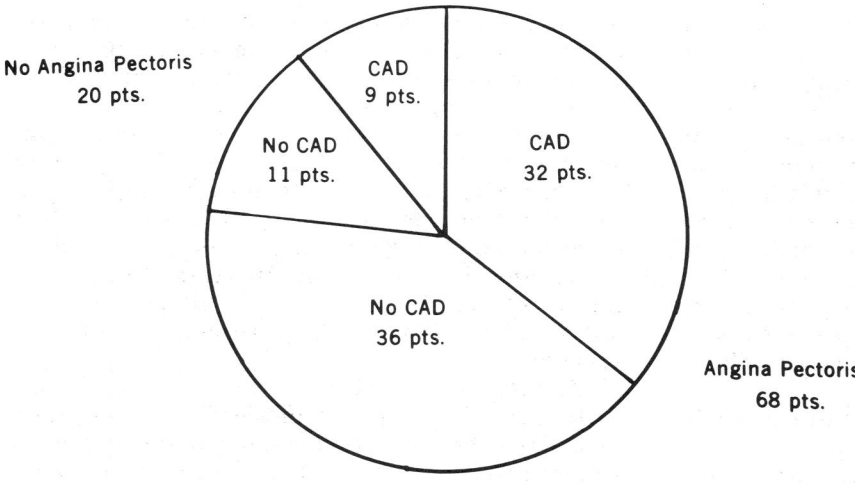

FIGURE 38-9 Aortic stenosis, angina pectoris, and coronary artery disease. In 88 patients with aortic stenosis the incidence of coronary artery disease was similar whether chest discomfort was present or absent. (*From R. E. Moraski, R. O. Russell, Jr., J. A. Mantle, and C. E. Rackley, Aortic Stenosis, Angina Pectoris, and Coronary Artery Disease, Catheterization and Cardiovascular Diagnosis, 2:157, 1976. Reproduced with permission.*)

and surgical procedures.[39] In patients with multivalvular involvement, rheumatic prophylaxis is in order, but this may not be necessary if aortic stenosis is the single lesion. For exertional chest pain nitrates should be cautiously administered, and patients should be warned about orthostatic hypotension and syncope. Although digitalis and diuretics would be indicated in left ventricular failure, left ventricular failure is due to mechanical obstruction, and surgical replacement of the aortic valve is indicated.

The physician should appreciate that depression of the contractile state and reduction of the cardiac output will diminish the intensity of the systolic murmur, and rarely the patient may present in advanced heart failure or cardiogenic shock without an audible murmur. Fluoroscopic detection of calcium in the area of the aortic valve should immediately alert one to aortic stenosis.

Although criteria for early valve replacement in the asymptomatic patient have not been delineated, the new noninvasive techniques of echocardiography and radionuclide scintigraphy can provide objective data on ventricular dimensions and function, in addition to simple radiographic estimates of heart size.[46,50] Heart size in pure aortic stenosis may not increase until significant depression of left ventricular function has developed. The increased incidence of sudden death after the development of symptoms, as well as the increased operative mortality with myocardial failure, emphasizes the need for the physician to proceed with surgery early in the patient's course.

In preparation for aortic valve replacement any elective surgery or dental work should be completed before cardiac surgery is performed. Electrolyte abnormalities should be corrected if the patient has been on diuretics. In elderly patients with calcific aortic stenosis, the radiation of the murmur into the carotid vessel may sometimes obscure underlying coronary carotid artery lesions. Therefore, noninvasive studies to detect disparity in flow through the carotids should be performed and, if necessary, carotid arteriography for the delineation of lesions.

Carotid arterial lesions can sometimes be corrected at the same procedure for aortic valve replacement.

Surgery

As noted in many studies, for example, the natural history study of Rapaport,[54] aortic stenosis has a significantly greater decline in survival than aortic incompetence, mitral stenosis, or mitral incompetence in patients followed from time of diagnosis. At least 50 percent of patients identified as having severe aortic stenosis with or without symptoms are dead in 5 years. Sudden death without significant preexisting symptoms occurs in about 20 percent of untreated patients, presumably from cardiac arrhythmia resulting from myocardial ischemia, or from cerebral ischemia sometimes manifested preterminally by syncopal attacks. Many patients with aortic stenosis suffer from angina pectoris, but the majority of patients in our surgical series had symptoms of pulmonary venous hypertension (dyspnea, orthopnea, and paroxysmal nocturnal dyspnea). These symptoms indicate reduction of left ventricular function and are often a prelude to death. Although the murmur and other ancillary findings of aortic stenosis may exist for a long time without symptoms, in many patients there is a point at which there is rapid progression of symptoms together with an important increase in the transvalvular gradient. As opposed to aortic incompetence (see below) ventricular function is preserved, for the most part, even in the presence of significant disability, and thus operative treatment effects a major improvement in quality of life and also in longevity.

Indications for Operation Asymptomatic patients with severe aortic stenosis and marked left ventricular hypertrophy (as evidenced by the chest roentgenogram and by electrocardiographic pattern of left ventricular hypertrophy with strain pattern) should be advised to undergo operation. Certainly, patients with symptoms from pulmonary venous hypertension should be advised to undergo operation promptly, as well as those with syncope or angina pectoris. It is usually stated that a peak trans-aortic valve gradient of greater than 50 mmHg is an indication for operation. However, a more precise rendering of the degree of aortic stenosis is obtained by measurement of the cardiac output along with the left ventricular aortic pressure gradient and calculating the aortic valve area by Gorlin's formula. Usually, operation is indicated in patients with aortic valve areas of 0.8 cm^2 or less. Occasionally, operation is indicated in patients with valve areas of 1.0 cm^2. It must be remembered that in patients with mild or moderate aortic valve incompetence associated with aortic stenosis the Gorlin formula will underestimate the true valve area.

The diagnosis of aortic stenosis can usually be based on the patient's history, the presence of a characteristic murmur and dampened carotid arterial pulses, and the radiologic identification of calcium in the aortic valve. Electrocardiographic evidence of left ventricular hypertrophy is helpful, but it is not present in all patients with important stenotic lesions. When the findings are not characteristic, measurement of systolic ejection times and the use of the echocardiogram may be helpful, the latter particularly to distinguish valvular aortic stenosis from discrete subvalvular or idiopathic hypertrophic subaortic stenosis. Cardiac catheterization is indicated in patients where there is a question of the diagnosis or the severity of the obstruction. Coronary arteriography is indicated for those patients over 40 years old because of possible coexisting coronary artery disease. When surgically correctable occlusive coronary arterial disease is demonstrated, coronary bypass grafting should be carried out at the time of replacement of the valve.

Operation The pathological alterations in the stenotic aortic valve are such that satisfactory results can rarely be obtained from incision of fused com-missures and debridement of the cusps. Commissurotomy can be done in aortic stenosis of the young. However, in all others the operation of choice is excision and replacement of the valve.

Various devices are available. The homograft aortic valve sewn freehand in the orthotopic position has performed quite well over a 3- to 7-year period.[55] However, in almost all patients we have noted a gradual degeneration of the valve, requiring reoperation between 7 and 10 years after implantation. Others have extended this period using antibiotic sterilization and preservation of fresh valve.[56,57]

Most institutions rely either on prosthetic devices, such as Bjork-Shiley, Lillehi-Caster, SJM, or Starr-Edwards prostheses, or on stent-mounted porcine xenografts, such as the Hancock or Carpentier-Edwards bioprostheses. Similar indications and caveats exist as for the mitral position. In patients unable to take anticoagulants, the stent-mounted xenograft seems appropriate. However, degeneration of this device certainly does occur. We and others have noted more rapid degeneration of the porcine xenografts in younger patients.[58] Additional problems exist with the xenograft, namely a less than optimal orifice-to-annulus ratio in the smaller valve sizes.[59]

Patients with prosthetic valves must receive anticoagulation therapy, but their prostheses may be expected to have good hemodynamic function and long-term durability.

The operation is performed via a median sternotomy. The left atrium is vented. The aorta is clamped after internal and external cooling, and cardioplegic solution is infused into the coronary ostia. The aortic valve is removed and the replacement device sutured in place using either continuous sutures, interrupted simple sutures, or horizontal mattress sutures (Fig. 38-10). Should associated procedures be necessary, such as coronary artery

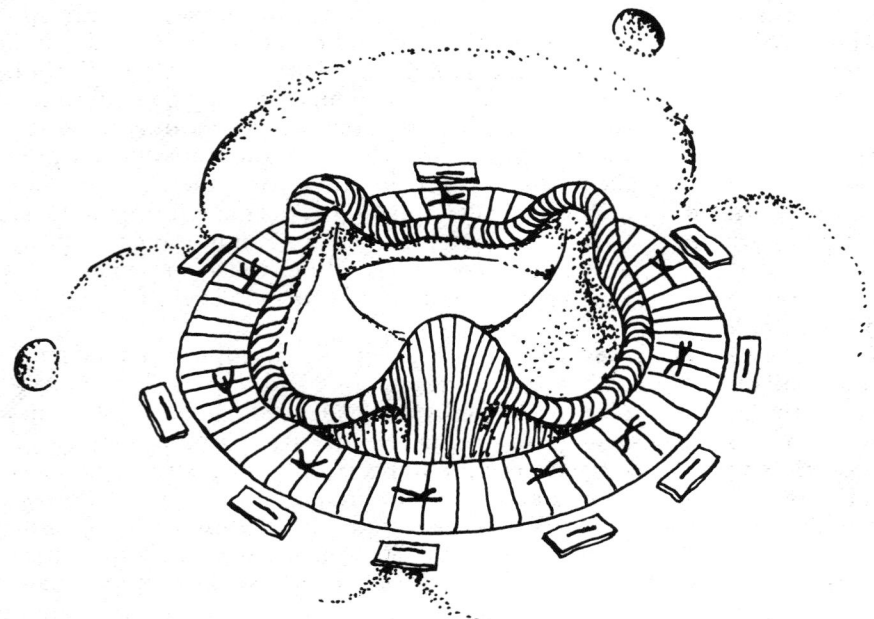

FIGURE 38-10 Technique for insertion of aortic xenograft using interrupted pledgeted mattress sutures.

bypass grafting, these are usually done with a single period of aortic cross-clamping. The usual precautions for ridding the heart of air are taken after the aortotomy is closed.

In patients with severe left ventricular hypertrophy, measures are taken to ensure a satisfactory perfusion pressure on release of the aortic cross-clamp to allow perfusion of both the subepicardial segment and the endocardial segment. When direct intermittent coronary perfusion or ischemic arrest was utilized for myocardial protection, subendocardial necrosis was an important finding in those patients with aortic stenosis who died after cardiopulmonary bypass. However, in the cardioplegic era this has been only a very infrequent event.

Postoperative Care Postoperative care is similar in general principles to that for patients undergoing operations on the mitral valve. It is generally simple, since nearly all patients have a good hemodynamic state after aortic valve replacement. Many patients have arterial hypertension, which may be some hazard because of the stress it places on the aortotomy and because of the increase it produces in left ventricular afterload. In these circumstances we decrease arterial pressure with nitroprusside infusion. Major cardiac arrhythmias (six or more premature ventricular contractions per minute) are aggressively treated either by infusion of potassium chloride to a serum level greater than 4 meq/liter, bolus or continuous infusion of lidocaine, or intramuscular doses of procainamide. We have found also that premature ventricular contractions are sometimes nicely suppressed with atrial pacing at between 90 and 100 beats per minute, using temporary fine-wire electrodes secured on the right atrial epicardium.[60]

Early Results The present operative mortality for primary isolated aortic valve replacement is between 2 percent and 3 percent. When cold potassium cardioplegia is used, the only major incremental risk factor has been New York Heart Association class (Fig. 38-11). Patients with advanced left ventricular failure have a higher risk of death than patients in New York Heart Association functional class III. The addition of coronary artery bypass grafting causes perhaps an additional 1 percent or 2 percent risk.[61] Thus, we believe that saphenous vein grafting at the time of aortic valve replacement is certainly justified. It is to be noted that aortic valve replacement can be conducted in a safe and satisfactory manner even in patients in the eighth decade, although in those patients tissues are fragile, and we have found that hemorrhage is an important cause of early postoperative mortality.

Late Results The medium-term survival for patients at the University of Alabama having aortic valve replacement using a Bjork-Shiley prosthesis is shown in Fig. 38-11. This actuarial survival is compared to data from a large series in which the Starr-Edwards ball-valve prosthesis was used,[62] and from another series in which the Hancock porcine xenograft was used.[63] As opposed to the situation seen in patients with aortic incompetence (Fig. 38-12), patients with aortic stenosis seem to have less deterioration in ventricular performance when operated upon and approach near-normal left ventricular contractile indexes postoperatively.[64,65] Thus, even in patients importantly symptomatic with aortic stenosis, a successful operation leads to good symptomatic recovery and quite satisfactory long-term survival. Late deaths are due to heart failure, complications of thromboembolism, myocardial infarction, and sudden death, the latter perhaps associated with an arrhythmia. The late survival of patients having a combined operation including aortic valve replacement and coronary artery bypass grafting is similar to that of patients having isolated aortic valve replacement.

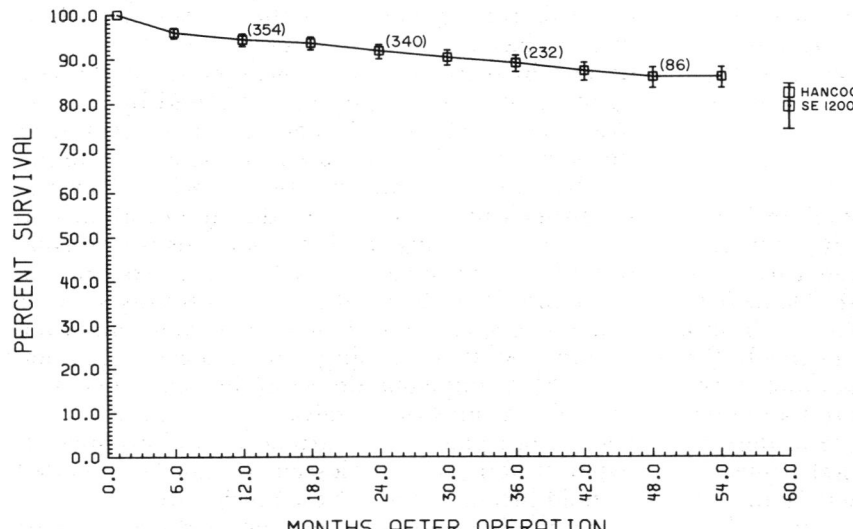

FIGURE 38-11 Actuarial survival of patients receiving aortic Bjork-Shiley prostheses at the University of Alabama. These data are compared to 5-year survival for the Hancock xenograft (Davila[63]) and for the Starr-Edwards silastic ball prosthesis (Macmanus[62]).

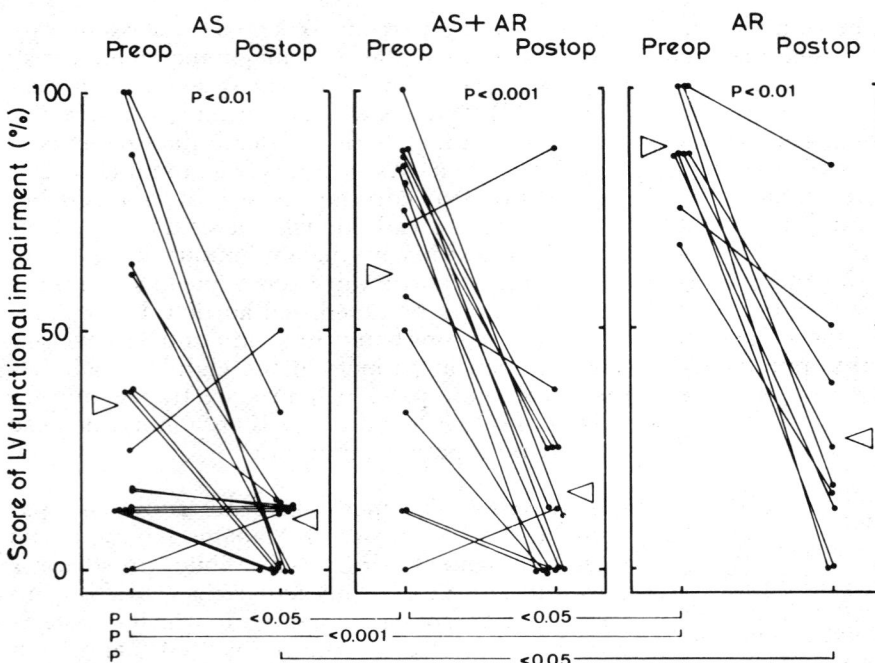

FIGURE 38-12 Change in multiple parameters of left ventricular impairment after aortic valve replacement in patients with aortic stenosis, mixed lesion, and aortic incompetence. (*From H. P. Karayenbuehl, M. Lurina, O. Hess, M. Rothlin, and A. Senning, Pre- and Postoperative Left Ventricular Contractile Function in Patients with Aortic Valve Disease, Br. Heart J., 41:204, 1979. Reproduced with permission.*)

Postoperative Management

The immediate postoperative management requires maintenance of cardiac and pulmonic function. During ambulation ventricular irritability may require antiarrhythmics for an elective 4- to 6-week period. Anticoagulation will depend on the type of prosthetic valve selected. A base-line cinefluorogram of the prosthetic valve should be obtained before discharge for future comparisons. Once the patient has been discharged from the hospital, periodic evaluations are in order to assess the function of the prosthetic valve for sharp clicks as well as the development of a diastolic murmur or any other changes suggesting impairment of the valve. Noninvasive techniques such as echocardiography and radionuclide scans can be used to follow ventricular function, specifically ejection fraction and end-diastolic and end-systolic volumes. Dysfunction of prosthetic devices can be suspected on the basis of evidence from heart sound recordings as well as periodic fluoroscopy to check for optimal positioning of the prosthetic valve.

Cost Effectiveness

A major consideration in management of aortic stenosis, as well as cost effectiveness in terms of money and health, is the selection of an optimal time for aortic valve replacement. Ideally, this should be performed before the patient has developed clinical symptoms, but patients can perform normally for many years. Advances in electrocardiographic techniques as well as radionuclide scans at rest and during exercise may provide early evidence of depression of myocardial function before clinical symptoms develop. Such information can be beneficial in both reducing the number of hospitalizations and selecting the optimal time for surgery.

Aortic Regurgitation

But when the semilunar valves, from any of the causes enumerated, became incapable of closing the mouth of the ventricle, a portion of the blood just sent into the aorta greater or less, according to the degree of the inadequacy of the valves turns back into the ventricle.

D. J. Corrigan, 1832[66]

Etiology

Although aortic regurgitation has been a long-recognized valvular cause of disturbed cardiac function, there has been a gradual change in the incidence of diseases that affect the integrity of the aortic valve. Several decades ago rheumatic fever and syphilis were generally accepted as major causes of aortic regurgitation, but the incidence of these diseases has decreased in recent years.[67–69] With the decline in these two infectious conditions the recognition of aortic regurgitation caused by connective tissue diseases and anatomic abnormalities of the aortic valve has increased (Table 38-1). Heritable disorders of connective tissue such as Marfan's syndrome can result in aortic dilatation with incompetence of the valve, and myxomatous transformation of the aortic valve may be a predisposing abnormality.[70] Arthritic disease conditions such as ankylosing spondylitis, Reiter's syndrome, and even rheumatoid arthritis can produce aortic regurgitation.[71–74] A congenital defect in the ventricular septum with a sinus of Valsalva aneurysm can lead to aortic regurgitation.[75] Chronic conditions such as hypertension and arteriosclerosis can be attended by mild incompetence of the aortic valve.[76]

Acute disruption of a normal or diseased aortic valve can lead to sudden aortic regurgitation. Dis-

**TABLE 38-1   Mechanisms of Chronic and
Acute Aortic Regurgitation**

1. Chronic mechanisms
   a. Rheumatic fever
   b. Syphilis
   c. Heritable disorders of connective tissue
      (1) Marfan's syndrome
      (2) Osteogenesis imperfecta
   d. Arthritic diseases
      (1) Ankylosing spondylitis
      (2) Reiter's syndrome
      (3) Rheumatoid arthritis
   e. Cystic medionecrosis of aorta
   f. Sinus of Valsalva aneurysm
   g. Hypertension
   h. Arteriosclerosis
   i. Myxomatous degeneration of valve
2. Acute mechanisms
   a. Dissection of aorta
   b. Bacterial endocarditis
   c. Rheumatic fever

section of the aorta, bacterial endocarditis, and acute rheumatic fever can produce sudden regurgitation across the aortic valve.[77,78] Aortic dissection may distort the annulus of the aortic valve, bacterial endocarditis can lead to leaflet perforation or paravalvular incompetence, and acute rheumatic fever can, although rarely, evert an aortic cusp.

Pathology

Aortic insufficiency results either from intrinsic disease of the cusps or from primary diseases of the ascending aorta. Additionally, shunts originating in the aorta may simulate aortic insufficiency.

Intrinsic Disease of Aortic Valve

Aortic insufficiency from acquired intrinsic diseases of the valve is most commonly of rheumatic or of bacterial inflammatory origin. Less common changes are those associated with rheumatoid arthritis, lupus erythematosus, and trauma.[79] The principal congenital disease is the congenital bicuspid aortic valve. In arachnodactyly, wherein the primary basis for aortic insufficiency usually is in the aorta, there may be an intrinsically prolapsed condition of the aortic cusps.

Rheumatic Disease

Rheumatic diseases of the aortic valve may cause pure aortic incompetence or incompetence may be associated with some degree of stenosis (see section on aortic stenosis). Pure aortic insufficiency of rheumatic origin results from fibrosis and contracture of the cusps.[76] The cusps become shorter than normal (Fig. 38-13). This may be of equal severity among the cusps or unequal so that one cusp undergoes greater contracture than the other two. The result is a malalignment of the cusps, allowing for incompetence of the valve. In pure rheumatic aortic incompetence, commissural fusion is either absent or

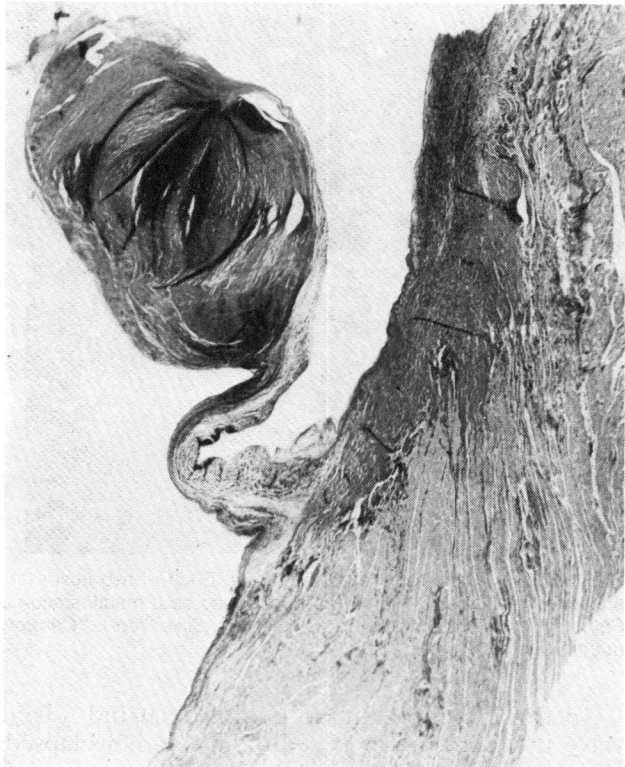

FIGURE 38-13   Low-power photomicrograph of an aortic cusp in chronic rheumatic aortic insufficiency. The distal one-half of the cusp is grossly thickened by fibrous tissue. Elastic tissue stain; ×5.

minimal. If contracture is coupled with fusion of two or three commissures, the effect is a combination of aortic stenosis and insufficiency.

Infectious Endocarditis

Infectious endocarditis of the aortic valve may involve a tricuspid aortic valve, but often the valve is bicuspid, either congenitally or acquired. The usual basis for incompetence is destruction of cusp tissue (Fig. 38-14). There may either be perforation of one or more cusps or detachment of a cusp at its aortic attachment. Atrioventricular conduction defects may be associated with aortic insufficiency caused by infectious endocarditis as the infectious process extends to the nearby conduction tissue.[80]

Trauma

Deceleration external blunt trauma may cause rupture of a cusp, but only rarely.[81] The usual basis for posttraumatic aortic insufficiency is a laceration of the aorta (see below).

Congenital Anomalies

There are two principal causes of intrinsic aortic incompetence associated with congenital disease, namely congenital bicuspid aortic valve and ventricular septal defect. Fenestration of aortic cusps, while common, is a rare cause of aortic regurgitation.[82] Myxomatous change may also be a cause of aortic incompetence.

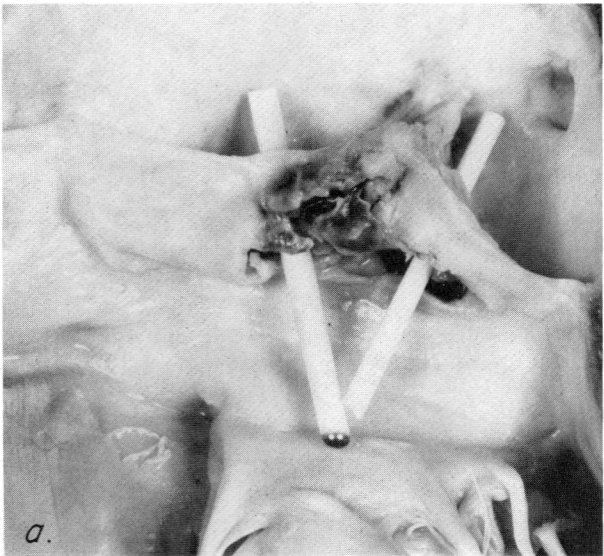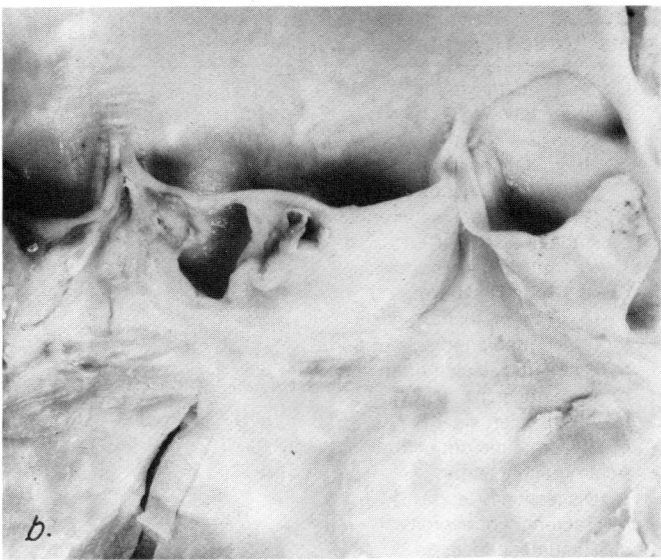

FIGURE 38-14 Bacterial endocarditis. *a.* Each of two cusps of the aortic valve shows perforation (probes) as part of active bacterial endocarditis. *b.* Perforation in an aortic cusp as a manifestation of bacteriologically healed bacterial endocarditis. [*From J. E. Edwards, Pathology of Aortic Incompetence, in M. D. Silver (ed.), "Cardiovascular Pathology," Churchill-Livingstone, New York, in press. Reproduced with permission.*]

In the incompetent congenital bicuspid aortic valve the larger cusp is redundant and prolapsed beyond the opposite cusp. Usually, incompetence of a congenital bicuspid valve is not apparent until early adult life. In an uncommon type of congenital bicuspid valve the raphe is represented by a thin strand of tissue running from near the free aspect of the larger cusp, on one hand, to the aortic wall, on the other. Rupture of the strand causes the larger cusp to lose much of its support so that it prolapses. This may account for the sudden appearance of major aortic regurgitation.[83]

In aortic incompetence associated with ventricular septal defect, the defect is closely related to the aortic root and valve. More commonly, the defect is of the supracristal type; it is less commonly infracristal.[84] The cause of the aortic incompetence appears to be an inadequate attachment of the aortic root to the cardiac skeleton. The aorta deviates to the right and the related cusp or cusps (usually the right, less commonly the left) are carried laterally with the displaced aorta and "tip." The result is malalignment of the cusps.

Myxomatous alteration of the aortic cusps ("floppy aortic valve") is usually associated with extensive cystic medial necrosis of the aorta. If aortic incompetence is present, its cause lies principally in the aorta. Nevertheless, an element of prolapse of a cusp may be either the only cause or a contributing one.

Primary Disease of Ascending Aorta
Primary disease of the aorta leading to aortic valvular insufficiency takes the form either of dilatation or laceration of the vessel.

Primary Dilatation Dilatation of the ascending aorta creates tension upon the individual cusps, causing them to be relatively short for closure of the dilated aortic root. One cause of this condition is aortitis, of which syphilitic aortitis is the classic example (Fig. 38-15).[85] Aortic changes associated with rheumatoid spondylitis[86] yield a similar picture, as

FIGURE 38-15 Aortic valve viewed from above in aortitis. Bowing of the cusps incident to dilatation of the aorta leaves a triangular defect thorough which regurgitation occurred. The commissures are not fused.

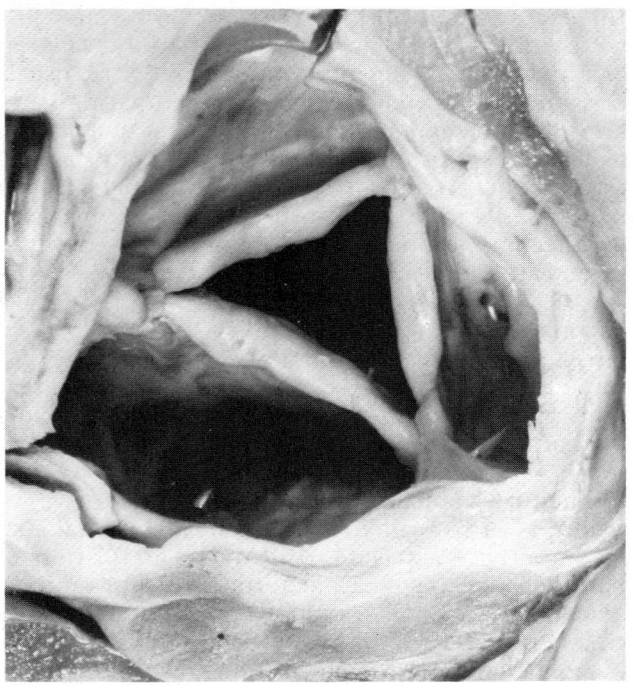

do various types of aortitis of unknown etiology. In rheumatoid arthritis, the root of the aorta may be affected, and inflammatory and fibrotic changes of the valve cusps may also be associated.[72] Unusually, in a person of advanced age the natural process of aortic dilatation with age may be of such proportion as to be responsible for aortic incompetence.

Extensive cystic medial necrosis of the aorta, either of the idiopathic type or associated with Marfan's syndrome, even in the absence of laceration of the aorta, is yet another cause of aortic incompetence (Fig. 38-16). In this condition a contributing factor to aortic incompetence may be the intrinsic changes of the cusps that allow the cusps to prolapse (Fig. 38-17) or, rarely, rupture.[70]

Laceration of the Aorta Laceration of the ascending aorta may complicate hypertension, extensive cystic medial necrosis, external blunt trauma, or, uncommonly, aortitis. It may be a localized process or lead to dissecting aneurysm.[87] If the primary laceration occurs near a commissural attachment of two cusps, the secondary retraction of aortic tissue

causes prolapse of the cusps at the related commissure[83] (Fig. 38-18*A* and 38-18*B*). The consequent malalignment of the cusps underlies the appearance of aortic insufficiency, which may appear suddenly.

In some cases of aortic laceration, the laceration lies below the upper aspect of a commissure and there is, additionally, the chance of tearing related cusps by retraction of the edges of the laceration[83] (Fig. 38-18*C*). Abnormal escape of blood from the aorta as occurs in various types of shunts may simulate aortic insufficiency, even though the valve is normal.[88]

Abnormal Physiology

In aortic regurgitation the diastolic flow of blood across the valve increases filling of the left ventricle, and thus a volume overload is imposed on the left ventricle (Fig. 38-19). The size of the regurgitant area, the diastolic pressure gradient across the valve, and the duration of diastole significantly influence the regurgitant volume.[89,90] The volume overload depends as much on the chronicity as the severity of the incompetence, since even a small regurgitant area of the valve can lead to a significant degree of aortic incompetence over a period of time.[91] Chronic aortic regurgitation produces a gradual increase in the end-diastolic volume of the left ventricle, since filling of the chamber derives from both the left atrium and the aorta. Total left ventricular stroke volume is increased in order to maintain the forward or effective stroke volume within the normal range. The chronicity of the leak across the aortic valve leads to compensatory dilatation of the left ventricle, which is accompanied by little if any elevation in the left ventricular end-diastolic pressure.[85] Diastolic compliance of the left ventricle is slowly increased due to slippage of myocardial fibers and other chronic mechanisms such as stress relaxation and creep.[92] The ventricular wall forces are maintained within the normal range by an increase in wall thickness and left ventricular mass, or hypertrophy.[89] This compensatory left ventricular hypertrophy tends to normalize systolic wall stress, or afterload.[86]

During the early years of chronic aortic regurgitation the increase in left ventricular stroke volume supports a normal forward cardiac output during rest and exercise. The ejection fraction or ratio of the left ventricular stroke volume to end-diastolic volume remains within or near the normal range. However, a gradual decline in the contractile state of the ventricular myocardium due to primary myocardial factors or secondary to lesions such as underlying coronary artery disease will result in a relatively greater increase in the end-systolic volume and a decline in the ejection fraction (Fig. 38-20). During this period of deterioration the left ventricular end-diastolic pressure will increase as the compliant properties, or elasticity, of the ventricle di-

FIGURE 38-16 Cystic medial necrosis of aorta in Marfan's syndrome. Exterior view of heart and aorta viewed from the left side. Marked dilatation of the ascending aorta. [*From J. E. Edwards, Pathology of Aortic Incompetence, in M. D. Silver (ed.), "Cardiovascular Pathology," Churchill-Livingstone, New York, in press. Reproduced with permission.*]

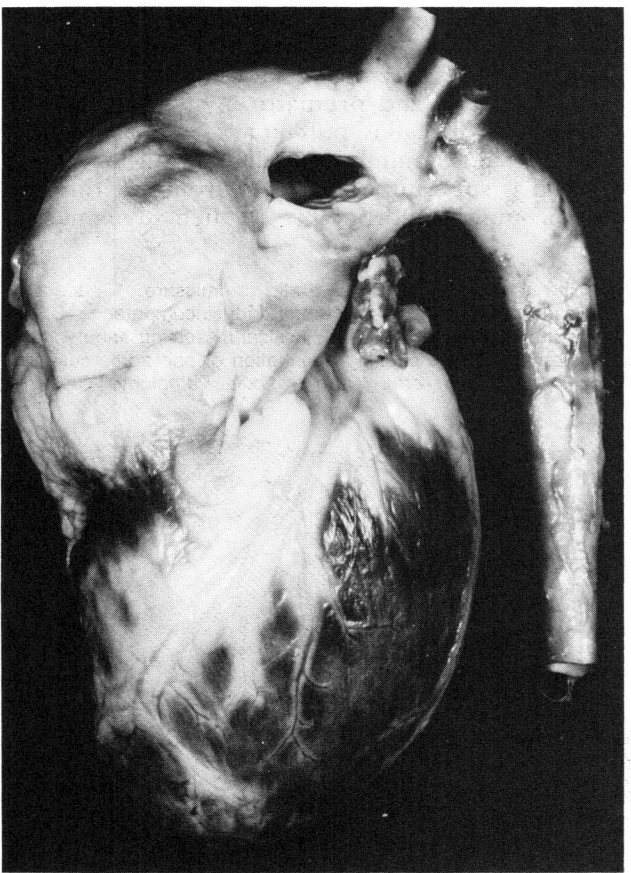

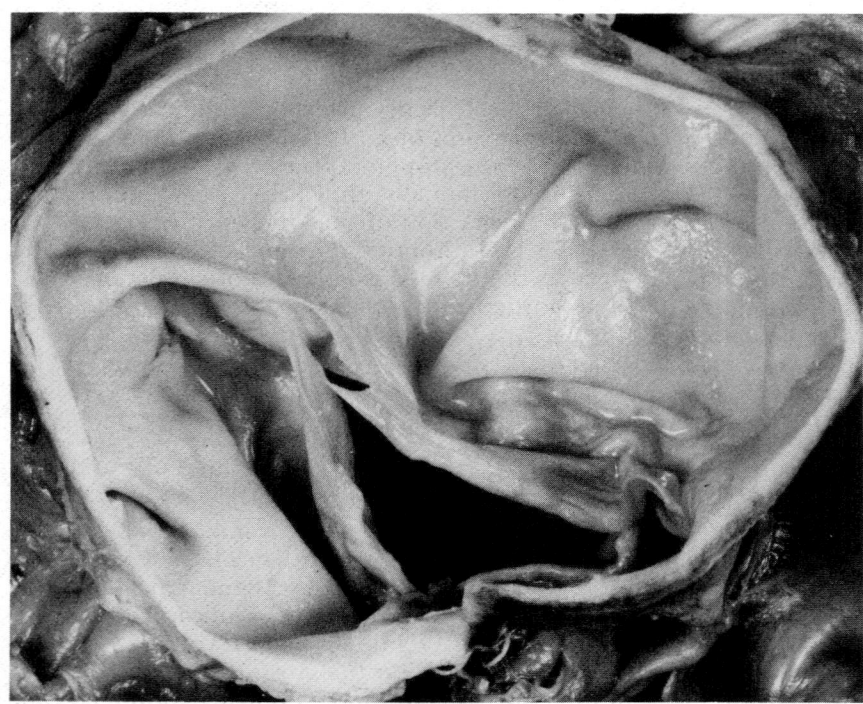

FIGURE 38-17 Interior of ascending aorta and aortic valve viewed from above in a case with extensive cystic medial necrosis of the aorta. Marked dilatation of aorta. The aortic cusps have been stretched and also show some features of prolapse. [*From J. E. Edwards, Pathology of Aortic Incompetence, in M. D. Silver (ed.), "Cardiovascular Pathology," Churchill-Livingstone, New York, in press. Reproduced with permission.*]

minish. The increase in end-systolic volume and decrease in diastolic compliance will elevate the left atrial pressure, eventually causing pulmonary hypertension. If the hypertrophy mechanism is exhausted in the course of further ventricular dilatation, systolic wall stress will rise significantly.[87]

In acute aortic regurgitation the hemodynamic changes in left ventricular function will be different from the chronic state if the damage occurs to a previously normal aortic valve. Under these conditions the regurgitation and volume overload will be suddenly imposed on a ventricle that is unable to dilate acutely and adapt to the increased filling. Left ventricular dilatation is limited as an acute mechanism by the increased thickness of the ventricular wall. Thus, marked elevation in left ventricular end-diastolic pressure and minimal ventricular dilatation accompany acute aortic regurgitation. The end-diastolic pressure may approach or even exceed left atrial pressure and prematurely close the mitral valve. This will lead to pulmonary venous hypertension and acute pulmonary edema. If acute regurgitation is superimposed on a chronically diseased and incompetent aortic valve, the hemodynamic dis-

FIGURE 38-18 Diagrammatic portrayal of consequences of laceration of the aorta in relation to an aortic commissure. *A.* Laceration without dissecting aneurysm. Retraction of the edges of the laceration allows for commissural prolapse and aortic incompetence. *B.* The process shown in *A* with regard to the aortic valve is the same, but there is the additional feature of classical dissecting aneurysm. *C.* Laceration of the aorta has been at a level just below the upper level of the commissure causing attenuation of one aortic cusp and rupture of the other. [*From J. E. Edwards, Pathology of Aortic Incompetence, in M. D. Silver (ed.), "Cardiovascular Pathology," Churchill-Livingstone, New York, in press. Reproduced with permission.*]

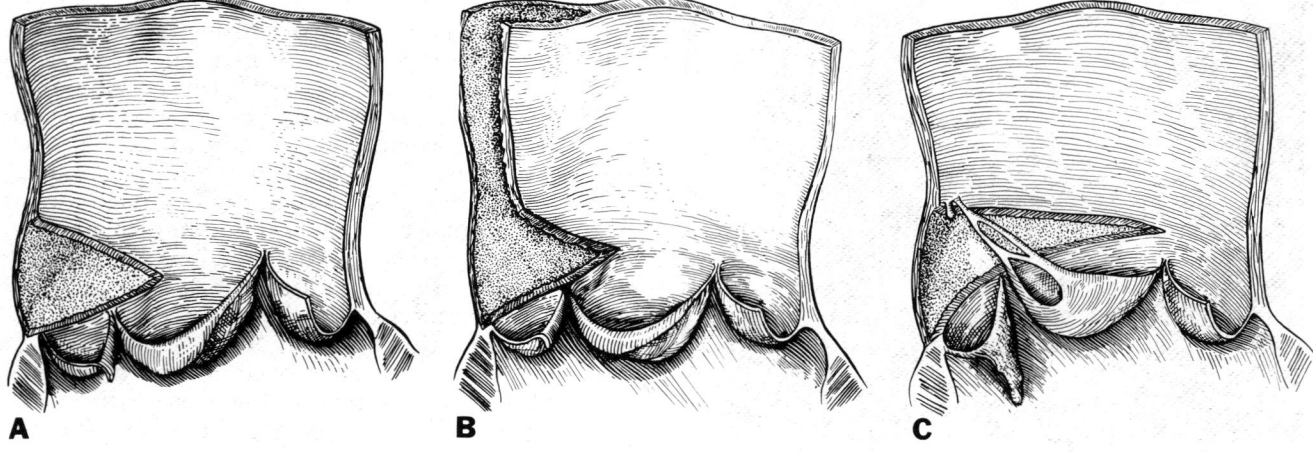

A   B   C

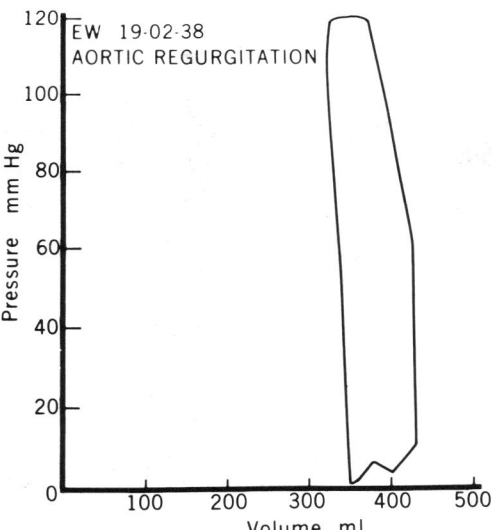

FIGURE 38-19 Left ventricular pressure-volume diagram in decompensated aortic regurgitation. The abnormal features of the loop are extreme displacement to the right due to an increase in end-diastolic volume and increased end-systolic volume indicative of depression of myocardial contractility. The isovolumic relaxation phase on the left-hand side of the pressure-volume loop is shortened due to early diastolic filling of the left ventricle from the aorta. The end-diastolic pressure is also abnormally elevated. [*From C. E. Rackley and W. P. Hood, Jr.: Aortic Valve Disease, in H. J. Levine (ed.), "Clinical Cardiovascular Physiology," Grune & Stratton, Inc., New York, 1976. Reproduced with permission.*]

turbance will depend on the extent of preexisting left ventricular dilatation and resultant changes in end-diastolic pressure and pulmonary capillary pressure.

Chronic aortic regurgitation with severe left ventricular dilatation can produce the largest left ventricular stroke volume seen in lesions affecting the left ventricle.[93] This large left ventricular stroke volume will elevate the mechanical pressure-volume work of the ventricle, and compensatory hypertrophy will further increase myocardial oxygen consumption.[96]

Clinical Manifestations

History

In slowly developing aortic incompetence with the attendant compensatory mechanisms of the left ventricle, the patient generally remains asymptomatic for many years. However, conditions affecting the aortic valve tend to be progressive and provide a potential site for bacterial endocarditis with further structural damage. Before symptoms of limited exercise performance develop, patients may be aware of palpitations and the circulatory effects of the large stroke volume and rapid diastolic runoff. These disturbances can be appreciated by prominent neck pulsations and awareness of the heartbeat, particularly while lying on the left side.[67] If cardiac irritability occurs, the patients may be particularly more inclined to notice such subtle disturb-

ances in rhythm because of the greatly increased left ventricular stroke volume.

Exertional chest pain may be noted by patients with severe aortic regurgitation, but angina pectoris may be less frequent than reported in studies.[69,94] Atypical features of the chest discomfort include occurrence at rest and a longer duration than the pain of coronary artery disease. Vasomotor symptoms such as flushing, sweating, and palpitations sometimes attend the chest pain in aortic regurgitation.[95] Rest angina and nocturnal chest pain have been attributed to the deleterious effects of bradycardia in severe aortic regurgitation.

The usual clinical manifestations of aortic regurgitation are symptoms of left ventricular failure, increased fatigue, dyspnea, orthopnea, and eventually paroxysmal nocturnal dyspnea. Left ventricular failure develops late in the course of aortic regurgitation unless acute valvular destruction is superimposed on a chronic lesion.

Atypical cardiac symptoms have been described in severe chronic aortic regurgitation and include neck and abdominal pain, postural dizziness, and

FIGURE 38-20 Left ventricular pressure, wall stress, and wall thickness in decompensated aortic regurgitation. Although the diastolic wall thickness is increased, there is a marked decrease in systolic wall thickening. This results in sustained elevation of the systolic wall stress, even though the left ventricular systolic pressure remains within the normal range. (——●——, stress; ——, pressure; ▲——▲, wall thickness.) [*From C. E. Rackley and W. P. Hood, Jr.: Aortic Valve Disease, in H. J. Levine (ed.), "Clinical Cardiovascular Physiology," Grune & Stratton, Inc., New York, 1976. Reproduced with permission.*]

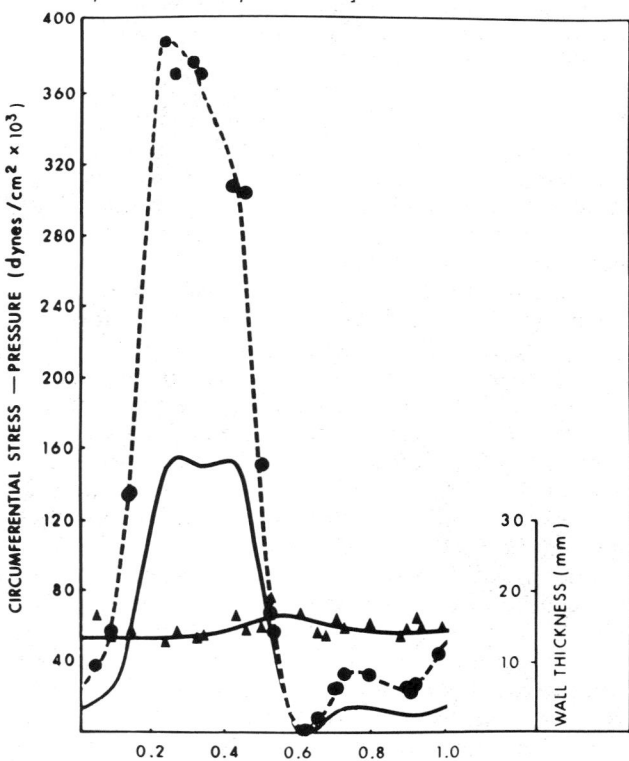

excessive sweating on the trunk.[95] The neck pain has been attributed to stretching of carotid sheath from the large left ventricular stroke volume, and the abdominal pain may be due to a similar mechanism in the aorta. Dizziness may be caused by disturbances in cerebral circulation with marked pressure changes and rapid diastolic runoff.[69]

Physical Examination

Chronic aortic regurgitation can present the most striking physical findings in the peripheral circulation of any valve lesion affecting the heart, and this is due to the large systolic stroke volume and rapid diastolic runoff. In the early phase of aortic regurgitation the physical findings, vital signs, and cardiac examination can all be normal except for the characteristic diastolic blowing murmur. The most striking physical findings occur in severe aortic regurgitation. While counting the heart rate, the marked increase in the pulse amplitude should alert the physician to the possibility of aortic regurgitation. A quick, rapid rise in the upstroke of the peripheral pulse is followed by a swift collapse of the diastolic pulse; this is known as Corrigan's pulse. The blood pressure is characteristically altered with a slightly increased systolic blood pressure and an abnormally low diastolic pressure. Sometimes the Korotkov sounds are audible to zero on the sphygmomanometer. If the pulse pressure does not exceed 50 percent of the peak systolic pressure, or if the diastolic pressure is above 70 mmHg, aortic regurgitation will not be hemodynamically severe unless advanced left ventricular failure has developed.[96]

Examination of the patient may reveal skin manifestations of a hyperdynamic state, such as increased sweating and flushing, to the extent that a hyperactive thyroid condition may be suspected. Skin changes from the connective tissue disorders associated with aortic valve disturbances can be appreciated, such as the yellowish linear streaks in the Ehlers-Danlos syndrome. The asthenic body habitus, long extremities, and arachnodactyly of the fingers are seen in Marfan's syndrome. A noticeable bobbing of the head with each cardiac pulsation has been described by deMusset. The eyes in aortic regurgitation may show the bluish tint in the sclera with osteogenesis imperfectus. Subluxation of the lens occurs in Marfan's syndrome, and pulsating retinal arteries suggest significant hemodynamic aortic regurgitation. Hemorrhages and exudates should also be sought as suggestive evidence of bacterial endocarditis. The mouth should be examined for a high arched palate in Marfan's syndrome.

The carotid vessels display the accentuated pulsatile motion due to the large stroke volume (Fig. 38-21). The neck veins will not be distended unless the patient has developed right ventricular failure. Rarely, the dilated aorta can compress the superior vena cava and produce distension of the neck veins. A tracheal tug may be noted with each heartbeat in conditions producing aneurysmal dilatation of the aortic arch.

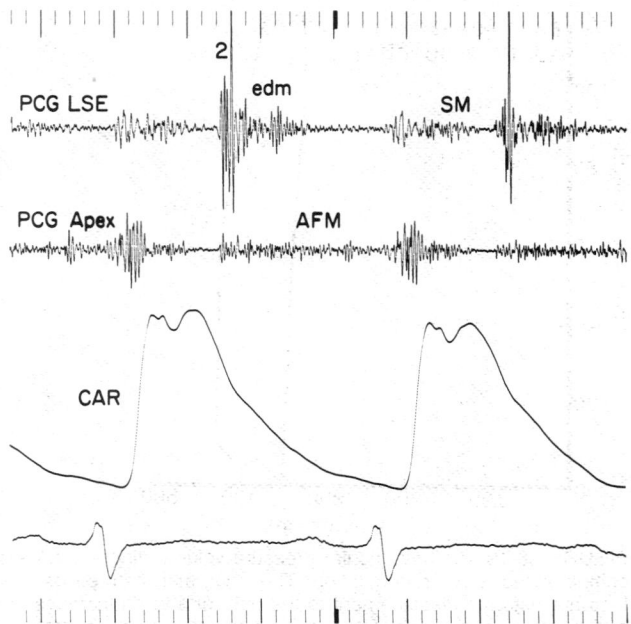

FIGURE 38-21 Phonocardiogram and carotid pulse recording in aortic regurgitation. At the left sternal edge a decrescendo diastolic murmur following the second sound (S2) is recorded. At the cardiac apex there is a low-frequency middiastolic and presystolic murmur (Austin Flint) culminating at the time of the first heart sound. The carotid arterial tracing shows a bisferious pattern in the absence of the dicrotic notch. (*Courtesy of Dr. Ernest Craige.*)

The chest deformity of pectus excavatum is another skeletal manifestation of Marfan's syndrome. Lungs remain clear unless pulmonary edema has developed. Severe dilatation of the left ventricle may result in compression of the lungs at the left base and produce the characteristic tubular breath sounds of consolidation designated as Ewart's sign.

Cardiac findings in aortic regurgitation will depend on the severity of the regurgitation, and heart size can vary from normal to extreme dilatation. If the heart size is normal and the apical impulse not abnormally displaced, mild aortic regurgitation is usually found.[68] Significant regurgitation and dilatation of the left ventricle will cause lateral and inferior displacement of the apical impulse, which also becomes diffuse and holosystolic.[97] Rarely, systolic vibrations can be appreciated over the second right interspace, but this does not necessarily indicate aortic stenosis, since ejection of a large stroke volume through a normal size aortic valve can generate turbulence and vibrations.

On auscultation, the first heart sound at the apex is preserved in pure aortic regurgitation, but it can be diminished if the PR interval on the electrocardiogram is prolonged or the heart rate is slow.[67] A systolic ejection click may be heard at the apex along the left sternal border and is probably related to sudden distension of the aorta. If the aortic regurgitation is sufficiently severe to produce a large systolic stroke volume, there will almost invariably be an audible ejection murmur along the left sternal border as well as at the apex and the second right interspace.[67,69] The aortic component of the second heart sound is preserved but can be diminished in the late stages of those conditions that cause scarring of the leaflet margins. The characteristic auscultatory finding in aortic regurgitation is the high-pitched diastolic blow heard best along the left sternal border. In the early stages of the disease the murmur can be best heard with the patient in the sitting position during full expiration. The intensity of the murmur partially reflects the severity of the regurgitation, but the duration of the diastolic blow correlates better with the hemodynamic abnormality.[69] Although the high-pitched diastolic blow is most characteristic of incompetence of the aortic valve, a musical or cooing murmur suggests eversion of one of the valve cusps.[98] Sometimes laceration of a leaflet or separation dislodgement of a leaflet from the annulus due to aortic dissection may generate a loud, coarse vibrating sound.

An early diastolic third heart sound or ventricular gallop is frequently audible in aortic regurgitation. If the murmur is loud and the peripheral findings of aortic regurgitation are marked, the third heart sound may reflect exaggerated early diastolic filling.[99] However, if the murmur is less prominent the third sound may indicate an abnormal reduction in the ejection fraction and myocardial failure.

In addition to the diastolic blow along the left sternal border there may be a rumbling diastolic murmur at the apex as described by Austin Flint. This diastolic murmur may be presystolic, middiastolic, or both.[69] This murmur has been attributed to functional mitral stenosis created by impingement of the aortic regurgitant flow on the anterior leaflet of the mitral valve. Echocardiography and simultaneous phonocardiography have demonstrated that the middiastolic component occurs when the mitral valve quickly closes after the rapid ventricular filling from the aorta and left atrium.[100] However, there is continued antegrade flow across the mitral valve due to incomplete left atrial emptying, and this creates turbulence in the antegrade stream responsible for the murmur. The location and duration of Austin Flint murmur may correspond to the severity of the aortic regurgitation since in mild regurgitation no murmur is heard. Moderate regurgitation may produce only the presystolic rumble, and severe regurgitation can generate the prolonged middiastolic to presystolic murmur.

In acute aortic regurgitation imposed on a normal left ventricle, the auscultatory findings and characteristics of the diastolic blow are distinctively different from the chronic condition.[101] Musical, cooing, or coarse vibrating qualities of the diastolic murmur may suggest leaflet laceration, eversion, or separation from the annulus (Fig. 38-22). In acute aortic regurgitation the mitral leaflet may close prematurely, and the first heart sound is diminished or absent. The diastolic murmur can even extend into early systole, since filling from the aorta can persist even though electrical depolarization of the ventricle has produced tension in the myocardium. A diastolic thrill may accompany the murmur in acute forms of aortic regurgitation.

Additional peripheral manifestations of aortic regurgitation have been ascribed to the large stroke volume and rapid diastolic runoff. Corrigan's pulse, which is the abruptly rising and collapsing pulsation, also may be seen in any high-output cardiac condition with a large stroke volume. Mueller's sign is the rhythmic pulsation of the uvula, and Quincke's sign is the arterial pulsation in the nailbeds with alternating redness and blanching during each heart beat. Duroziez's murmur is the systolic and diastolic murmur heard over the femoral artery with light pressure of the stethoscope. A disproportionate elevation in femoral systolic pressure has been designated Hill's sign.

With Marfan's syndrome, skeletal abnormalities in the extremities include high arches of the feet and hammer toes. Peripheral edema indicates right ventricular as well as left ventricular failure.

Chest Roentgenogram

The radiographic abnormality in aortic regurgitation is cardiac enlargement with dilatation of the left ventricle. As the volume overload on the left ventricle increases in the course of aortic regurgitation there is prominent elongation of the apex of the ventricle inferiorly and posteriorly.[106] Dilatation of the left ventricle may be attended by enlargement of the left atrium, and pulmonary venous congestion indicates cardiac decompensation. Dilatation of the ascending aorta is common in Marfan's syndrome and syphilitic aortitis, but in other causes of aortic regurgitation may not be a feature. Calcification of the aortic valve is unusual and should raise the question of combined aortic stenosis.

In acute aortic regurgitation in the absence of chronic left ventricular enlargement, heart size will be normal, yet pulmonary venous congestion and pulmonary edema are often present.

Electrocardiogram

The typical electrocardiographic changes in significant aortic regurgitation reflect left ventricular dilatation and hypertrophy, which are manifest by increased QRS amplitude with ST-T wave depression.[67,69] The rhythm is usually sinus with normal conduction, but prolonged AV conduction can occur in the late stages of aortic regurgitation.[102] The left ventricular volume overload pattern has been attributed to the early electrocardiographic changes in QRS prominence and tall precordial T waves.[103] Abnormalities in the P waves suggesting significant left atrial enlargement or development of atrial fibrillation should suggest combined mitral valve disease.

Special Laboratory Studies

Echocardiography Echocardiographic findings in aortic regurgitation can indicate volume overload on the ventricle with increased chamber dimensions.

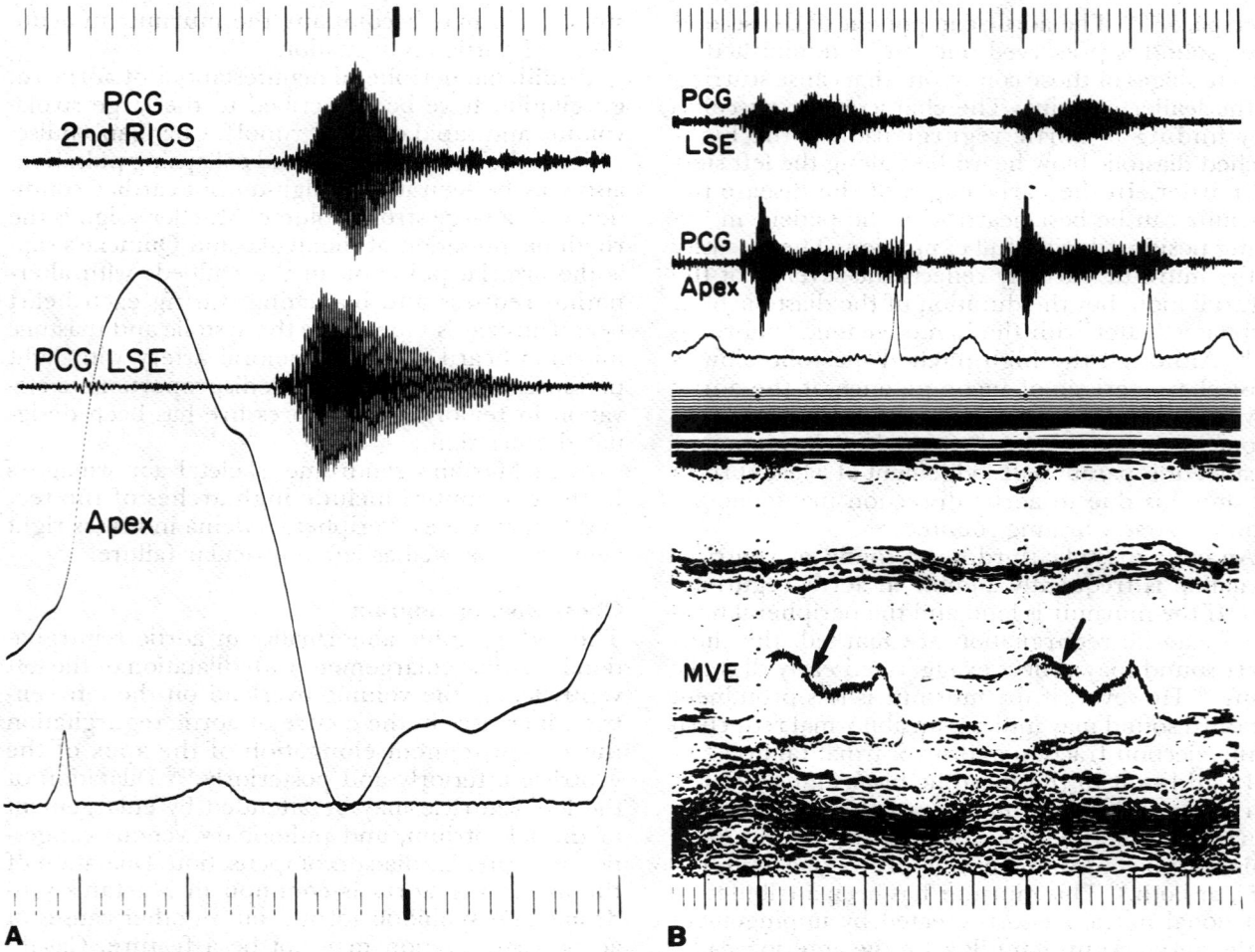

A

B

FIGURE 38-22   Phonocardiogram and echocardiogram in aortic regurgitation. *A.* The murmur is loudest at the left sternal edge with high-frequency and diminuendo configuration. The musical quality of the murmur is indicated by the pattern of the vibrations and suggests an everted cusp as the cause of the valvular incompetence. *B.* At slower paper speed the contrast in phonocardiographic appearance of the murmur at different precordial locations is evident. At left sternal edge (LSE) the early diastolic murmur has a diminuendo silhouette, and at the apex the murmur is of lower frequency and becomes accentuated prior to the next systole owing to the addition of an Austin Flint murmur. The vibrations of the anterior leaflet of the mitral valve coincide with the early diastolic murmur and not the Austin Flint murmur. (*Courtesy of Dr. Ernest Craige.*)

Disturbances in mitral valve motion due to regurgitant flow from the aortic valve can be recognized.[104,105] Echocardiographic changes in the aortic valve leaflets have not been specific or predictable. Rarely, the vegetations of bacterial endocarditis can be identified on the aortic leaflets.[106,107] Increased aortic dimensions may suggest a chronic basis for the regurgitation.[108]

End-diastolic and end-systolic dimensions can be measured from the echocardiogram to calculate chamber volume and left ventricular stroke volume.[109] The ejection fraction can be obtained by relating the total left ventricular stroke volume to the end-diastolic volume. Echocardiographic abnormalities of the mitral valve described in aortic regurgitation include diastolic fluttering of the anterior mitral valve leaflet, rapid diastolic closure rate of the mitral leaflet, premature closure of the mitral valve before the onset of the QRS complex, and, finally, thickening of the mitral leaflet[104,105] (Fig. 38-22B).

In acute aortic regurgitation diastolic oscillations in the aortic root or ventricular outflow tract suggest a flail leaflet as well as premature mitral valve closure.[110] As mentioned earlier, the vegetative lesion of bacterial endocarditis can sometimes be recognized, and reports have described the double lumen in the ascending aorta suggestive of aortic dissection.[108]

Pre- and postoperative echocardiographic studies have shown that a left ventricular end-systolic dimension greater than 55 mm can identify a high-risk group for mortality from surgery or congestive heart failure.[111] Ideally, aortic valve replacement should be undertaken before irreversible left ventricular dilatation has developed. The echocardiogram may provide an objective technique for recommendation of aortic valve replacement before symptoms of heart failure develop.

Cardiac Catheterization   Cardiac catheterization is advised in aortic regurgitation to document the presence of aortic valve incompetence and assess its severity, to evaluate left ventricular function, and to identify any additional cardiac abnormalities in the mitral valve as well as coronary artery anatomy (Fig. 38-23). The traditional angiographic method for assessing aortic regurgitation is the aortic root injection during cineangiography of the left ventricle and estimation of the regurgitation of contrast material into the left ventricle. The severity of aortic regurgitation detected by cineangiography has been based on an empirical grading system from minimal to severe regurgitation. Inconsistencies and disparities have been shown by this system when compared to quantitative angiocardiography.[112] Quantitative angiography can provide accurate determinations of end-diastolic and end-systolic volume. The left ventricular stroke volume can be related to the forward stroke volume determined by the Fick or indicator dilution technique to quantitate the regurgitant flow per beat across the aortic valve.[113] Studies have documented that quantitative angiography can provide more accurate assessment of regurgitation, and there are instances in which errors in clinical judgment have resulted from the empirical cineangiographic estimation of aortic regurgitation. In the visual angiographic assessment a dilated large left ventricular chamber may dilute the contrast material and result in the spurious grading of a minimal

amount of regurgitation across the valve, whereas regurgitation into a normal size left ventricular chamber may create an exaggerated impression of aortic regurgitation.

Although left ventricular end-diastolic pressure has been used as a hemodynamic index for assessing ventricular function, the end-diastolic pressure can be normal in chronic aortic regurgitation, similar to the volume overload in chronic mitral regurgitation.[89] This increased diastolic compliance in chronic volume overload is achieved by slippage of myocardial fibers as well as stress relaxation and creep.[114] Even if left ventricular end-diastolic pressure is moderately elevated, the increase in wall thickness and hypertrophy may result in a normal end-diastolic wall stress, or preload. The ejection fraction calculated from quantitative angiography remains a useful index of mechanical performance, but this value is artificially preserved in the volume overload of aortic valvular incompetence, since systolic ejection begins at a lower left ventricular pressure than normal.

Coronary arteriography is advised in all adults with aortic regurgitation whether there has been a history of chest pain or not. Underlying coronary artery disease can contribute to abnormalities in left ventricular function and will require surgical consideration at the time of aortic valve replacement.

FIGURE 38-23   Left ventricular pressure and volume in two patients with aortic regurgitation. The patient on the left enjoyed unrestricted activity without symptoms, whereas the patient on the right was extremely limited with left ventricular failure. For the patient on the left, end-diastolic volume (EDV) = 436; end-systolic volume (ESV) = 219; left ventricular stroke volume (LVSV) = 217; forward stroke volume (FSV) = 97; aortic regurgitation (AR) = 120; ejection fraction (EF) = 217/436 = 0.50; left ventricular weight (LVwt) = 474; left ventricular end-diastolic pressure (LVedp) = 8. For the patient on the right, EDV = 430; ESV = 329; LVSV = 101; FSV = 67; AR = 34; EF = 101/430 = 0.23; LVwt = 561; LVedp = 13. [From C. E. Rackley, W. P. Hood, Jr., B. R. Wilcox, and R. M. Peters, Quantitation of Myocardial Function in Valvular Heart Disease, in L. A. Brewer III (ed.), "Prosthetic Heart Valves," Charles C Thomas, Springfield, Illinois, 1969. Reproduced with permission.]

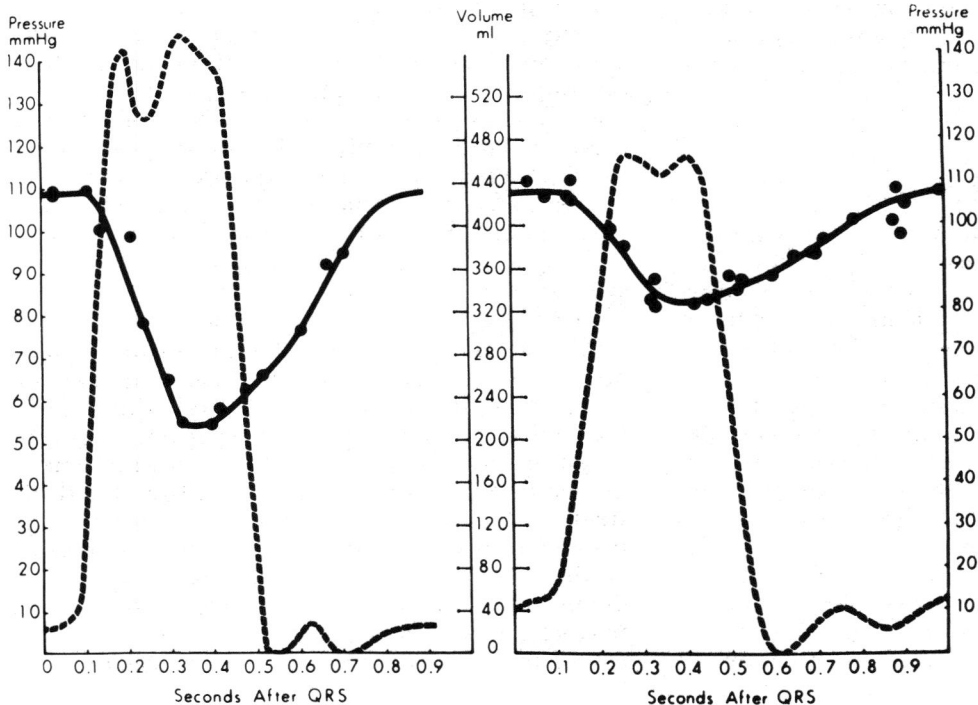

In acute aortic regurgitation the left ventricular end-diastolic volume is often normal or very slightly increased, yet the major hemodynamic change is marked elevation of the left ventricular end-diastolic pressure.[101] Severe elevation of end-diastolic pressure may cause premature closing of the mitral valve and create abnormal left atrial and pulmonary capillary pressures. Significant dilatation of the left ventricle and hypertrophy do not develop with acute aortic regurgitation, and if present under these circumstances usually indicate chronic overload on the left ventricle.

Radionuclide Studies Radionuclide angiography can now estimate left ventricular function in terms of resting and exercise ejection fraction.[115,116] Recently developed techniques suggest that blood pool imaging may be useful for noninvasive quantification of regurgitant flow in patients with valvular insufficiency.[117] Exercise studies in patients with aortic regurgitation have suggested that deterioration or decline of the ejection fraction during exercise may be an index of myocardial decompensation prior to the development of clinical symptoms.[115] Patients with aortic regurgitation and preservation of the contractile state demonstrated an increase in ejection fraction with exercise. Thus, radionuclide studies can provide physiological information on ventricular function both at rest and during exercise. Thallium scintigrams may identify perfusion defects in the myocardium and raise the possibility of underlying coronary artery disease.[118,119]

Graded Exercise Testing Exercise testing can be useful in the documentation of physical endurance as well as evaluation of atypical features in chronic aortic regurgitation.[120] This noninvasive technique can be employed in the follow-up of aortic regurgitation and in combination with radionuclide studies can provide additional information on cardiac performance during stress.

Natural History and Prognosis

In chronic aortic regurgitation the volume overload imposed on the left ventricle is usually well tolerated for long periods before the development of heart failure.[121] Three-fourths of patients with significant aortic regurgitation may survive 5 years, and 50 percent have been shown to live for 10 years after the diagnosis.[122] In mild to moderate aortic insufficiency as many as 85 to 95 percent of patients will survive for 10 years. However, once symptoms develop in aortic regurgitation there is fairly rapid deterioration. Patients developing congestive heart failure often die within 2 years after onset of symptoms, and the average survival after the development of angina pectoris is approximately 5 years.[117] Acute aortic regurgitation carries an extremely high mortality, progressing from acute pulmonary edema to refractory heart failure and cardiogenic shock.

Management

Medical

Prophylaxis against bacterial endocarditis is a primary responsibility in the care of the asymptomatic patient with aortic regurgitation. Not only should such prophylaxis be directed at dental care but any surgical instrumentation of the gastrointestinal or genitourinary tract should be adequately covered with antibiotics. Cardiac decompensation with left ventricular failure and pulmonary congestion requires standard treatment with digitalis, diuretics, and vasodilating agents. However, the physician must remember that the primary defect is mechanical, from the volume overload on the myocardium, and medical therapy alone will not restore the impaired ventricular performance.

An important clinical challenge in the treatment of aortic regurgitation is determining the optimal time of valve replacement. Ideally, the valve should be replaced before the clinical symptoms of heart failure develop. Previous efforts have utilized radiographic heart size, blood pressure, and electrocardiographic changes as predictors of future congestive heart failure or death within a predictable period. Results from serial echocardiographic evaluation of asymptomatic patients with aortic regurgitation suggest that an end-systolic dimension less than 50 mm should be followed at yearly intervals with an echocardiogram. If the asymptomatic patient has an end-systolic dimension of 50 to 54 mm, echocardiogram should be repeated every 4 to 6 months, and surgery is being advised for an end-systolic dimension of 55 mm or greater even in the absence of symptoms.[111] Radionuclide studies with the determination of ejection fraction and the demonstration of exercise-induced reduction of ejection fraction may be an additional index for advising valve replacement before development of symptoms.[115] Therefore, these two noninvasive techniques appear to be objective methods for detecting early deterioration of left ventricular function in chronic aortic regurgitation before the onset of symptoms and could establish a basis for valve replacement in asymptomatic patients.

Medical preparation for the patient undergoing aortic valve replacement involves stabilization of left ventricular function, control of arrhythmias, and correction of electrolyte disturbances. Vigorous measures to improve cardiac function with digitalis as well as elimination of all retained fluid with diuretics should be avoided since the drugs can present difficulties during anesthesia and postoperative surgical management. Patients should have dental repair or other elective surgical procedures performed prior to valve replacement in order to eliminate potential future sources of bacterial endocarditis. Acute aortic regurgitation from bacterial endocarditis will require valve replacement under antibiotic coverage if heart failure develops.[123]

Surgery

In a prospective study of patients with rheumatic aortic regurgitation, Spanuolo, Kloth, and associates[124] have shown that marked or moderate left ventricular enlargement (determined radiologically), electrocardiographic evidence of left ventricular hypertrophy (and ST-segment depression or T-wave inversion in V_6), systolic blood pressure over 140 mmHg, and diastolic blood pressure less than 40 mmHg are the four factors associated with a high risk of dying within 3 to 6 years, even though present in patients who were asymptomatic when first observed. Symptoms of angina pectoris indicate an even shorter life expectancy. Symptoms of dyspnea, paroxysmal nocturnal dyspnea, and orthopnea indicate a life expectancy of less than 1 year.

Patients with aortic regurgitation, little widening of the pulse pressure, and only mild left ventricular hypertrophy have a long life expectancy provided they do not develop the stigmata of high risk noted earlier. Recent studies (see below)[125] have indicated even these patients may develop left ventricular dysfunction and, when finally operated upon, have less than optimal late postoperative survival and less than satisfactory relief of symptoms.

In acute onset of aortic regurgitation, as may occur with ascending aortic dissection, rupture of a cusp, or infective endocarditis, the course is rapid and the response to medical management is poor. Additionally, the prognosis of patients with rheumatic aortic incompetence may differ from that of patients with connective tissue disease of the aortic valve, or from aortic incompetence associated with a congenital heart defect (e.g., ventricular septal defect or tetralogy of Fallot).

Present Indications for Treatment All patients with chronic aortic valve incompetence are advised to undergo operation when symptoms are present. Asymptomatic patients with the findings noted by Spanuolo and colleagues to characterize the cumulative high-risk category are also advised to have surgery. This is in hope of intervening before left ventricular dilatation and hypertrophy become massive and cardiac reserve is lost. In our experience, a graded exercise test is not an effective way to follow such patients. However, noninvasive studies such as serial echocardiograms[126] and left ventricular imaging using multigated radionuclide techniques[127] may offer objective criteria for decisions as to when to intervene in chronic aortic valve incompetence. As noted in the previous section, surgery is advised for an end-systolic dimension of 55 mm or greater even in the absence of symptoms. An additional index for operation may depend on demonstration by radionuclide imaging of an exercise-induced reduction in ejection fraction.

Acute aortic regurgitation, when associated with dissecting hematoma of the ascending aorta, or infective endocarditis is a more urgent indication for operation. In patients with more than mild heart failure due to endocarditis, valve replacement has been found to offer better early and long-term event-free survival than has medical treatment.[128] In aortic incompetence associated with aortic dissection, operation is considered to be urgent.[129] However, aortic valve replacement is not always necessary, this being one of the situations in which repair of the valve can be done. Another situation for which valve repair is offered is aortic valve incompetence associated with ventricular septal defect in young subjects.

At operation for severe noncalcific incompetence of the aortic valve the cusps commonly appear at first glance to be normal. Closer inspection reveals that they are slightly thickened. The free edges are rolled and the distance from the free margin to the aortic wall is shortened. Varying degrees of incompetence are found in patients with calcified stenotic valves whose cusps are sometimes shortened and immobile. The incidence of proximal aortic dilatation due to medical cystic necrosis appears to be increasing. In this condition the cusps are translucent. However, the aortic root is dilated and there is central incompetence. Dissecting aneurysms of the ascending aorta result in sudden onset of incompetence. The dissection proceeds down toward the sinuses of Valsalva and loosens the attachment of the cusps and thus renders them deformed and incompetent.

Surgical Technique In most cases a deformed and incompetent aortic valve is best treated by excision and replacement. In cases of aortic dissection competence can sometimes be restored by obliteration of the false channel and resuspension of the commissures.[130] This relieves the deformation of the cusps resulting from their loss of proper suspension secondary to the dissection.

For aortic valve incompetence associated with aortoannular ectasia with dilatation of the aortic root and aneurysm of the ascending aorta, we have found that composite Dacron tube–prosthetic valve replacement of the aortic valve and a portion of the ascending aorta has resulted in quite satisfactory early postoperative survival and good long-term function[131] (Fig. 38-24). The aortic valve is resected and the valve internal conduit is sutured in place at the aortic root. Small buttons of the Dacron tube are removed and the coronary ostia are sutured to them. The distal anastomosis of Dacron tube to the tubular portion of the ascending aorta is done within the aorta, and the residual aortic wall is wrapped around the conduit. This effectively removes the threat of subsequent further dilatation of the sinuses of Valsalva and has resulted in less blood loss during the operation.

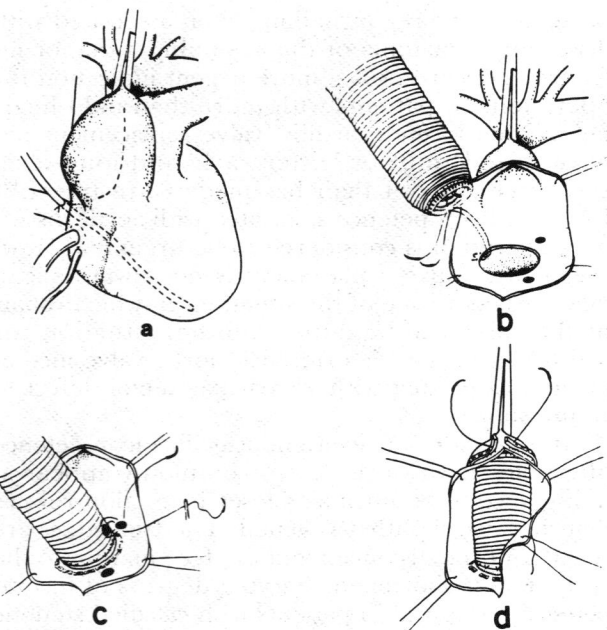

FIGURE 38-24 Technique for replacing the aortic valve and the proximal ascending aorta using a valved internal conduit. Modified from Kouchoukos. (*From N. T. Kouchoukos, R. B. Karp, and W. A. Lell, Replacement of the Ascending Aorta and Aortic Valve with a Composite Graft: Results in 25 Patients, Ann. Thorac. Surg., 24:140, 1977. Reproduced with permission.*)

Late Results The hospital mortality for patients having valve replacement for aortic valve incompetence is similar to that of patients having operation for aortic stenosis or a mixed lesion and is about 2 to 3 percent and between 3 and 5 percent if coronary artery bypass grafting is added. Recently, several investigators have shown that patients with aortic incompetence, even those asymptomatic or only functional class II or early class III, may have significant left ventricular dysfunction. This deterioration in myocardial performance probably plays a part in the slightly less satisfactory long-term results of aortic valve replacement in aortic regurgitation. Henry et al.[132] have shown that there is less satisfactory long-term survival in patients surviving aortic valve replacement for regurgitation as compared to those having valve replacement for aortic stenosis (Fig. 38-25). Noninvasive assessment of left ventricular function was performed using echocardiography or radionuclide imaging. For those reasons, many investigators now recommend earlier operation in patients with significant left ventricular volume overload from aortic regurgitation. When aortic regurgitation is associated with aneurysms of the ascending aorta, the recent surgical results (in our institution a 4 percent operative mortality) are improved over results of 10 years ago. The long-term postoperative survival of patients having aortic valve replacement and replacement of the ascending aorta is quite satisfactory.

Postoperative Management

After prosthetic aortic valve replacement patients should be seen every 6 or 12 months for follow-up assessment of competence of the aortic valve, to detect any regurgitation, and to assess prosthetic valve sounds. Left ventricular function can be followed by echocardiography and scintigraphy to assess cardiac performance. If the prosthetic valve requires anticoagulation therapy, this must be continued as well as antibiotic coverage for distal surgical procedures.

Cost Analysis

The emphasis on prophylactic antibiotic coverage to reduce or eliminate the possibility of bacterial endocarditis is extremely important in stabilizing the patient with chronic aortic regurgitation. The use of echocardiography and radionuclide studies may be significant factors in reducing costs for repeated hospitalization for heart failure. The optimal time for valve replacement can now possibly be identified

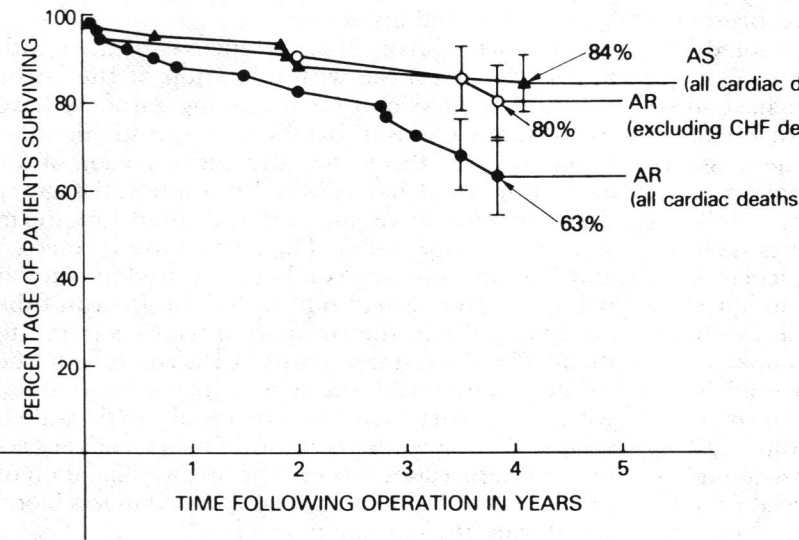

FIGURE 38-25 Actuarial survival following aortic valve replacement: aortic stenosis compared to aortic incompetence. (*From W. L. Henry, R. O. Bonow, D. R. Rosing, and S. E. Epstein, Observations on the Optimum Time for Operative Intervention for Aortic Regurgitation. II. Serial Echocardiographic Evaluation of Asymptomatic Patients, Circulation, 61:484, 1980. Reproduced with permission.*)

prior to irreversible depression of cardiac function. A delay in the decision for aortic valve replacement can be costly financially as well as preventing optimal postoperative benefit to the patient.

Combined Aortic Stenosis and Aortic Regurgitation

In the clinical presentation the majority of patients with aortic valve disease exhibit a combination of stenosis and insufficiency. In the stenotic aortic valve there frequently is a diastolic blow from the incomplete closure of the valve, and in predominant aortic regurgitation there is almost invariably a systolic murmur indicating turbulence across the aortic valve. Thus combined stenosis and regurgitation is a more common clinical finding in aortic valve disease. Symptoms of dyspnea and fatigue are most frequent and chest pain and syncope, although suggesting predominant aortic stenosis, are not specific in the combined lesion. Physical examination will reveal the influence of the combined lesion on the peripheral pulse, which may result in a near normal contour and pulse amplitude of the peripheral artery. The left ventricle is enlarged with the systolic and diastolic murmurs of the aortic valve, and frequently a diastolic rumble due to the Austin Flint murmur. Chest x-ray and cardiogram also demonstrate left ventricular hypertrophy. In the combined lesion, cardiac catheterization and angiography will demonstrate an increased end-diastolic volume, which can attain the largest size in any valvular lesion. However, the extent of increase in left ventricular mass or hypertrophy tends to be large in the combined lesion and may exceed that seen in pure aortic regurgitation.

Combined Aortic and Mitral Valve Disease

When mitral stenosis and insufficiency are combined with aortic valve disease similar symptoms of dyspnea and fatigue are common. A history of hemoptysis will suggest severe pulmonary venous hypertension due to mitral stenosis.

The detection and recognition of the diastolic rumble of mitral stenosis and the holosystolic murmur of mitral regurgitation can be easily obscured by the predominant murmurs of aortic stenosis and regurgitation. In predominant aortic stenosis the mitral stenosis murmur may be very difficult to identify. An aortic systolic murmur may be difficult to separate from a mitral regurgitation murmur, but radiation into the axilla does suggest a component of mitral regurgitation. Laboratory studies are particularly helpful in detecting the presence of associated mitral valve disease. Calcium in the area of the mitral valve would suggest mitral stenosis when murmurs of combined lesions are present. The echocardiogram can recognize the characteristic leaflet abnormality of mitral stenosis when this lesion is combined with aortic valve disease. Pressure measurements and angiography are particularly crucial in documenting associated mitral stenosis by recording the pressure gradient and demonstrating mitral regurgitation with left ventriculography in these patients.

Surgery

A number of patients with severe and progressing symptoms exhibit evidence of disease at both mitral and aortic valves. Our experience indicates that both valves can be replaced with a hospital mortality that is now between 5 and 10 percent, considerably less than the 22 percent reported for an earlier period. There has been marked subjective and objective improvement in surviving patients. When tricuspid replacement is added, the risk of the operation has been higher (about 20 percent), but even here the long-term results are considerably better than the life history of surgically untreated patients with triple valve disease. The increased use, when possible, of tricuspid annuloplasty rather than replacement has greatly improved the early results of operation in this group of patients.

Indications for Operation
Indication for operation in patients with involvement of aortic and mitral valves is usually NYHA class III status, but a number of patients present at a later stage of their disease. Atrial fibrillation is usually present and tricuspid involvement is somewhat more frequent than in left-sided, isolated valvular disease.

Operation
When hemodynamic derangement is significant at both valves, the decision to repair both is easily made, and the principles of surgical treatment are the same as when one valve alone requires attention. Median sternotomy is performed. With present techniques of myocardial preservation, using cold potassium cardioplegia, the operation can be done in an unhurried, precise manner with expectation of a quite low incidence of less than optimal cardiac performance. On cardiopulmonary bypass, the heart is cooled by the perfusate and by external cardiac cooling. The aorta is cross-clamped. The aorta is opened and cardioplegic solution is infused into each coronary orifice to attain a myocardial temperature of between 10 and 15°C (50 to 59°F). Reinfusion of the cardioplegic solution is done every 20 to 30 min, or when the myocardial temperature reaches 19 or 20°C (66 or 68°F). The aortic valve is resected and then attention is turned to the mitral valve. The left atrium is opened from the right side and the mitral valve is assessed and resected if necessary. The mitral prosthesis is inserted and the left atrium is left open while the aortic valve is then su-

tured in place. If there is also tricuspid valve disease, the right atrium is opened at this point and either annuloplasty or replacement is done. The aortotomy is then closed and reperfusion from the perfusate is allowed while the left atriotomy and right atriotomy are closed. The usual procedures are followed for removing all air from the heart and preventing air embolization as the heart begins to eject.

Occasionally, when the aortic valve is severely diseased and only about class II incompetence (on a scale of I to VI) is evident at the mitral valve without stenosis, attention to the mitral valve seems unnecessary. This is true even if left atrial pressure preoperatively was very high, since such pressure can result solely from severe pressure or volume overload of the left ventricle. After repair of the aortic valve disease, incompetence of the mitral valve usually regresses. However, when there is about class II incompetence of the aortic valve in the presence of severe disease at the mitral valve, the aortic valve incompetence often appears to be of greater magnitude after repair of the mitral valve and may contribute to poor postoperative performance. In these situations, therefore, replacement of both the mitral and aortic valve seems indicated.

Results

Long-term survival after replacement of either the aortic, the mitral, or both the aortic and mitral valve is only partially related to factors having to do with the device. Other factors more related to the preoperative condition of the patient, intraoperative events, and early postoperative events also have statistically significant association with late mortality.[133] Mainly patients having had previous valve replacement who need a second replacement, either because of xenograft degeneration, paraprosthetic leak, or other complications, do less well than patients having primary valve replacement. In our series patients having had left ventricular aneurysmectomy along with valve replacement have had less satisfactory long-term survival. However, there was no deleterious influence of ischemic heart disease in general, as suggested by the lack of any negative effect on long-term survival associated with coronary artery bypass grafting. Patients having lengthy periods of ischemic arrest had less good survival when the operation was done without potassium cardioplegia. It is anticipated that potassium cardioplegia will mute this effect. Finally, patients in whom treatment of ventricular arrhythmias was necessary in the early postoperative course were found to have less satisfactory survival than the group as a whole. This suggests that long-term antiarrhythmic therapy would be prudent in that group.

References

1. Stokes, W.: "The Diseases of the Heart and the Aorta," Hodges and Smith, Dublin, 1854, p. 139.
2. Monckeberg, J. G.: Der normale histologische Bau und die sklerose der aortenklappen, Virchows Arch. (Pathol. Anat.), 176:472, 1904.
3. Karsner, H. T., and Koletsky, S.: "Calcific Disease of Aortic Valves," J. B. Lippincott, Philadelphia, 1947.
4. Campbell, M., and Kauntze, R.: Congenital Aortic Valvular Stenosis, Br. Heart J., 15:179, 1953.
5. Roberts, W. C.: The Congenitally Bicuspid Aortic Valve: A Study of 85 Autopsy Cases, Am. J. Cardiol., 26:72, 1970.
*6. Glancy, D. L., and Epstein, S. E.: Differential Diagnosis of Type and Severity of Obstruction to Left Ventricular Outflow, Prog. Cardiovasc. Dis., 14:153, 1971. (121 references)
*7. Roberts, W. C.: The Structure of the Aortic Valve in Clinically Isolated Aortic Stenosis: An Autopsy Study of 162 Patients over 15 Years of Age, Circulation, 42:91, 1970. (6 references)
8. Roberts, W. C., Perloff, J. K., and Costantino, T.: Severe Valvular Aortic Stenosis in Patients over 65 Years of Age: A Clinicopathologic Study, Am. J. Cardiol., 27:497, 1971.
*9. Roberts, W. C.: Anatomically Isolated Aortic Valvular Disease: The Case against Its Being of Rheumatic Etiology, Am. J. Med., 49:151, 1970. (43 references)
10. Pomerance, A.: Pathogenesis of Aortic Stenosis and Its Relation to Age, Br. Heart J., 34:569, 1972.
*11. Edwards, J. E.: Pathology of Acquired Valvular Disease of the Heart, Seminars in Roentgenol., 14:96, 1979. (61 references)
12. Edwards, J. E.: On the Etiology of Calcific Aortic Stenosis, Circulation, 26:817, 1962.
13. Pomerance, A.: Cardiac Pathology and Systolic Murmurs in the Elderly, Br. Heart J., 30:687, 1968.
14. Pritzker, M. R., Ernst, J. D., Caudill, C., Wilson, C. S., Weaver, W. F., and Edwards, J. E.: Acquired Aortic Stenosis in Systemic Lupus Erythematosus, unpublished data.
15. Kavanaugh, G. J., Pruitt, R. D., and Edwards, J. E.: Coronary Embolism and Cystic Medial Necrosis of Ascending Aorta Associated with Calcific Aortic Stenosis, Proc. Mayo Clin., 33:222, 1958.
16. Levy, M. J., and Edwards, J. E.: Anatomy of Mitral Insufficiency, Prog. Cardiovasc. Dis., 5:119, 1962.
17. Moller, J. H., Nakib, A., and Edwards, J. E.: Infarction of Papillary Muscles and Mitral Insufficiency Associated with Congenital Aortic Stenosis, Circulation, 34:87, 1966.
18. Fukuda, T., Tadavarthy, S. M., and Edwards, J. E.: Dissecting Aneurysm of Aorta Complicating Aortic Valvular Stenosis, Circulation, 53:169, 1976.
19. Nakib, A., Lillehei, C. E., and Edwards, J. E.: The Degree of Coronary Atherosclerosis in Aortic Valvular Disease, Arch. Path., 80:517, 1965.
20. Kennedy, J. W., Twiss, R. D., Blackmon, J. R., and Dodge, H. T.: Quantitative Angiocardiography. III. Relationships of Left Ventricular Pressure, Volume, and Mass in Aortic Valve Disease, Circulation, 38:838, 1968.
21. Hood, W. P., Jr., Rackley, C. E., and Rolett, E. L.: Wall Stress in the Normal and Hypertrophied Human Left Ventricle, Am. J. Cardiol., 22:550, 1968.
22. Rackley, C. E., and Hood, W. P., Jr.: Aortic Valve

*This article is a review of the literature and contains additional references to the literature.

Disease, in H. J. Levine (ed.), "Clinical Cardiovascular Physiology," Grune & Stratton, New York, 1976, p. 493.

23. Stott, D. K., Marpole, D. G., Bristow, J. D., Kloster, F. E., and Griswold, H. E.: The Role of Left Atrial Transport in Aortic and Mitral Stenosis, *Circulation*, 41:1031, 1970.

24. Rackley, C. E., Hood, W. P., Jr., Rolett, E. L., and Young, D. T.: Left Ventricular End-Diastolic Pressure in Chronic Heart Disease, *Am. J. Med.*, 48:310, 1970.

25. Dodge, H. T., and Baxley, W. A.: Left Ventricular Volume and Mass and Their Significance in Heart Disease, *Am. J. Cardiol.*, 23:528, 1969.

26. Ross, J., Jr., and Braunwald, E.: Aortic Stenosis, *Circulation*, 38(suppl. 5):61, 1968.

27. Wood, P.: Aortic Stenosis, *Am. J. Cardiol.*, 1:553, 1958.

28. Rotman, M., Morris, J. J., Behar, V. W., Peter, R. H., and Kong, Y.: Aortic Valvular Disease: Comparison of Types and Their Medical and Surgical Management, *Am. J. Med.*, 51:241, 1971.

29. Kumpe, C. W., and Bean, W. B.: Aortic Stenosis: Study of the Clinical and Pathological Aspects of 107 Proved Cases. *Medicine (Baltimore)*, 27:139, 1948.

30. Moraski, R. E., Russell, R. O., Jr., Mantle, J. A., and Rackley, C. E.: Aortic Stenosis, Angina Pectoris, Coronary Artery Disease, *Catheterization and Cardiovasc. Diag.*, 2:157, 1976.

31. Baxley, W. A., Dodge, H. T., Rackley, C. E., Sandler, H., and Pugh, D.: Left Ventricular Mechanical Efficiency in Man with Heart Disease, *Circulation*, 55:564, 1977.

32. Hood, W. P., Jr., Thomson, W. J., Rackley, C. E., and Rolett, E. L.: Comparison of Calculations of Left Ventricular Wall Stress in Man from Thin-Walled and Thick-Walled Ellipsoidal Models, *Circ. Res.*, 24:575, 1969.

33. Holley, K. E., Bahn, R. C., McGoon, D. C., and Mankin, H. T.: Spontaneous Calcific Embolization Associated with Calcific Aortic Stenosis, *Circulation*, 27:197, 1963.

34. Flamm, M. D., Braiff, B. A., Kimball, R., and Hancock, E. W.: Mechanism of Effort Syncope in Aortic Stenosis, *Circulation*, 36(suppl. 2):II-109, 1967.

35. Schwartz, L. S., Goldfischer, J., Sprague, G. J., and Schwartz, S. P.: Syncope and Sudden Death in Aortic Stenosis, *Am. J. Cardiol.*, 23:647, 1969.

36. Baker, C., and Somerville, J.: Clinical Features and Surgical Treatment of Fifty Patients with Severe Aortic Stenosis, *Guys Hosp. Rep.*, 108:101, 1959.

37. Andersen, J. A., Hansen, B. F., and Lyngborg, K.: Isolated Valvular Aortic Stenosis, *Acta Med. Scand.*, 197:61, 1975.

38. Hancock, E. W.: The Ejection Sound in Aortic Stenosis, *Am. J. Med.*, 40:569, 1966.

39. Crawley, I. S., Morris, D. C., and Silverman, B. D.: Valvular Heart Disease, in J. W. Hurst, R. B. Logue, R. C. Schlant, and N. K. Wenger (eds.), "The Heart," 4th ed., McGraw-Hill Book Company, New York, 1978, p. 992.

40. Davison, E. T., and Friedman, S. A.: Significance of Systolic Murmurs in the Aged, *N. Engl. J. Med.*, 279:225, 1968.

41. Klatte, E. C., Tampas, J. P., Campbell, J. A., and Lurie, P. R.: The Roentgenographic Manifestations of Aortic Stenosis and Aortic Valvular Insufficiency, *Am. J. Roentgenol. Radium Ther. Nucl. Med.*, 88:57, 1962.

42. Myler, R. K., and Sanders, C. A.: Aortic Valve Disease and Atrial Fibrillation: Report of 122 Patients with Electrographic, Radiographic and Hemodynamic Observations, *Arch. Intern. Med.*, 121:530, 1968.

43. Feigenbaum, H.: "Echocardiography," Lea & Febiger, Philadelphia, 1976.

44. Johnson, M. L., Kisslo, J., Habersberger, P. G., and Wallace, A. G.: Echocardiographic Evaluation of Aortic Valvular Disease, *Circulation*, 47(suppl. 4):IV-46, 1973.

45. Radford, D. J., Bloom, K. R., Izukawa, T., Moes, C. A. F., and Rowe, R. D.: Echocardiographic Assessment of Bicuspid Aortic Valves: Angiographic and Pathological Correlates, *Circulation*, 53:80, 1976.

46. Johnson, G. L., Meyer, R. A., Schwartz, D. C., Korfhagen, J., and Kaplan, S.: Echocardiographic Evaluation of Fixed Left Ventricular Outlet Obstruction in Children; Pre- and Postoperative Assessment of Ventricular Systolic Pressures, *Circulation*, 56:299, 1977.

47. Hancock, E. W., and Fleming, P. R.: Aortic Stenosis. *Q. J. Med.*, 29:209, 1960.

48. Braunwald, E., Goldbatt, A., Aygen, M. M., Rockoff, D. S., and Morrow, A. G.: Congenital Aortic Stenosis. I. Clinical and Hemodynamic Findings in 100 Patients; Morrow, A. G., Goldbatt, A., Braunwald, E.: Congenital Aortic Stenosis. II. Surgical Treatment and the Results of Operation, *Circulation*, 27:426, 1963.

49. Rackley, C. E.: Quantitative Evaluation of Left Ventricular Function by Radiographic Techniques, *Circulation*, 54:862, 1976.

50. Borer, J. S., Bacharach, S. L., Green, M. V., Kent, K. M., Rosing, D. R., Seides, F., McIntosh, C. L., Conkle, D., Morrow, A. G., and Epstein, S. E.: Left Ventricular Function in Aortic Stenosis: Response to Exercise and Effects of Operation, *Am. J. Cardiol.*, 41:382, 1978.

51. Takeda, J., Warren, R., and Holzman, D.: Prognosis of Aortic Stenosis, *Arch. Surg.*, 87:931, 1963.

52. Dexter, L.: Evaluation of the Results of Cardiac Surgery, in A. M. Jones (ed.), "Modern Trends in Cardiology," Appleton-Century-Crofts, New York, 1969, vol. 2, p. 311.

53. Frank, S., Johnson, A., and Ross, J., Jr.: Natural History of Valvular Aortic Stenosis, *Br. Heart J.*, 35:41, 1973.

54. Rapaport, E.: Natural History of Aortic and Mitral Valve Disease, *Am. J. Cardiol.*, 35:221, 1975.

55. Karp, R. B., Kirklin, J. W., Kouchoukos, N. T., and Pacifico, A. D.: Comparison of Three Devices to Replace the Aortic Valve, *Circulation*, 50:II-163, 1974.

56. Thompson, R., Knight, E., Ahmed, M., Somerville, W., Towers, M., and Yacoub, M.: The Use of "Fresh" Unstented Homograft Valves for Replacement of the Aortic Valve: Analysis of 6½ Years Experience, *Circulation*, 56:837, 1977.

57. Barratt-Boyes, B. G., Roche, A. H. G., and Whitlock, R. M. L.: Six Year Review of the Results of Freehand Aortic Valve Replacement Using an Antibiotic Sterilized Homograft Valve, *Circulation*, 55:353, 1977.

*58. Geha, A. S., Laks, H., Stanel, H. C., Jr., Cornhill, J. F., Kilman, J. W., Buckley, M. J., and Roberts, W. C.: Late Failure of Porcine Valve Heterografts in Children, *J. Thorac. Cardiovasc. Surg.*, 78:351, 1979. (33 references)

*59. Chaitman, B. R., Bonan, R., Lepage, G., Tubau, J. F., David, P. R., Dyrda, I., and Grondin, C. M.: Hemodynamic Evaluation of the Carpentier-Edwards Porcine Xenograft, *Circulation*, 60:1170, 1979. (36 references)

60. Waldo, A. L., MacLean, W. A. H., Cooper, T. B., Kouchoukos, N. T., and Karp, R. B.: Use of Temporarily Placed Epicardial Atrial Wire Electrodes for the Diagnosis and Treatment of Cardiac Arrhythmias Following Open Heart Surgery, *J. Thorac. Cardiovasc. Surg.*, 76:500, 1978.

61. Richardson, J. W., Kouchoukos, N. T., Wright, J. O., III, and Karp, R. B.: Combined Aortic Valve Replacement and Myocardial Revascularization: Results in 220 Patients, *Circulation*, 59:75, 1979.

62. Macmanus, Q., Grunkemeier, G., Lambert, L. E., and Starr, A.: Non-Cloth-Covered Caged-Ball Prostheses, the Second Decade, *J. Thorac. Cardiovasc. Surg.*, 76:788, 1978.

*63. Davila, J. C., Magilligan, D. J., and Lewis, J. W.: Is The Hancock Porcine Valve the Best Cardiac Valve Substitute Today?, *Ann. Thorac. Surg.*, 26:303, 1978. (32 references)

64. Krayenbuehl, H. P., Lurina, M., Hess, O., Rothlin, M., and Senning, A.: Pre- and Postoperative Left Ventricular Contractile Function in Patients with Aortic Valve Disease, *Br. Heart J.*, 41:204, 1979.

65. Schwarz, F., Flameng, W., Langebartels, F., Sesto, M., Walter, P., and Schlepper, M.: Impaired Left Ventricular Function in Chronic Aortic Valve Disease: Survival and Function after Replacement by Bjork-Shiley Prosthesis, *Circulation*, 60:48, 1979.

66. Corrigan, D. J.: On Permanent Patency of the Mouth of the Aorta or Inadequacy of the Aortic Valves, *Edinburgh Med. Surg. J.*, XXXVII:225, 1832.

67. Segal, J., Harvey, W. P., and Hufnagel, C. L.: A Clinical Study of One Hundred Cases of Severe Aortic Insufficiency, *Am. J. Med.*, 21:200, 1956.

68. Stapleton, J. F., and Harvey, W. P.: A Clinical Analysis of Aortic Incompetence, *Postgrad. Med.*, 46:156, 1969.

69. Angloff, E.: Aortic Incompetence: Clinical Haemodynamic and Angiocardiographic Evaluation, *Acta Med. Scand.*, 193(suppl. 538):3, 1972.

*70. Read, R. C., Thal, A. P., and Wendt, V. E.: Symptomatic Valvular Myxomatous Transformation (The Floppy Valve Syndrome): A Possible Forme Fruste of the Marfan Syndrome, *Circulation*, 32:897, 1965. (69 references)

*71. Roberts, W. C., Hollingsworth, J. F., Bulkley, B. H., Jaffe, R. B., Epstein, S. E., and Stinson, E. B.: Combined Mitral and Aortic Regurgitation in Ankylosing Spondylitis: Angiographic and Anatomic Features, *Am. J. Med.*, 56:237, 1974. (11 references)

72. Bulkley, B. H., and Roberts, W. C.: Ankylosing Spondylitis and Aortic Regurgitation: Description of the Characteristic Cardiovascular Lesion from Study of Eight Necropsy Patients, *Circulation*, 48:1014, 1973.

73. Paulus, H. E., Pearson, C. M., and Pitts, W., Jr.: Aortic Insufficiency in Five Patients with Reiter's Syndrome: A Detailed Clinical and Pathologic Study, *Am. J. Med.*, 53:464, 1972.

74. Roberts, W. C., Kehoe, J. A., Carpenter, D. F., and Golden, A.: Cardiovascular Valvular Lesions in Rheumatoid Arthritis, *Arch. Intern. Med.*, 122:141, 1968.

75. Sakakibara, S., and Konno, S.: Congenital Aneurysm of the Sinus of Valsalva Anatomy and Classification, *Am. Heart J.*, 63:405, 1962.

76. Puchner, T. C., Huston, J. H., and Hellmuth, G. A.: Aortic Valve Insufficiency in Arterial Hypertension, *Am. J. Cardiol.*, 5:758, 1960.

77. Karp, R. B., and Carlson, D. E.: "Dissection of Aorta," F. A. Davis, Philadelphia, Cardiovascular Clinics, 1981, pp. 209–219.

78. Wilcox, B. R., Procter, H. J., Rackley, C. E., and Peters, R. M.: Early Surgical Treatment of Valvular Endocarditis, *J. Am. Med. Assoc.*, 200:820, 1967.

*79. Oh, W. M. C., Taylor, T. R., and Olsen, E. G. J.: Aortic Regurgitation in Systemic Lupus Erythematosus Requiring Aortic Valve Replacement, *Br. Heart J.*, 36:413, 1974. (13 references)

80. Wang, K., Gobel, F., Gleason, D. F., and Edwards, J. E.: Complete Heart Block Complicating Bacterial Endocarditis, *Circulation*, 46:939, 1972.

81. Spurny, O. M., and Hara, M.: Rupture of the Aortic Valve Due to Strain, *Am. J. Cardiol.*, 8:125, 1961.

82. Symbas, P. N., Walter, P. F., Hurst, J. W., and Schlant, R. C.: Fenestration of Aortic Cusps Causing Aortic Regurgitation, *J. Thor. Cardiovasc. Dis.*, 57:464, 1969.

83. Carter, J. B., Sethi, S., Lee, G. B., and Edwards, J. E.: Prolapse of Semilunar Cusps as Causes of Aortic Insufficiency, *Circulation*, 43:922, 1971.

*84. Tatsuno, K., Konno, S., and Sakakibara, S.: Ventricular Septal Defect with Aortic Insufficiency, *Am. Heart J.*, 85:13, 1973. (14 references)

85. Heggtveit, H. A.: Syphilitic Aortitis. A Clinicopathologic Autopsy Study of 100 Cases, 1950 to 1960, *Circulation*, 29:346, 1964.

86. Eversmeyer, W. H., Rosenstock, D., and Biundo, J. J., Jr.: Aortic Insufficiency with Mild Ankylosing Spondylitis in Black Men, *J. Am. Med. Assoc.*, 240:2652, 1978.

87. Murray, C. A., and Edwards, J. E.: Spontaneous Laceration of Ascending Aorta, *Circulation*, 47:848, 1973.

88. Edwards, J. E.: Lesions Causing or Simulating Aortic Insufficiency, *Cardiovasc. Clin.*, 5:128, 1973.

89. Brawley, R. K., and Morrow, A. G.: Direct Determination of Aortic Blood Flow in Patients with Aortic Regurgitation: Effects of Alterations in Heart Rate, Increased Ventricular Preload and Afterload, and Isoproterenol, *Circulation*, 35:32, 1967.

90. Judge, T. P., Kennedy, J. W., Bennett, L. J., Willis, R. E., Murray, J. A., and Blackman, J. R.: Quantitative Hemodynamic Effects of Heart Rate in Aortic Regurgitation, *Circulation*, 44:355, 1971.

91. Morrow, A. G., Brawley, R. K., and Braunwald, E.: Effects of Aortic Regurgitation on Left Ventricular Performance: Direct Determination of Aortic Blood Flow before and after Valve Replacement, *Circulation*, 31(suppl. 1):80, 1965.

92. Lingbach, A. J.: Heart Failure from the Point of

View of Quantitative Anatomy, *Am. J. Cardiol.*, 5:370, 1960.

93. Dodge, H. T., Kennedy, J. W., and Petersen, J.: Quantitative Angiocardiographic Methods in the Evaluation of Valvular Heart Disease, *Prog. Cardiovasc. Dis.*, 16:1, 1973.

94. Basta, L. L., Raines, D., Najjar, S., and Kioschos, J. M.: Clinical, Hemodynamic, and Coronary Angiographic Correlates of Angina Pectoris in Patients with Severe Aortic Valve Disease, *Br. Heart J.*, 37:150, 1975.

95. Harvey, W. P., Segal, J. P., and Hufnagel, C. A.: Unusual Clinical Features Associated with Severe Aortic Insufficiency, *Ann. Intern. Med.*, 47:27, 1957.

96. Cohn, L. H., Mason, D. T., Ross, J., Jr., Morrow, A. G., and Braunwald, E.: Preoperative Assessment of Aortic Regurgitation in Patients with Mitral Valve Disease, *Am. J. Cardiol.*, 19:177, 1967.

97. Conn, R. D., and Cole, J. S.: The Cardiac Apex Impulse: Clinical and Angiographic Correlations, *Ann. Int. Med.*, 75:185, 1971.

98. Groom, D., and Boone, J. A.: The Dove-Coo Murmur and Murmurs Heard at a Distance from the Chest Wall, *Ann. Intern. Med.*, 42:1214, 1955.

99. Porter, C. M., Baxley, W. A., Eddleman, E. E., Jr., Frimer, M., and Rackley, C. E.: Left Ventricular Dimensions and Dynamics of Filling in Patients with Gallop Heart Sounds, *Am. J. Med.*, 50:721, 1971.

*100. Fortuin, N. J., and Craige, E.: On the Mechanism of the Austin Flint Murmur, *Circulation*, 45:558, 1972. (33 references)

101. Wigle, E. D., and Labrosse, C. J.: Sudden, Severe Aortic Insufficiency, *Circulation*, 32:708, 1965.

102. Herbert, W. A.: Prolonged Atrioventricular Conduction and Aortic Insufficiency, *Thorax*, 25:577, 1970.

103. Selzer, A., Naruse, D. Y., York, E., Kahn, K. A., and Matthew, H. B.: Electrocardiographic Findings in Concentric and Eccentric Left Ventricular Hypertrophy, *Am. Heart J.*, 63:320, 1962.

104. Winsberg, F., Gabor, G. E., Hernberg, J. H., and Weiss, B.: Fluttering of the Mitral Valve in Aortic Insufficiency, *Circulation*, 41:225, 1970.

105. Pridie, R. B., Benham, M. B., and Oakley, C. M.: Echocardiography of the Mitral Valve in Aortic Valve Disease, *Br. Heart J.*, 33:296, 1971.

106. Wray, T. M.: The Variable Echocardiographic Features in Aortic Valve Endocarditis, *Circulation*, 52:658, 1975.

107. Stewart, J. A., Silimperi, D., Harris, P., Wise, N. K., Fraker, T. D., and Kisslo, J. A.: Echocardiographic Documentation of Vegetative Lesions in Infective Endocarditis: Clinical Implications, *Circulation*, 61:374, 1980.

*108. Gramiak, R., and Shah, P. M.: Echocardiography of the Normal and Diseased Aortic Valve, *Radiology*, 96:1, 1970. (11 references)

109. Troy, B. L., Pombo, J., and Rackley, C. E.: Measurement of Left Ventricular Wall Thickness and Mass by Echocardiography, *Circulation*, 45:602, 1972.

*110. Whipple, R. L., Morris, D. C., Felner, J. M., Merrill, A. J., and Miller, J. I.: Echocardiographic Manifestations of the Flail Aortic Valve Leaflet

Syndrome, *J. Clin. Ultrasound*, 5:417, 1977. (14 references)

*111. Henry, W. L., Bonow, R. O., Borer, J. S., Ware, J. H., Kent, K. M., Redwood, D. R., McIntosh, C. L., Morrow, A. G., and Epstein, S. E.: Observations on the Optimum Time for Operative Intervention for Aortic Regurgitation. I. Evaluation of the Results of Aortic Valve Replacement in Symptomatic Patients, *Circulation*, 61:471, 1980. (34 references)

112. Hunt, D., Baxley, W. A., Kennedy, J. W., Judge, T. P., Williams, J. E., and Dodge, H. T.: Quantitative Evaluation of Cineaortography in the Assessment of Aortic Regurgitation, *Am. J. Cardiol.*, 31:696, 1973.

113. Sandler, H., Dodge, H. T., Hay, R. E., and Rackley, C. E.: Quantitation of Valvular Insufficiency in Man by Angiocardiography, *Am. Heart J.*, 65:501, 1963.

114. Rackley, C. E., Dalldor, F. G., Hood, W. P., Jr., and Wilcox, B. R.: Sarcomere Length and Left Ventricular Function in Chronic Heart Disease, *Am. J. Med. Sci.*, 259:90, 1970.

115. Borer, J. S., Bacharach, S. L., Green, M. V., Kent, K. M., Henry, W. L., Rosing, D. R., Seides, S. F., Johnston, G. S., and Epstein, S. E.: Exercise-Induced Left Ventricular Dysfunction in Symptomatic and Asymptomatic Patients with Aortic Regurgitation: Assessment with Radionuclide Cineangiography, *Am. J. Cardiol.*, 42:351, 1978.

116. Borer, J. S., Bacharach, S. L., and Green, M. V.: Radionuclide Cineangiography at Rest and during Exercise in the Evaluation of Patients with Heart Disease, *Cardiovasc. Review & Repeats*, 1:31, 1980.

117. Baxter, R. H., Becker, L. C., Alderson, P. O., Rigo, P., Wagner, H. N., and Weisfeldt, M. L.: Quantification of Aortic Valvular Regurgitation in Dogs by Nuclear Imaging, *Circulation*, 61:404, 1980.

118. Ritchie, J. L., Zaret, B. L., Strauss, H. W., Pitt, B., Berman, D. S., Schelbert, H. R., Ashburn, W. L., Berger, H. J., and Hamilton, G. W.: Myocardial Imaging with Thallium-201: A Multicenter Study in Patients with Angina Pectoris or Acute Myocardial Infarction, *Am. J. Cardiol.*, 42:345, 1978.

119. Turner, J. D., Schwartz, K. M., Logic, J. R., Sheffield, L. T., Kansal, S., Roitman, D. I., Mantle, J. A., Russell, R. O., Jr., Rackley, C. E., and Rogers, W. J.: Detection of Residual Jeopardized Myocardium Three Weeks after Myocardial Infarction by Exercise Testing with Thallium-201 Myocardial Scintigraphy, *Circulation*, 61:729, 1980.

120. Sheffield, L. T., and Roitman, D.: Stress Testing Methodology, *Prog. Cardiovasc. Dis.*, 19:33, 1976.

*121. Goldschlager, N., Pfeifer, J., Cohn, K., Popper, R., and Selzer, A.: The Natural History of Aortic Regurgitation: A Clinical and Hemodynamic Study, *Am. J. Med.*, 54:577, 1973. (20 references)

122. Rapaport, E.: Natural History of Aortic and Mitral Valve Disease, *Am. J. Cardiol.*, 35:221, 1975.

123. Dismukes, W. E.: Management of Infective Endocarditis, in C. E. Rackley and A. N. Brest (eds.), "Critical Care Cardiology," F. A. Davis, Philadelphia, Cardiovascular Clinics, 1981, pp. 189–208.

124. Spagnuolo, M., Kloth, H., Taranta, A., Doyle, E., Pasternack, B.: Natural History of Rheumatic Aortic Regurgitation: Criteria Predictive of Death, Congestive Heart Failure, and Angina in Young Patients, *Circulation*, 44:368, 1971.

*125. Borer, J. S., Rosing, D. R., Kent, K. M., Bacharach, S. L., Green, M. W., McIntosh, C. J., Morrow, A. G., and Epstein, S. E.: Left Ventricular Function at Rest and during Exercise after Aortic Valve Replacement in Patients with Aortic Regurgitation, *Am. J. Cardiol.,* 44:1297, 1979. (19 references)

*126. Henry, W. L., Bonow, R. O., Rosing, D. R., and Epstein, S. E.: Observations on the Optimum Time for Operative Intervention for Aortic Regurgitation. II. Serial Echocardiographic Evaluation of Asymptomatic Patients, *Circulation,* 61:484, 1980. (29 references)

127. Borer, J. S., Bacharach, S. L., Green, M. V., Kent, K. M., Henry, W. L., Rosing, D. R., Seides, S. F., Johnston, G. S., and Epstein, S. E.: Exercise-Induced Left Ventricular Dysfunction in Symptomatic and Asymptomatic Patients with Aortic Regurgitation: Assessment with Radionuclide Cineangiography, *Am. J. Cardiol.,* 42:351, 1978.

*128. Richardson, J. V., Karp, R. B., Kirklin, J. W., and Dismukes, W. E.: Treatment of Infective Endocarditis: A Ten Year Comparative Analysis, *Circulation,* 58:589, 1978. (20 references)

129. Appelbaum, A., Karp, R. B., and Kirklin, J. W.: Ascending vs. Descending Aortic Dissections, *Ann. Surg.,* 183:296, 1976.

130. Koster, J. K., Jr., Cohn, L. H., Mee, R. B. B., and Collins, J. J., Jr.: Late Results of Operation for Acute Aortic Dissection Producing Aortic Insufficiency, *Ann. Thorac. Surg.,* 26:461, 1978.

131. Kouchoukos, N. T., Karp, R. B., and Lell, W. A.: Replacement of the Ascending Aorta and Aortic Valve with a Composite Graft: Results in 25 Patients. *Ann. Thorac. Surg.,* 24:14, 1977.

*132. Henry, W. L., Bonow, R. O., Borer, J. S., Kent, K. M., Ware, J. H., Redwood, D. R., Itscoitz, S. B., McIntosh, C. L., Morrow, A. G., and Epstein, S. E.: Evaluation of Aortic Valve Replacement in Patients with Valvular Aortic Stenosis, *Circulation,* 61:814, 1980. (39 references)

133. Williams, J. B., Karp, R. B., Kirklin, J. W., Kouchoukos, N. T., Pacifico, A. C., Zorn, G. L., Blackstone, E. H., Brown, R. N., Piantadose, S., and Bradley, E. L.: Considerations in Selection and Management of Patients Undergoing Valve Replacement with Glutaraldehyde-Fixed Porcine Bioprostheses, *Ann. Thorac. Surg.,* 30:247, 1980.

39

Mitral Valve Disease

Charles E. Rackley, M.D.
Jesse E. Edwards, M.D.
Robert B. Karp, M.D.
John W. Kirklin, M.D.

Mitral Stenosis

In examining the extraordinary dilatation of the body of the pulmonary vein, and its common openings, I perceived that the mouth of the left ventricle appeared very small and that it had an oval oblong shape.

Raymond Vieussens, 1715[1]

Etiology

Conditions which can impair flow through the mitral valve are rheumatic valvulitis, thrombus formation, atrial myxoma, bacterial vegetation, and calcium accumulation.[2-5] Rheumatic fever remains the most common and prevalent cause of mitral stenosis both in youngsters and adults. Outside the United States in the temperate zones, severe mitral stenosis can occur in children and adolescents.

Pathology

Mitral stenosis usually is the result of recurrent rheumatic endocarditis. The valvular leaflets and the chordae tendineae are affected by scarring with concomitant contracture (Fig. 39-1). An additional feature is that at each of the two junctional areas (the commissures) between the two major leaflets there is interadhesion between the two leaflets. This process, along with concomitant shortening of the chordae, causes the two interadherent leaflets to be held downward. The entire process is manifested by the leaflets' forming a funnel-shaped structure. The inlet to the funnel is at the level of the left atrial floor and is wider than the apex, which presents in the left ventricular cavity.

In the normal heart, blood flows freely through the mitral valve. It may flow through the principal orifice, that part of the opening which lies between the papillary muscles, or through multiple secondary orifices, which are the spaces between the chordae[6] (Fig. 39-2).

In rheumatic mitral stenosis, because of interchordal fusion, the secondary orifices are narrowed or obliterated and, by virtue of commissural fusion, the principal orifice is reduced in size. The anterior leaflet of the stenotic mitral valve frequently exhibits a deformity. Near its basal aspect the leaflet is convex toward the left atrium. It is possible that in early left ventricular diastole the deformity is buckled in the opposite direction and that this may account for the "opening snap" of mitral stenosis. Such movement does not affect the caliber of the effective orifice, which lies at a lower level. The deformity may

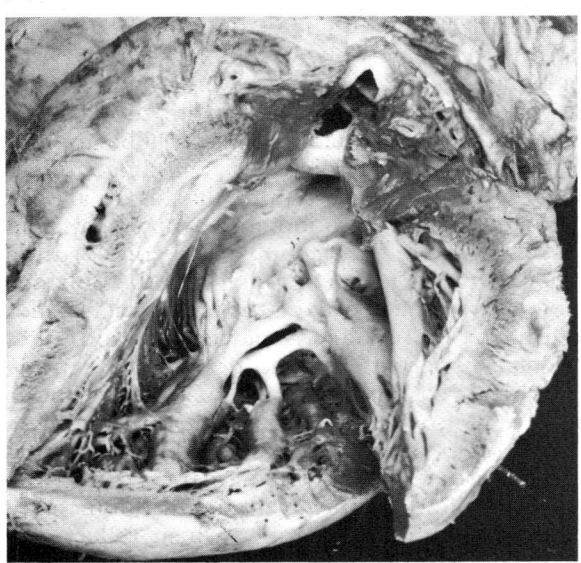

FIGURE 39-1 Mitral valve viewed from below in a case of mitral stenosis. The valve is converted into a funnel-shaped structure, the apex of which is in the left ventricle and is narrow.

contribute to closure of the valve as the prominence of the anterior leaflet is pressed against the base of the opposite leaflet during ventricular systole. Secondary effects of mitral stenosis include calcification of leaflet tissue, left atrial enlargement, and signs of pulmonary venous hypertension, including right ventricular hypertrophy.[7]

Fragmentation of leaflet tissue at calcific foci may lead to thrombosis upon the valvular surfaces and/or embolism of calcific material. Among the complications, thrombosis of the left atrial appendage and varying portions of the main left atrium are common, as is secondary systemic embolism.[8] Epi-

FIGURE 39-2 *A.* Diagrammatic portrayal of the normal mitral valve viewed from below. The principal orifice of the valve lies bounded anteriorly by the anterior leaflet, posteriorly by the posterior leaflet, and laterally by each papillary muscle and its related chordae. Secondary orifices lie in the spaces between the chordae tendineae and, for the most part, blood flowing through these orifices enters the left ventricle lateral to the respective papillary muscles. *B.* Diagrammatic portrayal of the stenotic mitral valve viewed from below. The principal orifice is narrow and, on the basis of commissural and chordal fusion, the secondary orifices are obliterated. (*From R. V. Bonnabeau, Jr., J. E. Stevenson, and J. E. Edwards, Obliteration of the Principal Orifice of the Stenotic Mitral Valve: A Rare Form of "Restenosis," J. Thorac. Cardiovasc. Surg., 49:264, 1965. Reproduced with permission.*)

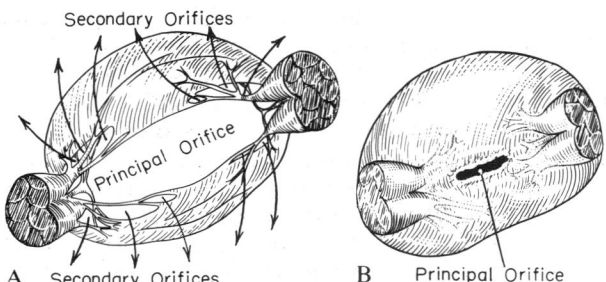

Secondary Orifices

Principal Orifice

A Secondary Orifices

B Principal Orifice

sodes of acute pulmonary edema and protracted right ventricular failure are common lethal complications.

Nonrheumatic mitral stenosis is rare in the adult. In the infant and child mitral stenosis results either from dysplasia of the valve or from the parachute deformity. Uncommonly, subjects with parachute mitral valve survive to adult life.[9,10]

Abnormal Physiology

The physiological abnormality produced by obstruction to mitral valve flow is a pressure gradient between the left atrium and left ventricle during diastolic filling. The pressure gradient is related to the orifice size and diastolic flow through the mitral valve. Mitral valve flow is determined by the cardiac output and duration of diastole. The diastolic pressure gradient across the mitral valve abnormally increases left atrial pressure and volume, which are further reflected to the pulmonary veins, capillaries, and, eventually, the pulmonary arteries. Elevation of left atrial pressure distends the chamber and pulmonary veins. If the pulmonary capillary pressure exceeds the oncotic pressure of the plasma proteins, pulmonary edema develops. Chronic elevation of left atrial pressure will lead to hyperplasia and hypertrophy of pulmonary arterioles. Ultimately, pulmonary vasoconstriction and hypertension develop. Eventually, right ventricular hypertrophy and dilatation result from significant pulmonary hypertension. In the early phase of mitral stenosis the pulmonary blood volume may be increased, but as noncompliant changes develop in the vessels there may be a reduction in pulmonary blood volume with a redistribution of the flow patterns from the base to the apex of the lung. Finally, the critical narrowing of the mitral orifice will reduce the cardiac output. In this manner, chronic mitral stenosis imposes a pressure overload on the left atrium, the pulmonary vascular tree, and the right ventricle.[11] Left ventricular function may gradually deteriorate as a result of diminished diastolic filling from the left atrium.[12,13]

Clinical Manifestations

History
Slightly over 50 percent of patients with recognized mitral stenosis recall a history of acute rheumatic fever, and thus the characteristic auscultatory findings detected for the first time during a medical examination may provide the initial history.[14] In symptomatic patients with mitral stenosis the most frequent complaints are dyspnea, fatigue, palpitations, and hemoptysis.[15,16] Less frequently the patients may present with hoarseness, chest pain, seizures, or a cerebral vascular accident from an embolus.

Dyspnea is the most prominent complaint in mitral stenosis and can be attributed to pulmonary venous hypertension.[15] When the mitral stenosis is mild, additional mechanical stress may be required to increase mitral valve flow and elevate left atrial and pulmonary venous pressures. Such conditions include the sudden development of atrial fibrillation with a rapid ventricular response, physical exertion, fever, emotional upsets, and pregnancy.[16,17] If excessive fluid has been retained during the day, a shift of the fluid at night from the trunk and lower extremities to the lungs can cause orthopnea and paroxysmal nocturnal dyspnea. However, it must be remembered that these symptoms of left ventricular failure are not specific for mitral stenosis. Fatigue is another clinical manifestation of mitral stenosis and occasionally may be more severe than dyspnea. Fatigue can be attributed to pulmonary hypertension and fixed vascular resistance. Right ventricular overload can produce hepatic congestion and peripheral edema, which contribute to easy tiring.

Hemoptysis is a significant symptom in mitral stenosis and is caused by pulmonary venous hypertension in the bronchial veins. Rupture of a bronchial vein and hemoptysis usually indicate severe mitral stenosis. Rarely, the bleeding may be massive and require emergency measures.[18]

Palpitations in mitral stenosis are often due to paroxysmal atrial fibrillation and left atrial enlargement.[16] Although the palpitations can be appreciated by the patient, sustained atrial fibrillation and a rapid ventricular response can cause or aggravate other symptoms such as dyspnea and fatigue.

Less frequent symptoms in mitral stenosis include chest pain, which can be due to pulmonary hypertension and pressure overload on the right ventricle; underlying coronary artery disease; or a pulmonary embolus.[19] Enlargement of the left atrium and compression of the recurrent laryngeal nerve can cause hoarseness. Central nervous system manifestations such as a seizure or stroke are usually due to embolic phenomena.[20]

Physical Examination

In the early stages of mitral stenosis abnormalities noted on the physical exam may be entirely limited to the heart. Pulmonary hypertension and right ventricular overload can create physical findings which reflect a reduced cardiac output, impaired tissue perfusion, right ventricular pressure overload, and systemic venous congestion. Vital signs in severe mitral stenosis may reveal a resting tachycardia, which is irregular if atrial fibrillation is present; increased respiratory rate; and a narrow pulse pressure due to reduced cardiac output and peripheral vasoconstriction. The general appearance of the patient may disclose the mitral facies with a malar flush and peripheral cyanosis. If right ventricular function is impaired, the neck veins will be distended. Right ventricular dilatation and failure are usually associated with a degree of tricuspid regurgitation, and this will produce a prominent v wave in the

neck veins. Impaired filling of the right ventricle is either due to hypertrophy or, rarely, secondary tricuspid stenosis, and can cause a prominent a wave in the jugular veins during atrial contraction. If pulmonary edema has developed, rales will be audible, but otherwise lungs remain clear. The characteristic findings of mitral stenosis on cardiac exam are the accentuated first heart sound, an opening snap, and a diastolic rumble. Inspection of the precordium may not reveal an apical impulse, and the only discernible activity may be along the left sternal border if significant pulmonary hypertension and right ventricular hypertrophy have developed.[21] Palpation in advanced mitral stenosis may detect an accentuated first sound at the apex, the opening snap, and vibrations from the diastolic rumble. Percussion often discloses a left ventricular apex within the midclavicular line. However, in the third interspace there may be dullness laterally, which reflects enlargement of the left atrium. Usually percussion is unremarkable to the right of the sternum, but if significant right ventricular enlargement or severe left atrial dilatation has developed there may be dullness to the right of the sternum. Auscultation characteristically reveals an accentuated first sound at the apex, and the opening snap after the second sound followed by a diastolic rumble.

The mechanism for the accentuation of the first heart sound in mitral stenosis is attributed to cessation of the upward motion of the valve, which has been depressed in the left ventricular chamber due to the diastolic gradient across the mitral valve[22–24] (Fig. 39-3). Factors which contribute to the intensity of the first sound are the mobility of the valve leaflet, the diastolic gradient across the valve, and the PR interval of the electrocardiogram.[25] The PR interval can be shortened by tachycardia, fever, and thyrotoxicosis. In severe mitral stenosis with loss of valve mobility, calcification of the leaflets, and associated mitral regurgitation, the first heart sound is not accentuated. Finally, the intensity of the first heart sound can vary with atrial fibrillation.

The opening snap is traditionally considered the most important physical sign of mitral stenosis[15] (Fig. 39-3). The sound occurs during the maximum excursion of the anterior leaflet of the mitral valve. The interval from the second heart sound to the opening snap can vary from 0.03 to 0.14 s and is influenced by the left atrial pressure.[26] The higher the left atrial pressure, the shorter will be the interval between aortic valve closure and the opening snap (2-OS). Critical mitral stenosis usually presents a 2-OS time less than 0.08 s. This time interval expressed as the (Q-1)-(2-OS) time has been used to determine the severity of mitral stenosis.[27] The time from the onset of the QRS complex on electrocardiogram to the generation of the first mitral sound (Q-S1) is delayed in mitral stenosis, and the 2-OS time reflects the left atrial pressure. Other factors such as valvular mobility, calcification, cardiac output, left ventricular systolic pressure, and relaxation

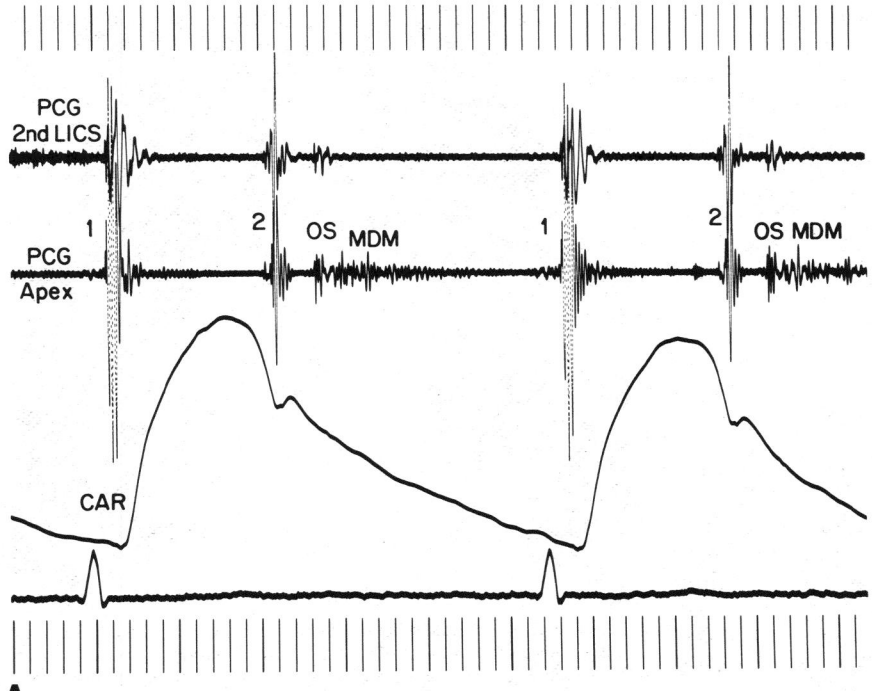

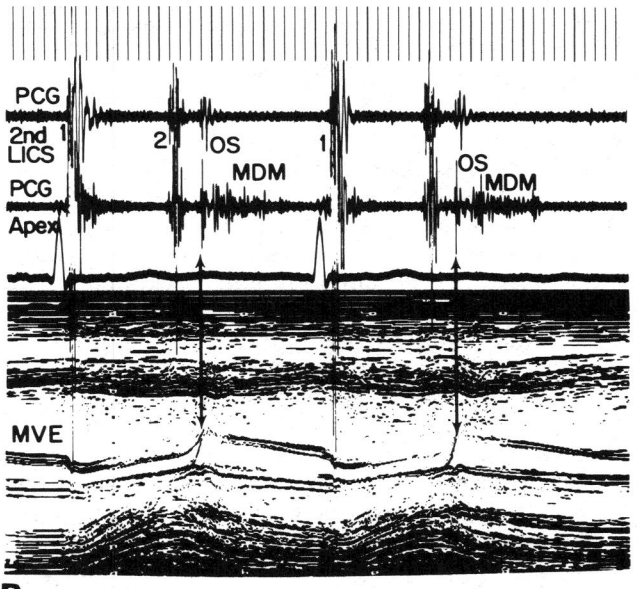

FIGURE 39-3 *A.* Phonocardiogram and carotid pulse recording in mitral stenosis and atrial fibrillation. A loud first sound (1), opening snap of the mitral valve occurs 0.11 s after the second heart sound, which is in turn followed by a low-frequency middiastolic murmur at the cardiac apex. *B.* The phonocardiogram on the same patient at a slower paper speed (50 mm/s) shows a relationship between the first heart sound and completion of closing movement of the mitral valve and, similarly, the opening snap accompanying the termination of the opening movement of the valve. (*Courtesy Dr. Ernest Craige.*)

of the left ventricle can influence the (Q-1)-(2-OS) time.[28,29]

An opening snap has been detected in other conditions, such as mitral regurgitation, ventricular sep-

tal defect, second- and third-degree heart block, tricuspid atresia with a large atrial septal defect, and tetralogy of Fallot after a Blalock-Taussig procedure.[30,31] An atrial myxoma can also produce an early diastolic sound similar in timing to the opening snap.[3] In addition to the mitral valve origin, opening snaps can be produced by the tricuspid valve in tricuspid stenosis, atrial septal defect, and Ebstein's anomaly.[32–34] Therefore, a tricuspid origin must be considered in the differential diagnosis of a mitral opening snap.

The opening snap is heard best with the diaphragm of the stethoscope at the apex, but sometimes it is audible along the left sternal border, at the base of the heart, and, rarely, in the suprasternal notch.[35] The opening snap must also be differentiated from a two-component second heart sound as well as a ventricular protodiastolic gallop. Sometimes inspiration will separate the aortic and pulmonary components of the second sound if an opening snap is present. Standing will increase the time from the aortic second sound to the opening snap by decreasing venous return and lowering left atrial pressure.[36] Exercise will shorten the 2-OS time by raising left atrial pressure. Usually the ventricular gallop sound is a low-pitched sound heard best at the apex with the bell of the stethoscope and occurs 0.12 s or later after the second sound. The ventricular gallop sound can be heard along the left sternal border, similar to radiation of an opening snap. If right ventricular dilatation and failure have developed due to severe pulmonary hypertension, the right ventricular gallop sound may be audible in the area of the apex, but this sound is usually located along the left sternal border.

A diastolic rumble is almost always present in mitral stenosis but can be difficult to detect at rest or can even diminish in the late stages of severe mitral stenosis with decreased mitral valve flow (Fig. 39-3). The murmur is low-pitched, is heard best with the bell of the stethoscope placed lightly on the chest wall, and becomes crescendo in the latter phase of diastole. Electrocardiographic studies on mitral valve motion have shown that the middiastolic rumble occurs as the mitral valve leaflets return toward the closed position despite continued flow.[37] This mechanism may also contribute to the presystolic accentuation of the rumble, which is augmented by atrial contraction.[38] However, there can be presystolic accentuation of the diastolic rumble with atrial fibrillation.[39]

The diastolic rumble of mitral stenosis may be localized to a small area at the apex of the left ventricle. Sometimes the murmur is audible only after the patient has turned to the left lateral decubitus position or has exercised in bed. A close correlation has not been documented between the loudness of the murmur and the severity of the mitral stenosis. However, middiastolic rumbles often occur with mild mitral stenosis, and a rumble which starts with the opening snap and continues to the first heart sound suggests more severe stenosis. In the late stages of mitral stenosis with significant reduction in cardiac output and diastolic flow across the mitral valve, the rumble may diminish or even disappear. Other causes of a mitral diastolic rumble include a left atrial myxoma, Blalock-to-left-atrial shunt, cor triatriatum, calcification of the mitral annulus, pericardial constriction of the AV groove around the mitral apparatus, and, finally, the Carey-Coombs murmur in acute rheumatic fever.[3,40–42] Aortic regurgitation may produce the Austin Flint murmur, which is a mitral rumble due to impingement of the aortic jet on the anterior leaflet of the mitral valve. Finally, the Graham Steell murmur of pulmonary insufficiency may be similar to that associated with aortic insufficiency, but peripheral signs will help differentiate between an aortic or pulmonary origin.[43]

Chest Roentgenogram (Fig. 39-4)

Radiographic changes produced by mitral stenosis are manifestations of left atrial hypertension and include left atrial enlargement, alterations in pulmonary venous pattern, prominence of the pulmonary arteries, and right ventricular enlargement. Some degree of left atrial enlargement is usually present with mitral stenosis and can often be detected on the posterior-anterior chest film.[44] Left atrial enlargement contributes to straightening of the left cardiac border, since the appendage occupies the position between the pulmonary artery segment and the left ventricle. Enlargement of the left atrium also occurs to the right of the spine and can be recognized as a double density along the right heart border. Finally, indentation from posterior

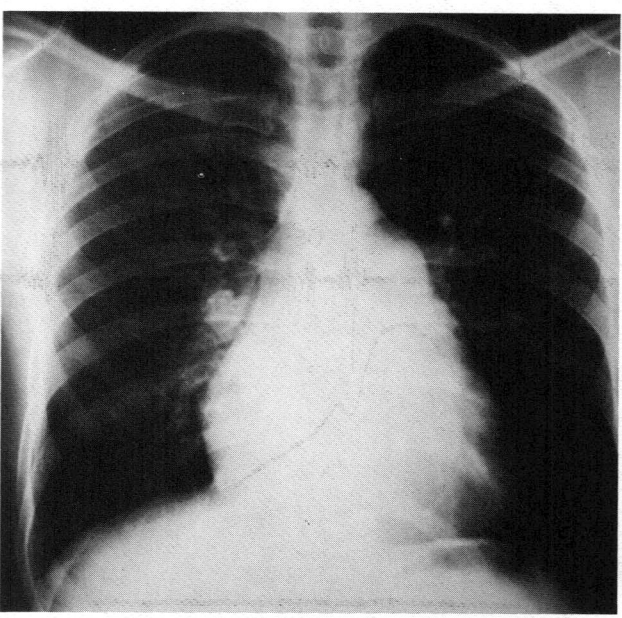

FIGURE 39-4 Chest roentgenogram of a patient with a calculated mitral valve area of 0.7 cm² and moderate pulmonary hypertension. Tricuspid regurgitation is evident on the physical examination, and the increase in the cardiac silhouette is due to right ventricular dilatation. Left atrial enlargement contributes to the heart shadow to the right of the spine and the left atrial appendage is seen along the left cardiac border.

atrial enlargement on the esophagus can be appreciated with a barium swallow.

With chronic pulmonary venous hypertension there is not only prominence of the vessels but also a redistribution of the flow toward the apexes of the lungs. When the elevated pulmonary capillary pressure exceeds the oncotic pressure of the plasma proteins, which ranges from 20 to 25 mmHg, fluid will accumulate in the interstitial space of the lungs.[45] These interlobular septal changes produce linear shadows perpendicular to the pleura at the bases of the lungs. These interlobular septal lines were described by Kerley, and the Kerley B lines are frequently identified with elevated capillary pressures at the costophrenic angle.[46] Kerley also described A lines in the upper lung fields and C lines in the lung bases, but these are infrequently seen. Pulmonary venous hypertension can redistribute blood flow to the upper lobes.[47] However, acute elevation of pulmonary venous pressure is more likely to cause pulmonary edema with both interstitial and alveolar extravasation of fluid.[48] However, it must be remembered that these chronic and acute radiographic changes of pulmonary venous hypertension are not specific for mitral stenosis but can result from left ventricular failure of any etiology.

Pulmonary arterial hypertension in mitral stenosis will enlarge the pulmonary arteries. This condition creates a pressure overload on the right ventricle, and eventually right ventricular dilatation and hypertrophy will be evidenced on the chest roentgenograms. Thus, the radiographic manifestations of left atrial enlargement, redistribution of pulmonary venous flow, interstitial edema, enlargement of pulmonary arteries, and right ventricular dilatation should suggest mitral stenosis but are not specific. In the absence of other valvular lesions the left ventricle remains of normal size and may become smaller in time.

Electrocardiogram (Fig. 39-5)

The electrocardiogram can provide evidence for underlying mitral stenosis but is not a reliable indicator of the severity of the lesion. Atrial fibrillation is common in mitral stenosis but can also occur with other cardiac disorders. The P wave is characteristically altered to produce a broad, notched wave most prominent in lead II with a conspicuous negative terminal deflection in lead V_1.[49] Atrial fibrillation can develop in any condition associated with left atrial enlargement as well as in the course of coronary artery disease and hypertensive heart disease.

Pulmonary hypertension can produce electrocardiographic evidence of right ventricular hypertrophy. This is usually manifested as rightward deviation of the QRS axis in the frontal frame. Unfortunately, correlation between electrocardiographic evidence of right ventricular hypertrophy and the degree of pulmonary hypertension or mitral valve area has not been a predictable one.[50,51] Finally, pulmonary hypertension from any etiology can result in right ventricular hypertrophy, and

atrial fibrillation can obscure the useful contribution of P-wave abnormalities.

Special Laboratory Studies

Echocardiography (See Chap. 95) The echocardiogram has become one of the most reliable noninvasive tools in the detection of mitral valve stenosis.[52–54] The most characteristic change is a decrease in the E-to-F slope of the anterior leaflet of the mitral valve, which results in the characteristic square-wave configuration on the echocardiogram. Additional echocardiographic abnormalities include abnormal posterior leaflet movement, decreased mitral valve motion, and thick echoes around the valve suggesting calcification. Echocardiograms can also delineate left atrial enlargement, right ventricular enlargement, and left ventricular dimensions. The E-to-F slope has been quantitated, and a value less than 10 mm/s is usually associated with severe mitral stenosis.[54]

The echocardiogram is also valuable in detecting nonrheumatic obstruction to mitral valve flow, and the most notable is a left atrial myxoma[55–57] (Fig. 39-6). The usual displacement of the anterior leaflet of the mitral valve can be demonstrated, plus the multiple echoes from the tumor.[55] The echocardiogram can sometimes outline the nidus of infection in bacterial endocarditis in the mitral valve.[58] Vegetations and calcium accumulations on the leaflets can be delineated by the echoes. Finally, the echocardiogram can be useful in following the clinical course of patients with mitral stenosis both before and after operative intervention.

Cardiac Catheterization Cardiac catheterization in mitral stenosis can provide measurements of the gradient across the mitral valve, measurements for the mitral valve area, response of pulmonary artery pressure to exercise, recognition of other valvular lesions, assessment of ventricular function, and delineation of coronary artery anatomy.

The mitral valve gradient is obtained by simultaneously recording the pulmonary capillary wedge pressure or the direct left atrial pressure and the left ventricular pressure. A determination of cardiac

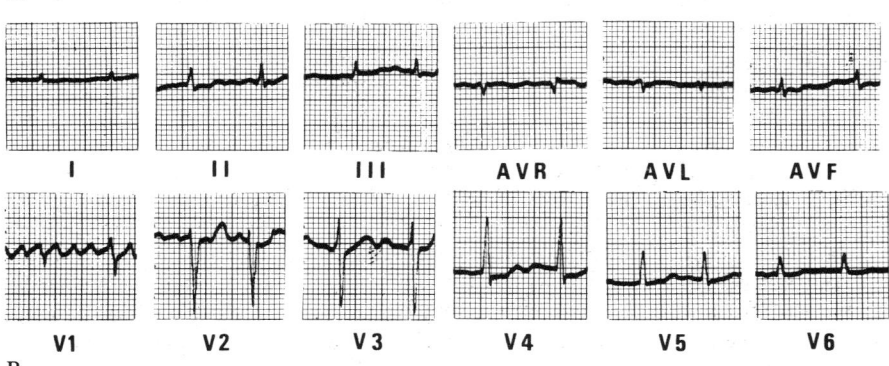

FIGURE 39-5 Electrocardiograms of a patient with mitral stenosis. The tracings were made 7 years apart, in which time the patient's symptoms and hemodynamic findings progressed. *A.* Left atrial abnormality and a +60° frontal QRS axis. *B.* Atrial fibrillation with coarse fibrillatory waves in a +85 percent frontal QRS axis.

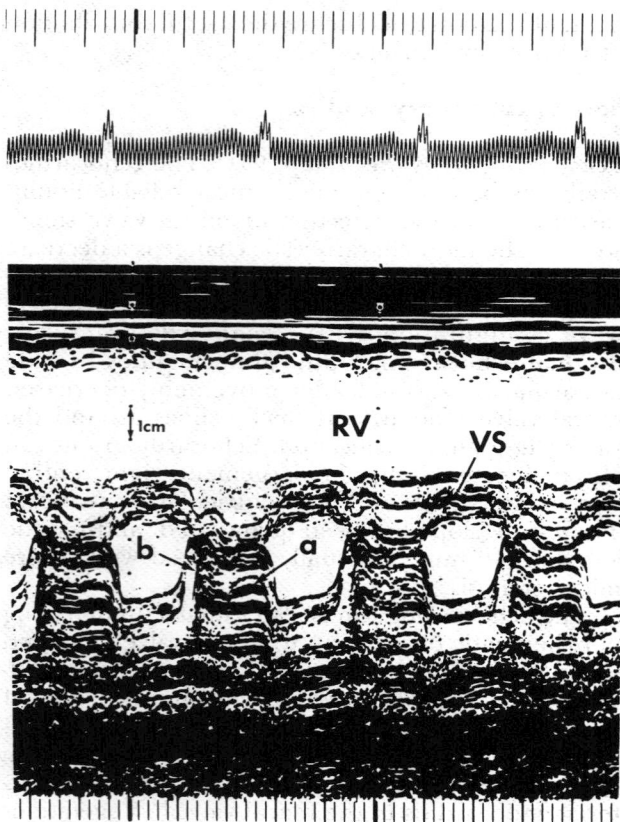

FIGURE 39-6 Echocardiogram of a left atrial myxoma. Arrow a points to the tumor, and arrow b points to the clear space, which is the time required for the tumor to move from the left atrium to the left ventricle. RV = right ventricle; VS = ventricular septum. (*Courtesy of Dr. Joel M. Felner.*)

output using the Fick principle or indicator dilution method is obtained at the time of mitral valve gradient recording. These measurements can be inserted into the hydraulic formula of Gorlin to calculate mitral orifice size.[59,60] The mitral valve area is directly proportional to the diastolic flow across the valve and inversely related to the square root of the pressure gradient. A range of values for mitral valve size can be derived from the same pressure gradient since diastolic flow will significantly influence the calculation. The normal mitral valve area is 4 to 6 cm², and hemodynamic abnormalities develop when the valve is reduced to 1.5 to 2.5 cm². Pulmonary congestion occurs when the valve size is reduced to 1.1 to 1.5 cm², and with a mitral valve size less than 1.0 cm² pulmonary hypertension, right ventricular failure, and reduced cardiac output are generally present.

Patients with symptoms of mitral stenosis generally present a capillary wedge pressure greater than 15 to 20 mmHg.[61] The pulmonary artery pressure in severe mitral stenosis can approach systemic blood pressure due to capillary hyperplasia and severe arteriolar vasoconstriction. If the pulmonary artery diastolic pressure greatly exceeds the wedge pressure, an increase in pulmonary vascular resistance will be calculated. However, in severe pulmonary hypertension, wedging the catheter may be technically difficult, and transseptal entry into the left atrium becomes necessary. Also, with excessive elevations of pulmonary artery pressure, cardiac output will fall. If the wedge pressure does not exceed 15 to 20 mmHg in symptomatic mitral stenosis, a form of exercise should be performed in the catheterization laboratory. The rise in pulmonary artery pressure may be striking, and the cardiac output response to exercise often is subnormal.

In addition to hemodynamic abnormalities of the mitral valve imposed on the left atrium and pulmonary vascular bed, left ventricular dysfunction has also been documented in isolated mitral stenosis.[12,62] Segmental and global wall motion abnormalities have been described, but the mechanism has not been clearly elucidated.[12,13,63,64] Besides the measurements of mitral valve gradient and cardiac output, left ventricular angiography is usually performed to detect mitral regurgitation. In adult patients coronary arteriography is done to delineate coronary anatomy, whether the patient has previously experienced chest pain, myocardial infarction, or not.

Cardiac catheterization may not be considered necessary in the young symptomatic female patient with isolated mitral stenosis documented by noninvasive techniques. However, catheterization should be undertaken if there is a disparity between symptoms and physical findings, if other valve lesions are present, and to determine the presence or absence of coronary artery disease. If there is suspicion of a left atrial myxoma that is not clearly resolved by echocardiography, as in silent mitral stenosis, cardiac catheterization is warranted.

Radionuclide Studies Radionuclide techniques can now provide information noninvasively during rest and exercise which can be useful in evaluating the patient with mitral stenosis before and after cardiac surgery. The heart rate, ejection fraction, end-diastolic volume, stroke volume, cardiac output, and diastolic filling rate have been measured before and after bicycle exercise in mitral stenosis.[65] Such noninvasively acquired quantitative information on the restriction of diastolic ventricular filling is clinically helpful, and alterations in these variables can be followed after mitral valve surgery in order to document the exercise-induced changes in cardiac performance as well as the benefits of surgery.

Exercise Testing Exercise testing in mitral stenosis can be employed to evaluate symptomatic response, assess functional capacity, and enhance auscultatory events. The blunted response of cardiac output to exercise has been described as the hemodynamic hallmark of mitral stenosis.[61] Hemodynamic measurements with exercise have been used to demonstrate the benefit of drugs such as propranolol by inhibition of tachycardias.[66–68]

Natural History and Prognosis

Rheumatic fever remains the most common cause of mitral stenosis worldwide. The average age of onset for acute rheumatic fever is 12 years of age, and a latent period of 19 years from the acute episode of rheumatic fever to detection of a murmur of mitral stenosis has been documented.[15] Thus, a patient experiencing rheumatic fever at age 12 will on an average exhibit findings of mitral stenosis at age 31. Cardiac symptoms usually develop in the fourth and fifth decade. Approximately 50 percent of patients develop symptoms gradually, while the remaining patients experience precipitation of symptoms by complications such as atrial fibrillation with a rapid ventricular response.[16]

The most common symptoms of dyspnea and fatigue can be attributed to pulmonary hypertension and right ventricular failure. Sudden increases in cardiac output from atrial fibrillation, fever, emotion, or pregnancy can abruptly elevate pulmonary capillary pressure and produce pulmonary edema. Chronic elevation of pulmonary capillary pressure can produce levels of pulmonary arterial hypertension that approach systemic values. Significant elevation of pulmonary arterial pressure is usually associated with a decline in cardiac output and a pressure overload on the right ventricle, which can lead to dilatation. At this stage hepatic congestion and peripheral edema often develop, and the typical picture of failure of the right side of the heart with neck vein distension, hepatic enlargement, ascites, and peripheral edema is seen. At this stage liver function abnormalities may be prominent. The usual physical findings are those of severe pulmonary hypertension, right ventricular failure, and jugular vein distension with *v* waves of tricuspid regurgitation. The electrocardiogram often exhibits atrial fibrillation and right ventricular hypertrophy. The chest x-ray will show enlarged pulmonary arteries with apical shunting and Kerley B lines. The prognosis at this advanced stage is poor but still may be improved with surgical intervention.

Approximately 40 to 50 percent of patients with mitral stenosis will experience atrial fibrillation, and this becomes more common in patients over the age of 40. The mechanism for atrial fibrillation involves both the enlarged left atrium from the chronic pressure overload and distension, as well as histologic changes that occur in the atrial wall. The onset of fibrillation may contribute to further left atrial dilatation. The physiological abnormality imposed on the left ventricle in mitral stenosis with the onset of atrial fibrillation is a rapid ventricular response, shortening of the diastolic filling period, elevation of left atrial pressure, and loss of atrial contraction with its contribution to ventricular filling. All these hemodynamic disturbances contribute to a reduction in cardiac output. Initially the atrial fibrillation may be paroxysmal or respond to drugs or cardioversion. However, as the atrial fibrillation becomes more chronic, there is also resistance to cardioversion.

One of the most hazardous complications of mitral stenosis is systemic embolization, and reports estimate the incidence from 9 to 20 percent.[69] Both age of the patient and history of atrial fibrillation appear associated with a high incidence of systemic emboli. However, the severity of the mitral stenosis, left atrial size, and heart failure do not consistently relate to embolic complications. Thus, systemic emboli may develop pre- and postoperatively during the course of mitral stenosis, and mitral stenosis should always be considered as a possible mechanism in the cause of systemic embolization, especially in a young female patient.[70] Neurological symptoms from a cerebral embolus can be the presenting manifestation of mitral stenosis.

Although bacterial endocarditis may be infrequent and isolated in mitral stenosis, a prolonged fever should always raise the possibility of valvular infection in a patient with known mitral stenosis. Rarely, the infected material can obstruct the mitral valve. Also, a left atrial myxoma should be considered in the presence of fever, arthralgias, anemia, and systemic emboli.

The prognosis and survival of patients with mitral stenosis will depend on the presence or absence of symptoms when first examined. In Rapaport's series of randomly selected patients, 80 percent were alive at 5 years follow-up and 60 percent survived 10 years[71] (Fig. 39-7). The average age at time of death in patients with medically managed mitral stenosis is 48 years.[72]

Management

Medical Management

The medical management of mitral stenosis cannot alter the obstruction of flow through the valve, and, therefore, efforts at prevention of recurrent rheumatic fever and bacterial endocarditis are important in the asymptomatic individual to retard further stenosis of the valve. With the onset of disturbances in atrial rhythm, such as atrial fibrillation, digitalis may control the ventricular response and slow the heart rate. In paroxysmal atrial fibrillation the digitalis may prevent recurrence of atrial irritability as well. An antiarrhythmic agent such as quinidine may be added to further suppress recurrences of atrial fibrillation, but a digitalis preparation should always be started prior to quinidine institution. If the fibrillation produces symptoms of pulmonary congestion, consideration should be given to immediate cardioversion. However, the longer the atrial fibrillation has been present, the less likely the patient is to remain in sinus rhythm after cardioversion.[73] If possible, digitalis should be withheld for 1 to 2 days before cardioversion. This is an important consideration in the emergent presentation of atrial fibrillation and pulmonary edema since one may pro-

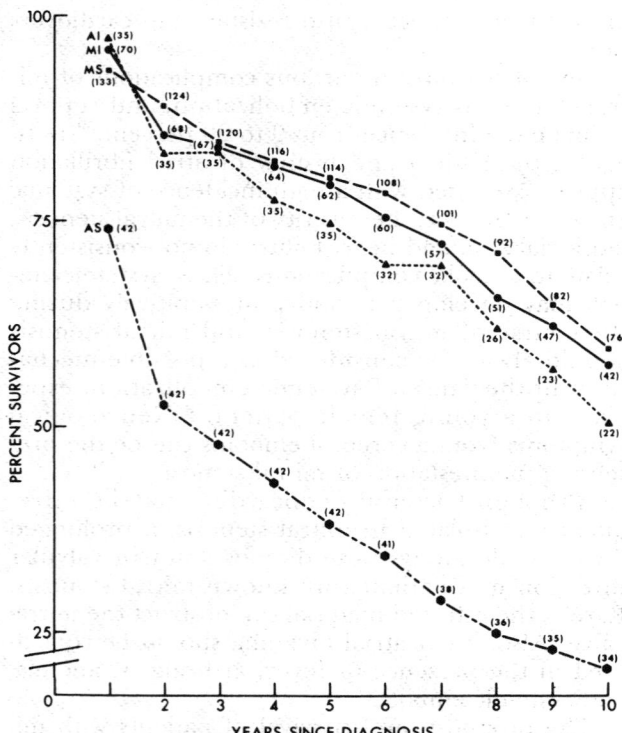

FIGURE 39-7 Actuarial survival in valvular heart disease treated medically, from time of diagnosis. (*From E. Rapaport, Natural History of Aortic and Mitral Valve Disease, Am. J. Cardiol., 35:221, 1975. Reproduced with permission.*)

ceed directly to cardioversion. If there is a history of a previous embolus, anticoagulation therapy for a 2-week period is desirable before efforts at cardioversion. After successful cardioversion, digitalis and quinidine are administered to prevent recurrences of atrial irritability. If the patient remains in atrial fibrillation, chronic quinidine administration is not needed, but if no contraindications are present, propranolol can slow the ventricular response.

A systemic embolus requires anticoagulation treatment, usually for a long period. An embolus to an extremity or to the mesenteric system requires consideration for surgical intervention and removal. However, a systemic embolus alone may not be an indication for mitral valve surgery since embolic phenomena can occur in milder forms of mitral stenosis. Progressive symptoms of dyspnea and fatigue due to pulmonary venous congestion require evaluation for surgical intervention in mitral stenosis.

If mitral valve surgery is planned, dental repair and any potential minor surgery should be corrected under antibiotic coverage. Previously used medications such as digitalis, diuretics, and anticoagulants should be reviewed and reduced or temporarily discontinued immediately prior to surgery. If the patient has been in chronic atrial fibrillation, the digitalis dose may be reduced or discontinued prior to surgery in order to eliminate postoperative

digitalis intoxication. If diuretics have been used, electrolytes should be checked and, if necessary, potassium restored. If the patient has been on long-term anticoagulation therapy for a previous embolus, it should be discontinued several days before surgery, and heparin can be substituted until the patient is taken to the operating room.

Surgical Management

Indications for Surgery For valvular heart disease, as in most other disease processes, the decision to intervene surgically is based on an appraisal of what is known concerning the natural history of the disease untreated or treated medically compared to the early and late results of surgical intervention. Analysis of the prognosis of patients with valvular heart disease treated medically is dependent on the stage of the disease at which the patient is first seen.[71] Three decades ago Oleson[72] reported that 20 percent of patients with mitral stenosis died within 1 year from the time that they were first seen. Within 10 years, 60 percent were dead. In the survivors there was progressive cardiac disability. This disability is usually gradual, although temporary plateaus of remarkable exercise tolerance occur. More recently, Rapaport[71] reported an 80 percent 5-year survival of patients followed from the time of first diagnosis (Fig. 39-7). It is apparent that the decision to intervene surgically must be based on the state of the disease process in any individual patient, and the New York Heart Association classification for functional disability is a convenient way to stratify these patients.

Because valve replacement is associated with more late complications than are reconstructive procedures, the decision to intervene surgically in mitral stenosis is partially based on the anticipated necessity of valve replacement versus reconstruction. In general, if there is a high probability of a reconstructive procedure, earlier operation is justified. In pure mitral stenosis, mitral commissurotomy is the procedure of choice. The commissurotomy can be done closed (without cardiopulmonary bypass) or open. In areas such as the Middle East and Far East where there is a relatively large group of patients with juvenile or third-decade pure mitral stenosis, closed commissurotomy remains the favored procedure. With certain exceptions, open commissurotomy has replaced the less precise closed method in the United States. At the present time, a mitral commissurotomy is offered to patients in functional classes II-B, III, and IV. These classes include the development of symptoms which interfere with a patient's productivity and enjoyment of life such as dyspnea, effort intolerance, and then, later, fluid retention, orthopnea, paroxysmal dyspnea, and, finally, weight loss. It is well known that the onset of atrial fibrillation in patients with mitral stenosis causes increased symptomatic distress. Thus, if atrial fibrillation becomes established or recurs after drug therapy or cardioversion, and the patient becomes increasingly symptomatic, operation is indicated. The occurrence of arterial thromboembolism in a patient with mitral stenosis is in general an indication for mitral commissurotomy. Perhaps the one clear-cut indication in the United States, at the present time, for closed commissurotomy is the presence of a pliable valve in a female with mitral stenosis who is pregnant and developing cardiac disability.

The feasibility of a mitral reconstructive procedure in mitral stenosis is based on preoperative assessment indicating a pliable mitral valve. Pliability is suggested by the presence of an opening snap, little or no calcification noted on echocardiography or cinefluoroscopy, and absent or mild mitral insufficiency. These patients are usually less than 50 years old and are most often in functional class II-B or III.

Preoperative evaluation usually includes typical findings on the electrocardiogram (in some cases) of P-mitrale and right ventricular hypertrophy, chest roentgenogram changes suggestive of pulmonary venous hypertension along with left atrial and right ventricular enlargement, and an echocardiogram showing an E-to-F slope typical of mitral stenosis. If these noninvasive studies point clearly to isolated mitral stenosis, and if the patient is less than 40 or 50 years old and angina is not present, it is entirely feasible to proceed to operation without cardiac catheterization.

Operation A median sternotomy incision is used routinely for the operation. The heart and the patient are cooled by the perfusate at the start of cardiopulmonary bypass. The aorta is cross-clamped and the heart is protected by multidose hypothermic potassium cardioplegia.[74] Thereafter, the left atrium is opened, with a flaccid heart and a clamped aorta, avoiding air and particulate embolization.

The mitral valve is studied for its suitability for mitral commissurotomy. If it is judged suitable, silk sutures are placed on the anterior and posterior leaflets for traction. An incision is made into the anterior lateral commissure just short of the edge of the valve ring. The chordae beneath the commissures go to both anterior and posterior leaflets and can be used as a guide to the commissures. When fused chordae exist beneath the commissure these may be separated carefully by sharp dissection in order to enlarge the orifice. A similar procedure is carried out at the posterior medial commissure. At times, when the chordae are short and the papillary muscles are scarred, the papillary muscle may be split between chordae to enlarge the orifice. Only if the leaflets are immobile or heavily calcified, or if the valve is found to be seriously incompetent after discontinuing cardiopulmonary bypass, is valve replacement utilized. At times, a larger mitral valve area can be achieved by incising areas within scarred commissures and making a secondary orifice for the

valve. The degree of residual incompetence can be assessed moderately well by filling the left ventricle with a cold saline solution. Should there be major incompetence, further reconstruction of the valve may be effected by using a remodeling procedure such as that suggested by Carpentier[75] or Duran[76] with excision of certain chordal or leaflet structures and insertion of a flexible annular ring (see below). Any thrombi present within the left atrium are removed, and the left atrial appendage is oversewn before discontinuing cardiopulmonary bypass. Strict precautions are taken to avoid air embolization as the aortic clamp is removed and the heart is refilled with blood. After cardiopulmonary bypass is discontinued, palpation of the left atrium at its roof and at the left posterior AV groove is used to assess any degree of residual mitral valve incompetence.

Postoperative Care The postoperative course of patients undergoing open mitral commissurotomy is similar to that of other patients undergoing cardiac operations.[77] When cardiac performance is suboptimal, infusion of blood or blood substitutes is used to maintain the mean left atrial pressure at levels of about 14 mmHg. If arterial blood pressure is higher than normal, reduction of left ventricular afterload is accomplished by the continuous intravenous infusion of nitroprusside. Efforts are made to maintain a sinus rhythm when possible, including the use of atrial pacing at a rate of about 110 beats per minute. Should these procedures fail to optimize cardiac performance as judged by indicator dilution measurement of cardiac output, small doses of inotropic agents such as dopamine, isoproterenol, or epinephrine can be used.

If the hemodynamic state is good, the patient is usually extubated a few hours after operation. If cardiac output has been low, a nasotracheal tube is utilized, and the patient is maintained on intermittent mandatory ventilation with moderate positive end-expiratory pressure. In any event, extubation is usually possible between 12 and 48 h after operation. Urine flow is monitored, and when less than 15 ml/h, interventions to optimize cardiac performance are utilized or a diuretic such as furosemide or mannitol is employed.

Generally, patients having mitral commissurotomy are given anticoagulation treatment for 10 days to 6 weeks postoperatively, using warfarin sodium begun about 48 h postoperatively.

Hospital Morbidity and Mortality The hospital mortality following open mitral commissurotomy is as low as that for closed commissurotomy and is approximately 1 percent. Morbidity is minimal and includes an occasional patient with an atrial or ventricular arrhythmia.

Late Results A number of patients may require reoperation from 5 to 20 years after commissurotomy. This deterioration has been estimated to be at a rate of 5 percent of patients per year.[78] Heger and Wann et al.[79] studied 18 patients 10 to 14 years after successful commissurotomy. At early restudy, mitral valve area increased from 0.9 cm^2 to 2.7 cm^2. Only 5 of the 18 patients had significant restenosis (average mitral valve area decreased from 2.7 cm^2 to 1.3 cm^2). This was associated with increased symptomatology. According to Higgs et al.[80] symptoms recurrent after commissurotomy more often result from factors other than restenosis. These include residual stenosis, mitral regurgitation, or other associated valvular or cardiac abnormalities.

Clearly, most patients experience marked symptomatic improvement after mitral commissurotomy and at 5 years the clinical status for the majority is NYHA functional class I or II.

Postoperative Management

Patients will require digitalis or propranolol after mitral valve surgery to prevent a rapid ventricular response if atrial fibrillation persists. If a prosthetic valve has been inserted, long-term anticoagulation will be required, and dental prophylaxis should be continued whether a commissurotomy was performed or prosthetic valve inserted. Since the patient may not fully achieve optimal return of function for 3 to 6 months after mitral valve surgery, noninvasive studies such as echocardiography and radionuclide exercise testing can be performed during the first 6 months after surgery to document the hemodynamic improvement as well as the patient's functional reserve.

Cost Analysis

In the asymptomatic patient with mitral stenosis, diligent rheumatic and endocardial prophylaxis can be most beneficial in retarding progression of the stenosis and preventing bacterial endocarditis. The goal of follow-up visits once or twice each year is to detect early symptoms as well as to gather noninvasive evidence of hemodynamic deterioration of the mitral lesion. Class II cardiac patients with symptoms on more than normal activity should be considered surgical candidates. An important consideration for mitral valve surgery can arise in the young female during her childbearing period when the stress of pregnancy produces symptoms of pulmonary congestion. In these individuals, careful thought has to be given to continued medical follow-up, a simple mitral commissurotomy, or the risk of mitral valve replacement with the need for long-term follow-up. If the patient remains asymptomatic, a conservative approach is probably justified, particularly in the younger individual; but for long-term benefits mitral valve surgery must be considered in a young woman with children who needs to perform physical tasks in properly caring for her youngsters. Thus, the cost consideration and risk-benefit ratio of continued medical therapy and surgical treatment must be directed toward preserva-

tion of function and prevention of heart failure and future complications.

Mitral Regurgitation

I have found perceptible purring tremor to be produced more frequently by regurgitation through the mitral valve than by any other valvular lesion—especially when the ventricle was hypertrophous and dilated by which the refluent current was rendered stronger.

James Hope, 1839[81]

Etiology

Although rheumatic fever has been considered a major cause of mitral regurgitation for many years, cardiac catheterization and noninvasive techniques have delineated a number of other conditions which can produce incompetence of the mitral valve apparatus.[82] Rheumatic fever remains a cause of mitral regurgitation, but frequently this lesion is in combination with stenosis of the mitral valve. The widespread use of echocardiography has identified mitral leaflet prolapse in many patients who otherwise would have not been examined by invasive techniques, and mitral leaflet prolapse may represent the most common mechanism for mitral regurgitation in the adult population.[83]

A variety of mechanisms must be considered in chronic or acute mitral regurgitation (Table 39-1). Other frequent causes of chronic mitral regurgitation besides rheumatic fever and mitral leaflet prolapse are coronary artery disease and left ventricular dilatation from any condition causing sufficient enlargement of the chamber.[84,85] The less common etiologies of chronic mitral regurgitation include calcified mitral annulus and connective tissue diseases such as Marfan's syndrome, Ehlers-Danlos syndrome, and pseudoxanthoma elasticum.[86-88] Papillary muscle dysfunction can result from coronary artery disease, infiltrative diseases, endocardial disorders, and inflammatory and myocardial diseases.[89-91] Several congenital heart diseases, such as

TABLE 39-1 Mechanisms of Chronic and Acute Mitral Regurgitation

1. Chronic mechanisms
   a. Rheumatic fever
   b. Mitral leaflet prolapse
   c. Coronary artery disease
   d. Left ventricular dilatation
   e. Calcified mitral annulus
   f. Heritable disorders of connective tissue
   g. Papillary muscle dysfunction
   h. Congenital heart disease
2. Acute mechanisms
   a. Rupture of chordae
   b. Rupture of papillary muscle
   c. Perforation of leaflet

corrected transposition of the great arteries, endocardial fibroelastosis, partial atrioventricular canal, and isolated cleft of the mitral leaflet, have associated mitral regurgitation.[92]

In acute mitral regurgitation, mechanisms involve rupture of the chordae, rupture of the papillary muscle, and perforation of the mitral valve leaflet. Ruptured chordae can result from bacterial endocarditis, mitral leaflet prolapse, trauma, and spontaneous rupture.[93,94] Papillary muscle rupture is most commonly produced by acute myocardial infarction, and perforation of the mitral valve is usually caused by bacterial endocarditis.

Therefore, etiologic mechanisms for mitral regurgitation include chronic and acute disorders as well as primary and secondary disturbances by diseases that affect the various components of the mitral apparatus.

Pathology

Mitral insufficiency may result from rheumatic endocarditis, bacterial endocarditis, myxomatous change, cardiomyopathy, failure, myocardial infarction, trauma, or undue restraint upon leaflets or chordae.[95,96]

Rheumatic Endocarditis

The same fundamental processes which result in rheumatic mitral stenosis may cause mitral insufficiency. The differences depend, in part, on fortuitous differences in physical orientation of the leaflets. Changes which tend to maintain the valve in a closed position cause mitral stenosis; those which cause the valve to be held open are associated with incompetence of the valve. The following structural patterns are found among cases of mitral insufficiency of rheumatic origin: (1) calcification of commissures (Fig. 39-8), (2) fibrous contracture of leaflet tissue, and (3) minor intrinsic valvular shortening with secondary distortion of the valve by the enlarged left atrium[97–98] (Fig. 39-9). The calcification which causes mitral insufficiency extends from one leaflet into the other across one or both of the commissures, keeping the two leaflets apart at the involved commissure or commissures. Fibrous contracture as a cause of mitral insufficiency is usually dominant at one commissure, but without fusion, shortening of valvular tissue is so great that the two leaflets cannot make complete contact.

Secondary distortion of the valvular tissue as a cause of major mitral insufficiency results from progressive enlargement of the left atrium from mitral insufficiency without commissural fusion. As the left atrium enlarges it causes the posterior leaflet to be displaced posteriorly. At the same time, the leaflet is restrained at the opposite end by the tensor apparatus. The result is that the posterior leaflet may lose its capacity to move as it becomes hamstrung over the base of the left ventricular wall. The pro-

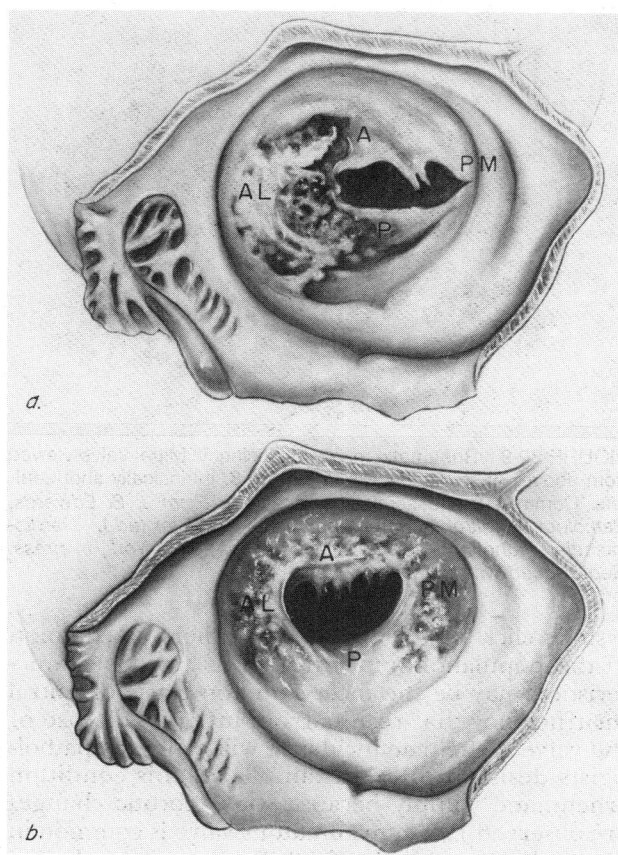

FIGURE 39-8 Anatomic types of rheumatic mitral insufficiency. Each unopened mitral valve viewed from above. In each, A = anterior, P = posterior leaflets of mitral valve, respectively; AL, PM = anterolateral and posteromedial commissures of mitral valve. a. Calcification and fusion of anterolateral commissure giving rise to the tear-drop type of mitral insufficiency. b. Calcification of the leaflets and commissures in continuity, yielding a wedding-ring type of mitral insufficiency. Some restriction of the orifice is present, but incompetence is predominant. [*From J. E. Edwards, Pathology of Mitral Incompetence, in M. D. Silver (ed.), "Cardiovascular Pathology," Churchill-Livingstone, New York, in press. Reproduced with permission.*]

gression leads to the situation wherein "mitral insufficiency begets mitral insufficiency."[99]

Bacterial Endocarditis (Fig. 39-10)

Bacterial endocarditis as a cause of mitral insufficiency is usually through its destructive effects leading to erosion or perforation of leaflets and/or rupture of chordae. Either of these processes may result from primary infection of the valve or secondarily from primary bacterial endocarditis of the aortic valve.[100] A less common cause of incompetence through bacterial endocarditis is through healing of those vegetations in the angle between the posterior leaflet and the left ventricular wall. This process results in immobilization of the posterior leaflet.[95]

Myxomatous Change (Figs. 39-11 through 39-14)

The myxomatous mitral valve, variously known as floppy or billowing valve and the mid- or mid-late

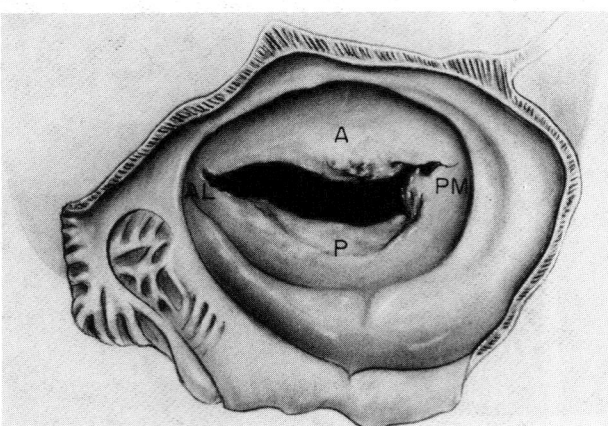

FIGURE 39-9   Rheumatic mitral insufficiency. Mitral valve viewed from above. Abbreviations as in Fig. 39-8. Intrinsically short leaflets. Commissures essentially unaffected. [*From J. E. Edwards, Pathology of Mitral Incompetence, in M. D. Silver (ed.), "Cardiovascular Pathology," Churchill-Livingstone, New York, in press. Reproduced with permission.*]

systolic click syndrome, among others, is common in the population and, through its various characteristics, may be the most common cause of mitral insufficiency that results from intrinsic disease of the valve. (The true incidence will evolve as pathologists desist in calling examples of this condition "rheumatic" simply because some fibrotic changes are observed.) The myxomatous valve is common in Marfan's syndrome, but in the vast majority of cases that syndrome is not identified.[101]

FIGURE 39-10   Healed bacterial endocarditis. Left side of heart shows major erosion of mitral valvular tissue and disappearance of many chordae.

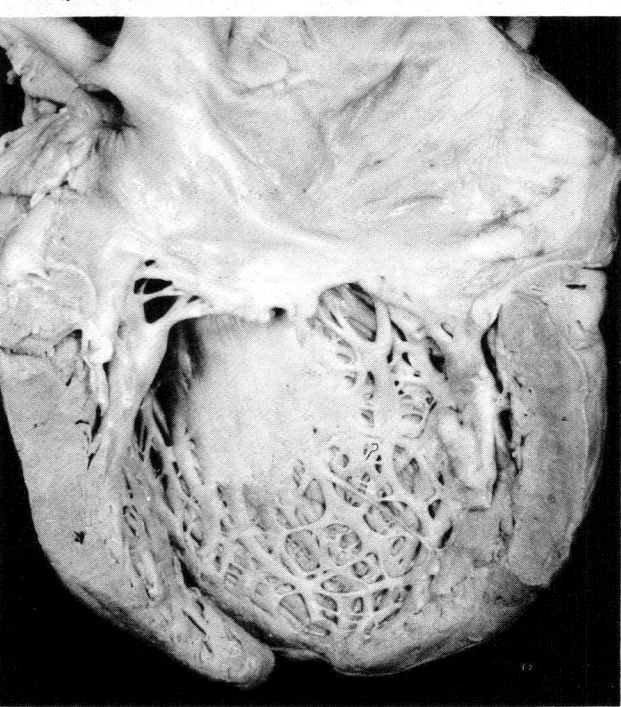

The basic process is an increase in size of the normally present mucinous layer of the valve, the so-called spongiosa[102] (Fig. 39-11). The mucinous layer invades and interrupts the continuity of the supporting fibrous layer of the leaflet, the fibrosa. From the resulting weakness of the leaflets, segments of the valve which lie between chordal insertions prolapse or hood abnormally toward the left atrium during ventricular systole. Part of the process of prolapse may result from weakness of chordae, which in some instances are elongated.

Secondary fibrotic changes of the leaflets occur in characteristic locations. There is fibroelastic thickening of the contact aspect of the leaflet. Fibrous tissue, predominantly collagenous, is deposited on the underaspect of prolapsing segments. The ultimate effect is that initially delicate, translucent leaflets may become opaque, thickened, and deformed[102] (Fig. 39-12). In spite of the fibrotic changes, the histologically identifiable intrinsic elements of the leaflet are maintained. This is one of the distinguishing characteristics from deforming rheumatic disease. Also, on gross examination there is no commissural fusion, a process common in the rheumatic valve. Elements of the posterior leaflet are more commonly involved than those of the anterior leaflet.[103]

A common secondary effect of myxomatous change of the mitral valve is fibrous deposits on the mural endocardium of the left ventricle as a response to friction by chordae[104] (Fig. 39-13). In some cases the fibrotic process may be extensive and result in incorporation of chordae into the fibrous tissue of the mural endocardium, as described by

FIGURE 39-11   Photomicrograph of posterior mitral leaflet from a 29-year-old man with myxomatous mitral valve. The spongiosa layer (S) is increased in thickness and invades and interrupts the fibrosa (F). There is fibrous thickening on the atrial aspect of the leaflet (A), as well as fibrous pad on the ventricular aspect under the fibrous layer. Elastic tissue stain; ×15. (*From R. G. Guthrie and J. E. Edwards, Pathology of the Myxomatous Mitral Valve. Nature, Secondary Changes and Complications, Minnesota Med., 59:637, 1976. Reproduced with permission.*)

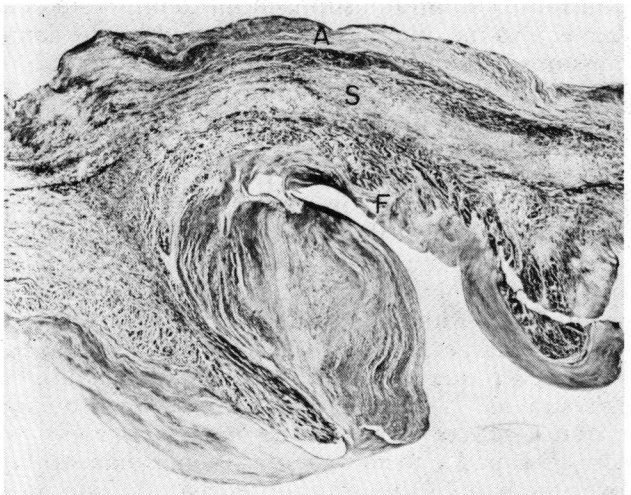

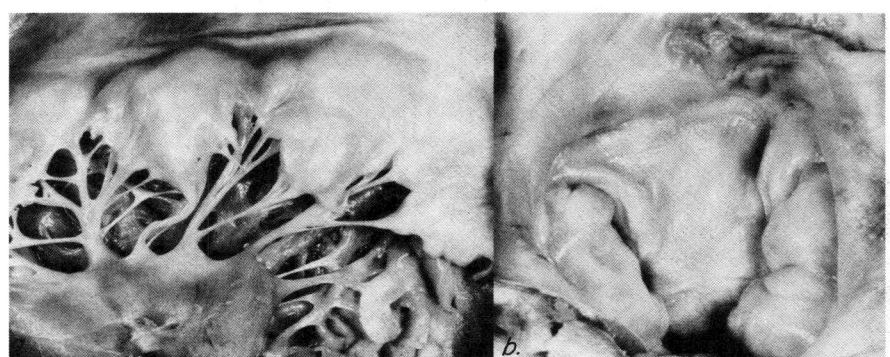

FIGURE 39-12 Photographs of the gross specimen from the case illustrated in Figure 39-11. *a.* The opened mitral valve shows characteristic interchordal hooding of the leaflets. *b.* The unopened mitral valve viewed from above showing unusual degrees of scalloping characteristic of the myxomatously altered mitral valve, the so-called floppy valve. (*From R. G. Guthrie and J. E. Edwards, Pathology of the Myxomatous Mitral Valve. Nature, Secondary Changes and Complications, Minnesota Med., 59:637, 1976. Reproduced with permission.*)

Salazar and Edwards.[104] If this happens, the effective length of the chorda becomes reduced.

In the uncomplicated state the myxomatous mitral valve is usually, but not universally, competent. In most cases of mitral insufficiency occurring in the myxomatous valve, the incompetence results from a complication of this process, such as bacterial endocarditis and, most commonly, noninfected "spontaneous" rupture of chordae (Fig. 39-14). It is now widely accepted that the usual basis for spontaneous rupture of the mitral chordae (to be distinguished from rupture of a papillary muscle) is the myxomatous valve.[102–105] When chordae rupture, the ones most commonly involved are those inserting into the central scallop of the posterior leaflet.

Cardiomyopathy

Even in the presence of a structurally normal mitral valve, incompetence may result from left ventricular failure for any reason, including congestive cardiomyopathy. The mechanical factors leading to the valvular malfunction include enlargement of the valvular orifice and distortion of the alignment of the tensor apparatus.[99] The primary form of the dilated type of endocardial fibroelastosis is comparable to the congestive cardiomyopathies in regard to its cause of mitral insufficiency.[106]

Obstructive cardiomyopathy (muscular subaortic stenosis) may be associated with mitral insufficiency. This is probably caused by the systolic anterior motion of the anterior mitral leaflet that occurs in this condition (see section on subaortic stenosis). The anatomic counterpart is fibrous thickening of the mural endocardium of the septal wall of the left ventricular outflow tract. Such thickening results from injury by contact of the anterior mitral leaflet with the mural endocardium.

Myocardial Infarction

Myocardial infarction may underlie mitral insufficiency in one of several ways, namely, (1) dilatation of the left ventricle in cases of extensive healed myocardial infarction (so-called ischemic congestive cardiomyopathy), (2) rupture of a papillary muscle complicating acute myocardial infarction, and (3) infarction of a nonruptured papillary muscle.

Rupture of a papillary muscle involves the posteromedial set of muscles more commonly than the anterior set by a ratio of 4:1.[107] The intensity of mitral insufficiency resulting from rupture of a papillary muscle depends upon whether an entire set or only isolated heads are involved.[108]

Infarction of a nonruptured papillary muscle with mitral insufficiency is usually associated with infarction of the adjacent free wall of the left ventricle (Fig. 39-15). According to clinical and experimental evidence, incompetence of the valve depends not only upon intrinsic dysfunction of the papillary muscle but also upon distortion of the papillary muscular function by asynergic contraction of the related free wall.[109]

Trauma

A traumatic cause of mitral insufficiency is through rupture of a papillary muscle. It is extremely rare that traumatic rupture of a papillary muscle is an

FIGURE 39-13 Left atrium and left ventricle in a case of myxomatous alteration of the mitral valve in a patient with Marfan's syndrome. Friction lesions upon the left ventricular endocardium have caused incorporation and functional shortening of the related chordae of the posterior mitral leaflet. (*From A. E. Salazar and J. E. Edwards, Friction Lesions of Ventricular Endocardium. Relation to Chordae Tendineae of Mitral Valve, Arch. Path., 90:364, 1970. Reproduced with permission.*)

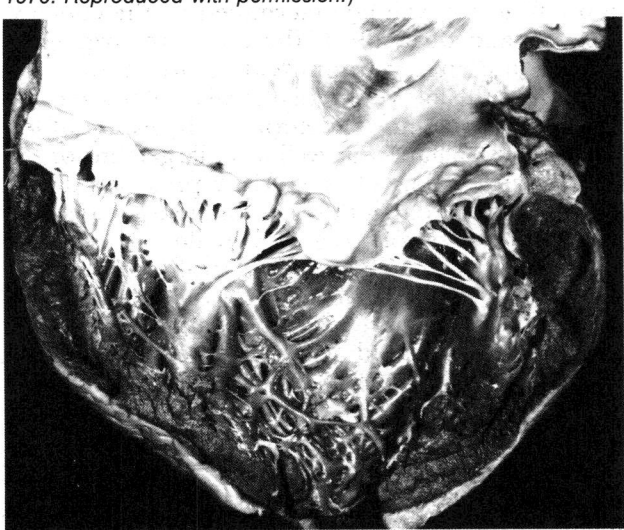

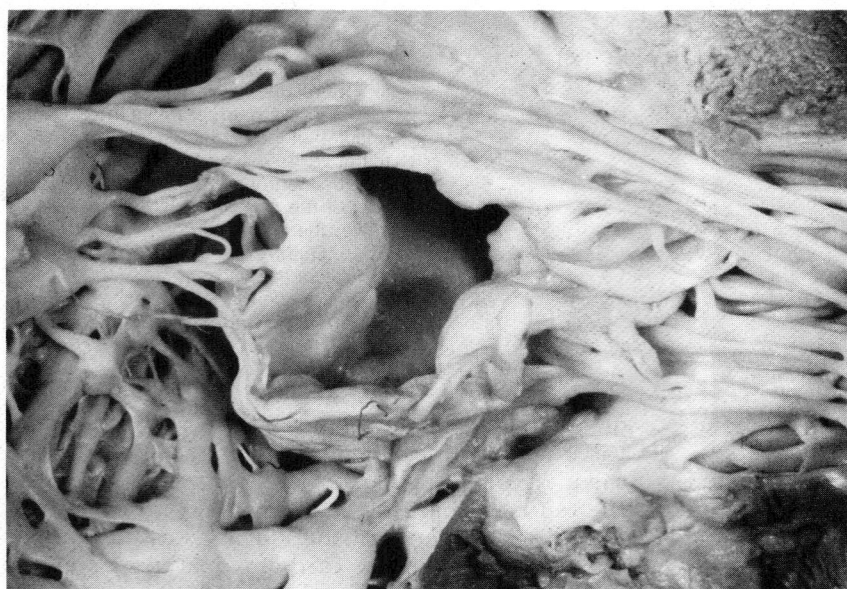

FIGURE 39-14 Myxomatous alteration of mitral valve with rupture of chordae to the posterior leaflet. The unopened mitral valve viewed from below. The central part of the posterior leaflet (lower center) shows fragments of ruptured chordae. The intact chordae are elongated and the leaflet tissue as seen through the orifice shows some prolapse and fibrous thickening as evidence of a preexisting myxomatous state. [*From J. E. Edwards, Pathology of Mitral Incompetence, in M. D. Silver (ed.), "Cardiovascular Pathology," Churchill-Livingstone, New York, in press. Reproduced with permission.*]

isolated cardiac injury. Accompanying lesions often are rupture of the ventricular septum and/or the wall of a chamber.

Undue Restraint upon Leaflets or Chordae

Undue restraint upon leaflets or chordae is a cause of mitral insufficiency. Most of the conditions contributing to this process have been covered in foregoing parts of this section (bacterial endocarditis and myxomatous mitral valve with extensive friction lesions). Among conditions not mentioned are Loeffler's endomyocardial fibrosis and lupus erythematosus.[110,111] In either of these conditions, but

FIGURE 39-15 Healed myocardial infarction involving the inferior wall of the left ventricle and related papillary muscles. The latter are atropic on the basis of coexistent infarction.

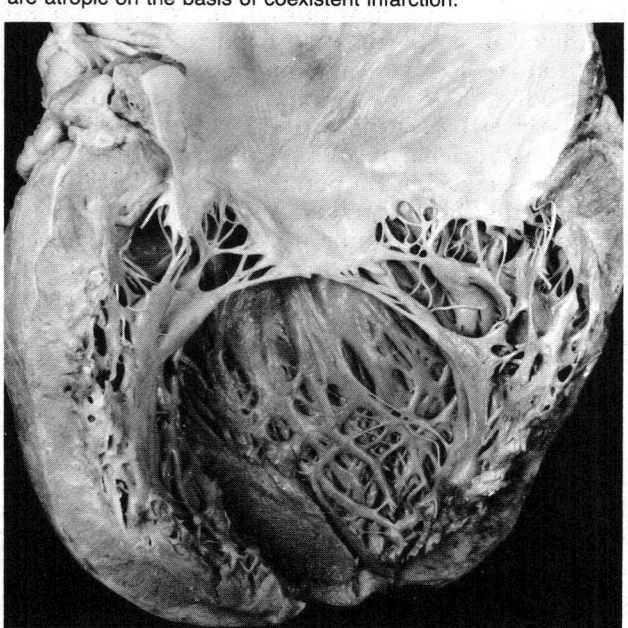

more commonly in the former, the posterior mitral leaflet may become immobilized by its adhesions to the left ventricular endocardium.

Calcification of the Mitral Ring

Calcification of the mitral ring is a common state in the elderly, particularly in the elderly female.[112] In the majority of instances it does not cause recognizable valvular dysfunction. When valvular malfunction results it usually takes the form of incompetence. This results from adhesions of the posterior mitral leaflet to the calcific mass (Fig. 39-16).

Abnormal Physiology

The basic mechanical abnormality producing mitral regurgitation is improper coaptation of the mitral leaflets during the systolic ejection phase. The hemodynamic burden imposed on the left ventricle and left atrium will be determined by the etiology, severity, and duration of the mitral regurgitation. In chronic rheumatic mitral regurgitation the amount of the left ventricular stroke volume ejected into the left atrium will determine the extent of left ventricular dilatation as well as enlargement of the left atrium.[113] The characteristic pressure abnormality in the left atrium is a prominent v wave produced by the systolic regurgitant flow of blood.[114] Although chronic rheumatic mitral regurgitation produces a volume overload on the left ventricle and left atrium, there will be elevation of pressure in the left atrium and pulmonary venous and capillary vessels. The compensatory mechanism to the volume-overloaded left ventricle in mitral regurgitation is dilatation of the chamber to accommodate the increase in left ventricular stroke volume and hypertrophy of the ventricular myocardium to maintain mechanical function.[115,116] The extent of

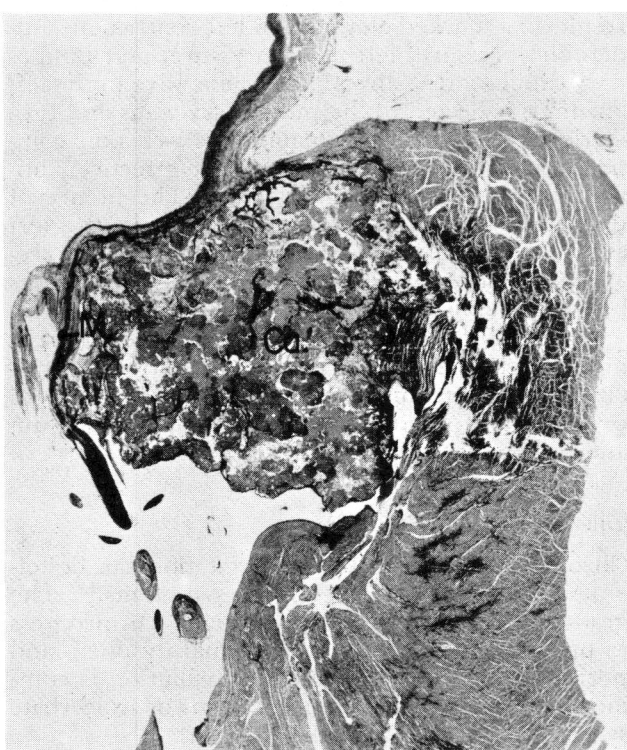

FIGURE 39-16 Calcification of mitral ring. Low-power photomicrograph showing calcific mass (Ca) at the junction of the left atrium and left ventricle. The posterior mitral leaflet (M) is in part adherent to the calcified mass, a process leading to its immobilization. Elastic tissue stain; ×4.

the increase in left ventricular wall thickness is determined by wall force or stress, and the myocardium hypertrophies in order to normalize systolic wall stress.[117] Furthermore, the compliance, or elastic properties, of the left ventricle and atrium increases in chronic mitral regurgitation, and pulmonary venous pressures are not elevated to the extreme degree encountered in mitral stenosis.

The increase in diastolic filling of the left ventricle in chronic mitral regurgitation is composed of the normal systolic output of the right ventricle plus the amount of blood regurgitated into the left atrium and pulmonary venous bed during the previous cardiac cycle (Fig. 39-17). This regurgitant volume is the basis for the volume overload on the left ventricle, and the v wave and elastic recoil of the left atrium contribute to the rapid early diastolic filling of the ventricle.[118] The augmentation of elastic properties of the left ventricle permits rapid diastolic filling from the increased volume without significant hemodynamic abnormalities. Normalization of the filling rate in patients with mitral regurgitation has shown that the protodiastolic gallop sound possesses the same hemodynamic characteristics as the physiological third sound in a young patient with a normal heart size.[119] Thus, the third heart sound in significant mitral regurgitation may not carry the same significance as impaired ventricular function under other conditions. The increased

ventricular compliance also results in minimal elevation of the left ventricular end-diastolic pressure in chronic mitral regurgitation. Left ventricular end-diastolic pressure may be only mildly elevated or sometimes retained within the normal range.[120] The systolic regurgitation of blood into the pulmonary venous bed is often tolerated without severe elevation of the pulmonary capillary or arterial pressure, and the lack of severe pulmonary hypertension in mitral regurgitation is in contrast to that encountered in pure mitral stenosis.

In the mitral leaflet prolapse syndrome the anatomic changes in the valve and abnormalities in ventricular wall motion can influence the degree of mitral regurgitation.[121,122] Anatomic abnormalities in the valve consist of thinning of the leaflet, elongation of the chordae, and excessive valve tissue, and sometimes there is dilatation of the mitral annulus.[123] The systolic click results from the abrupt deceleration of blood beneath the prolapsed leaflet and possible increased tension on the chordae. Abnormal systolic contraction patterns of the ventricle include hyperkinesis of localized areas, hypokinesis, akinesis, and cavity obliteration.[122,124] Despite these disturbances in left ventricular contraction, the end-diastolic pressure, volume, and mass are usually normal. Other pathophysiological mechanisms include myocardial ischemia, coronary spasm, and neurogenic mechanisms. A possible role of ischemia is suggested by a history of chest pain, arrhythmias, and electrocardiographic abnormalities. Mitral valve

FIGURE 39-17 Pressure-volume diagram in a patient with mitral regurgitation. There is a loss of the isovolumic contraction phase on the right side of the pressure-volume loop due to the mitral valve incompetence, and the early diastolic filling is initiated by the 40 mmHg v wave in the left atrium. [From C. E. Rackley, Value of Ventriculography in Cardiac Function and Diagnosis, in N. O. Fowler, M.D. (ed.), "Diagnostic Methods in Cardiology," F. A. Davis, Philadelphia, 1975, p. 283. Reproduced with permission.]

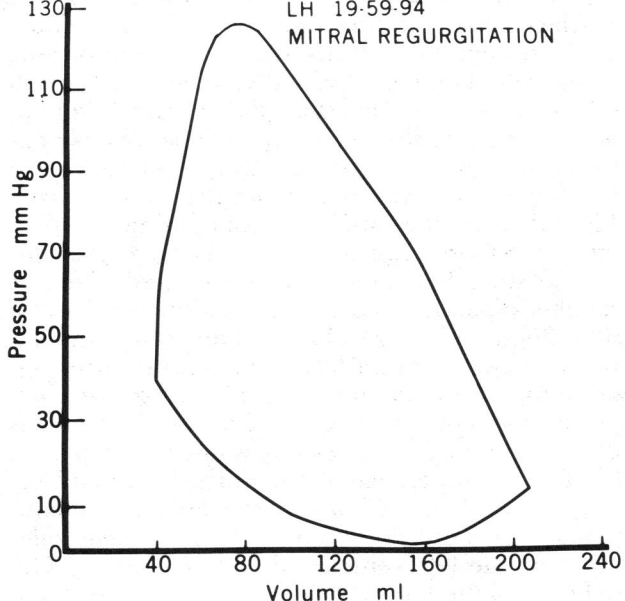

prolapse is a frequent finding in patients with angiographically documented coronary artery disease.[125,126] However, the low incidence of positive ergonovine tests suggests coronary spasm is not a mechanism for the pain or wall motion abnormalities.[127] Neurogenic mechanisms may play a role in mitral valve function and the genesis of arrhythmias.[128] Of the anatomic wall motion, perfusion, coronary artery, and neurogenic mechanisms in mitral leaflet prolapse, the abnormality of leaflet position appears most related to the degree of mitral regurgitation.

Mitral regurgitation in coronary artery disease can result from impaired papillary muscle function, abnormal ventricular wall motion, and significant dilatation of the ventricular chamber. In coronary artery disease significant mitral regurgitation requires a combination of abnormal posterior wall motion as well as dysfunction of the papillary muscle.[84] Lesions in the circumflex and right coronary arteries are most frequently associated with significant mitral regurgitation. After myocardial infarction an abnormally contracting segment greater than 17 percent will result in chronic dilatation of the left ventricle.[129] Only with rupture of a papillary muscle can mitral regurgitation be solely ascribed to this anatomic structure. In chronic coronary artery disease secondary mitral regurgitation due to dilatation of the ventricle will occur when the end-diastolic volume has dilated the left ventricle more than 50 percent of the normal value. Thus, several mechanisms are involved in the development of mitral regurgitation in coronary artery disease.

Significant dilatation of the left ventricle secondary to any extrinsic or intrinsic impairment of ventricular function can eventually lead to secondary mitral regurgitation.[85] Volume overload due to valvular incompetence as well as depression of the myocardial contractile state will eventually result in significant dilatation, downward displacement of the papillary muscle, and prevention of coarctation during systolic ejection. Primary myocardial disorders, ischemic cardiomyopathy, and volume overload will ultimately cause mitral regurgitation. In addition to the dilatation of the left ventricle in secondary mitral regurgitation, there may also be alterations in the shape of the ventricle from the characteristic ellipsoid to a more spheroid configuration, which can create more regurgitation.[116] Thus, as the contractile state becomes more depressed, further chamber dilatation and change to a spherical shape will influence the regurgitant volume across the mitral valve. Acute mitral regurgitation produces significantly different hemodynamic disturbances than the chronic type, since the valvular incompetence is often imposed on a previously normal ventricle. Sudden incompetence of the mitral valve and regurgitation of blood into the left atrium and pulmonary veins are not attended by immediate dilatation of the left ventricle or left atrium.[130] The inability of the left ventricle and atrium to dilate results in a marked elevation in left ventricular end-diastolic pressure, left atrial pressure, and pulmonary capillary pressure. The large v wave in the left atrium is reflected to the pulmonary veins and capillaries. Left ventricular dilatation is a chronic compensatory mechanism and cannot be effectively utilized in acute mitral regurgitation. The failure of dilatation and increased compliance in the left atrium to accommodate the regurgitant volume creates a pressure overload on the pulmonary venous bed and results in acute pulmonary edema.

Thus, the physiological mechanisms are different in the various etiologies of chronic mitral regurgitation, and acute mitral regurgitation produces both pressure and volume overload on the left atrium and pulmonary veins.

Clinical Manifestations

Chronic rheumatic mitral regurgitation can be tolerated for years without cardiac symptoms.[131] The gradual onset of dyspnea and fatigue can progress to orthopnea, paroxysmal nocturnal dyspnea, and peripheral edema.[132,133] Atrial fibrillation is common and may present as palpitations or exacerbate symptoms of left ventricular failure.

The symptoms in the mitral leaflet prolapse syndrome are most frequently palpitations, chest discomfort, fatigue, and anxiety.[121] Approximately 50 percent of the patients complain of palpitations, yet long-term monitoring may not confirm these complaints.[134] Atypical chest pain occurs in from one-third to one-half of patients, and occasionally is indistinguishable from angina pectoris. Fatigue, anxiety, and other psychological complaints are often present. The patients are female in more than two-thirds of instances.[83] Familial incidence can be striking in some individuals.

Mitral regurgitation encountered in coronary artery disease usually is attended by the typical symptoms of angina pectoris or with an acute myocardial infarction.[90,135] In chronic coronary artery disease with significant dilatation and depression of ventricular function, sometimes referred to as ischemic cardiomyopathy, symptoms are dyspnea, fatigue, orthopnea, and fluid retention. Chest pain may be minimal or absent in this stage of coronary artery disease.

In mitral regurgitation secondary to dilatation of the left ventricle, symptoms are those of left ventricular failure and consist of dyspnea, fatigue, orthopnea, and peripheral fluid retention. Systemic emboli from the left ventricle can create symptoms from the site of lodging.

In acute mitral regurgitation regardless of the mechanism of chordal or papillary muscle rupture or leaflet perforation, the symptoms are those of congestive heart failure or acute pulmonary edema. Rarely, the patient may experience minimal symptoms or even be asymptomatic with acute mitral regurgitation.

Therefore, symptoms in chronic mitral regurgitation may develop late in the course of the disease and are most commonly fatigue and dyspnea. Palpitations and chest pain suggest nonrheumatic forms of mitral regurgitation. Acute mitral regurgitation often presents as pulmonary edema.

Physical Examination

In rheumatic mitral regurgitation the vital signs may be normal, reveal atrial fibrillation, or reflect the changes in heart rate and respiration if left ventricular failure has developed. Atrial fibrillation frequently develops in the course of left atrial dilatation, but the chronic volume overload may be tolerated for long periods before development of heart failure and symptoms. Therefore, heart rate and blood pressure remain normal in many patients. With the development of failure of the right side of the heart secondary to left ventricular decompensation, the neck veins become distended. Pulmonary rales indicate left ventricular failure has developed.

Examination of the heart in chronic mitral regurgitation will generally reveal displacement of the apical impulse laterally due to dilatation, and there may be a hyperdynamic movement over a diffuse area. On palpation a lifting hyperdynamic apical impulse can be appreciated, but vibrations of the murmur will not be felt. Lateral to the left sternal border in the third interspace, systolic expansion of the left atrium can sometimes be palpated.[136] This lift is slightly more delayed than that of right ventricular hypertrophy and collapses more rapidly in systole.

The characteristic murmur of mitral regurgitation is a high-pitched systolic murmur that is typically holosystolic, beginning with the first sound and extending to the second sound at the apex.[137] The intensity is usually constant throughout the systolic ejection period, but variations can occur in early, mid, or late systole. The murmur usually radiates into the axilla and may radiate over the aortic outflow area. The murmur of rheumatic mitral regurgitation does not vary significantly during the respiratory cycle or with the variation of cardiac cycles in atrial fibrillation.[138]

The first heart sound is diminished in most cases of chronic mitral regurgitation.[139] The duration of systole may be shortened and result in the second sound occurring before pulmonary valve closure. This can produce a persistent expiratory splitting of the aortic and pulmonary components.[140] An early diastolic sound is frequently heard in mitral regurgitation and is most often the protodiastolic or ventricular gallop. Rarely an opening snap can be appreciated in pure mitral regurgitation.[139] If the mitral regurgitant murmur is harsh, suggesting a large regurgitant volume, the protodiastolic sound may occur with normal ventricular function.[119] However, in most instances of mitral regurgitation with a grade II murmur or less, the ventricular gallop sound indicates depressed left ventricular function. Sometimes, vibrations follow the gallop sound and indicate a flow rumble across the mitral valve.[141] Accentuation of the pulmonary second sound suggests pulmonary hypertension, which usually occurs with a right ventricular lift. The systolic murmur of tricuspid regurgitation can be audible at the left sternal border in right ventricular failure secondary to left ventricular decompensation. The murmur of tricuspid regurgitation is accentuated with inspiration and diminishes with expiration, whereas the mitral regurgitation murmur often remains unchanged during the respiratory cycle. The remaining physical findings in chronic mitral regurgitation depend on the development of chronic right ventricular failure. The amplitude of the peripheral pulse in long-standing mitral regurgitation is often reduced when heart failure has developed, and pulsus alternans may be detected. Additional findings with failure of the right side of the heart include hepatic enlargement, ascites, and peripheral edema.

In the mitral leaflet prolapse syndrome, additional features on physical examination involve anomalies of the chest wall, abnormalities in the precordial impulse, and the auscultatory complex of systolic click and late systolic murmur.[142] Patients are frequently asthenic and the majority are female. Vital signs do not reveal abnormalities. The chest wall may be thin with a decreased anteroposterior diameter; other chest wall abnormalities include pectus excavatum, scoliosis, and kyphosis. An abnormal apical impulse may sometimes be palpated with a systolic retraction or dip synchronous with the systolic click.[143] However, such findings are infrequent in the large number of patients with this disorder. The characteristic auscultatory findings are the systolic click, which may occur in early, mid-, or late systole, and the late systolic murmur[83,121,142,144] (Fig. 39-18). The systolic murmur can be holosystolic in about 10 percent of patients and there may be a crescendo pattern of the murmur up to the second sound. These auscultatory features of the prolapse leaflet syndrome can be influenced by changes in posture and physiological maneuvers, and by pharmacological agents to alter blood pressure.[145] Frequently the click or murmur may not be heard in the recumbent position but be brought out with standing (Fig. 39-19). Also, the click alone may be heard without the murmur, and physiological maneuvers may then bring out the late systolic murmur. Any maneuver which reduces the chamber size of the left ventricle will migrate the click and the onset of the murmur closer to the first sound earlier in systole. Likewise, the click and the murmur will occur later if ventricular cavity size is increased. Elevation of the systolic blood pressure will intensify the late systolic murmur, and reduction in the blood pressure will reduce the sound.

Mitral regurgitation murmurs associated with coronary artery disease may present in the patient without pain, during an episode of angina pectoris,

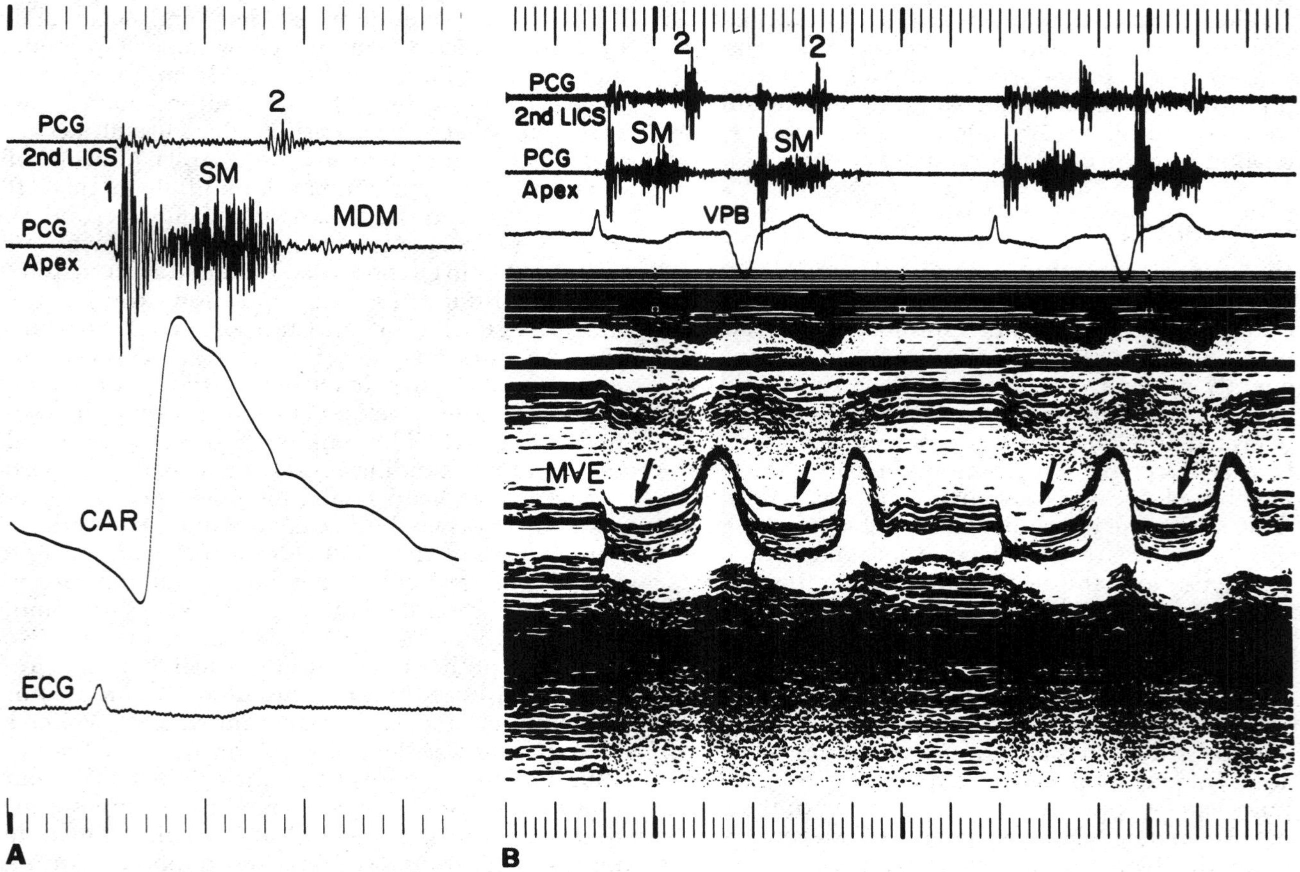

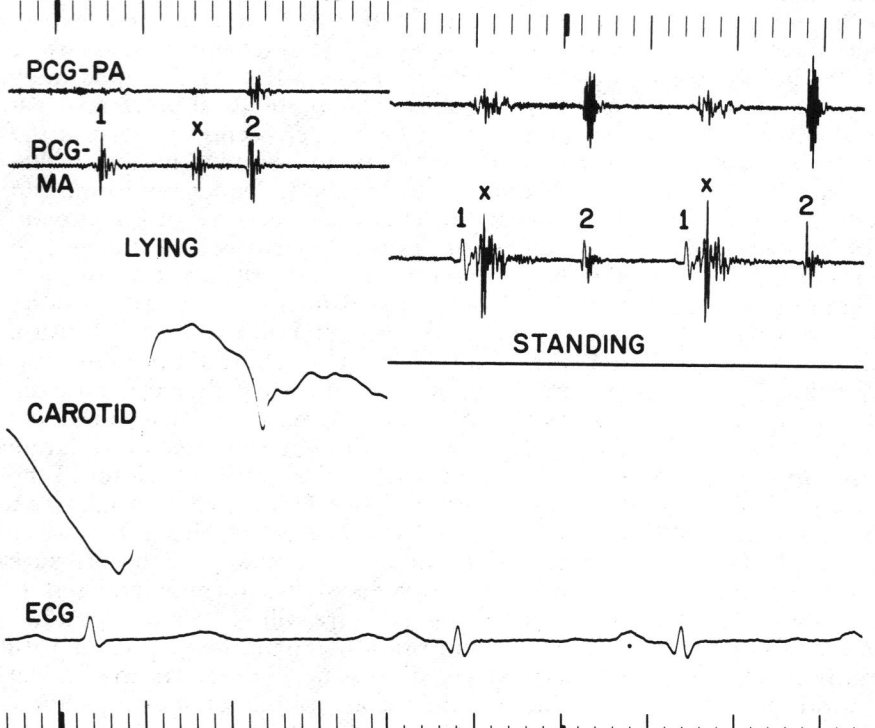

FIGURE 39-18 Mitral valve prolapse. *A.* The phonocardiogram demonstrates an intense high-frequency pansystolic murmur with accentuation in late systole. There is also a minimal middiastolic murmur (MDM). *B.* The echocardiogram demonstrates the hammock-shaped appearance of the valve leaflets (arrows), which coincide with the pansystolic murmur. The rhythm is atrial fibrillation with bigeminy. (*Courtesy of Dr. Ernest Craige.*)

FIGURE 39-19 Mitral valve prolapse. A late systolic click (x) moves to a position early in systole with standing. (*Courtesy of Dr. Ernest Craige.*)

with acute infarction, and in severe left ventricular failure.[85,90,135] The precordial findings may be unremarkable unless the ventricle has dilated, and then a sustained diffuse impulse can be appreciated. The mitral regurgitant murmur may occur in early, mid-, or late systole or be holosystolic with coronary artery disease.[146,147] Atrial gallops are common when the murmur of mitral regurgitation is caused by coronary artery disease. A ventricular gallop indicates significant depression of the mechanical function of the left ventricle. A ventricular gallop can be audible during an episode of angina, with acute infarction, or in chronic left ventricular failure. Finally, significant dilatation of the left ventricle is a result of myocardial scarring, and segmental contraction abnormalities can result in mitral regurgitation from left ventricular dilatation.

Mitral regurgitation can develop secondary to any condition producing significant dilatation of the ventricular chamber. Volume overload from aortic regurgitation, coronary artery disease with loss of contracting myocardium, and diffuse myocardial disease can create a degree of mitral regurgitation. Since the dilatation may occur as a result of reduction of the inotropic state of the ventricular myocardium, a ventricular gallop often accompanies secondary dilatation. The remaining causes of mitral regurgitation, such as connective tissue disorders, calcified mitral annulus, and congenital heart disease, produce murmurs that are holosystolic at the apex.

Acute mitral regurgitation produces characteristic findings on physical examination quite different from those observed in chronic mitral regurgitation.[148,149] Many of these patients present with acute pulmonary edema, and vital signs will reveal tachycardia, increased respiratory rate, and sometimes a fall in blood pressure. The neck veins may be significantly distended if the overload on the pulmonary vascular system has depressed right ventricular function. Pulmonary rales are diffuse. The precordial examination reveals a normal heart size with a hyperactive apical motion. A systolic thrill is often palpated at the apex. Rarely a thrill can be appreciated over the primary aortic area if the posterior leaflet has prolapsed with anterior direction of the regurgitant jet.[150] The murmur is extremely harsh, holosystolic, and heard not only at the apex but over the entire precordium with radiation into the axilla, back, and along the left sternal border. Rarely, such murmurs have even radiated to the top of the head.[151] An atrial gallop may be audible and a ventricular gallop is frequently present. Usually with the tachycardia only a summation gallop can be appreciated. The striking physical findings due to rupture of the chordae, papillary muscle, or perforation of the valve leaflet are in sharp contrast to the transient systolic murmur of myocardial ischemia in coronary artery disease. The mechanism of this murmur has been ascribed to papillary muscle dysfunction or decreased ventricular wall motion. If myocardial infarction is complicated by rupture of a papillary muscle, the systolic murmur becomes much harsher.

Chest Roentgenogram

In rheumatic mitral regurgitation left ventricular and left atrial enlargement is frequently present.[132] Left ventricular dilatation is suggested by apical displacement on the posterior-anterior view. The left atrium can attain enormous proportions and enlarge the left atrial appendage along the left cardiac border. Elevation of the left main stem bronchus can result from atrial enlargement, which appears as a double density along the right cardiac border.[152] Changes in the pulmonary venous pattern also develop with upper lobe shunting. However, these changes are not as marked as those seen in mitral stenosis, and in some instances the pulmonary vascular pattern may appear normal. On cardiac fluoroscopy calcium may be detected in the region of the mitral valve, but valvular calcification does not distinguish between mitral regurgitation and mitral stenosis. With severe mitral regurgitation, systolic pulsations can be detectable in the left atrium.

In the mitral leaflet prolapse syndrome the cardiac silhouette is usually normal, and the only abnormality may be the reduced posterior-anterior diameter of the chest.[153,154] In mitral regurgitation secondary to coronary artery disease, heart size can range from normal to dilatation of both the left ventricle and left atrium. Calcium can also be detected in the coronary arteries on fluoroscopy.

When mitral regurgitation is secondary to left ventricular dilatation due to extrinsic or intrinsic myocardial overloads, the left ventricular chamber is significantly dilated, and the left atrium may be enlarged as well. In mitral regurgitation secondary to calcification of the annulus, there will be prominence of the calcification even on the plain chest film and, at fluoroscopy, motion of the atrioventricular groove is apparent.

In acute mitral regurgitation the chest roentgenogram will often show pulmonary edema and a normal cardiac silhouette.[90,91] Disruption of the mitral valve apparatus often occurs with previously normal ventricular function.

Electrocardiogram

In chronic mitral regurgitation the electrocardiogram usually exhibits evidence of left ventricular and left atrial enlargement. If the patient remains in sinus rhythm atrial enlargement will be suggested by the prominent P terminal force in lead V_1.[155] In atrial fibrillation, atrial enlargement often is suggested by a coarse fibrillatory pattern.[156] The QRS voltage criteria for hypertrophy indicate left ventricular chamber enlargement, and right ventricular hypertrophy is much less common in mitral regurgitation than in mitral stenosis.

The mitral leaflet prolapse syndrome electrocardiographic abnormalities are frequent and manifest by ST-T wave changes, QT prolongation, and rhythm disturbances in both the atria and ventricles.

However, the most common abnormality is T-wave negativity in the inferior leads, and the ST segment may be slightly depressed as well.[121] QT-interval prolongation has been described, but no relationship exists to the syndrome of congenital deafness, arrhythmias, and sudden death.[157] Arrhythmias are frequently present on the resting electrocardiogram.[134,158] No relationship has been established between the severity of the prolapse and mitral regurgitation, systolic clicks, and ST-T segment abnormalities. One-third of patients have resting rhythm disturbances on the electrocardiogram, and ambulatory monitoring has documented premature ventricular contractions in 60 percent of these patients.[158] Rhythm disturbances include sinus arrhythmias, sinus arrest, atrial fibrillation, premature ventricular contractions, and ventricular tachycardia.

If coronary artery disease is the underlying mechanism in the production of mitral regurgitation, the electrocardiogram will often exhibit characteristic changes in the ST-T waves or Q-wave abnormalities of a previous myocardial infarction. Earlier descriptions of the papillary muscle dysfunction syndrome emphasized depression of the J junction and associated ST changes, but these are considered nonspecific ischemic manifestations which may occur with left ventricular hypertrophy, conduction defects, and digitalis.[159]

Mitral regurgitation due to significant dilatation of the left ventricle is usually associated with electrocardiographic voltage criteria and secondary ST-T wave changes of left ventricular hypertrophy. Diseases that may produce an infiltrative type of cardiomyopathy such as amyloid may exhibit loss of precordial R waves similar to an anterior infarction pattern.

In acute mitral regurgitation the electrocardiogram may display the changes of acute myocardial infarction, and in this situation inferior wall infarctions are more frequent than anterior infarctions.[90]

Special Laboratory Studies

Echocardiogram In chronic mitral regurgitation the echocardiogram can record the increased dimensions of the left ventricle and the left atrium. Increased systolic excursion of the posterior wall can be seen, but quantification of the mitral regurgitation is limited by this technique (Fig. 39-20).

One of the most significant contributions of echocardiography in mitral regurgitation is the recognition of the mitral leaflet prolapse syndrome[160-162] (Fig. 39-18). However, false-positive interpretation of the echocardiogram can result from improper positioning of the transducer and analysis of an artifact simulating mitral valve prolapse. The specific features of mitral leaflet prolapse include early to midsystolic posterior motion of the mitral leaflet or holosystolic prolapse of the leaflet. These deviations of the mitral leaflet are related to the C and D line of the mitral valve echo, which is produced by the systolic motion of the mitral apparatus. However, there are some suggestive features which are not necessarily specific for mitral valve prolapse. These include sagging of the mitral leaflets during systole, multiple echoes parallel to the mitral leaflet, and exaggerated leaflet mobility. Finally, echocardiographic mitral leaflet prolapse has been reported in

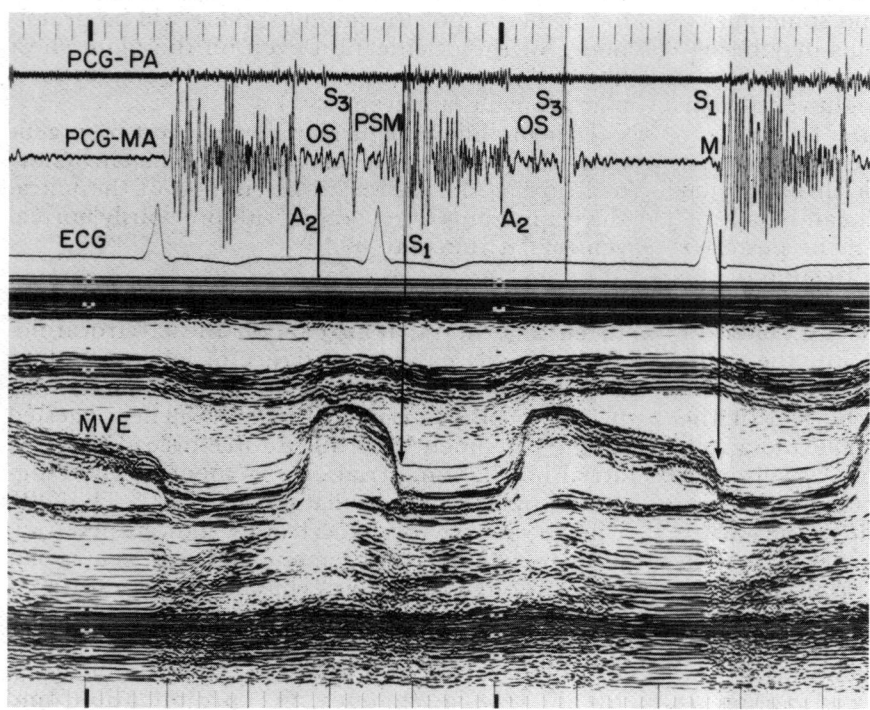

FIGURE 39-20 Phonocardiogram and echocardiogram in a patient with rheumatic heart disease, mitral regurgitation and stenosis, and atrial fibrillation. The echocardiogram is consistent with mitral stenosis. However, the pansystolic murmur is due to mitral regurgitation. There is a prominent presystolic murmur (PSM) after the short diastole but none following the longer diastoles. Cardiac catheterization in 1968 showed moderate mitral regurgitation but no stenosis. Repeat catheterization in 1978 showed severe mitral regurgitation, and mean left atrial pressure 28 mmHg and a *v* wave of 42 mmHg. (*Courtesy of Dr. Ernest Craige.*)

approximately 10 percent of patients in the absence of auscultatory abnormalities.[35]

In mitral regurgitation due to coronary artery disease, M-mode echocardiography is limited to detection of posterior wall motion abnormalities which may be involved in the mechanism of mitral regurgitation.[163] However, additional segment abnormalities in the ventricular contractile pattern cannot be reliably detected by the single-beam M-mode method. The two-dimensional echocardiogram can scan the ventricle for recognition of segmental changes.

In mitral regurgitation associated with diffuse left ventricular chamber enlargement, the echocardiogram can document increased diastolic dimensions and decreased systolic wall motion, indicating depression of the mechanical performance. Mitral valve motion can also be assessed in the dilated ventricle.

In acute mitral regurgitation the echocardiogram can detect several abnormal features which have been attributed to ruptured chordae or papillary muscle or perforated valve leaflet.[164] These findings include increased motion of the interventricular septum and posterior wall, increased diastolic excursion of the mitral valve, redundant systolic echoes, abnormal echoes at the level of the mitral valve representative of the flail chordae, systolic atrial expansion, systolic prolapse of the mitral leaflets, and, finally, densities on the mitral valve which may represent vegetative lesions.

Cardiac Catheterization Cardiac catheterization in mitral regurgitation is performed to confirm the diagnosis of mitral regurgitation and to assess ventricular function. In addition, catheterization techniques can identify certain etiologic mechanisms, recognize additional cardiac lesions and abnormalities, and evaluate coronary artery anatomy. Mitral regurgitation is demonstrated at catheterization by the injection of contrast material into the left ventricle and observing systolic regurgitation of the dye into the left atrium. However, direct injection into the left ventricle can be attended by ventricular irritability, and premature contractions of the ventricle may introduce spurious regurgitation into the left atrium.

Left ventricular function can be evaluated by measurement of the left ventricular end-diastolic pressure, quantitation of the mitral regurgitation, and calculation of the ejection fraction[116] (Fig. 39-21). Quantitative angiocardiography permits accurate assessment of mitral regurgitation from the determination of angiographic left ventricular stroke volume, which is obtained as the difference between end-diastolic volume and the end-systolic volume (Fig. 39-22). Forward stroke volume measured by the Fick or indicator dilution technique can be subtracted from the angiographic left ventricular stroke volume to yield the regurgitant volume per beat into the left atrium.[165] This calculation of mitral regur-

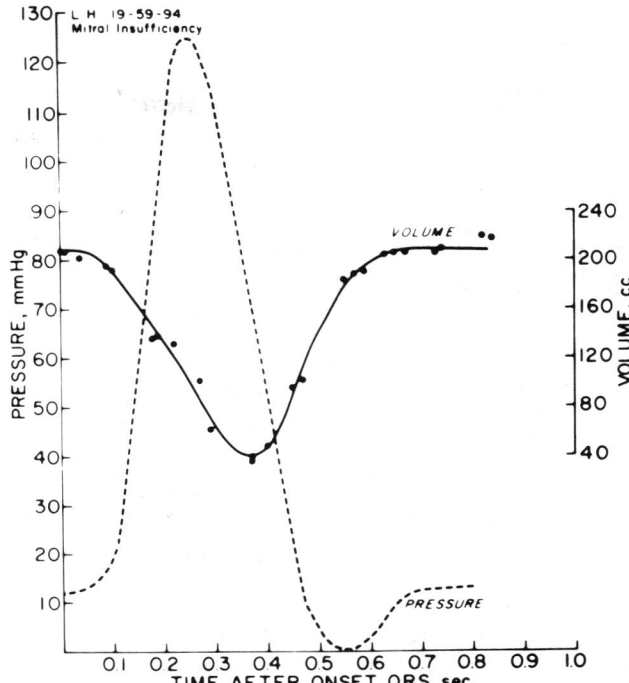

FIGURE 39-21 Left ventricular pressure and volume in a patient with mitral regurgitation. End-diastolic volume = 208; end-systolic volume = 42; left ventricular stroke volume = 166; forward stroke volume = 30; regurgitant stroke volume = 136; ejection fraction = 166/208 = 0.80; left ventricular weight in grams = 247; and left ventricular end-diastolic pressure = 14.

gitation assumes there is no regurgitation across the aortic valve. The ejection fraction is the relationship of the total left ventricular stroke volume to the end-diastolic volume. Although the end-diastolic volume may be significantly increased in chronic mitral regurgitation, the ejection fraction remains within or near the normal range until severe myocardial depression develops. At this advanced stage, further elevation of the ventricular end-diastolic pressure and left atrial pressure will be reflected to the pulmonary vasculature with increased pulmonary capillary and arterial pressures.[131,132] Rarely, severe mitral regurgitation and a giant left atrium can develop, with a normal left ventricular end-diastolic and left atrial pressure due to increased compliance of the ventricle and atrium.[166]

Quantitative angiographic techniques also permit calculation of left ventricular mass, which is a measure of hypertrophy of the ventricle.[167] From the Laplace relationship and measurements of chamber pressure, volume, and ventricular wall thickness, force or stress within the ventricular wall can be calculated throughout the cardiac cycle. Calculation of wall stress at end-diastole is equal to the preload of the ventricle, and wall stress calculation at the time of aortic valve opening is afterload.[120] These measurements of wall stress can be used to select the optimal time for mitral valve replacement and to predict the postoperative response.[168]

In the mitral leaflet prolapse syndrome the ma-

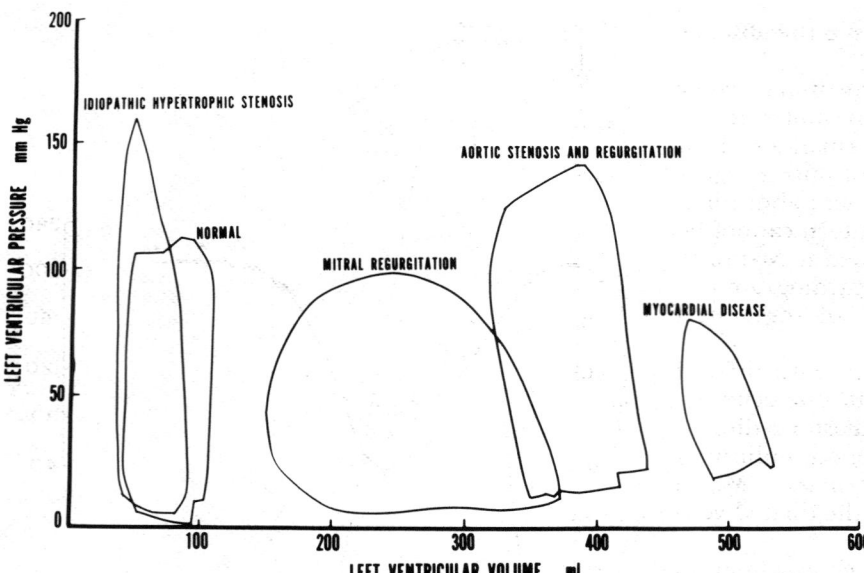

FIGURE 39-22 Pressure-volume diagrams for a normal subject and patients with idiopathic hypertrophic subaortic stenosis, mitral regurgitation, aortic stenosis and insufficiency, and a cardiomyopathy. Mitral regurgitation is present in all cardiac disease states as illustrated by loss of the isovolumic contraction phase. [*From C. E. Rackley, Value of Ventriculography in Cardiac Function and Diagnosis, in N. O. Fowler, M.D. (ed.), "Diagnostic Methods in Cardiology," F. A. Davis, Philadelphia, 1975, p. 283. Reproduced with permission.*]

jority of patients reveal normal hemodynamic measurements and minimal mitral regurgitation.[122,169] Left ventricular angiography from the right anterior oblique position provides an optimal view of the mitral apparatus for detection of mitral regurgitation and the prolapse scallops of the posterior leaflet. For the less common anterior leaflet prolapse, the left anterior oblique view is necessary. Contraction abnormalities of the left ventricle can also be assessed from the ventriculogram, but mitral leaflet prolapse commonly occurs without any detectable abnormalities in left ventricular contraction.[122,124,169] Coronary arteriography should be performed, since patients with mitral prolapse may have coronary artery disease, and, conversely, mitral prolapse is frequently observed in coronary artery disease, which probably illustrates a chance association between two common diseases.[121,125,126,169] Rarely, prolapse of the tricuspid valve can be demonstrated angiographically and can occur with an apparently normal mitral valve.

At catheterization in coronary artery disease, mitral regurgitation will frequently be demonstrated, but this is often minimal and cannot be clearly related to specific wall motion abnormalities or chamber dilatation (Fig. 39-23). In left ventricular failure from coronary artery disease, dilatation of the chamber alone can produce significant mitral regurgitation.[84] Wall motion abnormalities, particularly at the base of the papillary muscle, may play a role in mitral regurgitation.

In significant left ventricular dilatation due to either extrinsic volume overload or myocardial failure, secondary mitral regurgitation can develop (Fig. 39-24). There is slight enlargement of the left atrium, but the amount of mitral regurgitation is only mild to moderate.

In acute mitral regurgitation, left ventricular angiography will reveal massive regurgitation into the left atrium and pulmonary veins. Contraction of the previously normal left ventricle is vigorous, with systolic regurgitation into the left atrium and pulmonary veins.[130] Left ventricular end-diastolic pressure may be severely elevated with a large *v* wave in the left atrium that can be recorded from the pulmonary capillary wedge position. The Swan-Ganz catheter can be utilized clinically to confirm mitral regurgitation with papillary muscle rupture.[170] Occasionally the large *v* wave will not be detected from the pulmonary wedge position, and rupture of the ventricular septum must be excluded by comparing the oxygen content of blood samples from the right atrium and pulmonary artery.

Radionuclide Studies Radionuclide techniques can measure the ejection fraction in both the left and right ventricles of patients with mitral regurgitation. Scintigraphic techniques have been developed which provide estimates of left ventricular end-diastolic and systolic volumes in human beings.[171,172] Values for ejection fraction and ventricular volume at rest and during exercise can be obtained and radionuclide techniques can be repeated in the course of follow-up. Preliminary observations suggest that these radionuclide techniques can quantitate the amount of mitral regurgitation. Since coronary artery disease may be present in adult forms of mitral regurgitation, myocardial perfusion studies with selected radionuclides can identify areas of abnormal perfusion during exercise and at rest.

Other Studies Exercise testing can evaluate the functional reserve and assess symptoms in chronic mitral regurgitation. This can be useful, since significant left ventricular dilatation can develop in chronic mitral regurgitation without symptoms of pulmonary congestion. Documentation of a decline in exercise tolerance may provide information on

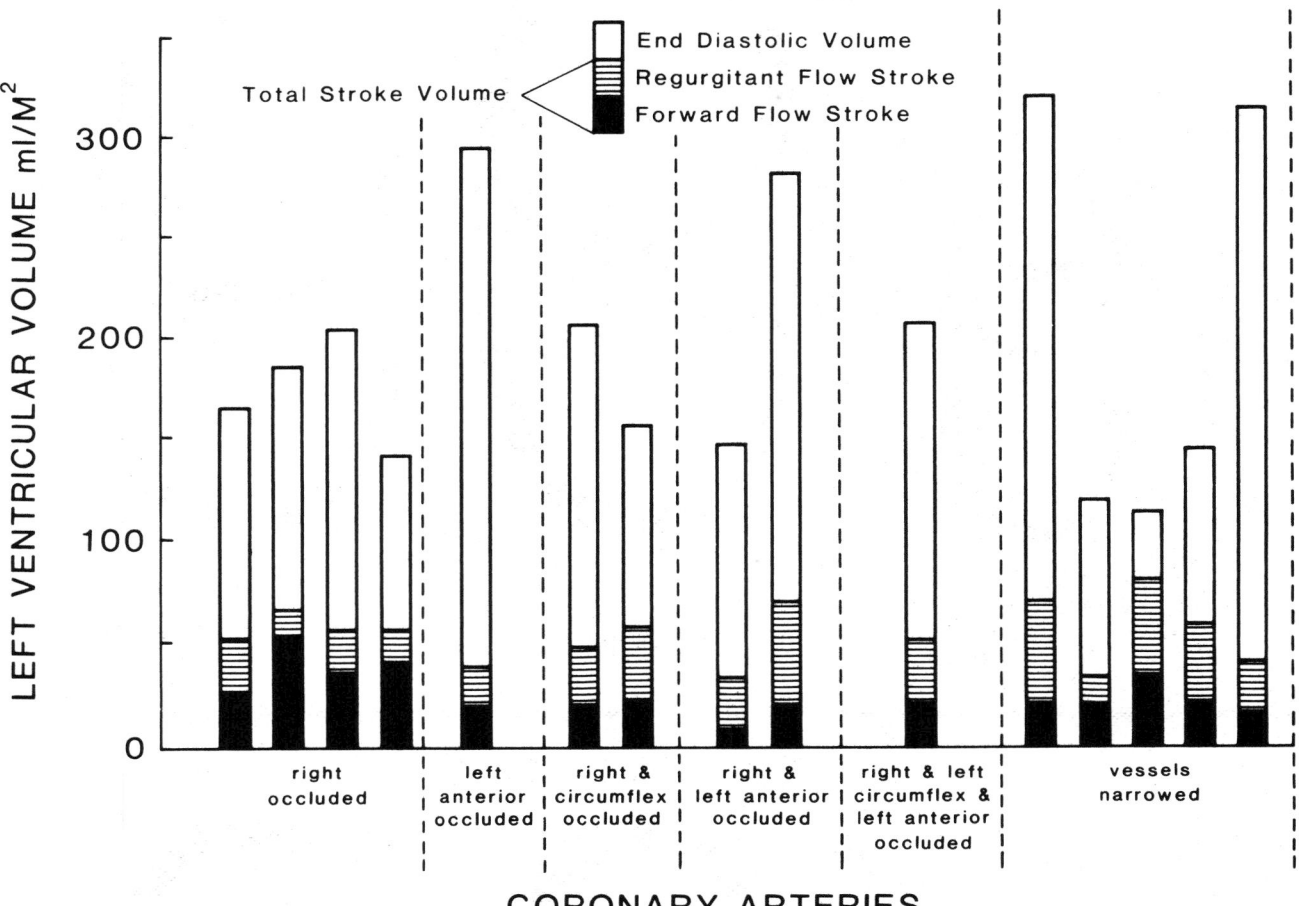

FIGURE 39-23 The left ventricular volume and coronary lesions in patients with mitral regurgitation. The total height of the bar is the end-diastolic volume, and the solid and slashed portion is the total left ventricular stroke volume. The mitral regurgitant stroke volume is indicated by the slashed area. (*From C. E. Rackley, H. D. Dear, W. A. Baxley, W. B. Jones, and H. T. Dodge, Left Ventricular Chamber Volume, Mass and Function in Severe Coronary Artery Disease, Circulation, 41:605, 1970. Reproduced with permission.*)

early deterioration of left ventricular performance. Since chest discomfort is unusual in chronic rheumatic mitral regurgitation, yet frequent in mitral valve prolapse, the possibility of underlying coronary artery disease can be further assessed with exercise stress testing.

Holter monitoring can be employed to document the presence and frequency of arrhythmias in mitral regurgitation and is particularly useful in the mitral leaflet prolapse syndrome.[158] Atrial and ventricular arrhythmias may occur in mitral valve prolapse more frequently than patients sometime recognize, and monitoring can provide the basis for therapeutic intervention and response.

Natural History and Prognosis

The history and prognosis of patients with mitral regurgitation will depend on the etiologic mechanism and left ventricular function.[131] In rheumatic mitral regurgitation the volume overload and compliant changes allow the patient to enjoy many years before development of left ventricular failure and

symptoms of pulmonary congestion. However, when the contractile state of the ventricular myocardium deteriorates, elevation of the left ventricular filling pressure will be reflected to the pulmonary capillaries with the eventual development of dyspnea, orthopnea, and pulmonary edema. There is a tendency in the course of chronic mitral regurgitation and left atrial enlargement to develop atrial fibrillation, which can be further complicated by systemic emboli.[155] However, embolization is less frequent in mitral regurgitation than in mitral stenosis.[133] Patients remain susceptible to endocarditis on the mitral valve, which can aggravate valvular incompetence and lead to acute mitral regurgitation with severe heart failure. Survival of patients with chronic mitral regurgitation treated medically has been shown to be similar to those with mitral stenosis. In a study of randomly selected patients 80 percent were alive at 5 years and 60 percent survived 10 years.[71]

Since detection of the mitral leaflet prolapse syndrome has increased due to the widespread use of echocardiography, the majority of individuals dis-

END-DIASTOLE

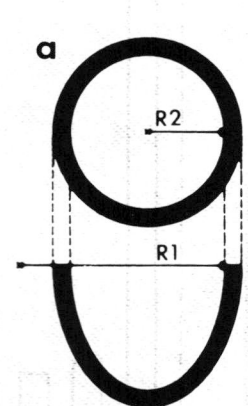
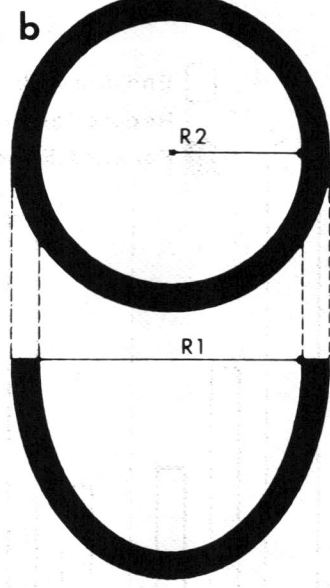
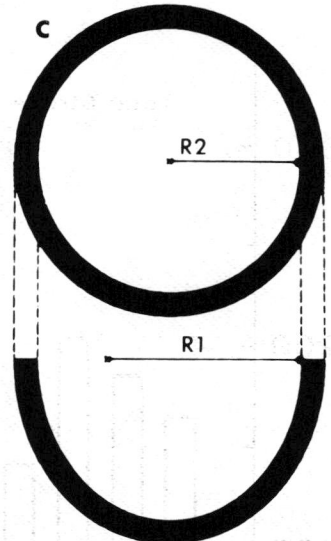

PATIENT I.D.
EDV =130. ML.   R1 =7.34 CM.
ESV = 42. ML.   R2 =2.77 CM.
E.F =0.67   R2/R1=0.37

PATIENT J.J.
EDV =616. ML.   R1 =10.11 CM.
ESV =262. ML.   R2 =4.79 CM.
E.F.=0.57   R2/R1=0.47

PATIENT L.C.
EDV =533. ML.   R1 =7.15 CM.
ESV =467. ML.   R2 =4.85 CM.
E.F.= 0.12   R2/R1=0.67

END-SYSTOLE

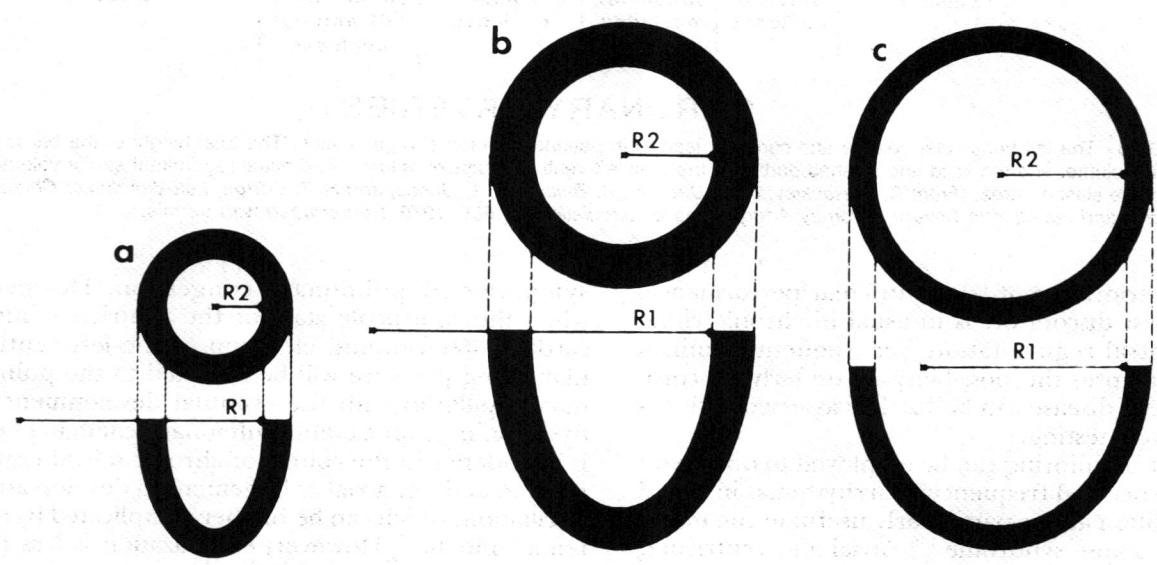

PATIENT I.D.
EDV =130. ML.   R1 =8.73 CM.
ESV = 42. ML.   R2 =1.75 CM.
E.F.=0.67   R2/R1=0.20

PATIENT J.J.
EDV =616. ML.   R1 =12.29 CM.
ESV =262. ML.   R2 = 3.29 CM.
E.F.=0.57   R2/R1= 0.26

PATIENT L.C.
EDV =533. ML.   R1 =7.38 CM.
ESV =487. ML.   R2 =4.57 CM.
E.F.=0.12   R2/R1=0.61

FIGURE 39-24 Exact-scale dimensions for cross-sections and longitudinal sections of the left ventricle in (a) a normal subject, (b) a patient with severe mitral regurgitation, and (c) a patient with decompensated volume overload. The patient with mitral regurgitation and preservation of mechanical performance maintains the ellipsoid configuration in diastole and systole with diastolic and systolic ratios of radii (R2/R1) similar to the normal subject. A more spherical configuration is apparent in diastole and systole in the patient with decompensated volume overload. In this patient the ejection fraction is extremely depressed, and the ratio of radii is approaching that of a sphere. EDV = end-diastolic volume; ESV = end-systolic volume; EF = ejection fraction; R1 and R2 are the radii of curvature. (From C. E. Rackley and W. P. Hood, Jr., Quantitative Angiographic Evaluation and Pathophysiologic Mechanisms in Valvular Heart Disease, Prog. Cardiovasc. Dis., 15:427, 1973. Reproduced with permission.)

covered with this entity are asymptomatic. Chest pain and palpitations cannot be related to any anatomical abnormalities, even when mitral leaflet prolapse is demonstrated. Thus, the prognosis is unusually good in the majority of patients with mitral valve prolapse, but sudden death, endocarditis, spontaneous rupture of chordae, and progressive mitral regurgitation are rare complications. In several series of patients with mitral prolapse, sudden death was recorded in 4 out of 387 patients.[142] Of valve replacements for isolated mitral regurgitation, 5 to 10 percent are for redundant mitral leaflets. However, fatigue, dyspnea, and other psychological complaints can be limiting and even disabling in some patients with mitral leaflet prolapse.

In mitral regurgitation due to coronary artery disease the course is usually determined by the extent of anatomic involvement of the coronary arteries and the state of left ventricular performance. Multivessel disease with depressed ejection fraction carries an increased yearly mortality in coronary artery disease, and this is probably independent of the presence or absence of secondary mitral regurgitation. Events are usually sudden death or acute myocardial infarction.

In conditions producing secondary mitral regurgitation, ventricular dilatation and heart failure are usually progressive and are the major determinants in the clinical course and prognosis.

In acute mitral regurgitation, regardless of the mechanism and structure disrupted in the mitral apparatus, the course is most frequently acute pulmonary edema and sometimes cardiogenic shock. These complications naturally carry a very high mortality, usually exceeding 60 to 80 percent. Rarely, a patient with ruptured chordae may not develop symptoms and continue normal activities for months or years before developing left ventricular failure.

Management

Medical

In chronic rheumatic mitral regurgitation prophylaxis for rheumatic fever and bacterial endocarditis are indicated. Atrial fibrillation requires control of the ventricular response with digitalis. If the left atrium is not enlarged significantly, thought should be given to cardioversion. Fatigue, dyspnea, and orthopnea suggest impairment of left ventricular function and are treated with digitalis and diuretics. However, it must be remembered that chronic mitral regurgitation is a form of high-output left ventricular failure, since total left ventricular output may be considerably higher than the normal forward cardiac output. Thus, optimal treatment requires correction of the mechanical defect, which is the mitral valve, and not the failing myocardium. Preload and afterload reducing agents have been used in the treatment of mitral regurgitation and other forms of chronic heart failure. Long-acting

nitrates and vasodilating agents such as hydralazine and prazosin have demonstrated hemodynamic improvement and symptomatic benefit.[168,173,174]

An important consideration in the management of patients with rheumatic mitral regurgitation is the optimal time for surgical replacement with a prosthetic valve. Ideally, surgery should be performed before clinical evidence of left ventricular failure. Echocardiographic left ventricular dimensions and radionuclide estimates of end-diastolic volume and ejection fraction may demonstrate significant dilatation and increased end-diastolic volume before clinical symtoms develop.[168] Exercise testing may further detect a decline in ejection fraction. Therefore, these measurements can assist the physician in advising prosthetic valve replacement before severe depression of myocardial contractility has developed.

In the mitral leaflet prolapse syndrome the majority of patients are asymptomatic and merely need reassurance. In those with palpitations, propranolol has been found to be particularly effective, but the evidence is not sufficient at present to recommend routine treatment of asymptomatic ectopic beats. In patients with chest pain as a primary symptom, even when coronary anatomy has been found to be normal, nitrates and propranolol may be required. Preliminary studies have shown that some of the rhythm disturbances and complaints respond to barbiturates through a central nervous system mechanism.[128]

Mitral regurgitation in coronary artery disease does not require specific treatment nor is there evidence at present to advocate prophylaxis for bacterial endocarditis. If heart failure has developed, digitalis, diuretics, and vasodilators are employed. Hydralazine has been shown to reduce the mitral regurgitation in both ischemic heart disease as well as nonischemic forms. If coronary artery bypass surgery is performed, the decision can be made during the operation to replace the mitral valve.

In mitral regurgitation due to ventricular dilatation, therapy is directed at the clinical heart failure with digitalis, diuretics, and vasodilating agents. Less common forms of mitral regurgitation such as calcification of the annulus and disorders of connective tissue do not require specific treatment unless heart failure develops, and then standard therapeutic measures are in order.

In the preoperative management of patients with mitral regurgitation there should be optimal control of cardiac rhythm, ventricular response, serum electrolytes, and blood-clotting mechanisms. Digitalis may be necessary to control the ventricular response in chronic atrial fibrillation, but this drug may be withheld immediately prior to cardiac surgery. Diuretics can be discontinued prior to surgery since blood volume will be adequately controlled during surgery, and hypovolemia is more of an anesthetic problem than a small degree of volume overload. Electrolytes, particularly potassium, should be maintained in the normal range. Anticoagulants should be discontinued several days before surgery, and if necessary intravenous heparin can be used if there has been recent embolus. Any elective surgery or dental work should be completed before cardiac surgery, since this will eliminate future sources for bacterial endocarditis.

Surgery

Presently, there are two areas of very active discussion relative to surgery for mitral valve incompetence. The first is consideration of earlier operation to improve hospital mortality and lengthen long-term survival. Creating a competent mitral valve in a patient with severe mitral valve incompetence significantly increases left ventricular wall stress and myocardial oxygen consumption, and may decrease ejection fraction. The presumed mechanism for this is an abrupt change in resistance to ejection. In fact, there are two resistances in parallel in a patient with mitral incompetence; one, the usual impedance imposed by systemic arterial resistance, and the second, the factor associated with retrograde ejection through the incompetent mitral valve into a compliant left atrium. The mathematical characterization of two resistances in parallel suggests that following operative elimination of the low-resistance circuit (i.e., retrograde ejection), there is imposed a greater impedance to left ventricular ejection.[175,176] In cases where the mitral incompetence has been allowed to progress, restoration of mitral valve competency may cause the volume overloaded ventricle to face a marked increase in impedance and wall stress. Indexes of contractility such as ejection fraction may drop, and left ventricular failure characterized early by low cardiac output and late by the congestive heart failure syndrome may supervene.[177]

The second consideration is associated with renewed interest in reconstructive rather than valve replacement procedures for a large number of patients with mitral valve incompetence. Pure rheumatic mitral valve incompetence, or incompetence associated with a floppy or myxomatous valve mild to moderate in severity, may be well tolerated for a long time. The onset of more severe symptoms may be associated with rupture of chordae tendineae, or a head of a papillary muscle, or increasing mitral annular dilatation, or left ventricular dysfunction. The natural history of medically treated rheumatic mitral incompetence is similar to that for mitral stenosis or aortic valve incompetence. The long-term survival of patients operated upon with mitral valve incompetence is very significantly related to their preoperative functional class, which to some degree is determined by the state of the left ventricular myocardium. Thus, it has been suggested that earlier operation would be appropriate in patients with mitral valve incompetence, particularly in those where a reconstructive procedure is feasible.[178]

Surgical Treatment A reparative procedure is done whenever the pathological condition of the valve permits it. Examples are some cases of myxomatous degeneration, some cases secondary to ischemic heart disease, those cases where a combination of commissurotomy and annuloplasty can be done for mixed mitral stenosis and incompetence, and some cases where there is a degenerative process localized to a portion of one or the other mitral leaflets. Reparative procedures have the advantage of avoiding the long-term risk of devices used to replace the mitral valve and the need for long-term anticoagulant therapy inherent in many of them. Disadvantages of a reparative procedure include some lack of certainty that total competence will be established and the difficulty in knowing before starting the repair whether sufficient valvular competence can be established to avoid valve replacement. We employ valve repair (rather than replacement) in about 20 percent of patients with pure incompetence.

Carpentier and his associates have made major contributions to the treatment of mitral incompetence by reparative techniques. Their careful studies of the pathology of mitral incompetence have generated various procedures required for its care. Like others,[179] Carpentier has stressed that annuloplasty is the basic technique required for most patients in whom mitral incompetence is repaired. Rather than a narrowing procedure, this is a plastic reconstruction of the leaflets and the annulus, using multiple-point fixation to a flexible ring (Fig. 39-25). Procedures on the leaflets themselves are indicated in certain circumstances, particularly in ruptured chordae to the central portion of the posterior leaflet, wherein one uses a quadrangular excision of that portion of the leaflet and combines it with ring annuloplasty (Fig. 39-26). Less frequently, in some lesions involving the anterior leaflet, similar excisions can be used, and occasionally a solitary perforation of either leaflet from bacterial endocarditis can be repaired.

Calcification and immobility of the leaflets are indications for replacement. Replacement of the mitral valve is required in cases of rheumatic involvement leading to severe mitral incompetence, mitral stenosis with loss of pliability of the leaflets, and various other causes of mitral incompetence, such as infective endocarditis and some cases of ischemic heart disease. Also, in occasional situations associated with idiopathic hypertrophic subaortic stenosis mitral valve replacement is needed for relief of left ventricular outflow tract obstruction or associated severe mitral regurgitation.

Surgical Technique The general technique for the operation is the same as described for mitral commissurotomy. The mitral valve is exposed after cooling the heart, cross-clamping the aorta, and introducing cold potassium cardioplegic solution. The valve is excised, taking care to leave sufficient residual valvular tissue for valve seating, and replacement is done inserting the device using either interrupted suture or continuous monofilament suture (Fig. 39-27). If there is associated coronary artery

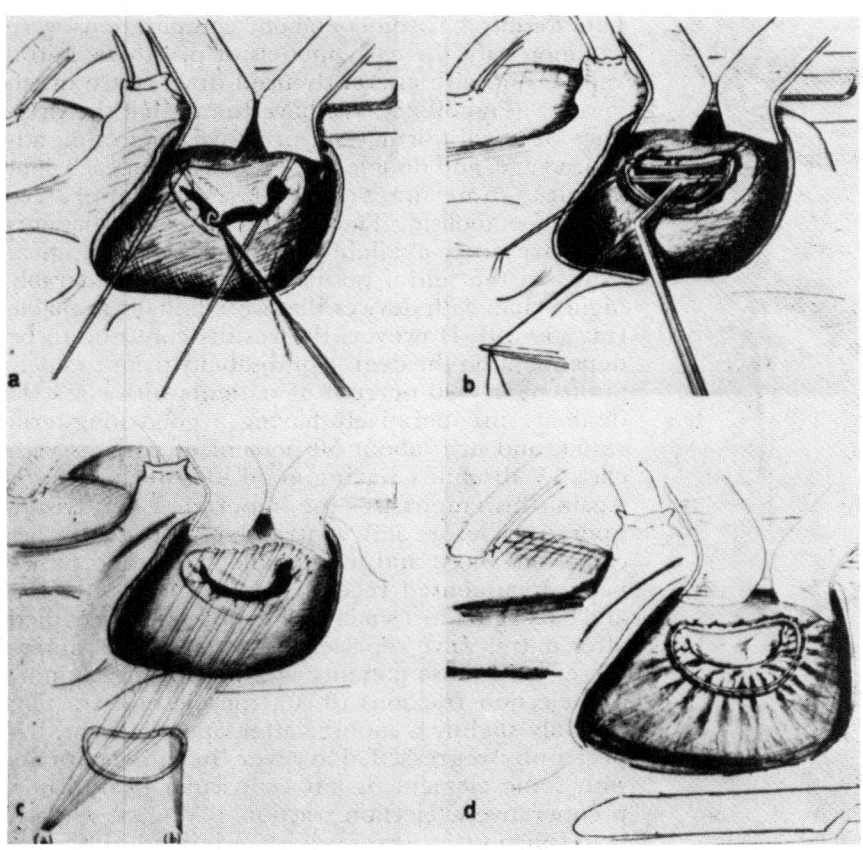

FIGURE 39-25 Repair of mitral insufficiency using the Carpentier ring for remodeling of the mitral annulus. [*From A. Carpentier, Plastic and Reconstructive Mitral Valve Surgery, in D. Kalmanson (ed.), "The Mitral Valve: A Pluridisciplinary Approach," Publishing Sciences Group, Inc., Littleton, Mass., 1976, p. 257. Reproduced with permission.*]

disease, saphenous vein grafts are used to bypass the obstructive lesion.

The Device A number of artificial and biological devices have been used to replace the mitral valve. Since most of those presently in use have been in patients for less than 10 years, the final evaluation of each is not yet possible. Most are durable and have given good long-term results. At present, unless anticoagulants are strongly contraindicated for the patient in question, we favor the Bjork-Shiley tilting disk valve prosthesis with a pyrolite occluder (Fig. 39-27). Long-term anticoagulant therapy is required. With less than optimal anticoagulation therapy, episodes of thromboembolism and occasionally thrombosis of the device have been reported (see below).

When anticoagulation therapy is contraindicated or particularly undesirable, as in children, young adult females, patients over 70 years old, or persons with a history of bleeding peptic ulcer disease, an alternative is the glutaraldehyde-preserved, stent-mounted porcine aortic valve xenograft. In contrast to the Bjork-Shiley prosthetic device there is some question as to the long-term durability of the biological devices, and the orifice size is not as large in relation to outside diameter as in the disk prosthesis. The incidence of thromboembolism has been low, but not totally absent. In some patients in whom there is chronic atrial fibrillation, anticoagulation

therapy may be indicated on that basis alone; thus the xenograft loses its advantage.

There have been equally good results with the Starr-Edwards silastic ball valve series 6300, the Lillehi-Caster tilting disk valve, and recently with the SJM bileaflet prosthesis. Although a further period of evaluation is necessary for all of these replacement devices, they certainly are superior to those available 10 years ago. Therefore, there is some reason to move forward in the natural history of an individual patient and recommend valve replacement sooner.

Hospital Morbidity and Mortality The risk of mitral valve replacement is related to the clinical condition of the patient prior to operation. In our experience, as of several years ago the risk of mitral valve replacement in patients with mitral incompetence was greater than that in patients with mitral stenosis or in the mixed lesion.[180,181] At the present time, the operative mortality seems very nearly similar in each group and is about 3 percent. In an experience with open operations in general for mitral valve disease, including replacement, the hospital risk has been zero for patients in New York Heart Association class II, 1.3 percent for patients in class III, but 24 percent in patients with advanced disability associated with New York Heart Association class IV. Morbidity in surviving patients is modest. Early thromboembolic complications are rare.

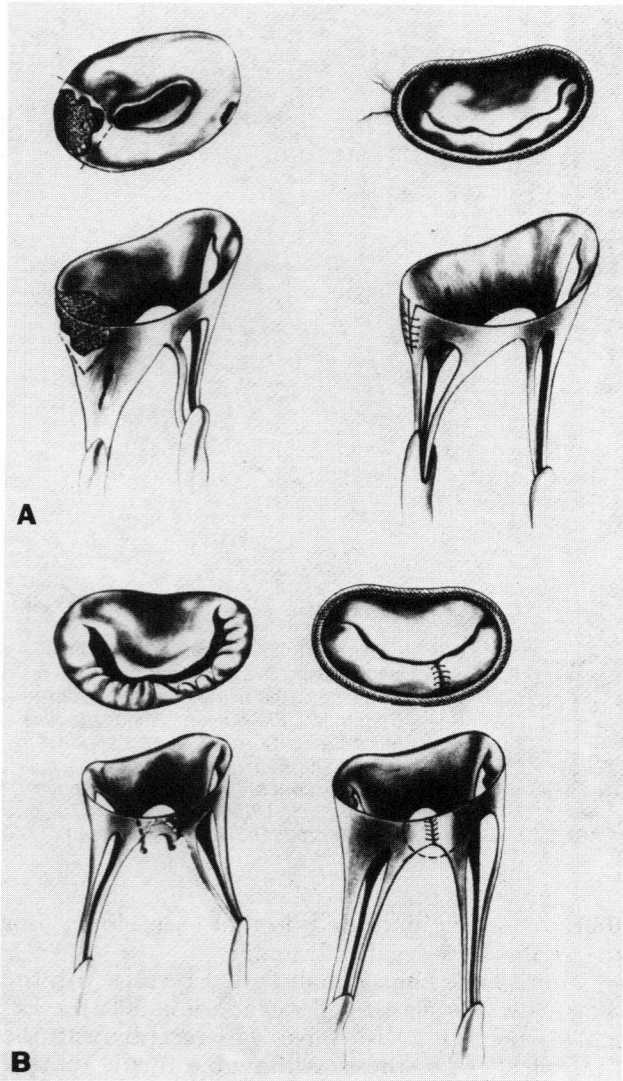

FIGURE 39-26 Repair of mitral insufficiency—Carpentier's methods. *A.* Resection of calcification. *B.* Quadrangular resection of prolapsed posterior leaflet secondary to ruptured chordae tendineae. Each repair is accompanied by ring annuloplasty. [*From A. Carpentier, Plastic and Reconstructive Mitral Valve Surgery, in D. Kalmanson (ed.), "The Mitral Valve: A Pluridisciplinary Approach," Publishing Sciences Group, Inc., Littleton, Mass., 1976, p. 534. Reproduced with permission.*]

There may be some pulmonary dysfunction early after mitral valve replacement, but prolonged tracheal intubation and ventilation are seldom indicated for greater than 24 h postoperatively.

Anticoagulation treatment is begun on the second day with Coumadin, and in patients with porcine xenografts it is continued for 6 weeks. In patients with prosthetic devices it is maintained indefinitely. Before hospital discharge, attempts are made to convert atrial fibrillation to a normal sinus mechanism either by drug therapy or electrical cardioversion. This is more successful in patients not having preoperative chronic atrial fibrillation of greater than 1-year duration.[182]

Late Results Thromboembolic complications were common with the early models of prosthetic mitral valves, but with currently used devices are much lower[183] (Fig. 39-28). We have found that the presence of atrial fibrillation, previous operation, advanced age, and double valve replacement each contribute some hazard to late postoperative thromboembolism. The survival rates for patients with presently available prosthetic or biological valves in the mitral position are also considerably higher than with devices that were initially available (Fig. 39-29). However, the results continue to be dependent on the degree of disability prior to operation, nearly 90 percent of patients with class III disability preoperatively having a good long-term result, and only about 50 percent of patients with class IV disability having good long-term results. Again, this emphasizes the importance of advising operation before left ventricular dysfunction becomes advanced and irreversible. This concept has been documented recently by Schuler, Peterson, and colleagues in a small number of patients studied after mitral valve replacement for mitral incompetence.[177] In those patients with preoperatively normal ejection fractions (0.70), the ejection fraction fell only slightly 6 months after operation and hypertrophy regressed. However, in those patients with some element of left ventricular dysfunction preoperatively (ejection fraction, 0.57), left ventricular function progressively deteriorated after surgery, and left ventricular hypertrophy did not regress. The authors concluded that left ventricular shortening likely had become partially dependent on systolic afterload reduction through a load impedance leak in the latter group. After a valve replacement, ejection fraction became markedly impaired and chamber dilatation and myocardial hypertrophy persisted in some patients.

Postoperative Management

If the patient remains in atrial fibrillation after hospital discharge, chronic digitalis administration will be required to control ventricular response. Anti-

FIGURE 39-27 Insertion of Bjork-Shiley mitral prosthesis using continuous monofilament suture.

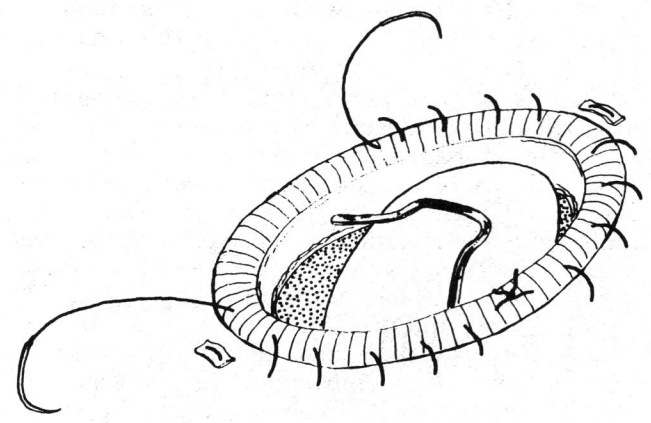

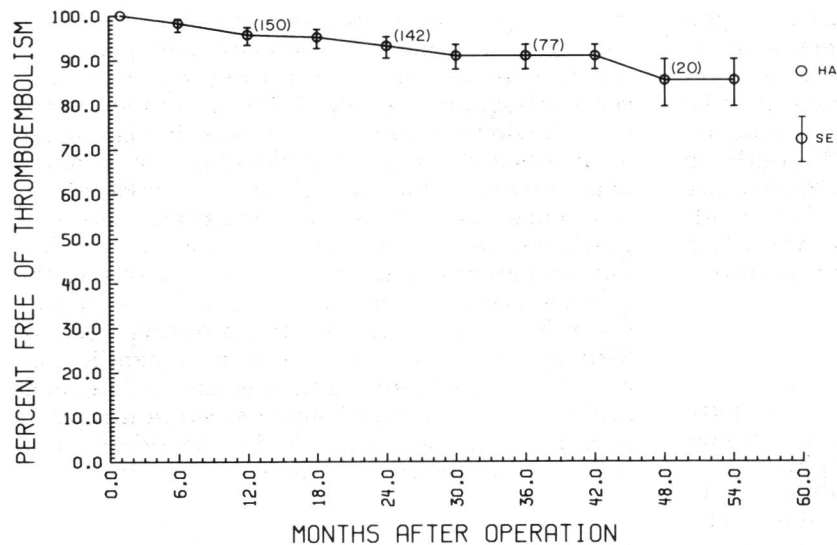

FIGURE 39-28 Actuarial freedom from thromboembolism in patients receiving Bjork-Shiley mitral prostheses at the University of Alabama in Birmingham. Those data are compared to 5-year freedom from thromboembolism to the Hancock xenograft from Davila and the Starr-Edwards (SE) from Macmanus. (*From J. C. Davila, D. J. Magilligan, and J. W. Lewis, Is the Hancock Porcine Valve the Best Cardiac Valve Substitute Today? Ann. Thorac. Surg., 26:303, 1978. From Q. Macmanus, G. Grunkemeier, L. E. Lambert, and A. Starr, Non-Cloth-Covered Caged-Ball Prostheses, the Second Decade, J. Thorac. Cardiovas. Surg., 76:788, 1978. Reproduced with permission.*)

FIGURE 39-29 Actuarial survival according to preoperative functional class over a 10-year period for patients having mitral valve replacement. (*From A. Starr, G. Grunkemeier, L. Lambert, J. E. Okies, and D. Thomas, Mitral Valve Replacement: A 10-Year Following of Non-Cloth-Covered vs. Cloth-Covered Caged-Ball Prostheses, Circulation, 54:III–47, 1976. Reproduced with permission.*)

Survival Curves for Starr-Edwards Mitral Valves*

Functional Classification

	valves	deaths
▲ 1 & 2	53	9
■ 3	183	37
● 4	32	12

%

*Operative Survivors Only

82%

75%

54%

p < .025

YEARS

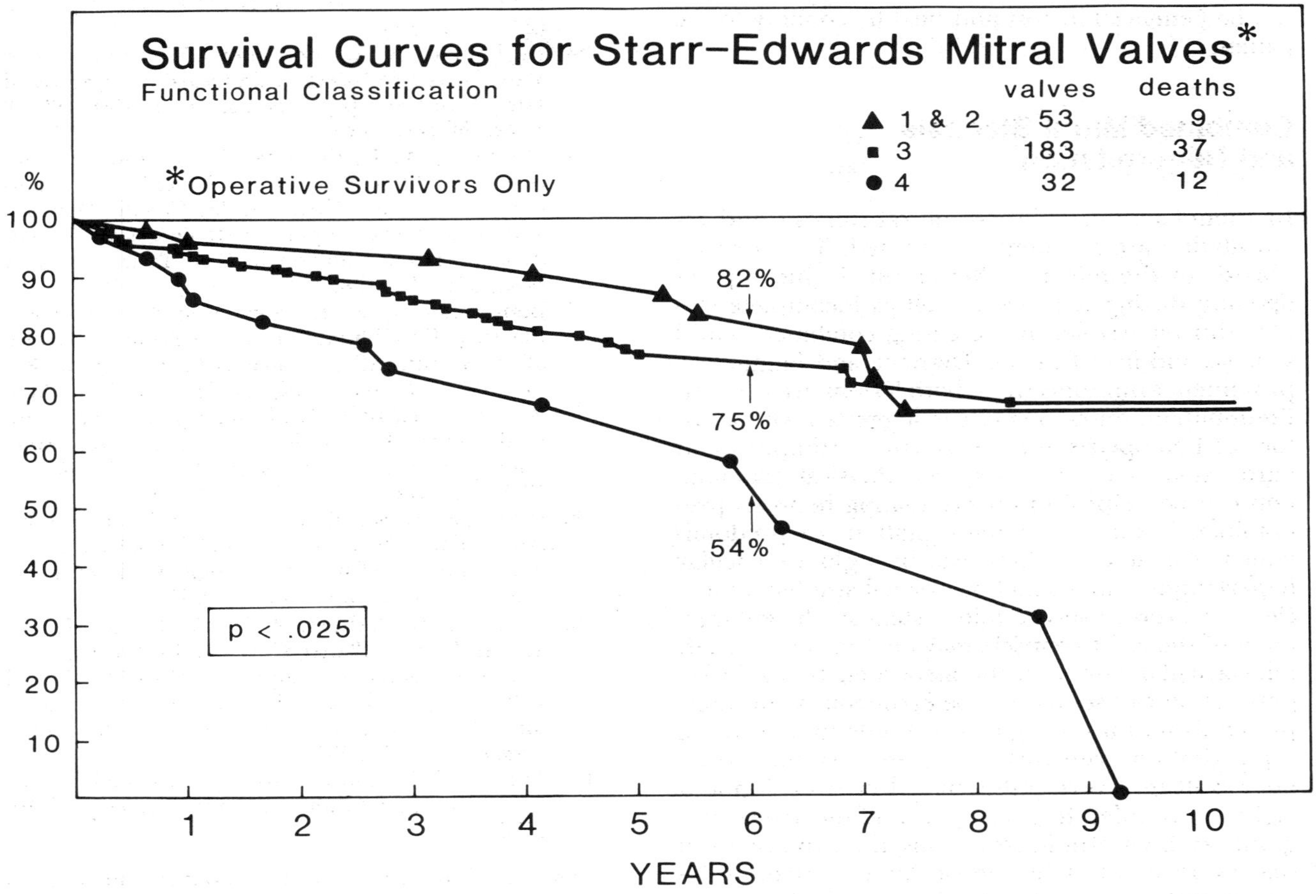

biotic coverage for dental work and elective surgical procedures remains important for prevention of endocarditis. Depending on the prosthetic valve inserted, long-term anticoagulation therapy may be necessary. Echocardiographic and radionuclide studies can be obtained every 6 to 12 months to evaluate ventricular size and function. Recurrence of symptoms or change in prosthetic valve sounds warrants cinefluorography of the valve, which can be compared to films taken before hospital discharge.

Cost Containment

Patients with chronic mitral regurgitation require periodic evaluations to assess cardiac function and to adjust medications. Emphasis on prophylaxis for rheumatic fever and bacterial endocarditis can obviously minimize these costly complications. The physician should be aware of noninvasive techniques to monitor ventricular size and performance, since many patients will eventually require mitral valve replacement, and the optimal time should be selected before heart failure and severe myocardial depression develop. Thus, prolonged medical treatment for symptoms of heart failure and mitral regurgitation can be costly not only in terms of expense to patients, but also in minimizing the eventual surgical benefit from valve replacement. Periodic evaluation of ventricular size and function can be beneficial in cost and health economy to the patient.

Combined Mitral Stenosis and Regurgitation

In rheumatic heart disease mitral stenosis and regurgitation are frequently combined. The scarring fibrosis of the mitral leaflet results in incomplete opening during diastole as well as incomplete closure during systole, thus creating combined mitral stenosis and insufficiency. Dyspnea and fatigue are prominent symptoms when both lesions are present. Predominant mitral stenosis is suggested with a history of hemoptysis and paroxysmal orthopnea and paroxysmal nocturnal dyspnea. Physical examination can be helpful in differentiating between predominant stenosis and regurgitation. In predominant mitral stenosis there will be right ventricular hypertrophy and a small or normal size left ventricle. However, in severe mitral stenosis the enlargement of the right ventricle may encroach on the left midclavicular line, and the associated tricuspid regurgitation can sometimes be erroneously misinterpreted as mitral regurgitation. Predominant mitral regurgitation even with a degree of stenosis does not result in severe pulmonary hypertension and right ventricular hypertropy. The electrocardiogram can be useful in separating the two lesions in that evidence of right ventricular hypertrophy favors mitral stenosis, whereas left ventricular hyper-

trophy suggests regurgitation. Similarly, left ventricular enlargement on the chest roentgenogram indicates predominant mitral regurgitation. The echocardiogram can help differentiate the lesions, since the slope of mitral valve motion in diastole can be quantitated and a range identified for predominant stenosis versus insufficiency. Increased left ventricular dimensions on echocardiography suggest predominant mitral regurgitation. Cardiac catheterization is important in both recording the gradient across the mitral valve as well as detecting regurgitation into the left atrium during left ventricular angiography. Medical management is similar, except vasodilating agents would not augment cardiac output in mitral stenosis. Surgical replacement of the mitral valve should be considered as in either stenosis or regurgitation.

References

1. Vieussens, R.: "Traite nouveau de la structure et des causes du mouvement naturel du coeur," Toulouse Guillemette, 1715, p. 101.
*2. Perloff, J. K., and Roberts, W. C.: The Mitral Apparatus. Functional Anatomy of Mitral Regurgitation, *Circulation*, 46:227, 1972. (54 references)
*3. Nasser, W. K., Davis, R. H., Dillon, J. C., Tavel, M. E., Helmen, C. H., Feigenbaum, H., and Fisch, C.: Atrial Myxoma. I. Clinical and Pathologic Features in Nine Cases, *Am. Heart J.*, 83:694, 1972. (22 references)
*4. Buchbinder, N. A., and Roberts, W. C.: Left-Sided Valvular Active Infective Endocarditis. A Study of Forty-Five Necropsy Patients, *Am. J. Med.*, 53:20, 1972. (56 references)
5. Hammer, W. J., Roberts, W. C., and deLeon, A. C., Jr.: "Mitral Stenosis" Secondary to Combined "Massive" Mitral Anular Calcific Deposits and Small, Hypertrophied Left Ventricles, Hemodynamic Documentation in Four Patients, *Am. J. Med.*, 64:371, 1978.
6. Bonnabeau, R. V., Jr., Stevenson, J. E., and Edwards, J. E.: Obliteration of the Principal Orifice of the Stenotic Mitral Valve: A Rare Form of "Restenosis," *J. Thorac. Cardiovasc. Surg.*, 49:264, 1965.
7. Wooley, C. F., Baba, N., Kilman, J. W., and Ryan, J. M.: Thrombotic Calcific Mitral Stenosis. Morphology of the Calcific Mitral Valve, *Circulation*, 49:1167, 1974.
8. Jordan, R. A., Scheifley, C. H., and Edwards, J. E.: Mural Thrombosis and Arterial Embolism in Mitral Stenosis. A Clinicopathologic Study of Fifty-One Cases, *Circulation*, 3:363, 1951.
9. Shone, J. D., Sellers, R. D., Anderson, R. C., Adams, P., Jr., Lillehei, C. W., and Edwards, J. E.: The Developmental Complex of "Parachute Mitral Valve," Supravalvular Ring of Left Atrium, Subaortic Stenosis, and Coarctation of Aorta, *Am. J. Cardiol.*, 11:714, 1963.
10. da Silva, C. L., and Edwards, J. E.: Parachute Mitral Valve in an Adult, *Arq. Bras. Cardiol.*, 26:149, 1973.

*This article is a review of the literature and contains additional references to the literature.

11. Kennedy, J. W., Yarnall, S. R., Murray, J. A., and Figley, M. M.: Quantitative Angiocardiography. IV. Relationships of Left Atrial and Ventricular Pressure and Volume in Mitral Valve Disease, *Circulation*, 41:817, 1970.

*12. Curry, G. C., Elliott, L. P., and Ramsey, H. W.: Quantitative Left Ventricular Angiocardiographic Findings in Mitral Stenosis; Detailed Analysis of the Anterolateral Wall of the Left Ventricle, *Am. J. Cardiol.*, 29:621, 1972. (27 references)

*13. Silverstein, D. M., Hansen, D. P., Ojiambo, H. P., and Griswold, H. E.: Left Ventricular Function in Severe Pure Mitral Stenosis as Seen at the Kenyatta National Hospital, *Am. Heart J.*, 99:727, 1980. (30 references)

14. Rowe, J. C., Bland, E. F., Sprague, H. B., and White, P. D.: The Course of Mitral Stenosis without Surgery: Ten and Twenty Year Perspectives, *Ann. Intern. Med.*, 52:741, 1960.

15. Wood, P.: An Appreciation of Mitral Stenosis, *Br. Med. J.*, 1:1051, 1954.

*16. Selzer, A., and Cohn, K. E.: Natural History of Mitral Stenosis: A Review, *Circulation*, 45:878, 1972.

17. Szekely, P., Turner, R., and Snaith, L.: Pregnancy and the Changing Pattern of Rheumatic Heart Disease, *Br. Heart J.*, 35:1293, 1973.

18. Schwartz, R., Meyerson, R. M., Lawrence, L. T., and Nichols, H. T.: Mitral Stenosis, Massive Pulmonary Hemorrhage and Emergency Valve Replacement, *N. Engl. J. Med.*, 272:755, 1966.

19. Ross, R. S.: Right Ventricular Hypertension as a Cause of Precordial Pain, *Am. Heart J.*, 61:134, 1961.

20. Baker, C. G., and Finnegan, T. R. L.: Epilepsy and Mitral Stenosis, *Br. Heart J.*, 19:159, 1957.

21. Mounsey, J. P. D.: Inspection and Palpation of the Cardiac Impulse, *Prog. Cardiovasc. Dis.*, 10:187, 1967.

22. Thompson, M. E., Shaver, J. A., Heidenreich, F. P., Leon, D. F., and Leonard, J. J.: Sound, Pressure and Motion Correlates in Mitral Stenosis, *Am. J. Med.*, 49:436, 1970.

*23. Luisada, A. A., MacCanon, D. M., Kumar, S., and Feigen, L. P.: Changing Views on the Mechanism of the First and Second Heart Sounds, *Am. Heart J.*, 88:503, 1974. (62 references)

24. Wooley, C. F., Klassen, K. P., Leighton, R. F., Goodwin, R. S., and Ryan, J. M.: Left Atrial and Left Ventricular Sound and Pressure in Mitral Stenosis, *Circulation*, 38:295, 1968.

25. Dack, S., Bleifer, S., Grishman, A., and Donoso, E.: Mitral Stenosis: Auscultatory and Phonocardiographic Findings, *Am. J. Cardiol.*, 5:815, 1960.

26. Mounsey, P.: The Opening Snap of Mitral Stenosis, *Br. Heart J.*, 15:135, 1953.

27. Wells, B.: The Assessment of Mitral Stenosis by Phonocardiography, *Br. Heart J.*, 16:261, 1954.

28. Rackley, C. E., Craig, R. J., McIntosh, H. D., and Orgain, E. S.: Phonocardiographic Discrepancies in the Assessment of Mitral Stenosis, *Arch. Intern. Med.*, 121:50, 1968.

29. Ebringer, R., Pitt, A., and Anderson, S. T.: Haemodynamic Factors Influencing Opening Snap Interval in Mitral Stenosis, *Br. Heart J.*, 32:350, 1970.

30. Nixon, P. G., Wooler, G. H., and Radigan, L. R.: The Opening Snap in Mitral Incompetence, *Br. Heart J.*, 22:395, 1960.

31. Millward, D. K., McLaurin, L. P., and Craige, E.: Echocardiographic Studies to Explain Opening Snaps in Presence of Non-stenotic Mitral Valves, *Am. J. Cardiol.*, 31:64, 1973.

32. Leatham, A., and Gray, I.: Auscultatory and Phonocardiographic Signs of Atrial Septal Defect, *Br. Heart J.*, 18:193, 1956.

*33. Vacca, J. B., Bussman, D. W., and Mudd, J. G.: Ebstein's Anomaly: Complete Review of 108 Cases, *Am. J. Cardiol.*, 2:210, 1958. (71 references)

*34. Perloff, J. K., and Harvey, W. P.: Clinical Recognition of Tricuspid Stenosis, *Circulation*, 22:346, 1960. (50 references)

35. Crawley, I. S., Morris, D. C., and Silverman, B. D.: Valvular Heart Disease, in J. W. Hurst, R. B. Logue, R. C. Schlant, and N. K. Wenger (eds.), "The Heart," 4th ed., McGraw-Hill Book Co., New York, 1978, p. 992.

36. Surawicz, B.: Effect of Respiration and Upright Position on the Interval between the Two Components of the Second Heart Sound and that between the Second Sound and Mitral Opening Snap, *Circulation*, 16:422, 1957.

37. Fortuin, N. J., and Craige, E.: Echocardiographic Studies of Genesis of Mitral Diastolic Murmurs, *Br. Heart J.*, 35:75, 1973.

38. Lakier, J. B., Pocock, W. A., Gale, G. E., and Barlow, J. B.: Haemodynamic and Sound Events Preceding First Heart Sound in Mitral Stenosis, *Br. Heart J.*, 34:1152, 1972.

39. Bonner, A. J., Jr., Stewart, J., and Travel, M. E.: "Presystolic" Augmentation of Diastolic Heart Sounds in Atrial Fibrillation, *Am. J. Cardiol.*, 37:427, 1976.

40. McGuire, L. B., Nolan, T. B., Reeve, R., and Dammann, J. F., Jr.: Cor Triatriatum as a Problem of Heart Disease, *Circulation*, 31:263, 1965.

41. Korn, D., DeSanctis, R. W., and Sell, S.: Massive Calcification of the Mitral Annulus, *N. Engl. J. Med.*, 267:900, 1962.

42. Spodick, D. H.: "Chronic and Constrictive Pericarditis," Grune & Stratton, Inc., New York, 1964.

43. McArthur, J. D., Sukumar, I. P., Munsi, S. C., Krishnaswami, S., and Cherian, G.: Reassessment of Graham Steell Murmur Using Platinum Electrode Technique, *Br. Heart J.*, 36:1023, 1974.

44. Chen, J. T. T., Behar, V. S., Morris, J. J., Jr., McIntosh, H. D., and Lester, R. G.: Correlation of Roentgen Findings with Hemodynamic Data in Pure Mitral Stenosis, *Am. J. Roentgenol. Radium Ther. Nucl. Med.*, 102:280, 1968.

45. Grainger, R. G.: Interstitial Pulmonary Edema and Its Radiographic Diagnosis: Signs of Pulmonary Venous and Capillary Hypertension, *Br. J. Radiol.*, 31:201, 1958.

46. Felson, B.: "Chest Roentgenology," W. B. Saunders Company, Philadelphia, 1973.

47. Chait, A.: Interstitial Pulmonary Edema, *Circulation*, 45:1323, 1972.

48. Meszaros, W. T.: Lung Changes in Left Heart Failure, *Circulation*, 47:859, 1973.

49. Saunders, J. L., Calatayud, J. B., Schulz, K. J., Maranhao, V., Gooch, A. S., and Goldberg, H.: Evaluation of ECG Criteria for P-Wave Abnormalities, *Am. Heart J.*, 74:757, 1967.

50. Lee, Y. C., Scherlis, L., and Singleton, R. T.: Mitral Stenosis: Hemodynamic, Electrocardiographic and

Vector Cardiographic Studies, *Am. Heart J.,* 69:559, 1965.

51. Walston, A., Harley, A., and Pipberger, H. V.: Computer Analysis of the Orthogonal Electrocardiogram and Vectorcardiogram in Mitral Stenosis, *Circulation,* 50:472, 1974.

52. Duchak, J. M., Chang, S., and Feigenbaum, H.: The Posterior Mitral Valve Echo and the Echocardiographic Diagnosis of Mitral Stenosis, *Am. J. Cardiol.,* 29:628, 1972.

53. Teicholz, L. E.: Echocardiography in Valvular Heart Disease, *Prog. Cardiovasc. Dis.,* 17:283, 1975.

54. Cope, G. D., Kisslo, J. A., Johnson, M. L., and Behar, V. S.: A Reassessment of the Echocardiogram in Mitral Stenosis, *Circulation,* 52:664, 1975.

55. Wolfe, S. B., Popp, R. L., and Feigenbaum, H.: Diagnosis of Atrial Tumors by Ultrasound, *Circulation,* 39:615, 1969.

56. McLarin, L. P., Gibson, T. C., Waider, W., Grossman, W., and Craige, E.: An Appraisal of Mitral Valve Echocardiograms Mimicking Mitral Stenosis in Conditions with Right Ventricular Pressure Overload, *Circulation,* 48:801, 1973.

57. Quinones, M. A., Gaash, W. H., Waisser, E., and Alexander, J. K.: Reduction in the Rate of Diastolic Descent of the Mitral Valve Echogram in Patients with Altered Left Ventricular Diastolic Pressure-Volume Relations, *Circulation,* 49:246, 1974.

58. Stewart, J. A., Silimperi, D., Harris, P., Wise, N. K., Fraker, T. D., and Kisslo, J. A.: Echocargraphic Documentation of Vegetative Lesions in Infective Endocarditis: Clinical Implications, *Circulation,* 61:374, 1980.

59. Gorlin, R., and Gorlin, S. G.: Hydraulic Formula for Calculation of the Area of the Stenotic Mitral Valve, Other Cardiac Valves and Central Circulatory Shunts, *Am. Heart J.,* 41:1, 1951.

60. Cohen, M. V., and Gorlin, R.: Modified Orifice Equation for the Calculation of Mitral Valve Area, *Am. Heart J.,* 84:839, 1972.

61. Hugenholtz, P. G., Ryan, T. J., Stein, S. W., and Abelmann, W. H.: The Spectrum of Pure Mitral Stenosis: Hemodynamic Studies in Relation to Clinical Disability, *Am. J. Cardiol.,* 10:773, 1962.

62. Bolen, J. L., Lopes, M. G., Harrison, D. C., and Alderman, E. L.: Analysis of Left Ventricular Function in Response to Afterload Changes in Patients with Mitral Stenosis, *Circulation,* 52:894, 1975.

63. Heller, S. J., and Carleton, R. A.: Abnormal Left Ventricular Contraction in Patients with Mitral Stenosis, *Circulation,* 42:1099, 1970.

64. Hildner, F. J., Javier, R. P., Cohen, L. S., Samet, P., Nathan, M. J., Yahr, W. Z., and Greenberg, J. J.: Myocardial Dysfunction Associated with Valvular Heart Disease, *Am. J. Cardiol.,* 30:319, 1972.

65. Newman, G. E., Bounous, P. E., Jones, R. H., and Saliston, D. C.: Noninvasive Assessment of Hemodynamic Effects of Mitral Valve Commissurotomy during Rest and Exercise in Patients with Mitral Stenosis, *J. Thorac. Cardiovasc. Surg.,* 78:750, 1979.

66. Bhathia, M. L., Shriuastava, S., and Roy, S. B.: Immediate Haemodynamic Effects of a Beta Adrenergic Blocking Agent, Propranolol, in Mitral Stenosis at Fixed Heart Rates, *Br. Heart J.,* 34:638, 1972.

67. Meister, S. G., Engel, T. R., Feitosa, G. S., Helfant, R. H., and Frankl, W. S.: Propranolol in Mitral Stenosis during Stress Rhythm, *Am. Heart J.,* 94:685, 1977.

68. Giuffrida, G., Bonzani, G., Betocchi, S., Piscione, F., Giudice, P., Miceli, D., Mazza, F., and Condorelli, M.: Hemodynamic Response to Exercise after Propranolol in Patients with Mitral Stenosis, *Am. J. Cardiol.,* 44:1076, 1979.

69. Abernathy, W. S., and Willis, P. W., III: Thromboembolic Complications of Rheumatic Heart Disease, *Cardiovasc. Clin.,* 5:131, 1973.

70. Kellogg, F., Lui, C. K., Fishman, W., and Larson, R.: Systemic and Pulmonary Emboli before and after Mitral Commissurotomy, *Circulation,* 24:263, 1961.

71. Rapaport, E.: Natural History of Aortic and Mitral Valve Disease, *Am. J. Cardiol.,* 35:221, 1975.

72. Olesen, K. H.: The Natural History of 271 Patients with Mitral Stenosis under Medical Treatment, *Br. Heart J.,* 24:349, 1962.

73. Upton, A. R. M., and Honey, M.: Electroconversion of Atrial Fibrillation after Mitral Valvotomy, *Br. Heart J.,* 33:732, 1971.

74. Kirklin, J. W., Conti, V. R., and Blackstone, E. H.: Prevention of Myocardial Damage during Cardiac Operations, *N. Engl. J. Med.,* 301:135, 1979.

75. Carpentier, A., Chauvaud, S., Fabiani, J. N., Deloche, A., Relland, J., Lessana, A., d'Allaines, C., Blondeau, P., Piwnica, A., and Dubost, Ch.: Reconstructive Surgery of Mitral Valve Incompetence, *J. Thorac. Cardiovasc. Surg.,* 79:338, 1980.

76. Duran, C. G., Pomar, J. L., Revuelta, J. M., Gallo, I., Poveda, J., Ochoteco, A., and Ubago, J. L.: Conservative Operation for Mitral Insufficiency: Critical Analysis Supported by Postoperative Hemodynamic Studies of 72 Patients, *J. Thorac. Cardiovasc. Surg.,* 69:326, 1980.

77. Kouchoukos, N. T., and Karp, R. B.: Management of the Postoperative Cardiovascular Surgical Patient, *Am. Heart J.,* 92:513, 1976.

78. Ellis, L. B., Singh, J. B., Morales, D. D., and Harken, D. E.: Fifteen to Twenty Year Study of One Thousand Patients Undergoing Closed Mitral Valvuloplasty, *Circulation,* 48:357, 1973.

79. Heger, J. J., Wann, L. S., Weyman, A. E., Dillon, J. C., and Feigenbaum, H.: Long-Term Changes in Mitral Valve Area after Successful Mitral Commissurotomy, *Circulation,* 59:443, 1979.

80. Higgs, L. M., Glancy, D. L., O'Brien, K. P., Epstein, S. E., and Morrow, A. G.: Mitral Restenosis an Uncommon Cause of Recurrent Symptoms Following Mitral Commissurotomy, *Am. J. Cardiol.,* 26:34, 1970.

81. Hope, J.: Signs of Disease of the Mitral Valve, in "A Treatise on the Diseases of the Heart," Churchill, London, 1839, p. 387.

*82. Silverman, M. E., and Hurst, J. W.: The Mitral Complex, *Am. Heart J.,* 76:399, 1968. (226 references)

*83. Barlow, J. B., and Pocock, W. A.: The Problem of Nonejection Systolic Clicks and Associated Mitral Systolic Murmurs: Emphasis on the Billowing Mitral Leaflet Syndrome, *Am. Heart J.,* 90:636, 1975. (173 references)

84. Rackley, C. E., Dear, H. D., Baxley, W. A., Jones, W. B., and Dodge, H. T.: Left Ventricular Chamber Volume, Mass, and Function in Severe Coronary Artery Disease, *Circulation,* 41:605, 1970.

85. Perloff, J. K., and Roberts, W. C.: The Mitral Ap-

paratus: Functional Anatomy of Mitral Regurgitation, *Circulation*, 46:227, 1972.

86. Rytand, D. A., and Lipsitch, L. S.: Clinical Aspects of Calcification of the Mitral Annulus Fibrosus, *Arch. Intern. Med.*, 78:544, 1946.

87. Roberts, W. C., Dangel, J. C., and Bulkley, B. H.: Nonrheumatic Valvular Cardiac Disease: A Clinicopathologic Survey of 27 Different Conditions Causing Valvular Dysfunction, in W. Likoff (guest ed.), "Valvular Heart Disease," *Cardiovasc. Clin.*, 5(2):333, 1973.

88. McKusick, V. A.: "Heritable Disorders of Connective Tissue," The C. V. Mosby Company, St. Louis, 1972.

89. Burch, G. E., DePasquale, N. P., and Phillips, J. H.: Clinical Manifestation of Papillary Muscle Dysfunction, *Arch. Intern. Med.*, 112:112, 1963.

90. Heikkila, J.: Mitral Incompetence Complicating Acute Myocardial Infarction, *Br. Heart J.*, 29:162, 1967.

91. DeBusk, R. F., and Harrison, D. C.: The Clinical Spectrum of Papillary-Muscle Disease, *N. Engl. J. Med.*, 281:1458, 1969.

92. Fowler, N. O., and Van der Mel-Kahn, J. M.: Indications for Surgical Replacement of the Mitral Valve; with Particular Reference to Common and Uncommon Causes of Mitral Regurgitation, *Am. J. Cardiol.*, 44:148, 1979.

93. Selzer, A., Kelly, J. J., Jr., Vannitamby, M., Walker, P., Gerbode, F., and Kerth, W. J.: The Syndrome of Mitral Insufficiency Due to Isolated Rupture of the Chordae Tendineae, *Am. J. Med.*, 43:822, 1967.

94. Sanders, C. A., Armstrong, P. W., Willerson, J. T., and Dinsmore, R. E.: Etiology and Differential Diagnosis of Acute Mitral Regurgitation, *Prog. Cardiovasc. Dis.*, 14:129, 1971.

*95. Edwards, J. E.: Pathology of Acquired Valvular Disease of the Heart, *Seminars in Roentgenol.*, 14:96, 1979. (61 references)

*96. Perloff, J. K., and Roberts, W. C.: The Mitral Apparatus. Functional Anatomy of Mitral Regurgitation, *Circulation*, 46:227, 1972. (54 references)

97. Burchell, H. B., and Edwards, J. E.: Rheumatic Mitral Insufficiency, *Circulation*, 7:747, 1953.

98. Levy, M. J., and Edwards, J. E.: Anatomy of Mitral Insufficiency, *Prog. Cardiovasc. Dis.*, 5:119, 1962.

99. Edwards, J. E., and Burchell, H. B.: Pathologic Anatomy of Mitral Insufficiency, *Proc. Mayo Clin.*, 33:497, 1958.

100. Edwards J. E.: Mitral Insufficiency Secondary to Aortic Valvular Bacterial Endocarditis, *Circulation*, 46:623, 1972.

101. Pomerance, A.: Ballooning Deformity (Mucoid Degeneration) of Atrioventricular Valves, *Br. Heart J.*, 31:343, 1969.

102. Guthrie, R. G., and Edwards, J. E.: Pathology of the Myxomatous Mitral Valve. Nature, Secondary Changes and Complications, *Minnesota Med.*, 59:637, 1976.

103. Ranganathan, N., Silver, M. D., Robinson, T. I., Kostuk, W. J., Felderhof, C. H., Patt, N. L., Wilson, J. K., and Wigle, E. D.: Angiographic Morphologic Correlation in Patients with Severe Mitral Regurgitation Due to Prolapse of the Posterior Mitral Leaflet, *Circulation*, 48:514, 1973.

104. Salazar, A. E., and Edwards, J. E.: Friction Lesions of Ventricular Endocardium. Relation to Chordae Tendineae of Mitral Valve, *Arch. Path.*, 90:364, 1970.

105. Goodman, D., Kimbiris, D., and Linhart, J. W.: Chordae Tendineae Rupture Complicating the Systolic Click–Late Systolic Murmur Syndrome, *Am. J. Cardiol.*, 33:681, 1974.

106. Moller, J. H., Lucas, R. V., Jr., Adams, P., Jr., Anderson, R. C., Jorgans, J., and Edwards, J. E.: Endocardial Fibroelastosis. A Clinical and Anatomic Study of 47 Patients with Emphasis on Its Relationship to Mitral Insufficiency, *Circulation*, 30:759, 1964.

107. Vlodaver, Z., and Edwards, J. E.: Rupture of Ventricular Septum or Papillary Muscle Complicating Myocardial Infarction, *Circulation*, 55:815, 1977.

108. Lee, K. S., Johnson, T., Karnegis, J. N., Quattlebaum, F. W., and Edwards, J. E.: Acute Myocardial Infarction with Long-Term Survival Following Papillary Muscle Rupture, *Am. Heart J.*, 79:258, 1970.

109. Tsakiris, A. G., Rastelli, G. C., Amorim, D., Titus, J. L., and Wood, E. H.: Effect of Experimental Papillary Muscle Damage on Mitral Valve Closure in Intact Anesthetized Dogs, *Proc. Mayo Clin.*, 45:275, 1970.

110. Hall, S. W., Jr., Theologides, A., From, A. H. L., Gobel, F. L., Fortuny, I. E., Lawrence, C. J., and Edwards, J. E.: Hypereosinophilic Syndrome with Biventricular Involvement, *Circulation*, 55:217, 1977.

111. Bulkley, B. H., and Roberts, W. C.: Systemic Lupus Erythematosus as a Cause of Severe Mitral Regurgitation. New Problem in an Old Disease, *Am. J. Cardiol.*, 35:305, 1975.

112. Pomerance, A.: Pathological and Clinical Study of Calcification of the Mitral Valve Ring, *Br. J. Clin. Path.*, 23:354, 1970.

113. Braunwald, E.: Mitral Regurgitation: Physiologic, Clinical and Surgical Considerations, *N. Engl. J. Med.*, 281:425, 1969.

114. Ross, J., Jr., Braunwald, E., and Morrow, A. G.: Clinical and Hemodynamic Observations in Pure Mitral Insufficiency, *Am. J. Cardiol.*, 2:11, 1958.

115. Dodge, H. T., and Baxley, W. A.: Left Ventricular Volume and Mass and Their Significance in Heart Disease, *Am. J. Cardiol.*, 23:528, 1969.

116. Rackley, C. E., and Hood, W. P., Jr.: Quantitative Angiographic Evaluation and Pathophysiologic Mechanisms in Valvular Heart Disease, in E. H. Sonnenblick and M. Lesch (eds.), "Valvular Heart Disease," Grune & Stratton, Inc., New York, 1975, p. 109.

117. Hood, W. P., Jr., Rackley, C. E., and Rolett, E. L.: Wall Stress in the Normal and Hypertrophied Human Left Ventricle, *Am. J. Cardiol.*, 22:550, 1968.

118. Rackley, C. E.: Value of Ventriculography in Cardiac Function and Diagnosis, in A. N. Brest (ed.), "Diagnostic Methods in Cardiology," *Cardiovasc. Clin.*, 6:3:283, 1975.

119. Porter, C. M., Baxley, W. A., Eddleman, E. E., Jr., Frimer, M., and Rackley, C. E.: Left Ventricular Dimensions and Dynamics of Filling in Patients with Gallop Heart Sounds, *Am. J. Med.*, 50:721, 1971.

120. Rackley, C. E., Hood, W. P., Jr., Rolett, E. L., and Young, D. T.: Left Ventricular End-Diastolic Pressure in Chronic Heart Disease, *Am. J. Med.*, 48:310, 1970.

121. Jeresaty, R. M.: Mitral Valve Prolapse-Click Syndrome, *Prog. Cardiovasc. Dis.*, 15:623, 1973.

122. Nutter, D. O., Wickliffe, C., Gilbert, C. A., Moody, C., and King, S. A.: The Pathophysiology of Idiopathic Mitral Valve Prolapse, *Circulation*, 52:297, 1975.

123. Bulkley, B. H., and Roberts, W. C.: Dilatation of the Mitral Annulus, *Am. J. Med.*, 59:457, 1975.

124. Gooch, A. S., Vicencio, F., Maranchao, V., and Goldberg, H.: Arrhythmias and Left Ventricle Asynergy in the Prolapsing Mitral Leaflet, *Am. J. Cardiol.*, 29:611, 1972.

125. Aranda, J. M., Befeler, B., Lazzara, R., Embi, A., and Marchado, H.: Mitral Valve Prolapse and Coronary Artery Disease, *Circulation*, 52:245, 1975.

126. Verani, M. S., Carroll, R. J., and Falsetti, H. L.: Mitral Valve Prolapse in Coronary Disease, *Am. J. Cardiol.*, 37:1, 1976.

127. Sabom, M. B., Curry, R. C, Jr., Pepine, C. J., Christie, L. G., and Conti, C. R.: Ergonovine Testing for Coronary Artery Spasm in Patients with Angiographic Mitral Valve Prolapse, *Cath. Cardiovasc. Diag.*, 4:265, 1978.

128. Coghlan, H. C., Phares, P., Cowley, M., Copley, D., and James, T. N.: Dysautonomia in Mitral Valve Prolapse, *Am. J. Med.*, 67:236, 1979.

129. Rackley, C. E., Russell, R. O., Jr., Mantle, J. A., and Rogers, W. J.: Modern Approach to the Patient with Acute Myocardial Infarction, in W. P. Harvey (ed.), "Current Problems in Cardiology," Yearbook Medical Publishers, Chicago, 1:10, 1977.

130. Klughaupt, M., Flamm, M. D., Hancock, E. W., and Harrison, D. C.: Nonrheumatic Mitral Insufficiency: Determination of Operability and Prognosis, *Circulation*, 39:307, 1969.

131. Selzer, A., and Katayama, F.: Mitral Regurgitation: Clinical Patterns, Pathophysiology, and Natural History, *Medicine (Baltimore)*, 51:337, 1972.

132. Bentivoglio, L., Urichio, J., and Goldberg, H.: Clinical and Hemodynamic Features of Advanced Rheumatic Mitral Regurgitation, *Am. J. Med.*, 30:372, 1961.

133. Ellis, L. B., and Ramirez, A.: The Clinical Course of Patients with Severe "Rheumatic" Mitral Insufficiency, *Am. Heart J.*, 78:406, 1969.

134. Winkle, R. A., Lopes, M. G., Fitzgerald, J. W., Goodman, D. J., Schroeder, J. S., and Harrison, D. C.: Arrhythmias in Patients with Mitral Valve Prolapse, *Circulation*, 52:73, 1975.

135. Brody, W., and Criley, J. M.: Intermittent Severe Mitral Regurgitation, *N. Engl. J. Med.*, 283:673, 1970.

136. Basta, L. L., Wolfson, P., Eckberg, D. L., and Abboud, F. M.: The Value of Left Parasternal Impulse Recordings in the Assessment of Mitral Regurgitation, *Circulation*, 48:1055, 1973.

137. Reichek, N., Shelburne, J. C., and Perloff, J. K.: Clinical Aspects of Rheumatic Valvular Disease, *Prog. Cardiovasc. Dis.*, 15:491, 1973.

138. Karliner, J. S., O'Rourke, R. A., Kearney, D. J., and Shabetai, R.: Haemodynamic Explanation of Why the Murmur of Mitral Regurgitation Is Independent of Cycle Length, *Br. Heart J.*, 35:397, 1973.

139. Perloff, J. K., and Harvey, W. P.: Auscultatory and Phonocardiographic Manifestations of Pure Mitral Regurgitation, *Prog. Cardiovasc. Dis.*, 5:172, 1962.

140. Perloff, J. K., and Harvey, W. P.: Mechanisms of Fixed Splitting of the Second Heart Sound, *Circulation*, 18:998, 1958.

141. Bleifer, S., Dack, S., Grishman, A., and Donoso, E.: The Auscultatory and Phonocardiographic Findings in Mitral Regurgitation, *Am. J. Cardiol.*, 5:836, 1960.

142. Devereux, R. B., Perloff, J. K., Reichek, N., and Josephson, M. E.: Mitral Valve Prolapse, *Circulation*, 54:3, 1976.

143. Epstein, E. J., and Coulshed, N.: Phonocardiogram and Apex Cardiogram in Systolic Click–Late Systolic Murmur Syndrome, *Br. Heart J.*, 35:260, 1973.

144. O'Rourke, R. A., and Crawford, M. H.: The Systolic Click–Murmur Syndrome: Clinical Recognition and Management, *Curr. Probl. Cardiol.*, 1(1):1, 1976.

145. Fontana, M. E., Wooley, C. G., Leighton, R. F., and Lewis, R. P.: Postural Changes in Left Ventricular and Mitral Valvular Dynamics in the Systolic Click–Late Systolic Murmur Syndrome, *Circulation*, 51:165, 1975.

146. Shelburne, J. C., Rubinstein, D., and Gorlin, R.: A Reappraisal of Papillary Muscle Dysfunction, *Am. J. Med.*, 46:862, 1969.

147. Holmes, A. M., Logan, W. F., and Winterbottom, T.: Transient Systolic Murmurs in Angina Pectoris, *Am. Heart J.*, 76:680, 1968.

148. Sanders, C. A., Austen, W. G., Harthorne, J. W., Dinsmore, R. E., and Scannell, J. G.: Diagnosis and Surgical Treatment of Mitral Regurgitation Secondary to Rupture Chordae Tendineae, *N. Engl. J. Med.*, 276:943, 1967.

149. Ronan, J. A., Jr., Steelman, R. B., DeLeon, A. C., Jr., Waters, T. J., Perlokk, J. K., and Harvey, W. P.: The Clinical Diagnosis of Acute Severe Mitral Insufficiency, *Am. J. Cardiol.*, 27:284, 1971.

150. Sleeper, J. C., Orgain, E. S., and McIntosh, H. D.: Mitral Insufficiency Simulating Aortic Stenosis, *Circulation*, 26:428, 1962.

151. Merendino, K. A., and Hessel, E. A.: The Murmur on Top of the Head in Acquired Mitral Insufficiency, *J. Am. Med. Assoc.*, 199:392, 1967.

152. Priest, E. A., Finlayson, J. K., and Short, D. S.: The X-Ray Manifestations in the Heart and Lungs of Mitral Regurgitation, *Prog. Cardiovasc. Dis.*, 5:219, 1962.

153. BonTempo, C. P., Ronan, J. A., DeLeon, A. C., and Twigg, H. L.: Radiographic Appearance of the Thorax in Systolic Click, Late Systolic Murmur Syndrome, *Am. J. Cardiol.*, 36:27, 1975.

154. Solomon, J., Shab, P. M., and Heinkle, R. A.: Thoracic Skeletal Abnormalities in Idiopathic Mitral Valve Prolapse, *Am. J. Cardiol.*, 36:32, 1975.

155. Bentivoglis, L. G., Uricchio, J. F., Waldow, A., Likoff, W., and Golberg, H.: An Electrocardiographic Analysis of Mitral Regurgitation, *Circulation*, 18:572, 1956.

156. Peter, R. H., Morris, J. J., Jr., and McIntosh, H. D.: Relationship of Fibrillatory Waves and P Waves in the Electrocardiogram, *Circulation*, 33:599, 1966.

157. Malcolm, A. D., Bougher, D. R., Kostuk, W. J., and Ahuja, S. P.: Clinical Features and Investigative Findings in Presence of Mitral Leaflet Prolapse, *Br. Heart J.*, 38:244, 1976.

158. DeMaria, A. N., Amsterdam, E. A., Vismara,

L. A., Neumann, A., and Mason, D. T.: Arrhythmias in the Mitral Valve Prolapse Syndrome, *Ann. Intern. Med.*, 84:656, 1976.

159. Burch, G. E., DePasquale, N. P., and Phillips, J. H.: The Syndrome of Papillary Muscle Dysfunction, *Am. Heart J.*, 75:399, 1968.

160. Popp, R. L., Brown, O. R., Silverman, J. F., and Harrison, D. C.: Echocardiographic Abnormalities in the Mitral Valve Prolapse Syndrome, *Circulation*, 49:428, 1974.

161. Burgess, J., Clark, R., Kamigaki, M., and Cohen, K.: Echocardiographic Findings in Different Types of Mitral Regurgitation, *Circulation*, 48:97, 1973.

162. DeMaria, A. N., King, J. F., Bogren, H. G., Lies, J. E., and Mason, D. T.: The Variable Spectrum of Echocardiographic Manifestations of the Mitral Valve Prolapse Syndrome, *Circulation*, 50:33, 1974.

163. Rackley, C. E., Russell, R. O., Jr., and Ratshin, R. A.: Hemodynamics of Acute Myocardial Infarction: Invasive and Noninvasive Studies. Proceedings of the William Likoff Symposium, New York, Dec. 14–16, 1973, in Henry I. Russek (ed.), "New Horizons in Cardiovascular Practice," University Park Press, Baltimore, 1975, p. 197.

164. Sweatman, T., Selzer, A., Kamageki, M., and Cohn, K.: Echocardiographic Diagnosis of Mitral Regurgitation Due to Rupture Chordae Tendineae, *Circulation*, 46:580, 1972.

165. Sandler, H., Dodge, H. T., Hay, R. E., and Rackley, C. E.: Quantitation of Valvular Insufficiency in Man by Angiocardiography. *Am. Heart J.*, 65:501, 1963.

166. Braunwald, E., and Awe, W. C.: The Syndrome of Severe Mitral Regurgitation with Normal Left Atrial Pressure, *Circulation*, 27:29, 1963.

167. Rackley, C. E., Dodge, H. T., Coble, Y. D., Jr., and Hay, R. E.: A Method for Determining Left Ventricular Mass in Man, *Circulation*, 29:666, 1964.

168. Mantle, J. A., Russell, R. O., Jr., Rogers, W. J., and Rackley, C. E.: Advances in the Treatment of Heart Failure, in C. E. Rackley and A. N. Brest (eds.), "Critical Care Cardiology," F. A. Davis, Philadelphia, Cardiovascular Clinics, 1981, pp. 49–64.

169. Scampardonis, G., Yang, S. S., Maranhao, V., Goldberg, H., and Gooch, A. S.: Left Ventricular Abnormalities in Prolapsed Mitral Leaflet Syndrome, *Circulation*, 48:287, 1973.

170. Rackley, C. E., Russell, R. O., Jr., Mantle, J. A., and Rogers, W. J.: Recognition of Acute Myocardial Infarction, in C. E. Rackley and R. O. Russell, Jr. (eds.), "Coronary Artery Disease: Recognition and Management," Futura Publishing Company, Mount Kisco, New York, 1979, p. 315.

171. Slutsky, R., Karliner, J., Ricci, D., Kaiser, R., Pfisterer, M., Gordon, D., Peterson, K., and Ashburn,

W.: Left Ventricular Volumes by Gated Equilibrium Radionuclide Angiography: A New Method, *Circulation*, 60:556, 1979.

172. Dehmer, G. J., Lewis, S. E., Hillis, L. D., Twieg, D., Falkoff, M., Parkey, R. W., and Willerson, J. T.: Nongeometric Determination of Left Ventricular Volumes from Equilibrium Blood Pool Scans, *Am. J. Cardiol.*, 45:293, 1980.

173. Greenberg, B. H., Masie, B. M., Brundage, B. H., Botvinick, E. H., Parmley, W. W., and Chatterjee, K.: Beneficial Effects of Hydrazaline in Severe Mitral Regurgitation, *Circulation*, 58:273, 1978.

174. Miller, R. R., Awan, N. A., Maxell, K. S., and Mason, D. T.: Sustained Reduction of Cardiac Impedance and Preload in Congestive Heart Failure with the Antihypertensive Vasodilator Prazosin, *N. Engl. J. Med.*, 297:303, 1977.

175. Mantle, J. A., Hood, W. P., Jr., Kouchoukos, N. T., Karp, R. B., Zisserman, D., and Rackley, C. E.: Physiologic Basis for Afterload Reduction Following Mitral Valve Replacement, *Am. J. Cardiol.*, 41:420, 1978.

176. Eckberg, D. L., Gault, J. H., Bouchard, R. L., Karliner, J. S., and Ross, J., Jr.: Mechanics of Left Ventricular Contraction in Chronic Severe Mitral Regurgitation, *Circulation*, 47:1252, 1973.

177. Schuler, G., Peterson, K. L., Johnson, A., Francis, G., Dennish, G., Utley, J., Ashburn, W., and Ross, J., Jr.: Temporal Response of Left Ventricular Performance to Mitral Valve Surgery, *Circulation*, 59:1218, 1979.

178. Kirklin, J. W.: Replacement of Mitral Valve for Mitral Incompetence, *Surgery*, 72:827, 1972.

179. Reed, G. E., Tice, D. A., and Clauss, R. H.: Asymmetric Exaggerated Mitral Annuloplasty: Repair of Mitral Insufficiency with Hemodynamic Predictability, *J. Thorac. Cardiovasc. Surg.*, 49:752, 1965.

180. Allen, W. B., Karp, R. B., and Kouchoukos, N. T.: Mitral Valve Replacement, *Arch. Surg.*, 109:642, 1974.

181. Kirklin, J. W., and Pacifico, A. C.: Surgery for Acquired Valvular Heart Disease, *N. Engl. J. Med.*, 288:133, 1973.

182. Hansen, J. F., Anderson, E. D., Olesen, K. H., Steiness, E., Lyngborg, K., Andersen, J. D., Efsen, F., Henningsen, P., and Wennevold, A.: DC Conversion of Atrial Fibrillation after Mitral Valve Operation, *Scand. J. Thorac. Cardiovasc. Surg.*, 13:267, 1979.

183. Williams, J. B., Karp, R. B., Kirklin, J. W., Kouchoukos, N. T., Pacifico, A. C., Zorn, G. L., Jr., Blackstone, E. H., Brown, R. N., Piantadose, S., and Bradley, E. L.: Considerations in Selection and Management of Patients Undergoing Valve Replacement with Glutaraldehyde-Fixed Porcine Bioprostheses, *Ann. Thorac. Surg.*, 30:247, 1980.

40

Tricuspid and Pulmonary Valve Disease

Charles E. Rackley, M.D.
Jesse E. Edwards, M.D.
Robert B. Karp, M.D.
John W. Kirklin, M.D.

I wish to plead for the admission among the recognized auscultatory signs of disease of a murmur due to pulmonary regurgitation occurring independently of disease or deformity of the valves, and as the result of long-continued excess of blood pressure in the pulmonary artery.

Graham Steell, 1888[1]

Etiology

Tricuspid stenosis is most commonly caused by rheumatic fever and is associated with mitral stenosis. However, stenosis of the tricuspid valve has been reported in the carcinoid syndrome, endocardial fibroelastosis, endomyocardial fibrosis, and systemic lupus erythematosus. Right atrial myxomas can obstruct the tricuspid orifice and produce the hemodynamic condition of tricuspid stenosis.[2,3]

Tricuspid regurgitation is most often functional and secondary to right ventricular dilatation and failure.[4] Any condition producing left ventricular failure and/or pulmonary hypertension can eventually cause tricuspid regurgitation. Isolated tricuspid regurgitation is rare, and infectious endocarditis is the most common cause.[5] Less common mechanisms involve trauma, myocardial infarction, prolapsed leaflet, and congenital abnormalities such as atrial septal defect and Ebstein's anomaly.

Acquired pulmonary valvular lesions generally lead to incompetence, but rarely an inflammatory process can produce stenosis and regurgitation of the pulmonary valve. Severe pulmonary hypertension can produce pulmonary incompetence as encountered in mitral stenosis, chronic lung disease, and pulmonary emboli. Inflammatory lesions such as endocarditis, rheumatic fever, and even tuberculosis can result in pulmonary regurgitation.[6,7] Tumors such as sarcomas and myxomas can also involve the valve.[8] Previous cardiac surgery on congenital pulmonary valvular lesions can result in pulmonary incompetence. Finally, mediastinal lesions such as tumor, aneurysm, and constrictive pericarditis can compress the pulmonary artery and simulate stenosis of the valve. (See Table 40-1.)

Pathology

The tricuspid valve may be stenotic or, more commonly, incompetent.[9] A variety of causes exist for tricuspid valvular dysfunction.

Rheumatic

The most common basis for tricuspid stenosis is rheumatic disease. The changes in the tricuspid valve are characterized by fibrosis with contracture of the leaflets and commissural fusion; the former leads to tricuspid regurgitation, the latter to stenosis (Fig. 40-1). It should be emphasized that the stenotic element of the rheumatic tricuspid valve is intrinsically minor and would usually go undetected were it not for the high flow across the valve incident to the coexistent regurgitation. In our view, whenever the tricuspid valve is involved by rheumatic disease, there is always coinvolvement of the left-sided valves, an observation in agreement with that of Clawson.[10]

Flammang and associates found that 9.5 percent of cases requiring surgical replacement of both the mitral and aortic valves exhibited rheumatic involvement of the tricuspid valve.[11] Among cases having mitral commissurotomy, the incidence of clinically evident tricuspid disease was 3 percent. In a series of 217 autopsied cases of rheumatic heart disease, Cooke and White found 47 cases (22 percent) in which the tricuspid valve was also involved by rheumatic disease.[12]

Carcinoid Tumor (See Chap. 60)

In about 10 percent of cases of malignant carcinoid tumor (usually primary in the ileum) with extensive metastases, the tricuspid and pulmonary valves may be affected (Fig. 40-2). The changes are those of deposits of fibrous tissue on the surfaces of these valves. Fibrous plaques may also be deposited on the endocardial surfaces of the right atrium and ventricle and on the intima of the coronary sinus and pulmonary artery.[13] The hemodynamic effects result from the rigidity and contracture of the fibrous tissues deposited on the valves. In the tricuspid valve, the major functional effect is regurgitation, while the pulmonary valve, if affected, may be both stenotic and incompetent.

TABLE 40-1   Acquired Lesions of the Pulmonary Valve

1. Pulmonary hypertension with pulmonary regurgitation
   a. Mitral stenosis
   b. Chronic lung disease
   c. Pulmonary emboli
2. Inflammatory lesions
   a. Endocarditis
   b. Rheumatic fever
   c. Tuberculosis
3. Tumors
   a. Sarcoma
   b. Myxoma
4. Previous surgery on congenital lesions
5. Mediastinal lesions
   a. Tumor
   b. Aneurysm
   c. Constrictive pericarditis

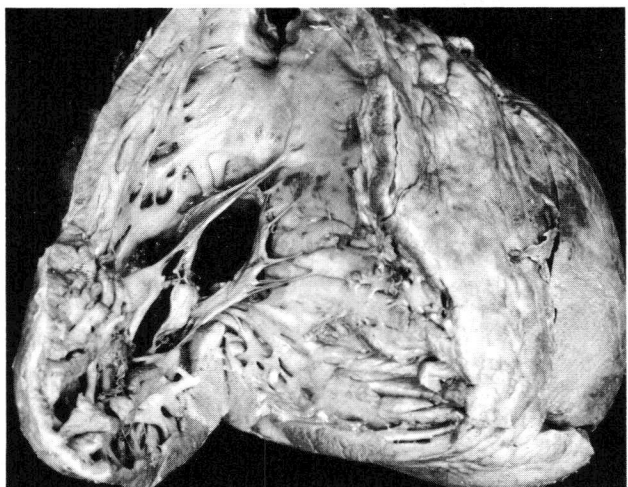

FIGURE 40-1 Tricuspid valve from below in chronic rheumatic endocarditis. Although the chordae are relatively uninvolved, there is fusion of the leaflets at the commissures creating a narrowed and fixed orifice. The valve is both stenotic and incompetent.

Congestive Cardiac Failure

The most common type of tricuspid regurgitation is the so-called secondary type resulting from enlargement of the orifice incident to congestive cardiac failure with right ventricular dilatation, while the structure of the valve is intrinsically normal. The process may be reversible with return of competence of the right ventricle.[14,15]

Infectious Endocarditis

In infectious endocarditis the basis for tricuspid regurgitation may, in part, be improper apposition of the leaflets by interposed vegetations. Major degrees of tricuspid regurgitation on an infectious basis result most commonly from rupture of chordae tendineae.

Trauma

The classical background for traumatic tricuspid insufficiency is external blunt trauma (including sudden deceleration), most commonly an automobile accident. Gerry and associates described two cases of rupture of a tricuspid papillary muscle resulting from external cardiopulmonary resuscitation.[16]

The main basis for traumatic tricuspid regurgitation is rupture of one or several elements of the tensor apparatus, with rupture of a papillary muscle being more common than rupture of chordae. Less commonly, there is laceration of leaflet tissue and, in an occasional case, more than one of the anatomic elements of the valve is affected.[17,18] Stephenson and associates described an uncommon case in which traumatic tricuspid regurgitation and ruptured ventricular septum coexisted.[19]

Tolerance of tricuspid regurgitation of traumatic origin varies, with tolerance for 39 years reported.[20–23] Those cases with rupture of a papillary muscle tend to tolerate the tricuspid regurgitation less than do those in which the trauma resulted in rupture of chordae.[21] Among cases of tricuspid regurgitation resulting from rupture of chordae, a traumatic background is more common than is bacterial endocarditis.[24]

Myocardial Infarction

Except for cases involving chronic congestive cardiac failure, myocardial infarction is not a common cause of tricuspid regurgitation.[25] Direct results of myocardial infarction causing tricuspid insufficiency are uncommon and have been described from aneurysmal dilatation of the right ventricle and a rare case of rupture of a right ventricular papillary muscle.[25–28]

Prolapse

Varying degrees of prolapse of the tricuspid valve are commonly present and usually associated with identified prolapse of the mitral valve. Nevertheless, instances of tricuspid insufficiency on this basis, though described, are uncommon.[29]

Congenital Anomalies

Among the primary diseases of the tricuspid valve that cause incompetence are Ebstein's malformation

FIGURE 40-2 Diagrammatic portrayal of the effects of the carcinoid syndrome on the heart. Insert shows pulmonary stenosis. The leaflets of the tricuspid valve are thickened. The valve is predominantly incompetent. Fibrous plaques are deposited on the lining of the right ventricle and pulmonary trunk. (*From J. E. Edwards, Effects of Malignant Noncardiac Tumors upon the Cardiovascular System, Cardiovasc. Clin., 4:282, 1971. Reproduced with permission.*)

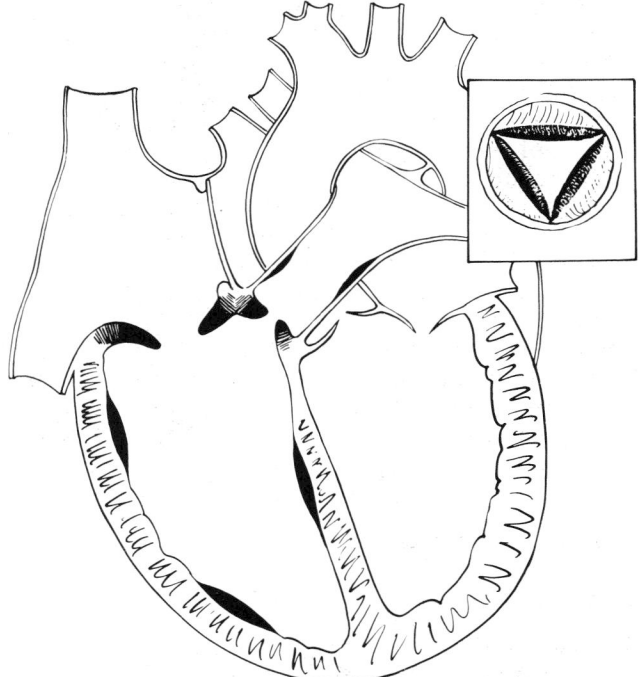

and valvular dysplasia. These are discussed in detail in Chap. 36.

Pulmonary Valve

Acquired diseases of the pulmonary valve are uncommon, while abnormalities in or near this valve are among the common types of congenital heart disease (see Chap. 36).

Acquired pulmonary stenosis and/or incompetence is one of the consequences of the valvular changes complicating the carcinoid syndrome[30] (Fig. 40-2).

Pathophysiology

In tricuspid stenosis the hemodynamic disturbance is an elevation of the right atrial pressure and decreased diastolic flow across the valve, which results in a reduced cardiac output.[31,32] The approximate area of the normal tricuspid valve is 7 cm^2, and estimates suggest that impairment of right ventricular filling occurs when valve area is reduced below 1.5 cm^2. The level of the right atrial pressure is a critical factor in the production of systemic venous pressure elevation and the development of peripheral edema. Elevation of the mean right atrial pressure above 10 mmHg is often associated with clinical development of edema. Atrial fibrillation produces a higher mean right atrial pressure in tricuspid stenosis than is present with sinus rhythm and normal atrial contraction. The hemodynamic abnormalities in tricuspid stenosis are also influenced by the frequently coexisting mitral stenosis. Tricuspid valve obstruction and reduced right ventricular flow have been proposed as mechanisms which protect against severe pulmonary hypertension.

In tricuspid regurgitation the systolic regurgitation into the right atrium elevates right atrial pressure.[33] This regurgitation produces prominent v waves reflected in the venous system, and once the right atrial pressure exceeds 10 mmHg, peripheral edema often develops.

In acquired pulmonary valve lesions regurgitation is the most frequent disturbance. Regurgitation can be secondary to pulmonary hypertension or a primary disturbance in the leaflets preventing adequate coaptation. The consequence of pulmonary regurgitation is a volume overload on the right ventricle which can be superimposed on hypertrophied myocardium if pulmonary hypertension was preexistent. Isolated pulmonary valvular insufficiency can be tolerated for a long period without cardiac decompensation.[34]

Clinical Manifestations

History

Dyspnea and fatigue are the most frequent symptoms in tricuspid stenosis, but the development of

significant tricuspid stenosis may diminish the paroxysmal symptoms of dyspnea, pulmonary edema, and hemoptysis in mitral stenosis by preventing the increase in pulmonary congestion and hypertension.[2,3] Patients with tricuspid stenosis occasionally complain of prominent pulsations in the neck which often precede the development of peripheral edema late in the course.

Since tricuspid regurgitation usually accompanies left ventricular failure or mitral stenosis, the symptoms are those of dyspnea, orthopnea, and peripheral edema, but paroxysmal nocturnal dyspnea may be surprisingly infrequent.[35] Tricuspid regurgitation in these conditions may ameliorate the pulmonary symptoms and provide a physiological basis for the clinical contention that right heart failure alleviates symptoms of left heart failure. If the isolated tricuspid regurgitation is due to bacterial endocarditis, the symptoms of a febrile illness may be attended by fatigue and peripheral accumulation of fluid.

In acquired pulmonary valvular lesions the clinical manifestations depend on the severity of the impaired valve as well as the extent of the underlying disease. Isolated pulmonary regurgitation can be tolerated without symptoms. Severe pulmonary hypertension may not only cause dyspnea and fatigue but also syncope. Inflammatory lesions may be attended by additional febrile manifestations with infectious sites in the lungs in addition to those in the valve structure. The carcinoid syndrome is typically characterized by episodes of facial flushing, increased intestinal activity, diarrhea, and bronchial spasm. Tumors involving the pulmonary valve may exert pressure from expansion and metastases which affect the lungs and the heart.

Physical Examination

Tricuspid stenosis is frequently associated with mitral stenosis and aortic regurgitation, and the vital signs often reflect the peripheral changes seen in this condition. The neck vessels in tricuspid stenosis may display the large venous a wave indicative of impaired right ventricular diastolic filling. In the majority of patients with tricuspid stenosis the a waves in the neck will be of moderate height or giant, sometimes reaching the mandible.[2,3] Simultaneous palpation of the opposite carotid vessel may be necessary to time the venous pulse wave and to document the rise of the a wave simultaneously with the first heart sound. The v wave is small and the y descent is insignificant.

On precordial examination the presence or absence of right ventricular hypertension is important since severe pulmonary hypertension and right ventricular hypertrophy render tricuspid stenosis a less likely lesion. With inspiration, the first heart sound may be slightly enhanced and often split. The split in the two components of the first sound is due to delay of closure both in the stenotic mitral valve and the tricuspid valve. Auscultation of the second heart sound is important to identify the pulmonary component, which may indicate pulmonary hypertension. Respiratory variations in splitting of the pulmonary sound may be absent in tricuspid stenosis since right ventricular filling remains fairly constant throughout the respiratory cycle. The characteristic auscultatory finding in tricuspid stenosis is the diastolic rumble heard best at the lower left sternal border.[2,3,36] If sinus rhythm is present, the murmur will be presystolic, but if atrial fibrillation has developed the murmur may be early or middiastolic. The most effective differentiation from mitral stenosis is the influence of respiration on the murmur, since the inspiratory phase will markedly accentuate the diastolic rumble of tricuspid stenosis (Fig. 40-3). The augmentation of the rumble in tricuspid stenosis with inspiration, Carvallo's sign, is due to the augmented venous return to the right atrium as well as an increase in right ventricular filling.[37] Although an opening snap in tricuspid stenosis can be recorded by intracardiac phonocardiography, this sound is rarely appreciated at the clinical level.

In tricuspid regurgitation atrial fibrillation is quite common, and the neck veins will reveal a prominent v wave which is generated from regurgitation into the right atrium.[35] The v wave is more gradual in upstroke than the sharp rise of the a wave, but simultaneous auscultation of the first heart sound is the best method for timing venous pulsations. The characteristic auscultatory finding is a holosystolic murmur at the left sternal border which is augmented during inspiration. Frequently the murmur of mitral regurgitation is also present, but respiration exerts a predominant influence on tricuspid regurgitation with little change in the mitral murmur.

In patients with acquired lesions of the pulmonary valve, vital signs may reflect left ventricular failure or respiratory distress of a febrile condition. A prominent v wave will be present in the jugular pulse if right ventricular failure has developed secondary to tricuspid regurgitation. Even though right ventricular hypertrophy may have been preexistent from pulmonary hypertension, a waves are rarely observed in the neck veins once incompetence

of the pulmonary valve has developed. Increased right ventricular activity can be palpated along the left sternal border, and if pulmonary hypertension is present the pulmonary second sound will be markedly accentuated. The pulmonary insufficiency murmur may be difficult to distinguish from the murmur of aortic regurgitation. The systemic blood pressure and peripheral pulse findings of aortic regurgitation can be helpful.

Chest Roentgenogram

In tricuspid stenosis, prominence of the right atrium without significant pulmonary artery enlargement or pulmonary hypertension is the most characteristic finding.[2] Some degree of right atrial enlargement is present in tricuspid regurgitation, but there will also be accompanying right ventricular enlargement.[35] In pulmonary valvular insufficiency the pulmonary artery may be quite prominent.[34]

Electrocardiogram

In tricuspid stenosis a helpful electrocardiographic finding is the characteristic P wave of right atrial enlargement in the absence of right ventricular hypertrophy.[2,36] In tricuspid regurgitation, atrial fibrillation is quite common without other consistent features.[35] With pulmonary valvular lesions there are no characteristic changes in the electrocardiogram other than preexisting pulmonary hypertension, P mitrale, and right-axis deviation with mitral stenosis.

Special Laboratory Studies

The difficulty in identifying the tricuspid valve is a major limitation in the application of echocardiography, but characteristic stenotic patterns of the tricuspid valve can sometimes be recorded. In tricuspid regurgitation the systolic prolapse can occasionally be identified, as well as a vegetative lesion on the valve.[38] Increased right ventricular dimensions indicate impaired right ventricular function and the likelihood of secondary tricuspid regurgitation. Contrast echocardiography with peripheral venous injection can identify back-and-forth movement across the tricuspid valve.[39] If the pulmonary valve can be identified, leaflet motion, vegetative lesion, or tumor can sometimes be delineated in the pulmonary valvular area.

Cardiac Catheterization

To confirm tricuspid stenosis at catheterization, simultaneous pressures must be recorded in the right atrium and right ventricle.[31] The normal gradient across the tricuspid valve is less than 1 mmHg, and, therefore, small gradients will not be detected if a pullback pressure is recorded from the right ventricle to the right atrium. Cardiac output can be measured and orifice size calculated. The area of

FIGURE 40-3 Phonocardiogram in a patient with tricuspid stenosis. Striking features are the prominent tricuspid component of the first sound (T_1) in comparison to the mitral component (m), and the late diastolic murmur which increases during the inspiratory phase (ip) of respiration.

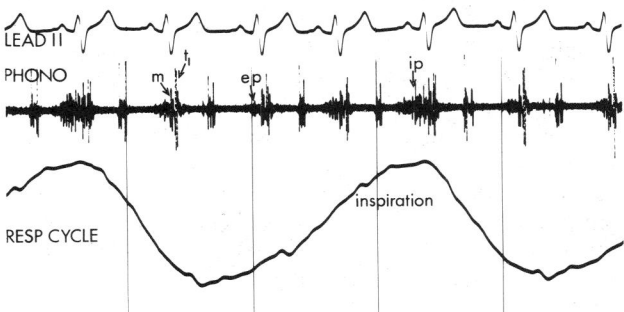

the tricuspid valve in significant stenosis is less than 1.5 cm², and in severe stenosis it is less than 1 cm².

Angiographic documentation of tricuspid regurgitation is difficult to obtain, since the catheter overrides the tricuspid valve and ventricular irritability from a right ventricular injection can induce artifactual tricuspid regurgitation. A prominent *v* wave in the right atrium suggests tricuspid regurgitation. Indicator dilution curves have been used with simultaneous injection into the right ventricle and sampling in the right atrium and femoral artery to demonstrate early appearance in the right atrium.[33]

Pulmonary insufficiency cannot be easily demonstrated angiographically, but an aortic root injection can be useful to eliminate aortic regurgitation as a cause of the diastolic murmur. Rarely, intracardiac phonocardiography has been used to detect the diastolic murmur in the right ventricular outflow tract.

Natural History and Prognosis

In tricuspid stenosis the symptoms are primarily those of mitral stenosis, but a conspicuous absence of paroxysmal aggravation of pulmonary congestion in the presence of peripheral edema should alert one to the possible coexistence of tricuspid stenosis. Thus, tricuspid stenosis may hinder the development of the characteristic symptoms of mitral stenosis and mislead the physician into underestimating the severity of mitral stenosis.

In tricuspid regurgitation the symptoms and course are primarily related to the left heart conditions, which produce a pressure or volume overload on the right ventricle. The eventual development of tricuspid regurgitation indicates severe right ventricular failure. In acute bacterial endocarditis of the tricuspid valve the type of organism will also significantly influence the course and response to therapy.

In pulmonary valve lesions the course will be more prolonged if there is long-standing pulmonary hypertension due to mitral stenosis or chronic lung disease. Inflammatory conditions and tumors which affect the valve usually involve a much shorter course.

Management

Medical

In tricuspid stenosis the usual precautionary measures for antibiotic coverage and prevention of endocarditis apply. Peripheral edema will not respond to the usual measurements of digitalis and diuretics, and this emphasizes the clinical necessity to recognize underlying tricuspid stenosis with mitral stenosis.

In tricuspid regurgitation, the treatment of right ventricular failure will involve digitalis and diuretic therapy of left ventricular failure. If right heart failure is due to mitral stenosis, early surgical intervention is the best management.

In pulmonary lesions antibiotic prophylaxis is required, and if pulmonary emboli are involved, anticoagulation will be useful. Treatment of pulmonary hypertension will require management of left heart failure, correction of mitral stenosis or the use of vasodilating agents which have been effective in lowering pulmonary artery pressure.

Surgery

Pathology of the tricuspid valve in association with involvement of the aortic or mitral valve occurs in 10 to 15 percent of patients with chronic rheumatic heart disease. In the Mediterranean, Middle East, and Far East the incidence is probably higher. The valve leaflets are thickened and the commissures are fused and usually ill-defined. The chordae very seldom may be fused and shortened. If such is the case, the tricuspid valve is usually rendered both stenotic and incompetent.

Patients with disease of the mitral valve commonly exhibit signs and symptoms of tricuspid valve incompetence. In many such cases the leaflets of the tricuspid valve appear normal and incompetence is believed to be caused by malfunction of the valve due to severe right ventricular hypertension or dilatation of the right ventricle. In all but the mildest cases of this functional tricuspid regurgitation, we believe that operative treatment of the incompetence is quite helpful in the early and late postoperative period. Annuloplasty is performed in this situation. When there is some stenosis as well as incompetence, recent experience has suggested that tricuspid commissurotomy along with annuloplasty is quite successful.

Operation

Tricuspid annuloplasty is done in a fashion similar to that described for the mitral valve. In general there are two techniques. One is insertion of the Carpentier flexible ring, which is modified to avoid the area of the septal leaflet intimately related to the atrioventricular node and His bundle. The insertion of the flexible ring narrows and helps to remodel the dilated annulus. The second and equally satisfactory procedure is the use of a DeVega annuloplasty stitch,[40] which effectively narrows the lateral two-thirds of the tricuspid annulus (Fig. 40-4).

Replacement of the tricuspid valve is only infrequently indicated. The indications are a severely deformed, stenotic, and incompetent valve. The preferred device is a low-profile prosthesis or xenograft. The valve is inserted, taking care to place sutures at the base of the septal leaflet rather than encompassing the annulus in the area of the septum, thus avoiding harm to the conduction system.

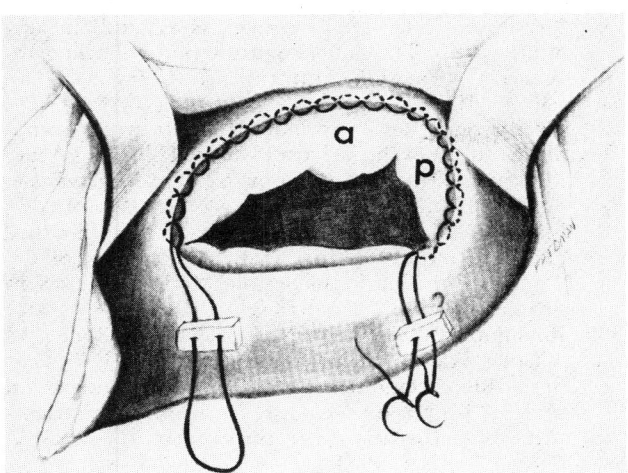

FIGURE 40-4 DeVega tricuspid annuloplasty. (*From P. N. West and C. S. Weldon, Reconstructive Valve Surgery, Ann. Thorac. Surg., 25:167, 1978. Reproduced with permission.*)

Postoperative Care

After tricuspid replacement or reconstruction patients frequently have a tendency to retain fluid. Diuretic treatment is indicated for several months. If a prosthetic device has been used, long-term anticoagulation therapy is mandatory.

Results

The operative risk for a patient undergoing operation on the tricuspid valve combined with replacement of one or both of the left-sided valves depends on the cardiac disability and on whether an annuloplasty is possible or valve replacement is necessary. At present, the risk for annuloplasty is 10 to 12 percent when associated with left-sided cardiac valve replacement, and when tricuspid valve replacement is necessary it is 15 to 20 percent. In general, after annuloplasty the tricuspid valve remains competent. However, to some extent this depends on the level

of systolic pressure in the right ventricle and pulmonary artery. The long-term results of triple-valve replacement are shown in Fig. 40-5.

References

1. Steell, G.: The Murmur of High-Pressure in the Pulmonary Artery, *Medical Chronicle*, IX:182, 1888.
2. Perloff, J. K., and Harvey, W. P.: Clinical Recognition of Tricuspid Stenosis, *Circulation*, 22:346, 1960.
3. Kitchin, A., and Turner, R.: Diagnosis and Treatment of Tricuspid Stenosis, *Br. Heart J.*, 26:354, 1964.
4. McMichael, J., and Shillingford, J. P.: The Role of Valvular Incompetence in Heart Failure, *Br. Med. J.*, 1:537, 1957.
5. Glancy, D. L., Marcus, F. I., Cuadra, M., Ewy, G. A., and Roberts, W. C.: Isolated Organic Tricuspid Valvular Regurgitation, *Am. J. Med.*, 46:989, 1969.
6. Espino Vela, J., Contreros, R., and Rustrian Sosa, F.: Rheumatic Pulmonary Valve Disease, *Am. J. Cardiol.*, 23:12, 1969.
7. Roberts, W. C., and Buchbinder, N. A.: Right Sided Valvular Infective Endocarditis, *Am. J. Med.*, 53:7, 1972.
8. Seymour, J., Emaneul, R., and Patterson, N.: Acquired Pulmonary Stenosis, *Br. Heart J.*, 30:776, 1968.
*9. Edwards, J. E.: The Spectrum and Clinical Significance of Tricuspid Regurgitation, *Practical Cardiol.*, 6:86, 1980. (36 references)
10. Clawson, B. J.: Rheumatic Heart Disease. An Analysis of 796 Cases, *Am. Heart J.*, 20:454, 1940.
11. Flammang, D., Juamin, P., and Kremer, R.: Organic Tricuspid Pathology in Rheumatic Valvulopathies, *Acta Cardiol.*, 30:155, 1975.
12. Cooke, W. T., and White, P. D.: Tricuspid Stenosis: With Particular Reference to Diagnosis and Prognosis, *Br. Heart J.*, 3:147, 1941.

*This article is a review of the literature and contains additional references to the literature.

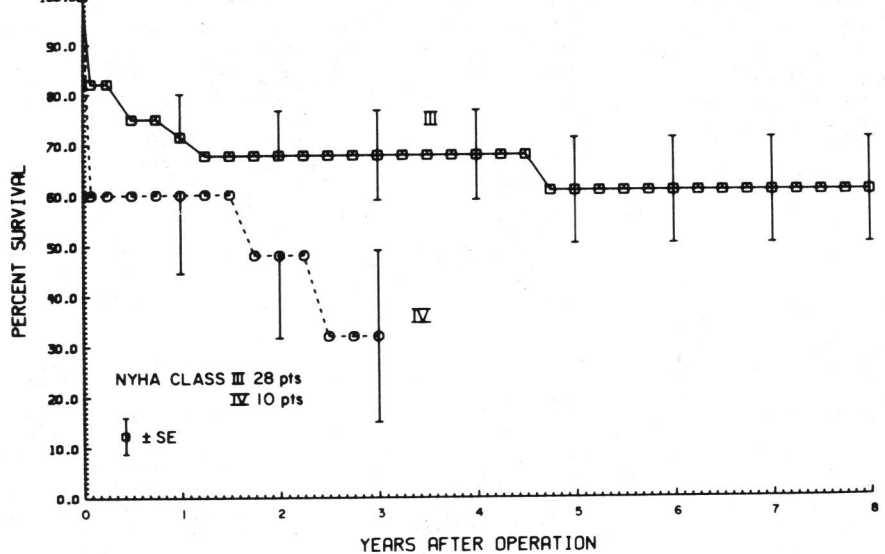

FIGURE 40-5 Actuarial survival according to preoperative functional class for patients receiving tricuspid valve replacement. (*From L. W. Stephenson, N. T. Kouchoukos, and J. W. Kirklin, Triple Valve Replacement: An Analysis of Eight Years Experience, Ann. Thorac. Surg., 23:327, 1977. Reproduced with permission.*)

13. Ludwig, J.: Cardiac Vein Involvement in Carcinoid Syndrome. Possible Evidence of Retrograde Blood Flow in Cardiac Veins in Tricuspid Insufficiency, *Am. J. Clin. Path.*, 55:617, 1971.

14. McMichael, J., and Shillingford, J. P.: The Role of Valvular Incompetence in Heart Failure, *Br. Med. J.*, 1:537, 1957.

15. Boucek, R. J., Jr., Graham, T. P., Morgan, J. P., Atwood, G. F., and Boerth, R. C.: Spontaneous Resolution of Massive Congenital Tricuspid Insufficiency, *Circulation*, 54:795, 1976.

16. Gerry, J. L., Jr., Bulkley, B. H., and Hutchins, G. M.: Rupture of the Papillary Muscle of the Tricuspid Valve. A Complication of Cardiopulmonary Resuscitation and a Rare Cause of Tricuspid Insufficiency, *Am. J. Cardiol.*, 40:825, 1977.

17. Jahnke, E. J., Jr., Nelson, W. P., Aaby, G. V., and FitzGibbon, G. M.: Tricuspid Insufficiency. The Result of Nonpenetrating Cardiac Trauma, *Arch. Surg.*, 95:880, 1967.

18. VanGilder, J. E., Jain, A. C., Weiss, R. B., Bowyer, A. F., and Tarnay, T. J.: Traumatic Right Ventricular Aneurysm Presenting as Tricuspid Regurgitation, *W. Va. Med. J.*, 75:93, 1979.

19. Stephenson, L. W., MacVaugh, H., III, and Kastor, J. A.: Tricuspid Valvular Incompetence and Rupture of the Ventricular Septum Caused by Nonpenetrating Trauma, *J. Thorac. Cardiovasc. Surg.*, 77:768, 1979.

20. Brandenburg, R. O., McGoon, D. C., Campeau, L., and Giuliani, E. R.: Traumatic Rupture of the Chordae Tendineae of the Tricuspid Valve. Successful Repair Twenty-Four Years Later, *Am. J. Cardiol.*, 18:911, 1966.

21. Morgan, J. R., and Forker, A. D.: Isolated Tricuspid Insufficiency, *Circulation*, 43:559, 1971.

22. Marvin, R. F., Schrank, J. P., and Nolan, S. P.: Traumatic Tricuspid Insufficiency, *Am. J. Cardiol.*, 32:723, 1973.

23. Croxson, M. S., O'Brien, K. P., and Lowe, J. B.: Traumatic Tricuspid Regurgitation. Long-Term Survival, *Br. Heart J.*, 33:750, 1971.

24. Grubier, M., Denis, B., and Martin-Noel, P.: Les Ruptures de cordages tricuspidiens, *Coeur Med. Int.*, 15:215, 1976.

25. Collins, R., and Daly, J. J.: Tricuspid Incompetence Complicating Acute Myocardial Infarction, *Postgrad. Med. J.*, 53:51, 1977.

26. Zone, D. D., and Botti, R. E.: Right Ventricular Infarction with Tricuspid Insufficiency and Chronic Right Heart Failure, *Am. J. Cardiol.*, 37:445, 1976.

27. McAllister, R. G., Jr., Friesinger, G. C., and Sinclair-Smith, B. C.: Tricuspid Regurgitation Following Inferior Myocardial Infarction, *Arch. Intern. Med.*, 136:95, 1976.

28. Eisenberg, S., and Suyemoto, J.: Rupture of a Papillary Muscle of the Tricuspid Valve Following Acute Myocardial Infarction. Report of a Case, *Circulation*, 30:588, 1964.

29. Maranhao, V., Gooch, A. S., Yang, S. S., Sumathisena, D. R., and Goldberg, H. H.: Prolapse of the Tricuspid Leaflets in the Systolic Murmur-Click Syndrome, *Cath. Cardiovasc. Diag.*, 1:81, 1975.

30. Rossignol, B., Machecourt, J., Denis, B., Roche, J., N'Golet, A., Morena, H., and Martin-Noel, P.: Cardiopathie carcinoide secondaire à une tumeur du grele. À propos d'un cas associat insuffisance tricuspidienne et insuffisance pulmonaire, *Arch. Mal. Coeur.*, 70:1221, 1977.

31. Killip, T., and Lukas, D. S.: Tricuspid Stenosis: Physiologic Criteria for Diagnosis and Hemodynamic Abnormalities, *Circulation*, 16:3, 1957.

32. El-Sherif, N.: Rheumatic Tricuspid Stenosis: A Haemodynamic Correlation, *Br. Heart J.*, 33:16, 1971.

33. Hansing, C. E., and Rowe, G. G.: Tricuspid Insufficiency: A Study of Hemodynamics and Pathogenesis, *Circulation*, 45:793, 1972.

34. Holmes, J. C., Fowler, N. O., and Kaplan, S.: Pulmonary Valvular Insufficiency, *Am. J. Med.*, 44:851, 1968.

*35. Salazar, E., and Levine, H. D.: Rheumatic Tricuspid Regurgitation: The Clinical Spectrum, *Am. J. Med.*, 33:111, 1962. (61 references)

36. Killip, T., and Lukas, D. S.: Tricuspid Stenosis: Clinical Features in Twelve Cases, *Am. J. Med.*, 24:836, 1958.

37. Rivero-Carvallo, J. M.: El diagnóstica de la estenosis tricúspides, *Arch. Inst. Cardiol. Mexico*, 20:1, 1950.

38. Chandraratna, P. A., Lopez, J. M., Fernandex, J. J., and Cohen, L. S.: Echocardiographic Detection of Tricuspid Valve Prolapse, *Circulation*, 51:823, 1975.

39. Lieppe, W., Behar, V. S., Scallion, R., and Kisslo, J. A.: Detection of Tricuspid Regurgitation with Two-Dimensional Echocardiography and Peripheral Vein Injections, *Circulation*, 57:128, 1978.

40. DeVega, N. G., deRabago, G. P., Castillon, L., Moreno, P. T., Fraile, J., and Batanero, J.: Immediate Results Six Months and One Year Later of the Surgical Treatment of Valvulotomy by Means of a New Original Technique, *Rev. Esp. Cardiol.*, 25:555, 1972.

41

Factors Influencing Atherogenesis

Russell Ross, Ph.D.

The Lesions of Atherosclerosis

Atherosclerosis is not a single disease entity. The lesions of atherosclerosis take different forms, depending upon their anatomic site; the age, genetic, and physiological status of the affected individual; and, presumably, upon the so-called risk factors to which each individual may have been exposed. Examination of atherosclerotic lesions with modern techniques of cell and molecular biology has revealed that each lesion contains significant elements of three cellular phenomena. These are smooth-muscle proliferation; formation by the proliferated cells of large amounts of connective tissue matrix including collagen, elastic fibers, and proteoglycans; and accumulation of intracellular and extracellular lipid.[1] In each instance, the relative degree to which each of the cells responds to different atherogenic stimuli determines the unique combination that defines the type and the extent of the resulting lesion.

The lesions of atherosclerosis occur principally within the innermost layer of the artery wall, the intima. They include the fatty streak, the fibrous plaque, and the so-called complicated lesions.[2] (See Chap. 45.) Secondary changes have been noted in the media of the artery underlying the lesion, principally in association with the more advanced lesions of atherosclerosis (Fig. 41-1).

The Fatty Streak (See Fig. 45-1)

The process of atherosclerosis begins in childhood with the development of flat, lipid-rich lesions called *fatty streaks*. These lesions consist of a small increase in the number of smooth-muscle cells, together with some macrophages within the arterial intima. Both of these cell types contain deposits of cholesterol and cholesterol oleate. Fatty streaks can be found in the aorta shortly after birth and appear in increasing numbers between the ages of 8 and 18 years. Fatty streaks appear in the coronary arteries at about age 15 and continue to increase in amount in these vessels through the third decade of life.[3]

The lesions are yellowish and sessile in appearance and cause little to no obstruction of the affected artery and no clinical sequelae. The fatty streak is ubiquitous in young people and even in those populations that do not appear to develop severe atherosclerosis. This observation suggests that lipid deposition does not inevitably lead to the advanced lesions of atherosclerosis, but that a number of other factors, as yet largely hypothetical, are associated with the progression of the lesions and with the development of the more complex form of atherosclerosis, the fibrous plaque.

The Fibrous Plaque (See Fig. 45-2)

More advanced lesions begin to develop around the age of 25 in those populations in which there is a high incidence of atherosclerosis and its clinical sequelae. The fibrous plaque is grossly white in appearance and becomes elevated so that it may protrude into the lumen of the artery. If this lesion progresses sufficiently, it can occlude the lumen and compromise the vascular supply of the involved tissue. The principal change that occurs within the arterial intima during the development of the fibrous plaque consists of proliferation of smooth-muscle cells. These cells usually form a fibrous cap due to the deposition by the cells of new connective tissue

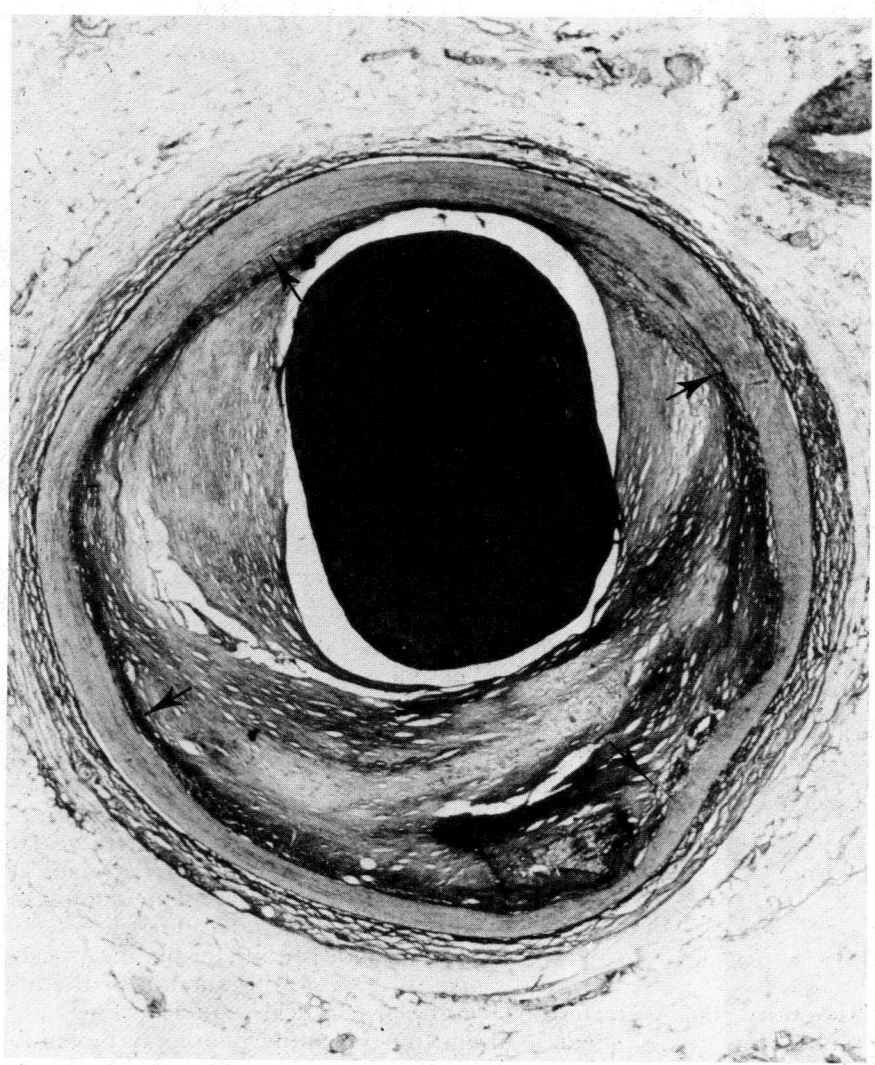

FIGURE 41-1 This is a classical light micrograph of a cross section of a coronary artery that contains a large atherosclerotic lesion. The lumen of the artery is relatively small. The original lumen is indicated by the arrows. In this preparation, it is virtually impossible to see cellular detail and, in particular, to determine the type of cells involved in the formation of the lesion.

matrix and to the accumulation of intracellular and extracellular lipids. This fibrous cap covers a deeper deposit of varying amounts of extracellular lipid and cell debris[4] (Fig. 41-2).

It has been suggested that fibrous plaques are derived from fatty streaks that continue the process of cell proliferation, lipid accumulation, and connective tissue formation, and that the deep core of lipid and cell debris results from inadequate blood supply and cell necrosis. Such a relationship has not been proved but has been questioned, since although fatty streaks in young individuals are often found in the same anatomic location in the coronary and extracranial cerebral arteries as fibrous plaques in older individuals, fatty streaks can also occur in anatomic sites that are different from those in which fibrous plaques appear. The reasons for these differences are not understood. It has been suggested that in those instances where their location is different, the fatty streaks may have simply regressed and disappeared; whereas in the instances where the anatomic location is the same, lesion progression has occurred. This remains a matter of controversy. There is a lesion that is generally accepted as a forerunner of the fibrous plaque. This is known as the *fibromusculoelastic lesion* of the intima, which consists of proliferated smooth-muscle cells surrounded by connective tissue which contains little to no lipid.[5]

The Advanced (Complicated) Lesion (See Figs. 45-3 and 45-5)

The complicated lesions of atherosclerosis occur in increasing frequency with increasing age. The fibrous plaque can become vascularized both from the luminal as well as its medial aspects. In the complicated lesion, the necrotic "lipid-rich core" increases in size and often becomes calcified. The lesions may become increasingly complex as a result of hemorrhage and calcification, and the intimal surface may disintegrate and ulcerate and become involved with thrombotic episodes that may lead to

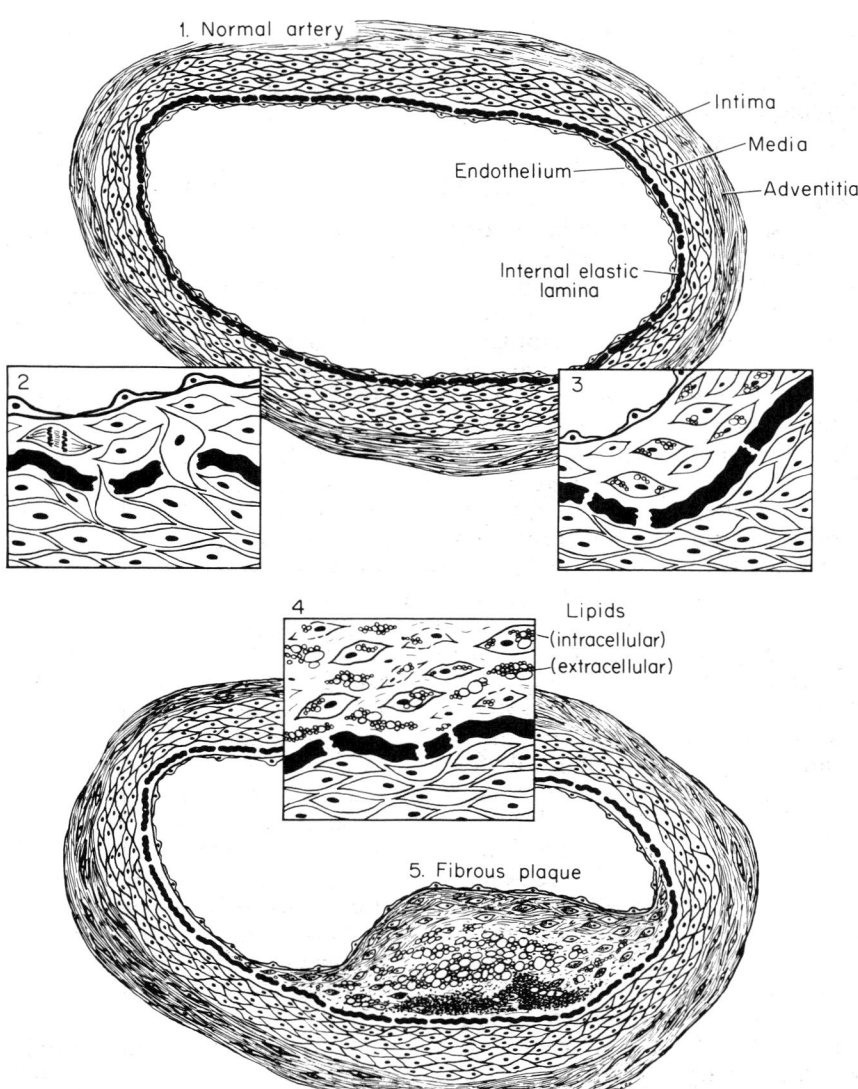

FIGURE 41-2 A series of possible stages in the development of the various lesions of atherosclerosis. (1) The appearance of a normal muscular artery and its component layers: the intima bounded by endothelium and internal elastic lamina, the media, and adventitia. In children and young adults the intima is thin and contains only an occasional smooth-muscle cell; with age it slowly and uniformly increases in thickness and cell content. It is important to note that there are no fibroblasts present in either the intima or the media of mammalian arteries. Fibroblasts are found only in the adventitia. (2) The first phase of a developing lesion in atherosclerosis; a focal thickening of the intima consists of an increase in smooth-muscle cells and extracellular matrix. Smooth-muscle cells are shown proliferating within the intima; two are in the process of migrating through fenestrae of the internal elastic lamina. Subsequent to or possibly concomitant with intimal smooth-muscle proliferation, accumulation of intercellular lipid deposits (3) or extracellular lipid (4), or both, occur resulting in a fatty streak. A fibrous plaque (5) may result from a continued accumulation of a connective tissue cap covering increased numbers of smooth-muscle cells laden with lipids, extracellular lipid, and cell debris overlying a deeper extracellular pool of lipid. A complicated lesion may form as a result of continuing cell degeneration, ingress of blood constituents, and calcification superimposed upon the elements present in the fibrous plaque. Observations made at necropsy and experiments such as those described in the text suggest that this may represent the sequence of events that occurs in humans. *(From J. A. Glomset and R. Russell, Atherosclerosis and the Arterial Smooth Muscle Cell,* Science, *180:1332, 1973. Reproduced with permission of author and publisher).*

occlusive disease. Such thrombi may then organize and further increase the thickness of the plaque while progressively reducing the size of the arterial lumen. It is not uncommon that as the intimal lesions progress, the number of smooth-muscle cells in the underlying media decreases and the media undergoes atrophy, which can sometimes result in aneurysmal changes rather than lead to thrombotic occlusion of the artery.

There is quite a range of variability in the degree of severity of the lesions of atherosclerosis in different arteries. Recognition that the components of smooth-muscle proliferation, connective tissue formation, and lipid accumulation represent the key elements of the developing lesions of atherosclerosis has led to the utilization of a number of models of experimentally induced atherosclerosis to study this process in different animal species.

Experimentally Induced Atherosclerosis

Four species have been widely used in studying atherogenesis: rabbits, chickens, swine, and nonhuman primates. Most early work was performed in rabbits; however, swine and nonhuman primates are generally considered to develop lesions that correspond more closely with those that occur in human beings. A great deal of new information has been gained from studies of swine and primates, although rabbits continue to provide important data in terms of understanding a number of cellular phenomena. Atherosclerosis has been induced in most animal models by a high-fat, high-cholesterol diet. A principal shortcoming of this approach, however, is that to produce more advanced lesions, it is necessary to maintain animals on such diets for years. Even though it is possible to induce the lesions in a relatively short period (1 to 3 years in the monkey), it is not clear that the lesions produced in this manner actually simulate those that may require 20 to 30 years to form in human beings. On the other hand, the rate at which lesions form in humans is not entirely clear, since some may progress more rapidly than had heretofore been considered to be possible.[6]

Other approaches to studying the smooth-muscle proliferative changes associated with atherosclerosis have included endothelial injury resulting from mechanical injury from varying types of intra-arterial catheters;[7,8] chemically induced injury (from sources such as chronic hypercholesterolemia[9] or chronic homocystinemia[10]); immune-type injuries[11] (from exposure to antigen-antibody complexes); and, more recently, virally induced injury in diseases such as Marek's disease.[12] Each of these animal models has its shortcomings; however, important new information has been obtained from these approaches, particularly when they can be studied in correlation with in vitro models using cell culture techniques. The latter have permitted in-depth studies of endothelium, smooth muscle, macrophages, and platelets. The interrelationships among these cells and among observations resulting from in vivo studies of atherogenesis and cell culture are discussed later in this chapter.

Hypotheses of Atherogenesis

Historical View of Atherogenesis

Atherosclerosis has been recognized in humans for thousands of years. Lesions of atherosclerosis were identified in Egyptian mummies as early as the fifteenth century B.C. Long[13] has discussed the development of clinical-pathological correlations that evolved during the era when autopsy examination permitted the development of an understanding between the degree of atherosclerosis and the incidence of myocardial infarction and stroke. In the mid-nineteenth century, Virchow[14] proposed the idea that some form of injury to the artery wall associated with an inflammatory response resulted in what was then considered to be a degenerative lesion of atherosclerosis. This idea was subsequently modified by Anitschkow[15] and further included the role of platelets and thrombogenesis in atherosclerosis, as expanded by Duguid[16] in 1948. Many of the modern views of atherogenesis stem from the work of John French,[17] who noted that the structural integrity of the endothelial lining of the artery represented a key element in the maintenance of normal arterial function, and that alterations in endothelial integrity might precede a sequence of events that led to the various forms of the lesions of atherosclerosis. Thus, over the years a number of theories concerning the etiology and pathogenesis of atherosclerosis have been developed. At least

three of these deserve elaboration and comment. These are the response to injury hypothesis, the monoclonal hypothesis, and the lipogenic hypothesis.

The Response to Injury Hypothesis

One basis for the *response to injury hypothesis* of atherosclerosis[1,9,18] lies in the marked similarity observed by many investigators between the ubiquitous fibromusculoelastic lesions noted at autopsy and a similar lesion that can be induced in a number of animal species, including nonhuman primates, rabbits, and swine, after different forms of arterial endothelial injury.

The hypothesis (Fig. 41-3) states that some form of "injury" to the endothelium results in either structural and/or functional alterations in the endothelial cells. Factors such as chronic hypercholesterolemia;[9] increased shear stress from the flow of blood over the endothelial cells, as may occur at branch points or bifurcations in arteries in hypertension;[19] and dysfunction induced by toxins or other injurious agents may lead to changes in the nature of the permeability barrier established by the endothelial cells. In the normal artery, the endothelial cells form a continuous monolayer that regulates the passage of substances from the plasma to the underlying artery wall. Injury to the endothelial cells may alter their permeability characteristics and change endothelial cell-cell or endothelial cell–connective tissue relationships, permitting hemodynamic forces to induce focal endothelial cell detachment and thus permit interactions to occur between elements from the blood and the wall of the artery.

Not only do the endothelial cells play an important role as a permeability barrier, but they also form a thromboresistant surface that promotes the continuous flow of blood throughout the vascular tree. The thromboresistant character of the endothelium appears to be due principally to two factors produced by the cells. Both of these have been identified but their physiological roles are relatively poorly understood. They are the cell surface glycoproteins and proteoglycans that form the surface coat of the endothelial cells, and a prostaglandin derivative, prostacycline (PGI_2).[20] Prostacycline is one of the most potent vasodilatory agents thus far isolated and is a potent inhibitor of platelet aggregation. Both endothelial cells and smooth-muscle cells are capable of synthesizing prostacycline; however, endothelial cells appear to make this prostaglandin derivative in greater quantities. This is discussed in greater detail below.

Injury to the endothelium that results in alterations in permeability would permit plasma constituents such as lipoproteins to have more ready access to the artery wall. Endothelial dysfunction could also alter the thromboresistant character of the lumen of the artery so that platelets could interact

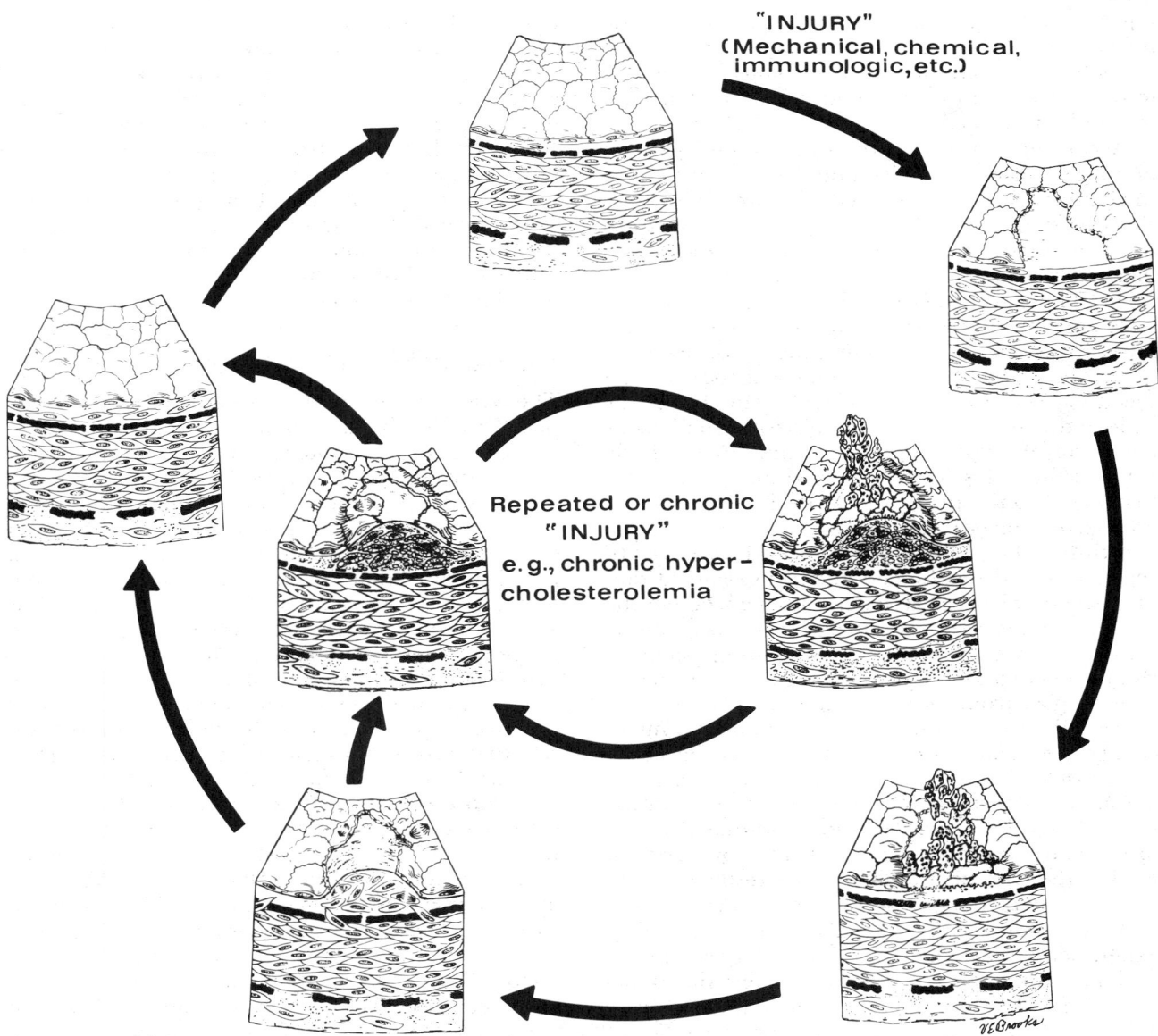

FIGURE 41-3   This diagram represents the essence of the response-to-injury hypothesis of atherosclerosis. In the response-to-injury hypothesis, two different cyclic events may occur. The outer, or regression, cycle may represent common single occurrences in all individuals in whom endothelial injury leads to desquamation, platelet adherence, aggregation, and release, followed by intimal smooth-muscle proliferation and connective tissue formation. If the injury is a single event, the lesions may go on to heal and regression occur. The inner, or progression, cycle demonstrates the possible consequences of repeated or chronic endothelial injury such as may occur in chronic hyperlipidemia. In this instance, lipid deposition as well as continued smooth-muscle proliferation may occur after recurrent sequences of proliferation and regression, and these may lead to complicated lesions that calcify. Such lesions could go on to produce clinical sequelae such as thrombosis and infarction. *(From L. Harker and R. Russell, Hyperlipidemia and Atherosclerosis,* Science, *193:1094, 1976. Reproduced with permission of author and publisher).*

directly at sites of endothelial injury. If the injury were sufficiently severe, the endothelial cells might desquamate and be lost into the bloodstream, leading to exposure of the underlying connective tissue to platelets and to other elements in the circulation. The response to injury hypothesis suggests that the interaction between platelets and the subendothelial connective tissue, principally collagen, results in platelet adherence, aggregation, and release of contents normally stored within the granules of the platelets. The exposure of the artery wall at sites of injury to factors derived from the platelets, together with components from the plasma, such as lipoproteins and hormones, would then lead to focal proliferation of arterial smooth-muscle cells. According to the hypothesis, this smooth-muscle proliferation would be derived from two sources: preexisting intimal smooth-muscle cells and medial smooth-muscle cells that are attracted to, and migrate and proliferate within, the intima at sites of injury. Such a local stimulus could also lead to the formation of new connective tissue matrix constituents by the proliferating smooth-muscle cells and to the deposition of lipids both within and around the proliferated cells.

According to this hypothesis, if the injury to the endothelium were a self-limited event and endothelial integrity were restored, the proliferative lesions might be capable of regressing. If this were the case, the lesions would be reversible, and if they had not reached a critical size, would be clinically silent. There is evidence both in experimental animals and in human beings that the lesions of atherosclerosis can, under certain conditions, regress.[21]

On the other hand, if the injury at focal sites in the artery wall is either long-standing or chronically repeated over periods of many years, the lesions could continue to progress, become increasingly complex in terms of their composition, and eventually lead to the principal clinical sequelae of atherosclerosis, myocardial infarction, and cerebral infarction. The capacity of the endothelium to regenerate and restore endothelial integrity at sites of injury may be critical in determining whether the lesions of atherosclerosis enlarge, remain relatively constant in size, or regress. The superimposition of risk factors that might possibly affect this balance by providing a chronic source of injury, or by somehow altering the normal tissue response to injury, might change the balance so that lesions would be slowly progressive. As an example, the increased levels of plasma low-density lipoproteins associated with hypercholesterolemia may provide a source of injury to the endothelial cells and may also convert what might otherwise be a limited tissue response to injury to frank progressive lesions of atherosclerosis.

This hypothesis has stimulated a great deal of experimental work that has led to an increase in our understanding of factors that determine the capacity of the endothelial cells to maintain themselves as an integral continuous cell layer, and to studies of those factors that control the growth of endothelium. Of equal importance, many studies have elucidated the factors that modify the capacity of arterial smooth-muscle cells to form connective tissue proteins, to synthesize and metabolize lipids and lipoproteins, and to proliferate in response to different mitogenic factors.

One of the more important observations that has resulted from examination of this hypothesis is the discovery that platelets contain a potent mitogen, the platelet-derived growth factor, that is stored in the platelets.[22] It has been suggested that this factor may play an important role in inducing the intimal smooth-muscle proliferative response seen in experimentally induced atherosclerosis and in atherosclerosis in human beings. This is discussed in greater detail below.

A number of important questions have arisen concerning the factors that promote proliferation of smooth-muscle and endothelial cells and the mech-anisms whereby lesions of atherosclerosis may regress. Relatively little is known concerning the factors responsible for the turnover of connective tissue matrix within the artery wall or concerning the mechanisms responsible for removing either this matrix or cholesterol from lesions. The response to injury hypothesis has provided explanations for some of these phenomena. However, much remains to be learned, for example, with respect to the capacity of endothelium and smooth muscle to bind and to metabolize the different types of lipoproteins. These will be discussed below.

The Monoclonal Hypothesis

The *monoclonal hypothesis* of atherosclerosis was proposed by Benditt and Benditt.[23] This hypothesis suggests that each lesion of atherosclerosis is derived from a single smooth-muscle cell and that this cell serves as the progenitor for all of the proliferating cells within the lesion. The hypothesis is based upon the Lyon, or inactive X chromosome, hypothesis, which suggests that only one of the two X chromosomes present in each adult female somatic cell is active. Except for early stages of embryogenesis, the progeny of each cell expresses the same inactive X chromosome as its parent cell. In a sense, therefore, all female individuals are a mosaic, since their tissues are made up of "patches" of genetically identical cells that have either an active maternal or an active paternal X chromosome. This observation makes little to no metabolic difference, since both X chromosomes code for similar enzymes. However, the Benditts took advantage of the fact that a special case exists for the enzyme glucose-6-phosphate dehydrogenase (G6PD). The genes for this enzyme are located in the X chromosome and in humans can occur in two forms of isoenzyme that can be separated by paper electrophoresis. Some black females have been found to be heterozygous for these two isoenzymes so that they represent a mosaic of the two isoenzymes in various somatic cell populations. Consequently, it is possible to distinguish different cell patches within this mosaic by identification of the appropriate isoenzyme. This was originally taken advantage of by Lindner and Gartler,[24] who examined multiple samples of uterine leiomyomas and found that they were composed of cells that contained the same active X chromosome, whereas comparable samples of normal myometrium contained a mixture of cells derived from both types of progenitor cells. Studies of some other tumors have demonstrated similar phenomena, and in some cases there are data supporting the notion that all the cells of a given tumor originate from a single cell and are therefore monoclonal.[25]

More recently, Benditt and others have referred to this character of lesions as *monotypic*. Additional research has produced data that both support and negate this hypothesis. Pearson et al.[26] observed that the majority of atherosclerotic lesions examined from a series of autopsied black females contained either one or the other of the two isoenzymes of G6PD, but that fatty streaks from these individuals and the noninvolved, or normal, arterial tissue contained both isoenzymes and therefore did not appear to be monotypic. Thomas et al. examined the lesion and nonlesion areas of arteries from black females at autopsy in a slightly different manner and obtained data that are at variance with the data supporting the hypothesis and which have been interpreted differently.[27] Thomas et al. examined multiple samples of lesions versus nonlesion areas and found a much higher percentage of both isoenzymes within lesions than had been reported in the earlier studies.

The Benditts[28] have interpreted their data to signify that since each lesion of atherosclerosis is monotypic and is presumably derived from a single smooth-muscle cell, each lesion is a benign neoplasm that may have occurred as a result of cell transformation by agents such as viruses or chemicals. These are interesting possibilities that deserve to be tested further. Fialkow[25] has pointed out that the observation of a single enzyme phenotype in a lesion does not necessarily imply a clonal origin for such a lesion. He stresses that each lesion could arise from a population of genetically identical cells that contained the same isoenzyme rather than from a single cell. These two possibilities could not be distinguished from one another using the single technique of paper electrophoresis. In the artery wall, the possibility of a monoclonal origin would presumably depend on the mosaic composition of the artery wall and therefore the distribution of cells with one or the other isoenzyme within the normal intima or media. Unfortunately, relatively little is known concerning the distribution of isoenzymes within the artery, and the possibility that sparsely distributed, single progenitor cells in the normal intima could give rise to smooth-muscle cell patches that are appreciably larger than those in the media deserves to be explored. If lesion development were characterized by repeated cycles of cell death and growth, according to Fialkow, "repetitive sampling could lead to a single enzyme phenotype, despite multicellular origin."[25] It is therefore possible that under those circumstances, clonal selection with evolution toward a single enzyme phenotype within the lesion could conceivably occur in some kinds of hyperplastic responses. Therefore it is not clear whether the lesions of atherosclerosis are derived from a single cell, from a population of cells of identical phenotype, or some combination of these events.

The monoclonal hypothesis has been an important development in the study of atherosclerosis since it has raised many questions concerning the cellular origin of the lesions and has stimulated a great deal of new thought and research. Whether the lesions are hyperplastic or are neoplastic remains to be determined.

The Lipogenic Hypothesis

Both lesion initiation and lesion progression in atherosclerosis appear somehow to be associated in many individuals with markedly increased elevations of plasma low-density lipoproteins (LDL). The accumulation of lipid within proliferated smooth-muscle cells, within macrophages in the lesions, and within the extracellular connective tissue matrix are common findings, particularly in the lesions of atherosclerosis.[29] The presence of elevated levels of LDL suggest that cholesterol internalization and esterification by cells may be accelerated to such a degree that proliferated smooth-muscle cells within lesions become filled with cholesterol oleate. Many of the cells may go on to become necrotic and may release their lipid into the extracellular spaces. In the presence of excess plasma LDL, which is relatively rich in cholesterol linoleate, the debris may be a mixture of both types of cholesteryl esters.

Some studies have suggested that there are factors present in LDL in hyperlipemic animals that, in themselves, may promote proliferation from smooth-muscle cells and the production of new connective tissue components by these cells.[30] Thus, a sequence of events involving injury to the endothelium by chronic elevated levels of LDL and continuing progression of lesions of atherosclerosis by exposure to elevated levels of LDL [and presumably by decreased levels of high-density lipoproteins (HDL)—see Chap. 42, "Cholesterol Metabolism"] could provide a sequence of events leading to the development of advanced lesions of atherosclerosis. This hypothesis might explain how some fatty streaks could progress to become fibrous plaques but fails to take into account many of the other components of the lesions of atherosclerosis, in particular, the basis for explaining, in addition to the proliferative response of smooth-muscle cells, other phenomena such as the stimulation of new connective tissue formation.

It is possible that the different lesions of atherosclerosis may occur by any of the mechanisms suggested in these different hypotheses or by different combinations of them. It is also clear that as many aspects of our understanding of the biology of smooth muscle and endothelium continue to be expanded, new factors that have not been anticipated may be revealed that may play a role in the pathogenesis of atherosclerosis.

The Role of Risk Factors

A number of risk factors of atherosclerosis have become reasonably well established on the basis of their relationship in epidemiologic studies to the incidence of clinically manifest disease. Unfortunately, there is no basis for comparison between risk factors and the severity or extent of the lesions of atherosclerosis. Among many factors that are considered to be important are hyperlipidemia, hypertension, cigarette smoking, male sex, and diabetes mellitus. These have in general been associated with an increased incidence of fibrous plaques and their sequelae. The associations are relatively strong when they are made on a group basis comparison, although all of the studies have demonstrated a high degree of variability among individuals within even the most homogeneous of groups.[31]

Hyperlipidemia

Dietary lipids are considered to be one of the most important environmental agents responsible for severe atherosclerosis and for the high frequency of atherosclerotic disease in industrially developed parts of the world. Saturated fats became associated with increased incidence of atherosclerosis when it was found that they elevated the concentration of plasma cholesterol; however, the specific contributions of cholesterol, saturated fats, polyunsaturated fats, and total fats in atherosclerosis are still unclear. It has not been possible to demonstrate an unequivocal association between ingestion of dietary cholesterol and plasma cholesterol levels or the incidence and prevalence of coronary disease within population groups when they are analyzed on an individual basis. Unfortunately, there is a great deal of variation from individual to individual in terms of dietary intake of fats and plasma cholesterol levels on a daily basis. There is also intrinsic variation in plasma cholesterol levels among individuals who consume the same diet and respond differently to it. This has increased the difficulty in relating this factor to the incidence of atherosclerosis but does not negate the clear association between hyperlipidemia and atherosclerosis that has been demonstrated by numerous epidemiologic studies.

There is little question, however, that dietary cholesterol directly affects the levels of plasma cholesterol.[32] However, only recently has it been suggested that dietary cholesterol may affect the incidence of atherosclerosis by altering the profile of plasma lipoproteins and possibly by changing the structural or functional properties of these lipoproteins.[33] Increased dietary cholesterol generally results in an increase in LDL cholesterol with a lesser increase in HDL cholesterol. The role of these two lipoproteins in atherogenesis is not clear, although it has been suggested that elevated HDL may be protective, whereas the reverse is true for elevated LDL. (See Chap. 42.)

Unfortunately, there are many differences in the ways in which animals and humans respond to dietary cholesterol, and there are limits to the extent to which information concerning responses in experimental animals to dietary intake can be applied to human beings. Nevertheless, the epidemiologic association between the increased incidence of atherosclerosis and increased intake of fat is very strong. The means by which these fats affect the incidence of atherosclerosis at the cellular and molecular levels remain to be elucidated, as indicated in the discussions of the various hypotheses of atherogenesis.

Hypertension

Hypertension has been established unequivocally as an associated risk factor in that individuals with elevated blood pressure show accelerated atherogenesis, an increased incidence of coronary heart disease, and in particular, increased incidence of cerebrovascular disease. The effects of hypertension appear to be independent of other risk factors in an epidemiologic sense; however, it does not appear to be a primary cause of advanced atherosclerosis in those populations in which the incidence of clinically manifest atherosclerosis is less than average.

The means by which hypertension induces atherogenesis are not clear, although there are many humoral mediators of blood pressure which may participate in this process. For example, renin and other hypertensive agents may induce cellular changes that lead to atherogenesis. Fry[19] and his colleagues, as well as others, have suggested that the increased shear stress of the flow of blood, particularly in hypertensive individuals, at selected anatomic sites within the arterial tree may result in focally altered endothelium and in the development of atherosclerotic lesions very much as suggested in the response to injury hypothesis discussed earlier.

Cigarette Smoking

Cigarette smoking provides perhaps the strongest and most consistent correlation with the increased incidence of atherosclerotic disease and appears to be a major contributor to increased risk of disease, generally in combination with other risk factors. Unfortunately, there is relatively little information concerning the means by which cigarette smoking exerts an impact at the cellular level. Early studies suggested that carbon monoxide might be a causative agent; however, these have not been confirmed. Becker[34] has recently identified agents derived from cigarette smoke that may be injurious to the artery wall. It has also been suggested that inhalation of cigarette smoke may result in the exposure of arterial cells to mutagens that transform the smooth-muscle cells and result in the stimulation of their proliferation. Apparently, cessation of cigarette smoking decreases the risk for development of the clinical sequelae of atherosclerosis and possibly may augment regression of lesions. Further research is clearly required to identify the factors in cigarette smoke that are responsible for its cardiovascular effects and for determining the mechanisms by which it alters cellular metabolism.

Male Sex

Perhaps one of the best-documented and most consistent risk factors for coronary atherosclerosis is male sex. This differential is accentuated in non-white populations, and it has been suggested that females have a decreased incidence because of a protective function exerted by estrogens. Paradoxically, unfortunately, large doses of estrogenic hormones appear to increase cardiovascular mortality in men who have had one myocardial infarct and among men under treatment for prostatic cancer. Consequently, the reason for the sex difference is not understood and remains to be elucidated.

Diabetes

Another risk factor known to be associated with increased incidence of atherosclerosis and myocardial infarction is diabetes mellitus. The mechanisms involved are poorly understood. There is, unfortunately, no consistency in the evidence related to whether elevated concentrations of plasma cholesterol and lipoproteins occur in diabetics whose concentrations of blood and urine glucose are carefully regulated. There does appear to be some evidence suggesting a decreased concentration of HDL cholesterol in diabetics and a high prevalence of hypertension associated with hyperglycemia. The basic mechanisms associated with the proliferation of smooth-muscle-type cells in the mesangium of the kidney in renal complications of diabetes and in increased thickness of capillary basement membrane in diabetics with microvascular disease may bear some similarity to smooth-muscle proliferation in atherogenesis. However, the alterations in the arterial tree in diabetics that precede the lesions of atherogenesis are not well documented and are poorly understood.

Although a great deal of new information, to be discussed below, has evolved concerning our understanding of endothelial cells, smooth-muscle cells, platelets, and the interactions among these cells, the specific role of each of the risk factors that are associated with increased incidence of atherosclerosis on an epidemiologic basis remains, for the most part, to be investigated and elucidated. This information will be critical if we are to proceed with the development of improved means of diagnosis, prevention, and intervention in this disease process.

Cellular Modulations in Atherosclerosis

Endothelium

The Barrier Role

Endothelial cells provide a selective permeability barrier, a blood-compatible interphase, and a thromboresistant lining to the artery wall, and are metabolically active. A number of studies of endothelial permeability using various tracer molecules have demonstrated the presence of pinocytotic vesicles, transendothelial channels, and intracellular clefts in different kinds of endothelium. The junctional complexes between endothelial cells and the artery wall appear to be functionally dynamic structures that can respond to stimuli such as changes in blood pressure and pharmacologic agents. The surface components, at the molecular level, of the endothelial cells appear to influence the selective permeability of the endothelium.[35,36] Endothelial cells have been shown by the Steins[37] to be capable of transporting plasma lipoproteins of given sizes into the artery wall via vesicles. Thus, molecules like HDL would be transported, but larger lipoproteins the size of VLDL (very low density lipoproteins) or chylomicrons would have difficulty in crossing the endothelial barrier without some kind of alteration of these lipid-rich particles.

The disruption of this barrier has been shown, in a number of experimental animals, to result in opportunities that permit interactions between platelets and the artery wall at sites of endothelial injury resulting in the formation of an intimal smooth-muscle proliferative response. Stemerman and Ross[7] observed that if endothelial cells were removed by abrasion with an intraarterial catheter, sites of exposure of the subendothelial connective tissue were quickly coated with a "carpet" of degranulated platelets (Fig. 41-4). The interaction of products released from the platelets and plasma constituents at such sites of endothelial injury precedes a sequence of events that begins with focal smooth-muscle migration and proliferation and that eventually leads to the develoment of a fibromusculoelastic lesion. If this mechanical injury is modified by the addition of a high-fat, high-cholesterol diet to the experiment, then the hyperlipemic animals whose endothelium has been mechanically injured develop intimal proliferative lesions essentially identical to fibrous plaques. In the normocholesterolemic animals, such endothelial injury leads to a fibromusculoelastic proliferative lesion that, over a period of 6 months, may undergo regression, whereas in hypercholesterolemic animals, the lesions become slowly progressive and show no signs of regression (Figs. 41-5 and 41-6).

Ross and Harker[9] observed that monkeys that received no mechanical injury but that were only fed a high-fat, high-cholesterol diet for a year or longer showed signs of endothelial injury as determined morphologically and by measurements of endothelial cell turnover at selected sites in the arterial tree.

The intimal smooth-muscle proliferation seen to accompany disruption of the endothelial cell barrier has been shown to be associated with the interaction between platelets and the exposed subendothelium at such sites of injury. This will be discussed below.

Endothelial Cell Culture

Arterial endothelial cells have been successfully cultured from a number of species, including the cow, rabbit, swine, nonhuman primate, and human being.[38,39] Endothelial cells from each of these species demonstrate a number of common characteristics. They grow, as they do in vivo, in a unique, continuous monolayer, and unlike cells such as smooth muscle or fibroblasts, appear to be truly "contact inhibited." That is, the cells become quies-

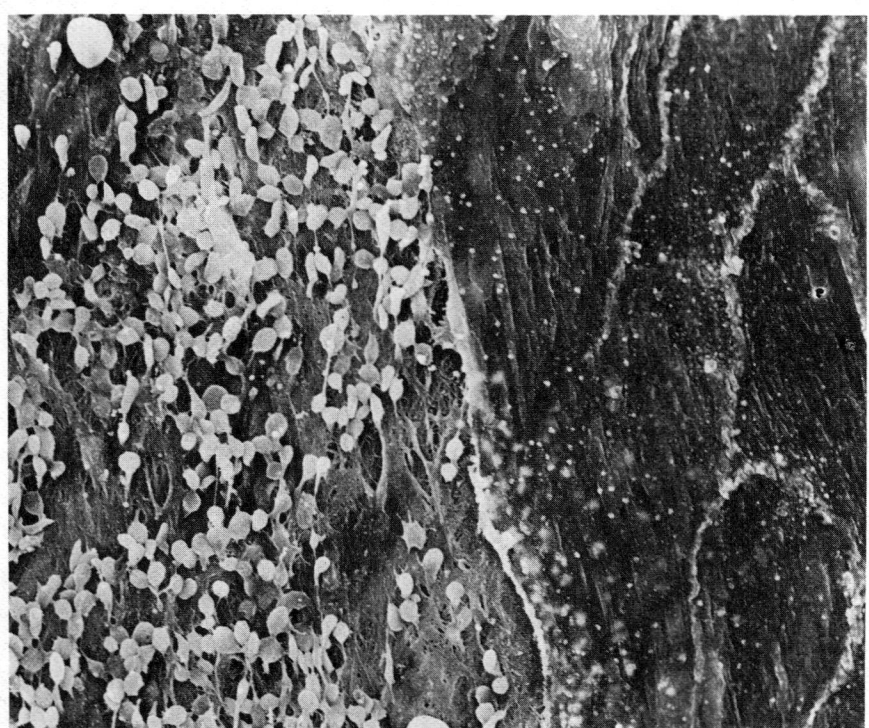

FIGURE 41-4 This is a scanning electron micrograph presenting a surface view of an artery in which the endothelial cells shown on the right have been removed with a catheter in the left portion of the micrograph. This scanning electron micrograph demonstrates platelets, seen as the small ovoid bodies which have attached to the subendothelial connective tissue that was exposed upon injury to the endothelium. These platelets tend to adhere to the exposed connective tissue and to one another, and in the process of doing so, release their intracellular contents.

cent when they remain in contact and become confluent. If the monolayer is disrupted, for example, by wounding, the cells are stimulated to synthesize new DNA and to proliferate and restore the continuity of the monolayer. Only those cells in the culture next to the margins of the wound appear to undergo DNA synthesis and proliferation, whereas those in the monolayer at a distance from the wound appear to remain relatively quiescent. This peculiar characteristic of the growth of endothelium is so strikingly different from that of smooth-muscle cells that it has been suggested that these two different cell types are under different sets of controls of their growth and that somehow cell-cell contact appears to be important in determining the state of quiescence of endothelial cells. Endothelial cells grown in culture have been shown to be capable of forming a number of connective tissue matrix macromolecules including particular types of collagen;[40] of transporting lipids; of synthesizing prostacycline,[41] factor VIII,[42] and angiotensin-converting enzyme;[43] and in maintaining many aspects of their differentiated phenotype through several passages.

Endothelial-Derived Growth Factor
Recently, endothelial cells have been shown to be capable of forming a mitogen or growth factor in culture. This substance, termed the *endothelial-derived growth factor,* appears to be a potent molecule in terms of its capacity to stimulate cells such as fibroblasts and smooth muscle to proliferate.[44] Endothelial cells in culture release this factor into the medium after they have been exposed to plasma or

to serum-free medium. Thus far, studies of this factor show that it appears to have a number of characteristics different from those of the platelet-derived growth factor (to be discussed below). It is not as yet known whether it is formed by endothelial cells in vivo. This observation could have potential importance in atherogenesis; however, the studies are too early in their development for this to be clear.

Smooth Muscle

Smooth-Muscle Proliferation
Smooth-muscle cells have long been recognized to possess a number of features important to normal arterial function, including their capacity to contract, to maintain arterial tonus, and to synthesize connective tissue proteins. Perhaps the most important phenomenon associated with the smooth-muscle cell is the process of cell proliferation in atherogenesis. Since intimal smooth-muscle proliferation is an important early feature in atherogenesis, the factors responsible for this proliferative response are under intensive investigation in vivo and in vitro. In cell culture, it is well known that serum provides all of the factors necessary for smooth-muscle proliferation. Arterial smooth-muscle cells from a large number of species can be grown in culture and are able to maintain their differentiated phenotype under these conditions.[45,46]

Ross and coworkers,[22] together with several other laboratories,[47,48] have demonstrated that the prin-

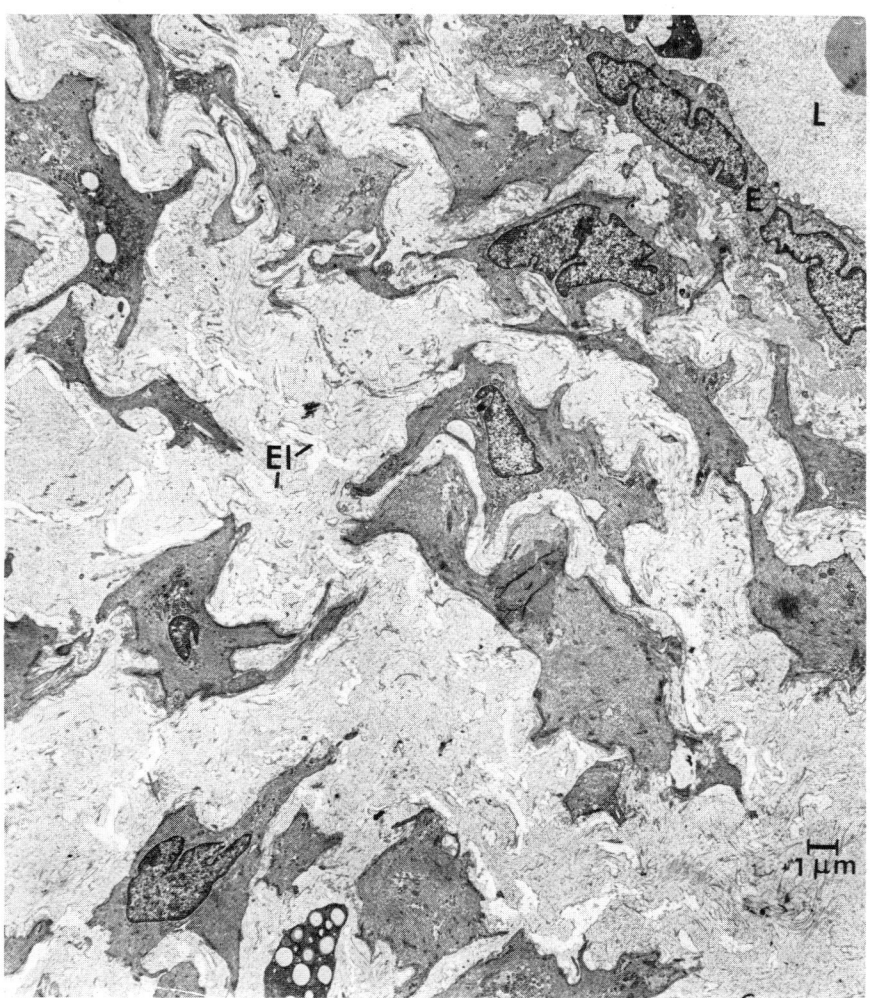

FIGURE 41-5 Electron micrograph of part of the intima from the right iliac artery of a macaque 3 months after the endothelium was removed with an intravascular balloon catheter. The lumen (L) is to the upper right. Endothelial cells cover the markedly thickened intima which contains large numbers of smooth-muscle cells surrounded by a matrix of small elastic fibers (EI), collagen, and proteoglycan.

cipal mitogenic component present in whole blood serum and missing in cell-free, plasma-derived serum and responsible for the proliferation of arterial smooth-muscle cells in culture is a mitogen derived from the platelet, the *platelet-derived growth factor*. The observation that smooth-muscle proliferation in culture is stimulated principally by this mitogen led to a series of studies to examine the role of platelets in in vivo–induced smooth-muscle proliferation.

As described above, several forms of endothelial injury result in adherence of platelets at sites of injury. Platelet adherence is followed by degranulation and release into the artery wall of material stored in the platelet granules. Together with plasma constituents, these platelet products have far-reaching effects upon the smooth-muscle cells of the artery wall.

Harker et al.[10] demonstrated that in homocystinuria, a genetic disease of childhood commonly associated with marked increased incidence of arteriosclerosis, platelets appear to interact at sites where the endothelium has somehow been injured by increased levels of plasma homocysteine. Harker et al.[10] demonstrated this association by measuring the survival of autologous ^{51}Cr-labeled platelets in homocystinuric children and observed that the greater the levels of plasma homocysteine, the greater the decrease in platelet survival. As a result of these observations, they developed an animal model of homocystinuria by chronically infusing homocysteine in baboons. In this model they showed a similar correlation between elevated levels of plasma homocysteine and decreased levels of platelet survival (or increased platelet utilization). When they maintained the baboons on a homocystinemic regimen for 3 months, they observed an increased incidence of missing endothelial cells by morphometric examination of whole-mount preparations of the aorta. Their studies established a correlation between the amounts of injured endothelium, decrease in platelet survival, and the formation of proliferative smooth-muscle atherosclerotic lesions at the sites of endothelial injury. Harker and his colleagues[10] went on to demonstrate that if they administered one of two pharmacologic agents to the homocystinemic baboons that could inhibit platelet interactions with the injured artery

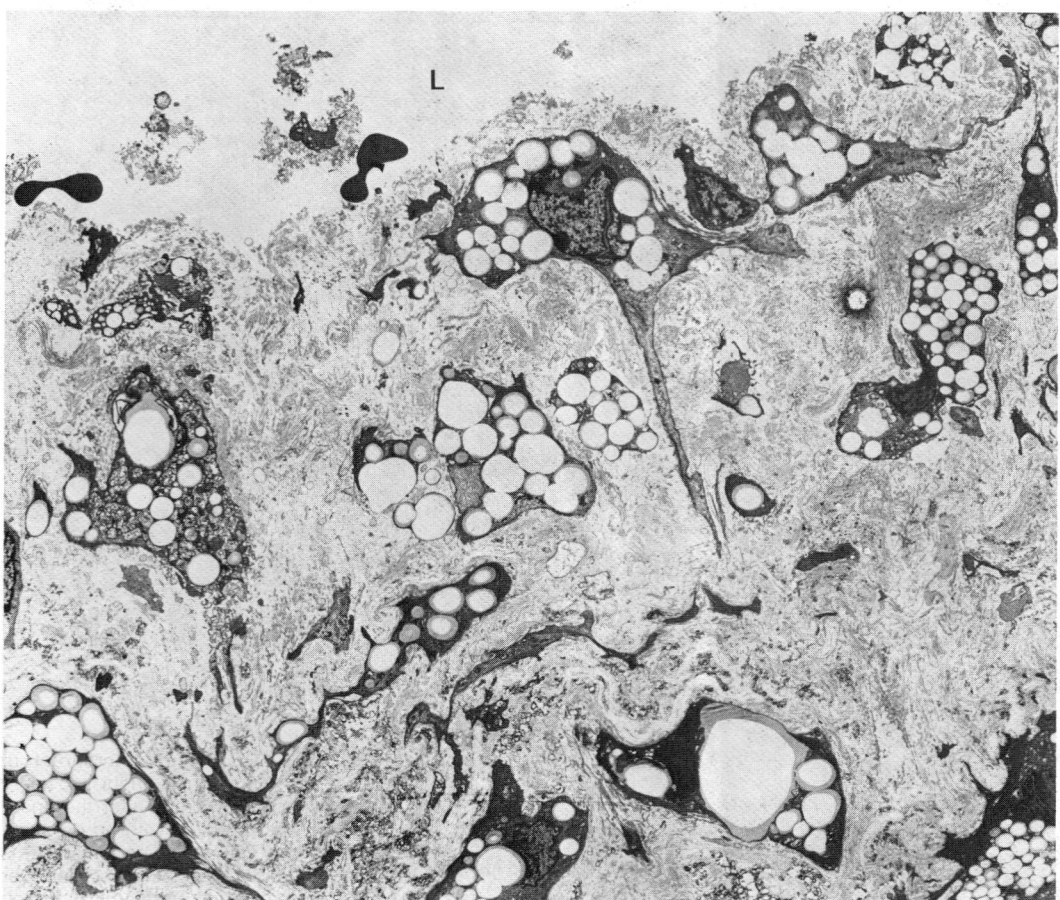

FIGURE 41-6 Electron micrograph of a portion of an intimal lesion in the iliac artery of a monkey on a hyperlipidemic diet 6 months after balloon injury. Most of the smooth-muscle cells in the lesion contain large lipid deposits. The cells are surrounded by small globular membranous deposits in the connective tissue. An endothelial cover is lacking at the luminal surface (L) at the crest of the lesion.

wall, they could prevent the intimal smooth-muscle proliferative lesions that otherwise developed. One of these agents, dipyridamole, returned platelet survival to normal levels and is known because of its capacity to inhibit platelet phosphodiesterase activity and to inhibit platelet adherence. The other agent, sulfinpyrazone, appeared to somehow protect the endothelial cells, since the sulfinpyrazone-treated homocystinemic baboons demonstrated fewer areas of endothelial injury. In both approaches, platelet survival levels were normalized, and the proliferative lesions of atherosclerosis were prevented. These were the first data to correlate a requirement for platelet function with experimentally induced atherosclerosis.

Other approaches to examining these same phenomena were taken by Moore and his colleagues[49] and by Friedman et al.[50] In both of their studies, atherosclerosis was induced in rabbits by injuring the endothelium with an intraarterial catheter. In each case, the investigators induced a thrombocytopenia by administration of a specific antiplatelet antiserum. The animals made thrombocytopenic in this manner had no proliferative atherosclerotic lesions, whereas the control animals had extensive lesions.

Using a different approach, Fuster and his colleagues[51] examined the incidence of atherosclerosis in the aortas of swine fed a high-fat, high-cholesterol diet. They were able to study the role of platelets in these swine by trying to induce atherosclerosis with a high-cholesterol diet in a group of swine that were homozygous for von Willebrand's disease, as compared with a group of normal swine. The swine with severe von Willebrand's disease contained essentially no factor VIII—von Willebrand's factor—in their plasma. Normally this factor is required for platelet adherence and release. The control animals on the high-lipid diet developed extensive proliferative lesions of atherosclerosis, whereas the von Willebrand's swine developed intimal infiltrates of lipid but no smooth-muscle proliferative lesions. In the absence of the von Willebrand's factor, platelet interactions may be somewhat inhibited in the hypercholesterolemic von Willebrand swine.

All of these studies point to the importance of

platelet interactions at sites of endothelial alterations that precede the formation of experimentally induced proliferative lesions of atherosclerosis.

Lipid Metabolism

Since lipids are essential components of all cells, it is not surprising that they are involved in a number of cell functions and metabolic processes, as they represent the principal constituent of all cell membranes. Both the plasma membrane and the internal membranous compartments of all cells, including smooth muscle, are composed of phospholipids, proteins, and cholesterol, principally unesterified cholesterol. Esterified cholesterol is found in smooth muscle only under abnormal conditions. Accumulations of cholesteryl ester in smooth-muscle cells and macrophages lead to the development of foam cells found in the lesions of atherosclerosis. Recent experiments have shown that smooth-muscle cells can acquire cholesterol both by de novo synthesis[52] and from an exogenous source of cholesterol-carrying lipoproteins.[53] Such a dual mechanism may help the cell to protect itself against possible deficits in cholesterol.

Smooth-muscle and many other cells can also protect themselves against excess cholesterol. The mechanism that has evolved for this purpose is the surface-located, high-affinity LDL receptor.[54,55] These receptors bind LDL, and the cell then internalizes the bound LDL by the process of endocytosis and transports it to lysosomes where the LDL is degraded and free cholesterol is liberated for use by the cell. If the cell is exposed to excess LDL, there is a feedback inhibitory pathway in the cell that inhibits the synthesis of LDL receptors. In addition, the presence within the cell of excess cholesterol provides a signal that inhibits cholesterol synthesis by the rate-limiting intracellular enzyme, HMG-CoA reductase (hydroxymethylglutarylcoenzyme A reductase).

Under normal circumstances, sterol balance in the cell maintains a given receptor level for LDL at the cell surface. In this way the requirements for extracellular cholesterol are met by concentrations of plasma LDL that are not atherogenic. Increased concentrations of plasma LDL may alter the endothelial barrier and bring large amounts of LDL in direct contact with the smooth-muscle cell which may ingest much of the LDL by bulk-phase endocytosis, bypassing the high-affinity receptor mechanism, and leading to increased esterification and storage of cholesteryl esters and the development of foam cells.

LDL have been said to play a mitogenic role for smooth-muscle cells in culture. Wissler and his colleagues[30] have observed that LDL derived from hyperlipemic monkeys was mitogenic in explant cultures of aorta as compared to LDL from normolipemic monkeys. The means by which this LDL acts as a mitogen is not clear; however, there do appear to be differences between LDL from nor-molipemic versus hyperlipemic donors in terms of their effects on smooth muscle and endothelium. The elucidation of the effects of hyperlipemic LDL may be important in understanding the basis of the atherogenic effect of hyperlipidemia.

Genetic defects in cellular metabolism of lipoprotein are relatively common and will be discussed in Chap. 42.

Evidence is accumulating in favor of the notion that HDL, in contrast to LDL, is a negative factor in the development of atherosclerosis. Two mechanisms have been proposed to explain how HDL might be a deterrent against atherosclerosis. The first suggests that HDL augments the removal of cholesterol from cells such as smooth muscle. The second mechanism involves the apparent ability of HDL to influence the binding and absorption of LDL by cells such as smooth muscle. However, neither of these mechanisms has been shown to be responsible for control of cellular cholesterol. Further information concerning the nature of the lipoproteins and their effects on cells and potential roles in atherogenesis is discussed in Chap. 42.

The Macrophage

Macrophages are commonly found in early lesions of atherosclerosis as well as in advanced lesions like the fibrous plaque. These cells could conceivably play several roles in lesion progression and possibly in regression as well. In tissue culture, macrophages have been shown to release a mitogen as potent as that derived from platelets into the culture medium.[56] Such a growth factor, if formed in vivo, could conceivably be important in lesion progression.

Macrophages have long been known to be largely responsible for tissue debridement. There is increasing evidence in experimental studies and in human beings[21] that some lesions of atherosclerosis are capable of regression. The potential role of the macrophage in this phenomenon remains to be elucidated.

Platelets

The Platelet-Derived Growth Factor

The platelet-derived growth factor is a mitogen that is stored in the alpha granule of the platelets and which has been purified to homogeneity. It has a molecular weight of approximately 32,000 and is a highly cationic (pI 9.8), stable, disulfide-bonded protein. This growth factor is extremely potent, as it will cause proliferation of all susceptible cells in culture at a level of 5 ng/ml of culture medium (equivalent to addition of 5% whole blood serum). As discussed earlier in this chapter, platelet-derived growth factor is the principal mitogen in whole blood serum to which cells characteristically respond by cell proliferation. Exposure of susceptible cells to this factor results in a sequence of events that includes binding of the molecule to the surface of the cells. This then causes the cell to undergo cell cycle traverse leading to DNA synthesis and cell multiplication.

The platelet-derived growth factor stimulates a number of phenomena upon exposure to smooth-muscle cells in addition to DNA synthesis. It causes increases in pinocytosis, protein synthesis, RNA synthesis, and lipid metabolism. Chait et al.[53] have observed that exposure of arterial smooth-muscle cells to this growth factor results in increased binding of LDL to the cells due to the formation of an increased number of high-affinity receptors for LDL at the cell surface. This increased binding of LDL permits the cells to utilize exogenous sources of cholesterol for cell multiplication more effectively. Habenicht et al.[52] have demonstrated that this mitogen also stimulates increased cholesterol synthesis by cells if an exogenous source of cholesterol is not available to them. Davies and Ross[57] observed that smooth-muscle cells exposed to the platelet-derived growth factor undergo a marked increase in the rate of endocytosis of tracer molecules. In other words, exposure to this mitogen results in an increase in a number of cellular activities, many of which are associated with cell proliferation and with new protein synthesis, and therefore with connective tissue formation.[58] Thus, exposure to this factor could potentially provide the trigger that results in the initiation of all of the components of a proliferative lesion. Although the factor is clearly operative in cell culture, there are as yet no data to determine whether this factor is operative in vivo. The role of functional platelets in inducing experimental atherosclerosis in vivo is unquestioned. The role of the platelet-derived growth factor in stimulating mitogenesis in cell culture is also clear. The question remains as to whether this factor is active in vivo.

Prostaglandins

A great deal has been learned during the past 10 years about a new category of substances, the prostaglandins, that may play critical roles in the metabolism of platelets, endothelium, and smooth muscle. All three cell types are capable of converting the fatty acid, arachidonic acid, into prostaglandin endoperoxides. Studies of these endoperoxides identified a number of unstable intermediates in the metabolic pathway of arachidonic acid that lead to the formation of two important end products: thromboxane A_2 (formed by platelets) and prostacycline (formed by endothelium and smooth muscle). Understanding these two end products has greatly expanded our view of the role potentially played by platelets in thrombosis and by endothelium and smooth muscle in prevention of thrombosis and potentially atherosclerosis.

Arachidonic acid is derived either from linolenic acid, an essential fatty acid in the membranes of cells, or from arachidonic acid in the diet. Thromboxane A_2 is a powerful vasoconstrictor and, therefore, is capable of stimulating smooth-muscle contraction and platelet aggregation. It has a short half-life (30 s) and breaks down spontaneously into a stable substance, thromboxane B_2. A number of inhibitors of thromboxane synthesis markedly reduce platelet aggregation. These include aspirin and indomethacin.[59,60]

Prostacycline (PGI_2) is the principal product of cycloxygenase activity in the walls of arteries and veins. Endothelium and smooth muscle synthesize PGI_2 from arachidonic acid and may also be able to synthesize this prostaglandin derivative from endoperoxides released from platelets. PGI_2 is also unstable and is an extremely potent vasodilator, as well as an inhibitor of platelet aggregation.

It is possible that an imbalance in the relative amounts of thromboxane A_2 versus PGI_2 may provide part of the explanation of the involvement of platelets in cardiovascular diseases. Since platelets contain thromboxane synthetase, the enzyme responsible for synthesis of thromboxane A_2, and since inhibition of the activity of this enzyme does not interfere with cycloxygenase activity, it has been speculated that platelets could potentially donate endoperoxides to endothelial cells which can then use them as substrates for PGI_2 production. Therefore, attempts are being made to develop specific inhibitors of thromboxane synthesis that would not affect PGI_2 production by cells of the blood vessel wall.

Prostaglandin biosynthesis may be important not only in thrombosis (in terms of platelet adherence and aggregation) but also in prevention of atherogenesis (by formation of PGI_2). This had led to speculation that alterations in the contents of fatty acids in the diet might offer some protection against the development of atherosclerosis. Populations that consume diets principally composed of marine animals often replace arachidonic acid, the normal substrate for prostaglandin synthesis, with eicosapentaenoic acid. This fatty acid is not completely metabolized by platelets and, instead, produces a relatively inert form of thromboxane, thromboxane A_3. Eicosapentaenoic acid appears to inhibit the capacity of platelets to metabolize arachidonic acid. When eicosapentaenoic acid is exposed to cells of the blood vessel, they will form an analogue of prostacycline, PGI_3. PGI_3 appears to be as effective as PGI_2 in preventing platelet aggregation and in inducing vasodilatation. Thus, further studies of the role of this fatty acid derived from marine animals could have implications for individuals who consume a marine diet in terms of being protected against atherogenesis. Clearly, there is much to be learned in prostaglandin metabolism before the agents that have thus far been discovered, and those that are yet undiscovered, can be understood, both in atherogenesis and in protection against this disease process.

The Role of Research at the Cellular Level in Diagnosis, Treatment, and Prevention

The field of atherosclerosis research has changed dramatically within the last decade. The emphasis in our understanding the pathogenesis of this disease process has shifted to probing the fundamental roles of the cells of the artery wall as well as those in the blood, particularly the platelet. The development of cell biology, experimental pathology, and immunology has provided tools that should lead to new approaches to diagnosis, intervention, and prevention.

If, for example, it can be demonstrated unequivocally that the platelet-derived growth factor plays a role in either the initiation of the lesions of atherosclerosis and/or in their progression, and if it can be demonstrated that there are higher levels of this factor in the circulation in individuals who are actively forming lesions or who are at increased risk, then the development of a radioimmunoassay to detect the presence of this factor in the plasma would be significant in that it could be used in the diagnosis of patients who are at increased risk. Similarly, the efficacy of different pharmacologic agents or other modes of intervention could be determined with the use of such a radioimmunoassay. Other approaches to understanding the role of platelets in atherogenesis involve the use of radiolabeled platelets or the development of means to maintain endothelial integrity. As a consequence, future research at the cellular and molecular levels could provide important diagnostic tools that may be of use clinically.

The process of atherogenesis is a highly complex one, involving many cellular interactions as well as interactions between cells and constituents in the fluid phase of the blood, the plasma. The importance of these interactions will undoubtedly be modified by the genetic makeup of each individual. Consequently, the differences in susceptibility from individual to individual to each of the risk factors and at the cellular level to the different various components considered to be important in atherogenesis will have to be understood if we are to make further progress, not only in diagnosis and treatment, but ultimately in prevention.

References

*1. Ross, R., and Glomset, J. A.: The Pathogenesis of Atherosclerosis, *N. Engl. J. Med.*, 295:369, 420, 1976. (131 references)

2. McGill, H. C., Jr.: Atherosclerosis: Problems in Pathogenesis, *Atherosclerosis Rev.*, 2:27, 1977.

3. Bierman, E. L., and Ross, R.: Aging and Atherosclerosis, *Atherosclerosis Rev.*, 2:79, 1977.

4. Geer, J. C., and Haust, M. D.: "Monographs on Atherosclerosis," S. Karger, Basel, Switzerland, 1972, vol. 2, p. 1.

5. "Arteriosclerosis: A Report by the National Heart and Lung Institute Task Force on Arteriosclerosis," DHEW Publication (NIH) 72-219, vol. 2, 1971.

6. Debakey, M. E.: "Atherosclerosis Reviews," Raven Press, New York, 1976, vol. 3, p. 1.

7. Stemerman, M. B., and Ross, R.: Experimental Atherosclerosis. I. Fibrous Plaque Formation in Primates, an Electron Microscope Study, *J. Exp. Med.*, 136:769, 1972.

8. Bjorkerud, S., and Bondjers, G.: Arterial Repair and Atherosclerosis after Mechanical Injury. I. Permeability and Light Microscopic Characteristics of Endothelium in Non-atherosclerotic and Atherosclerotic Lesions, *Atherosclerosis*, 13:355, 1971.

9. Ross, R., and Harker, L.: Hyperlipidemia and Atherosclerosis, *Science*, 193:1094, 1976.

10. Harker, L., Ross, R., Slichter, S., and Scott, C.: Homocystine-Induced Arteriosclerosis: The Role of Endothelial Cell Injury and Platelet Response in Its Genesis, *J. Clin. Invest.*, 58:731, 1976.

11. Minick, C. R., and Murphy, G. E.: Experimental Induction of Atheroarteriosclerosis by the Synergy of Allergic Injury to Arteries and Lipid-Rich Diet. II. Effect of Repeatedly Injected Foreign Protein in Rabbits Fed a Lipid-Rich, Cholesterol-Poor Diet, *Am. J. Pathol.*, 73:265, 1973.

12. Fabricant, C. G., Fabricant, J., Litrenta, M. M., and Minick, C. R.: Virus-Induced Atherosclerosis, *J. Exp. Med.*, 148:335, 1978.

13. Long, E. R.: "Arteriosclerosis. A Survey of the Problem," The Macmillan Company, New York, 1933, p. 19.

14. Virchow, R.: "Gesammelte Adhandlungen zur Wissenschaftlichen Medicin," Meidinger Sohn and Company, Frankfurt-am-Main, 1856, p. 458.

15. Anitschkow, H. H.: "Cowdry's Arteriosclerosis," 2d ed., Macmillan, New York, 1967, p. 21.

16. Duguid, J. B.: Thrombosis as a Factor in the Pathogenesis of Coronary Atherosclerosis, *J. Pathol. Bacteriol.*, 58:207, 1948.

17. French, J. E.: Atherosclerosis in Relation to the Structure and Function of the Arterial Intima, with Special Reference to the Endothelium, *Intern. Rev. Exp. Pathol.*, 5:253, 1966.

*18. Ross, R., and Glomset, J.: Atherosclerosis and the Arterial Smooth Muscle Cell, *Science*, 180:1332, 1973. (32 references)

19. Fry, D. L.: "Cerebrovascular Diseases," Raven Press, New York, 1976, p. 77.

20. Moncada, S., Higgs, H. A., and Vane, J. R.: Human Arterial and Venous Tissue Generate Prostacycline, a Potent Inhibitor of Platelet Aggregation, *Lancet*, 2:18, 1977.

*21. Wissler, R. W., and Vesselinovitch, D.: Studies of Regression of Advanced Atherosclerosis in Experimental Animals and Man, *Ann. N.Y. Acad. Sci.*, 275:363, 1976. (51 references)

22. Ross, R., Glomset, J., Kariya, B., and Harker, L.: A Platelet-Dependent Serum Factor That Stimulates the Proliferation of Arterial Smooth Muscle Cells *in Vitro*, *Proc. Natl. Acad. Sci.*, 71:1207, 1974.

23. Benditt, E. P., and Benditt, J. M.: Evidence for a Monoclonal Origin of Human Atherosclerotic Plaques, *Proc. Natl. Acad. Sci.*, 70:1753, 1973.

24. Lindner, D., and Gartler, S. M.: Glucose-6-Phosphate Dehydrogenase Mosaicism: Utilization as a

*This article is a review of the literature and contains additional references to the literature.

Cell Marker in the Study of Leiomyomas, *Science*, 150:67, 1965.

25. Fialkow, P.: The Origin and Development of Human Tumors Studied with Cell Markers, *N. Engl. J. Med.*, 291:26, 1974.

26. Pearson, T. A., Wang, A., Solez, K., and Heptinstall, R. H.: Clonal Characteristics of Fibrous Plaques and Fatty Streaks from Human Aortas, *Am. J. Pathol.*, 81:379, 1975.

27. Thomas, W. A., Reiner, J. M., Janakidevi, K., and Lee, K. T.: Population Dynamics of Arterial Cells during Atherogenesis. X. Study of Monotypism in Atherosclerotic Lesions of Black Women Heterozygous for Glucose-6-Phosphate Dehydrogenase, *Exp. Mol. Pathol.*, 31:327, 1979.

*28. Benditt, E. P.: "Atherosclerosis Reviews," Raven Press, New York, 1978, vol. 3, p. 77. (Extensively referenced)

29. Geer, J. C., McGill, H. C., Jr., and Strong, J. P.: The Fine Structure of Human Atherosclerotic Lesions, *Am. J. Pathol.*, 38:263, 1961.

*30. Wissler, R. W.: "Biochemistry of Atherosclerosis," Marcel Dekker, New York, 1979, vol. 7, p. 345. (Extensively referenced)

31. McGill, H.: Risk Factors for Atherosclerosis, *Adv. Exp. Med. Biol.*, 104:273, 1977.

32. Grundy, S. M.: "Nutrition, Lipids, and Coronary Heart Disease," Raven Press, New York, 1979, p. 89.

33. McGill, H. C., Jr.: The Relationship of Dietary Cholesterol to Serum Cholesterol Concentration and to Atherosclerosis in Man, *Am. J. Clin. Nutr.*, 32 (suppl.):2664, 1979.

34. Becker, C. G., Dubin, T., and Widemann, H. P.: Hypersensitivity to Tobacco Antigen, *Proc. Natl. Acad. Sci.*, 73:1712, 1976.

35. Simionescu, N., Simionescu, M., and Palade, G. E.: Permeability of Muscle Capillaries to Small Heme-Peptides. Evidence for the Existence of Patent Transcendothelial Channels, *J. Cell Biol.*, 64:586, 1975.

36. Renkin, E. M.: Multiple Pathways of Capillary Permeability, *Circ. Res.*, 41:735, 1977.

37. Stein, Y., and Stein, O.: "Biochemistry of Atherosclerosis," Marcel Dekker, New York, 1979, vol. 7, p. 313.

38. Gimbrone, M. A., Jr.: "Progress in Hemostasis and Thrombosis," Grune & Stratton, New York, 1976, vol. 3, p. 1.

39. Jaffe, E. A., Nachman, R. L., Becker, C. G., and Minick, C. R.: Culture of Human Endothelial Cells Derived from Umbilical Veins, *J. Clin. Invest.*, 52:2745, 1973.

40. Jaffe, E. A., Adelman, B., and Minick, C. R.: Synthesis of Basement Membrane by Cultured Human Endothelial Cells, *Circulation*, 51(suppl. 2):11, 1975.

41. Moncada, S., Higgs, E. A., and Vane, J. R.: Human Arterial and Venous Tissue Generate Prostacyclin, a Potent Inhibitor of Platelet Aggregation, *Lancet*, 2:18, 1977.

42. Jaffe, E. A., Hoyer, L. W., and Nachman, R. L.: Synthesis of Antihemophilic Factor Antigen by Cultured Human Endothelial Cells, *J. Clin. Invest.*, 52:2757, 1973.

43. Gimbrone, M. A., Jr., and Alexander, R. W.: Angiotensin II Stimulation of Prostaglandin Production in Cultured Human Vascular Endothelium, *Science*, 189(abstract):219, 1975.

44. Gajdusek, C., DiCorleto, P., Ross, R., and Schwartz, S.: An Endothelial Cell Derived Growth Factor, *J. Cell Biol.*, 85:467, 1980.

45. Ross, R., and Kariya, B.: "Handbook of Physiology—Circulation, Vascular Smooth Muscle," American Physiological Society, Bethesda, Maryland, 1980, p. 69.

46. Chamley-Campbell, J., Campbell, G. R., and Ross, R.: The Smooth Muscle Cell in Culture, *Physiol. Rev.*, 59:1, 1979.

47. Kohler, N., and Lipton, A.: Platelets as a Source of Fibroblast Growth-Promoting Activity, *Exp. Cell Res.*, 87:297, 1974.

48. Heldin, C.-H., Wasteson, A., and Westermark, B.: Partial Purification and Characterization of Platelet Factors Stimulating the Multiplication of Normal Human Glial Cells, *Exp. Cell Res.*, 109:429, 1977.

49. Moore, A., Friedman, R. J., Singal, D. P., Gauldie, J., and Blajchman, M.: Inhibition of Injury Induced Thromboatherosclerotic Lesions by Antiplatelet Serum in Rabbits, *Thromb. Diath. Haemorr.*, 35:70, 1976.

50. Friedman, R. J., Stemerman, M. B., Wenz, B., Moore, S., Gauldie, J., Gent, M., Tiell, M. L., and Spaet, T. H.: The Effect of Thrombocytopenia on Experimental Atherosclerotic Lesion Formation in Rabbits. Smooth Muscle Cell Proliferation and Reendothelialization, *J. Clin. Invest.*, 60:1191, 1977.

51. Fuster, V., Bowie, E. J. W., Lewis, J. C., Fass, D. N., Owen, C. A., Jr., and Brown, A. L.: Resistance to Arteriosclerosis in Pigs with von Willebrand's Disease. Spontaneous and High Cholesterol Diet-Induced Arteriosclerosis, *J. Clin. Invest.*, 61:722, 1978.

52. Habenicht, A., Glomset, J., and Ross, R.: Relation of Cholesterol and Mevalonic Acid to the Cell Cycle in Smooth Muscle and Swiss 3T3 Cells Stimulated to Divide by Platelet-Derived Growth Factor, *J. Biol. Chem.*, 255:5134, 1980.

53. Chait, A., Ross, R., Albers, J., and Bierman, E.: Platelet Derived Growth Factor Stimulates Low Density Lipoprotein Receptor Activity, *Proceedings of the National Academy of Sciences (USA)*, 77:4084, 1980.

54. Brown, M. S., Faust, J. R., and Goldstein, J. L.: Role of the Low Density Lipoprotein Receptor in Regulating the Content of Free and Esterified Cholesterol in Human Fibroblasts, *J. Clin. Invest.*, 55:783, 1975.

55. Goldstein, J. L., and Brown, M. S.: The Low-Density Lipoprotein Pathway and Its Relation to Atherosclerosis, *Ann. Rev. Biochem.*, 46:879, 1977.

56. Leibovich, S. J., and Ross, R.: A Macrophage-Dependent Factor That Stimulates the Proliferation of Fibroblasts *in Vitro*, *Am. J. Pathol.*, 84:501, 1976.

57. Davies, P. F., and Ross, R.: Mediation of Pinocytosis in Cultured Arterial Smooth Muscle and Endothelial Cells by Platelet-Derived Growth Factor, *J. Cell Biol.*, 79:663, 1978.

58. Burke, J., and Ross, R.: "International Review of Connective Tissue Research," Academic Press, Inc., New York, 1979, vol. 8, p. 119.

59. Moncada, A., and Vane, J. R.: Arachidonic Acid Metabolites and the Interactions between Platelets and Blood-Vessel Walls, *N. Engl. J. Med.*, 300:1142, 1979.

60. Moncada, S., and Vane, J. R.: Mode of Action of Aspirin-like Drugs, *Adv. Intern. Med.*, 24:1, 1979.

42

Cholesterol Metabolism

John A. Glomset, M.D.

There is now substantial evidence that dysbalance of cholesterol in arteries, in the plasma, and perhaps in the body as a whole is an important contributing factor in atherogenesis. Chemical analyses have shown that cholesterol and cholesteryl ester are quantitatively important constituents of atherosclerotic lesions in humans (Chap. 41). Familial hypercholesterolemia is known to be associated with severe premature atherosclerotic disease. A wealth of prospective epidemiologic data (Chap. 34) has shown that the risk of developing clinical signs of coronary heart disease correlates positively with the concentration of plasma low-density lipoproteins (LDL, β-lipoproteins) but negatively with the concentration of plasma high-density lipoproteins (HDL, α-lipoproteins). Finally, experimentally induced hypercholesterolemia in animals has been repeatedly shown to be associated with arterial disease.

This evidence has focused attention on the factors that control the metabolism of cholesterol and has stimulated attempts to prevent or treat atherosclerosis by altering cholesterol balance or changing the concentrations of specific plasma lipoproteins. While the efficacy of this approach remains to be established, it seems clear that the role of cholesterol must be considered in treatment and, ultimately, prevention of atherosclerosis. Some knowledge of the metabolism of cholesterol and plasma lipoproteins is therefore essential for those involved in the management of vascular disease, and there is a need to follow developments in the field because understanding is expanding rapidly. This chapter will present a brief overview of aspects of the metabolism of cholesterol and plasma lipoproteins that seem closely related to atherosclerosis, focusing on current information about cholesterol balance in the body as a whole, in the plasma, and in tissues, then describing several conditions of cholesterol dysbalance known to lead to premature vascular disease.

Cholesterol Balance in the Body as a Whole: The Enterohepatic Circulation

Several facts should be kept in mind when considering cholesterol balance in the body as a whole. (1) Cholesterol is critical for the function of all animal cells. (2) All of the cholesterol required can be provided by biosynthesis. (3) Though there is thus no dietary requirement for cholesterol, absorbed dietary cholesterol reduces the need for cholesterol bio-

synthesis. (4) Most cells cannot degrade cholesterol, but 1.0 to 1.5 g cholesterol must be synthesized or provided each day to compensate for a constant daily loss by desquamation and excretion in the feces.

Cholesterol is important for the function of all animal cells because it is a key constituent of cell membranes. Apparently, its hydrophobic character and compact, wedgelike shape allow it to intercalate between molecules of membrane phospholipid and influence membrane permeability and fluidity. Cholesterol is also a precursor of several critical compounds. Liver cells convert it into bile acids; cells of the adrenal cortex, ovary, and testis convert it into steroid hormones; and cells of the skin can convert it into skin sterols and vitamin D.

The cholesterol that is required for cell function is synthesized by a multistep pathway present in all nucleated animal cells. This pathway uses two carbon units (acetylcoenzyme A) formed from carbohydrate or lipid and is regulated by a rate-limiting enzyme, hydroxymethylglutarylcoenzyme A (HMG-CoA) reductase.[1] Alternatively, most cells can take up cholesterol from the extracellular fluid by mechanisms mediated by receptors on the cell surface. When they do, a feedback mechanism diminishes the activity of HMG-CoA reductase and thereby decreases the formation of cholesterol from acetyl CoA.

The cholesterol that is formed each day contributes to several different pools of cellular and extracellular sterol[2] and balances a constant daily loss from these pools. About half of the cholesterol lost is converted into biologic detergents (bile acids) by an enzymic pathway present only in hepatocytes. This pathway is initiated by a rate-limiting enzyme, 7α-hydroxylase, under feedback control by bile acids.[3] The net effect of the pathway is to modify both the ring structure and side chain of the cholesterol molecule to produce a group of planar molecules that are hydrophilic on one side, hydrophobic on the other.[4]

The bile acids formed by hepatocytes stimulate formation of hepatocyte phospholipid, whereupon the cells secrete a mixture of bile acids, phospholipid, and unesterified cholesterol into biliary canaliculi. The amount of cholesterol secreted in this way is limited, since cholesterol is only sparingly soluble in aqueous media, and only a small amount can be solubilized in bile by being included in aggregates of bile acid and phospholipid referred to as *mixed micelles*. When the amount of cholesterol present in these micelles approaches saturation, cholesterol tends to precipitate, and the risk of developing cholesterol-rich gallstones rises.[5]

After a fatty meal, when bile is squirted into the intestinal lumen, the bile acids and bile phospholipids facilitate the partial hydrolysis of dietary triglyceride and promote absorption of the hydrolytic products by cells of the proximal intestinal mucosa. The bile phospholipid is partially hydrolyzed also, and both it and bile unesterified cholesterol are absorbed by the same cells that absorb the dietary triglyceride. All three components are then converted into special lipid-protein complexes, called *lipoproteins,* which transport triglyceride to adipose tissue. Finally, most of the phospholipid and cholesterol is returned to the liver to complete part of the enterohepatic circulation of biliary lipids. The bile acids are returned to the liver by a different route. They are actively absorbed toward the distal end of the small intestine and returned to the liver complexed with albumin in the portal circulation.

With each enterohepatic cycle of bile acid, phospholipid, and unesterified cholesterol, a fraction of the bile acids and cholesterol escapes absorption and is altered by intestinal bacteria and ultimately excreted in the feces. Though the fraction lost during one pass of the enterohepatic circulation is small, the cumulative daily loss is substantial because biliary components cycle between the liver and intestine as often as 10 times per day. Indeed, excretion by this route accounts for the bulk of the daily loss of cholesterol from the body.

As mentioned earlier, biosynthetic mechanisms can readily compensate for the daily loss of cholesterol. Alternatively, dietary cholesterol, absorbed and transported to the liver with biliary cholesterol, can meet the same need. The dietary cholesterol reaching the liver contributes to intracellular pools; this is followed by a reduction in the activity of hepatic HMG-CoA reductase and a decrease in cholesterol biosynthesis.[4] Conversion of cholesterol to bile acids continues, however, since the activity of 7α-hydroxylase is regulated downward, not by cholesterol but by bile acids in the enterohepatic circulation.

It is important to realize that intake and absorption of dietary cholesterol may not always be completely balanced by decreased biosynthesis or increased excretion of cholesterol. For complete balance to occur, all processes involved would have to be precisely interregulated. Since feeding cholesterol-rich diets can lead to extreme hypercholesterolemia in laboratory animals, including nonhuman primates, and significantly increase plasma cholesterol levels in humans as well, it is apparent that this interregulation is often not effective.

Cholesterol Balance in Plasma: Metabolism of Plasma Lipoproteins

To appreciate the factors that contribute to cholesterol balance in the plasma, it is important to understand that (1) essentially all of the cholesterol in plasma is associated with lipoproteins; (2) both unesterified and esterified cholesterol are present, and they play very different roles in relation to lipoprotein structure; (3) though the bulk of the cholesterol in a typical sample of plasma is esterified, most of the cholesterol that enters plasma is unesterified; (4) this unesterified cholesterol is mainly associated with the surface of large lipoproteins whose primary function is to transport triglyceride of dietary or endogenous origin to peripheral tissues; and (5) the unesterified cholesterol is subsequently converted to cholesteryl ester in the plasma and leaves the plasma in the interior of very different lipoproteins.

The role of cholesterol in lipoprotein structure is schematically illustrated in Fig. 42-1. Most plasma lipoproteins are spherical complexes of phospholipid, unesterified cholesterol, triglyceride, cholesteryl ester, and specific proteins called *apolipoproteins.* The lipid constituents by themselves are at best only slightly soluble in water. When present in lipoproteins, however, the phospholipid, unesterified cholesterol, and apolipoproteins form a thin surface film that solubilizes the lipoprotein complex. They do this because they are in part hydrophilic, part hydrophobic. The phospholipids have a charged polar group at one end of the molecule, two fatty acid chains at the other. The unesterified cholesterol has a hydroxyl group at one end of the ring structure and an aliphatic chain at the other. Thus, both types of molecules orient spontaneously with respect to the aqueous environment of the complex. The charged or hydroxyl ends orient outward to form a hydrophilic "face" that interacts with water. The fatty acid or aliphatic ends orient toward the oily interior "core" that contains the almost completely hydrophobic molecules, triglyceride and cholesteryl ester. In this way the hydrophilic components of the lipoprotein are maximally exposed to water, whereas exposure of the hydrophobic components to water is minimal.

Several classes of lipoprotein in plasma share this general structure, including chylomicrons, very low density lipoproteins (VLDL; prebeta lipoproteins), intermediate-density lipoproteins (IDL), LDL, and HDL.[7] Chylomicrons are the largest of the lipo-

FIGURE 42-1 Schematic diagram of the structure of plasma lipoproteins. A thin film of surface lipid and protein maintains the solubility of the lipoprotein particle. The film is essentially one molecule thick, and the lipids are oriented perpendicularly to the aqueous environment. The inset shows the approximate molecular dimensions of the major surface components, seen in cross section.

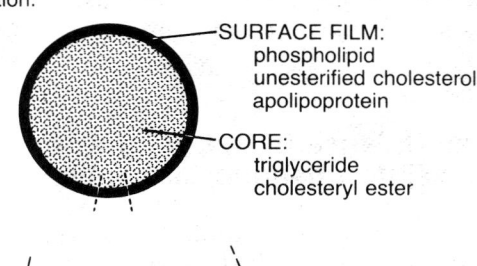

SURFACE FILM:
phospholipid
unesterified cholesterol
apolipoprotein

CORE:
triglyceride
cholesteryl ester

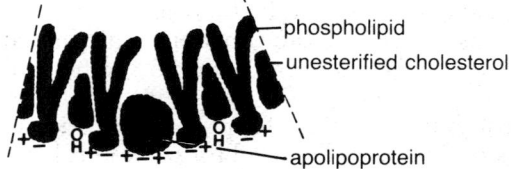

phospholipid

unesterified cholesterol

apolipoprotein

proteins (100 to 200 nm in diameter) and also the richest in triglyceride. They are the lipoproteins mentioned previously that are formed by cells of the intestinal mucosa from absorbed dietary triglyceride and contribute to the enterohepatic circulation. The phospholipid and unesterified cholesterol required for the surface film are derived from absorbed components of bile and diet. When more cholesterol is absorbed than is required for the surface film, it is esterified by an intracellular enzyme called acyl CoA:cholesterol acyltransferase (ACAT).[8] The cholesteryl ester formed is then included with triglyceride and other hydrophobic lipids such as vitamin A ester in the oily chylomicron core.

The apolipoproteins of the chylomicron surface seem to play an important metabolic role. Apolipoprotein B seems particularly necessary, as patients who lack it can neither form nor secrete chylomicrons.[9] As will be discussed later, another chylomicron apolipoprotein, apolipoprotein A, seems to play a role in the ultimate removal of chylomicron surface components from the circulation.

Once chylomicrons are formed, they are secreted into the intestinal lymph and transported to the bloodstream via the thoracic duct. During passage through the lymph and blood, apolipoprotein A and some of the chylomicron phospholipid are lost from the chylomicron surface, and there is a gain of unesterified cholesterol and various apolipoproteins through transfer from HDL and other lipoproteins already in the circulation.[10,11] These apolipoproteins play a major role in directing subsequent steps in chylomicron metabolism. Apolipoprotein C II activates an enzyme called *lipoprotein lipase* (LPL),[12] which is synthesized and secreted by cells such as adipocytes and muscle cells, and is thought subsequently to adsorb to the lumenal surface of nearby capillary endothelial cells.[13] Chylomicrons rapidly adsorb to the same surface and are there attacked by the adsorbed LPL. This leads to hydrolysis of most of the chylomicron triglyceride and release of

free fatty acids (Fig. 42-2). The free fatty acids cross the endothelium and are taken up and reesterified by subjacent adipocytes to form adipose tissue triglyceride. This triglyceride subsequently becomes a principal source of energy during exercise or fasting. It is then hydrolyzed by a hormone-sensitive intracellular lipase, whereupon fatty acids are released to the extracellular fluid, form complexes there with albumin, and circulate to other tissues where they are oxidized.

Though action of LPL on chylomicrons leads to hydrolysis of the bulk of the chylomicron triglyceride, the remaining constituents of the chylomicron are relatively unaffected. They are released from the site of chylomicron adsorption on capillary endothelial cells and reenter the circulation as particles called *chylomicron remnants*.[14] One type of remnant seems to be nearly spherical, though considerably smaller than the parent chylomicron. It has a core, which contains the remainder of the chylomicron triglyceride and the bulk of the original cholesteryl ester and vitamin A ester.[15] Since it is smaller than the original chylomicron, only a fraction of the original chylomicron phospholipid, unesterified cholesterol, and apolipoprotein is required for its surface film. Once released into the plasma, it normally circulates only briefly. Apparently apolipoproteins on its surface—apolipoprotein B and apolipoprotein E, which transfers to chylomicrons in the circulation—promote its immediate removal by hepatocytes. The latter contain enzymes that hydrolyze the triglyceride, cholesteryl ester, and other remnant components. The cholesterol and phospholipid, taken up by hepatocytes, contribute to the enterohepatic circulation of biliary phospholipid and cholesterol, and can be used to form bile once again or can be incorporated into hepatic membranes or lipoproteins.

A second type of chylomicron remnant for which evidence has recently been obtained[16,17] is composed of the remaining surface components of the original

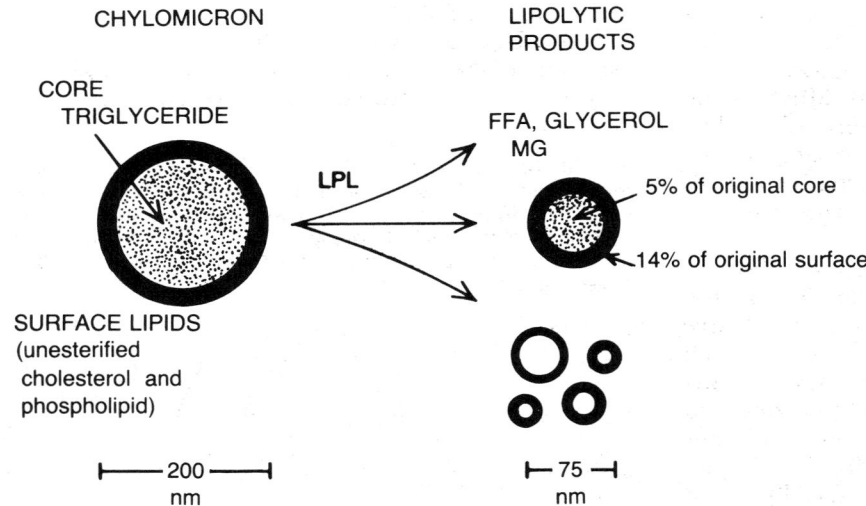

CHYLOMICRON

CORE
TRIGLYCERIDE

LPL

SURFACE LIPIDS
(unesterified
cholesterol and
phospholipid)

├── 200 ──┤
nm

LIPOLYTIC
PRODUCTS

FFA, GLYCEROL
MG

5% of original core

14% of original surface

├─ 75 ─┤
nm

FIGURE 42-2 Schematic diagram showing effects of the action of lipoprotein lipase (LPL) on chylomicrons. LPL hydrolyzes the triglyceride of chylomicrons, forming free fatty acids (FFA), monoglyceride (MG), and glycerol. This greatly diminishes the volume of the interior core of the chylomicron without substantially affecting the surface components. The nonhydrolyzed remainder of the core and a fraction of the original surface form a particle referred to as a *chylomicron remnant*. The bulk of the original surface lipid interacts with high-density lipoproteins (HDL) or forms disk-shaped or vesicle-shaped particles that lack a core. Action of lecithin:cholesterol acyltransferase (LCAT) on this lipid converts it to cholesteryl ester.

chylomicron, but no core. The surface components appear to form bilayered disks, vesicles, or multilamellar particles, in which each layer has the thickness of the surface film of a typical spherical lipoprotein. Unlike the core remnants mentioned above, these "surface remnants" of chylomicrons are not removed from the plasma directly but are metabolized through interaction with HDL (see below).

VLDL resemble chylomicrons in that they consist mainly of triglyceride, but are smaller, 30 to 80 nm in diameter, and are principally formed by hepatocytes. Hepatocytes synthesize VLDL triglyceride from dietary carbohydrate or from lipid taken up from the plasma. They provide the triglyceride with a surface film of phospholipid, unesterified cholesterol, and apolipoproteins B, C, and E. Then they secrete the VLDL into the bloodstream, whereupon the VLDL adsorb onto the surface of capillary endothelial cells as chylomicrons do and are attacked by LPL. Whether VLDL thus contribute free fatty acids to adipose tissue or muscle normally depends on the caloric state. In the fed state, and particularly when carbohydrates are being ingested in excess of caloric requirements, LPL activity in adipose tissue is high, VLDL adsorb to adipose tissue capillaries and are attacked, and the free fatty acids released are converted to adipose tissue triglyceride. During fasting, however, the activity of adipose tissue LPL is low, and VLDL are instead metabolized by muscle. In this circumstance, the free fatty acids released are used directly as a source of energy.

Core remnants of VLDL released from the capillary endothelium seem to circulate much longer in plasma than do chylomicron core remnants. Rather than being taken up immediately by the liver, they are successively converted to IDL and LDL over the course of hours to days.[18] How this conversion occurs is not completely known, but the lipoproteins in these two density classes are smaller and denser than VLDL and contain a much lower content of triglyceride, cholesteryl ester, and apolipoproteins C and E. LDL, normally the major carriers of cholesterol in the plasma of fasting subjects, are thus remnants of VLDL, formed in the course of triglyceride transport. After circulating in the plasma for 3 to 4 days, the LDL are removed by cells whose receptors recognize apolipoprotein B. Much of the LDL is thus returned to the liver where it is hydrolyzed,[19] and its components become available for the synthesis of bile or new VLDL. Alternatively, LDL can be taken up and hydrolyzed by peripheral cells, as will be discussed later.

HDL are involved in the metabolism of all of the lipoproteins mentioned above. Smaller (6 to 12 nm in diameter) and denser than LDL, HDL are thought to be derived from precursors synthesized by the liver and intestinal mucosa.[20] These precursors include the apolipoprotein A and phospholipid mentioned earlier that dissociate from chylomicrons in the circulation. They also include disk-shaped particles composed of a bilayer of surface lipid and apolipoproteins A and E, which are directly secreted by the liver and perhaps also by the intestinal mucosa.[21]

Once disk-shaped "nascent" HDL appear in plasma, they react with a plasma enzyme of hepatic origin called lecithin:cholesterol acyltransferase (LCAT).[22] This enzyme, activated by the principal apolipoprotein component of HDL, apolipoprotein A I,[23] catalyzes the conversion of surface unesterified cholesterol and phospholipid to cholesteryl ester. This conversion apparently occurs on the surface of the disk, but most of the cholesteryl ester formed leaves the surface and either penetrates between the layers of the disk to form a core or is transferred to VLDL, IDL, and LDL by a cholesteryl ester exchange protein.[24,25] Thus LCAT converts the disk-shaped nascent HDL into spherical particles and contributes cholesteryl ester to all other plasma lipoproteins.

To appreciate the potential role of the LCAT reaction in human plasma lipoprotein metabolism, it is important to realize that the surface remnants of chylomicrons and VLDL mentioned earlier apparently can interact with HDL and provide phospholipid and unesterified cholesterol for the LCAT reaction (Fig. 42-3).[26,27] The cholesteryl ester formed can then be transferred to lipoproteins that contain apolipoprotein B or E,[24] whereupon the latter can mediate the removal of cholesteryl ester (and other lipoprotein components) from the plasma.

In summary, the metabolism of plasma triglyceride is closely interdigitated with that of cholesterol. There are two major pathways of triglyceride transport. One involves chylomicrons, which carry triglyceride of dietary origin from the intestinal mucosa to adipose tissue; the other involves VLDL, which mainly carry triglyceride from the liver to adipose tissue or muscle. Unesterified cholesterol and phospholipid are required for both pathways because they contribute to the surface film of the triglyceride-rich lipoproteins. After the triglyceride of the large lipoproteins is hydrolyzed by LPL, most of the surface lipid is converted to cholesteryl ester by action of LCAT on HDL and then transferred to LDL, IDL, and VLDL by the plasma cholesteryl ester exchange protein. Finally, most of the plasma cholesteryl ester is apparently returned to the liver.

FIGURE 42-3 Role of high-density lipoproteins (HDL) in cholesterol transport. Action of lecithin:cholesterol acyltransferase (LCAT) on HDL converts disk-shaped particles into spherical particles that contain cholesteryl ester (CE) in an interior core. The core CE is subsequently transferred out of HDL to other lipoproteins and perhaps to cells.

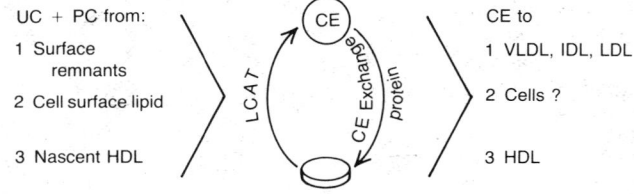

Thus, there also are two major pathways of cholesterol transport, which are interrelated through the combined action of LPL, LCAT, and cholesteryl ester exchange protein. One involves the enterohepatic circulation, the other is a smaller loop involving the liver and peripheral tissues.

Cholesterol Balance in Peripheral Cells

Unlike the cholesterol in plasma, the cholesterol of peripheral cells is mainly unesterified and located in membranes. Since the cholesterol is only slightly soluble in water and not degraded to CO_2 or water-soluble products by most cells, the mechanisms involved in the biosynthesis of cellular cholesterol or in the uptake of the cholesterol from the extracellular fluid must be regulated and/or balanced by mechanisms of cholesterol removal. As will be discussed below, there is evidence that different cells regulate cholesterol metabolism somewhat differently. Most cells appear to take up lipoprotein cholesterol from the medium instead of synthesizing cholesterol from acetyl CoA. However, different receptors for different plasma lipoproteins appear to be involved, and different mechanisms appear to control receptor activity.

By far the most is known about the regulation of cholesterol metabolism in human skin fibroblasts in culture. Studies have shown that these cells have high-affinity receptors on the cell surface that recognize and bind lipoproteins that contain apolipoproteins B or E.[28] In vitro binding of lipoproteins to these receptors is usually followed by a process of internalization in which coated segments of plasma membrane containing the bound lipoproteins pinch off into the cell to form endocytotic vacuoles. The vacuoles then fuse with intracellular organelles (lysosomes) that are richly supplied with hydrolytic enzymes, whereupon the enzymes attack the lipoproteins, releasing hydrolytic products that cross the lysosomal membrane and become available to biosynthetic pathways in the cytoplasm. Uptake of lipoprotein cholesterol by this mechanism reduces the requirement for cholesterol biosynthesis from acetyl CoA and leads to a diminution in the activity of HMG-CoA reductase. Cholesterol taken up in excess of cellular requirements is esterified by an intracellular ACAT enzyme. Accumulation of cholesteryl ester is limited, however, because uptake of lipoproteins also leads to a reduction in the number of lipoprotein receptors associated with the cell surface. Other important mechanisms for maintaining cholesterol balance within fibroblasts apparently involve HDL. There is evidence that HDL can bind to the cell surface and interfere with the uptake of LDL.[29] In addition, HDL appear able to remove cholesterol from preloaded fibroblasts by a process that involves equilibration of cellular and HDL unesterified cholesterol.[30] This process of equilibration may be influenced by the LCAT reaction, which controls the level of unesterified cholesterol in the plasma and in the plasma membranes of cells such as erythrocytes. Similar effects of HDL on cholesterol metabolism in arterial smooth-muscle cells may account for the inverse relation between the concentration of HDL in plasma and the risk of developing atherosclerotic heart disease.[31]

Cells such as fibroblasts take up LDL when they are stimulated to divide.[32] This presumably provides the cells with cholesterol and other lipids that can be used for new membrane formation. However, cells that form steroid hormones have a special requirement for cholesterol. Thus, adrenal cortical cells take up LDL by a receptor-mediated process that is stimulated by adrenocorticotropic hormone (ACTH), and the cholesterol introduced into the cell by this process clearly becomes available for synthesis of corticosteroid hormones.[33] Other steroid hormone–forming cells may have receptors that recognize apolipoprotein A I, the principal apolipoprotein of HDL. Evidence for this has been obtained for the rat testis and ovary,[34] though more evidence is needed about the role of HDL in steroid hormone formation in humans.

A different kind of lipoprotein receptor has been demonstrated for macrophages.[35] These cells lack receptors for normal LDL but have receptors that recognize modified LDL (LDL covalently modified by the inclusion of acidic groups, or LDL complexed with natural acidic substances), and also a special kind of lipoprotein, referred to as *B VLDL,* that accumulates in the plasma of animals fed cholesterol-rich diets.[36] This is of special interest since studies of the interaction of B VLDL with macrophages in culture have shown that uptake of lipoprotein cholesterol leads to accumulation of intracellular cholesteryl ester and gives the macrophages the appearance of the foam cells seen in the lesions of atherosclerosis. Apparently, a large excess of cholesteryl ester accumulates within the cells because the lipoprotein receptors are not down-regulated following the uptake of lipoproteins.

When macrophages rich in cholesteryl ester are incubated with HDL, however, there is a rapid loss of cholesteryl ester from the cells and a corresponding increment in the content of HDL unesterified cholesterol in the medium. Apparently, this occurs because there is a rapid turnover of intracellular cholesteryl esters owing to the combined action of an intracellular ACAT and a cytoplasmic cholesteryl ester hydrolase. The unesterified cholesterol formed by the hydrolase equilibrates with cell-surface unesterified cholesterol, which can equilibrate with HDL. As long as the content of unesterified cholesterol in HDL is kept low, the HDL act as a "sink" for cellular unesterified cholesterol and thus cause a net hydrolysis of intracellular cholesteryl ester.

In summary, cholesterol balance in peripheral cells is closely related to the metabolism of plasma lipoproteins. Cholesterol-rich remnants of VLDL and possibly chylomicrons are apparently recognized and taken up not just by fibroblasts but also by many other types of cells, including arterial smooth-muscle cells. HDL that contain apolipoprotein E can also be taken up by cells, but the fate of other HDL remains unclear, at least in humans. Evidence is accumulating that HDL facilitate cholesterol removal from cells. This type of function may be of particular importance in macrophages that take up altered lipoproteins and accumulate intracellular cholesteryl ester without down-regulating the lipoprotein receptor.

Cholesterol Dysbalance

Cholesterol dysbalance can be defined in terms of atherosclerosis as a condition of cholesterol accumulation in arterial cells caused by increased uptake or decreased removal of cholesterol. The most well known and dramatic example of this in humans is seen in patients homozygous for familial hypercholesterolemia. These patients have high levels of LDL in the plasma and correspondingly high levels of plasma cholesterol (on the order of 800 mg/dl), accompanied by xanthomatosis and severe coronary heart disease that can occur even in early childhood. The pioneering studies of Brown and Goldstein[37] established that patient skin fibroblasts lack the receptor that recognizes normal LDL and thus take up and degrade LDL only by nonspecific mechanisms related to bulk-phase endocytosis (pinocytosis). Other cells apparently lack these receptors also, and it appears that general absence of receptors for normal LDL leads to the increased concentration of LDL in plasma. Studies of the skin fibroblasts of patients heterozygous for familial hypercholesterolemia support this possibility, since these fibroblasts have an intermediate number of receptors for LDL, while the level of LDL in the plasma also is intermediate.[38] Conceivably, therefore, different genetically determined forms of the LDL receptor might lead to different levels of LDL in the plasma in the general population. That a variety of defects related to the LDL receptor may indeed occur is suggested by the recent discovery[39] of a patient who appears to have an abnormality involving LDL internalization.

A major question, not yet answered at a molecular level, is why high concentrations of LDL in the plasma associated with defective LDL-receptor activity should be accompanied by intracellular deposition of cholesteryl esters in atherosclerotic lesions. It was formerly thought that patient arterial cells might be overproducing cholesterol and that this might lead to accumulation of intracellular cholesterol in foam cells.[40] However, another possibility is that the foam cells reflect the activity of a receptor similar to that demonstrated in macrophages. This seems more likely at present since evidence is lacking that absence of the usual LDL receptor directly

compromises arterial cell function. Indeed, high concentrations of other lipoproteins associated with very different conditions appear to be atherogenic. For example, a second inborn error associated with severe vascular disease involves cholesterol-rich lipoproteins that appear to be either VLDL or chylomicron remnants. This inborn error, variously referred to as *type III hyperlipoproteinemia, broad beta disease,* or *dysbetalipoproteinemia,* was formerly thought to be a monogenic disorder. Recent evidence has indicated, however, that it results from the combined action of two abnormal genes, one associated with increased concentrations of triglyceride-rich VLDL and one associated with an unusual distribution of isoforms of apolipoprotein E, detectable by electrophoresis.[41] When both genes are present in the same individual, there is an increased concentration of cholesterol-rich "VLDL" in the plasma, apparently because these lipoproteins are defectively cleared by the liver.[42] Furthermore, distinctive tuberous xanthomata develop on exposed areas of the extremities, and there is premature atherosclerosis.

A third inborn error associated with vascular disease is referred to as *familial combined hyperlipidemia* because the concentrations of plasma triglyceride and plasma cholesterol are both elevated.[43] Cholesterol-rich VLDL and IDL both accumulate in this disease for reasons that are still poorly understood. However, as in the case of the first two diseases, both xanthomatosis and atherosclerosis accompany the defect.

In contrast to this, other inborn errors of plasma lipoprotein metabolism associated with hyperlipoproteinemia show a much weaker correlation with vascular disease. This is true for familial hypertriglyceridemia, a disease characterized by elevated concentrations of VLDL,[44] and for familial hyperchylomicronemia, a disease characterized by defective action of LPL. Thus, it appears that disorders of plasma lipoprotein metabolism associated with premature vascular disease share three features: (1) the presence of elevated concentrations of cholesterol-rich VLDL, IDL, or LDL; (2) xanthomatosis; and (3) foam cells in arterial lesions. The fact that these features occur irrespective of the cause of the hyperlipidemia suggests that it is the effect of the hyperlipidemia that is critical. This possibility is supported by observations of diet-induced hypercholesterolemia in animals, which indicate that elevated concentrations of either LDL or cholesterol-rich VLDL (chylomicron remnants?) can lead to vascular disease.[45]

Since foam cells rich in cholesteryl ester are found in all of these conditions, increasing attention is being focused on the role of macrophages and other phagocytic cells in arterial disease. It seems possible that phagocytic cells accumulate at sites of injury in both skin and arteries and take up large amounts of β migrating lipoproteins by a mechanism unrelated to the normal LDL receptor. The possibility clearly needs to be explored that the resulting accumulation of intracellular cholesteryl ester interferes with the normal tissue response to injury and leads to or exacerbates arterial disease.

A final major question related to cholesterol dysbalance is whether more subtle forms of hyperlipidemia have effects on the arterial wall analogous to those of the more exaggerated conditions discussed above. The epidemiologic studies of normal populations discussed in Chap. 34 suggest that indeed this may be the case, and this finding has stimulated attempts to prevent or treat atherosclerosis by decreasing the concentrations of VLDL, IDL, and LDL, or by increasing the concentration of HDL. Lacking precise knowledge of the many different factors that regulate the concentrations of these lipoproteins, investigators have used relatively simple forms of intervention thought to be compatible with a prolonged treatment period. This is the basis for the recommendation to decrease the dietary intake of animal products, which are rich in cholesterol and saturated fat. Measures of this type have been tested in adult males thought to be at high risk of developing coronary heart disease; in most cases they have led to a reduction of about 15 percent in the concentration of total plasma cholesterol, presumably by decreasing the amount of cholesterol entering plasma in chylomicrons. Whereas the efficacy of this type of intervention is still controversial (see Chap. 43), adequate testing remains to be carried out. Definitive judgment may have to await intervention trials initiated in young adults and carried out effectively for many years. In addition, better methods will certainly be required to lower the concentrations of "atherogenic" plasma lipoproteins, while increasing the concentration of others.

Summary

The argument presented in this chapter is that cholesterol balance should be considered at three interrelated levels. Cholesterol balance in the body as a whole is largely determined by events related to the enterohepatic circulation. Cholesterol balance in the plasma is largely determined by events related to the transport of exogenous and endogenous triglyceride. Cholesterol balance in cells is largely determined by interregulated rates of cholesterol biosynthesis, uptake, and efflux. Cholesterol balance at these three levels is interrelated because (1) the enterohepatic circulation of biliary lipid is closely interdigitated with the metabolism and transport of dietary triglyceride, (2) cholesterol-rich lipoprotein remnants that are the principal source of cholesterol for hepatic and peripheral cells are produced in the course of the metabolism of triglyceride-rich lipoproteins, and (3) HDL seem to be involved both in the regulation of cholesterol balance in the plasma and in cells.

Nonetheless, critical questions remain to be answered. We still understand only incompletely the factors that regulate absorption and excretion of cholesterol by the intestine. Similarly, the hepatic mechanisms that interrelate uptake of lipoprotein cholesterol with secretion of biliary cholesterol and bile acid have yet to be adequately defined. Finally, the most critical question is how cholesterol dysbalance affects cell function. This question must clearly be answered if we are to understand the role of cholesterol in atherogenesis.

References

*1. Brown, M. S., and Goldstein, J. L.: Multivalent Feedback Regulation of HMG CoA Reductase, a Control Mechanism Coordinating Isoprenoid Synthesis and Cell Growth, *J. Lipid Res.,* 1980.

2. Goodman, De W. S., Noble, R. P., and Dell, R. B.: Three-Pool Model of the Long-Term Turnover of Plasma Cholesterol in Man, *J. Lipid Res.* 14:178, 1973.

*3. Myant, N. B., and Mitropoulos, K. A.: Cholesterol 7 α-hydroxylase, *J. Lipid Res.* 18:135, 1977. (115 references)

*4. Small, D. M.: The Formation of Gallstones, *Adv. Intern. Med.,* 16:243, 1970. (77 references)

*5. Bennion, L. J., and Grundy, S. M.: Risk Factors for the Development of Cholelithiasis in Man, *N. Engl. J. Med.,* 299:1161, 1221, 1978. (140 references)

6. Andersen, J. M., and Dietschy, J. M.: Regulation of Sterol Synthesis in 16 Tissues of Rat, *J. Biol., Chem.,,* 252:3646, 1977.

*7. Smith, L. C., Pownell, H. J., and Gotto Se, A. M.: Lipoproteins Structure and Metabolism, *Ann. Rev. Biochem.,* 47:751, 1978. (181 references)

8. Norum, K. R., Lilljeqvist, A. C., Helgerud, P., Normann, E., Mo, A., and Selbekk, B.: Esterification of Cholesterol in Human Small Intestine: The Importance of Acyl-CoA:Cholesterol Acyltransferase, *Europ. J. Clin. Invest.,* 9:55, 1979.

*9. Kayden, H. J.: Abetalipoproteinemia, *Ann. Rev. Med.,* 23:285, 1972. (48 references)

10. Havel, R. J., Kane, J. P., and Kashyap, M. D.: Interchange of Apolipoproteins between Chylomicrons and High Density Lipoproteins during Alimentary Lipemia in Man, *J. Clin. Invest.,* 52:32, 1973.

11. Imaizumi, K., Havel, R. J., Fainaru, M., and Vigne, J.-L.: Origin and Transport of the A-I and Arginine-Rich Apolipoproteins and Mesenteric Lymph of Rats, *J. Lipid Res.,* 19:1038, 1978.

*12. Nilsson-Ehle, P., Garfinkel, A. S., and Schotz, M. C.: Lipolytic Enzymes and Plasma Lipoprotein Metabolism, *Ann. Rev. Biochem.,* 49:667, 1980. (155 references)

*13. Scrow, R. O., Blanchette-Mackie, E. J., and Smith, L. C.: Role of Capillary Endothelium in the Clearance of Chylomicrons, *Circ. Res.,* 39:149, 1976. (103 references)

14. Redgrave, T. G.: Formation of Cholesteryl Ester–Rich Particulate Lipid during Metabolism of Chylomicrons, *J. Clin. Invest.,* 49:465, 1970.

*This article is a review of the literature and contains additional references to the literature.

15. Mjøs, O. D., Faergeman, O., Hamilton, R. L., and Havel, R. J.: Characterization of Remnants Produced during the Metabolism of Triglyceride-Rich Lipoproteins of Blood Plasma and Intestinal Lymph in the Rat, *J. Clin. Invest.*, 56:603, 1975.

16. Glomset, J. A., Norum, K. A., Nichols, A. V., King, W. C., Mitchell, C. D., Applegate, K. R., Gong, E. L., and Gjone, E.: Plasma Lipoproteins in Familial Lecithin Cholesterol Acyltransferase Deficiency. Effects of Dietary Manipulation, *Scand. J. Clin. Invest.*, 35:3, 1975.

17. Eisenberg, S., and Olivecrona, T.: Very Low Density Lipoprotein. Fate of Phospholipids, Cholesterol, and Apolipoprotein C during Lipolysis in Vitro, *J. Lipid Res.*, 20:614, 1979.

*18. Eisenberg, S.: Very-Low-Density Lipoprotein Metabolism, in S. Eisenberg (ed.), "Lipoprotein Metabolism," S. Karger, Basel, Switzerland, 1979, p. 139. (Extensively referenced)

*19. Steinberg, D.: Origin, Turnover and Fate of Plasma Low-Density Lipoprotein, in S. Eisenberg (ed.), "Lipoprotein Metabolism," S. Karger, Basel, Switzerland, 1979, p. 166. (Extensively referenced)

*20. Glomset, J. A.: High Density Lipoproteins in Human Health and Disease, in M. D. Siperstein, and G. H. Stollerman (eds.), "Advances in Internal Medicine," Year Book Medical Publishers, Inc., Chicago, 1980, vol. 25. (Extensively referenced)

21. Green, P. H., Tall, A. R., and Glickman, R. M.: Rat Intestine Secretes Discoid High Density Lipoproteins, *J. Clin. Invest.*, 61:528, 1978.

*22. Glomset, J. A.: The Plasma Lecithin:Cholesterol Acyltransferase Reaction, *J. Lipid Res.*, 9:155, 1968. (83 references)

23. Fielding, C. J., Shore, V. G., and Fielding, P. E.: A Protein Cofactor of Lecithin:Cholesterol Acyltransferase, *Biochem. Biophys. Res. Commun.*, 46:1493, 1972.

24. Zilversmit, D. B., Hughes, L. B., and Balmer, J.: Stimulation of Cholesterol Ester Exchange by Lipoprotein-Free Rabbit Plasma, *Biochim. Biophys. Acta*, 409:393, 1975.

25. Chajek, T., and Fielding, C. J.: Isolation and Characterization of a Human Serum Cholesteryl Ester Transfer Protein, *Proc. Natl. Acad. Sci. USA*, 75:3445, 1978.

26. Norum, K. R., Glomset, J. A., Nichols, A. V., Forte, T., Albers, J. J., King, W. C., Mitchell, C. D., Applegate, K. R., Gong, E. L., Cabana, V., and Gjone, E.: Plasma Lipoproteins in Familial Lecithin:Cholesterol Acyltransferase Deficiency: Effects of Incubation with Lecithin:Cholesterol Acyltransferase in Vitro, *Scand. J. Clin. Lab. Invest.*, 35:31, 1975.

27. Eisenberg, S., Patsch, J. R., Olivecrona, T., and Gotto, A. M., Jr.: Effects of Lipolysis on Human High Density Lipoproteins (HDL), *Circulation*, 58:11, 1978.

*28. Brown, M. S., and Goldstein, J. L.: Receptor-Mediated Control of Cholesterol Metabolism, *Science*, 191:150, 1976. (38 references)

29. Stein, O., and Stein, Y.: High Density Lipoproteins Reduce the Uptake of Low Density Lipoproteins by Human Endothelial Cells in Culture, *Biochim. Biophys. Acta*, 431:363, 1976.

30. Verdery, R. B., Nist, C., and Fujimoto, W.: Effect of HDL_3 and LCAT on Cholesterol Balance in Quiescent Fibroblasts, to be published.

31. Miller, G. J., and Miller, N. E.: Plasma-High-Density-Lipoprotein Concentration and Development of Ischaemic Heart-Disease, *Lancet*, 1:16, 1975.

32. Chait, A., Ross, R., Albers, J., and Bierman, E.: Platelet Derived Growth Factor Stimulates Low Density Lipoprotein Receptor Activity, *Proc. Natl. Acad. Sci. USA*, 77:4084, 1980.

33. Faust, J. R., Goldstein, J. L., and Brown, M. S.: Receptor-Mediated Uptake of Low Density Lipoprotein and Utilization of Its Cholesterol for Steroid Synthesis in Cultured Mouse Adrenal Cells, *J. Biol. Chem.*, 252:4861, 1977.

34. Andersen, J. M., and Dietschy, J. M.: Regulation of Sterol Synthesis in 16 Tissues of Rat. II. Role of Rat and Human High and Low Density Lipoproteins and of Rat Chylomicron Remnants, *J. Biol. Chem.*, 252:3652, 1977.

35. Goldstein, J. L., Ho, Y. K., Brown, M. S., Innerarity, T. L., and Mahley, R. W.: Cholesteryl Ester Accumulation in Macrophages Resulting from Receptor-Mediated Uptake and Degradation of Hypercholesterolemic Canine β–Very Low Density Lipoproteins, *J. Biol. Chem.*, 255:1839, 1980.

*36. Mahley, R. W.: Alterations in Plasma Lipoproteins Induced by Cholesterol Feeding in Animals Including Man, in J. M. Dietschy, A. M. Gotto, Jr., and J. A. Ontko (eds.), "Disturbances in Lipid and Lipoprotein Metabolism," American Physiological Society, Bethesda, Maryland, 1978, p. 181. (Extensively referenced)

37. Goldstein, J. L., and Brown, M. S.: Familial Hypercholesterolemia: Identification of a Defect in the Regulation of 3-Hydroxy-3-Methylglutaryl Coenzyme A Reductase Activity Associated with Overproduction of Cholesterol, *Proc. Acad. Sci. USA*, 70:2804, 1973.

38. Brown, M. S., and Goldstein, J. L.: Expression of the Familial Hypercholesterolemia Gene in Heterozygotes: Mechanism for a Dominant Disorder in Man, *Science*, 185:61, 1974.

39. Brown, M. S., and Goldstein, J. L.: Analysis of a Mutant Strain of Human Fibroblasts with a Defect in the Internalization of Receptor-Bound Low Density Lipoprotein, *Cell*, 9:663, 1976.

*40. Goldstein, J. L., and Brown, J. S.: The Low-Density Lipoprotein Pathway and Its Relation to Atherosclerosis, *Ann. Rev. Biochem.*, 46:897, 1977. (126 references)

41. Utermann, G., Vogelberg, K. H., Steinmetz, A., Schoenborn, W., Pruin, N., Jaeschke, M., Hees, M., and Canzler, H.: Polymorphism of Apolipoprotein E. II. Genetics of Hyperlipoproteinemia Type III, *Clin. Genet.* 15:37, 1979.

42. Chait, A., Albers, J. J., Brunzell, J. D., and Hazzard, W. R.: Type-III Hyperlipoproteinaemia ("Remnant Removal Disease"): Insight into the Pathogenic Mechanism, *Lancet*, 1:1176, 1977.

43. Goldstein, J. L., Schrott, H. G., Hazzard, W. R., Bierman, E. L., and Motulsky, A. G.: Hyperlipidemia in Coronary Heart Disease. II. Genetic Analysis of Lipid Levels in 176 Families and Delineation of a New Inherited Disorder, Combined Hyperlipidemia, *J. Clin. Invest.*, 52:1544, 1973.

*44. Havel, R. J.: Classification of the Hyperlipidemias, *Ann. Rev. Med.*, 28:195, 1977. (94 references)

45. Zilversmit, D. B.: A Proposal Linking Atherogenesis to the Interaction of Endothelial Lipoprotein Lipase with Triglyceride-Rich Lipoproteins, *Circ. Res.*, 33:633, 1973.

INDEX

Index